SAUNDERS MEDICAL AND NURSING DICTIONARIES
AND VOCABULARY AIDS

Dorland's Illustrated Medical Dictionary

Dorland's Pocket Medical Dictionary

Cole: The Doctor's Shorthand

Jablonski: Illustrated Dictionary of Eponymic Syndromes
and Diseases

Leader & Leader: Dictionary of Comparative Pathology and
Experimental Biology

Miller–Keane: Encyclopedia and Dictionary of Medicine
and Nursing

Sloane: The Medical Word Book – A Spelling and Vocabulary
Guide to Medical Transcription

Encyclopedia and Dictionary of Medicine and Nursing

By

BENJAMIN F. MILLER, M.D.

and

CLAIRE BRACKMAN KEANE, R.N., B.S., M.Ed.

with 138 illustrations, including 16 color plates

W. B. SAUNDERS COMPANY · Philadelphia · London · Toronto

W. B. Saunders Company: West Washington Square
Philadelphia, Pa. 19105

12 Dyott Street
London, WC1A 1DB

833 Oxford Street
Toronto, Ontario M8Z 5T9, Canada

Encyclopedia and Dictionary of Medicine and Nursing   ISBN 0-7216-6355-9

Print No: 9   8   7   6

Publisher's Foreword

Behind every encyclopedia/dictionary lie immense labor, high purpose and great hope. Whether that labor has been well done, purpose fulfilled and hope justified is a determination to be made only by the reader. As Johnson so bluntly put it in the Preface to his *Dictionary of the English Language*, "The value of a work must be estimated by its use; it is not enough that a dictionary delights the critic, unless at the same time, it instructs the learner."

Therefore as the reader considers the pages to follow and whether their millions of individual letters have been well put together, he should know what philosophy has animated this work and what use has been foreseen for it.

Its philosophy can be simply put. Especially in a time of expanding details of knowledge, the first requirement for teaching, learning and communication by scientists and professional persons is the existence of an agreed-upon vocabulary of terms. Indeed the first and vital step in learning any discipline is mastery and understanding of its language. It is the intent of this *Encyclopedia and Dictionary of Medicine and Nursing* to provide precisely such an authoritative vocabulary for students and learners of all ages and degrees in the nursing and paramedical sciences.

Although a dictionary must have authority, it may not pretend to dictate. The language of science has not descended to us in a state of uniformity and perfection. Words are like their authors; when they are not gaining strength, they are generally losing it.

In fine, the purpose of an encyclopedia/dictionary is to afford a body of knowledge built upon usage — not upon fixed canons of philology. The skill of such a work lies in its understanding of usage, its reasoned selection of terms, its accuracy and usefulness of definition and its rational adjudication of conflict in terminology. These characters in the work have had their achievement through a variety of means.

The Authors: Creation of this reference source has involved the special knowledge and assistance of many people; but the carrying out of its essential concepts has been the responsibility of its two authors, Benjamin F. Miller, M.D., and Claire Brackman Keane, R.N.

Dr. Miller's sudden death occurred after he had completed work on this manuscript of the Encyclopedia/Dictionary but before he could see it brought to print. He would have relished seeing the printed work, for Dr. Miller was, above all, a bookish man. He felt that "a good book is the best of friends, the same today and forever."

His professional life was given to clinical investigation to which he made significant contribution as Director of the May Institute and whose findings he applied dynamically to the practice of internal medicine, especially the management of cardiovascular disease. At the same time he somehow found time for both the reading and writing of books. His experience as Editor-in-Chief of the *Modern Medical Encyclopedia* honed to a sharp edge his innate capacity to present complex matters in concise and readily understandable form. The Golden Press has graciously allowed adaptation of some of the entries of his *Encyclopedia* for use in the present work.

Dr. Miller was fortunate above all in his coauthor, Claire Brackman Keane, who brought to the work long and thoughtful experience in nursing education, nursing service and textbook authorship. To her critical mind every word was a new and unavoidable challenge. To selection and definition she brought a capacious memory and a sharp sense of what constitutes relevance and usefulness of detail.

The Consultants: Accuracy of the work has demanded not only contemporaneity of content but provision of altogether new definitions keeping pace with the great advances in the sciences which comprise the mosaic of medicine, such as the swift-moving disciplines of genetics, neuroscience, molecular biology, pharmacology, biochemistry and microbiology. Here both authors and publisher have been fortunate in being able to consult with the foremost authors of basic-science texts in English. It is a pleasure to record that the response to calls for counsel and specific advices was always prompt and helpful. To his writers of books in all areas of medicine, nursing and their supporting sciences the publisher owes a debt of gratitude that cannot be repaid but is reflected in the authority of the work here presented.

The Sources: These have been many and varied; but the authors have freely called upon two splendid lexicons for help—the current editions of *Dorland's Illustrated Medical Dictionary* and *Dorland's Pocket Medical Dictionary.* Occasionally entries from these two dictionaries have been sharpened or simplified or revised, in these instances the dictionaries providing a sure entry point for such elaboration and modification.

In one area the authors alone have been responsible for the framing of suitable entries. These are the encyclopedic terms. Their purpose has been to provide a full picture of the nature of disease and disease process, and of the principles of nursing management. Tables too are an important part of the useful encyclopedic character of the work, and their formulations have been checked and rechecked against original sources to secure an error-free compendium of specific data.

Illustrations: The drawing of fresh figures for the work has been under the supervision of Grant Lashbrook, Art Director of the Saunders Company; and the 16 anatomic plates in color represent a distillation of morphologic knowledge useful to both the beginning student and the experienced nurse and physician.

Typography: The alphabet is an extraordinarily ancient and ingenious device for communication and storage of information, and even the present-day forms of its letters derive from Roman and Arabic sources. Hence it is appropriate that typography (an expression of the alphabet) be traditional and conservative. Design of this book has been in the hands of Lorraine Battista, who has given just care to its openness, legibility and attractiveness. Such a small device as beginning each subentry on a new line consults not economy but the convenience of the reader and pleasantness of the page.

Comparative Brevity: Partly by concision of expression, partly by tough-minded selection and partly by ignoring useless accretions of the past this Encyclopedia/Dictionary has been kept modest in size. It is not, in the Duke of Gloucester's phrase, "another damned, thick, square book," but rather an inviting book in large format whose consultation will be rewarding and may justify the hopes with which its preparation was attended.

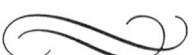

Finally, the use of this book of words will be assisted by appreciation of the essential fact that words are not things-in-themselves—they are rather *signs* of things, whose validity and use rest upon convention, the purpose of lexicography being the codification and clarification of these conventions. Again we may quote Johnson: "I am not yet so lost in lexicography as to forget that *words are the daughters of earth, and that things are the sons of heaven*. Language is only the instrument of science, and words are but the signs of ideas: I wish, however, that the instrument might be less apt to decay and that signs might be permanent, like the things which they denote."

W. B. SAUNDERS COMPANY

Contents

Notes on the Use of This Book

Cross References

Words set in SMALL CAPITALS denote cross references. They are used liberally, and the reader is well advised to turn to the term so noted, because he will find important additional information there. For example, within the definition for *rejection* there is a cross reference to TRANSPLANTATION, because the problem of rejection is discussed fully in the encyclopedic definition for *transplantation*. In the *pregnancy* definition a cross reference to ABORTION shows the reader that a fuller discussion of that subject is given at *abortion*.

Compound Terms

Terms composed of a noun modified by a descriptive or eponymic designation are defined under the adjective or eponym when logic dictates. Thus, the definition for *plastic surgery* appears at *plastic*, not at *surgery*. *Parkinson's disease* is defined at *Parkinson's*, not at *disease*. *Boric acid* is defined at *boric*, not at *acid*.

In certain cases, when the logical placement of the full definition seems less clear-cut, a summary definition is given as a subentry under the noun entry, and a cross reference directs the reader to the complete definition at the modifying term. This is done, for example, in the *balance* entry, where the subentry for *acid-base balance* gives a one-sentence definition and a cross reference to the main definition in the A's. *Bell's palsy* is treated similarly, with the full definition at *Bell's* and a short definition and cross reference at *palsy*.

It is hoped that this system will save the reader time and effort by giving the full information where he is most likely to look for it.

Pronunciation

The pronunciation of words is indicated by a simple phonetic respelling in parentheses. Diacritical markings to distinguish vowel sounds are used only when necessary.

An unmarked vowel ending a syllable is long (ba′be).

An unmarked vowel in a syllable ending with a consonant is short (ab-dukt′).

A long vowel in a syllable that must end with a consonant is indicated by a macron (be-hāv′yer).

A short vowel that constitutes or ends a syllable is marked with a breve (ĕ-de′mah; ab′stĭ-nens).

The syllable *ah* is used for the sound of *a* in open, unaccented syllables (ah-bor′shun).

The primary accent in a word is indicated by a bold face, single accent. The secondary accent is indicated by a light face, double accent.

Abbreviations

Abbreviations used in the text of the definitions are few and fairly obvious. They include

adj. (adjective)	It. (Italian)
Fr. (French)	L. (Latin)
Ger. (German)	pl. (plural)
Gr. (Greek)	

In elaboration of entries that are themselves abbreviations, the words "abbreviation for" have been omitted.

A

A. accommodation; ampere; anode (anodal); anterior; axial.

a [L.] *arte'ria* (artery).

a- word element [L.], *without; not.*

Å angstrom.

A₂ aortic second sound (see HEART SOUNDS).

A.A. achievement age; Alcoholics Anonymous.

aa [L. pl.] *arte'riae* (arteries).

a̅a̅ [Gr.] *an'a* (of each), in prescriptions.

A.A.A.S. American Association for the Advancement of Science.

A.A.I.N. American Association of Industrial Nurses.

A.A.P.B. American Association of Pathologists and Bacteriologists.

A.A.P.M.R. American Academy of Physical Medicine and Rehabilitation.

ab [L.] preposition, *from.*

ab- word element [L.], *from; off; away from.*

abacterial (a″bak-te're-al) free from bacteria.

abalienation (ab″āl-yĕ-na'shun) derangement of the mental faculties.

abarognosis (ah-bar″og-no'sis) loss of sense of weight.

abarthrosis (ab″ar-thro'sis) abarticulation.

abarticular (ab″ar-tik'u-ler) not affecting a joint; at a distance from a joint.

abarticulation (ab″ar-tik″u-la'shun) 1. diarthrosis. 2. a dislocation.

abasia (ah-ba'ze-ah) inability to walk because of defective coordination. adj., **aba'sic, abat'ic.**
   a.-asta'sia, astasia-abasia.
   a. atac'tica, abasia with uncertain movements. **choreic a.,** abasia due to paralysis of the limbs. **paralytic a.,** abasia due to paralysis.
   paroxysmal trepidant a., spastic a., abasia caused by paralysis of the legs in attempting to stand.
   trembling a., a. trep'idans, abasia due to trembling of the legs.

abatement (ah-bāt'ment) decrease in severity of a pain or symptom.

abaxial (ab-ak'se-al) not situated in the axis of the body.

abd., abdom. abdomen, abdominal.

abdomen (ab-do'men) the portion of the body between the thorax and the pelvis. adj., **abdom'inal.** Within this part of the body is the abdominal cavity, which is separated from the chest area by the diaphragm. The cavity, which is lined with a membrane known as the peritoneum, contains the stomach, large and small intestines, liver, spleen, pancreas, kidneys, appendix, gallbladder, urinary bladder and other structures.
   acute a., surgical a., medical jargon for an acute condition within the abdomen demanding immediate operation.

abdomin(o)- (ab-dom'ĭ-no) word element, *abdomen.*

abdominoanterior (ab-dom″ĭ-no-an-tēr'e-or) with the abdomen directed toward the anterior surface of the maternal body; said of the fetus in utero.

abdominocentesis (ab-dom″ĭ-no-sen-te'sis) paracentesis of the abdomen (see also abdominal PARACENTESIS).

abdominocystic (ab-dom″ĭ-no-sis'tik) pertaining to the abdomen and gallbladder.

abdominohysterectomy (ab-dom″ĭ-no-his″tĕ-rek'-to-me) hysterectomy through an abdominal incision.

abdominohysterotomy (ab-dom″ĭ-no-his″tĕ-rot'o-me) hysterotomy through an abdominal incision.

abdominoposterior (ab-dom″ĭ-no-pos-tēr'e-or) with the abdomen directed toward the posterior surface of the maternal body; said of the fetus in utero.

abdominoscopy (ab-dom″ĭ-nos'ko-pe) examination of the abdomen.

abdominous (ab-dom'ĭ-nus) having a prominent abdomen.

abdominovaginal (ab-dom″ĭ-no-vaj'ĭ-nal) pertaining to the abdomen and vagina.

abduce (ab-dūs') to abduct, or draw away.

abducens (ab-du'senz) [L.] drawing away.
   a. muscle, the lateral rectus muscle of the eyeball which abducts the eye.
   a. nerve, the sixth cranial nerve; it arises from the pons and supplies the lateral rectus muscle of the eyeball, allowing for motion. Paralysis of the nerve causes diplopia (double vision).

abducent (ab-du'sent) abducting.

abduct (ab-dukt') to draw away from a center or median line.

1

abduction (ab-duk′shun) the act of abducting; the state of being abducted.

abductor (ab-duk′tor) that which abducts.

abenteric (ab″en-ter′ik) situated elsewhere than in the intestine.

abepithymia (ab″ep-ĭ-thi′me-ah) paralysis of the solar plexus.

aberratio (ab″er-a′she-o) [L.] aberration.

aberration (ab″er-a′shun) 1. deviation from the normal or usual. 2. imperfect refraction or focalization of a lens.
  chromatic a., unequal refraction by a lens of light rays of different lengths passing through it, producing a blurred image and a display of colors.
  dioptric a., spherical a., inability of a spherical lens to bring all rays of light to a single focus.

aberrometer (ab″er-om′ĕ-ter) an instrument for determining the amount of aberration.

a-beta-lipoproteinemia (a-ba″tah-lip″o-pro″te-in-e′me-ah) a condition characterized by the lack of beta-lipoproteins in the blood.

abevacuation (ab″e-vak″u-a′shun) incomplete evacuation.

abiatrophy (ab″e-at′ro-fe) 1. premature and endogenous loss of vitality. 2. a condition due to an inborn defect, but not clinically evident until some time after maturity; also used more generally to designate any disorder with late onset.

abiogenesis (ab″e-o-jen′ĕ-sis) production of life from matter not alive. adj., **abiogenet′ic, abiog′-enous.**

abionergy (ab″e-on′er-je) abiotrophy.

abiosis (ab″e-o′sis) absence or deficiency of life. adj., **abiot′ic.**

abiotrophy (ab″e-ot′ro-fe) loss of early ability to function normally because of innate constitutional weakness leading to ultimate breakdown.

abirritant (ab-ir′ĭ-tant) diminishing irritation; soothing.

abirritation (ab-ir″ĭ-ta′shun) diminished irritability; atony.

abiuret (ah-bi′u-ret) not giving the biuret reaction.

ablactation (ab″lak-ta′shun) weaning.

ablate (ab-lāt′) to remove, especially by cutting.

ablatio (ab-la′she-o) [L.] detachment.
  a. ret′inae, detachment of the retina.

ablation (ab-la′shun) removal, especially by cutting.

ablepharon (a-blef′ah-ron) total or partial absence of the eyelids. adj., **ableph′arous.**

ablepsia (a-blep′se-ah) blindness.

abluent (ab′lu-ent) detergent; cleansing.

abnerval (ab-ner′val) passing from a nerve through a muscle.

abneural (ab-nu′ral) away from the central nervous system.

abnormality (ab″nor-mal′ĭ-te) 1. the state of being unlike the usual condition. 2. a malformation.

abocclusion (ab″ŏ-kloo′zhun) occlusion in which the mandibular teeth are not in contact with the maxillary teeth.

aborad (ab-o′rad) away from the mouth.

aboral (ab-o′ral) opposite to, or remote from, the mouth.

abort (ah-bort′) to arrest prematurely a disease or developmental process.

abortifacient (ah-bor″tĭ-fa′shent) 1. causing abortion. 2. an agent that induces abortion.

abortion (ah-bor′shun) termination of pregnancy before the fetus is viable. In the strictest medical sense, the words abortion and miscarriage both refer to the termination of pregnancy before the fetus is capable of survival outside the uterus. In general language, however, abortion refers to deliberate (and often criminal) termination of pregnancy, while miscarriage connotes a spontaneous or natural loss of the fetus. Since there is some confusion as to the exact meanings of these terms, care should be exercised in the use of the word abortion when discussing this condition with a lay person.

It is rare for a fetus to survive if it weighs less than 1000 Gm., or if the pregnancy is terminated before 20 weeks of gestation. When a live infant is born between the 20th and 35th weeks of pregnancy the term premature termination of pregnancy, or premature birth, is used.

NURSING CARE. The role of the nurse in the control of abortion is twofold: she must help in the prevention of criminal abortions by taking an active part in the education of the public as to their hazards, and she must assist in the treatment of the patient and employ palliative measures once abortion—spontaneous, therapeutic or criminal—has occurred.

The social, religious and cultural aspects of abortion must be considered in the teaching of the patient and her family. The nurse should always avoid sitting in judgment of the patient and should examine closely her own attitudes toward the moral implications of contraception and birth control, as well as her feelings about abortion. Whenever a pregnancy must be terminated, there will usually be some guilt feelings on the part of the patient. She may feel that she could have been more careful during her pregnancy, or, if the abortion is induced, she may feel that she has participated in and given consent to the destruction of her child even though the pregnancy was of very short duration.

The type of treatment necessary and the complications to be avoided in abortion will depend on whether the abortion was spontaneous, induced under sterile conditions for therapeutic reasons or performed illegally by a criminal abortionist or the patient herself. In any case of criminal abortion the nurse must be prepared to assist in prompt diagnosis and immediate treatment of a dangerously ill patient. A sterile pelvic set with speculum and forceps, gloves and lubricant should be on hand. Culture tubes and equipment for taking blood samples must be readily available.

In the early care of the patient, prevention of

hemorrhage and shock are of primary concern. The patient's vital signs and blood pressure are observed carefully and recorded. The number of perineal pads used during a given period will help determine the amount of blood loss. Restlessness, excessive thirst and extreme pallor are also noted as signs of excessive bleeding. It is often necessary to elevate the foot of the bed to alleviate the symptoms of shock; however, this should not be done without a physician's order.

Elevation of body temperature usually indicates the presence of infection. This is especially likely to occur in an abortion that has been performed illegally. Measures aimed at reducing the body temperature may be called for, including sponge baths, ice packs and ice caps, or the use of an ice mattress.

Intravenous fluids and blood transfusions are employed to replace blood and body fluids lost. The rate of flow, kind and amount of fluid given and the patient's reaction to the infusion are observed and recorded.

Since acute renal failure is a common complication of septic abortion, the patient's intake and output must be measured and recorded. The amount and peculiar characteristics of the urine should also be noted on the patient's record.

During the convalescent period the patient may show a need to talk with an interested, objective listener who will not sit in judgment of her actions. By listening to her patient and showing a willingness to help her with her problem, the nurse may find an excellent opportunity for educating the patient, and thus preventing future abortions as a means of controlling the size of the family.

complete a., a complete expulsion of all the products of conception.

criminal a., termination of pregnancy by illegal interference. Contrary to popular belief, most illegally induced abortions are performed on married women, most often among the desperate indigent mothers of several children who feel that the economic burden of another child would be more than the family could bear. Most therapeutic abortions take place in private hospitals, whereas more patients who have had illegal abortions are admitted to county and state institutions that provide care for the economically underprivileged or indigent.

The exact number of criminal abortions performed in this country cannot be recorded because many go unreported; research has shown that there is an alarming increase in the practice of criminal abortions. In spite of the discovery of antibiotics and improved medical techniques, the mortality is tragically high because most of these patients wait until too late to seek medical attention. The high rate of maternal deaths from criminal abortion can also be attributed to the drastic and often incredibly unsanitary measures used to terminate the pregnancy. The most frequent complications of criminal abortion are severe hemorrhage, sepsis, renal failure and septic shock.

early a., abortion within the first 12 weeks of pregnancy.

habitual a., spontaneous abortion occurring in three or more successive pregnancies.

incomplete a., abortion in which parts of the products of conception are retained in the uterus.

induced a., abortion brought on intentionally by medication or instrumentation.

inevitable a., abortion in which termination cannot be prevented.

missed a., retention of a dead embryo for more than 2 weeks.

septic a., abortion in which there is infection of the tissue of the uterus.

spontaneous a., abortion occurring naturally. It has been estimated that 10 to 12 per cent of all pregnancies end in spontaneous abortion. Habitual aborters are uncommon, but they account for the high percentage of abortions of this type. The woman who has repeated abortions should have a comprehensive examination to determine the cause of this disorder. Hormonal imbalances, especially those involving the progestational hormones, and emotional and psychologic disturbances frequently play an important role in spontaneous abortion. Early prenatal care, under the supervision of an obstetrician, may prevent spontaneous termination of pregnancy.

When spontaneous abortion does occur, the patient should notify her physician at once in order to prevent serious complications that may develop. Any material such as clots or bits of tissue should be saved for laboratory examination. Hemorrhage, shock and infection are the most frequent hazards of spontaneous abortion. Treatment usually consists of DILATION AND CURETTAGE to remove tissues that may be retained in the uterus. If the abortion is complete, the attending physician may consider a surgical procedure unnecessary. In any event the patient should consult her physician at the first sign of bleeding or cramping during pregnancy.

therapeutic a., abortion induced legally by a qualified physician for medical or other reasons. Some people, because of religious or ethical convictions, feel that destroying a life is never justified, and that abortions should therefore never be permitted. Others believe that the life of a mother, with all that it means to her present and future children, should not be sacrificed or endangered for the sake of maintaining the life of an unborn infant whose chances of survival may be slim.

The decision to perform an abortion places a heavy responsibility on the physician. In most hospitals a committee of several recognized authorities or specialists must agree that an abortion is necessary before it may be performed. When an abortion is deemed essential, and is performed under hospital conditions by a qualified surgeon, the operation, by a procedure called curettage, is relatively simple and safe. Recent advances in medical sciences have almost eliminated the need for induced abortions as a means of safeguarding the mother's life. The most common indications for such a procedure are hypertensive, renal or heart disease. Therapeutic abortion is sometimes performed in this country if the fetus is abnormal or because of neurologic or psychologic disease.

abortive (ah-bor′tiv) 1. incompletely developed. 2. abortifacient.

abortus (ah-bor′tus) a dead or nonviable fetus (weighing less than 17 ounces, or 500 Gm., at birth).

abrachia (ah-bra′ke-ah) congenital absence of the arms.

abrachiocephalia (ah-bra″ke-o-sĕ-fa′le-ah) a developmental anomaly with absence of the head and arms.

Abrami's disease (ah-brahm′ēz) acquired hemolytic jaundice.

abrasion (ah-bra′zhun) a wound caused by rubbing or scraping the skin or mucous membrane. A "skinned knee" and a "floor burn" are common examples. To treat the injury, the wound should be washed, a mild antiseptic such as hydrogen peroxide applied and the wound covered with sterile gauze. If there is much oozing, a thin film of boric acid ointment will help prevent the gauze from sticking to the wound.

abrasive (ah-bra′siv) 1. causing abrasion. 2. an agent that produces abrasion.

abreaction (ab″re-ak′shun) the release of tension and anxiety associated with the emotional reliving of past, especially repressed, events (catharsis).

abreuography (ab″roo-og′rah-fe) photofluorography.

abruptio (ah-brup′she-o) [L.] separation.
 a. placen′tae, premature separation of a normally situated placenta (see also PLACENTA).

abscess (ab′ses) a localized collection of pus in a cavity formed by the disintegration of tissue. Abscesses are usually caused by specific microorganisms that invade the tissues, often by way of small wounds or breaks in the skin. An abscess is a natural defense mechanism in which the body attempts to localize an infection and "wall off" the microorganisms so they cannot spread throughout the body. As the microorganisms destroy the tissue, an increased supply of blood is rushed to the area. The cells, bacteria and dead tissue accumulate in a clump of cream-colored liquid, which is the pus. The accumulating pus and the adjacent swollen, inflamed tissues press against the nerves, causing pain. The concentration of blood in the area causes redness. The abscess sometimes "comes to a head" (localizes) by itself and breaks through the skin or other tissues, allowing the pus to drain.
 A skin abscess, no matter how small, should never be squeezed since pressure against the inflamed tissues is likely to spread the infection. Small abscesses frequently drain and heal themselves; larger abscesses and internal abscesses should always be treated by a physician, who may find it necessary to incise the abscess to allow for drainage of the exudate. Sulfonamide drugs and some of the antibiotics often help combat the infection.
 alveolar a., a localized suppurative inflammation of tissues about the apex of the root of a tooth.
 arthrifluent a., a wandering abscess originating in a diseased joint.
 Bezold's a., subperiosteal abscess of the temporal bone.
 Brodie's a., a circumscribed abscess in bone, caused by hematogenous infection, that becomes a chronic nidus of infection.
 cold a., one of slow development and with little inflammation, usually tuberculous.
 diffuse a., a collection of pus not enclosed by a capsule.
 miliary a., one composed of numerous small collections of pus.
 milk a., abscess of the breast occurring during lactation.
 perianal a., one beneath the skin of the anus and the anal canal.
 phlegmonous a., one associated with acute inflammation of the subcutaneous connective tissue.
 primary a., one formed at the seat of the infection.
 stitch a., one developed about a stitch or suture.
 thecal a., one in the sheath of a tendon.
 wandering a., one that burrows through the tissues, moving from place to place.

abscissa (ab-sis′ah) one of the lines in a graph along which are plotted the units of one of the factors considered in the study, as time in a time-temperature study. The other line is called the ordinate.

abscission (ab-sish′un) removal of a part or growth by cutting.

absent-mindedness (ab′sent-mīnd″ed-nes) preoccupation to the extent of being unaware of one's immediate surroundings.

absorb (ab-sorb′) to attract and incorporate other material, as through a membrane.

absorbefacient (ab-sor″bĕ-fa′shent) causing absorption.

absorbent (ab-sorb′ent) 1. characterized by absorption. 2. a solid that attracts other material and incorporates it into its substance.

absorption (ab-sorp′shun) the act of taking up or in by specific chemical or molecular action; especially the passage of liquids or other substances through a surface of the body into body fluids and tissues, as in the absorption of the end products of DIGESTION into the villi that line the intestine.

absorptive (ab-sorp′tiv) having the power of absorption.

abstergent (ab-ster′jent) 1. cleansing or detergent. 2. a cleansing agent.

abstinence (ab′stĭ-nens) a refraining from the use or indulgence in food, stimulants or coitus.
 a. syndrome, withdrawal.

abstraction (ab-strak′shun) 1. the mental process of forming abstract ideas. 2. a state synonymous with absent-mindedness.

abtorsion (ab-tor′shun) a turning outward of both eyes.

abulia (ah-bu′le-ah) inability to perform acts voluntarily or to make decisions. adj., **abu′lic.**

abulomania (ah-bu″lo-ma′ne-ah) mental disease with loss of will power.

abutment (ah-but′ment) the anchorage tooth for a bridge.

Ac chemical symbol, *actinium.*

a.c. [L.] *an′te ci′bum* (before meals).

acacia (ah-ka′shah) the dried gummy exudate from stems and branches of species of Acacia, prepared as a mucilage or syrup. It is used as a suspending agent for drugs in pharmaceutical preparations, as an emollient and demulcent and, in solution, as in an intravenous infusion in shock.

acalcicosis (ah-kal″sĭ-ko′sis) a condition due to deficiency of calcium in the diet.

acalculia (a″kal-ku′le-ah) inability to do mathematical calculations.

acampsia (a-kamp′se-ah) rigidity of a part or limb.

acanth(o)- (ah-kan′tho) word element [Gr.], *sharp spine; thorn.*

acantha (ah-kan′tha) a spinous process of a vertebra.

acanthaceous (ak″an-tha′shus) bearing prickles.

acanthesthesia (ah-kan″thes-the′ze-ah) a sensation of a sharp point pricking the body.

Acanthocephala (ah-kan″tho-sef′ah-lah) a phylum of elongate, mostly cylindrical organisms parasitic in the intestines of all classes of vertebrates.

acanthocephaliasis (ah-kan″tho-sef″ah-li′ah-sis) infection with worms of the phylum Acanthocephala.

Acanthocephalus (ah-kan″tho-sef′ah-lus) a genus of parasitic worms (phylum Acanthocephala).

Acanthocheilonema (ah-kan″tho-ki″lo-ne′mah) a genus of long, threadlike worms; also called Dipetalonema.
   A. per′stans, a species often infecting man.

acanthocyte (ah-kan′tho-sīt) an erythrocyte with protoplasmic projections giving it a thorny appearance.

acanthokeratodermia (ah-kan″tho-ker″ah-to-der′me-ah) hyperkeratosis.

acantholysis (ah″kan-thol′ĭ-sis) loss of cohesion between the cells of the prickle cell layer and between it and the layer above.
   a. bullo′sa, epidermolysis bullosa.

acanthoma (ak″an-tho′mah) a tumor in the prickle cell layer of the skin.

acanthosis (ak″an-tho′sis) hypertrophy or thickening of the prickle cell layer of the skin. adj., **acanthot′ic.**
   a. ni′gricans, a dermatosis with roughness and increased pigmentation, either generalized or in the axillae or body folds.

acanthrocyte (ah-kan′thro-sīt) acanthocyte.

acapnia (ah-kap′ne-ah) decrease of carbon dioxide in the blood. adj., **acap′nic.**

acarbia (ah-kar′be-ah) decrease of bicarbonate in the blood.

acardia (ah-kar′de-ah) a developmental anomaly with absence of the heart.

acardiacus (ah″kar-di′ah-kus) [L.] having no heart.

acardius (ah-kar′de-us) a fetal monster without a heart.

acariasis (ak″ah-ri′ah-sis) infestation with mites.

acaricide (ah-kar′ĭ-sīd) an agent that destroys mites.

acarid (ak′ah-rid) a tick or mite of the order Acarina.

Acarina (ak″ah-ri′nah) an order of arthropods (class Arachnoidea), including mites and ticks.

acarinosis (ah-kar″ĭ-no′sis) any disease caused by mites.

acarodermatitis (ak″ah-ro-der″mah-ti′tis) skin inflammation due to bites of parasitic mites (acarids).
   a. urticarioi′des, grain itch.

acarology (ak″ah-rol′o-je) the scientific study of mites and ticks.

acarophobia (ak″ah-ro-fo′be-ah) morbid dread or delusion of infestation by mites.

Acarus (ak′ah-rus) a genus of arthropods (order Acarina), including mites.
   A. folliculo′rum, *Demodex folliculorum.*
   A. scab′iei, *Sarcoptes scabiei.*

acaryote (ah-kār′e-ōt) non-nucleated.

acatalasemia (a″kat-ah-la-se′me-ah) deficiency of catalase in the blood.

acatalasia (a″kat-ah-la′ze-ah) congenital absence of catalase from the body cells.

acatalepsy (ah-kat′ah-lep″se) 1. lack of understanding. 2. uncertainty. adj., **acatalep′tic.**

acathexia (ak″ah-thek′se-ah) inability to retain bodily secretions. adj. **acathec′tic.**

A.C.C. American College of Cardiology.

accelerator (ak-sel′er-a″tor) [L.] an agent or apparatus that increases the rate at which something occurs or progresses.
   serum prothrombin conversion a., clotting factor VII.
   serum thrombotic a., a factor in serum that has procoagulant properties and the ability to induce blood CLOTTING.
   thromboplastin generation a., a heat-labile component in plasma which appears to influence the rate of formation of thromboplastin.

accelerin (ak-sel′er-in) clotting factor V.

acceptor (ak-sep′tor) a substance that unites with another substance.
   hydrogen a., the molecule accepting hydrogen in an oxidation-reduction reaction.

accessory (ak-ses′o-re) supplementary or affording aid to another similar and generally more important thing.
   a. nerve, the eleventh cranial nerve; it originates in the medulla oblongata and provides motion for the sternocleidomastoid and trapezius muscles of the neck. Called also spinal accessory nerve.

accipiter (ak-sip′ĭ-ter) a facial bandage with tails like the claws of a hawk.

acclimation (ak-lī-ma′shun) the process of becoming accustomed to a new climate, soil and conditions.

accommodation (ah-kom″o-da′shun) adjustment, especially adjustment of the eye for seeing objects at various distances. This is accomplished by the ciliary muscle, which controls the LENS of the eye, allowing it to flatten or thicken as is needed for distant or near vision.

absolute a., the accommodation of either eye separately.

amplitude of a., the total amount of accommodative power of the eye; the difference in refractive power of the eye when adjusted for near and for far vision. The amplitude diminishes as age increases because elasticity of the lens is decreased. Called also range of accommodation.

histologic a., changes in morphology and function of cells following changed conditions.

negative a., adjustment of the eye for long distances by relaxation of the ciliary muscle.

positive a., adjustment of the eye for short distances by contraction of the ciliary muscle.

a. reflex, the coordinated changes that occur when the eye adapts itself for near vision; they are constriction of the pupil, convergence of the eyes and increased convexity of the lens.

accouchement (ah-kōōsh-maw′) [Fr.] childbirth; delivery; labor.

a. force, forcible delivery with the hand.

accretion (ah-kre′shun) accumulation of matter in a part.

acelomate (ah-se′lo-māt) having no coelom or body cavity.

acenocoumarol (ah-se″no-koo′mah-rol) a compound used as an anticoagulant.

acentric (a-sen′tric) having no center; in genetics, designating an apparent pair of sister chromatids without a centromere.

acephalia (ah″sĕ-fa′le-ah) a developmental anomaly with absence of the head.

acephalobrachia (ah-sef″ah-lo-bra′ke-ah) a developmental anomaly with absence of the head and arms.

acephalocardia (ah-sef″ah-lo-kar′de-ah) a developmental anomaly with absence of the head and heart.

acephalocardius (ah-sef″ah-lo-kar′de-us) a fetal monster without a head or heart.

acephalochiria (ah-sef″ah-lo-ki′re-ah) a developmental anomaly with absence of the head and hands.

acephalocystis racemosa (ah-sef″ah-lo-sis′tis ra-se-mo′sah) a hydatid mole of the uterus.

acephalogaster (ah-sef″ah-lo-gas′ter) a fetal monster without a head or stomach.

acephalogastria (ah-sef″ah-lo-gas′tre-ah) a developmental anomaly with absence of the head, chest and stomach.

acephalopodia (ah-sef″ah-lo-po′de-ah) a developmental anomaly with absence of the head and feet.

acephalopodius (ah-sef″ah-lo-po′de-us) a fetal monster without a head or feet.

acephalorachia (ah-sef″ah-lo-ra′ke-ah) a developmental anomaly with absence of the head and vertebral column.

acephalostomia (ah-sef″ah-lo-sto′me-ah) a developmental anomaly with absence of the head, with the mouth aperture on the upper aspect of the fetal body.

acephalothoracia (ah-sef″ah-lo-tho-ra′se-ah) a developmental anomaly with absence of the head and thorax.

acephalous (ah-sef′ah-lus) headless.

acephalus (ah-sef′ah-lus) a fetal monster without a head.

acervuloma (ah-ser″vu-lo′mah) a meningioma containing psammoma bodies.

acervulus (ah-ser′vu-lus), pl. *acer′vuli* [L.] a little heap.

a. cer′ebri, sandy matter about the pineal gland and other parts of the brain.

acescence (ah-ses′ens) sourness.

acestoma (ah″ses-to′mah) a mass of granulations.

acetabular (as″ĕ-tab′u-lar) pertaining to the acetabulum.

acetabulectomy (as″ĕ-tab″u-lek′to-me) excision of the acetabulum.

acetabuloplasty (as″ĕ-tab′u-lo-plas′te) plastic repair of the acetabulum.

acetabulum (as″ĕ-tab′u-lum) the cup-shaped cavity in the coxa, receiving the head of the femur.

acetaldehyde (as″et-al′de-hīd) a colorless volatile liquid, CH_3CHO, found in freshly distilled spirits, that produces profound narcosis and deleterious aftereffects.

acetaminophen (as″et-am′ĭ-no-fen″) a compound used as an analgesic and antipyretic.

acetanilid (as″ĕ-tan′ĭ-lid) a white powder, slightly soluble in water, used as an analgesic and antipyretic, particularly in combination with other drugs in various proprietary preparations such as headache remedies. Habituation may occur and the drug is little used because its continued use may lead to methemoglobinemia.

acetarsol, acetarsone (as″et-ar′sol), (as″et-ar′sōn) an arsenical compound occasionally used to destroy parasites in amebiasis and vaginitis caused by *Trichomonas vaginalis.* In excessive doses it may damage kidneys or liver.

acetate (as′ĕ-tāt) a salt of acetic acid.

acetazolamide (as″et-ah-zol′ah-mīd) a diuretic of the carbonic anhydrase inhibitor type, useful in the treatment of cardiac edema. It is also used to reduce intraocular pressure in the treatment of glaucoma. Side effects of the drug are minor but an electrolyte imbalance with potassium depletion may occur.

Acetest (as′ĕ-test) a test for acetone in urine, utilizing tablets impregnated with chemicals. Urine is dropped on the tablet, which is then held against a color chart for comparison. If acetone is present, the tablet will have a purplish color.

acetic (ah-se′tik, ah-set′ik) pertaining to vinegar or its acid; sour.

a. acid, a short-chain, saturated fatty acid, the characteristic component of vinegar. It has the odor of vinegar and a sharp acid taste. A 36.5 per cent solution of acetic acid is used topically as a caustic and rubefacient. A dilute acetic acid solution (6 per cent) may be used as an antidote to alkali. Glacial acetic acid is a 99.4 per cent solution.

aceticoceptor (ah-se″tĭ-ko-sep′tor) a side chain having an affinity for the acetic acid radical.

acetimeter (as″ĕ-tim′ĕ-ter) an instrument for measuring the acetic acid in a fluid.

acetoacetic acid (ah-se″tō-ah-se′tik) one of the KETONE BODIES formed in the body in metabolism of certain substances, particularly in the liver in the combustion of fats. It is present in the body in increased amounts in abnormal conditions such as diabetes mellitus and starvation.

Acetobacter (ah-se″to-bak′ter) a genus of Schizomycetes important in completion of the carbon cycle and in production of vinegar.

acetomeroctol (as″ĕ-to-mer-ok′tol) an antiseptic for prevention and control of superficial skin infections.

acetone (as′ĕ-tōn) a compound, $CH_3.CO.CH_3$, with solvent properties and characteristic odor, obtained by fermentation or produced synthetically; it is a by-product of acetoacetic acid. Acetone is one of the KETONE BODIES produced in abnormal amounts in DIABETES MELLITUS. (See also KETOSIS).
   a. bodies, acetone, acetoacetic acid and beta-oxybutyric acid, being intermediates in fat metabolism. Also called ketone bodies.

acetonemia (as″ĕ-to-ne′me-ah) ketonemia.

acetonitrile (as″ĕ-to-ni′trĭl) methyl cyanide, CH_3CN, a colorless acid.

acetonuria (as″ĕ-to-nu′re-ah) ketonuria.

acetophenazine (as″ĕ-to-fen′ah-zēn) a compound used as a tranquilizer.

acetophenetidin (as″ĕ-to-fĕ-net′ĭ-din) a white crystalline powder with antipyretic properties but primarily used as an analgesic in the relief of common aches and pains such as headache, neuralgia and dysmenorrhea. Called also phenacetin. The drug must be used with caution because its continued overdose can lead to serious renal and hematologic complications. Preparations of acetophenetidin must be labeled with the following warning: Do not take regularly for more than 10 days unless directed to do so by a physician.

acetrozoate sodium (as″ĕ-tro′zo-āt so′de-um) a radiopaque medium for roentgenographic visualization of blood vessels and kidneys.

acetyl (as′ĕ-til) the monovalent radical, CH_3CO, a combining form of acetic acid.
   a. peroxide, a powerful oxidizing agent.
   a. sulfisoxazole, a sulfanilamide used an an anti-infective.

acetylaniline (as″ĕ-til-an′ĭ-lin) acetanilid.

acetylation (ah-set″ĭ-la′shun) introduction of an acetyl radical into an organic molecule.

acetyl-beta-methylcholine (as″ĕ-til-ba″tah-meth″il-ko′lēn) methacholine.

acetylcarbromal (as″ĕ-til-kar-bro′mal) a sedative

drug used primarily to relieve tension and anxiety and as a daytime sedative.

acetylcholine (as″ĕ-til-ko′lēn) a reversible acetic acid ester of choline, normally present in many parts of the body and having important physiologic functions, such as the transmission of nerve impulses; used as a parasympathomimetic agent.
   a. chloride, an agent that rapidly produces miosis, or contraction of the pupil; used in cataract surgery and iridectomy.

acetylcholinesterase (as″ĕ-til-ko″lin-es′ter-ās) an enzyme having a higher affinity for acetylcholine than for any other ester (see also CHOLINESTERASE).

acetyldigitoxin-α (as″ĕ-til-dij″ĭ-tok′sin al′fah) an oral digitalis preparation derived from lanatoside, used to improve function of the failing heart. It provides a more rapid curve of action than digitoxin and is less completely absorbed, but is not actually less toxic.

acetylene (ah-set′ĭ-lēn) a colorless, combustible gas, C_2H_2, with an unpleasant odor.

acetylphenylhydrazine (as″ĕ-til-fen″il-hi′drah-zēn) an erythrocyte depressant now seldom used in the treatment of polycythemia.

acetylsalicylic acid (ah-sēt′il-sal-ĭ-sil′ik) aspirin, a commonly used analgesic, antipyretic and antirheumatic drug. It is available in pure form or in combination with a variety of drugs.

A.C.G. American College of Gastroenterology.

Ac-G accelerator globulin (clotting factor V).

ACH adrenocortical hormone.

ACh acetylcholine.

achalasia (ak″ah-la′ze-ah) failure to relax of the smooth muscle fibers of the gastrointestinal tract at any junction of one part with another; especially failure of the lower esophagus to relax with swallowing.
   The cause of achalasia is unknown, but anxiety and emotional tension seem to aggravate the condition and precipitate attacks. As the condition progresses there is dilatation of the esophagus above the constriction and absence of peristalsis in the area.
   SYMPTOMS. The patient complains of a feeling of fullness in the sternal region; vomiting frequently occurs, and there may be aspiration of the esophageal contents into the respiratory passages. As a result of this aspiration the patient may develop pneumonia or atelectasis.
   Diagnosis is confirmed by x-ray studies using barium and by visual examination of the area by esophagoscope.
   TREATMENT. Conservative treatment of mild cases consists of advising the patient to eat a bland diet that is low in bulk. Very large meals should be avoided and all foods should be eaten slowly with frequent drinking of fluids during the meal. To reduce the possibility of aspiration of esophageal contents during sleep, the patient is instructed to sleep with his head and shoulders elevated.
   For severe constriction surgical relief may be necessary. The incision, which includes the lower

esophagus and upper stomach wall, is made down to but not through the intestinal mucosa. This allows for stretching of the mucosa to accommodate food passing through. Approach is made through an incision into the chest; thus, preoperative care and postoperative care are the same as for elective chest surgery (see also THORACIC SURGERY).

AChE acetylcholinesterase.

ache (āk) continuous pain, as opposed to sharp pangs or twinges. An ache can be either dull and constant, as in some types of backache, or throbbing, as in some types of headache and toothache.

acheilia (ah-ki′le-ah) a developmental anomaly with absence of the lips.

acheiria (ah-ki′re-ah) 1. a developmental anomaly with absence of the hands. 2. a sensation as of loss of the hands, seen in hysteria.

acheiropodia (ah-ki″ro-po′de-ah) a developmental anomaly characterized by absence of both hands and feet.

Achilles tendon (ah-kil′ēz) the strong tendon at the back of the heel that connects the calf muscles to the heel bone. The name is derived from the legend of the Greek hero Achilles, who was vulnerable only in one heel. Tapping the Achilles tendon normally produces the Achilles REFLEX, or ankle jerk. Failure or exaggeration of this reflex indicates disease or injury to the nerves of the leg muscles or of a part of the spinal cord.

achillobursitis (ah-kil″o-bur-si′tis) inflammation of the bursae about the Achilles tendon.

achillodynia (ah-kil″o-din′e-ah) pain in the Achilles tendon.

achillorrhaphy (ak″il-lor′ah-fe) suturing of the Achilles tendon.

achillotenotomy (ah-kil″o-ten-ot′o-me) incision of the Achilles tendon.

achlorhydria (a″klor-hi′dre-ah) absence of hydrochloric acid from gastric juice; associated with PERNICIOUS ANEMIA, stomach cancer and pellagra.

achloropsia (a″klo-rop′se-ah) blindness to green colors.

acholia (a-ko′le-ah) absence of bile secretion. adj., **acho′lic**.

acholuria (ak″o-lu′re-ah) absence of bile pigments from the urine.

achondroplasia (a-kon″dro-pla′ze-ah) a disorder of cartilage formation in the fetus, leading to a type of dwarfism. adj., **achondroplas′tic**.

achoresis (ak″o-re′sis) diminution of the capacity of an organ.

Achorion (ah-ko′re-on) Trichophyton.

achrestic (ah-kres′tik) caused not by absence of a necessary substance, but by inability to utilize such a substance.

achroacyte (ah-kro′ah-sīt) a colorless cell or leukocyte.

achroacytosis (ah-kro″ah-si-to′sis) excessive development of lymph cells (colorless cells).

achroiocythemia (ah-kroi″o-si-the′me-ah) deficiency or lack of hemoglobin in the erythrocytes.

achroma (ah-kro′mah) absence of color.

achromacyte (ah-kro′mah-sīt) a decolorized erythrocyte.

achromasia (a″kro-ma′ze-ah) lack of normal skin pigment.

achromat (ak′ro-mat″) a person who is color-blind.

achromatic (ak″ro-mat′ik) 1. producing no discoloration, or staining with difficulty. 2. pertaining to achromatin. 3. refracting light without decomposing it into its component colors.

achromatin (ah-kro′mah-tin) the faintly staining groundwork of a cell nucleus.

achromatocyte (ak″ro-mat′o-sīt) a decolorized erythrocyte.

achromatolysis (ah-kro″mah-tol′ĭ-sis) disorganization of cell achromatin.

achromatophil (a″kro-mat′o-fil, ak″ro-mat′o-fil) not easily stainable.

achromatopia (ah″kro-mah-to′pe-ah) defective visual perception of colors.

achromatosis (ah-kro″mah-to′sis) any disease marked by deficiency of pigmentation.

achromatous (a-kro′mah-tus) colorless.

achromaturia (a-kro″mah-tu′re-ah) colorless state of the urine.

achromia (a-kro′me-ah) absence of normal color.

achromocyte (ah-kro′mo-sīt) a red cell artifact that stains more faintly than intact erythrocytes.

achromodermia (ah-kro″mo-der′me-ah) colorless state of the skin.

achromophil (ah-kro′mo-fil) achromatophil.

achromotrichia (ah-kro″mo-trik′e-ah) loss of color of the hair.

Achromycin (ak″ro-mi′sin) trademark for preparations of tetracycline hydrochloride, a broad-spectrum antibiotic.

achylanemia (a-ki″lah-ne′me-ah) a condition in which gastric achylia is associated with simple or hypochromic anemia.

achylia (a-ki′le-ah) absence of chyle.
  a. gas′trica, absence of hydrochloric acid and enzymes from the gastric secretion.
  a. pancreat′ica, deficiency of enzymes secreted by the pancreas.

achylous (a-ki′lus) deficient in chyle.

achymia (a-ki′me-ah) deficiency of chyme.

acicular (ah-sik′u-lar) needle-shaped.

acid (as′id) 1. sour. 2. a substance that yields hydrogen ions in solution and from which hydrogen may be displaced by a metal to form a salt. All acids react with bases to form salts and water (neutralization). Other properties of acids include a sour taste and the ability to cause certain dyes to undergo a color change. A common example of this is the ability of acids to change litmus paper from blue to red.

Acids play a vital role in the chemical processes that are a normal part of the functions of the cells and tissues of the body. A stable balance between acids and bases in the body is essential to life. (See also ACID-BASE BALANCE.) For the various acids, see under the specific name, such as acetic acid.

amino a., any one of a class of organic compounds containing the amino and the carboxyl group, occurring naturally in plant and animal tissues and forming the chief constituents of protein. (See also AMINO ACID.)

bile a's, organic compounds—glycocholic acid and taurocholic acid—formed in the liver and secreted in the bile.

a. burn, injury to tissues caused by an acid, such as sulfuric acid or nitric acid. Emergency first aid for an acid burn of the skin includes (1) immediate and thorough washing of the burn with water; (2) calling a physician; and (3) continued bathing of the burn in water until the physician arrives. (See also BURN.)

fatty a., any monobasic aliphatic acid containing only carbon, hydrogen and oxygen. (See also FATTY ACID.)

inorganic a., an acid containing no carbon atoms.

keto a's, compounds containing the groups CO (carbonyl) and COOH (carboxyl).

nucleic a's, substances that constitute the prosthetic groups of the nucleoproteins and contain phosphoric acid, sugars and purine and pyrimidine bases. See also NUCLEIC ACIDS.

organic a., an acid containing the carboxyl group, COOH.

a. phosphatase, a phosphatase that is active in an acid environment.

acidaminuria (as"id-am"ĭ-nu're-ah) excess of amino acid in the urine.

acid-ash diet a special diet prescribed for the purpose of lowering the urinary pH so that alkaline salts will remain in solution. The diet may be given to aid in the elimination of fluid in certain kinds of edema, in the treatment of some types of urinary tract infection and to inhibit the formation of alkaline urinary calculi. Meat, fish, eggs and cereals are emphasized; fruits, vegetables and milk may be forbidden or restricted.

acid-base balance the maintenance of a normal balance between the acidity and alkalinity of the body fluids located within the extracellular and intracellular compartments. Since most of the normal metabolic processes of the body produce acids as their end products, the body must work continuously to maintain this delicate balance. Chemical buffers, principally bicarbonates, phosphates and salts of proteins, help in the neutralization process. The kidneys and lungs also participate in this mechanism because of their control of the availability of the ELECTROLYTES that are essential to proper functioning of the buffer system.

The term pH is used to indicate the acidity or alkalinity of a solution; for serum a pH of 7.35 to 7.45 is considered neutral; a decrease in the pH indicates ACIDOSIS, whereas an increase indicates ALKALOSIS. A favorable pH is essential to the functioning of living cells; a pH of below 6 or above 8 is generally fatal.

The most important abnormalities in acid-base balance involve the bicarbonate buffer and result in changes in the electrolyte structure of the body fluids. These changes are usually caused by renal dysfunction, loss of gastric secretions or excess metabolic acids in the extracellular fluid, as occurs in starvation and uncontrolled diabetes mellitus. Respiratory disorders may also produce a change in the acid-base balance by altering the output or input of carbon dioxide which is dissolved as carbonic acid in the blood.

acidemia (as"ĭ-de'me-ah) abnormal acidity of the blood.

acid-fast (as'id-fast) not readily decolorized by acids after staining; said of bacteria, especially *Mycobacterium tuberculosis.*

acidifier (ah-sid'ĭ-fi"er) an agent that causes acidity; a substance used to increase gastric acidity.

acidity (ah-sid'ĭ-te) 1. the quality of being acid; the power to unite with positively charged ions or with basic substances. 2. excess acid quality, as of the gastric juice.

acidocyte (ah-sid'o-sīt) an acidophilic cell (eosinophil).

acidophilic (as"ĭ-do-fil'ik) 1. easily stained with acid dyes. 2. growing best on acid media.

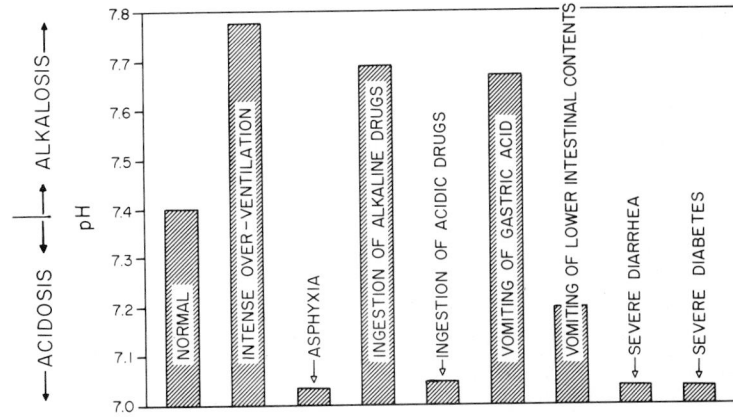

pH of the body fluids in various acid-base disorders. (From Guyton, A. C.: Function of the Human Body. 3rd ed. Philadelphia, W. B. Saunders Co., 1969.)

acidophilism (as″ĭ-dof′ĭ-lizm) the state produced by acidophilic adenoma of the pituitary gland, resulting in ACROMEGALY.

acidophilous (as″ĭ-dof′ĭ-lus) acidophilic.

acidosis (as″ĭ-do′sis) a pathologic condition resulting from accumulation of acid or depletion of the alkaline reserve (bicarbonate content) in the blood and body tissues, and characterized by increase in hydrogen ion concentration (decrease in pH). The normal pH of the blood is about 7.4 (slightly alkaline) and is maintained at that level by chemical buffers and normal functioning of the kidneys and lungs. The opposite of acidosis is ALKALOSIS.
Uncorrected acidosis causes disorientation, coma and death. Treatment consists of intravenous or oral administration of sodium bicarbonate or sodium lactate solutions and removal of the underlying cause of the condition.
compensated a., a condition in which the compensatory mechanisms have returned the pH toward normal.
diabetic a., a metabolic acidosis produced by accumulation of ketones in uncontrolled diabetes mellitus.
hypercapnic a., respiratory acidosis.
hyperchloremic a., renal tubular acidosis.
metabolic a., acidosis resulting from accumulation in the blood of keto acids (derived from fat metabolism) at the expense of bicarbonate, thus diminishing the body's ability to neutralize these acids. This type of disturbance in the acid-base balance usually occurs in diabetes mellitus or starvation. Dyspnea, with deep, periodic breathing (as the body attempts to remove carbon dioxide), and a fruity-smelling breath (caused by acetone) are among the symptoms of metabolic acidosis.
renal tubular a., a metabolic acidosis resulting from impairment of the reabsorption of bicarbonate by the renal tubules, the urine being alkaline.
respiratory a., acidosis due to retention of carbonic acid as carbon dioxide when disorders of the respiratory tract restrict its release from the lungs, causing interference with the bicarbonate buffer system.
starvation a., a metabolic acidosis due to accumulation of ketones following a severe caloric deficit.

acid-proof (as′id-prōōf) acid-fast.

acidulous (ah-sid′u-lus) moderately sour.

acidum (as′ĭ-dum) [L.] acid.

aciduric (as″ĭ-du′rik) capable of growing in extremely acid media.

acinetic (as″ĭ-net′ik) akinetic.

aciniform (ah-sin′ĭ-form) grapelike.

acinitis (as″ĭ-ni′tis) inflammation of the acini of a gland.

acinose, acinous (as′ĭ-nōs), (as′ĭ-nus) made up of acini.

acinus (as′ĭ-nus), pl. *ac′ini* [L.] one of the smallest lobules of a compound gland.

acladiosis (ah-klad″e-o′sis) an ulcerative skin disease caused by a fungus of the genus Acladium.

Acladium (ah-kla′de-um) a genus of fungus sometimes infecting man.

aclasis (ak′lah-sis) pathologic continuity of structure, as in chondrodystrophy.
diaphyseal a., imperfect formation of bone in the cartilage between the diaphysis and epiphysis; dyschondroplasia.

acleistocardia (ah-klīs″to-kar′de-ah) an open state of the foramen ovale.

acme (ak′me) the critical stage or crisis of a disease.

acne (ak′ne) a disorder of the skin with eruption of papules or pustules; more particularly, acne vulgaris.
a. che′loidique, keloid folliculitis.
a. congloba′ta, conglobate a., a staphylococcal infection of the skin leading to formation of cutaneous and subcutaneous abscesses and keloidal scarring.
a. indura′ta, acne vulgaris with deep-seated, destructive lesions.
keloid a., keloid folliculitis.
a. necrot′ica, acne varioliformis.
a. papulo′sa, acne vulgaris with the formation of papules.
a. rosa′cea, rosacea.
a. variolifor′mis, a skin disease with reddish brown papulopustular umbilicated lesions, usually on the brow or scalp, leading to scarring.
a. vulga′ris, a skin condition, usually occurring in adolescence, with comedones (blackheads), papules, nodules and pustules on the face, neck and upper part of the trunk.
At the beginning stages of adulthood, there is an increase in hormonal activity and glandular secretion, including increased production of sebum from the sebaceous glands in the skin. In girls this may be more pronounced at the time of the menstrual period. Certain foods also cause an increase in the activity of the sebaceous glands, the worst offenders being chocolate, nuts, sharp cheeses and fatty foods. If a hair follicle opening on the surface of the skin is small or is clogged by dirt or heavy cosmetics, the fatty material made by the sebaceous glands accumulates, and a "bump" appears under the skin, or a whitehead or blackhead (comedo) shows on the surface. The dark color of blackheads is caused not by dirt but by the discoloring effect of air on the fatty material in the clogged follicle. If this substance becomes infected, as it often does, a pimple results. The temptation to squeeze the unsightly pimple should be resisted. A squeeze can break the membrane around the pimple and spread the infection to the surrounding tissue. The result is more pimples, scars and pits.
This story is all too familiar to young people. It is not enough to be reminded that "you'll grow out of it," although this is generally true. Acne does tend to disappear with maturity. If the adolescent is excessively troubled with this condition, the scars may be mental as well as physical.
TREATMENT. The first step is to discover and eliminate any food that encourages acne. The skin must be kept clean, particularly in the areas where acne is most apt to appear, such as the face, chest and back. With plain soap, fairly hot water and a clean washcloth, the skin is washed, but not scrubbed so hard as to cause injury, and then rinsed with cold water. Sometimes the physician may recommend an antibacterial soap. Towels should

be changed at least daily. Hair should be shampooed frequently, and hairbrush, comb and powder puff should be kept scrupulously clean. All creams and greasy lotions should be avoided, and the follicles should not be plugged with heavy makeup or "pore-closing" beauty aids.

Blackheads are removed with a comedo extractor after the skin has been soaked in warm sudsy water to loosen them. Extractors can be purchased at most drugstores, and should be used instead of fingers. If the blackhead comes out easily, the spot should be touched with rubbing alcohol (70 per cent). If it does not, it should be left alone for a while.

Severe cases of acne require more intensive and complicated treatment, which only a physician can provide. Some cases require therapy by a dermatologist.

When acne has left permanent, disfiguring scars, there are medical techniques that can remove or improve the blemishes. One method is planing with a rotary, high-speed brush. This removes the outer layer of pitted skin, leaving the growing layer and the layers containing the glands and hair follicles. New epithelium grows from the layers underneath; it is rosy at first and gradually becomes normal in color. The technique has also been used successfully in removing some types of disfigurations resulting from accidents. This so-called "sand-paper surgery" or dermabrasion is recommended only for selected cases of acne. It must be performed by a qualified specialist.

acnegenic (ak″ne-jen′ik) producing acne.

acneiform (ak-ne′ĭ-form) resembling acne.

acoelomate (a-se′lo-māt) without a coelom or body cavity.

aconite (ak′o-nīt) dried tuberous root of *Aconitum napellus;* used as a counterirritant and local anesthetic.

aconitine (ah-kon′ĭ-tin) an alkaloid that is the active principle of aconite.

acorea (ah″ko-re′ah) absence of the pupil.

acoria (ah-ko′re-ah) insatiable appetite.

acormus (ah-kor′mus) a fetal monster with a rudimentary trunk.

acouesthesia (ah-koo″es-the′ze-ah) acoustic sensibility.

acoumeter (ah-koo′mě-ter) an instrument for measuring the accuracy or acuteness of the hearing.

acoustic (ah-koos′tik) relating to sound or hearing.

acoustics (ah-koos′tiks) the science of sound and hearing.

acoustogram (ah-koos′to-gram) the graphic tracing of the curves of sounds produced by motion of a joint.

A.C.P. American College of Pathologists; American College of Physicians.

acquired (ah-kwīrd′) incurred as a result of factors acting from or originating outside the organism; not inherited.

A.C.R. American College of Radiology.

acragnosia (ak″rag-no′ze-ah) lack of sensory recognition of a limb.

acral (a′kral) affecting the extremities.

acrania (a-kra′ne-ah) partial or complete absence of the cranium.

acranius (a-kra′ne-us) fetal monster in which the cranium is absent or rudimentary.

acridine (ak′rĭ-dēn) a crystalline alkaloid from anthracene, the basis of certain dyes.

acriflavine (ak″rĭ-fla′vin) an antiseptic dye used for application to mucous membranes; average strength is 1:1000 to 1:8000 solution

acritical (a-krit′ĭ-kal) having no crisis.

acro- (ak′ro) word element [Gr.], *extreme; top; extremity.*

acroagnosis (ak″ro-ag-no′sis) acragnosia.

acroanesthesia (ak″ro-an″es-the′ze-ah) anesthesia of the extremities.

acroasphyxia (ak″ro-as-fik′se-ah) lack of circulation in the digits.
  chronic a., acrocyanosis.

acrobrachycephaly (ak″ro-brak″e-sef′ah-le) abnormal height of the skull, with shortness of its anteroposterior dimension.

acrocentric (ak″ro-sen′trik) having the centromere toward one end of the replicating chromosome.

acrocephalia (ak″ro-sě-fa′le-ah) acrocephaly.

acrocephalic (ak″ro-sě-fal′ik) having a high, pointed head, with a vertical index of 77 or more.

acrocephalosyndactyly (ak″ro-sef″ah-lo-sin-dak′tĭ-le) acrocephaly associated with webbing of the fingers or toes.

acrocephaly (ak″ro-sef′ah-le) a high, pointed condition of the top of the skull.

acrochordon (ak″ro-kor′don) a pedunculated growth of skin occurring principally on the neck, upper chest and axillae in women of middle age or older.

acrocinesis (ak″ro-si-ne′sis) acrokinesia.

acrocyanosis (ak″ro-si″ah-no′sis) cyanosis and bluish or red discoloration of the digits.

acrodermatitis (ak″ro-der″mah-ti′tis) inflammation of the skin of the hands or feet.
  a. atroph′icans chron′ica, chronic atrophic a., chronic inflammation of the skin of the extremities, leading to atrophy of the cutis.
  enteropathic a., a familial disorder, occurring chiefly in infants, with localized eruption, and associated with disorders of the gastrointestinal tract.

acrodermatosis (ak″ro-der″mah-to′sis) an eruption on the skin of the hands and feet.

acrodynia (ak″ro-din′e-ah) erythredema polyneuropathy.

acroedema (ak″ro-ě-de′mah) edema of the hand or foot.

acroesthesia (ak″ro-es-the′ze-ah) 1. exaggerated sensitiveness. 2. pain in the extremities.

acrognosis (ak″rog-no′sis) sensory recognition of a limb.

acrohyperhidrosis (ak″ro-hi″per-hĭ-dro′sis) excessive sweating of the hands and feet.

acrohypothermy (ak″ro-hi′po-ther″me) abnormal coldness of the hands and feet.

acrokeratosis (ak″ro-ker″ah-to′sis) a condition involving the skin of the extremities, with the appearance of horny growths.

acrokinesia (ak″ro-ki-ne′se-ah) abnormal motility or movement of the extremities.

acrolein (ak-ro′le-in) a volatile liquid from the decomposition of glycerin.

acromacria (ak″ro-mak′re-ah) acromegaly.

acromegaly (ak″ro-meg′ah-le) abnormal enlargement of the facial features, hands and feet, resulting from overproduction of the growth-stimulating hormone of the PITUITARY GLAND. The condition is relatively rare and occurs in adults. In children overproduction of growth hormone stimulates growth of long bones and results in GIGANTISM, in which the child grows to exaggerated heights. With adults, however, growth of the long bones has already stopped, so that the bones most affected are those of the face, the jaw and the hands and feet.

Overproduction of growth hormone is most often due to a tumor of the pituitary, and in such cases the condition is treated by surgical removal of the tumor or radiotherapy, or a combination of the two.

acromelalgia (ak″ro-mel-al′je-ah) erythromelalgia.

acromicria (ak″ro-mi′kre-ah) abnormal smallness of the facial features, hands and feet.

acromio- (ah-kro′me-o) word element [Gr.], *acromion.*

acromioclavicular joint (ah-kro″me-o-klah-vik′u-lar) the point at which the clavicle joins with the acromion.

acromiohumeral (ah-kro″me-o-hu′mer-al) pertaining to the acromion and humerus.

acromion (ah-kro′me-on) the lateral extension of the spine of the scapula, forming the highest point of the shoulder. adj., **acro′mial.**

acromionectomy (ah-kro″me-on-ek′to-me) resection of the acromion.

acromiothoracic (ah-kro″me-o-tho-ras′ik) pertaining to the acromion and thorax.

acromphalus (ah-krom′fah-lus) 1. bulging of the navel as the first stage of umbilical hernia. 2. the center of the navel.

acroneuropathy (ak″ro-nu-rop′ah-the) a familial neuropathy affecting the distal parts of the extremities and producing anesthetic ulcers.

acronyx (ak′ro-niks) an ingrowing nail.

acropachy (ak′ro-pak″e) clubbing of the fingers.

acropachyderma (ak″ro-pak″e-der′mah) thickening of the skin over the face, scalp and extremities, together with deformities of the long bones.

acroparalysis (ak″ro-pah-ral′ĭ-sis) paralysis of the extremities.

acroparesthesia (ak″ro-par″es-the′ze-ah) an abnormal sensation, such as tingling, numbness, pins and needles, in the digits.

acropathy (ak-rop′ah-the) any disease of the extremities.

acrophobia (ak″ro-fo′be-ah) morbid fear of heights.

acroposthitis (ak″ro-pos-thi′tis) inflammation of the prepuce.

acroscleroderma (ak″ro-skle″ro-der′mah) sclerodactylia; scleroderma of the fingers and toes.

acrosclerosis (ak″ro-sklĕ-ro′sis) scleroderma involving the extremities and distal portions of the head and face, accompanied by Raynaud's phenomenon.

acrotism (ak′ro-tizm) defect or failure of the pulse.

A.C.S. American Cancer Society; American Chemical Society; American College of Surgeons.

ACTH adrenocorticotropic hormone, a hormone produced by the anterior lobe of the PITUITARY GLAND that stimulates the cortex of the ADRENAL GLAND to secrete its hormones, including corticosterone. If production of ACTH falls below normal, the adrenal cortex decreases in size, and production of the cortical hormones declines. Called also adrenocorticotropin and corticotropin.

ACTH is prescribed to stimulate the adrenal glands in the treatment of some allergies, including asthma, and it has anti-inflammatory properties that sometimes help in the treatment of rheumatoid arthritis. It has been used experimentally in a large number of disorders.

Actidil (ak′tĭ-dil) trademark for preparations of triprolidine, an antihistamine.

actin (ak′tin) a protein occurring in filaments in muscle which, acting along with myosin particles, is responsible for the contraction and relaxation of muscle.

actinic (ak-tin′ik) producing chemical action; said of rays of light beyond the violet of the spectrum.

actinism (ak′tĭ-nizm) the chemical property of light rays.

actinium (ak-tin′e-um) a chemical element, atomic number 89, atomic weight 227, symbol Ac. (See table of ELEMENTS.)

actino- (ak′tĭ-no) word element [Gr.], *ray; radiation.*

actinobacillosis (ak″tĭ-no-bas″ĭ-lo′sis) infection due to actinobacilli.

Actinobacillus (ak″tĭ-no-bah-sil′us) a genus of Schizomycetes capable of infecting cattle and other domestic animals, but rarely man.

A. mall′ei, the causative agent of glanders, a disease of horses that is communicable to man.

actinochemistry (ak″tĭ-no-kem′is-tre) the chemistry of radiant energy.

actinodermatitis (ak″tĭ-no-der″mah-ti′tis) dermatitis from exposure to x-rays.

actinogen (ak-tin′o-jen) any radioactive substance.

actinogenesis (ak″tĭ-no-jen′ĕ-sis) the formation or production of actinic rays.

actinogenic (ak″tĭ-no-jen′ik) producing rays, especially actinic rays.

actinology (ak″tĭ-nol′o-je) 1. the study of radiant energy. 2. the science of the chemical effects of light.

actinolyte (ak-tin′o-līt) an apparatus for concentrating the rays of electric light in phototherapy.

actinometer (ak″tĭ-nom′ĕ-ter) an instrument for measuring the penetrating power of x-rays.

Actinomyces (ak″tĭ-no-mi′sēz) a genus of Schizomycetes.
   A. bo′vis, a gram-positive microorganism causing actinomycosis in cattle.
   A. israe′li, the microorganism causing actinomycosis in humans.

actinomyces (ak″tĭ-no-mi′sēz) an organism of the genus Actinomyces. adj., **actinomycet′ic.**

actinomycete (ak″tĭ-no-mi′sēt) a moldlike microorganism occurring as elongated, frequently filamentous cells, with a branching tendency.

actinomycin (ak″tĭ-no-mi′sin) an antibiotic derived from *Streptomyces antibioticus;* it is active against many bacteria and fungi. There are several forms: actinomycin A is a bright red bacteriostatic; actinomycin B is colorless and bactericidal; actinomycin C is employed during the rejection crisis after kidney transplantation; actinomycin D is used in the management of certain cancers.

actinomycoma (ak″tĭ-no-mi-ko′mah) a tumor formed in actinomycosis.

actinomycosis (ak″tĭ-no-mi-ko′sis) a fungus infection involving the deeper tissues of the skin and mucous membranes and caused by a fungus of the genus Actinomyces (specifically *A. israeli*). The head and neck are most often involved, the lesions beginning as painless, tumor-like masses around the jaw and neck. Later these masses break down and begin to suppurate with discharge of the exudate through a network of sinuses extending through the skin. The source of infection is unknown, although the mouth is thought to be the portal of entry because the fungi are often found in decayed teeth and in the tonsillar crypts of persons who are otherwise normal.
   The infection progresses slowly, without remission, and without at first seeming to affect the general health of the patient. If it is not treated successfully the condition may eventually be fatal.
   Treatment is usually with sulfonamide drugs or penicillin. X-ray therapy may be employed for local lesions and in some cases corticosteroids may help eliminate the infection.

actinon (ak′tĭ-non) a radioactive isotope of radon, symbol An.

actinotherapy (ak″tĭ-no-ther′ah-pe) treatment of disease by rays of light, especially ultraviolet rays.

actinotoxemia (ak″tĭ-no-tok-se′me-ah) toxemia from tissue destruction caused by x-rays or other radioactivity.

action (ak′shun) the accomplishment of an effect, whether mechanical or chemical, or the effect so produced.
   cumulative a., the sudden and markedly increased action of a drug after administration of several doses.
   reflex a., an involuntary response to a stimulus conveyed to the nervous system and reflected to the periphery, passing below the level of consciousness (see also REFLEX).

activator (ak′tĭ-va″tor) a substance that makes another substance active or that renders an inactive enzyme capable of exerting its proper effect.
   plasminogen a., a substance that activates plasminogen and converts it into plasmin.
   tissue a., fibrinokinase.

active transport (ak′tiv trans′port) the movement of substances, particularly electrolyte ions, across the cell membranes and epithelial layers, usually against a concentration gradient. For example, under normal circumstances more potassium ions are present within the cell and more sodium ions extracellularly. The process of maintaining these normal differences in electrolytic composition between the intracellular fluids is active transport. The process differs from simple diffusion or osmosis in that it requires the expenditure of metabolic energy.

activity (ak-tiv′ĭ-te) the quality or process of exerting energy or of accomplishing an effect.
   displacement a., irrelevant activity produced by an excess of one of two conflicting drives in a person.
   enzyme a., the catalytic effect exerted by an enzyme, expressed as units per milligram of enzyme (*specific* activity) or molecules of substrate transformed per minute per molecule of enzyme (*molecular* activity).
   optical a., the ability of a chemical compound to rotate the plane of polarization of plane-polarized light.

actomyosin (ak″to-mi′o-sin) the system of actin filaments and myosin particles constituting muscle fibers and responsible for the contraction and relaxation of muscle.

acuity (ah-ku′ĭ-te) acuteness or clearness.

acumeter (ah-koo′mĕ-ter) acoumeter.

acuminate (ah-ku′mĭ-nāt) sharp-pointed.

acupressure (ak′u-presh″er) compression of a blood vessel by inserted needles.

acupuncture (ak′u-pungk″tūr) therapeutic insertion of needles.

acus (a′kus) a needle or needle-like process.

acute (ah-kūt′) 1. sharp. 2. having severe symptoms and a short course.

acyanotic (ah-si″ah-not′ik) not characterized or accompanied by cyanosis.

acyesis (ah″si-e′sis) 1. sterility in a woman. 2. absence of pregnancy.

Acylanid (as″il-an′id) trademark for acetyldigi-toxin-α, a digitalis preparation derived from lana-toside.

acystia (a-sis′te-ah) congenital absence of the bladder.

acystinervia (a-sis″tǐ-ner′ve-ah) paralysis of the bladder.

A.D. [L.] *au′ris dex′tra* (right ear).

ad [L.] preposition, *to.*

A.D.A. American Dental Association; American Diabetes Association; American Dietetics Asso-ciation.

adactylia (a″dak-til′e-ah) congenital absence of the fingers or toes.

Adam's apple a subcutaneous prominence at the front of the throat produced by the thyroid cartilage of the LARYNX.

adamantine (ad″ah-man′tin) pertaining to the enamel of the teeth.

adamantinoma (ad″ah-man″tǐ-no′mah) amelo-blastoma.

adamantoblast (ad″ah-man′to-blast) ameloblast.

adamantoblastoma, adamantoma (ad″ah-man″to-blas-to′mah), (ad″ah-man-to′mah) amelo-blastoma.

Adams-Stokes disease (ad′amz stōks) a condi-tion characterized by sudden attacks of uncon-sciousness, with or without convulsions, which frequently accompanies heart block; called also Adams-Stokes syndrome and Stokes-Adams dis-ease.

adaptation (ad″ap-ta′shun) adjustment, especial-ly of the pupil to light, or of an organism to environ-mental conditions.
  color a., 1. changes in visual perception of color with prolonged stimulation. 2. adjustment of vision to degree of brightness or color tone of illumina-tion.
  dark a., adaptation of the eye to vision in the dark or in reduced illumination.

adaptometer (ad″ap-tom′ě-ter) an instrument for measuring the time required for adaptation of the pupil.
  color a., an instrument to demonstrate adaptation of the eye to color or light.

addict (ad′ikt) a person exhibiting addiction.

addiction (ah-dik′shun) physiologic or psychologic dependence on some agent (e.g., alcohol, drug), with a tendency to increase its use (see also DRUG ADDICTION).

addictologist (ad″ik-tol′o-jist) a physician special-izing in the study and treatment of addiction.

Addis count (ad′is) a count of the cells in 10 cc. of urinary sediment as a means of calculating total urinary sediment in a 12-hour specimen.

Addison's disease (ad′ǐ-sunz) a disease caused by the underfunctioning of the ADRENAL GLANDS,

named for Thomas Addison, the 19th-century English physician who first identified it. Addison's disease is comparatively rare, and although it is known to be due to a failure of the adrenal glands, the cause of this failure is not always certain. Tuberculosis of the adrenals accounts for less than half the cases, and idiopathic atrophy of the glands for most of the rest.

An early symptom of the disease is a darkening of the pigmentation of the skin and the membranes of the mouth. The patient then becomes increasingly weak; he may lose weight and suffer attacks of diarrhea and vomiting; there is often a lowering of blood pressure accompanied by changes in the con-stituents of the blood, especially the electrolyte balance.

The isolation of cortisone, a hormone of the adrenal cortex that can be extracted from the adrenals of animals, greatly improved the prognosis of the disease. With proper administration of corti-sone or allied hormones and an adequate intake of sodium chloride, patients with Addison's disease now have a good chance of being maintained in good health.

addisonian crisis (ad″ǐ-so′ne-an) symptoms of fatigue, nausea and vomiting and weight loss accompanying an acute attack of Addison's dis-ease.

addisonism (ad′ǐ-sun-izm″) symptoms seen in pulmonary tuberculosis, resembling Addison's dis-ease.

adduct (ah-dukt′) to draw toward a center or median line.

adduction (ah-duk′shun) the act of adducting; the state of being adducted.

adductor (ah-duk′tor) that which adducts.

Ademol (ad′e-mol) trademark for a preparation of flumethiazide, a diuretic and antihypertensive.

adenalgia (ad″ě-nal′je-ah) pain in a gland.

adenase (ad′e-nās) an enzyme found in spleen, pancreas and liver.

adenasthenia (ad″en-as-the′ne-ah) deficient glan-dular activity.
  a. gas′trica, deficient glandular secretion in the stomach.

adendric (ah-den′drik) without dendrites.

adenectomy (ad″ě-nek′to-me) excision of a gland.

adenectopia (ad″ě-nek-to′pe-ah) displacement of a gland.

adenemphraxis (ad″ě-nem-frak′sis) obstruction of the duct of a gland.

adenia (a-de′ne-ah) any one of various conditions of unknown etiology chiefly affecting lymph nodes; called also lymphoma.

adeniform (ah-den′ǐ-form) gland-shaped.

adenine (ad′ě-nīn) a purine present in nucleopro-teins of cells of plants and animals. Adenine and guanine are essential components of NUCLEIC ACIDS. The end product of the metabolism of ade-nine in man is URIC ACID.

adenitis (ad″ě-ni′tis) inflammation of a gland.

adenization (ad″ĕ-nī-za′shun) assumption of an abnormal glandlike appearance.

adeno- (ad′ĕ-no) word element [Gr.], *gland.*

adenoacanthoma (ad″ĕ-no-ak″an-tho′mah) adenocarcinoma.

adenoameloblastoma (ad″ĕ-no-ah-mel″o-blas-to′mah) ameloblastoma with formation of ductlike structures in place of or in addition to the typical odontogenic pattern.

adenoangiosarcoma (ad″ĕ-no-an″je-o-sar-ko′mah) an angiosarcoma with glandular elements.

adenoblast (ad′ĕ-no-blast″) 1. a gland cell, secretory or excretory. 2. an embryonic forerunner of gland tissue.

adenocarcinoma (ad″ĕ-no-kar″sĭ-no′mah) a carcinoma with glandular elements.

adenocele (ad′ĕ-no-sēl″) a cystic adenomatous tumor.

adenocellulitis (ad″ĕ-no-sel″u-li′tis) inflammation of a gland and the cellular tissue around it.

adenocystoma (ad″ĕ-no-sis-to′mah) adenoma blended with cystoma.

adenocyte (ad′ĕ-no-sīt″) a mature secretory cell of a gland.

adenodynia (ad″ĕ-no-din′e-ah) pain in a gland.

adenoepithelioma (ad″ĕ-no-ep″ĭ-the″le-o′mah) a tumor composed of glandular and epithelial elements.

adenogenous (ad″ĕ-noj′ĕ-nus) originating from glandular tissue.

adenography (ad″ĕ-nog′rah-fe) anatomy, physiology, histology and pathology of glands.

adenohypophysis (ad″ĕ-no-hi-pof′ĭ-sis) the anterior or glandular portion of the hypophysis cerebri (see also PITUITARY GLAND).

adenoid (ad′ĕ-noid) 1. resembling a gland. 2. in the plural, hypertrophy of the glandular tissue that normally exists in the nasopharynx of children and is known as the pharyngeal tonsil. Enlargement of this tissue may cause obstruction of the outlet from the nose so that the child breathes chiefly through the mouth, or the eustachian tube may be blocked, with pain in the ear or a sense of pressure resulting. It also may prepare the way for infections of the middle ear and occasionally interferes with hearing.

Prolonged obstruction by enlarged adenoids produces a typical "adenoid facies." The child appears to be dull and apathetic, and has some degree of nutritional deficiency and hearing loss, and some delay in growth and development.

Surgical excision of the enlarged tissue is called adenoidectomy.

adenoidectomy (ad″ĕ-noi-dek′to-me) surgical excision of the adenoids. The operation is usually performed in conjunction with tonsillectomy since both the adenoids and palatine tonsils tend to become enlarged after repeated infections of the throat. The preoperative and postoperative care in adenoidectomy is similar to that in TONSILLECTOMY and is described under that heading.

adenoiditis (ad″ĕ-noi-di′tis) inflammation of the adenoids.

adenolipoma (ad″ĕ-no-lĭ-po′mah) a mixed adenoma and lipoma.

adenology (ad″ĕ-nol′o-je) the sum of knowledge regarding glands.

adenolymphitis (ad″ĕ-no-lim-fi′tis) lymphadenitis; inflammation of lymph nodes.

adenolymphoma (ad″ĕ-no-lim-fo′mah) adenoma of a lymph node.

adenoma (ad″ĕ-no′mah) an epithelial tumor composed of glandular tissue.

　acidophilic a., a tumor arising from the acidophilic cells of the anterior lobe of the pituitary gland; called also eosinophilic adenoma. Such tumors produce ACROMEGALY and GIGANTISM.

　basophilic a., a tumor arising from the basophilic cells of the anterior lobe of the pituitary gland.

　chromophobe a., a tumor arising from the chromophobe cells of the anterior lobe of the pituitary gland.

　a. des′truens, adenocarcinoma.

　eosinophilic a., a tumor arising from the eosinophilic cells of the anterior lobe of the pituitary gland.

　a. seba′ceum, a yellowish tumor on the face, containing a mass of yellowish glands.

　a. sim′plex, glandular hyperplasia.

adenomalacia (ad″ĕ-no-mah-la′she-ah) undue softness of a gland.

adenomatosis (ad″ĕ-no″mah-to′sis) the formation of adenomas in glandular tissue.

adenomatous (ad″ĕ-no′mah-tus) pertaining to or resembling adenoma.

adenomere (ad′ĕ-no-mēr″) the blind terminal portion of the glandular cavity of a developing gland, being the functional portion of the organ.

adenomyofibroma (ad″ĕ-no-mi″o-fi-bro′mah) a fibroma containing both glandular and muscular elements.

adenomyoma (ad″ĕ-no-mi-o′mah) a tumor made up of endometrium and muscle tissue, found in the uterus, or more frequently in the uterine ligaments.

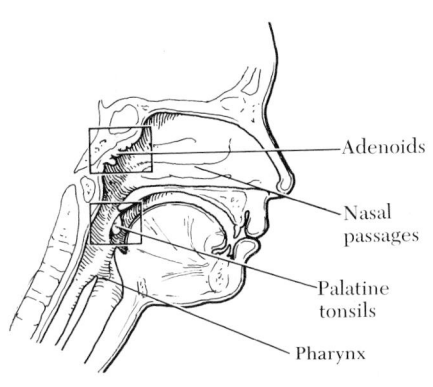

Adenoids.

Adenoids

Nasal passages

Palatine tonsils

Pharynx

adenomyomatosis (ad"ĕ-no-mi"o-mah-to'sis) the presence of multiple adenomyomas.

adenomyometritis (ad"ĕ-no-mi"o-mĕ-tri'tis) endometriosis.

adenomyosarcoma (ad"ĕ-no-mi"o-sar-ko'mah) adenosarcoma containing striated muscle.

adenomyosis (ad"ĕ-no-mi-o'sis) invasion of the muscular wall of an organ (e.g., stomach, uterus) by glandular tissue.

adenomyositis (ad"ĕ-no-mi"o-si'tis) endometriosis.

adenomyxoma (ad"ĕ-no-mik-so'mah) a tumor composed of glandular and mucous tissue.

adenomyxosarcoma (ad'ĕ-no-mik"so-sar-ko'-mah) a sarcoma containing glandular elements.

adenopathy (ad"ĕ-nop'ah-the) any disease of glands.

adenopharyngitis (ad"ĕ-no-far"in-ji'tis) inflammation of tonsils and pharynx.

adenosarcoma (ad"ĕ-no-sar-ko'mah) adenoma blended with sarcoma.

adenosclerosis (ad"ĕ-no-sklĕ-ro'sis) hardening of a gland.

adenosine (ah-den'o-sēn) a nucleoside containing adenine, a pentose sugar and phosphoric acid, which functions as a coenzyme in the metabolic functions of the cell. Adenosine plays a role in the activation of fatty acids and amino acids, and in "energy trapping" in the metabolism of carbohydrates. Nucleosides such as adenosine are believed to be intermediates in the synthesis or degradation of NUCLEIC ACIDS.
 a. diphosphate, a compound containing two phosphoric acids, formed by hydrolysis of adenosine triphosphate, with release of one high-energy bond; abbreviated ADP.
 a. monophosphate, adenosine containing only one phosphoric acid; abbreviated AMP.
 a. triphosphate, a compound containing three phosphoric acids, with one low- and two high-energy bonds; abbreviated ATP.

adenosis (ad"ĕ-no'sis) any disease of a gland.

adenotome (ad'ĕ-no-tōm") an instrument for incising glands.

adenotomy (ad"ĕ-not'o-me) incision of a gland.

adenotonsillectomy (ad"ĕ-no-ton"sĭ-lek'to-me) removal of the tonsils and adenoids.

adenotyphus (ad"ĕ-no-ti'fus) typhus with lesions chiefly in the mesenteric lymph nodes.

adenovirus (ad"ĕ-no-vi'rus) a virus causing infection of the upper respiratory tract, less virulent than the viruses causing influenza.

adenylic acid (ad"ĕ-nil'ik) a component of nucleic acid, consisting of adenine, ribose and phosphoric acid, found in muscle, yeast and other material.

adermia (ah-der'me-ah) defect or absence of the skin.

ADH antidiuretic hormone.

adhesion (ad-he'zhun) union of two surfaces that are normally separate; also, any fibrous band that connects them. Surgery within the abdomen sometimes results in adhesions from scar tissue. As an organ heals, fibrous scar tissue forms around the incision. This scar tissue may cling to the surface of adjoining organs, causing them to kink. Adhesions are usually painless and cause no difficulties, although occasionally they produce obstruction or malfunction by distorting the organ. They can also occur following peritonitis and other inflammatory conditions. They may occur in the pleura, in the pericardium and around the pelvic organs, in addition to the abdomen. Surgery is sometimes recommended to relieve adhesions.

adhesiotomy (ad-he"ze-ot'o-me) surgical division of adhesions.

adhesive (ad-he'siv) pertaining to, characterized by or causing close adherence of adjoining surfaces. 2. a substance that causes close adherence of adjoining surfaces.

adiadochokinesia (ah-di"ah-do"ko-ki-ne'ze-ah) inability to perform fine, rapidly repeated, coordinated movements.

adiaphoresis (ah-di"ah-fo-re'sis) deficiency of the perspiration.

adiaphoria (ah-di"ah-fo're-ah) nonresponse to stimuli as a result of previous similar stimuli.

adiapneustia (ah-di"ap-nūs'te-ah) defect or absence of perspiration.

adiastole (a-di-as'to-le) absence of diastole.

adicity (ah-dis'ē-te) valence.

Adie's syndrome (a'dēz) a syndrome consisting of a pathologic pupil reaction (pupillotonia), the most important element of which is a myotonic condition on accommodation; the pupil on the affected side contracts to near vision more slowly than does the pupil on the opposite side, and it also dilates more slowly. The affected pupil does not usually react to light (direct or indirect), but it may do so in an abnormal fashion. Certain tendon reflexes are absent or diminished, but there are no motor or sensory disturbances, nor are there demonstrable changes indicative of disease of the nervous system.

adip(o)- (ad'ĭ-po) word element [L.], *fat.*

adipectomy (ad"ĭ-pek'to-me) excision of adipose tissue.

adiphenine (ad"ĭ-fen'ēn) a drug used as an anticholinergic and antispasmodic.

adipic (ah-dip'ik) pertaining to fat.

adipocele (ad'ĭ-po-sēl") a hernia containing fat.

adipocellular (ad"ĭ-po-sel'u-lar) composed of fat and connective tissue.

adipocere (ad'ĭ-po-sēr") a waxy substance from bodies long dead.

adipofibroma (ad"ĭ-po-fi-bro'mah) a fibrous tumor with fatty elements.

adipogenous (ad"ĭ-poj'ĕ-nus) producing fat.

adipoid (ad'ĭ-poid) fatlike; lipoid.

adipokinesis (ad″i-po-ki-ne'sis) the mobilization of fat in the body.

adipokinin (ad″ĭ-po-ki'nin) a factor from the anterior pituitary that accelerates mobilization of stored fat.

adipolysis (ad″ĭ-pol'ĭ-sis) the digestion of fats.

adipoma (ad″ĭ-po'mah) lipoma; a fatty tumor.

adiponecrosis (ad″ĭ-po-nĕ-kro'sis) necrosis of fatty tissue.
  a. neonato'rum, a. subcuta'nea, alteration of subcutaneous fat thought to be caused by obstetric trauma, in newborn infants.

adipopexis (ad″ĭ-po-pek'sis) the fixation or storing of fat.

adipose (ad'ĭ-pōs) fatty.

adiposis (ad″ĭ-po'sis) a condition marked by deposits or degeneration of fatty tissue.
  a. cerebra'lis, fatness from cerebral pituitary disease.
  a. doloro'sa, a painful condition due to pressure on nerves caused by fatty deposits.
  a. hepat'ica, fatty degeneration of liver.
  a. tubero'sa, adiposis dolorosa in which the fatty degeneration occurs in nodular masses.

adipositis (ad″ĭ-po-si'tis) inflammation of adipose tissue.

adiposity (ad″ĭ-pos'ĭ-te) obesity.

adiposogenital dystrophy (ad″ĭ-po-so-jen'ĭ-tal dis'tro-fe) abnormal distribution of fat (obesity) accompanied by underdevelopment of the genitalia. The condition is caused by damage to certain parts of the HYPOTHALAMUS, with a decrease in the secretion of gonadotropic hormones from the anterior lobe of the PITUITARY GLAND. Treatment depends on the primary cause of the condition, usually a tumor or infection involving the hypothalamus. Called also adiposogenital syndrome and Fröhlich's syndrome.

adiposuria (ad″ĭ-po-su're-ah) the occurrence of fat in the urine.

adipsia (a-dip'se-ah) abnormal avoidance of drinking.

aditus (ad'ĭ-tus), pl. *ad'itus* [L.] an entrance or opening; used in anatomic nomenclature for various passages in the body.

adjuvant (ad'joo-vant) 1. assisting or aiding. 2. a substance that aids another, such as an auxiliary remedy.

adnerval, adneural (ad-ner'val), (ad-nu'ral) toward a nerve.

adnexa (ad-nek'sah) [L., pl.] appendages; accessory organs, as of the eye (*adenx'a oc'uli*) or uterus (*adnex'a u'teri*). adj., **adnex'al.**

adnexopexy (ad-nek'so-pek″se) surgical fixation of the oviduct and ovary.

adolescence (ad″o-les'ens) the period between the onset of PUBERTY and beginning adulthood. adj., **adoles'cent.** During adolescence, boys and girls undergo the extensive physical changes of puberty; these changes sometimes create emotional difficulties. The adolescent has two main problems: he must adjust himself to the changes in his body; and he must also adjust himself socially—that is, he must learn to live independently, and to be responsible for himself.

Adolescents are usually extremely sensitive about their appearance. They should never be ridiculed on account of it, and great care should be taken to avoid causing them embarrassment. For example, nicknames like "Chubby" and "Skinny," which imply some physical peculiarity, should be avoided as far as possible, however affectionately intended. Adolescents may be particularly sensitive about their weight. They often go through a temporary stage of being overweight or underweight, and it is usually a matter of time before the situation rights itself. Good nutrition is very important at this stage. Adolescence is a period of exceptionally rapid growth and strenuous exercise, and young people's bodies need especially good and complete diets if they are to develop properly. Their food must be rich in protein to make new muscle and body tissue, minerals for the growth of bones, vitamins for good general health and enough supplementary carbohydrates and fat to provide energy. For more detailed information about the value of different foods, see NUTRITION.

Many adolescents are susceptible to ACNE, BOILS and other skin complaints; this is mainly because the level of new hormones pouring into the blood is not yet stabilized, and the normal lubricating oil produced by the sebaceous glands in the skin thickens and forms plugs in the hair follicles. Bacteria find a ready home in these fatty plugs, and the follicular pores become infected, with the formation of pimples and boils.

adoral (ad-o'ral) 1. situated near the mouth. 2. directed toward the mouth.

ADP adenosine diphosphate.

adren(o)- (ah-dre'no) word element [L.], *adrenal glands.*

adrenal (ah-dre'nal) 1. near the kidney. 2. of or produced by the adrenal glands.
  a. gland, a small endocrine gland that rests on top of each kidney; called also suprarenal gland. Like other endocrine glands, the two adrenals secrete hormones into the blood, which carries them to various parts of the body where they exert their effects. Each adrenal gland is actually a gland within a gland: the outer shell, or cortex, and the inner core, or medulla.
  CORTEX. The adrenal cortex plays a vital role in the chemistry of the body. Its hormones, known as corticosteroids, are divided into three groups: GLUCOCORTICOIDS (cortisol, or hydrocortisone, cortisone and corticosterone), MINERALOCORTICOIDS (aldosterone and desoxycorticosterone, and also corticosterone) and androgens. Progesterone and estrogen are also present in the adrenal secretion in small amounts.
  The glucocorticoids help control the metabolism of protein, fat and carbohydrate. The mineralocorticoids influence the concentration of sodium and potassium in body fluids, exerting an important role in general fluid and electrolyte balance. If both adrenal cortices are removed or cease to func-

tion, the patient cannot live long unless he receives supportive adrenocortical hormones.

Like other endocrine glands, the cortex is under the control of the PITUITARY GLAND. The pituitary exercises its control by way of its adrenocorticotropic hormone, familiarly known as ACTH, which stimulates the cortex to secrete its hormones.

Diseases of the adrenal cortex are serious but rare. They cause the cortex to overproduce or underproduce its hormones. Two of the commonest of these rare diseases are ADDISON'S DISEASE (underproduction of hormones) and CUSHING'S SYNDROME (overproduction of hormones).

MEDULLA. The two hormones produced by the adrenal medulla are epinephrine (Adrenaline) and norepinephrine (noradrenaline). Their secretion is controlled by the HYPOTHALAMUS. The actions of these two hormones are similar and they are referred to as "sympathomimetic" agents because they mimic the actions of the sympathetic nervous system. They affect automatic responses of the body such as cardiac activity, gastrointestinal motility, dilatation of the pupil of the eye and various metabolic activities. Epinephrine affects the conversion of glycogen in the liver into glucose, greatly increases the metabolic rate and increases the cardiac output. Norepinephrine causes vascular constriction, thereby raising the arterial pressure. In general, it can be said that these hormones have almost exactly the same effects as direct sympathetic stimulation except that the hormonal effects are more prolonged.

Hyperfunction of the adrenal medulla is usually due to a tumor (PHEOCHROMOCYTOMA) and the chief symptom is hypertension.

a. insufficiency, hypofunction of the adrenal gland, particularly the cortex, leading to symptoms of weakness and loss of sodium, chloride and water. See also ADDISON'S DISEASE.

adrenalectomy (ah-dre"nah-lek'to-me) surgical excision of an adrenal gland. This procedure is indicated when a disorder of the adrenal gland,

such as CUSHING'S SYNDROME and PHEOCHROMOCYTOMA, causes an overproduction of adrenal hormones. In some instances of severe Cushing's syndrome, total bilateral adrenalectomy is performed. Adrenalectomy also has been advocated for therapy of some cases of metastatic breast cancer.

Adrenaline (ah-dren'ah-lin) trademark for epinephrine, an adrenergic agent.

adrenalism (ah-dren'ah-lizm) ill health due to adrenal dysfunction.

adrenalitis (ah-dre"nal-i'tis) inflammation of the adrenal glands.

adrenergic (ad"ren-er'jik) activated or transmitted by epinephrine; said of nerve fibers that liberate sympathin at a synapse when a nerve impulse passes, i.e., the sympathetic fibers.

a. agent, a substance that duplicates most of the effects of stimulation of the sympathetic nervous system.

a.-blocking agent, a drug that blocks the secretion of epinephrine and norepinephrine at the postganglionic nerve endings of the sympathetic nervous system. By blocking these adrenergic substances, which cause constriction of blood vessels and increased cardiac output, adrenergic-blocking agents produce a dilatation of the blood vessels and a decrease in cardiac output. They are classified as antihypertensive drugs. Guanethidine sulfate and methyldopa are examples of adrenergic-blocking agents. During therapy with these drugs, patients should avoid strenuous exercise, which is likely to produce a sudden drop in the blood pressure. Another difficulty to be expected with these drugs is postural hypotension.

adrenocortical (ah-dre"no-kor'tĭ-kal) pertaining to or arising from the cortex of the adrenal gland.

a. hormone, one of the steroids produced by the adrenal cortex (see also CORTICOSTEROID).

adrenocorticomimetic (ah-dre"no-kor"tĭ-ko-mimet'ik) having effects similar to those of hormones of the adrenal cortex.

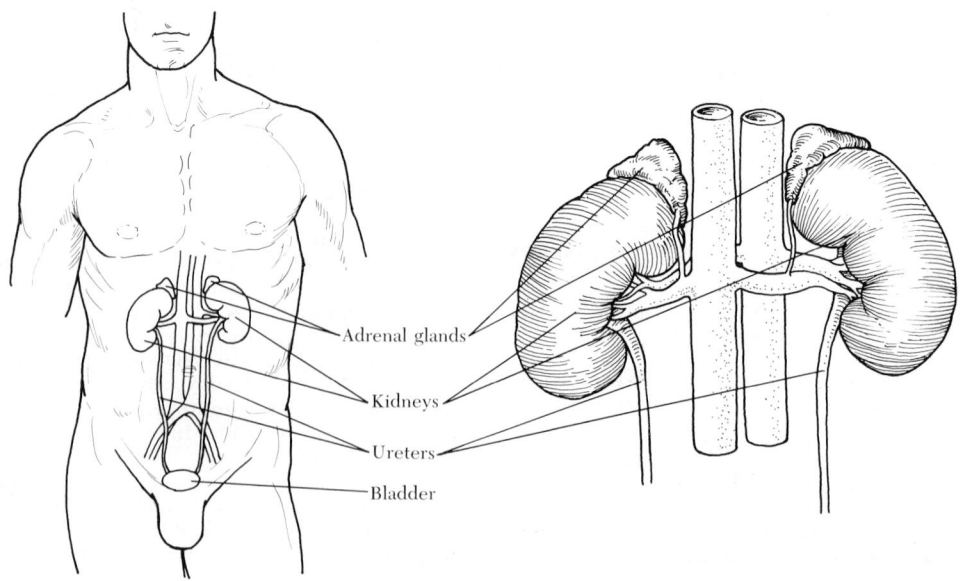

Adrenal glands.

adrenocorticosteroid (ah-dre″no-kor″tĭ-ko-ste′-roid) a hormone elaborated by the adrenal cortex (see also CORTICOSTEROID).

adrenocorticotrophic (ah-dre″no-kor″tĭ-ko-trof′-ik) adrenocorticotropic.

adrenocorticotrophin (ah-dre″no-kor″tĭ-ko-trof′-in) adrenocorticotropic hormone (see also ACTH).

adrenocorticotropic (ah-dre″no-kor″ti-ko-trōp′ik) having a stimulating effect on the adrenal cortex.
   a. hormone, a hormone of the anterior lobe of the pituitary gland that stimulates the action of the adrenal cortex (see also ACTH).

adrenocorticotropin (ah-dre″no-kor″tĭ-ko-tro′pin) adrenocorticotropic hormone (see also ACTH).

adrenogenital syndrome (ah-dre″no-jen′ĭ-tal) a group of symptoms associated with alterations of the sex characters and due to abnormally increased production of androgens by the adrenal glands. The term most commonly applies to the development of masculine traits in the female or premature puberty in male children. The condition may be congenital, in which case it is due to an inherited defect of the adrenal gland, or acquired, developing as a result of a tumor or hyperplasia of the adrenals.
   SYMPTOMS. Females with the congenital form may be reared as boys because of masculinization of the external genitalia. Males may show sexual prococity, with development of the reproductive organs, appearance of pubic hair and excessive body growth in early childhood. In acquired adrenogenital syndrome there is appearance of masculine secondary sex characters in the female, and precocious puberty in the male.
   TREATMENT. When an adrenal tumor is the underlying cause of the disorder, it is removed surgically. Other treatment consists of administration of corticoids such as cortisone and prednisone. Estrogen therapy is successful in some cases.

adrenoglomerulotropin (ah-dre″no-glo-mer″u-lo-tro′pin) a hormone that stimulates production of aldosterone by the adrenal cortex.

adrenolytic (ah-dre″no-lit′ik) antagonizing the action of epinephrine or of the adrenal gland.

adrenomegaly (ah-dre″no-meg′ah-le) abnormal enlargement of the adrenal gland.

adrenopathy (ad″ren-op′ah-the) any disease of the adrenal glands.

Adrenosem (ah-dren′o-sem) trademark for preparations of carbazochrome salicylate, a hemostatic agent.

adrenotropism (ad″ren-ot′ro-pizm) predominance of the adrenal glands in the endocrine constitution.

ADS antidiuretic hormone (substance).

adsorb (ad-sorb′) to attract and retain other material on the surface.

adsorbent (ad-sorb′ent) 1. pertaining to or characterized by adsorption. 2. a substance that attracts other materials or particles to its surface.
   gastrointestinal a., a substance, usually a powder, taken to adsorb gases, toxins and bacteria in the stomach and intestines. Examples include activated charcoal and kaolin.

adsorption (ad-sorp′shun) the action of a substance in attracting and holding other materials or particles on its surface.

adtorsion (ad-tor′shun) a turning inward of both eyes.

adult (ah-dult′) having attained full growth or maturity, or an organism that has done so.

adulteration (ah-dul″ter-a′shun) addition of an impure, cheap or unnecessary ingredient to cheat, cheapen or falsify a preparation.

advancement (ad-vans′ment) detachment of a portion of tissue, especially muscle, and reattachment at an advanced point, as is done with an eye muscle for correction of strabismus.
   capsular a., attachment of Tenon's capsule in front of its normal position.

adventitia (ad″ven-tish′e-ah) the outer coat of an organ or structure, especially the outer coat of an artery.

adventitious (ad″ven-tish′us) not normal to a part.

adynamia (ad″dĭ-na′me-ah) lack of normal or vital powers. adj., **adynam′ic.**

aec- for words beginning thus, see those beginning, *ec-*.

Aedes (a-e′dēz) a genus of mosquitoes, including approximately 600 species.
   A. aegyp′ti, the mosquito that transmits the causative organisms of yellow fever and dengue.

aeg- for words beginning thus, see those beginning *eg-*.

aeration (a″er-a′shun) the exchange of carbon dioxide for oxygen by the blood in the lungs.

aeriform (ār′ĭ-form, a-er′ĭ-form) resembling air; gaseous.

aero- (a′er-o) word element [Gr.], *air; gas.*

Aerobacter (a″er-o-bak′ter) a genus of Schizomycetes that includes two species, *A. aero′genes* and *A. cloa′cae.*

aerobe (a′er-ōb) a microorganism that lives and grows in the presence of free oxygen. adj., **aero′bic.**
   facultative a., a microorganism that can live in the presence of oxygen, but does not require it.
   obligate a., one that cannot live without oxygen.

aerobiology (a″er-o-bi-ol′o-je) the study of the distribution of living organisms (microorganisms) by the air.

aerobion (a″er-o′be-on) an aerobe.

aerobiosis (a″er-o-bi-o′sis) life requiring free oxygen.

aerocele (a′er-o-sēl) a tumor formed by air filling an adventitious pouch, such as laryngocele and tracheocele.
   epidural a., a collection of air between the dura mater and the wall of the vertebral column.

aerocolpos (a″er-o-kol′pos) distention of the vagina with gas.

aerocoly (a″er-o′ko-le) distention of the colon with gas.

aerodermectasia (a″er-o-der″mek-ta′ze-ah) subcutaneous or surgical emphysema.

aerodontalgia (a″er-o-don-tal′je-ah) pain in the teeth due to lowered atmospheric pressure at high altitudes.

aerodromophobia (a″er-o-dro″mo-fo′be-ah) morbid dread of traveling by air.

aerodynamics (a″er-o-di-nam′iks) the science of air or gases in motion.

aeroembolism (a″er-o-em′bo-lizm) obstruction of a blood vessel by air or gas.

aerogastrocolia (a″er-o-gas″tro-ko′le-ah) air or gas in the stomach and colon.

aerogen (a′er-o-jen″) a gas-producing bacillus.

aerogenesis (a″er-o-jen′ĕ-sis) formation or production of gas.

aerogram (a′er-o-gram″) a roentgenogram of an organ after injection with air or gas.

aerohydrotherapy (a″er-o-hi″dro-ther′ah-pe) therapeutic use of air and water.

aeromammography (a″er-o-mah-mog′rah-fe) roentgenography of the mammary gland after injection of air or other gas.

aeroneurosis (a″er-o-nu-ro′sis) a functional nervous disorder occurring in aviators.

aero-otitis (a″er-o-o-ti′tis) barotitis.

aeropathy (a″er-op′ah-the) bends (decompression sickness).

aerophagia (a″er-o-fa′je-ah) habitual swallowing of air.

aerophilous (a″er-of′ĭ-lus) requiring air for proper growth.

aerophobia (a″er-o-fo′be-ah) 1. morbid dread of drafts of air. 2. morbid dread of being up in the air.

aerophyte (a′er-o-fīt″) a microorganism that lives upon air.

aeroplethysmograph (a″ero-o-plĕ-thiz′mo-graf) an apparatus for graphically recording the expired air.

aerosinusitis (a″er-o-si″nŭ-si′tis) barosinusitis.

aerosol (a′er-o-sol″) a colloid system in which solid or liquid particles are suspended in a gas, especially a suspension of a drug or other substance to be dispensed in a fine spray or mist.

Aerosporin (a″er-o-spōr′in) trademark for a preparation of polymyxin B sulfate.

aerostatics (a″er-o-stat′iks) the science of air or gases at rest.

aerotherapy (a″er-o-ther′ah-pe) treatment of disease by air.

aerothorax (a″er-o-tho′raks) pneumothorax.

aerotitis (a″er-o-ti′tis) barotitis.

aerotonometer (a″er-o-to-nom′ĕ-ter) a device used in measuring the tension of the blood gases.

aes-, for words beginning thus, see those beginning *es-*.

Æsculapius (es″cu-la′pe-us) the god of healing in Roman mythology. The staff of Æsculapius, a rod or staff with a snake entwined around it, is a symbol of medicine and is the official insignia of the American Medical Association (see also CADUCEUS).

aet- for words beginning thus, see those beginning *et-*.

afebrile (a-feb′rīl) without fever.

affect (af′ekt) emotional tone or feeling.

affection (ah-fek′shun) a morbid condition or diseased state.

affective (ah-fek′tiv) pertaining to emotional tone or feeling.
   a. psychosis, a severely disabling disorder of mood or emotional feeling, with profound effect upon thought and behavior. The disorder is characterized by changes in mood from manic to depressive, or the patient may exhibit the manic or the depressive reaction only, or variants of the two moods. (See also PSYCHOSIS).

afferent (af′er-ent) conducting toward a center or specific site of reference.
   a. nerve, any nerve that transmits impulses from the periphery toward the central nervous system (see also NEURON).

affinity (ah-fin′ĭ-te) attraction; a tendency to seek out or unite with another object or substance.
   chemical a., the force that unites atoms of different substances.
   elective a., the force that causes union of a substance with one substance rather than another.

afibrinogenemia (a-fi″brin-o-jĕ-ne′me-ah) absence or deficiency of fibrinogen in the circulating blood. Congenital afibrinogenemia—complete absence of fibrinogen—is a rare anomaly that is inherited. Acquired afibrinogenemia is actually a deficiency of fibrinogen (*hypofibrinogenemia*) and often is a serious complication in obstetrics, the primary cause being excessive maternal use of fibrinogen during an abnormal pregnancy. The condition may be seen in association with malignancies of the bone and prostate, and with leukemia. It also may follow transfusion of incompatible blood and sometimes may complicate thoracic and abdominal surgery.
   SYMPTOMS. As would be expected in a deficiency of fibrinogen, which plays an important role in the blood clotting mechanism, the chief symptom is generalized bleeding, external or internal. In obstetric or surgical patients suffering from this condition there is frequently sudden and uncontrollable hemorrhage.
   TREATMENT. Fibrinogen is administered intravenously to supply the body with this essential substance; transfusions of whole blood may also be indicated. In patients with cancer of the prostate the fibrinogen level often returns to normal after administration of estrogens. In obstetric patients the fibrinogen level returns to normal after the uterus has been emptied.

afterbirth (af'ter-berth") the special tissues associated with the development of a fetus in the uterus that are expelled after the birth of a baby. These are the PLACENTA, or the structure attached to the wall of the uterus through which nourishment passes from the mother to the fetus, and the UMBILICAL CORD, which attaches the fetus to the placenta.

afterbrain (af'ter-brān) metencephalon.

afterhearing (af"ter-hēr'ing) hearing of sounds after the stimulus has ceased.

afterimage (af'ter-im"ij) a retinal impression remaining after cessation of the stimulus causing it.

afterpain (af'ter-pān") pain that follows expulsion of the placenta, due to contraction of the uterus.

afterperception (af"ter-per-sep'shun) perception of aftersensations.

aftersensation (af"ter-sen-sa'shun) sensation persisting after cessation of the stimulus that caused it.

aftersound (af'ter-sownd") sensation of a sound after cessation of the stimulus causing it.

aftertaste (af'ter-tāst") sensation of taste continuing after the stimulus has ceased.

A-G ratio the ratio of albumin to globulin in blood serum, plasma or urine.

Ag chemical symbol, *silver* (L. argentum).

agalactia (ag"ah-lak'she-ah) absence or failure of secretion of milk.

agammaglobulinemia (a"gam-ah-glob"u-lin-e'-me-ah) absence or severe deficiency of the plasma protein gamma globulin. There are three main types: transient, congenital and acquired. The transient type occurs in early infancy, because gamma globulins are not produced in the fetus and the gamma globulins derived from the maternal blood are soon depleted. This temporary deficiency of gamma globulin lasts for the first 6 to 8 weeks, until the infant begins to synthesize the protein. Congenital agammaglobulinemia is a rare condition, occurring in males, and resulting in decreased production of antibodies. Acquired agammaglobulinemia is secondary to other disorders and is usually a hypogammaglobulinemia, that is, a deficiency rather than total absence of this plasma protein. It is often secondary to malignant diseases such as leukemia, myeloma and lymphoma, and to diseases associated with hypoproteinemia such as nephrosis and liver disease. Some of the patients have a family history of rheumatoid arthritis or allergies. This seems to indicate the presence of genetic factors in the development of agammaglobulinemia.

SYMPTOMS. Because gamma globulin is so important in the production of antibodies and thus in the body's ability to defend itself against infection, it follows that a deficiency or absence of gamma globulin would result in severe and recurrent infections. The infections are usually bacterial rather than viral in origin and are extremely difficult to eliminate. The condition is often complicated by local damage to tissues because of scarring and repeated infection. Disorders of connective tissue such as scleroderma, arthritis and lupus erythematosus are also frequent complications.

TREATMENT. Replacement therapy with human gamma globulin is effective in preventing severe infections. The aim is to maintain the gamma globulin level above 150 mg. per 100 ml. of blood. The patient is given an initial dose of 0.2 Gm. per kilogram of body weight and a maintenance dose of 0.1 Gm. per kilogram every 4 weeks. Antibiotics are also given and are continued until all signs of infection have disappeared.

aganglionic (a-gang"gle-on'ik) lacking ganglion cells.

aganglionosis (ah-gang"gle-on-o'sis) congenital absence of parasympathetic ganglion cells.

agar (ag'ar) a dried hydrophilic, colloidal substance extracted from various species of red algae. It is used in cultures for bacteria and other microorganisms. Because of its bulk it is also used in medicines to promote peristalsis and relieve constipation.

agastria (ah-gas'tre-ah) absence of the stomach.

agastric (ah-gas'trik) having no stomach.

agastroneuria (ah-gas"tro-nu're-ah) lack of nervous tonicity in the stomach.

age (āj) the duration, or the measure of time of the existence of a person or object.

 achievement a., proficiency in study expressed in terms of the chronologic age of a normal child showing the same degree of attainment.

 chronologic a., the actual measure of time elapsed since a person's birth.

 mental a., the age level of mental ability of a person as gauged by standard intelligence tests.

aged (a'jed) persons of advanced age. It is convenient for statisticians to define everyone 65 or over as "aged"; however, there is no known definite age at which individuals become "old." There are nearly 18 million Americans 65 years of age or older. This is almost 10 per cent of the entire United States population of the mid-1960's, in contrast to 1900, when only about 4 per cent of the people in the United States lived to be more than 65. Improvements in public health, nutrition, surgery, drugs and medical care since 1900 have added years to the life expectancy in the United States. According to present figures, the average white, male American who has reached the age of 65 will live for another dozen years, and the average woman will live for another 14.

CAUSES OF THE AGING PROCESS. The reasons why we age are complex and only partially understood. It is evident that the aging process is a combination of many factors.

The body is constantly replacing its worn-out cells, literally by the millions, every day of our lives. As the years pass, this rate of replacement slows down very gradually, beginning at about the time the body has reached its full growth. This is such a gradual change, in fact, that in some of the body's functions there is remarkably little difference between people in their forties and those in their sixties. The part of the body that ages least, and maintains its vigor into the latest years, is the brain.

Hereditary factors play a part in determining how durable a person may be. It is known, for example, that people born to long-living parents and grandparents tend to be longer-lived themselves. It is also believed that the capacity to withstand or adjust to such stresses and strains of living as disease, infection and worry comes in part from hereditary make-up.

The progress of aging may also be hastened by environment, disease, emotional stress and such lifetime habits as boredom, laziness or faulty diet. The physical exhaustion and malnutrition of poverty are two prime causes of early aging.

EFFECTS OF AGING.   Old age brings certain physical changes as a normal aspect of aging. They may be discomforting, even limiting, but they are not necessarily incapacitating. The body has less strength and less endurance as it ages, and needs more repair work. Its speed of reaction and its agility are slowed. The basal metabolism, or rate of energy production in the body cells, is gradually lowered, so that people tire more easily, and are more sensitive to weather changes. Sexual desire and ability decline although they need never entirely end for either sex. The capacity to bear children ends in women with MENOPAUSE, but many men apparently retain their reproductive function into the late years. Those who never used eyeglasses usually need them in later years, or their regular glasses will need changing to bifocals (see also PRESBYOPIA). Hearing changes also come with greater age. Older people hear low tones fairly well, but their ability to perceive the high tones declines. The capacity of tissue and bone to repair itself is slowed, as is cellular growth and division. Bones are more brittle. Skin becomes drier and loses some of its elasticity. Artificial teeth may become necessary. Few people reach the age of 65 with a full set of natural teeth.

Much of the disability and discomfort that used to be considered a part of normal aging can now be prevented with proper medical care and health habits.

DISEASES OF OLD AGE.   No disease is caused by old age, but certain diseases are more likely to occur in old age. ARTHRITIS, CATARACT, CORONARY OCCLUSION (heart attack), CEREBRAL VASCULAR ACCIDENT (stroke), DIABETES MELLITUS, SENILITY and others are diseases that tend to develop after decades of living. Worry, poor habits such as overeating, malnutrition and lack of proper preventive attention to early signs very likely accelerate onset of these diseases of the aged.

In the majority of cases, the disease originates during the middle years. This is why the habit of periodic health examinations is so important and becomes increasingly important after middle age.

AGE AND MENTAL POWERS.   In most people aging has little effect upon mental powers. It is one of the joys of old age that long after the body slows down and begins to limit physical activity, the mind can continue to seek and explore.

In older persons memory of recent events declines while important memories from long ago remain intact. This has been found to be largely a matter of interest and attention rather than an inability to remember. If the memory changes at all, it tends to become more accurate. Older people do not learn new things as quickly as younger people, but once something has been learned, they remem-

ber it better and more accurately. Older persons have the further benefit of long experience and seasoned judgment to apply to the solution of new problems.

SOME RULES OF HEALTH AND HYGIENE FOR THE AGED

Periodic Health Examinations.   The diseases that make invalids of old people, such as diabetes mellitus and heart disease, begin unnoticed in middle age; with regular checkups they can be detected in their early stages when they are easier to treat. The physician can also give good advice on exercise, diet and rest needs through the years.

Proper Nutrition.   Poor eating habits may stem from childhood but they begin to have their effects as people grow older. Poor nutrition has been demonstrated to have a definite adverse effect upon mental and physical vigor. Proper food can prolong life as well as preserve the strength and ability to fight off disease. Good nutrition is a vital aspect of successful aging.

Many older people subsist on poor diets because they live alone and the preparation of proper meals requires too much effort. Some suffer from poor teeth or dentures that interfere with chewing. Others are victims of poor diet habits or lack of interest, or, in some cases, misinformation.

The aged need the same nutrients as those that must be supplied at any age. They must have all basic food elements every day, and this means not overloading the menu with any single type of food. The only kind of food that can be safely reduced in the diet is fat. Because of a gradual decrease in the amount of fat-digesting enzymes in the digestive tract of an older person, the aging body manages fat less well. In general, the older person's diet tends to include too little of the foods that supply vitamin C, iron, vitamin A, vitamin B (thiamine) and vitamin B_2 (riboflavin).

Some older people believe that acid-containing foods such as citrus fruits and tomatoes, which are prime sources of vitamin C, cause acidity in the body. Actually, these acid-containing fruits are excellent alkalizers and rich sources of necessary vitamins and minerals as well, and should be included in the diet. Another common mistake is the belief that milk is only for children. It is an excellent food for adults too. Milk (whole or skimmed) contains protein, calcium and riboflavin, and is readily digested and tolerated by most people of all ages.

If an older person has difficulty chewing, some foods will have to be chopped, strained or cooked soft for his special requirements, but foods with important nutrient values must not be eliminated from the diet. (See also NUTRITION.)

Exercise.   Proper exercise promotes good circulation and appetite, and helps to maintain good mental and physical functioning. Older people should be as active as possible, although never to the point of strain or exhaustion.

Rest.   Rest becomes increasingly important in the later years. It is of great value to rest for half an hour after meals, and at intervals during the day. Older people whose work does not permit them to lie down should take advantage of "breaks" or rest periods to relax as completely as possible, with their feet elevated, perhaps on a chair, if at all feasible.

Avoidance of Inactivity.   Following an illness, when the physician says it is time to get out of bed, his instructions should be followed. A prolonged unnecessary stay in bed is harmful at all ages but especially in later years.

RETIREMENT PROBLEMS.   Although many people look forward to retirement, it is not uncommon to hear of someone who, having worked hard all his life with that goal in mind, begins to fail mentally and physically the moment he actually reaches it. Successful retirement depends on far more than money in the bank. There must be a reserve of interests that make life worth living. Hobbies and recreational activities are important because they can be continued in later years. As Dr. George Lawton, an authority on gerontology, the scientific study of aging, puts it: "To grow old successfully, a man must learn to push around, not his body, but his mind. If his speed, strength, and endurance decline with the years, then he must train in advance skills which will hold up with age and even improve."

agenesia (ah"jĕ-ne'ze-ah) 1. imperfect development. 2. sterility or impotence.

agenesis (a-jen'ĕ-sis) absence of an organ due to nonappearance of its primordium in the embryo.

agenitalism (a-jen'ĭ-tal-izm") a eunuch-like condition due to lack of secretion of the testes.

agenosomia (ah-jen"o-so'me-ah) imperfect development of reproductive organs.

agent (a'jent) a person or substance by which something is accomplished.
  alkylating a., a compound with two or more end (alkyl) groups that combine readily with other molecules.
  chelating a., a compound that combines with metals to form weakly dissociated complexes in which the metal is part of a ring, and used to extract certain elements from a system.
  chimpanzee coryza a., respiratory syncytial virus.
  Eaton a., one of the pleuropneumonia-like organisms that cause primary atypical pneumonia.
  surface-active a., any substance capable of altering the physicochemical nature of surfaces and interfaces; an example is a detergent. Called also surfactant.

ageusia (ah-gu'ze-ah) absence of the sense of taste.

agger (aj'er), pl. *ag'geres* [L.] an elevation.
  a. na'si, an elevation at the anterior free margin of the middle nasal concha.

agglutinable (ah-gloo'tĭ-nah-bl) capable of agglutination.

agglutinant (ah-gloo'tĭ-nant) 1. acting like glue. 2. a substance that promotes union of parts.

agglutination (ah-gloo"tĭ-na'shun) collection of separate particles into clumps or masses; especially the clumping together of bacteria by the action of certain antibodies. adj., **agglutina'tive.**
  group a., agglutination of an organism by an agglutinin specific for other organisms.
  platelet a., clumping together of platelets due to the action of platelet agglutinins.

agglutinator (ah-gloo'tĭ-na"tor) something that agglutinates; an agglutinin.

agglutinin (ah-gloo'tĭ-nin) a specific antibody formed in the blood in response to the presence of an invading agent and capable of causing a clumping together (agglutination) of cells. Agglutinins are proteins (GAMMA GLOBULINS) and function as part of the immune mechanism of the body. When the invading agents that bring about the production of agglutinins are bacteria, the agglutinins produced bring about agglutination of the bacterial cells.
  Erythrocytes also may agglutinate when agglutinins are formed in response to the entrance of noncompatible blood cells into the bloodstream. A transfusion reaction is an example of the result of agglutination of blood cells brought about by agglutinins produced in the recipient's blood in response to incompatible or foreign cells (the donor's blood). Anti-Rh agglutinins are produced in cases of Rh incompatibility and can result in a condition known as ERYTHROBLASTOSIS FETALIS when the maternal blood is Rh negative and the fetal blood is Rh positive (see also RH FACTOR).
  cold a., one that acts only at low temperature.
  group a., one that has a specific action on certain organisms, but will agglutinate other species as well.
  H a., one produced by the motile strain of an organism.
  immune a., a specific agglutinin found in the blood after recovery from the disease or injection of the microorganism.
  incomplete a., *blocking antibody.*
  leukocyte a., one that is directed against neutrophils and other leukocytes.
  normal a., a specific agglutinin found in the blood of an animal or of man that has neither had the disease nor been injected with the causative organism.
  O a., one produced by the nonmotile strain of an organism.
  partial a., one present in agglutinative serum which acts on organisms closely related to the specific antigen, but in a lower dilution.
  platelet a., one that is directed against platelets.
  warm a., an incomplete antibody that sensitizes and reacts optimally with erythrocytes at 37° C.

agglutinogen (ag"loo-tin'o-jen) a substance (antigen) that stimulates the animal body to form agglutinin (antibody).

agglutinoid (ah-gloo'tĭ-noid) an agglutinin that has lost the power to produce clumping, although it can still unite with its agglutinogen.

agglutinum (ah-gloo'tĭ-num) the agglutinable part of a bacillus.

aggregation (ag"rĕ-ga'shun) 1. massing or clumping of materials together. 2. a clumped mass of material.
  familial a., the occurrence of more cases of a given disorder in close relatives of a person with the disorder than in control families.
  platelet a., platelet agglutination.

aglaucopsia (ah"glaw-kop'se-ah) inability to distinguish green tints.

aglossia (ah-glos'e-ah) congenital absence of the tongue.

aglossostomia (ah"glos-o-sto'me-ah) a developmental anomaly with absence of the tongue and the mouth opening.

aglucone (a-gloo'kōn) aglycone.

aglutition (ag″loo-tish′un) inability to swallow.

aglycemia (a″gli-se′me-ah) absence of sugar from the blood. (See also HYPOGLYCEMIA).

aglycone (a-gli′kōn) the noncarbohydrate portion of a glycoside molecule.

aglycosuric (ah-gli″ko-su′rik) free from glycosuria.

agnathia (ag-na′the-ah) congenital absence of the lower jaw.

agnogenic (ag″no-jen′ik) of unknown origin.

agnosia (ag-no′ze-ah) inability to recognize the import of sensory impressions.
  acoustic a., auditory a., inability to recognize the significance of sounds.
  finger a., loss of ability to indicate one's own or another's fingers.
  tactile a., inability to recognize familiar objects by touch or feel.
  time a., loss of comprehension of the succession and duration of events.
  visual a., inability to recognize familiar objects by sight.

-agogue (ah-gog′) word element [Gr.], *something that leads or induces.*

agonad (ah-go′nad) an individual having no sex glands (gonads).

agonal (ag′ŏ-nal) pertaining to death or extreme suffering.

agonist (ag′o-nist) a muscle that in moving a part is resisted by a muscle that relaxes.

agony (ag′o-ne) 1. death struggle. 2. extreme suffering.

agoraphobia (ag″o-rah-fo′be-ah) fear of open or public spaces.

-agra (ag′rah) word element [Gr.], *attack; seizure.*

agranulocyte (a-gran′u-lo-sīt″) a nongranular leukocyte.

agranulocytosis (a-gran″u-lo-si-to′sis) an acute disease in which there is a sudden drop in the production of leukocytes, leaving the body defenseless against bacterial invasion. A great majority of the cases of agranulocytosis are caused by sensitization to drugs or chemicals that affect the bone marrow and thereby depress the formation of granulocytes.
  SYMPTOMS.   The first manifestations of this disorder are usually produced by a severe infection and include high fever, chills, prostration and ulcerations of mucous membrane such as in the mouth, rectum or vagina. Laboratory tests reveal a profound leukopenia (low leukocyte count).
  TREATMENT.   Treatment is aimed at immediate withdrawal of the drug or chemical causing the disorder, and control of infection. In most cases control can be achieved by the administration of antibiotics, usually penicillin, streptomycin or oxytetracycline. If the bone marrow is not irreparably damaged, the prognosis is good, with proper treatment, and the patient will recover as the production of granulocytes resumes. Rarely, the leukocyte-producing tissues are damaged beyond repair, and death ensues.

agranuloplastic (a-gran″u-lo-plas′tik) able to form nongranular cells.

agranulosis (a-gran″u-lo′sis) agranulocytosis.

agraphia (a-graf′e-ah) loss of ability to express thoughts in writing.

ague (a′gu) 1. malaria. 2. a chill.

A.H.A.   American Heart Association; American Hospital Association.

AHF antihemophilic factor (clotting factor VIII).

AHG antihemophilic globulin (clotting factor VIII).

ahypnia (ah-hip′ne-ah) sleeplessness; insomnia.

aichmophobia (āk″mo-fo′be-ah) morbid dread of pointed instruments.

ailurophobia (i-lu″ro-fo′be-ah) morbid fear of cats.

ainhum (ān′hum) a condition of unknown origin, occurring chiefly in dark-skinned races, leading to spontaneous amputation of the fourth or fifth toe.

air (ār) the gaseous mixture that makes up the atmosphere.
  complemental a., the volume of air, in excess of normal, that can be taken into the lungs by forced inspiration.
  factitious a., nitrous oxide.
  reserve a., supplemental a.
  residual a., the volume of air remaining in the lungs after forced expiration.
  supplemental a., the volume of air, in excess of normal, that can be expelled from the lungs by forced expiration.
  tidal a., the volume of air inhaled and exhaled in quiet breathing.

airway (ār′wa) 1. the passage by which air enters and leaves the lungs. 2. a mechanical device used for securing unobstructed respiration during general anesthesia or other occasions in which the patient is not ventilating or exchanging gases properly.
  ORAL AIRWAY.   This is a rubber or plastic hollow tube inserted into the mouth and back of the throat to prevent the tongue from slipping back into the throat and closing off the passage of air.
  ENDOTRACHEAL TUBE.   This inflatable tube is inserted into the mouth or nose and passed down into the trachea. It is used for the administration of anesthetics and may be left in place after the completion of surgery until the patient no longer is in danger of asphyxiation. The endotracheal tube can be connected to a mechanical respirator when necessary.
  TRACHEOSTOMY.   This involves a surgical incision into the trachea to relieve obstruction of the respiratory tract above the level of the incision. A metal or plastic tracheostomy tube is inserted into the incision. (See also TRACHEOSTOMY.)

akaryocyte (ah-kar′e-o-sīt″) erythrocyte.

akathisia (ak″ah-the′ze-ah) a condition marked by motor restlessness and anxiety.

akinesia (a″ki-ne′ze-ah) 1. abnormal absence or poverty of movements. 2. the temporary paralysis of a muscle by the injection of procaine.
  a. al′gera, paralysis due to the intense pain of muscular movement.

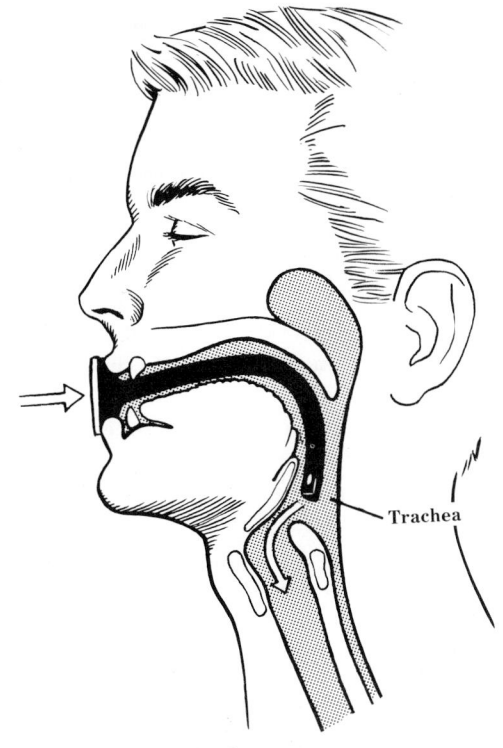

Oral airway.

akinesthesia (ah-kin″es-the′ze-ah) absence of movement sense.

akinetic (a″ki-net′ik) affected with akinesia.

Akineton (a″ki-ne′ton) trademark for preparations of biperiden, an anticholinergic used in the treatment of Parkinson's disease and certain forms of spasticity.

Al chemical symbol, *aluminum.*

ala (a′lah), pl. *a′lae* [L.] a winglike process. adj., **a′late.**
   a. na′si, the cartilaginous flap on the outer side of either nostril.

alalia (ah-la′le-ah) impairment of the ability to speak.

alanine (al′ah-nēn, al′ah-nin) a naturally occurring, nonessential amino acid.

alar (a′lar) 1. pertaining to or like a wing. 2. pertaining to the axilla.

alarm reaction (ah-larm′) the response of the adrenal cortex in times of stress or emergency, resulting in the production of certain adrenocortical hormones (corticosteroids); called also stress response. The exact mechanism is not known; it is believed that the release of epinephrine from the adrenal medulla triggers the production of ACTH, which in turn stimulates the adrenal cortex to release its hormones. Another theory is that the corticosteroids are released independently of ACTH and are a direct response to impulses from the sympathetic nervous system. The corticosteroids provide the body with glucose and amino acids for energy and tissue repair, elevate the blood pressure and help maintain a normal fluid and electrolyte balance.

alastrim (ah-las′trim) a contagious eruptive fever resembling smallpox.

alba (al′bah) [L.] white.

Albamycin (al′bah-mi″sin) trademark for preparations of novobiocin, an antibiotic.

albedo (al-be′do) [L.] whiteness.
   a. ret′inae, paleness of the retina due to edema caused by transudation of fluid from the retinal capillaries.

Albers-Schönberg disease (al′berz shān′berg) a rare hereditary, congenital condition in which there are bandlike areas of condensed bone at the epiphyseal lines of long bones and condensation of the edges of smaller bones. Fractures occur frequently and deformities of the head, chest or spine develop. There is no treatment and the prognosis is unfavorable. Called also osteopetrosis and marble bones.

albicans (al′bĭ-kans) [L.] white.

albinism (al′bĭ-nizm) congenital absence of normal pigmentation in the body (hair, skin, eyes).

albino (al-bi′no) a person affected with albinism.

albinuria (al″bĭ-nu′re-ah) whiteness of the urine.

albocinereous (al″bo-sĭ-ne′re-us) containing both white and gray matter.

Albright's syndrome (awl′brīts) a group of symptoms, including distortion of bone with fibrous changes in the bone marrow spaces, brownish pigmentation of the skin and precocious puberty in females, of unknown cause. Called also polyostotic fibrous dysplasia. The bone lesions may cause the bones to become bowed or shortened,

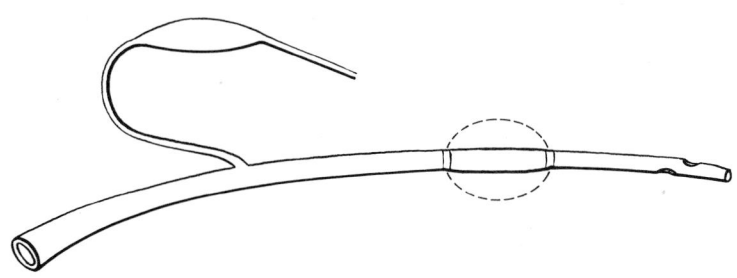

Endotracheal tube.

resulting in difficulty in walking, and may make them more susceptible to fractures. Treatment is concerned with the complications of the disorder — fractures and deformities. Corrective orthopedic surgery is often indicated.

albuginea (al″bu-jin′e-ah) 1. a tough, whitish layer of fibrous tissue investing a part or organ. 2. the tunica albuginea.

albumen (al-bu′men) albumin.

albumin (al-bu′min) a simple protein found in most animal and vegetable tissues; it is soluble in water and coagulable by heat. Albumin is a plasma protein, formed principally in the liver and constituting about four-sevenths of the 6 to 8 per cent protein concentration in the plasma. Albumin is responsible for much of the osmotic force of the blood, and thus is a very important factor in regulating the exchange of water between the plasma and the intercellular compartment (space between the cells). Because of hydrostatic pressure, water is forced through the walls of the capillaries into the tissue spaces. This flow of water continues until the osmotic pull of protein (albumin) molecules causes it to stop. A drop in the amount of albumin in the plasma leads to an increase in the flow of water from the capillaries into the intercellular compartment. This results in an increase in tissue fluid which, if severe, becomes apparent as edema. Albumin serves also as a transport substance.

The presence of albumin in the urine (albuminuria) indicates malfunction of the kidney, and may accompany kidney disease or heart failure. A person with severe renal disease may lose as much as 20 to 30 Gm. of plasma proteins in the urine in one day.

The normal amount of albumin in the blood is 4.5 to 5.5 Gm. per milliliter of serum. A decrease in serum albumin may, as stated, occur with severe disease of the kidney. Other conditions such as liver disease, malnutrition and extensive burns may result in serious decrease of plasma proteins.

    a.-globulin ratio, the ratio of albumin to globulin in blood serum, plasma or urine.

    egg a., the white of eggs.

    normal human serum a., a sterile solution of the serum albumin constituent from healthy donors.

    radioiodinated serum a., normal human serum albumin treated with iodine-131, used for measuring blood volume and cardiac output.

    serum a., albumin of the blood.

albuminate (al-bu′mĭ-nāt) a compound of albumin with a base.

albuminemia (al-bu″mĭ-ne′me-ah) excess of albumin in the blood.

albuminiferous (al-bu″mĭ-nif′er-us) yielding albumin.

albuminimeter (al-bu″mĭ-nim′ĕ-ter) an instrument for determining the proportion of albumin present.

albuminocholia (al-bu″mĭ-no-ko′le-ah) presence of protein in the bile.

albuminoid (al-bu′mĭ-noid) 1. resembling albumin. 2. an albumin-like substance; the term is sometimes applied to scleroproteins.

albuminolysin (al-bu″mĭ-nol′ĭ-sin) a lysin that splits up albumins.

albuminolysis (al-bu″mĭ-nol′ĭ-sis) the splitting up of albumins.

albuminometer (al-bu″mĭ-nom′ĕ-ter) a laboratory device for quantitative determination of albumin in a fluid, such as urine.

albuminoptysis (al-bu″mĭ-nop′tĭ-sis) albumin in the sputum.

albuminorrhea (al-bu″mĭ-no-re′ah) excessive excretion of albumins.

albuminosis (al-bu″mĭ-no′sis) abnormal excess of albuminous elements.

albuminous (al-bu′mĭ-nus) charged with or resembling albumin.

albuminuria (al-bu″mĭ-nu′re-ah) the presence in the urine of serum albumin or serum globulin. adj., **albuminu′ric.**

    adventitious a., that not due to renal disease.

    orthostatic a., albuminuria on assuming the erect position.

Albumisol (al-bu′mĭ-sol) trademark for a preparation of normal human serum albumin.

albumose (al′bu-mōs) a primary product of the digestion of a protein; further digestion converts albumoses into peptones.

    Bence Jones a., Bence Jones protein.

albumosemia (al″bu-mo-se′me-ah) albumose in the blood.

albumosuria (al″bu-mo-su′re-ah) albumose in the urine.

    Bence Jones a., myelopathic a., multiple myeloma.

Alcaligenes (al″kah-lij′ĕ-nēz) a genus of Schizomycetes found in the intestines of vertebrates or in dairy products.

alcapton (al-kap′ton) a class of substances with an affinity for alkali, found in the urine and causing the condition known as alcaptonuria. The compound commonly found, and most commonly referred to by the term, is homogentisic acid.

alcaptonuria (al-kap″to-nu′re-ah) excretion in the urine of homogentisic acid and its oxidation products as a result of a genetic disorder of phenylalanine-tyrosine metabolism.

alcohol (al′ko-hol) 1. a colorless, volatile liquid obtained by fermentation of carbohydrates by yeast. 2. a compound of hydrocarbon with hydroxyl (OH).

    absolute a., alcohol free from water and impurities.

    benzyl a., a colorless liquid used as a local anesthetic.

    cetyl a., a solid alcohol used in making ointment bases.

    denatured a., ethyl alcohol made unfit for consumption by the addition of substances known as denaturants. Although it should never be taken internally, denatured alcohol is widely used on the skin as a cooling agent and skin disinfectant.

    ethyl a., the major ingredient of alcoholic beverages; called also ethanol and grain alcohol. It is sometimes used medically to stimulate the appetite of convalescent, weak or elderly patients.

isopropyl a., a transparent, volatile colorless liquid used as a rubbing compound; called also isopropanol.

methyl a., a mobile, colorless liquid used as a solvent; called also wood alcohol or methanol. It is a useful fuel, but is poisonous if taken internally. Consumption may lead to blindness or death.

phenylethyl a., an alcohol used as an antibacterial and preservative.

primary a., an alcohol that on oxidation forms a corresponding aldehyde and acid having the same number of carbon atoms.

propyl a., a colorless fluid of alcoholic taste and fruity odor.

stearyl a., a mixture of solid alcohols, used as an ingredient of various pharmaceutic or cosmetic preparations.

wood a., methyl alcohol.

alcoholemia (al″ko-hol-e′me-ah) alcohol in the blood.

alcoholic (al″ko-hol′ik) 1. containing or pertaining to alcohol. 2. a person addicted to alcohol.

alcoholism (al′ko-hol″izm) drunkenness (acute alcoholism); or long-continued, excessive consumption of alcohol (chronic alcoholism). Generally, the term refers to chronic alcoholism. The chronic alcoholic is a person who drinks compulsively and in such a way that his drinking is damaging to himself, to his way of life and to those about him. It is the compulsive character of his drinking that sets the alcoholic apart from the heavy or occasionally excessive drinker. His craving for alcohol is deeply rooted, and he cannot govern that craving even if he is aware of its destructive consequences.

CAUSES. There is no accepted explanation to account for the fact that one person becomes an alcoholic while another does not. Generally speaking, a person is more likely to become an alcoholic if his environment emphasizes drinking, presenting it as a fashionable, or indeed indispensable, social pastime. Also, the heavy social drinker has a good chance of becoming an alcoholic. Psychologic factors play an important role in the development of alcoholism in an individual. Unresolved conflicts, loneliness, financial difficulties or marital problems may contribute to alcoholism.

Once a person becomes an alcoholic, whatever the cause or causes, he has something in common with all other alcoholics: he cannot stop drinking by a simple act of will. It is the recognition of this fact that forms the basis of modern treatment for alcoholics. The alcoholic is regarded not as depraved or weak but as sick. He is unable to cure himself. His problem is not moral but medical.

COMPLICATIONS. Alcoholism is all the more a medical matter because it is often complicated by other diseases which afflict both body and mind. Nervous and mental disorders are common in the alcoholic. DELIRIUM TREMENS (DT's) is an acute condition that is particularly apt to occur if the alcoholic is suddenly deprived of drink. The body trembles and there are frightening hallucinations. In KORSAKOFF'S SYNDROME, the memory is impaired, sometimes permanently. Deterioration of the powers of reasoning is a real possibility in alcoholics. In alcoholic polyneuritis, there may be persistent nerve changes. Cirrhosis of the liver, in which the liver becomes swollen with fatty and fibrous tissue, is not limited to alcoholics but often does occur in those with alcoholism of several years' standing. Alcoholic amblyopia, or dimness of vision, is a result of alcohol's toxic effect on the optic nerve. The heart and kidneys may be impaired as an indirect result of alcoholism. Gastric disturbances, excessive bowel activity and circulatory disorders may affect the alcoholic. The chronic alcoholic may suffer from severe malnutrition including vitamin deficiencies. Habitual drinking usually lowers the resistance to infectious diseases such as pneumonia.

TREATMENT. There is no simple remedy for alcoholism. To be helped, the alcoholic must drastically alter his approach to life and destroy a pattern of habits that has been firmly established, perhaps for years. He must stop drinking altogether, for there is little possibility that he will recover the ability to take a drink or two with restraint. Successful treatment is possible only if the alcoholic wants to stop drinking, and this happens only when he has been brought to recognize the seriousness of his condition and the prospect of help. Since he has probably created many difficulties and problems in his life, he will feel guilty and despondent, wishing more for oblivion than for rehabilitation. Condemnation, sermonizing and the like will only reinforce his conviction that life is not worth the trouble.

The first step is to place the alcoholic under the care of a competent physician. He will recommend one or more of the following modes of treatment:

Vitamin and Other Nutritional Therapy. Some of the diseases that complicate alcoholism are due to nutritional deficiencies because the alcoholic often eats improperly or not at all.

Tranquilizers and Sedatives. These are used during withdrawal of alcohol to aid in relaxation and sleep.

Hospitalization. This is advised when withdrawal must be subject to controlled conditions, when the patient's health is bad or when the patient is a criminal risk.

Disulfiram (Antabuse). This is a compound that renders the body so sensitive to alcohol that one drink produces breathlessness, flushing, rapid heartbeat and later nausea, vomiting and fall in blood pressure. Although far from a cure, it is useful in abolishing impulsive drinking. In some cases it is possible through long-continued use of disulfiram to create in the alcoholic, by means of reflex conditioning, a lasting aversion to alcohol. The preparation must be administered only under a doctor's supervision and with the full knowledge and consent of the patient.

Alcoholics Anonymous. A.A. is an organization of individuals who have conquered or are trying to conquer their own habitual drinking. From their own experiences, these people have learned how to encourage and stimulate others in their desire to stop drinking. Meetings and discussions provide the individual with an opportunity to air his own problems as well as to learn from the experiences of others. Hundreds of thousands of alcoholics have been helped by A.A. since the organization was founded in 1935, and membership today totals about 350,000. Help in locating a local group and information about A.A. and alcoholism can be obtained from Alcoholics Anonymous, P.O. Box 459, Grand Central Station, New York, N.Y. 10017.

Psychotherapy. This is advisable when a personality disorder is at the root of the problem.

NURSING CARE. Education of the public as to

the true nature of alcoholism as an illness is the responsibility of the nurse as well as other members of the health team. She should also evaluate her own feelings toward alcoholism and avoid a self-righteous and disdainful attitude toward the alcoholic. Although alcoholics can be and often are difficult patients to care for, they are suffering from a serious and crippling illness that affects their physical well-being, family life, economic status and social relationships.

Hospital treatment of alcoholism is often necessary and alcoholic patients are sometimes admitted to a medical unit if no other facilities are available. They are often boisterous and belligerent and may disrupt the routine of the unit, but their acute illness demands all the attention afforded any patient in this condition. During the acute state of alcoholism the patient requires serenity and physical rest. Attendants must be alert for early symptoms of withdrawal from alcohol as the patient is denied the drug. These symptoms include irritability, insomnia or extreme restlessness. Convulsions and delirium tremens can usually be avoided if adequate sedation is given when the withdrawal symptoms first appear. If delirium tremens does occur, the patient becomes truly frightened and terrified by auditory or visual hallucinations. He must be reassured and offered emotional support and understanding during these trying times.

Adequate fluid intake and a high-protein, high-vitamin diet are necessary because most acute alcoholics are dehydrated and poorly nourished. An accurate record of intake and output of fluids should be kept during the acute phase of this illness.

Diversional activities, such as reading, watching television and visiting with other patients, help relieve the boredom and restlessness felt by the alcoholic during his convalescence. The alcoholic is likely to feel shame and remorse during this time and often indicates a desire to talk with someone about his problems. The nurse must do much more than merely tolerate his presence. She should be a good listener, allowing him to express his feelings and anxieties without fear of reprisal or reprimand. An attitude of understanding will do much toward helping the alcoholic seek help in coping with his problem.

alcoholometer (al″ko-hol-om′ĕ-ter) an instrument for determining the amount of alcohol present.

alcoholuria (al″ko-hol-u′re-ah) the presence of alcohol in the urine.

alcoholysis (al″ko-hol′ĭ-sis) a process analogous to hydrolysis, but in which alcohol takes the place of water.

Aldactone (al-dak′tōn) trademark for a preparation of spironolactone, an aldosterone antagonist used as a diuretic.

aldehyde (al′dĕ-hīd) any of a large class of chemical compounds derived from the primary alcohols by oxidation and containing the monovalent group —CHO.

aldopentose (al″do-pen′tōs) any one of a class of sugars that contain five carbon atoms and an aldehyde group (—CHO).

aldose (al′dōs) a sugar containing an aldehyde group (—CHO).

aldosterone (al-dos′ter-ōn) an electrolyte-regulating hormone of the adrenal cortex; the principal MINERALOCORTICOID.

aldosteronism (al-dos′ter-ōn-izm″) an abnormality of electrolyte metabolism due to excessive secretion of aldosterone.

primary a., hypersecretion of aldosterone by the adrenal cortex, with excessive loss of potassium and generalized muscular weakness.

secondary a., abnormally high levels of aldosterone in the urine as the result of some other disease, such as heart failure or renal or hepatic disease.

aldosteronoma (al-dos″ter-o-no′mah) an aldosterone-secreting adrenocortical tumor.

Aldrich syndrome (awl′drich) chronic eczema, chronic suppurative otitis media, anemia and thrombocytopenic purpura, transmitted as a sex-linked recessive by an unaffected female to the male.

alecithal (ah-les′ĭ-thal) having no distinct yolk.

alemmal (ah-lem′al) having no neurolemma.

Aleppo boil (ah-lep′o) cutaneous leishmaniasis, a type of ulcer or sore caused by *Leishmania tropica*, which is usually transmitted by a bite from the sandfly. The lesion is characterized by cutaneous granulation which has a tendency to become chronic. It occurs principally in Asian and African countries and is known by various names, such as Delhi sore, Baghdad sore, oriental sore.

alethia (ah-le′the-ah) inability to forget.

aleukemia (ah″lu-ke′me-ah) aleukemic leukemia.

aleukia (ah-lu′ke-ah) 1. aleukemic leukemia. 2. absence of blood platelets.

aleukocytosis (ah-lu″ko-si-to′sis) diminished proportion of leukocytes in the blood.

Alevaire (al′ĕ-vār) trademark for a mucolytic solution that is administered by nebulizer in respiratory disorders.

alexia (ah-lek′se-ah) visual aphasia.

alexic (ah-lek′sik) 1. pertaining to alexia. 2. having the properties of an alexin.

alexin (ah-lek′sin) complement.

aleydigism (ah-li′dig-izm) absence of secretion of the interstitial cells of the testis (Leydig cells).

Alflorone (al′flo-rōn) trademark for preparations of fludrocortisone, a synthetic corticoid.

ALG antilymphocyte globulin.

algae (al′je) a group of plants living in the water, including all seaweeds, and ranging in size from microscopic cells to fronds hundreds of feet long.

algefacient (al″jĕ-fa′shent) cooling or refrigerant.

algesia (al-je′ze-ah) sensitiveness to pain; hyperesthesia. adj., **alge′sic, alget′ic.**

algesimetry (al″jĕ-sim′ĕ-tre) measurement of sensitivity to pain.

algesthesis (al″jes-the′sis) a painful sensation.

-algia (al′je-ah) word element [Gr.], *pain.*

algicide (al'ji-sīd) 1. destructive to algae. 2. an agent that destroys algae.

algid (al'jid) chilly; cold.

alginate (al'ji-nāt) a salt of alginic acid, a colloidal substance from brown seaweed; used, in the form of calcium, sodium or ammonium alginate, as foam, clot or gauze for absorbable surgical dressings.

algo- (al'go) word element [Gr.], *pain; cold.*

algogenic (al"go-jen'ik) 1. causing pain. 2. lowering temperature.

algometer (al-gom'ĕ-ter) a device used in testing the sensitiveness of a part.

algometry (al-gom'ĕ-tre) estimation of the sensitivity to painful stimuli.

algophobia (al"go-fo'be-ah) morbid dread of pain.

algor (al'gor) chill or rigor; coldness.
  a. mor'tis, the cooling of the body after death, which proceeds at a definite rate, influenced by the environmental temperature and protection of the body.

Alidase (al'ĭ-dās) trademark for a preparation of hydraluronidase for injection, used as a spreading agent to promote diffusion and hasten absorption.

alienia (ah"li-e'ne-ah) absence of the spleen.

aliform (al'ĭ-form) shaped like a wing.

aliment (al'ĭ-ment) food; nutritive material.

alimentary (al"ĭ-men'tar-e) pertaining to or caused by food, or nutritive material.
  a. canal, all the organs making up the route taken by food as it passes through the body from mouth to anus; called also digestive tract. (See also DIGESTIVE SYSTEM.)

alimentation (al"ĭ-men-ta'shun) giving or receiving of nourishment.

alimentology (al"ĭ-men-tol'o-je) the science of nutrition.

alinasal (al"ĭ-na'zal) pertaining to either of the cartilaginous flaps of the nose.

aliphatic (al"ĭ-fat'ik) pertaining to or derived from fat; having an open-chain structure.

aliquot (al'ĭ-kwot) 1. a sample that is representative of the whole. 2. a number that will divide another without a remainder; e.g., 2 is an aliquot of 6.

alizarin (ah-liz'ah-rin) a red coloring principle obtained from coal tar or madder, the root of the herb *Rubia tinctoria.*

alkalemia (al"kah-le'me-ah) abnormal alkalinity of the blood.

alkali (al'kah-li) any one of a class of compounds such as sodium hydroxide that form salts with acids and soaps with fats; a base, or substance capable of neutralizing acids. Other properties include a bitter taste and the ability to turn litmus paper from red to blue. Alkalis play a vital role in maintaining the normal functioning of the body chemistry. (See also ACID-BASE BALANCE and BASE.)

  a. reserve, the ability of the combined buffer systems of the blood to neutralize acid. The pH of the blood normally is slightly on the alkaline side, between 7.35 and 7.45. Since the principal buffer in the blood is bicarbonate, the alkali reserve essentially is represented by the plasma bicarbonate concentration. However, hemoglobin, phosphates and other bases also act as buffers against acids. A lowered alkali reserve means a state of acidosis; increased reserve indicates alkalosis. Measurement of the alkali reserve is done by means of the CARBON DIOXIDE COMBINING POWER, expressed as the number of milliliters of carbon dioxide that can be bound as bicarbonate by 100 ml. of blood plasma. Normal values range from 53 to 78 ml. of carbon dioxide, sometimes stated as 53 to 78 volumes per cent.

alkali-ash diet a therapeutic diet prescribed to dissolve uric acid and cystine urinary calculi. This type of diet changes the urinary pH so that certain salts are kept in solution and excreted in the urine. Emphasis is placed on fruits, vegetables and milk. Meat, eggs, bread and cereals are restricted.

alkalimetry (al"kah-lim'ĕ-tre) measurement of alkalinity of a compound or of the alkali in a mixture.

alkaline (al'kah-līn) having the reactions of an alkali.
  a. phosphatase, a phosphatase that is active in an alkaline environment.

alkalinity (al"kah-lin'ĭ-te) 1. the quality of being alkaline. 2. the combining power of a base, expressed as the maximum number of equivalents of acid with which it reacts to form a salt.

alkalinuria (al"kah-lin-u're-ah) an alkaline condition of the urine.

alkalization (al"kah-lĭ-za'shun) the act of making alkaline.

alkalizer (al"kah-līz'er) an agent that causes alkalization.

alkaloid (al'kah-loid) one of a large group of organic, basic substances found in plants. They are usually bitter in taste and are characterized by powerful physiologic activity. Examples are morphine, cocaine, atropine, quinine, nicotine and caffeine. The term is also applied to synthetic substances that have structures similar to plant alkaloids, such as procaine.

alkalosis (al"kah-lo'sis) a pathologic condition resulting from accumulation of base or loss of acid without comparable loss of base in the body, and characterized by decrease in hydrogen ion concentration (increase in pH).
  Alkalosis is the opposite of ACIDOSIS. Although the blood is normally slightly alkaline, a drastic shift of the acid-base balance toward alkalinity can produce serious symptoms, including shallow or irregular respirations, prickling or burning sensation in the fingers, toes or lips, muscle cramps and, in severe cases, convulsions.
  compensated a., a condition in which compensatory mechanisms have returned the pH toward normal.

hypokalemic a., a metabolic alkalosis due to losses of potassium level.

metabolic a., a disturbance in which the acid-base status shifts toward the alkaline side because of changes in the fixed (nonvolatile) acids and bases. It frequently results from excessive vomiting in which hydrochloric acid is lost from the stomach, or from loss of acids or potassium in the urine in renal or endocrine disease.

respiratory a., a state due to excess loss of carbon dioxide from the body, due to HYPERVENTILATION.

alkapton (al-kap′tōn) alcapton.

alkaptonuria (al-kap″to-nu′re-ah) alcaptonuria.

alkavervir (al″kah-ver′vir) a mixture of alkaloids extracted from *Veratrum viride,* used to lower blood pressure.

alkyl (al′kil) the radical that results when an aliphatic hydrocarbon loses one hydrogen atom.

alkylate (al′kĭ-lāt) to treat with an alkylating agent.

alkylating agent (al′kĭ-lāt-ing) a synthetic compound containing two or more end (alkyl) groups that combine readily with other molecules. Their action seems to be chiefly on the deoxyribonucleic acid (DNA) in the nucleus of the cell. They are used in chemotherapy of cancer although they do not damage malignant cells selectively, but also have a toxic action on normal cells. Locally they cause blistering of the skin and damage to the eyes and respiratory tract. Systemic toxic effects are nausea and vomiting, reduction in both leukocytes and erythrocytes and hemorrhagic tendencies. Among the agents of this group used in therapy are the NITROGEN MUSTARDS, including mechlorethamine hydrochloride, chlorambucil and triethylenemelamine, and busulfan and cyclophosphamide.

all(o)- (al′o) word element [Gr.], *other; deviating from normal.*

allachesthesia (al″ah-kes-the′ze-ah) allocheiria.

allantochorion (ah-lan″to-ko′re-on) the allantois and chorion as one structure.

allantoid (ah-lan′toid) 1. sausage-shaped. 2. pertaining to the allantois.

allantoin (ah-lan′to-in) a crystalline substance from allantoic fluid and fetal urine.

allantoinuria (ah-lan″to-ĭ-nu′re-ah) allantoin in the urine.

allantois (ah-lan′to-is) a ventral outgrowth of the hindgut of the early embryo, which is a conspicuous component of the developing umbilical cord. adj., **allanto′ic.**

allele (ah-lēl′) one of two or more alternative forms of a gene at the same site in a chromosome, which determine alternative characters in inheritance. adj., **allel′ic.**

silent a., one that produces no detectable effect.

allelomorph (ah-le′lo-morf) allele.

allelotaxis (ah-le″lo-tak′sis) development of an organ from several embryonic structures.

Allen's law (al′enz) the more carbohydrates a diabetic takes, the less he utilizes.

allergen (al′er-jen) a substance capable of inducing hypersensitivity. Almost any substance in the environment can become an allergen. The list of known allergens — that is, substances to which individual patients have become sensitive — includes plant and tree pollens, spores of mold, animal hairs, dust, foods, feathers, dyes, soaps, detergents, cosmetics, plastics, some valuable medicines, including penicillin, and even sunlight. Allergens can enter the body by being inhaled, swallowed, touched or injected. The allergen is not directly responsible for the allergic reaction, but sets off the chain of events that brings it about.

When a foreign substance enters the body, the system reacts by producing ANTIBODIES that attack the substance and render it harmless. When their work is done, the antibodies attach themselves to tissue surfaces, where they remain in reserve, ready to be called into action if the same substance should enter the body again. Should the substance do so, the antibodies again enter into the immune reaction which is part of the body's valuable natural defense against invading disease germs.

A variety of allergic reactions can take place almost anywhere in the body; the cells affected may be destroyed or injured, and they release chemicals such as heparin, leukotaxine and especially histamine that cause systemic symptoms characteristic of an ALLERGY which may range from sneezing and slight local edema to fatal ANAPHYLACTIC SHOCK.

allergist (al′er-jist) a physician specializing in the diagnosis and treatment of allergic conditions.

allergization (al″er-jĭ-za′shun) active sensitization by introduction of allergens into the body.

allergologist (al″er-gol′o-jist) one who specializes in allergology.

allergology (al″er-gol′o-je) the science dealing with problems of hypersensitivity.

allergy (al′er-je) an abnormal and individual hypersensitivity to substances that are ordinarily harmless. For example, the pollen of plants is not generally harmful, yet many people are acutely sensitive to its presence in the atmosphere. adj., **aller′gic.**

An allergy cannot occur on the first contact with a potential ALLERGEN because antibodies have not yet been produced by the body. It may occur on the second contact, when antibodies have been produced and are in reserve in the body tissues, but it does not necessarily do so. In some cases, it may not occur until late in life when, after repeated contact with the allergen, a person suddenly develops a sensitivity.

COMMON ALLERGIES. The most common allergies affect the respiratory passages and the skin, although other areas such as the digestive tract, nervous system, joints, kidneys and blood vessels can be affected. HAY FEVER symptoms are stuffed-up and running nose, spasms of sneezing and itching and watery eyes. ASTHMA is an allergy characterized by shortness of breath, coughing and wheezing. The allergies of the skin include URTICARIA (hives), or itchy swellings, and ECZEMA, an itchy rash. CONTACT DERMATITIS, a rash similar to eczema, occurs as a result of direct contact of the skin with the allergen. Skin eruptions resulting from INSECT BITES AND STINGS and from contact with poisonous plants, such as POISON IVY, OAK AND SUMAC, also are true allergic reactions. Not everyone is sensitive to poison ivy, oak or sumac, and some people are comparatively unaffected by mosquito and other insect bites. Usually the stings of bees and wasps will produce more severe reactions in the allergic than in the nonallergic person. Some people react so strongly that the whole system is affected, and there is a risk of their suffering ANAPHYLACTIC SHOCK.

Emotional factors also have a role in allergy. There is as yet no evidence that allergy can be caused by emotional upset, but it is known that anxiety, fear, anger and strong excitement may set off an allergic attack.

TREATMENT. In most cases allergy is dealt with by identifying the responsible allergen and then avoiding it. In some instances, the victim himself knows what is causing his suffering, but usually it is more difficult to track down. In order to identify the harmful substance, a series of tests conducted by a physician may be necessary. The tests are not foolproof, but they are usually successful. In some cases they reveal not only the guilty substance but the degree of sensitivity to it.

A minute quantity of various suspected allergens is applied to the skin of the patient's forearm, either to the skin surface by means of a saturated adhesive patch (patch test) or under the skin by injection or by applying the substance to a small scratch (scratch test). (See also SKIN TEST.) When the substance so applied is the offending allergen, a mild allergic reaction takes place at the test site. As many as 30 tests may be necessary before the allergen or allergens are identified, so the test series may be an inconvenience to the patient, but it is certainly worthwhile if it means the end to allergic discomfort. The tests are not painful.

In some cases it is not an easy matter to avoid the offending substance. Hay fever and asthma sufferers sometimes have to move to a different locale at certain seasons to escape an airborne allergen. If an important food such as milk is the offender, the doctor may have to design a special diet. If the allergen is animal hair from a household pet, the pet may have to be given away.

An allergy that is resistant to cure may be controlled with medication. Some useful medications are ANTIHISTAMINES, EPINEPHRINE, ephedrine, aminophylline and varieties of steroids of the cortisone and ACTH type. In many instances the patient can be cured of the allergy by a series of desensitization treatments, in which the patient is exposed to gradually increasing amounts of the allergen until his resistance is built up to immunity. The series is time consuming. A new "one-shot" treatment that may eliminate this inconvenience is being evaluated.

More information concerning allergy can be obtained by writing to the Allergy Foundation of America, 801 Second Avenue, New York, N.Y. 10017.

allobarbital (al″o-bar′bĭ-tal) diallylbarbituric acid, an intermediate-acting sedative.

allocheiria (al″o-ki′re-ah) reference of a sensation to the side opposite to that to which the stimulus is applied.

allochezia (al″o-ke′ze-ah) discharge of nonfecal matter by the anus, or of fecal matter by an abnormal passage.

allochromasia (al″o-kro-ma′ze-ah) change in color of hair or skin.

allocinesia (al″o-si-ne′ze-ah) performance of a movement on the side of the body opposite to that directed.

allodiploidy (al″o-dip′loi-de) the state of having two sets of chromosomes derived from different ancestral species.

allodromy (ah-lod′ro-me) disturbed rhythm of the heart.

alloerotism (al″o-er′o-tizm) direction of libido toward others or toward objects outside one's self.

allolalia (al″o-la′le-ah) any defect of speech of central origin.

allomorphism (al″o-mor′fizm) existence of the same substance in different forms.

alloplasia (al″o-pla′ze-ah) heteroplasia.

alloplastic (al″o-plas′tik) pertaining to the open, direct and unmodified expression of impulses outwardly into the environment.

alloplasty (al′o-plas″te) plastic repair of the human body with other than human tissue.

alloploidy (al″o-ploi′de) the state of having any number of chromosome sets derived from different ancestral species.

allopolyploidy (al′o-pol′e-ploi″de) the state of having more than two sets of chromosomes derived from different ancestral species.

allopsychic (al″o-si′kik) pertaining to another's mind or psyche.

REACTIONS TO DIAGNOSTIC SKIN TESTS

1. Short ragweed + +
2. Giant ragweed +
3. Sagebrush + + +
4. Russian thistle + + + +
5. Control —
6. Bluegrass +
7. Timothy +

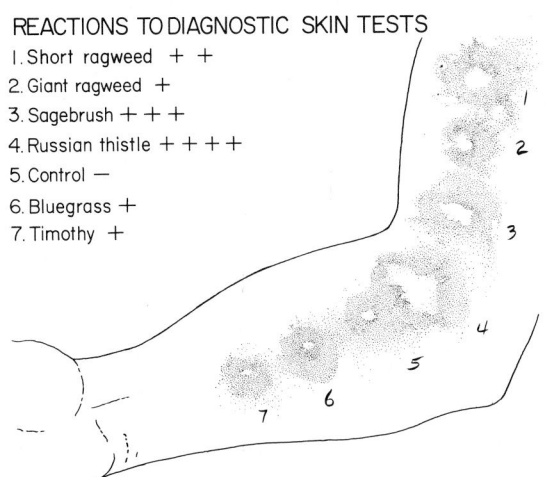

The results of a scratch test. In this case, the patient has reacted violently to Russian thistle and badly to sagebrush and short ragweed. The control and the other tests show no reaction. (Courtesy of Abbott Laboratories.)

allopurinol (al″o-pūr′ĭ-nol) a drug that inhibits uric acid production and reduces serum and urinary uric acid levels; used in prevention of acute attacks of gout.

allorhythmia (al″o-rith′me-ah) irregularity of the pulse.

allorphine (al′or-fēn) nalorphine hydrochloride, a narcotic antagonist.

allosome (al′o-sōm) a chromosome that differs from an ordinary chromosome; a sex chromosome.

allotherm (al′o-therm) an organism whose body temperature changes with its environment.

allotriogeustia (ah-lot′re-o-gōōs′te-ah) perverted sense of taste.

allotropic (al″o-trop′ik) 1. exhibiting allotropism. 2. concerned with others: said of a type of personality that is more preoccupied with others than with self.

allotropism (ah-lot′ro-pizm) existence of an element in two or more distinct forms.

allotropy (ah-lot′ro-pe) 1. allotropism. 2. direction of one's interest more toward others than toward one's self.

alloxan (ah-lok′san) a substance capable of causing diabetes mellitus in experimental animals when administered orally or parenterally.

alloxuremia (ah-lok″su-re′me-ah) the presence of purine bases in the blood.

alloxuria (al″ok-su′re-ah) the presence of purine bases in the urine.

alloy (al′oi) a mixture obtained by fusing metals together.

alogia (ah-lo′je-ah) inability to speak, due to a nerve lesion.

aloin (al′o-in) a mixture of active principles obtained from the plant aloe, used as a cathartic.

alopecia (al″o-pe′she-ah) loss of hair; baldness. The cause of simple baldness is not yet fully understood, although it is known that the tendency to become bald is limited almost entirely to males, runs in certain families and is more common in certain racial groups than in others. Baldness is often associated with aging. The maintenance of general good health may help postpone the onset of baldness; however, it is impossible to cure ordinary baldness once it has occurred.

    androgenetic a., hair loss, dependent on androgen secretion, in hereditarily predisposed persons.

    a. area′ta, hair loss in sharply defined areas, usually the scalp.

    a. cap′itis tota′lis, loss of all the hair from the scalp.

    a. cicatrisa′ta, a disease marked by various sized and shaped patches of alopecia with atrophy of the scalp in the areas.

    a. congenita′lis, complete or partial absence of the hair at birth.

    female-pattern a., loss of scalp hair in girls or women, analogous to male-pattern alopecia, but more benign.

    a. heredita′ria, hereditary loss of hair.

    a. limina′ris, hair loss at the hairline along the front and back edges of the scalp.

    male-pattern a., loss of scalp hair genetically determined and androgen-dependent, beginning with frontal recession and progressing symmetrically to leave ultimately only a sparse peripheral rim of hair.

    a. medicamento′sa, hair loss due to ingestion of a drug.

    symptomatic a., a. symptomat′ica, loss of hair due to systemic or psychogenic causes, such as general ill health, infections of the scalp or skin, nervousness or a specific disease such as typhoid fever, or to stress. The hair may fall out in patches, or there may be diffuse loss of hair instead of complete baldness in one area.

    a. tota′lis, loss of hair from the entire scalp.

    a. universa′lis, loss of hair from the entire body.

alpha (al′fah) first letter of the Greek alphabet, α; used in names of chemical compounds to distinguish the first in a series of isomers, or to indicate position of substituting atoms or groups.

    a. particles, a type of emission produced by the disintegration of a radioactive substance. The atoms of radioactive elements such as uranium and radium are very unstable; they are continuously breaking apart with explosive violence and emitting particulate and nonparticulate types of radiation. The alpha particles, consisting of two protons and two neutrons, have an electrical charge and form streams of tremendous energy when they are released from the disintegrating atoms. These streams of energy (alpha rays) are used to advantage in the treatment of various malignancies. (See also RADIATION and RADIOTHERAPY.)

Alphadrol (al′fah-drol) trademark for a preparation of fluprednisolone, a corticosteroid and anti-inflammatory agent.

alphaprodine (al″fah-pro′dēn) a compound used as an analgesic and narcotic.

ALS antilymphocyte serum.

alseroxylon (al″ser-ok′sĭ-lon) a purified extract of *Rauwolfia serpentina*, used as an antihypertensive, tranquilizer and sedative.

altitude sickness (al′tĭ-tūd) a syndrome caused by exposure to altitude high enough to cause significant hypoxia, or lack of oxygen. At high altitudes the atmospheric pressure is decreased and consequently arterial oxygen content is also lowered.

    Acute altitude sickness may occur after a few hours' exposure to a high altitude. Mental functions may be affected, and there may be lightheadedness and breathlessness. Eventually headache and prostration may occur. Older persons and those with pulmonary or cardiovascular disease are most likely to be affected. After a few hours or days of acclimation the symptoms will subside.

    Chronic altitude sickness (sometimes called Monge's disease or Andes disease) occurs in those living in the high Andes above 15,000 feet. It resembles POLYCYTHEMIA, but is completely relieved if the patient is moved to sea level.

alum (al′um) a substance used, in the form of colorless crystals or white powder, as a styptic or hemostatic because of its astringent action. It also may be given by mouth to induce vomiting. Large doses may cause gastrointestinal disturbances.

aluminosis (ah-loo″mĭ-no′sis) a lung disease of alum workers.

aluminum (ah-loo′mĭ-num) a chemical element, atomic number 13, atomic weight 26.982, symbol Al. (See table of ELEMENTS.)

a. **acetate solution,** a prepartion of aluminum subacetate and glacial acetic acid, used for its antiseptic and astringent action on the skin; called also Burow's solution.

a. **chloride,** a deliquescent, crystalline powder used topically as an astringent solution.

a. **hydroxide gel,** an aluminum preparation, available in suspension or in dried form, used as an antacid in the treatment of peptic ulcer and gastric hyperacidity.

a. **phosphate gel,** a water suspension of aluminum phosphate and some flavoring agents; used as a gastric antacid, astringent and demulcent.

a. **sulfate,** a compound used as an astringent solution.

a. **subacetate,** a compound used as an astringent, diluted with water.

Alurate (al′ūr-āt) trademark for a preparation of aprobarbital, an intermediate-acting sedative and hypnotic.

alveolalgia (al″ve-o-lal′je-ah) pain in the socket of an extracted tooth.

alveolectomy (al″ve-o-lek′to-me) surgical excision of part of the alveolar process.

alveolodental (al-ve″o-lo-den′tal) pertaining to teeth and the alveolar process.

alveolotomy (al″ve-o-lot′o-me) incision of the alveolar process.

alveolus (al-ve′o-lus), pl. *alve′oli* [L.] a little hollow, as the socket of a tooth, a follicle of an acinous gland or one of the thin-walled chambers of the lungs (pulmonary alveoli), surrounded by networks of capillaries through whose walls exchange of carbon dioxide and oxygen takes place. adj., **alve′olar.**

dental alveoli, the cavities or sockets of either jaw, in which the roots of the teeth are embedded.

alveus (al′ve-us), pl. *al′vei* [L.] a canal or trough.

Alvodine (al′vo-dīn) trademark for preparations of piminodine ethanesulfonate, a narcotic analgesic.

alymphia (ah-lim′fe-ah) absence or lack of lymph.

alymphocytosis (a-lim″fo-si-to′sis) deficiency of lymphocytes in the blood.

Am chemical symbol, *americium.*

A.M.A. American Medical Association.

amacrine (am′ah-krīn) 1. without long processes. 2. a branched retinal structure, considered a modified nerve cell.

Amadil (am′ah-dil) trademark for a preparation of acetaminophen, an analgesic and antipyretic.

amalgam (ah-mal′gam) a compound of mercury with another metal.

emotional a., an unconscious attempt to bind, neutralize, deny or counteract anxiety.

amastia (ah-mas′te-ah) congenital absence of one or both mammary glands.

amaurosis (am″aw-ro′sis) loss of sight without apparent lesion of the eye, from disease of the optic nerve, retina, spine or brain.

a. fu′gax, sudden temporary or fleeting blindness.

a. partia′lis fu′gax, sudden transitory partial blindness.

amaurotic (am″aw-rot′ik) pertaining to, or of the nature of, amaurosis.

a. **familial idiocy,** a group of disorders of infancy or childhood that tend to occur in families and are due to a defect of lipid metabolism. Tay-Sachs disease is the infantile form, and is probably the most common of these rare disorders. It occurs mainly in Jewish children, and is characterized by severe idiocy and blindness that is usually complete by the second year. The late infantile form is called Bielschowsky's disease. Spielmeyer-Vogt disease is the juvenile form; it begins at about 8 years and may or may not include blindness. In all forms, there is deposition of lipid in all nerve cells, producing a progressive and unremitting paralysis, usually of the spastic type. There is no cure and the prognosis is extremely poor. Death usually occurs between the ages of 14 and 18.

ambenonium (am″be-no′ne-um) a chemical used as a cholinesterase inhibitor or to increase muscular strength in myasthenic patients.

ambidextrous (am″bĭ-deks′trus) using either hand for the performance of certain tasks.

ambilateral (am″bĭ-lat′er-al) pertaining to or affecting both sides.

ambilevous (am″bĭ-le′vus) awkward at using both hands.

ambiopia (am″be-o′pe-ah) diplopia.

ambisexual (am″bĭ-seks′u-al) pertaining to both sexes.

ambivalence (am-biv′ah-lens) simultaneous existence of conflicting emotional attitudes toward a goal, object or person. adj., **ambiv′alent.**

amblyacousia (am″ble-ah-ku′se-ah) dullness of hearing.

amblyaphia (am″ble-a′fe-ah) bluntness of the sense of touch.

amblygeustia (am″ble-goos′te-ah) dullness of the sense of taste.

Amblyomma (am″ble-om′ah) a genus of ticks, comprising approximately 100 species, which are vectors of various disease-producing organisms.

A. **america′num,** a species of ticks widely distributed in the United States and Central and South America; a vector of Rocky Mountain spotted fever.

A. **cajennen′se,** a tick widely distributed in North, Central and South America; a vector of São Paulo fever, a form of typhus.

A. **macula′tum,** a tick widely distributed in the United States and Central and South America.

A. **va′rium,** a species of Amblyomma, including the largest tick known.

amblyopia (am″ble-o′pe-ah) dimness of vision not due to organic defect or refractive errors. adj., **amblyop′ic.**

color a., dimness of color vision due to toxic or other influences.

amblyoscope (am'ble-o-skōp") an instrument for training an amblyopic eye to take part in vision.

ambo (am'bo) ambon.

amboceptor (am'bo-sep"tor) the body that is thought to join the complement to the animal or bacterial cell.

Ambodryl (am'bo-dril) trademark for preparations of bromodiphenhydramine, an antihistamine.

ambon (am'bon) the edge of the socket in which the head of a long bone is lodged.

ambotoxoid (am"bo-tok'soid) a mixture of the soluble products of bacteria which have been lysed by a bacteriophage, with a filtrate from a culture of the organism.

ambulant, ambulatory (am'bu-lant), (am'bu-lah-tor"e) walking or able to walk; not confined to bed.

ambutonium (am"bu-to'ne-um) a chemical used as an anticholinergic or an antispasmodic or to reduce gastric acid secretion.

ameba (ah-me'bah), pl. *ame'bae, ame'bas* [L.] a minute, one-celled protozoan. The common laboratory example is *Amoeba proteus.* The usual cause of human amebic infection is *Entamoeba histolytica.*

amebiasis (am"e-bi'ah-sis) infection with amebas, especially with *Entamoeba histolytica* (see also AMEBIC DYSENTERY).

amebic (ah-me'bik) pertaining to, or of the nature of, an ameba.
 a. dysentery, a form of dysentery caused by *Entamoeba histolytica* and spread by contaminated food, water and flies; called also amebiasis. Amebic dysentery was once thought to be a purely tropical disease, but it is now known that many cases occur throughout the United States. Symptoms are diarrhea, fatigue and intestinal bleeding. Complications include involvement of the liver, liver abscess and pulmonary abscess. For treatment several drugs are available, for example, emetine hydrochloride and chloroquine, which may be used singly or in combination.

amebicide (ah-me'bĭ-sīd) destructive to amebas.

amebocyte (ah-me'bo-sīt) a cell showing ameboid movement.

ameboid (ah-me'boid) resembling an ameba.

ameboidism (ah-me'boid-izm) performance of ameba-like movements.

ameboma (am"e-bo'mah) a tumor-like mass caused by granulomatous reaction in the intestines in amebiasis.

amelia (ah-me'le-ah) a developmental anomaly with absence of the limbs.

amelification (ah-mel"ĭ-fĭ-ka'shun) the develop- ment of ameloblasts into enamel.

ameloblast (ah-mel'o-blast) a cell that takes part in forming dental enamel.

ameloblastoma (ah-mel"o-blas-to'mah) a locally invasive, highly destructive tumor of the jaw.
 pituitary a., craniopharyngioma.

amelodentinal (am"ĕ-lo-den'tĭ-nal) pertaining to dental enamel and dentin.

amelogenesis (ah-mel"o-jen'ĕ-sis) formation of dental enamel.
 a. imperfec'ta, imperfect formation of enamel, resulting in brownish coloration and friability of the teeth.

amelogenic (am"ĕ-lo-jen'ik) forming enamel.

amelus (am'ĕ-lus) an individual exhibiting amelia.

amenorrhea (a-men"o-re'ah) absence of the menses. adj., **amenorrhe'al.** Primary amenorrhea refers to absence of the onset of menstruation at puberty. It may be caused by underdevelopment or malformation of the reproductive organs, or by glandular disturbances. When menstruation has begun and then ceases, the term secondary amenorrhea is used. The most common cause is usually a disturbance of the endocrine glands concerned with the menstrual process. General ill health, a change in climate or living conditions, emotional shock or, frequently, either the hope or fear of becoming pregnant can sometimes stop the menstrual flow.

amensalism (a-men'sal-izm) interaction between coexisting populations of different species, one of which is adversely affected and the other unaffected.

amentia (a-men'she-ah) lifelong intellectual retardation or subnormality, usually due to lack of development of adequate brain tissue.
 nevoid a., amentia with nevus formation on face and scalp.

American Nurses' Association A.N.A., the national organization and official spokesman for registered nurses. The A.N.A. was founded in 1896 and exists for the purposes of improving the standards of nursing and promoting the general welfare of professional nurses. The association is a federation of 54 local organizations in the 50 states, District of Columbia, Panama Canal Zone, Puerto Rico and the Virgin Islands. The local organizations serve to implement the goals and carry out the functions of the national organization. The official publication of the A.N.A. is the *American Journal of Nursing.* Offices of the organization are located at 10 Columbus Circle, New York, N.Y. 10019.

americium (am"er-ish'e-um) a chemical element, atomic number 95, atomic weight 243, symbol Am. (See table of ELEMENTS.)

ametria (ah-me'tre-ah) congenital absence of the uterus.

ametropia (am"ĕ-tro'pe-ah) a condition of the eye in which parallel rays fail to come to a focus on the retina. adj., **ametrop'ic.**

amicrobic (ah"mi-kro'bic) not produced by microorganisms.

amicron (ah-mi'kron) a particle so small it cannot be seen with the ultramicroscope.

amidase (am'ĭ-dās) a deamidizing ferment.

amide (am'īd) any compound derived from ammonia by substitution of an acid radical for hydrogen.

amido (am'ĭ-do) the monovalent radical NH_2 united with an acid radical.

amidopyrine (am″ĭ-do-pi'rēn) aminopyrine.

Amigen (am'ĭ-jen) trademark for protein hydrolysate preparation for intravenous injection.

amimia (a-mim'e-ah) loss of ability to imitate or mimic or to use appropriate gestures, due to a disorder of the language center of the brain.

amine (am'in, ah'mēn) an organic compound containing nitrogen.

amino (am'ĭ-no, ah-me'no) the monovalent radical NH_2, when not united with an acid radical.

    a. acid, any one of a class of organic compounds containing the amino (NH_2) and the carboxyl (COOH) group, occurring naturally in plant and animal tissues and forming the chief constituents of protein.

    More than 20 different amino acids are commonly found in proteins. Some of them can be produced within the body, but there are eight that the human organism cannot manufacture; these essential amino acids must be provided by protein foods in the diet. The essential amino acids are isoleucine, leucine, lysine, methionine, phenylalanine, threonine, tryptophan and valine. Histidine and arginine, which may be manufactured in the body under certain circumstances, are also sometimes considered essential.

    Protein foods that provide large amounts of essential amino acids are known as complete proteins and include proteins from animal sources, such as meat, eggs, fish and milk. Proteins that cannot supply the body with all the essential amino acids are known as incomplete proteins; these are the vegetable proteins most abundantly found in peas, beans and certain forms of wheat.

aminoacetic acid (ah-me'no-ah-se'tik) glycine.

aminoacidemia (am″ĭ-no-as″ĭ-de'me-ah) the presence of amino acids in the blood.

aminoaciduria (am″ĭ-no-as″ĭ-du're-ah) the presence in the urine of amino acids.

p-aminobenzoic acid (par″ah-am″ĭ-no-ben-zo'ik) a member of the B group of vitamins, a growth factor for certain organisms, and used in the treatment of certain rickettsial infections, including scrub typhus; called also PABA.

ε-aminocaproic acid (ep'sĭ-lon am″ĭ-no-kah-pro'-ik) a synthetic amino acid that is a potent inhibitor of fibrinolysis, plasminogen activator and plasmin.

aminoglutethimide (am″ĭ-no-gloo-teth'ĭ-mīd) a compound used in the treatment of most forms of epilepsy.

aminogram (am-i'no-gram) a graphic representation of the pattern of amino acids present in a substance, as determined quantitatively.

aminolysis (am″ĭ-nol'ĭ-sis) the splitting up of amines.

aminometradine, aminometramide (am″ĭ-no-met'rah-dēn), (am″ĭ-no-met'rah-mīd) a compound used to increase urine formation and in treatment of edema of heart failure.

aminopentamide (am″ĭ-no-pen'tah-mīd) a compound used as an anticholinergic and applied locally to the eye for dilatation of the pupil.

aminophylline (am″ĭ-no-fil'in) a mixture of theophylline and ethylenediamine; used as a smooth muscle relaxant, myocardial stimulant and diuretic. Administration of the drug may be by mouth, intramuscularly, intravenously or rectally. If given too rapidly by vein it may produce circulatory collapse. Intramuscular administration should be performed with caution because aminophylline is very irritating to the tissues. It also may cause gastric or urinary irritation when taken by mouth. Dose depends on the route of administration and the effect desired.

aminopterin (am″in-op'ter-in) a folic acid antagonist and antimetabolite used in the treatment of leukemia.

aminopyrine (am″ĭ-no-pi'rēn) white odorless crystals used as an analgesic and antipyretic, somewhat more potent than aspirin. This drug must be given with caution because it may cause a sudden serious and even fatal leukopenia and agranulocytosis. This reaction in hypersensitive persons can occur without warning and after they have taken the drug previously without incident. Aminopyrine was formerly used in many patent medicines dispensed as "headache preparations," but because of its toxicity, it is now dispensed only by prescription.

aminosis (am″ĭ-no'sis) excessive formation of amino acids in the body.

Aminosol (ah-me'no-sol) trademark for an amino acid preparation for intravenous injection.

aminotrate (am'ĭ-no-trāt″) trolnitrate, a vasodilator used in the treatment of angina pectoris.

aminuria (am″ĭ-nu're-ah) the presence of amines in the urine.

amisometradine (am-i″so-met'rah-dēn) a compound used as diuretic.

amitosis (am″ĭ-to'sis) direct cell division; simple cleavage of the nucleus without the formation of a spireme spindle figure or chromosomes. adj., **amitot'ic.**

amitriptyline (am″ĭ-trip'tĭ-lēn) a compound used as an antidepressant.

ammeter (am'me-ter) an instrument for measuring in amperes the strength of a current flowing in a circuit.

ammoaciduria (am″o-as″ĭ-du're-ah) the presence of ammonia and amino acids in the urine.

ammonia (ah-mo'ne-ah) a colorless alkaline gas, NH_3, with a pungent odor and acrid taste, and soluble in water.

ammoniate (ah-mo'ne-āt) to combine with ammonia.

ammoniated mercury (ah-mo'ne-āt″ed mer'ku-re) a compound used as an antiseptic skin and ophthalmic ointment. It should be applied with caution as excessive use may irritate the skin and cause a dermatitis.

ammoniemia (ah-mo″ne-e'me-ah) the presence of ammonia or its compounds in the blood.

ammonium (ah-mo'ne-um) a hypothetical radical,

NH$_4$, forming salts analogous to those of the alkaline metals.

a. acetate, a compound used as a diaphoretic and diuretic.

a. bromide, a crystalline compound used as a central nervous system depressant.

a. carbonate, a mixture of ammonium compounds used as a liquefying expectorant in the treatment of chronic bronchitis and similar lung disorders. It is sometimes used as a reflex stimulant in "smelling salts" because of the strong ammonia odor it gives off.

a. chloride, colorless or white crystals, with a cool, salty taste, used as an expectorant because it liquefies bronchial secretions. In the body it is changed to urea and hydrochloric acid, and thus is useful in acidifying the urine and increasing the rate of urine flow. Excessive dosage may produce ACIDOSIS.

a. iodide, a compound used as a resolvent and expectorant.

a. mandelate, a compound used as a urinary antiseptic.

ammoniuria (ah-mo″ne-u′re-ah) excess of ammonia in the urine.

amnalgesia (am″nal-je′ze-ah) abolition of pain and memory of a painful procedure by the use of drugs or hypnosis.

amnesia (am-ne′ze-ah) pathologic impairment of memory. adj., **amnes′tic.** Amnesia is usually the result of physical damage to areas of the brain from injury, disease or alcoholism. It may also be caused by a decreased supply of blood to the brain, a condition that may accompany senility. Another cause is psychologic. A shocking or unacceptable situation may be too painful to remember, and the situation is then retained only in the subconscious mind. The technical term for this is repression.

Rarely is the memory completely obliterated. When amnesia results from a single physical or psychologic incident, such as a concussion suffered in an accident or a severe emotional shock, the victim may forget only the incident itself, he may be unable to recall events occurring before or after the incident or the order of events is confused, with recent events imputed to the past and past events to recent times. In another form, only certain isolated events are lost to memory.

Amnesia victims usually have a good chance of recovery if there is no irreparable brain damage. The recovery is often gradual, the memory slowly reclaiming isolated events while others are still missing. Psychotherapy may be necessary when the amnesia is due to a psychologic reaction.

Amnesia takes different forms depending upon the area of the brain affected and how extensive the damage is. In auditory amnesia, or word deafness, the patient is unable to interpret spoken language. Words come to him as a jumble of sounds which he is unable to associate meaningfully with ideas. Similarly, in visual amnesia, or word blindness, the written language is forgotten. Tactile amnesia is the inability to recognize once familiar objects by the sense of touch.

amniocentesis (am″ne-o-sen-te′sis) transabdominal perforation of the amniotic sac for the purpose of obtaining a sample of amniotic fluid. This is a relatively new procedure and is safely done only by trained personnel and in well equipped medical centers.

The usual indication for amniocentesis is the suspected occurrence of ERYTHROBLASTOSIS FETALIS, which results from incompatibility of the fetal and maternal blood. In order to forestall the effects of erythroblastosis the physician needs to know how much destruction of the fetal cells is taking place while the fetus is in utero. Samples of amniotic fluid obtained by amniocentesis are analyzed for concentrations of protein and bilirubin. The higher the concentration the stronger the evidence that erythrocytes are being destroyed.

The physician obtains the sample of amniotic fluid through a long pudendal needle that is introduced into the mother's abdomen and then guided through the uterine wall and into the amniotic cavity between the fetus and the placenta. Local anesthesia may be used and the patient must be cautioned not to move during the procedure lest the needle become displaced.

Following the amniocentesis the patient is observed for changes in blood pressure. Hemorrhage from the placenta must be considered a possibility if the blood pressure begins to drop. Increased fetal activity or other signs of fetal distress such as changes in the fetal heart rate must be reported to the physician at once as they may warrant immediate measures such as delivery of the infant if it is considered to be viable.

amniochorial (am″ne-o-ko′re-al) pertaining to amnion and chorion.

amniogenesis (am″ne-o-jen′ĕ-sis) the development of the amnion.

amniography (am″ne-og′rah-fe) roentgenography of the gravid uterus.

amnion (am′ne-on) the innermost membrane enclosing the developing fetus and the fluid in which it is bathed.

a. nodo′sum, a nodular condition of the fetal surface of the amnion, observed in oligohydramnios associated with absence of the kidneys in the fetus.

amnionitis (am″ne-o-ni′tis) inflammation of the amnion.

amniorrhea (am″ne-o-re′ah) escape of the amniotic fluid.

amniorrhexis (am″ne-o-rek′sis) rupture of the amnion.

amnioscope (am′ne-o-skōp″) an instrument that, by passage through the abdominal wall into the amniotic cavity, permits direct visualization of the fetus in utero.

amniote (am′ne-ōt) any animal with amnion.

amniotic (am″ne-ot′ik) pertaining to the amnion.

a. fluid, the albuminous fluid contained in the amniotic sac and secreted by the amnion; called also liquor amnii and "waters." The fetus floats in the amniotic fluid, which serves as a cushion against injury from sudden blows or movements and helps maintain a constant body temperature for the fetus. Normally the amniotic fluid is clear and slightly alkaline. Discoloration or excessive cloudiness of the fluid may indicate fetal distress or disease, as in erythroblastosis fetalis in which the amniotic fluid is usually a greenish yellow color. The amount varies from 500 to 1500 ml.

An excessive amount of amniotic fluid is called polyhydramnios; the amount may be as much as several gallons. The cause of this condition is unknown but it frequently accompanies multiple pregnancy or some congenital defect of the fetus, especially hydrocephalus and meningocele.

An abnormally small amount of amniotic fluid is referred to as oligohydramnios. In this condition there may be less than 100 ml. of fluid present. The cause is unknown. The condition may produce pressure deformities of the fetus, such as clubfoot or torticollis (wryneck). Adhesions may result from direct contact of the fetus with the amnion.

Recently a technique for removal of a sample of amniotic fluid from the pregnant uterus, called AMNIOCENTESIS, has been developed. The sample is then tested for bilirubin pigments and protein concentration to determine the severity of erythroblastosis.

a. sac, the sac enclosing the fetus suspended in the amniotic fluid.

amniotome (am′ne-o-tōm) an instrument for cutting the fetal membranes.

amniotomy (am″ne-ot′o-me) surgical rupture of the fetal membranes.

amobarbital (am″o-bar′bĭ-tal) one of the barbiturates, used as a short-acting hypnotic and sedative. Effects develop rapidly and the drug is eliminated more quickly than other barbiturates. Regular use may lead to habituation and overdosage can produce narcosis and death.

amodiaquine (am″o-di′ah-kwin) a chemical used to suppress malaria and to treat malaria due to *Plasmodium falciparum* or liver abscess due to ameba.

Amoeba (ah-me′ba) ameba.

amolanone (ah-mo′lah-nōn) a chemical used for parasympathetic blockade, relaxation of spasm of the urinary tract and as a topical anesthetic, particularly for urologic diagnostic procedures.

amorph (a′morf) an amorphous mutant gene.

amorphism (a-mor′fizm) state of being amorphous.

amorphous (ah-mor′fus) having no definite form; shapeless.

amotio (ah-mo′she-o) [L.] a removing.
a. ret′inae, detachment of the retina.

AMP adenosine monophosphate.

amp. ampere, ampule.

ampere (am′pēr) a unit of electric current strength, the current yielded by one volt of electromotive force against one ohm of resistance.

Amphedroxyn (am″fe-drok′sin) trademark for a preparation of methamphetamine, an adrenergic, central nervous system stimulant.

amphetamine (am-fet′ah-mēn) a white crystalline powder used as a central nervous system stimulant. It is odorless and has a slightly bitter taste.

Amphetamine has the temporary effect of increasing energy and apparent mental alertness. It is used in some cases of mental depression and alcoholism, in the chronic rigidity following encephalitis, in attacks of narcolepsy and to control the appetite in the overweight. It is also used to overcome the depressant effects of barbiturates.

Caution must be exercised in using amphetamine in persons hypersensitive to stimulants, those suffering from coronary or cardiovascular disease or hypertension or women in the early stages of pregnancy. The drugs should be used only with a doctor's prescription and never by normal persons as "pep pills" to increase their working capacity.

amphi- (am′fe) word element [Gr.], *both; on both sides.*

amphiarthrosis (am″fe-ar-thro′sis) a joint in which the surfaces are connected by disks of fibrocartilage, as between vertebrae.

Amphibia (am-fib′e-ah) a class of animals living both on land and in water.

amphiblastula (am″fĭ-blas′tu-lah) a blastula resulting from unequal segmentation.

amphibolic (am″fĭ-bol′ik) 1. uncertain. 2. having both an anabolic and catabolic function.

amphicelous (am″fĭ-se′lus) concave on either side or end.

amphicentric (am″fĭ-sen′trik) beginning and ending in the same vessel.

amphichroic, amphichromatic (am″fĭ-kro′ik), (am″fĭ-kro-mat′ik) affecting both red and blue litmus.

amphicrania (am″fĭ-kra′ne-ah) headache affecting both sides of the head.

amphicyte (am′fĭ-sīt) one of the cells forming the capsule surrounding a spinal ganglion.

amphicytula (am″fĭ-sit′u-lah) the ovum in its cytula stage.

amphidiarthrosis (am″fĭ-di″ar-thro′sis) a joint having the nature of both ginglymus and arthrodia, as that of the lower jaw.

amphigastrula (am″fĭ-gas′troo-lah) the gastrula resulting from unequal segmentation, the cells of the two hemispheres being of unequal size.

amphigonadism (am″fĭ-gon′ah-dizm) possession of both ovarian and testicular tissue.

amphimixis (am″fĭ-mik′sis) 1. intermingling of hereditary units of sperm and ovum in the fertilized ovum. 2. in psychiatry, association of libido or sexual energy with both urethral and genital regions.

amphimorula (am″fĭ-mor′u-lah) the morula resulting from unequal segmentation, the cells of the two hemispheres being of unequal size.

amphithymia (am″fĭ-thi′me-ah) a mental state characterized by both depression and elation.

amphitrichous (am-fit′rĭ-kus) having flagella at each end.

amphocyte (am′fo-sīt) a cell staining with either acid or basic dyes.

ampholyte (am′fo-līt) an organic or inorganic substance capable of acting as either an acid or a base.

amphophil (am'fo-fil) an amphophilic cell or element.

amphophilic (am″fo-fil'ik) staining with either acid or basic dyes.

amphoric (am-for'ik) pertaining to a bottle; resembling the sound made by blowing across the neck of a bottle.

amphoteric (am″fo-ter'ik) capable of acting as both an acid and a base; capable of neutralizing either bases or acids.

amphotericin B (am″fo-ter'ĭ-sin b) an antifungal antibiotic used to treat deep-seated mycotic infections, especially histoplasmosis. It is of no benefit in the treatment of bacterial infections. It may be applied topically or administered intravenously. Toxic effects from the drug have not been clearly established but anorexia, chills, fever and headache may occur. Renal damage with evidence of renal tubular acidosis occurs, but usually clears when the drug is discontinued.

amphotericity (am″fo-ter-is'ĭ-te) the power to unite with either positively or negatively charged ions, or with either basic or acid substances.

amphoterism (am-fo'ter-izm) the possession of both acid and basic properties.

amphotony (am-fot'o-ne) hypertonia of the entire autonomic nervous system.

ampicillin (am″pĭ-sil'in) a broad-spectrum penicillin of synthetic origin, used in treatment of a number of infections, and available in oral preparations as well as ampules for intramuscular injections. It is active against many of the gram-negative pathogens, in addition to the usual gram-positive ones that are affected by penicillin.

amplification (am″plĭ-fĭ-ka'shun) the process of making larger, as the increase of an auditory or visual stimulus, as a means of improving its perception.

amplitude (am'plĭ-tūd) largeness, fullness; wideness or breadth of range or extent.
 a. of accommodation, the total amount of accommodative power of the eye.

amprotropine (am″pro-tro'pēn) an anticholinergic drug that acts like atropine in its depression of the parasympathetic impulses, but is much less potent. It is used in the treatment of peptic ulcer and cases of hypermotility of the intestinal tract, and is available in combination with a barbiturate.

ampule (am'pūl) a small, hermetically sealed glass flask, e.g., one containing medication for parenteral administration.

ampulla (am-pul'ah), pl. *ampul'lae* [L.] a flasklike dilatation of a tubular structure, especially of the expanded ends of the semicircular canals of the ear.
 a. chy'li, receptaculum chyli.
 a. duc'tus deferen'tis, the enlarged and tortuous distal end of the ductus deferens.
 Henle's a., ampulla ductus deferentis.
 hepatopancreatic a., ampulla of Vater; a flasklike cavity in the major duodenal papilla into which the common bile duct and pancreatic duct open.

Lieberkühn's a., the blind termination of the lacteals in the villi of the intestines.
 ampul'lae membrana'ceae, the dilatations at one end of each of the three semicircular ducts.
 ampul'lae os'seae, the dilatations at one of the ends of the semicircular canals.
 phrenic a., the dilatation at the lower end of the esophagus.
 a. of rectum, the dilated portion of the rectum just proximal to the anal canal.
 a. of Thoma, one of the small terminal expansions of an interlobar artery in the pulp of the spleen.
 a. of uterine tube, the longest and widest portion of the uterine tube, between the infundibulum and the isthmus of the tube.
 a. of Vater, hepatopancreatic ampulla; the term "ampulla of Vater" is often mistakenly used instead of "papilla of Vater," or major duodenal papilla.

amputation (am″pu-ta'shun) the removal of a limb or other appendage or outgrowth of the body. Amputation is sometimes necessary in cases of cancer, infection and gangrene. It may be necessary after irreparable traumatic injury to a limb. Blood vessel disorders such as arteriosclerosis, often secondary to diabetes mellitus, account for the greatest percentage of leg amputations.

Many amputees adjust quickly to the loss, but in some cases there are emotional difficulties. If the patient is properly prepared for the amputation, the chances of psychologic repercussions are reduced. It is best that the patient learn as much as possible about the amputation itself, the therapy that follows and the PROSTHESIS, if one is to be used. If possible, he should talk to someone who has had a similar amputation.

A program of rehabilitation should follow soon after amputation. If a limb has been removed, the stump may be prepared for an artificial replacement. The remaining muscles are strengthened and, in the case of lower-limb amputation, the stump is made to shrink so that it will fit into the socket of the artificial leg.

NURSING CARE. The nurse's role in psychologic preparation of a patient for amputation includes education in regard to fitting and use of a prosthesis as well as emotional support and understanding. The physician usually explains the types of prostheses available and the treatments necessary before the limb is fitted on the stump; however, the nurse must also be prepared to encourage the patient in his period of adjustment to the artificial limb.

Preoperative Care. Prior to surgery the affected limb is shaved and thoroughly cleansed with an antiseptic. Special wrapping of the limb with sterile towels is sometimes ordered by the surgeon.

Postoperative Care. The most frequent danger after amputation is hemorrhage. The stump is usually elevated on a pillow and watched closely for signs of fresh bleeding. *A large tourniquet is kept at the bedside at all times during the postoperative period.* Special exercises are usually ordered to prevent contractures of the muscles leading to the stump. Infection is always a danger and must be avoided by careful dressing and handling of the stump to prevent the entrance of bacteria into the wound.

A sensation called phantom pain is often experienced by patients after amputation. This phenomenon is characterized by a feeling of pain in the limb that has been amputated and is a result of irritation of the nerve endings at the site of the stump. The pains are sometimes quite disturbing to the patient unless he is told that they do occur and that he need not doubt his sanity or feel that the nursing staff doubts their existence. Narcotics may be administered as ordered to relieve the phantom pains. In extreme cases surgery may be necessary to alleviate irritation of the nerve endings causing the sensation.

Chopart's a., amputation of the foot, with the calcaneus, talus and other parts of the tarsus being retained.

congenital a., absence of a limb at birth, attributed to constriction of the part by an encircling band during intrauterine development.

a. in contiguity, amputation at a joint.

a. in continuity, amputation of a limb elsewhere than at a joint.

diaclastic a., amputation in which the bone is broken by osteoclast and the soft tissues divided by an écraseur.

Dupuytren's a., amputation of the arm at the shoulder joint.

Gritti-Stokes a., amputation of the leg at the knee through condyles of the femur.

Hey's a., amputation of the foot between the tarsus and metatarsus.

interpelviabdominal a., amputation of the thigh with excision of the lateral portion of the pelvic girdle.

interscapulothoracic a., amputation of the arm with excision of the lateral portion of the shoulder girdle.

Lisfranc's a., amputation of the foot between the metatarsus and tarsus.

racket a., one in which there is a single longitudinal incision continuous below with a spiral incision on either side of the limb.

spontaneous a., loss of a part without surgical intervention.

Syme's a., disarticulation of the foot with removal of both malleoli.

Trippier's a., amputation of the foot through the calcaneus.

Amsustain (am'sus-tān) trademark for a preparation of dextroamphetamine; an adrenergic, central nervous system stimulant.

amusia (a-mu'ze-ah) loss of ability to produce (motor amusia) or to recognize (sensory amusia) musical sounds.

A.M.W.A. American Medical Writers' Association.

amydricaine (ah-mi'dri-kān) a compound used as a surface or spinal anesthetic agent.

amyelia (a"mi-e'le-ah) absence of the spinal cord in a fetal monster.

amyelineuria (ah-mi"ĕ-lin-u're-ah) defective function of the spine.

amyelinic (ah-mi"ĕ-lin'ik) without myelin.

amyelonic (ah-mi"ĕ-lon'ik) 1. having no spinal cord. 2. having no marrow.

amyelus (ah-mi'ĕ-lus) a fetal monster with no spinal cord.

amygdala (ah-mig'dah-lah) 1. a tonsil. 2. a lobule of the cerebellum. 3. almond.

amygdalin (ah-mig'dah-lin) a glycoside from bitter almonds.

amygdaline (ah-mig'dah-lin) 1. like an almond. 2. pertaining to tonsils.

amygdalolith (ah-mig'dah-lo-lith") a calculus in a tonsil.

amyl nitrite (am'il ni'trīt) a vasodilator often used in the treatment of ANGINA PECTORIS because of its quick relief of the pain. Presumably it relaxes the smooth muscles of the coronary arteries, bringing about dilation of these blood vessels. The drug is dispensed in pearls that are crushed and inhaled. It acts very quickly and its effects are brief. The blood pressure is lowered by amyl nitrite, and the patient should be sitting when inhaling its vapors. Irregular pulse, headache and dizziness may occur. If these symptoms prove troublesome, the physician should be notified.

amyl(o)- (am'ĭ-lo) word element [Gr.], *starch.*

amylaceous (am"ĭ-la'shus) composed of or resembling starch.

amylase (am'ĭ-lās) an enzyme that catalyzes the hydrolysis of starch into simpler compounds.

amylene (am'ĭ-lēn) a poisonous hydrocarbon; a dangerous anesthetic.

a. hydrate, clear, colorless liquid used as a vehicle in pharmacy.

amylobarbitone (am"ĭ-lo-bar'bĭ-tōn) amobarbital.

amylogenesis (am"ĭ-lo-jen'ĕ-sis) the formation of starch. adj., **amylogen'ic.**

amyloid (am'ĭ-loid) 1. starchlike; amylaceous. 2. an optically homogeneous, waxy, translucent glycoprotein that is deposited intercellularly in a variety of conditions.

amyloidosis (am"ĭ-loi-do'sis) the deposition in various tissues of amyloid. This glycoprotein is almost insoluble and once it infiltrates the tissues they become waxy and nonfunctioning. Primary amyloidosis is thought to be due to some obscure metabolic disturbance in which there is an abnormal protein in the plasma; the tissues most often affected are cardiac and smooth and skeletal muscle tissue. Secondary amyloidosis is related to chronic suppuration, especially those types associated with tuberculosis, lung abscess, osteomyelitis or bronchiectasis; the most common sites of deposition are the spleen, kidney, liver and adrenal cortex.

The symptoms of amyloidosis appear insidiously and progress slowly. They depend on the specific organ affected, and frequently in secondary amyloidosis they are overshadowed by symptoms of the disease causing the disorder. Primary systemic amyloidosis is treated symptomatically; there is no cure, and death usually occurs within 3 years of the onset. Heart failure is the most common cause of death. Secondary amyloidosis is best treated by eliminating the underlying cause. This includes control of suppuration by effective use of antibiotic drugs. There has been a reduction in incidence of secondary amyloidosis in recent years because of the development of drugs that are successful in controlling infection and suppuration.

amylolysis (am"ĭ-lol'ĭ-sis) digestive change of starch into sugar. adj., **amyloly'tic.**

amylopectinosis (am″ĭ-lo-pek′tĭ-no′sis) a form of hepatic glycogen disease resulting from deficiency of glycogen brancher enzyme and associated with a form of cirrhosis of the liver.

amylopsin (am″ĭ-lop′sin) a pancreatic enzyme that converts starch to maltose.

amylorrhea (am″ĭ-lo-re′ah) the presence of an abnormal amount of starch in the stools.

amylose (am′ĭ-lōs) any carbohydrate other than a glucose or saccharose.

amylosis (am′ĭ-lo′sis) amyloidosis.

amylum (am′ĭ-lum) [L.] starch.

amyocardia (ah-mi″o-kar′de-ah) weakness of the heart muscle.

amyoplasia (ah-mi″o-pla′ze-ah) lack of muscle formation or development.
  a. congen′ita, generalized lack in the newborn of muscular development and growth, with contracture and deformity at most joints.

amyostasia (ah-mi″o-sta′ze-ah) nervous tremor of the muscles.

amyosthenia (ah-mi″os-the′ne-ah) failure of muscular strength.

amyosthenic (ah-mi″os-then′ik) 1. characterized by amyosthenia. 2. an agent that diminishes muscular power.

amyotonia (ah-mi″o-to′ne-ah) atonic condition of the muscles.
  a. congen′ita, a rare congenital disease of children marked by general hypotonia of the muscles (Oppenheim's disease).

amyotrophia (ah-mi″o-tro′fe-ah) amyotrophy.

amyotrophic lateral sclerosis (ah-mi″o-trof′ik lat′er-al sklĕ-ro′sis) a type of motor disorder of the nervous system in which there is destruction of the anterior horn cells and pyramidal tract. The cause is unknown. Early symptoms include weakness of the hands and arms, difficulty in swallowing and talking and weakness and spasticity of the legs. As the disorder progresses there is increased spasticity and atrophy of the muscles, with loss of motor control and overactivity of the reflexes. There is no known specific or effective treatment. Although there may be periods of remission, the disease usually progresses rapidly, death ensuing in 2 to 5 years in most cases.

amyotrophy (ah″mi-ot′ro-fe) a painful condition with wasting and weakness of muscle, commonly involving the deltoid muscle.

Amytal (am′ĭ-tal) trademark for amobarbital, a short-acting hypnotic and sedative.

amyxia (ah-mik′se-ah) absence of mucus.

amyxorrhea (ah-mik″so-re′ah) absence of mucous secretion.

An chemical symbol, *actinon.*

An. anisometropia, anode.

A.N.A. American Nurses' Association.

ana (an′ah) [Gr.] of each, used in prescription writing; abbreviated a̅a̅.

ana- (an′ah) word element [Gr.], *upward; again; backward; excessively.*

anabasis (ah-nab′ah-sis) the stage of increase in a disease.

anabiosis (an″ah-bi-o′sis) restoration of life processes after their apparent cessation.

anabolism (ah-nab′o-lizm) the constructive phase of metabolism, in which the body cells synthesize protoplasm for growth and repair. adj., **anabol′ic.** The manner in which this synthesis takes place is directed by the genetic code carried by the molecules of deoxyribonucleic acid (DNA). The "building blocks" for this synthesis of protoplasm are obtained from amino acids and other nutritive elements in the diet.

anacatharsis (an″ah-kah-thar′sis) violent and continued vomiting.

anachlorhydria (an″ah-klōr-hi′dre-ah) diminished hydrochloric acid in the gastric juice.

anachoresis (an″ah-ko-re′sis) preferential collection or deposit of particles at a site, as of bacteria or metals that have localized out of the bloodstream in areas of inflammation.

anachronobiology (an″ah-kron″o-bi-ol′o-je) the study of the constructive effects (growth, development, maturation) of time on a living organism.

anacidity (an″ah-sid′ĭ-te) abnormal lack or deficiency of acid.
  gastric a., achlorhydria.

anaclisis (an″ah-kli′sis) the process of a sexual drive becoming attached to and exploiting nonessential self-preservative trends such as eating and defecation.

anaclitic (an″ah-klit′ik) dependent upon another; characterized by libido depending on another instinct, such as hunger.

anacousia (an″ah-koo′ze-ah) anakusis.

anacroasia (an″ah-kro-a′ze-ah) inability to understand language, due to cerebral disease.

anacrotism (ah-nak′rŏ-tizm) the occurrence of one or more indentations on the ascending limb of the sphygmogram. adj., **anacrot′ic.**

anaculture (an′ah-kul″tūr) a bacterial whole culture treated with formalin and incubated; used for prophylactic vaccination.

anadenia (an″ah-de′ne-ah) defect of glandular action.

anadicrotism (an″ah-dik′ro-tizm) the occurrence of two indentations on the ascending limb of the sphygmogram. adj., **anadicrot′ic.**

anadipsia (an″ah-dip′se-ah) intense thirst.

anadrenalism (an″ah-dre′nal-izm) absence or failure of adrenal function.

anaerobe (an-a′er-ōb) an organism that lives and grows in the absence of molecular oxygen. adj., **anaero′bic.**
  facultative a., an organism that can live without molecular oxygen, but does not require its absence.

obligate a., an organism that cannot live in the presence of molecular oxygen.

anaerobiosis (an-a″er-o-bi-o′sis) life without free oxygen.

anaerogenic (an-a″er-o-jen′ik) suppressing the formation of gas by gas-producing bacteria.

anaerophyte (an-a′er-o-fīt″) a vegetable anaerobic microorganism.

anaerosis (an″a-er-o′sis) interruption of the respiratory function.

anagenesis (an″ah-jen′ĕ-sis) regeneration of tissue.

anakatadidymus (an″ah-kat″ah-did′ĭ-mus) a twin fetal monster, separate above and below, but united in the trunk.

anakusis (an″ah-ku′sis) deafness due to a nervous or central lesion.

anal (a′nal) relating to the anus.

analbuminemia (an″al-bu″mĭ-ne′me-ah) deficiency of serum albumins in the blood.

analeptic (an″ah-lep′tik) 1. a drug that acts as a stimulant to the central nervous system, such as caffeine and amphetamine. 2. a restorative medicine.

Analexin (an″ah-lek′sin) trademark for preparations of phenyramidol, an analgesic.

analgesia (an″al-je′ze-ah) 1. absence of sensibility to pain. 2. reduction or abolition of the response to painful stimuli.

 continuous caudal a., continuous injection of an anesthetic solution into the sacral canal to relieve the pain of childbirth (see also CAUDAL ANESTHESIA).

 infiltration a., paralysis of the nerve endings at the site of operation by subcutaneous injection of an anesthetic.

 surface a., local analgesia produced by an anesthetic applied to the surface of such mucous membranes as those of the eye, nose, throat, larynx and urethra.

analgesic (an″al-je′sik) 1. relieving pain. 2. pertaining to analgesia. 3. a drug that relieves pain.

analgia (an-al′je-ah) painlessness. adj., **anal′gic.**

analogous (ah-nal′o-gus) 1. serving a similar function, but not arising from common rudiments and not similar in basic plan and development. 2. having similar properties.

analogue (an′ah-log) 1. a part resembling another in function, but not in structure. 2. one of two or more chemical compounds having similar properties, but different atomic structure.

analogy (ah-nal′o-je) 1. resemblance in function between organs of different origin. 2. similarity in properties of two or more chemical compounds.

analysand (ah-nal′ĭ-sand) a person undergoing psychoanalysis.

analysis (ah-nal′ĭ-sis) 1. separation into component parts. 2. psychoanalysis.

 chromosome a., determination of the number and types of chromosomes in a cell.

 qualitative a., determination of the nature of the constituents of a compound.

 quantitative a., determination of the proportionate quantities of the constituents of a compound.

 vector a., analysis of a moving force to determine both its magnitude and its direction, e.g., analysis of the scalar electrocardiogram to determine the magnitude and direction of the electromotive force for one complete cycle of the heart.

anamnesis (an″am-ne′sis) the past history of a patient.

anamnestic (an″am-nes′tik) 1. pertaining to anamnesis. 2. aiding the memory.

anamniotic (an″am-ne-ot′ik) having no amnion.

ananabolic (an″an-ah-bol′ik) characterized by absence of anabolism.

anangioplasia (an-an″je-o-pla′ze-ah) imperfect formation of blood vessels in a part.

anapeiratic (an″ah-pi-rat′ik) due to excessive use or overexercise.

anaphase (an′ah-fāz) the third stage of division of the nucleus of a cell in either meiosis or mitosis.

anaphia (an-a′fe-ah) lack or loss of the sense of touch.

anaphoresis (an″ah-fo-re′sis) diminished activity of the sweat glands.

anaphoria (an″ah-fo′re-ah) the tendency to tilt the head downward, with visual axes deviating upward, on looking straight ahead.

anaphrodisia (an″af-ro-diz′e-ah) absence or loss of sexual desire.

anaphrodisiac (an″af-ro-diz′e-ak) 1. repressing sexual desire. 2. a drug that represses sexual desire.

anaphylactic shock (an″ah-fi-lak′tik) a serious and profound state of shock brought about by hypersensitivity (anaphylaxis) to an ALLERGEN, such as a drug, foreign protein or toxin. Insect bites and stings in hypersensitive persons may produce anaphylactic shock. Early symptoms are typical of an allergic reaction, e.g., sneezing, edema or itching at the site of injection or sting. The symptoms increase in severity very rapidly and progress to dyspnea, cyanosis and shock. The blood pressure drops rapidly, the pulse becomes weak and thready, and convulsions and loss of consciousness may occur. Severe anaphylactic shock can be fatal if immediate emergency measures are not taken.

PREVENTION AND TREATMENT. Prevention of anaphylactic shock requires a thorough knowledge of the person's history and various allergies. If there is a history of allergy, a sensitivity test should be done before he receives injections of animal serum or other proteins or drugs. Any person who has been given an injection of animal serum or an antigen should be watched closely for 30 minutes after the injection. If early symptoms of a reaction occur, a physician should be notified immediately.

 The drug most often used to counteract the effects of anaphylactic shock is epinephrine. Further treatment is aimed at combating shock and relieving dyspnea. In some cases tracheostomy may be necessary.

NURSING CARE. Because of the serious nature of anaphylactic shock, alertness to this possibility is required in the administration of drugs and foreign proteins. Immunizing agents are particularly dangerous to hypersensitive persons. If a patient says he has a history of an allergy the medication should be withheld until the physician is notified.

Nursing measures that may be taken to combat shock once the reaction takes place include placing the patient in Trendelenburg position and maintaining body heat. An emergency tray containing needle, syringe and epinephrine should be kept on hand, and a tracheostomy set should be readily available.

anaphylactogen (an″ah-fi-lak′to-jen) a substance that produces anaphylaxis.

anaphylactogenesis (an″ah-fi-lak″to-jen′ĕ-sis) the production of anaphylaxis.

anaphylatoxin (an″ah-fi″lah-tok′sin) the poisonous substance in anaphylaxis.

anaphylatoxis (an″ah-fi″lah-tok′sis) the reaction produced by an anaphylatoxin.

anaphylaxis (an″ah-fi-lak′sis) an unusual or exaggerated reaction of the organism to foreign protein or other substances.
  acquired a., that in which sensitization is known to have been produced by administration of a foreign protein.
  active a., that produced by injection of a foreign protein.
  antiserum a., passive anaphylaxis.
  heterologous a., passive anaphylaxis induced by transfer of serum from an animal of a different species.
  homologous a., passive anaphylaxis induced by transfer of serum from an animal of the same species.
  indirect a., that induced by an animal's own protein modified in some way.
  passive a., that resulting in a normal person from injection of serum of a sensitized person.
  psychic a., liability to development of neurotic symptoms as result of early psychic trauma.
  reverse a., that following injection of antigen, succeeded by injection of antiserum.

anaplasia (an″ah-pla′ze-ah) an irreversible alteration in adult cells toward more primitive (embryonic) cell types.

anaplastic (an″ah-plas′tik) 1. restoring a lost or absent part. 2. characterized by anaplasia or reversed development.

anaplasty (an′ah-plas″te) plastic or restorative surgery.

anapnograph (an-ap′no-graf) a device for registering the speed and pressure of the respired air current.

anapophysis (an″ah-pof′ĭ-sis) an accessory vertebral process.

anaptic (an-ap′tik) pertaining to or characterized by loss of the sense of touch.

anarithmia (an″ah-rith′me-ah) inability to count, due to a lesion of the brain.

anarthria (an-ar′thre-ah) lack of the faculty of speech because of impairment of speech organs and their innervation.
  a. litera′lis, stuttering.

anasarca (an″ah-sar′kah) accumulation of great amounts of fluid in all the body tissues.

anastalsis (an″ah-stal′sis) 1. an upward-moving wave of contraction without a preceding wave of inhibition, occurring in the alimentary canal in addition to the peristaltic wave. 2. styptic action.

anastaltic (an″ah-stal′tik) styptic; highly astringent.

anastole (ah-nas′to-le) retraction, as of the lips of a wound.

anastomosis (ah-nas″to-mo′sis) 1. communication between two tubular organs. 2. surgical or pathologic formation of a connection between two normally distinct structures. adj., **anastomot′ic**.
  arteriovenous a., anastomosis between an artery and a vein.
  crucial a., an arterial anastomosis in the upper part of the thigh.
  heterocladic a., one between branches of different arteries.
  intestinal a., establishment of a communication between two formerly distant portions of the intestine.

anat. anatomy.

anatomic, anatomical (an″ah-tom′ik), (an″ah-tom′ĭ-kal) pertaining to anatomy, or to the structure of the body.

anatomist (ah-nat′o-mist) one skilled in anatomy.

anatomy (ah-nat′o-me) the science dealing with the form and structure of living organisms.
  comparative a., description and comparison of the form and structure of different animals.
  developmental a., embryology.
  gross a., macroscopic a., that dealing with structures visible with the unaided eye.
  microscopic a., histology.
  morbid a., pathologic a., anatomy of diseased tissues.
  radiologic a., x-ray anatomy.
  special a., anatomy devoted to study of a single type or species of organism.
  topographic a., that devoted to determination of relative positions of various body parts.
  x-ray a., study of organs and tissues based on their visualization by x-rays in both living and dead bodies.

anatoxin (an″ah-tok′sin) toxoid.

anatricrotism (an″ah-trik′ro-tizm) the occurrence of three indentations on the ascending limb of the sphygmogram. adj., **anatricrot′ic**.

anatriptic (an″ah-trip′tik) a medicine applied by rubbing.

anatropia (an″ah-tro′pe-ah) upward deviation of the visual axis of one eye when the other eye is fixing.

anaxon (an-ak′son) a nerve cell devoid of an axon.

anazoturia (an-az″o-tu′re-ah) decreased urea in the urine.

anchorage (ang′kŏ-rāj) surgical fixation of a displaced viscus.

anchylo- for words beginning thus, see those beginning *ankylo-*.

ancipital (an-sip'ĭ-tal) two-edged.

anconad (ang'ko-nad) toward the elbow or olecranon.

anconal (ang'ko-nal) pertaining to the elbow.

anconitis (an"ko-ni'tis) inflammation of the elbow joint.

ancylo- for words beginning thus, see also those beginning *ankylo-*.

Ancylostoma (an"sĭ-los'to-mah) a genus of nematode parasites.

A. america'num, *Necator americanus.*

A. brazilien'se, a species parasitic in dogs and cats in tropical and subtropical regions; also reported in man.

A. cani'num, the common hookworm of dogs and cats.

A. duodena'le, a common HOOKWORM, parasitic in the small intestine.

ancylostomiasis (an"sĭ-los"to-mi'ah-sis) infection by worms of the genus Ancylostoma or by other hookworms (*Necator americanus*).

Ancylostomidae (an"sĭ-lo-sto'mĭ-de) a family of nematode parasites having two ventrolateral cutting plates at the entrance to a large buccal capsule, and small teeth at its base; the hookworms.

andr(o)- (an'dro) word element [Gr.], *male; masculine.*

andriatrics (an"dre-at'riks) the branch of medicine dealing with diseases of men.

andrin (an'drin) any one of the androgens of the testes.

androgen (an'dro-jen) any substance that stimulates male characteristics. The two main androgens are androsterone and testosterone. adj., **androgen'ic.**

The androgenic hormones are internal endocrine secretions circulating in the bloodstream and manufactured mainly by the testes under stimulation from the PITUITARY GLAND. To a lesser extent, androgens are produced by the adrenal glands in both sexes, as well as by the ovaries in women. Thus women normally have a small percentage of male hormones, in the same way that men's bodies contain some female sex hormones, the estrogens.

The androgens are responsible for the secondary sex characteristics, such as the beard and the deepening of the voice at puberty. They also stimulate the growth of muscle and bones throughout the body and thus account in part for the greater strength and size of men as compared to women.

android (an'droid) resembling a man.

andrology (an-drol'o-je) the science of man or human nature.

andromerogon (an"dro-mer'o-gon) an organism produced by andromerogony and containing only the paternal set of chromosomes.

andromerogony (an"dro-mer-og'o-ne) development of a portion of a fertilized ovum containing the male pronucleus only.

androphobia (an"dro-fo'be-ah) morbid dread of the male sex.

androphonomania (an"dro-fo"no-ma'ne-ah) a morbid impulse to homicide.

androstane (an'dro-stān) the hydrocarbon nucleus, $C_{19}H_{32}$, from which androgens are derived.

androstanediol (an"dro-stān'de-ol) an androgen, $C_{19}H_{32}O_2$, prepared by reducing androsterone.

androstene (an'dro-stēn) an unsaturated cyclic hydrocarbon, $C_{19}H_{30}$, forming the nucleus of testosterone and certain other androgens.

androstenediol (an"dro-stēn'de-ol) a crystalline androgenic steroid, $C_{19}H_{30}O_2$.

androsterone (an-dros'tĕ-rōn) an androgenic hormone, $C_{19}H_{30}O_2$, occurring in urine or prepared synthetically.

Anectine (an-ek'tin) trademark for preparations of succinylcholine, a skeletal muscle relaxant.

anemia (ah-ne'me-ah) a deficiency in the blood, either in quality or in quantity. There are numerous forms of anemia. Usually the term refers to a decrease in the number of erythrocytes (red blood cells) or a reduction in hemoglobin.

Anemia is not a disease; it is a symptom of a number of different diseases or disorders. It may be caused by poor diet, loss of blood, industrial poisons, diseases of the bone marrow or any of several other conditions. Careful diagnosis is very important, since treatment varies according to the cause of the anemia.

SYMPTOMS. Mild degrees of anemia often cause only slight and vague symptoms, perhaps nothing more than a lack of energy. The anemic person may also become fatigued more often and more easily. In more severe cases of anemia, exertion causes actual shortness of breath. This may be accompanied by pounding of the heart and a rapid pulse and heart action. These symptoms are caused by the inability of anemic blood to supply the body tissues with enough oxygen.

Pallor, particularly in the palms of the hands, the fingernails and the conjunctiva (the lining of the eyelids), may also indicate anemia. In very advanced cases, swelling of the ankles and other evidence of heart failure may appear.

DIAGNOSIS. Anemia is diagnosed by means of blood tests. A sample of the patient's blood is examined under a microscope, and the number, size, color and shape of the erythrocytes are determined; the amount of hemoglobin in the sample is also measured. If these studies of the blood indicate signs of anemia, other tests, such as STERNAL PUNCTURE or other bone marrow examination, may be necessary.

A thorough physical examination is also done to evaluate the person's state of general health and to rule out possible sources of blood loss.

COMMON CAUSES OF ANEMIA

Loss of Blood. If there is massive bleeding from a wound or other lesion, the body may lose enough blood to cause severe anemia. This acute anemia is often accompanied by shock. Immediate transfusions are generally required to replace the lost blood. Chronic blood loss, such as excessive menstrual flow or slow loss of blood from an ulcer or cancer of the stomach or intestines, may also lead to anemia.

These anemias disappear when the cause has been found and corrected. To help the blood rebuild itself, the physician may prescribe medicines containing iron, which is necessary to build hemoglobin, and foods with high iron content, such as kidney and navy beans, liver, spinach and whole-wheat bread.

Diet Deficiency.   Anemia may develop if the diet does not provide enough iron, protein, vitamin B_{12} and other vitamins and minerals needed in the production of hemoglobin and the formation of erythrocytes. The combination of poor diet and chronic loss of blood makes for particular susceptibility to severe anemia. For example, a child suffering from hookworm, living on an inadequate diet, is doubly likely to suffer from anemia.

A good basic diet is the best way to combat diet-deficiency anemia (see also NUTRITION). So-called "blood tonics" containing iron or other vitamins or minerals are not necessary unless the physician prescribes them.

NURSING CARE.   Rest is one of the first considerations in the care of the patient with anemia. Mild exercise is usually desirable but overexertion places an added and unnecessary strain on the heart and lungs.

Observation for signs of blood loss through the intestinal tract or urinary tract may assist the physician in his diagnosis of the cause of anemia. Tarry stools or hazy brown urine should be recognized as evidence of internal bleeding and should be reported.

Combating a lack of appetite and disinterest in food may be a nursing problem in patients with anemia. Fatigue, weakness or soreness of the mouth must be considered as contributing factors. The patient may need to overcome poor eating habits developed through ignorance or indifference to the nutritional values of food.

Special mouth care is required when mouth and gums are tender and bleed easily. Brushing of the teeth is usually too traumatic and frequent cleansing of the mouth with cotton-tipped applicators dipped in a mild mouthwash can be substituted. The lips are kept lubricated with mineral oil or some other emollient to prevent dryness and cracking.

Extra warmth in the form of blankets and warm clothing usually must be provided because many anemia patients suffer from poor circulation and are easily chilled. The poor circulation also brings about decreased sensitivity to heat and these patients may be burned if care is not taken with hot water bottles and heating pads.

achrestic a., anemia due to inability to utilize a necessary factor present in the body.

aplastic a., anemia due to disease of the bone marrow—a tumor or cancer—or to destruction of bone marrow by certain agents, particularly chemical compounds of various sorts. Treatment consists of removal of the cause, if possible, regular transfusions and sometimes injections of cortisone. The prognosis is not good. (See also APLASTIC ANEMIA.)

Cooley's a., thalassemia.

essential a., idiopathic anemia.

hemolytic a., anemia caused by increased destruction of erythrocytes, resulting from Rh incompati-

bility (see RH FACTOR), mismatched blood transfusions, industrial poisons or hypersensitivity to certain antibiotics and tranquilizers, or secondary to some other disease. Jaundice may be a symptom, in addition to the usual symptoms of anemia. Treatment includes blood transfusions and sometimes splenectomy. (See also HEMOLYTIC ANEMIA.)

hypochromic a., anemia in which the decrease in hemoglobin is proportionally much greater than the decrease in number of erythrocytes.

hypoplastic a., anemia due to incapacity of blood-forming organs.

idiopathic a., that due to disease of the blood or the blood-producing organs.

a. lymphat'ica. Hodgkin's disease.

macrocytic a., anemia in which the erythrocytes are much larger than normal.

Mediterranean a., thalassemia.

megaloblastic a., anemia characterized by the presence of megaloblasts in the bone marrow.

microcytic a., anemia characterized by decrease in size of the erythrocytes.

myelopathic a., myelophthisic a., anemia due to destruction or crowding out of hematopoietic tissues by space-occupying lesions.

normocytic a., anemia characterized by proportionate decrease in hemoglobin, packed red cell volume, and number of erythrocytes per cubic millimeter of blood.

pernicious a., a serious anemia that results from lack of secretion by the gastric mucous membrane of a factor (intrinsic factor) essential to formation of erythrocytes and absorption of vitamin B_{12}. This deficiency may be secondary to an illness or idiopathic, that is, from unknown causes. Treatment consists of regular administration, usually by injection, of vitamin B_{12}, which must be continued for life. (See also PERNICIOUS ANEMIA.)

primary a., that due to disease of the blood-forming organs.

secondary a., that due to some cause other than disease of the blood-forming organs.

sickle cell a., a genetically determined defect of hemoglobin synthesis associated with poor physical development and skeletal anomalies, occurring usually in Negroes. (See also SICKLE CELL ANEMIA.)

anemic (ah-ne'mik) pertaining to anemia.

anemophobia (an"ĕ-mo-fo'be-ah) morbid fear of wind or draughts.

anencephalohemia (an"en-sef"ah-lo-he'me-ah) insufficient supply of blood to the brain.

anencephaly (an"en-sef'ah-le) a developmental anomaly with absence of neural tissue in the cranium.

anenzymia (an"en-zi'me-ah) absence of an enzyme normally present in the body.

a. catala'sea, congenital absence of the enzyme catalase.

anephrogenesis (a"nef-ro-jen'ĕ-sis) failure of embryonic development of kidney tissue.

anepia (an-e'pe-ah) inability to speak.

anergasia (an"er-ga'se-ah) a behavioral disorder due to organic lesions of the central nervous system.

anergy (an'er-je) a total loss of reactivity. adj., **aner'gic.**

anerythropsia (an″er-ĭ-throp′se-ah) inability to distinguish red colors.

anesthecinesia (an-es″the-sĭ-ne′ze-ah) combined sensory and motor paralysis.

anesthesia (an″es-the′ze-ah) loss of feeling or sensation. Artificial anesthesia may be produced by a number of agents capable of bringing about partial or complete loss of sensation (see also ANESTHETIC).

NURSING CARE. The patient recovering from general anesthesia must be watched constantly until he has reacted. The vital signs and blood pressure are checked regularly; any sudden change is reported immediately. The patient must be observed to see that the airway is clear at all times. If vomiting occurs, the head is turned to the side to prevent aspiration of vomitus into the respiratory tract.

In addition to the physical effects of general anesthesia, the emotional and psychologic aspects must also be considered. Fear of being "put to sleep" or rendered unconscious is common among patients. During recovery from anesthesia noise should be kept at a minimum, as all sounds may be exaggerated to the patient. It is important to remember that conversations held within hearing of the patient may be misunderstood by him since he is not capable of interpreting words and phrases clearly as long as he is under the effects of the anesthetic. When the patient is awakening from general anesthetia he may be extremely restless, attempting to get out of bed or even striking out at those around him because he is afraid and disoriented.

Patients who have had local anesthesia of the throat for diagnostic procedures or minor surgery should not be given food or liquids until the effects of the anesthesia have worn off and the gag reflex has returned. Otherwise these substances may be aspirated into the respiratory tract.

Some local anesthetics produce violent allergic reactions or anaphylactic shock in certain hypersensitive persons; for this reason, skin tests are done before these drugs are administered. An emergency tray containing hypodermic needles, syringes and ampules of a stimulant such as epinephrine should be on hand whenever a local anesthetic is to be used.

basal a., narcosis produced by preliminary medication so that the inhalation of anesthetic necessary to produce surgical anesthesia is greatly reduced.

block a., that produced by blocking transmission of impulses through a nerve.

caudal a., injection of an anesthetic into the sacral canal to relieve the pain of childbirth (see also CAUDAL ANESTHESIA).

central a., lack of sensation caused by disease of the nerve centers.

closed a., that produced by continuous rebreathing of a small amount of anesthetic gas in a closed system with an apparatus for removing carbon dioxide.

crossed a., loss of sensation on one side of the face and loss of pain and temperature sense on the opposite side of the body.

dissociated a., dissociation a., loss of perception of certain stimuli while that of others remains intact.

electric a., anesthesia induced by passage of an electric current.

endotracheal a., anesthesia produced by introduction of a gaseous mixture through a tube inserted into the trachea.

frost a., abolition of feeling or sensation as a re-

sult of topical refrigeration produced by a jet of a highly volatile liquid.

general a., a state of unconsciousness and insusceptibility to pain, produced by an anesthetic agent.

infiltration a., local anesthesia produced by injection of the anesthetic solution directly into the tissues.

inhalation a., anesthesia produced by the respiration of a volatile liquid or gaseous anesthetic agent.

insufflation a., anesthesia produced by introduction of a gaseous mixture into the trachea through a slender tube.

local a., that confined to a limited area.

mixed a., that produced by use of more than one anesthetic agent.

open a., general inhalation anesthesia in which there is no rebreathing of the expired gases.

peripheral a., lack of sensation due to changes in the peripheral nerves.

rectal a., anesthesia produced by introduction of the anesthetic agent into the rectum.

refrigeration a., local anesthesia produced by chilling the part to near freezing temperature.

regional a., insensibility caused by interrupting the sensory nerve conductivity of any region of the body; it may be produced by (1) field block, encircling the operative field by means of injections of a local anesthetic; or (2) nerve block, making injections in close proximity to the nerves supplying the area.

segmental a., loss of sensation in a segment of the body due to a lesion of a single nerve root.

spinal a., 1. anesthesia due to a spinal lesion. 2. anesthesia produced by injection of the agent beneath the membrane of the spinal cord.

splanchnic a., block anesthesia for visceral operation by injection of the anesthetic agent into the region of the celiac ganglia.

surgical a., that degree of anesthesia at which operation may safely be performed.

tactile a., loss of the sense of touch.

topical a., that produced by application of a local anesthetic directly to the area involved.

twilight a., twilight sleep.

anesthesimeter (an″es-thĕ-sim′ĕ-ter) 1. an instrument for testing the degree of anesthesia. 2. a device for regulating the amount of anesthetic given.

Anesthesin (ah-nes′the-sin) trademark for a preparation of ethyl aminobenzoate, a topical anesthetic.

anesthesiologist (an″es-the″ze-ol′o-jist) a specialist in anesthesiology.

anesthesiology (an″es-the″ze-ol′o-je) that branch of medicine concerned with administration of anesthetics and the condition of the patient while under anesthesia.

anesthesiophore (an″es-the′ze-o-fōr″) the group of atoms in a molecule which produces the anesthetic action.

anesthetic (an″es-thet′ik) 1. lacking feeling or sensation. 2. an agent that produces anesthesia. There are two types of anesthetics: general anesthetics, which produce a sound sleep; and regional anesthetics, which render a specific area insensible to pain.

GENERAL ANESTHETICS. The inhalant types are the most widely used general anesthetics. Ether, one of the best known, is administered by means of a face mask in amounts controlled by the anesthetist.

Chloroform is now little used principally because it may damage the liver. Nitrous oxide, so-called laughing gas, is used for short surgical procedures, or, in the case of long operations, before the patient is given ether. Nitrous oxide is also used by dentists for extractions, especially when the patient is allergic to or has a distaste for a local anesthetic such as procaine.

Cyclopropane and halothane are more recently discovered inhalants, as is ethylene, a gas that produces a light sleep resembling that caused by nitrous oxide.

Intravenous anesthetics are also used for light general anesthesia or in advance of an inhalant anesthetic. The best known of these is a barbiturate, thiopental sodium (Pentothal sodium).

Some anesthetics are administered rectally, for example, paraldehyde, which is often prescribed for alcoholics, psychotics and extremely apprehensive patients. Given in the form of a light enema, the substance is absorbed into the system and takes effect rapidly.

REGIONAL ANESTHETICS. Regional anesthetics are administered by injection or by topical application to the skin or mucous membranes. Spinal anesthetics are injected into the subarachnoid space of the spinal canal. For short procedures, procaine is the anesthetic of choice; for longer ones, tetracaine or dibucaine is used. This type of regional anesthesia may be used for operations on the lower part of the body.

A variant of spinal anesthesia is caudal anesthesia, which is used in childbirth. The anesthetic, usually procaine, is dripped in through a needle inserted into the spinal canal at the sacrum. In continuous caudal anesthesia, the needle is left in place throughout the delivery while the anesthetic drips in gradually. (See also CAUDAL ANESTHESIA.)

Various local anesthetics are used for operations on the skin or the tissues immediately beneath, and in dentistry for many tooth fillings and most extractions. Cocaine was once popular for this type of minor surgery, but today it has been replaced by derivatives such as procaine. After injection, the sensory nerves in the area become insensitive and may remain so for several hours.

In some parts of the body where a main nerve is accessible, the anesthetic is injected directly into or adjacent to that nerve, in this way desensitizing all the adjacent tissue. This is called nerve block or block anesthesia, and is often used in dental surgery on the lower jaw.

Certain anesthetics have enough penetrating power to relieve pain when they are applied directly to a body surface, a technique known as topical (or surface) anesthesia. One such anesthetic, butacaine sulfate, is often applied to the surface of the eye before eye operations. Tetracaine is also used on the eye, as well as on membranes of the nose and throat. Some surface anesthetics, such as benzocaine, can be safely applied directly on wounds and ulcers for the relief of pain.

OTHER TECHNIQUES. The search continues for other anesthetics that will be safe, agreeable, quick and effective. In some cases hypnosis has been used successfully without the necessity of any anesthetic substance whatsoever. There have also been experiments with electric anesthesia.

Another technique is cooling of the body, either wholly or in part. In hypothermia, the temperature of the entire body is lowered. The patient is first anesthetized by a general anesthetic and is then placed for about an hour in an ice blanket, through which cold alcohol circulates. At the resulting low temperature, the heart action and other body functions are slowed to a very low rate. Although this has an anesthetic effect, the real purpose is to permit heart and blood vessel operations with greater general safety, and particularly with less danger of hemorrhage.

Similar means are used to lower the temperature of specific parts of the body, such as the foot in cases of amputation. A tourniquet is employed to reduce the circulation, and then cold is applied by ice packs or an electrical unit until the operative area is desensitized. This type of local anesthetic is called refrigeration anesthesia and although the idea is not entirely new, it is now being used in new ways.

anesthetist (ah-nes′thĕ-tist) one who administers anesthetics.

anesthetization (ah-nes″thĕ-tĭ-za′shun) production of anesthesia.

anethole (an′e-thōl) a colorless or faintly yellow liquid used as a flavoring agent for drugs and to expel secretions from the air passages and to stimulate intestinal peristalsis.

aneuploidy (an″u-ploi′de) the state of having chromosomes in a number that is not an exact multiple of the haploid number.

aneuria (ah-nu′re-ah) deficiency of nervous energy.

aneurin (ah-nu′rin) thiamine (vitamin B$_1$).

aneurysm (an′u-rizm) a sac formed by dilatation of the walls of a blood vessel, usually an artery, and filled with blood. adj., **aneurys′mal**. There are two types of aneurysms: true aneurysm, in which the wall of the sac consists of one or more of the layers that make up the wall of the blood vessel, and false aneurysm, in which all the layers of the vessel are ruptured and the blood is retained by surrounding tissues.

Aneurysms occur when the blood vessel wall becomes weakened, by either a physical injury to the vessel, a congenital defect or a disease. They may occur in any vein or artery, but they most commonly are located in the abdomen or chest. Certain infections may attack and weaken the tissues of the blood vessels; however, atherosclerosis is a common cause. A less common cause is syphilis. A person may have a small aneurysm for years without being aware of it; such aneurysms are often identified only accidentally, on x-ray examination for another purpose. An aneurysm may form a pulsating tumor which can be painful to the sufferer, especially if it is large enough to press against some other organ in the body.

Aneurysms tend to increase in size, and there is a risk of rupture. If rupture occurs in the heart or brain or any other vital organ of the body, the results can be very serious.

Great advances are being made in surgical methods of repairing aneurysms. If an aneurysm occurs in a small blood vessel, the vessel can be tied off and the flow of blood transferred to another vessel. There is also a more complex operation which involves removing the segment of widened blood vessel and replacing it with a plastic graft or an artery or vein from a vascular bank. This is a serious operation, but more physicians are recommending it when there is a danger that the aneurysm may rupture or may produce dangerous effects from blood clots.

arteriovenous a., simultaneous rupture of an artery and vein, the blood being retained in the surrounding tissue.

berry a., a small outpouching of the inner lining of a blood vessel, usually at an angle of bifurcation of the cerebral arteries.

cirsoid a., dilatation and tortuous lengthening of part of an artery.

compound a., one in which some of the layers of the wall of the vessel are ruptured and some merely dilated.

dissecting a., one in which rupture of the inner coat has permitted blood to escape between layers of the vessel wall.

fusiform a., a spindle-shaped aneurysm.

mixed a., compound aneurysm.

racemose a., cirsoid aneurysm.

sacculated a., a saclike aneurysm.

varicose a., one formed by rupture of an aneurysm into a vein.

aneurysmectomy (an"u-riz-mek'to-me) excision of an aneurysm.

aneurysmoplasty (an"u-riz'mo-plas"te) plastic repair of an artery for aneurysm.

aneurysmorrhaphy (an"u-riz-mor'ah-fe) suture of an aneurysm.

anfractuosity (an-frak"tu-os'i-te) a cerebral sulcus.

anfractuous (an-frak'tu-us) convoluted; sinuous.

angi(o)- (an"je-o) word element [Gr.], *vessel (channel).*

angiectasis (an"je-ek'tah-sis) dilatation of a vessel.

angiectomy (an"je-ek'to-me) excision of part of a blood or lymph vessel.

angiitis (an"je-i'tis) inflammation of the coats of a vessel, chiefly blood or lymph vessels.

angina (an'ji-nah, an-ji'nah) any disease marked by spasmodic suffocative attacks, especially angina pectoris.

agranulocytic a., agranulocytosis.

a. cru'ris, intermittent lameness with cyanosis of the affected limb; due to arterial obstruction.

intestinal a., generalized cramping abdominal pain occurring shortly after a meal and persisting for one to three hours, due to ischemia of the smooth muscle of the bowel.

a. ludovi'ci, Ludwig's a., **a. lud'wigi,** purulent inflammation around the submaxillary gland.

a. parotid'ea, mumps.

a. pec'toris, acute pain in the chest caused by interference with the supply of oxygen to the heart. Most sufferers from angina pectoris can readily distinguish it from other pains in the chest, such as might be caused by indigestion or coronary thrombosis, for the pain is usually of an unmistakable nature. It is generally described as a feeling of tightness, strangling, heaviness or suffocation. The pain is usually concentrated on the left side, beginning just under the sternum; it sometimes radiates to the neck, throat and lower jaw and down the left arm, and, more rarely, to the stomach, back or across to the right side of the chest.

Angina pectoris is more common in men than in women, and in older than in younger people. It is not a disease in itself, but a symptom of underlying diseases which interfere with the supply of oxygen to the heart. Usually the direct cause is a narrowing or obstruction of the coronary arteries carrying blood to the heart muscle. The pain is precipitated by activity which puts additional strain on the heart. It is most often brought on by strenuous exercise, especially exercise taken out of doors, in cold weather or after a heavy meal. It can also be caused by emotional excitement, by digestion of a heavy meal or by any activity that subjects the heart to particular stress. Attacks sometimes occur in the night. Such attacks are known as nocturnal angina, and are thought to result from disturbing dreams.

The pain seldom lasts more than 15 minutes, often less, and is usually relieved by remaining motionless. Several medicines bring immediate relief from angina pectoris; nitroglycerin (glyceryl trinitrate) is the one most commonly prescribed, and amyl nitrite is another. These drugs should be taken only on a physician's instructions.

Angina pectoris is a warning that the heart is under special stress and needs relief before damage occurs. A person who suffers from angina pectoris should be under a physician's care. For any pain in the chest the doctor should be consulted. If angina is diagnosed, the doctor will try to discover and treat the underlying complaint, which is usually primary or secondary atherosclerosis of the coronary arteries.

Meanwhile the patient should try to protect himself from attacks by avoiding the situations in which they occur. He should take note of the conditions which most often bring on his attacks and regulate his life accordingly. He should avoid tiring himself, getting overexcited and taking unnecessarily strenuous exercise. He should, of course, keep with him at all times the medicine prescribed by his doctor for relieving any attack that should occur.

NURSING CARE. An attitude of calmness and efficiency is most important when caring for a person suffering from an attack of angina pectoris. His pain produces emotional reactions and the strongest of these is fear. Most of these patients know that their pain is resulting from an insufficient supply of oxygen to the heart and they frequently have a feeling of impending death. The nurse must secure the confidence of the patient by her willingness to stay with him during the attack and by her reassurance that the pain will eventually subside. It usually helps to raise the patient to a sitting position so that he may breathe without difficulty. The prompt administration of nitroglycerin or the specific drug ordered by the physician usually shortens the attack and relieves pain. Above all, the nurse must remember that her presence can do much to reassure the patient and help him relax, thus lessening the severity of the attack.

Vincent's a., necrotizing ulcerative gingivitis; inflammation of the gingivae and oral mucous membrane, with tenderness and bleeding of the gums, sore throat and mouth, swelling of the lymph nodes of the neck, fever, offensive breath and pain on swallowing. Called also TRENCH MOUTH.

anginoid (an'jĭ-noid) resembling angina.

anginophobia (an"jĭ-no-fo'be-ah) morbid dread of angina pectoris.

anginose (an'jĭ-nōs) characterized by angina.

angioblast (an'je-o-blast") the earliest formative tissue from which blood cells and blood vessels arise. adj., **angioblast'ic**.

angioblastoma (an"je-o-blas-to'mah) a blood vessel tumor arising from the meninges of the brain and spinal cord; called also angioblastic meningioma.

angiocardiogram (an"je-o-kar'de-o-gram") the film produced by angiocardiography.

angiocardiography (an"je-o-kar"de-og'rah-fe) roentgenography of the heart and great vessels after introduction of an opaque contrast medium into a blood vessel or one of the cardiac chambers.

angiocardiokinetic (an"je-o-kar"de-o-ki-net'ik) pertaining to movements of the heart and blood vessels.

angiocardiopathy (an"je-o-kar"de-op'ah-the) disease of the heart and blood vessels.

angiocarditis (an"je-o-kar-di'tis) inflammation of the heart and blood vessels.

angiocholecystitis (an"je-o-ko"le-sis-ti'tis) inflammation of the gallbladder and bile ducts.

angioclast (an'je-o-klast") a forceps for compressing a bleeding artery.

angiodermatitis (an"je-o-der"mah-ti'tis) inflammation of the vessels of the skin.

angio-edema (an"je-o-ĕ-de'mah) angioneurotic edema.

angioendothelioma (an"je-o-en"do-the"le-o'mah) hemangioendothelioma.

angiofibroma (an"je-o-fi-bro'mah) angioma containing fibrous tissue.

angiogenesis (an"je-o-jen'ĕ-sis) the development of blood vessels in the embryo.

angioglioma (an"je-o-gli-o'mah) a form of vascular glioma.

angiogram (an'je-o-gram") a roentgenogram of a blood vessel.

angiography (an"je-og'rah-fe) roentgenography of vessels of the body (arteriography, lymphangiography or phlebography).

angiohemophilia (an"je-o-he"mo-fil'e-ah) a congenital hemorrhagic diathesis with bleeding from the skin and mucosal surfaces, due to abnormal blood vessels with or without platelet defects or deficiencies of clotting factor VIII or IX.

angiohyalinosis (an"je-o-hi"ah-lĭ-no'sis) hyaline degeneration of the muscular coat of blood vessels.

angioid (an'je-oid) resembling blood vessels.

angioinvasive (an"je-o-in-va'siv) tending to invade the walls of blood vessels.

angiokeratoma (an"je-o-ker"ah-to'mah) angioma blended with keratoma of the skin.
    a. cor'poris diffu'sum, a condition marked by dark purple lesions on the trunk, associated with cardiovascular disease, renal abnormalities and hypertension.

angiokinetic (an"je-o-ki-net'ik) vasomotor.

angiolipoma (an"je-o-lĭ-po'mah) angioma containing fatty tissue.

angiolith (an'je-o-lith") a calcareous deposit in the wall of a blood vessel.

angiology (an"je-ol'o-je) scientific study or description of the blood and lymph vessels.

angiolupoid (an"je-o-lu'poid) a tuberculous skin lesion consisting of small, oval red plaques.

angiolymphoma (an"je-o-lim-fo'mah) a tumor made up of lymph vessels.

angiolysis (an"je-ol'ĭ-sis) retrogression or obliteration of blood vessels, as in embryologic development.

angioma (an"je-o'mah) a tumor made up of blood or lymph vessels. adj., **angiom'atous**.
    a. caverno'sum, cavernous a., an erectile tumor.
    hereditary hemorrhagic a., a condition marked by unexplained bleeding and angiomatous lesions of skin and mucous membrane.
    a. serpigino'sum, a skin disease marked by minute vascular points arranged in rings on the skin.
    telangiectatic a., an angioma made up of dilated blood vessels.

angiomalacia (an"je-o-mah-la'she-ah) softening of the walls of the vessels.

angiomatosis (an"je-o-mah-to'sis) the presence of multiple angiomas.
    hemorrhagic familial a., hereditary hemorrhagic angioma.
    a. of retina, diseased retinal blood vessels with subretinal hemorrhages.

angiomegaly (an"je-o-meg'ah-le) enlargement of blood vessels, especially a condition of the eyelid marked by great increase in its volume.

angiometer (an"je-om'ĕ-ter) an instrument for measuring the diameter and tension of blood vessels.

angiomyoma (an"je-o-mi-o'mah) angioma blended with myoma.

angiomyoneuroma (an"je-o-mi"o-nu-ro'mah) glomangioma.

angiomyosarcoma (an"je-o-mi"o-sar-ko'mah) angioma blended with myoma and sarcoma.

angioneurectomy (an"je-o-nu-rek'to-me) resection of all elements of the spermatic cord except the vas deferens with its artery and vein, for cure of enlarged prostate.

angioneuroma (an"je-o-nu-ro'mah) glomangioma.

angioneuromyoma (an"je-o-nu"ro-mi-o'mah) glomangioma.

angioneurosis (an"je-o-nu-ro'sis) any neurosis affecting primarily the blood vessels; a disorder of the vasomotor system, as angioparalysis or angiospasm.

angioneurotic (an"je-o-nu-rot'ik) caused by or of the nature of an angioneurosis.
  a. edema, a local condition characterized by the sudden and temporary appearance of large edematous areas (wheals) of the skin and mucous membranes accompanied by intense itching; called also giant hives and angio-edema. It may be an acute or chronic inflammatory reaction and is of allergic, neurotic or unknown origin. Common causes are food, drugs, insect bites, parasitic infection and emotional disturbances.

angioparalysis (an"je-o-pah-ral'ĭ-sis) vasomotor paralysis of blood vessels.

angiopathy (an"je-op'ah-the) any disease of the vessels.

angioplany (an'je-o-plan"e) abnormality in position, course or structure of a vessel.

angioplasty (an'je-o-plas"te) plastic repair of blood vessels or lymphatic channels.

angiopoiesis (an"je-o-poi-e'sis) the formation of blood vessels. adj., **angiopoiet'ic.**

angiorrhaphy (an"je-or'ah-fe) suture of a blood vessel.

angiosarcoma (an"je-o-sar-ko'mah) a malignant tumor of vascular tissue; called also hemangiosarcoma.

angiosclerosis (an"je-o-sklĕ-ro'sis) hardening of the walls of blood vessels.

angioscotoma (an"je-o-sko-to'mah) a defect in the visual field caused by the shadow of the retinal blood vessels.

angiosialitis (an"je-o-si"ah-li'tis) inflammation of a salivary gland duct.

angiospasm (an'je-o-spazm") spasmodic contraction of the walls of a blood vessel. adj., **angiospas'tic.**

angiostrongyliasis (an"je-o-stron"jĭ-li'ah-sis) infection by nematodes of the genus Angiostrongylus.

Angiostrongylus (an"je-o-stron'jĭ-lus) a genus of nematode parasites.
  a. cantonen'sis, a species reported in cases of human meningoencephalitis in Hawaii and in other areas in the Pacific and in Asia.
  a. vaso'rum, a species of worms parasitic in the pulmonary arteries of dogs.

angiotelectasis (an"je-o-tel-ek'tah-sis) dilatation of blood vessels.

angiotensin (an"je-o-ten'sin) a vasoconstrictor substance found in the blood.

angiotitis (an"je-o-ti'tis) inflammation of the vessels of the ear.

angiotome (an'je-o-tōm") one of the segments of the vascular system of the embryo.

angiotomy (an"je-ot'o-me) incision of a blood vessel or lymphatic channel.

angiotonase (an"je-o-to'nās) an enzyme formed by the kidneys that activates angiotensin.

angiotonic (an"je-o-ton'ik) increasing vascular tension.

angiotonin (an"je-o-to'nin) angiotensin.

angiotribe (an'je-o-trīb") a strong forceps for crushing tissue containing an artery, for the purpose of checking hemorrhage.

angiotripsy (an'je-o-trip"se) hemostasis by means of an angiotribe.

angiotrophic (an"je-o-trof'ik) pertaining to the nutrition of vessels.

angle (ang'gl) the space or figure formed by two diverging lines, measured as the number of degrees one would have to be moved to coincide with the other.
  acromial a., that between the head of the humerus and the clavicle.
  alpha a., that formed by intersection of the visual axis with the optic axis.
  cardiodiaphragmatic a., that formed by the junction of the shadows of the heart and diaphragm in posteroanterior roentgenograms of the heart.
  costovertebral a., the angle formed on either side of the vertebral column between the last rib and the lumbar vertebrae.
  filtration a., a. of the iris, the angle between the iris and cornea at the periphery of the anterior chamber of the eye, through which the aqueous humor readily permeates.
  a. of jaw, the junction of the lower edge with the posterior edge of the lower jaw.
  meter a., the angle formed by intersection of the visual axis and the perpendicular bisector of the line joining the centers of rotation of the two eyes when viewing a point one meter distant (small meter angle) or the angle formed by intersection of the visual axes of the two eyes in the midline at a distance of one meter (large meter angle).
  optic a., visual angle.
  a. of pubis, that between the pubic bones at the symphysis.
  sternoclavicular a., that between the sternum and the clavicle.
  visual a., the angle between two lines passing from the extremities of an object seen, through the nodal point of the eye, to the corresponding extremities of the image of the object seen.

angstrom (ang'strom) the unit of wavelength, equivalent to 0.1 millimicron (10^{-7} mm.); abbreviated Å.

angulation (ang"gu-la'shun) the formation of a sharp obstructive angle as in the intestine, the ureter or similar tubes.

angulus (ang'gu-lus), pl. **an'guli** [L.] angle; used in names of anatomic structures or landmarks.

anhedonia (an"he-do'ne-ah) inability to experience pleasure.

anhematopoiesis, anhematosis (an-hem″ah-to-poi-e′sis), (an″hem-ah-to′sis) defective blood formation.

anhemolytic (an″he-mo-lit′ik) not destructive to blood cells.

anhidrosis (an″hĭ-dro′sis) absence of sweating.

anhidrotic (an″hĭ-drot′ik) 1. checking the flow of sweat. 2. an agent that suppresses perspiration.

anhydrase (an-hi′drās) an enzyme that catalyzes the removal of water from a compound.
  carbonic a., an enzyme that catalyzes the decomposition of carbonic acid into carbon dioxide and water, facilitating transfer of carbon dioxide from tissues to blood and from blood to alveolar air.

anhydration (an″hi-dra′shun) the condition of not being hydrated.

anhydremia (an″hi-dre′me-ah) diminution of the fluid content of the blood.

anhydride (an-hi′drīd) a compound derived from an acid by removal of a molecule of water.

anhydrochloric (an″hi-dro-klōr′ik) characterized by absence of hydrochloric acid.

anhydromyelia (an″hi-dro-mi-e′le-ah) deficiency of the fluid of the spinal cord.

anhydrous (an-hi′drus) containing no water.

anideus (ah-nid′e-us) a parasitic monster fetus consisting of a shapeless mass of flesh.

anidrosis (an″ĭ-dro′sis) anhidrosis.

anileridine (an″ĭ-ler′ĭ-dēn) a compound used as a narcotic, analgesic or sedative.

aniline (an′ĭ-lin) an amine from coal tar and indigo.

anilinophil (an″ĭ-lin′o-fil) a cell that stains readily with aniline dyes. adj., **anilinoph′ilous.**

anilism (an′ĭ-lizm) aniline poisoning.

anility (ah-nil′ĭ-te) the state of being like an old woman.

anima (an′ĭ-mah) in psychology, a term for the unconscious, or inner being, of the individual, as opposed to the persona, the personality he presents to the outside world.

animal (an′ĭ-mal) a living organism having sensation and power of voluntary movement.
  a. bite, a wound caused by the bite of an animal (see also BITE).
  control a., an untreated animal otherwise identical in all respects to one that is used for purposes of experiment, used for checking results of treatment.

animalcule (an″ĭ-mal′kūl) a minute animal organism.

animation (an″ĭ-ma′shun) the quality of being full of life.
  suspended a., temporary suspension or cessation of the vital functions.

anion (an′i-on) an ion carrying a negative charge; the element that in electrolysis passes to the positive pole.

aniridia (an″ĭ-rid′e-ah) congenital absence of the iris.

anis(o)- (an-i′so) word element [Gr.], *unequal.*

aniseikonia (an″ĭ-si-ko′ne-ah) inequality of the retinal images of the two eyes.

anisochromatic (an-i″so-kro-mat′ik) not of the same color throughout.

anisocoria (an-i″so-ko′re-ah) inequality in size of the pupils of both eyes.

anisocytosis (an-i″so-si-to′sis) the presence in the blood of erythrocytes showing abnormal variations in size.

anisohypercytosis (an-i″so-hi″per-si-to′sis) increase in leukocytes, with abnormality in the proportion of the various forms of neutrophils.

anisohypocytosis (an-i″so-hi″po-si-to′sis) decrease in leukocytes, with abnormality in the proportion of the various forms.

anisokaryosis (an-i″so-kar″e-o′sis) inequality in the size of the nuclei of cells.

anisoleukocytosis (an-i″so-lu″ko-si-to′sis) abnormality in the proportion of various forms of leukocytes in the blood.

anisomastia (an-i″so-mas′te-ah) inequality of the breasts.

anisometropia (an-i″so-mĕ-tro′pe-ah) inequality in the refractive power of the two eyes, of considerable degree. adj., **anisometrop′ic.**

anisonormocytosis (an-i″so-nor″mo-si-to′sis) normal number of leukocytes with abnormal proportion of various forms of neutrophils.

anisopiesis (an-i″so-pi-e′sis) difference in blood pressure recorded in corresponding arteries on the right and left sides of the body.

anisopoikilocytosis (an-i″so-poi″kī-lo-si-to′sis) the presence in the blood of erythrocytes of varying sizes and abnormal shapes.

anisospore (an-i′so-spōr) a spore that unites with another to form an adult.

anisosthenic (an-i″sos-then′ik) not having equal power; said of muscles.

anisotonic (an-i″so-ton′ik) having different osmotic pressure; not isotonic.

anisotropic (an-i″so-trop′ik) 1. having unlike properties in different directions. 2. doubly refracting, or having a double polarizing power.

anisotropy (an″i-sot′ro-pe) the quality of being anisotropic.

anisuria (an″i-su′re-ah) alternating oliguria and polyuria.

ankle (ang′kl) the part of the leg just above the foot; the joint between the leg and the foot. The ankle joint is a hinge joint and is formed by the junction of the tibia and fibula with the talus, or ankle bone. The bones are cushioned by cartilage and connected by a number of ligaments, tendons and muscles that strengthen the joint and enable it to be moved.
  Because it is in almost constant use, the ankle is particularly susceptible to injuries, such as SPRAIN

and FRACTURE. It is also often one of the first joints to be affected by ARTHRITIS or GOUT.

Edema or swelling of the tissues around the ankles is a fairly common occurrence in overweight people and pregnant women and is usually relieved by elevating the feet. It may, however, be a symptom of serious heart or renal disease.

a. jerk, plantar extension of the foot elicited by a tap on the Achilles tendon, preferably while the patient kneels on a bed or chair, the feet hanging free over the edge; called also Achilles reflex and triceps surae reflex.

ankyl(o)- (ang'kĭ-lo) word element [Gr.], *bent; crooked; in the form of a loop; adhesion.*

ankyloblepharon (ang″kĭ-lo-blef'ah-ron) fusion of the eyelids.

ankylocheilia (ang″kĭ-lo-ki'le-ah) adhesion of the lips.

ankyloglossia (ang″kĭ-lo-glos'e-ah) tongue-tie; abnormal shortness of the frenulum of the tongue, resulting in limitation of its motion.

a. superior, extensive adhesion of the tongue to the palate.

ankylopoietic (ang″kĭ-lo-poi-et'ik) producing ankylosis.

ankyloproctia (ang″kĭ-lo-prok'she-ah) stricture of the anus.

ankylosed (ang'kĭ-lōsd) affected with ankylosis.

ankylosis (ang″kĭ-lo'sis) abnormal immobility and consolidation of a joint. Ankylosis may be caused by destruction of the membranes that line the joint or by faulty bone structure. It is most often a result of chronic rheumatoid arthritis, in which the affected joint tends to assume the least painful position and may become more or less permanently fixed in it.

Artificial ankylosis, locking of a joint by surgical

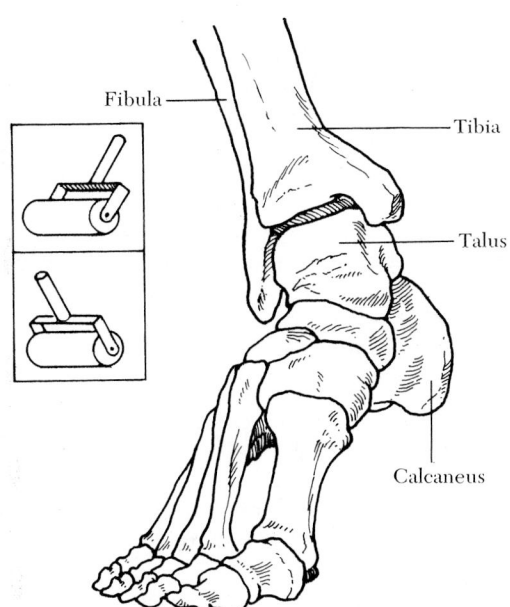

Ankle.

operation, is sometimes done in treatment of a severe joint condition.

extracapsular a., false a., that caused by rigidity of surrounding parts.

intracapsular a., that caused by rigidity of structures within the joint.

spurious a., extracapsular ankylosis.

true a., that in which motion is prevented by bony or fibrous union of the participating bones.

ankylotia (ang″kĭ-lo'she-ah) closure of the external meatus of the ear.

ankylotome (ang-kil'o-tōm) a knife for operating for tongue-tie.

ankyroid (ang'kĭ-roid) hooklike.

anlage (an'lah-geh), pl. *anla'gen* [Ger.] primordium.

anneal (ah-nēl') to soften a material, as a metal, by controlled heating and cooling, to make its manipulation easier.

annectent (ah-nek'tent) connecting; joining together.

Annelida (ah-nel'ĭ-dah) a phylum of metazoan invertebrates, the segmented worms, including leeches.

annular (an'u-lar) ring-shaped.

annulorrhaphy (an″u-lor'ah-fe) suture of a hernial ring or sac.

annulus (an'u-lus), pl. *an'nuli* [L.] a small ring or encircling structure; also spelled anulus.

anococcygeal (a″no-kok-sij'e-al) pertaining to anus and coccyx.

anode (an'ōd) the electrode by which electric current enters a cell, apparatus or body. adj., **ano'dal.**

anodontia (an″o-don'she-ah) congenital absence of some or all of the teeth.

anodyne (an'o-dīn) 1. relieving pain. 2. a medicine that eases pain.

anodynia (an″o-din'e-ah) freedom from pain.

anoetic (an″o-et'ik) not subject to conscious attention.

anoia (ah-noi'ah) idiocy.

anomalopia (ah-nom″ah-lo'pe-ah) a slight anomaly of visual perception.

color a., a minor deviation of color vision, without loss of ability to distinguish the four primary colors.

anomaloscope (ah-nom'ah-lo-skōp″) an apparatus used to detect anomalies of color vision.

anomaly (ah-nom'ah-le) deviation from normal. adj., **anom'alous.**

developmental a., absence, deformity or excess of body parts as the result of faulty development of the embryo.

anomia (ah-no'me-ah) loss of power of naming objects or of recognizing names.

anonychia (an″o-nik'e-ah) absence of the nails.

Anopheles (ah-nof′ĕ-lēz) a widely distributed genus of mosquitoes, comprising over 300 species, many of which are important vectors of MALARIA.

anophthalmos (an″of-thal′mos) congenital absence of the eyeballs.

anoplasty (a′no-plas″te) plastic repair of the anus.

anopsia (an-op′se-ah) 1. suppression of vision in one eye. 2. hypertropia.

anorchid (an-or′kid) a person with no testes or with cryptorchidism (undescended testes).

anorchism (an-or′kizm) congenital absence of one or both testes.

anorectic (an″o-rek′tik) 1. pertaining to anorexia. 2. an agent that diminishes the appetite for food.

anorectocolonic (a″no-rek″to-ko-lon′ik) pertaining to the anus, rectum and colon.

anorectum (a″no-rek′tum) the distal portion of the digestive tract, including the entire anal canal and the distal 2 cm. of the rectum. adj., **anorec′tal.**

anorexia (an″o-rek′se-ah) lack or loss of appetite for food. APPETITE is psychologic, dependent on memory and associations, as compared with hunger, which is physiologically aroused by the body's need for food. Anorexia can be brought about by unattractive food, surroundings or company.
 a. nervo′sa, loss of appetite due to emotional states, such as anxiety, irritation, anger and fear.

anorexic (an″o-rek′sik) anorectic.

anorexigenic (an″o-rek″sĭ-jen′ik) 1. producing anorexia. 2. an agent that diminishes or controls the appetite.

anorthography (an″or-thog′rah-fe) impairment of the ability to write.

anorthopia (an″or-tho′pe-ah) asymmetrical or distorted vision.

anorthosis (an″or-tho′sis) absence of erectility.

anoscope (a′no-skōp) a speculum or endoscope used in direct visual examination of the anal canal.

anoscopy (a-nos′ko-pe) examination of the anal canal with an anoscope.

anosigmoidoscopy (a″no-sig-moi″dos′ko-pe) visual examination of the anus and sigmoid by means of a speculum.

anosmia (an-oz′me-ah) absence of the sense of smell. adj., **anosmat′ic, anos′mic.**

anosognosia (an″o-sog-no′ze-ah) failure to recognize one's own disease or defect.

anosphrasia (an″os-fra′ze-ah) anosmia.

anospinal (a″no-spi′nal) pertaining to the anus and spinal cord.

anostosis (an″os-to′sis) defective formation of bone.

anotia (an-o′she-ah) a developmental anomaly with absence of the ears.

anotus (an-o′tus) a fetus without ears.

anovaginal (a″no-vaj′ĭ-nal) pertaining to the anus and vagina.

anovarism (an-o′var-izm) absence of the ovaries.

anovesical (a″no-ves′ĭ-kal) pertaining to the anus and bladder.

anovular, anovulatory (an-ov′u-lar), (an-ov′u-lah-tor″e) not associated with ovulation.

anoxemia (an″ok-se′me-ah) lack of sufficient oxygen in the blood. adj., **anoxe′mic.**

anoxia (an-ok′se-ah) absence or deficiency of oxygen, as reduction of oxygen in body tissues below physiologic levels. The condition is accompanied by deep respirations, cyanosis, increased pulse rate and impairment of coordination. adj., **anox′ic.**
 ambient a., diminished oxygen content of the surrounding atmosphere.
 anemic a., reduction of oxygen in body tissues because of diminished oxygen-carrying capacity of the blood.
 anoxic a., reduction of oxygen in body tissues due to interference with the oxygen supply.
 histotoxic a., condition resulting from diminished ability of cells to utilize available oxygen.
 stagnant a., condition due to interference with the flow of blood and its transport of oxygen.

anoxybiosis (an-ok″se-bi-o′sis) anaerobiosis.

ansa (an′sah), pl. *an′sae* [L.] a looplike structure.
 a. cervica′lis, a nerve loop in the neck attached in front and above to the hypoglossal nerve and behind to the upper cervical spinal nerves. Its hypoglossal attachment is misleading since this part of the loop ultimately rejoins the upper spinal nerves.
 a. of Henle, Henle's loop.
 a. hypoglos′si, ansa cervicalis.
 a. lenticula′ris, a tract between the crusta and the lenticular nucleus.
 an′sae nervo′rum spina′lium, loops of spinal nerves joining the anterior spinal nerves.
 a. peduncula′ris, the portion of the brain to the ventral side of the thalamus.

Ansolysen (an″so-li′sen) trademark for preparation of pentolinium tartrate, used as an antihypertensive.

ansotomy (an-sot′o-me) incision of the ansa lenticularis for treatment of tremor.

Antabuse (an′tah-būs) trademark for a preparation of disulfiram, used in the treatment of alcoholism.

antacid (ant-as′id) 1. counteracting acidity. 2. an agent that counteracts acidity. Substances that act as antacids include sodium bicarbonate, aluminum hydroxide gel, magnesium hydroxide, magnesium trisilicate, magnesium oxide and calcium carbonate. They are often used in the treatment of peptic ULCER.

antagonist (an-tag′o-nist) an agent (muscle, drug) that exerts an action opposite to that of another.

antalgesic (ant″al-je′sik) analgesic.

antalgic (ant-al′jik) analgesic.

antalkaline (ant-al′kah-lĭn) counteracting alkalinity.

antaphrodisiac (ant″af-ro-diz′e-ak) an agent that allays the sexual impulse.

antazoline hydrochloride (ant-az′o-lēn) a drug that blocks the action of histamine, which is present in large amounts in individuals hypersensitive and suffering from various allergies. The drug relieves the symptoms of itching, nasal and conjunctival edema and inflammation and urticaria of skin allergies. Another antazoline compound is antazoline phosphate which is also an antihistamine.

Both drugs are likely to produce drowsiness, excessive dryness of the mouth and throat, lassitude and other side effects of an antihistaminic drug. They are available in tablet form and in a 0.5 per cent solution to be used as eye drops or in a nebulizer.

ante (an′te) [L.] preposition, *before*.

ante- (an′te) word element [L.], *before* (in time or space).

antebrachium (an″te-bra′ke-um) the forearm. adj., **antebra′chial.**

antecedent (an″te-se′dent) a precursor.
plasma thromboplastic a., PTA; clotting factor XI.

antecurvature (an″te-kur′vah-tūr) a slight anteflexion.

antefebrile (an″te-feb′ril) preceding fever.

anteflexion (an″te-flek′shun) the bending of an organ so that its top is thrust forward.

antelocation (an″te-lo-ka′shun) displacement of an organ forward.

antemetic (ant″e-met′ik) antiemetic.

ante mortem (an′te mor′tem) [L.] before death.

antemortem (an″te-mor′tem) performed or occurring before death.

antenna (an-ten′ah) one of the appendages on the head of arthropods.

Antepar (an′te-par) trademark for a preparation of piperazine citrate and piperazine phosphate, an anthelmintic.

antepartal (an″te-par′tal) occurring before childbirth.

ante partum (an′te par′tum) [L.] before parturition.

antepartum (an″te-par′tum) performed or occurring before parturition.

antephase (an′te-fāz) the portion of interphase immediately preceding mitosis, when energy is being produced and stored for mitosis and chromosome reproduction is taking place.

anteposition (an″te-po-zish′un) forward displacement, as of the uterus.

antepyretic (an″te-pi-ret′ik) before the stage of fever.

anterior (an-tēr′e-or) situated at or directed toward the front; opposite of posterior.

a. chamber, the part of the aqueous humor-containing space of the eyeball between the cornea and the iris.

antero- (an′ter-o) word element [L.], *anterior; in front of.*

anterograde (an′ter-o-grād″) extending or moving forward.

anteroinferior (an″ter-o-in-fēr′e-or) situated in front and below.

anterolateral (an″ter-o-lat′er-al) situated in front and to one side.

anteromedian (an″ter-o-me′de-an) situated in front and on the midline.

anteroposterior (an″ter-o-pos-tēr′e-or) directed from the front toward the back.

anterosuperior (an″ter-o-su-pēr′e-or) situated in front and above.

anteversion (an″te-ver′zhun) the tipping forward of an entire organ.

anteverted (an″te-vert′ed) tipped or bent forward.

anthelix (ant′he-liks) antihelix.

anthelmintic (ant″hel-min′tik) 1. destructive to worms. 2. an agent destructive to worms. Examples of anthelmintic drugs include: piperazine and hexylresorcinol for the treatment of the roundworm *Ascaris lumbricoides;* quinacrine hydrochloride and aspidium oleoresin for the treatment of tapeworms; and oxytetracycline hydrochloride and emetine hydrochloride for protozoan infection such as amebic dysentery.

Many anthelmintic drugs are toxic and should be given with care. The toxic effects of a specific drug should be known prior to administration and the patient observed carefully for these effects after the drug is given.

anthocyanin (an″tho-si′ah-nin) the red pigment of beet root.

anthophobia (an″tho-fo′be-ah) morbid dislike of flowers.

anthorisma (an″tho-riz′mah) a diffuse swelling.

anthracemia (an″thrah-se′me-ah) 1. asphyxia, as from carbon monoxide poisoning. 2. the presence of *Bacillus anthracis* in the blood.

anthracene (an′thrah-sēn) a crystalline hydrocarbon, $C_{14}H_{10}$, from coal tar.

anthracia (an-thra′se-ah) a disease marked by formation of carbuncles.

anthracin (an′thrah-sin) a poisonous compound from cultures of the organism causing anthrax.

anthracoid (an′thrah-koid) resembling anthrax.

anthracometer (an″thrah-kom′ĕ-ter) an instrument for measuring carbon dioxide in the air.

anthraconecrosis (an″thrah-ko-nĕ-kro′sis) degeneration of tissue into a black mass.

anthracosilicosis (an″thrah-ko-sil″ĭ-ko′sis) a

lung disease due to inhalation of coal dust and fine particles of silica.

anthracosis (an"thrah-ko'sis) a lung disease due to inhalation of coal dust not containing silica (see also PNEUMOCONIOSIS).

anthracotherapy (an"thrah-ko-ther'ah-pe) treatment with charcoal.

anthralin (an'thrah-lin) a yellowish brown crystalline powder used topically in eczema.

anthraquinone (an"thrah-kwin'ōn) a yellow substance from anthracene, used in the manufacture of certain dyes.

anthrax (an'thraks) an infectious disease of cattle, horses, mules, sheep and goats, due to *Bacillus anthracis;* sometimes acquired by man through contact with infected animals or their byproducts, such as carcasses or skins.
  Anthrax in humans usually occurs as a malignant pustule or malignant edema of the skin. In rare instances it can affect the lungs if the spores of the bacillus are inhaled, or it can involve the intestinal tract when infected meat is eaten. The condition often is accompanied by hemorrhage, as the exotoxins from the bacillus attack the endothelium of small blood vessels. The condition is treated by the use of antibiotics such as penicillin, the tetracyclines and chloramphenicol. The disorder is also known by a variety of names, including woolsorters' disease, ragpickers' disease and charbon.
  cutaneous a., anthrax due to lodgment of the causative organisms in wounds or abrasions of the skin, producing swelling in various parts of the body.
  fulminant a., a form characterized by sudden onset and rapidly fatal course.
  pulmonary a., infection of the respiratory tract resulting from inhalation of dust or animal hair containing spores of *Bacillus anthracis.*

anthropo- (an'thro-po) word element [Gr.], *man (human being).*

anthropocentric (an"thro-po-sen'trik) with a human bias; considering man the center of the universe.

anthropogeny (an"thro-poj'ĕ-ne) development or evolution of man.

anthropoid (an'thro-poid) resembling a man.

Anthropoidea (an"thro-poi'de-ah) a suborder of Primates, including monkeys, apes and man, characterized by a larger and more complicated brain than the other suborders.

anthropokinetics (an"thro-po-ki-net'iks) study of the total human being in action, including biological and physical, psychologic and sociologic aspects.

anthropology (an"thro-pol'o-je) the science that treats of man.
  criminal a., that branch of anthropology that treats of criminals and crimes.
  cultural a., that branch of anthropology that treats of man in relation to his fellows and to his environment.

physical a., that branch of anthropology that treats of the physical characteristics of man.

anthropometer (an"thro-pom'e-ter) an instrument especially designed for measuring various dimensions of the body.

anthropometry (an"thro-pom'e-tre) the science that deals with the measurement of the size, weight and proportions of the human body.

anthropomorphism (an"thro-po-mor'fizm) the attribution of human characteristics to nonhuman objects.

anthropophagy (an"thro-pof'ah-je) cannibalism.

anthropophilic (an"thro-po-fil'ik) preferring human beings to animals; said of certain mosquitoes.

anthropophobia (an"thro-po"fo'be-ah) morbid dread of society.

anthropozoonosis (an"thro-po-zo"o-no'sis) a disease of either animals or man that may be transmitted from one species to the other.

anthydropic (ant"hi-drop'ik) relieving dropsy.

anthypnotic (ant"hip-not'ik) preventing sleep.

anthysteric (ant"his-ter'ik) relieving hysteria.

anti- (an'ti, an'te) word element [Gr.], *counteracting; effective against.*

antiabortifacient (an"te-ah-bor"ti-fa'shent) 1. preventing abortion or promoting gestation. 2. an agent that prevents abortion or promotes successful gestation.

antiagglutinin (an"te-ah-gloo'ti-nin) a substance that opposes the action of an agglutinin.

antialexin (an"te-ah-lek'sin) a substance that opposes the action of an alexin.

antiamboceptor (an"te-am"bo-sep'tor) a substance that opposes the action of an amboceptor.

antiamebic (an"te-ah-me'bik) 1. destroying or suppressing the growth of amebas. 2. an agent that destroys or suppresses the growth of amebas.

antianemic (an"te-ah-ne'mik) counteracting anemia.

antiantibody (an"te-an'ti-bod"e) a substance that counteracts the effect of an antibody.

antiarrhythmic (an"te-ah-rith'mik) 1. preventing or alleviating cardiac arrhythmias. 2. an agent that prevents or alleviates cardiac arrhythmias.

antiarthritic (an"te-ar-thrit'ik) 1. effective in treatment of arthritis. 2. an agent used in treatment of arthritis.

antibacterial (an"ti-bak-te're-al) 1. checking the growth of bacteria. 2. an agent that checks the growth of bacteria.

antibechic (an"ti-bek'ik) 1. relieving cough. 2. an agent that relieves cough.

antibiosis (an"ti-bi-o'sis) an association between two populations of organisms that is detrimental to one of them.

antibiotic (an"ti-bi-ot'ik) a chemical compound produced by and obtained from certain living cells, especially lower plant cells, such as bacteria, yeasts and molds, or an equivalent synthetic compound, which is antagonistic to some other form of life, especially pathogenic or noxious organisms. Their action is biostatic or biocidal.

Penicillin, the first widely used antibiotic, was accidentally discovered in 1929 by Sir Alexander Fleming when bacteria in a laboratory dish were killed by mold spores floating in the air. In World War II it prevented many deaths from wound infection and disease. When penicillin was found to be ineffective against many types of disease, especially those caused by viruses, worldwide search in soil and other natural sources yielded new medicines such as chlortetracycline hydrochloride (Aureomycin), chloramphenicol and oxytetracycline (Terramycin), called the broad-spectrum antibiotics because they are effective against a wide range of bacterial infections, and also some viruses. Some antibiotics are now produced synthetically.

The antibiotics have now largely controlled pneumonia, mastoiditis and peritonitis, have reduced the danger of many other diseases and are frequently used to prevent infection in surgery and injury. They are powerful substances and should never be used except under a physician's care. Unless an antibiotic is properly prescribed, pathogenic organisms can develop resistance to the drug, and then the value of this weapon against disease is destroyed.

antibiotin (an″tǐ-bi′o-tin) avidin, a protein that renders biotin inactive.

antiblennorrhagic (an″tǐ-blen″o-raj′ik) preventing or relieving gonorrhea.

antibody (an′tǐ-bod″e) a protein that is produced in the body in response to invasion by a foreign agent (ANTIGEN), and that reacts specifically with it.

Antibodies are part of the body's natural defense against invasion by foreign substances. Each antibody is effective only against the particular antigen that stimulates its production. Almost all the antibodies are formed in the lymph nodes, spleen, bone marrow and lymphoid tissue. They are usually proteins and are GAMMA GLOBULIN molecules.

The reaction of the body to the entrance of antigens is called the antigen-antibody reaction. Once the body responds to the invasion and begins to produce the antibodies it can continue to do so for many weeks to several years. Thus is it possible for immunity to last for many months or years.

Antibodies are classified according to their behavior on electrophoresis, ultracentrifugation and immunoelectrophoresis, and also according to the mode of their observed action, as agglutinins, amboceptors, antienzymes, antitoxins, bacteriolysins, blood group antibodies, cytotoxins, hemolysins, opsonins and precipitins.

anaphylactic a., a substance formed as a result of the first injection of a foreign protein and responsible for the anaphylactic symptoms following the second injection of the same protein.

blocking a., incomplete a., inhibiting a., an antibody that combines with an antigen without causing visible reaction, but preventing another antibody from combining with the antigen.

neutralizing a., one that reduces or destroys infectivity of a homologous infectious agent by partial or complete destruction of the agent.

protective a., one responsible for immunity to an infectious agent observed in passive immunity.

sensitizing a., anaphylactic antibody.

antibrachium (an″tǐ-bra′ke-um) antebrachium, or forearm.

anticachectic (an″tǐ-kah-kek′tik) 1. preventing or relieving cachexia. 2. an agent that prevents or relieves cachexia.

anticalculous (an″tǐ-kal′ku-lus) suppressing the formation of calculi.

anticariogenic (an″tǐ-kār″e-o-jen′ik) effective in suppressing caries production.

anticatarrhal (an″tǐ-kah-tahr′al) counteracting catarrh.

anticholagogue (an″tǐ-ko′lah-gog) an agent that inhibits secretion of bile. adj., **anticholagog′ic.**

anticholinergic (an″tǐ-ko″lin-er′jik) blocking the passage of impulses through the parasympathetic nerves; parasympatholytic.

anticholinesterase (an″tǐ-ko″lin-es′ter-ās) a substance that inhibits the action of cholinesterase.

anticoagulant (an″tǐ-ko-ag′u-lant) any substance that inhibits the blood clotting mechanism. Anticoagulant drugs are administered to maintain the blood in a fluid state, thereby preventing abnormal, or pathologic clotting. Heparin and the bishydroxycoumarin derivatives (Dicumarol and warfarin sodium) are examples of anticoagulant drugs.

Patients receiving anticoagulant therapy must be watched closely for signs of spontaneous bleeding. These include hematuria, petechiae on the head and body, bleeding gums or tarry stools.

Initially, the patient is hospitalized and the prothrombin time of his blood is determined daily before the dose of anticoagulant is administered. After the patient is discharged from the hospital, prothrombin time tests are performed periodically for the entire duration of anticoagulant therapy. The drugs may be given for a period of weeks or indefinitely. While taking the drug the patient is instructed to carry an emergency supply of oral vitamin K in the event that spontaneous bleeding should occur.

anticoagulin (an″tǐ-ko-ag′u-lin) a substance that suppresses, delays or nullifies coagulation of the blood.

anticomplement (an″tǐ-kom′plě-ment) a substance that counteracts a complement.

anticonvulsant (an″tǐ-kon-vul′sant) 1. inhibiting convulsions. 2. an agent that suppresses convulsions. Drugs that act as anticonvulsants include diphenylhydantoin (Dilantin), mephenytoin (Mesantoin) and trimethadione (Tridione). They are used in the treatment of epilepsy and in psychomotor and myoclonic seizures.

anticus (an-ti′kus) anterior.

anticytolysin (an″tǐ-si-tol′ǐ-sin) a substance that counteracts cytolysin.

anticytotoxin (an″tǐ-si″to-tok′sin) a substance that counteracts cytotoxin.

antidepressant (an″tǐ-de-pres′ant) 1. effective against depressive illness. 2. an agent that is effective against depressive psychologic illness. The many antidepressant drugs used in the treatment of the various psychologic depressions include amitriptyline (Elavil), desipramine hydrochloride (Norpramin, Pertofrane), imipramine hydrochloride (Tofranil), isocarboxazid (Marplan) and nialamide (Niamid).

antidiarrheal (an″tĭ-di″ah-re′al) 1. counteracting diarrhea. 2. an agent that counteracts diarrhea.

antidinic (an″tĭ-din′ik) relieving giddiness or vertigo.

antidipsia (an″tĭ-dip′se-ah) aversion to the ingestion of fluids.

antidiuresis (an″tĭ-di″u-re′sis) the suppression of secretion of urine by the kidneys.

antidiuretic (an″tĭ-di″u-ret′ik) 1. pertaining to or causing suppression of urine. 2. an agent that causes suppression of urine.

   a. hormone, a hormone that suppresses the secretion of urine; vasopressin, which has a specific effect on the epithelial cells of the renal tubules, stimulating the reabsorption of water independently of solids, and resulting in concentration of urine. It is secreted by the posterior lobe of the PITUITARY GLAND. Abbreviated ADH.

antidote (an′tĭ-dōt) an agent that counteracts a poison. adj., **antido′tal.**
   chemical a., one that neutralizes the poison by changing its chemical nature.
   mechanical a., one that prevents absorption of the poison.
   physiologic a., one that counteracts the effects of the poison by producing other effects.
   universal a., a mixture formerly recommended as an antidote when the exact poison is not known. There is, in fact, no known universal antidote. Activated charcoal is now being used for many poisons.

antidromic (an″tĭ-drom′ik) conducting impulses in a direction opposite to the normal.

antidysenteric (an″tĭ-dis″en-ter′ik) counteracting dysentery.

antiedemic (an″te-ĕ-dem′ik) 1. counteracting or relieving edema. 2. an agent that counteracts or relieves edema.

antiemetic (an″te-e-met′ik) 1. useful in the treatment of vomiting. 2. an agent that relieves vomiting.

antienzyme (an″te-en′zīm) a substance that counteracts an enzyme.

antiepileptic (an″te-ep″ĭ-lep′tik) 1. combating epilepsy. 2. a remedy for epilepsy.

antiepithelial (an″te-ep″ĭ-the′le-al) destructive to epithelial cells.

antiesterase (an″te-es′ter-ās) an agent that counteracts the activity of esterolytic enzymes.

antifebrile (an″tĭ-feb′ril) counteracting fever.

antifebrin (an″tĭ-feb′rin) acetanilid.

antifertilizin (an″tĭ-fer″tĭ-li′zin) a substance on the surface of a spermatozoon that reacts with a

substance on the surface of the ovum (fertilizin), thus binding the spermatozoon to the ovum.

antifibrinolysin (an″tĭ-fi″brĭ-nol′ĭ-sin) antiplasmin.

antifibrinolytic (an″tĭ-fi″brĭ-no-lit′ik) inhibiting fibrinolysis.

antifungal (an″tĭ-fung′gal) 1. checking the growth of fungi. 2. an agent that checks the growth of fungi.

antigalactic (an″tĭ-gah-lak′tik) diminishing secretion of milk.

antigen (an′tĭ-jen) any substance not normally present in the body which, when introduced into it, stimulates production of an ANTIBODY that reacts specifically with it. adj., **antigen′ic.** Antigens are almost always of protein composition; for example, the structures of bacteria and viruses and the toxins they elaborate are protein. Other antigens include proteins in human or animal serum used for immunization and blood cells of donors who have a blood type incompatible with that of the recipient.
   The antigen-antibody reaction that occurs is a chemical reaction between the antigen molecules and the antibody molecules. Several different types of specific reactions can take place, including neutralization of those antigens that are toxins; agglutination or clumping of antigens such as bacteria so that they are rendered harmless, or the clumping of erythrocytes in a transfusion reaction; and lysis, or rupture of the cell membrane of the antigen. Opsonification refers to a specific reaction in which the antibodies (opsonins) prepare the bacteria so that they can be destroyed more easily by phagocytes.
   flagellar a., H antigen.
   Forssman a., a heterophil antigen discovered in guinea pig tissues, which produced in rabbits antibodies that lysed sheep erythrocytes in the presence of complement.
   H a. (Ger. *Hauch,* film), the antigen that occurs in the flagella of motile bacteria.
   heterophil a., one capable of stimulating the production of antibodies that react with tissues from other animals or even plants.
   isophil a., one occurring within a species, but not in all individuals of the species, e.g., human blood group antigens.
   O a. (Ger. *ohne Hauch,* without film), the antigen that occurs in the bodies of bacteria.
   partial a., an antigen that does not produce antibody formation, but gives specific precipitation when mixed with the antibacterial immune serum.
   V a., Vi a., an antigen contained in the sheath of a bacterium, as *Salmonella typhosa* (the typhoid bacillus), and giving greater virulence to the strain containing it.

antigenicity (an″tĭ-jĕ-nis′ĭ-te) ability of a substance to stimulate antibody formation.

antiglobulin (an″tĭ-glob′u-lin) a precipitin that precipitates globulin.

antigoitrogenic (an″tĭ-goi″tro-jen′ik) inhibiting the development of goiter.

antihallucinatory (an″tĭ-hah-lu′sĭ-nah-to″re) preventing the occurrence of hallucinations.

antihelix (an″tĭ-he′liks) the curved ridge opposite the helix of the ear.

antihelmintic (an″tĭ-hel-min′tik) anthelmintic.

antihemolysin (an″tĭ-he-mol′ĭ-sin) a substance that counteracts hemolysin.

antihemophilic (an″tĭ-he″mo-fil′ik) 1. effective against the bleeding tendency in hemophilia. 2. an agent that counteracts the bleeding tendency in hemophilia.

   a. factor, AHF, one of the clotting factors, deficiency of which causes classic, sex-linked hemophilia; called also factor VIII and antihemophilic globulin. It is available in a preparation for preventive and therapeutic use.

antihemorrhagic (an″tĭ-hem″o-raj′ik) 1. exerting a hemostatic effect and counteracting hemorrhage. 2. an agent that prevents or checks hemorrhage.

antihistamine (an″tĭ-his′tah-min) a drug that counteracts the effects of histamine, a normal body chemical that is believed to cause the symptoms of persons who are hypersensitive to various allergens. Antihistamines are used to relieve the symptoms of allergic reactions, especially hay fever and other allergic disorders of the nasal passages. Some antihistamines have an antinauseant action that is useful in the relief of motion sickness. Others have a sedative and hypnotic action and may be used as tranquilizers.

   Patients for whom an antihistamine has been prescribed should be warned of the side effects of these drugs, including drowsiness, dizziness and muscular weakness. These side effects present a special hazard in driving an automobile or operating heavy machinery. Other side effects include dryness of the mouth and throat and insomnia.

antihistaminic (an″tĭ-his″tah-min′ik) 1. counteracting the pharmacologic effects of histamine. 2. an antihistamine.

antihormone (an″tĭ-hōr′mōn) a substance that counteracts a hormone.

antihydropic (an″tĭ-hi-drop′ik) effective in relieving or preventing dropsy.

antihypercholesterolemic (an″tĭ-hi″per-ko-les′-ter-ol-e″mik) 1. effective against hypercholesterolemia. 2. an agent that prevents or relieves hypercholesterolemia.

antihypertensive (an″tĭ-hi″per-ten′siv) 1. effective against hypertension. 2. an agent that prevents or relieves high blood pressure.

anti-icteric (an″te-ik-ter′ik) relieving icterus, or jaundice.

anti-immune (an″te-ĭ-mūn′) preventing immunity.

anti-infective (an″te-in-fek′tiv) 1. counteracting infection. 2. a substance that counteracts infection.

anti-inflammatory (an″te-in-flam′ah-to-re) counteracting or suppressing inflammation.

antiketogenic (an″tĭ-ke″to-jen′ik) preventing or suppressing the development of ketones (ketone bodies) and preventing development of ketosis.

antileukocytic (an″tĭ-lu″ko-sit′ik) destructive to leukocytes.

antilewisite (an″tĭ-lu′ĭ-sīt) dimercaprol, a chelating agent used in poisoning with arsenic, gold and mercury.

antilobium (an″tĭ-lo′be-um) the tragus of the ear.

antilogia (an″tĭ-lo′je-ah) a combination of contradictory symptoms, rendering diagnosis uncertain.

antilysin (an″tĭ-li′sin) an antibody that inactivates a lysin.

antilysis (an″tĭ-li′sis) inhibition of lysis.

antimalarial (an″tĭ-mah-la′re-al) 1. therapeutically effective against malaria. 2. an agent that is therapeutically effective against malaria.

antimere (an′tĭ-mēr) one of the segments of the body bounded by planes at right angles to the long axis of the body.

antimetabolite (an″tĭ-mē-tab′o-līt) a substance exerting its desired effect perhaps by replacing or interfering with the utilization of an essential metabolite.

antimetropia (an″tĭ-mē-tro′pe-ah) hyperopia of one eye, with myopia in the other.

antimicrobic (an″tĭ-mi-kro′bik) checking the growth of microbes.

antimicrobiosis (an″tĭ-mi″kro-bi-o′sis) suppression of the growth of microorganisms.

antimongoloid (an″tĭ-mon′go-loid) opposite to that characteristic of Down's syndrome (mongolism), e.g., antimongoloid slant of the palpebral fissures.

antimony (an′tĭ-mo″ne) a chemical element, atomic number 51, atomic weight 121.75, symbol Sb. (See table of ELEMENTS.) Antimony compounds are used in medicine as anti-infective agents in the treatment of tropical diseases, especially those of protozoan origin. All antimony compounds are potentially poisonous and must be used with caution.

   a. potassium tartrate, a compound used in treatment of parasitic infections, e.g., schistosomiasis or leishmaniasis.

antimorphic (an″tĭ-mor′fik) in genetics, antagonizing or inhibiting normal activity (antimorphic mutant gene).

antimycotic (an″tĭ-mi-kot′ik) destructive to fungi.

antinarcotic (an″tĭ-nar-kot′ik) relieving narcotism.

antinauseant (an″tĭ-naw′se-ant) 1. counteracting nausea. 2. an agent that counteracts nausea.

antineoplastic (an″tĭ-ne″o-plas′tik) inhibiting the maturation and proliferation of malignant cells.

antinephritic (an″tĭ-nĕ-frit′ik) effective against nephritis.

antineuralgic (an″tĭ-nu-ral′jik) relieving neuralgia.

antineuritic (an″tĭ-nu-rit′ik) relieving neuritis.

antinion (an-tin′e-on) the frontal pole of the head.

antiopsonin   (an″te-op′so-nin) a substance that counteracts opsonins.

antiovulatory   (an″te-ov′u-lah-to″re) suppressing ovulation.

antioxidant   (an″te-ok′sĭ-dant) a substance that in small amount will inhibit the oxidation of other compounds.

antioxidation   (an″te-ok″sĭ-da′shun) prevention of oxidation.

antiparalytic   (an″tĭ-par″ah-lit′ik) relieving paralytic symptoms.

antiparasitic   (an″tĭ-par″ah-sit′ik) 1. destroying parasites. 2. an agent that destroys parasites.

antiparasympathomimetic   (an″tĭ-par″ah-sim″-pah-tho-mi-met′ik) producing effects that resemble those of interruption of the parasympathetic nerve supply.

antipathic   (an″tĭ-path′ik) opposite in nature.

antipediculotic   (an″tĭ-pĕ-dik″u-lot′ik) 1. effective against lice and in treatment of pediculosis. 2. an agent that is effective against lice.

antipepsin   (an″tĭ-pep′sin) an antienzyme that counteracts pepsin.

antiperistalsis   (an″tĭ-per″ĭ-stal′sis) upward waves of contraction sometimes occurring normally in the lower ileum, competing with the normal downward peristalsis and retarding passage of intestinal contents into the cecum. adj., **antiperistalt′ic.**

antiphlogistic   (an″tĭ-flo-jis′tik) 1. diminishing inflammation. 2. an agent that diminishes inflammation.

antiphthisic   (an″tĭ-tiz′ik) antituberculotic.

antiplasmin   (an″tĭ-plaz′min) a principle in the blood that inhibits plasmin.

antiplastic   (an″tĭ-plas′tik) unfavorable to healing.

antiprotease, antiproteolysin   (an″tĭ-pro′te-ās), (an″tĭ-pro″te-o-li′sin) antiplasmin.

antiprothrombin   (an″tĭ-pro-throm′bin) a substance that retards the conversion of prothrombin into thrombin.

antiprotozoan   (an″tĭ-pro″to-zo′an) effective against protozoa.

antipruritic   (an″tĭ-proo-rit′ik) 1. preventing or relieving itching. 2. an agent that counteracts itching.

antipyic   (an″tĭ-pi′ik) preventing suppuration.

antipyretic   (an″tĭ-pi-ret′ik) 1. effective against fever. 2. an agent that relieves fever. Cold packs, aspirin and quinine are all antipyretics. Antipyretic drugs dilate the blood vessels near the surface of the skin, thereby allowing more blood to flow through the skin, where it can be cooled by the air. Also, an antipyretic can increase perspiration, the evaporation of which cools the body.

antipyrine   (an″tĭ-pi′rēn) a crystalline analgesic and antipyretic compound.

antipyrotic   (an″tĭ-pi-rot′ik) 1. effective in the treatment of burns. 2. an agent used in the treatment of burns.

antirabic   (an″tĭ-ra′bik) 1. used to prevent development of rabies. 2. an agent used to prevent rabies.

antirachitic   (an″tĭ-rah-kit′ik) therapeutically effective against rickets.

antiradiation   (an″tĭ-ra″de-a′shun) capable of counteracting the effects of radiation; effective against radiation injury.

antirheumatic   (an″tĭ-roo-mat′ik) counteracting rheumatism.

antirickettsial   (an″tĭ-rĭ-ket′se-al) effective against rickettsiae.

antiscabious   (an″tĭ-ska′be-us) counteracting scabies.

antiscorbutic   (an″tĭ-skor-bu′tik) counteracting scurvy.

antisepsis   (an″tĭ-sep′sis) prevention of sepsis by destruction of microorganisms and infective matter.

antiseptic   (an″tĭ-sep′tik) any substance that inhibits the growth of bacteria, in contrast to a germicide, which kills bacteria outright. Antiseptics are not considered to include antibiotics, which are usually taken internally. The term antiseptic includes disinfectants, although most disinfectants are too strong to be applied to body tissue and are generally used to clean inanimate objects such as floors and bathroom fixtures.

Antiseptics are divided into two types: physical and chemical. The most important physical antiseptic is heat, applied by boiling, autoclaving, flaming or burning. These are among the oldest and most effective methods of disinfecting contaminated objects, water and food.

Antiseptics have many applications. They are used in treating wounds and infections, in sterilizing, as before an operation, and in general hygiene. Antiseptics also have an application in the preservation of food and in the purification of sewage. The wide variety of antiseptics, their strength and the speed at which they work are all factors that influence the choice of which one to use for a specific job.

urinary a., a drug that is excreted mainly by way of the urine and performs its antiseptic action in the bladder. These drugs may be given before examination of or operation on the urinary tract, and they are sometimes used to treat urinary tract infections.

antiserotonin   (an″tĭ-se″ro-to′nin) a substance capable of antagonizing or inhibiting the action of serotonin.

antiserum   (an″tĭ-se′rum) a serum containing antibodies. It may be obtained from an animal that has been subjected to the action of antigen either by injection into the tissues or blood or by infection. (See also IMMUNITY and IMMUNIZATION.)

antisialagogue   (an″tĭ-si-al′ah-gog) an agent that inhibits the flow of saliva.

antisialic   (an″tĭ-si-al′ik) checking the flow of saliva.

antispasmodic, antispastic   (an″tĭ-spaz-mod′ik),

(an″tĭ-spas′tik) 1. preventing or relieving spasms. 2. an agent that prevents or relieves spasms.

antistalsis (an″tĭ-stal′sis) antiperistalsis.

Antistine (an-tis′tin) trademark for preparations of antazoline, an antihistamine.

antistreptococcic (an″tĭ-strep″to-kok′sic) counteracting streptococcal infection.

antisudoral (an″tĭ-soo′dor-al) counteracting sweating.

antisympathetic (an″tĭ-sim″pah-thet′ik) 1. producing effects resembling those of interruption of the sympathetic nerve supply. 2. an agent that produces effects resembling those of interruption of the sympathetic nerve supply.

antisyphilitic (an″tĭ-sif″ĭ-lit′ik) counteracting syphilis.

antithenar (an″tĭ-the′nar) placed opposite to the palm or sole.

antithrombin (an″tĭ-throm′bin) a principle in the blood that inhibits thrombin.

antithromboplastin (an″tĭ-throm″bo-plas′tin) a substance that interferes with thromboplastin and inhibits coagulation of blood.

antithyroid (an″tĭ-thi′roid) suppressing thyroid activity.

antitoxin (an″tĭ-tok′sin) a particular kind of antibody produced in the body in response to the presence of a toxin (see also IMMUNIZATION). adj., antitox′ic.
  diphtheria a., preparation from the blood serum or plasma of healthy animals immunized against diphtheria toxin, used as a passive immunizing agent.
  gas gangrene a., a sterile solution of antitoxic substances from blood of healthy animals immunized against gas-producing organisms of the genus Clostridium.
  scarlet fever streptococcus a., sterile solution of antitoxic substances from blood serum of healthy animals immunized against toxin produced by the streptococcus considered the cause of scarlet fever.
  tetanus a., preparation from the blood serum or plasma of healthy animals immunized against tetanus toxin, used as a passive immunizing agent.

antitragus (an″tĭ-tra′gus) a projection on the ear opposite the tragus.

antitrichomonal (an″tĭ-trik″o-mo′nal) 1. destructive to Trichomonas. 2. an agent that is destructive to Trichomonas.

antitrope (an′tĭ-trōp) one of two structures that are similar but oppositely oriented, like a right and a left glove.

antitrypsin (an″tĭ-trip′sin) an antienzyme counteracting the action of trypsin. adj., antitryp′tic.

antitryptase (an″tĭ-trip′tās) antiplasmin.

antituberculotic (an″tĭ-tu-ber″ku-lot′ik) counteracting tuberculosis.

antitussive (an″tĭ-tus′iv) 1. effective against cough. 2. an agent that suppresses coughing.

antivenereal (an″tĭ-vĕ-ne′re-al) counteracting venereal disease.

antivenin (an″tĭ-ven′in) a material used to neutralize the venom of a poisonous animal.
  black widow spider a., an antitoxin to the venom of a black widow spider (Latrodectus mactans).
  a. (Crotalidae) polyvalent, a preparation containing globulins effective in neutralizing venoms of most pit vipers (rattlesnake, copperhead, water moccasin, fer-de-lance) throughout the world.

antiviral (an″tĭ-vi′ral) 1. effective against viruses. 2. an agent effective against viruses.

antixerotic (an″tĭ-ze-rot′ik) preventing dryness.

antizymotic (an″tĭ-zi-mot′ik) counteracting enzymes.

antodontalgic (ant″o-don-tal′jik) relieving toothache.

antorphine (an-tor′fēn) nalorphine hydrochloride, a derivative of morphine, used as a narcotic antagonist.

antr(o)- (an′tro) word element [L.], chamber; cavity; often used with specific reference to the maxillary antrum or sinus.

antrectomy (an-trek′to-me) excision of an antrum.

Antrenyl (an′trĕ-nil) trademark for a preparation of oxyphenonium, an anticholinergic.

antritis (an-tri′tis) inflammation of an antrum, especially of the antrum of Highmore (maxillary sinus).

antroatticotomy (an″tro-at″ĭ-kot′o-me) atticoantrotomy.

antrocele (an′tro-sēl) accumulation of fluid in the maxillary antrum (sinus).

antrodynia (an″tro-din′e-ah) pain in the antrum.

antronasal (an″tro-na′zal) pertaining to maxillary antrum (sinus) and nasal fossa.

antroscope (an′tro-skōp) an instrument for inspecting antrum of Highmore (maxillary sinus).

antrostomy (an-tros′to-me) incision of an antrum with drainage.

antrotomy (an-trot′o-me) incision of an antrum.

antrotympanic (an″tro-tim-pan′ik) pertaining to the tympanic (mastoid) antrum and tympanum.

antrotympanitis (an″tro-tim″pah-ni′tis) inflammation of the tympanic (mastoid) antrum and tympanum.

antrum (an′trum), pl. an′tra [L.] a cavity or chamber. adj., an′tral.
  a. of Highmore, maxillary sinus.
  mastoid a., an air space in the mastoid portion of the temporal bone communicating with the middle ear and the mastoid cells.
  a. maxilla′re, maxillary a., maxillary sinus.
  pyloric a., a. pylor′icum, the proximal, expanded portion of the pyloric part of the stomach.
  tympanic a., a. tympan′icum, mastoid antrum.

Anturane (an'tu-rān) trademark for a preparation of sulfinpyrazone, a uricosuric agent used in the management of gout.

anuclear (a-nu'kle-ar) having no nucleus.

anulus (an'u-lus), pl. *an'uli* [L.] alternate spelling of *annulus;* used in names of certain ringlike or encircling structures of the body.

anuresis (an"u-re'sis) complete suppression of urine secretion by the kidneys. adj., **anuret'ic.**

anuria (ah-nu're-ah) diminution of urine secretion to 100 ml. or less in 24 hours. adj., **anu'ric.**

anus (a'nus) the opening of the rectum on the body surface.
   imperforate a., congenital absence of the normal opening of the rectum.

anvil (an'vil) incus; the middle of the three bones of the ear.

anxietas (ang-zi'ĕ-tas) [L.] anxiety; unrest.
   a. tibia'rum, a condition of restlessness leading to constant change of position of the legs.

anxiety (ang-zi'ĕ-te) a feeling of uneasiness, apprehension or dread. This may be rational, such as the anxiety about making good in a new job, about one's own or someone else's illness, about passing an examination or about moving to a new community. People also feel realistic anxiety about world dangers, such as the possibility of nuclear war, and about social and economic changes that may affect their livelihood or way of living. Modern mass communications tend to intensify normal anxieties about large issues by dramatizing minor incidents as though they were major crises.

A certain amount of unrealistic and irrational anxiety also is part of most people's experience. Some degree of generalized anxiety seems to be an unavoidable part of the human personality, since life is full of uncertainties and human beings have an awareness of past and future. Certain periods of life also generate increased anxiety; adolescence and middle age are especially anxious times for many. Persons who spend much of their time alone are likely to suffer more anxiety than those who live and work with others.

Most persons find healthy ways to deal with their normal quota of anxiety. They seek out friends and interesting activities; they take their minds off their own anxious feelings by listening to and doing things for other people. The enjoyment of art, music and literature, especially when it is shared, is an antidote to anxiety. The physical activity of games and sports, preferably with companions and out of doors, is one of the best antidotes. A good walk often dissipates an anxious mood.

Overindulgence in alcohol does not alleviate anxiety but only makes it worse. When a cause of anxiety is real, then the healthy step is to take realistic measures against it; for example, a real anxiety about money should be dealt with by improving money management or income or both.

When anxiety is chronic and not traceable to any specific cause, or when it interferes with normal activity, then it is neurotic, and the sufferer is in need of some wholesome self-examination and possibly expert help.

Anxiety that needs attention can often be readily recognized by family or friends or by the family physician. Parents should be alert to symptoms of anxiety in their children. For instance, a child may develop compulsive habits, like overeating, or he may lose his appetite for no apparent reason. He may seem to want to spend an abnormal amount of time on his own; he may have difficulty with his schoolwork, or he may develop frequent headaches or stomachaches as a result of anxiety about school or friends. In a younger child, excessive thumb-sucking or an unusual attachment to a particular plaything can sometimes be a sign of the kind of anxiety that needs professional help. Any important change in a young child's life, such as moving to a new home or the illness or absence of a parent, can give rise to behavior problems stemming from anxiety. Similarly in adults, insomnia, recurrent headaches or the development of compulsive habits may be signs of chronic anxiety.

Whether it is purely psychologic or arises from a real situation, severe anxiety can often be controlled by the proper use of medications, such as tranquilizers, under a physician's care. PSYCHOTHERAPY is frequently the most effective method to relieve cases of chronic anxiety.

   a.-equivalent, translation of anxiety into a kind of emotional activity, e.g., the experiencing or expression of angry feelings.
   free-floating a., fear in the absence of known cause for anxiety.
   a. neurosis, a neurosis characterized by anxiety or extreme fear without apparent cause. Anxiety is regarded as pathologic when the individual cannot control his emotions and the anxiety interferes with effectiveness in living and the achievement of desired goals or satisfactions. The neurosis may be manifest as organic pain or physical illness.
   separation a., apprehension due to removal of significant persons or familiar surroundings, common in infants 6 to 10 months old.

aorta (a-or'tah), pl. *aor'tae* [Gr.], *aor'tas* the great artery arising from left ventricle (see also CIRCULATORY SYSTEM).
   abdominal a., the part of the descending aorta below the diaphragm.
   ascending a., the proximal segment of the aorta, from the orifice of the heart to the arch.
   descending a., the distal segment of the aorta, extending from the arch to the point of bifurcation into the common iliac arteries.
   thoracic a., the part of the descending aorta above the diaphragm.

aortalgia (a"or-tal'je-ah) pain in the region of the aorta.

aortarctia (a"or-tark'she-ah) narrowing of the aorta.

aortectasia (a"or-tek-ta'ze-ah) dilatation of the aorta.

aortic (a-or'tik) pertaining to the aorta.
   a. bodies, small groups of chromophil cells on either side of the aorta in the region of the inferior mesenteric artery which act as chemoreceptors.
   a. valve, a semilunar valve that guards the orifice between the left ventricle and the aorta.

aortitis (a"or-ti'tis) inflammation of aorta.

aortoclasia (a-or"to-kla'ze-ah) rupture of the aorta.

aortogram (a-or′to-gram) the film produced by aortography.

aortography (a″or-tog′rah-fe) roentgenography of the aorta after introduction into it of a contrast material.

aortolith (a-or′to-lith) a calculus in the aorta.

aortomalacia (a-or″to-mah-la′she-ah) softening of the aorta.

aortopathy (a″or-top′ah-the) noninflammatory disease of the aorta.

aortorrhaphy (a″or-tor′ah-fe) suture of the aorta.

aortosclerosis (a-or″to-sklĕ-ro′sis) sclerosis of the aorta.

aortostenosis (a-or″to-stĕ-no′sis) narrowing of the aorta.

aortotomy (a″or-tot′o-me) incision of the aorta.

Apamide (ap′ah-mīd) trademark for a preparation of acetaminophen, an analgesic and antipyretic.

apancreatic (ah-pan″kre-at′ik) 1. not pertaining to the pancreas. 2. due to absence of the pancreas.

apandria (ap-an′dre-ah) aversion to men.

apanthropy (ap-an′thro-pe) aversion to human society.

aparalytic (ah″par-ah-lit′ik) characterized by absence of paralysis.

aparthrosis (ap″ar-thro′sis) diarthrosis.

apathic (ah-path′ik) without sensation or feeling.

apathism (ap′ah-thizm) slowness of response to stimuli.

apathy (ah′pah-the) reactive absence of emotions. adj., **apathet′ic.**

APC abbreviation for acetylsalicylic acid, acetophenetidin and caffeine, used as an analgesic or antipyretic.

APE anterior pituitary extract.

apepsia (ah-pep′se-ah) cessation or failure of digestive function.
  a. nervo′sa, anorexia nervosa.

aperient (ah-pe′re-ent) 1. mildly cathartic. 2. a gentle purgative.

aperistalsis (ah″per-ĭ-stal′sis) absence of peristaltic action.

apertura (ap″er-tu′rah), pl. *apertu′rae* [L.] aperture.

aperture (ap′er-tūr) an opening.
  numerical a., an expression of the measure of efficiency of a microscope objective.

apex (a′peks), pl. *a′pices* [L.] the pointed end of a cone-shaped part. adj., **ap′ical.**
  root a., the terminal end of the root of the tooth.

Apgar score (ap′gar) a method for determining an infant's condition at birth by scoring the heart rate, respiratory effort, muscle tone, reflex irritability and color.

A.P.H.A. American Public Health Association.

aphacia (ah-fa′se-ah) aphakia.

aphagia (ah-fa′je-ah) loss of the power of swallowing.

aphagopraxia (ah-fa″go-prak′se-ah) inability to swallow.

aphakia (ah-fa′ke-ah) absence of the lens of an eye, occurring congenitally or as a result of trauma or surgery. adj., **apha′kic.**

aphalangia (ah″fah-lan′je-ah) absence of fingers or toes.

aphasia (ah-fa′ze-ah) disturbance or loss of ability to comprehend, elaborate or express speech concepts. adj., **apha′sic.**
  amnestic a., inability to remember words.
  ataxic a., aphasia in which the patient knows what he wishes to say, but cannot utter the words.
  auditory a., loss of ability to comprehend spoken language.
  Broca's a., ataxic aphasia.
  conduction a., aphasia due to a lesion of the pathway between the sensory and motor speech centers.
  jargon a., paraphasia; aphasia characterized by misuse of words.
  mixed a., combined motor and sensory aphasia.
  motor a., loss of ability to express one's thoughts in speech or writing.
  sensory a., inability to comprehend spoken (auditory aphasia) or written (visual aphasia) language.
  visual a., loss of ability to comprehend written language.

aphasiology (ah-fa″ze-ol′o-je) scientific study of aphasia and specific neurologic lesions producing it.

aphemia (ah-fe′me-ah) loss of the power of speech due to a central lesion.

aphephobia (af″ĕ-fo′be-ah) morbid dread of being touched.

aphonia (a-fo′ne-ah) loss of the voice; inability to produce vocal sounds.
  a. clerico′rum, loss of the voice from overuse, as by clergymen.

aphonic (a-fon′ik) 1. pertaining to aphonia. 2. without audible sound.

aphose (ah′fōz) any subjective visual sensation due to absence or interrruption of light sensation.

aphosphorosis (ah-fos″fo-ro′sis) a condition caused by deficiency of phosphorus in the diet.

aphotic (a-fōt′ik) without light; totally dark.

aphrasia (ah-fra′ze-ah) inability to speak.
  a. parano′ica, stubborn and willful silence.

aphrenia (ah-fre′ne-ah) 1. dementia. 2. unconsciousness.

aphrodisiac (af″ro-diz′e-ak) 1. arousing sexual desire. 2. a drug that arouses sexual desire.

aphtha (af′thah), pl. *aph′thae* [L.] a whitish spot. adj., **aph′thous.**

aphthosis (af-tho′sis) a condition marked by presence of aphthae.

aphylaxis (ah″fi-lak′sis) absence of phylaxis or immunity. adj., **aphylac′tic.**

apicectomy (a″pĭ-sek′to-me) apicoectomy.

apicitis (a″pĭ-si′tis) inflammation of the apex of the lung or of the root of a tooth.

apicoectomy (a″pĭ-ko-ek′to-me) excision of the apical portion of the root of a tooth through an opening in overlying tissues of the jaw.

apicolysis (a″pĭ-kol′ĭ-sis) collapse of the apex of the lung, with obliteration of the apical cavity.

apituitarism (ah″pĭ-tu′ĭ-tar-izm″) absence of a functioning pituitary gland.

A.P.L. anterior pituitary-like.

aplacental (a″plah-sen′tal) having no placenta.

aplanatic (ap″lah-nat′ik) correcting or not affected by spherical aberration.

aplasia (ah-pla′ze-ah) absence of an organ due to failure of development of the embryonic primordium.

aplastic (a-plas′tik) pertaining to or characterized by aplasia; having no tendency to develop into new tissue.

   a. anemia, the medical name given to anemia caused by disease of the bone marrow, which produces most of the blood cells. In addition to the usual symptoms of anemia, there is frequently bleeding from the nose and mouth and "black and blue" spots on the skin.

   Aplastic anemia may be caused by a tumor or cancer of the bone marrow, or by destruction of the bone marrow by other agents, including excessive radiation; some antibiotics; sulfonamides; phenylbutazone; mephytoin; insecticides or weed killers; benzene; certain hair dyes; and medicines containing heavy metals such as gold, mercury and bismuth. The physician will question the patient very closely about possible contact with such substances, since determining the cause of the disorder may be crucial in treating it.

   Aplastic anemia is serious, and should be treated in a hospital. The most effective treatment is removal of the cause, if possible. Regular transfusions of blood are almost always necessary. In some cases, injections of cortisone have appeared to relieve the condition.

   Individual cases of aplastic anemia vary a great deal, and may respond to treatment so successfully that transfusions can be stopped. Generally, however, the outlook for a patient with aplastic anemia is not good, although better than was thought in the past.

   See also ANEMIA for nursing care.

apnea (ap′ne-ah) 1. temporary cessation of breathing. 2. asphyxia. adj., **apne′ic.**

apneumia (ap-nu′me-ah) a developmental anomaly with absence of the lungs.

apneusis (ap-nu′sis) sustained inspiratory effort, even to the point of asphyxia. adj., **apneu′stic.**

apo- (ap′o) word element [Gr.], *away from; separated.*

apochromatic (ap″o-kro-mat′ik) free from chromatic aberration.

apocrine (ap′o-krin) denoting that type of glandular secretion in which the secretory products become concentrated at the free end of the secreting cell and are thrown off, along with the portion of the cell where they have accumulated, as in the mammary gland; cf. holocrine and merocrine.

apodia (ah-po′de-ah) a developmental anomaly with absence of the feet.

apoenzyme (ap″o-en′zīm) the portion of the enzyme that requires the presence of coenzyme to become a complete enzyme.

apoferritin (ap″o-fer′ĭ-tin) a colorless protein occurring in the mucosal cells of the small intestine, forming a compound with iron called ferritin, which has been implicated in the regulation of iron absorption in the gastrointestinal tract.

apogee (ap′o-je) the state of greatest severity of a disease.

apolar (ah-po′lar) having neither poles nor processes; without polarity.

apolepsis (ap″o-lep′sis) suppression of a natural secretion.

apomorphine (ap″o-mor′fēn) an alkaloid from morphine.

   a. hydrochloride, a crystalline alkaloid that is a prompt and effective emetic; used to produce vomiting in certain kinds of poisoning.

aponeurectomy (ap″o-nu-rek′to-me) excision of an aponeurosis.

aponeurorrhaphy (ap″o-nu-ror′ah-fe) suture of an aponeurosis.

aponeurosis (ap″o-nu-ro′sis), pl. *aponeuro′ses* [Gr.] a sheetlike tendon attaching or investing muscles. adj., **aponeurot′ic.**

aponeurositis (ap″o-nu-ro-si′tis) inflammation of an aponeurosis.

aponeurotomy (ap″o-nu-rot′o-me) incision of an aponeurosis.

apophylaxis (ap″o-fi-lak′sis) decrease in the phylactic power of the blood.

apophyseal (ap″o-fiz′e-al) pertaining to an apophysis.

apophysis (ah-pof′ĭ-sis), pl. *apoph′yses* [Gr.] any outgrowth or swelling, especially a bony outgrowth that has never been entirely separated from the bone of which it forms a part, such as a process, tubercle or tuberosity.

apoplectoid (ap″o-plek′toid) resembling a stroke or seizure.

apoplexy (ap′o-plek″se) copious extravasation of blood into an organ; often used alone to designate such extravasations into the brain (cerebral apoplexy) after rupture of an intracranial blood vessel; stroke. (See also CEREBRAL VASCULAR ACCIDENT.) adj., **apoplec′tic.**

aposia (ah-po′ze-ah) absence of thirst.

apositia (ap″o-sish′e-ah) disgust or loathing for food. adj., **aposit′ic.**

apostasis (ah-pos′tah-sis) 1. an abscess. 2. an exfoliation.

apostema (ap″o-ste′ma) an abscess.

aposthia (ah-pos′the-ah) absence of the prepuce.

apothecaries' weights and measures (ah-poth′-ĕ-ka″rēz) a system used for measuring and weighing drugs and solutions. This system of measurement was brought to the United States from England during the colonial period; it is gradually being replaced by the metric system.

In the apothecaries' system fractions are used to designate portions of a unit of measure: e.g., one-fourth grain is written gr. 1/4. The fraction 1/2 is written ss.

There are two symbols in this system which are sometimes confused and always must be written clearly. These are the symbols for drams and ounces. Small Roman numerals are used after the symbols. For example, ʒiss reads drams one and one-half; ℥iii reads ounces three. (See also Table of Weights and Measures in the Appendix.)

apothecary (ah-poth′ĕ-ka″re) a person who compounds and dispenses drugs.

apotripsis (ap″o-trip′sis) removal of a corneal opacity.

apparatus (ap″ah-ra′tus) 1. mechanical appliances used in diagnosis, therapy or experimentation. 2. the complex parts which unite in any function.

Abbe-Zeiss a., a device for counting blood corpuscles.

Golgi a., an irregular complex of parallel membranes and vesicles in a cell, thought to play a role in its secretory activity.

Wangensteen's a., a nasal suction apparatus connected with a duodenal tube for aspirating gas and fluid from stomach and intestine.

appendage (ah-pen′dij) a less important portion of an organ, or an outgrowth, such as a tail.

appendectomy (ap″en-dek′to-me) excision of the vermiform appendix.

appendicectasis (ah-pen″dĭ-sek′tah-sis) dilatation of the vermiform appendix.

appendicitis (ah-pen″dĭ-si′tis) inflammation of the vermiform appendix. Appendicitis is a serious disease, usually requiring surgery. When performed early by a competent surgeon, the operation is comparatively simple and safe. When the appendix becomes inflamed and infected, rupture may occur within a matter of hours. Rupture of the appendix leads to PERITONITIS, one of the most serious of all diseases, although its danger has been reduced by antibiotics.

CAUSE. If the tubelike appendix becomes plugged by a hard bit of fecal matter or by intestinal worms, or becomes inflamed from other causes, normal drainage cannot take place. The appendix then becomes susceptible to bacterial infection. Streptococci, *Escherichia coli* (colon bacilli) and other types of germs multiply and cause inflammation which will spread into the peritoneal cavity unless (1) the body's defenses overcome the infection or (2) a surgeon removes the infected appendix before it ruptures.

There are usually three main symptoms: (1) nausea, (2) abdominal pain, which may localize in the lower right abdomen over the appendix area and (3) mild fever in adults, sometimes high fever in young children. There may also be vomiting, constipation or diarrhea.

DIAGNOSIS. The physician looks for positive evidence of an inflamed appendix. There may be tenderness over the appendix when pressure is exerted there. Sometimes pain is experienced in the region of the appendix during an examination through the rectum, or through the vagina in a female. A laboratory test, the leukocyte count, is also helpful in making the diagnosis. The physician always searches for other diseases that are sometimes mistaken for appendicitis, such as gallbladder attacks or kidney infection on the right side. The onset of pneumonia, rheumatic fever or dia-

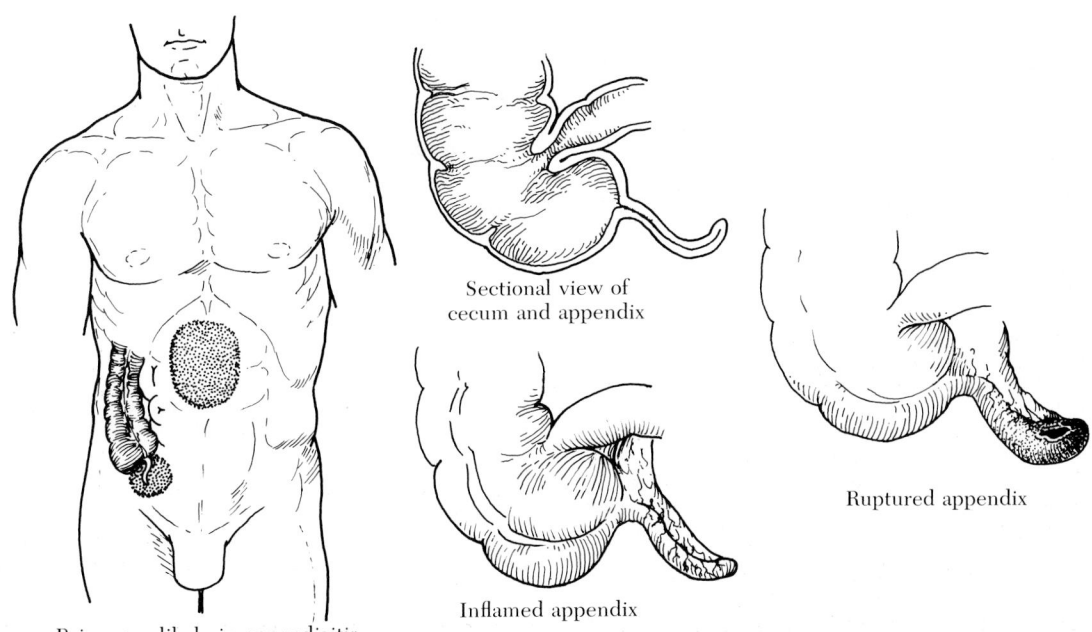

Sectional view of cecum and appendix

Inflamed appendix

Ruptured appendix

Pain areas likely in appendicitis

betic coma may imitate appendicitis. In women, there is the possibility of a ruptured ECTOPIC PREGNANCY, a twisted ovarian cyst or a hemorrhaging ovarian follicle at the middle of the menstrual cycle.

NURSING CARE. When appendicitis is suspected because of symptoms exhibited by the patient, a physician should be notified immediately. The patient should lie down and remain as quiet as possible. It is best to give him nothing by mouth, and because of the danger of aggravating the condition and possibly causing rupture of the appendix, cathartics and laxatives are contraindicated. Applications of heat are contraindicated for the same reasons. After the patient has been seen by the physician and a diagnosis of appendicitis has been established, surgical removal of the appendix (appendectomy) will probably be performed as soon as possible. Routine PREOPERATIVE CARE is then indicated.

appendicolithiasis   (ah-pen″dĭ-ko-lĭ-thi′-ah-sis) formation of calculi in the vermiform appendix.

appendicolysis   (ah-pen″dĭ-kol′ĭ-sis) surgical separation of adhesions binding the appendix.

appendicopathy   (ah-pen″dĭ-kop′ah-the) any disease of the vermiform appendix.

appendicosis   (ah-pen″dĭ-ko′sis) a noninflammatory lesion of the appendix.

appendicostomy   (ah-pen″dĭ-kos′to-me) surgical creation of an opening into the vermiform appendix.

appendicular   (ap″en-dik′u-lar) 1. pertaining to an appendix or appendage. 2. pertaining to the limbs.

appendix   (ah-pen′diks), pl. *appen′dices.* [L.] 1. a slender outgrowth or appendage. 2. the vermiform appendix, a small appendage near the juncture of the small intestine and the large intestine (ileocecal valve). An apparently useless structure, it can be the source of a serious illness, APPENDICITIS. adj., **appendic′eal.**

apperception   (ap″er-sep′shun) conscious perception of a sensory stimulus.

appestat   (ap′pĕ-stat) a center in the hypothalamus thought to control the appetite.

appetite   (ap′ĕ-tīt) the desire for food. It is stimulated by the sight, smell or thought of food and accompanied by the flow of saliva in the mouth and gastric juice in the stomach. The stomach wall also receives an extra blood supply in preparation for its digestive activity.

Appetite is psychologic, dependent on memory and associations, as compared with hunger, which is physiologically aroused by the body's need for food. Appetite can be discouraged by unattractive food, surroundings or company, and by emotional states such as anxiety, irritation, anger and fear.

Chronic loss of appetite is known as anorexia. It may be a symptom of physical disorders, or it may be related to emotional disturbances, in which case it is known as anorexia nervosa. Excessive appetite may be an indication of metabolic disorders or may be caused by emotional disturbances. This latter condition is especially common among children, particularly girls, who may develop a habit of compulsive eating to compensate for a feeling of insecurity.

apposition   (ap″o-zish′un   the placement or position of adjacent structures or parts so that they can come into contact.

apprehension   (ap″re-hen′shun) 1. perception and understanding. 2. anticipatory fear or anxiety.

approximal   (ah-prok′sĭ-mal) close together.

apraxia   (ah-prak′se-ah) impairment of the ability to use objects correctly.
   amnestic a., loss of ability to carry out a movement on command due to inability to remember the command.
   motor a., loss of ability to make proper use of an object.
   sensory a., loss of ability to make proper use of an object due to lack of perception of its purpose.

Apresoline   (ah-pres′o-lēn) trademark for preparations of hydralazine hydrochloride, an antihypertensive drug.

aprobarbital   (ap″ro-bar′bĭ-tal) a crystalline powder, an intermediate-acting sedative and hypnotic.

aproctia   (ah-prok′she-ah) imperforation of the anus.

aprosopia   (ap″ro-so′pe-ah) a developmental anomaly with partial or complete absence of the face.

aptyalism   (ap-ti′ah-lizm) deficiency or absence of saliva.

apus   (a′pus) a fetal monster without one or both feet.

apyogenous   (ah″pi-oj′ĕ-nus) not caused by pus.

apyretic   (ah″pi-ret′ik) without fever.

apyrexia   (ah-pi-rek′se-ah) absence of fever.

apyrogenic   (ah-pi″ro-jen′ik) not producing fever.

aq. [L.] *aq′ua* (water).
   aq. dest., *aq′ua destilla′ta* (distilled water).

aqua   (ak′wah) [L.] 1. water, H_2O. 2. a saturated solution of a volatile oil or other aromatic or volatile substance in purified water.

aquaphobia   (ak″wah-fo′be-ah) morbid fear of water.

aqueduct   (ak′wĕ-dukt″) any canal or passage.
   cerebral a., a cavity of the midbrain connecting the third and fourth ventricles and containing cerebrospinal fluid.
   a. of cochlea, a foramen in the temporal bone for a vein from the cochlea.
   a. of Fallopius, the canal for the facial nerve in pars petrosa of the temporal bone.
   sylvian a., a. of Sylvius, ventricular a., a canal connecting the third and fourth ventricles of the brain.

aqueous   (a′kwe-us) water; prepared with water.
   a. humor, the fluid produced in the eye, occupying the anterior and posterior chambers, and diffusing out of the eye into the blood; regarded as lymph of the eye, its composition varies from that of lymph in the body generally.

aquocapsulitis   (ak″wo-kap″su-li′tis) serous inflammation of the iris.

arachnephobia (ah-rak″ně-fo′be-ah) arachnophobia.

Arachnida (ar-ak′nĭ-dah) a class of animals of the phylum Arthropoda, including 12 orders, comprising such forms as spiders, scorpions, ticks and mites.

arachnidism (ah-rak′nĭ-dizm) poisoning from a spider bite.

arachnitis (ar″ak-ni′tis) arachnoiditis.

arachnodactyly (ah-rak″no-dak′tĭ-le) extreme length and slenderness of the fingers or toes, seen in Marfan's syndrome.

arachnoid (ah-rak′noid) 1. resembling a spider's web. 2. the delicate membrane interposed between the dura mater and the pia mater, and with them constituting the meninges.

arachnoiditis (ah-rak″noid-i′tis) inflammation of the arachnoid membrane.

arachnophobia (ah-rak″no-fo′be-ah) morbid fear of spiders.

arachnopia (ah-rak″no-pi′ah) the pia mater and arachnoid membrane together.

Aralen (ar′ah-len) trademark for a preparation of choroquine, an antimalarial used also in treatment of amebic abscess and lupus erythematosus.

Aramine (ar′ah-min) trademark for a preparation of metaraminol, a sympathomimetic and vasopressor.

Aran-Duchenne disease (ar-ahn′ du-shen′) myelopathic muscular atrophy.

araphia (ah-ra′fe-ah) failure of closure of the neural tube, the spinal cord developing as a flat plate. adj., **ara′phic.**

arbor (ar′bor), pl. *arbo′res* [L.] a tree.
   a. vi′tae, 1. treelike outlines seen on median section of the cerebellum. 2. a series of ridges within cervix uteri.

arborescent (ar″bo-res′ent) branching like a tree.

arborization (ar″bor-ĭ-za′shun) a collection of branches, as the branching terminus of a nerve-cell process.

arborvirus, arbovirus (ar″bor-vi′rus), (ar″bo-vi′rus) a group of viruses that are transmitted to man by mosquitoes and ticks. (See also VIRUS.)

A.R.C. American Red Cross.

arc (ark) a part of the circumference of a circle, or a regularly curved line.
   binauricular a., the arc across the top of the head from one auricular point to the other.
   reflex a., the circuit traveled by impulses producing a reflex action: receptor organ, afferent nerve, nerve center, efferent nerve, effector organ in a muscle. (See also REFLEX.)

arcate (ar′kāt) curved; bow-shaped.

arch (arch) a structure of bowlike or curved outline.

abdominothoracic a., the lower boundary of the front of the thorax.
   a. of aorta, the curving portion between the ascending aorta, giving rise to the truncus brachiocephalicus, the left common carotid and the left subclavian artery.
   aortic a's, a series of five pairs of arterial arches of the embryo in the region of the neck.
   branchial a's, four pairs of mesenchymal and later cartilaginous arches of the fetus in the region of the neck.
   dental a., the curving structure formed by the crowns of the teeth in their normal position, or by the residual ridge after loss of the teeth.
   a's of foot, the longitudinal and transverse arches of the foot. The longitudinal arch comprises the pars medialis, formed by the calcaneus, talus and the navicular, cuneiform and the first three tarsal bones; and the pars lateralis formed by the calcaneus, the cuboid bone and the lateral two metatarsal bones. The transverse arch comprises the navicular, cuneiform, cuboid and five metatarsal bones.
   lingual a., a wire appliance that conforms to the lingual aspect of the dental arch, used to secure movement of the teeth in orthodontic work.
   mandibular a., the first branchial arch, being the rudiment of the maxillary and manidibular regions.
   neural a., vertebral arch.
   palatal a., the arch formed by the roof of the mouth from the teeth on one side to those on the other.
   pubic a., the arch formed by the conjoined rami of the ischium and pubis of the two sides of the body.
   pulmonary a's, the most caudal of the aortic arches, which become the pulmonary arteries.
   tendinous a., a linear thickening of fascia over some part of a muscle.
   vertebral a., the dorsal bony arch of a vertebra, enclosing the cerebrospinal nervous system; it is composed of the laminae and pedicles of a vertebra.
   zygomatic a., the arch formed by the processes of the zygomatic and temporal bones.

arch(i)- (ar′ke) word element [Gr.], *ancient; beginning; first; original.*

archebiosis, archegenesis (ar″ke-bi-o′sis), (ar″ke-jen′ě-sis) abiogenesis.

archencephalon (ark″en-sef′ah-lon) the primitive brain from which the midbrain and forebrain develop.

archenteron (ark-en′ter-on) the central cavity that is the provisional gut in the gastrula; the primitive digestive cavity of the embryo.

archeokinetic (ar″ke-o-ki-net′ik) relating to the primitive type of motor nerve mechanism as seen in the peripheral and ganglionic nervous systems.

archesporium (ar″ke-spo′re-um) the cell giving rise to spore mother cells.

archetype (ar′kě-tīp) in psychology, a type unconsciously considered to be the universal standard or ideal.

archinephron (ar″kĭ-nef′ron) the pronephros.

archineuron (ar″kĭ-nu′ron) the neuron at which efferent impulse starts.

archipallium (ar″kĭ-pal′e-um) that portion of the pallium, or gray matter, which phylogenetically is the first to show the characteristic layering of the cellular elements.

architis (ar-ki′tis) proctitis.

arciform (ar′sĭ-form) arcuate.

arctation (ark-ta′shun) narrowing of an opening or canal.

arcuate (ar′ku-āt) bent like a bow.

arcuation (ar″ku-a′shun) a bending or curvature.

arcus (ar′kus), pl. *ar′cus* [L.] arch; bow.
 a. adipo′sus, arcus senilis.
 a. juveni′lis, an opaque line partially encircling the margin of the cornea, occurring congenitally in children.
 a. seni′lis, an opaque line partially surrounding the margin of the cornea, usually occurring bilaterally in persons of 50 years or older as a result of lipoid degeneration.

area (a′re-ah), pl. *a′reae, areas* [L.] a limited space or plane surface.
 association a's, areas of the cerebral cortex not themselves functionally differentiated, but connected with other centers and the neothalamus by numerous fibers.
 Broca's a., an area in the left (or right) inferior frontal gyrus; called also area subcallosa and Broca's center. It is the cortical area controlling the motor aspects of speech.
 Brodmann's a's, specific occipital and preoccipital areas of the cerebral cortex, identified by number, which are considered to be the seat of specific functions of the brain.
 germinal a., a. germinati′va, the part of the ovum where the embryo is formed.
 Kiesselbach's a., an area on the anterior part of the nasal septum, richly supplied with capillaries, and a common site of epistaxis (nosebleed).
 motor a., the ascending frontal and ascending parietal convolutions of the brain where the nerve centers for motion are thought to be situated.
 projection a's, the areas of the cerebral cortex that are concerned in the sensory and motor functions of the brain.
 psychomotor a., the area of the cerebral cortex concerned with the initiation of motor impulses.
 silent a., an area of the brain in which pathologic conditions may occur without producing symptoms.
 a. subcallo′sa, Broca's area.
 vocal a., the part of the glottis between the vocal cords.

arecoline (ah-rek′o-lin) a compound used as a parasympathomimetic agent.

areflexia (ah″re-flek′se-ah) absence of the reflexes.

areola (ah-re′o-lah), pl. *are′olae* [L.] a narrow zone surrounding a central area, e.g., the darkened area surrounding the nipple of the mammary gland.
 Chaussier's a., the indurated area encircling a malignant pustule.

areolar (ah-re′o-lar) 1. containing minute spaces. 2. pertaining to an areola.

areometer (ar″e-om′ĕ-ter) hydrometer.

Arfonad (ar′fon-ad) trademark for a preparation of trimethaphan, a ganglion-blocking agent and antihypertensive.

Argas (ar′gas) a genus of arthropods parasitic in poultry and other birds and sometimes man.

Argasidae (ar-gas′ĭ-de) a family of arthropods made up of the soft-bodied ticks.

argentaffin (ar-jen′tah-fin) staining readily with silver.

argentaffinoma (ar″jen-taf″fĭ-no′mah) a tumor arising from argentaffin cells, most frequently in the terminal ileum or the appendix; called also carcinoid.

argentum (ar-jen′tum) [L.] silver (symbol Ag).

argillaceous (ar″jĭ-la′shus) composed of clay.

arginase (ar′jĭ-nās) an enzyme of the liver that splits arginine.

arginine (ar′jĭ-nin) a basic amino acid produced by the hydrolysis or digestion of proteins.

argininosuccinic acid (ar″jĭ-ne′no-suk-sin″ik) a compound normally formed in urea formation in the liver, but not normally present in urine.

argininosuccinicaciduria (ar″jĭ-ne″no-suk-sin″-ik-as″ĭ-du′re-ah) excretion in the urine of argininosuccinic acid, a feature of an inborn error of metabolism marked also by mental retardation.

argon (ar′gon) a chemical element, atomic number 18, atomic weight 39.948, symbol Ar. (See table of ELEMENTS.)

argyria (ar-jĭ′re-ah) discoloration of skin and mucous membranes from excessive use of silver salts.

argyric (ar-jĭ′rik) pertaining to silver.

argyrism (ar′jĭ-rizm) argyria.

Argyrol (ar′jĭ-rol) trademark for a preparation of mild silver protein that is used as an antiseptic on mucous membranes.

argyrophil (ar-ji′ro-fil) easily impregnated with silver.

argyrosis (ar″jĭ-ro′sis) argyria.

arhigosis (ah″rĭ-go′sis) inability to perceive cold.

arhinia (ah-rin′e-ah) a developmental anomaly with absence of the nose.

arhythmia (ah-rith′me-ah) arrhythmia.

ariboflavinosis (a-ri″bo-fla″vĭ-no′sis) deficiency of RIBOFLAVIN (vitamin B₂) in the diet, a condition marked by lesions in the corners of the mouth, on the lips and around the nose and eyes, malaise, weakness, weight loss and, in severe cases, corneal or other eye changes and seborrheic dermatitis.

Aristocort (ah-ris′to-cort) trademark for a preparation of triamcinolone, a prednisolone derivative used as an anti-inflammatory steroid.

arithmomania (ah-rith″mo-ma′ne-ah) a psychoneurotic compulsion to count objects, with concern for accuracy or significant numbers.

Arlidin (ar′lĭ-din) trademark for preparation of nylidrin, a peripheral vasodilator.

arm (arm) 1. the upper extremity, from shoulder to elbow; often used to denote the entire extremity, from shoulder to wrist. 2. an armlike part, e.g., the portion of the chromatid extending in either direction from the centromere of a mitotic chromosome.
    brawny a., a hard, swollen condition of the arm following mastectomy.

armamentarium (ar″mah-men-ta′re-um) the entire equipment of a practitioner, such as medicines, instruments, books.

arnica (ar′nĭ-kah) dried flowerheads of *Arnica montana,* used as an alcoholic extract or tincture as a skin irritant.

aromatic (ar″o-mat′ik) 1. having a spicy fragrance. 2. a stimulant, spicy medicine. 3. pertaining to or derived from the benzene ring; having a closed-chain structure.

arrector (ah-rek′tor), pl. *arrecto′res* [L.] an erector muscle.

arrest (ah-rest′) sudden cessation or stoppage.
    cardiac a., sudden cessation of beating of the heart (see also CARDIAC ARREST).
    epiphyseal a., arrest of the longitudinal growth of bone by surgical fusion of the epiphysis and diaphysis.
    maturation a., interruption of the process of development, as of blood cells, before the final stage is reached.

arrheno- (ah-re′no) word element [Gr.], *male; masculine.*

arrhenoblastoma (ah-re″no-blas-to′mah) a rare ovarian tumor that causes development of masculine qualities.

arrhinia (ah-rin′e-ah) arhinia.

arrhythmia (ah-rith′me-ah) variation from the normal rhythm, especially of the heartbeat. adj., **arrhyth′mic.**
    sinus a., irregularity of the heartbeat dependent on interference with the impulses originating at the sinoatrial node.

arseniasis (ar″sĭ-ni′ah-sis) arsenical poisoning.

arsenic (ar′sĕ-nik) a chemical element, atomic number 33, atomic weight 74.92, symbol As. (See table of ELEMENTS.) Arsenic compounds have been widely used in medicine; however, they have been replaced for the most part by antibiotics, which are less toxic and equally effective. Some of the arsenicals are used for infectious diseases, especially those caused by protozoa, and some skin disorders and blood dyscrasias also are treated with arsenic compounds. Since arsenic is highly toxic it must be administered with caution. The antidote for arsenic poisoning is DIMERCAPROL (BAL).
    a. trioxide, white a., white, odorless powder used as an irritant and escharotic.

arsenical (ar-sen′ĭ-kal) 1. pertaining to arsenic. 2. a compound containing arsenic.

arsenoblast (ar-sen′o-blast) the male element of a zygote; a male pronucleus.

arsenotherapy (ar″sĕ-no-ther′ah-pe) treatment with arsenic and arsenical compounds.

arsine (ar′sēn) a toxic gas, compounds of which have been used in warfare.

arsphenamine (ars-fen′ah-min) a light yellow powder containing 30 to 32 per cent of arsenic; used intravenously in syphilis, yaws and other protozoan infections.

arsthinol (ars′thĭ-nol) an arsenical preparation used for the treatment of intestinal amebiasis and yaws.

Artane (ar′tān) trademark for preparations of trihexyphenidyl hydrochloride, used as an anticholinergic and in treatment of Parkinson's disease.

artefact (ar′tĕ-fakt) artifact.

arterectomy (ar″ter-ek′to-me) excision of an artery.

arteria (ar-te′re-ah), pl. *arter′riae* [L.] artery.
    a. luso′ria, an abnormally situated vessel in the region of the aortic arch.

arterial (ar-te′re-al) pertaining to an artery or to the arteries.

arterialization (ar-te″re-al-ĭ-za′shun) the conversion of venous into arterial blood by the absorption of oxygen.

arteriarctia (ar-te″re-ark′she-ah) contraction of the lumen of an artery.

arteriasis (ar″tĕ-ri′ah-sis) degeneration of the walls of an artery.

arteriectasis (ar-te″re-ek′tah-sis) dilatation of an artery.

arteriectomy (ar-te″re-ek′to-me) excision of an artery.

arterio- (ar-te′re-o) word element [L., Gr.], *artery.*

arteriogram (ar-te′re-o-gram″) 1. a tracing of the arterial pulse. 2. a roentgenogram of an artery.

arteriography (ar-te″re-og′rah-fe) roentgenography of an artery or arterial system after injection of a contrast medium in the bloodstream.
    catheter a., roentgenography of vessels after introduction of contrast material through a catheter inserted into an artery.
    selective a., roentgenography of a specific vessel that is opacified by medium introduced through a catheter passed through the aorta to the site of origin of the vessel.

arteriol(o)- (ar-te″re-o′lo) word element [L.], *arteriole.*

arteriola (ar-te″re-o′lah), pl. *arterio′lae* [L.] arteriole.
    arterio′lae rec′tae re′nis, branches of the arteries of the kidney going to the renal pyramids.

arteriole (ar-te′re-ōl) a minute arterial branch. adj., **arterio′lar.**

  postglomerular a., a branch of the renal vascular system that conveys blood away from a glomerulus.

arteriolith (ar-te′re-o-lith″) a chalky concretion in an artery.

arteriolitis (ar-te″re-o-li′tis) inflammation of arterioles.

arteriology (ar-te″re-ol′o-je) sum of knowledge regarding the arteries.

arteriolonecrosis (ar-te″re-o″lo-ně-kro′sis) necrosis or destruction of arterioles.

arteriolosclerosis (ar-te″re-o″lo-sklě-ro′sis) thickening of the walls of the arterioles. adj., **arteriolosclerot′ic.**

arteriomalacia (ar-te″re-o″mah-la′she-ah) softening of the arterial wall.

arteriometer (ar-te″re-om′ě-ter) an instrument for measuring changes in the caliber of a beating artery.

arteriomotor (ar-te″re-o-mo′tor) causing dilation or constriction of arteries.

arteriomyomatosis (ar-te″re-o-mi″o-mah-to′sis) growth of muscular fibers in the walls of an artery, causing thickening.

arterionecrosis (ar-te″re-o-ně-kro′sis) necrosis of arteries.

arteriopathy (ar-te″re-op′ah-the) any disease of an artery.

  hypertensive a., involvement of the smaller arteries and arterioles, associated with hypertension and characterized by hypertrophy of the tunica media of the vessels.

arterioplasty (ar-te′re-o-plas″te) plastic repair of an artery.

arteriopressor (ar-te″re-o-pres′or) increasing arterial blood pressure.

arteriorrhaphy (ar-te″re-or′ah-fe) suture of an artery.

arteriorrhexis (ar-te″re-o-rek′sis) rupture of an artery.

arteriosclerosis (ar-te″re-o-sklě-ro′sis) thickening and loss of elasticity of the coats of the arteries, with inflammatory changes; popularly called hardening of the arteries. adj., **arteriosclerot′ic.**

  TYPES OF ARTERIOSCLEROSIS. Strictly speaking, there are two main types of arteriosclerosis: arteriosclerosis proper, in which the hardening is the result of fibrous and mineral deposits in the middle layer of the artery wall, and atherosclerosis, in which fatty and other substances collect in the inner lining of the arteries to form what are known as atheromatous plaques. These plaques encroach upon the passageway and gradually obstruct the flow of blood. Of the two types, atherosclerosis is by far the more common and more serious condition. When hardening of the arteries is referred to, in most cases it is atherosclerosis that is meant. For practical purposes, however, it is useful to group

arteriosclerosis and atherosclerosis together, and to speak of them as one disease.

  Arteriosclerosis is today one of the major killers and disablers in the United States. It is estimated that one million deaths a year can be traced to this source. It is a major cause of heart disease and of CEREBRAL VASCULAR ACCIDENT (stroke). Hardening of the arteries is common in middle and old age.

  CAUSES. The exact causes of arteriosclerosis are not yet known. However, several factors are thought to contribute to the disease. Heredity appears to play some part, since men in certain families have been found to be more susceptible than the average. The fact that women are seldom affected by arteriosclerosis before menopause suggests that the sex hormones have a connection with the disease. Arteriosclerosis may also arise in connection with other diseases. Persons suffering from DIABETES MELLITUS are especially susceptible and tend to develop the disease earlier in life than nondiabetics. Other conditions which may lead to arteriosclerosis include HYPERTENSION, hypothyroidism and certain disorders of metabolism, such as gout.

  One factor being investigated is the relationship of CHOLESTEROL, a fatty substance found in most tissues in the body, to atherosclerosis. There is evidence that a high cholesterol level in the blood often accompanies arteriosclerosis. Also, cholesterol levels appear to be higher when the fat in the diet contains an excess of saturated fatty acids, which are found in significant quantities in such foods as milk, dairy products, eggs and meat fats. For this reason, the American Heart Association has recommended that people balance their intake of these foods with foods containing unsaturated and polyunsaturated FATS. Unsaturated fats are found abundantly in vegetable oils; fish and poultry are also good sources. In recent years some extravagant claims have been made for food products which contain unsaturated fats.

  SYMPTOMS. The symptoms of arteriosclerosis depend on which arteries are most affected. Early symptoms may include coldness or numbness in the feet, dizziness, shortness of breath, headache and a tendency to tire easily. If the arteries in the legs are affected, there may be cramps, aches and sharp pains after even slight exercise. If the arteries that supply the brain are affected, mental symptoms, such as loss of memory, may develop. The symptoms of KIDNEY disease may follow hardening of the renal arteries and especially the arterioles.

  ARTERIOSCLEROSIS As A CAUSE OF OTHER DISEASES. As a major cause of HEART disease and other disorders, arteriosclerosis may manifest itself in various ways. If the coronary arteries, which supply blood to the heart muscle, are partly blocked, the result may be ANGINA PECTORIS, a pain or feeling of tightness in the chest. Sometimes the roughened lining of an affected artery can cause the blood to clot as it flows past. The blood flow may be obstructed, or the clot may break away from the artery wall and be carried through the bloodstream until it lodges and blocks the flow of blood elsewhere. More frequently an atheromatous plaque is the site of the formation of a blood clot. If this occurs in the coronary arteries, it can cause a CORONARY OCCLUSION or CORONARY THROMBOSIS, often called a heart attack. If the arteries supplying the brain are blocked suddenly, a cerebral thrombosis, or CEREBRAL VASCULAR ACCIDENT (stroke), can result. If the clot has formed in an artery of the neck, it can sometimes be removed surgically. In the arteries leading to, or in, the legs, a blockage, or peripheral thrombosis, can cut off circulation to the affected limb.

TREATMENT AND PREVENTION. At present there is no treatment that can reverse the effects of advanced arteriosclerosis. Once they have become hardened, there is no way to make the walls of the arteries more elastic or to get rid of the minerals and fats that have accumulated inside them. Instead, treatment concentrates on preventing the condition from becoming worse, or on allowing other arteries to enlarge as they make up for some of the lost blood supply. Nitroglycerin and related medicines help relieve the pain of angina pectoris. Chronic reduction of circulation by narrowing or weakening of the abdominal aorta or distal arteries in the lower extremities often can be corrected by vascular surgery and replacement of the diseased arterial segment. In cases of thrombosis it is sometimes possible to remove the clot by surgery.

Because of the suspected relationship between blood cholesterol and the development of arteriosclerosis, the patient may be placed on a diet low in cholesterol and saturated fats.

Rest and relaxation are also important. Regular exercise will probably be prescribed by the physician and should be followed. Smoking should be stopped or greatly curtailed. If the legs are seriously involved, shoes and clothing must be properly fitted to avoid blocking circulation further, and the feet should be carefully protected from cold, dampness and infection. Several drugs that may be helpful in treating arteriosclerosis are still in the experimental stage. Diseases such as diabetes mellitus, hypertension and gout that predispose to arteriosclerosis should be treated and controlled to slow their effect on the arteries.

Since the causes of arteriosclerosis are not fully understood, it is not certain whether taking precautions can prevent the onset of the disease. In part, the disease may be a natural effect of aging. However, avoiding obesity is very important for good health in general, and seems to help retard arteriosclerosis as well. Men over 35 should take special care to control their weight and their intake of the saturated fats found in meat and dairy products. Several small meals a day are probably better than one or two large ones.

Mönckeberg's a., arteriosclerosis characterized by calcification of the middle coat (tunica media) of the artery.

a. oblit'erans, arteriosclerosis in which proliferation of the intima has caused complete obliteration of the lumen of the artery.

arteriospasm (ar-te're-o-spazm″) spasm of an artery.

arteriostenosis (ar-te″re-o-stĕ-no′sis) constriction of an artery.

arteriosympathectomy (ar-te″re-o-sim″pah-thek′to-me) periarterial sympathectomy.

arteriotomy (ar-te″re-ot′o-me) incision of an artery.

arteriotony (ar-te″re-ot′o-ne) blood pressure.

arteriovenous (ar-te″re-o-ve′nus) pertaining to both artery and vein.

arterioversion (ar-te″re-o-ver′zhun) eversion of the cut end of an artery to arrest hemorrhage.

arteritis (ar″ter-i′tis) inflammation of an artery.

a. defor′mans, chronic endarteritis.

a. oblit′erans, endarteritis obliterans.

rheumatic a., generalized inflammation of arterioles and arterial capillaries occurring in rheumatic fever.

temporal a., inflammation involving the temporal artery, with painful nodular swellings along the vessel.

a. verruco′sa, arteritis marked by projections from the wall into the lumen of the blood vessel.

artery (ar′ter-e) a vessel through which the blood passes away from the heart to various parts of the body. The wall of an artery consists typically of an outer coat (tunica adventitia), a middle coat (tunica media) and an inner coat (tunica intima). (For named arteries of the body, see the table.)

end a., one that undergoes progressive branching without development of channels connecting with other arteries.

arthr(o)- (ar′thro) word element [Gr.], *joint; articulation.*

arthragra (ar-thrag′rah) gouty pain in a joint.

arthral (ar′thral) pertaining to a joint.

arthralgia (ar-thral′je-ah) pain in a joint.

arthrectomy (ar-threk′to-me) excision of a joint.

arthritid (ar′thrī-tid) a skin eruption of gouty origin.

arthritis (ar-thri′tis) inflammation of a joint. adj., **arthrit′ic.** The term covers more than 100 different types of joint diseases, the most common types being RHEUMATOID ARTHRITIS and OSTEOARTHRITIS. Arthritis also may arise as a side effect of a number of diseases, including tuberculosis, syphilis, gonorrhea and viral diseases such as measles and influenza.

Rheumatism is a general term for arthritis and is often applied to almost any pain in the joints or muscles. Of every 100 patients who go to clinics complaining of "rheumatism," about 40 have rheumatoid arthritis, 30 have osteoarthritis and about 15 are found to have rheumatic diseases of the muscles; the remaining 15 have miscellaneous conditions such as GOUT.

Arthritis and its related diseases are one of the chief causes of chronic disability in the United States. The disorder may strike anyone, although it is comparatively rare in those under the age of 25. Of those who live beyond middle age, almost all develop some degenerative changes in bones and joints; however, only about one person in ten develops symptoms.

SYMPTOMS. The symptoms of rheumatoid arthritis are usually mild with a gradual onset. The incidence in the general population is 2 to 3 per cent; female patients outnumber males almost 2:1. Usual age of onset is between 20 and 40 years. Early symptoms include malaise, fever, weight loss and morning stiffness of the joints. One or more joints may become swollen, painful and inflamed. The symptoms may come and go at intervals, leaving no disability. If the disease progresses, there is degeneration of the joint with permanent changes that produce deformities and immobility.

Osteoarthritis is most likely to occur in the large

(Text continued on page 87)

TABLE OF ARTERIES

COMMON NAME*	NA EQUIVALENT†	ORIGIN*	BRANCHES*	DISTRIBUTION
accompanying a. of sciatic nerve. see *sciatic a.*				
acromiothoracic a. see *thoracoacromial a.*				
alveolar a., inferior	a. alveolaris inferior	maxillary a.	dental, mylohyoid branches, mental a.	lower teeth, gums, mandible, lower lip, chin
alveolar a's, anterior superior	aa. alveolares superiores anteriores	infraorbital a.	dental branches	incisors and canine teeth of upper jaw, maxillary sinus
alveolar a., posterior superior	a. alveolaris superior posterior	maxillary a.	dental branches	molar and premolar teeth of upper jaw, maxillary sinus, buccinator muscle
angular a.	a. angularis	facial a.		lacrimal sac, inferior portion of orbicular muscle of eye, nose
aorta	aorta	left ventricle		
abdominal aorta	aorta abdominalis	lower portion of descending aorta, from aortic hiatus of diaphragm to bifurcation into common iliac a's	inferior phrenic, lumbar, median sacral, superior and inferior mesenteric, middle suprarenal, renal, and testicular or ovarian a's, celiac trunk	
arch of aorta	arcus aortae	continuation of ascending aorta	brachiocephalic trunk, left common carotid and left subclavian a's; continues as descending (thoracic) aorta	
ascending aorta	aorta ascendens	proximal portion of aorta, arising from left ventricle	right and left coronary a's; continues as arch of aorta	
descending aorta. see *thoracic aorta; abdominal aorta*	aorta descendens	continuation of arch of aorta		

* a. = artery; a's = (pl.) arteries.
† a. = [L.] arteria; aa. = [L. (pl.)] arteriae.

	NA Term	Origin	Branches	Distribution
aorta (*continued*) thoracic aorta	aorta thoracica	proximal portion of descending aorta, continuing from arch of aorta to aortic hiatus of diaphragm	bronchial, esophageal, pericardiac and mediastinal branches, superior phrenic a's, posterior intercostal a's [III-XI], subcostal a's; continues as abdominal aorta	
appendicular a.	a. appendicularis	ileocolic a.		vermiform appendix
arcuate a. of foot	a. arcuata pedis	dorsalis pedis a.	deep plantar branch and dorsal metatarsal a's	foot, including toes
arcuate a's of kidney	aa. arcuatae renis	interlobar a.	interlobar a's and straight arterioles of kidney	parenchyma of kidney
auditory a., internal. see *a. of labyrinth*				
auricular a., deep	a. auricularis profunda	maxillary a.		skin of auditory meatus, tympanic membrane, temporomandibular joint
auricular a., posterior	a. auricularis posterior	external carotid a.	auricular and occipital branches, stylomastoid a.	middle ear, mastoid cells, auricle, parotid gland, digastric and other muscles
axillary a.	a. axillaris	continuation of subclavian a.	subscapular branches, and highest thoracic, thoracoacromial, lateral thoracic, subscapular, and anterior and posterior circumflex humeral a's	upper limb, including shoulder and axilla, and chest
basilar a.	a. basilaris	from junction of right and left vertebral a's	pontine branches, and anterior inferior cerebellar, labyrinthine, superior cerebellar and posterior cerebral a's	brain stem, internal ear, cerebellum, posterior part of cerebrum
brachial a.	a. brachialis	continuation of axillary a.	profunda brachii, superior and inferior ulnar collateral, radial and ulnar a's	shoulder, arm, forearm and hand
brachial a, deep. see *profunda brachii a.*				
brachial a., superficial	a. brachialis superficialis	variant brachial a., taking a more superficial course than usual	see *brachial a.*	see *brachial a.*
brachiocephalic trunk	truncus brachiocephalicus	arch of aorta	right carotid and right subclavian a's	right side of head and neck, right upper limb
buccal a.	a. buccalis	maxillary a.		buccinator muscle, mucous membrane of mouth

TABLE OF ARTERIES — *Continued*

COMMON NAME*	NA EQUIVALENT†	ORIGIN*	BRANCHES*	DISTRIBUTION
a. of bulb of penis	a. bulbi penis	internal pudendal a.		bulbourethral gland and bulb of penis
a. of bulb of urethra. see *a. of bulb of penis*				
a. of bulb of vestibule of vagina	a. bulbi vestibuli [vaginae]	internal pudendal a.		bulb of vestibule of vagina and Bartholin glands
carotid a.	a. carotis communis	brachiocephalic trunk (right), arch of aorta (left)	external and internal carotid a's	see *carotid a., external* and *carotid a., internal*
carotid a., external	a. carotis externa	carotid a.	superior thyroid, ascending pharyngeal, lingual, facial, sternocleidomastoid, occipital, posterior auricular, superficial temporal and maxillary a's	neck, face, skull
carotid a., internal	a. carotis interna	carotid a.	caroticotympanic branches, and ophthalmic, posterior communicating, anterior choroid, anterior cerebral and middle cerebral a's	middle ear, brain, hypophysis, orbit, choroid plexus of lateral ventricle
caudal a. see *sacral a., median*				
celiac trunk	truncus celiacus	abdominal aorta	left gastric, common hepatic and splenic a's	esophagus, stomach, duodenum, spleen, pancreas, liver, gallbladder
central a. of retina	a. centralis retinae	ophthalmic a.		retina
cerebellar a., inferior, anterior	a. cerebelli inferior anterior	basilar a.	a. of labyrinth	lower anterior cerebellar cortex, inner ear
cerebellar a. inferior, posterior	a. cerebelli inferior posterior	vertebral a.		lower part of cerebellum, medulla, choroid plexus of fourth ventricle
cerebellar a., superior	a. cerebelli superior	basilar a.		upper part of cerebellum, midbrain, pineal body, choroid plexus of third ventricle
cerebral a., anterior	a. cerebri anterior	internal carotid a.	cortical (orbital, frontal, parietal) and central branches and anterior communicating a.	orbital, frontal and parietal cortex and corpus callosum

cerebral a., middle	a. cerebri media	internal carotid a.	cortical (orbital, frontal, parietal, temporal) and central (striate) branches	orbital, frontal, parietal and temporal cortex, and basal ganglia
cerebral a., posterior	a. cerebri posterior	terminal bifurcation of basilar a.	cortical (temporal, occipital, parieto-occipital), central and choroid branches	occipital and temporal lobes, basal ganglia, choroid plexus of lateral ventricle, thalamus, midbrain
cervical a., ascending	a. cervicalis ascendens	inferior thyroid a.	spinal branches	muscles of neck, vertebrae, vertebral canal
cervical a., deep	a. cervicalis profunda	costocervical trunk		deep neck muscles
cervical a., transverse	a. transversa colli	subclavian a.	deep and superficial branches	trapezius, muscles and lymph nodes of neck, rhomboid and latissimus dorsi muscles
choroid a., anterior	a. choroidea anterior	internal carotid a.		choroid plexus of lateral ventricle, hippocampus, fimbria
ciliary a's, anterior	aa. ciliares anteriores	ophthalmic and lacrimal a's	episcleral and anterior conjunctival a's	iris, conjunctiva
ciliary a's, posterior, long	aa. ciliares posteriores longae	ophthalmic a.		iris, ciliary processes
ciliary a's, posterior, short	aa. ciliares posteriores breves	ophthalmic a.		choroid coat of eye
circumflex femoral a., lateral	a. circumflexa femoris lateralis	profunda femoris a.	ascending, descending and transverse branches	hip joint, thigh muscles
circumflex femoral a., medial	a. circumflexa femoris medialis	profunda femoris a.	deep, ascending, transverse and acetabular branches	hip joint, thigh muscles
circumflex humeral a., anterior	a. circumflexa humeri anterior	axillary a.		shoulder joint and head of humerus, long tendon of biceps, tendon of greater pectoral muscle
circumflex humeral a., posterior	a. circumflexa humeri posterior	axillary a.		deltoid, shoulder joint, teres minor and triceps muscles
circumflex iliac a., deep	a. circumflex ilium profunda	external iliac a.	ascending branch	psoas, iliac, sartorius, tensor fasciae latae, and oblique and transverse abdominal muscles, and adjacent skin
circumflex iliac a., superficial	a. circumflexa ilium superficialis	femoral a.		inguinal nodes, skin of thigh and abdomen
circumflex a. of scapula	a. circumflexa scapulae	subscapular a.		subscapular muscle, shoulder joint, teres major and minor muscles
coccygeal a., see *sacral a., median*				

TABLE OF ARTERIES — *Continued*

COMMON NAME*	NA EQUIVALENT†	ORIGIN*	BRANCHES*	DISTRIBUTION
colic a., left	a. colica sinistra	inferior mesenteric a.		descending colon
colic a., middle	a. colica media	superior mesenteric a.		transverse colon
colic a., right	a. colica dextra	superior mesenteric a.		ascending colon
colic a., right, inferior. see *ileocolic a.*				
colic a., superior accessory. see *colic a., middle*				
collateral a., middle	a. collateralis media	profunda brachii a.		triceps muscle and elbow joint
collateral a., radial	a. collateralis radialis	profunda brachii a.		brachioradial and brachial muscles
collateral a., inferior ulnar	a. collateralis ulnaris inferior	brachial a.		arm muscles at back of elbow
collateral a., superior ulnar	a. collateralis ulnaris superior	brachial a.		elbow joint and triceps muscle
communicating a., anterior	a. communicans anterior cerebri	anterior cerebral a.		interconnects anterior cerebral a's
communicating a., posterior	a. communicans posterior cerebri	internal carotid and posterior cerebral a's		hippocampus, thalamus
conjunctival a's, anterior	aa. conjunctivales anteriores	anterior ciliary a's		conjunctiva
conjunctival a's, posterior	aa. conjunctivales posteriores	medial palpebral a.		lacrimal caruncle, conjunctiva
coronary a., left	a. coronaria sinistra	left aortic sinus	anterior interventricular and circumflex branches	left ventricle, left atrium
coronary a., right	a. coronaria dextra	right aortic sinus	posterior interventricular branch	right ventricle, right atrium
costocervical trunk	truncus costocervicalis	subclavian a.	deep cervical and highest intercostal a's	deep neck muscles, intercostal spaces
cremasteric a.	a. cremasterica	inferior epigastric a.		cremaster muscle, coverings of spermatic cord
cystic a.	a. cystica	right branch of hepatic a., proper		gallbladder
deep brachial. see *profunda brachii a.*				
deep a. of clitoris	a. profunda clitoridis	internal pudendal a.		clitoris
deep a. of penis	a. profunda penis	internal pudendal a.		corpus cavernosum penis

Common Name	NA Term	Origin	Branches	Distribution
deep femoral a. see *profunda femoris a.*				
deep lingual a. see *profunda linguae a.*				
deferential a. see *a. of ductus deferens*				
dental a's, anterior superior. see *alveolar a's, anterior superior*				
dental a., inferior. see *alveolar a., inferior*				
dental a., posterior superior. see *alveolar a., posterior superior*				
diaphragmatic a., inferior. see *phrenic a., inferior*				
diaphragmatic a's, superior. see *phrenic a's, superior*				
digital a's, collateral. see *digital a's, palmar, proper*				
digital a's of foot, common. see *metatarsal a's, plantar*				
digital a's of foot, dorsal	aa. digitales dorsales pedis	dorsal metatarsal a's		dorsum of toes
digital a's of hand, dorsal	aa. digitales dorsales manus	dorsal metacarpal a's		dorsum of fingers
digital a's, palmar, common	aa. digitales palmares communes	superficial palmar arch	proper palmar digital a's	fingers
digital a's, palmar, proper	aa. digitales palmares propriae	common palmar digital a's		fingers
digital a's, plantar, common	aa. digitales plantares communes	plantar metatarsal a's	proper plantar digital a's	toes
digital a's, plantar, proper	aa. digitales plantares propriae	common plantar digital a's		toes
dorsal a. of clitoris	a. dorsalis clitoridis	internal pudendal a.		clitoris
dorsal a. of foot. see *dorsalis pedis a.*				
dorsal a. of nose	a. dorsalis nasi	ophthalmic a.		skin of dorsum of nose

TABLE OF ARTERIES—*Continued*

COMMON NAME*	NA EQUIVALENT†	ORIGIN*	BRANCHES*	DISTRIBUTION
dorsal a. of penis	a. dorsalis penis	internal pudendal a.		glans, corona and prepuce of penis
dorsalis pedis a.	a. dorsalis pedis	continuation of anterior tibial a.	lateral and medial tarsal, and arcuate a's	foot, including toes
a. of ductus deferens	a. ductus deferentis	umbilical a.	ureteric branches	ureter, bladder, ductus deferens, seminal vesicles
duodenal a. see *pancreaticoduodenal a., inferior*				
epigastric a., external. see *circumflex iliac a., deep*				
epigastric a., inferior	a. epigastrica inferior	external iliac a.	pubic branch, cremasteric a., a. of round ligament of uterus	cremaster and abdominal muscles, peritoneum
epigastric a., superficial	a. epigastrica superficialis	femoral a.		skin of abdomen, inguinal lymph nodes
epigastric a., superior	a. epigastrica superior	internal thoracic a.		abdominal muscles, diaphragm, skin, peritoneum
episcleral a's	aa. episclerales	anterior ciliary a.		iris, ciliary processes
ethmoidal a., anterior	a. ethmoidalis anterior	ophthalmic a.	anterior meningeal a.	dura mater, nose, frontal sinus, skin, anterior ethmoidal cells
ethmoidal a., posterior	a. ethmoidalis posterior	ophthalmic a.		posterior ethmoidal cells, dura mater, nose
facial a.	a. facialis	external carotid a.	ascending palatine, submental, inferior and superior labial and angular a's; tonsillar and glandular branches	face, tonsil, palate, submandibular gland
facial a., deep. see *maxillary a.*				
facial a., transverse	a. transversa faciei	superficial temporal a.		parotid gland, masseter muscle, skin of face
fallopian a. see *uterine a.*				
femoral a.	a. femoralis	continuation of external iliac a.	superficial epigastric, superficial circumflex iliac, external pudendal, profunda femoris and descending genicular a's	lower abdominal wall, external genitalia, lower limb
femoral a., deep. see *profunda femoris a.*				

TABLE OF ARTERIES — *Continued*

COMMON NAME*	NA EQUIVALENT†	ORIGIN*	BRANCHES*	DISTRIBUTION
hypogastric a. see *iliac a., internal*				
ileal a's	aa. ilei	superior mesenteric a.		ileum
ileocolic a.	a. ileocolica	superior mesenteric a.	appendicular a.	ileum, cecum, vermiform appendix, ascending colon
iliac a., common	a. iliaca communis	abdominal aorta	internal and external iliac a's	pelvis, abdominal wall, lower limb
iliac a., external	a. iliaca externa	common iliac a.	inferior epigastric, deep circumflex iliac a's	abdominal wall, external genitalia, lower limb
iliac a., internal	a. iliaca interna	continuation of common iliac a.	iliolumbar, obturator, superior gluteal, inferior gluteal, umbilical, inferior vesical, uterine, middle rectal and internal pudendal a's	wall and viscera of pelvis, buttock, reproductive organs, medial aspect of thigh
iliolumbar a.	a. iliolumbalis	internal iliac a.	iliac and lumbar branches, lateral sacral a's	pelvic muscles and hip bones, fifth lumbar vertebra, sacrum
infraorbital a.	a. infraorbitalis	maxillary a.	anterior superior alveolar a's	maxilla, maxillary sinus, upper teeth, lower eyelid, cheek, side of nose
innominate a. see *brachiocephalic trunk*				
intercostal a., highest	a. intercostalis suprema	costocervical trunk	posterior intercostal a's I and II	first and second intercostal spaces, vertebral column, back muscles
intercostal a's, posterior, I and II	aa. intercostales posteriores [I et II]	highest intercostal a.	dorsal and spinal branches	first and second intercostal spaces, back muscles, vertebral column
intercostal a's, posterior, III–XI	aa. intercostales posteriores [III–XI]	thoracic aorta	dorsal, lateral, and lateral cutaneous branches	body wall of thorax
interlobar a's of kidney	aa. interlobares renis	renal a.	arcuate a's of kidney	lobes of kidney
interlobular a's of kidney	aa. interlobulares renis	arcuate a's of kidney		renal glomeruli
interlobular a's of liver	aa. interlobulares hepatis	right or left branch of proper hepatic a.		between lobules of liver
interosseous a., anterior	a. interossea anterior	posterior or common interosseous a.	median a.	deep muscles of fingers and long flexor muscle of thumb, radius, ulna
interosseous a., common	a. interossea communis	ulnar a.	anterior and posterior interosseous a's	deep structures of forearm
interosseous a., posterior	a. interossea posterior	common interosseous a.	recurrent interosseous a.	superficial and deep muscles on back of forearm
interosseous a., recurrent	a. interossea recurrens	posterior or common interosseous a.		back of elbow joint

Term	NA	Origin	Branches	Distribution
intestinal a's	aa. intestinales	vessels arising from superior mesenteric a. and supplying intestines; they include pancreaticoduodenal, jejunal, iliac, ileocolic and colic a's		
jejunal a's	aa. jejunales	superior mesenteric a.		jejunum
labial a., inferior	a. labialis inferior	facial a.		lower lip
labial a., superior	a. labialis superior	facial a.	septal and alar branches	upper lip and nose
a. of labyrinth	a. labyrinthi	basilar or anterior inferior cerebellar a.	vestibular and cochlear branches	internal ear
lacrimal a.	a. lacrimalis	ophthalmic a.	lateral palpebral a.	lacrimal gland, eyelids, conjunctiva
laryngeal a., inferior	a. laryngea inferior	inferior thyroid a.		larynx, upper part of trachea, esophagus
laryngeal a., superior	a. laryngea superior	superior thyroid a.		larynx
lingual a.	a. lingualis	external carotid a.	suprahyoid, sublingual, dorsal lingual, profunda linguae branches	tongue, sublingual gland, tonsil, epiglottis
lingual a., deep. see *profunda linguae a.*				
lumbar a's	aa. lumbales	abdominal aorta	dorsal and spinal branches	abdominal wall, vertebrae, lumbar muscles, renal capsule
lumbar a., lowest	a. lumbalis ima	median sacral a.		sacrum, greatest gluteal muscle
malleolar a., anterior, lateral	a. malleolaris anterior lateralis	anterior tibial a.		ankle joint
malleolar a., anterior, medial	a. malleolaris anterior medialis	anterior tibial a.		ankle joint
mammary a., external. see *thoracic a., lateral*				
mammary a., internal. see *thoracic a., internal*				
mandibular a. see *alveolar a., inferior*				
masseteric a.	a. masseterica	maxillary a.		masseter muscle
maxillary a.	a. maxillaris	external carotid a.	pterygoid branches; deep auricular, anterior tympanic, inferior alveolar, middle meningeal, masseteric, deep temporal, buccal, posterior superior alveolar, infraorbital, descending palatine, and sphenopalatine a's, and a. of pterygoid canal	both jaws, teeth, muscles of mastication, ear, meninges, nose, paranasal sinuses, palate

Table of Arteries—*Continued*

COMMON NAME*	NA EQUIVALENT†	ORIGIN*	BRANCHES*	DISTRIBUTION
maxillary a., external. see *facial a.*				
maxillary a., internal. see *maxillary a.*				
median a.	a. mediana	anterior interosseous a.		median nerve, muscles of front of forearm
meningeal a., anterior	a. meningea anterior	anterior ethmoidal a.		dura mater of anterior cranial fossa
meningeal a., middle	a. meningea media	maxillary a.	frontal, parietal, anastomotic, accessory meningeal, and petrous branches, and superior tympanic a.	cranial bones, dura mater of brain
meningeal a., posterior	a. meningea posterior	ascending pharyngeal a.		bones and dura mater of posterior cranial fossa
mental a.	a. mentalis	inferior alveolar a.		skin and muscles of chin
mesenteric a., inferior	a. mesenterica inferior	abdominal aorta	left colic, sigmoid and superior rectal a's	descending colon, rectum
mesenteric a., superior	a. mesenterica superior	abdominal aorta	inferior pancreaticoduodenal, jejunal, ileal, ileocolic, right colic and middle colic a's	small intestine, proximal half of colon
metacarpal a's, dorsal	aa. metacarpeae dorsales	dorsal carpal rete and radial a.	dorsal digital a's	dorsum of fingers
metacarpal a's, palmar	aa. metacarpeae palmares	deep palmar arch		lumbrical and interosseous muscles, bones of fingers
metatarsal a's, dorsal	aa. metatarseae dorsales	arcuate a. of foot	dorsal digital a's	dorsum of foot, including toes
metatarsal a's, plantar	aa. metatarseae plantares	plantar arch	perforating branches, common and proper plantar digital a's	plantar surface of toes
musculophrenic a.	a. musculophrenica	internal thoracic a.		diaphragm, abdominal and thoracic walls
nasal a's, posterior lateral and septal	aa. nasales posteriores laterales et septi	sphenopalatine a.		structures bounding nasal cavity, nasal septum, adjacent sinuses
nutrient a's of humerus	aa. nutriciae humeri	brachial and deep brachial a's		substance of humerus
obturator a.	a. obturatoria	internal iliac a.	pubic, acetabular, anterior and posterior branches	pelvic muscles, hip joint

Term	Latin	Arises from	Branches	Distribution
obturator a., accessory	a. obturatoria accessoria	name given to obturator a. when it arises from inferior epigastric instead of internal iliac a.		
occipital a.	a. occipitalis	external carotid a.	auricular, meningeal, mastoid, descending, occipital and sternocleidomastoid branches	muscles of neck and scalp, meninges, mastoid cells
ophthalmic a.	a. ophthalmica	internal carotid a.	lacrimal and supraorbital a's, central a. of retina, ciliary, posterior and anterior ethmoidal, palpebral, supratrochlear and dorsal nasal a's	eye, orbit, adjacent facial structures
ovarian a.	a. ovarica	abdominal aorta	ureteric branches	ureter, ovary, uterine tube
palatine a., ascending	a. palatina ascendens	facial a.		soft palate, portions of wall of pharynx, tonsil, auditory tube
palatine a., descending	a. palatina descendens	maxillary a.	greater and lesser palatine a's	palate, tonsil
palatine a., greater	a. palatina major	descending palatine a.		hard palate
palatine a's, lesser	aa. palatinae minores	descending palatine a.		soft palate and tonsil
palpebral a's, lateral	aa. palpebrales laterales	lacrimal a.		eyelids, conjunctiva
palpebral a's, medial	aa. palpebrales mediales	ophthalmic a.	posterior conjunctival a's	eyelids
pancreaticoduodenal a., inferior	a. pancreaticoduodenalis inferior	superior mesenteric a.		pancreas, duodenum
pancreaticoduodenal a., superior	a. pancreaticoduodenalis superior	gastroduodenal a.		pancreas, duodenum
perforating a's	aa. perforantes	profunda femoris a.		adductor, hamstring and gluteal muscles, femur
pericardiacophrenic a.	a. pericardiacophrenica	internal thoracic a.		pericardium, diaphragm, pleura
perineal a.	a. perinealis	internal pudendal a.		perineum, skin of external genitalia
peroneal a.	a. peronea	posterior tibial a.	perforating, communicating, calcaneal, and lateral and medial malleolar branches, calcaneal rete	lateral side and back of ankle, deep calf muscles
pharyngeal a., ascending	a. pharyngea ascendens	external carotid a.	posterior meningeal, pharyngeal, inferior tympanic branches	pharynx, soft palate, ear, meninges; cranial nerves, muscles of head
phrenic a., great. see *phrenic a., inferior*				
phrenic a., inferior	a. phrenica inferior	abdominal aorta	superior suprarenal a's	diaphragm, suprarenal gland
phrenic a's, superior	aa. phrenicae superiores	thoracic aorta		upper surface of vertebral portion of diaphragm
plantar a., lateral	a. plantaris lateralis	posterior tibial a.	plantar arch, plantar metatarsal a's	sole of foot, toes

TABLE OF ARTERIES—*Continued*

COMMON NAME*	NA EQUIVALENT†	ORIGIN*	BRANCHES*	DISTRIBUTION
plantar a., medial	a. plantaris medialis	posterior tibial a.	deep and superficial branches	muscles and joints of foot, skin of medial aspect of sole and toes
popliteal a.	a. poplitea	continuation of femoral a.	lateral and medial superior genicular, middle genicular, sural, lateral and medial inferior genicular, anterior and posterior tibial a's; articular rete of knee, patellar rete	knee and calf
princeps pollicis a.	a. princeps pollicis	radial a.	radialis indicis a.	sides and palmar aspect of thumb
principal a. of thumb. see *princeps pollicis a.*				
profunda brachii a.	a. profunda brachii	brachial a.	nutrient to humerus, deltoid branch, middle and radial collateral a's	humerus, muscles and skin of arm
profunda femoris a.	a. profunda femoris	femoral a.	medial and lateral circumflex femoral a's, perforating a's	thigh muscles, hip joint, gluteal muscles, femur
profunda linguae a.	a. profunda linguae	termination of lingual a.		side and tip of tongue
a. of pterygoid canal	a. canalis pterygoidei	maxillary a.		roof of pharynx, auditory tube
pudendal a's, external	aa. pudendae externae	femoral a.	anterior scrotal or anterior labial branches, inguinal branches	external genitalia, medial thigh muscles
pudendal a, internal	a. pudenda interna	internal iliac a.	posterior scrotal or posterior labial branches, inferior rectal, perineal, urethral a's, a. of bulb of penis or vestibule, deep a. of penis or clitoris, dorsal a. of penis or clitoris	external genitalia, anal canal, perineum
pulmonary trunk	truncus pulmonalis	right ventricle	right and left pulmonary a's	conveys unaerated blood toward lungs
pulmonary a., left	a. pulmonalis sinistra	pulmonary trunk	numerous branches named according to segments of lung to which they distribute unaerated blood	left lung
pulmonary a., right	a. pulmonalis dextra	pulmonary trunk	numerous branches named according to segments of lung to which they distribute unaerated blood	right lung

radial a.	a. radialis	brachial a.	palmar carpal, superficial palmar and dorsal carpal branches; recurrent radial a., princeps pollicis a., deep palmar arch	forearm, wrist, hand
radial a., collateral. see collateral a., radial				
radial a. of index finger. see radialis indicis a.				
radialis indicis a.	a. radialis indicis	princeps pollicis a.		both sides of index finger
radiate a's of kidney. see interlobular a's of kidney				
ranine a. see profunda linguae a.				
rectal a., inferior	a. rectalis inferior	internal pudendal a.		rectum, levator ani and external sphincter muscles, overlying skin
rectal a., middle	a. rectalis media	internal iliac a.		rectum, vagina
rectal a., superior	a. rectalis superior	inferior mesenteric a.		rectum
recurrent a., radial	a. recurrens radialis	radial a.		brachioradial and brachial muscles, elbow joint
recurrent a., tibial, anterior	a. recurrens tibialis anterior	anterior tibial a.		anterior tibial muscle and long extensor muscle of toes; knee joint, skin of lower leg
recurrent a., tibial, posterior	a. recurrens tibialis posterior	anterior tibial a.		knee joint, tibiofibular joint
recurrent a., ulnar	a. recurrens ulnaris	ulnar a.	anterior and posterior branches	elbow joint, adjacent skin, and muscles
renal a.	a. renalis	abdominal aorta	ureteric branches, inferior suprarenal a., interlobar a's	kidney, suprarenal gland, ureter
a. of round ligament of uterus	a. ligamenti teretis uteri	inferior epigastric a.		round ligament of uterus
sacral a's, lateral	aa. sacrales laterales	iliolumbar a.	spinal branches	structures about coccyx and sacrum
sacral a., median	a. sacralis mediana	central continuation of abdominal aorta, beyond origin of common iliac a's	lowest lumbar a.	sacrum, coccyx, rectum
scapular a., transverse. see suprascapular a.				
sciatic a.	a. comitans nervi ischiadici	inferior gluteal a.		accompanies sciatic nerve

TABLE OF ARTERIES – *Continued*

COMMON NAME*	NA EQUIVALENT†	ORIGIN*	BRANCHES*	DISTRIBUTION
sigmoid a.'s	aa. sigmoideae	inferior mesenteric a.		sigmoid colon
spermatic a., external. see *cremasteric a.*				
sphenopalatine a.	a. sphenopalatina	maxillary a.	posterior lateral and septal nasal a's	structures adjoining nasal cavity, nasopharynx
spinal a., anterior	a. spinalis anterior	vertebral a.		anterior portion of spinal cord
spinal a., posterior	a. spinalis posterior	vertebral a.		posterior portion of spinal cord
splenic a.	a. lienalis	celiac trunk	pancreatic and splenic branches; left gastroepiploic and short gastric a's	spleen, pancreas, stomach, greater omentum
straight arterioles of kidney	arteriolae rectae renis	arcuate a's of kidney		renal pyramids
stylomastoid a.	a. stylomastoidea	posterior auricular a.	mastoid and stapedial branches, posterior tympanic a.	middle ear walls, mastoid cells, stapedius
subclavian a.	a. subclavia	brachiocephalic trunk (right), arch of aorta (left)	vertebral, internal thoracic a's, thyrocervical and costocervical trunks	neck, thoracic wall, spinal cord, brain, meninges, upper limb
subcostal a.	a. subcostalis	thoracic aorta		upper abdominal wall
sublingual a.	a. sublingualis	lingual a.	dorsal and spinal branches	sublingual gland, side of tongue, floor of mouth
submental a.	a. submentalis	facial a.		tissues under chin
subscapular a.	a. subscapularis	axillary a.	thoracodorsal and circumflex scapular a's	scapular region
supraorbital a.	a. supraorbitalis	ophthalmic a.		forehead, superior muscles of orbit, upper eyelid, frontal sinus
suprarenal a., inferior	a. suprarenalis inferior	renal a.		suprarenal gland
suprarenal a., middle	a. suprarenalis media	abdominal aorta		suprarenal gland
suprarenal a's, superior	aa. suprarenales superiores	inferior phrenic a.		suprarenal gland
suprascapular a.	a. suprascapularis	thyrocervical trunk	acromial branch	clavicle and scapula, shoulder joint, muscles
supratrochlear a.	a. supratrochlearis	ophthalmic a.		anterior part of scalp
sural a's	aa. surales	popliteal a.		muscles of popliteal fossa and calf, adjacent skin
sylvian a. see *cerebral a., middle*				
tarsal a., lateral	a. tarsea lateralis	dorsalis pedis a.		muscles and joints of tarsus

tarsal a's, medial	aa. tarseae mediales	dorsalis pedis a.		skin and joints of medial aspect of foot
temporal a's, deep	aa. temporales profundae	maxillary a.		temporal muscle, pericranium, subjacent bone
temporal a., middle	a. temporalis media	superficial temporal a.		temporal muscle
temporal a., superficial	a. temporalis superficialis	external carotid a.	parotid, anterior auricular, frontal and parietal branches; transverse facial, zygomatico-orbital, middle temporal a's	parotid gland, auricle, scalp, skin of face, masseter muscle
testicular a.	a. testicularis	abdominal aorta	ureteric branches	ureter, epididymis, testis
thoracic a., highest	a. thoracica suprema	axillary a.		intercostal, serratus anterior, greater and lesser pectoral muscles
thoracic a., internal	a. thoracica interna	subclavian a.	mediastinal, thymic, bronchial, sternal, perforating, lateral costal and anterior intecostal branches; pericardiacophrenic, musculophrenic, superior epigastric a's	anterior thoracic wall, mediastinal structures, diaphragm
thoracic a., lateral	a. thoracica lateralis	axillary a.	mammary branches	pectoral muscles, mammary gland
thoracoacromial a.	a. thoracoacromialis	axillary a.	clavicular, pectoral, deltoid and acromial branches	pectoral, deltoid, subclavius muscles, acromion
thoracodorsal a.	a. thoracodorsalis	subscapular a.		subscapular and teres major and minor muscles
thyrocervical trunk	truncus thyrocervicalis	subclavian a.	inferior thyroid, suprascapular and transverse cervical a's	deep neck, including thyroid gland, scapular region
thyroid a., inferior	a. thyroidea inferior	thyrocervical trunk	pharyngeal, esophageal, tracheal and glandular branches; inferior laryngeal, ascending cervical a's	larynx, esophagus, trachea, neck muscles, thyroid gland
thyroid a., lowest. see *thyroidea ima a.*				
thyroid a., superior	a. thyroidea superior	external carotid a.	hyoid, sternocleidomastoid, superior laryngeal, cricothyroid muscular and glandular branches	muscles of hyoid bone, larynx, thyroid gland, pharynx
thyroidea ima a.	a. thyroidea ima	arch of aorta, brachiocephalic trunk or right carotid a.		thyroid gland
tibial a., anterior	a. tibialis anterior	popliteal a.	posterior and anterior tibial recurrent a's, lateral and medial anterior malleolar a's, lateral and medial malleolar retes	leg, ankle, foot
tibial a., posterior	a. tibialis	popliteal a.	fibular circumflex branch; peroneal, medial plantar, lateral plantar a's	leg, foot, including heel

TABLE OF ARTERIES—*Continued*

COMMON NAME*	NA EQUIVALENT†	ORIGIN*	BRANCHES*	DISTRIBUTION
transverse a. of face. see *facial a., transverse*				
transverse a. of neck. see *cervical a., transverse*				
transverse a. of scapula. see *suprascapular a.*				
tympanic a., anterior	a. tympanica anterior	maxillary a.		lining membrane of middle ear
tympanic a., inferior	a. tympanica inferior	ascending pharyngeal a.		medial wall of middle ear
tympanic a., posterior	a. tympanica posterior	stylomastoid a.		posterior part of tympanic membrane, secondary tympanic membrane
tympanic a., superior	a. tympanica superior	middle meningeal a.		tensor tympani muscle lining membrane of meatus
ulnar a.	a. ulnaris	brachial a.	palmar carpal, dorsal carpal and deep palmar branches; ulnar recurrent and common interosseous a's; superficial palmar arch	forearm, wrist, hand
ulnar a., collateral, inferior. see *collateral a., ulnar, inferior*				
ulnar a., collateral, superior. see *collateral a., ulnar, superior*				
umbilical a.	a. umbilicalis	internal iliac a.	a. of ductus deferens, superior vesical a's	ductus deferens, seminal vesicles, testes, urinary bladder, ureter
urethral a.	a. urethralis	internal pudendal a.		urethra
uterine a.	a. uterina	internal iliac a.	ovarian and tubal branches; vaginal a.	uterus, vagina, round ligament of uterus, uterine tube, ovary
vaginal a.	a. vaginalis	uterine a.		vagina, fundus of bladder
vertebral a.	a. vertebralis	subclavian a.	spinal and meningeal branches; posterior inferior cerebellar, basilar, anterior and posterior spinal a's	muscles of neck, vertebrae, spinal cord, cerebellum, cerebrum
vesical a., inferior	a. vesicalis inferior	internal iliac a.		bladder, prostate, seminal vesicles
vesical a's, superior	aa. vesicales superiores	umbilical a.		bladder, urachus, ureter
zygomatico-orbital a.	a. zygomaticoorbitalis	superficial temporal a.		orbicular muscle of eye

and weight-bearing joints. It is a degenerative disorder that is commonly secondary to other joint diseases. Another common form of osteoarthritis affects the joints of the fingers; this form usually occurs in women. Osteoarthritis is much less crippling than severe rheumatoid arthritis because it does not cause the two bone surfaces to fuse and immobilize the joint. Osteoarthritis usually responds well to treatment and though there is no cure the symptoms may be greatly relieved.

TREATMENT. Early treatment of rheumatoid arthritis can be effective in preventing crippling deformities. Also, a great deal can be done to relieve the pain of both diseases, rheumatoid arthritis and osteoarthritis. However, at this time there is no specific cure for either form. Since there are as many as a hundred different rheumatic diseases, accurate diagnosis is the first step toward proper treatment. The kind of treatment necessary may differ widely from case to case, and what is helpful in one case may be useless or even harmful in another.

Among the basic elements of treatment for both rheumatoid arthritis and osteoarthritis are physical therapy to preserve the function of the joints and muscles, medication to control the course of the disease and ease the pain and a regimen of rest and special exercises. In some cases psychotherapy is used.

Physical Therapy. The application of heat to the affected joints is generally helpful in both types of arthritis. For dry heat, a therapeutic heat lamp is often the most convenient method, although hot water bottles or electric heating pads may also be used. For treatment of the hands, paraffin baths may be preferred. Wet heat can be applied either by hot tub baths with the water temperature not exceeding 102° F., or by means of a towel dipped in hot water, wrung out and applied to the joint.

Exercises and Rest. Special exercises are often prescribed, taking into account the type and severity of the case, the joints affected and many other factors. Reduction of weight may be necessary in osteoarthritis patients to lighten the stress on the affected joints. However, there is no diet that can cure or materially lessen the effects of arthritis. A normal, healthful diet that maintains average body weight is the best measure the average arthritic can adopt.

Another important aspect of physical therapy for the arthritic is proper rest. Ten to twelve hours a day of sleep and bed rest is frequently recommended for the patient with rheumatoid arthritis. In these rest periods the patient must be careful to keep his joints as straight as possible. Sometimes complete bed rest is essential during periods of severe inflammation.

Medication. There are several medications that are used in treating arthritis. The selection and dosage of medicines in each individual case must be made by the physician, and continued under his care so that possible side effects can be noted at an early stage.

The cheapest, safest, and among the most useful medicines in treating arthritis are the salts of salicylic acid. The most common of these are aspirin and sodium salicylate. Since there is some evidence that salicylates may have a beneficial effect on the disease aside from relieving pain, they should be taken on a regular basis as prescribed by a physician. For those who suffer stomach upset or other side effects from aspirin, coated tablets or antacid mixtures of aspirin are available.

Most patent medicines sold "for the relief of arthritic pain" are expensive mixtures whose basic ingredient is aspirin or a closely related compound. In almost all cases the same effect can be achieved by aspirin, which is much less expensive.

In recent years hormones such as cortisone have been used with excellent results in treating some cases of rheumatoid arthritis. These substances

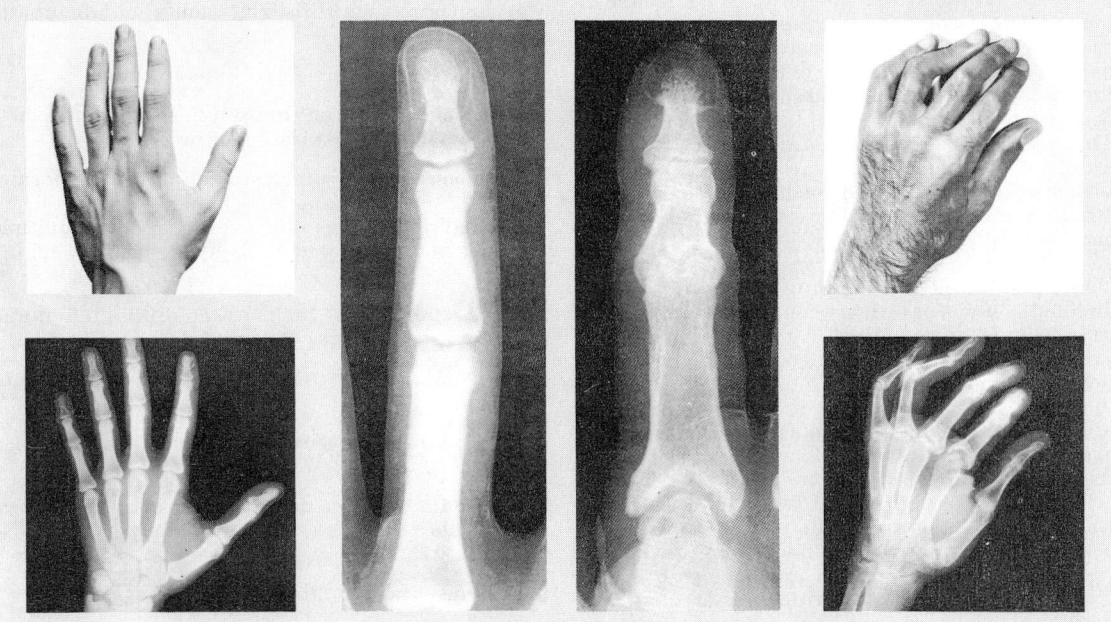

Arthritis of the fingers. Left, normal hand and finger. Right, arthritic hand and finger, with ankylosis, or "locking" of the joint by bone and scar tissue. (Courtesy of Bergman Associates.)

reduce the effect of inflammation in the joint, thus decreasing the pain, swelling and stiffness. These hormones may also produce adverse effects such as decalcification and weakness of the bones, gastric ulcer and abrupt changes of mood.

The use of hormones in cases of osteoarthritis is strictly limited. In a few cases when osteoarthritis in a large joint such as the knee threatens to disable the patient, it may be helpful to inject cortisone or its analogues directly into the affected joint. However, the effect of these injections tends to wear off, and it may be necessary to repeat them periodically.

Compounds of gold have been used for many years in treating rheumatoid arthritis. The gold compound, given by injection, acts to modify the course of the disease, and treatment must continue over a relatively long period of time. The gold may produce harmful reactions in some people, and those receiving it should have frequent medical examinations.

Several other drugs are available for therapy.

Although much is still unknown about rheumatoid arthritis and osteoarthritis, it has been observed that emotional disturbances can provoke or aggravate the diseases. There is also some evidence that certain psychologic types of people are more likely to have rheumatoid arthritis. Why this is so is still not understood, but in treating a patient with arthritis the doctor will take these facts into account. He may recommend psychotherapy or simply advise sufferers to try to avoid emotional upsets.

In the early stages of arthritis many patients fear that they may become severely crippled. The emotional strain of this worrying may in itself have a harmful effect on the course of the disease. It should be noted that modern surgery can benefit even some greatly deformed or crippled joints.

Frauds and Fallacies in Treatment. Arthritis is so widespread that it is a natural haven for charlatans and promoters of miraculous "cures." The fact that the symptoms normally come and go makes the work of those who prey on arthritics even easier. If a natural disappearance of symptoms happens to coincide with one of these "treatments," the promoter can be assured of a sincere and enthusiastic testimonial from a satisfied patient. The Arthritis Foundation estimated in 1959 that arthritics were spending more than $250 million a year on misrepresented medicines, devices and other treatments. Most of these are worthless; some are potentially dangerous.

NURSING CARE. Prevention of permanent disability resulting from crippling deformities of the affected joints is of primary concern in the nursing care of an arthritic patient. A regimen of rest and exercise is aimed at prevention of permanent fixation of the joints and loss of muscle tone. Although the exercises are important in strengthening the muscles and keeping the joints mobile, they can be overdone in some cases and care should be taken that fatigue and exhaustion are avoided.

Proper positioning of the joints and frequent changes of position while the patient is at rest in bed or sitting up are most effective in preventing complications. Since motion produces pain in the affected joints, many arthritics resist changing position; however, it is no kindness to allow the patient to lie in bed with his joints flexed and unmoved for long periods of time. Explaining the need for periodic motion and good posture at all times often makes the patient more cooperative.

Emotional support and an attitude of understanding and sympathy frequently are necessary in dealing with the arthritic patient. He is often irritable and difficult to get along with, and understandably so, when one considers his constant discomfort and limited activity during the acute phases of his disease. The exact effect of emotional disturbances on the course of arthritis is not yet fully understood, but it is known that a relaxed and emotionally serene person is less likely to suffer from severe and painful flare-ups of this disorder.

Promotion of general health aids in the prevention of infections and other debilitating factors which tend to aggravate arthritis and increase the severity of its symptoms.

The Self-Help Device Office of the Institute of Physical Medicine and Rehabilitation, 400 East 34th Street, New York, N.Y. 10016, can supply information on specially designed self-help devices for arthritics. The office is maintained by a grant received from the Arthritis Foundation.

The Arthritis Foundation, 1212 Avenue of the Americas, New York, N.Y. 10036, has more than 80 local chapters throughout the United States. The foundation supports a broad program of education and research, and publishes a wide variety of literature on arthritis. This foundation also helps finance improvement of local facilities for treating arthritis.

acute a., arthritis marked by pain, heat, redness and swelling.

acute rheumatic a., swelling, tenderness and redness of many joints of the body, often accompanying rheumatic fever.

gonococcal a., severe pain and swelling of the joints resulting from infection by *Neisseria gonorrhoeae.*

hypertrophic a., rheumatoid arthritis marked by hypertrophy of the cartilage at the edge of the joints; osteoarthritis.

suppurative a., inflammation of a joint with a serous, serofibrinous or purulent effusion and destruction of articular tissue.

arthritism   (ar'thrī-tizm) gouty or rheumatic diathesis.

arthrocele (ar'thro-sēl) a joint swelling.

arthrocentesis (ar"thro-sen-te'sis) puncture of a joint cavity with aspiration of fluid.

arthrochalasis (ar"thro-kal'ah-sis) abnormal relaxation or flaccidity of a joint.

a. mul'tiplex congen'ita, overflaccidity of multiple joints, not associated with hyperelasticity of the skin.

arthrochondritis (ar"thro-kon-dri'tis) inflammation of the cartilages of a joint.

arthroclasia (ar"thro-kla'ze-ah) manipulation of a joint.

arthrodesis (ar"thro-de'sis) surgical fusion of a joint.

arthrodia (ar-thro'de-ah) a type of synovial joint that allows only a gliding motion; called also gliding joint.

arthrodynia (ar"thro-din'e-ah) arthralgia.

arthrodysplasia (ar"thro-dis-pla'ze-ah) any abnormality of joint development.

arthroempyesis (ar"thro-em"pi-e'sis) suppuration within a joint.

arthroendoscopy (ar″thro-en-dos′ko-pe) inspection of the interior of a joint with an endoscope.

arthrography (ar-throg′rah-fe) roentgenography of a joint.

air a., pneumoarthrography.

arthrogryposis (ar″thro-gri-po′sis) 1. persistent flexion of a joint. 2. tetanoid spasm.

arthrokleisis (ar″thro-kli′sis) ankylosis.

arthrolith (ar′thro-lith) a calculus deposit within a joint.

arthrology (ar-throl′o-je) scientific study or description of the joints.

arthrolysis (ar-throl′i-sis) mobilization of an ankylosed joint.

arthrometer (ar-throm′e-ter) an instrument for measuring the angles of movements of joints.

arthronosos (ar″thro-no′sos) any disease of a joint.

arthropathy (ar-throp′ah-the) any joint disease.

Charcot's a., neurogenic a., osteoarthritis with joint enlargement due to trophic disturbance, affecting ankle, knee, hip, spine or hand.

osteopulmonary a., clubbing of fingers and toes, and enlargement of ends of the long bones, in cardiac or pulmonary disease.

arthrophyte (ar′thro-fit) abnormal growth in a joint cavity.

arthroplasty (ar′thro-plas″te) plastic repair of a joint.

arthropod (ar′thro-pod) an individual of the phylum Arthropoda.

Arthropoda (ar-throp′o-dah) a phylum of the animal kingdom including bilaterally symmetrical animals with segmented bodies bearing jointed appendages; embracing the largest number of known animals, with at least 740,000 species, divided into 12 classes.

arthrosclerosis (ar″thro-skle-ro′sis) stiffening or hardening of the joints.

arthrosis (ar-thro′sis) 1. an articulation. 2. disease of a joint.

arthrosteitis (ar″thros-te-i′tis) inflammation of the bony structures of a joint.

arthrostomy (ar-thros′to-me) incision of a joint with drainage.

arthrosynovitis (ar″thro-sin″o-vi′tis) inflammation of the synovial membrane of a joint.

arthrotomy (ar-throt′o-me) incision of a joint.

arthroxesis (ar-throk′se-sis) scraping of joints.

articular (ar-tik′u-lar) pertaining to a joint.

articulare (ar-tik″u-la′re) the point of intersection of the dorsal contours of the articular process of the mandible and the temporal bone.

articulate (ar-tik′u-lāt) 1. to unite by joints; to join. 2. united by joints. 3. capable of expressing one's self orally.

articulatio (ar-tik″u-la′she-o), pl. *articulatio′nes* [L.] an articulation or joint.

articulation (ar-tik″u-la′shun) 1. the place of union or junction between two or more bones of the skeleton. 2. enunciation of words and sentences.

articulator (ar-tik′u-la″tor) a device for effecting a jointlike union.

dental a., a device that simulates movements of the temporomandibular joints or mandible, used in dentistry.

articulo mortis (ar-tik′u-lo mor′tis) at the point or moment of death.

artifact (ar′ti-fakt) a structure or appearance that is not natural, but is due to manipulation (man-made).

artificial (ar″ti-fish′al) made by art; not natural or pathologic.

a. limb, a replacement for a natural limb (see also PROSTHESIS).

a. organ, a mechanical device that can substitute temporarily or permanently for a body organ. The development of artificial organs represents one of the outstanding achievements of contemporary medicine. The field of organ substitution has progressed rapidly over a brief span of years. Most of the artificial organs in use today are hospital devices that are connected temporarily to patients in order to do the work of an organ that is either disabled or undergoing surgery. Recent advances in electronics (principally the development of the transistor and the low-drain battery), together with advances in surgical techniques, have made possible the development of miniature artificial organs that can be surgically implanted in a patient and function independently for long periods.

The development of artificial organs has paved the way for other medical advances in the field of organ TRANSPLANTATION, the replacement of a disabled organ with a healthy living organ from a "donor." The surgical techniques of artificial organ implantation and living organ transplantation have much in common. Also, it is often necessary to use an artificial organ to temporarily take over the functions of an organ undergoing transplantation surgery.

The heart-lung machine is a surgery aid that permits previously impossible operations on the heart, lungs and great vessels, and also allows other kinds of surgery to be performed on seriously weakened patients without fear of heart failure. The "heart" of the machine is a pump that draws blood from the patient, routes it through a "lung" chamber, where the blood is exposed to oxygen, and then pumps the oxygenated blood back through the patient's circulatory system. During this procedure, the temperature, pressure and chemistry of the blood are carefully controlled.

Cardiac patients suffering from heart block (a defect in the transmission of nerve impulses between the separate pumping chambers of the heart) are kept alive with an electronic heart stimulator called the artificial PACEMAKER. The device is also used in certain cardiac operations in which heart block is a possible complication. A compact version of the hospital pacemaker can be surgically implanted in the chest of a patient. Miniature pacemakers of this kind are keeping thousands of heart block victims alive today.

Researchers in cardiac disease are experimenting with several types of artificial hearts. It is hoped that a mechanical pump implanted permanently in a patient can match the output of a normal heart. Another experimental device along similar lines is called a "booster heart," designed to reduce the work load of the left ventricle.

Artificial heart valves are also used to replace those damaged by disease. The mitral valve, which controls the passage of blood between the left atrium and left ventricle, is often impaired by rheumatic fever. Some cardiac disorders impair the aortic valve, which controls blood flow from the heart to the body. Artificial aortic and mitral valves have been successfully implanted in human hearts. Damaged blood vessels (which in the past could be replaced only by a difficult procedure of transplantation from donors who had died suddenly) are now replaced with tubes made of Teflon or Dacron.

Normal kidneys filter waste products from the blood, expelling these substances in the urine. When the kidneys fail, waste products can build up in the blood to poisonous levels, causing uremia. The only treatment available for this condition is the artificial kidney. A simple filtering device, the artificial kidney takes blood from the patient and circulates it through a coil of cellophane tubing which is immersed in a "rinsing" fluid. The process is complete only after all the patient's blood has been purified. (See also KIDNEY and PERITONEAL DIALYSIS.) Uremia patients must undergo the lengthy treatment frequently; they are almost entirely dependent upon hospital equipment. It may soon be possible, however, for uremia patients to lead normal lives thanks to a miniature artificial kidney now under development. Like the pacemaker and other internal organ substitutes, the new kidney will be implanted by surgery and will function on its own for long periods.

a. respiration, any method of forcing air into and out of the lungs to start breathing in a person whose breathing has stopped. Artificial respiration can be given with no equipment whatsoever, so that it is an ideal emergency first-aid procedure.

WHEN TO GIVE IT. Artificial respiration can save a life whenever breathing has stopped but heartbeat has not, as in near-drowning, electric shock, choking, gas poisoning, drug poisoning, injury to the chest or suffocation from other causes. Usually one can tell that breathing has stopped by noting the lack of up-and-down movement of the chest. Often the cause of the stoppage of breathing is obvious, as when a drowning person is pulled out of the water. But sometimes it is impossible to tell what stopped the breathing—accident or disease—and therefore whether artificial respiration would or would not be helpful. In such cases, the rule to follow is: when in doubt, give artificial respiration, and continue if possible until a physician takes charge.

WHAT TO DO. To be effective, artificial respiration must be begun immediately. A person dies in minutes after his breathing stops. A delay of seconds may be the difference between life and death. That is why it is so important to learn how to apply artificial respiration before an accident happens.

At the same time artificial respiration is begun someone should call a doctor or the local fire department, but if there is no one to send, artificial respiration should be given in preference to going for help.

Any obstruction in the victim's mouth that would interfere with the passage of air—mud, sand, chewing gum or displaced false teeth, for example—is removed immediately. Clothing that is tight around the neck is loosened.

Once begun, artificial respiration should be continued until the victim begins to breathe regularly by himself, until a physician takes charge or until it is obvious that the victim will not revive. Do not give up easily. Victims have recovered as long as 4 hours after artificial respiration was started. If cardiac arrest or weakness occurs, a second person who knows how should give CARDIAC MASSAGE. If only one person is present, he should provide both alternately.

When the victim has revived, he is kept quiet, covered to prevent chills and given other first aid for SHOCK.

METHODS. There are three methods of artificial respiration: the mouth-to-mouth method, the chest pressure–arm lift (Silvester) method and the back pressure-arm lift (Holger-Nielsen) method.

The mouth-to-mouth technique is recognized by

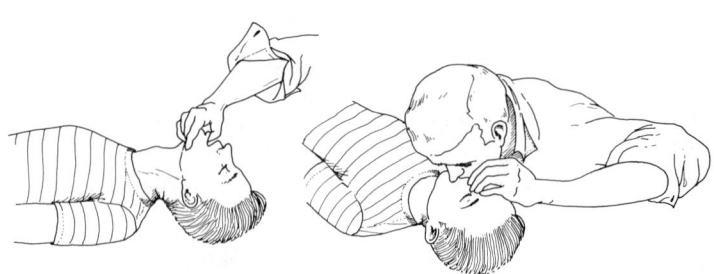

Place the victim on his back. Remove foreign matter from his mouth. Tilt his head back by lifting with one hand under his neck and pushing on his forehead with the other hand. Pull or push the jaw into jutting-out position and maintain it.

Cover the victim's mouth with your mouth, pinch his nostrils shut and blow vigorously about 12 times a minute. If the victim is a small child, place your mouth tightly over his mouth and nose and blow gently about 20 times a minute. After each blow, remove your mouth; if no air is exhaled by the victim, recheck the head and jaw positions.

authorities as the most effective method that can be given by an individual. Some persons feel squeamish at the thought of using it, but in an emergency such doubts usually vanish. Anyone who hesitates about putting his mouth on another person's, even in an emergency, can place a handkerchief over the victim's mouth. Air will pass readily through the cloth.

The other two methods are recommended only (1) if a person cannot bring himself to use the mouth-to-mouth technique, (2) if circumstances (such as a severe mouth injury in the victim) prevent him from using it or (3) if he feels more familiar with another method at the time of the emergency.

aryl- (ar′il) prefix, *a chemical radical belonging to the aromatic series.*

arytenoid (ar″ĭ-te′noid) shaped like a jug or pitcher, as the arytenoid cartilages or arytenoid muscles of the larynx.

arytenoidectomy (ar″ĭ-te-noi-dek′to-me) excision of an arytenoid cartilage.

arytenoiditis (ar″ĭ-te-noi-di′tis) inflammation of the arytenoid muscles or cartilage.

arytenoidopexy (ar″ĭ-te-noi′do-pek″se) surgical fixation of arytenoid cartilage or muscle.

A.S. [L.] *au′ris sinis′tra* (*left ear*).

As chemical symbol, *arsenic.*

ASA acetylsalicylic acid (aspirin).

asbestiform (as-bes′ti-form) resembling asbestos.

asbestos (as-bes′tos) fibrous magnesium and calcium silicate, a nonburning compound used in roofing and insulating materials.

asbestosis (as″bes-to′sis) lung disease caused by inhalation of asbestos fibers (see also PNEUMOCONIOSIS).

ascariasis (as″kah-ri′ah-sis) infection with Ascaris.

ascaricide (as-kar′ĭ-sīd) a drug destructive to ascarids. adj., **ascarici′dal.**

ascarid (as′kah-rid) an organism (worm) of the genus Ascaris.

Ascaris (as′kah-ris) a genus of nematode parasites found in the intestines of man and other vertebrates.

A. lumbricoi′des, a species widely distributed about the world; also called giant intestinal roundworm. (See also WORMS.)

A. su′is, a species morphologically similar to *A. lumbricoides,* but commonly found in pigs.

Aschheim-Zondek test (ash′hīm tson′dek) AZ test; a biologic test for pregnancy. Injection of urine from a pregnant woman into immature female mice produces marked changes in the appearance of their ovaries within 100 hours. The test is 95 to 99 per cent accurate. (See also PREGNANCY TESTS.)

Aschoff's bodies (ash′ofs) submiliary collections of cells and leukocytes in the interstitial tissues of the heart in rheumatic myocarditis; called also Aschoff's nodules.

ascites (ah-si′tēz) abnormal accumulation of fluid in the peritoneal cavity, sometimes resulting in considerable and uncomfortable distention of the abdomen. adj., **ascit′ic.** Ascites can be caused by many conditions, including cirrhosis of the liver, heart and kidney disease and inflammation and tumors within the abdominal cavity.

NURSING CARE. The position most comfortable for the patient is with the head of the bed elevated to facilitate breathing. When the patient is lying on his side a small pillow is used to support the rib cage. Skin care is given frequently to prevent the breakdown of edematous tissue associated with ascites.

Sodium restriction and diuretics are usually necessary as a part of the treatment of ascites. Potassium may be given to replace that lost through the kidneys. Intake and output must be measured and recorded accurately.

PARACENTESIS may be done to remove excess fluid from the abdominal cavity. The patient should void immediately before the procedure so as to eliminate the danger of injury to the urinary bladder. The amount and character of the fluid removed is observed and recorded on the patient's chart. The site of the puncture should be covered with a dry dressing after the procedure and observed periodically for drainage and signs of infection.

chylous a., the presence of milky fluid containing globules of fat in the peritoneal cavity owing to rupture of the thoracic duct or to extravasation through its wall.

Ascomycetes (as″ko-mi-se′tēz) a genus of fungi.

ascorbate (as-kor′bāt) a derivative of ascorbic acid.

ascorbic acid (as-kor′bik) vitamin C, called also cevitamic acid; a substance found in many fruits and vegetables, especially citrus fruits, such as oranges and lemons, and tomatoes. Ascorbic acid is an essential element of the diet; lack of vitamin C can lead to SCURVY or to less severe conditions, such as delayed healing of wounds. Solutions of ascorbic acid deteriorate very rapidly and the vitamin is not stored in the body to any extent. Large doses of commerical preparations of ascorbic acid may cause gastrointestinal irritation. There is no general agreement as to the normal and therapeutic daily requirements of vitamin C. It is believed that ascorbic acid requirements in stress are abnormally high. Under moderate stress circumstances authorities recommend about 300 mg. daily.

ascospore (as′ko-spōr) a spore contained or produced in an ascus.

ascus (as′kus) the spore case of certain fungi.

-ase (ās) suffix used in forming the name of an enzyme, affixed to the name of the substrate (luciferase) or to a term indicating the general nature of the substrate (proteinase), the type of reaction effected (hydrolase) or a combination of these (transaminase).

asemasia (as″e-ma′ze-ah) inability to make or comprehend signs or tokens of communication.

asepsis (a-sep′sis) absence of septic matter; freedom from infection or infectious material. adj., **asep′tic.**

MEDICAL ASEPSIS. Medical asepsis refers to destruction of organisms after they leave the body. This technique is used in the care of patients with infectious diseases to prevent reinfection of the patient and to avoid the spread of infection from one person to another. This is achieved by ISOLATION TECHNIQUE in which the objects in the patient's environment are protected from contamination or disinfected as soon as possible after contamination.

SURGICAL ASEPSIS. Surgical asepsis refers to destruction of organisms before they enter the body. It is used in caring for open wounds and in surgical procedures. In surgical asepsis an object may be sterile (free from microorganisms) or unsterile. Measures that can be taken to provide surgical asepsis include absolute sterilization of all instruments, linens or other inanimate objects that may come in contact with the surgical wound. The surgeon and his assistants wash their hands thoroughly for at least 5 minutes, using a special germicidal soap, and then don surgical gloves and other outer clothing to avoid contamination of the wound. In some operating rooms the air supply is specially treated so that organisms present can be destroyed. All equipment and other inanimate objects in the operating room must be kept clean and periodically treated with a disinfectant.

asexual (a-seks'u-al) without sex; not pertaining to sex.

asexualization (a-seks"u-al-ĭ-za'shun) castration.

asialia (ah"si-a'le-ah) aptyalism.

asiderosis (ah"sid-er-o'sis) deficiency of iron reserve of the body.

asitia (ah-sish'e-ah) loathing of food.

asparagine (ah-spar'ah-jēn) a white crystalline amino acid found in most plants and converted in the human body to aspartic acid and ammonia.

aspartic acid (ah-spar'tik) a dibasic amino acid, derivable from asparagine, produced by pancreatic digestion; it is actively anticoagulant.

aspect (as'pekt) 1. that part of a surface viewed from a particular direction. 2. the look or appearance.
  dorsal a., that surface of a body viewed from the back or from above.
  ventral a., that surface of a body viewed from the front or from below.

aspergilloma (as"per-jil-o'mah) a tumor-like mass formed by growth of the fungus, frequently observed in the lungs in aspergillosis.

aspergillosis (as"per-jil-o'sis) infection caused by Aspergillus.

Aspergillus (as"per-jil'us) a genus of fungi (molds), several species of which are endoparasitic and probably pathogenic.

aspermia (ah-sper'me-ah) absence of semen or spermatozoa.

asphyxia (as-fik'se-ah) a condition in which there is a deficiency of oxygen in the blood and an increase in carbon dioxide in the blood and tissues. The symptoms include irregular and disturbed respirations, or a complete absence of breathing, and pallor or cyanosis. Asphyxia may occur whenever there is an interruption in the normal exchange of oxygen and carbon dioxide between the lungs and the outside air. Some common causes are drowning, electric shock, lodging of a foreign body in the air passages, inhalation of smoke and poisonous gases and trauma to or disease of the lungs or air passages. Treatment includes immediate remedy of the situation by ARTIFICIAL RESPIRATION and removal of the underlying cause whenever possible.

asphyxiate (as-fik'se-āt) to deprive of oxygen for utilization by the tissues.

aspidium (as-pid'e-um) the dried products of a genus of plants known as male fern.
  a. oleoresin, a dark green, thick liquid used as a vermifuge or anthelmintic in the treatment of tapeworm infection. It is toxic in large doses and may cause violent symptoms such as vomiting, weakness, convulsions, coma, permanent blindness, jaundice and kidney damage. This drug is contraindicated in heart disease, liver and kidney disorders and ulcerations of the gastrointestinal tract, and is seldom used today.

aspirate (as'pĭ-rāt) to withdraw fluid by negative pressure, or suction.

aspiration (as"pĭ-ra'shun) 1. the act of breathing or drawing in. Pathologic aspiration of vomitus or mucus into the respiratory tract may occur when a person is unconscious or under the effects of a general anesthesia. This can be avoided by keeping the head turned to the side and removing foreign material such as vomitus, mucus or blood from the air passages. 2. withdrawal of fluid by an aspirator. The method is widely used in hospitals, especially during surgery, to drain the area of the body being operated on and keep it clear of excess fluids. Sometimes after extensive surgery, suction drainage under the skin is used to speed the healing process.

aspirator (as"pĭ-ra'tor) an instrument for evacuating fluid by suction.

aspirin (as'pĭ-rin) acetylsalicylic acid, a common drug generally used to relieve pain and reduce fever, and specifically prescribed for rheumatic and arthritic disorders. Indiscriminate use of the drug may lead to toxic symptoms such as gastrointestinal disorders, ringing in the ears, headache and, in severe toxicity, depression of the heart rate.

asplenia (ah-sple'ne-ah) absence of the spleen.

asporogenic (as"po-ro-jen'ik) not producing spores.

asporous (ah-spo'rus) having no true spores.

assay (as'a) determination of the purity of a substance or the amount of any particular constituent of a mixture.
  biological a., determination of the potency of a drug or other substance by comparing the effects it has on animals with those of a reference standard.

assimilation (ah-sim"ĭ-la'shun) 1. conversion of absorbed material into the substance of the absorbing body. 2. psychologically, absorption of new experiences into the existing psychologic makeup.

association (ah-so"se-a'shun) 1. close relation in

time or space. 2. in psychiatry, the continuing development and expansion of ideas.

a. areas, areas of the cerebral cortex not themselves functionally differentiated, but connected with other centers and the neothalamus by numerous fibers.

free a., oral expression of one's ideas as they arrive spontaneously; a method used in psychoanalysis.

astasia (as-ta′ze-ah) motor incoordination with inability to stand. adj., **astat′ic.**

a.-aba′sia, hysterical inability or refusal to stand or walk because of fear of falling. Other use of the legs is normal.

astatine (as′tah-tēn) a chemical element, atomic number 85, atomic weight 210, symbol At. (See table of ELEMENTS.)

asteatosis (as″te-ah-to′sis) deficiency or absence of sebum.

aster (as′ter) a cluster of raylike filaments extending from each daughter centriole at the beginning of division of the nucleus of a cell.

astereognosis (ah-ster″e-og-no′sis) inability to recognize familiar objects by feeling their shape.

asterixis (as″ter-ik′sis) a motor disturbance marked by intermittency of sustained contraction of groups of muscles; called liver flap because of its occurrence in coma associated with liver disease, but observed also in other conditions.

asternal (a-ster′nal) not joined to the sternum.

asternia (ah-ster′ne-ah) a developmental anomaly with absence of the sternum.

asteroid (as′ter-oid) star-shaped.

Asterol (as′ter-ol) trademark for preparations of diamthazole, an antifungal.

asthen(o)- (as′thĕ-no) word element [Gr.], *weak; weakness.*

asthenia (as-the′ne-ah) debility; loss of strength. adj., **asthen′ic.**

neurocirculatory a., a symptom complex characterized by the occurrence of breathlessness, giddiness, a sense of fatigue, pain in the region of the precordium and palpitation. It occurs chiefly in soldiers in active war service, though it is also seen in civilians, and is a form of NEUROSIS.

tropical anhidrotic a., a condition due to generalized absence of sweating in conditions of high temperature, characterized by a tendency to overfatigability, irritability, anorexia, inability to concentrate and drowsiness, with headache and vertigo.

asthenocoria (as″thĕ-no-ko′re-ah) sluggishness of the pupillary light reflex.

asthenometer (as″thĕ-nom′ĕ-ter) a device used in measuring muscular asthenia.

asthenopia (as″thĕ-no′pe-ah) impairment of vision, with pain in the eyes, back of the head and the neck. adj., **asthenop′ic.**

accommodative a., asthenopia due to strain of the ciliary muscle.

muscular a., asthenopia due to weakness of the external ocular muscles.

asthenospermia (as″thĕ-no-sper′me-ah) reduced motility of spermatozoa in the semen.

asthma (az′mah) a disease of the bronchi, technically known as bronchial asthma, characterized by dyspnea, wheezing and a sense of constriction of the chest. adj., **asthmat′ic.** A chronic disease, it strikes the sufferer periodically rather than constantly. Attacks vary greatly in frequency, duration and intensity, ranging from occasional periods of wheezing and slight dyspnea to severe attacks that almost cause suffocation. An acute attack that persists for days or weeks is called status asthmaticus.

Extrinsic asthma is due to an allergy to antigens; usually the offending allergens are suspended in the air, but occasionally food or drugs taken by the patient may be the inciting factors. More than half the cases of asthma are of this type. Intrinsic asthma is usually secondary to chronic and recurrent infections of the bronchi, sinuses or tonsils and adenoids. There is evidence that this type of asthma develops from a hypersensitivity to the bacteria causing the infection.

Some cases of bronchial asthma appear to be due chiefly to nervous tension and often improve when the patient's emotional problems are solved. This may require psychotherapy. Even cases of asthma that have a physical cause are apt to become worse if the patient is emotionally disturbed or tense. For this reason asthma is usually included among diseases of psychologic origin, known as psychosomatic illnesses.

SYMPTOMS. Typically, an attack of asthma is characterized by dyspnea and a wheezing type of respiration. The patient usually sits upright and leans forward so as to use all of the muscles of respiration. Cyanosis is rare except in severe attacks. The end of the attack is usually indicated by a productive cough in which the patient expectorates a considerable quantity of thick, tenacious, mucoid sputum.

TREATMENT. The treatment of asthma begins with attempts to determine the substance or substances to which the person is allergic. After the allergens have been discovered the patient must make every effort to avoid them.

Drugs used in the treatment of asthma are given primarily for the relief of symptoms. As yet there is no cure for asthma. Bronchodilators such as epinephrine and aminophylline may be used to enlarge the bronchioles, thus relieving respiratory embarrassment. Other drugs that thin the secretions and help the patient cough up the mucus obstructing his air passages (expectorants) may also be prescribed.

The patient with status asthmaticus is very seriously ill and must receive special attention and medication to avoid excessive strain on the heart and severe respiratory difficulties.

NURSING CARE. Relief of respiratory difficulties can be obtained best by supporting the patient in a sitting position during an acute attack, administering oxygen as ordered and providing a quiet and restful atmosphere. Special filters or air conditioning systems may be used to remove dust, pollen and other allergens from the patient's environment.

Protection of the patient from sources of emotional excitement frequently lessens the severity of the attack. Since asthma is a psychosomatic illness, the emotions of the patient play a very important part in the severity and frequency of asthmatic attacks. It is essential that the nurse know her patient well and carefully observe his reaction to various stimuli, such as noise, individual visitors and hospital routine, so that she may help the patient avoid the things that upset him.

cardiac a., a term applied to breathing difficulties due to pulmonary edema in heart disease.

astigmatism (ah-stig′mah-tizm) an error of refraction in which parallel light rays fail to come to focus on the retina, owing to differences in curvature in various meridians of the refractive surfaces (cornea and lens) of the eye. adj., **astigmat′ic.** The exact cause of astigmatism is not known. Common types of astigmatism seem to run in families and are believed to be inherited. Probably everyone has some astigmatism, since it is rare to find perfectly shaped curves in the cornea and lens. The defect may not be serious enough to make treatment necessary; however, corrective lenses may be needed when the refractive error is troublesome.

compound a., that in which the two principal meridians are both hyperopic (compound hyperopic astigmatism) or myopic (compound myopic astigmatism), but in varying degrees.

corneal a., that due to the presence of abnormal curvatures on the anterior or posterior surface of the cornea.

hyperopic a., that in which the light rays are brought to a focus behind the retina.

irregular a., that in which the refraction varies even in one principal meridian, making correction by lenses impossible.

lenticular a., astigmatism due to defect of the crystalline lens.

mixed a., that in which one principal meridian is hyperopic and the other myopic.

myopic a., that in which the light rays are brought to a focus in front of the retina.

regular a., that in which the refraction changes gradually in power from one principal meridian of the eye to the other, the two meridians always being at right angles; this condition is further classified as being against the rule when the meridian of greatest refractive power tends toward the horizontal, with the rule when it tends toward the vertical, and oblique when it lies 45 degrees from the horizontal and vertical.

astigmometer (as″tig-mom′ĕ-ter) an apparatus used in measuring astigmatism.

astomia (ah-sto′me-ah) congenital atresia of the mouth. adj., **asto′matous.**

astomus (ah-sto′mus) a fetal monster exhibiting astomia.

astragalectomy (ah-strag″ah-lek′to-me) excision of the astragalus.

astragalus (ah-strag′ah-lus) talus.

astraphobia (as″trah-fo′be-ah) morbid fear of lightning.

astringent (ah-strin′jent) 1. causing contraction and arresting discharges. 2. an agent that arrests discharges. Astringents act as protein precipitants; they arrest discharge by causing shrinkage of tissue.

Some astringents, such as tannic acid, have been used in treating diarrhea; others, such as boric acid and sodium borate, help relieve the symptoms of inflammation of the mucous membranes of the throat or conjunctiva of the eye. Skin preparations such as shaving lotions often contain astringents such as aluminum acetate that help to reduce oiliness and excessive perspiration. Witch hazel is a common household astringent used to reduce swelling. Styptic pencils, used to stop bleeding from small cuts, contain astringents. Zinc oxide and calamine are astringents used in lotions, powders and ointments to relieve itching and chafing in various forms of dermatitis. Astringents have some bacteriostatic properties, though they are not generally used as antiseptics.

astroblast (as′tro-blast) a cell that develops into an astrocyte.

astroblastoma (as″tro-blas-to′mah) a rare, malignant tumor of the nervous system.

astrocyte (as′tro-sīt) 1. a star-shaped cell of the neuroglia. 2. a bone cell.

astrocytoma (as″tro-si-to′mah) a tumor of the central nervous system, usually slowly growing, consisting of astrocytes.

astroglia (ah-strog′le-ah) neuroglia tissue made up of astrocytes.

astrosphere (as′tro-sfēr) a structure made up of a group of radiating fibrils that converge toward the centrosome and continue in the centrosphere of a cell.

asymbolia (ah″sim-bo′le-ah) loss of ability to understand symbols, as words, figures, gestures, signs.

asymphytous (ah-sim′fĭ-tus) separate or distinct; not grown together.

asymptomatic (a″simp-to-mat′ik) showing no symptoms.

asynchronism (a-sin′kro-nizm) occurrence at different times.

asynclitism (ah-sin′klĭ-tizm) oblique presentation of the head in parturition.

asyndesis (ah-sin′dĕ-sis) a disorder of thinking in which related elements of a thought cannot be welded together in a whole.

asynechia (ah″sĭ-nek′e-ah) absence of continuity of structure.

asynergia (a″sin-er′je-ah) failure of cooperation among muscle groups that is necessary for execution of movement.

asynesia (ah″sĭ-ne′ze-ah) dullness of intellect.

asynovia (ah″sĭ-no′ve-ah) absence or insufficiency of synovia.

asyntaxia (a″sin-tak′se-ah) lack of proper and orderly embryonic development.

asystole (a-sis′to-le) imperfect or incomplete systole.

At chemical symbol, *astatine.*

at. atomic.

Atabrine (at′ah-brin, at′ah-brēn) trademark for quinacrine, an antimalarial and anthelmintic preparation.

atactic (ah-tak′tik) pertaining to or characterized by ataxia; marked by incoordination or irregularity.

atactilia (ah″tak-til′e-ah) loss of the sense of touch.

ataractic (at″ah-rak′tik) 1. pertaining to or characterized by ataraxia. 2. an agent that induces ataraxia.

ataralgesia (at″ar-al-je′ze-ah) combined sedation and analgesia intended to abolish mental distress and pain attendant on surgical procedures.

Atarax (at′ah-raks) trademark for preparations of hydroxyzine hydrochloride, a tranquilizer.

ataraxia (at″ah-rak′se-ah) a state of detached serenity without depression of mental faculties or impairment of consciousness.

atavism (at′ah-vizm) inheritance of characters from remote ancestors. adj., **atavis′tic.**

ataxia (ah-tak′se-ah) incoordination occurring in the absence of apraxia, paresis, rigidity, spasticity or involuntary movement. adj., **atac′tic, atax′ic.**
  Friedreich′s a., hereditary a., the spinal form of hereditary sclerosis (see also FRIEDREICH′S ATAXIA).
  locomotor a., tabes dorsalis.
  a.-telangiectasia, a heredofamilial, progressive ataxia, associated with oculocutaneous telangiectasia, sinopulmonary disease with frequent respiratory infections and abnormal eye movements.

ataxiamnesic (ah-tak″se-am-ne′sik) characterized by ataxia and amnesia.

ataxiaphasia (ah-tak″se-ah-fa′ze-ah) ability to utter words, but not sentences.

ataxophemia (ah-tak″so-fe′me-ah) lack of coordination of speech muscles.

ataxy (ah-tak′se) ataxia.

atel(o)- (at′ĕ-lo) word element [Gr.], *incomplete; imperfectly developed.*

atelectasis (at″ĕ-lak′tah-sis) a collapsed or airless state of the lung, which may be acute or chronic, and may involve all or part of the lung. adj., **atelectat′ic.** The primary cause of atelectasis is obstruction of the bronchus serving the affected area. In fetal atelectasis the lungs fail to expand normally at birth. This condition may be due to a variety of causes, including prematurity (and may accompany HYALINE MEMBRANE DISEASE), diminished nervous stimulus to breathing and crying, fetal hypoxia from any cause, including oversedation of the mother during labor and delivery and obstruction of the bronchus by a mucous plug.
  SYMPTOMS. In acute atelectasis in which there is sudden obstruction of the bronchus, there may be pain in the affected side, dyspnea and cyanosis, elevation of temperature, a drop in blood pressure or shock. In the chronic form of atelectasis the patient may experience no symptoms other than gradually developing dyspnea and weakness.
  X-ray examination may show a shadow in the area of collapse. If an entire lobe is collapsed, the x-ray will show the trachea, heart and mediastinum deviated toward the collapsed area, with the diaphragm elevated on that side.
  TREATMENT. Atelectasis in the newborn is treated by suctioning the trachea to establish an open airway and by the administration of oxygen (40 per cent concentration). High concentrations of oxygen given over a prolonged period tend to promote atelectasis and may lead to the development of retrolental fibroplasia in premature infants.
  Acute atelectasis is treated by removing the cause whenever possible. To accomplish this, coughing (sometimes using a cough-inducing machine), suctioning and BRONCHOSCOPY may be employed. Detergent aerosols, used with a mist-producing apparatus, may be administered at regular intervals. Chronic atelectasis usually requires surgical removal of the affected segment or lobe of lung. Antibiotics are given to combat the infection that almost always accompanies secondary atelectasis.
  acquired a., compression or collapse of previously expanded pulmonary alveoli attending some underlying disease of the lungs.
  congenital a., that present at (primary atelectasis) or immediately after birth (secondary atelectasis).
  primary a., that in which the alveoli have never been expanded with air.
  secondary a., that in which resorption of the contained air has led to collapse of the alveoli.

atelia (ah-te′le-ah) incompleteness; imperfection due to failure to develop completely.

ateliosis (ah-te″le-o′sis) a condition characterized by failure to develop completely. adj., **ateliot′ic.**

atelocardia (at″ĕ-lo-kar′de-ah) imperfect development of the heart.

atelocephaly (at″ĕ-lo-sef′ah-le) imperfect development of the skull. adj., **atelocephal′ic.**

atelomyelia (at″ĕ-lo-mi-e′le-ah) imperfect development of the spinal cord.

athelia (ah-the′le-ah) congenital absence of the nipples.

athermic (ah-ther′mik) without rise of temperature.

athermosystaltic (ah-ther″mo-sis-tal′tik) not contracting under the action of cold or heat.

atherogenesis (ath″er-o-jen′ĕ-sis) formation of atheromatous lesions in arterial walls. adj., **atherogen′ic.**

atheroma (ath″er-o′mah) an abnormal mass of fatty or lipid material existing as a discrete deposit in an arterial wall. adj., **atherom′atous.**

atheromatosis (ath″er-o″mah-to′sis) the presence of multiple atheromas.

atheronecrosis (ath″er-o-nĕ-kro′sis) necrosis accompanying atherosclerosis.

atherosclerosis (ath″er-o-sklĕ-ro′sis) a condition characterized by degeneration and hardening of the walls of the arteries and sometimes the valves of the heart, related especially to thickening of the tunica intima (intimal layer). (See also ARTERIOSCLEROSIS.)

atherosis (ath″er-o′sis) atheromatosis.

athetoid (ath′ĕ-toid) 1. resembling athetosis. 2. affected with athetosis.

athetosis (ath″ĕ-to′sis) repetitive involuntary, slow gross movements.

athlete's foot (ath′lēts) a fungus infection of the skin of the foot; called also tinea pedis. Athlete's foot causes itching and often blisters and cracks, usually between the toes. Causative agents are *Candida albicans, Epidermophyton floccosum* and species of *Trichophyton*, which thrive on warmth and dampness.

If not arrested, athlete's foot can cause a rash and itching in other parts of the body as well. It is likely to be recurrent, since the fungus survives under the toenails and reappears when conditions are favorable. Although athlete's foot is usually little more than an uncomfortable nuisance, its open sores provide excellent sites for more serious infections. Early treatment and medical advice insure correct diagnosis and prevention of complications. Specific diagnosis is made by microscopic examination or culture of skin scrapings for the fungus.

Prevention of athlete's foot includes keeping the feet dry and open to the air as much as possible, especially the areas between the toes. Small cotton pads may be used between the toes if this area is difficult to keep dry. A dusting powder may be used on the feet and sprinkled in the shoes to reduce the accumulation of moisture.

For treatment, there are a number of compounds that can be applied locally for both the acute and chronic stages. Resistant cases may need x-ray or grenz-ray therapy (by a specialist).

athrepsia (ah-threp′se-ah) marasmus. adj., **athrep′tic.**

athrombia (ah-throm′be-ah) defective clotting of the blood.

athymia (ah-thi′me-ah) 1. dementia. 2. absence of functioning thymus tissue.

athymism (ah-thi′mizm) the condition induced by removal of the thymus.

athyreosis (ah-thi″re-o′sis) athyria. adj., **athyreot′ic.**

athyria (ah-thi′re-ah) absence of functioning thyroid tissue.

atlantal (at-lan′tal) pertaining to the atlas.

atlas (at′las) the uppermost segment of the backbone on which the occipital bone sits.

atloaxoid (at″lo-ak′soid) pertaining to atlas and axis.

atlodymus (at-lod′ĭ-mus) a fetal monster with two heads and one body.

atmos (at′mos) atomsphere (2).

atmosphere (at′mos-fēr) 1. the entire gaseous envelope surrounding the earth, extending to an altitude of 10 miles. 2. a unit of pressure, equivalent to that on a surface at sea level, being about 15 lb. per square inch, or equivalent to that of a column of mercury 760 mm. high.

atmospheric (at″mos-fer′ik) of or pertaining to the atmosphere.

a. pressure, the pressure exerted by the atmosphere, about 15 lb. to the square inch at sea level.

at. no. atomic number.

atocia (ah-to′se-ah) sterility in the female.

atom (at′om) the smallest particle of an element that has all the properties of the element. adj., **atomic.** There are two main parts of an atom: the nucleus and the electron cloud. The nucleus is made up of protons, which carry a positive electrical charge, and (except in hydrogen) neutrons, which contain one proton and one electron and carry no electrical charge. The electron cloud is made up of particles called electrons, which carry a negative electrical charge and move in orbits or "shells" around the nucleus. Different atoms have different numbers of protons, neutrons and electrons in their makeup.

In a chemical change atoms do not break up but act as individual units. The chemical behavior of an atom is controlled by the number and spatial arrangement of electrons in orbit around the nucleus. The atoms of radioactive elements are very unstable and are capable of emitting nuclear particles in a stream or "ray." These are called radiations. (See also ELEMENT and RADIATION.)

The atomic number of an element is the number of free protons (those not in neutrons) in the nucleus; it is equal to the net positive charge of the nucleus.

The atomic weight is the weight of an atom of a substance as compared with the weight of an atom of oxygen, which is taken as 16.

atomization (at″om-ĭ-za′shun) the act or process of breaking up a liquid into a fine spray.

atomizer (at′om-iz″er) an instrument for dispensing liquid in a fine spray.

atonia, atony (ah-to′ne-ah), (at′o-ne) absence or lack of normal tone. adj., **aton′ic.**

atopen (at′o-pen) an allergen.

atopic (ah-top′ik) 1. displaced. 2. pertaining to atopy.

atopy (at′o-pe) a clinical hypersensitivity state that is subject to hereditary influences; included are hay fever, asthma and eczema.

atoxic (ah-tok′sik) not poisonous; not due to a poison.

atoxigenic (a-tok″sĭ-jen′ik) not producing or elaborating toxins.

ATP adenosine triphosphate.

atraumatic (a″traw-mat′ik) not producing injury or damage.

atresia (ah-tre′ze-ah) absence of a normal opening. adj., **atret′ic.**

a. a′ni, imperforation of the anus.

aortic a., absence of the opening from the left ventricle of the heart into the aorta.

follicular a., a. follic′uli, absence of an opening in an ovarian follicle which retains a blighted ovum.

tricuspid a., absence of the opening between the right atrium and right ventricle.

atrial (a′tre-al) pertaining to an atrium.
  a. septal defect, a congenital heart defect, failure of closure of the foramen ovale.

atrichia (ah-trik′e-ah) absence of hair.

atrichosis (at″rĭ-ko′sis) complete congenital lack of hair.

atrichous (ah-trik′us) 1. having no hair. 2. having no flagella.

atriomegaly (a″tre-o-meg′ah-le) abnormal enlargement of an atrium of the heart.

atrionector (a″tre-o-nek′tor) the sinoatrial node.

atrioseptopexy (a″tre-o-sep′to-pek″se) surgical correction of a defect in the interatrial septum.

atrioseptoplasty (a″tre-o-sep′to-plas″te) plastic repair of the interatrial septum.

atrioventricular (a″tre-o-ven-trik′u-lar) pertaining to the atrium and ventricle.
  a. node, a mass of cardiac muscle fibers lying on the right lower part of the interatrial septum of the heart. Its function is the transmission of the cardiac impulse from the sinoatrial node to the muscular walls of the ventricles. The conductive system is organized so that transmission is slightly delayed at the atrioventricular node, thus allowing time for the atria to empty their contents into the ventricles before the ventricles begin to contract.

atrium (a′tre-um), pl. *a′tria* [L.] an external chamber, or entrance hall, especially the upper chamber (a′trium cor′dis) on either side of the heart, transmitting to the ventricle of the same side blood received (left a′trium) from the pulmonary veins and (right a′trium) from the venae cavae.

atrophia (ah-tro′fe-ah) [L.] atrophy.

atrophoderma (at″ro-fo-der′mah) atrophy of the skin.

atrophy (at′ro-fe) decrease in size of a normally developed organ or tissue; wasting. adj., **atroph′ic.**
  acute yellow a., atrophy and yellow discoloration of the liver, with jaundice.
  disuse a., atrophy of a tissue or organ as a result of its inactivity or diminished function.
  myelopathic muscular a., progressive muscular wasting due to degeneration of cells of the anterior horns of the spinal cord, beginning usually in the small muscles of the hands, but in some cases (scapulohumeral type) in those of the upper arm and shoulder, and progressing slowly to the muscles of the lower extremity.
  progressive neuromuscular a., progressive neuropathic (peroneal) muscular a., muscular atrophy due to degeneration of the cells of the posterior columns of the spinal cord and of the peripheral nerves, beginning in the muscles supplied by the peroneal nerves, and progressing slowly to involve the muscles of the hands and arms.

atropine (at′ro-pēn) a poisonous parasympatholytic alkaloid of belladonna, used in a variety of conditions. Actions include decrease of secretions, increased heart rate and rate of respirations and relaxation of smooth muscle tissue. It may be used to dilate pupils, for general cerebral stimulation, for relief of gastrointestinal cramps and hypermotility and locally to relieve pain. In various combinations with other drugs, atropine may be administered orally or intramuscularly, or applied topically. Atropine methylnitrate and atropine sulfate are soluble compounds of atropine, with similar uses.
  a. poisoning, severe toxic reaction due to overdosage of atropine. Symptoms include dryness of mouth, thirst, difficulty in swallowing, dilated pupils, tachycardia, fever, delirium, stupor and a rash on the face, neck and upper trunk. Treatment consists of gastric suction or the inducement of vomiting to remove the poison from the stomach; the stomach is then washed with 2 to 4 liters of water containing activated charcoal. The lavage is followed with a solution of 30 Gm. of sodium sulfate in 200 ml. of water which is left in the stomach. Barbiturates may be used to control excitability. There may be a need for treatment of respiratory difficulty. Measures also are taken to reduce the high body temperature.

A.T.S. antitetanus serum.

attenuation (ah-ten″u-a′shun) 1. the act of thinning or weakening. 2. the alteration of the virulence of a pathogenic microorganism by passage through another host species.

attic (at′ik) a small upper space of the middle ear, containing the head of the malleus and the body of the incus.

atticoantrotomy (at″ĭ-ko-an-trot′o-me) surgical exposure of the attic and mastoid antrum.

atticotomy (at″ĭ-kot′o-me) incision into the attic.

attitude (at′ĭ-tūd) 1. a posture or position of the body; in obstetrics, the position of the fetus in the uterus. 2. a pattern of mental views established by cumulative prior experience.

attraction (ah-trak′shun) the force or influence by which one object is drawn toward another.
  capillary a., the force that causes a liquid to rise in a fine-caliber tube.

at. wt. atomic weight.

atypia (a-tip′e-ah) deviation from the normal or typical state.

A.U. 1. Angstrom unit. 2. both ears.

Au chemical symbol, *gold* (L. *aurum*).

audi(o)- (aw′de-o) word element [L.], *hearing.*

audile (aw′dil) pertaining to hearing.

audioanalgesia (aw″de-o-an″al-je′ze-ah) reduction or abolition of pain by listening to recorded music to which has been added a background of so-called white sound.

audiogenic (aw″de-o-jen′ik) produced by sound.

audiogram (aw′de-o-gram″) a graphic record of the findings by audiometry.

audiology (aw″de-ol′o-je) the science concerned with the sense of hearing.

audiometer (aw″de-om′ĕ-ter) an apparatus used in audiometry.

audiometry (aw″de-om′ĕ-tre) measurement of the acuity of hearing for the various frequencies of sound waves.

audiosurgery (aw″de-o-ser′jer-e) surgery of the ear.

audition (aw-dish′un) perception of sound; hearing.
   chromatic a., chromesthesia.

auditory (aw′dĭ-to″re) pertaining to the ear or the sense of hearing.
   a. nerve, the eighth cranial nerve; called also VESTIBULOCOCHLEAR NERVE and acoustic nerve.

augnathus (awg-nath′us) a fetal monster with a double lower jaw.

aula (aw′lah) the forward part of the third ventricle of the brain.

aura (aw′rah) a peculiar sensation preceding the appearance of more definite symptoms. An epileptic aura precedes the convulsive seizure and may involve visual disturbances, dizziness, numbness or any of a number of sensations which the patient may find difficult to describe exactly. In epilepsy the aura serves a useful purpose in that it warns the patient of an impending attack and gives him time to seek privacy and a safe place to lie down before the seizure actually begins.
   A migraine aura sometimes precedes migraine headache, warning the patient that an attack is imminent. When it occurs the patient should lie down in a quiet, darkened room. A warm bath before lying down sometimes increases relaxation and helps to prevent a severe attack.

aural (aw′ral) 1. pertaining to the ear. 2. pertaining to an aura.

aurantiasis (aw″ran-ti′ah-sis) yellowness of skin caused by intake of large amounts of food containing carotene.

aureomycin (aw″re-o-mi′sin) trademark for chlortetracycline hydrochloride, a broad-spectrum antibiotic effective against many different types of microorganisms.

auriasis (aw-ri′ah-sis) chrysiasis.

auric (aw′rik) pertaining to gold.

auricle (aw′rĭ-kl) 1. the flap of the ear. 2. the ear-shaped appendage of either atrium of the heart; sometimes used incorrectly to designate the entire atrium.

auricula (aw-rik′u-lah), pl. *auric′ulae* [L.] auricle.

auricular (aw-rik′u-lar) pertaining to an auricle or ear.

auricularis (aw-rik″u-la′ris) [L.] pertaining to the ear.

auriculotemporal (aw-rik″u-lo-tem′po-ral) pertaining to the ear and the temporal bone.

auriculoventricular (aw-rik″u-lo-ven-trik′u-lar) atrioventricular.

auripuncture (aw′rĭ-pungk″tūr) puncture of the tympanic membrane; called also myringotomy.

auris (aw′ris), pl. *au′res* [L.] ear.

auriscope (aw′rĭ-skōp) an instrument for examining the ear.

aurotherapy (aw″ro-ther′ah-pe) use of gold salts in treatment of disease.

aurothioglucose (aw″ro-thi″o-gloo′kōs) a gold preparation used in treating rheumatoid arthritis.

aurothioglycanide (aw″ro-thi″o-gli′kah-nīd) a gold preparation used in treating rheumatoid arthritis.

aurum (aw′rum) [L.] gold (symbol Au).

auscultate (aw′skul-tāt) to examine by auscultation.

auscultation (aw″skul-ta′shun) listening to sounds produced within the body by various organs as they perform their functions.

auscultatory (aw-skul′tah-to″re) pertaining to auscultation.

aut(o)- (aw′to) word element [Gr.], *self*.

autacoid (aw′tah-koid) any internal secretion.

autarcesis (aw-tar′sĕ-sis) normal ability of body cells to resist infection. adj., **autarcet′ic.**

autism (aw′tizm) morbid self-absorption with extreme withdrawal and failure to relate to other persons. adj., **autis′tic.**
   childhood a., a form of autism in children that is characteristic of schizophrenia; called also childhood schizophrenia. The autistic child responds chiefly to his inner thoughts and cannot relate to his environment. He often appears immature and mentally retarded.
   early infantile a., an emotional illness characterized by early failure to relate emotionally to parents and others.

autoagglutination (aw″to-ah-gloo″tĭ-na′shun) clumping together of a persons's cells due to a substance present in his own serum.

autoagglutinin (aw″to-ah-gloo′tĭ-nin) a factor in serum capable of causing clumping together of the subject's own cellular elements.

autoamputation (aw″to-am″pu-ta′shun) spontaneous detachment from the body and elimination of an appendage or an abnormal growth, such as a polyp.

autoantibody (aw″to-an′tĭ-bod″e) an antibody or antibody-like factor supposedly directed against components native to the tissues of the organism in which it is found.

autoantigen (aw″to-an′tĭ-jen) a substance that stimulates production of antibody in the organism in which it occurs.

autoantitoxin (aw″to-an″tĭ-tok′sin) antitoxin produced by the body itself.

autocatalysis (aw″to-kah-tal′ĭ-sis) 1. catalysis in which a product of the reaction hastens or intensifies the catalysis. 2. the process in mitosis by which a chromosome brings about the synthesis of an exact replica immediately beside itself.

autochthonous (aw-tok′tho-nus) originating in the same area in which it is found.

autocinesis (aw″to-si-ne′sis) autokinesis.

autoclasis (aw-tok′lah-sis) destruction of a part by influences within itself.

autoclave (aw′to-klāv) a self-locking apparatus for the sterilization of materials by steam under pressure. The autoclave allows steam to flow around each article placed in the chamber. The vapor penetrates cloth or paper used to package the articles being sterilized. Autoclaving is one of the most effective methods for destruction of all types of microorganisms. The amount of time and degree of temperature necessary for sterilization depend on the articles to be sterilized and whether they are wrapped or left directly exposed to the steam.

autocytolysin (aw″to-si-tol′ĭ-sin) autolysin.

autocytolysis (aw″to-si-tol′ĭ-sis) autolysis.

autodigestion (aw″to-di-jes′chun) dissolution of tissue by its own secretions.

autodiploidy (aw″to-dip′loi-de) the state of having two sets of chromosomes as the result of doubling of the haploid set.

autoecholalia (aw″to-ek″o-la′le-ah) insane repetition of one's own words.

autoeczematization (aw″to-ek-zem″ah-tĭ-za′-shun) the spread, at first locally and later more generally, of lesions from an originally circumscribed focus of eczema.

autoerotism (aw″to-er′o-tizm) erotic behavior directed toward one's self. adj., **autoerot′ic.**

autogenesis (aw″to-jen′ĕ-sis) 1. spontaneous generation. 2. origination within the organism. adj., **autog′enous.**

autograft (aw′to-graft) a graft transferred from one part of the patient's body to another part.

autographism (aw-tog′rah-fizm) dermographia.

autohemagglutination (aw″to-hem″ah-gloo″tĭ-na′shun) agglutination of erythrocytes by a factor produced in the subject's own body.

autohemagglutinin (aw″to-hem″ah-gloo′tĭ-nin) a substance produced in a person's body that causes agglutination of his own erythrocytes.

autohemolysin (aw″to-he-mol′ĭ-sin) a hemolysin produced in the body of an animal which causes destruction of its own erythrocytes.

autohemolysis (aw″to-he-mol′ĭ-sis) hemolysis of the blood cells of an individual by his own serum.

autohemotherapy (aw″to-he″mo-ther′ah-pe) treatment by administration of the patient's own blood.

autohypnosis (aw″to-hip-no′sis) self-induced hypnosis.

autoimmune disease (aw″to-ĭ-mūn′) disease due to immunologic action of one's own cells or antibodies on components of the body.

autoimmunization (aw″to-im″u-nĭ-za′shun) production in an organism of reactivity to its own tissues.

autoinoculation (aw″to-ĭ-nok″u-la′shun) inoculation with a virus from one's own body.

autointoxication (aw″to-in-tok″sĭ-ka′shun) poisoning by uneliminated material (toxins) formed within the body.

autoisolysin (aw″to-i-sol′ĭ-sin) a substance that lyses the corpuscles of the individual in which it is formed and also those of other individuals of the same species.

autokeratoplasty (aw″to-ker′ah-to-plas″te) corneal grafting with tissue from the other eye.

autokinesis (aw″to-ki-ne′sis) voluntary motion. adj., **autokinet′ic.**

autolesion (aw″to-le′zhun) a self-inflicted injury.

autologous (aw-tol′o-gus) related to self; belonging to the same organism.

autolysate (aw-tol′ĭ-sāt) a substance produced by autolysis.

autolysin (aw-tol′ĭ-sin) a lysin originating in an organism and capable of destroying its own cells and tissues.

autolysis (aw-tol′ĭ-sis) the disintegration of cells or tissues by endogenous enzymes. adj., **autolyt′ic.**

automatic (aw″to-mat′ik) spontaneous; done involuntarily.

automatism (aw-tom′ah-tizm) mechanical, repetitive motor behavior performed unconsciously.
    command a., uncritical response to commands, as in hypnosis and certain mental states.

automysophobia (aw″to-mi″so-fo′be-ah) insane dread of personal uncleanness.

autonomic (aw″to-nom′ik) not subject to voluntary control.
    a. nervous system, the branch of the nervous system that works without conscious control. The voluntary nervous system governs the striated or skeletal muscles, whereas the autonomic nervous system governs the glands, the cardiac muscle and the smooth muscles, such as those of the digestive system, the respiratory system and the skin. The autonomic nervous system is divided into two subsidiary systems, the sympathetic system and the parasympathetic system.

autonomotropic (aw″to-nom″o-trop′ik) having an affinity for the autonomic nervous system.

autopathy (aw-top′ah-the) a disease without apparent external causation.

autopepsia (aw″to-pep′se-ah) digestion of stomach wall by its own secretion.

autophagy (aw-tof′ah-je) eating or biting of one's own flesh.

autophilia (aw″to-fil′e-ah) pathologic self-esteem; narcissism.

autophobia (aw″to-fo′be-ah) morbid dread of solitude.

autophony (aw-tof′o-ne) the sensation of abnormal loudness of one's own voice.

autoplasmotherapy (aw″to-plaz″mo-ther′ah-pe) therapeutic injection of one's own plasma.

autoplastic (aw″to-plas′tik) pertaining to the indirect modification and adaptation of impulses prior to their outward expression.

autoplasty (aw′to-plas″te) plastic repair of diseased or injured parts with tissue from another region of the body.

autoploidy (aw″to-ploi′de) the state of having two or more chromosome sets as the result of redoubling of the haploid set.

autopolyploidy (aw″to-pol″ĭ-ploi′de) the state of having more than two chromosome sets as a result of redoubling of the chromosomes of a haploid individual or cell.

autoprecipitin (aw″to-pre-sip′ĭ-tin) a substance that precipitates the serum of the animal in which it was developed.

autoprothrombin (aw″to-pro-throm′bin) an activation product of prothrombin.

autopsy (aw′top-se) examination of a body after death to determine the actual cause of death; called also postmortem examination and necropsy. An autopsy is ordered by a coroner or medical examiner whenever the cause of death is unknown or the death takes place under suspicious circumstances. Unless an autopsy is demanded by public authorities, it cannot be performed without the permission of the next of kin of the deceased. However, an autopsy examination is always undertaken in a dignified and respectful manner, and leading religious authorities are in favor of it when it is requested by the attending physician. Autopsies are also valuable sources of medical knowledge.

autopsychic (aw″to-si′kik) pertaining to one's ideas concerning his own personality.

autoradiogram (aw″to-ra′de-o-gram″) the film produced by autoradiography.

autoradiography (aw″to-ra″de-og′rah-fe) the recording, on specially sensitized film, of radiation emitted by the tissue itself, especially after purposeful introduction into it of radioactive material.

autoregulation (aw″to-reg″u-la′shun) control of certain phenomena by factors inherent in a situation; usually restricted to the circulatory system.

autoscopy (aw-tos′ko-pe) the visual hallucination of one's self.

autosensitization (aw″to-sen″sĭ-tĭ-za′shun) development of sensitivity to one's own serum or tissues.

autosepticemia (aw″to-sep″tĭ-se′me-ah) septicemia from poisons developed within the body.

autoserodiagnosis (aw″to-se″ro-di″ag-no′sis) diagnostic use of autoserum.

autoserotherapy (aw″to-se″ro-ther′ah-pe) treatment by autoserum.

autoserum (aw″to-se′rum) serum prepared from the patient's own blood.

autosite (aw′to-sīt) a fetal monster capable of independent life, on or in which a parasitic twin lives.

autosome (aw′to-sōm) one of the 22 pairs of chromosomes in man not concerned with determination of the sex of the subject.

autosplenectomy (aw″to-sple-nek′to-me) extirpation of the spleen by progressive fibrosis and shrinkage.

autostimulation (aw″to-stim″u-la′shun) stimulation of an animal with antigenic material from its own tissues.

autosuggestion (aw″to-sug-jes′chun) suggestion arising in one's self.

autotomography (aw″to-to-mog′rah-fe) a method of body-section roentgenography involving movement of the patient instead of the x-ray tube.

autotopagnosia (aw″to-top-ag-no′se-ah) inability to orient correctly different parts of the body.

autotoxin (aw″to-tok′sin) a toxin developed within the body.

autotransfusion (aw″to-trans-fu′zhun) 1. the forcing of blood into vital parts by bandaging or elevating the limbs. 2. reinfusion of a patient's own blood.

autotransplantation (aw″to-trans″plan-ta′shun) transfer of tissue from one part of the body to another part.

autotroph (aw′to-trōf) an autotrophic organism.

autotrophic (aw″to-trof′ik) capable of synthesizing necessary nutrients if water, carbon dioxide, inorganic salts and a source of energy are available.

autovaccination (aw″to-vak″sĭ-na′shun) injection of autovaccine.

autovaccine (aw″to-vak′sēn) a vaccine prepared from the patient's own tissues or secretions.

autoxidation (aw″tok-sĭ-da′shun) the spontaneous reaction of a compound with molecular oxygen at room temperature.

auxanology (awk″sah-nol′o-je) the science of growth.

auxesis (awk-se′sis) increase in size; growth. adj., **auxet′ic.**

auxin (awk′sin) a chemical substance present in plants that is capable of accelerating the growth of cells.

auxocardia (awk″so-kar′de-ah) 1. diastole. 2. enlargement of the heart.

auxodrome (awk′so-drōm) the course of growth of a child as plotted on a specially devised graph.

auxology (awk-sol′o-je) the science of the growth of organisms.

auxotherapy (awk″so-ther′ah-pe) substitution therapy.

auxotroph (awk′so-trōf) an auxotrophic organism.

auxotrophic (awk″so-trof′ik) requiring a growth factor; used especially with reference to a mutation that causes such a requirement.

A.V. atrioventricular.

av. avoirdupois.

avascular (a-vas'ku-lar) not vascular; bloodless.

avascularization (a-vas"ku-lar-ĭ-za'shun) expulsion of blood, as by bandaging.

Avertin (ah-ver'tin) trademark for tribromoethanol, used in the induction phase of anesthesia.

avidin (av'ĭ-din) a protein in egg white which combines with biotin to render the latter inactive.

avirulence (a-vir'u-lens) lack of strength or virulence; lack of competence of an infectious agent to produce pathologic effects. adj., **avir'- ulent.**

avitaminosis (a-vi"tah-mĭ-no'sis) disease due to deficiency of vitamins in the diet. adj., **avitaminot'- ic.**

Avogadro's law (av-o-gad'rōz) equal volumes of perfect gases at the same temperature and pressure contain the same number of molecules.
 A's number, the number of particles of the type specified by the chemical formula of a certain substance in 1 gram-molecule of the substance.

avoidance (ah-void'ans) a conscious or unconscious human reaction defensively intended to escape anxiety, conflict, danger, fear or pain.

avoir. avoirdupois.

avoirdupois (av'er-dŭ-poiz") a common system of weight used in English-speaking countries for all commodites except drugs, precious stones and precious metals. (See also Table of Weights and Measures in the Appendix.)

avulsion (ah-vul'shun) the tearing away of a structure or part.
 phrenic a., extraction of a portion of the phrenic nerve.

axilla (ak-sil'ah), pl. *axil'lae* [L.] the armpit.

axillary (ak'sĭ-ler"e) of or pertaining to the armpit.

axio- (ak"se-o) word element [L., Gr.] denoting relation to an axis; in dentistry, used in special reference to the long axis of a tooth.

axioplasm (ak'se-o-plazm") the amorphous material of an axon in which the nerve fibers are buried.

axis (ak'sis), pl. *ax'es* [L., Gr.] 1. a straight line through a center. 2. the second cervical vertebra. adj., **ax'ial, ax'ile.**
 brain a., the brain stem.
 celiac a., a thick branch from the abdominal aorta.
 cerebrospinal a., the central nervous system.
 a.-cylinder, axon.
 dorsoventral a., one passing from the back to the belly surface of the body.
 electrical a. of heart, the resultant of the electromotive forces within the heart at any instant.
 frontal a., an imaginary line running from right to left through the center of the eyeball.
 a. of heart, a line passing through the center of the base of the heart and the apex.
 optic a., 1. a straight line joining the central points of curvature of the corneal (anterior pole) and scleral (posterior pole) spheres of the eye. 2. the visual axis.
 sagittal a., an imaginary line extending through the eye from before backward.

 visual a., a line from the point of vision of the retina to the object of vision.

axite (ak'sīt) a terminal filament of an axon.

axodendrite (ak"so-den'drīt) a nonmedullated side-fibril of an axon.

axolemma (ak"so-lem'ah) the limiting membrane surrounding the cytoplasm of the axon.

axolysis (ak-sol'ĭ-sis) degeneration of an axon.

axon (ak'son) the long outgrowth of the body of a nerve cell which conducts impulses from the body toward the next neuron; sometimes spelled axone. (See also NEURON.)

axoneme (ak'so-nēm) a slender axial filament, such as the axial thread of a chromosome, or that forming the central core of a flagellum or cilium.

axoneuron (ak"so-nu'ron) a nerve cell of the central nervous system.

axonotmesis (ak"son-ot-me'sis) damage to nerve fibers causing complete peripheral degeneration, but not disturbing the epineurium and intimate supporting structures of the nerve, so that regeneration of fibers occurs, with spontaneous recovery.

axophage (ak'so-fāj) a glia cell occurring in excavations in the myelin in myelitis.

axoplasm (ak'so-plazm) axioplasm.

axopodium (ak"so-po'de-um) a more or less permanent type of pseudopodium, long and needlelike, characterized by an axial rod, composed of a bundle of fibrils inserted near the center of the body of the cell.

axospongium (ak"so-spun'je-um) the network structure of the substance of an axon.

axostyle (ak'so-stīl) a supporting structure embedded along the longitudinal axis in the cytoplasm of a parasitic flagellate (Mastigophora).

Ayerza's disease (ah-yer'thaz) a form of erythremia marked by chronic cyanosis, chronic dyspnea, chronic bronchitis, bronchiectasis, hepatosplenomegaly and hyperplasia of bone marrow, and associated with sclerosis of the pulmonary artery.

AZ test Aschheim-Zondek test (for pregnancy).

Az. azote (nitrogen).

azacyclonol (a"zah-si'klo-nol) a compound used as a tranquilizer.

azaleine (ah-za'le-in) fuchsin.

azapetine (a"zah-pet'ēn) a compound used as an adrenergic-blocking agent and to dilate peripheral blood vessels.

azaserine (a"zah-ser'ēn) an agent used in treatment of acute leukemia.

azoospermia (a"zo-o-sper'me-ah) absence of spermatozoa in the semen.

azote (a'zōt) nitrogen.

azotemia (az"o-te'me-ah) the presence of nitrogen-containing compounds in the blood; uremia. adj., **azote'mic.**

azotenesis (az″o-tĕ-ne′sis) a disease due to excess nitrogen in system.

Azotobacter (ah-zo″to-bak′ter) a genus of Schizomycetes.

azotometer (az″o-tom′ĕ-ter) an instrument for measuring urea in urine.

azotorrhea (az″o-to-re′ah) discharge of abnormal quantities of nitrogenous matter in the stools.

azoturia (az″o-tu′re-ah) excess of urea in the urine.

azure (azh′ūr) a methylthionine dye.

azuresin (azh″u-rez′in) a complex combination of azure A dye and carbacrylic cation-exchange resin used as a diagnostic aid in detection of gastric secretion.

azurophil (azh-u′ro-fil) an element that stains easily with azure dye.

azurophilia (azh″u-ro-fil′e-ah) a condition in which the blood contains cells having azurophil granules.

azygogram (az′ĭ-go-gram″) the film obtained by azygography.

azygography (az″ĭ-gog′rah-fe) roentgenography of the azygous venous system.

azygos (az′ĭ-gos) any unpaired part.
  a. vein, a vein beginning in the abdomen as a continuation of the ascending lumbar vein which is a tributary of the inferior vena cava. The azygos vein and its tributaries serve as vessels for the return of blood from the thorax to the superior vena cava. The azygos vein also serves as a connecting link, through the ascending lumbar vein, between the venae cavae returning blood from above and below the heart.

azygous (az′ĭ-gus) having no fellow; unpaired.

azymia (a-zim′e-ah) absence of enzyme.

azymic (ah-zim′ik) not giving rise to fermentation.

B

B chemical symbol, *boron.*

B. Bacillus.

B.A. Bachelor of Arts.

Ba chemical symbol, *barium.*

Babes-Ernst granules (bah'bāz ernst) metachromatic granules, present in many bacterial cells.

Babinski reflex (bah-bin'ske) a reflex action of the toes, indicative of abnormalities in the motor control pathways leading from the cerebral cortex and widely used as a diagnostic aid in disorders of the central nervous system. It is elicited by a firm stimulus (usually scraping) on the sole of the foot, which results in dorsiflexion of the great toe and fanning of the smaller toes. Normally such a stimulus causes all the toes to bend downward. Called also Babinski's sign.

baby (ba'be) an infant (birth to 2 years).
   blue b., an infant born with cyanosis due to a congenital heart lesion or to congenital atelectasis.
   "**cloud b.,**" an apparently well infant who, because of viruses and bacteria in the respiratory tract or elsewhere, is able to contaminate the surrounding atmosphere and thus be responsible for nursery epidemics of staphylococcal infection.

Bacillaceae (bas″ĭl-la'se-e) a family of Schizomycetes.

bacillary (bas'ĭ-ler″e) pertaining to bacilli or to rodlike structures.

bacillemia (bas″ĭ-le'me-ah) the presence of bacilli in the blood.

bacilli (bah-sil'i) plural of *bacillus.*

bacillicide (bah-sil'ĭ-sīd) an agent that destroys bacilli.

bacilliform (bah-sil'ĭ-form) shaped like a bacillus.

bacillogenous (bas″ĭ-loj'ĕ-nus) caused by bacilli.

bacillophobia (bah-sil″o-pho'be-ah) morbid dread of microbes.

bacillosis (bas″ĭ-lo'sis) infection with bacilli.

bacillotherapy (bah-sil″o-ther'ah-pe) treatment with bacilli or bacteria.

bacilluria (bas″ĭ-lu're-ah) bacilli in the urine.

Bacillus (bah-sil'us) a genus of Schizomycetes containing several species only a small proportion of which are pathogenic.
   B. an'thracis, the causative agent of anthrax.
   B. co'li, *Escherichia coli.*
   B. dysente'riae, *Shigella dysenteriae.*
   B. enterit'idis, *Salmonella enteritidis.*
   B. lep'rae, *Mycobacterium leprae.*

   B. pneumo'niae, *Klebsiella pneumoniae.*
   B. pyocya'neus, *Pseudomonas aeruginosa.*
   B. tet'ani, *Clostridium tetani.*
   B. ty'phi, B. typho'sus, *Salmonella typhi.*
   B. welch'ii, *Clostridium perfringens.*

bacillus (bah-sil'us), pl. *bacilli* [L.] 1. a rod-shaped bacterium; any spore-forming, rod-shaped microorganism of the order Eubacteriales. 2. an organism of the genus Bacillus.
   Bang's b., *Brucella abortus.*
   Battey bacilli, unclassified mycobacteria that may produce tuberculosis-like disease in man.
   Bordet-Gengou b., *Bordetella pertussis.*
   Calmette Guérin b., an organism of the strain *Mycobacterium tuberculosis* var. *bovis,* rendered completely avirulent by cultivation for many years on bile-glycerol-potato medium and used as a vaccine against tuberculosis (see BCG VACCINE).
   coliform b., *Escherichia coli* and related organisms, including *Aerobacter aerogenes.*
   colon b., *Escherichia coli.*
   Friedländer's b., *Klebsiella pneumoniae.*
   Gärtner's b., *Salmonella enteritidis.*
   glanders b., *Actinobacillus mallei.*
   Hansen's b., *Mycobacterium leprae.*
   Klebs-Löffler b., *Corynebacterium diphtheriae.*
   Koch-Weeks b., *Haemophilus aegyptius.*
   paratyphoid b., any species of the genus Salmonella that causes paratyphoid fever.
   Pfeiffer's b., *Haemophilus influenzae.*
   tetanus b., *Clostridium tetani.*
   tubercle b., *Mycobacterium tuberculosis.*
   typhoid b., *Salmonella typhi.*

bacitracin (bas″ĭ-tra'sin) an antibiotic substance produced in ordinary culture media by an aerobic, gram-positive, spore-forming bacillus found in a contaminated wound, and named for the patient, Margaret Tracy; useful in a wide range of infections, applied topically or given intramuscularly.
   zinc b., the zinc salt of bacitracin, used in an ointment as a topical antibacterial agent.

backache (bak'āk) any pain in the back, usually the lower part. The pain is often dull and continuous, but sometimes sharp and throbbing.
   Backache, or lumbago, is one of the commonest ailments and can be caused by a wide variety of disorders, some serious and some not. Occasionally backache is a symptom of spinal arthritis, peptic ulcer, enlargement of the pancreas, SCIATICA, diseases of the kidney or other serious disorders, but usually backache is caused simply by strain of the back in such a way that the bones, ligaments, nerves or muscles of the spine are compressed or stretched. A sudden action, using muscles that are already fatigued or out of condition, is particularly likely to cause acute strain. In such cases, rest and time usually bring recovery, although a physician should always be consulted. A very sharp and persistent pain, following the use of unusual force against something—for example, when trying to

open a jammed window—could indicate a slipped DISK or SACROILIAC strain.

TREATMENT. Aspirin and a heating pad or hot, wet towels may temporarily relieve backache, but persistent pain requires a thorough examination, perhaps including x-ray examination, for the disorders of the back are not only many in number, but often difficult to identify.

backbone (bak'bōn) the rigid column formed by the vertebrae.

back-cross (bak'cros) a mating between a heterozygote and a homozygote.

    double b., the mating between a double heterozygote and a homozygote.

backflow (bak'flo) abnormal backward flow of fluids; regurgitation.

    pyelovenous b., drainage from the renal pelvis into the venous system occurring under certain conditions of back pressure.

Bact. bacterium.

bacter(io) (bak-te're-o) word element [G.], *bacteria*.

bacteremia (bak″ter-e'me-ah) the presence of bacteria in the blood.

bacteria (bak-te're-ah) plural of *bacterium*. adj., **bacte'rial.**

bactericidal (bak-tēr″ĭ-si'dal) destructive to bacteria.

bactericide (bak-tēr'ĭ-sīd) an agent that destroys bacteria.

bacterid (bak'ter-id) a skin condition due to hypersensitivity to a bacterial infection.

bacteriemia (bak-tēr″e-e'me-ah) bacteremia.

bacterioagglutinin (bak-te″re-o-ah-gloo'tĭ-nin) an agglutinin formed by the action of bacteria.

bacteriocidin (bak-te″re-o-si'din) a bactericidal substance present in the blood.

bacterioclasis (bak-te″re-ok'lah-sis) the breaking up of bacteria into fragments.

bacteriodiagnosis (bak-te″re-o-di″ag-no'sis) diagnosis by bacteriologic examination of tissues or fluids.

bacteriogenic (bak-te″re-o-jen'ik) caused by bacteria.

bacteriologist (bak-te″re-ol'o-jist) an expert in the study of bacteria.

bacteriology (bak-te″re-ol'o-je) the scientific study of bacteria. adj., **bacteriolog'ic.**

bacteriolysin (bak-te″re-ol'ĭ-sin) a substance formed in the blood as a result of infection, and capable of destroying the bacteria causing the infection.

bacteriolysis (bak-te″re-ol'ĭ-sis) the destruction of bacteria. adj., **bacteriolyt'ic.**

bacterio-opsonin (bak-te″re-o-op-so'nin) an opsonin that acts on bacteria.

bacteriophage (bak-te're-o-fāj″) a virus that destroys bacteria; several varieties exist, and usually each attacks only one kind of bacteria. Certain types of bacteriophages attach themselves to the cell membrane of the bacterium and instill a charge of DNA into the cytoplasm. DNA carries the genetic code of the virus, so that rapid multiplication of the virus can and does take place inside the bacterium. The growing viruses act as parasites, using the metabolism of the bacterial cell for growth and development. Eventually the bacterial cell bursts, releasing many more viruses capable of destroying similar bacteria.

bacteriophagia (bak-te″re-o-fa'je-ah) destruction of bacteria by a cell or an organism.

bacteriophobia (bak-te″re-o-fo'be-ah) morbid fear of bacteria.

bacterioprecipitins (bak-te″re-o-pre-sip'ĭ-tins) precipitins occurring in the serum treated with bacteria.

bacterioprotein (bak-te″re-o-pro'te-in) a toxalbumin formed by bacteria.

bacteriosis (bak-te″re-o'sis) a bacterial disease.

bacteriostatic (bak-te″re-o-stat'ik) arresting the growth of bacteria.

bacteriotoxin (bak-te″re-o-tok'sin) a toxin destructive to bacteria. adj., **bacteriotox'ic.**

bacteriotrypsin (bak-te″re-o-trip'sin) a proteolytic enzyme produced by *Vibrio comma*.

Bacterium (bak-te're-um) a former name for a genus of Schizomycetes (order Eubacteriales).
    B. aerugino'sum, *Pseudomonas aeruginosa.*
    B. co'li, *Escherichia coli.*
    B. pes'tis bubon'icae, *Pasteurella pestis.*
    B. son'nei, *Shigella sonnei.*
    B. tularen'se, *Pasteurella tularensis.*
    B. typho'sum, *Salmonella typhi.*

bacterium (bak-te're-um), pl. *bacte'ria* [L., Gr.] a nonspore-forming or nonmotile microorganism; applied loosely to any microorganism of the order Eubacteriales and popularly called germ. Bacteria are one-cell organisms visible only through a microscope. There are many varieties, only some of which cause disease; most are nonpathogenic, and many are useful.

Bacteria are forms of plant life, and are found almost everywhere. They reproduce about every 20 minutes, and would soon overrun the world if there were not other types of bacteria waiting to feed on them.

Bacteria are classified in three basic groups according to their shape. The rod-shaped bacteria are called bacilli, spiral-shaped bacteria spirilla and dot-shaped bacteria cocci. The last-named may appear in pairs (diplococci), in chains like strings of beads (streptococci) or in clusters that resemble a bunch of grapes (staphylococci).

The great majority of bacteria coexist peacefully with mankind. Many are necessary to plant life. For example, certain bacteria in the soil convert dead matter such as leaves into humus, which is rich in the nitrates essential to plant growth. Other bacteria have the ability to take atmospheric nitrogen from the air and convert it to nutrients usable by plants.

Helpful bacteria existing in the human intestine

feed on other microscopic organisms that might be harmful. They also produce some vitamins, including the vitamin B complex and vitamins C and K.

Most pathogenic bacteria that invade the body produce toxins. The body's defenses fight back against the invader by rushing leukocytes (white blood cells) and antitoxins to the area of infection; some of the leukocytes engulf the bacteria while the antitoxins neutralize the poisons. The extra blood supply contributes to the inflammatory process. The resulting fever and pain also help by enforcing rest and thus conserving the body's energies to fight off the invader.

DISEASES CAUSED BY BACTERIA. The different kinds of bacteria tend to affect different organs and systems of the body, producing infectious diseases, each with its own group of symptoms.

Staphylococci are generally found on the surface of the skin. When they invade the body tissue, for instance through a cut, they usually produce a local infection with inflammation and pus. Occasionally a strain of staphylococcus develops that can cause an infection affecting more than a local area of the body, but this is relatively rare.

The diseases produced by streptococci are often more serious. Streptococci tend to resist localization and may spread through the bloodstream. Among the diseases caused by streptococci are streptococcal sore throat, RHEUMATIC FEVER and SCARLET FEVER.

PNEUMONIA, MENINGITIS and GONORRHEA are produced by different types of diplococci. The pneumococcus, which produces pneumonia, has its special effect on the lungs; the meningococcus has an affinity for the coverings, or meninges, of the brain and spinal cord. Both types of bacteria enter the body via the respiratory tract. The gonorrhea bacteria (gonococci) are usually spread by coitus.

CHOLERA, caused by a spirillum and spread by unsanitary water supplies, was formerly a dread epidemic disease. SYPHILIS, like gonorrhea, is spread most often by coitus. It also is caused by a spirillum.

Bacilli are responsible for many serious diseases, including PLAGUE, DIPHTHERIA, LEPROSY, TUBERCULOSIS and TYPHOID FEVER. Prevention and control of the spread of many infectious diseases can be accomplished through IMMUNIZATION and proper sanitary conditions.

acid-fast b., one that is not readily decolorized by acids after staining, especially *Mycobacterium tuberculosis.*

coliform bacteria, *Escherichia coli* and related organisms, including *Aerobacter aerogenes.*

lactic acid bacteria, bacteria that, in suitable media, produce fermentation of carbohydrate materials to form lactic acid.

bacteriuria (bak-te″re-u′re-ah) bacteria in the urine.

bacteroid (bak′ter-oid) resembling a bacterium.

Bacteroidaceae (bak″tĕ-roi-da′se-e) a family of Schizomycetes (order Eubacteriales).

Bacteroides (bak″tĕ-roi′dez) a genus of Bacteroidaceae, occurring as normal intestinal flora.

bacteruria (bak″ter-u′re-ah) bacteriuria.

baculiform (bah-ku′lĭ-form) rod-shaped.

bag (bag) 1. a sac or pouch. 2. an inflatable rubber pouch for inserting in a part, for the purpose of dilating it.

Barnes's b., an hourglass-shaped rubber bag for dilating the cervix uteri.

colostomy b., a receptable worn over the stoma by a colostomy patient, to receive the fecal discharge.

Douglas b., a receptacle for the collection of expired air, permitting measurement of respiratory gases.

micturition b., a receptacle used for urine by ambulatory patients with urinary incontinence.

Politzer b., a soft bag of rubber for inflating the eustachian tube.

Voorhees b., a rubber bag to be inflated with water to dilate the cervix uteri.

b. of waters, the membranes enclosing the amniotic fluid and the developing fetus in utero.

bagassosis (bag″ah-so′sis) a lung disease due to inhalation of dust from the residue of cane after extraction of sugar (bagasse).

Baker's cyst (ba′kerz) a swelling about the knee, due to escape of synovial fluid in popliteal bursitis.

BAL dimercaprol (British antilewisite), a chelating agent used in poisoning with arsenic, gold and mercury.

balance (bal′ans) 1. an instrument for weighing. 2. harmonious adjustment of different elements or parts.

acid-base b., the proportion of acid and base required to keep the blood and body fluids neutral (see also ACID-BASE BALANCE).

fluid b., the state of the body in relation to ingestion and excretion of water, electrolytes and colloids.

inhibition-action b., the balance maintained in every person between emotional feelings and response to them.

nitrogen b., the state of the body in regard to ingestion and excretion of nitrogen. In negative nitrogen balance the amount of nitrogen excreted is greater than the quantity ingested. In positive nitrogen balance the amount excreted is smaller than the amount ingested.

semimicro b., a device for determining weight, sensitive to variations of 0.01' mg.

water b., fluid balance.

balaneutics (bal″ah-nu′tiks) the science of giving baths.

balanic (bah-lan′ik) pertaining to the glans penis or glans clitoridis.

balanitis (bal″ah-ni′tis) inflammation of the glans penis.

gangrenous b., infection of the glans penis by a combination of microorganisms, leading to its ulceration and rapid destruction.

balanoblennorrhea (bal″ah-no-blen″o-re′ah) gonorrheal balanitis.

balanoposthitis (bal″ah-no-pos-thi′tis) inflammation of glans penis and prepuce.

balanopreputial (bal″ah-no-pre-pu′she-al) pertaining to glans penis and prepuce.

balanorrhagia (bal″ah-no-ra′je-ah) gonorrheal balanitis.

balantidiasis (bal″an-tĭ-di′ah-sis) infection with organisms of the genus Balantidium.

Balantidium (bal″an-tid′e-um) a genus of ciliated protozoa, including many species found in the intestine in vertebrates and invertebrates.

B. co′li, a species found in the large intestine of man, causing diarrhea and secondary complications.

Balarsen (bah-lar′sen) trademark for preparations of arsthinol, an arsenical used in the treatment of intestinal amebiasis and yaws.

baldness (bawld′nes) total or partial loss or absence of hair; called also ALOPECIA. Baldness is a common condition that occurs much more often in men than in women. Ordinary baldness is usually a permanent and incurable condition; symptomatic baldness occurs as a result of some other condition or disorder and usually is temporary.

Balkan frame (bawl′kan) an apparatus for continuous extension in treatment of fractures of the femur, consisting of an overhead bar, with pulleys attached, by which the leg is supported in a sling.

ball (bawl) a globular structure, or sphere.

ballism (bal′izm) quick jerking or shaking movements seen in chorea.

ballistocardiogram (bah-lis″to-kar′de-o-gram″) the record produced by ballistocardiography.

ballistocardiograph (bah-lis″to-kar′de-o-graf″) the apparatus used in ballistocardiography.

ballistocardiography (bah-lis″to-kar″de-og′rah-fe) graphic recording of forces imparted to the body by cardiac ejection of blood.

ballistophobia (bah-lis″to-fo′be-ah) morbid dread of missiles.

ballottement (bah-lot′maw) [FR.] a diagnostic maneuver, involving pressure on an organ, as the uterus or kidney, and noting the impact when it rebounds.

balm (bahm) 1. a balsam. 2. a soothing or healing medicine.

balneology (bal″ne-ol′o-je) the science dealing with baths and bathing.

balneotherapeutics (bal″ne-o-ther″ah-pu′tiks) scientific study of the use of baths in the treatment of disease.

balneotherapy (bal″ne-o-ther′ah-pe) use of baths in the treatment of disease.

balsam (bawl′sam) a semifluid, fragrant, resinous, vegetable juice. It is used in various preparations to treat irritated or denuded areas of the skin and mucous membranes. Stains from these preparations are extremely difficult to remove. Friar's balsam, called also tincture of benzoin, is used as a

USE OF STERILE GAUZE SQUARE

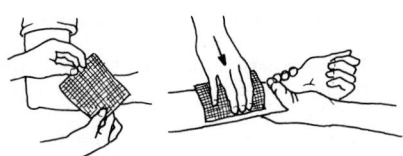

To cover wound
Fasten square over wound with tape or bandage.

To stop bleeding
Place square over wound and press down firmly.

USE OF ROLLER BANDAGE

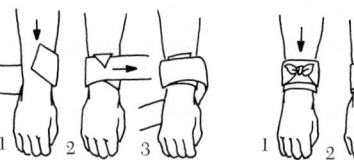

To anchor bandage
1. Place end on bias.
2. Fold down corner of end over first winding. 3. Cover corner with subsequent windings.

To fasten final end
1. Split into two ends and tie. 2. Or fasten with tape.

To bandage ankle
Wrap bandage around instep several times, then wind it twice around ankle, and bring it down under instep again.

USE OF ROLLER BANDAGE (CONTINUED)

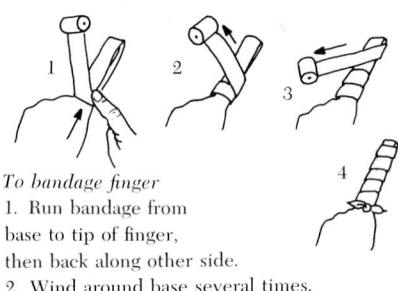

To bandage finger
1. Run bandage from base to tip of finger, then back along other side.
2. Wind around base several times.
3. Wind to tip of finger and back to base.
4. Split end and tie.

USE OF TRIANGULAR BANDAGE

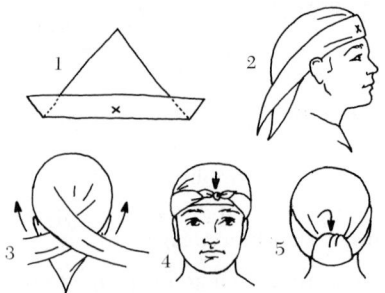

To bandage head
1. Fold 2-inch hem. 2. Place with hem side out, point of triangle at rear, and hem passing above ears. 3. Cross ends at back of head. 4. Bring to front and tie. 5. Tuck point of triangle under hem, or pin in place.

protective. Balsam of Peru or Peruvian balsam mildly stimulates cell proliferation and is used as a dressing for wounds. Tolu balsam is used as an ingredient in many cough syrups.

Bamberger-Marie disease (bahm'ber-ger mah-re') hypertrophic osteoarthropathy.

bancroftosis (ban"krof-to'sis) infection with *Wuchereria bancrofti*.

band (band) a strip that constricts or binds a part. In dentistry, a thin strip of metal formed to encircle horizontally the crown of a natural tooth or its root.

bandage (ban'dij) a strip or piece of gauze or other fabric for wrapping or covering any part of the body. Bandages may be used to stop the flow of blood, to provide a safeguard against contamination or to hold a medicated dressing in place. They may also be used to hold a splint in position or otherwise immobilize an injured part of the body to prevent further injury and to facilitate healing.

APPLICATION OF BANDAGES. In applying a bandage: (1) If the skin is broken a sterile pad or several thicknesses of gauze should be placed over the wound before tape or bandaging material is applied over the pad to hold it in place. Adhesive tape is never applied directly on a wound. (2) The bandage should not be made so tight that it interferes with circulation. A pressure bandage should be applied

only for the purpose of arresting hemorrhage. (3) A bandage does not have to look well to be effective; in an emergency, that the bandage serves its purpose is more important than its appearance.

cravat b., one that is made by bringing the point of a triangular bandage to the middle of the base and then folding lengthwise to the desired width.

demigauntlet b., a bandage that covers the hand, but leaves the fingers uncovered.

figure-of-8 b., one in which the turns cross each other like the figure 8.

gauntlet b., one that covers the hands and fingers like a glove.

plaster b., a bandage stiffened with a paste of plaster of paris.

pressure b., one for applying pressure, for the purpose of arresting hemorrhage; pressure is applied directly over the wound.

roller b., a strip of sterilized gauze rolled tightly into a spool. Commercial roller bandage is usually several yards long and is available in various widths. In an emergency, strips may be torn from a sheet or piece of yard goods and rolled. When more than a few inches of length is needed, rolling is essential for quick and clean bandaging.

tailed b., a square piece of cloth cut or torn into strips from the ends toward the center, with as large a center left as necessary. The bandage is centered over a compress on the wound and the

USE OF TRIANGULAR BANDAGE
(CONTINUED)

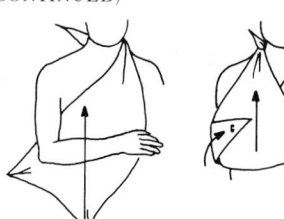

To make arm sling

Place triangle as shown so point extends a little beyond elbow. Bring lower end around arm and up. Tie ends behind neck. Pin point of triangle to front. Be sure fingers are visible and wrist is higher than elbow.

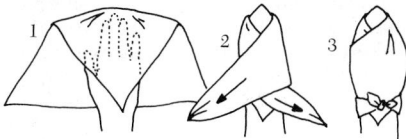

To bandage hand (or foot)

1. Place hand on triangle and fold as shown.
2. Cross ends over back of hand. 3. Wrap ends once around wrist and tie. Foot is bandaged in same way.

USE OF CRAVAT BANDAGE

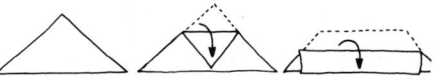

Fold triangle twice to make wide cravat. To vary width, vary number and width of folds.

USE OF CRAVAT BANDAGE (CONTINUED)

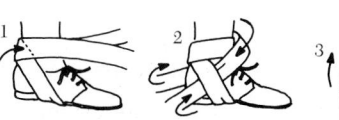

To bandage sprained ankle

1. Loosen shoelaces. With middle of cravat under shoe in front of heel, cross ends behind ankle and bring to front. 2. Cross ends and wrap them under and around diagonal parts of bandage. 3. Pull ends to front and tie.

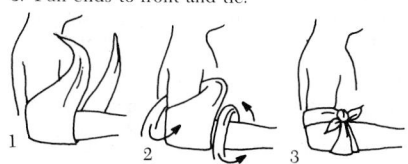

To bandage elbow (or knee)

1. Place middle of wide cravat under elbow of bent arm. 2. Cross ends and wind one around arm above elbow. 3. Tie.

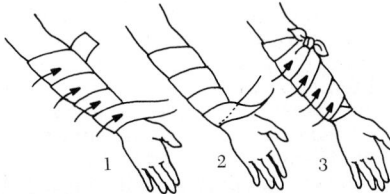

To bandage forearm (or lower leg)

1. Starting with end above wound, wind cravat diagonally over and past wound. 2. When wound is under middle of cravat, twist cravat and wind it back upward. 3. Tie ends above wound. Repeat, each time overlapping previous winding, until desired area is covered.

ends are then tied separately. A four-tailed bandage is useful for wounds of the nose and chin.

triangular b., one made by folding or cutting a large square of cloth diagonally. It may form a sling for an injured arm, or can be folded several times into a cravat of any desired width.

bank (bank) a place of storage for such materials as blood (blood bank), or for other human tissue (bone bank, eye bank, skin bank, etc.) to be used in reparative surgery.

Banthine (ban'thīn) trademark for preparations of methantheline bromide, an antispasmodic and anticholinergic.

Banti's disease (ban'tēz) a disease of the spleen with splenomegaly and pancytopenia, now considered secondary to portal hypertension.

Banting, (ban'ting) Sir Frederick Grant (1891–1941). Canadian scientist. Born in Allison, Ontario, and educated at the University of Toronto, Banting undertook research on the internal secretion of the pancreas, and in 1921, with Charles Herbert Best, he discovered insulin. Banting and J. J. R. Macleod shared the Nobel prize for medicine in 1923. The Banting Research Foundation was established in 1924, and the Banting Institute was opened at Toronto in 1930. Banting was knighted in 1934.

bar (bahr) 1. a structure that hinders or impedes. 2. a unit used in measuring pressure, equivalent to that of a column of mercury about 750 mm. high per square centimeter.

median b., a fibrotic formation across the neck of the prostate, producing obstruction of the urethra.

baragnosis (bar"ag-no'sis) impairment of the ability to perceive differences in weight or pressure.

barber's itch a contagious infection of the hair follicles on the face and neck, caused by staphylococci; called also SYCOSIS BARBAE.

barbital (bahr'bi-tahl) a long-acting barbiturate.

b. sodium, soluble b., a white, odorless, bitter powder, more soluble than barbital, used similarly.

barbituism (bahr-bit'u-izm) a toxic condition produced by use of barbital and its derivatives.

barbiturate (bahr-bit'u-rāt) one of a group of organic compounds derived from barbituric acid, and commonly described as "sleeping pills." Available by prescription only, barbiturates may be used to induce sedation or sleep. The many types of barbiturates vary in their strength and in the rapidity and duration of their effect. In varying degrees, all serve to depress the central nervous system, depress respiration, affect the heart rate and decrease blood pressure and temperature.

Barbiturates in the proper dosage may be helpful in several ways. As a sedative, a barbiturate such as phenobarbital, which is slowly absorbed by the system, may relieve tension, anxiety and insomnia. Certain types of pruritus respond to the soothing effects of barbiturates. Dentists sometimes prescribe a mild dose to allay acute fear in an unusually apprehensive patient before dental work is begun. Barbiturates have proved effective in the controlling of epileptic convulsions.

Sometimes for brief operations a quick-acting barbiturate such as thiopental sodium (Pentothal sodium) may be used as an intravenous anesthetic. In essence, this has the effect of a powerful sleeping pill. The so-called "truth serum" is in reality a barbiturate adjusted to produce a state of semiconsciousness, much like a hypnotic trance.

Since barbiturates can become habit-forming, they should be used only by the person for whom they have been prescribed and only according to specific directions.

Barbiturate overdose can be fatal and should be treated with utmost promptness. It produces heavy, unnatural sleep, or a state resembling acute intoxication. A physician or the emergency pulmotor squad of the police or fire department should be called immediately. Until professional help arrives, the victim should be made to vomit by sticking a finger down his throat, but only if he is awake; he should be kept warm and his breathing should be facilitated by removing constricting clothing and proper positioning. (See also POISONING.)

barbituric acid (bahr"bi-tu'rik) a compound, $C_4H_4N_2O_3$, the parent substance of BARBITURATES.

barbiturism (bahr-bit'u-rizm) barbituism.

barbotage (bahr"bo-tahzh') [Fr.] repeated alternate injection and withdrawal of fluid with a syringe, as in administration of an anesthetic agent into the subarachnoid space.

baresthesia (bar"es-the'ze-ah) sensibility for weight or pressure.

baresthesiometer (bar"es-the"ze-om'ĕ-ter) an instrument for estimating the sense of weight or pressure.

barium (ba're-um) a chemical element, atomic number 56, atomic weight 137.34, symbol Ba. (See table of ELEMENTS.)

b. sulfate, a fine, white, bulky powder, used as an opaque medium for x-ray examination of the digestive tract.

b. test, x-ray examination using a barium mixture to help locate disorders in the esophagus, stomach, duodenum and the small and large intestines. Such conditions as peptic ulcer, benign or malignant tumors, colitis or enlargement of organs that might be causing pressure on the stomach may be readily identified with the use of barium tests.

Barium sulfate is a harmless chalky compound that does not permit x-rays to pass through it. Taken before or during an examination, it causes the intestinal tract to stand out in silhouette when viewed through a fluoroscope or seen on an x-ray film.

Two main types of tests are conducted with the use of barium: the barium meal and the barium enema.

BARIUM MEAL. The patient, who has fasted since the previous evening, reports to the x-ray laboratory in the morning. He swallows a substance known as the "barium meal" (barium sulfate mixed with water and perhaps a flavoring). By fluoroscopy the radiologist watches the barium pass through the esophagus into the stomach, with the patient positioned so that the stomach and duodenum can be seen in various profiles. Then x-ray films are taken. If the small bowel is being studied it may be necessary to take additional x-rays during subsequent hours as the barium progresses through the digestive tract. The test is therefore often referred to as a "G.I. series" (gastrointestinal series). The patient is given no food until the series is completed.

The barium mixture may be constipating, and sometimes a laxative is given afterward. The patient is told to expect white barium in his stool during the following few days.

BARIUM ENEMA. The barium enema is valuable in examining the colon. The patient is given no food after a light evening meal. He may be given a cathartic to clear the colon of its contents, and an enema is usually given the morning of the test.

On the examination table, the patient is asked to relax on his side as the rectal tube is inserted. He is then helped to turn on his back. He is examined

under the fluoroscope while the barium is being injected. For better views, the patient may be asked to turn from side to side. Usually enough of the barium mixture is administered to fill the entire colon. The films are taken, and the patient is allowed to evacuate in the bathroom. After another x-ray film is taken the test is finished.

barognosis (bar″og-no′sis) the faculty by which weight is recognized.

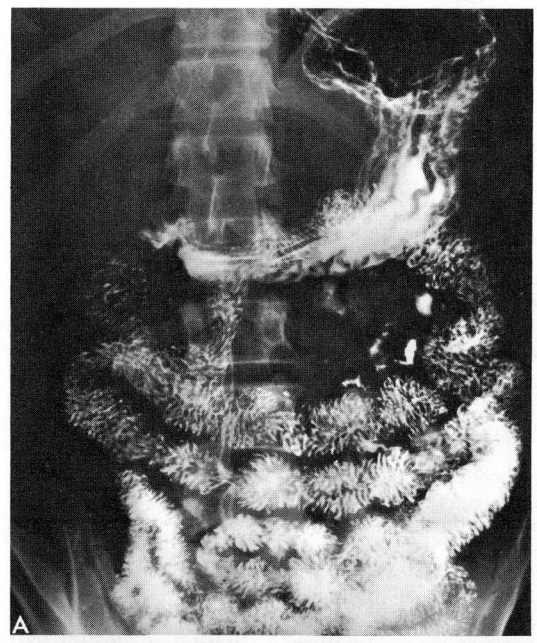

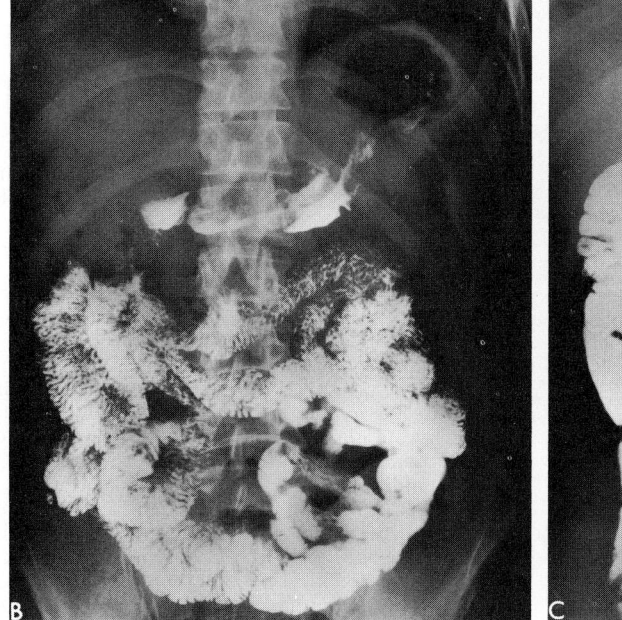
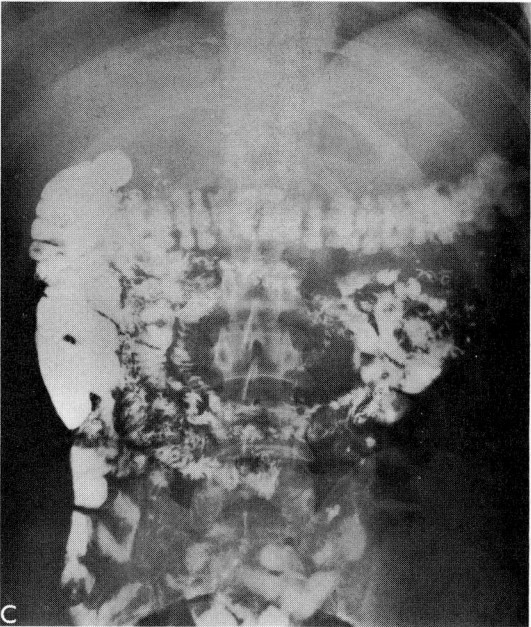

Frequent-interval film and fluoroscopy method for examination of the small intestine. *A*, At 1 hour after administration of the barium; *B*, at 2 hours; *C*, at 3 hours. (From Meschan, I.: Radiographic Positioning and Related Anatomy. Philadelphia, W. B. Saunders Co., 1968.)

barometer (bah-rom′ĕ-ter) an instrument indicating the atmospheric pressure.

   aneroid b., one containing no mercury or other fluid, making use of a chamber in which the air is partially exhausted.

baro-otitis (bar″o-o-ti′tis) barotitis.

baroreceptor (bar″o-re-sep′tor) a sensory nerve terminal that is stimulated by changes in pressure.

baroscope (bar′o-skōp) a delicate or highly sensitive form of barometer.

barosinusitis (bar″o-si″nŭ-si′tis) pain in the sinus due to rapid changes in atmospheric air pressure.

barotaxis (bar″o-tak′sis) the orientation of living organisms in response to pressure.

barotitis (bar″o-ti′tis) a morbid condition due to exposure to differing atmospheric pressures (see also BENDS).

   b. me′dia, a symptom complex due to difference between the atmospheric pressure of the environment and air pressure in the inner ear.

barotrauma (bar″o-traw′mah) injury due to pressure, as to structures of the ear, in high-altitude flyers, owing to differences between atmospheric and intratympanic pressures.

Barr body (bahr) sex chromatin; observed in cells of the normal female, considered to be the remnant of the inactive X chromosome.

Bartholin cyst (bar′to-lin) a type of retention cyst, affecting the Bartholin glands, and usually developing as a consequence of an earlier infection of the glands.

   B. glands, two small glands, one on each side of the vaginal wall, that secrete mucus; their ducts open on the vulva; called also the vulvovaginal glands. Their exact function is not clear but they are believed to secrete large amounts of mucus during sexual excitement, thereby providing lubrication for the vagina during coitus. The Bartholin glands are homologues of the bulbourethral glands in the male.

bartholinitis (bar″to-lin-i′tis) inflammation of the Bartholin glands.

Barton, (bar′ton) Clara (1821–1912). Founder and first president of American National Red Cross. Born in North Oxford, Massachusetts, she distributed supplies for the relief of wounded soldiers during the Civil War, and at its close organized a bureau of records in Washington to aid in the search of missing men. She assisted in organizing military hospitals when the Franco-Prussian War started in 1870, and began at once to establish an American Red Cross Society upon her return to the United States in 1873.

Bartonella (bar″to-nel′lah) a genus of Microtatobiotes.

   B. bacilliform′is, the etiologic agent of the anemic and eruptive types of human bartonellosis (Carrión's disease).

Bartonellaceae (bar″to-nel-la′se-e) a family of Microtatobiotes occurring as pathogenic parasites in the erythrocytes of man and other animals.

bartonellemia (bar″to-nel-le′me-ah) the presence in the blood of organisms of the genus Bartonella.

bartonellosis (bar″to-nel-lo′sis) infection by microorganisms of the genus Bartonella (Carrión's disease).

baruria (bah-ru′re-ah) high specific gravity of the urine.

baryesthesia (bar″e-es-the′ze-ah) baresthesia.

barylalia (bar″e-la′le-ah) indistinct, thick speech, resulting from a lesion of the central nervous system. ’

baryphonia (bar″e-fo′ne-ah) deepness and hoarseness of the voice.

basal (ba′sal) pertaining to a base; fundamental; in physiology, pertaining to the lowest possible level, resting level.

   b. metabolism test, a method of measuring the body's expenditure of energy by recording its rate of oxygen intake and consumption. The test is sometimes used to determine whether the THYROID GLAND, a major regulator of body activity, is functioning properly.

   METABOLISM is the series of chemical processes by which the body uses nutritive elements for building body tissues and producing heat and energy. Oxygen is essential to the metabolic processes. Basal refers to the state of the body when it is most completely at rest but not asleep. Basal metabolism is the minimal rate at which the body must produce energy to continue its essential life processes, such as maintaining temperature and circulation of the blood. The standard basal metabolism test determines this rate by measuring how much oxygen the person is taking into his body from the air he breathes, calculated according to his size and weight.

   So that the patient may be at complete rest, the test is usually done in the morning, after a good night's sleep and before the day's activities have begun. The patient takes no food for at least 12 hours before the test, so that digestive activity will not affect the metabolic rate. The patient is asked to avoid exercise and excitement the night before, have a light supper and go to bed early. For the standard test based on oxygen intake, the patient lies on his back and breathes through a mask. The rate at which he takes in oxygen determines how much energy his body is generating. From this his basal metabolic rate (BMR) is calculated.

   The BMR is usually expressed as a percentage that indicates how far it varies from the average. For example, a BMR of plus 15 would mean that the patient's basal metabolism rate was 15 per cent higher than the average for someone of his age, sex and size. A variation between plus 20 and minus 20 is considered within a normal range. A reading above the normal range may indicate overactivity of the thyroid gland, or hyperthyroidism; one below normal usually indicates a thyroid deficiency, or hypothyroidism.

   The basal metabolic rate also can be determined by use of a metabolic scale designed to make highly accurate measurements of the patient's weight while he is lying in his hospital bed. The measurement is taken during a period of 30 to 60 minutes when no food or liquids are taken in and there is no output of urine or feces. Thus the very small amount of weight lost through the evaporation of water from the lungs and skin (insensible weight loss) can be measured. The amount of insensible weight loss is proportional to the metabolic rate. By measuring the weight lost in 1 hour, and multiplying this amount in grams by 54.4, the basal metabolic rate can be calculated.

base (bās) the lower part of an object, or the broadest part of a conical or pyramidal structure. 2. the main ingredient of a compound. 3. a substance that yields hydroxyl ions and reacts with an acid to form salt and water. In the chemical processes of the body bases are essential to the maintenance of a normal ACID-BASE BALANCE. Excessive concentration of bases in the body fluids leads to ALKALOSIS.

    purine b., a group of compounds of which purine is the base, including uric acid, adenine, xanthine and theobromine.

Basedow's disease (bas'ĕ-dōz) exophthalmic goiter.

basement membrane (bās'ment) the delicate layer underlying the epithelium of mucous membranes and secreting glands.

baseosis (ba″se-o'sis) alkalosis.

basic (ba'sik) 1. pertaining to a base. 2. capable of uniting with negatively charged ions or with acid substances.

basicity (ba-sis'ĭ-te) the quality of being basic; the power to unite with negatively charged ions or with acid substances.

basidium (bah-sid'e-um), pl. *basid'ia* [L.] the clublike spore-producing organ of certain of the higher fungi.

basihyoid (ba″se-hi'oid) the body of the hyoid bone.

basilad (bas'ĭ-lad) toward the base.

basilar (bas'ĭ-lar) pertaining to the base.

basilateral (ba″sĭ-lat'er-al) pertaining to the base and side.

basilemma (ba″sĭ-lem'ah) 1. basement membrane. 2. neuroglia.

basiloma (bas″ĭ-lo'mah) a basal cell carcinoma.

basion (ba'se-on) the midpoint of the anterior border of the foramen magnum.

basiotripsy (ba'se-o-trip″se) cranioclasis.

basiphobia (ba″sĭ-fo'be-ah) morbid dread of walking.

basis (ba'sis) a foundation or base; especially the principal ingredient of a medication (prescription). In anatomic nomenclature, used as a general term to designate the base of a structure or organ, or the part opposite to or distinguished from the apex.

basisphenoid (ba″sĭ-sfe'noid) an embryonic bone that becomes the back part of the body of the sphenoid.

basocyte (ba'so-sīt) a cell staining readily with alkaline dyes; a basophilic leukocyte.

basocytopenia (ba″so-si″to-pe'ne-ah) deficiency of basophilic leukocytes of the blood.

basocytosis (ba″so-si-to'sis) excess of basophilic leukocytes of the blood.

baso-erythrocyte (ba″so-ĕ-rith'ro-sīt) an erythrocyte containing basophil granules.

basopenia (ba″so-pe'ne-ah) basocytopenia.

basophil (ba'so-fil) 1. a cell or other element staining readily with basic dyes. 2. a medium-sized leukocyte with a two-lobed nucleus, and cytoplasm containing large granules that stain a deep blue, normally constituting 0.5 per cent of the leukocytes of the blood.

basophile (ba'so-fil) 1. basophil. 2. basophilic.

basophilia (ba″so-fil'e-ah) 1. degeneration of erythrocytes with formation of basophilic granules (blue dots). 2. abnormal increase in the basophilic leukocytes of the blood.

basophilic (ba″so-fil'ik) staining readily with alkaline dyes.

basophilism (ba-sof'ĭ-lizm) abnormal increase of basophilic cells.

    pituitary b., Cushing's syndrome, including vascular hypertension, hirsutism, obesity and osteoporosis.

basoplasm (ba'so-plazm) the portion of the cytoplasm that stains easily with alkaline dyes.

bath (bath) application of water or other medium to the body for cleansing or therapeutic purposes, especially immersion of a considerable portion or a particular part of the body.

    colloid b., a bath prepared by adding soothing agents to the bath water, for the purpose of relieving skin irritation and pruritus. The patient is dried by patting rather than rubbing the skin. Care must be taken to avoid chilling.

    contrast b., alternate immersion of a part in hot water and ice water.

    cool b., one in water from 60 to 75° F.

    emollient b., a bath in a soothing and softening liquid, used in various skin disorders.

    hot b., one in water from 98 to 112° F.

    sitz b., immersion of only the hips and buttocks. Sitz baths are used to relieve pain and discomfort following rectal surgery, cystoscopy or vaginal surgery; they also may be ordered for patients with cystitis or infections within the pelvic cavity. Temperature for a hot sitz bath is started at 95° and gradually increased to 105 to 110° F.; the patient must be watched for fatigue and faintness, and an attendant must remain within calling distance. Cool compresses to the head or cool drinks during the bath promote comfort and relieve faintness.

    sponge b., one in which the patient's body is not immersed but is wiped with a wet cloth or sponge. Sponge baths are most often employed for reduction of body temperature in the presence of a fever, in which case the water used is ice cold and may contain alcohol to increase evaporation of moisture from the skin.

    tepid b., one in water 85 to 92° F.

    warm b., one in water 90 to 104° F.

    whirlpool b., one in which the water is kept in constant motion by mechanical means. It has a gentle massaging action that promotes relaxation.

bathophobia (bath″o-fo′be-ah) morbid dread of depths or looking down from high places, with fear of falling.

bathrocephaly (bath″ro-sef′ah-le) external bulging of the pars squamosa of the occipital bone, producing steplike deformity of the skull.

bathy- (bath′e) word element [Gr.], *deep*.

bathyanesthesia (bath″e-an″es-the′ze-ah) loss of deep sensibility.

bathyesthesia (bath″e-es-the′ze-ah) deep sensibility; the sensibility in the parts of the body beneath the surface.

bathyhyperesthesia (bath″ĭ-hi″per-es-the′ze-ah) abnormally increased sensitiveness of deep body structures.

bathyhypesthesia (bath″ĭ-hi″pes-the′ze-ah) abnormally diminished sensitiveness of deep body structures.

bathypnea (bath″ĭ-ne′ah) deep breathing.

Bayle's disease (bālz) progressive general paresis.

Bazin's disease (bah-zaz′) tuberculosis indurativa, chronic tuberculosis of the skin, characterized by indurated nodules.

BCG vaccine bacille Calmette Guérin vaccine, a tuberculosis vaccine, containing living, avirulent, bovine-strain tubercle bacilli (*Mycobacterium tuberculosis* var. *bovis*). The vaccine is administered by a special technique using a multiple-puncture disk. It cannot be given when the patient is reactive to tuberculin, when acute infectious disease is present or when there is any skin disorder. It offers some protection against tuberculosis, but cannot be relied on for total control of the disease. In a high percentage of cases the vaccine causes local ulcers at the site of administration. Public health officials in this country recommend the use of BCG vaccine only for those persons living in communities having a high rate of tuberculosis cases. After vaccination with BCG, the patient will have a positive response to the tuberculin test.

Be chemical symbol, *beryllium*.

beaker (bēk′er) a round laboratory vessel of various materials, usually with parallel sides and often with a pouring spout, of a capacity ranging from 1 to hundreds of milliliters.

beat (bēt) a throb, as of the heart or pulse (see also HEARTBEAT).
  apex b., the beat felt over the apex of the heart, usually in the fifth left intercostal space.
  ectopic b., a heartbeat originating at some point other than the sinoatrial node.
  premature b., an extrasystole.

bechic (bek′ik) 1. relieving a cough. 2. an agent for relief of cough.

Bechterew's disease (bek-ter′yefs) rheumatoid arthritis of the spine.

bed (bed) a supporting structure, especially a structure for supporting the body during sleep.
  b. cradle, a device made of metal or wood and placed on the bed for the purpose of supporting the weight of the top covers to prevent their coming in contact with the patient's body. Cradles vary in size according to their intended purpose and can be used over the entire body or over one or more extremities.
  fracture b., a bed for the use of patients with broken bones.
  Gatch b., a bed fitted with jointed springs, which may be adjusted to various positions.
  nail b., the surface covered by the nail of a finger or toe.

bedbug (bed′bug) a bug of the genus Cimex, a flattened, oval, reddish insect that inhabits houses, furniture and neglected beds and feeds on man, usually at night.

bedpan (bed′pan) a shallow vessel used for defecation or urination by patients confined to bed.

bedsore (bed′sōr) an ulcerlike sore caused by prolonged pressure of the patient's body against the bed (see also DECUBITUS ULCER).

MEDICATED BATHS

TYPE	PURPOSE	PREPARATION
Mustard	To stimulate peripheral circulation and promote muscle relaxation	Mustard is dissolved in tepid water and added to bath water. For adult use 1 tsp. dry mustard to 1 gal. water; for child use ½ tsp. dry mustard to 1 gal. water
Oatmeal	As soothing agent in skin disorders	3 cups oatmeal boiled in 2 qt. water. Add 1 cup sodium bicarbonate (baking soda) and pour in cheesecloth bag. Tie bag securely and put in bath water; use swirling action to mix thoroughly
Paraffin	To apply heat to inflamed joints; especially useful in the treatment of arthritis	Melt 3 to 4 lb. paraffin with 1 lb. petrolatum; take care to *keep away from open flame*. Cool mixture until a thin crust appears on the surface
Saline (salt)	As stimulant to skin, to lessen pain of sprains and contusions	Mix sodium chloride in sufficient water to make 2% solution (8 lb. table salt to 30 gal. water)
Sodium bicarbonate	To relieve pruritus in various skin disorders	Dissolve sodium bicarbonate (baking soda) in hot water and add to bath to make a 5% solution (20 lb. sodium bicarbonate to 30 gal. water)

bed-wetting (bed'wet-ing) enuresis. Most small children wet their beds occasionally; although it is a nuisance it is no cause for alarm. Only when a child persists in regularly wetting his bed after the age of 6, when he can reasonably be expected to have stopped, or when a child who has stopped bed-wetting reverts to it, should a physical or emotional disorder be sought.

bee sting injury caused by the venom of a bee. The pain from a bee sting can be relieved by sodium bicarbonate, a few drops of ammonia or calamine lotion; a cold compress also has a soothing effect. The skin should not be scratched as this may lead to infection. The insect's "stinger" should be scraped out with a fingernail or removed with tweezers held flat against the skin. If the pain or swelling persists, or if the sting is on the tongue or in the mouth, a physician should be consulted at once. Symptoms of a severe allergic reaction, such as collapse or swelling of the body, indicate ANAPHYLACTIC SHOCK and require that medical help be sought immediately.

behavior (be-hāv'yer) the manner in which an individual acts or performs. adj., **behav'ioral.**
  automatic b., automatism.
  invariable b., activity whose character is determined by innate structure, such as reflex action.
  variable b., behavior that is modified by individual experience.

behaviorism (be-hāv'yer-izm) a theory of psychology based upon a purely objective observation and analysis of human and animal behavior without reference to the complexities and nuances of psychoanalytic depth psychology.

Behring's law (ba'ringz) blood and serum of an immunized person, when transferred to another subject, will render the latter immune.

bejel (bej'el) a nonvenereal disease similar to yaws, occurring in the Middle East and caused by an organism indistinguishable from *Treponema pallidum.*

bel (bel) a unit of sound intensity.

belching (belch'ing) the eructation of gas.

belemnoid (bĕ-lem'noid) 1. dart-shaped. 2. the styloid process.

Bell's palsy (belz) neuropathy of the facial nerve, resulting in paralysis of the muscles of the face, usually on one side. The victim usually is unable to close his mouth, so that he drools and cannot whistle. If he is unable to close the eye on the affected side, it may become tearful and inflamed.

Facial palsy is often no more than a temporary condition lasting a few days or weeks. Occasionally the paralysis results from a tumor pressing on the nerve, or from physical trauma to the nerve. In this event, recovery will depend on the success in treating the tumor or injury. More often, however, the cause is unknown. In many cases the deformity can be reduced by plastic surgery.

belladonna (bel"ah-don'ah) powdered leaf of the plant *Atropa belladonna,* called also deadly nightshade. This plant is the main source of the alkaloids atropine and hyoscyamine, to which its properties are due. Belladonna acts through parasympathetic blockade and is used in the management of peptic ulcer and other gastrointestinal disorders.

Overdosage may lead to mydriasis (dilatation of the pupils), dryness of the mouth, elevated temperature and delirium.
  b. poisoning, a severe toxic condition due to overdosage of belladonna or accidental ingestion of large amounts of the drug. Symptoms include dryness of the mouth, thirst, dilated pupils, flushed skin or rash on the face, neck and upper trunk, tachycardia, fever, delirium and stupor. Treatment consists of removal of the poison from the stomach by inducing vomiting or gastric suction. This is followed by gastric lavage with water containing activated charcoal and an instillation of a solution of 200 ml. of water and 30 Gm. of sodium sulfate. Barbiturates such as Seconal are administered to reduce excitability. Respiratory difficulties may require administration of oxygen or in extreme cases tracheostomy. Measures are also taken to reduce high body temperature and maintain an adequate blood pressure.

belly (bel'e) 1. the abdomen. 2. the prominent, fleshy part of a bulging muscle.

bemegride (bem'ĕ-grīd) a drug used as an analeptic in the treatment of barbiturate poisoning. The drug may cause muscle twitching and convulsions; if so, it is discontinued and thiopental is given as an antidote. Bemegride is administered intravenously.

benactyzine (ben-ak'tĭ-zēn) a compound used as an anticholinergic and ataractic; it is contraindicated in patients with severe psychosis.

Benadryl (ben'ah-dril) trademark for diphenhydramine, an antihistamine.

Bence Jones protein (bens jōnz) a low-molecular-weight, heat-sensitive urinary protein found in patients with multiple myeloma.

bendroflumethiazide (ben"dro-floo"mĕ-thi'ah-zīd) a compound used as a diuretic and antihypertensive. It enhances the excretion of sodium and chloride.

bends (bendz) decompression sickness; a condition resulting from a too-rapid decrease in atmospheric pressure, as when a deep-sea diver is brought too hastily to the surface. The term bends is derived from the bodily contortions its victims undergo when atmospheric pressure is abruptly changed from a high pressure to a relatively lower one. Aqualung divers and underwater construction workers are particularly susceptible to this condition. A form of altitude sickness suffered by aviators who ascend too rapidly to high altitudes is similar to bends. Bends may also be a complication in a type of oxygen therapy called HYPERBARIC OXYGENATION, in which the patient is placed in a high-pressure chamber to increase the oxygen content of his blood. Nursing personnel, physicians and the patient within the chamber must be protected from bends when they emerge from the high-pressure chamber.
  CAUSE. The phenomenon of bends is explained in terms of a law of physics: The greater the atmospheric pressure, the greater the amount of gas that can be dissolved in a liquid. The gas involved in bends is the air we breathe, composed chiefly of nitrogen and oxygen. Under normal atmospheric

pressure (about 15 lb. per square inch), nitrogen is present in the blood in dissolved form. If the atmospheric pressure is substantially increased, a proportionately greater amount of nitrogen will be dissolved in the blood. The same is true of oxygen, and this is the basis for hyperbaric oxygenation in the treatment of oxygen deficiency.

The increase in pressure causes no ill effects. Nor will there be any ill effects if the pressure is gradually brought back to normal. When the decrease in pressure is slow, the nitrogen escapes safely from the blood as it passes through the lungs to be exhaled. If the pressure drops abruptly back to normal, the nitrogen is suddenly released from its state of solution in the blood and forms bubbles. Although the body is now under normal air pressure, expanding bubbles of nitrogen are present in the circulation and force their way into the capillaries, blocking the normal passage of the blood. This blockage (or embolism) starves cells dependent on a constant supply of oxygen and other blood nutrients. Some of these cells may be nerve cells located in the limbs or in the spinal cord. When they are deprived of blood, an attack of bends occurs.

The oxygen in the blood reacts similarly when abnormal pressure is abruptly relieved. But because oxygen is dissolved more easily than nitrogen, and because some of the oxygen combines chemically with hemoglobin, the oxygen released in decompression forms fewer bubbles, and is therefore less troublesome.

SYMPTOMS AND TREATMENT. The symptoms of bends include joint pain, dizziness, staggering, visual disturbances, dyspnea and itching of the skin. Partial paralysis occurs in severe cases; collapse and insensibility are also possible. Only rarely is the condition itself fatal, although a diver while in this condition may suffer a fatal accident unless he is rescued.

Bends is treated by placing the victim in a decompression chamber where the air pressure is at the level to which he was originally exposed. If the victim is a diver, this is the pressure at the depth where he was working. Pressure in the chamber is then reduced to normal at a safe rate.

Benedict's solution   (ben'ĕ-dikts) a chemical solution used to determine the presence of glucose in the urine; called also Benedict's reagent. It is prepared by dissolving 173 Gm. of sodium citrate and 100 Gm. of anhydrous sodium carbonate in 800 ml. of water; the solution is filtered and to the filtrate is added 17.3 Gm. of copper sulfate in 100 ml. of water. Water is then added to make a total of 1 liter of prepared solution.

B's test, a laboratory test for determining the presence of sugar in the urine. Eight drops of urine and 5 ml. of Benedict's solution are mixed in a test tube and then held over a flame and allowed to boil for 5 minutes. The color of the solution after boiling determines the amount of sugar present. Blue indicates no glucose; green a trace, or 1 plus; yellow, up to 0.5 per cent or 2 plus; orange, 0.5 to 1.5 per cent or 3 plus; red, 1.5 per cent and over or 4 plus.

Benemid   (ben'ĕ-mid) trademark for probenecid, used mainly in the treatment of chronic gout and also for some forms of arthritis.

benign   (be-nīn') not recurrent or tending to progress.

Benoquin   (ben'o-kwin) trademark for a preparation of monobenzone, a melanin-inhibiting agent.

benoxinate   (ben-ok'sĭ-nāt) an agent used as a surface anesthetic for the eye.

Benson's disease   (ben'sunz) a condition of unknown origin, sometimes occurring with age, characterized by small, dustlike, glistening particles in the vitreous.

bentonite   (ben'to-nīt) a fine, odorless powder used in preparing pharmaceutical agents for external use.

benzaldehyde   (ben-zal'dĕ-hīd) a colorless, strongly refractive liquid, used chiefly as a flavoring agent.

benzalkonium chloride   (ben″zal-ko'ne-um klo'rīd) a mixture of alkyldimethyl-benzylammonium chlorides; a topical antiseptic.

Benzedrex   (ben'zĕ-dreks) trademark for an inhalant used in shrinking nasal mucosa.

Benzedrine   (ben'zĕ-drēn) trademark for amphetamine, a central nervous system stimulant.

benzene   (ben'zēn) a liquid hydrocarbon, C_6H_6, from coal tar.
  b. hexachloride, a powerful insecticide.
  b. ring, the closed hexagon of carbon atoms in benzene, from which the different benzene compounds are derived by replacement of the hydrogen atoms.

benzestrol   (ben-zes'trol) a synthetic estrogenic compound, used in the treatment of menopausal symptoms, to depress lactation, to relieve the symptoms of prostatic cancer and in the relief of certain forms of vaginitis.

benzethonium   (ben″zĕ-tho'ne-um) an ammonium derivative used as a local anti-infective.

benzhexol   (benz-hek'sol) trihexyphenidyl, used as an anticholinergic and in treatment of Parkinson's disease.

benzhydramine   (benz-hi'drah-mēn) diphenhydramine, an antihistamine.

benzidine   (ben'zĭ-dēn) a compound used as a test for traces of blood (benzidine test).

benzin   (ben'zin) a liquid obtained from petroleum, a solvent for rubber, fats, oils, etc.

benzoate   (ben'zo-āt) a salt of benzoic acid.

benzoated   (ben'zo-āt″ed) charged with benzoic acid.

benzocaine   (ben'zo-kān) a crystalline compound used topically as a local anesthetic.

benzoic acid   (ben-zo'ik) a white or yellowish crystalline substance used primarily as a mild antiseptic, e.g., in combination with salicylic acid in the preparation of Whitefield's ointment for treatment of fungus infections of the skin. The sodium salt of benzoic acid, sodium benzoate, is used as a liver function test and a preservative for food and various pharmaceutical preparations.

benzoin (ben'zo-in, ben-zo'in) the balsamic resin from *Styrax benzoin*, used as a local antiseptic and as a stimulant to promote healing. Benzoin acts as an expectorant and thus is sometimes used in steam inhalations in treating respiratory disorders.

benzol (ben'zŏl) benzene.

benzonatate (ben-zo'nah-tāt) a compound used as an antitussive. it depresses cough without affecting respiration. The capsule should be swallowed immediately so that it does not dissolve in the mouth.

benzononatine (ben-zo"no-na'tin) benzonatate.

benzpyrinium (benz"pi-rin'e-um) a compound that acts as a cholinergic, blocking the action of cholinesterase and thus prolonging the action of acetylcholine. It has much the same actions and effects as physostigmine and neostigmine but is considered less toxic. The drug is contraindicated in urinary obstruction, mechanical intestinal obstruction and asthma since it may induce asthmatic reaction. It is given intramuscularly, never intravenously. The antidote for severe reaction is atropine.

benztropine (benz'tro-pēn) a compound used as an anticholinergic and antihistamine and to reduce the tremors of Parkinson's disease.

benzyl (ben'zil) the hydrocarbon radical, C_7H_7.
  b. alcohol, a colorless liquid used as a local anesthetic.
  b. benzoate, a clear, oily liquid used externally for scabies and pediculosis.

benzylpenicillin (ben'zil-pen-ĭ-sil'in) penicillin G.

beriberi (ber"e-ber'e) an endemic form of polyneuritis due to an unbalanced diet, chiefly a lack of vitamin B_1, or thiamine. The disease is more common in the Orient where refined rice is the main staple in the diet; however, improved refining processes and dietary habits have decreased the incidence of this disease.

In the United States, mild forms of the disease sometimes occur in persons who are on extremely restricted diets. Alcoholics, who tend to decrease food intake drastically during periods of drinking, may show signs of beriberi. The disease also occurs in persons whose diet consists of highly refined and overcooked food.

berkelium (ber-ke'le-um) a chemical element, atomic number 97, atomic weight 247, symbol Bk. (See table of ELEMENTS.)

Berubigen (be-roo'bĭ-jen) trademark for preparations of vitamin B_{12}.

berylliosis (bĕ-ril"e-o'sis) a morbid condition caused by exposure to fumes or finely divided dust of beryllium salts, involving lungs, skin, subcutaneous tissues, lymph nodes, liver and other organs.

beryllium (bĕ-ril'e-um) a chemical element, atomic number 4, atomic weight 9.012, symbol Be. (See table of ELEMENTS.)

Besnier-Boeck disease (bez'ne-a bek) Boeck's sarcoid.

Best's disease (bests) congenital degeneration of the macula lutea of the retina.

bestiality (bes-te-al'ĭ-te) sexual connection with an animal.

beta (ba'tah) second letter of the Greek alphabet, β; used in names of chemical compounds to distinguish one of two or more isomers or to indicate position of substituting atoms or groups.
  b. particles, negatively charged particles emitted by radioactive elements. These particles are the result of the disintegration of neutrons, their source being the unstable atoms of radioactive metals such as radium and uranium. There are three general types of emissions from radioactive substances: alpha and beta particles and gamma rays. Beta particles are less penetrating than gamma rays and may be used to treat certain conditions on or near the surface of the body. (See also RADIATION and RADIOTHERAPY.)

betacism (ba'tah-sizm) excessive use of the b sound in speaking.

Betadine (ba'tah-dēn) trademark for preparations of povidone-iodine, which have a longer antiseptic action than most iodine solutions.

betaine hydrochloride (be'tah-in) an agent used as a lipotropic agent and as a substitute for hydrochloric acid in achlorhydria.

beta-ketobutyric acid (ba"tah-ke"to-bu-tir'ik) acetoacetic acid.

Betalin (ba'tah-lin) trademark for preparations of the vitamin B complex.

betamethasone (ba"tah-meth'ah-sōn) a crystalline corticosteroid.

betanaphthol (ba"tah-naf'thol) a pale, crystalline powder with a faint, phenol-like odor, used as an intestinal antiseptic and vermifuge.

beta-oxybutyric acid (ba"tah-ok"se-bu-tir'ik) a compound produced in abnormal amounts in diabetes mellitus; considered one of the KETONE BODIES, although it does not contain the carbonyl group typical of their structure.

betatron (ba'tah-tron) an apparatus for accelerating electrons to millions of electron volts by magnetic induction.

Betaxin (be-tak'sin) trademark for preparations of thiamine hydrochloride, used as a vitamin supplement.

betazole (ba'tah-zōl) an analogue of histamine used in place of it to stimulate gastric secretion during gastric analysis. There is no accompanying fall in blood pressure with the administration of betazole as there is with histamine. Epinephrine should be on hand at the time betazole is given in the event an untoward reaction occurs.

bethanechol (bĕ-tha'nĕ-kol) a choline derivative used as a parasympathomimetic agent and in the treatment of abdominal distention or urinary retention. Hypotension and dyspnea may occur as side effects; if they do, the patient is placed in Fowler's position and atropine is usually administered.

bev. billion electron volts (3.82×10^{-11} gram (small) calorie, or 1.6×10^{-3} erg).

Bevidox (bev′ĭ-doks) trademark for a solution of vitamin B_{12}.

bezoar (be′zōr) a mass formed in the stomach by compaction of repeatedly ingested material that does not pass into the intestine.

BFP biologic false positive reaction; a positive finding in serologic tests for syphilis when syphilis does not exist.

Bi chemical symbol, *bismuth.*

bi- (bi) word element [L.], *two.*

biarticular (bi″ar-tik′u-lar) affecting two joints.

bibasic (bi-ba′sik) doubly basic.

bibliotherapy (bib″le-o-ther′ah-pe) use of books and reading in treatment of nervous disorders.

bicameral (bi-kam′er-al) having two chambers or cavities.

bicapsular (bi-kap′su-lar) having two capsules.

bicarbonate (bi-kar′bon-āt) a salt containing two equivalents of carbonic acid and one of a basic substance.
   blood b., plasma b., the bicarbonate of the blood plasma, an index of the alkali reserve.
   b. of soda, sodium bicarbonate.

bicaudal, bicaudate (bi-kaw′dal), (bi-kaw′dāt) having two tails.

bicellular (bi-sel′u-lar) made up of two cells.

bicephalus (bi-sef′ah-lus) a two-headed monster.

biceps (bi′seps) a muscle having two heads. The biceps muscle of the arm flexes and supinates the forearm; the biceps muscle of the thigh flexes and rotates the leg laterally and extends the thigh.

bichloride (bi-klo′rīd) a chloride containing two equivalents of chlorine.

biciliate (bi-sil′e-āt) having two cilia.

bicipital (bi-sip′ĭ-tal) having two heads; pertaining to a biceps muscle.

biconcave (bi-kon′kāv) having two concave surfaces.

bicontaminated (bi″kon-tam′ĭ-nāt″ed) infected by two different types of organisms.

biconvex (bi-kon′veks) having two convex surfaces.

bicornuate (bi-kor′nu-āt) having two horns, or cornua.

bicorporate (bi-kor′po-rāt) having two bodies.

bicoudate (bi-koo′dāt) twice bent; said of catheters.

bicuspid (bi-kus′pid) 1. having two cusps. 2. pertaining to the bicuspid (mitral) valve. 3. a premolar tooth.

bicuspidate (bi-kus′pĭ-dāt) having two cusps or projections.

b.i.d. [L.] *bis in di′e* (twice a day).

biduous (bid′u-us) lasting two days.

Bielschowsky's disease (be″el-show′skēz) late infantile amaurotic familial idiocy.

Bielschowsky-Jansky disease (be″el-show′ske yan′ske) amaurotic familial idiocy.

bifid (bi′fid) cleft into two parts.

bifocal eyeglasses (bi-fo′kal) eyeglasses in which each lens is made up of two segments of different refractive powers, or strength. Generally, the upper part of the lens is used for ordinary or distant vision, and the smaller, lower section for near vision, for close work such as reading or sewing. Bifocal eyeglasses are often prescribed for PRESBYOPIA, which may occur as part of the aging process. For advanced cases of presbyopia, and for special purposes such as watchmaking, trifocal glasses are available.

biforate (bi-fo′rāt) having two perforations or foramina.

bifurcate (bi-fur′kāt) divided into two branches.

bifurcation (bi″fur-ka′shun) 1. division into two branches. 2. the point at which division into two branches occurs.

bilateral (bi-lat′er-al) having or pertaining to two sides.

bile (bīl) a clear yellow or orange fluid produced by the liver. It is concentrated and stored in the gallbladder until needed for digestion, especially for emulsification of fats. The bile salts emulsify fats by breaking up large fat globules into smaller ones so that they can be acted on by the fat-splitting enzymes of the intestine and pancreas. A healthy liver produces bile according to the body's needs and does not require stimulation by drugs. Infection or disease of the liver, inflammation of the gallbladder or gallstones can interfere with the flow of bile.
   b. acids, glycocholic acid and taurocholic acid, formed in the liver and secreted in the bile.
   b. ducts, the canals or passageways that conduct bile. There are three bile ducts: the hepatic duct drains bile from the liver; the cystic duct is an extension of the gallbladder and conveys bile from the gallbladder. These two ducts may be thought of as branches which drain into the "trunk," or common bile duct. The common bile duct passes through the wall of the small intestine at the duodenum and joins with the pancreatic duct to form the hepatopancreatic ampulla, or ampulla of Vater. At the opening into the small intestine there is a sphincter that automatically controls the flow of bile into the intestine.
   The bile ducts may become obstructed by GALLSTONES, benign or malignant tumors or a severe local infection. Various disorders of the GALLBLADDER or bile ducts are often diagnosed by CHOLECYSTOGRAPHY and CHOLANGIOGRAPHY, i.e., x-ray examination of the gallbladder and bile ducts, using a special contrast medium so that these hollow structures can be clearly outlined on the x-ray film.
   b. pigment, any one of the coloring matters of the bile; they are bilirubin, biliverdin, bilifuscin, biliprasin, choleprasin, bilihumin and bilicyanin.

bilharziasis (bil″har-zi′ah-sis) a chronic disease

caused by infection with schistosome (blood fluke) eggs and adults; called also SCHISTOSOMIASIS. The disease is sometimes known as "snail fever" because the parasitic worms develop and multiply within a snail. The disease is widespread in Egypt, Africa, the West Indies and the northern part of South America. It is second only to malaria as man's most serious parasitic infection.

bili- (bil'ĭ) word element [L.], *bile.*

biliary (bil'e-a″re) pertaining to the bile, to the bile ducts or to the gallbladder.
    b. tract, the liver and gallbladder, and their various ducts.

bilicyanin (bil″ĭ-si'ah-nin) a blue pigment derived by oxidation from biliverdin.

bilifulvin (bil″ĭ-ful'vin) an impure bilirubin.

bilifuscin (bil″ĭ-fus'in) one of a class of compounds related to the bile pigments (but produced in constructive metabolism in the body); chiefly responsible for the color of the feces.

biligenesis (bil″ĭ-jen'ĕ-sis) production of bile.

biligenic (bil″ĭ-jen'ik) producing bile.

bilihumin (bil″ĭ-hu'min) an insoluble ingredient of gallstones.

bilin (bi'lin) the main constituent of the bile, composed chiefly of the sodium salts of normal bile acids.

biliousness (bil'yus-nes) malaise with constipation, headache and indigestion, attributed to excessive bile production.

biliprasin (bil″ĭ-pra'sin) a green pigment from gallstones.

bilirachia (bil″ĭ-ra'ke-ah) the presence of bile pigments in the spinal fluid.

bilirubin (bil″ĭ-roo'bin) an orange bile pigment produced by the breakdown of hemoglobin and excreted by the liver cells. Failure of the liver cells to excrete bile, or obstruction of the BILE DUCTS, can cause an increased amount of bilirubin in the body fluids and thus lead to obstructive JAUNDICE.
    Another type of jaundice results from excessive destruction of erythrocytes (hemolytic jaundice). The more rapid the destruction of red blood cells and the degradation of hemoglobin, the greater the amount of bilirubin in the body fluids.
    Laboratory tests for the determination of bilirubin content in the blood are of value in diagnosing liver dysfunction and in evaluating hemolytic anemias. Bilirubin may be classified as indirect ("free" or unconjugated) while en route to the liver from its site of formation by reticuloendothelial cells, and direct (bilirubin diglucuronide) after its conjugation in the liver.
    Normally the body produces a total of about 260 mg. of bilirubin per day. Almost 99 per cent of this is excreted in the feces; the remaining 1 per cent is excreted in the urine as UROBILINOGEN. A test for bilirubin in the blood is called the van den Bergh test. Normal range for this test is 0.0 to 0.1 mg. per 100 ml. of serum for direct bilirubin, and 0.2 to 1.4 mg. per 100 ml. of serum for total bilirubin. The only preparation required for the van den Bergh test is that the patient be in a fasting state when the blood is drawn.

bilirubinemia (bil″ĭ-roo″bĭ-ne'me-ah) the presence of bilirubin in the blood.

bilirubinuria (bil″ĭ-roo″bĭ-nu're-ah) the presence of bilirubin in the urine.

biliuria (bil″e-u're-ah) the presence of bile acids in the urine.

biliverdin (bil″ĭ-ver'din) one of the substances formed from bilirubin by oxidation.

Billroth's operation (bil'rōts) gastrectomy.

bilobate (bi-lo'bāt) having two lobes.

bilobular (bi-lob'u-lar) having two lobules.

bilocular (bi-lok'u-lar) having two compartments.

bimanual (bi-man'u-al) with both hands.

bimastoid (bi-mas'toid) pertaining to both mastoid processes.

binary (bi'nah-re) made up of two elements, or of two radicals that act as elements.
    b. fission, the halving of the nucleus and then of the cytoplasm of the cell, as in protozoa.

binaural (bi-naw'ral, bin-aw'ral) pertaining to both ears.

binauricular (bin″aw-rik'u-lar) pertaining to both auricles.

binder (bīnd'er) a large band, usually made of muslin, worn around the abdomen or chest for support.
    breast b., one used to give support and hold the breasts firmly in proper position.
    scultetus b., one applied to the abdomen from below upward, with each tail firmly tucked at the base of the opposite tail; the last tail is pinned in place with a safety pin in vertical position.
    T b., one used to hold perineal or rectal dressings in place.
    double T b., one used for male patients to hold perineal or rectal dressings in place.

binocular (bin-ok'u-lar) pertaining to both eyes.

binomial (bi-no'me-al) composed of two names or terms.

binotic (bin-ot'ik) binaural.

binovular (bin-ov'u-lar) derived from two ova.

binucleate (bi-nu'kle-āt) having two nuclei.

binucleation (bi″nu-kle-a'shun) formation of two nuclei within a cell without division of the cytoplasm into two daughter cells.

binucleolate (bi-nu'kle-o-lāt) having two nucleoli.

bio- (bi'o) word element [Gr.], *life; living.*

bio-assay (bi″o-as'a) biological assay.

bioastronautics (bi″o-as″tro-naw'tiks) scientific study of effects of space and interplanetary travel on biologic systems.

biocatalyst (bi″o-kat'ah-list) an enzyme.

biochemistry (bi″o-kem'is-tre) the study of chemical reactions occurring in living organisms.

biocidal (bi″o-si′dal) causing the death of living organisms.

bioclimatology (bi″o-kli″mah-tol′o-je) scientific study of effects on living organisms of conditions of natural environment (rainfall, daylight, temperature, etc.) prevailing in specific regions of the earth.

biocolloid (bi″o-kol′oid) a colloid from animal or vegetable tissue.

biocycle (bi″o-si′kl) the sequence of certain rhythmically repeated phenomena observed in living organisms.

biodegradable (bi″o-de-grād′ah-bl) susceptible of degradation by biological processes, as by bacterial or other enzymatic action.

biodynamics (bi″o-di-nam′iks) the doctrine or science of living force.

bioelectricity (bi″o-e″lek-tris′ĭ-te) electrical phenomena apparent in living cells.

bioflavonoid (bi″o-fla′vo-noid) a generic term for a group of compounds widely distributed in plants and concerned with maintenance of a normal state of the walls of small blood vessels.

biogenesis (bi″o-jen′ĕ-sis) the origination of living organisms only from organisms already living.

biogeography (bi″o-je-og′rah-fe) the scientific study of the geographic distribution of living organisms.

biokinetics (bi″o-ki-net′iks) the science of movement of living organisms.

biological (bi″o-loj′ĭ-kal) 1. pertaining to biology. 2. a medicinal preparation made from living organisms and their products; these include serums, vaccines, antigens and antitoxins.
  b. clock, the physiologic mechanism that governs the rhythmic occurrence of certain biochemical, physiologic and behavioral phenomena in living organisms.

biologist (bi-ol′o-jist) a specialist in biology.

biology (bi-ol′o-je) scientific study of living organisms. adj., biolog′ic, biolog′ical.
  molecular b., study of the biochemical and biophysical aspects of structure and function of genes and other subcellular entities, and of such specific proteins as hemoglobins, enzymes and hormones; it provides knowledge of cellular differentiation and metabolism and of comparative evolution.
  radiation b., scientific study of the effects of ionizing radiation on living organisms.

bioluminescence (bi″o-lu″mĭ-nes′ens) emission of light by an organism as a consequence of the oxidation of some substrate in the presence of an enzyme.

biolysis (bi-ol′ĭ-sis) decomposition of organic matter by living organisms.

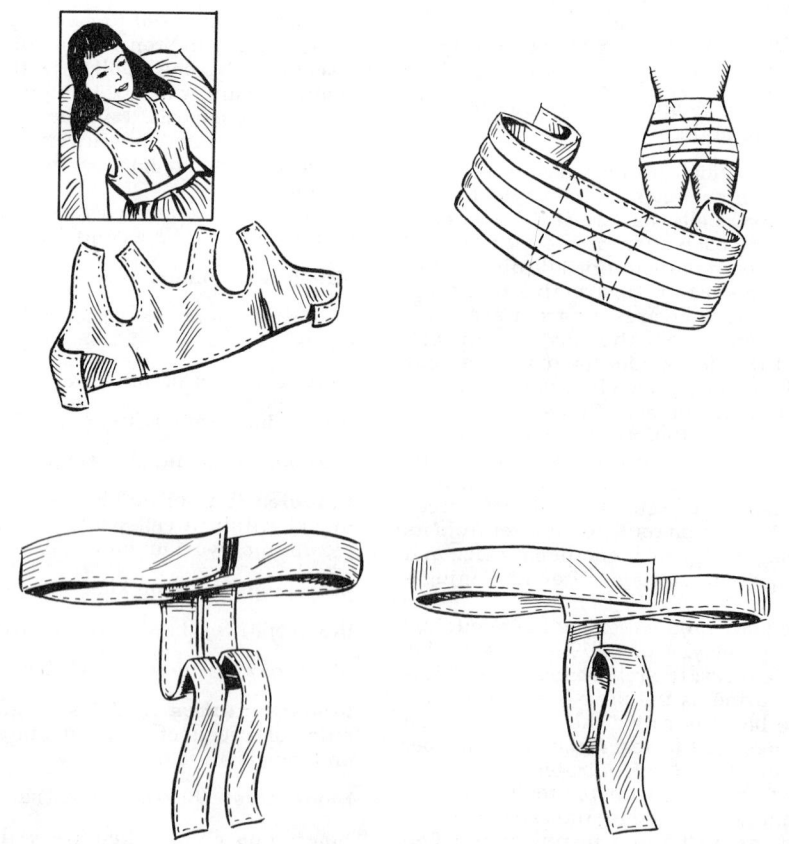

Binders: top left, breast; top right, abdominal; bottom left, double T; bottom right, T.

biolytic (bi″o-lit′ik) 1. pertaining to biolysis. 2. destructive to life.

biomass (bi′o-mas) the entire assemblage of living organisms of a particular region, considered collectively.

biomathematics (bi″o-math″ĕ-mat′iks) mathematics as applied to the phenomena of living things.

biome (bi′ōm) a large, distinct, easily differentiated community of organisms arising as a result of complex interactions of physical and biotic environmental factors.

biomechanics (bi″o-mĕ-kan′iks) the science of mechanics as applied to the living body.

biometeorology (bi″o-me″te-or-ol′o-je) scientific study of effects on living organisms of the extraorganic aspects (temperature, humidity, barometric pressure, rate of air flow, and air ionization) of the physical environment, whether natural or artificially created, and also their effects in closed ecological systems, as in satellites or submarines.

biometer (bi-om′ĕ-ter) an instrument for measuring carbon dioxide given off by living tissue.

biometrics, biometry (bi″o-met′riks), (bi-om′ĕ-tre) the application of statistical methods to biological facts.

biomicroscope (bi″o-mi′kro-skōp) a microscope for examining living tissue.

biomicroscopy (bi″o-mi-kros′ko-pe) observation by microscope of a living cell or tissue in its functional state.

biomutation (bi″o-mu-ta′shun) the modification produced in an organism when injected into the animal body.

bion (bi′on) an individual living organism.

bionecrosis (bi″o-nĕ-kro′sis) necrobiosis.

bionergy (bi-on′er-je) the vital energy that underlies all organic life.

bionics (bi-on′iks) scientific study of functions, characteristics and phenomena observed in the living world and application of knowledge gained therefrom in the world of machines.

bionomics (bi″o-nom′iks) ecology.

bionomy (bi-on′o-me) the science of the laws of life.

bionucleonics (bi″o-nu″kle-on′iks) scientific study of biological applications of radioactive and rare stable isotopes.

biophore (bi′o-fōr) an early name for one of the submicroscopic particles in a cell that manifest specific functions.

biophylactic (bi″o-fi-lak′tik) guarding or preserving life.

biophysics (bi″o-fiz′iks) the physics of vital processes.

biophysiology (bi″o-fiz″e-ol′o-je) the portion of biology including organogenesis, morphology and physiology.

bioplasia (bi″o-pla′ze-ah) the storing up of food energy in the form of growth.

bioplasm (bi′o-plazm) the more vital or essential part of protoplasm. adj., **bioplas′mic.**

bioplast (bi′o-plast) 1. an independently existing mass of living substance. 2. a living cell.

bioplastic (bi′o-plas′tik) aiding in growth.

biopoiesis (bi″o-poi-e′sis) the origin of life from inorganic matter.

biopsy (bi′op-se) examination of tissue removed from the living body. Biopsies are usually done to determine whether a tumor is malignant or benign; however, a biopsy may be a useful diagnostic aid in other disease processes such as infections.
    aspiration b., needle biopsy.
    excision b., biopsy of tissue removed from the body by surgical cutting.
    needle b., biopsy of material obtained from an internal organ by means of a hollow needle inserted through the body wall and into the affected part.
    sponge b., examination of material (particles of tissue and tissue juices) absorbed in a sponge rubbed over a lesion or over mucous membrane, the entire sponge being stained and sectioned.
    sternal b., examination of samplings of bone marrow removed from the sternum by puncture or aspiration (see also STERNAL PUNCTURE).

biorheology (bi″o-re-ol′o-je) study of deformation and flow of matter in living systems and in materials directly derived from them.

bios (bi′os) any one of a group of growth factors for single-celled organisms such as yeast. Bios occurs in yeast, leaves of plants, bran and the outer coating of seeds.
    b. I, inositol.
    b. II, biotin.

bioscopy (bi-os′ko-pe) examination with respect to viability or to the extinction of life.

biose (bi′ōs) a disaccharide.

bioset (bi′o-set) a grouping of biological components.

biospectrometry (bi″o-spek-trom′ĕ-tre) the spectrometry of matter in living tissue.

biospectroscopy (bi″o-spek-tros′ko-pe) the spectroscopy of living tissue.

biosphere (bi′o-sfēr) the regions of the known universe in which the environment supports the existence of living organisms.

biostatic (bi″o-stat′ik) inhibiting the growth and reproduction of living organisms.

biostatistics (bi″o-stah-tis′tiks) collected numerical data relating to living organisms.

biosynthesis (bi″o-sin′thĕ-sis) creation of a compound by physiologic processes in a living organism.

biotaxis (bi″o-tak′sis) 1. the selecting and arranging powers of living cells. 2. systematic classification of organisms.

biotaxy (bi″o-tak′se) biotaxis (1).

biotelemetry (bi″o-tel-em′ĕ-tre) registration and measurement of certain vital phenomena occurring in living organisms remote from the measuring device.

biotherapy (bi″o-ther′ah-pe) treatment by means of living organisms and their products, including vaccines, immune serum, blood transfusion.

biotic (bi-ot′ik) pertaining to living organisms.

biotics (bi-ot′iks) the science of the qualities of living organisms.

biotin (bi′o-tin) a member of the vitamin B complex, required by or occurring in all forms of life.

biotomy (bi-ot′o-me) vivisection.

biotoxication (bi″o-tok″sĭ-ka′shun) intoxication due to a poison derived from a living organism.

biotoxicology (bi″o-tok″sĭ-kol′o-je) scientific study of poisons produced by living organisms, their cause, detection and effects, and treatment of conditions produced by them.

biotoxin (bi″o-tok′sin) a poisonous substance produced by and derived from a living organism (plant or animal).

biotransformation (bi″o-trans″for-ma′shun) conversion of a material by natural processes occurring in a living organism.

biotrepy (bi-ot′rĕ-pe) study of the body by means of its reactions to chemical substances.

biotripsis (bi″o-trip′sis) wearing away of the skin, seen in the aged.

biotropism (bi-ot′ro-pizm) a decrease in resistance that allows a latent infection to become active or a saprophytic germ to become virulent.

biotype (bi′o-tīp) a group of individuals having the same fundamental constitution.

biovular (bi-ov′u-lar) binovular.

bipara (bip′ah-rah) secundipara; a woman who has had two pregnancies that resulted in viable offspring; para II.

biparental (bi″pah-ren′tal) derived from two parents, male and female.

biparous (bip′ah-rus) producing two at a birth.

bipenniform (bi-pen′ĭ-form) doubly feather-shaped.

biperiden (bi-per′ĭ-den) an anticholinergic used in the treatment of Parkinson's disease and certain other forms of spasticity. Side effects are minor and include dryness of the mouth, blurring of vision, drowsiness and nausea. Biperiden is contraindicated in patients with epilepsy and should be given with great care to patients with glaucoma.

bipolar (bi-po′lar) 1. having two poles. 2. pertaining to both poles.

bipotentiality (bi″po-ten″she-al′ĭ-te) ability to develop in either of two different ways.

biramous (bi-ra′mus) having two branches.

birefractive (bi″re-frak′tiv) doubly refractive.

birefringence (bi″re-frin′jens) the quality of transmitting light unequally in different directions.

birth (berth) a coming into being; the act or process of being born.

b. canal, the canal through which the fetus passes in birth.

b. certificate, a written, authenticated record of the birth of a child, required by state laws throughout the United States. After a birth is registered, a birth certificate is issued which represents legal proof of parentage, age and citizenship, and is of great personal and legal importance. A birth certificate is required for many legal and business or personal transactions. Whether the child is born at home or at the hospital, the physician, midwife or other attendant must report the birth to the local or state registrar. The report becomes a permanent record, and a certificate is issued to the parents. If a child dies during birth, an immediate report and certification of the birth and death are required, containing a statement of the cause of death.

b. control, the concept of limiting the size of families. The movement of that name began in modern times as a humanitarian reform to conserve the health of mothers and the welfare of children, especially among the poor. More recently it has been superseded by the term "planned parenthood," which means planning the arrival of children to correspond with the desire and resources of the married couple and provide greater happiness for the children. (See also CONTRACEPTION.) Planned parenthood is concerned not only with controlling fertility but also with overcoming apparent sterility in those couples who want a child and have been unsuccessful in having one.

multiple b., the birth of two or more offspring produced in the same gestation period.

premature b., expulsion of the fetus from the uterus before termination of the normal gestation period, but after independent existence has become a possibility. (See also PREMATURE INFANT.)

b. rate, the number of births during one year for the total population (crude birth rate), for the female population (refined birth rate) or for the female population of childbearing age (true birth rate).

birthmark (berth′mark) a congenital blemish or spot on the skin, usually visible at birth or shortly after. Those appearing later occur at the location of a skin defect present at birth. The cause is unknown.

epidermal b., the result of a flaw in pigmentation of the skin. NEVI (moles) are examples of this type.

physiologic b., a small, irregular bluish red patch in the occipital region. It is frequently present at birth and persists throughout adult life.

vascular b., one caused by an unusual clustering of small blood vessels near the surface of the skin; called also HEMANGIOMA. These birthmarks include "strawberry" or "raspberry" marks, "port-wine stains" and an elevated type called cavernous hemangiomas.

bisacodyl (bis-ak′o-dil) a drug used as a laxative.

bisacromial (bis″ah-kro′me-al) pertaining to the two acromions.

bisalbuminemia (bis″al-bu″mĭ-ne′me-ah) a congenital anomaly with two electrophoretically distinct albumins in the serum.

bisection (bi-sek′shun) division into two parts.

bisexual (bi-seks′u-al) 1. having gonads of both

sexes; hermaphrodite. 2. having both active (male) and passive (female) sexual interests and characteristics.

bisferious (bis-fe're-us) dicrotic; having two beats.

bishydroxycoumarin (bis"hi-drok"se-koo'mah-rin) a white crystalline powder used as an anticoagulant. It interferes with the production, in the liver, of prothrombin, so that the prothrombin content of the blood is decreased and the prothrombin time is lengthened. It prevents clotting within the blood vessels and reduces the formation of emboli and thrombi, and is used in the treatment of coronary thrombosis and thrombophlebitis and in the prevention of emboli. Average dose depends on the results of a daily prothrombin time test and varies greatly from one patient to another. In overdosage, which can be accompanied by severe hemorrhage, intravenous injections of vitamin K and transfusions of whole fresh blood may be necessary to restore the normal prothrombin content of the blood.

bisiliac (bis-il'e-ak) pertaining to the two ilia.

bis in die (bis in de'a) [L.] twice a day; abbreviated b.i.d.

bismuth (biz'muth) a chemical element, atomic number 83, atomic weight 208.980, symbol Bi. (See table of ELEMENTS.)
  b. glycolylarsanilate, glycobiarsol, used in treatment of amebiasis.
  b. sodium triglycollamate, a double salt of sodium bismuthyl triglycollamate and disodium triglycollamate, used as a suppressant for lupus erythematosus and in treatment of chronic sore throat.
  b. subcarbonate, a basic salt used topically in lotions and ointments, and internally as an astringent, protective and adsorbent.
  b. subgallate, a bright yellow, amorphous powder, applied locally in skin diseases.
  b. subnitrate, a white, slightly hygroscopic powder, sometimes used as a gastrointestinal astringent.

bismuthosis (biz"muth-o'sis) a state of chronic poisoning from the misuse of bismuth.

bistoury (bis'too-re) a long, narrow surgical knife used in opening sinuses and fistulas, incisioning abscesses, etc.

Bistrimate (bis'tri-māt) trademark for a preparation of bismuth sodium triglycollamate, used as a suppressant for lupus erythematosus and in treatment of chronic sore throat.

bistrium (bis'tre-um) trademark for hexamethonium, a ganglion-blocking agent and antihypertensive.

bisulfate (bi-sul'fāt) an acid sulfate; one with twice the proportion of acid found in a normal sulfate.

bite (bīt) 1. seizure with the teeth. 2. a wound or puncture made by an insect. 3. in dentistry, the occlusion of the teeth, or an imprint of the teeth or gums in some plastic material, used in making artificial dentures.
  ANIMAL BITE. Any animal bite that breaks the skin should be treated rapidly and with care. The wound should be washed at once with soap and

water. A physician should be consulted so that necessary steps may be taken to prevent the development of RABIES.

Every effort should be made to catch an animal that has bitten someone, so that it may be confined and examined by the health department for signs of rabies. Whenever possible the animal should be caught alive because evidence of rabies disappears rapidly after death. If the animal is not caught, the bitten person is given antirabies treatment immediately.

HUMAN BITE. Any human bite that penetrates the skin should be considered dangerous. The wound should be washed immediately with soap and water and a physician should be consulted. Antibiotics may be needed as there is a serious danger of infection, a danger that is more serious with human bites than with animal bites since many of the organisms carried by animals do not affect humans.

bitemporal (bi-tem'po-ral) pertaining to both temples or temporal bones.

biteplate (bīt'plāt) an appliance worn in the palate as a diagnostic or therapeutic adjunct in orthodontics or prosthodontics.

bite-wing (bīt'wing) a film used in making roentgenograms of the teeth, having a flange to be held between the jaws and permitting production of images of both the upper and lower teeth.

bitrochanteric (bi-tro"kan-ter'ik) pertaining to both trochanters.

bitumen (bĭ-too'men) a natural or artificial solid or dry petroleum product.

bituminosis (bĭ-too"mi-no'sis) a form of PNEUMOCONIOSIS due to dust from soft coal.

biuret (bi'u-ret) a crystalline compound formed by heating urea.
  b. reaction, a chemical test used to demonstrate the presence of protein.

bivalent (bi-va'lent, biv'ah-lent) having a valence of two.

biventral (bi-ven'tral) having two bellies.

bizygomatic (bi-zi"go-mat'ik) pertaining to the two zygomatic bones.

Bk chemical symbol, *berkelium.*

black eye a bruise of the tissue around the eye marked by discoloration, swelling and pain. Cold compresses, if applied immediately, help to slow the bleeding under the skin and thus reduce swelling and discoloration. Later, warm wet towels should be applied in order to hasten the absorption of discoloring fluids. Any of the complications of a bruise, such as a clot, may develop, in which case medical attention will be necessary. A black eye resulting from an unusually violent blow may be accompanied by injury to the skull or damage to the eye itself.

blackhead comedo; a plug of fatty material (sebum) in the orifice of a hair follicle. The color of blackheads is caused not by dirt but by the discoloring effect of air on the sebum in the clogged pore. Infection may cause the comedo to develop into a pustule or boil. See also ACNE VULGARIS.

blackout temporary loss of vision and momentary unconsciousness. Blackout refers specifically to a condition which sometimes occurs in aviators resulting from increased acceleration, which causes a decrease in blood supply to the brain cells. The term can also refer to other forms of temporary loss of consciousness and to FAINTING, as well as to temporary loss of memory and to certain forms of vertigo.

black-water fever a dangerous and poorly understood complication of malaria, especially of the falciparum type, characterized by the passage of dark red to black urine, severe toxicity and high mortality, especially for Europeans.

bladder (blad′er) a membranous sac, especially that into which urine drains. The urinary bladder is a hollow container with muscular walls. It is joined to the kidneys by the ureters and to the exterior of the body by the urethra. Urine passes to the bladder from the kidneys every few seconds, and it remains there until it is voided. Voiding occurs when the sphincters (circular muscles) at the juncture of the bladder and urethra are relaxed and the muscular walls of the bladder contract, forcing the urine out. In the adult the sphincters can prevent urination even when the bladder is uncomfortably full, but in children full bladder control is slow to develop. BED-WETTING may normally continue to the age of 3 or 4 years.

DISORDERS OF THE BLADDER. Infections of the bladder are fairly common, especially in women and girls, since the female urethra is shorter than that of the male and permits easier entry of infectious agents. Most infections yield readily to treatment with antibiotics.

Inflammation of the bladder, or CYSTITIS, may be caused by many different agents, and can vary greatly in seriousness. Its most usual symptoms are a persistent desire to urinate, and a burning sensation at urination.

Various deformations of the bladder are found. The most common and least serious is the formation of an outpocketing or diverticulum. The pocket may be caused by pressure from inside the bladder, when for some reason the urine is obstructed, or it may have existed from birth.

An abnormal opening in the bladder causes a fistula, which conducts escaping urine to other parts of the body, or to the exterior through the skin. The most common varieties are those in which the fistulas lead into the intestine or directly into the vagina (vesicovaginal fistula). They occur sometimes after childbirth or after diverticulitis of the colon. The condition may be remedied by surgery.

Stones (calculi) may form in the bladder and often lead to painful and difficult urination. They are usually caused by obstructions in the mouth of the bladder, brought about, for example, by an enlarged prostate. If necessary, they can be removed by surgery.

Tumors may also form in the bladder, especially in later life. These may be benign or cancerous. The benign tumors do not spread, but may require removal to relieve other symptoms. The most common symptom of tumor of the bladder is the presence of blood in the urine unaccompanied by pain. In malignancy, surgery is likely to be necessary.

Atonic baldder is a condition marked by paralysis of the motor nerves of the bladder without any evidence of a lesion of the central nervous system. Cord bladder refers to defective bladder function from a lesion in the nervous system, as myelitis or tabes dorsalis. Neurogenic bladder refers to any disturbance of the bladder due to a lesion of the nervous system.

SURGERY OF THE BLADDER. The two most common types of major surgery of the bladder are cystotomy and cystectomy. Cystotomy is surgical incision into the bladder for removal of bladder stones or as a part of the surgical procedure known as suprapubic PROSTATECTOMY.

Tumors of the bladder are the most frequent indication for surgery of the bladder. Large tumors involving several layers of the bladder wall require partial or complete removal of the bladder. Cystectomy is done when widespread malignant disease or severe physical trauma has destroyed much of the bladder wall. Removal of the entire bladder requires diversion of the urinary flow by transplantation of the ureters to the surface of the abdomen (ureterostomy) or to the bowel (ureteroenterostomy).

Small, superficial tumors of the bladder may be treated by fulguration, with the use of a cystoscope and an electric cautery. Normally, after fulguration there is minimal bleeding and the patient is usually allowed to go home within a few days.

Cystostomy is an operation in which an opening is made through the abdominal wall for draining of the bladder.

Nursing Care. In any type of surgery of the bladder or ureters it is extremely important that there be constant maintenance of the flow of urine. Urine is secreted by the kidneys continuously and normally dribbles in a constant stream down the ureters into the bladder. If for any reason the flow of urine from the ureters is obstructed, there is a damming up of urine in the kidney and hydronephrosis results. To be aware of this eventuality it is necessary to observe carefully and at frequent intervals any drainage from CATHETERS inserted before or after surgery. Should there be evidence of obstruction to the urine flow the surgeon should be notified at once.

The urine is also observed for signs of hemorrhage, presence of clots or bits of tissue and unusual odor or concentration. These observations are important in the preoperative as well as the postoperative period. The amount of urinary output must be measured with extreme care and recorded accurately.

Infection is always a possibility after surgery of the urinary system. To guard against this complication care must be taken in the handling of catheters or other drainage tubes. If dressings are applied they should be changed frequently to reduce the hazard of infection and the unpleasant odor that usually is caused by the leakage of urine.

The intake of fluids is prescribed by the physician as part of the treatment and the fluids should be considered medication. Explaining to the patient and his family the need to restrict or force fluids usually insures their cooperation.

Providing for adequate collection and disposal of urine for patients with total cystectomy depends on the type of surgery done and the devices chosen by the surgeon. The patient with a ureterostomy needs much support emotionally and psychologically during the period of adjustment to his new way of life. When ureteroenterostomy has been done a program of control of the rectal sphincter is carried out. This requires patience and tact on the part of the nurse. She must also be alert to signs of urinary infections in these patients because the danger of contamination of the ureters and kidneys by intestinal bacteria is always present.

Blalock-Taussig operation (bla′lok taw′sig) surgical creation of a shunt between the subclavian artery and the pulmonary artery for treatment of congenital pulmonary stenosis.

blanch (blanch) to become pale.

blast (blast) 1. an immature stage in cellular development before appearance of the definitive characteristics of the cell; used also as a word termination. 2. the wave of air pressure produced by the detonation of high-explosive bombs or shells or by other explosions; it causes pulmonary damage and hemorrhage (lung blast, blast chest), laceration of abdominal viscera, ruptured eardrums and effects on the nervous system.

blast(o)- (blas′to) word element [Gr.], *a bud* or *sprout*.

blastema (blas-te′mah) 1. the primitive substance from which cells are formed. 2. a group of cells that will give rise to a new individual, in asexual reproduction, or to an organ or part, in either normal development or regeneration.

blastocoele (blas′to-sēl) the fluid-filled cavity of the mass of cells (blastula) produced by cleavage of a fertilized ovum.

blastocyst (blas′to-sist) the thin-walled cystic blastula produced in development of many mammals, including man.

blastocyte (blas′to-sīt) an undifferentiated embryonic cell.

blastocytoma (blas″to-si-to′mah) a tumor composed of undifferentiated embryonic tissue.

blastoderm (blas′to-derm) 1. the cellular cap at the animal pole of yolk-rich eggs. 2. the disk consisting of the primary germ layers.

blastodisk (blas′to-disk) the convex structure formed by the blastomeres at the animal pole of an ovum undergoing incomplete cleavage.

blastogenesis (blas″to-jen′ĕ-sis) 1. reproduction by gemmation. 2. transmission of characters by germ plasm.

blastolysis (blas-tol′ĭ-sis) destruction of the germ substance.

blastoma (blas-to′mah) 1. a true tumor; a tumor, not teratogenous, that exhibits an independent localized growth. 2. blastocytoma.

blastomatosis (blas″to-mah-to′sis) the presence of numerous blastomas.

blastomere (blas′to-mēr) one of the cells produced by cleavage of a fertilized ovum.

Blastomyces (blas″to-mi′sēz) a genus of yeast-like fungi; pathogenic for man and animals.

B. brasilien′sis, the fungus that causes South American blastomycosis.

B. dermatit′idis, the fungus that causes North American blastomycosis.

blastomycosis (blas″to-mi-ko′sis) infection with organisms of the genus Blastomyces.

North American b., an infection caused by *Blastomyces dermatitidis*, marked by suppurating tumors in the skin (cutaneous blastomycosis) or by lesions in the lungs, bones, subcutaneous tissues, liver, spleen and kidneys (systemic blastomycosis).

South American b., a systemic fungal disease caused by *Blastomyces brasiliensis*. The disease occurs in Central and South America and is especially prevalent in Brazil. Infection may involve the nasopharynx and oropharynx, skin, lymph nodes, lungs, gastrointestinal tract, liver and spleen. Amphotericin B is the specific drug used for treatment. All untreated cases are fatal.

blastula (blas′tu-lah) the spherical structure produced by cleavage of a fertilized ovum, consisting of a single layer of cells surrounding a fluid-filled cavity (blastocoele); it follows the morula stage.

blastulation (blas″tu-la′shun) the formation of the blastula.

bleb (bleb) a blister.

bleeder (blēd′er) 1. the popular term for a person who bleeds freely, especially one suffering from a condition in which the blood fails to clot properly (see also HEMOPHILIA). 2. a large blood vessel divided during surgery.

bleeding (blēd′ing) 1. the escape of blood, as from an injured vessel. (See also HEMORRHAGE.) 2. the purposeful withdrawal of blood from a vessel of the body; venesection; phlebotomy.

functional b., bleeding from the uterus when no organic lesions are present.

implantation b., that occurring at the time of implantation of the fertilized ovum in the uterine wall.

occult b., escape of blood in such small quantity that it can be detected only by chemical tests.

placentation b., escape of blood from the uterine vessels being eroded and tapped by the developing placenta during the early weeks of pregnancy.

b. time, the time required for a small pinpoint wound to cease bleeding. If done properly, the test can be helpful in determining the functional capacity of platelets and of vasoconstriction. The Ivy method is generally considered to be the most accurate: a blood pressure cuff is placed on the arm and a pressure of 40 mm. of mercury is maintained. A small puncture wound is made on the inner surface of the forearm. Normally, bleeding will cease in 3 to 6 minutes. A prolonged bleeding time is found in patients with vascular abnormalities, with deficiencies in the platelet count, and with conditions in which there is a deficiency of fibrinogen.

blennogenic (blen″o-jen′ik) producing mucus.

blennoid (blen′oid) resembling mucus.

blennorrhagia (blen″o-ra′je-ah) 1. any discharge of mucus. 2. gonorrhea.

blennorrhea (blen″o-re′ah) a discharge from the mucous surfaces, especially a gonorrheal discharge from the urethra or vagina; gonorrhea.

inclusion b., an inflammatory condition of the conjunctiva, urethra or cervix, caused by a filterable virus and characterized by the presence of large basophilic inclusion bodies.

blennostasis (blĕ-nos'tah-sis) diminution of mucous secretion. adj., **blennostat'ic.**

blennothorax (blen"o-tho'raks) mucus in the chest.

blennuria (blen-u're-ah) mucus in the urine.

blephar(o)- (blef'ah-ro) word element [Gr.], *eyelid; eyelash.*

blepharadenitis (blef"ar-ad"ĕ-ni'tis) blepharoadenitis.

blepharal (blef'ar-al) pertaining to the eyelids.

blepharectomy (blef"ar-ek'to-me) excision of an eyelid.

blepharism (blef'ah-rizm) spasm of the eyelid.

blepharitis (blef'ah-ri'tis) inflammation of the edges of the eyelid margins.
  angular b., inflammation involving the outer angle of the eyelids.
  squamous b., seborrhea of eyelid margins, with formation of little plates of dried secretion on the eyelashes.
  ulcerative b., a condition characterized by loss of eyelashes and the appearance of small ulcerated pockets on the eyelid margin.

blepharoadenitis (blef"ah-ro-ad"ĕ-ni'tis) inflammation of the meibomian glands of the eyelids.

blepharoatheroma (blef"ah-ro-ath"er-o'mah) an encysted tumor or sebaceous cyst of an eyelid.

blepharochalasis (blef"ah-ro-kal'ah-sis) acquired atrophy of the skin of the upper eyelid.

blepharoconjunctivitis (blef"ah-ro-kon-junk"ti-vi'tis) inflammation of the eyelids and conjunctiva.

blepharoncus (blef"ar-ong'kus) a tumor on the eyelid.

blepharophimosis (blef"ah-ro-fi-mo'sis) diminution in the overall size of the opening between the eyelids.

blepharoplasty (blef'ah-ro-plas"te) plastic repair of an eyelid.

blepharoplegia (blef"ah-ro-ple'je-ah) paralysis of an eyelid.

blepharoptosis (blef"ar-op-to'sis) drooping of an upper eyelid.

blepharorrhaphy (blef"ah-ror'ah-fe) suture of an eyelid.

blepharospasm (blef'ah-ro-spazm") spasm of the orbicular muscle of the eye.

blepharostat (blef'ah-ro-stat") an instrument for holding the eyelids apart.

blepharostenosis (blef"ah-ro-stĕ-no'sis) blepharophimosis.

blepharosynechia (blef"ah-ro-sĭ-nek'e-ah) growing together of the eyelids.

blepharotomy (blef"ah-rot'o-me) incision of an eyelid.

blind (blīnd) not having the sense of sight.
  b. spot, the place where the optic nerve enters the retina of the eye. The blind spot, which is a normal part of the eye, is devoid of rods and cones and therefore is not sensitive to light.

blindness (blīnd'nes) inability to see; legally, less than 20/200 vision with eyeglasses (vision of 20/200 is the ability to see only at 20 feet what the normal eye can see at 200 feet). It is estimated that there are more than 350,000 legally blind persons in the United States. Of these, over half are 65 or older.
  CAUSES. A major cause of blindness is CATARACT, clouding of the lens of the eye. Removal of the clouded lens from the eye restores sight to most cataract patients.
  A second major cause is chronic GLAUCOMA, an increase in the fluid pressure inside the eyeball. This disease, which can usually be cured or controlled if discovered and treated early enough, often causes no pain and gives no warning. People over 35 are more susceptible to glaucoma than younger persons, and there is a familial tendency toward the disease.
  DETACHMENT OF RETINA is a condition in which pieces of the retina become separated from the underlying tissues. It once led to incurable blindness, but now can often be repaired by a delicate surgical operation.
  Scarring of the cornea may result from a local infection and can usually be checked by medical treatment. If it becomes so severe as to interfere seriously with vision, the condition may require a cornea transplant.
  TRACHOMA, a virus infection of the conjunctiva, was once a major cause of blindness in the United States, and still is in many of the developing countries. Sulfonamide drugs and antibiotics can halt the disease.
  In the last 30 years, two of the greatest causes of blindness in newborn children have been virtually eliminated. One, ophthalmia neonatorum, is caused by gonococci and is transmitted to the infant during passage through the birth canal. The practice of instilling silver nitrate in the eyes of every child at the time of birth has greatly reduced its incidence. The second disease, retrolental fibroplasia, was found to occur most often in premature infants. Investigation proved excessive administration of oxygen during the neonatal period to be the cause of this disorder. With revised procedures in the administration of oxygen to newborn infants the incidence of retrolental fibroplasia has decreased greatly.
  Blindness may also come as an effect of various infectious diseases, including scarlet fever, smallpox and syphilis. Modern techniques of immunization and the development of antibiotics have brought most of these diseases under control. There is still grave danger to the sight of the child whose mother contracts rubella (German measles) during the early months of pregnancy.
  About 3 per cent of all cases of blindness in the United States are the result of accidental injury on the job.
  Some cases of blindness are caused by hereditary factors. Little is known about this aspect of heredity, but an increasing amount of research is being done.

The National Society for the Prevention of Blindness estimates that more than half of all cases of blindness could be prevented or cured with our present knowledge. An eye examination every 2 years is recommended for early detection and prompt treatment.

EDUCATION AND TRAINING.   Today a blind person is no longer thought of as helpless or dependent on others for everything. New methods of education and recreation have made it possible for more than half the blind children in school to attend schools with children having normal eyesight. Many colleges provide special funds to enable blind students to hire readers and tape recorders to help them in their studies.

The Library of Congress, in Washington, D.C., lends records and recording machines without charge to the blind, and maintains a wide selection of recordings. Tape-recorded textbooks and other educational material are available from a private organization, Recording for the Blind, 121 East 58th Street, New York, N.Y. 10022.

Those of working age who are legally blind are entitled to special counseling, vocational training and placement through joint state and federal programs. Other programs provide work for blind people who are home-bound, visiting teachers for those who want to learn to read and write Braille and recreation facilities, including swimming pools and bowling alleys.

The American Foundation for the Blind publishes many excellent pamphlets to help those who must deal with the special problems involved in blindness.

NURSING CARE.   The patient who is blind often presents a special challenge to the nurse assigned to his care. She must strive to know her patient well and quickly learn his degree of dependence and his attitude toward his loss of vision. Her handling of the situation will depend on whether the patient has been deprived of his sight recently or has been blind for several years. If she is helping him to adjust to a recent loss of vision she must delicately balance sympathy with a sincere desire to help him adjust to a new life in which he must learn again the simple activities of daily living. A patient who has been blind for years and has adjusted to his handicap most often wishes to be treated as any other patient.

Feeding the Blind Patient. A blind person should be told what different types of food he has on his tray. Before he is given hot foods or iced liquids he should be warned that they are hot or cold. Liquids are usually easier for the blind patient to handle if they are served in a cup, without a straw. The cup is placed in his hand so that he can drink from it himself. Solid foods are given to the patient in the same manner in which the nurse would eat them herself, with variety and combining of foods that go well together. The patient should be allowed to feed himself "finger foods" and liquids.

The Ambulatory Patient. When walking with a blind patient it is best to hold his arm and walk at his side. Directions are given in advance so that he will know to turn to the left or right or go down steps, as well as how many steps. The prevention of accidents is an important part of the care of the blind patient who is up and about. Aside from the physical effects of bumping into objects or falling over them, the blind person also suffers from a loss of self-confidence and security if he cannot move about safely and independently. Doors should be kept closed or completely open. They must never

be left ajar. If it is necessary to move a piece of furniture in the patient's room, he should be told of its new location.

Other rules that should be observed in caring for the blind include:

1. Remember that the person is blind, not deaf. There is no reason to shout at him or address him as if he were a child or mentally retarded. Speak normally and naturally.

2. Speak to the blind person as you enter his room and do not touch him until after you have spoken to him. Otherwise he may be startled or frightened if he has not heard you enter his room.

3. When you leave the room tell the patient you are going. He will not then resume the conversation later and find that he is talking to someone who is not there.

4. Pity is neither expected nor appreciated by the blind. They want to be treated as normal people, and would rather ask for help than have someone do everything for them. It is important to remember that there are no such things as "extra senses of blindness," which many people mistakenly believe blind people are given to compensate for their loss of sight. Whatever a blind person has learned about living with his blindness he has accomplished through hard work and determination.

color b., deviation from normal perception of color (see also COLOR BLINDNESS).

night b., defective vision in conditions of diminished illumination (see also NIGHT BLINDNESS).

snow b., dimness of vision, usually temporary, due to the glare of the sun upon snow.

blister (blis′ter) a collection of serous, bloody or watery fluid under the skin.
   fever b., herpes febrilis.

block (blok) 1. an obstruction or stoppage. 2. regional anesthesia.
   bundle-branch b., a form of HEART BLOCK involving obstruction in one of the branches in the bundle of His.
   field b., production of anesthesia in an area by injection of an anesthetic agent at points around its perimeter.
   heart b., a condition in which the passage of the electrical stimulation between the atrium and ventricle is interrupted so that they beat independently of each other (see also HEART BLOCK).
   mental b., obstruction to thought or memory, particularly that produced by emotional factors.
   nerve b., interruption of transmission of impulses by injection of an anesthetic agent in close proximity to the nerve.
   paravertebral b., infiltration of the cervicothoracic ganglion with procaine hydrochloride.

Blockain (blok′ān) trademark for a preparation of propoxycaine hydrochloride, a local anesthetic.

blocking (blok′ing) 1. interruption of an afferent nerve pathway, as by injection of an anesthetic. 2. repression of an idea from consciousness due to a mental conflict.

blood (blud) the fluid that circulates through the heart, arteries and veins. Blood is the chief means of transport within the body. It transports oxygen from the lungs to the body tissues, and carbon dioxide from the tissues to the lungs. It carries foods from the digestive system to the tissues, removes waste products to the kidneys and carries fluid to and from the tissues, helping to maintain the fluid balance of the body.

In an emergency, blood cells and antibodies carried in the blood are brought to a point of infection, or blood-clotting substances are carried to a break in a blood vessel. The blood distributes hormones from the endocrine glands to the organs they influence. And it helps in the regulation of body temperature by carrying excess heat from the interior of the body to the surface layers of the skin, where the heat is dissipated to the surrounding air.

Blood varies in color from a bright red in the arteries to a duller red in the veins. The total quantity of blood within an individual depends upon his body weight. A person who weighs 150 lbs. has about 5 quarts of blood in his body.

Blood is composed of two main parts: (1) plasma, the fluid portion, consisting mainly of water in which are dissolved the substances carried by the blood to and from the tissues; and (2) solid particles, including blood cells and blood platelets, suspended in the fluid.

PLASMA. The plasma accounts for about 55 per cent of the total volume of the blood. It consists of about 92 per cent water, 7 per cent proteins and less than 1 per cent inorganic salts, organic substances other than proteins, dissolved gases, hormones, antibodies and enzymes. Plasma from which the fibrinogen has been removed is called serum.

Dissolved in the plasma are many important proteins such as serum albumin, gamma globulin and fibrinogen. Serum albumin is important in the nutrition of the body. It probably originates in the liver, as does the fibrinogen. Fibrinogen is essential in the clotting process. Gamma globulin, which is formed in the lymphoid tissues and reticuloendothelial system, contains almost all of the antibodies important in establishing immunity.

BLOOD CELLS AND PLATELETS. The suspended particles of the blood comprise the other 45 per cent of the total volume of blood. They include erythrocytes (red blood cells), leukocytes (white blood cells) and platelets (thrombocytes). The red and white blood cells are also known as corpuscles (Latin for "little bodies").

Erythrocytes (Red Blood Cells). The great majority of the cells in the blood are red blood cells. There are about 5 million red blood cells in a speck of blood the size of a pinhead, and about 35 trillion of them in the average adult. Although microscopic in size, these cells have a total surface area almost the size of a football gridiron. This vast surface area is important in the blood's task of carrying oxygen from the lungs to the tissues, because the exchange of oxygen in both places takes place across the cell surfaces and must be accomplished quickly as the blood flows by.

The erythrocytes owe their oxygen-carrying ability to the protein *heme,* which contains iron and gives the blood its red color. Heme combines with another protein, globin, and forms HEMOGLOBIN, a major part of the red blood cell. Hemoglobin has the special ability of attracting and forming a loose connection with free oxygen, and its presence enables blood to absorb some 60 times the amount of oxygen that the plasma by itself absorbs.

Red blood cells are stored in the SPLEEN, which acts as a reservoir for the blood system and discharges the cells into the blood as required. The spleen also discharges extra red blood cells into the blood during emergencies such as hemorrhage or shock.

Red blood cells originate in the red bone marrow of the ribs, sternum, skull, pelvic bone, vertebrae and the ends of the long bones of the limbs. The average red cell has a life of 110 to 120 days. It then disintegrates, and is removed in the spleen and the liver. About 180 million red blood cells are destroyed every minute. Since the number of cells in the blood remains more or less constant, this means that about 180 million red blood cells are manufactured every minute. The hemoglobin of destroyed cells is decomposed and carried to the liver. There the iron is stored and the rest of the chemicals are passed on to be excreted from the body in the bile, the feces and the urine.

Leukocytes (White Blood Cells). The leukocytes are the body's primary defense against infections. They have no hemoglobin and thus are colorless and, unlike red blood cells, they can move about under their own power. White blood cells are larger than red blood cells and fewer in number. Normally the blood has about 8000 white blood cells per cubic millimeter.

Of the several types of leukocytes, the neutrophils are the most numerous, forming about 70 per cent of the total number; lymphocytes make up about 20 per cent of the total. The neutrophils, the lymphocytes and most other white blood cells are phagocytic – that is, they have the ability to engulf and destroy bacteria. Leukocytes multiply rapidly when the body is invaded by bacteria. The cells migrate rapidly to the site of the infection, surround the bacteria and overwhelm them. Under a microscope, as many as 15 or 20 bacteria can be seen within a single white blood cell. Leukocytes originate in the red bone marrow, except for the lymphocytes, which are formed in lymphoid tissue.

Platelets. Platelets are small, clear, disk-shaped bodies about one-third the size of red blood cells or even smaller, which initiate blood clotting and are concerned in contraction of a clot. When they encounter a leak in a blood vessel, they disintegrate and adhere to the edges of the injured tissue. There are about 25,000 platelets per cubic millimeter of blood.

BLOOD CHEMISTRY TESTS. Chemical analyses of various substances in the blood are done to determine certain changes and disturbances in the body's functioning. These tests may be useful in diagnosis and treatment of diseases, and may also be used to measure the progress of a patient recovering from a disease.

Glucose is a simple sugar, the end product of carbohydrate digestion, and a normal constituent of blood. A normal fasting level for glucose would be between 70 and 90 mg. per 100 ml. Unusually high levels of glucose in the blood (hyperglycemia) may indicate such diseases as diabetes mellitus, an overactive thyroid gland or an overactive pituitary gland. Low levels of blood sugar (hypoglycemia) may be caused by disorders of the kidneys or liver, an underactive pituitary gland or hyperinsulinism, an uncommon condition in which too much insulin is produced. A GLUCOSE TOLERANCE TEST analyzes the liver's efficiency in absorbing and storing glucose.

Iron determinations frequently are used to identify and differentiate certain anemias. In cases of iron deficiency, a test of the blood's iron-binding capacity can indicate the extent to which the patient will be helped by increasing his intake of iron, either in his diet or by taking iron preparations.

Protein tests are used in the diagnosis of numerous disturbances in the body. In electrophoresis, the different proteins are separated and their amounts determined and compared; the varying patterns of high and low levels point toward particular disorders and courses of treatment.

Blood urea nitrogen (BUN) tests measure the blood's content of urea, one of the nitrogenous waste products of the body's protein metabolism (see also UREA NITROGEN). Normally urea is excreted by the kidneys and given off in the urine. When the kidneys are affected by disease, they may fail to remove enough urea from the blood; tests will then show a high level of blood urea nitrogen. Unusually low levels may be caused by liver disease. Measurement of nonprotein NITROGEN (NPN) may also be used as a test of kidney function, after severe injury or extended infection or when the body is overloaded with fluid; a high level of NPN may indicate poisoning, hormonal disorders or shock.

Bilirubin tests measure the orange pigment, called bilirubin, found in the bile. When the bile flow is impaired or the liver is not functioning properly, bilirubin appears in excessive amounts in the blood and may cause jaundice. The icteric index is another test for measuring the extent of jaundice.

CALCIUM in the blood plays an important role in blood clotting, in the functioning of nerves and muscles and in the growth and maintenance of teeth and bones. Calcium determinations are significant in measuring the activity of the parathyroid glands and the body's supply of vitamin D, and in identifying certain bone diseases. Tests for phosphate may also be done, since the relationship of phosphate and calcium in the blood is important in the diagnosis of some bone diseases and parathyroid conditions. Alkaline phosphatase tests measure an enzyme related to the building up and breaking down of bone tissue, which is also found in the liver.

Tests for chloride, potassium and sodium are used for patients who have suffered severe injuries or illnesses, or who have undergone extensive surgery, especially when intravenous administration of ELECTROLYTES is necessary.

pH is the term used to indicate the relative acidity and alkalinity of blood plasma. The pH may reflect an imbalance in the body's chemistry. Results of its measurement are expressed in pH numbers taken from a standard scale. pH 7.0 indicates a state of neutrality. Values below 7 indicate acidity and values above 7 alkalinity. In addition to pH measurement (and sometimes instead of it), tests may be made for carbon dioxide, which plays an important part in relation to acidity in the body. (See also ACID-BASE BALANCE.)

   central b., blood from the pulmonary venous system; sometimes applied to blood obtained from chambers of the heart or from bone marrow.

   citrated b., blood treated with sodium citrate to prevent its coagulation.

   cord b., that contained in the umbilical vessels at the time of delivery of the fetus.

   defibrinated b., blood incapable of clotting because the fibrin has been removed.

   occult b., that which has escaped from tissues in such small amounts as to be detectable only by chemical tests or by microscopic examination.

   peripheral b., that circulating through vessels remote from the heart.

   whole b., that from which none of the elements has been removed.

blood-brain barrier the barrier that prevents or delays the entry into brain tissue of certain substances in the blood. Presumably it consists of the walls of the blood vessels of the central nervous system and the surrounding glial membranes.

blood clotting, coagulation see CLOTTING.

blood count the number of blood cells in a given sample of blood, usually expressed as the number of cells in a cubic millimeter of blood. A differential white cell count determines the number of various types of leukocytes in a sampling of blood. The cell count is useful in the diagnosis of various blood dyscrasias, infections or other abnormal conditions of the body and is one of the most common tests done on the blood. For normal ranges and significance of changes in the blood count see the table of normal values under BLOOD.

blood poisoning septicemia.

blood pressure the pressure of the blood against the walls of the blood vessels. The term usually refers to the pressure of the blood within the arteries, or arterial blood pressure. This pressure is determined by several factors, including the pumping action of the heart, the resistance to the flow of blood in the arterioles, the elasticity of the walls of the main arteries, the quantity of blood within the blood vessels and the blood's viscosity, or thickness.

The pumping action of the heart refers to how hard the heart pumps the blood (force of heartbeat) and how much blood it pumps and how efficiently it does the job. Contraction of the heart, which forces blood through the arteries, is the phase known as systole. Relaxation of the heart between contractions is called diastole.

The main arteries leading from the heart have walls with strong elastic fibers capable of expanding and absorbing the pulsations generated by the heart. At each pulsation the arteries expand and absorb the momentary increase in blood pressure. As the heart relaxes in preparation for another beat, the aortic valves close to prevent blood from flowing back to the heart chambers, and the artery walls spring back, forcing the blood through the body between contractions. In this way the arteries act as dampers on the pulsations and thus provide a steady flow of blood through the blood vessels.

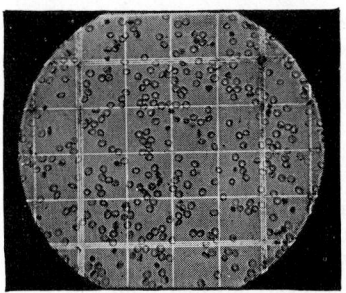

Spencer Bright Line blood counting chamber. Blood count is made by determining the number of cells in squares on the microscopic slide. (From Davidsohn, I., and Henry, J. B.: Todd-Sanford Clinical Diagnosis by Laboratory Methods. 14th ed. Philadelphia, W. B. Saunders Co., 1969.)

COMMON HEMATOLOGIC
DETERMINATIONS: NORMAL VALUES*

Unless otherwise stated, venous blood is used for determination in all cases.

Measurement	Normal Value	Clinical Significance
BLEEDING TIME Duration of bleeding from standard puncture wound of skin	Duke method: 1-4 min. Ivy method: 2-3 min.	Measures platelet function and integrity of vessel wall. Time is prolonged in thrombocytopenic purpura and other disorders.

BONE MARROW, DIFFERENTIAL CELL COUNT	Range %	Average %	Differential counts used in diagnosing various blood disorders, including leukemias, pernicious and other megaloblastic anemias, and thrombocytopenic disorders.
Myeloblasts	0.3-5.0	2.0	
Promyelocytes	1.0-8.0	5.0	
Myelocytes: neutrophilic	5.0-19.0	12.0	
eosinophilic	0.5-3.0	1.5	
basophilic	0.0-0.5	0.3	
Metamyelocytes	13.0-32.0	22.0	
Polymorph neutrophils	7.0-30.0	20.0	
Polymorph eosinophils	0.5-4.0	2.0	
Polymorph basophils	0.0-0.7	0.2	
Lymphocytes	3.0-17.0	10.0	
Plasma cells	0.0-2.0	0.4	
Monocytes	0.5-5.0	2.0	
Reticulum cells	0.1-2.0	0.2	
Megakaryocytes	0.03-3.0	0.4	
Pronormoblasts	1.0-8.0	4.0	
Normoblasts	7.0-32.0	18.0	

CLOT RETRACTION Time and extent of contraction of undisturbed clot	Clot is decreased by ½ within an hour after clotting	Dependent on platelet function. In thrombocytopenic purpura retraction is delayed and incomplete.
COAGULATION (CLOTTING) TIME (LEE-WHITE) Time required for formation of solid clot in whole blood. Values vary according to number and size of test tubes used in performing test.	6-17 min. (glass tubes) 19-60 min. (siliconized tubes)	Prolonged time indicates coagulation defects. Heparin administration will affect results..
CORPUSCULAR VALUES OF ERYTHROCYTES MCH (mean corpuscular hemoglobin). Content of hemoglobin in average individual red cell	29 ± 2 micromcg.	Increased in macrocytic (e.g., pernicious) anemia; low in hypochromic anemia
MCHC (mean corpuscular hemoglobin concentration). Average hemoglobin concentration per 100 ml. packed red cells.	34 ± 2 Gm./100 ml.	Same as above
MCV (mean corpuscular volume). Average volume of individual red cells.	87 ± 5 cu. microns	Same as above

---

*From Nursing Clinics of North America, 4:551–553, 1969.

Because of this, there are actually two blood pressures within the blood vessels during one complete beat of the heart; a higher blood pressure during systole (contraction phase) and a lower blood pressure during diastole (relaxation phase). These two blood pressures are known as the systolic pressure and the diastolic pressure, respectively.

MEASUREMENT OF THE BLOOD PRESSURE. The blood pressure is usually measured in the artery of the upper arm, with a sphygmomanometer. This consists of a rubber cuff connected to a glass tube containing a column of mercury. Alongside the glass tube are numbers that indicate the height of the column of mercury in millimeters (25 mm. equals 1 inch). In some sphygmomanometers the mercury column is replaced by a gauge. The rubber cuff is wrapped about the patient's arm, and then air is pumped into the cuff by means of a rubber bulb. As the pressure inside the rubber cuff increases, the flow of blood through the artery is momentarily checked. The pressure within the cuff causes the mercury to rise or the gauge's needle to move.

A stethoscope is then placed over the artery at the elbow and the air pressure within the cuff is slowly released. The pressure begins to fall slowly. As soon as blood begins to flow through the artery again, tapping sounds can be heard through the stetho-

COMMON HEMATOLOGIC DETERMINATIONS: NORMAL VALUES—*Continued*

Measurement	*Normal Value*	*Clinical Significance*
RED CELL OSMOTIC FRAGILITY Red cells suspended in NaCl become spheroidal and more fragile, and eventually burst. Test measures increases in fragility, leading to hemolysis.	Hemolysis begins in 0.45-0.39% NaCl Hemolysis complete in 0.33-0.30% NaCl	Fragility increased in hereditary spherocytosis and in hemolytic jaundice; decreased in obstructive jaundice.
RETICULOCYTE COUNT Measures number of cells being delivered by marrow to blood; hence is a measure of effective erythropoiesis.	0.5-1.5% of red cells or 25,000-75,000/cu. mm.	Used to test effectiveness of treatment in pernicious anemia and recovery of bone marrow in aplastic anemias; also to check effect of radioactive substances on workers. Count increased in hemolytic anemias and decreased in aplastic and pernicious anemias.

SEDIMENTATION RATE (ESR)
The ESR is the rapidity with which red blood cells settle out of unclotted blood in 1 hour. It is a rough measure of abnormal concentrations of fibrinogen and serum globulins.
	Westergren method:
	  Males 0-15 mm./hr.
	  Females 0-20 mm./hr.
	Wintrobe method:
	  Males 0-6.5 mm./hr.
	  Females 0-15 mm./hr.
		Increased rate is nonspecific response to inflammation or tissue damage. Increase occurs in pregnancy and in infectious and inflammatory diseases.

WHITE CELL (LEUKOCYTE) COUNT (WBC) Venous or capillary blood used. Sample is diluted and counted in a counting chamber using a microscope, to give the total cell count. Differential counting is done on a stained smear.		Total increased in infections; decreased in agranulocytosis and chemical toxicities. Differential count helpful in diagnosing various infections, allergic conditions, leukemias and other disorders.

Total: 5000-10,000/cu. mm.

Differential:

Myelocytes	0%	0/cu. mm.
Juvenile neutrophils	3-5%	150-400/cu. mm.
Segmented neutrophils	54-62%	3000-5800/cu. mm.
Lymphocytes	24-33%	1500-3000/cu. mm.
Monocytes	3-7%	285-500/cu. mm.
Eosinophils	1-3%	50-250/cu. mm.
Basophils	0-0.75%	15-50/cu. mm.

(Infants and children have greater relative numbers of lymphocytes and monocytes)

scope. This is the pulse. When the first tapping sound is heard, the systolic pressure is noted.

As the air pressure continues to escape from the cuff, the tapping sounds grow louder. A point is reached at which the sounds change suddenly to very soft and then disappear entirely. The point on the mercury column at which the sound disappears entirely is the diastolic pressure.

The blood pressure is usually written and spoken of as one number over another—for example, 120/80, or "one-twenty over eighty." The first number represents the systolic pressure and the second is the diastolic pressure, both recorded in millimeters of mercury.

The blood pressure can vary considerably between the sexes, among different age groups and even between two persons of the same age and sex. At birth, the systolic blood pressure is about 80 mm. of mercury. In young people it varies normally from 100 to 140 mm., and in people at 60 years of age from 140 to about 170 mm.

Blood pressure also varies according to the time of day and the kind of activity a person is engaged in. It is usually lowest just before awakening in the

COMMON HEMATOLOGIC DETERMINATIONS: NORMAL VALUES—*Continued*

Measurement	Normal Value	Clinical Significance
FIBRINOGEN LEVEL IN PLASMA	200-400 mg./100 ml.	Fibrinogen is necessary in blood clotting. Deficiency may indicate severe liver disease; it may also be congenital.
HEMATOCRIT (HCT) Volume of erythrocytes expressed as percentage of volume of whole blood in a sample. Measurement is done after centrifugation of blood from vein or from finger prick (microhematocrit).	Males: 47.0 ± 7 Females: 42.0 ± 5	Often used to indicate the red blood cell count. Low value indicates anemia; high value polycythemia or hemoconcentration.
HEMOGLOBIN Capillary blood used and measurement done by matching standard samples or by using a photometer.	Males: 16.0 ± 2.0 Gm./100 ml. Females: 14.0 ± 2.0 Gm./100 ml. Children: 11.2-16.5 Gm./100 ml. Newborn: 16.5-19.5 Gm./100 ml.	Hemoglobin is the chief component of red blood cell and acts as oxygen carrier. Values are decreased in anemias, particularly iron-deficiency type; also in hemolytic disease of newborn. Increased in polycythemia and hemoconcentration.
PLATELET COUNT Capillary or venous blood used. Counting done in a hemacytometer. Values vary according to method used.	150,000-450,000/cu. mm.	Platelet deficiency leads to prolonged bleeding time or impaired clot retraction. Platelet count is used in distinguishing hemorrhagic diseases. Values low in thrombocytopenia.
PROTHROMBIN TIME (PT) Elapsed time between addition of calcium to a plasma sample and the presence of a visible clot.	11.0-12.5 sec. (one-stage method)	Indirect test of clotting ability. Used to control administration of anticoagulant drugs.
PROTHROMBIN UTILIZATION Measures prothrombin lost during coagulation, and thereby the amount of thrombin formed.	Over 80% consumed in 1 hour	Tests ability to form thromboplastin and gives information about first stage of coagulation.
RED CELL (ERYTHROCYTE) COUNT (RBC) Venous or capillary blood may be used. Diluted blood is counted with a counting chamber, using a microscope	Males: 5.4 ± 0.8 million/cu. mm. Females: 4.8 ± 0.6 million/cu. mm. Children: 4.5-5.1 million/cu. mm.	Decreased in anemias; increased in hemoconcentration and polycythemia.

morning. Strenuous physical activity can increase the systolic blood pressure 60 to 80 mm. above normal. Excitement, nervous tension or fright raises the systolic blood pressure. Increased weight tends to lead to increased blood pressure. See also HYPERTENSION and HYPOTENSION.

blood transfusion see TRANSFUSION.

blood type the phenotype of erythrocytes defined by one or more antigenic determinants. Under the usual system of blood typing there are four main blood types or blood groups: A, B, O and AB. The ABO blood typing system was first introduced in 1900 by Karl Landsteiner and is still generally used today as the basis for transfusing whole blood. It is now known, however, that many different antigens exist in the red blood cells, and that as many as 11 or more different antigenic systems of grouping blood can be recognized. Even within the ABO system numerous subgroups of the main groups exist.

The Rh factor must also be considered in blood typing. This system of differentiating blood types is very complex; eight principal variants of the Rh factor are known, and there are others not yet identified and grouped. For practical purposes there are two main groups of Rh types. Persons with the Rh factor present in the blood are referred to as Rh positive. Those without are Rh negative. (See also RH FACTOR.)

Correct typing and crossmatching of blood are extremely important clinically in the prevention of transfusion reactions. To determine the blood type, a sample of blood is taken and mixed with specially prepared sera. One serum, anti-A agglutinin, causes blood of group A to agglutinate (the cells clump together); another serum, anti-B agglutinin, causes blood of group B to agglutinate. Thus, if anti-A serum alone causes clumping, the blood is type A; if anti-B serum alone causes clumping, it is group B. If both cause clumping, the blood group is AB, and if it is not clumped by either it is identified as Group O.

blood vessel a channel for carrying blood; an artery, vein or capillary.

Blount's disease (bluntz) aseptic necrosis of the medial condyle of the tibia, sometimes causing lateral bowing of the legs.

blowpipe (blo'pīp) a tube through which a current of air is forced upon a flame to concentrate and intensify the heat.

blue baby an infant born with cyanosis, with a bluish color that is due to abnormally low concentration of oxygen in the circulating blood. The term is commonly used to designate an infant born with congenital atelectasis or with one or more defects of the heart and great vessels (see also CONGENITAL HEART DEFECT).

blue dome cyst a benign retention cyst of the breast that is bluish and usually is the result of chronic mastitis, which causes obstruction of the ducts of the mammary glands. It is found most commonly in childless women at menopause.

Blumberg's sign (blum'bergz) pain on abrupt release of steady pressure over the site of a suspected abdominal lesion, indicative of peritonitis.

Blutene (bloo'tēn) trademark for a preparation of tolonium, a heparin-inhibiting compound used to control small hemorrhages.

B.M.A. British Medical Association.

BMR basal metabolic rate.

BNA Basle Nomina anatomica, a system of anatomic nomenclature adopted at the annual meeting of the German Anatomic Society in 1895.

body (bod'e) 1. a mass of matter. 2. the trunk of a vertebrate animal, considered apart from the limbs.

  acetone b's, ketone bodies.

  alcapton b's, a class of substances with an affinity for alkali, found in the urine and causing the condition known as alcaptonuria. The compound commonly found, and most commonly referred to by the term, is homogentisic acid.

  alloxur b's, compounds of purines secreted in the urine in certain conditions and considered end products of albuminous catabolism.

  amygdaloid b., a small mass of subcortical gray matter within the tip of the temporal lobe, anterior to the inferior horn of the lateral ventricle of the brain.

  aortic b's, small groups of chromophil cells on either side of the aorta in the region of the inferior mesenteric artery which act as chemoreceptors.

  asbestos b's, golden yellow bodies of various shapes in sputum, lung secretions and feces of patients with asbestosis.

  Aschoff's b's, submiliary collections of cells and leukocytes in the interstitial tissues of the heart in rheumatic myocarditis; called also Aschoff's nodules.

  asteroid b., an irregularly star-shaped inclusion body found in the giant cells in sarcoidosis and other diseases.

  Barr b., sex chromatin; a mass of chromatin situated at the periphery of the nucleus of cells of normal females, but not observed in those of normal males, derived from an inactive X chromosome.

  carotid b's, masses of chromaffin cells located on the wall of each internal carotid artery that act as chemoreceptors.

  ciliary b., the thickened part of the vascular tunic of the eye, connecting the choroid and iris.

  Donovan b's, *Donovania granulomatis*.

  elementary b., 1. a blood platelet. 2. an inclusion body.

  fimbriate b., corpus fimbriatum.

BLOOD TYPES

SERUM OF GROUP	AGGLUTININ IN SERUM	REACTION TO RECIPIENT'S BLOOD CELLS			
		O	A	B	AB
O	Anti-A and Anti-B	−	+	+	+
A	Anti-B	−	−	+	+
B	Anti-A	−	+	−	+
AB	None	−	−	−	−

*− = No clumping; + = clumping.

foreign b., a mass of material that is not normal to the place where it is found.

geniculate b., corpus geniculatum.

geniculate b's, lateral, two forebrain eminences, one on each side, marking the termination of the optic tract.

geniculate b's, medial, two forebrain eminences, one on each side of the midbrain, concerned with hearing.

Howell-Jolly b's, small, round or oval bodies seen in erythrocytes when stains are added to fresh blood and found in various anemias and leukemias and after splenectomy.

immune b., amboceptor.

inclusion b's, round, oval or irregular-shaped bodies occurring in the protoplasm of nuclei of cells of the body, as in disease caused by filterable virus infection such as rabies, smallpox, herpes, etc.

ketone b's, intermediate products of fat metabolism, including acetone, acetoacetic acid and beta-oxybutyric acid (see also KETONE BODIES).

Leishman-Donovan b's, oval bodies found in the spleen in chronic dysentery and certain other diseases.

mamillary b's, two small eminences on the inferior surface of the forebrain behind the site of attachment of the stalk of the pituitary gland.

Negri b's, oval or round bodies in the nerve cells of animals dead of rabies.

Nissl b's, large granular protein bodies that stain with basic dyes, forming the substance of the reticulum of the cytoplasm of a nerve cell. Ribonucleoprotein is one of the main constituents.

olivary b's, oval prominences on the sides of the anterior pyramids of the medulla oblongata.

pineal b., a small, conical structure attached by a stalk to the posterior wall of the third ventricle of the cerebrum (see also PINEAL GLAND).

pituitary b., pituitary gland.

psammoma b., a spherical, laminated mass of calcareous material occurring in both benign and malignant epithelial and connective tissue tumors, and sometimes associated with chronic inflammation.

quadrigeminal b's, corpora quadrigemina.

striate b., corpus striatum.

trachoma b's, minute bodies in the epithelial cells of the conjunctiva in trachoma.

vertebral b., the forward, weight-bearing portion of a vertebra, separated from vertebral bodies above and below by intervertebral disks.

vitelline b., yolk nucleus.

vitreous b., the gelatinous mass filling the posterior four-fifths of the eyeball, behind the diaphragm formed by the lens and ciliary body.

wolffian b., mesonephros.

Boeck's sarcoid (beks) a type of multiple benign sarcoid characterized by its superficial nature and showing a predilection for the face, arms and shoulders.

boil (boil) a local infection of the skin containing pus and showing on the surface as a reddened, tender swelling; a type of skin abscess. Called also *furuncle.* Boils occur most frequently on the neck and buttocks, although they may develop wherever friction or irritation, or a scratch or break in the skin, allows the bacteria resident on the surface to penetrate the outer layer of the skin. A carbuncle is a group of interconnected boils and is more serious than a simple boil.

CAUSE. When bacteria gain entrance into the skin, the infection settles in the hair follicles or the sebaceous glands. To combat the infection, large numbers of leukocytes travel to the site and attack the invading bacteria. Some bacteria and white cells are killed and they and their liquefied products form pus. The body's defenses may succeed in overcoming the invaders so that the boil subsides by itself, or the pus may build up pressure against the skin surface so that it ruptures, drains and heals.

Boils may afflict healthy persons but often their appearance is a sign that the resistance is low, usually as a result of poor nutrition or illness. Persons suffering from dermatitis or untreated *diabetes mellitus* are particularly susceptible to boils.

TREATMENT. In most cases, a single boil is not serious and will respond to careful treatment, but there are some important exceptions. Medical attention is necessary if the patient is an infant, a young child or an elderly person. A boil on or above the upper lip, on the nose or scalp or in the outer ear can be very serious because in these areas infection has easy access to the brain. Other danger zones are the armpit, the groin and the breast of a woman who is nursing. If bacteria from a boil enter the bloodstream, septicemia may result.

bolometer (bo-lom′ĕ-ter) 1. an instrument for measuring the force of the heartbeat. 2. an instrument for measuring minute degrees of radiant heat.

boloscope (bo′lo-skōp) an apparatus for locating metallic foreign bodies in the tissues.

bolus (bo′lus) a rounded mass, such as (1) a large pill, (2) a quantity of food entering the esophagus at one swallow, (3) a quantity of opaque medium introduced into an artery at one time in arteriography, (4) a cushion used in bolstering the position of a patient for roentgenography or (5) a rounded pad used to apply pressure to a wound.

alimentary b., the mass of food, made ready by mastication, that enters the esophagus at one swallow.

bond (bond) the linkage between atoms or radicals of a chemical compound, or the symbol representing this linkage and indicating the valence of the atoms or radicals, as H.O.H or H—O—H; Ca:O or Ca=O; HC:CH or HC≡CH.

bone (bōn) the hard, tough, elastic tissue that forms the skeleton, composed principally of calcium salts. There are 206 separate bones in the human body. Collectively they form the SKELETAL SYSTEM, a structure bound together by ligaments at the joints and set in motion by the muscles, which are secured to the bones by means of tendons. Bones, ligaments, muscles and tendons are the tissues of the body responsible for supporting and moving the body.

Some bones have chiefly a protective function. An example is the skull, which encloses the brain, the back of the eyeball and the inner ear. Some, such as the pelvis, are mainly supporting structures. Other bones, such as the jaw and the bones of the fingers, are concerned chiefly with movement. The MARROW contained in bones manufactures the blood cells. The bones themselves act as a storehouse of calcium, which must be maintained at a certain level in the blood for the body's normal chemical functioning.

STRUCTURE AND COMPOSITION. Bone is not uniform in structure but is composed of several layers of different materials. The outermost layer, the periosteum, is a thin, tough membrane of fibrous tissue. It gives support to the tendons that secure the muscle to the bone and also serves as a protective sheath. This membrane encloses all bones completely except at the joints where there is a layer of cartilage. Beneath the periosteum lie the dense, hard layers of bone tissue called compact bone. Its composition is fibrous rather than solid and it gives bone its resiliency. Encased within these layers is the tissue that makes up most of the volume of bone, called cancellous or spongy bone because it contains little hollows like those of a sponge. The innermost portion of the bone is a hollow cavity containing marrow. Blood vessels course through every layer of bone, carrying nutritive elements, oxygen and other products. Bone tissue also contains a large number of nerves. The basic chemical in bone, which gives bone its hardness and strength, is calcium phosphate.

DEVELOPMENT. Cartilage forms the major part of bone in the very young; this accounts for the great flexibility and resiliency of the infant skeleton. Gradually, calcium phosphate collects in the cartilage, and it becomes harder and more brittle. Some of the cartilage cells break loose, so that channels develop in the bone shaft. Blood vessels enter the channels, bearing with them small cells of connective tissue, some of which become osteoblasts, cells that form true bone. The osteoblasts enter the hardened cartilage, forming layers of hard, firm bone. Other cells, called osteoclasts, work to tear down old or excess bone structure, allowing the osteoblasts to rebuild with new bone. This renewal continues throughout life, although it slows down with age.

Cartilage formation and the subsequent replacement of cartilage by hard material is the mechanism by which bones grow in size. During the period of bone growth, cartilage grows over the hardened portion of bone. In time, this layer of cartilage hardens as calcium phosphate is added, and a fresh layer grows over it, and it too hardens. The process continues until the body reaches full growth. Long bones grow in length because of special cross-sectional layers of cartilage located near the flared ends of the bone. These harden and new cartilage is produced by the same process as previously described.

BONE DISORDERS. FRACTURE, a break in the bone, is the most common injury to the bone; it may be closed, with no break in the skin, or open, with penetration of the skin and exposure of portions of the broken bone.

OSTEOPOROSIS is excessive brittleness and porosity of bone in the aged. OSTEOMYELITIS is a bone infection similar to a boil on the skin, but much more serious because the infection can destroy the bone and invade other body tissues. OSTEOMALACIA is the term used for RICKETS when it occurs in adults. In these diseases there is softening of the bones, due to inadequate concentration of calcium or phosphorus in the body. The usual cause is deficiency of vitamin D, which is required for utilization of calcium and phosphorus by the body.

In osteitis fibrosa cystica, bone is replaced by fibrous tissue because of abnormal calcium metabolism. The condition usually is due to overactivity of the parathyroid glands.

OSTEOMA refers to abnormal new growth, either benign or malignant, of the tissue of the bones. Although it is not common, it may occur in any of the bones of the body, and at any age.

ankle b., talus.

cancellous b., bone containing many empty spaces, the calcified matrix being arranged in trabeculae rather than lamellae.

carpal b., one of the eight bones composing the carpus, or wrist.

cartilage b., bone that replaces a provisional cartilaginous model.

cheek b., zygoma.

collar b., clavicle.

compact b., bone containing no empty spaces, being made up of lamellae which fit closely together.

cortical b., the solid portion of the shaft of a bone that surrounds the marrow cavity.

ear b's, the incus, malleus and stapes.

flat b., one of greater width and length than thickness, often consisting of two layers of compact bone separated by a layer of cancellous bone and usually bent or curved.

haunch b., ilium.

heel b., calcaneus.

hip b., os coxae, which comprises the ilium, ischium and pubis.

hyoid b., a horseshoe-shaped bone situated at the base of the tongue, just below the thyroid cartilage.

incisive b., a separate bone in the upper jaw of the fetus which later fuses with the maxilla on either side.

innominate b., hip bone.

jaw b., the mandible or maxilla, especially the mandible.

jugal b., zygoma.

lingual b., hyoid bone.

long b., one whose length far exceeds its breadth and thickness.

malar b., zygoma.

marble b's, osteopetrosis.

mastoid b., the mastoid process of the temporal bone.

membrane b., bone that develops directly within sheet of mesenchyma.

metacarpal b., one of the five bones composing the metacarpus.

metatarsal b., one of the five bones composing the metatarsus.

occipital b., the unpaired bone constituting the back and part of the base of the skull.

pelvic b., hip bone.

petrous b., the petrous portion of the temporal bone; pars petrosa.

pneumatic b., bone that contains air-filled spaces.

premaxillary b., incisive bone.

pterygoid b., pterygoid process.

pubic b., the anterior portion of the hip bone; called also pubis.

rider's b., an ossification sometimes seen in the tendon of the adductor muscle of the thigh in those who ride on horseback.

sesamoid b's, small bones embedded in tendons or joint capsules, occurring mainly in hands and feet.

shin b., tibia.

short b., one of approximately equal length, width and thickness.

solid b., compact bone.

spongy b., cancellous bone.

TABLE OF BONES, LISTED BY REGIONS OF THE BODY

REGION	NAME	TOTAL NUMBER
Axial skeleton		
Skull		21
	(eight paired—16)	
	inferior nasal concha	
	lacrimal	
	maxilla	
	nasal	
	palatine	
	parietal	
	temporal	
	zygomatic	
	(five unpaired—5)	
	ethmoid	
	frontal	
	occipital	
	sphenoid	
	vomer	
Ossicles of each ear		6
	incus	
	malleus	
	stapes	
Lower jaw		
	mandible	1
Neck		
	hyoid	1
Vertebral column		26
	cervical vertebrae (7)	
	(atlas)	
	(axis)	
	thoracic vertebrae (12)	
	lumbar vertebrae (5)	
	sacrum (5 fused)	
	coccyx (4–5 fused)	
Chest		
	sternum	1
	ribs (12 pairs)	24

REGION	NAME	TOTAL NUMBER
Upper limb (×2)		64
Shoulder	scapula	
	clavicle	
Upper arm	humerus	
Lower arm	radius	
	ulna	
Wrist	carpal (8)	
	(capitate)	
	(hamate)	
	(lunate)	
	(pisiform)	
	(scaphoid)	
	(trapezium)	
	(trapezoid)	
	(triquetral)	
Hand	metacarpal (5)	
Fingers	phalanges (14)	
Lower limb (×2)		62
Pelvis	hip bone (1)	
	(ilium)	
	(ischium)	
	(pubis)	
Thigh	femur	
Knee	patella	
Leg	tibia	
	fibula	
Ankle	tarsal (7)	
	(calcaneus)	
	(cuboid)	
	(cuneiform, medial)	
	(cuneiform, intermediate)	
	(cuneiform, lateral)	
	(navicular)	
	(talus)	
Foot	metatarsal (5)	
Toes	phalanges (14)	

TABLE OF BONES

COMMON NAME*	NA EQUIVALENT†	REGION	DESCRIPTION	ARTICULATIONS
astragalus. see *talus*				
atlas	atlas	neck	first cervical vertebra, ring of bone supporting the skull	with occipital b. and axis
axis	axis	neck	second cervical vertebra, with thick process (odontoid process) around which first cervical vertebra pivots	with atlas above and third cervical vertebra below
calcaneus	calcaneus	foot	the "heel bone," of irregularly cuboidal shape, largest of the tarsal bones	with talus and cuboid b.
capitate b.	o. capitatum	wrist	third from thumb side of 4 bones of distal row of carpal b's.	with second, third and fourth metacarpal b's, and hamate, lunate, trapezoid and scaphoid b's
carpal b's	oss. carpi	wrist	see *capitate, hamate, lunate, pisiform b's, scaphoid, trapezium, trapezoid and triquetral b's*	
clavicle	clavicula	shoulder	elongated, slender, curved bone (collar bone) lying horizontally at root of neck, in upper part of thorax	with sternum and ipsilateral scapula and cartilage of first rib
coccyx	o. coccygis	lower back	triangular bone formed usually by fusion of last 4 (sometimes 3 or 5) (coccygeal) vertebrae	with sacrum
concha, inferior nasal	concha nasalis inferior	skull	thin, rough plate of bone attached by one edge to side of each nasal cavity, the free edge curling downward	with ethmoid and ipsilateral lacrimal and palatine b's and maxilla
cuboid b.	o. cuboideum	foot	pyramidal bone, on lateral side of foot, in front of calcaneus	with calcaneus, lateral cuneiform b., fourth and fifth metatarsal b's, occasionally with navicular b.
cuneiform b., intermediate	o. cuneiforme intermedium	foot	smallest of 3 cuneiform b's, located between medial and lateral cuneiform b's	with navicular, medial and lateral cuneiform b's and second metatarsal b.
cuneiform b., lateral	o. cuneiforme laterale	foot	wedge-shaped bone at lateral side of foot, intermediate in size between medial and intermediate cuneiform b's	with cuboid, navicular, intermediate cuneiform b's and second, third and fourth metatarsal b's

*b. = bone; b's = (pl.) bones.
†o. = os; oss. = (L. pl.) ossa.

TABLE OF BONES—*Continued*

COMMON NAME*	NA EQUIVALENT†	REGION	DESCRIPTION	ARTICULATIONS
cuneiform b., medial	o. cuneiforme mediale	foot	largest of 3 cuneiform b's, at medial side of foot	with navicular, intermediate cuneiform and first and second metatarsal b's
epistropheus. see *axis*				
ethmoid b.	o. ethmoidale	skull	unpaired bone in front of sphenoid b. and below frontal b., forming part of nasal septum and superior and medial conchae of nose	with sphenoid and frontal b's, vomer, and both lacrimal, nasal and palatine b's, maxillae and inferior nasal conchae
fabella		knee	sesamoid b. in lateral head of gastrocnemius muscle	with femur
femur	femur	thigh	longest, strongest, heaviest bone of the body (thigh b.)	proximally with hip b., distally with patella and tibia
fibula	fibula	leg	lateral and smaller of 2 bones of leg	proximally with tibia, distally with tibia and talus
frontal b.	o. frontale	skull	unpaired bone constituting anterior part of skull	with ethmoid and sphenoid b's, and both parietal, nasal, lacrimal and zygomatic b's and maxillae
hamate b.	o. hamatum	wrist	most medial of 4 bones of distal row of carpal b's	with fourth and fifth metacarpal b's and lunate, capitate and triquetral b's
hip b.	o. coxae	pelvis and hip	broadest bone of skeleton, composed originally of 3 bones which become fused together in acetabulum: *ilium*, broad, flaring, uppermost portion; *ischium*, thick, three-sided part behind and below acetabulum and behind obturator foramen; *pubis*, consisting of body (expanded anterior portion), inferior ramus (extending backward and fusing with ramus of ischium) and superior ramus (extending from body to acetabulum)	with femur, anteriorly with its fellow (at symphysis pubis), posteriorly with sacrum
humerus	humerus	arm	long bone of upper arm	proximally with scapula, distally with radius and ulna
hyoid b.	o. hyoideum	neck	U-shaped bone at root of tongue, between mandible and larynx	none; attached by ligaments and muscles to skull and larynx
ilium	o. ilium	pelvis	see *hip b.*	
incus	incus	ear	middle ossicle of chain in the middle ear, so named because of its resemblance to an anvil	with malleus and stapes
innominate b. see *hip b.*				

Term	Location	Description	Articulates with
ischium / o. ischii	pelvis	see *hip b.*	
lacrimal b. / o. lacrimale	skull	thin, uneven scale of bone near rim of medial wall of each orbit	with ethmoid and frontal b's, and ipsilateral inferior nasal concha and maxilla
lunate b. / o. lunatum	wrist	second from thumb side of 4 bones of proximal row of carpus	with radius, and capitate, hamate, scaphoid and triquetral b's
malleus	ear	most lateral ossicle of chain in middle ear, so named because of its resemblance to a hammer	with incus; fibrous attachment to tympanic membrane
mandible / mandibula	lower jaw	horseshoe-shaped bone carrying lower teeth	with temporal b's
maxilla	skull (upper jaw)	paired bone, below orbit and at either side of nasal cavity, carrying upper teeth	with ethmoid and frontal b's, vomer, fellow maxilla, and ipsilateral inferior nasal concha and lacrimal, nasal, palatine and zygomatic b's
maxilla, inferior. see *mandible*			
maxilla, superior. see *maxilla*			
metacarpal b's / oss. metacarpalia	hand	five miniature long bones of hand proper, slightly concave on palmar surface	first—trapezium and proximal phalanx of thumb; second—third metacarpal b., trapezium, trapezoid, capitate and proximal phalanx of index finger (second digit); third—second and fourth metacarpal b's, capitate and proximal phalanx of middle finger (third digit); fourth—third and fifth metacarpal b's, capitate, hamate and proximal phalanx of ring finger (fourth digit); fifth—fourth metacarpal b., hamate b. and proximal phalanx of little finger (fifth digit)
metatarsal b's / oss. metatarsalia	foot	five miniature long bones of foot, concave on plantar and slightly convex on dorsal surface	first—medial cuneiform b., proximal phalanx of great toe, and occasionally with second metatarsal b.; second—medial, intermediate and lateral cuneiform b's, third and occasionally with first metatarsal b. and proximal phalanx of second toe; third—lateral cuneiform b., second and fourth metatarsal b's and proximal phalanx of third toe; fourth—lateral cuneiform b., cuboid b., third and fifth metatarsal b's and proximal phalanx of fourth toe; fifth—cuboid b., fourth metatarsal b. and proximal phalanx of fifth toe

TABLE OF BONES—*Continued*

COMMON NAME*	NA EQUIVALENT†	REGION	DESCRIPTION	ARTICULATIONS
multangulum majus. see *trapezium*; *trapezoid*				
nasal b.	o. nasale	skull	paired bone, the two uniting in median plane to form bridge of nose	with frontal and ethmoid b's, fellow of opposite side and ipsilateral maxilla
navicular b.	o. naviculare	foot	bone at medial side of tarsus, between talus and cuneiform b's	with talus and 3 cuneiform b's, occasionally with cuboid b.
occipital b.	o. occipitale	skull	unpaired bone constituting back and part of base of skull	with sphenoid b. and atlas and both parietal and temporal b's
os magnum. see *capitate b.*				
palatine b.	o. palatinum	skull	paired bone, the two forming posterior portion of bony palate	with ethmoid and sphenoid b's, vomer, fellow of opposite side, and ipsilateral inferior nasal concha and maxilla
parietal b.	o. parietale	skull	paired bone between frontal and occipital b's, forming superior and lateral parts of skull	with frontal, occipital, sphenoid, fellow parietal and ipsilateral temporal b's
patella	patella	knee	small, irregularly rectangular compressed (sesamoid) bone over anterior aspect of knee (kneecap)	with femur
phalanges (proximal middle and distal phalanges)	oss. digitorum (phalanx proximalis, phalanx media and phalanx distalis)	fingers and toes	miniature long bones, two only in thumb and great toe, three in each of other fingers and toes	proximal phalanx of each digit with corresponding metacarpal or metatarsal b., and phalanx distal to it; other phalanges with phalanges proximal and distal (if any) to them
pisiform b.	o. pisiforme	wrist	medial and palmar of 4 bones of proximal row of carpal b's	with triquetral b.
pubic b.	o. pubis	pelvis	see *hip b.*	
radius	radius	forearm	lateral and shorter of 2 bones of forearm	proximally with humerus and ulna; distally with ulna and lunate and scaphoid b's
ribs	costae	chest	12 pairs of thin, narrow, curved long bones, forming posterior and lateral walls of chest	all posteriorly with thoracic vertebrae; upper 7 pairs (true ribs) with sternum; lower 5 pairs (false ribs) by costal cartilages, with rib above or (lowest 2—floating ribs) unattached anteriorly.

Term	Latin	Location	Description	Articulates with
sacrum	o. sacrum	lower back	wedge-shaped bone formed usually by fusion of 5 vertebrae below lumbar vertebrae, constituting posterior wall of pelvis	with fifth lumbar vertebra above, coccyx below, and with ilium at each side
scaphoid	o. scaphoideum	wrist	most lateral of 4 bones of proximal row of carpal b's	with radius, trapezium and trapezoid, capitate and lunate b's
scapula	scapula	shoulder	wide, thin, triangular bone (shoulder blade) opposite second to seventh ribs in upper part of back	with ipsilateral clavicle and humerus
sesamoid b's	oss. sesamoidea	chiefly hands and feet	small, flat, round bones related to joints between phalanges or between digits and metacarpal or metatarsal b's; include also 2 at knee (fabella and patella)	
sphenoid b.	o. sphenoidale	base of skull	unpaired, irregularly shaped bone, constituting part of sides and base of skull and part of lateral wall of orbit	with frontal, occipital and ethmoid b's, vomer and both parietal, temporal, palatine and zygomatic b's
stapes	stapes	ear	most medial ossicle of chain in middle ear, so named because of its resemblance to a stirrup	with incus; ligamentous attachment to fenestra vestibuli
sternum	sternum	chest	elongated flat bone, forming anterior wall of chest, consisting of 3 segments: *manubrium* (topmost segment), *body* (in youth composed of 4 separate segments joined by cartilage) and *xiphoid process* (lowermost segment)	with both clavicles and upper 7 pairs of ribs
talus	talus	ankle	the "ankle bone," second largest of tarsal b's	with tibia, fibula, calcaneus and navicular b.
tarsal b's	oss. tarsi	ankle and foot	see *calcaneus, cuboid, intermediate, lateral and medial cuneiform b's, navicular b. and talus*	
temporal b.	o. temporale	skull	irregularly shaped bone, one on either side, forming part of side and base of skull, and containing middle and inner ear	with occipital, sphenoid, mandible, and ipsilateral parietal and zygomatic b's
tibia	tibia	leg	medial and larger of 2 bones of lower leg (shin b.)	proximally with femur and fibula, distally with talus and fibula
trapezium	o. trapezium	wrist	most lateral of 4 bones of distal row of carpal b's	with first and second metacarpal b's and trapezoid and scaphoid b's
trapezoid b.	o. trapezoideum	wrist	second from thumb side of 4 bones of distal row of carpal b's	with second metacarpal b. and capitate, trapezium and scaphoid b's
triquetral b.	o. triquetrum	wrist	third from thumb side of 4 bones of proximal row of carpal b's	with hamate, lunate and pisiform b's and articular disk

TABLE OF BONES — *Continued*

COMMON NAME*	NA EQUIVALENT†	REGION	DESCRIPTION	ARTICULATIONS
turbinate b., inferior. see *concha, inferior nasal*				
ulna	ulna	forearm	medial and longer of 2 bones of forearm	proximally with humerus and radius, distally with radius and articular disk
vertebrae (cervical, thoracic [dorsal], lumbar, sacral and coccygeal)	vertebrae (vertebrae cervicales, vertebrae thoracicae, vertebrae lumbales, vertebrae sacrales, vertebrae coccygeae)	back	separate segments of vertebral column; about 33 in the child; uppermost 24 remain separate as true, movable vertebrae; the next 5 fuse to form the sacrum; the lowermost 3-5 fuse to form the coccyx	except first cervical (atlas) and fifth lumbar, each vertebra articulates with adjoining vertebrae above and below; the first cervical articulates with the occipital b. and second cervical vertebra (axis); the fifth lumbar with the fourth lumbar verbetra and sacrum; the thoracic vertebrae articulate also with the heads of the ribs
vomer	vomer	skull	thin bone forming posterior and posteroinferior part of nasal septum	with ethmoid and sphenoid b's and both maxillae and palatine b's
zygomatic b.	o. zygomaticum	skull	bone forming hard part of cheek and lower, lateral portion of rim of each orbit	with frontal and sphenoid b's and ipsilateral maxilla and temporal b.

squamous b., the upper forepart of the temporal bone, forming an upright plate.

supraoccipital b., the part of the occipital bone behind the foramen magnum, distinct in early childhood.

sutural b's, variable and irregularly shaped bones in the sutures between the bones of the skull.

tarsal b., one of the seven bones composing the tarsus.

temporal b., one of the two irregular bones forming part of the lateral surfaces and base of the skull, and containing the organs of hearing.

thigh b., femur.

turbinated b., nasal concha.

tympanic b., the part of the temporal bone surrounding the middle ear.

wormian b's, sutural bones.

bone marrow (mar'o) the soft spongelike material in the cavities of bones, which has as its principal function the manufacture of erythrocytes, leukocytes and platelets. (See also MARROW.)

bonelet (bōn'let) an ossicle, or small bone.

Bonine (bo'nēn) trademark for preparations of meclizine hydrochloride, an antihistamine and antinauseant.

Boophilus (bo-of'ĭ-lus) a genus of ticks primarily parasitic on cattle.

boot (bōōt) a covering for the foot.

Gibney b., an adhesive tape support used in treatment of sprains and other painful conditions of the ankle, the tape being applied in a basket-weave fashion with strips placed alternately under the sole of the foot and around the back of the leg.

Unna's paste b., a dressing for varicose ulcers, consisting of a paste made from gelatin, zinc oxide and glycerin, and spiral bandages. The entire leg is covered with paste and bandage, applied in alternate layers until they make a rigid boot.

borate (bōr'āt) a salt of boric acid.

borax (bōr'aks) sodium borate.

borborygmus (bor"bor-ig'mus) the sound of flatus in the intestines.

Bordetella (bor"dě-tel'ah) a genus of Schizomycetes.

B. parapertussis, the causative agent of parapertussis.

B. pertussis, the causative agent of whooping cough (pertussis).

boric acid (bōr'ik) a crystalline powder, formerly used as a household antiseptic for treating minor irritations of the skin and eyes. Because the powder is highly poisonous when taken internally, and since other antiseptics are more effective, boric acid is no longer recommended. Boric acid ointment (for external use only) is occasionally helpful in cases of mild skin irritations or in keeping a gauze dressing from sticking to a wound.

borism (bōr'izm) poisoning by a boron compound.

Bornholm disease (born'hōm) epidemic pleurodynia, an epidemic disease marked by a sudden attack of pain in the chest or epigastrium, fever of brief duration and a tendency to recrudescence on the third day; called also devil's grip, epidemic myalgia and epidemic myositis.

boron (bōr'on) a chemical element, atomic number 5, atomic weight 10.811, symbol B. (See table of ELEMENTS.)

Borrelia (bo-rel'e-ah) a genus of Schizomycetes.

B. recurren'tis, a causative agent of relapsing fever, transmitted by the human body louse.

B. vincen'tii, a species occurring in large numbers with a fusiform bacillus in trench mouth (Vincent's angina).

boss (bos) a roundish eminence.

bosselated (bos'ě-lāt"ed) covered with bosses.

Bothriocephalus (both"re-o-sef'ah-lus) Diphyllobothrium, a genus of TAPEWORMS.

botryoid (bot're-oid) shaped like a bunch of grapes.

botuliform (bot-u'lĭ-form) sausage-shaped.

botulin (bot'u-lin) a toxin sometimes found in imperfectly preserved or canned meats and vegetables.

botulism (bot'u-lizm) an extremely severe form of food poisoning, caused by ingestion of the preformed exotoxin of *Clostridium botulinum*, sometimes found in improperly canned or bottled food or improperly preserved meat or fish.

The symptoms are headache, weakness, constipation and nerve paralysis, which causes difficulty in seeing, breathing and swallowing. Death is usually due to paralysis of the respiratory organs.

This is a highly dangerous form of food poisoning, and to prevent it home canning and preserving of all nonacid foods—that is, all foods other than fruits and tomatoes—must be done according to proper specific directions.

bougie (boo'zhe) a long instrument for introduction, usually through a natural orifice, into a body channel such as the esophagus or urethra for the purpose of dilating its lumen.

armed b., a bougie with a piece of caustic attached to its end.

bulbous b., a bougie with a bulb-shaped tip.

filiform b., a bougie of very small diameter.

soluble b., a bougie composed of a substance that becomes fluid at body temperature.

bougienage (boo"zhě-nahzh') passage of a bougie.

bouquet (boo-ka') a structure resembling a cluster of flowers.

Bourneville's disease (boor'ně-vēz) tuberous sclerosis.

bouton (boo-taw') [Fr.] a knoblike swelling or enlargement.

boutonneuse fever (boo-ton-ez') a form of rickettsial infection endemic in southern Europe and northern Africa, transmitted by the dog tick.

bovine (bo'vīn) pertaining to, characteristic of or derived from the ox (cattle).

bowel (bow'el) the intestine.

Bowen's disease (bo'enz) a precancerous condition characterized by scaly skin lesions resembling psoriasis and showing microscopic changes in the epidermal cells.

bowleg (bo'leg) a deformity in which the space between the knees is abnormally large; genu varum.

Boyle's law (boilz) at a constant temperature the volume of a perfect gas varies inversely as the pressure, and the pressure varies inversely as the volume.

B.P. 1. blood pressure. 2. boiling point. 3. British Pharmacopoeia, a publication of the General Medical Council, describing and establishing standards for medicines, preparations, materials and articles used in the practice of medicine, surgery or midwifery.

Br chemical symbol, *bromine.*

brace (brās) a device, usually made of metal or leather, applied to the body, particularly the trunk and lower extremities, to support the weight of the body, to correct deformities, to prevent deformities or to control involuntary movements, such as occur in spastic conditions. In some cases bracing is needed after remedial surgery. Back braces are used to treat certain kinds of backache.
    Dental braces are used to support the teeth or to change their position in treatment of malocclusion.

brachi(o)- (bra'ke-[o]) word element [L., Gr.], *arm.*

brachial (bra'ke-al) pertaining to the arm.
    b. plexus, a nerve plexus originating from the ventral branches of the last four cervical and the first thoracic spinal nerves. It gives off many of the principal nerves of the shoulder, chest and arms.

brachialgia (bra″ke-al'je-ah) pain in the arm.

brachiation (bra″ke-a'shun) locomotion in a position of suspension by means of the hands and arms, as by monkeys swinging from branch to branch.

brachiocephalic (bra″ke-o-sĕ-fal'ik) pertaining to the arm and head.

brachiocrural (bra'ke-o-kroo'ral) pertaining to the arm and leg.

brachiocubital (bra″ke-o-ku'bĭ-tal) pertaining to the arm and forearm.

brachiocyllosis (bra″ke-o-sil-o'sis) crookedness of the arm.

brachium (bra'ke-um), pl. *bra'chia* [L.] 1. the arm; specifically the arm from shoulder to elbow. 2. any armlike process or structure.
    b. conjuncti'vum cerebel'li, the superior peduncle of the cerebellum, a fibrous band extending from each hemisphere of the cerebellum upward over the pons, the two joining to form the sides and part of the roof of the fourth ventricle.
    b. pon'tis, the brachium of the pons, the middle peduncle of the cerebellum.

brachy- (brak'e) word element [Gr.], *short.*

brachybasia (brak″e-ba'ze-ah) a slow, shuffling, short-stepped gait.

brachycardia (brak″e-kar'de-ah) bradycardia.

brachycephalic (brak″e-sĕ-fal'ik) having a cephalic index over 80.

brachycephaly (brak″e-sef'ah-le) anteroposterior shortening and increased height of the skull.

brachycheilia (brak″e-ki'le-ah) shortness of the lip.

brachydactylia (brak″e-dak-til'e-ah) abnormal shortness of the fingers and toes.

brachygnathia (brak″ig-na'the-ah) abnormal shortness of the mandible.

brachymetacarpia (brak″e-met″ah-kar'pe-ah) abnormal shortness of the metacarpal bones.

brachymetropia (brak″e-mĕ-tro'pe-ah) myopia.

brachypellic (brak″e-pel'ik) having a short oval pelvis.

brachyphalangia (brak″e-fah-lan'je-ah) abnormal shortness of one of the phalanges.

Bradford frame (brad'ford) a rectangular structure of gas pipe across which are stretched two strips of canvas, used for patients with fractures or disease of the hip or spine.

brady- (brad'e) word element [Gr.], *slow.*

bradyacusia (brad″e-ah-ku'ze-ah) dullness of hearing.

bradycardia (brad″e-kar'de-ah) abnormal slowness of the heart rate and pulse, usually less than 60 beats per minute. The condition may occur following an infectious or febrile disease or it may be a symptom of a disorder of the conduction system of the heart. It sometimes occurs with increased intracranial pressure, obstructive jaundice and myxedema.
    A heart rate and pulse of less than 60 beats per minute can occur in normal persons, particularly during sleep. Trained athletes usually have a slow pulse and heart rate.

bradyesthesia (brad″e-es-the'ze-ah) dullness of perception.

bradyglossia (brad″e-glos'e-ah) abnormal slowness of utterance.

bradykinesia (brad″e-kin-ne'ze-ah) abnormal slowness of movement.

bradykinin (brad″e-ki'nin) a kinin composed of a chain of amino acids liberated by the action of trypsin or certain snake venoms on a globulin of blood plasma.

bradylalia (brad″e-la'le-ah) slow utterance due to a central nervous system lesion.

bradylexia (brad″e-lek'se-ah) abnormal slowness in reading.

bradylogia (brad″e-lo'je-ah) abnormal slowness of speech.

bradymenorrhea (brad″e-men″o-re'ah) menstruation of unusually long duration.

bradypepsia (brad″e-pep'se-ah) abnormally slow digestion.

bradyphagia (brad″e-fa'je-ah) abnormal slowness of eating.

bradyphasia (brad″e-fa′ze-ah) slow utterance of speech.

bradyphemia (brad″e-fe′me-ah) slowness of speech.

bradyphrasia (brad″e-fra′ze-ah) slowness of speech due to mental defect.

bradypnea (brad″e-ne′ah) abnormal slowness of breathing.

bradyspermatism (brad″e-sper′mah-tizm) abnormally slow ejaculation of semen.

bradysphygmia (brad″e-sfig′me-ah) abnormal slowness of the pulse.

bradystalsis (brad″e-stal′sis) delayed or slow peristalsis.

bradytocia (brad″e-to′she-ah) slow parturition.

bradyuria (brad″e-u′re-ah) slow discharge of urine.

brain (brān) the mass of soft, spongy, pinkish gray nerve tissue occupying the cranial cavity, consisting of the cerebrum, cerebellum, pons and medulla oblongata and connecting at its base with the spinal cord. The human brain weighs about 3 lb.

The brain is made up of billions of nerve cells, intricately connected with each other. It contains centers (groups of NEURONS and their connections) which control many involuntary functions, such as circulation, temperature regulation and respiration, and interpret sensory impressions received from the eyes, ears and other sense organs. Consciousness, emotion, thought and reasoning are functions of the brain. It also contains centers or areas for associative memory which allow for recording, recalling and making use of past experiences.

CEREBRUM. The largest and main portion of the brain, the cerebrum is made up of an outer coating, or cortex, of gray cells, several layers deep, which covers the cerebral hemispheres. The cortex is the thinking and reasoning brain, the intellect, as well as the part of the brain that receives information from the senses and directs the conscious movements of the body.

In appearance the cortex is rather like a relief map, with one very deep valley (longitudinal fissure) dividing it lengthwise into symmetrical halves, and each of the halves again divided by two major valleys and many shallower folds. The longitudinal fissure runs from the brow to the back of the head, and deep within it is a bed of matted white fibers, the corpus callosum, which connects the left and right halves of the brain hemispheres.

The major folds of the cortex divide each hemisphere of the cerebrum into four sections or lobes: the occipital lobe at the back of the skull, the parietal lobe at the side, the frontal lobe at the forehead and the temporal lobe at the temple.

The Senses. The major senses of sight and hearing are well mapped in the cortex; the center for vision is at the back, in the occipital lobe, and the center for hearing is at the side, in the temporal lobe. Two other areas have been carefully explored; these are the sensory and motor areas for the body, which parallel each other along the fissure of Rolando.

In the sensory strip are located the brain cells that register all sensations. In the motor strip are the nerves that control the voluntary muscles. In both, the parts of the body are represented in an orderly way.

It is in the sensory areas of the brain that all perception takes place. Here sweet and sour, hot and cold and the form of an object held in the hand are recognized. Here are sorted out the sizes, colors, depth and space relationships of what the eye sees, and the timbre, pitch, intensity and harmony of what the ear hears. The significance of these perceptions is interpreted in the cortex and other parts

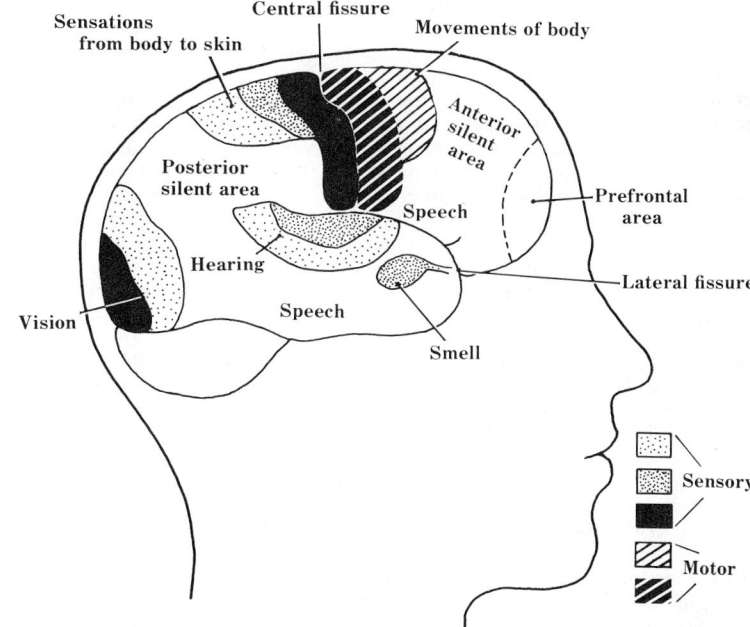

Projection areas of the brain.

of the brain. A face is not merely seen; it is recognized as familiar or interesting or attractive. Remembering takes place at the same time as perception, so that other faces seen in the past, or experiences linked to that face are called up. Emotions may also be stirred. For this type of association the cortex draws on other parts of the brain by way of the communicating network of nerves.

A large part of the cortex that remains unmapped is thought to be involved in associative response. Factual knowledge and technical skills depend upon a background of experience and relationships between one kind of thing and another. Whether the mind is daydreaming, thinking rationally or experiencing a surge of emotion, it draws upon an intensely personal and private background of association. The richer a person's life is in experiences that have made their imprint on thought and feeling, the richer will be the patterns upon which the conscious mind can draw.

Until recently, the frontal lobe, which particularly distinguishes man's brain from that of the lower orders, was thought to be an associative area. It was called a "silent" area because it seemed to have no specific function. This appears to be true for most of the frontal area, but it has been learned that in the frontal lobe, close to the small center for the sense of smell, is the center for speech.

Memory.   In the temporal lobe, near the auditory area, is a recently discovered center for memory. This center appears to be a storehouse where memories are filed. When this area alone is stimulated, a particular event, a piece of music or an experience long forgotten or deeply buried is brought to the individual's mind, complete in every detail, This is a very mechanical type of memory; when the stimulation is removed the memory ends. When it is applied again, the memory begins again, not where it left off, but from the beginning. (See also MEMORY.)

BRAIN STEM.   This is the stemlike portion of the brain made up of the diencephalon, midbrain, pons and medulla oblongata.

Thalamus.   Beneath the cortex, deep within the cerebral hemispheres, lies the thalamus. This organ is a relay station for body sensations; it also integrates these sensations on their way to the cortex. The thalamus is an organ of crude consciousness and of sensations of rough contact and extreme temperatures, either hot or cold. It is principally here that pain is felt. In the thalamus, responses are of the all-or-nothing sort; even mild stimuli would be felt as acutely painful if they were not graded and modified by the cortex.

Hypothalamus.   Below the thalamus, at the base of the cerebrum, is the HYPOTHALAMUS. This organ, no larger than a lump of sugar, takes part in such vital activities as the ebb and flow of the body's fluids and the regulation of metabolism, blood sugar levels and body temperature. It directs the body's many rhythms, including those of activity and rest, appetite and digestion, sexual desire and menstrual and reproductive cycles. The hypothalamus is also the body's emotional brain. It is the integrating center of the autonomic NERVOUS SYSTEM, with its sympathetic and parasympathetic branches, and is situated close to the pituitary gland.

Midbrain.   Just below the thalamus is the short narrow pillar of the midbrain. This contains a center for visual reflexes, such as moving the head and eyes, as well as a sound-activated center, obsolete in man, for pricking up the ears.

Medulla Oblongata.   Below the midbrain is the medulla oblongata, the continuation upward of the spinal cord. In the medulla, the great trunk nerves, both motor and sensory, cross over, left to right and right to left, producing the puzzling phenomenon by which the left hemisphere of the cerebrum controls the right half of the body, while the right hemisphere controls the left half of the body. This portion of the brain also contains the centers that activate the heart, blood vessels and respiratory system.

CEREBELLUM.   The cerebellum, or "little brain," is attached to the back of the brain stem, under the curve of the cerebrum. It is connected, by way of the midbrain, with the motor area of the cortex and with the spinal cord, as well as with the SEMICIRCULAR CANALS, the organs of balance.

The function of the cerebellum appears to be to blend and coordinate motion of the various muscles involved in voluntary movements. It does not direct these movements; that is the function of the cortex. The cortex, however, operates in terms of movements, not of muscles. As a conscious function the cortex may, for example, direct the arm to pick up a glass of water; the cerebellum, which operates entirely below the level of consciousness, then translates this instruction into detailed actions by the 32 different muscles in the hand, plus several more in the arm and shoulder. When the cerebellum is injured, the patient's movements are jerky and uncoordinated.

CRANIAL NERVES.   From the brain stem there emerge on their separate pathways the CRANIAL NERVES. They arise within the skull and, with one important exception, the VAGUS NERVE, serve the head and neck.

PROTECTION OF THE BRAIN.   The brain is protected by the bony skull and by three layers of membranes, the meninges. Between the middle and inner layer is a space filled with CEREBROSPINAL FLUID, which serves as a shock absorber. The same system of membranes and fluid protects the spinal cord.

The brain is protected from harmful substances in the bloodstream by a barrier of some kind (the blood-brain barrier) that keeps some of the substances out of the brain entirely and delays the entry of others for hours or even days after they have penetrated the rest of the body.

DISORDERS OF THE BRAIN.   In spite of protection of the brain by the skull and membranes and by the blood-brain barrier, a number of functional disorders and diseases may affect the brain.

Concussion or fracture of the skull may occur as a result of a severe shock or blow to the head. An interruption to the flow of blood to the brain may result from hemorrhage from one of the blood vessels serving the brain, or an obstruction caused by formation of a thrombus. Cerebral vascular accident (stroke) occurs when brain cells are deprived of their supply of blood.

Several diseases attack the brain specifically, including epilepsy, meningitis and encephalitis.

Hydrocephalus, or "water on the brain," is caused by an abnormal accumulation of cerebrospinal fluid in the head.

Cerebral palsy is a name given to a motor disorder that results in inability to control muscle movement. It is usually the result of brain damage before, during or immediately after birth.

Many diseases that originate in other parts of the body may affect the brain and nerves. Rabies and tetanus (lockjaw) are two examples of diseases that can cause brain damage. Others are syphilis, rheumatic fever and alcoholism.

Brain Abscess. Brain abscess is a localized suppurative lesion within the intracranial cavity. The majority of cases are secondary to middle ear infections. Other causes include compound fracture of the skull with contamination of the brain tissue, sinusitis and infections of the face, lung or heart. Symptoms include fever, malaise, irritability, severe headache, convulsions, vomiting and other signs of intracranial hypertension. Treatment consists of surgical removal of the infected area and administration of antibiotic drugs.

Brain Tumor. Any abnormal growth within the skull creates a special problem because it is in a confined space and will press on normal brain tissue and interfere with the functions of the body controlled by the affected parts. This is true whether the tumor itself is benign or malignant. Fortunately, the functions of certain areas of the brain are well known, and a disturbance of some specific function guides physicians readily to the affected area. If diagnosed early, a benign tumor often can be removed surgically with a good chance of recovery. Malignant tumors are more difficult to remove.

The causes of brain tumor are not known. It is not a common disease, but it can occur at any age, and it can appear in any part of the brain. It may originate in the brain or may metastasize from a tumor in another part of the body.

The symptoms of brain tumor vary. Headache together with nausea is sometimes the first sign. The headache can be general or localized in one part of the head, and the pain is usually intense. Vomiting can be significant if it is sudden and without nausea. Disturbances of vision, loss of coordination in movement, weakness and stiffness on one side of the body are also possible symptoms. Loss of sight, hearing, taste or smell may result from brain tumor. A tumor can also cause a distortion of any of these senses, such as seeing flashes at the sides of the field of vision, or smelling odors or hearing sounds that do not exist. It can affect the ability to speak clearly or to understand the speech of others. Varying degrees of weakness or paralysis in the arms or legs may appear. A tumor may cause convulsions.

Changes in personality or mental ability are rare in cases of brain tumor. When such changes occur they may take the form of lapses of memory or absent-mindedness, mental sluggishness or loss of initiative.

Brain tumor is treated surgically. As a result of recent progress in the methods of brain surgery, many cases of brain tumor can now be operated on successfully.

BRAIN SURGERY. There are two types of brain surgery—that which corrects damage to the brain itself, and that which seeks to remedy a condition in another part of the body. The first type includes operations to relieve tumors, brain injuries, abscesses and infections, hydrocephalus and PARKINSON'S DISEASE. The second includes surgery for severe neuralgia and MENIÈRE'S DISEASE.

Nursing Care. Diagnostic tests and examinations are usually done preoperatively to locate the tumor or other disorder of the brain. During this time the patient's symptoms should be noted carefully so that his condition before and after surgery can be compared. Things to be observed include: personality and speech characteristics, vision, paralysis or weakness in one or more areas and incontinence.

Immediately before surgery the patient's unit is prepared for his return from the operating room or recovery room. There should be assembled at the bedside a suction apparatus with catheters, a padded tongue depressor, equipment for measuring blood pressure and other vital signs, a lumbar puncture set and a tray with syringes and needles and emergency drugs such as caffeine sodium benzoate and amobarbital. The bed is made so that the patient's head is at the foot of the bed to facilitate observation of the operative site and the changing of dressings. Side rails are applied to the bed.

Postoperatively, the patient will require constant attendance during the first 24 hours. Observations should include checking and recording the vital signs as ordered, usually every 15 minutes until they stabilize and then every 2 hours. The dressings are checked for drainage and if necessary reinforced with sterile dressings and towels. A clear, yellowish drainage may indicate leakage of cerebrospinal fluid and should be reported immediately. The pupils are observed for irregularity in size or fixation with failure to respond to light. The level of consciousness is determined periodically as is the patient's reaction to stimuli.

As the patient progresses he is allowed a diet as tolerated and may be ambulatory if the surgeon deems this advisable.

brainwashing mental conditioning of a captive subject to secure attitudes conformable to the wishes of the captors.

branchial (brang'ke-al) pertaining to, or resembling, gills.
b. arches, four pairs of mesenchymal and later cartilaginous arches of the fetus in the region of the neck.
b. clefts, the clefts between the branchial arches of the embryo, formed by rupture of the membrane separating corresponding entodermal pouch and ectodermal groove.
b. cyst, a cyst formed deep within the neck from an incompletely closed branchial cleft. The branchial arches develop during the first 2 months of embryonic life and are separated by four clefts, which correspond to the gills of a fish. As the fetus develops, these arches grow to form structures within the head and neck. Two of the arches grow together and enclose the cervical sinus, a cavity in the neck. A branchial cyst may develop within the cervical sinus. Called also branchiogenic or branchiogenous cyst.

branchiogenic (brang″ke-o-jen′ik) derived from a branchial cleft.

Branham's sign (bran'hamz) closure of an arteriovenous fistula by digital pressure results in slowing of the pulse, increased diastolic pressure and disappearance of the heart murmur.

brash (brash) a burning sensation in the stomach.
weaning b., diarrhea in infants occurring as a result of weaning.

Braxton Hicks contractions (braks′ton hiks) light, irregular contractions of the uterus throughout pregnancy, often mistaken for true labor, and sometimes referred to as "false labor." These contractions are more frequent during the later stages of pregnancy and may be stimulated by the descent of the head of the infant into the pelvic inlet. Braxton Hicks contractions are not regular and rhythmic as are true labor contractions.

breast (brest) the mammary gland. In women the breasts are secondary sex organs with the function of producing milk after childbirth. The term breast is less commonly used to refer to the breasts of the human male, which neither function nor develop.

At the tip of each breast is an area called the areola, usually reddish in color; at the center of this area is the nipple. About 20 separate lactiferous ducts empty into a depression at the top of the nipple. Each duct leads from alveoli within the breast called lobules, where the milk is secreted. Along their length, the ducts have widened areas that form reservoirs in which milk can be stored. The ducts and lobules form the glandular tissue of which the breasts are chiefly composed. Connective tissue covers the glandular tissue and is itself sheathed in a layer of fatty tissue. The fatty tissue gives the breast its smooth outline and contributes to its size and firmness.

ABNORMALITIES AND DISORDERS OF THE BREAST. Amastia is the absence of one or both breasts at birth. Hypomastia is abnormal smallness of the breasts. Hypertrophy of the breasts, abnormal enlargement of the breasts, is often a symptom of an endocrine disorder. Enlargement of the breasts in the male is called gynecomastia and is a not uncommon occurrence during adolescence. Polymastia is the presence of more than two breasts; it is more common in men than in women.

MASTITIS, inflammation of the breast, may occur in a variety of forms and in varying degrees of severity. Persistent cases may require mastectomy, but usually medical treatment suffices.

Breast Tumor. Benign tumors are growths of breast tissue that metastasize but, if removed, do not recur. The most common of these is fibroadenoma, which is found most frequently in women between 21 and 25, although it can develop during and after menopause. This tumor grows rapidly during pregnancy, is seldom painful and can be removed surgically. Another benign breast tumor is intraductal papilloma. It occurs most frequently in women between 35 and 55. Its symptoms are discharge of blood or fluid containing blood from the nipples when the breast is compressed.

Breast cancer is one of the two most common types of cancer among women. Malignant tumors are rare among men, but can occur, usually in those between the ages of 50 and 60.

Breast cancer first appears as a small, painless lump, most frequently in the outer, upper portion of the breast. If the lump is near the surface, there is often a visible dimpling of the skin. If a malignant tumor is suspected, a biopsy is usually done to confirm the diagnosis. Surgery is usually indicated for malignant tumors, and is often followed by radiation therapy and sometimes by administration of hormones.

Recent improvements in x-ray techniques have made it possible to diagnose breast tumors in the beginning stages; however, the interpretation of the films must be done by an experienced radiologist. The term used for x-ray study of the breast is mammography. Another technique involves the use of infrared rays and is called thermography.

SELF-EXAMINATION OF THE BREAST. Women should train themselves to perform a simple self-examination of the breasts, described in the accompanying diagrams. The best time for this is just after menstruation when the breasts are normally soft. If any lump in the breast can be felt, a physician should be consulted immediately.

SURGERY OF THE BREAST. Surgical operations of the breast may be done for a variety of reasons. Mammoplasty refers to reconstructive surgery of the breast and is usually done for the purpose of reducing the size of large, pendulous breasts. Mastectomy is surgical removal of breast tissue and is most often done to treat cancer of the breast. Simple mastectomy is the surgical removal of breast tissue only; radical mastectomy involves removal of the entire breast and neighboring tissues such as the underlying pectoral muscles and axillary lymph nodes.

Nursing Care. The psychologic aspects of surgery of the breast must always be considered. The breast is a symbol of femininity, motherhood and sexual attractiveness; thus, a surgical procedure involving its partial or complete removal will always bring about some degree of emotional upheaval for the patient. Many women, out of fear of mutilation or even death, resist surgical treatment of the breast even though the procedure may be necessary to save their lives. The patient should be reassured that modern prostheses and specially designed brassieres eliminate many of the outward signs of the loss of a breast.

Before the operation the surgeon usually explains the procedure to the patient and her family, stressing the need for surgery and the type of operation that will be performed. Diagnostic tests, such as x-ray examination and electrocardiography, are done to determine the extent of metastasis, if any,

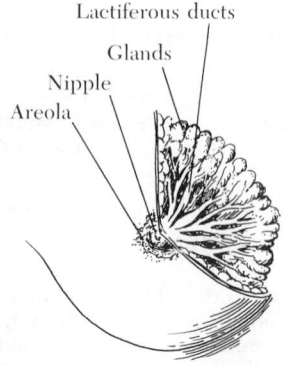
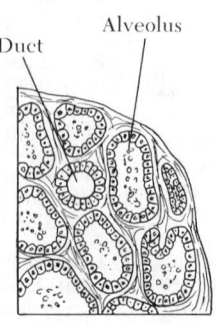
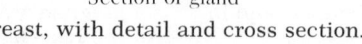
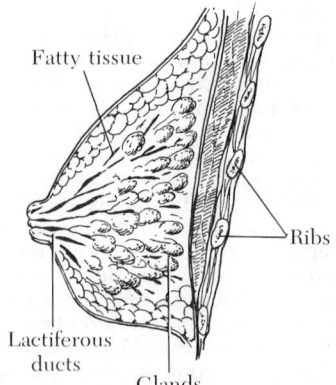

Breast, with detail and cross section.

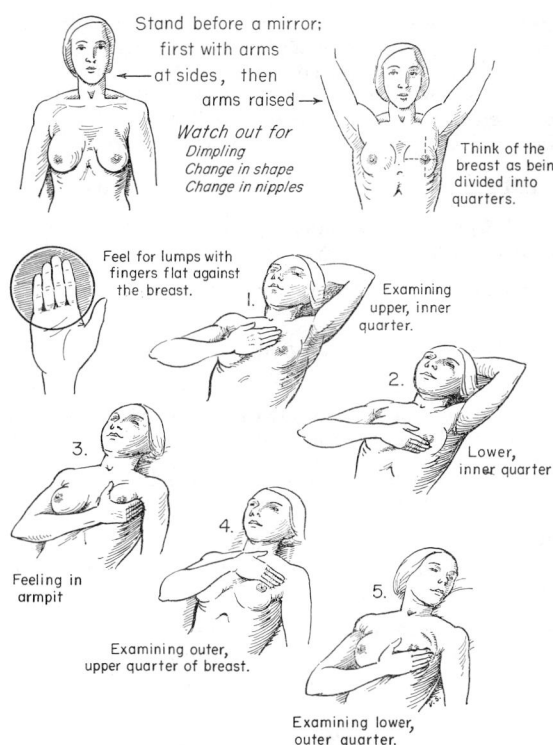

Stand before a mirror; first with arms at sides, then arms raised →

Watch out for
*Dimpling
Change in shape
Change in nipples*

Think of the breast as being divided into quarters.

Feel for lumps with fingers flat against the breast.

1. Examining upper, inner quarter.

2. Lower, inner quarter

3.

4. Feeling in armpit

Examining outer, upper quarter of breast.

5. Examining lower, outer quarter.

Self-examination of the breast. (From Dowling, H. F., and Jones, T.: That the Patient May Know. Philadelpha, W. B. Saunders Co., 1959.)

and to rule out heart disease. If there is doubt that the tumor is malignant, a biopsy is performed in the operating room so that, if cancer is present, mastectomy may be performed immediately. Since there is danger of spreading malignant cells once the tumor has been incised for biopsy, most surgeons prefer to perform the necessary surgery as soon as the sample tissue has been removed, examined and found to be malignant. For this reason, preoperative physical preparation of the skin should include complete cleansing and shaving of the entire breast and axilla.

After the operation dressings must be checked at frequent intervals for signs of excessive bleeding. The patient is placed on her back immediately after surgery; however, it is important to turn the patient gently, and to inspect the back on the operative side frequently to be sure blood is not seeping through. Although the dressings will be snug to reduce the loss of blood, they should not be so tight as to restrict circulation. Numbness and tingling or paralysis of the arm or hand should be reported at once.

Pulmonary complications are prevented by having the patient cough and breathe deeply at frequent intervals. This may produce discomfort in the operative site but is necessary. Pain may be quite severe the first few days after surgery, requiring frequent administration of analgesics as ordered by the physician.

Most surgeons wish to have the patient out of bed and walking the first day after mastectomy. Loss of balance is quite common immediately after this operation because of reduction in body weight on one side of the chest and restriction of arm movement on the affected side. The patient will need assistance and supervision while getting up and walking until she has adjusted to this change in her body structure.

Special exercises are essential to recovery from mastectomy. They are begun as soon as ordered by the surgeon and should be continued after the patient has returned home. Combing and brushing the hair, buttoning clothes at the back, "wall climbing" with the fingers and arm-swinging exercises are all useful in preserving muscle tone and preventing contracture of the joints. The pamphlet "Help Yourself to Recovery," published by the American Cancer Society, is a useful guide for the patient during the convalescent period.

breast feeding the method of feeding a baby with milk directly from the mother's breasts rather than from a bottle. Most physicians agree that breast feeding is usually better for baby and mother physically and emotionally, although there are conditions in which bottle feeding proves more satisfactory; sometimes a combination of both methods is the best solution.

ADVANTAGES. Breast milk is easily digested by the baby, for whom nature especially made it. It is safe and clean and contains practically everything the baby needs during the first months of his life. Babies who are breast fed are less susceptible to certain types of infections than bottle-fed babies. Also, the act of nursing helps to satisfy some of their emotional needs.

For the mother, nursing causes contraction of the muscles of the uterus, encouraging its rapid return to normal size. It makes her feel close to the baby, satisfying her emotional needs. It is less expensive and is not dependent on obtaining supplies. Nursing mothers need not gain any weight even though they eat well and drink a quart of milk a day (skimmed milk is suitable and is less fattening than whole milk). If the mother does not gain weight, and if she wears a good supporting brassiere, the appearance of her breasts is not appreciably altered. Nursing does not interfere with her health.

DISADVANTAGES AND OBJECTIONS. There are disadvantages to breast feeding as far as the mother is concerned. Her freedom is restricted and she cannot go away for days at a time, although it is possible to supplement breast feeding with a formula.

Women who feel a real revulsion toward the act of nursing a baby (and not just an objection on the grounds that it will be a nuisance) should not force themselves to do so. Nursing is a little better than bottle feeding, but there is not enough difference to matter significantly.

NURSING THE BABY. Breast feeding can be a very simple and satisfactory way to feed a baby. The mother should be relaxed about it, because tension or fatigue can inhibit the milk supply.

The breasts require little care. Just before each feeding, the hands are washed and the nipple (or nipples if both breasts are used at each feeding) is cleansed with some sterile cotton moistened in warm water that has been sterilized by boiling.

The mother can lie on one side while she nurses, holding the baby close to her in the curve of her arm. Or she can sit in a comfortable chair with a pillow at her back and one foot on a stool so that her knee will help support the baby; her curved arm will support his back. If the nipple or a finger is touched to the infant's lips or cheek, he will turn his head toward the breast on the same side and open his mouth to grasp the nipple. The mother should be sure to touch the baby on the side toward which she wants him to turn. This is an instinctive reaction, and trying to turn the baby's face toward the breast by pushing against the opposite cheek will not work. It is usually necessary for the mother to hold the breast back from the baby's nose with her free hand so that it will not interfere with his breathing.

As a rule, the baby nurses at one breast at a feeding, and the breasts are alternated with each feeding. In this way the breast is emptied completely; this prevents the milk from diminishing. Some babies nurse rapidly and some slowly. They usually get most of the milk during the first few minutes, but should be allowed to continue. The average nursing time is 15 to 20 minutes at first, but after 2 to 3 weeks, when the milk begins to flow more rapidly and the baby sucks more efficiently, the time may be reduced to as little as 10 minutes.

Menstruation usually does not interfere with nursing. Also, nursing is not, as some believe, an effective contraceptive measure.

breath (breth) the air taken in and expelled by the expansion and contraction of the thorax.

breathing (brēth'ing) the alternate inspiration and expiration of air into and out of the lungs (see also RESPIRATION).

glossopharyngeal b., respiration unaided by the primary or ordinary accessory muscles of respiration, the air being "swallowed" rapidly into the lungs by use of the tongue and the muscles of the pharynx.

intermittent positive pressure b., IPPB, active inflation of the lungs during inspiration under positive pressure from a cycling valve; a principle used in the operation of certain types of RESPIRATORS.

Breckinridge, (brek'in-rij) Mary (1881–1965) American nurse, founder of the Frontier Nursing Service, a primarily midwifery service for women in remote areas of Kentucky. The Service, originally the Kentucky Committee for Mothers and Babies, was founded in 1925.

Breda's disease (bra'dahz) yaws.

breech (brēch) the buttock.

b. presentation, buttock-first presentation of the fetus in labor (see also PRESENTATION).

bregma (breg'mah) the junction of the coronal and sagittal sutures. adj., **bregmat'ic.**

bretylium (bre-til'e-um) an ammonium derivative used as a sympathetic nerve blockade and as an antihypertensive.

brevicollis (brev'ĭ-kol'is) shortness of the neck.

Brevital (brev'ĭ-tal) trademark for a preparation of methohexital, an ultra-short-acting barbiturate.

bridge (brij) a structure joining two other parts or organs, especially a structure bearing one or more artificial teeth, attached to natural teeth in the jaw.

fixed b., a partial denture retained with crowns or inlays cemented to the natural teeth.

removable b., a partial denture retained by attachments which permit its removal.

Bright's disease (brīts) any one of a group of kidney diseases attended with albuminuria and edema. The diseases are commonly referred to collectively as NEPHRITIS. The name Bright's disease is derived from a description of the diseases published in 1827 by Richard Bright, an English physician.

Brill's disease (brilz) recrudescent typhus.

Brill-Symmers disease (bril sim'erz) giant follicular lymphadenopathy.

Brill-Zinsser disease (bril zin'ser) recrudescent typhus.

brim (brim) the edge of the superior strait of the pelvis.

brisement (brēz-maw') [Fr.] a crushing, especially the breaking up of an ANKYLOSIS.

Bristamin (bris'tah-min) trademark for a preparation of phenyltoloxamine, an antihistamine.

British antilewisite dimercaprol, a chelating agent used against poisoning with arsenic, gold and mercury.

British thermal unit B.T.U., a unit of heat being the amount necessary to raise the temperature of one pound of water from 39 to 40° F., generally considered the equivalent of 252 calories.

Broca's area (bro'kahz) an area in the left (or right) inferior frontal gyrus; called also area subcallosa and Broca's center. It is the cortical area that controls the motor aspects of speech.

Brock syndrome (brok) middle lobe syndrome.

Brodmann's areas (brod'manz) specific occipital and preoccipital areas of the cerebral cortex, identified by number, which are considered to be the seat of specific functions of the brain.

bromated (bro'māt-ed) charged with bromine.

bromatology (bro"mah-tol'o-je) the science of foods and diet.

bromatotherapy (bro"mah-to-ther'ah-pe) dietotherapy.

bromatoxism (bro"mah-tok'sizm) poisoning by food.

bromhidrosis (bro"mĭ-dro'sis) the secretion of foul-smelling perspiration.

bromide (bro'mīd) a binary compound of bromine. Many of these compounds have a depressant effect on the nervous system and can be used as sedatives. Since bromides are slowly eliminated and may cumulate in the body to reach toxic amounts, their use is of questionable value and many hospital formularies have omitted them. Patent medicines and drugs sold over the counter frequently contain bromides, and bromide poisoning (BROMISM) is relatively common.

bromidrosis (bro"mĭ-dro'sis) bromhidrosis.

bromine (bro'mēn) a chemical element, atomic number 35, atomic weight 79.909, symbol Br. (See table of ELEMENTS.)

bromism (bro'mizm) poisoning by bromine or its compounds. This condition occurs when the bromine concentration in the body fluids is high enough to have a toxic and depressant action on the central nervous system. The toxic level varies with each individual and is also somewhat dependent on chloride intake because the bromide ion and the chloride ion are equally absorbed and distributed throughout the same fluid compartments. This means that in a person with a limited salt intake bromine accumulates more quickly and severe poisoning can occur after ingestion of an amount of bromine that would be relatively harmless for a person with a normal or high salt intake.

Many cases of bromism result from indiscriminate use of patent medicines advertised as "nerve tonics" and "headache remedies" containing bromide. The early symptoms may be similar to the symptoms for which the patient is taking the patent medicine, and correct diagnosis and treatment of the condition may be delayed. The symptoms of bromine poisoning are headache, irritability, emotional instability, malaise, and mental aberrations such as hallucinations, amnesia and disorientation.

Treatment consists of immediate curtailment of bromine ingestion and efforts to eliminate the substance from the body. Mercurial diuretics aid in bromine removal. Enteric-coated tablets of ammonium and sodium chloride are prescribed if they are not contraindicated by cardiac or renal disease. The removal of bromine from the system may take as long as several months. In severe, acute poisoning the bromine may be removed by DIALYSIS.

When an emotional disturbance or mental illness is the primary cause of bromism, psychotherapy is indicated.

bromisovalum (brōm″i-so-val′um) a gentle, quick-acting sedative and hypnotic of moderately long action. It does not belong to the barbiturate group. Long-term use can lead to BROMISM.

bromochlorotrifluoroethane (bro″mo-klo″ro-tri-flu″o-ro-eth′ān) halothane, a general anesthetic.

bromoderma (bro″mo-der′mah) a skin eruption due to use of bromides.

bromodiphenhydramine (bro″mo-di″fen-hi′drah-min) compound used as an antihistamine.

bromohyperhidrosis (bro″mo-hi″per-hĭ-dro′sis) excessive fetid perspiration.

bromo-iodism (bro″mo-i′o-dizm) poisoning by bromides and iodides.

bromomania (bro″mo-ma′ne-ah) mania induced by misuse of bromides.

bromomenorrhea (bro″mo-men″o-re′ah) profuse, foul-smelling menstruation.

brompheniramine (brōm″fen-ir′ah-mēn) a pyridine derivative used as an antihistamine.

Bromsulphalein (brom-sul′fah-lin) trademark for sulfobromophthalein, a dye used in testing liver function; abbreviation BSP. In the laboratory test, the dye is introduced into the circulatory system and a blood sample is withdrawn 30 or 45 minutes later, depending on the dose injected. The parenchymal cells remove almost all of the dye within this time if they are functioning normally. The rate of removal is influenced by the blood flow through the portal circulation, the functioning capacity of the liver cells and the patency of the biliary tract.

The patient must be in a fasting state for the test. A blood sample is taken, and then the Bromsul-phalein is given by vein very slowly. The amount given is determined by body weight (2 or 5 mg. per kilogram of body weight). While the dye is being administered the patient should be watched closely for signs of an allergic reaction. Thirty minutes after the injection (or 45 minutes if 5 mg. per kilogram of body weight was given) a blood sample is taken from a vein in the opposite arm. Normally the liver cells remove about 95 per cent of the dye in that period of time, leaving about 5 per cent in the circulating blood.

Bromural (brōm-u′ral) trademark for preparations of bromisovalum, a sedative and hypnotic.

bronchadenitis (brongk″ad-ĕ-ni′tis) inflammation of the bronchial glands.

bronchi (brong′ki) plural of *bronchus*.

bronchial (brong′ke-al) pertaining to the bronchi.
  b. asthma, asthma.
  b. tree, the bronchi and their branching structures.

bronchiarctia (brong″ke-ark′she-ah) bronchostenosis.

bronchiectasis (brong″ke-ek′tah-sis) a chronic dilatation of the bronchi or bronchioles, accompanied by paroxysmal coughing and copious purulent exudate.

Bronchiectasis can restrict the activities of the patient, but its seriousness depends upon the patient's general health and the extent of the condition. Its complications derive from the intermittent bouts of pneumonia and bronchitis to which the sufferer is prone, and the general lowering of resistance. It is one of the most frequent causes of hemoptysis.

Bronchiectasis can be congenital, but it is more likely to be secondary to other conditions such as chronic sinus infection or asthma, an aftereffect of whooping cough, lung abscess, pneumonia or tuberculosis or caused by a foreign body in the respiratory tract.

SYMPTOMS. The most immediate symptom of bronchiectasis is persistent coughing. The coughing may be mild, often occurring when the patient first gets up in the morning. In severe cases, the coughing becomes more violent as the walls of the bronchial tubes thicken and secrete quantities of mucus. The muscles may become so weak that even violent coughing fails to expel the mucus. Pus may also be secreted, and the cilia destroyed. In advanced cases the sputum and breath may become foul-smelling, and the patient may suffer loss of appetite, anemia, fever, intermittent attacks of pneumonia and a general lowering of resistance to infection.

TREATMENT. To maintain the strength and general health of the patient, fresh air and sunshine, a good diet and plenty of rest are essential. A move to a mild climate may be of great benefit. Cigarette smoking should be stopped. If the disease is fairly well localized, it may be relieved by surgery. Penicillin or other antibiotics are sometimes useful, particularly in controlling other infections, which may weaken the patient and further lower his resistance.

An expectorant cough medicine may be prescribed. The patient should be warned against overuse of the sedative type of cough remedy which suppresses coughing. When the chest becomes severely congested, it is helpful for the patient to lie down with the thorax lower than the rest of the body, and allow the bronchial tubes to drain by gravity (postural drainage). In advanced cases, the patient may wish to make this a daily practice, for as long as 30 minutes each day.

Although no cures for this ailment have been found, bronchiectasis has been decreasing in the United States in recent years. Health authorities attribute this in part to the vaccines that have been developed against whooping cough, measles and influenza.

NURSING CARE. Avoidance of secondary infections of the respiratory tract is essential in the prevention of complications. Mouth care before meals and after postural drainage helps overcome halitosis and a subsequent loss of appetite.

POSTURAL DRAINAGE is the term to describe the procedure done to facilitate drainage of stagnant and purulent secretions collected in the bronchial tree. The exact position of the patient for this procedure depends on the location of the disorder in the lung. While the patient is in an "upside down" position, with the thorax lower than the rest of the body, he is instructed to cough up the secretions. Clapping the chest with the cupped hand has been found to be beneficial in dislodging the tenacious mucus. This should be done by a person trained in the technique.

bronchiloquy (brong-kil'o-kwe) high-pitched pectoriloquy due to lung consolidation.

bronchiocele (brong'ke-o-sēl") dilatation or swelling of a bronchiole.

bronchiogenic (brong"ke-o-jen'ik) bronchogenic.

bronchiole (brong'ke-ōl) one of the successively smaller channels into which the segmental bronchi divide within the bronchopulmonary segments. adj., **bronchi'olar.**
  respiratory b., one of the final branches of the bronchioles, communicating directly with the alveolar ducts.

bronchiolectasis (brong"ke-o-lek'tah-sis) chronic dilatation of bronchioles.

bronchiolitis (brong"ke-o-li'tis) inflammation of the bronchioles.

bronchiolus (brong-ko'o-lus), pl. *bronchi'oli* [L.] bronchiole.

bronchiospasm (brong'ke-o-spazm") spasmodic narrowing of the bronchi.

bronchiostenosis (brong"ke-o-stĕ-no'sis) bronchostenosis.

bronchismus (brong-kiz'mus) bronchial spasm.

bronchitis (brong-ki'tis) inflammation of the bronchi. Bronchitis can be either acute or chronic; an acute case occasionally develops into a chronic one. If the inflammation reaches the bronchioles and the alveoli, the condition is bronchopneumonia (see also PNEUMONIA).

ACUTE BRONCHITIS. Acute bronchitis is most commonly encountered in small children and in old people, though it can attack anyone of any age. In its mild form it is often referred to as a "cold on the chest," but as it progresses downward into the lungs, it can develop into a serious disease. Children have small bronchi that are obstructed more easily than those of adults.

Symptoms of acute bronchitis include chest pain, fever, general listlessness and considerable coughing. The cough starts as a dry cough but then becomes productive. The disease runs its course in about 10 days, but in some cases the symptoms may linger on for several weeks.

If the bronchitis is bacterial in origin, recovery may be hastened by the administration of penicillin or other antibiotics. If the cause is viral, antibiotics are of no value in most cases. After the symptoms have disappeared, the patient must still take care of himself and avoid fatigue in order to avoid a relapse.

Acute bronchitis may follow childhood diseases such as measles and whooping cough. Tracheobronchitis, or inflammation of the trachea and bronchi, occurs most often in infants and children. Treatment of this, as well as of croup, includes steam inhalations, sometimes medicated with detergent solutions such as Alevaire, which liquefy and loosen respiratory secretions, to help in their removal.

CHRONIC BRONCHITIS. Chronic bronchitis usually attacks the middle-aged and the elderly. Although it may follow a series of attacks of acute bronchitis or another related disease such as influenza or tonsillitis, it may appear without apparent cause. The disease may come about gradually from inhaling irritants such as dust and fumes and from the heavy use of tobacco. The so-called smoker's cough is actually chronic bronchitis in most cases. Bronchitis may be present only in the winter, but if it returns each year, it is classified as chronic.

Chronic bronchitis is a stubborn disease that interferes with the air flow from the lungs, causes shortness of breath, induces constant coughing and expectoration and breeds infection in the bronchial tubes.

Treatment consists of the use of antibiotics and of medication designed to loosen the phlegm in the bronchi to induce easier breathing. POSTURAL DRAINAGE helps in removal of secretions from the lungs. A vaporizer in the bedroom is sometimes helpful.

Chronic bronchitis makes its victims more vulnerable to heart disease (the heart has to work harder as the respiration breaks down) as well as to other more serious lung diseases. It is not uncommon for one pulmonary disease to follow another, and sometimes two may be present simultaneously, making diagnosis and treatment difficult. Chronic bronchitis is frequently associated with emphysema, bronchiectasis and pneumoconiosis, a chronic fibrous condition of the lungs caused by inhalation of special dusts. It is also sometimes accompanied by pulmonary fibrosis, another chronic disease in which the lung tissue becomes fibrous, causing contraction of the chest and symptoms resembling those of chronic asthma.

bronchoadenitis (brong"ko-ad"ĕ-ni'tis) bronchadenitis.

bronchobiliary (brong"ko-bil'e·a"re) pertaining to or communicating with a bronchus and the biliary tract.

bronchoblennorrhea (brong"ko-blen"o-re'ah) chronic bronchitis with copious thick sputum.

bronchocavernous (brong″ko-kav′er-nus) both bronchial and cavernous.

bronchocele (brong′ko-sēl) 1. localized dilatation of a bronchus. 2. goiter.

bronchoclysis (brong-kok′lĭ-sis) instillation of a medicated solution into the bronchi.

bronchoconstriction (brong″ko-kon-strik′shun) bronchostenosis.

bronchoconstrictor (brong″ko-kon-strik′tor) 1. narrowing the lumina of the air passages of the lungs. 2. an agent that causes constriction of the bronchi.

bronchodilatation (brong″ko-dil″ah-ta′shun) dilatation of a bronchus.

bronchodilator (brong″ko-di-la′tor) 1. expanding the lumina of the air passages of the lungs. 2. an agent that causes dilatation of the bronchi. The drug aminophylline acts as a bronchodilator by virtue of its ability to relax smooth muscle tissue, thereby relieving spasms of the bronchial muscles and resulting in enlargement of the lumina of the bronchi.

bronchoesophageal (brong″ko-e-sof″ah-je′al) pertaining to or communicating with a bronchus and the esophagus.

bronchoesophagology (brong″ko-e-sof″ah-gol′o-je) the branch of medicine concerned with the air passages (bronchi) and esophagus.

bronchoesophagoscopy (brong″ko-e-sof″ah-gos′-ko-pe) instrumental examination of the bronchi and esophagus.

bronchogenic (brong″ko-jen′ik) originating in the bronchi.

bronchogram (brong′ko-gram) the film obtained at bronchography.

bronchography (brong-kog′rah-fe) roentgenography of the lungs after instillation of an opaque medium in the bronchi.

broncholith (brong′ko-lith) a bronchial calculus.

broncholithiasis (brong″ko-lĭ-thi′ah-sis) formation of calculi in the bronchi.

bronchology (brong-kol′o-je) the study of diseases of the bronchial tree.

bronchomotor (brong″ko-mo′tor) affecting the caliber of the bronchi.

bronchopathy (brong-kop′ah-the) disease of the bronchi.

bronchophony (brong-kof′o-ne) the sound of the voice as heard through the stethoscope applied over a healthy bronchus.

bronchoplasty (brong′ko-plas″te) plastic repair of a bronchus.

bronchoplegia (brong″ko-ple′je-ah) paralysis of the bronchial tubes.

bronchopleural (brong″ko-ploor′al) pertaining to a bronchus and the pleura, or communicating with a bronchus and the pleural cavity.

bronchopneumonia (brong″ko-nu-mo′ne-ah) in-

flammation of the bronchi and lungs (see also PNEUMONIA).

bronchopneumopathy (brong″ko-nu-mop′ah-the) noninflammatory disease of the bronchi and lung tissue.

bronchopulmonary (brong″ko-pul′mo-ner″e) pertaining to the bronchi and lungs.
  b. segment, one of the smaller divisions of the lobe of a lung, separated from others by a connective tissue septum and supplied by its own branch of the bronchus leading to the particular lobe.

bronchorrhagia (brong″ko-ra′je-ah) hemorrhage from the bronchi.

bronchorrhaphy (brong-kor′ah-fe) suture of a bronchus.

bronchorrhea (brong″ko-re′ah) bronchitis with profuse expectoration.

bronchoscope (brong′ko-skōp) an endoscope especially designed for passage through the trachea to permit inspection of the interior of the tracheobronchial tree.

bronchoscopy (brong-kos′ko-pe) inspection of the interior of the tracheobronchial tree with a bronchoscope. Bronchoscopy is used as a diagnostic aid or as treatment. The physician may examine the interior of the bronchi and take a biopsy of tissue or a sample of secretions. He may also use the bronchoscope to locate and remove foreign bodies or mucous plugs that are obstructing the air passages.
  NURSING CARE. Food and fluids are withheld for 8 hours before bronchoscopy is performed. The patient should brush his teeth and wash out his mouth carefully before the procedure to lessen the danger of introducing bacteria from the mouth into the bronchi. Dentures are removed and any loose teeth are brought to the attention of the physician. A mild sedative such as one of the barbiturates may be given prior to the bronchoscopy. This medication plus instructions to the patient and a full explanation of what is going to be done will help him relax and make the passing of the bronchoscope into the bronchi easier and less traumatic.
  After bronchoscopy fluids and food are withheld until the effects of the local anesthetic have worn off and the gag reflex has returned completely. The patient must be observed for signs of bleeding from the throat and respiratory embarrassment. Since swelling of the larynx may necessitate a tracheostomy, the equipment should be readily at hand. The patient should be kept quiet and discouraged from talking or coughing.

bronchosinusitis (brong″ko-si″nŭ-si′tis) coexisting infection of paranasal sinuses and lower respiratory passages.

bronchospasm (brong′ko-spazm) bronchial spasm; spasmodic contraction of the muscular coat of the smaller divisions of the bronchi, such as occurs in asthma.

bronchospirography (brong″ko-spi-rog′rah-fe) the graphic recording of breathing in one lung or lobe.

bronchospirometry (brong″ko-spi-rom′ĕ-tre) determination of the function of the lungs by measurement of tidal volume, vital capacity, maximum breathing capacity and oxygen consumption.

differential b., measurement of the function of each lung separately.

bronchostaxis (brong″ko-stak′sis) bleeding from the bronchial wall.

bronchostenosis (brong″ko-stĕ-no′sis) stricture or abnormal diminution of the caliber of a bronchial tube.

spasmodic b., a spasmodic contraction of the walls of the bronchi.

bronchostomy (brong-kos′to-me) surgical creation of an opening through the chest wall into the bronchus.

bronchotetany (brong″ko-tet′ah-ne) spasm of the bronchi, causing dyspnea.

bronchotomy (brong-kot′o-me) incision of a bronchus.

bronchotracheal (brong″ko-tra′ke-al) pertaining to the bronchi and trachea.

bronchovesicular (brong″ko-vĕ-sik′u-ler) bronchial and vesicular.

bronchus (brong′kus), pl. *bron′chi* [L.] one of the larger passages conveying air to (right or left main bronchus) and within the lungs (lobar and segmental bronchi). (See also RESPIRATION.)

brontophobia (bron″to-fo′be-ah) morbid fear of thunder.

bronze diabetes (bronz di″ah-be′tēz) a primary disorder of iron metabolism, with deposits of iron-containing pigments in the body tissues, and often with pigmentation of the skin, diabetes mellitus and cirrhosis of the liver; called also hemochromatosis and iron storage disease.

brow (brow) the forehead, or either lateral half thereof.

Brown-Séquard's syndrome (brown-sa-karz′) paralysis of motion on one side of the body and of sensation on the other, due to a lesion involving one side of the spinal cord.

Broxolin (brok′so-lin) trademark for a preparation of glycobiarsol, used in amebiasis.

Brucella (broo-sel′ah) a genus of Schizomycetes.

B. abor′tus, the causative agent of contagious abortion in cattle and the commonest cause of BRUCELLOSIS in man.

B. meliten′sis, the causative agent of classic Malta fever (undulant fever or BRUCELLOSIS).

B. su′is, a species found in swine that is capable of producing severe disease in man.

brucella (broo-sel′ah), pl. *brucel′lae* an organism of the genus Brucella.

brucellar (broo-sel′ar) pertaining to brucellae.

brucellemia (broo″sel-e′me-ah) the presence of brucellae in the blood.

brucellergen (broo-sel′er-jen) an antigen ob-

tained from Brucella; used in testing for brucella infection.

brucellosis (broo″sel-o′sis) a generalized infection marked by remittent undulant fever, malaise, headache and anemia, caused by various species of Brucella. It is transmitted to man from domestic animals such as pigs, goats and cattle, especially through infected milk or contact with the carcass of an infected animal.

The disease is also called undulant fever because one of the major symptoms in man is a fever that fluctuates widely at regular intervals. The symptoms in the beginning stages are difficult to notice and include loss of weight and increased irritability. As the illness advances, headaches, chills, diaphoresis and muscle aches and pains appear. It is possible for these symptoms to persist for years, either intermittently or continuously, although most patients recover completely within 2 to 6 months. Diagnosis is confirmed by blood tests.

Treatment consists of bed rest, antibiotics and a high intake of vitamins.

Prevention is best accomplished by the pasteurization of milk and a program of testing, vaccination and elimination of infected animals.

Brudzinski's sign (brood-zin′skēz) 1. in meningitis, bending the patient's neck produces flexion of the ankle, knee and hip. 2. in meningitis, passive flexion of the lower limb on one side causes a similar movement in the opposite limb.

Brugia (broo′je-ah) a genus of nematode parasites of the superfamily Filarioidea.

B. mala′yi, a species, morphologically distinguishable from *Wuchereria bancrofti,* also found in cases of elephantiasis.

bruise (brōōz) a large, blotchy superficial discoloration due to hemorrhage into the tissues from ruptured blood vessels beneath the skin surface, without the skin itself being broken; called also CONTUSION.

bruit (brōōt) [Fr.] a sound or murmur, especially an abnormal one.

aneurysmal b., a blowing sound heard over an aneurysm.

placental b., an auscultatory sound heard over the placenta in pregnancy.

bruxism (bruk′sizm) grinding of the teeth.

B.S. Bachelor of Science.

BSA bovine serum albumin.

bsp Bromsulphalein, a dye used in the study of liver function.

B.T.U., B.Th.U. British thermal unit.

buba (boo′bah) yaws.

bubo (bu′bo) a tender, enlarged lymph node, resulting from absorption of infective material and occurring in various diseases, e.g., lymphogranuloma venereum, plague, syphilis, gonorrhea, chancroid.

indolent b., a syphilitic bubo with no tendency to break down.

inguinal b., painful swelling of the inguinal lymph nodes, which sometimes become matted together.

bubonalgia (bu″bo-nal′je-ah) pain in the groin.

bubonic (bu-bon′ik) pertaining to buboes.
  b. plague, a highly contagious and severe fever caused by the bacillus *Pasteurella pestis* carried in infected rats and transmitted to man by fleas (see also PLAGUE).

bubonocele (bu-bon′o-sēl) incomplete inguinal hernia.

bucardia (bu-kar′de-ah) cor bovinum; extreme enlargement of the heart.

buccal (buk′al) pertaining to the mouth, especially to the inner surface of the cheeks.

bucco- (buk′ko) word element [L.] denoting relationship to the cheek.

buclizine (bu′klĭ-zēn) a compound used as an antihistamine and antinauseant.

bucnemia (buk-ne′me-ah) inflammatory swelling of the leg.

bud (bud) 1. a small protuberance on a plant from which growth occurs. 2. a structure resembling the bud of a plant, especially a protuberance in the embryo from which an organ or part develops.
  limb b., one of the four lateral swellings appearing in vertebrate embryos, which develop into the two pairs of limbs.
  tail b., the primordium of the caudal appendage.
  taste b's, end organs in the tongue receiving stimuli which give rise to the sense of taste.
  ureteric b., a hollow bud arising from the mesonephric duct, which develops into the ureter.
  b. of urethra, the enlarged proximal part of the corpus spongiosum.

budding (bud′ing) gemmation; development of a new organism from a protuberance on the body of the parent, a form of asexual reproduction.

Buerger's disease (ber′gerz) a disease affecting the medium-sized blood vessels, particularly the arteries of the legs, which can cause severe pain and in serious cases lead to gangrene; called also thromboangiitis obliterans, a term that refers to the clotting, pain and inflammation occurring in this disease and to the fact that it can obliterate, or destroy, blood vessels.
  The cause of this violent reaction has been thought to be excessive use of tobacco over a long period of time. The number of cases has diminished strikingly in recent years.
  The intense pain that is a symptom of the disease is caused by the formation of blood clots, or THROMBOSIS, in the lining of the arterial blood vessels.
  When the clots grow larger, the blood flow slows and may stop entirely. Since every part of the body depends on the continuous flow of blood, affected areas such as fingers and toes, for example, soon begin to atrophy or develop ulcers. If the causes of the disease are not completely arrested, amputation may be necessary.
  To treat the disease, the patient must stop smoking at once and entirely. This generally results in the partial healing of the affected membrane with a renewed flow of blood. However, more blood may have to be brought to damaged tissue by surgical methods of channeling detours or making canals in the clot itself.

  Special exercises called BUERGER-ALLEN EXERCISES are sometimes used to empty the engorged blood vessels and stimulate collateral circulation. These exercises can be done at home by the patient and are usually prescribed to be done several times during the day. The patient is also instructed to avoid wearing any tight clothing such as tight girdles, rolled garters, constricting belts and other items that may impair circulation. He should also avoid sitting or standing in one position for long periods of time. Care should be used in the selection of shoes and stockings so that they fit properly and do not cause pressure against the blood vessels. The patient should be told to avoid walking barefoot or otherwise subjecting himself to the hazards of trauma to the feet and legs. Should such an accident occur, no matter how minor it may seem, he must notify the physician so that treatment may be begun and infection and ulceration can be prevented.

Buerger-Allen exercises (ber′ger al′en) specific exercises intended to improve circulation to the feet and legs. The lower extremities are elevated to a 45 to 90 degree angle and supported in this position until the skin blanches (appears dead white). The feet and legs are then lowered below the level of the rest of the body until redness appears (care should be taken that there is no pressure against the back of the knees); finally, the legs are placed flat on the bed for a few minutes. The length of time for each position varies with the patient's tolerance and the speed with which color change occurs. Usually the exercises are prescribed so that the legs are elevated for 2 to 3 minutes, down 5 to 10 minutes, and then flat on the bed for 10 minutes.

buffer (buf′er) a substance that, by its presence in solution, increases the amount of acid or alkali necessary to produce unit change in pH.

buffy coat (buf′e) the thin yellowish layer of leukocytes overlying the packed erythrocytes in centrifuged blood.

bulb (bulb) 1. any rounded mass. 2. the medulla oblongata. adj., **bul′bar.**
  b. of aorta, the enlargement of the aorta at its point of origin from the heart.
  auditory b., the membranous labyrinth and cochlea.
  end b., the bulbous peripheral extremity of a sensory nerve.
  gustatory b's, taste buds.
  hair b., the bulbous expansion at the lower end of a hair root.
  Krause's b's, Krause's corpuscles.
  medullary b., medulla oblongata.
  olfactory b., the bulblike extremity of the olfactory nerve on the under surface of each anterior lobe of the cerebrum.
  b. of penis, bulb of urethra.
  taste b's, taste buds.
  b. of urethra, the proximal part of the corpus spongiosum.
  b. of vestibule, vestibulovaginal b., one of two masses of erectile tissue, situated one on either side of the vaginal orifice.

bulbiform (bul′bĭ-form) bulb-shaped.

bulbitis (bul-bi′tis) inflammation of the bulb of the urethra.

bulbonuclear (bul″bo-nu′kle-ar) pertaining to the medulla oblongata and its nuclei.

bulbourethral (bul″bo-u-re′thral) pertaining to the bulb of the urethra.

b. glands, two glands embedded in the substance of the sphincter of the male urethra, just posterior to the membranous part of the urethra. Their secretion, which is slippery and viscous, lubricates the urethra. Called also bulbocavernous glands and Cowper's glands.

bulbous (bul′bus) resembling a bulb.

bulbus (bul′bus), pl. *bul′bi* [L.] bulb.

b. aor′tae, bulb of the aorta.
b. carot′icus, carotid sinus.
b. oc′uli, the bulb, or globe, of the eye.
b. olfacto′rius, olfactory bulb.
b. ure′thrae, bulb of the urethra.
b. vestib′uli vagi′nae, bulb of the vestibule.

bulimia (bu-lim′e-ah) insatiable hunger. adj., **bulim′ic.**

bulla (bul′ah) pl., *bul′lae* [L.] a bladder, or bubble, especially a large blister or cutaneous vesicle filled with serous fluid. adj., **bul′lous.**

BUN blood urea nitrogen (see UREA NITROGEN).

bundle (bun′dl) a collection of units.

ground b., that part of the white matter of the spinal cord bordering the gray matter.
b. of His, a muscular band connecting the atria with the ventricles of the heart; called also atrioventricular bundle.
Keith's b., a bundle of fibers in the wall of the atrium of the heart between the venae cavae; called also sinoatrial bundle.
Thorel's b., a bundle of muscle fibers in the heart connecting the sinoatrial and atrioventricular nodes.
b. of Vicq d'Azyr, a bundle of white fibers around the base of the anterior nucleus of the optic thalamus.

bunion (bun′yun) a swelling of the bursa mucosa of the first joint below the base of the great toe. Bunions are almost always caused by wearing shoes that are too tight and that force the toes together. They are also often associated with flat or weak feet. In mild cases, the pain can be relieved by heat, and the condition will clear by itself after properly fitting shoes have been worn for some time. In more severe cases a physician should be consulted; he may recommend special corrective shoes or a simple surgical operation (bunionectomy) to correct the condition.

bunionectomy (bun″yun-ek′to-me) excision of a bunion.

bunionette (bun″yun-et′) a bunion-like enlargement of the joint of the little toe due to pressure over the lateral surface of the foot.

buphthalmos (būf-thal′mos) abnormal distention and enlargement of the eyeball in infancy.

bur (bur) a form of drill used for creating openings in bone or similar hard material.

buret, burette (bu-ret′) a glass tube with a capacity of the order of 25 to 100 ml. and graduation intervals of 0.05 to 0.1 ml., with stopcock attachment, used to deliver an accurately measured quantity of liquid.

burn (burn) injury caused by contact with dry heat (fire), moist heat (steam or liquid), chemicals, electricity, lightning or the ultraviolet rays of the sun.

Burns are classified according to degree. A first-degree burn involves a reddening of the skin area. In a second-degree burn, the skin is blistered. a third-degree burn is the most serious type, involving damage to the deeper layers of the skin. In some cases the growth cells of the tissues in the area may be destroyed.

All burns are dangerous if not properly cared for right away. In addition to the danger of infection from contamination of the burned area, the possibility of shock is a major hazard in any serious burn. If a large enough area of the body is affected, an otherwise minor or first-degree burn may have serious consequences.

It is difficult to determine the depth of a burn at first glance, but any burn involving more than 10 per cent of the body area is usually considered serious. First-degree and second-degree burns often occur together. In second-degree and third-degree burns, the danger of infection from contamination of the burned area is great.

IMMEDIATE TREATMENT. The following steps should be taken for prompt and effective treatment of the various types of burns.

Major Burns. If a person's clothing or hair is on fire, water, milk or other noninflammable liquid should be poured on the victim if the liquid is *immediately* available in sufficient quantities. Otherwise, the flames should be smothered with a coat, rug or blanket.

The victim of a serious burn should lie down to lessen shock, and a physician should be called. The head and chest should be kept lower than the rest of the body, and the legs should be elevated, if possible. In shock, the liquid part of the blood rushes to the burned area, and there may not be enough left to maintain normal function of the heart, brain and other vital organs. Therefore these organs should be lowered so that gravity will help send them a supply of blood.

With attention to cleanliness to prevent contamination, dry dressings of sterile gauze are applied over the burned areas. If sterile dressings are not available, at least four layers of clean cotton cloth should be used. To protect the burn from air, the dressings are covered with a layer of tightly woven cloth; protecting a burn from air helps to relieve pain, and the application of a sterile dressing reduces the danger of infection. In case of an extensive burn, the victim should be wrapped in a clean sheet and transported to a hospital.

Attempts should *not* be made to remove clothing from a burned area; the clothing should be cut around the area. Absorbent cotton, oily substances and antiseptics are *not* used on a burn. Blisters are *not* opened or disturbed in any way.

If the victim is conscious and can swallow, he is given fluids to quench his thirst. If medical aid is not available quickly, he should be given, at 15 minute intervals, a solution of ½ teaspoonful of salt and ½ teaspoonful of sodium bicarbonate (baking soda) dissolved in a quart of water. This is discontinued if it causes nausea.

Minor Burns. For a small first-degree burn, the reddened area is immersed in clean cold water or ice cubes are applied. This relieves the pain. Or a sterile gauze pad or clean cloth soaked in a solution of 2 tablespoonfuls of sodium bicarbonate (baking soda) dissolved in a quart of lukewarm water is applied and bandaged loosely. Or a paste of baking soda and water, or petroleum jelly, may be applied and covered with sterile gauze.

Even first-degree burns are extremely serious if they involve a large area. They should receive prompt medical attention. Death may result if a first-degree burn covers as much as two-thirds of

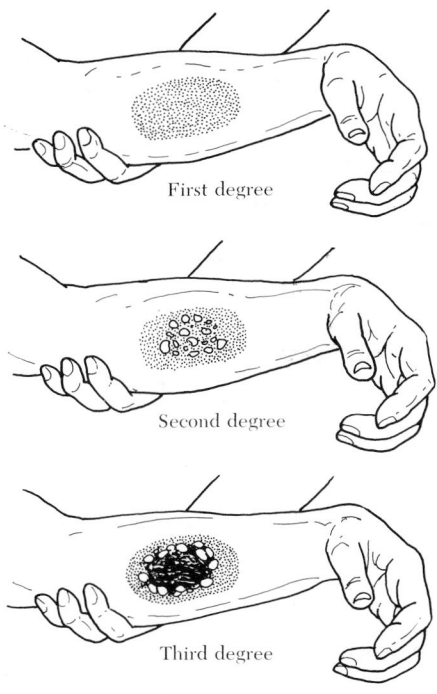

First degree

Second degree

Third degree

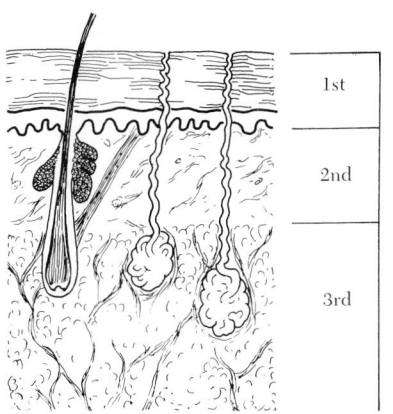

1st

2nd

3rd

First-degree burns damage the epidermis; second-degree burns damage both epidermis and dermis; third-degree burns damage the epidermis, dermis and subcutaneous tissue.

the body area. On a child such burns are dangerous on a smaller area of the skin.

Chemical and Other Burns. For chemical burns, such as those caused by acids, the affected area should be bathed immediately with water, using plenty of water and continuing bathing the area until all of the chemical has been washed away. A physician should be called and first-aid treatment should be given as for any similar heat burn. If the burned area is extensive, the victim should lie down and be treated for shock.

If the area affected is the eye, it is held open and flushed gently but thoroughly with water. Then it is covered with a sterile dressing and medical aid is sought immediately.

In electrical burns, shock is the main danger. It may be necessary to use artificial respiration. This should be begun as soon as contact with the current has been broken. A person struck by lightning also requires artificial respiration if the shock has been severe enough to interfere with normal breathing.

Safety measures in the home and on the job are extremely important in the prevention of burns.

HOSPITAL TREATMENT. The burned areas of the body may be treated by one of two methods: the open method in which no dressings are applied and the wound is left uncovered; and the closed method in which the wound is covered with dressings and various medications such as sterile petrolatum or nitrofurazone (Furacin) ointment are applied. Before either of these methods is employed the entire burned area is thoroughly cleansed with a mild antiseptic or antibacterial soap and water.

In recent years there has been interest in the use of 0.5 per cent silver nitrate in the treatment of burns. The dressings on the wound are soaked in this solution periodically so that the dressings are kept wet at all times. The dressings are changed every 12 to 24 hours, depending on the amount of drainage from the wound. Those who advocate this method believe that it reduces infection and fever and promotes healing with a minimum of scarring.

Nursing Care. Prevention of shock and avoiding contamination of the wound are of immediate concern. The principal causes of death from burns are the initial shock suffered by the victim and infection of the wound. Nursing measures aimed at avoiding these problems include: protection of the patient from loss of body heat; careful and accurate taking and recording of the vital signs; and extreme care in handling equipment, dressings or other articles that come in contact with the wound.

An accurate record of intake and output is of primary importance. Since large amounts of the body fluids and many essential minerals and salts are lost through open wounds caused by burns, it is imperative to keep a record of fluids lost through the kidneys or intestinal tract (by emesis or diarrhea). Observations should include not only the amount lost but also the color, concentration, unusual odor or any other characteristic of the patient's urine.

A high-protein diet with supplemental vitamins and minerals is used to aid the body in its repair of damaged tissue. Ingenuity and imagination must be used in convincing the patient that he must eat all of his meals as well as the between-meal feedings prepared for him.

Proper positioning and exercises are necessary to prevent permanent and crippling contractions of the skeletal muscles (CONTRACTURES). Even though motion may be painful for the patient he must be helped to understand that the muscles must be gently stretched and used every day if they are to be kept in a good state of tone and functioning normally.

Burow's solution　(boor'ovz) a preparation of albumin subacetate and glacial acetic acid; used for its antiseptic and astringent action on the skin. Called also aluminum acetate solution.

bursa　(bur'sah), pl. *bur'sae, bursas* [L.] a small fluid-filled sac that allows one part of a joint to move easily over another part or over other structures. Bursae function to facilitate the gliding of muscles or tendons over bony or ligamentous surfaces. They are numerous and are found throughout the body; the most important are located at the shoulder, elbow, knee and hip. Inflammation of a bursa is known as BURSITIS.

　　b. anseri'na, one under the insertion of the sartorius and gracilis muscles.

　　b. muco'sa, synovial b., any membranous sac that secretes synovia.

bursalogy　(bur-sal'o-je) the study of bursae.

bursectomy　(bur-sek'to-me) excision of a bursa.

bursitis　(bur-si'tis) inflammation of a bursa. The bursa of the shoulder is most commonly affected, but inflammation may develop in almost any bursa in the body. Excessive use of the joint or chilling or a draft on the joint may be the cause.

Acute bursitis comes on suddenly; severe pain and limitation of motion of the affected joint are the principal symptoms. Resting the joint in a sling and applications of moist heat frequently are sufficient treatment. In some cases it may be necessary to aspirate fluid and calcium salts from the inflamed area. Steroids, such as cortisone, hydrocortisone and ACTH, injected into the joint, may be effective in relieving acute attacks. X-ray therapy is also frequently effective.

Chronic bursitis may follow the acute attacks. There is continued pain and limitation of motion around the joint. X-ray examination will usually reveal the deposit of calcium salts. If rest, heat and medications do not relieve the condition, x-ray therapy or surgery may be required to remove the calcium deposits or free the area of chronic inflammation.

bursolith　(būr'so-lith) a calculus in a bursa.

bursopathy　(būr-sop'ah-the) any disease of a bursa.

bursotomy　(bur-sot'o-me) incision of a bursa.

Busse-Buschke disease　(boos'ĕ boosh'ke) cryptococcosis.

busulfan　(bu-sul'fan) an alkylating agent that acts selectively on the bone marrow, depressing granulocyte formation, and therefore used in the treatment of myelocytic (granulocytic) leukemias. Side effects include nausea and vomiting, and heavy doses may lead to excessive bone marrow depression. Complete blood counts (including platelet counts) must be done frequently while the drug is being administered and are used as a guide to dosage and effects on bone marrow production.

butabarbital　(bu″tah-bar'bĭ-tal) a short- to intermediate-acting barbiturate.

butacaine sulfate　(bu'tah-kān) a colorless, odorless, crystalline powder; used instead of cocaine for topical anesthesia in the eye and on mucous membranes.

butamben　(bu-tam'ben) butyl aminobenzoate, a topical anesthetic.

butane　(bu'tān) an anesthetic hydrocarbon, C_4H_{10}.

Butazolidin　(bu″tah-zol'ĭ-din) trademark for a preparation of phenylbutazone, an analgesic and antipyretic.

Butesin　(bu-te'sin) trademark for a preparation of butyl aminobenzoate, a topical anesthetic.

butethamine　(bu-teth'ah-mēn) an agent used as a local anesthetic.

Butisol　(bu'tĭ-sol) trademark for preparations of butabarbital, a short- to intermediate-acting barbiturate.

buttock　(but'ok) either of the two fleshy masses formed by the gluteal muscles, on the posterior aspect of the lower trunk.

butyl　(bu'til) a hydrocarbon radical, C_4H_9.

　　b. aminobenzoate, a white crystalline powder used as a topical anesthetic. Excessive amounts may be absorbed if applied to broken skin and can produce systemic toxic effects. The drug is available in powder, ointment or suppository forms.

butylene　(bu'tĭ-lēn) a gaseous hydrocarbon, C_4H_8.

butyraceous　(bu″tĭ-ra'shus) resembling butter.

butyrate　(bu'tĭ-rāt) a salt of butyric acid.

Butyribacterium　(bu-ti″re-bak-te're-um) a genus of Schizomycetes occurring as nonpathogenic parasites in the intestinal tract.

butyric acid　(bu-tir'ik) a saturated fatty acid found in butter.

butyrin　(bu'tĭ-rin) a yellowish fat, the chief constituent of butter.

butyroid, butyrous　(bu'tĭ-roid), (bu'tĭ-rus) resembling butter.

byssaceous　(bis-sa'shus) composed of fine, flaxlike threads.

byssinosis　(bis″ĭ-no'sis) a lung disease due to inhalation of cotton dust.

C

C chemical symbol, *carbon*.

C. Celsius, or less correctly, centigrade.

Ca chemical symbol, *calcium*.

cacanthrax (kak-an'thraks) anthrax.

cacesthesia (kak″es-the'ze-ah) disordered sensibility.

caché (kah-sha') [Fr.] a lead cone used for applying a radioactive substance.

cachet (kah-sha') [Fr.] a wafer or capsule for medicines.

cachexia (kah-kek'se-ah) a state of malnutrition, emaciation and debility, usually in the course of a chronic illness. adj., **cachec'tic.**
  pituitary c., that due to diminution or absence of pituitary function.

cachinnation (kak″ĭ-na'shun) excessive or hysterical laughter.

cacodyl (kak'o-dil) a poisonous arsenical compound.

cacogenics (kak″o-jen'iks) deterioration of the physical and moral properties of a race resulting from the mating and propagation of inferior individuals. adj., **cacogen'ic.**

cacogeusia (kak″o-gu'se-ah) a bad taste.

cacomelia (kak″o-me'le-ah) congenital deformity of a limb.

cacoplastic (kak″o-plas'tik) susceptible of imperfect organization only.

cacorhythmic (kak″o-rith'mik) marked by irregularity of rhythm.

cacosmia (kak-oz'me-ah) foul odor; stench.

cacotrophy (kak-ot'ro-fe) malnutrition.

cacumen (kah-ku'men), pl. *cacu'mina* [L.] 1. the top or apex of an organ. 2. the part of the cerebellum below the declivis; called also culmen.

cadaver (kah-dav'er) a dead body.

cadmium (kad'me-um) a chemical element, atomic number 48, atomic weight 112.40, symbol Cd. (See table of ELEMENTS.)
  c. sulfide, a light yellow or orange powder used, in a 1 per cent suspension, in treatment of seborrheic dermatitis of the scalp (dandruff).

caduceus (kah-du'se-us) the wand of Hermes or Mercury; used as a symbol of the medical profession and as the emblem of the Medical Corps of the U.S. Army. Another symbol of medicine is the staff of Æsculapius, which is the official insignia of the American Medical Association.

cae- for words beginning thus, see also those beginning *ce-*.

caelotherapy (se″lo-ther'ah-pe) the therapeutic use of religion and religious symbols.

caffeine (kaf'ēn, kaf'e-in) a white powder, slightly soluble in water and having a bitter taste, found in coffee and tea. It is an alkaloid and acts as a central nervous system stimulant and a mild diuretic.
  citrated c., a white, odorless powder, mixture of caffeine and citric acid.
  c. sodium benzoate, a mixture of equal parts of anhydrous caffeine and sodium benzoate, used as a central nervous system stimulant; overdosage may produce nervousness and wakefulness.

caffeinism (kaf'ēn-izm) a morbid state induced by excessive use of coffee or tea.

Caffey's disease (kaf'fēz) infantile cortical hyperostosis.

cainotophobia (ki-no″to-fo'be-ah) morbid dread of anything new.

caisson disease (ka'son) decompression sickness, a condition suffered by underwater workers and caused by too-rapid decrease in atmospheric pressure. The condition is named after the pressurized, watertight compartments (caissons) in which underwater construction men work. The main symptoms are dizziness, staggering, muscle spasms, difficulty in breathing, abdominal pain, and partial paralysis. Caisson disease is a form of BENDS.

Cal. large calorie (kilogram calorie).

cal. small calorie (gram calorie).

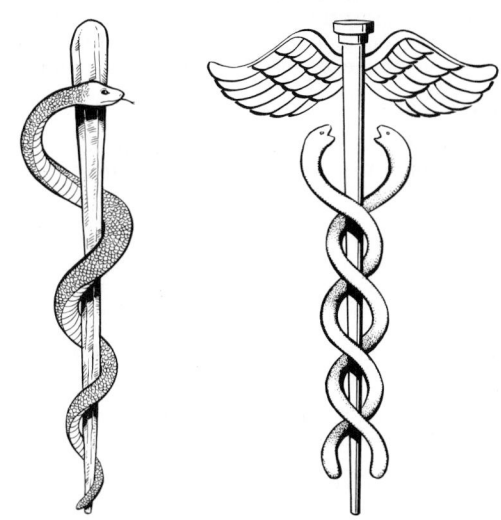

Staff of Æsculapius.   Caduceus.

calamine (kal′ah-mīn) a mixture of zinc and ferric oxides, used topically in lotions and ointments.

calcaneo-apophysitis (kal-ka″ne-o-ah-pof″ĭ-si′-tis) inflammation of the posterior part of the calcaneus, marked by pain and swelling.

calcaneodynia (kal-ka″ne-o-din′e-ah) pain in the heel.

calcaneum, calcaneus (kal-ka′ne-um), (kal-ka′-ne-us) the irregular quadrangular bone at the back of the tarsus; called also heel bone and os calcis.

calcar (kal′kar) a spur.
  c. a′vis, a white elevation in the floor of the posterior horn of the lateral ventricle; called also hippocampus minor.

calcareous (kal-kār′e-us) containing lime; chalky.

calcarine (kal′kar-in) 1. spur-shaped. 2. pertaining to the calcar avis.

calcariuria (kal-kār″e-u′re-ah) the presence of lime salts in the urine.

calcemia (kal-se′me-ah) excessive calcium in the blood.

calcibilia (kal″sĭ-bil′e-ah) the presence of calcium in the bile.

calcicosis (kal″sĭ-ko′sis) a lung disease due to inhalation of marble dust.

calciferol (kal-sif′er-ol) activated ergosterol, used in treating vitamin D deficiency.

calcific (kal-sif′ik) forming lime.

calcification (kal″sĭ-fĭ-ka′shun) the deposit of calcium salts in a tissue. The normal absorption of calcium is facilitated by parathyroid hormone and by vitamin D. When there are increased amounts of parathyroid hormone in the blood (as in hyperparathyroidism), there is deposition of calcium in the alveoli of the lungs, the renal tubules, the thyroid gland, the gastric mucosa and the arterial walls. Normally calcium is deposited in the bone matrix to insure stability and strength of the bone. In OSTEOMALACIA there is decalcification of bone because of a failure of calcium and phosphorus to be deposited in the bone matrix.

calcine (kal′sīn) to reduce to a dry powder.

calcinosis (kal″sĭ-no′sis) a condition characterized by abnormal deposition of calcium salts in the tissues.
  c. circumscrip′ta, a condition marked by calcifications occurring only in subcutaneous fat.
  c. universa′lis, calcinosis in which calcifications appear in other connective tissues, as well as in subcutaneous fat.

calciokinesis (kal″se-o-ki-ne′sis) mobilization of calcium stored in the body.

calcipenia (kal″sĭ-pe′ne-ah) deficiency of calcium in the system.

calcipexy (kal′sĭ-pek″se) fixation of calcium in the tissues. adj., **calcipec′tic, calcipex′ic.**

calciphilia (kal″sĭ-fil′e-ah) a tendency to calcification.

calciphylaxis (kal″sĭ-fi-lak′sis) the formation of calcified tissue in response to administration of a challenging agent after induction of a hypersensitive state.

calciprivia (kal″sĭ-priv′e-ah) deprivation or loss of calcium.

calcitonin (kal″sĭ-to′nin) a polypeptide, thought to be a secretion of the thyroid gland, which lowers both calcium and phosphate in the plasma.

calcium (kal′se-um) a chemical element, atomic number 20, atomic weight 40.08, symbol Ca. (See table of ELEMENTS.) Calcium is the most abundant mineral in the body. In combination with phosphorus it forms calcium phosphate, the dense, hard material of the bones and teeth.
  A constant level of a small amount of calcium in the blood is required for certain important body functions, including maintenance of the heartbeat, clotting of blood (in which it is considered clotting factor IV) and normal functioning of muscles and nerves.
  The body obtains calcium from food sources. Milk and cheese are the readiest sources, and other dairy products are rich in calcium. Molasses, turnip greens and dandelion greens also provide calcium. In addition, vitamin D is necessary to put the calcium to use.
  Calcium deficiency diseases may be due to an insufficient amount of calcium food sources in the diet, to a lack of vitamin D or occasionally to a disorder of the parathyroid glands.
  The most familiar calcium deficiency disease is rickets, in which the bones and teeth soften. Calcium deficiency may also impair blood clotting and cause nervous and muscular disturbances. Tetany, a disorder characterized by convulsive muscle cramps, is due to underactivity of the parathyroid glands, which causes the level of blood calcium to fall.
  c. bromide, a hydrated salt, containing 84 to 94 per cent calcium bromide; used in asthma and convulsive disorders.
  c. carbonate, a compound occurring naturally in bones, shells, etc.; also prepared artificially and used as an antacid.
  c. carbonate, precipitated, a white, microcrystalline powder used as an antacid.
  c. chloride, a deliquescent compound used as an electrolyte replenisher.
  c. cyclamate, an odorless, white crystalline compound formerly used as a noncaloric sweetener.
  c. disodium edetate, EDTA, a white soluble powder that acts as a chelating agent; that is, it draws certain metals from their combination with tissues and alters them so that they become more soluble and less toxic, and accelerates their elimination from the body. Called also calcium disodium versenate. EDTA is used chiefly in the treatment of lead poisoning. It is administered intravenously in saline or dextrose solution. It is not to be confused with DISODIUM EDETATE which is used specifically to remove calcium and lower blood calcium levels.
  c. gluconate, used to replenish calcium in the body.
  c. glycerophosphate, a fine, white, odorless powder used in bone diseases.
  c. hydroxide, an astringent compound used topically in solution or lotions.

c. lactate, a white, almost odorless compound used as an electrolyte replenisher.

c. mandelate, a white, odorless powder used as a urinary antiseptic.

c. oxalate, a compound occurring in the urine in crystals and in certain calculi.

c. oxide, lime.

c. pantothenate, a calcium salt of the dextrorotatory isomer of pantothenic acid, used as a growth-promoting vitamin.

c. phosphate, dibasic, a white, odorless powder, used to replenish calcium in the body.

c. phosphate, tribasic, a compound used as an antacid and source of calcium.

c. sulfate, a compound of calcium and sulfate. Dry calcium sulfate has been used as an absorbent dressing for ulcers and wounds; calcium sulfate dihydrate, or plaster of paris, is used in dressings to support or immobilize parts.

calciuria (kal″se-u′re-ah) calcium in the urine.

calcospherite (kal″ko-sfēr′īt) a small calcareous body found in tumors, nerve tissue, etc.

calculifragous (kal″ku-lif′rah-gus) breaking up calculi in the bladder.

calculogenesis (kal″ku-lo-jen′ĕ-sis) the formation of calculi.

calculosis (kal″ku-lo′sis) a condition characterized by the presence of calculi.

calculus (kal′ku-lus), pl. *cal′culi* [L.] a small hard mass formed chiefly in the hollow organs of the body or their passages. Called also stones, as in kidney stones (see also KIDNEY) and GALLSTONES. adj., **cal′culous.**

  biliary c., a gallstone.

  dendritic c., an irregular, branching calculus formed in the renal pelvis and calices.

  dental c., an adherent, calcified mass of bacteria, fungi, desquamated epithelial cells and food debris, formed on the surface of teeth and dental appliances.

  renal c., a calculus occurring in the kidney.

  urinary c., a calculus in any part of the urinary tract.

  vesical c., one in the urinary bladder.

calefacient (kal″ĕ-fa′shent) causing a sensation of warmth.

calf (kaf) the fleshy back part of the leg below the knee.

caliber (kal′ĭ-ber) the diameter of a canal or tube.

calibrator (kal″ĭ-bra′ter) a device for measuring the caliber of a canal or tube.

calicectasis (kal″i-sek′tah-sis) dilatation of a calix of the kidney.

calicectomy (kal″i-sek′to-me) excision of a calix of the kidney.

calices (kal′ĭ-sēs) plural of *calix.*

caliculus (kah-lik′u-lus) a small, bud- or cup-shaped structure.

California disease coccidioidomycosis.

californium (kal″ĭ-fōr′ne-um) a chemical element, atomic number 98, atomic weight 249, symbol Cf. (See table of ELEMENTS.)

calipers (kal′ĭ-perz) a two-bladed instrument used in taking measurements.

calisthenics (kal″is-then′iks) systematic exercise for attaining strength and gracefulness.

calix (ka′liks), pl. *cal′ices* [L.] a cuplike structure, such as one of the recesses of the kidney pelvis receiving the summits of the renal pyramids. adj., **calice′al.**

callosity (kah-los′ĭ-te) a callus (1).

callosum (kah-lo′sum) corpus callosum.

callous (kal′us) of the nature of a callus; hard.

callus (kal′us) 1. an acquired, localized area of thickening of the stratum corneum, resulting from continued physical trauma. 2. fibrous tissue formed by condensation of granulation tissue at the site of fracture, in which fibrocartilage and hyaline cartilage form, sealing the ends of the bone together (provisional callus) and being ultimately replaced by mature bone (permanent callus).

calmative (kal′mah-tiv, kah′mah-tiv) 1. having a calming or sedative effect. 2. an agent that has a calming or sedative effect.

calomel (kal′o-mel) a heavy white powder, mercurous chloride, used rarely as a cathartic. It increases peristalsis and glandular secretions, especially of bile. It is also used rarely as an intestinal antiseptic and to reduce edema, or in an ointment as a local antibacterial agent.

calor (kal′er) [L.] heat.

caloric (kah-lor′ik) pertaining to heat.

caloricity (kal″o-ris′ĭ-te) the power of the body of developing heat.

calorie (kal′o-re) a unit of measurement of heat. One calorie is the amount of heat required to raise the temperature of 1 kilogram of water by 1 degree Celsius (C.) (This is about the same as the amount of heat required to raise the temperature of 1 lb. of water by 4 degrees Fahrenheit.) It is possible to calculate the amount of energy contained in a certain food by measuring the amount of heat units, or calories, in that food. Every bodily process—the building up of cells, motion of the muscles, the maintenance of body temperature—requires energy, and the body derives this energy from the food it consumes. Digestive processes reduce food to usable "fuel," which the body "burns" in the complex chemical reactions that sustain life.

The amount of energy required for these chemical processes varies. Factors such as weight, age, activity and metabolic rate determine a person's daily calorie requirement. Nutrition experts have computed daily calorie requirements in terms of age and other factors. These tabulations serve only as guides; they cannot, of course, embrace all individual variations.

AVERAGE CALORIE REQUIREMENTS

Adult male	2900 calories
Adult female	2000 calories
Adolescent male	3400 calories
Adolescent female	2400 calories
Retired male	2200 calories
Retired female	1600 calories

CALORIE CHART

FOOD AND MEASURES*	APPROXIMATE CALORIES	FOOD AND MEASURES*	APPROXIMATE CALORIES	FOOD AND MEASURES*	APPROXIMATE CALORIES
Apple, baked, 1 large and 2 tbs. sugar	200	Cream, light, 2 tbs.	65	Peas, canned, ½ cup	65
fresh, 1 large	100	heavy, 2 tbs.	120	fresh, shelled, ¾ cup	100
Asparagus, fresh or canned, 5 stalks, 5 in. long	15	whipped, 3 tbs.	100	Pepper, green, 1 medium	20
Avocado, ½ 4-in. pear	265	Custard, ½ cup	130	Pie, apple, 3-in. sector	200
				mincemeat, 3-in. sector	300
Bacon, 2-3 long slices, cooked	100	Eggs, medium	75	Pineapple, fresh, 1 slice, ¾ in. thick	50
Banana, 1 medium, 6 in. long	90	Eggplant, 3 slices, 4 in. diam., ½ in. thick, raw	50	canned, unsweetened, 1 slice, ½ in. thick, 1 tbs. juice	50
Beans, lima, fresh or canned, ½ cup	100	Flour, 1 tbs., unsifted	35	juice, unsweetened, 1 cup	135
green or yellow, fresh or canned, ½ cup	25	Frankfurter	125	Pork chop, lean, 1 medium	200
canned with pork, ½ cup	175			Potato chips, 8-10 large	100
Beef (cooked), corned, 1 slice 4 by 1½ in. by 1 in.	100	Gelatin, fruit flavored, ready to serve, ½ cup	85	Potato salad with mayonnaise, ½ cup	200
hamburger, 3 oz.	300	Grapefruit juice, unsweetened, 1 cup	100	Potatoes, mashed, ½ cup	100
round, lean, 1 medium slice (2 oz.)	125	Grape juice, ½ cup	80	sweet, ½ medium	100
sirloin lean, 1 average slice (3 oz.)	250	Griddle cake, 4 in. diam.	75	white, 1 medium	100
tongue, 2 oz.	125			Prunes, dried, 4 medium	100
Beets, fresh or canned, 2, 2-in. in diam.	50	Halibut, 1 piece, 3 by 1⅜ by 1 in.	100	Pumpkin, ½ cup	50
Bread, corn (1 egg), 1, 2-in. square	120	Ham, lean, 1 slice, 4¼ by 4 by ½ in.	265	Raisins, ¼ cup	90
rye, 1 slice, ½ in. thick	70–75	Hominy grits, cooked, ¾ cup	100	Rice, cooked, ¾ cup	100
white, enriched, 1 slice, average	75			Rutabagas, ½ cup	30
whole wheat, 100%, 1 slice average	75	Ice cream, ½ cup	200	Salad dressing, French, 1 tbs.	90
Broccoli, 3 stalks, 5½ in. long	100	Ice cream soda, fountain size	325	mayonnaise, 1 tbs.	100
Brussels sprouts, 6 sprouts, 1½ in. diam.	50			Salmon, canned, ½ cup	100
Butter, 1 tbs.	95	Jellies and jams, 1 rounded tbs.	100	Sauerkraut, ½ cup	15
				Soup, condensed, 11-oz. can, mushroom	360
Cabbage, cooked, ½ cup	40	Lamb, roast, 1 slice, 3½ by 4½ by ⅛ in.	100	tomato	230
raw, 1 cup	25	Lettuce, 2 large leaves	5	vegetable	200
Cake, angel, 1/10 large cake		Liver, 1 slice, 3 by 3 by ½ in.	100	Spaghetti, cooked, ¾ cup	100
choc, or vanilla, with icing 2 by 1½ by 2 in.	155 200	Liverwurst, 2 oz.	130	Spinach, cooked, ½ cup	20
cupcake (med.), choc. icing	250	Macaroni, cooked, ¾ cup	100	Squash, summer, cooked, ½ cup	20
Cantaloupe, ½ 5½-in. melon	50	Maple syrup, 1 tbs.	70	winter, cooked, ½ cup	50
Carrot, 4 in. long	25	Margarine, 1 tbs.	100	Sugar, brown, 1 tbs.	50
Cauliflower, ¼ of head, 4½ in. in diam.	25	Milk, buttermilk, 1 cup	85	granulated, 1 tbs.	50
Celery, 2 stalks	15	condensed, 1½ tbs.	100	Tapioca, uncooked, 1 tbs.	50
Cheese, American cheddar, 1 cube 1⅛ in. square	110	evaporated, ½ cup	160	Tomato juice, 1 cup	60
cottage, 5 tbs.	100	skim, 1 cup	85	Tomatoes, canned, ½ cup	25
cream, 2 tbs.	100	whole, 1 cup	170	fresh, 1 medium	30
Chicken, ½ med. broiler	270	yogurt, plain, 1 cup	120–160	Tuna fish, canned, ¼ cup, drained	100
Chocolate, milk, sweetened 1 oz.	140	Mushrooms, 10 large	10	Turnip, 1, 1¾ in. diam.	25
malted milk, fountain size	460	Noodles, cooked, ¾ cup	75	Veal, roast, 1 slice, 3 by 3¾ by ½ in.	120
syrup, ¼ cup	200				
Cocoa, half milk, half water, 1 cup	150	Oatmeal, cooked, ¾ cup	110	Waffle, 6 in. in diam.	250
Cod steak, 1 piece, 3½ by 2 by 1 in.	100	Oil, corn, cottonseed, olive, peanut, 1 tbs.	100	Wheat flakes, ¾ cup	100
Cola soft drinks, 6-oz. bottle	75	Olives, green, 6 medium	50	**Alcoholic Beverages**	
Collards, ½ cup, cooked	50	ripe, 4-5 medium	50	Beer, 8 oz.	120
Corn, ½ cup	70	Onions, 3-4 medium	100	Gin, 1½ oz.	120
Corn flakes, 1 cup	80	Orange, 1 medium	80	Rum, 1½ oz.	150
Cracker, graham, 1 square	35	juice, 1 cup	125	Whisky, 1½ oz.	150
saltine, 2-in. square	15	Parsnip, 7 in. long	100	Wines	
		Peach, fresh, 1 medium	50	champagne, 4 oz.	120
		canned in syrup, 2 lg. halves, 3 tbs. juice	100	port, 1 oz.	50
		Peanut butter, 1 tbs.	100	sherry, 1 oz.	40
		Peanuts, shelled, 10	50	table, red or white, 4 oz.	95
		Pear, fresh, 1 medium	50		
		canned in syrup, 3 halves, 3 tbs. juice	100		

*1 cup equals 8 ounces (oz.); 3 teaspoons (tsp.) equal 1 tablespoon (tbs.); 4 tablespoons (tbs.) equal ¼ cup.
Courtesy of the Metropolitan Life Insurance Company.

From its daily intake of energy foods, the body uses only the amount it needs for energy purposes. The remainder is stored as fat; hence the utility of calorie counting in weight control. If the average adult male consumes more than his 2900-calorie daily requirement, he will gain weight. However, if he consumes less than 2900 calories, the body will supplement its energy sources by drawing upon fat which the body has stored away, and he will lose weight.

A person can usually gain or lose weight as he wishes by keeping to a daily diet with a calorie count above or below his daily requirement.

gram c., small calorie.

kilogram c., large calorie.

large c., the calorie used in metabolic studies, being the amount of heat required to raise the temperature of 1 kg. of water 1 degree Celsius (C.).

small c., the amount of heat required to raise the temperature of 1 Gm. of water 1 degree Celsius (C.).

standard c., small calorie.

calorifacient (kah-lor″ĭ-fa′shent) heat-producing.

calorific (kal″o-rif′ik) producing heat.

calorigenic (kah-lor″ĭ-jen′ik) 1. generating heat. 2. increasing the rate of oxidation of tissue cells.

calorimeter (kal″o-rim′ĕ-ter) a laboratory device for the rapid measurement of the heat evolved in any system.

calorimetry (kal″o-rim′ĕ-tre) measurement of the actual heat eliminated or stored in any system.

calvaria, calvarium (kal-va′re-ah), (kal-va′re-um) the domelike superior portion of the cranium, comprising superior portions of the frontal, parietal and occipital bones.

Calvé-Perthes disease (kal-va′ per′tēz) osteochondrosis of the epiphysis at the head of the femur.

calx (kalks) 1. calcium oxide, or lime. 2. the hindmost part of the foot; the heel.

calyculus (kah-lik′u-lus) caliculus.

Calymmatobacterium (kah-lim″mah-to-bak-te′-re-um) a genus of Schizomycetes made up of gram-negative rods.

calyx (ka′liks) calix.

camera (kam′er-ah), pl. *cam′erae* [L.] a cavity or chamber.

Camoquin (kam′o-kwin) trademark for a preparation of amodiaquine, an antimalarial.

camphor (kam′fer) a ketone derived from a cinnamon tree, *Cinnamomum camphora*, or produced synthetically, used locally as an analgesic and antipruritic agent.

camphorate (kam′fer-āt) to combine with camphor.

camptocormia (kamp″to-kor′me-ah) a static deformity characterized by forward flexion of the trunk.

camptodactylia (kamp″to-dak-til′e-ah) a claw-like condition of the hand or foot.

camptospasm (kamp′to-spazm) camptocormia.

canal (kah-nal′) a relatively narrow tubular passage in the body.

Alcocks's c., a sheath of the obturator fascia containing the internal pudendal artery.

alimentary c., the digestive tube from mouth to anus.

anal c., the most distal portion of the digestive tract.

atrioventricular c., the common canal connecting the primitive atrium and ventricle; it sometimes persists as a congenital anomaly.

birth c., the canal through which the fetus passes in birth.

carotid c., one in the pars petrosa of the temporal bone, transmitting the internal carotid artery.

femoral c., the cone-shaped medial part of the femoral sheath lateral to the base of Gimbernat's ligament.

haversian c., one of the anastomosing channels of the haversian system in compact bone, containing blood and lymph vessels, nerves and marrow.

Hunter's c., a triangular canal in the great adductor muscle of the thigh, transmitting the femoral artery and vein and the saphenous nerve.

infraorbital c., a small canal running obliquely through the floor of the orbit, transmitting the infraorbital artery and nerve.

inguinal c., a space at the lower margin on either side between the layers composing the abdominal wall, through which passes the round ligament of the uterus in the female, and the spermatic cord in the male.

medullary c., the cavity of a long bone, containing the marrow.

pulp c., the hollow part of the root of a tooth, containing the pulp.

sacral c., the continuation of the spinal canal in the sacrum.

Schlemm's c., the venous sinus of the sclera, a circular canal at the junction of the sclera and cornea.

semicircular c's, long canals in the labyrinth of the ear (see also SEMICIRCULAR CANALS).

spinal c., vertebral c., the canal through the vertebrae, transmitting the spinal cord.

Volkmann's c's, canals in the subperiosteal layer of bones communicating with haversian canals.

canaliculus (kan″ah-lik′u-lus), pl. *canalic′uli* [L.] a small canal or channel. adj., **canalic′ular.**

bile canaliculi, fine tubular channels forming a three-dimensional network within the parenchyma of the liver.

lacrimal c., the short passage in an eyelid, beginning at the lacrimal point and draining tears from the lacrimal lake to the lacrimal sac; called also lacrimal duct.

mastoid c., a small channel in the temporal bone transmitting the auricular branch of the vagus nerve.

canalis (kah-na′lis), pl. *cana′les* [L.] a canal or channel.

canalization (kan″al-ĭ-za′shun) the formation of canals in a mass of tissue by the anastomosis and progressive dilation of organizing capillary channels.

canaloplasty (kah-nal′o-plas″te) plastic reconstruction of a passage, as of the external acoustic meatus.

canavanine   (kah-nav'ah-nin) a naturally occurring amino acid, isolated from soybean meal.

cancellate (kan'sel-āt) having a lattice-like structure.

cancellous (kan'sĕ-lus) of a reticular, spongy, or
lattice-like structure; used mainly of bone tissue.

cancellus   (kan-sel'us), pl. *cancel'li* [L.] the
lattice-like structure in bone.

cancer   (kan'ser) any malignant tumor. adj.,
can'cerous. Cancer is a neoplastic disease in which
there is new growth of abnormal cells. Normally
the cells that compose body tissues grow in response to a normal stimulus. Worn-out body cells
are regularly replaced by new cell growth which
stops when the cells are replaced; new cells form to
repair tissue damage and stop forming when
healing is complete. Why they stop forming is unknown, but clearly the body in its normal processes
regulates cell growth. In cancer, cell growth is un-
regulated. The cells continue to reproduce until
they form a mass of tissue known as a tumor. Not
all tumors are malignant; those which are noncancerous are referred to as benign tumors. Benign
tumors vary in size, and may grow so large that they
obstruct organs or cause ulceration and bleeding.
They are encapsulated, do not metastasize and usually can be removed by surgery without difficulty.

Malignant tumors grow in a disorganized fashion,
interrupting body functions and robbing normal
cells of their food and blood supply. The malignant
cells may spread to other parts of the body by (1)
direct extension into adjacent tissue, (2) permeation along lymphatic vessels, (3) traveling in the
lymph stream to the lymph nodes, (4) entering the
blood circulation and (5) invasion of a body cavity
by diffusion.

CAUSES.   Cancer is many different diseases and
no one factor can be pinpointed as the cause of the
various types of malignant growths. Environmental, hereditary and biologic influences seem to
play an important part. There are known to be certain agents that can divert cells from their normal
growth pattern, causing them to become malignant. These cancer-causing agents are called carcinogens, and include both chemical and physical
irritants. Examples include irradiation (including
prolonged exposure to sunlight), some synthetic
dyes, various metallic dusts, and certain by-products of petroleum. Chemicals suspected of being
carcinogens include asbestos, arsenic, nickel, coal
tar and substances found in some insecticides. Certain chemicals found in cigarette smoke and
atmospheric pollution are also considered carcinogens.

Hormones are also known to be involved in cancer. Research has shown that breast cancer can be
caused in mice by injecting them with certain hormones. At the same time, hormones can be extremely useful in the treatment of certain kinds of
cancer.

The occurrence of types of cancer varies from
one country to another. Stomach cancer is common in Ireland and Japan but rare in Ecuador and
Indonesia. Breast cancer, common in the United
States, is rare in Japan. And in the United States
mortality from stomach cancer has declined since
World War II, but the reason for the decline is
unknown.

Viruses have been shown to cause cancer in laboratory animals, although there is still no evidence
that they can cause cancer in man. If viruses were
proved to cause cancer in man, this would offer the
possibility of preparing a vaccine against the disease.

CLASSIFICATION.   Cancers are divided into two
large groups: SARCOMAS and CARCINOMAS. Sarcomas are of mesenchymal origin and affect such
tissues as the bones and muscles. They tend to
grow rapidly and to be very destructive. The carcinomas are of epithelial origin and make up the
great majority of the glandular cancers and cancers of the breast, stomach, uterus, skin and tongue.

Precancers. Some potentially dangerous cancers appear first in the form of harmless changes in
the body's tissues. Their danger lies in the fact
that they have a tendency to become malignant.
Hence they are known as precancers. Among these
are sores that appear as thickened white patches
(leukoplakia) in the mouth and on the vulva, some
moles and any chronically irritated area on the skin
or the mucous membranes of the mouth and tongue. Polyps also are possible precancers, as are
some forms of lymphomas.

Hodgkin's Disease. This disease is generally
considered a form of cancer. It usually afflicts
young people, causing a progressive enlargement of
the lymph nodes, in most cases starting in the neck,
groin or armpit. Treatment may be by surgery,
radiotherapy, use of certain chemicals or a combination of these (see HODGKIN'S DISEASE).

Leukemias. In these diseases, abnormal leukocytes are produced in enormous quantities. The
leukemias respond to much the same treatment as
cancer and are commonly considered cancers (see
LEUKEMIA).

SYMPTOMS OF CANCER.   There are seven early
warning signs of cancer. *These signs do not
necessarily signify cancer, but should they occur,
a physician should be consulted and an examination is advisable.* Other symptoms depend on location and type of malignancy present.

EARLY DANGER SIGNS OF CANCER

1. Any lump or thickening, especially in the breast,
   lip or tongue.
2. Any irregular or unexplained bleeding. Blood in
   the urine or bowel movements. Blood or bloody
   discharge from the nipple or any body opening.
   Unexplained vaginal bleeding or discharge, or
   any bleeding after the menopause.
3. A sore that does not heal, particularly around the
   mouth, tongue or lips, or anywhere on the skin.
4. Noticeable changes in the color or size of a wart,
   mole or birthmark.
5. Loss of appetite or continual indigestion.
6. Persistent hoarseness, cough or difficulty in
   swallowing.
7. Persistent change in normal elimination (bowel
   habits).

*Special Note: Pain is not usually an early warn-
ing sign of cancer.*

Stomach cancer: continued lack of appetite;
persistent indigestion; pain after eating; loss of
weight; vomiting; anemia.

Cancer of the rectum: changes in bowel habits, such as periods of constipation followed by episodes of diarrhea; abdominal cramps and a sensation of incomplete elimination or a feeling that there is a mass in the rectum; rectal pain and bleeding.

Cancer of the uterus: increased or irregular vaginal discharges; return of vaginal bleeding after the menopause; bleeding between menstrual periods or after coitus.

Cancer of the breast: painless lumps in the breast; bleeding or discharging from the nipple. Many kinds of lumps in the breast are innocent, but since this form of cancer is now the leading cause of death from cancer among women, any breast nodule or tumor should be examined by a physician.

Skin cancer: sores and ulcers that do not heal; sudden changes in color, size and texture in moles, warts, scars and birthmarks.

Lung cancer: a persistent cough that lasts beyond 2 weeks; wheezing or other noises in the chest; coughing up of blood or bloody sputum; shortness of breath not caused by obvious exertion, such as climbing stairs or running; chest ache or pain.

Cancer of the mouth, tongue and lips: any sore that does not heal in 2 weeks; any white patch taking the place of the normal pink color of the tongue or inside of the mouth; hoarseness lasting more than 2 weeks.

Cancer of the larynx: persistent hoarseness.

Kidney, bladder and prostate cancers: bloody urine or reddish or pink urine; difficulty in starting urination; increasing frequency of urination during the night.

Brain tumors and cancers: headaches; changes in vision; dizziness; nausea and vomiting; paralysis.

DIAGNOSIS. The detection of cancer can be accomplished by a number of tests and examinations. By palpation, a tumor can be felt as a lump or nodule below the surface of the skin or mucous membrane. By visualization of the hollow organs with instruments such as the cystoscope, proctoscope, or bronchoscope, abnormal growths of cells can be seen. Laboratory examination of the cells removed by BIOPSY can determine whether a tumor is malignant or benign. This test is considered the most accurate and dependable aid to diagnosis of cancer.

The PAPANICOLAOU SMEAR TEST is used for diagnosing early cancers of the uterine cervix, mouth, bronchi, stomach and other organs lined with mucous membrane. In this technique washings or scrapings from the mucous membrane are removed by the physician, placed on a glass slide and sent to a laboratory for cytologic examination. Radiologic studies, using x-ray films and fluoroscopy, can reveal tumors which may not be detected by other means. In addition to gastrointestinal studies, chest x-rays and pyelography, radiologic studies for cancer include angiography and mammography. Radioisotopes and photoscanners may be used to locate tumors of the brain, pancreas, thyroid, liver and kidney. In this method the radioactive compound is introduced into the body orally or by injection. The compound travels through the body and localizes in a specific organ. Special instruments are used to trace and "photograph" the abnormal collection of radioisotopes, thereby pinpointing the location of the tumor.

There is at present no general chemical test of the blood by which malignant growths can be distinguished from benign. The blood can be tested chemically for cancer of the prostate and for a rare malignancy of the bone marrow called multiple myeloma. A blood count can also help in the diagnosis of leukemias.

TREATMENT. The present methods of treating cancer are surgery, radiation and chemotherapy. Surgical removal of the tumor is aimed at removal of all cancerous tissue and is most frequently successful if undertaken when the growth is still small and localized. The goal of radiotherapy is also the complete destruction of all malignant tissue. Radiation damages tissue, particularly tissue that is growing. Since malignant tissue grows rapidly, it is more readily destroyed than normal body tissue.

The type of radiation to be used is determined by the radiologist, depending upon the nature and location of the cancerous growth. He may use x-rays or gamma rays. Gamma rays are similar in nature to x-rays, but they are usually more powerful and penetrating. If the cancer is accessible, this deep radiation therapy may not be necessary. In some cases, radiation sources in the form of radium or radioisotopes can be embedded directly in the cancer and removed when the desired dose has been delivered.

Of the chemicals and drugs used in treating cancer, the most widely used are compounds known as the nitrogen mustards. These are composed of various combinations of carbon, hydrogen, chlorine and nitrogen, and are similar in some respects to the poisonous mustard gas used in World War I. Their effect is to shrink and otherwise retard the growth of the cancer. These and other compounds such as folic acid antagonists, corticosteroids, purine analogues, alkaloids and alkylating agents have been found particularly valuable in treating leukemias and Hodgkin's disease, and have been helpful in some cases of cancer of the ovaries and advanced lung cancer. Researchers are constantly testing other substances, a number of which are showing promise. Radioactive iodine, mixed in water and given orally, has been used to help treat some rare cancers of the thyroid gland. An antibiotic, actinomycin D, used together with surgery and radiation, has been of value in children treated for a kidney cancer known as Wilms' tumor.

Also of use in treating cancer are various hormones. Female hormones have been found effective in some cases of cancer of the prostate, and male hormones are frequently helpful in treating cancer of the breast.

NURSING CARE. Physical care of the patient with uncontrollable cancer involves all nursing measures necessary to keep the patient in as good a state of general health as is possible under the circumstances. Each patient will have individual problems, such as loss of appetite, listlessness or mental depression, inability to relax or sleep and loss of interest in the world around him. Knowing the patient, his background, his personality and his attitude toward his illness will be of invaluable help in serving each individual patient's nursing problems.

Cleanliness and medical asepsis can do much to eliminate the side effects of necrosis and tissue damage which sometimes accompany malignant growths. Frequent irrigations of the affected area and adequate changing of dressings are essential to the patient's comfort and the prevention of infection.

Specific nursing procedures for patients having surgery or radiation therapy will depend on the type of treatment used and the location of the malignancy. (See also RADIOTHERAPY.)

Emotional support of the patient during his illness demands emotional maturity and a positive attitude. The nurse cannot presume that her responsibilities cease once she has attended to the patient's physical needs. Even though the patient may have received treatment early and has a good chance of surviving his present illness, he still may have many fears and anxieties about his future and his ability to resume his former activities. In cases of uncontrollable or advanced cancer fear of pain, disfigurement and death are not uncommon. When the patient turns to the nurse for comfort and moral support she must draw her strength from a deep and well-founded philosophy of life and do what she can to make his remaining days serene and meaningful.

canceremia (kan″ser-e′me-ah) the presence of cancer cells in the blood.

cancericidal (kan″ser-ĭ-si′dal) destructive to cancer cells.

cancerogenic (kan″ser-o-jen′ik) carcinogenic.

cancerology (kan″ser-ol′o-je) the study of cancer.

cancerophobia (kan″ser-o-fo′be-ah) carcinophobia; morbid dread of cancer.

cancriform (kang′krĭ-form) resembling cancer.

cancroid (kang′kroid) 1. cancer-like. 2. a skin cancer of a low grade of malignancy.

cancrum (kang′krum) [L.] canker.
  c. o′ris, gangrenous stomatitis.
  c. puden′di, noma pudendi; destructive ulceration of the external genitalia in the female.

Candeptin (kan-dep′tin) trademark for a preparation of candicidin, an antibiotic and antifungal compound.

candicidin (kan″dĭ-si′din) an antibiotic and antifungal compound derived from Streptomyces, used to treat vaginitis due to Candida infection.

Candida (kan′dĭ-dah) a genus of yeastlike fungi that produce mycelia, but not ascospores.
  C. al′bicans, a species that causes human infection.

candidemia (kan″dĭ-de′me-ah) the presence in the blood of fungi of the genus Candida.

candidiasis (kan″dĭ-di′ah-sis) infection by fungi of the genus Candida.

candle (kan′dl) a unit of luminous intensity equal to the intensity of light from a ⅞-inch sperm candle burning at the rate of 120 grains an hour.
  international c., a unit equal to the intensity of light from 5 square millimeters of platinum at the temperature of solidification.

canine (ka′nīn) 1. pertaining to or characteristic of dogs. 2. pertaining to a canine tooth (cuspid).

canker (kang′ker) an ulceration, especially of the lip or oral mucosa.

Cannabis (kan′ah-bis) a genus of plants, hemp.
  C. in′dica, an Asiatic variety of common hemp; preferred for medicinal use.
  C. sati′va, the common hemp; it has narcotic and antispasmodic properties. Common names are marijuana and hashish.

cannabism (kan′ah-bizm) habituation to the use of hemp derivatives.

cannula (kan′u-lah) a small tubular instrument for insertion into the body, its lumen being usually occupied by a trocar during insertion.

cannulate (kan′u-lat) to penetrate with a cannula, which may be left in place.

cannulation (kan″u-la′shun) introduction of a cannula into a tubelike organ or body cavity.

canthectomy (kan-thek′to-me) excision of a canthus.

canthitis (kan-thi′tis) inflammation of a canthus.

cantholysis (kan-thol′ĭ-sis) surgical section of a canthus or canthal ligament.

canthoplasty (kan′tho-plas″te) plastic repair of a canthus.

canthorrhaphy (kan-thor′ah-fe) suture of a canthus.

canthotomy (kan-thot′o-me) incision of a canthus.

canthus (kan′thus), pl. *can′thi* [L.] the angular junction of the eyelids at either corner of the eyes. adj., **can′thal.**

Cantil (kan′til) trademark for a preparation of mepenzolate bromide, an anticholinergic and antispasmodic used in hypermotility of the lower bowel.

capacitor (kah-pas′ĭ-tor) a device for holding and storing charges of electricity.

capacity (kah-pas′ĭ-te) the power of receiving and holding, usually expressed numerically as the measure of such ability.
  functional residual c., the amount of gas remaining in the lung at the resting expiratory level.
  heat c., thermal capacity.
  inspiratory c., the maximal amount of gas that can be inspired from the resting expiratory level.
  thermal c., the amount of heat absorbed by a body in being raised 1 degree C.
  total lung c., the amount of gas contained in the lung at the end of a maximal inspiration.
  vital c., a measure of the volume of air that can be exhaled from the lungs by forceful effort after a maximal inspiration.

capillarectasia (kap″ĭ-lār″ek-ta′ze-ah) dilatation of capillaries.

Capillaria (kap″ĭ-la′re-ah) a genus of nematode parasites.
  C. hepat′ica, a species parasitic in animals, including man.

capillariomotor (kap″ĭ-lār″e-o-mo′tor) pertaining to control of the caliber of the capillaries.

capillaritis (kap″ĭ-lār-i′tis) inflammation of the capillaries.

capillarity (kap″ĭ-lār′ĭ-te) the action by which the surface of a liquid where it is in contact with a solid, as in a small-caliber, or capillary, tube, is elevated or depressed.

capillary (kap′ĭ-ler″e) 1. hairlike. 2. one of the minute blood vessels interposed between arterioles and venules, or a similar channel conveying lymph. The exchange of necessary substances and fluids between the blood and the tissues takes place through the capillary walls. (See CIRCULATORY SYSTEM.) The walls consist of thin endothelial cells through which dissolved substances and the body fluids can pass. At the arterial end, the blood pressure within the capillary is higher than the pressure in the surrounding tissues, and the blood fluid and some dissolved solid substances pass outward through the capillary wall. At the venous end of the capillary, the pressure within the tissues is higher and waste material and fluids from the tissues pass into the capillary, to be carried away for disposal.

capitular (kah-pit′u-lar) pertaining to the head of a bone.

capitulum (kah-pit′u-lum), pl. *capit′ula* [L.] a small boss on the surface of a bone, as on the humerus.

Capla (kap′lah) trademark for a preparation of mebutamate, a mild tranquilizer and antihypertensive agent.

capnohepatography (kap″no-hep″ah-tog′rah-fe) radiography of the liver after intravenous injection of carbon dioxide gas.

capotement (kah-pōt-maw′) [Fr.] a splashing sound heard in dilatation of the stomach.

cappa (kap′ah) a layer of gray matter of the corpora quadrigemina.

capping (kap′ing) the provision of a protective or obstructive covering.
  pulp c., the covering of an exposed dental pulp with some material to provide protection against external influences.

Capsebon (kap′se-bon) trademark for a suspension of cadmium sulfide, used in treatment of dandruff.

capsicum (kap′sĭ-kum) dried ripe fruit of species of *Capsicum frutescens;* a powerful local stimulant.

capsula (kap′su-lah), pl. *cap′sulae* [L.] capsule.

capsulation (kap″su-la′shun) enclosure in a capsule.

capsule (kap′sūl) an enclosing structure, as (1) a membrane or saclike structure enclosing an organ or part; (2) a small, soluble container for medicine; (3) the envelope surrounding certain bacteria. adj., **cap′sular.**
  articular c., the saclike envelope that encloses the cavity of a synovial joint by attaching to the circumference of the articular end of each involved bone.

  bacterial c., a gelatinous envelope surrounding a bacterial cell which is associated with the virulence of pathogenic bacteria; usually polysaccharide, but sometimes polypeptide.
  Bowman's c., malpighian capsule.
  c's of the brain, two layers of white matter in the substance of the brain; external capsule and internal capsule.
  external c., the layer of white fibers forming the outer border of the corpus striatum.
  Glisson's c., a sheath of connective tissue enclosing the hepatic artery, hepatic duct and portal vein.
  c. of heart, pericardium.
  internal c., a broad band of white matter separating the lentiform nucleus from the thalamus and caudate nucleus.
  joint c., the capsular ligament of a joint.
  c. of lens, the transparent sac enclosing the lens of the eye.
  malpighian c., a two-layered cellular envelope enclosing the tuft of capillaries constituting the glomerulus of the kidney.
  renal c., the fibrous or the fatty material enveloping the kidney, the inner fibrous layer being continuous with the lining of the renal sinus.
  suprarenal c., adrenal gland.
  Tenon's c., the connective tissue enclosing the eyeball.

capsulectomy (kap″su-lek′to-me) excision of a capsule, as of the renal capsule or the capsule of the lens.

capsulitis (kap″su-li′tis) inflammation of a capsule.

capsulolenticular (kap″su-lo-len-tik′u-lar) pertaining to the capsule and lens.

capsuloma (kap″su-lo′mah) a capsular tumor of the kidney.

capsuloplasty (kap′su-lo-plas″te) plastic repair of a joint capsule.

capsulorrhaphy (kap″su-lor′ah-fe) suture of a joint capsule.

capsulotomy (kap″su-lot′o-me) incision of a capsule, as that of the lens or of a joint.

captodiamine (kap″to-di′ah-mēn) a compound used as a sedative and tranquilizer.

captodramin (kap″to-dram′in) captodiamine.

caput (kap′ut), pl. *cap′ita* [L.] the head or headlike object or part.
  c. medu′sae, the pattern presented by congested cutaneous veins about the umbilicus in obstruction of the portal vein.
  c. succeda′neum, edema sometimes occurring in and under the fetal scalp during labor.

caramiphen (kah-ram′ĭ-fen) an agent used in parasympathetic blockade, as an antispasmodic and in treatment of Parkinson's disease.

carbachol (kar′bah-kol) white or yellowish crystals, a parasympathomimetic (cholinergic) agent used to relieve intraocular pressure in GLAUCOMA.

carbamazepine (kar″bam-az′ĕ-pin) a compound used as an anticonvulsant.

carbamide (kar-bam′īd) urea in anhydrous, lyophilized, sterile powder form; injected intravenously in dextrose or invert sugar solution to induce diuresis.

carbamylcholine chloride (kar″bah-mil-ko′lēn) carbachol.

carbarsone (kar′bar-sōn) an arsenical compound used in amebic dysentery.

carbazochrome salicylate (kar-baz′-o-krom) a hemostatic agent used for control of capillary oozing and bleeding during and after surgery. It does not affect blood clot formation and is not effective in massive hemorrhage. Its therapeutic status as a systemic hemostatic agent has not yet been established.

carbetapentane (kar-ba″tah-pen′tān) a compound used as an antitussive agent.

carbethyl salicylate (kar-beth′il) salicylic ethyl ester carbonate, used as an analgesic and antiarthritic agent.

carbinoxamine (kar″bin-ok′sah-mēn) a pyridine derivative used as an antihistamine.

Carbocaine (kar′bo-kān) trademark for preparations of mepivacaine hydrochloride, a local anesthetic.

carbocholine (kar″bo-ko′lēn) carbachol.

carbohemoglobin (kar″bo-he″mo-glo′bin) a combination of carbon dioxide and hemoglobin.

carbohydrase (kar″bo-hi′drās) an enzyme that catalyzes the hydrolysis of carbohydrates.

carbohydrate (kar″bo-hi′drāt) a compound of carbon, hydrogen and oxygen, the latter two in the proportions of water, synthesized by green plants. Carbohydrates in food are an important and immediate source of energy for the body; 1 Gm. of carbohydrate yields 4 calories. They are present, at least in small quantities, in most foods, but the chief sources are the sugars and starches. The sugars include granulated sugar, maple sugar, honey and molasses. The simple sugars (monosaccharides) include glucose, called also dextrose or grape sugar, and fructose, called also levulose or fruit sugar. Galactose is a simple sugar produced by the digestion or hydrolysis of lactose (milk sugar). The double sugars (disaccharides) include sucrose, which is found in sugar cane or sugar beet, maltose or malt sugar, and lactose or milk sugar. All ripe fruits and many vegetables contain some natural sugars. The starches are present in such foods as rice, wheat and potatoes.

Carbohydrates may be stored in the body as glycogen for future use. If they are eaten in excessive amounts, however, the body changes them into fats and stores them in that form.

carbolic acid (kar-bol′ik) a powerful antiseptic and germicide; called also phenol. It can be irritating to the skin, so it is seldom used as an antiseptic today. Carbolic acid is highly poisonous and should be properly labeled and stored to avoid accidental poisoning.

carbolism (kar′bo-lizm) phenol (carbolic acid) poisoning.

carbolize (kar′bo-līz) to impregnate with phenol (carbolic acid).

carboluria (kar″bo-lu′re-ah) phenol (carbolic acid) in the urine.

carbometer (kar-bom′ĕ-ter) an instrument for determining the proportion of carbon dioxide exhaled with the breath.

carbon (kar′bon) a chemical element, atomic number 6, atomic weight 12.011, symbol C. (See table of ELEMENTS.)
c. cycle, the steps by which carbon is extracted from the atmosphere, incorporated in the body of living organisms and ultimately returned to the air.

carbon dioxide an odorless, colorless gas, CO_2, used with oxygen to stimulate respiration and in solid form as an escharotic.
c. d. combining power, the ability of blood plasma to combine with carbon dioxide; indicative of the ALKALI RESERVE and a measure of the acid-base balance of the blood. In determination of the carbon dioxide combining power, actually the plasma bicarbonate is measured, since it is virtually impossible to determine the plasma carbon dioxide concentration in a clinical laboratory.

In a normal acid-base balance the ratio of carbonic acid to base bicarbonate is 1 to 20. This balance is maintained by a system of buffer substances, the most important of which is the carbonic acid-bicarbonate buffer system. Since a determination of the plasma bicarbonate will indicate whether this system is functioning normally, it is of help in diagnosing metabolic ACIDOSIS or ALKALOSIS. In the presence of metabolic acidosis the carbon dioxide combining power is decreased; in alkalosis it is increased. This test is of no value in diagnosing respiratory alkalosis or acidosis.

Normal range for this test is 53 to 78 volumes of carbon dioxide per 100 ml. of serum. Blood for the test is obtained by venipuncture and no special preparation of the patient is necessary.

carbon monoxide (a colorless, odorless, tasteless gas, CO, formed by incomplete combustion of carbon; rapidly fatal because it forms a stable compound with hemoglobin. Carbon monoxide is present in the exhaust of gasoline engines, in the smoke of wood and coal fires, in manufactured gas such as that used in the household, and wherever carbon burns without a sufficient supply of oxygen.
c. m. poisoning, poisoning by carbon monoxide; one of the most common types of gas poisoning. When carbon monoxide is inhaled, it comes in contact with the blood and combines with hemoglobin. Since carbon monoxide combines more readily with hemoglobin than does oxygen, it takes the place of oxygen in the erythrocytes, and the tissues are thus deprived of their normal oxygen supply. Death from asphyxia results if a large enough quantity of carbon monoxide is inhaled.
SYMPTOMS AND TREATMENT. The symptoms of carbon monoxide poisoning are dizziness, headache, weakness, shortness of breath, possibly nausea and then unconsciousness. The skin becomes pink in color.

Emergency treatment consists of opening doors and windows, and turning off the source of the gas, if possible. The victim should be dragged or carried out into the air. If breathing has stopped or is irregular, ARTIFICIAL RESPIRATION should be undertaken immediately. The police or fire department or the hospital should be called and the nature of the accident described so that emergency equipment to administer oxygen may be rushed to the scene. The victim is kept lying down.

PREVENTION. Cases of carbon monoxide poisoning are usually accidental. It should be remembered that carbon monoxide has no odor and its presence may not be detected unless other gases, such as exhaust fumes from an automobile motor, are also escaping. Care should be taken to ensure proper ventilation of working and sleeping areas. It is extremely dangerous to leave an automobile motor running in a closed garage. Stoves and furnaces should be kept in good repair. Burners using gas, especially in a bedroom, should have a ventilator pipe to carry the exhaust to the outside.

carbon tetrachloride a clear, colorless, mobile liquid; anthelmintic and insecticide, and toxic to the liver, kidney and heart when taken in excessive doses.

carbonate (kar′bon-āt) a salt of carbonic acid.

carbonemia (kar″bo-ne′me-ah) excess of carbon dioxide in the blood.

carbonic acid (kar-bon′ik) aqueous solution of carbon dioxide, H_2CO_3.
  c. anhydrase, an enzyme that catalyzes the decomposition of carbonic acid into carbon dioxide and water, facilitating transfer of carbon dioxide from tissues to blood and from blood to alveolar air.

carbonize (kar′bo-nīz) to convert into charcoal or carbon.

carbonometry (kar″bo-nom′ĕ-tre) measurement of carbon dioxide in the breath.

carbonuria (kar″bo-nu′re-ah) excretion of urine containing carbon dioxide or other carbon compounds.

carbonyl (kar′bo-nil) the bivalent radical, =CO.
  c. chloride, phosgene, a poisonous gas developed for war use.

carboxyhemoglobin (kar-bok″se-he″mo-glo′bin) a combination of carbon monoxide and hemoglobin.

carboxyl (kar-bok′sil) the monovalent radical, —COOH, found in nearly all organic acids.

carboxylase (kar-bok′sĭ-lās) an enzyme that splits carbon dioxide from carboxyl groups.

carboxymyoglobin (kar-bok″se-mi″o-glo′bin) a compound formed from myoglobin on exposure to carbon monoxide.

carboxypeptidase (kar-bok″se-pep′tĭ-dās) an exopeptidase that acts only on the peptide linkage of a terminal amino acid containing a free carboxyl group.

carboxypolypeptidase (kar-bok″se-pol″e-pep′tĭ-dās) an enzyme that causes splitting off of a free carboxyl group from a polypeptide.

carbromal (kar-bro′mal) white, odorless, crystalline powder, used as a nerve sedative and somnifacient.

carbuncle (kar″bung-kl) a hard, pus-filled and painful inflammation. Carbuncles are similar to BOILS, but are larger and more deeply rooted and have several openings. They are often a symptom of general poor health.

Like boils, carbuncles are caused by pus-forming bacteria. These organisms are often present on the skin but are unable to do any damage unless resistance is lowered by such conditions as irritating friction, cuts, poor health, nutritional deficiency or diabetes mellitus.

Treatment includes administration of antibiotics and incision and drainage when necessary to remove exudate. Efforts are made to determine the cause of the carbuncles so that it can be eliminated.
  malignant c., anthrax.
  renal c., a massive parenchymal suppuration due to bacterial metastasis following vascular thrombosis or infarction of the kidney.

carbunculosis (kar-bung″ku-lo′sis) formation of numerous carbuncles.

carcass (kar′kas) a dead body; generally applied to other than a human body.

Carcholin (kar′ko-lin) trademark for a preparation of carbachol, used to relieve intraocular pressure in glaucoma.

carcinogen (kar-sin′o-jen) a substance that causes cancer. adj., **carginogen′ic.**

carcinogenesis (kar″sĭ-no-jen′ĕ-sis) production of cancer.

carcinogenicity (kar″sĭ-no-jĕ-nis′ĭ-te) the ability to produce cancer.

carcinoid (kar′sĭ-noid) a yellow, circumscribed tumor occurring in the small intestine, appendix, stomach or colon; called also argentaffinoma.

carcinolysis (kar″sĭ-nol′ĭ-sis) destruction of cancer cells.

carcinoma (kar″sĭ-no′mah) a malignant tumor made up of connective tissue enclosing epithelial cells. A form of CANCER, carcinoma makes up the majority of the cases of malignancy of the breast, uterus, intestinal tract, skin and tongue.
  alveolar c., carcinoma in which the cells appear in groups, enclosed in connective tissue.
  basal cell c., a cutaneous cancer of relatively low-grade malignancy, arising from the basal layers of the epidermis.
  bronchogenic c., carcinoma of the lung.
  cylindrical cell c., carcinoma in which the cells are cylindrical or nearly so.
  epidermoid c., squamous cell carcinoma.
  giant cell c., carcinoma containing many giant cells.
  c. in si′tu, carcinoma that has not invaded adjoining tissues, but is still confined to its site of origin.
  prickle cell c., squamous cell carcinoma.
  scirrhous c., carcinoma with a hard structure composed of connective tissue alveoli filled with masses of cells that have no vessels or ground substance.
  squamous cell c., a rapidly growing and readily metastasizing carcinoma originating in the epidermis, particularly the prickle cell layer.

sweat gland c., a rare skin tumor arising from the sweat glands, having a metastatic tendency between that of basal cell and that of squamous cell carcinoma.

carcinomatosis (kar″sĭ-no″mah-to′sis) the development of multiple carcinomas.

carcinomatous (kar″sĭ-no′mah-tus) of carcinoma or cancer.

carcinophilia (kar″sĭ-no-fil′e-ah) special affinity for cancerous tissue. adj., **carcinophil′ic.**

carcinophobia (kar″sĭ-no-fo′be-ah) morbid dread of cancer.

carcinosarcoma (kar″sĭ-no-sar-ko′mah) a mixed tumor containing the elements of carcinoma and sarcoma.

embryonal c., a rapidly developing sarcoma of the kidneys, made up of embryonal elements, and occurring chiefly in children before the fifth year; called also Wilms' tumor.

carcinosis (kar″sĭ-no′sis) widespread dissemination of cancer throughout the body.

miliary c., that marked by development of numerous nodules resembling miliary tuberculosis.

cardamom (kar′dah-mom) the fruit of *Elettaria cardamomum,* source of a seed and oil used as flavoring agents.

Cardarelli's sign (kar-dar-el′ēz) pulsation of the laryngotracheal tube synchronous with the pulse, visible and palpable when the larynx is displaced to the left by pressure on the thyroid cartilage; observed in aortic aneurysm.

cardi(o)- (kar′de-o) word element [Gr.], *heart.*

cardia (kar′de-ah) the upper orifice of the stomach.

cardiac (kar′de-ak) pertaining to the heart or to the upper orifice of the stomach.

c. arrest, sudden and often unexpected stoppage of effective heart action. Either the periodic impulses which trigger the coordinated heart muscle contractions cease or ventricular fibrillation or flutter occurs in which the individual muscle fibers have a rapid irregular twitching. If resuscitation is not undertaken within minutes of the occurrence of cardiac arrest, permanent damage to other organs will result from insufficient blood supply, and the death of the individual is probable. Resuscitation involves not only use of CARDIAC MASSAGE (external or internal), but also ARTIFICIAL RESPIRATION by the mouth-to-mouth method or by mechanical respirator. The use of a defibrillator or artificial pacemaker will depend on the cause of the arrest, usually determined by electrocardiography.

c. catheterization, passage of a long, fine catheter through a blood vessel into the chambers of the heart, as an aid in diagnosis of various heart disorders and anomalies. This procedure is carried out under direct visualization with a FLUOROSCOPE. Samples of blood are taken from the right and left chambers of the heart and from the pulmonary artery, and later tested for measurement of the hematocrit and oxygen saturation. Pressures with-

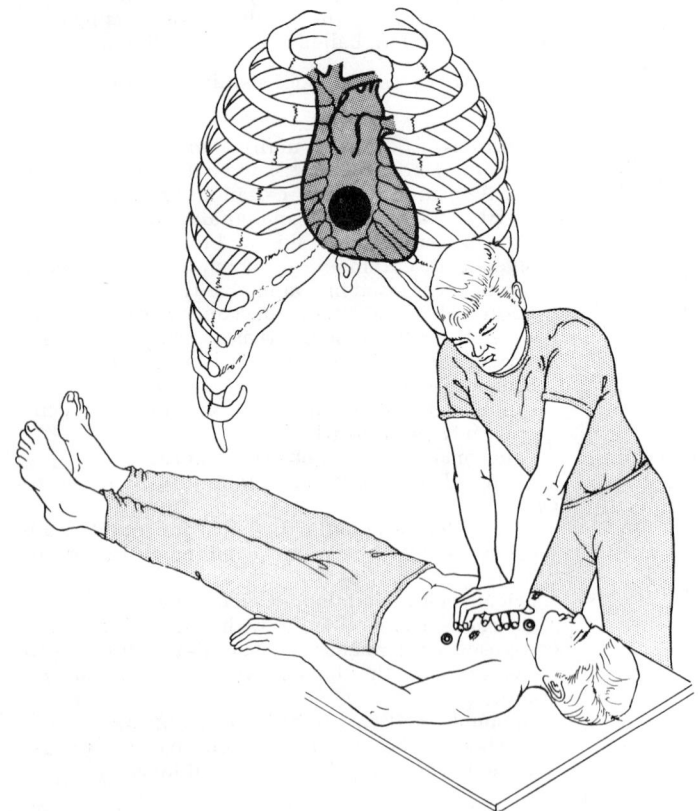

Closed-chest cardiac massage. Heavy circle in heart drawing shows area of application of force. Circles on supine figure show points of application of electrodes for defibrillation. (From Brainerd, H., et al.: Current Diagnosis and Treatment. Los Altos, Calif., Lange Medical Publications, 1967.)

in the heart chambers are also measured and recorded. The findings obtained from these tests help determine valvular insufficiencies and stenosis, deformities of the heart chambers and pulmonary artery and other disorders and malfunctions of the heart.

c. massage, a medical procedure performed as an emergency measure to empty the ventricles of the heart in an effort to circulate the blood, and also to stimulate the heart so that it will resume its pumping action. In both external and internal cardiac massage mouth-to-mouth resuscitation must be carried out at the same time the heart is being massaged. If available, an automatic resuscitator with mask and rebreathing bag can be used.

CLOSED OR EXTERNAL CARDIAC MASSAGE. This closed-chest method of cardiopulmonary resuscitation is a rhythmic massage of the heart between the lower sternum in the front and the vertebral column in the back. It is a drastic measure that should be undertaken only by trained personnel because of the risk of causing injuries such as rib fractures, damage to the heart and liver and puncture of the lungs or blood vessels that can lead to internal bleeding, fat emboli and other serious complications. The following statement by the American Heart Association describes the correct technique and ways to avoid such complications.

Injuries can be kept to an acceptable minimum if the resuscitator is trained to open the airway adequately, apply expired air ventilation, locate the correct pressure point for closed-chest manual heart compression (lower half of the sternum), and position himself to the side of the victim who should be on a solid surface. Pressure should be applied through the heel of the hand and the sternum pushed in toward the spine about 4 or 5 cm. in adults. The proper positioning of the hands over the correct pressure point reduces the likelihood of injuries. Successful resuscitation can be performed by one person giving both artificial ventilation and circulation, although two qualified persons are preferable. The risk of such complications is acceptably small and the anticipated benefits are great enough to warrant the prompt application of closed-chest cardiopulmonary resuscitation by well-trained individuals in instances of suspected cardiac arrest. Since it is estimated that irreversible changes to the central nervous system occur 4 to 6 minutes after cardiac arrest, resuscitation efforts must be begun promptly after the recognition of cardiac arrest.

OPEN OR INTERNAL CARDIAC MASSAGE. This involves a surgical incision directly over the heart and manual massage of the heart or stimulation with an electric current.

cardialgia　(kar″de-al′je-ah) pain in the epigastrium.

cardianeuria　(kar″de-ah-nu′re-ah) deficiency of tone in the heart.

cardiataxia　(kar″de-ah-tak′se-ah) incoordination of heart movements.

cardio-accelerator　(kar″de-o-ak-sel′er-a″tor) an agent that quickens the heart's action.

cardio-angiology　(kar″de-o-an″je-ol′o-je) study of the heart and blood vessels.

cardiocele　(kar′de-o-sēl″) hernial protrusion of the heart through the diaphragm.

cardiocentesis　(kar″de-o-sen-te′sis) surgical puncture of the heart.

cardiochalasia　(kar″de-o-kah-la′ze-ah) relaxation

or incompetence of the cardiac orifice of the stomach.

cardiocirrhosis　(kar″de-o-sĭ-ro′sis) cirrhosis of the liver associated with heart disease.

cardioclasis　(kar″de-ok′lah-sis) rupture of the heart.

cardiodiaphragmatic　(kar″de-o-di″ah-frag-mat′-ik) pertaining to the heart and the diaphragm.

cardiodilator　(kar″de-o-di′la-tor) an instrument for dilating the cardia.

cardiodiosis　(kar″de-o-di-o′sis) dilatation of the cardiac orifice of the stomach.

cardiodynamics　(kar″de-o-di-nam′iks) study of the forces involved in the heart's action.

cardiodynia　(kar″de-o-din′e-ah) pain in the region of the heart.

cardiogenesis　(kar″de-o-jen′ĕ-sis) development of the heart in the embryo.

cardiogenic　(kar″de-o-jen′ik) originating in the heart.

cardiogram　(kar′de-o-gram″) a record produced by cardiography (see also ELECTROCARDIOGRAM).

cardiograph　(kar′de-o-graf″) an instrument for recording the heart movements.

cardiography　(kar″de-og′rah-fe) the graphic recording of a physical or functional aspect of the heart, e.g., electrocardiography, kinetocardiography, phonocardiography, vibrocardiography.

apex c., graphic recording of low-frequency pulsations at the anterior chest wall over the apex of the heart.

ultrasonic c., echocardiography.

Cardio-green　(kar′de-o-grēn″) trademark for a preparation of indocyanine green, a dye used to test cardiovascular function.

cardiohepatic　(kar″de-o-hĕ-pat′ik) pertaining to heart and liver.

cardio-inhibitor　(kar″de-o-in-hib′ĭ-tor) an agent that restrains the heart's action.

cardiokinetic　(kar″de-o-ki-net′ik) 1. exciting or stimulating the heart. 2. an agent that excites or stimulates the heart.

cardiolith　(kar′de-o-lith) a calculus in the heart.

cardiologist　(kar″de-ol′o-jist) a specialist in the study and treatment of heart disease.

cardiology　(kar″de-ol′o-je) study of the heart and its functions.

cardiolysin　(kar″de-ol′ĭ-sin) a lysin that acts on the heart muscle.

cardiolysis　(kar″de-ol′ĭ-sis) the separation of adhesions constricting the heart.

cardiomalacia　(kar″de-o-mah-la′she-ah) softening of the heart substance.

cardiomegaly　(kar″de-o-meg′ah-le) hypertrophy of the heart.

cardiometer (kar″de-om′ĕ-ter) an instrument for estimating the power of the heart's action.

cardiomotility (kar″de-o-mo-til′ĭ-te) motility of the heart.

cardiomyoliposis (kar″de-o-mi″o-lĭ-po′sis) fatty degeneration of the heart muscle.

cardiomyopathy (kar″de-o-mi-op′ah-the) a subacute or chronic disorder of heart muscle, often with involvement of the endocardium and sometimes of the pericardium.

cardionector (kar″de-o-nek′tor) a structure that regulates the heartbeat, i.e., the sinoatrial node or the bundle of His.

cardionephric (kar″de-o-nef′rik) pertaining to the heart and kidney.

cardioneural (kar″de-o-nu′ral) pertaining to the heart and nervous system.

cardioneurosis (kar″de-o-nu-ro′sis) functional neurosis marked by cardiac symptoms.

cardio-omentopexy (kar″de-o-o-men′to-pek″se) suture of a portion of the omentum to the heart.

cardiopalmus (kar″de-o-pal′mus) palpitation of the heart.

cardiopathy (kar″de-op′ah-the) a morbid condition of the heart.

cardiopericardiopexy (kar″de-o-per″ĭ-kar′de-o-pek″se) surgical establishment of adhesive pericarditis, for relief of coronary disease.

cardiopericarditis (kar″de-o-per″ĭ-kar-di′tis) inflammation of the heart and pericardium.

cardiophobia (kar″de-o-fo′be-ah) morbid dread of heart disease.

cardiophone (kar′de.o-fōn″) an instrument for making audible the sound of the heart muscle.

cardioplasty (kar′de-o-plas″te) plastic repair of the opening between the esophagus and the stomach.

cardioplegia (kar″de-o-ple′je-ah) interruption of myocardial contraction, as by use of chemical compounds or cold in cardiac surgery.

cardiopneumatic (kar″de-o-nu-mat′ik) pertaining to the heart and the lungs.

cardiopneumograph (kar″de-o-nu′mo-graf) a machine for registering cardiopneumatic movements.

cardioptosis (kar″de-o-to′sis) downward displacement of the heart.

cardiopulmonary (kar″de-o-pul′mo-ner″e) pertaining to the heart and lungs.

cardiopuncture (kar″de-o-pungk′tūr) cardiocentesis.

cardiopyloric (kar″de-o-pi-lor′ik) pertaining to the cardia and pylorus.

cardiorenal (kar″de-o-re′nal) pertaining to the heart and kidneys.

cardiorrhaphy (kar″de-or′ah-fe) suture of the heart.

cardiorrhexis (kar″de-o-rek′sis) rupture of the heart.

cardiosclerosis (kar″de-o-sklĕ-ro′sis) fibroid induration of the heart.

cardioscope (kar′de-o-skōp″) cardiophone.

cardiospasm (kar′de-o-spazm″) spasm of the cardiac sphincter (gastroesophageal sphincter) of the stomach.

cardiosphygmograph (kar″de-o-sfig′mo-graf) an instrument for recording movements of the heart and pulse.

cardiosplenopexy (kar″de-o-splen′o-pek″se) suture of the parenchyma of the spleen to the denuded surface of the heart for revascularization of the myocardium.

cardiosymphysis (kar″de-o-sim′fĭ-sis) obliteration of the pericardium by adhesions.

cardiotachometer (kar″de-o-tah-kom′e-ter) an instrument that records the heart rate continuously for hours or days.

cardiotherapy (kar″de-o-ther′ah-pe) the treatment of diseases of the heart.

cardiotomy (kar″de-ot′o-me) surgical incision of the heart.

cardiotonic (kar″de-o-ton′ik) having a tonic effect on the heart.

cardiotoxic (kar″de-o-tok′sik) poisonous to the heart.

cardiovalvular (kar″de-o-val′vu-lar) pertaining to the valves of the heart.

cardiovalvulotome (kar″de-o-val′vu-lo-tōm″) an instrument for incising the mitral valve.

cardiovascular (kar″de-o-vas′ku-lar) pertaining to the heart and blood vessels.

carditis (kar-di′tis) inflammation of the heart; myocarditis.

cardivalvulitis (kar″dĭ-val″vu-li′tis) inflammation of the heart valves.

Cardrase (kar′drās) trademark for a preparation of ethoxzolamide, a diuretic used mainly in edema, glaucoma and epilepsy.

caries (ka′re-ēz) decay, as of bone or teeth.

   dental c., a destructive process causing decalcification of the tooth enamel and leading to continued destruction of enamel and dentin, and cavitation of the tooth.

   Decayed and infected teeth can be the source of other infections throughout the body, and decayed or missing teeth can interfere with the proper chewing of food, leading to nutrition deficiencies, or to disorders of digestion.

   CAUSES. The causes of tooth decay are not completely understood, but certain facts are known. Tooth decay seems to be a disease of civilization, possibly associated with refined foods. A lack of dental cleanliness is also closely associated with tooth decay.

   Decay occurs where bacteria and food adhere to

the surface of the teeth, especially in pits or crevices, and form plaques. It is believed that the action of the bacteria on sugars and starches creates lactic acid, which can quickly and permanently dissolve the enamel that covers the teeth. The acid produced in just half an hour when sugar comes into contact with the plaque is enough to begin the process of dissolving tooth enamel. In most people this process and its resulting decay occur whenever sweet foods are eaten. It is for this reason that sweet or starchy foods between meals and at bedtime can be so harmful to the teeth unless the teeth are thoroughly brushed and rinsed immediately afterward.

Decay that is not treated will progress through the tooth enamel and the dentin just below it into the pulp of the tooth, which contains the nerves. When it reaches the pulp, it can cause intense pain. There is no relief until the pulp dies or is removed, or the tooth is extracted.

TREATMENT. The only treatment for tooth decay is regular dental care. Enamel that has been destroyed does not grow back. The decay must be removed, and the cavity filled. The fillings, or restorations, may be of gold foil, baked porcelain, synthetic cements, silver amalgam or cast gold inlays.

When decay has reached the pulp of a tooth, it may be necessary to extract the tooth. Whenever possible, however, the exposed pulp is re-covered, or capped, and the tooth is then filled. New techniques of root canal therapy are saving many teeth that would formerly have been lost.

PREVENTION. There is no cure for tooth decay. Prevention is the only real answer to the problem. This means scrupulous cleanliness. The teeth should be thoroughly brushed at least once a day, and preferably after every meal. Dental floss or tape should be used to remove any particles of food from between the teeth. If teeth cannot be brushed after every meal, the mouth should be thoroughly rinsed with water.

Diet, too, plays a most important part in the prevention of tooth decay. Sugars and starches (the carbohydrates) should be limited, especially between meals. This applies particularly to those which are sticky and tend to cling to the teeth.

FLUORIDATION of drinking water is also proving effective in combating tooth decay. In communities where fluoride is not added to the water supply, a dentist may apply a fluoride solution directly to a child's teeth. Fluoride drops or tablets may also be prescribed in small amounts, to be mixed with milk or other fluids, but this treatment must always be carefully supervised by a doctor or dentist.

c. sic′ca, a form of bone or joint decay unaccompanied by enlargement, swelling or abscess formation in surrounding tissues, often caused by *Mycobacterium tuberculosis.*

carina (kah-ri′nah), pl. *cari′nae* [L.] a ridgelike structure.

c. tra′cheae, a downward and backward projection of the lowest tracheal cartilage, forming a ridge between the openings of the right and left principal bronchi.

c. urethra′lis vagi′nae, the median ridge on the anterior wall of the vagina.

cariogenic (kār″e-o-jen′ik) conducive to caries.

carisoprodol (kar″i-so′pro-dol) a drug used as an analgesic and skeletal muscle relaxant.

carminative (kar-min′ah-tiv) 1. relieving flatulence. 2. an agent that relieves flatulence.

carnivorous (kar-niv′o-rus) eating flesh.

carnophobia (kar″no-fo′be-ah) aversion to meat diet.

carotenase (kar-ot′ē-nās) an enzyme that converts carotene into vitamin A.

carotene (kar′o-tēn) a lipochrome or coloring pigment in carrots, tomatoes and other vegetables, egg yolk, milk fat and other substances; in the body it can be converted into vitamin A.

carotenemia (kar″o-tĕ-ne′me-ah) the presence of carotene in the blood.

carotenoid (kah-rot′ĕ-noid) 1. resembling carotene. 2. a compound resembling carotene.

carotenosis (kar″o-tĕ-no′sis) deposition of carotene in tissues, especially the skin.

caroticotympanic (kah-rot″ĭ-ko-tim-pan′ik) pertaining to the carotid canal and tympanum.

carotid (kah-rot′id) relating to the carotid artery, the principal artery of the neck (see table of ARTERIES).

c. bodies, masses of chromaffin cells located on the wall of each internal carotid artery that act as chemoreceptors.

c. sinus, the dilated portion of the carotid artery at its point of bifurction into the internal and external carotid arteries just above the upper border of the thyroid cartilage of the trachea. Its wall contains special nerve endings, and stimulation of these nerves or changes in pressure in and on the sinus initiate changes in the heart rate and blood pressure.

c. sinus syndrome, a group of symptoms related to stimulation of nerve endings in, or pressure on, the carotid sinus. In certain susceptible persons the carotid sinus is too easily stimulated and symptoms are produced by sudden turning of the head or the wearing of a tight collar. The syndrome is characterized by a history of transient attacks of numbness or weakness of the face, arm or leg, headache and in some cases aphasia. There also may be some mental confusion, loss of vision or fainting at the time of the attack.

Diagnosis can be confirmed by a gentle massage of the carotid sinus area, which will cause an attack. Drugs used to terminate attacks or to prevent their occurrence include atropine sulfate, ephedrine sulfate with phenobarbital and amphetamine sulfate.

carotidynia (kah-rot″ĭ-din′e-ah) pain caused by pressure on the carotid artery.

carotin (kar′o-tin) carotene.

carpal (kar′pal) pertaining to the carpus, or wrist.

c. tunnel, the osseofibrous passage for the median nerve and the flexor tendons.

c. tunnel syndrome, pain, numbness and tingling of the fingers due to compression of the median nerve where it passes under a carpal ligament. The disorder is found most often in middle-aged women. Excessive wrist movements, arthritis, hypertrophy of the bone and connective tissue in ACROMEGALY and swelling of the wrist can produce the carpal tunnel syndrome. Treatment is usually conservative and consists of splinting the wrist to immobilize it for several weeks until the irritation of the median nerve has healed. In severe cases surgical resection of the carpal ligament is helpful.

carpectomy (kar-pek′to-me) excision of a carpal bone.

carphology (kar-fol′o-je) involuntary picking at the bedclothes, seen in states of great exhaustion and severe fever.

carpometacarpal (kar″po-met″ah-kar′pal) pertaining to the carpus and metacarpus.

carpoptosis (kar″po-to′sis) wristdrop.

carpus (kar′pus) the eight bones composing the articulation between the hand and the forearm; the WRIST.

carrier (kār′e-er) an agent by which something is carried, especially an individual harboring pathogenic microorganisms and capable of transmitting them to others.

  chronic c., one who has recovered from a disease or, though he has never had the disease, still carries the organisms in his body.

  healthy c., a person who has never had the disease, but carries the infecting organism in his body.

  hemophiliac c., the female transmitter of classic sex-linked hemophilia, who may show only a clotting factor deficiency.

  incubatory c., one in the incubation period of an infectious disease, who will soon manifest the symptoms.

  typhoid c., a carrier of live typhoid germs which frequently grow in the gallbladder and are excreted in the feces. Usually public health laws prevent such individuals from working in food industries, such as processing and packing plants and restaurants.

Carrión's disease (kar-e-ōnz′) an infectious disease of South America due to *Bartonella bacilliformis,* and transmitted by sandflies, lice and ticks; an acute febrile anemia (Oroya fever) is followed by the appearance of a nodular cutaneous eruption (verruga peruana).

cartilage (kar′tĭ-lij) a specialized fibrous connective tissue; the gristle or white elastic substance attached to articular bone surfaces and forming parts of the skeleton.

  alar c's, the cartilages of the wings of the nose.

  aortic c., the second costal cartilage on the right side.

  arthrodial c., articular c., that lining the articular surfaces of bones.

  arytenoid c's, two pyramid-shaped cartilages of the larynx.

  connecting c., that connecting the surfaces of an immovable joint.

  costal c's, cartilages between the true ribs and the sternum.

  cricoid c., a ringlike cartilage forming the lower and back part of the larynx.

  diarthrodial c., articular cartilage.

  elastic c., cartilage whose matrix contains yellow elastic fibers.

  ensiform c., xiphoid process.

  fibrous c., fibrocartilage.

  floating c., a detached portion of semilunar cartilage in the knee joint.

  hyaline c., cartilage with a glassy, translucent appearance, the matrix and embedded collagenous fibers having the same index of refraction.

  ossifying c., temporary cartilage.

  permanent c., cartilage that does not normally become ossified.

  reticular c., elastic cartilage.

  semilunar c., one of the two interarticular cartilages of the knee joint.

  temporary c., cartilage that is normally destined to become changed into bone.

  thyroid c., the shield-shaped cartilage of the larynx.

  yellow c., elastic cartilage.

cartilaginous (kar″tĭ-laj′ĭ-nus) consisting of cartilage.

cartilago (kar″tĭ-lah′go), pl. *cartilag′ines* [L.] cartilage.

caruncle (kar′ung-kl) a small fleshy eminence, often abnormal.

  hymenal c's, mucosal tags at the vaginal orifice, supposedly relics of the ruptured hymen.

  lacrimal c., the red eminence at the medial angle of the eye.

  sublingual c., an eminence on either side of the frenulum of the tongue (frenulum linguae), on which the major duct of the sublingual gland and the duct of the submandibular gland open.

  urethral c., a polypoid growth usually near the meatus of the urethra in females, sometimes causing difficulty in voiding.

caruncula (kah-rung′ku-lah), pl. *carun′culae* [L.] caruncle.

caryo- (kār′e-o) for words beginning thus, see those beginning *karyo-.*

cascara (kas-kār′ah) husk, bark.

  c. sagra′da, dried bark of *Rhamnus purshiana,* used as a stimulant cathartic.

case (kās) a particular instance of disease; as a case of leukemia; sometimes used incorrectly to designate the patient with the disease.

casease (ka′se-ās) a bacterial enzyme capable of dissolving albumin.

caseation (ka″se-a′shun) the conversion of tissue by degeneration into a dry, amorphous mass like cheese.

casein (ka′se-in) the phosphoprotein found in milk.

caseinogen (ka″se-in′o-jen) the precursor of casein.

caseous (ka′se-us) cheeselike.

cassette (kah-set′) [Fr.] a light-proof housing for x-ray film, containing front and back intensifying screens, between which the film is placed.

cast (kast) an object molded to shape, as (1) a mass of molded plastic material produced by effusion into a body passage, especially such masses in the urine, named according to the constituents, as epithelial, fatty, hyaline, mucous, waxy, etc., or (2) a rigid dressing molded to the body while pliable, and hardening as it dries to give a firm support. These cases are usually made of crinoline impregnated with plaster of paris and are applied (a) to immobilize a part while healing takes place, or (b) to correct a deformity of the musculoskeletal system.

NURSING CARE. If the patient is confined to bed after a plaster of paris cast is applied, it is necessary to provide a firm mattress protected by a waterproof material. Several small pillows should be available for placing under the curves of the cast to prevent remolding or cracking of the plaster and to provide adequate support of the patient. When handling a wet cast only the palm or flat of the hand is used so that the fingertips will not make indentations that might produce pressure against the patient's skin.

While the cast is drying it is left uncovered to allow sufficient circulation of air around it. The parts of the body not included in the cast are covered with a sheet or light blanket to avoid chilling. Extreme heat should not be used to hasten drying as this may produce burns under the cast. The patient is turned frequently to insure proper drying and to avoid prolonged pressure on any one area.

Parts of the cast that may become soiled by urine or feces can be covered with a plastic material which can be changed as necessary. To minimize crumbling of the edges and irritation of the skin around and under the cast, a strip of stockinette or adhesive tape is applied so that the rim of the cast is thoroughly covered. Observation of the patient for signs of impaired circulation or pressure against a nerve is extremely important. Any numbness, recurrent pain, or tingling should be reported at once. If an extremity is enclosed in a cast it should be elevated to reduce swelling. Cyanosis or blanching of the fingers or toes extending from a cast usually indicates impaired blood flow which may lead to serious complications if not corrected immediately.

castor oil (kas′tor) oil obtained from the castor bean plant; it has an irritant effect on the intestines and acts as a powerful purgative. Castor oil is a powerful CATHARTIC, and should not be used as a treatment for constipation or any digestive disorder. It is used primarily in the preparation of the bowel for diagnostic tests and surgery. Its unpleasant taste and texture can be disguised if it is given in iced orange juice.

castrate (kas′trāt) 1. to subject to excision of the gonads. 2. an individual whose gonads have been removed.

castration (kas-tra′shun) excision of the gonads, especially in the male, rendering the individual incapable of reproduction.
   female c., removal of the ovaries, or bilateral OOPHORECTOMY.
   male c., removal of the testes, or bilateral ORCHIECTOMY. It may be employed in therapy of metastatic cancer of the prostate.

casualty (kaz′u-al-te) 1. an accidental or other injury. 2. a person suffering accidental or other injury.

casuistics (kaz″u-is′tiks) the recording and study of cases of disease.

cat-scratch disease an infection most frequently acquired through the scratch of a cat. It is a sterile regional lymphadenitis.

The disease is probably caused by a virus that is found between the claws of cats and kittens. Here the virus usually does no harm to the cat, and the animal appears healthy, but a scratch may transfer it to a human being.

In half the cases, after several days there is a persistent sore at the site of the scratch, and fever and other symptoms of infection may develop. There is also swelling of the lymph nodes draining the infected part.

In milder cases, the symptoms soon disappear, with no aftereffects. Sometimes the attack is more serious and the glands may require surgical incision and drainage. The disease is generally mild and lasts for about 2 weeks. In rare cases, it may persist for a period of up to 2 years.

No specific remedy exists for cat-scratch disease, although certain antibiotics appear to shorten its course. The main treatment consists simply of keeping the patient as comfortable as possible. The disease can, however, usually be prevented by avoiding cat scratches or by thoroughly washing and disinfecting any scratch that does occur.

catabasis (kah-tab′ah-sis) the stage of decline of a disease. adj., **catabat′ic.**

catabiosis (kat″ah-bi-o′sis) the natural decline of vital phenomena in a cell. adj., **catabiot′ic.**

catabolin (kah-tab′o-lin) a product of destructive metabolism; a catabolite.

catabolism (kah-tab′o-lizm) destructive metabolism; the process by which an organism reconverts living, organized substances into simpler compounds, with release of energy for its use (see also METABOLISM). adj., **catabol′ic.**

catabolite (kah-tab′o-līt) a compound produced in catabolism.

catachronobiology (kat″ah-kron″o-bi-ol′o-je) the study of the deleterious effects of time on a living system.

catacrotism (kah-tak′rŏ-tizm) the occurrence of one or more indentations on the descending limb of the sphygmogram. adj., **catacrot′ic.**

catadicrotism (kat″ah-di′krŏ-tizm) the occurrence of two indentations on the descending limb of the sphygmogram. adj., **catadicrot′ic.**

catadioptric (kat″ah-di-op′trik) pertaining to both refraction and reflection of light.

catagenesis (kat″ah-jen′ĕ-sis) involution or retrogression.

catalase (kat′ah-lās) a crystalline enzyme that specifically catalyzes the decomposition of hydrogen peroxide and is found in almost all cells except certain bacteria.

catalepsy (kat′ah-lep″se) a condition in which the entire body or the limbs remain passively in any position in which placed. The patient with catalepsy may remain in one position for minutes, days or even longer. adj., **catalep′tic.**

Catalepsy may occur in several mental illnesses. It is most common and indeed considered typical in cases of catatonic SCHIZOPHRENIA. The patient may sit with his hands flat on his knees and his head bowed, or may remain in an awkward and uncomfortable position. He is not necessarily unaware of what is going on, but he does not respond. This apathetic condition may end as suddenly as it begins.

Treatment depends on the underlying disturbance and requires psychiatric examination. It may consist of PSYCHOTHERAPY, medications, SHOCK THERAPY or a combination of methods.

NURSING CARE. Regular skin care and exercise of the muscles and joints are necessary to prevent circulatory complications in the patient with catalepsy. Attention must also be given to his nutritional status and an adequate diet provided. Even though the patient may not be able to respond to spoken directions or conversation and is physically unable to move, he cannot be left in one position for long periods of time any more than can the patient who is physically paralyzed. The cataleptic's mental state is such that he cannot recognize numbness or pain, nor can he communicate his need for attention.

Care must be used in conversations held within the patient's hearing. His total apathy does not mean that he cannot hear or see what is going on around him. Sometimes it is of great help to this type of patient to have someone sit quietly beside him so that he is aware that someone cares and is genuinely interested in his welfare. Above all, he should not be ignored simply because he is quiet and undemanding of the staff's time and attention.

A sudden change in the patient's condition, with increased activity, may indicate his progression from one state of extreme emotion to another. Restlessness or talkativeness usually do not indicate that a cataleptic's mental condition has dramatically improved. When the patient becomes more active the nurse should be alert to the possibility of suicide and attempts at self-mutilation. A person who has exhibited symptoms as severe as catalepsy is very ill and will need continued and long-term care to help him overcome his serious emotional problems.

cataleptiform   (kat″ah-lep′tĭ-form) resembling catalepsy.

catalysis (kah-tal′ĭ-sis) influence on a chemical reaction by small quantities of a substance which does not enter into the reaction but persists unchanged. adj., **catalyt′ic.**

catalyst (kat′ah-list) a substance capable of promoting or altering the speed of a chemical reaction, but one that does not take part in it.

catalyze (kat′ah-līz) to promote the occurrence or influence the velocity of a chemical reaction.

catamenia   (kat″ah-me′ne-ah) menstruation.

catamnesis (kat″am-ne′sis) the medical history of a patient from the date on which he is discharged from treatment to a follow-up visit.

cataphasia (kat″ah-fa′ze-ah) speech disorder with constant repetition of a word or phrase.

cataphora (kah-taf′ŏ-rah) a state resembling sleep, with loss of feeling and voice.

cataphoresis (kat″ah-fo-re′sis) introduction of medicinal ions or charged particles through the unbroken skin, by means of an electric field.

cataphoria (kat″ah-fo′re-ah) the tendency to tilt the head upward, the visual axes deviating downward on looking straight ahead.

cataphrenia (kat″ah-fre′ne-ah) mental debility of the dementia type which tends to recovery.

cataphylaxis (kat″ah-fi-lak′sis) movement of leukocytes and antibodies to the site of an infection.

cataplasia (kat″ah-pla′ze-ah) atrophy with tissues reverting to earlier conditions.

cataplexy (kat′ah-plek″se) a sudden, temporary loss of muscular tone, causing collapse.

cataract (kat′ah-rakt) opacity of the lens of the eye.

CAUSES AND SYMPTOMS. Cataract may result from injuries to the eye, exposure to great heat or radiation or inherited factors. The great majority of cases, however, are senile cataracts, which are apparently a part of the aging process of the human body.

Blurred and dimmed vision are often the first symptoms of cataract. The patient may find that he needs a brighter reading light, or must hold objects closer to his eyes. The continued clouding of the lens may cause double vision. Finally, a need for frequent changes of eyeglasses may be caused by the presence of cataract. These symptoms do not necessarily indicate cataract, but if any of them are present, an ophthalmologist should be consulted immediately.

TREATMENT. The only known effective treatment for cataract is surgery. No ointments or drops can dissolve a cataract. The surgical method removes the entire clouded lens from the eye (cataract extraction). Loss of the lens is later compensated for by special eyeglasses or contact lenses.

While removal of a cataract is a delicate operation, it is more than 95 per cent successful in restoring sight. A cataract can be removed at any time, despite the former belief that it had to become mature or "ripe."

NURSING CARE. *Preoperative Care.* The patient having a cataract extraction will require little special care other than attention to his need to feel comfortable and at home in the hospital environment. He may have extremely poor vision which will demand special attention to safety hazards in his environment. Side rails should be applied to his bed, foot stools and other low objects must be removed to prevent his falling over them while out of bed. The surgeon usually orders eye drops at frequent intervals prior to surgery. These are mydriatics, which dilate the pupil and should be given with extreme care and accuracy.

Postoperative Care. The patient should be instructed to avoid sudden movements, sneezing or coughing, or squeezing the eyelids together as these motions place stress on the suture line. Most surgeons now allow these patients out of bed the first postoperative day. However, the nurse should be sure of the physician's orders before allowing physical activity for the patient having a cataract extraction.

after-c., secondary cataract.

capsular c., opacification of the capsule of the lens, often associated with degeneration of subcapsular lens fibers.

cortical c., opacification involving lens fibers just beneath the capsule and beginning at the periphery of the lens.

hypermature c., one in which the entire lens has become opaque and the cortex (the softer external part of the lens) liquid, allowing the lens nucleus (the harder internal part) to sink downward by gravity.

lenticular c., one occurring in the lens proper.

mature c., one in which the whole lens substance is involved.

secondary c., a condition sometimes following extracapsular extraction of a cataractous lens, due to density of the capsular remains or proliferation of the capsular epithelium.

senile c., the cataract of old persons.

cataracta (kat″ah-rak′tah) [L.] cataract.

catarrh (kah-tahr′) a term formerly used to indicate inflammation of a mucous membrane with free discharge. adj., **catar′rhal.**

catathymia (kat″ah-thi′me-ah) a psychic disorder marked by perseveration.

catatonia (kat″ah-to′ne-ah) a form of SCHIZO-PHRENIA marked by conspicuous motor disturbances (retardation and stupor, or excessive activity and excitement). adj., **cataton′ic.**

catatricrotism (kat″ah-tri′krŏ-tizm) the occurrence of three indentations in the descending limb of the sphygmogram. adj., **catatricrot′ic.**

catatropia (kat″ah-tro′pe-ah) downward turning of the visual axis.

catechol (kat′ĕ-kol) a compound, 1,2-dehydroxybenzene, used for dyeing and as a reagent.

catecholamine (kat″ĕ-kol-am′in) a compound of catechol and an amine, having a sympathomimetic action; examples include epinephrine and norepinephrine.

Catenabacterium (kah-te″nah-bak-te′re-um) a genus of Schizomycetes found in the intestinal tract.

catgut (kat′gut) absorbable suture material prepared from submucous connective tissue of the small intestine of healthy sheep.

catharsis (kah-thar′sis) a purging or cleansing, especially the emotional reliving of past (repressed) events as a means of releasing tension and anxiety.

cathartic (kah-thar′tik) 1. promoting defecation. 2. an agent that promotes defecation; sometimes classified according to increasing intensity of their actions as laxatives, purgatives and drastics.

lubricant c., one that acts by softening the feces and reducing friction between them and the intestinal wall.

saline c., one that increases fluidity of intestinal contents by retention of water by osmotic forces, and indirectly increases motor activity.

stimulant c., one that directly increases motor activity of the intestinal tract.

cathepsin (kah-thep′sin) an intracellular protein-splitting enzyme that acts in an essentially neutral medium.

catheter (kath′ĕ-ter) a tubular instrument of rubber, plastic, metal or other material, used for draining or injecting fluids through a body passage.

Urethral catheters are used to drain urine from the bladder. They may be inserted for the purpose of withdrawing a sample of urine for laboratory analysis, or as indwelling catheters in cases of urinary incontinence. Indwelling catheters are sometimes employed to prevent fullness of the bladder following bladder surgery, or to prevent pressure against the suture line and contamination of the operative site during and after vaginal and perineal surgery. (See also CATHETERIZATION.)

Ureteral catheters are inserted directly into the ureters. These are extremely small catheters and require skilled handling. They are inserted by the

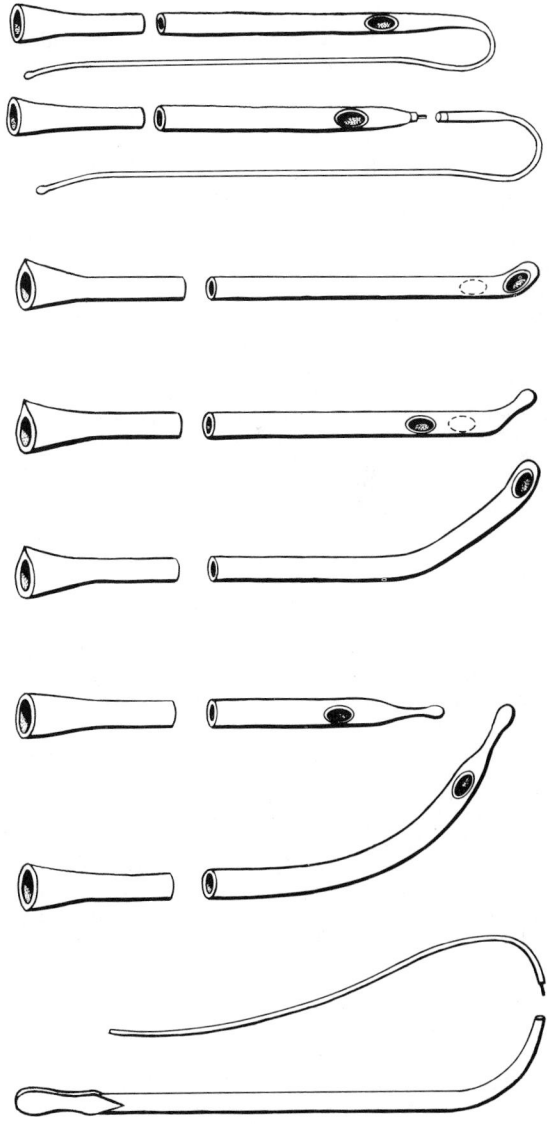

Urethral catheters.

urologist and aid in the diagnosis and treatment of disorders of the kidney and urinary tract.

A nasal catheter may be used to administer OXY-GEN. Nasogastric tubes, such as the Levin tube and the Miller-Abbott tube, are inserted into the stomach or small intestine for diagnosis and treatment of disorders of the gastrointestinal tract. TUBE FEEDINGS, which may be necessary when a patient cannot or will not take fluids and food by mouth, are administered via a nasogastric tube.

Catheters are also used for the introduction of fluids into the veins (as in intravenous feedings), and for withdrawal of blood samples from the major blood vessels and chambers of the heart (see also CARDIAC CATHETERIZATION). When x-ray studies are made of the heart and blood vessels (angiocardiography), the radiopaque material is injected by way of a catheter inserted into a blood vessel.

elbowed c., a catheter bent at an angle near the beak; used principally in cases of enlarged prostate.

eustachian c., an instrument for dilating the eustachian tube.

female c., a short catheter for the female bladder.

indwelling c., one that is held in position in the urethra.

prostatic c., one with a short angular tip.

self-retaining c., a catheter constructed so that it remains in the bladder, effecting constant drainage.

winged c., one with two projections on the end to retain it in the bladder.

catheterization (kath″ĕ-ter-ĭ-za′shun) passage of a catheter into a body channel or cavity. (See also CARDIAC CATHETERIZATION.) The most common usage of the term is in reference to the introduction of a catheter via the urethra into the urinary bladder. This is often a nursing procedure, one that demands strict adherence to the principles of medical and surgical asepsis so that pathogenic microorganisms are not introduced into the urinary system. Since the urinary tract is normally sterile, any break in technique during the insertion of a catheter, or in the care of an indwelling catheter that is left in the bladder for a period of time, may result in a serious infection.

NURSING CARE. As stated above, catheterization is a sterile procedure. The nurse must wear sterile gloves, use sterile equipment, drape the patient so as to provide a sterile field on which to work and avoid contamination of the catheter before it is inserted.

If the catheterization is done to obtain a sample of urine for laboratory analysis, the urine is collected in a sterile container; 60 to 100 ml. is considered adequate for most tests. When an indwelling catheter is inserted for continuous drainage, a specially designed catheter such as the Foley catheter with an inflatable balloon, or a mushroom-tipped catheter is used to avoid its accidental removal from the bladder.

Before the catheter is introduced, the area surrounding the urinary meatus is thoroughly cleansed with a mild antiseptic. In some institutions the procedure includes irrigation of the urethra with a mild antiseptic prior to insertion of the catheter, or use of an antibiotic ointment to lubricate the tip of the catheter. These measures reduce the possibility of transferring microorganisms from the external genitalia and urethra into the bladder.

Once the catheter has been inserted, special care must be given to the drainage tubing to guard against tension on the catheter or kinking of the tubing, which may obstruct the flow of urine. Catheters should never be pinned to the bed clothes as this may result in accidental removal or unnecessary pulling when the patient moves about in bed. The tubing leading from the catheter to the collecting bottle must *always* be kept below the level of the bladder to avoid backflow of urine and introduction of bacteria into the urinary tract. When changing the tubing, or disconnecting it for irrigations or to empty the drainage bottle, the nurse must be careful to avoid contamination of the catheter and inside of the tubing. Cleansing the open end of the catheter and the end of the connecting tubing with 70 per cent alcohol is recommended as a means of reducing the possibility of contamination. The urine may be collected by way of an open drainage system (in which there is more danger of infection) or a closed drainage system. The type of system used will depend on hospital policy and the instructions from the attending physician.

Nursing care must also include attention to the area surrounding the urinary meatus. At least twice daily, or more often if necessary, the genital area should be washed gently with soap and water and dried thoroughly. Crusts and secretions around the catheter may be removed by gentle wiping with a gauze or cotton square saturated with a mild antiseptic. These measures will reduce the possibility of infection and insure the comfort of the patient by eliminating unpleasant odors and irritation.

catheterize (kath′ĕ-ter-īz″) to introduce a catheter into a body cavity, usually into the urinary bladder for the withdrawal of urine.

cathexis (kah-thek′sis) attachment of psychic or emotional energy to an object or idea.

cathode (kath′ōd) the negative electrode by which the electric current leaves a cell, apparatus or body.

Cathomycin (kath′o-mi″sin) trademark for preparations of novobiocin, an antibiotic.

cation (kat′i-on) an electropositive element; the element that in electrolysis passes to the negative pole.

catoptrophobia (kat″op-tro-fo′be-ah) morbid dread of mirrors.

cauda (kaw′da), pl. *cau′dae* [L.] a tail or tail-like appendage.

c. equi′na, the sheaf of roots of the lower spinal nerves descending from their point of attachment to the spinal cord to the site of emergence of the nerves from the spinal canal.

caudad (kaw′dad) toward a cauda or toward the posterior or distal end.

caudal (kaw′dal) pertaining to a cauda or to the posterior or distal end.

c. anesthesia, a type of regional anesthesia used in childbirth in which the anesthetizing solution, usually procaine, is injected into the caudal area of the spinal canal through the lower end of the sacrum. It affects the caudal nerve roots, and renders the cervix, vagina and perineum insensitive to pain. In continuous caudal anesthesia, the needle is left in place throughout the delivery and the anesthetic is allowed to drip in gradually. Care must be taken to ensure that the solution does not enter higher in the spinal canal, and use of the procedure requires constant attendance by an obstetrician or trained anesthetist. It is used in only a small percentage of patients.

caudate (kaw′dat) having a tail.

caudatum (kaw-da′tum) the caudate nucleus.

caul (kawl) a part of the amnion that sometimes envelops the head of the fetus at birth.

cauliflower ear (kaw′lĭ-flow″er) a thickened and deformed ear caused by the accumulation of fluid and blood clots in the tissue following repeated injury. It is most commonly seen in boxers, for whom it is almost an occupational hazard. A cauliflower ear will not recover its normal shape but it can be restored to normal by means of plastic surgery.

caumesthesia (kaw″mes-the′ze-ah) a condition in which a patient experiences a sense of burning heat, unrelated to the temperature.

causalgia (kaw-zal′je-ah) persistent, diffuse and burning pain associated with trophic skin changes in the hand or foot following injury of the part. The syndrome may be aggravated by the slightest stimuli or it may be intensified by the emotions. Causalgia usually begins several weeks after the initial injury and the pain is described as intense, with the patient sometimes taking elaborate precautions to avoid any stimulus he knows to be capable of causing a flare-up of symptoms. He often will go to great extremes to protect the affected limb and becomes preoccupied with such protection.

Any one of a variety of injuries to the hand, foot, arm or leg can lead to causalgia, but in most cases there has been some injury to the median or the sciatic nerve. Sympathectomy may be necessary to eliminate the severe pain, and in the majority of cases it is quite successful. Psychotherapy may be necessary when emotional instability is suspected. Emotional problems may have been present before the initial injury, or they may result from the intense suffering characteristic of severe causalgia.

caustic (kaws′tik) 1. burning or escharotic. 2. a burning or escharotic compound.

cauterant (kaw′ter-ant) a caustic material or application.

cauterization (kaw″ter-ĭ-za′shun) application of a caustic or of a hot instrument.

cautery (kaw′ter-e) 1. application of a caustic, or of a burning substance or instrument, for the destruction of tissue. 2. a hot instrument or caustic substance used to destroy tissue.

caverna (ka-ver′nah), pl. *caver′nae* [L.] a general term to designate a cavity.

cavernitis (kav″er-ni′tis) inflammation of the corpus cavernosum.

cavernoma (kav″er-no′mah) hemangioma.

cavernositis (kav″er-no-si′tis) cavernitis.

cavernostomy (kav″er-nos′to-me) open drainage of a tuberculous cavity of the lung.

cavernous (kav′er-nus) containing hollow spaces.

cavitary (kav′ĭ-ta″re) characterized by the presence of a cavity or cavities.

cavitas (kav′ĭ-tas), pl. *cavita′tes* [L.] cavity.

cavitation (kav″ĭ-ta′shun) the formation of a cavity, or empty place.

cavitis (ka-vi′tis) inflammation of a vena cava.

cavity (kav′ĭ-te) a hollow or space, especially a space within the body or one of its organs. In dentistry, the lesion produced by CARIES.
  abdominal c., the part of the body cavity between the diaphragm above and the pelvis below.
  amniotic c., the cavity of the amnion.
  cranial c., the space enclosed by the bones of the cranium.
  glenoid c., the cavity in the head of the scapula for articulation with the humerus.
  marrow c., medullary c., the cavity of a bone that contains the bone marrow.
  nasal c., the mucosa-lined cavity at either side of the nasal septum, within the nose.
  oral c., the cavity of the mouth, bounded by the jaw bones and associated structures (muscles and mucosa).
  pelvic c., the space within the walls of the pelvis.
  pericardial c., the potential space between the epicardium and the parietal layer of the serous pericardium.
  peritoneal c., the potential space between parietal and the visceral peritoneum.
  pleural c., the potential space between the parietal and the visceral pulmonary pleura.
  pulp c., the pulp-filled central chamber in the crown of a tooth.
  serous c., any cavity, like that enclosed by the peritoneum or pleura, not communicating with the outside of the body, the lining membrane of which secretes a watery fluid.
  thoracic c., the portion of the ventral body cavity situated between the neck and the diaphragm.

cavum (ka′vum), pl. *ca′va* [L.] cavity.

cavus (ka′vus) [L.] hollow.

CBC complete blood cell count (see also BLOOD COUNT).

cc. cubic centimeter.

C.D. curative dose.

C.D.$_{50}$ median curative dose; that which abolishes symptoms in 50 per cent of the cases.

Cd chemical symbol, *cadmium.*

Cd. caudal.

Ce chemical symbol, *cerium.*

cebocephalia (se″bo-sĕ-fa′le-ah) a monkey-like deformity of the head, with the eyes close together and the nose flat.

cebocephalus (se″bo-sef′ah-lus) a fetal monster exhibiting cebocephalia.

cecal (se'kal) pertaining to the cecum.

cecectomy (se-sek'to-me) excision of the cecum.

cecitis (se-si'tis) inflammation of the cecum.

ceco- (se'ko) word element [L.], *cecum.*

cecocoloplicopexy (se"ko-ko"lo-pli'ko-pek"se) fixation of the cecum and ascending colon to the posterior abdominal wall, by means of the parietal peritoneum, to prevent torsion.

cecocolostomy (se"ko-ko-los'to-me) anastomosis of the cecum to a formerly remote portion of the colon.

cecoileostomy (se"ko-il"e-os'to-me) ileocecostomy; anastomosis of the ileum to the cecum.

Cecon (se'kon) trademark for preparations of ascorbic acid (vitamin C).

cecopexy (se'ko-pek"se) fixation of the cecum to the abdominal wall.

cecorectal (se"ko-rek'tal) pertaining to the cecum and rectum.

cecorrhaphy (se-kor'ah-fe) suture of the cecum.

cecosigmoidostomy (se"ko-sig"moi-dos'to-me) anastomosis of the cecum to the sigmoid colon.

cecostomy (se-kos'to-me) surgical creation of an artificial opening into the cecum.

cecotomy (se-kot'o-me) incision of the cecum.

cecum (se'kum) 1. the proximal part of the large intestine just distal to the ileum. 2. any blind pouch or cul-de-sac.

Cedilanid (se"dĭ-lan'id) trademark for a preparation of a crystalline digitalis glycoside (lanatoside C); used in heart failure and cases of cardiac arrhythmia.

Cel. Celsius.

-cele (sēl) word element [Gr.], *hernia.*

celi(o)- (se'le-o) word element [Gr.], *abdomen; through the abdominal wall.*

celiac (se'le-ak) pertaining to the abdomen.
  c. disease, a comparatively uncommon disease of the digestive system, in which there is an inability to digest and utilize fats, starches and sugars. It is usually thought of as a children's disease but symptoms may persist into adult life. The condition is closely related to SPRUE and may be identical with it.
  CAUSE. The causes of celiac disease are not precisely known. Recent studies have indicated that persons suffering from the disease may have a sensitivity to the gluten of wheat and rye, because of a deficiency in the enzymes that help to metabolize these substances. There is also strong evidence that the disease is associated with hereditary factors.
  SYMPTOMS. The disease is characterized by flatulence and by large, very foul-smelling, bulky, frothy and pale-colored stools containing much fat. There are recurrent attacks of diarrhea, with pos-

sible accompanying stomach cramps, alternating with constipation. The abdomen is swollen as in serious malnutrition. The child becomes weak, undernourished and anemic, and his growth is stunted. He is irritable, has little appetite and may refuse to eat. Occasionally the reverse is true, and the patient may eat voraciously but with no gain in weight.
  TREATMENT. Treatment usually depends on a diet high in protein and free from gluten and fat. Fruit sugars are used to replace the milk sugars and other sugars, and the main content of the diet is made up of milk protein or skimmed milk, the white of eggs, lean meat, fish, liver and protein-rich vegetables such as peas and beans. After the patient has done well on this for 6 months, a full diet is gradually achieved by adding one food at a time. The last foods to be added are starchy foods. While on the diet the patient is given vitamin supplements, especially vitamin B complex, to combat the anemia and nutritional deficiencies.
  Full recovery from this disease may take 1 to 2 years, and relapses may occur if the diet is disregarded. During severe relapses, intravenous feeding may be necessary to combat acidosis, dehydration and symptoms of starvation.
  Death from uncomplicated celiac disease is rare, and the symptoms usually disappear in later childhood and adolescence, although in a few cases the condition may continue in some degree. The recovery may be permanent, or the symptoms may reappear in the third to sixth decade of life, with the onset of adult celiac disease.

celialgia (se"le-al'je-ah) pain in the abdomen.

celiectasia (se"le-ek-ta'ze-ah) excessive size of the abdominal cavity.

celiectomy (se"le-ek'to-me) 1. excision of the celiac branches of the vagus nerve. 2. excision of an abdominal organ.

celiocentesis (se"le-o-sen-te'sis) puncture of the abdomen.

celioma (se"le-o'mah) a tumor of the abdomen.

celiomyalgia (se"le-o-mi-al'je-ah) pain in the abdominal muscles.

celiomyositis (se"le-o-mi"o-si'tis) inflammation of the abdominal muscles.

celioparacentesis (se"le-o-par"ah-sen-te'sis) puncture of the abdomen.

celiopathy (se"le-op'ah-the) any abdominal disease.

celiopyosis (se"le-o-pi-o'sis) suppuration in the abdominal cavity.

celiorrhaphy (se"le-or'ah-fe) suture of the abdominal wall.

celioscope (se'le-o-skōp") an endoscope for examining a body cavity, especially the abdominal cavity.

celioscopy (se"le-os'ko-pe) examination of a body cavity, especially the abdominal cavity, through a celioscope.

celiotomy (se"le-ot'o-me) opening of the abdominal cavity through an incision in its wall; laparotomy.

vaginal c., incision into the abdominal cavity through the vagina.

cell (sel) the basic unit in the organization of living substance. Although cells may be widely differentiated and highly specialized in their function, they all have the same basic structure; that is, they have an outer covering called the membrane, a main substance called the cytoplasm and a control center called the nucleus. The cytoplasm and the substance of the nucleus (nucleoplasm or karyoplasm) are collectively referred to as protoplasm.

Cell membranes are capable of selection in the passage of substances into and out of the cell. These substances can pass through a cell membrance by DIFFUSION, by active transport and by pinocytosis, a mechanism by which the membrane engulfs some of the extracellular fluid and its contents. Another method of ingestion by the cell is phagocytosis, whereby the cell ingests large particles such as a bacterium or a particle of degenerating tissue. Gases such as oxygen and carbon dioxide readily pass through the cell membrane. Because of this semipermeability of the cell membrane it is possible for cells to receive nutrition and dispose of waste products.

Metabolism of the cell, which includes all the physical and chemical reactions within the cell, takes place in the protoplasm. These reactions are essential to the life of the cell and the normal functioning of the body. They include the synthesis of protein, lipid secretion, oxidation with release of energy and the release of glucose from glycogen stores of the cells.

The control center of the cell is the nucleus. The chemical reactions of cellular metabolism are controlled in the nucleus, and it is this part of the cell that contains DEOXYRIBONUCLEIC ACID (DNA) which effects reproduction of the cell. The nucleus, then, influences growth, repair and reproduction of the cell.

Cells of the body are organized into tissues and tissues into organs. The fluid within the cell (60 to 90 per cent of the protoplasm is water) is called intracellular fluid. The fluid surrounding the cell and within the tissues is called interstitial fluid or tissue fluid. The molecules and ions in these fluids are essential to the life of the cell. (See also FLUIDS and ELECTROLYTES.)

argentaffin c's, cells containing cytoplasmic granules capable of reducing silver compounds, located throughout the gastrointestinal tract, chiefly in the basilar portions of the gastric glands and the crypts of Lieberkühn.

basal c., an early keratinocyte, present in the basal layer of the epidermis.

beta c's, cells in the pancreas that make up most of the bulk of the islands of Langerhans; they contain granules that are soluble in alcohol.

Betz c's, large pyramidal ganglion cells forming a layer of the gray matter of the brain.

blast c., the least differentiated blood cell type.

blood c., one of the formed elements of the blood (see also BLOOD).

bone c., a nucleated cell in the lacunae of bone.

chromaffin c's, cells whose cytoplasm shows fine brown granules when stained with potassium bichromate, occurring in the adrenal medulla and in scattered groups in various organs and throughout the body.

cleavage c., one of the cells derived from the fertilized ovum by mitosis; a blastomere.

daughter c., a cell formed by division of a mother cell.

foam c., a cell with a vacuolated appearance due to the presence of complex lipoids; seen in xanthoma.

ganglion c., a large nerve cell, especially one of those of the spinal ganglia.

Gaucher's c., a large cell characteristic of Gaucher's disease, with eccentrically placed nuclei and fine wavy fibrils parallel to the long axis of the cell.

germ c., one that, under suitable conditions, will contribute to the formation of a new individual of the species; an egg cell or sperm cell.

giant c., a large, multinuclear cell.

glia c's, branching cells constituting the reticulum of neuroglia.

Golgi's c's, nerve cells with short processes in the posterior horns of the spinal cord.

granular c., one containing granules, such as a keratinocyte in the stratum granulosum of the epidermis, when it contains a dense collection of darkly staining granules.

heart failure c's, iron-containing, rust-colored cells found in the sputum of patients with long-standing heart failure.

HeLa c's, the first continuously cultured carcinoma cells, used in studies of life processes.

interstitial c's, the cells of the connective tissue of the ovary or testis which furnish the internal secretion of those structures.

islet c's, cells composing the islands of Langerhans.

juxtaglomerular c's, specialized cells, containing secretory granules, located in the tunica media of the afferent glomerular arterioles.

Kupffer's c's, large star-shaped or pyramidal cells along the walls of the venous capillaries of the liver.

L.E. c., a mature neutrophilic polymorphonuclear leukocyte with a large phagocytic vacuole containing partially digested and lysed nuclear material, characteristic of lupus erythematosus.

Leydig's c's, interstitial cells of the testis.

Lipshütz c., centrocyte.

lutein c's, the enlarged follicular cells of the ovary seen after rupture of an ovarian follicle.

lymph c., a leukocyte from lymph.

lymphoid c., a mononuclear cell in lymphoid tissue which ultimately is concerned with humoral or cellular immunologic reactivity.

mast c., a connective tissue cell capable of elaborating basophilic, metachromatic cytoplasmic granules that contain histamine, heparin and, in some species, serotonin.

mastoid c's, hollow spaces of various size and shape in the mastoid process of the temporal bone, communicating with the mastoid antrum and lined with a continuation of its mucous membrane.

mother c., a cell that divides to form new cells.

myeloma c., a cell found in bone marrow and sometimes in peripheral blood in multiple myeloma.

nerve c., any cell of a nerve, nerve center or ganglion.

olfactory c's, a set of specialized cells of the

mucous membrane of the nose; the receptors for smell.

Pick's c's, round, oval or polyhedral cells with foamy, lipid-containing cytoplasm found in the bone marrow and spleen in Niemann-Pick disease.

pigment c's, cells containing granules of pigment.

plasma c., plasmocyte; a mononuclear cell of the bone marrow, responsible, in part, for the manufacture of antibodies.

prickle c., a dividing keratinocyte in the stratum germinativum of the epidermis, with delicate radiating process connecting with other similar cells.

primordial germ c's, the earliest germ cells, at first located outside the gonad.

Purkinje's c's, large branched cells of the middle layer of the brain.

reticuloendothelial c., one of the RETICULOENDO-THELIAL SYSTEM.

reticulum c., one of the primitive mesenchymal cells forming the framework of lymph nodes, bone marrow and spleen, which may differentiate into myeloblast, lymphoblast or monoblast.

sickle c., a crescentic or sickle-shaped erythrocyte, the abnormal shape caused by the presence of varying proportions of hemoglobin S (see also SICKLE CELL ANEMIA).

signet c., a globular, vacuolated cell, with the flattened nucleus pushed to the periphery, producing a resemblance to a signet ring.

somatic c's, the cells of the somatoplasm; undifferentiated body cells.

squamous c's, epithelial cells that are flat, like scales.

stellate c., a star-shaped cell, particularly a glia cell having a large number of filaments extending in all directions.

Sternberg's giant c's, Sternberg-Reed c's, giant, polyploid mesenchymal cells with hyperlobulated nuclei and multiple large nucleoli characteristic of Hodgkin's disease.

stipple c., an erythrocyte containing granules that take a basic or bluish stain with Wright's stain.

target c., an abnormally thin erythrocyte showing, when stained, a dark center and a peripheral ring of hemoglobin, separated by a pale, unstained zone containing less hemoglobin, occurring in various chronic anemias.

tart c., a histiocyte or monocytoid reticuloendothelial cell containing a second, characteristic nucleus, usually in the cytoplasm filling the concavity of the major nucleus.

taste c's, cells in the taste buds associated with the nerves of taste.

totipotential c., a cell that is capable of developing into any variety of body cell.

visual c's, the neuroepithelial element of the retina.

wandering c's, mononuclear phagocytic cells that are components of the reticuloendothelial system.

cell division the process by which cells reproduce.
   direct c.d., amitosis.
   indirect c. d., mitosis.

cellular (sel′u-lar) pertaining to, or made up of, cells.

cellularity (sel″u-lar′ĭ-te) the state of a tissue or organ relative to its constituent cells.

cellulicidal (sel″u-lĭ-si′dal) destroying cells.

cellulitis (sel″u-li′tis) a diffuse inflammatory process within solid tissues, characterized by edema, redness, pain and interference with function. It may be caused by infection with streptococci, staphylococci or other organisms.

Cellulitis usually occurs in the loose tissues beneath the skin, but may also occur in tissues beneath mucous membranes or around muscle bundles or surrounding organs.

ERYSIPELAS, a surface cellulitis of the skin, is characterized by patches of skin that are red with sharply defined borders and that feel hot to the touch. Other types of skin cellulitis are also characterized by hot red patches, but the borders are less clearly defined. Red streaks extending from the patch indicate that the lymph vessels have been infected. Ludwig's angina is a cellulitis of the tissues of the floor of the mouth and neck, in the area around the submaxillary gland. Orbital cellulitis is an acute inflammation of the eye socket. Pelvic cellulitis involves the tissues surrounding the uterus and is called parametritis.

Cellulitis is potentially dangerous but usually can be treated successfully with antibiotics or sulfonamides. Any cellulitis on the face must be given special attention because the infection may extend directly to the cavernous sinuses of the brain.

cellulofibrous (sel″u-lo-fi′brus) partly cellular and partly fibrous.

celluloid (sel′u-loid) a plastic compound of pyroxylin and camphor.

celluloneuritis (sel″u-lo-nu-ri′tis) inflammation of nerve cells.

cellulose (sel′u-lōs) the structural form of polysaccharides in plants, acting as a support for plant tissues.
   oxidized c., an absorbable oxidation product of cellulose, applied locally to stop bleeding.

celology (se-lol′o-je) the study of hernias.

Celontin (se-lon′tin) trademark for a preparation of methsuximide, an anticonvulsant.

celoschisis (se-los′kĭ-sis) fissure of the abdominal wall.

celoscope (se′lo-skōp) celioscope.

celosomia (se″lo-so′me-ah) a developmental anomaly characterized by fissure or absence of the sternum, with hernial protrusion of the viscera.

celothelioma (se″lo-the″le-o′mah) mesothelioma.

celozoic (se″lo-zo′ik) inhabiting the intestinal canal of the body; said of parasites.

Celsius thermometer (sel′se-us) centigrade thermometer on which the ice point is at 0 and the normal boiling point of water is at 100 degrees (100° C.), with the interval between these two established points divided into 100 equal units. The abbreviation 100° C. should be read "one hundred degrees Celsius."

cement (se-ment′) a substance supporting or connecting other structures, or in which they may be embedded.
   dental c., cementum.
   muscle c., the myoglia.

cementicle (se-men′tĭ-kl) a small, discrete globular mass of dentin in the region of a tooth root.

cementoblast (se-men′to-blast) a large cuboidal cell active in the formation of cementum.

cementoblastoma (se-men″to-blas-to′mah) an odontogenic fibroma whose cells are developing into cementoblasts and in which there is only a small proportion of calcified tissue.

cementoclasia (se-men″to-kla′ze-ah) destruction by disease of the cementum of a tooth root.

cementocyte (se-men′to-sīt) a cell found in lacunae of cellular cementum, frequently having long processes radiating from the cell body toward the periodontal surface of the cementum.

cementogenesis (se-men″to-jen′ĕ-sis) development of cementum on the root dentin of a tooth.

cementoma (se″men-to′mah) an odontogenic fibroma in which the cells have developed into cementoblasts and which consists largely of cementum.

cementosis (se″men-to′sis) proliferation of cementum.

cementum (se-men′tum) calcified tissue of mesodermal origin covering the root of a tooth.

cenesthesia (sen″es-the′ze-ah) the sense or feeling of consciousness. adj., **cenesthe′sic, cenesthet′ic.**

cenophobia (sen″o-fo′be-ah) cenotophobia.

cenosis (se-no′sis) a morbid discharge. adj., **cenot′ic.**

cenosite (se′no-sīt) a parasite able to live apart from its host.

cenotophobia (se-no″to-fo′be-ah) morbid fear of new things or new ideas.

cenotype (sen′o-tīp) the original from which other types have arisen.

censor (sen′sor) the psychic influence which prevents unconscious thoughts and wishes coming into consciousness.

Cent. centigrade.

center (sen′ter) a point from which a process starts, especially a plexus or ganglion giving off nerves that control a function.
  accelerating c., one in the medulla oblongata that accelerates action of the heart.
  auditory c., one in the first temporosphenoidal convolution of the brain, concerned with the sense of hearing.
  Broca's c., speech center.
  cardio-inhibitory c., one in the medulla oblongata that depresses heart action.
  germinal c., the area in lymphoid tissue where mitotic figures are observed, differentiation and formation of lymphocytes occur and elements related to antibody synthesis are found.
  gustatory c., the cerebral center supposed to control taste.
  heat-regulating c., the center for the control of body temperature.
  nerve c., a collection of nerve cells in the central nervous system that are associated together in the performance of some particular function.
  c. of ossification, the place in bones at which ossification begins.
  pneumotaxic c., a special group of cells in the midbrain that is responsible for periodic inhibition of the respiratory center.
  reflex c., a nerve center at which afferent sensory impressions are converted into efferent motor impulses.
  respiratory c., a special group of cells in the medulla and pons from which impulses pass to the diaphragm and rib muscles, resulting in their regular and coordinated contraction.
  speech c., one in the left (or right) inferior frontal gyrus concerned with the motor aspects of speech.
  visual c., the center that regulates the power of vision, located in the occipital lobe, especially in the cuneus.
  Wernicke's c., the speech center in the cortex of the left temporo-occipital convolution.
  word c., one concerned with the recognition of words, different areas being involved for recognition of written and of spoken words.

-centesis (sen-te′sis) word element [Gr.], *puncture and aspiration of.*

centi- (sen′tĭ) word element [L.], *hundred;* usually used in naming units of measurement to indicate one-hundredth (10^{-2}) of the unit designated by the root with which it is combined, e.g., centigram.

centigrade (sen′tĭ-grād) having 100 gradations (steps or degrees), as the Celsius temperature scale (thermometer).

centigram (sen′tĭ-gram) one-hundredth of a gram; abbreviated cg.

centiliter (sen′tĭ-le″ter) one-hundredth of a liter; abbreviated cl.

centimeter (sen′tĭ-me″ter) one-hundredth of a meter; abbreviated cm.
  cubic c., a unit of mass, being that of a cube each side of which measures 1 cm.; abbreviated cm.³, cu. cm. or cc.

centinormal (sen″tĭ-nor′mal) one-hundredth of normal strength.

centrad (sen′trad) toward a center.

central (sen′tral) pertaining to a center; located at the midpoint.
  c. nervous system, the portion of the NERVOUS SYSTEM consisting of the brain and spinal cord.

centrencephalic (sen″tren-sĕ-fal′ik) pertaining to the center of the encephalon.

centric (sen′trik) pertaining to a center.

centriciput (sen-tris′ĭ-put) the head, excluding occiput and sinciput; the midhead.

centrifugal (sen-trif′u-gal) moving away from a center.

centrifugation (sen-trif″u-ga′shun) the process of separating materials from solution by rotating vessels containing the solution at high speed.

centrifuge (sen′trĭ-fūj) 1. to rotate, in a suitable container, at extremely high speed, to cause the deposition of solids in solution. 2. a laboratory device for subjecting substances in solution to relative centrifugal force up to 25,000 times gravity.

centrilobular (sen″trĭ-lob′u-lar) pertaining to the central portion of a lobule.

centriole (sen′tre-ōl) a minute cell within the centrosome.

centripetal (sen-trip′ĕ-tal) moving toward a center.

centro- (sen′tro) word element [L., Gr.] indicating relationship to a center or to a central location.

centrocyte (sen′tro-sīt) a cell containing in its protoplasm granules that stain with hematoxylin.

centrokinesia (sen″tro-ki-ne′se-ah) movement originating from central stimulation.

centrolecithal (sen″tro-les′ĭ-thal) having the yolk in the center.

centromere (sen′tro-mēr) the clear region at the point of junction of the arms of a replicating chromosome; called also kinetochore.

centrosclerosis (sen″tro-sklĕ-ro′sis) osteosclerosis of the marrow cavity of a bone.

centrosome (sen′tro-sōm) a specially differentiated region of cytoplasm near the nucleus of a cell.

centrosphere (sen′tro-sfēr) a clear, homogeneous zone surrounding the centrosome of a cell.

centrostaltic (sen″tro-stal′tik) pertaining to a center of motion.

centrum (sen′trum), pl. *cen′tra* [L.] a center.
c. commu′ne, the solar plexus.

cephal(o)- (sef′ah-lo) word element [Gr.], *head.*

cephalad (sef′ah-lad) toward the head.

cephalalgia (sef″al-al′je-ah) pain in the head; headache.

cephaledema (sef″al-ĕ-de′mah) edema of the head.

cephalemia (sef″al-e′me-ah) congestion of the head or brain.

cephalhematocele (sef″al-he-mat′o-sēl) a collection of blood under the pericranium, communicating with the sinuses of the dura mater.

cephalhematoma (sef″al-he″mah-to′mah) a localized effusion of blood beneath the periosteum of the skull of a newborn infant, due to disruption of the vessels during birth.

cephalic (sĕ-fal′ik) pertaining to the head.
c. index, 100 times the maximal breadth of the skull divided by its maximal length.

cephalin (sef′ah-lin) 1. a monaminomonophosphatide in brain tissue, nerve tissue and yolk of egg. 2. a crude phospholipid usually extracted from brain tissue, used as a clotting agent in blood coagulation work.

c.-cholesterol flocculation test a liver function test based upon alterations in serum proteins; called also Hanger's test. The purpose of the test is to distinguish between jaundice due to liver disease and obstructive jaundice. When the liver cells are damaged they are unable to make certain changes in the serum proteins. Serum from the blood of a patient with liver damage shows distinct flocculation (collects in small lumps) when combined with a reagent. The reagent in this test is an emulsion of cholesterol, cephalin and water. The emulsion is mixed with dilute serum and then checked at 24 and 48 hours for signs of flocculation. Normally flocculation will be negative; normal range for the test is negative to 2 plus.
Preparation of the patient requires fasting from midnight the evening before the test. Venous blood is used for the test.

cephalitis (sef″ah-li′tis) encephalitis.

cephalocele (sĕ-fal′o-sēl) protrusion of a part of the cranial contents.

cephalocentesis (sef″ah-lo-sen-te′sis) surgical puncture of the head.

cephalodynia (sef″ah-lo-din′e-ah) pain in the head.

cephalogaster (sef″ah-lo-gas′ter) the anterior portion of the enteric canal of the embryo.

cephalogyric (sef″ah-lo-ji′rik) pertaining to turning motions of the head.

cephalohematoma (sef″ah-lo-he″mah-to′mah) cephalhematoma.

cephalohemometer (sef″ah-lo-he-mom′ĕ-ter) an instrument for measuring intracranial blood pressure.

cephaloma (sef″ah-lo′mah) a soft or encephaloid tumor.

cephalomelus (sef″ah-lom′ĕ-lus) a double monster with a limb attached to the head.

cephalometer (sef″ah-lom′ĕ-ter) an instrument for measuring the head.

cephalometry (sef″ah-lom′ĕ-tre) determination of the dimensions of the head and face.

cephalomotor (sef″ah-lo-mo′tor) pertaining to motions of the head.

cephalonia (sef″ah-lo′ne-ah) idiocy with enlargement of the head and sclerosis of the brain.

cephalopathy (sef″ah-lop′ah-the) any disease of the head.

cephalopelvic (sef″ah-lo-pel′vik) pertaining to the fetal head and maternal pelvis.

cephalothoracic (sef″ah-lo-tho-ras′ik) pertaining to the head and thorax.

cephalothoracopagus (sef″ah-lo-tho″rah-kop′ah-gus) a double fetal monster joined at the head and thorax.

cephalotomy (sef″ah-lot′o-me) craniotomy.

cephalotractor (sef″ah-lo-trak′tor) obstetrical forceps.

cephalotribe (sef′ah-lo-trīb″) an instrument for crushing the fetal head.

cephalotripsy (sef′ah-lo-trip″se) the crushing of the fetal head to facilitate delivery.

cephalotropic (sef″ah-lo-trop′ik) having an affinity for brain tissue.

cephalotrypesis (sef″ah-lo-tri-pe′sis) trephination of the skull.

ceptor (sep′tor) a nerve process that receives impulses from an adjoining neuron.

cera (se′rah) [L.] wax.

cerasine (ser′ah-sin) a cerebroside occurring in brain tissue.

cerate (sēr′āt) an oily substance for external application, compounded with fat or wax, or both.

ceratin (ser′ah-tin) keratin.

ceratitis (ser″ah-ti′tis) keratitis.

cerato- (ser′ah-to) for words beginning thus, see also those beginning *kerato-*.

Ceratophyllus (ser-ah-tof′ĭ-lus) a genus of fleas.

cercaria (ser-ka′re-ah), pl. *cerca′riae* [Gr.] the final, free-swimming larval stage of a trematode parasite.

cerclage (ser-klahzh′) [Fr.] encirclement with a ring or loop, as for correction of an incompetent cervix uteri or fixation of the adjacent ends of a fractured bone.

cercus (ser′kus) a bristle-like structure.

cerebellar (ser″ĕ-bel′ar) pertaining to the cerebellum.

cerebellitis (ser″ĕ-bel-i′tis) inflammation of the cerebellum.

cerebellum (ser″ĕ-bel′um) that part of the hindbrain lying dorsal to the pons and medulla oblongata, comprising a median portion (the vermis) and a cerebellar hemisphere on each side; the cerebellum is concerned with coordination of movements. (See also BRAIN.)

cerebral (ser′ĕ-bral, sĕ-re′bral) pertaining to the cerebrum.

c. cortex, the outer layer of gray matter of the brain, which governs thought, reasoning, memory, sensation and voluntary movement. (See also BRAIN.)

c. palsy, partial paralysis and lack of muscle coordination resulting from a defect, injury or disease of the nerve tissue contained within the skull. The defects are generally thought to be caused at or near the time of birth and may be due to a lack of oxygen, premature delivery, blood type incompatibility, head injury or infections of the brain or the meninges.

SYMPTOMS. The defect may affect one or more areas of the brain and produce a variety of muscular disorders. The largest majority of cerebral palsy cases are of three forms: (1) spastic type in which there are exaggerated stretch reflexes, muscle spasm and increased deep tendon reflexes; (2) athetoid, with purposeless, uncontrollable movements and muscle tension; and (3) atactic, in which the child has poor balance, poor coordination and a staggering gait. Visual, hearing and speech defects may be present. Mental retardation may or may not be a manifestation of the brain damage.

Often the parents or pediatrician can observe indications of cerebral palsy when an infant is only a few months old, but in mild cases the diagnosis may not be made until age 2 or 3.

TREATMENT. Treatment varies according to the nature and extent of brain damage. Muscle relaxants may help reduce spasms. Anticonvulsant drugs are necessary when seizures are among the symptoms of the disorder. Orthopedic surgery, casts, braces and traction can be used to correct some types of disability associated with cerebral palsy. Early muscle training and special exercises often help the child lead a useful, productive life. If muscle training is not begun early, extensive rehabilitation may be necessary to correct faulty habits and poor muscle patterns established by the child. However, it is never too late for a complete evaluation of the condition of a patient with cerebral palsy. A rehabilitation program can produce good results later in life as well as in childhood.

c. vascular accident, a disorder of the blood vessels of the brain resulting in impaired blood supply to parts of the brain. Cerebral vascular accident is also called "stroke" or cerebral apoplexy.

CAUSES. There are three main causes of cerebral vascular accident—cerebral thrombosis, cerebral embolism and cerebral hemorrhage. The onset of the stroke differs somewhat according to cause, but thereafter the symptoms are the same.

Cerebral Thrombosis. A thrombus is a blood clot that forms within a blood vessel. A clot in an artery supplying the brain gradually cuts off the blood supply to that particular area of the brain and a stroke occurs. Most often a thrombus occurs because of some damage to the wall of the vessel (see also THROMBOSIS). A frequent cause of blood vessel damage is atherosclerosis, in which plaques of fatty material are deposited on the smooth inner lining of the arteries. Though this may occur at any age, it is most common in middle-aged and elderly persons.

Cerebral Embolism. An embolus is a plug that has entered the bloodstream. It can consist of air, fat or other material introduced into the circulatory system, or it can be, and is more often, a detached portion of a thrombus that settles in one of the arteries of the brain.

Cerebral Hemorrhage. This is the rupturing of a blood vessel, usually an artery, in the brain. The hemorrhage is frequently associated with pre-existing HYPERTENSION. There is often weakening of the blood vessel as well. Healthy arteries can withstand considerable pressure because of their elasticity. However, in elderly persons the elastic tissue of the arteries becomes hard and brittle in a condition known as ARTERIOSCLEROSIS. This tends to raise the blood pressure and also to weaken the blood vessel wall. In younger persons, the effects of syphilis or weakening of the walls of the blood vessels (ANEURYSM) may cause cerebral hemorrhage.

SYMPTOMS. The onset of a cerebral vascular accident differs according to the cause. There may be preliminary symptoms of cerebral thrombosis several days or hours before the stroke. The patient may suffer dizzy spells, suddenly forget what he is saying in the middle of a sentence, become clumsy or stumble without cause. Usually no pain accompanies these symptoms, which may be very mild.

A cerebral embolism usually comes on without prior warning. The patient simply becomes speechless, or paralyzed, or lapses suddenly into unconsciousness. In such cases, the patient usually has a history of heart disease.

A person who suffers a cerebral hemorrhage feels the symptoms of cerebral thrombosis; in addition he may have violent headaches and ringing in the ears, and he may feel dizzy or nauseated immediately before the stroke occurs. A cerebral hemorrhage may follow undue exertion, such as a straining bowel movement, heavy eating or coughing.

TREATMENT AND REHABILITATION. Whatever the cause, the results of a cerebral vascular accident are the same and depend upon the portion of the brain involved, as well as the extent and severity of the damage. The patient may suffer a mild to severe paralysis of an arm or leg, or both, without losing consciousness; less often, he may lapse suddenly into a coma which may continue until death. Coma is more likely to develop in cerebral hemorrhage.

The first few days after the stroke are the critical period. Even if a patient recovers satisfactorily from the initial stroke, and he often does, he is usually paralyzed in at least a part of one side of his body. If one complete side is involved, this is called hemiplegia. The paralysis occurs because the usual site for cerebral thrombosis, embolism or hemorrhage is in a part of the brain that controls movements of the body. If the right side of the brain is affected, the left side of the body is paralyzed, and vice versa. In addition, there is usually a speech disturbance if the paralysis affects the right side

of the body in a right-handed person or the left side of the body in a left-handed person. Bladder or bowel disturbances occur in many cases. Emotional disturbances are also encountered and they often persist for a long time.

As early as possible, the patient should begin a course of PHYSICAL THERAPY to regain the use of his limbs. If such rehabilitation is delayed, chances for a complete recovery decrease.

Aftereffects. The ultimate amount of recovery possible depends upon many factors – the severity and location of the stroke, the general physical health of the patient, his age, his will and desire for recovery and the attitude and help given him by his family. A great many patients make a complete recovery, even from the most incapacitating strokes, and can return to full-time work. Many patients, however, may be left with some residual effects in an arm or a leg; sometimes there is some impairment of speech. If physical therapy is begun soon enough many of these aftereffects can be greatly reduced, if not eliminated.

NURSING CARE. The plan of care is based on the individual patient's symptoms and needs. Daily changes in the nursing care will be necessary as the patient progresses from the acute phase (immediately after the accident) to the chronic phase.

During the acute phase the patient is likely to have difficulty breathing because of impairment of the swallowing mechanism, with resultant accumulation of saliva and mucus in the throat and mouth. In order to maintain a patent airway the head and neck should be positioned so that the chin is slightly elevated and does not rest on the chest. Keeping the head turned to one side will avoid aspiration of fluid into the lungs. If the patient is turned on his side he should be turned onto the affected side. Suctioning equipment and a mechanical airway may be needed if paralysis of the throat is severe.

The vital signs are taken and recorded at frequent intervals night and day. An elevated tempera-

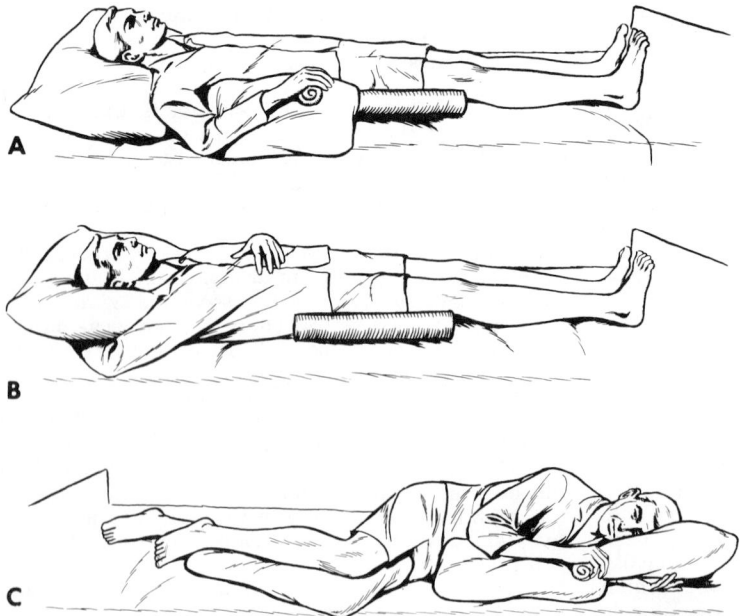

Positioning in cerebral vascular accident. *A*, A pillow is placed next to the body on the weak side. The weak arm is placed on the pillow. Make sure that the elbow points away from the body and that the lower arm and hand are placed alongside the body and about 12 inches away from it. A rolled napkin or small towel is placed under the weak hand to keep the fingers open. Note trochanter roll along affected side to keep hip from rotating. *B*, The affected arm is tucked under the pillow with hand flattened to prevent curling of the fingers. *C*. in this side-lying position, a pillow is used to support the weak arm. Another pillow is used to support the weak leg. (From Strike Back at Stroke. Washington, D.C., U.S. Government Printing Office.)

ture, with decrease in the pulse and respiratory rates, indicates a poor prognosis.

To avoid complications such as circulatory stasis and hypostatic pneumonia, the patient is turned at least every 2 to 3 hours. He must be taught how to cough in spite of his partial paralysis, and should be encouraged to breathe deeply so that the lungs are expanded adequately.

Frequent turning also will help prevent such complications as DECUBITUS ULCERS, kidney stones and CONTRACTURES. Another measure that helps avoid contractures is putting the affected joints through their full range of motion at least once daily. No written order is necessary for these exercises. When establishing a schedule for turning the patient and administering passive exercises of the joints, one must bear in mind that the patient needs rest and quiet, no matter how severe his condition may be. The exercises can be given during the bed bath or immediately afterward so that the patient is disturbed as infrequently as possible (see also EXERCISE).

Proper positioning is of paramount importance if orthopedic deformities are to be avoided. Devices such as the footboard, bed cradle, sandbags and trochanter roll are used to keep the body in good alignment at all times. There must be adequate support of the affected limbs so that there is not undue strain on the shoulder and hip joints. When turning the patient and positioning the limbs all motions should be gentle and unhurried. Whenever possible two persons, one on each side of the bed, should turn the patient, to reassure the patient that he will not roll off the bed and to avoid undesirable pulling and tugging at the patient.

Each time a nursing procedure is necessary the patient should be told what is going to be done to him. Even though he may appear unable to understand, or at least unable to respond to the spoken word, it is wrong to assume that he does not hear what is being said. For this reason one should be careful in conversations held within the patient's hearing. It is extremely rude to talk "about" the patient in his presence, implying that he is not able to react emotionally and therefore could not be interested in the things being said about him. Actually, the patient with a cerebral vascular accident may be more easily upset emotionally than another patient would.

If the physician approves of early ambulation, the patient should be allowed to sit up on the side of the bed and learn to balance himself before getting out of bed. Once again the movements should be gentle and slow while the patient gains confidence in handling his affected limbs.

Physical therapy is begun as soon as the physician gives his permission. Although the physical therapist usually is responsible for extensive exercises given the patient, the nursing staff must be familiar with the goals of physical therapy and work in cooperation with the physical therapist.

Nutrition is maintained by whatever means necessary, depending on the patient's ability to chew, handle food in his mouth and swallow. In some cases TUBE FEEDING may be the only method by which food is administered. If the patient is able to swallow, but has difficulty moving the food about in his mouth, he should be turned to the affected side while he is being fed. Rinsing the mouth after meals and frequent mouth care help eliminate accumulation of food in the mouth and halitosis.

The lips should be kept lubricated with cold cream or mineral oil to keep them from drying and cracking.

INCONTINENCE of urine and feces sometimes accompanies a cerebral vascular accident. A regular schedule of offering the bedpan, especially after each meal, may help establish a routine of elimination. It is also helpful to get the patient up to the bathroom or to a bedside commode whenever this is possible. In any event the patient must be kept clean and dry and skin care must be given frequently to avoid pressure areas and decubitus ulcers. Fecal impaction and urinary retention may occur and can be avoided by intelligent observation and recording of bowel movements and urinary output. The physician may order an enema to be given periodically if constipation becomes a problem.

Rehabilitation of the patient begins the moment he enters the hospital. This means that all measures taken to maintain bodily functions and to avoid complications are aimed at the ultimate goal of getting the patient back to a state as near normal as possible. His reaction to his illness, his family's attitude, the quality of care he receives and the attitude of those caring for him will greatly affect the eventual outcome of his illness. There may be a tendency on the part of nurses and the patient's family to do everything for the patient when he seems so helpless and handicapped. Certainly he should be helped with the things he cannot do for himself, but total dependence on others can become very demoralizing and for the patient's sake he must be encouraged to help himself. This may be a slow and demanding process, requiring much patience and optimism. One can begin by providing the means by which the patient can gradually begin to bathe, feed and dress himself.

Special equipment, such as an overbed table made of cardboard or plywood, can be used so that the patient can reach the bath water, toilet articles and other things he needs. His food should be prepared and arranged on his tray so that he can handle it without great difficulty. If his first movements are awkward and messy, no mention should be made of this and he must never be made to feel that he has caused an inconvenience to anyone through his efforts to help himself.

There has been much interest in the rehabilitation of cerebral vascular accident patients in recent years and there is a wealth of information and help available for the stroke victim and his family. Pamphlets dealing with the special problems of this illness are readily available from the American Heart Association and the American Red Cross. Centers for speech therapy, vocational rehabilitation and homemaker services are located in many communities. The local health department can provide information as to the location of these centers and services they provide.

cerebralgia (ser″ĕ-bral′je-ah) pain in the head.

cerebrasthenia (ser″ĕ-bras-the′ne-ah) asthenia complicated with brain disorders.

cerebration (ser″ĕ-bra′shun) functional activity of the brain.
   unconscious c., mental action of which the person is unconscious.

cerebritis (ser″ĕ-bri′tis) inflammation of the cerebrum.

cerebroid (ser′ĕ-broid) resembling brain substance.

cerebrology (ser″ĕ-brol′o-je) the scientific study of the brain.

cerebroma (ser″ĕ-bro′mah) an abnormal mass of brain tissue outside the cranium.

cerebromalacia (ser″ĕ-bro-mah-la′she-ah) abnormal softness of the brain.

cerebromeningitis (ser″ĕ-bro-men″in-ji′tis) inflammation of the brain and its covering membranes.

cerebronic acid (ser″ĕ-bron′ik) a saturated monohydroxy acid, from phrenosin.

cerebropathy (ser″ĕ-brop′ah-the) any brain disease.

cerebrophysiology (ser″ĕ-bro-fiz″e-ol′o-je) physiology of the brain.

cerebropontile (ser″ĕ-bro-pon′tīl) pertaining to the cerebrum and pons.

cerebropsychosis (ser″ĕ-bro-si-ko′sis) any cerebral disorder characterized by mental aberration.

cerebrosclerosis (ser″ĕ-bro-sklĕ-ro′sis) abnormal hardness of the brain.

cerebrose (ser′ĕ-brōs) a compound derived from brain substance; brain sugar.

cerebroside (sĕ-re′bro-sīd) a compound of a nitrogenous base, a long-chain fatty acid and a sugar, found chiefly in nerve tissue.

cerebrosis (ser″ĕ-bro′sis) any brain disease.

cerebrospinal (ser″ĕ-bro-spi′nal) pertaining to the brain and spinal cord.

c. fluid, the fluid in the subarachnoid spaces surrounding the brain and spinal cord, and in the ventricles of the brain. The fluid is formed continuously by the choroid plexus in the ventricles, and, so that there will not be an abnormal increase in amount and pressure, it is reabsorbed into the blood by the arachnoid villi at approximately the same rate at which it is produced.

The cerebrospinal fluid aids in the protection of the brain, spinal cord and meninges by acting as a watery cushion surrounding them to absorb the shocks to which they are exposed. There is a blood-cerebrospinal fluid barrier that prevents harmful substances, such as metal poisons, some pathogenic organisms and certain drugs from passing from the capillaries into the cerebrospinal fluid.

The normal cerebrospinal fluid pressure is 5 mm. of mercury (100 mm. of water) when the individual is lying in a horizontal position on his side. Fluid pressure may be increased by a brain tumor or by hemorrhage or infection in the cranium. HYDROCEPHALUS, or excess fluid in the cranial cavity, can result from either excessive formation or poor absorption of cerebrospinal fluid. Blockage of the flow of fluid in the spinal canal may result from a tumor, blood clot or severance of the spinal cord. The pressure remains normal or decreases below the point of obstruction but increases above that point.

Cell counts, bacterial smears and cultures of samples of cerebrospinal fluid are done when an inflammatory process or infection of the meninges is suspected. Since the cerebrospinal fluid contains nutrient substances such as glucose, proteins and sodium chloride, and also some waste products such as urea, it is believed to play a role in metabolism. The major constituents of cerebrospinal fluid are water, glucose, sodium chloride and protein, and changes in their concentrations are helpful in diagnosis of brain diseases.

Samples of cerebrospinal fluid may be obtained by SPINAL PUNCTURE, in which a hollow needle is inserted between two lumbar vertebrae (below the lower end of the spinal cord), or into the cisterna cerebellomedullaris just below the occipital bone

TYPICAL SPINAL FLUID FINDINGS

CONDITION	WBC	RBC	TOTAL PROTEIN	GLUCOSE	COLLOIDAL-GOLD TEST	SEROLOGY
Normal	0–5	0	20–40 mg 100 ml	60–80% of blood glucose	0000000000-0	Neg.
Bacterial infection	200 or more (polys)	0	Elevated	Lowered	Not done	Not done
Viral infection	100 or more (lymphs)	0	Normal to slightly elevated	Normal	Not done	Not done
Tuberculous infection	50–100 (lymphs)	0	Elevated	Lowered	Not done	Not done
CNS syphilis	10–60 (lymphs)	0	Normal to slightly elevated	Normal	Luetic: 0123100000-0 Paretic: 5555542100-0	Pos.
Multiple sclerosis	0–5	0	Normal to slightly elevated	Normal	5555542100-0	Neg.
Tumor	Normal	0	Elevated	Normal	Not done	Not done
Hemorrhage	Influenced by mixture with blood		Markedly elevated, owing to presence of blood	Not accurate, owing to presence of blood	Not done	Not done

Source: Charles M. Poser, M.D., University of Kansas Medical Center, Kansas City, Kans. From French, R. M.: Nurse's Guide to Diagnostic Procedures. 3rd ed. New York, McGraw-Hill Book Co., 1971.

of the skull (cisternal puncture). Pressure of the cerebrospinal fluid is measured by a manometer attached to the end of the needle after it has been inserted.

cerebrotomy (ser″ĕ-brot′o-me) anatomy or dissection of the brain.

cerebrotonia (ser″ĕ-bro-to′ne-ah) a psychic type characterized by predominance of restraint, inhibition and desire for concealment; considered typical of an ectomorph.

cerebrum (ser′ĕ-brum) the main portion of the brain occupying the upper part of the cranium; the two cerebral hemispheres, united by the corpus callosum, form the largest part of the central nervous system in man. (See also BRAIN.)

cerium (se′re-um) a chemical element, atomic number 58, atomic weight 140.12, symbol Ce. (See also table of ELEMENTS.)
    c. oxalate, a mixture of the oxalates of cerium, neodymium, praseodymium, lanthanum and other associated elements; used as an antiemetic.

Cer-o-cillin (ser′o-sil″in) trademark for preparations of penicillin O for parenteral administration.

ceroma (se-ro′mah) a tumor that has undergone amyloid (waxy) degeneration.

ceruloplasmin (sĕ-roo″lo-plaz′min) an alpha globulin of the blood, being the form in which 96 per cent of the plasma copper is transported.

cerumen (sĕ-roo′men) a waxy secretion of the glands of the external acoustic meatus; ear wax. adj., **ceru′minous.**

ceruminolysis (sĕ-roo″mĭ-nol′ĭ-sis) dissolution or disintegration of cerumen in the external acoustic meatus.

ceruminosis (sĕ-roo′mĭ-no′sis) excessive secretion of cerumen.

cervic(o)- (ser′vĭ-ko) word element [L.], *neck; cervix.*

cervical (ser′vĭ-kal) pertaining to the neck or to the cervix.
    c. plexus, a network of nerve fibers formed by the first four cervical nerves and supplying the structures in the region of the neck. One important branch is the phrenic nerve, which supplies the diaphragm.
    c. rib, a supernumerary rib arising from a cervical vertebra.
    c. rib syndrome, pain over the shoulder, often extending down the arm or radiating up the back of the neck, due to compression of the nerves and vessels between a cervical rib and the anterior scalene muscle.
    c. vertebrae, the seven vertebrae closest to the skull, constituting the skeleton of the neck.

cervicectomy (ser′vĭ-sek′to-me) excision of the cervix uteri.

cervicitis (ser″vĭ-si′tis) inflammation of the cervix uteri.

cervicocolpitis (ser″vĭ-ko-kol-pi′tis) inflammation of the cervix uteri and vagina.

cervicofacial (ser″vĭ-ko-fa′shal) pertaining to the neck and face.

cervicoplasty (ser′vĭ-ko-plas″te) plastic surgery on the neck.

cervicovesical (ser″vĭ-ko-ves′ĭ-kal) relating to the cervix uteri and bladder.

cervix (ser′viks), pl. *cer′vices* [L.] a neck or neck-like part of an organ. The term used alone often refers to the cervix uteri.
    incompetent c., a cervix uteri that is abnormally prone to dilate before termination of the normal period of gestation, resulting in premature expulsion of the fetus.
    c. u′teri, the narrow lower end of the uterus extending into the vagina and serving as a passageway between the two organs.
    Cervical cancer is surpassed only by breast cancer as a cause of female cancer deaths in the United States. Its victims are usually women over 40. One of the first warning signs of cervical cancer is vaginal bleeding between menstrual periods, after coitus or after menopause is established. There may also be increased vaginal discharge. The PAPANICO-LAOU SMEAR TEST should be done routinely every year in women over 30 to rule out the possibility of cervical malignancy. This test identifies cancer in its earliest stages while the malignancy is still capable of relatively easy eradication. Treatment may include surgery or radiotherapy or both.
    Cervical erosion refers to ulceration of the surface epithelium of the cervix resulting from trauma (as in childbirth) or infection. The condition is treated by cauterization and douches. Although the condition is not serious, it should be treated promptly to avoid possible development of malignancy in later years. Cervical lacerations are likely to occur during childbirth. Most small lacerations heal by themselves; more extensive tears in the cervix may require surgical repair. Cervical polyps are fleshy growths that may form on the cervix, causing bleeding. They are removed surgically.
    c. ves′icae, the neck of the bladder.

cesarean section (sĕ-sa′re-an) delivery of a fetus by incision through the abdominal wall and uterus. The procedure takes its name from the Latin word *caedere,* to cut, and has no relation to the birth of Caesar as is sometimes believed. Indications for cesarean section include dystocia, toxemia, hemorrhage from abruptio placentae or placenta praevia, fetal distress and breech presentation.

cesium (se′ze-um) a chemical element, atomic number 55, atomic weight 132.905, symbol Cs. (See table of ELEMENTS.)

cesticidal (ses″tĭ-si′dal) destructive to the platyhelminths, or cestodes.

cestode (ses′tōd) a tapeworm; an organism of the class Cestoidea.

cestodology (ses″to-dol′o-je) the scientific study of cestodes.

cestoid (ses′toid) resembling a tapeworm.

Cestoidea (ses-toi′de-ah) a class of animals of the phylum Platyhelminthes, characterized by a noncellular cuticular layer covering their bodies and generally having a segmented body with a special holdfast segment to the anterior end; the tapeworms.

cetylpyridinium (se″til-pi″rĭ-din′e-um) a pyridine derivative used as a local anti-infective.

Cevalin (se′vah-lin) trademark for preparations of ascorbic acid.

Cevex (se′veks) trademark for a liquid preparation of ascorbic acid.

Ce-vi-sol (se′vi-sol) trademark for a preparation of ascorbic acid.

cevitamic acid (se″vi-tam′ik) ascorbic acid.

Cf chemical symbol, *californium*.

cg. centigram.

C.G.S. centimeter-gram-second, the metric units of linear measurement, weight and time.

Chaddock's sign (chad′oks) dorsiflexion of the big toe when the foot is stroked around the lateral malleolus and along the dorsum laterally.

Chadwick's sign (chad′wiks) bluish discoloration of the vestibule and vaginal wall, due to venous congestion, and sometimes a sign of pregnancy.

chafing (chāf′ing) irritation of the skin by friction, usually from clothing or the rubbing together of body surfaces, such as the thighs, when they are damp with perspiration. The skinfolds of the obese are particularly subject to chafing. Tight shoes, badly fitting brassieres and other clothing that binds all cause chafing. Babies are particularly susceptible.

The irritation can usually be cleared up by keeping the parts dry, using a plain talcum powder and, if necessary, substituting clothing that does not bind or rub. In some cases, a sterile dressing may be necessary to help relieve the rubbing. The best prevention is to keep the skin clean and dry and to wear clothing that fits properly.

Chagas' disease, Chagas-Cruz disease (chag′-as), (chag′as kruz) trypanosomiasis due to *Trypanosoma cruzi* (see also South American TRYPANOSOMIASIS).

chain (chān) a collection of objects linked together in linear fashion, or end to end, as the assemblage of atoms or radicals in a chemical compound, or an assemblage of individual bacterial cells.

chalazion (kah-la′ze-on) a cyst or tumor on the eyelid caused by an infection of a sebaceous (oil) gland. A chalazion can sometimes be treated at home with the application of hot compresses, but while this method is usually successful with a sty, a similar infection that has not yet formed a cyst, chalazion often requires incision and drainage, performed by a physician. Called also meibomian cyst.

chalcosis (kal-ko′sis) copper deposits in tissue.

chalicosis (kal″ĭ-ko′sis) lung disease from inhalation of stony particles.

chalybeate (kah-lib′e-āt) impregnated with iron.

chamaecephalic (kam″e-sĕ-fal′ik) having a low, flat head, with a vertical index of 70 or less.

chamber (chām′ber) an enclosed space.

anterior c., the part of the aqueous humor-containing space of the eyeball between the cornea and iris.

hyperbaric c., an enclosed space in which gas (oxygen) can be raised to greater than atmospheric pressure (see also HYPERBARIC OXYGENATION).

ionization c., an enclosure containing two or more electrodes between which an electric current may be passed when the enclosed gas is ionized by radiation; used for determining the intensity of x-rays and other rays.

posterior c., that part of the aqueous humor-containing space of the eyeball between the iris and the lens.

vitreous c., the vitreous humor-containing space in the eyeball, bounded anteriorly by the lens and ciliary body and posteriorly by the posterior wall of the eyeball.

chancre (shang′ker) the primary lesion of SYPHILIS, caused by *Treponema pallidum* and followed by constitutional syphilis.

A true chancre begins as a papule which breaks down into a reddish ulcer. It is generally firm and accompanied by little or no pain. Although most frequently located on the external genitalia, it may be on the lips or fingers. In women, a chancre is sometimes concealed in the internal genitalia where it may not be seen or felt. Two or three may develop simultaneously.

A chancre heals of its own accord without treatment, thus leading many persons infected with syphilis to believe they are cured. They are not, and if adequate medical treatment is not begun at this early and curable stage of syphilis, the disease will progress, doing irreparable damage.

chancroid (shang′kroid) a nonsyphilitic venereal sore caused by *Haemophilus ducreyi*. As in syphilis, the first symptom of the disease may be the appearance of a sore, but the sore is soft, as distinguished from the hard chancre of syphilis.

Chancroid is almost always spread by sexual contact, but in rare instances it may be transmitted indirectly from soiled dressings or towels. Three to five days after exposure one or more small soft sores appear on or near the external genitalia. These sores soon develop into ulcers with irregular edges and surrounding areas which become red and swollen. In many cases, the infection spreads to the lymph nodes of the groin, causing swelling and tenderness.

Chancroid is successfully treated with sulfonamides or the antibiotics tetracycline and streptomycin.

chancrous (shang′krus) of the nature of chancre.

chappa (chap′ah) a disease of South Africa resembling syphilis or yaws.

character (kar′ak-ter) 1. a separate and distinct trait exhibited by an individual. 2. the sum of observable attributes of a material or of an individual.

dominant c., one that can develop through the agency of a single gene.

mendelian c's, in genetics, the separate and distinct traits exhibited by an animal or plant and dependent on the genetic constitution of the organism.

primary sex c., one directly concerned in the reproductive function of the individual.

recessive c., one that must be carried in the gene from each parent to become apparent in the offspring.

secondary sex c., one typical of the sex, but not directly concerned in the reproductive function of the individual.

sex-linked c., one transmitted by a gene carried in the sex chromosome and appearing only in individuals of one sex.

charcoal (char′kōl) carbon prepared by burning organic material.

activated c., the residue of destructive distillation of various organic materials, treated to increase its adsorptive power; used in gas masks, in emergency treatment of poisoning by certain drugs and also as a decolorizer.

purified animal c., charcoal prepared from bone and purified by removal of materials dissolved by hot hydrochloric acid and water; adsorbent and decolorizer.

Charcot's disease (shar-kōz′) neurogenic arthropathy.

Charcot-Marie-Tooth disease (shar-ko′ mah-re′ tōōth) progressive neuropathic (peroneal) muscular atrophy.

charlatan (shar′lah-tan) a pretender to knowledge or skills not possessed; in medicine, a quack.

charley horse a minor muscle disorder resulting from the violent use of a muscle or group of muscles in strenuous work or play. It usually occurs when muscles that have not been conditioned for hard use are put under a strain, with the result that some of the muscle fibers are strained or may actually tear. It is characterized by soreness, stiffness and pain which often comes on very suddenly. Heat, particularly from warm baths, helps the condition, and aspirin is useful in relieving the pain. If the pain persists for several days, there may be some other muscle injury and a physician should be consulted.

chart (chart) a record of data in graphic or tabular form.

genealogical c., a graph showing various descendants of a common ancestor, used to indicate those affected by genetically determined disease.

Snellen's c., a chart printed with block letters in gradually decreasing sizes, used in testing distance vision.

charting (chart′ing) the keeping of a clinical record of the important facts about a patient and the progress of his illness. The patient's chart most often contains a medical history, results of a physical examination, laboratory reports, results of special diagnostic tests performed and the observations of the nursing staff and the particular treatments and medications administered to the patient.

The nursing staff is primarily responsible for recording data on the nurses' notes, the graphic chart of the vital signs and the medication sheet if one is required by the hospital or institution. At the time of the patient's admission entries should be made in the nurses' notes containing special observations made by the person admitting the patient, symptoms and complaints stated by the patient and any special characteristics such as allergies or drug idiosyncrasies and problems of vision or hearing necessitating special precautions. The patient's temperature, pulse, respiratory rate, and blood pressure are also taken and recorded at this time.

The daily clinical record to be kept on the nurses' notes should include individual reaction of the patient to tests or treatments administered; treatments or tests omitted, the reason for the omission and to whom this was reported; dressings changed, the amount and type of drainage and the condition of the wound; medications given or omitted, drug effects and reason for omission of a drug; changes in the patient's condition or behavior, and complaints volunteered by the patient. Other special sheets may be included in the patient's chart which require notation by the nursing staff. These include the graphic record of the patient's vital signs, intake and output records or records of fluids administered intravenously.

Notations made by the nurse and kept in the patient's chart vary from hospital to hospital; it is the responsibility of the nurse to become familiar with the routine of the institution in which she is working and to maintain the patient's chart with intelligence and clarity. The chart or clinical record is considered a legal document and may be used as evidence in court.

chauffage (sho-fahzh′) [Fr.] application of a low-heated cautery near a body part.

chaulmoogra oil (chawl-moo′grah) an antiinfective used principally in the treatment of leprosy; also effective in certain types of arthritis. Because of its toxicity and tendency to cause local skin and mucous membrane irritation, it has been replaced by antibiotics and modern chemotherapeutic agents and is rarely used in the United States.

chaulmoogric acid (chawl-moo′grik) a cyclic fatty acid, from chaulmoogra oil.

Ch.B. [L.] *Chirur′giae Baccalau′reus* (Bachelor of Surgery).

cheek (chēk) a fleshy, rounded protuberance, especially the fleshy portion of either side of the face.

cleft c., a developmental anomaly characterized by an abnormal fissure.

cheil(o)- (ki′lo) word element [Gr.] *lip.*

cheilectropion (ki″lek-tro′pe-on) eversion of the lip.

cheilitis (ki-li′tis) inflammation of a lip.

actinic c., c. actin′ica, involvement of the lips after exposure to actinic rays, with pain and swelling, and development of a scaly crust on the vermilion border.

cheilognathopalatoschisis (ki″lo-na″tho-pal″ah-tos′kĭ-sis) cleft of the lip, upper jaw and hard and soft palates.

cheiloplasty (ki′lo-plas″te) plastic repair of a lip.

Cheilopoda (ki-lop′o-dah) Chilopoda.

cheilopodiasis (ki″lo-po-di′ah-sis) chilopodiasis.

cheilorrhaphy (ki-lor′ah-fe) suture of the lip.

cheilosis (ki-lo′sis) a fissured condition of the lips and angles of the mouth.

cheilotomy (ki-lot′o-me) incision of the lip.

cheir(o)- (ki′ro) word element [Gr.], *hand.* See also words beginning *chir(o)-.*

cheiralgia (ki-ral′je-ah) pain in the hand.

cheirarthritis (ki″rar-thri′tis) inflammation of the joints of the hand and fingers.

cheirokinesthesia (ki″ro-kin″es-the′ze-ah) the subjective perception of movements of the hand, especially in writing.

cheiroplasty (ki′ro-plas″te) plastic surgery on the hand.

cheiropompholyx (ki′ro-pom′fo-liks) a skin disease with peculiar vesicles on the palms and soles.

cheirospasm (ki′ro-spazm) writers' cramp.

chelate (ke′lāt) to combine with a metal in weakly dissociated complexes in which the metal is part of a ring; by extension, applied to a chemical compound in which a metallic ion is sequestered and firmly bound into a ring within the chelating molecule.

Chel-iron (kēl′i-ern) trademark for preparations of ferrocholinate, an iron preparation used as a hematinic.

cheloid (ke′loid) keloid.

chemexfoliation (kem″eks-fo″le-a′shun) removal of epidermis and part of dermis by chemicals applied to the body surface.

chemical (kem′ĭ-kal) 1. pertaining to chemistry. 2. a substance produced by the forces or operations of chemistry.

chemicocautery (kem″ĭ-ko-kaw′ter-e) cauterization by chemical means.

cheminosis (kem″ĭ-no′sis) a disease due to chemical agents.

chemist (kem′ist) an expert in chemistry.

chemistry (kem′is-tre) the science that treats of the elements and atomic relations of matter, and of the various compounds of the elements.
   colloid c., the scientific study of colloids.
   inorganic c., the scientific study of compounds not containing carbon.
   organic c., the scientific study of carbon-containing compounds.

chemoantigen (ke″mo-an′tĭ-jen) a chemical compound capable of acting as an antigen.

chemoautotrophic (ke″mo-au″to-trof′ik) a term applied to bacteria that can synthesize their cell constituents from carbon dioxide by means of energy derived from inorganic reactions.

chemobiotic (ke″mo-bi-ot′ik) a compound of a chemotherapeutic agent and an antibiotic.

chemodectoma (ke″mo-dek-to′mah) any tumor of the chemoreceptor system, e.g., a carotid body tumor.

chemokinesis (ke″mo-ki-ne′sis) increased activity of an organism caused by a chemical substance.

chemoluminescence (ke″mo-loo″mĭ-nes′ens) 1. radiation that produces chemical action. 2. luminescence produced by the direct transformation of chemical energy.

chemolysis (ke-mol′ĭ-sis) chemical decomposition.

chemomorphosis (ke″mo-mor-fo′sis) change of form due to chemical action.

chemopallidectomy (ke″mo-pal″ĭ-dek′to-me) destruction of tissue of the globus pallidus by a chemical agent.

chemoprophylaxis (ke″mo-pro″fĭ-lak′sis) prevention of disease by chemical means.

chemopsychiatry (ke″mo-si-ki′ah-tre) the treatment of mental and emotional disorders by the use of drugs.

chemoreceptors (ke″mo-re-sep′tor) special cells or organs adapted for excitation by chemical substances and located outside the central nervous system. There are chemoreceptors in the large arteries of the thorax and the neck; these are called carotid and aortic bodies. These receptors are responsive to changes in the oxygen, carbon dioxide and hydrogen ion concentration in the blood. When oxygen concentration falls below normal in the arterial blood, the chemoreceptors send impulses to stimulate the respiratory center so that there will be an increase in alveolar ventilation, and consequently, an increase in the intake of oxygen by the lungs.
   Other chemoreceptors are the taste buds, which are sensitive to chemicals in the mouth, and the olfactory cells of the nose, which detect certain chemicals in the air.

chemoreflex (ke″mo-re′fleks) a reflex resulting from chemical action.

chemosensitive (ke″mo-sen′sĭ-tiv) sensitive to chemical stimuli.

chemoserotherapy (ke″mo-se″ro-ther′ah-pe) treatment of infection by means of drugs and serum.

chemosis (ke-mo′sis) edema of conjunctiva of the eye.

chemosterilant (ke″mo-ster′ĭ-lant) a chemical compound that upon ingestion causes sterility of an organ.

chemosurgery (ke″mo-ser′jer-e) the destruction of tissue by chemical agents; originally applied to chemical fixation of malignant, gangrenous or infected tissue, with use of frozen sections to facilitate systematic microscopic control of its excision.

chemosynthesis (ke″mo-sin′thĕ-sis) the building up of chemical compounds under the influence of chemical stimulation, specifically the formation of carbohydrates from carbon dioxide and water as a result of energy derived from chemical reactions.

chemotaxis (ke″mo-tak′sis) the movement of an organism in response to a chemical concentration gradient.

chemotherapy (ke″mo-ther′ah-pe) the treatment of illness by chemical means; that is, by medication. adj., **chemotherapeu′tic.** The term was first applied to the treatment of infectious diseases, but it now is used to include treatment of mental illness and cancer with drugs.

chenopodium oil (ke″no-po′de-um) an anthelmintic drug, particularly useful in the treatment of hookworm, pinworm and roundworm infections.

cherubism (cher′u-bism) a facial appearance produced by fibrous dysplasia of the jaws.

chest (chest) the part of the body enclosed by the ribs and sternum, especially its anterior aspect.
   flail c., one whose wall moves paradoxically with respiration, owing to multiple fractures of the ribs.
   funnel c., depression of the sternum and rib cartilage; PECTUS EXCAVATUM.
   pigeon c., prominence of the sternum and rib cartilage; PECTUS CARINATUM.

Cheyne-Stokes respiration (chān stōks) breathing characterized by rhythmic waxing and waning of the depth of respiration; the patient breathes deeply for a short time and then breathes very slightly or stops breathing altogether. The pattern occurs over and over again every 45 seconds to 3 minutes. Periodic breathing of this type is caused by disease affecting the respiratory center, usually heart failure or brain damage.

chiasm (ki′azm) a crossing or decussation.
   optic c., a structure in the forebrain formed by the junction of fibers of the optic nerves from the medial portions of the retina.

chiasma (ki-az′mah) chiasm.
   c. formation, the cytologic basis of genetic recombination, or crossing over.

chickenpox (chik′en-poks) an acute communicable disease of childhood, caused by a virus, with mild constitutional symptoms and a maculopapular vesicular skin eruption; called also varicella. It is a common childhood disease, and is rarely severe. Although there is no preventive inoculation for chickenpox, one attack usually gives immunity.
   The varicella virus is usually spread either by contact with blisters, or by droplet infection. The incubation period is 2 to 3 weeks. The period of contagion lasts about 2 weeks, beginning 2 days before the rash appears. The same virus that causes chickenpox also causes HERPES ZOSTER (shingles); the differences in the two diseases probably reflect differences in the response to the virus.
   SYMPTOMS. Chickenpox may begin with a slight fever, headache, backache and loss of appetite. At the same time, or a day or two later, small red spots appear, usually on the back and chest first. Within a few hours the spots enlarge and a vesicle filled with a clear fluid appears in the center of each spot, surrounded by an area of reddened skin. After a day or two, the fluid turns yellow and a crust or scab forms. This crust peels off in from 5 to 20 days. During this period the patient experiences severe itching.
   The vesicles do not appear all at once, but in crops, the number of crops depending on the severity of the case. Usually the eruptions are con-

centrated on the back and chest, with only a few appearing on the arms, legs and face, but in severe cases they may cover almost all of the body.
   TREATMENT. Most cases of chickenpox are mild and require no special treatment except rest in bed and forcing fluids during the fever stage. For severe itching, emollient baths, calamine lotion or other applications offer some relief. Since scratching the scabs may result in permanent scars and opens the way for other infections, the child's fingernails should be cut short and his hands washed often. Petrolatum applied to the sores reduces itching, keeps the scabs soft and reduces the possibility of scarring. The clothes and bedding should be kept fresh and clean.
   The child should be kept in bed during the period of acute illness and isolated during the period of communicability, or until about 12 days after the first appearance of the blisters. Isolation need not last until the scabs are gone.

chigger (chig′er) the six-legged red larva of the mite *Trombicula alfreddugési,* known as harvest mite and red bug; its bite produces a wheal on the skin that is accompanied by intense itching.

chigoe (chig′o) the sand flea, *Tunga penetrans,* of tropical America and the southern United States. The pregnant female flea burrows into the skin of the feet and legs of man, causing intense irritation and resulting in ulceration if untreated.

chilblain (chil′blān) a localized painful erythema of the fingers, toes or ears produced by excessive exposure to cold; pernio. The basic cause of chilblain is sensitivity to cold, sometimes resulting from circulatory disturbances, which may be corrected in part by exercise and proper diet; severe cases require medical attention. Extreme heat or cold applications should not be applied directly to chilblains. This condition should not be confused with FROSTBITE, another type of skin damage caused by exposure to cold.

child (chīld) the human young, from infancy to puberty.

childbed (chīld′bed) the puerperal state or period.
   c. fever, puerperal fever.

childbirth (chīld′berth) expulsion or delivery of an infant (see also LABOR).

chill (chil) a feeling of cold, with convulsive shaking of the body. A true chill, or rigor, results from an increase in chemical activity within the body and usually ushers in a considerable rise in body temperature. The pallor and coldness of a chill, and the goose flesh that often accompanies it, are caused by constriction of the peripheral blood vessels. Chills are symptomatic of a wide variety of diseases. They usually do not accompany well localized infections.
   NURSING CARE. During a chill sufficient heat should be applied to maintain normal body temperature. Since the patient will most likely begin to have a sharp rise in body temperature immediately after or during the chill, it is best to use only a light blanket and several hot water bottles of moderate temperature to alleviate the sensation of cold. In addition to this the patient's temperature should

be taken every 30 minutes until it is stabilized or further orders are obtained from the physician.

Chilomastix (ki″lo-mas′tiks) a genus of parasitic protozoa.

C. mesnil′i, a species sometimes found in the human intestine.

Chilopoda (ki-lop′o-dah) a class of the phylum Arthropoda embracing the centipedes.

chilopodiasis (ki″lo-po-di′ah-sis) the presence of a centipede of the class Chilopoda in a body cavity.

chimera (ki-me′rah) an organism whose body contains different cell populations derived from different zygotes of the same or different species, occurring spontaneously or produced artificially.

heterologous c., one in which the foreign cells are derived from an organism of a different species.

homologous c., one in which the foreign cells are derived from an organism of the same species, but of a different genotype.

isologous c., one in which the foreign cells are derived from a different organism having the identical genotype, as from an identical twin.

radiation c., an organism that has been subjected to heavy radiation and later received injection of cells from nonirradiated donors.

chimerism (ki′mer-izm) the presence in an organism of cells derived from different zygotes of the same or different species.

chin (chin) the anterior prominence of the lower jaw; the mentum.

chiniofon (kin′e-o-fon) a bitter, slightly odorous, canary yellow powder; amebicide.

chionablepsia (ki″o-nah-blep′se-ah) snow blindness.

chir(o)- (ki″ro) word element [Gr.], *hand.* See also words beginning *cheir(o)-.*

chiropodist (ki-rop′ŏ-dist) a specialist in treating minor ailments of the feet; called also podiatrist. Chiropodists are not graduate physicians and their activity should be restricted entirely to the treatment of corns, ingrown toenails and other minor foot conditions.

chiropractic (ki″ro-prak′tik) a system of treating disease by manipulation of the vertebral column. Chiropractic is based on the theory that most diseases are caused by pressure on the nerves because of faulty alignment of bones, especially the vertebrae, and that the nerves are thus prevented from transmitting to various organs of the body the neural impulses for proper functioning. Medical science has never found a scientific basis for this theory.

Acting on this theory, the chiropractor manipulates various parts of the spine in treating the complaint. If the patient is suffering from a displaced vertebra, the manipulation may bring relief. If he has some other disorder or disease, however, manipulation will have little if any effect.

Chiropractors are licensed to practice in 44 states and the District of Columbia. They are not physicians and hence are forbidden by law to dispense prescription medicines.

chiropractor (ki″ro-prak′tor) a specialist in chiropractic.

chirospasm (ki′ro-spazm) writers' cramp; cheirospasm.

chirurgenic (ki″rer-jen′ik) induced by or occurring as the result of a surgical procedure.

chirurgery (ki-rer′jer-e) surgery.

chitin (ki′tin) a nitrogen-containing polysaccharide constituting the shells of crustaceae and the structural substance of insects and fungi.

Chlamydia (klah-mid′e-ah) a genus of the family Chlamydiaceae, order Rickettsiales, occurring as two species, both pathogenic for man.

C. oculogenita′lis, the agent causing inclusion conjunctivitis.

C. tracho′matis, the causative agent of trachoma.

Chlamydiaceae (klah-mid″e-a′se-e) a family of the order Rickettsiales parasitic in warm-blooded animals.

chlamydospore (klam′ĭ-do-spōr″) 1. the reproductive organ of certain fungi, enclosed by two envelopes. 2. a spore that is covered.

chloasma (klo-az′mah) hyperpigmentation in circumscribed areas of the skin; melanoderma.

c. gravida′rum, chloasma occurring in pregnancy.

c. hepat′icum, discoloration of the skin allegedly due to disorder of the liver.

c. uteri′num, chloasma occurring during menstruation, in pregnancy or at the time of the menopause.

chlophedianol (klo″fĕ-di′ah-nol) a compound used as a cough depressant.

chloracne (klōr-ak′ne) an acneiform eruption, caused by chlorine.

chloral (klo′ral) a colorless, oily liquid, trichloracetic aldehyde, prepared by the mutual action of alcohol and chlorine.

c. hydrate, a hypnotic and sedative with mild action as a pain reliever but used most commonly to induce sleep. It is given when barbiturates are not desirable, as in patients who have poor kidney function and who might have difficulty excreting barbiturates, or in the elderly, who react poorly to barbiturates. It is also used for patients undergoing withdrawal from alcohol, morphine or barbiturates, and in cases of delirium tremens. Overdoses can be extremely poisonous.

Chloral hydrate is available in liquid and in capsule form. It may be habit forming. It should not be given with alcohol.

chloralism (klo′ral-izm) poisoning from habitual use of chloral.

chlorambucil (klōr-am′bu-sil) a nitrogen mustard derivative used as an antineoplastic agent.

chloramphenicol (klōr″am-fen′ĭ-kol) a broad-spectrum antibiotic with specific therapeutic activity against rickettsiae and many different bacteria. Side effects include serious, even fatal, blood dyscrasias in certain patients. Frequent blood tests are recommended during therapy.

chloranemia (klo″rah-ne′me-ah) idiopathic hypochromic anemia.

chlorate (klo'rāt) a salt of chloric acid.

chlorbutol (klōr'bu-tol) chlorobutanol.

chlorcyclizine (klōr-si'klĭ-zēn) a white, odorless or almost odorless powder used as an antihistamine.

chlordiazepoxide (klōr"di-a"ze-pok'sīd) a tranquilizing drug.

chloremia (klo-re'me-ah) 1. chlorosis. 2. the presence of excessive chlorides in the blood.

Chloretone (klo'rĕ-tōn) trademark for a preparation of chlorobutanol, a hypnotic and preservative, with a moderate antiseptic action.

chlorhydria (klōr-hi'dre-ah) excess of hydrochloric acid in the stomach.

chloride (klo'rīd) a salt of hydrochloric acid; any binary compound of chlorine in which the latter carries a negative charge of electricity.

chloridemia (klo"rĭ-de'me-ah) chlorides in the blood.

chloridimetry (klo"rĭ-dim'ĕ-tre) measurement of the chloride content of a fluid.

chloriduria (klo"rĭ-du're-ah) excess of chlorides in the urine.

chlorinated (klo'rĭ-nāt"ed) charged with chlorine.

chlorination (klo"rĭ-na'shun) the addition of chlorine to water or sewage to kill germs. Liquid chlorine has been found to be the most effective water disinfectant, and is almost invariably used in the United States for the purification of both public water supplies and swimming pools. This addition of chlorine is harmless, since enough chlorine to affect the health of those using the chlorinated water would also make the water too unpalatable to drink.

chlorine (klo'rēn) a gaseous chemical element, atomic number 17, atomic weight 35.453, symbol Cl. (See table of ELEMENTS.) It is a disinfectant, decolorizer and irritant poison. It is used for disinfecting, fumigating and bleaching, either in an aqueous solution or in the form of chlorinated lime.

chlorisondamine (klōr"i-son'dah-mēn) a compound used to produce ganglionic blockade and to reduce blood pressure.

chlorite (klo'rīt) a salt of chlorous acid; disinfectant and bleaching agent.

chlormerodrin (klōr-mer'o-drin) a mercurial diuretic.

chlormezanone (klōr-mez'ah-nōn) an agent used as a muscle relaxant and tranquilizer.

chloro-anemia (klo"ro-ah-ne'me-ah) chlorosis.

chloroblast (klo'ro-blast) an erythroblast.

chlorobutanol (klo"ro-bu'tah-nol) colorless or white crystals with a moderate antiseptic action, used as a preservative for solutions and as a hypnotic.

chloroform (klo'ro-form) a colorless, mobile liquid with a characteristic odor and sweet taste; solvent, anesthetic and counterirritant.

chloroleukemia (klo"ro-lu-ke'me-ah) myelogenous leukemia in which no specific tumor masses are observed at autopsy, but the body organs and fluids show a definite green color.

chlorolymphosarcoma, chloroma (klo"ro-lim"-fo-sar-ko'mah), (klo-ro'mah) a malignant, green-colored tumor arising from myeloid tissue.

Chloromycetin (klo"ro-mi-se'tin) trademark for preparations of chloramphenicol, a broad-spectrum antibiotic.

chloromyeloma (klo"ro-mi"ĕ-lo'mah) chloroma with multiple growths in bone marrow.

chloropenia (klo"ro-pe'ne-ah) deficiency in chlorine.

chlorophane (klo'ro-fān) a green-yellow pigment from the retina.

chlorophenothane (klo"ro-fe'no-thān) a compound of DDT used in a lotion as an insecticide in pediculosis and scabies.

chlorophyll (klo'ro-fil) the green photosynthetic pigment contained in many vegetable organisms.

chloroplast (klo'ro-plast) the photosynthetic unit of a plant cell, containing all the chlorophyll.

chloroprivic (klo"ro-pri'vik) relating to lack or loss of chlorides.

chloroprocaine (klo"ro-pro'kān) a compound used as a local or epidural anesthetic.

chloropsia (klo-rop'se-ah) a defect of vision in which objects appear green.

chloroquine (klo'ro-kwin) an antimalarial compound, used also in amebic abscess and lupus erythematosus.

chlorosarcoma (klo"ro-sar-ko'mah) chloroma.

chlorosis (klo-ro'sis) a disorder, generally of pubescent females, characterized by greenish yellow discoloration of the skin and hypochromic erythrocytes; related to iron deficiency.

chlorothen (klo'ro-then) a pyridine derivative used as an antihistamine.

chlorothiazide (klo"ro-thi'ah-zīd) a diuretic drug that also has an antihypertensive effect. Possible side effects include potassium depletion and other electrolyte imbalances; bone marrow depression with a lowering of the platelet and leukocyte counts, agranulocytosis and aplastic anemia are rare side reactions.

chlorotrianisene (klo"ro-tri-an'ĭ-sēn) a synthetic estrogenic compound.

chlorpheniramine (klōr"fen-ir'ah-mēn) a pyridine derivative used as an antihistamine.

chlorphenoxamine (klōr"fen-ok'sah-mēn) an agent used as an antihistamine and to reduce muscular rigidity.

chlorpromazine (klōr-pro'mah-zēn) a phenothiazine used as an antiemetic in motion sickness; used also as a mild sedative and as a tranquilizer, in the control of agitated patients. It is available for oral or intramuscular administration. Side effects include drowsiness and slight hypotension. In prolonged therapy the patient should be observed for jaundice.

chlorpropamide (klōr-pro′pah-mīd) an oral hypoglycemic drug useful in the treatment of diabetes mellitus in the adult whose condition is stabilized. The drug is contraindicated in patients with impairment of renal, thyroid or hepatic function. Dosage is individually adjusted.

chlorprophenpyridamine (klōr″pro-fen-pi-rid′-ah-mēn) chlorpheniramine.

chlorquinaldol (klōr-kwin′al-dol) a bactericide and fungicide for application to the skin.

chlortetracycline hydrochloride (klōr″tet-rah-si′klēn) a broad-spectrum antibiotic effective against both gram-positive and gram-negative microorganisms. It is available in capsules and in ampules for intravenous injection. Side effects include gastrointestinal disturbances, especially diarrhea.

chlorthalidone (klōr-thal′ĭ-dōn) a compound used as a diuretic and antihypertensive.

Chlor-Trimeton (klōr-tri′mĕ-ton) trademark for preparations of chlorpheniramine, an antihistamine.

chloruresis (klōr″u-re′sis) excretion of chlorides in the urine.

chloruria (klo-ru′re-ah) excess chlorides in the urine.

chlorzoxazone (klōr-zok′sah-zōn) a drug used as a skeletal muscle relaxant.

Ch.M. [L.] *Chirur′giae Ma′gister* (Master of Surgery).

choana (ko-a′nah), pl. *choa′nae* [L.] the posterior cavity of the nose.

Choanotaenia (ko-a″no-te′ne-ah) a genus of tapeworm.

chokes (chōks) a burning sensation in the substernal region, with uncontrollable coughing, occurring during decompression.

chol(o)- (ko′lo) word element [Gr.], *bile.*

cholagogue (ko′lah-gog) an agent that stimulates gallbladder contraction.

cholalic acid (ko-lal′ik) an acid formed in the liver from cholesterol that plays, with other bile acids, an important role in digestion; called also cholic acid.

cholaligenic (ko-lal″ĭ-jen′ik) forming cholalic acid from cholesterol.

Cholan (ko′lan) trademark for preparations of dehydrocholic acid.

cholangiogastrostomy (ko-lan″je-o-gas-tros′to-me) anastomosis of a bile duct to the stomach.

cholangiogram (ko-lan′je-o-gram″) the film obtained by cholangiography.

cholangiography (ko-lan″je-og′rah-fe) x-ray examination of the bile ducts, using a radiopaque dye as a contrast medium. In the intravenous method, the dye is administered intravenously and is excreted by the liver into the bile ducts. X-ray films are taken at 10-minute intervals as the dye is excreted via the cystic, hepatic and common bile ducts into the intestinal tract. The excretion is usually completed within 4 hours. Preparation of the patient for the intravenous method requires restriction of fluids to concentrate the dye and also cleansing of the intestinal tract with castor oil and enemas so that fecal material and gas will not obscure the biliary tract.

Sometimes cholangiography is done after surgery of the gallbladder and biliary tract. In this method the radiopaque dye is injected directly into a tube that has been left in the biliary tract since the time of surgery. Films are taken immediately after the dye is injected. If no obstruction is present, the biliary structures fill readily and rapidly empty into the intestinal tract.

When it is necessary for the surgeon to locate gallstones or other obstructive conditions at the time that surgery is being performed, the dye may be injected directly into the bile ducts. Films are taken in the operating room and obstructions not otherwise discernible can be located and corrected while the patient is still anesthetized. This procedure may also be performed in the x-ray department prior to the contemplated surgery to evaluate the cause of jaundice.

cholangiohepatoma (ko-lan″je-o-hep″ah-to′mah) a tumor containing abnormally mixed masses of liver cell cords and bile ducts.

cholangiole (ko-lan′je-ōl) one of the fine terminal elements of the bile duct system.

cholangiolitis (ko-lan″je-o-li′tis) inflammation of the cholangioles.

cholangioma (ko-lan″je-o′mah) a tumor of the bile ducts.

cholangiostomy (ko″lan-je-os′to-me) incision of a bile duct with drainage.

cholangiotomy (ko″lan-je-ot′o-me) incision of a bile duct.

cholangitis (ko″lan-ji′tis) inflammation of a bile duct.

cholate (ko′lāt) a salt or ester of cholic acid.

chole- (ko′le) word element [Gr.], *bile.*

cholecalciferol (ko″le-kal-sif′er-ol) an oil-soluble antirachitic vitamin.

cholecystagogue (ko″le-sis′tah-gog) an agent that promotes evacuation of the gallbladder.

cholecystalgia (ko″le-sis-tal′je-ah) biliary colic.

cholecystectasia (ko″le-sis″tek-ta′ze-ah) distention of the gallbladder.

cholecystectomy (ko″le-sis-tek′to-me) excision of the gallbladder (see also surgery of the GALL-BLADDER).

cholecystenterostomy (ko″le-sis″ten-ter-os′to-me) formation of a new communication between the gallbladder and the intestine.

cholecystic (ko"le-sis'tik) pertaining to the gall-bladder.

cholecystitis (ko"le-sis-ti'tis) inflammation of the GALLBLADDER, acute or chronic.

ACUTE CHOLECYSTITIS. The most frequent cause of acute cholecystitis is GALLSTONES. Other causes include typhoid fever and a malignant tumor obstructing the biliary tract. The inflammation may be secondary to a systemic staphylococcal or streptococcal infection.

The symptoms of a mild inflammation may be very slight and include indigestion, moderate pain and tenderness in the upper right quadrant of the abdomen that is usually aggravated by deep breathing, malaise and a low-grade fever. When gallstones or other disorders cause complete obstruction of the bile ducts the symptoms are much more extreme. The pain becomes unbearable, the temperature may rise to 104° F. and there is nausea and vomiting.

Treatment of acute cholecystitis may entail either cholecystectomy or cholecystostomy. In some cases the surgery may be postponed until the attack subsides, the initial treatment consisting of administration of antibiotics and parenteral fluids and, after a period of no oral intake, administration of a special gallbladder diet.

CHRONIC CHOLECYSTITIS. Chronic cholecystitis progresses more slowly than acute cholecystitis, but it also is usually the result of gallstones or other conditions that lead to obstruction of the bile ducts and impaired gallbladder function. It is the most common disorder of the gallbladder.

The characteristic symptom of chronic cholecystitis is indigestion manifested by discomfort after eating, with flatulence and nausea. If the meal has been larger than usual, or high in fat content, the symptoms are more pronounced and there is eructation (belching) and regurgitation. There may also be vomiting and some pain in the upper right quadrant of the abdomen. It is not unusual for patients to suffer repeated episodes before seeking medical attention. Neglect of the situation may lead to permanent damage to the gallbladder and liver.

Diagnosis of cholecystitis is aided by the use of CHOLECYSTOGRAPHY, x-ray examination after administration of a radiopaque dye that is concentrated by the gallbladder.

The preferred treatment of chronic cholecystitis with gallstones is cholecystectomy. If surgery is contraindicated for some reason, then the symptoms may be controlled to some extent by low-fat diet, restriction of alcohol intake and spacing of meals so that large amounts of food are avoided and there is not a long interval between meals.

cholecystocholangiogram (ko"le-sis"to-ko-lan'-je-o-gram") a roentgenogram of the gallbladder and bile ducts.

cholecystoduodenostomy (ko"le-sis"to-du"o-dĕ-nos'to-me) formation of an opening between the gallbladder and duodenum.

cholecystogastrostomy (ko"le-sis"to-gas-tros'-to-me) formation of an opening between the gallbladder and stomach.

cholecystogram (ko"le-sis'to-gram) a roentgenogram of the gallbladder.

cholecystography (ko"le-sis-tog'rah-fe) roentgenologic examination of the gallbladder, using a

radiopaque dye as contrast medium. The purpose of the examination is to determine the ability of the gallbladder to fill, concentrate bile and empty. The dye is administered in tablets the evening before the x-ray films are made.

Preparation of the patient requires enemas and a mild cathartic to cleanse the intestinal tract of fecal material and gas which can prevent adequate visualization of the gallbladder. The evening before the test the patient is given a fat-free meal. The tablets are administered after the meal, usually at 5-minute intervals until six tablets have been taken. The patient is then given nothing by mouth until the x-ray filming is completed.

In the morning films are made of the gallbladder, which should be filled with the dye. The patient is then given a fatty meal to stimulate emptying of the gallbladder and further x-ray films are made to evaluate the functioning of the gallbladder.

cholecystojejunostomy (ko"le-sis"to-je-ju-nos'to-me) formation of an opening between the gallbladder and jejunum.

cholecystokinin (ko"le-sis"to-ki'nin) a hormone secreted in the small intestine, which stimulates contraction of the gallbladder.

cholecystolithiasis (ko"le-sis"to-lĭ-thi'ah-sis) the presence of stones in the gallbladder.

cholecystopathy (ko"le-sis-top'ah-the) disease of the gallbladder.

cholecystorrhaphy (ko"le-sis-tor'ah-fe) suture of the gallbladder.

cholecystostomy (ko"le-sis-tos'to-me) incision of the gallbladder with drainage.

cholecystotomy (ko"le-sis-tot'o-me) incision of the gallbladder.

choledochal (kol'e-dok"al) pertaining to the common bile duct.

choledochectomy (kol"e-do-kek'to-me) excision of part of the common bile duct.

choledochitis (kol"e-do-ki'tis) inflammation of the common bile duct.

choledocho- (ko-led'ŏ-ko) word element [Gr.], *common bile duct.*

choledochoduodenostomy (ko-led"ŏ-ko-du"o-dĕ-nos'to-me) anastomosis of the common bile duct to the duodenum.

choledochoenterostomy (ko-led"ŏ-ko-en"ter-os'-to-me) anastomosis of the common bile duct to the intestine.

choledochogastrostomy (ko-led"ŏ-ko-gas-tros'-to-me) anastomosis of the common bile duct to the stomach.

choledochojejunostomy (ko-led"ŏ-ko-je-ju-nos'to-me) anastomosis of the common bile duct to the jejunum.

choledocholithiasis (ko-led"ŏ-ko-lĭ-thi'ah-sis) calculi in the common bile duct.

choledocholithotomy (ko-led"ŏ-ko-lĭ-thot'o-me) incision of the common bile duct for removal of a stone.

choledocholithotripsy (ko-led″ŏ-ko-lith′o-trip″se) crushing of a gallstone in the common bile duct.

choledochoplasty (ko-led′ŏ-ko-plas″te) plastic repair of the common bile duct.

choledochostomy (ko″led-o-kos′to-me) incision of the common bile duct with drainage.

choledochotomy (ko″led-o-kot′o-me) incision of the common bile duct.

Choledyl (kōl′ĕ-dil) trademark for a preparation of oxtriphylline, used for treatment of the pain of angina pectoris and in asthma.

cholehemia (ko″le-he′me-ah) bile in the blood.

choleic (ko-le′ik) pertaining to the bile.

cholelith (ko′lĕ-lith) gallstone.

cholelithiasis (ko″le-lĭ-thi′ah-sis) the presence of GALLSTONES. adj., **cholelith′ic.**

cholelithotomy (ko″le-lĭ-thot′o-me) incision of the biliary tract for removal of gallstones.

cholelithotripsy, cholelithotrity (ko″le-lith′o-trip″se), (ko″le-lĭ-thot′rĭ-te) crushing of a gallstone.

cholemesis (ko-lem′ĕ-sis) vomiting of bile.

cholemia (ko-le′me-ah) bile or bile pigment in the blood. adj., **chole′mic.**

cholemimetry (ki″le-mim′ĕ-tre) measurement of bile pigment in the blood.

cholepathia (ko″le-path′e-ah) disease of the biliary tract.
 c. spas′tica, spasmodic contraction of the bile ducts.

choleperitoneum (ko″le-per″ĭ-to-ne′um) bile in the peritoneum.

choleprasin (ko″le-pra′sin) one of the pigments of bile.

cholera (kol′er-ah) an acute enteritis characterized by a superficial sloughing necrosis of the epithelial lining of the gut. The term usually refers specifically to Asiatic cholera, caused by *Vibrio comma.*
 INCIDENCE. Immunization and modern methods of sanitation have all but eliminated cholera epidemics in the United States and Europe, but they are still a danger in many other parts of the world, e.g., in the tropics, and particularly in India. Travelers to cholera-ridden areas should protect themselves by vaccination, but this does not provide complete immunity. The local drinking water should be boiled and uncooked foods avoided. Food should be protected from flies, and fruits and vegetables peeled and the rinds discarded.
 TRANSMISSION. *Vibrio comma,* a spiral microorganism, is carried in the cholera victim's feces, urine and vomitus, and transmitted to others in contaminated water or food. Once it has reached the intestines, the intestinal lining becomes inflamed and the passages distended with a thin, watery fluid.
 SYMPTOMS. Symptoms begin to appear at any time from a few hours to 5 days after contact; the usual incubation period is 3 days. When the disease is at its peak, diarrhea and vomiting occur with such frequency and abundance that dehydration results very rapidly. The skin is cyanotic and shriveled, the eyes are sunken and the voice is feeble. There may be painful muscular cramps throughout the body.
 TREATMENT. Since alkaline substances are lost in the vomitus and feces, acidosis as well as dehydration must be combated. The fluids and electrolytes are replaced by intravenous infusions. Acid intoxication may require intravenous administration of sodium bicarbonate.
 NURSING CARE. Measures must be taken to maintain normal body temperature because of the loss of body heat, which often causes the body temperature to drop to as low as 70 degrees. Warmth by blankets, hot-water bottles and electric pads may be necessary. Antiemetic drugs are given to reduce vomiting.
 Victims of cholera (and proved carriers of the disease) should be isolated. The vomitus, urine and feces of the patient must be promptly and thoroughly disinfected. Eating utensils, dishes and all other contaminated articles must be disinfected or burned. (See also COMMUNICABLE DISEASE and ISOLATION TECHNIQUE.)
 c. infan′tum, a noncontagious diarrhea occurring in infants; formerly common in the summer months.
 c. mor′bus, an acute gastroenteritis with diarrhea, cramps and vomiting.

choleraic (kol″ĕ-ra′ik) pertaining to cholera.

choleresis (ko-ler′ĕ-sis) the output of bile by the liver.

choleretic (ko″ler-et′ik) 1. increasing the output of bile by the liver. 2. an agent that stimulates an increase in the output of bile by the liver.

choleriform (ko-ler′ĭ-form) resembling cholera.

cholerine (kol′er-ēn) a relatively mild form of cholera.

cholerophobia (kol″er-o-fo′be-ah) morbid fear of cholera.

cholerrhagia (ko″lĕ-ra′je-ah) an excessive flow of bile.

cholerythrin (ko-ler′ĭ-thrin) bilirubin.

cholestasis (ko″le-sta′sis) retention and accumulation of bile in the liver, due to factors within (intrahepatic cholestasis) or outside the liver (extrahepatic cholestasis). adj., **cholestat′ic.**

cholesteatoma (ko″lĕ-ste″ah-to′mah) a cystic mass with a lining of stratified squamous epithelium, filled with desquamating debris frequently including cholesterol; sometimes associated with chronic infection of the middle ear (cholesteatoma tympani).

cholesterase (ko-les′ter-ās) an enzyme that splits up cholesterol.

cholesteremia (ko-les″ter-e′me-ah) cholesterolemia.

cholesterin (ko-les′ter-in) cholesterol.

cholesterinemia (ko-les″ter-in-e′me-ah) cholesterolemia.

cholesterinuria (ko-les″ter-in-u′re-ah) cholesteroluria.

cholesteroderma (ko-les″ter-o-der′mah) xanthoderma.

cholesterol (ko-les′ter-ol) the principal animal sterol, occurring in faintly yellow, pearly leaflets or granules in all animal tissues.

Research has suggested the possibility that eating foods high in cholesterol may be a contributing factor in heart and circulatory disease, particularly in the formation of fatty deposits in the arteries (atherosclerosis). However, the reason why such deposits form is still unknown. Some investigators believe that the fatty deposits accumulate from an excess of fatty particles in the blood brought about by eating foods rich in cholesterol. Others reject this theory and claim that no relationship exists between the amount of cholesterol eaten and the amount of cholesterol found in the blood.

It is also thought that the saturated fats found in animal fat, which are low in linoleic acid, may contribute to the formation of cholesterol in the body. Experiments have indicated that unsaturated fats (called also polyunsaturates), which are high in linoleic acid, help to reduce the amount of cholesterol in the blood. These unsaturated fats are found in large quantities in vegetable oils such as corn oil.

The body's own normal production of cholesterol is essential to the functioning of certain systems, for example, the nervous system. The medical approach in controlling tendencies to atherosclerosis and high blood pressure is to keep cholesterol formation in the body at its lowest normal levels.

It seems likely that a relationship exists between tension and the cholesterol level of the blood. When a person is under stress, his cholesterol level tends to rise. It is also known that the obese usually have higher than normal levels of cholesterol in their blood, and that they are more subject to coronary occlusion ("heart attack") than are lean people. As a result, the American Heart Association has suggested that reducing the amount of food containing large amounts of cholesterol, and maintaining the weight within reasonable limits, are possible ways of preventing atherosclerosis and decreasing the risk of coronary occlusion.

BLOOD CHOLESTEROL. A laboratory test for determination of the blood cholesterol level is often included in liver function studies because the liver plays an important role in the metabolism of cholesterol and an unusually high blood cholesterol may indicate liver disease. It also may be indicative of the metabolic rate since the cholesterol level tends to be low in hyperthyroidism and high in hypothyroidism. The normal ranges for blood cholesterol tests are: Cholesterol esters, from 95 to 200 mg. per 100 ml. of serum; total cholesterol, from 135 to 260 mg. per 100 ml. of serum. The patient must be in a fasting state for this test.

cholesterolemia (ko-les″ter-ol-e′me-ah) cholesterol in the blood.

cholesteroluria (ko-les″ter-ol-u′re-ah) cholesterol in the urine.

cholesterosis (ko-les″ter-o′sis) deposition of cholesterol in abnormal quantities.
    c. cu′tis, xanthomatosis.

choletherapy (ko″le-ther′ah-pe) use of bile as a medicine.

choleuria (ko″le-u′re-ah) choluria.

cholic acid (ko′lik, kol′ik) an acid formed in the liver from cholesterol that plays, with other bile acids, an important role in digestion; called also cholalic acid.

choline (ko′lēn) a quaternary ammonium compound that is an essential component of the diet of mammals and is therefore included among the vitamins. It is derivable from many animal and some vegetable tissues. It prevents the deposition of fat in the liver and is required for the synthesis of acetylcholine, a compound concerned with the transmission of nerve impulses at the myoneural junction.

Synthetic preparations of choline derivatives are used as parasympathetic stimulants and act to increase the heart rate, contract smooth muscle tissue, contract the pupil of the eye and increase secretions of most of the glands.

choline-acetylase (ko″lēn-ah-set′ĭ-lās) an enzyme that brings about the synthesis of acetylcholine.

cholinergic (ko″lin-er′jik) 1. activated or transmitted by acetylcholine; applied to nerve fibers that liberate acetylcholine at a synapse when a nerve impulse passes, i.e., the parasympathetic fibers. 2. an agent that resembles acetylcholine or simulates its action.

cholinesterase (ko″lin-es′ter-ās) an enzyme that splits acetylcholine into acetic acid and choline. This enzyme is present throughout the body, but is particularly important at the myoneural junction where the nerve fibers terminate and become embedded in muscle fibers. Acetylcholine, which is formed when a nerve impulse reaches a myoneural junction, acts as a stimulant to the muscle fibers, causing them to contract. Immediately after acetylcholine has sparked a contraction it must be removed so that the muscle fiber will repolarize, or recharge itself; otherwise, it would not be ready to contract the next time it is stimulated. Cholinesterase performs this service by splitting acetylcholine into its components, thus rendering it ineffective. The end products of the metabolism of acetycholine (acetic acid and choline) are eventually resynthesized into acetylcholine, which can once again act as a stimulant.

The drugs neostigmine, physostigmine and pyridostigmine combine chemically with cholinesterase to deactivate it. Some authorities believe that the muscular weakness of MYASTHENIA GRAVIS is due to excessive amounts of cholinesterase at the myoneural junction. They base this theory on the fact that the symptoms of this disorder respond to the administration of these drugs. The relief is only temporary and lasts no more than several hours in most cases.

cholinolytic (ko″lin-o-lit′ik) 1. blocking the action of acetylcholine or of cholinergic substances. 2. an agent that blocks the action of acetylcholine or of cholinergic substances.

cholinomimetic (ko″lin-o-mi-met′ik) having an action similar to that of choline.

cholochrome (ko′lo-krōm) a bile pigment.

Cholografin (ko″lo-gra′fin) trademark for preparations of iodipamide, used in cholecystography.

cholohemothorax (ko"lo-he"mo-tho'raks) bile and blood in the thorax.

chololithiasis (ko"lo-lĭ-thi'ah-sis) cholelithiasis.

cholorrhea (ko"lo-re'ah) profuse secretion of bile.

choloscopy (ko-los'ko-pe) examination of the biliary tract.

cholothorax (ko"lo-tho'raks) a pleural effusion containing bile.

choluria (ko-lu're-ah) bile in the urine.

chondodendron tomentosum extract (kon"do-den'dron to"men-to'sum) a curare derivative used as a strong muscle relaxant.

chondr(o)- (kon'dro) word element [Gr.], *cartilage.*

chondral (kon'dral) pertaining to cartilage.

chondralgia (kon-dral'je-ah) pain in a cartilage.

chondrectomy (kon-drek'to-me) excision of a cartilage.

chondric (kon'drik) pertaining to cartilage.

chondrification (kon"drĭ-fĭ-ka'shun) development of cartilage.

chondrin (kon'drin) a protein, resembling gelatin, from cartilage; considered to be a mixture of gelatin and mucin.

chondrio- (kon'dre-o) word element [Gr.], *cartilage; granule.*

chondriome (kon'dre-ōm) the entire complement of chondriosomes in a cell.

chondriosome (kon'dre-o-sōm") one of the particles constantly found in protoplasm, distinguishable by their greater degree of refractivity.

chondritis (kon-dri'tis) inflammation of a cartilage.

chondroadenoma (kon"dro-ad"ĕ-no'mah) an adenoma containing cartilaginous elements.

chondroangioma (kon"dro-an"je-o'mah) an angioma containing cartilaginous elements.

chondroblast (kon'dro-blast) an immature cartilage-producing cell.

chondroblastoma (kon"dro-blas-to'mah) a benign tumor arising from young chondroblasts in the epiphysis of a bone.

chondrocalcinosis (kon"dro-kal"sĭ-no'sis) a condition resembling gout, resulting from calcification of articular plate of a joint.

chondroclast (kon'dro-klast) a giant cell concerned in absorption and removal of cartilage.

chondrocostal (kon"dro-kos'tal) pertaining to ribs and costal cartilages.

chondrocranium (kon"dro-kra'ne-um) the embryonic skull from the seventh week to the middle of the third month, when it is a unified cartilaginous mass without clear boundaries indicating the limits of future bones.

chondrocyte (kon'dro-sīt) a mature cartilage-producing cell.

chondrodermatitis (kon"dro-der"mah-ti'tis) an inflammatory process involving cartilage and skin.

chondrodynia (kon"dro-din'e-ah) pain in a cartilage.

chondrodysplasia (kon"dro-dis-pla'ze-ah) dyschondroplasia.

chondrodystrophia, chondrodystrophy (kon"-dro-dis-tro'fe-ah), (kon"dro-dis'tro-fe) a disorder of cartilage formation.

chondroendothelioma (kon"dro-en"do-the"le-o'mah) an endothelioma containing cartilage tissue.

chondroepiphysitis (kon"dro-ep"ĭ-fiz-i'tis) inflammation of epiphyses and cartilages.

chondrofibroma (kon"dro-fi-bro'mah) a chondroma with fibrous elements.

chondrogen (kon'dro-jen) the substance regarded as the basis of cartilage.

chondrogenesis (kon"dro-jen'ĕ-sis) formation of cartilage.

chondrogenic (kon"dro-jen'ik) giving rise to or forming cartilage.

chondroid (kon'droid) resembling cartilage.

chondroitin sulfuric acid (kon-dro'ĭ-tin sul-fur'-ik) a compound of high molecular weight in skin and connective tissue and, combined with collagen, constituting 20 to 40 per cent of cartilage.

chondroituria (kon"dro-ĭ-tu're-ah) chondroitin sulfuric acid in the urine.

chondrolipoma (kon"dro-lĭ-po'mah) a tumor containing cartilaginous and fatty tissue.

chondrology (kon-drol'o-je) the study of cartilages.

chondrolysis (kon-drol'ĭ-sis) dissolution of cartilage.

chondroma (kon-dro'mah) a hyperplastic growth of cartilaginous tissue. It may remain in the interior or substance of a cartilage or bone (true chondroma, or enchondroma), or may develop on the surface of a cartilage and project under the periosteum of a bone (ecchondroma, or ecchondrosis).

chondromalacia (kon"dro-mah-la'she-ah) abnormal softening of cartilage.

chondromatosis (kon"dro-mah-to'sis) formation of multiple chondromas.
    synovial c., a rare condition in which cartilage is formed in the synovial membrane of joints, tendon sheaths or bursae, sometimes becoming detached and producing a number of loose bodies.

chondrometaplasia (kon"dro-met"ah-pla'-ze-ah) a condition characterized by metaplastic activity of the chondroblasts.

chondromucin, chondromucoid (kon"dro-mu'-sin), (kon"dro-mu'koid) a compound of chondroitin sulfuric acid and mucin forming the intercellular substance of cartilage.

chondromyoma (kon″dro-mi-o′mah) myoma with cartilaginous elements.

chondromyxoma (kon″dro-mik-so′mah) myxoma with cartilaginous elements.

chondromyxosarcoma (kon″dro-mik″so-sar-ko′-mah) a sarcoma containing cartilaginous and mucous tissue.

chondro-osseous (kon″dro-os′e-us) composed of cartilage and bone.

chondro-osteodystrophy (kon″dro-os″te-o-dis′tro-fe) 1. eccentro-osteochondrodysplasia. 2. lipochondrodystrophy.

chondropathology (kon″dro-pah-thol′o-je) pathology of the cartilages.

chondropathy (kon-drop′ah-the) disease of cartilage.

chondroplasia (kon″dro-pla′ze-ah) the formation of cartilage by specialized cells (chondrocytes).

chondroplast (kon′dro-plast) chondroblast.

chondroplasty (kon′dro-plas″te) plastic repair of cartilage.

chondroporosis (kon″dro-po-ro′sis) the formation of sinuses or spaces in cartilage.

chondroprotein (kon″dro-pro′te-in) a protein occurring in cartilage.

chondrosarcoma (kon″dro-sar-ko′ma) sarcoma with cartilaginous elements.

chondrosis (kon-dro′sis) the formation of cartilage.

chondrosteoma (kon″dros-te-o′mah) osteoma with cartilaginous elements.

chondrosternal (kon″dro-ster′nal) pertaining to costal cartilages and sternum.

chondrosternoplasty (kon″dro-ster′no-plas″te) surgical correction of pectus excavatum (funnel chest).

chondrotomy (kon-drot′o-me) incision of a cartilage.

chondroxiphoid (kon″dro-zif′oid) pertaining to the xiphoid process.

chondrus (kon′drus) sun-bleached plant of *Chondrus crispus* or *Gigartina mamillosa;* used as a protective agent for the skin.

chord (kord) cord.

chorda (kor′dah), pl. *chor′dae* [L.] a cord or sinew. adj., **chor′dal.**
   c. mag′na, Achilles tendon.
   chor′dae tendin′eae, tendinous strings joining the papillary muscles of the heart with the valves.
   c. umbilica′lis, umbilical cord.
   c. voca′lis, vocal cord.

Chordata (kor-da′tah) a phylum that includes the vertebrates and the animals that have a notochord.

chordate (kor′dāt) an individual of the phylum Chordata.

chordee (kor′de) downward deflection of the penis, due to a congenital anomaly (hypospadias) or to infection.

chorditis (kor-di′tis) inflammation of vocal or spermatic cords.

chordoma (kor-do′mah) a tumor developed from embryonic remains of the notochord.

chordotomy (kor-dot′o-me) surgical division of a nerve tract of the spinal cord.

chorea (ko-re′ah) a nervous disease in which there are involuntary and irregular movements. adj., **chore′ic.**
   chronic c., Huntington's chorea.
   c. gravida′rum, a rare form of chorea seen in pregnancy.
   hereditary c., Huntington's c., a progressive hereditary affection, marked by irregular movements, speech disturbance and dementia.
   Sydenham's c., ordinary and uncomplicated chorea; it is one of the clinical manifestations of rheumatic fever.

choreiform (ko-re′ĭ-form) resembling chorea.

choreoathetosis (ko″re-o-ath″ĕ-to′sis) a morbid condition characterized by choreic and athetoid movements.

chorioadenoma (ko″re-o-ad″ĕ-no′mah) adenoma of the chorion.

chorioallantois (ko″re-o-ah-lan′to-is) an extra-embryonic sac of some vertebrate embryos, formed by fusion of the chorion and allantois.

chorioamnionitis (ko″re-o-am″ne-o-ni′tis) bacterial infection of the fetal membranes.

chorioangioma (ko″re-o-an″je-o′mah) hydatid mole.

choriocapillaris (ko″re-o-kap″ĭ-la′ris) the second or capillary layer of the choroid.

choriocarcinoma (ko″re-o-kar″sĭ-no′mah) a tumor formed from malignant proliferation of the epithelium of the chorionic villi.

choriocele (ko′re-o-sēl″) protrusion of the chorion through an aperture.

chorioepithelioma (ko″re-o-ep″ĭ-the″le-o′mah) choriocarcinoma.

choriogenesis (ko″re-o-jen′ĕ-sis) the development of the chorion.

chorioid (ko′re-oid) choroid.

chorioma (ko″re-o′mah) choriocarcinoma.

choriomeningitis (ko″re-o-men″in-ji′tis) inflammation of the meninges and choroid plexus.
   lymphocytic c., a specific viral infection of the meninges and choroid plexus with an increased number of lymphocytes in the cerebrospinal fluid and infiltrating the membranes.
   pseudolymphocytic c., a benign, aseptic lymphocytic meningitis, with virus in the cerebrospinal fluid, and with severe headache, drowsiness, irritability and vomiting.

chorion (ko′re-on) the outermost of the fetal membranes.

c. frondo'sum, the part of the chorion covered by villi.

c. lae've, the smooth membranous part of the chorion.

chorionic (ko″re-on'ik) pertaining to the chorion.

c. gonadotropin, a hormone with properties similar to those of luteinizing hormone that is secreted in large amounts by the placenta during gestation. It stimulates the formation of interstitial cells in the testes of the fetus and causes the secretion of testosterone. It is found in substantial amounts in human pregnancy urine (see PREGNANCY TESTS). It is used in treatment of underdevelopment of the gonads.

chorionitis (ko″re-o-ni'tis) scleroderma; inflammation of the corium of the skin.

chorioretinitis (ko″re-o-ret″i-ni'tis) inflammation of the choroid and retina.

chorioretinopathy (ko″re-o-ret″i-nop'ah-the) a noninflammatory process involving both the choroid and retina.

chorista (ko-ris'tah) an error of development characterized by separation.

choristoma (ko″ris-to'mah) a mass of histologically normal tissue in an abnormal location.

choroid (ko'roid) one of the vascular coats of the eye. It contains an abundant supply of blood vessels and a large amount of brown pigment which serves to reduce reflection or diffusion of light when it falls on the retina. Adequate nutrition of the eye is dependent upon blood vessels in the choroid.

c. plexus, the ependyma lining the ventricles of the brain with the vascular fringes of the pia mater invaginating them; concerned with formation of the cerebrospinal fluid.

choroidea (ko-roi'de-ah) choroid.

choroideremia (ko-roi″der-e'me-ah) absence of the choroid.

choroiditis (ko″roi-di'tis) inflammation of the choroid.

choroidocyclitis (ko-roi″do-si-kli'tis) inflammation of the choroid and ciliary processes.

choroidoiritis (ko-roi″do-i-ri'tis) inflammation of the choroid and iris.

choroidoretinitis (ko-roi″do-ret″i-ni'tis) inflammation of the choroid and retina.

Christian-Weber disease (kris'chan web'er) nodular nonsuppurative panniculitis.

Christmas disease (kris'mas) a hereditary hemorrhagic diathesis clinically similar to hemophilia A (classic hemophilia) but due to deficiency of clotting factor IX; called also hemophilia B.

chrom(o)- (kro'mo) word element [Gr.], *color.*

chromaffin (kro-maf'in) taking up and staining strongly with chromium salts; said of certain cells occurring in the adrenal and coccygeal glands and the carotid bodies, along with the sympathetic nerves, and in various organs.

chromaffinoblastoma (kro-maf″i-no-blas-to'mah) a tumor containing embryonic chromaffin cells.

chromaffinoma (kro-maf″i-no'mah) any tumor containing chromaffin cells.

medullary c., pheochromocytoma.

chromaffinopathy (kro-maf″i-nop'ah-the) a disease of the chromaffin cells.

chromagogue (kro'mah-gog) tending to eliminate pigments.

chromaphil (kro'mah-fil) chromaffin.

chromat(o)- (kro'mah-to) word element [Gr.], *color; chromatin.*

chromate (kro'māt) a salt of chromium trioxide (chromic acid).

chromatic (kro-mat'ik) 1. pertaining to color; stainable with dyes. 2. pertaining to chromatin.

chromatid (kro'mah-tid) either of the two long, thin, parallel strands held together at one spot (the centromere), constituting a replicating chromosome in a dividing cell.

chromatin (kro'mah-tin) the DNA-containing chromosomal substance of the nucleus of a cell.

sex c., a mass of chromatin situated at the periphery of the nucleus, which is present in normal females, but not in normal males.

chromatin-negative (kro'mah-tin-neg'ah-tiv) lacking sex chromatin; characteristic of the nuclei of cells in a normal male.

chromatinolysis (kro″mah-ti-nol'i-sis) chromatolysis.

chromatinorrhexis (kro-mat″i-no-rek'sis) splitting up of chromatin.

chromatin-positive (kro'mah-tin-poz'i-tiv) containing sex chromatin; characteristic of the nuclei of cells in a normal female.

chromatism (kro'mah-tizm) abnormal pigmentation.

chromatodysopia (kro″mah-to-dis-o'pe-ah) imperfect perception of colors.

chromatogenous (kro″mah-toj'ĕ-nus) producing color or coloring matter.

chromatogram (kro-mat'o-gram) the record produced by chromatography.

chromatography (kro″mah-tog'rah-fe) chemical analysis by determining reactions apparent on adsorption of the substance on different materials contained in a vertical glass tube.

paper c., chromatography using paper treated with various chemicals instead of an adsorption column.

chromatokinesis (kro″mah-to-ki-ne'sis) movement of chromatin during the life and division of a cell.

chromatolysis (kro″mah-tol'i-sis) 1. disintegration of the chromatin of cell nuclei. 2. disappearance of the Nissl bodies of a nerve cell as the result of a noxious influence.

chromatometer (kro″mah-tom'ĕ-ter) an instrument for measuring color or color perception.

chromatopathy (kro″mah-top′ah-the) a skin disease marked by a disorder of pigmentation.

chromatophil (kro-mat′o-fil) a cell or structure that stains easily. adj., **chromatophil′ic.**

chromatophore (kro-mat′o-fōr) a pigment-containing cell.

chromatopsia (kro″mah-top′se-ah) perversion of color vision, in which objects are seen as abnormally colored.

chromatoptometry (kro″mah-top-tom′ĕ-tre) measurement of color perception.

chromatosis (kro″mah-to′sis) abnormal deposition of pigment, as in the skin.

chromaturia (kro″mah-tu′re-ah) abnormal coloration of the urine.

chromesthesia (kro″mes-the′ze-ah) association of color sensations with sensations of taste, hearing and smell.

chromhidrosis (krōm″hĭ-dro′sis) secretion of colored sweat.

chromic acid (kro′mik) chromium trioxide.

chromicize (kro′mĭ-sīz) to treat with chromium.

chromidiosis (kro-mid″e-o′sis) outflow of chromatin from the nucleus to the cytoplasm of a cell.

chromidium (kro-mid′e-um), pl. *chromid′ia,* a grain of extranuclear chromatin in the cytoplasm of a cell.

chromidrosis (kro″mĭ-dro′sis) chromhidrosis.

chromium (kro′me-um) a chemical element, atomic number 24, atomic weight 51.996, symbol Cr. (See table of ELEMENTS.)
   c. trioxide, chromic acid, a powerful caustic used for removal of warts and other foreign growths. In dilute solutions it may be used as an astringent wash and for the treatment of Vincent's angina.

chromoblast (kro′mo-blast) an embryonic cell that develops into a pigment cell.

chromoblastomycosis (kro″mo-blas″to-mi-ko′sis) a chronic fungal infection of the skin, producing wartlike nodules or papillomas that may or may not ulcerate.

chromocrinia (kro″mo-krin′e-ah) secretion or excretion of coloring matter.

chromocyte (kro′mo-sīt) a colored cell.

chromocytometer (kro″mo-si-tom′ĕ-ter) an instrument for measuring the hemoglobin of the erythrocytes.

chromodacryorrhea (kro″mo-dak″re-o-re′ah) the shedding of colored tears.

chromodermatosis (kro″mo-der″mah-to′sis) any skin disease with pigmentation.

chromogen (kro′mo-jen) a precursor of coloring matter.

chromogene (kro′mo-jēn) a gene located on a chromosome.

chromogenesis (kro″mo-jen′ĕ-sis) the formation of color or pigment.

chromogenic (kro″mo-jen′ik) producing color or pigment.

chromolipoid (kro″mo-lip′oid) lipochrome.

chromolysis (kro-mol′ĭ-sis) chromatolysis.

chromoma (kro-mo′mah) a malignant tumor supposed to be derived from chromatophore cells.

chromomere (kro′mo-mēr) 1. a beadlike granule of chromatin found in a chromosome. 2. granulomere.

chromometry (kro-mom′ĕ-tre) measurement of coloring matter.

chromonema (kro″mo-ne′mah), pl. *chromone′mata* [Gr.] the threadlike structure of a chromosome.

chromopectic (kro″mo-pek′tik) pertaining to, characterized by or promoting chromopexy.

chromopexy (kro′mo-pek″se) the fixation of pigment, especially by the liver in the formation of bilirubin.

chromophane (kro′mo-fān) a retinal pigment.

chromophil (kro′mo-fil) any easily stainable structure.

chromophobe (kro′mo-fōb) any cell, structure or tissue that does not stain readily; applied especially to the nonstaining cells of the anterior lobe of the pituitary gland.

chromophobia (kro″mo-fo′be-ah) 1. the quality of staining poorly with dyes. 2. morbid aversion to colors.

chromophore (kro′mo-fōr) any chemical group whose presence gives a decided color to a compound and which unites with certain other groups (auxochromes) to form dyes; called also color radical.

chromophoric (kro″mo-fōr′ik) bearing color.

chromophose (kro′mo-fōz) a subjective sensation of color.

chromophytosis (kro″mo-fi-to′sis) skin discoloration due to a vegetable parasite; tinea versicolor.

chromoplasm (kro′mo-plazm) the easily staining portion of a cell nucleus.

chromoplastid (kro″mo-plas′tid) a protoplasmic pigment granule.

chromoprotein (kro″mo-pro′te-in) a conjugated protein that contains a colored prosthetic group, for example, the red hemoglobin of higher animals.

chromopsia (kro-mop′se-ah) chromatopsia.

chromoptometer (kro″mop-tom′ĕ-ter) an instrument for measuring color perception.

chromoradiometer (kro″mo-ra″de-om′ĕ-ter) an instrument for measuring x-ray dosage.

chromoscopy (kro-mos′ko-pe) 1. the testing of color vision. 2. the diagnosis of renal function by the color of urine following the administration of dyes.

gastric c., diagnosis of gastric function by the color of the gastric contents: a test for achylia gastrica.

chromosome (kro'mo-sōm) one of several small dark-staining and more or less rod-shaped bodies which appear in the nucleus of a cell at the time of cell division. adj., **chromoso'mal.** They contain the genes, or hereditary factors, and are constant in number in each species. Chromosomes are composed of DEOXYRIBONUCLEIC ACID (DNA) that is loosely bound with protein. There are 46 chromosomes in each human cell, 22 pairs of autosomes and two *sex chromosomes*, which are associated with the determination of sex. In the female the sex chromosomes are called X chromosomes; they are identical and are designated as XX. In the male the sex chromosomes are not identical and they are designated as X and Y. (See also HEREDITY.)

CLASSIFICATION. Human chromosomes are difficult to classify into exactly 23 pairs; for practical purposes however, the so-called Denver Classification is frequently used. The chromosomes are categorized according to size and divided into seven groups identified by the letters A to G, beginning with the largest chromosomes and progressing to the smallest. The word karyotype is used to identify this classification. The karyotyping of chromosomes is useful in determining whether or not they are normal in number and structure.

CHROMOSOMAL ERRORS. Abnormalities in the number and structure of chromosomes in the human cell recently have become the subject of much research and widespread interest. In 1959 it was shown that children with DOWN'S SYNDROME (mongolism) have an extra chromosome per cell. Since that time chromosomal aberrations in number or structure have been shown to be a significant cause of mental and physical defects.

Trisomy is the term used to describe the state of having an extra chromosome, that is, three per cell instead of the usual pair. If a chromosome is missing, the individual is said to be monosomic for that particular chromosome.

The causes of chromosomal errors are not completely understood. In some conditions such as Down's syndrome late maternal age seems to be a factor. Other factors may include the predisposition of chromosomes to nondisjunction (failure to separate during meiosis), exposure to radiation and viruses.

homologous c's, chromosomes that are identical in size and shape, have identical chrommomeres along their length, and contain similar genes, which undergo synapsis during meiosis and separate, one going to either pole.

Philadelphia c., an abnormal chromosome observed in the leukocytes of patients with chronic myelocytic leukemia.

sex c's, the chromosomes responsible for determination of the sex of the individual that develops from a zygote.

somatic c., one in a diploid (tissue) cell of the body.

X c., an accessory chromosome carried in both the sperm and ovum, being the female-determining factor.

Y c., an accessory chromosome occurring only in the sperm, being the male-determining factor.

chromotoxic (kro"mo-tok'sik) due to toxic action on hemoglobin.

chromotropic (kro"mo-trop'ik) attracting color or pigment.

chron(o)- (kron'o) word element [Gr.], *time*.

chronaxie (kro'nak-se) chronaxy.

chronaximeter (kro"nak-sim'ĕ-ter) an instrument for measuring chronaxy.

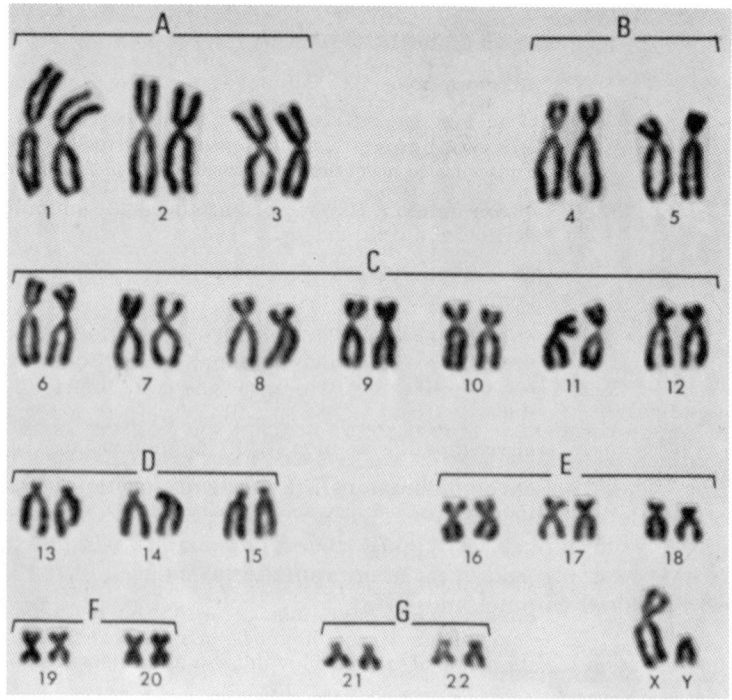

Human metaphase chromosomes from a leukocyte culture, arranged in a standard classification known as a karyotype. (Courtesy of D. H. Carr; from Thompson, J. S., and Thompson, M. W.: Genetics in Medicine. Philadelphia, W. B. Saunders Co., 1966.)

chronaxy (kro'nak-se) the time required for excitation of a neural element by a definite stimulus; the minimum time at which a current just double the rheobase will excite contraction.

chronic (kron'ik) persisting for a long time; applied to a morbid state, designating one showing little change or extremely slow progression over a long period.

chronobiology (kron″o-bi-ol'o-je) the study of the duration of life.

chronograph (kron'o-graf) an instrument for recording small intervals of time.

chronoscope (kron'o-skōp) an instrument for measuring small intervals of time.

chronotropic (kron″o-trop'ik) affecting the time or rate.

chronotropism (kro-not'ro-pizm) interference with regularity of a periodical movement, such as the heart's action.

chrotoplast (kro'to-plast) a skin cell.

chrys(o)- (kris'o) word element [Gr.], *gold*.

chrysarobin (kris″ah-ro'bin) a mixture of neutral principles derived from Goa powder; used in treatment of various skin diseases.

chrysiasis (krī-si'ah-sis) deposition of gold in living tissue.

chrysoderma (kris″o-der'mah) permanent pigmentation of the skin due to gold deposit.

chrysophoresis (kris″o-fo-re'sis) the distribution to various parts of the body of particles of gold administered therapeutically, by macrophages and polymorphonuclear leukocytes.

Chrysops (kris'ops) a genus of flies of worldwide distribution; commonly known as deerflies, they are important vectors of various organisms, e.g., *Pasteurella tularensis* and *Loa loa*.

chrysotherapy (kris″o-ther'ah-pe) treatment with gold salts.

chthonophagia (thon″o-fa'je-ah) eating clay or dirt; geophagy.

Chvostek's sign, Chvostek-Weiss sign (vos'-teks), (vos'tek vīs) a spasm of the facial muscles resulting from tapping the muscles or the branches of the facial nerve; seen in tetany.

chylangioma (ki-lan″je-o'mah) a tumor of intestinal lymph vessels filled with chyle.

chyle (kīl) the product of intestinal digestion absorbed into the lymphatic system through the lacteals and conveyed through the thoracic duct to empty into the venous system at the root of the neck.

chylemia (ki-le'me-ah) chylous material in the blood.

chylidrosis (ko″lī-dro'sis) chylous perspiration.

chylifaction, chylification (ki″lī-fak'shun), (ki″-lī-fī-ka'shun) formation of chyle.

chyliform (ki'lī-form) resembling, but not containing, chyle.

chylocele (ki'lo-sēl) distention of the tunica vaginalis testis with effused chyle.

chyloderma (ki″lo-der'mah) dilatation of the scrotal lymphatics.

chylology (ki-lol'o-je) the study of chyle.

chylomediastinum (ki″lo-me″de-ah-sti'num) effused chyle in the mediastinum.

chylomicron (ki″lo-mi'kron) a particle of emulsified fat, about 1 micron in diameter, found in the blood during the digestion of fat.

chylomicronemia (ki″lo-mi″kro-ne'me-ah) the presence of chylomicrons in the blood.

chylopericardium (ki″lo-per″ĭ-kar'de-um) effused chyle in the pericardium.

chyloperitoneum (ki″lo-per″ĭ-to-ne'um) effused chyle in the peritoneal cavity.

chylopneumothorax (ki″lo-nu″mo-tho'raks) effused chyle and air in the pleural cavity.

chylopoiesis (ki″lo-poi-e'sis) the formation of chyle.

chylothorax (ki″lo-tho'raks) effused chyle in the pleural cavity.

chylous (ki'lus) of the nature of or containing chyle.

chyluria (ki-lu're-ah) the presence of chyle in the urine, giving it a milky appearance.

Chymar (ki'mar) trademark for preparations of chymotripsin, used as an anti-inflammatory agent.

chymase (ki'mās) an enzyme of the gastric juice that hastens the action of the pancreatic juice.

chyme (kīm) the gruel-like material produced by action of the gastric juice on ingested food and discharged through the pylorus into the duodenum.

chymification (ki″mĭ-fī-ka'shun) conversion of food into chyme.

chymosin (ki-mo'sin) rennin.

chymotrypsin (ki″mo-trip'sin) an endopeptidase with action similar to that of trypsin, produced in the intestine by activation of chymotrypsinogen; a product crystallized from an extract of the pancreas of the ox is used clinically as an anti-inflammatory agent.

chymotrypsinogen (ki″mo-trip-sin'o-jen) the inactive precursor of chymotrypsin, the form in which it is secreted by the pancreas.

Ci abbreviation for *curie* recommended by the International Commission on Radiological Units and Measurements.

cib. [L.] *ci'bus* (food).

cicatrectomy (sik″ah-trek'to-me) excision of a cicatrix.

cicatricial (sik″ah-trish′al) pertaining to a cicatrix.

cicatrix (sik′ah-triks, sĭ-ka′triks), pl. *cica′trices* [L.] the mark or fibrous tissue left after the healing of a wound; a scar.

cicatrization (sik″ah-trĭ-za′shun) the formation of permanent fibrous tissue in the healing of a wound; scarring.

-cide (sīd) word element [L.], *destruction or killing* (homicide); *an agent that kills or destroys* (germicide). adj., **-ci′dal.**

cilia (sil′e-ah) [L.] 1. plural of cilium. 2. eyelashes.

ciliariscope (sil′e-ar″ĭ-skōp) an instrument for examining the ciliary region of the eye.

ciliarotomy (sil″e-ar-ot′o-me) surgical division of the ciliary zone for glaucoma.

ciliary (sil′e-er″e) pertaining to cilia or the eyelashes and to certain structures of the eye.
  c. body, the organ connecting choroid and iris, made up of the ciliary muscle and the ciliary processes. These processes radiate from the ciliary muscle and give attachment to ligaments supporting the lens of the eye.
  c. glands, glands of the conjunctiva.
  c. muscle, the muscle that forms the main part of the ciliary body and functions in accommodation of the eye.
  c. reflex, the movement of the pupil in accommodation.

ciliate (sil′e-āt) a protozoan of the subphylum Ciliophora, characterized by the presence of cilia throughout its life.

ciliated (sil′e-āt″ed) provided with cilia.

ciliectomy (sil″e-ek′to-me) excision of the roots of the eyelashes.

Ciliophora (sil′e-of′o-rah) a subphylum of Protozoa, including two major groups, the ciliates and suctorians, and distinguished from the other subphyla by the presence of cilia at some stage in the existence of the member organisms.

cilium (sil′e-um), pl. *cil′ia* [L.] a hair or slender hairlike process, e.g., the fine projections from the surfaces of ciliated cells.

Cillobacterium (sil′o-bak-te′re-um) a genus of Schizomycetes found in the intestinal tract and occasionally associated with purulent infections.

cillosis (sil-o′sis) spasmodic quivering of the eyelid.

cimbia (sim′be-ah) a white band running across the ventral surface of the crus cerebri.

Cimex (si′meks) a genus of arthropods (order Hemiptera), including blood-sucking insects—the bedbugs and allied forms.
  C. lectula′rius, the common bedbug; other species are limited to tropical and subtropical areas and feed on other animals as well as man.

cinchona (sin-ko′nah) the dried bark of the stem or root of various species of *Cinchona;* used medically as an appetite stimulant.

cinchonine (sin′ko-nēn) an alkaloid obtained from cinchona.

cinchonism (sin′ko-nizm) poisoning from cinchona bark or its alkaloids.

cinchophen (sin′ko-fen) an analgesic and antipyretic; its uses are similar to those of aspirin. It is little used because of the danger of liver damage in hypersensitive patients.

cineangiocardiography (sin″e-an″je-o-kar″de-og′rah-fe) the photographic recording of fluoroscopic images of the heart and great vessels by motion picture techniques.

cineangiography (sin″e-an″je-og′rah-fe) the photographic recording of fluoroscopic images of the blood vessels by motion picture techniques.

cinefluorography (sin″ĕ-floo′or-og′rah-fe) photography, by motion picture techniques, of the shadow images appearing on the fluoroscopic screen.

cinematics (sin″ĕ-mat′iks) kinematics.

cinematoradiography (sin″ĕ-mah-to-ra″de-og′-rah-fe) the recording of x-ray images by motion picture techniques; cinefluorography.

cinemicrography (sin″ĕ-mi-krog′rah-fe) the making of motion pictures of a small object through the lens system of a microscope.

cineol (sin′e-ol) eucalyptol.

cineplasty (sin′e-plas″te) kineplasty.

cineradiography (sin″ĕ-ra″de-og′rah-fe) the photographic recording by motion picture techniques of x-ray images.

cinerea (sĭ-ne′re-ah) the gray matter of the nervous system.

cineritious (sin″ĕ-rish′us) ashen gray in color.

cineroentgenofluorography (sin″ĕ-rent″gen-o-floo″or-og′rah-fe) cineradiography.

cinesi- for words beginning thus, see those beginning *kinesi-.*

cineto- for words beginning thus, see those beginning *kineto-.*

cingulectomy (sing″gu-lek′to-me) bilateral extirpation of the anterior half of the gyrus cinguli.

cingulum (sing′gu-lum), pl. *cingula* [L.] a bundle of association fibers partly encircling the corpus callosum not far from the median plane, interrelating the cingulate and hippocampal gyri.

cingulumotomy (sing″gu-lum-ot′o-me) the creation of lesions in the cingulum of the frontal lobe for relief of intractable pain.

cionectomy (si″o-nek′to-me) uvulectomy.

cionitis (si″o-ni′tis) uvulitis.

cionotomy (si″o-not′o-me) uvulotomy.

circadian (ser″kah-de′an) pertaining to a period of about 24 hours; applied especially to the rhythmic repetition of certain phenomena in living organisms at about the same time each day.

circle (ser′kl) a round or continuous structure.

Berry's c's, charts with circles on them for testing stereoscopic vision.

Minsky's c., a device for the graphic recording of eye lesions.

sensory c., a body area within which it is impossible to distinguish separately the impressions arising from two sites of stimulation.

c. of Willis, a loop of vessels near the base of the brain.

circulation (ser-ku-la′shun) movement in a circle, returning to the point of origin, as the circulation of the blood (see also CIRCULATORY SYSTEM).

collateral c., that carried on through secondary channels after obstruction of the principal channel supplying the part.

coronary c., that within the muscular tissue of the heart.

extracorporeal c., circulation of blood outside the body, as through an artificial kidney or a heart-lung apparatus.

fetal c., circulation of blood through the body of the fetus and to and from the placenta through the umbilical cord (see also FETAL CIRCULATION).

portal c., a general term denoting the circulation of blood through larger vessels from the capillaries of one organ to those of another; applied especially to the passage of blood from the gastrointestinal tract and spleen through the portal vein to the liver.

pulmonary c., the flow of blood from the right ventricle through the pulmonary artery to the lungs, where carbon dioxide is exchanged for oxygen, and back through the pulmonary vein to the left atrium.

systemic c., the flow of blood from the left ventricle through the aorta, carrying oxygen and nutrient material to all the tissues of the body, and returning through the superior and inferior venae cavae to the right atrium.

c. time, the time required for blood to flow between two given points. It is determined by injecting a substance into a vein and then measuring the time required for it to reach a specific site, for example, the tongue or the lungs.

circulatory (ser′ku-lah-tor″e) pertaining to circulation.

c. collapse, shock; circulatory insufficiency without congestive heart failure.

c. system, the major system concerned with the movement of blood and lymph; it consists of the heart, blood vessels and lymph vessels. The circulatory system transports to the tissues and organs of the body the oxygen, nutritive substances, immune substances, hormones and chemicals necessary for normal function and activities of the organs; it also carries away waste products and carbon dioxide. It equalizes body temperature and helps maintain normal water and electrolyte balance.

An adult has an average of 5 quarts of blood in his body; the circulatory system carries this entire quantity on one complete circuit through the body every minute. In the course of 24 hours, 7200 quarts of blood passes through the heart.

The rate of blood flow through the vessels depends upon several factors: force of the heartbeat, rate of the heartbeat, venous return and control of the arterioles and capillaries by chemical, neural and thermal stimuli.

PULMONARY AND SYSTEMIC CIRCULATION. There are in reality two independent circulatory systems within the body, each with its own pump inside the sheathing of the heart. In one of these systems, called the pulmonary circulation, the right side of the heart pumps blood through the lungs. In the lungs, the blood gives up its carbon dioxide and absorbs a fresh supply of oxygen. The reoxygenated blood then flows to the left side of the heart, and is pumped out again to all the systems and organs of the body. This major circulatory system is called the systemic circulation.

The circulation of blood through the fetus bypasses the pulmonary circuit (see also FETAL CIRCULATION).

ARTERIAL SYSTEM. Blood pumped from the left side of the heart enters the aorta, the main arterial trunk of the systemic circulation. The aorta, which is about 1 inch in diameter, arches upward and toward the left side of the body. Just above the heart two coronary arteries branch off from the aorta. These arteries supply the muscles of the heart with blood.

Branching from the top of the aortic arch are three large arteries which supply the upper part of the body, the brachiocephalic trunk, which divides into the right carotid and right subclavian arteries, and the left carotid and left subclavian arteries. The carotid arteries supply the head and neck; the subclavian arteries supply the arms. The aorta then turns downward and passes through the trunk of the body, close to the vertebral column. Smaller arteries branch off from the aorta to supply the lungs, stomach, spleen, pancreas, kidneys, intestines and other organs of the body. At about the level of the umbilicus, the aorta divides into two branches, the two iliac arteries, which supply the vessels of the pelvic organs and the legs.

The arteries so far named are the main conducting arteries. They consist of a smooth inner lining covered largely by elastic fibers that absorb the pulsations of the heart. As the heart beats the elastic arterial walls damp the strong pulsations into a more nearly constant blood pressure.

Distributing arteries branch out from the conducting arteries. These arteries are composed largely of muscle fibers that encircle the smooth inner lining of the blood vessels and have the ability to contract and relax. The distributing arteries in turn branch out into arterioles, or little arteries, which are barely visible to the eye. The elastic walls of the arterioles and distributing arteries are under the control of the AUTONOMIC NERVOUS SYSTEM. The arterioles lead directly to the capillaries.

Blood passes through the aorta at the speed of about 15.6 inches per second when the body is at rest, and at a faster rate when it is active. As the blood spreads through the distributing arteries and arterioles, its speed gradually diminishes. By the time the blood has reached the capillaries, it has slowed to a speed about one-eightieth of that in the arteries.

CAPILLARIES. The complex network of innumerable and microscopically small capillaries distributed throughout the tissues supplies blood to all cells in the body. Each capillary is about 10 microns in diameter, about the size of a single blood cell, and the blood cells must make their way through the capillaries in single file.

Despite their minute size, the capillaries have a vast total area. The capillary "lake" can be called the climax of the circulatory system, for it is here that the vital work of the circulatory system is carried out. Nutrients leaving the blood capillaries enter the capillary lake, a collection of tissue fluid which bathes each cell. From there the nutrients permeate the walls of the cells. Waste products of cell metabolism enter the capillary lake and eventually pass through the capillary wall and into the blood circulation. The capillary walls are selective; i.e., they permit the exchange of special nutrients and chemicals and bar the passage of unwanted substances. For example, the cells making up the walls of the capillaries in the brain bar the passage of many substances that might injure the brain cells, and the capillaries in the placenta also act as a barrier against substances that might be harmful to the developing fetus.

VENOUS SYSTEM. From the capillaries the blood returns to the heart via the veins, which together make up the venous system. The blood flows from the capillaries to minute venules, and then to the veins, in a network of blood vessels of ever increasing size that parallels in reverse the branching of the arterial system. The walls of the veins, however, are thinner, less elastic and less muscular than those of the arteries. And whereas the arteries are for the most part buried deep within the body for protection, the venous system has many superficial veins that run close to the surface of the skin. If an arterial blood vessel is cut, the blood flows from the cut in spurts, whereas blood from a cut vein flows steadily.

The blood returning to the heart collects into two main veins. Blood returning from the arms, head and upper chest flows into the superior vena cava; blood returning from the rest of the body flows into the inferior vena cava. Both these veins return the blood to the right side of the heart.

The blood from the lower part of the body must return to the heart against the force of gravity, since all the pressure built up by the heart has been dissipated in the capillaries. This is accomplished in several ways. The veins themselves contain one-way venous valves which work in pairs. When the blood is flowing in the correct direction, the venous valves are pressed against the walls of the veins, permitting unobstructed flow. If the blood should tend to flow backward, however, the venous valves fall open and press against each other, effectively stopping the backward flow of blood. The blood is "milked" upward toward the heart principally by the massaging action of the abdominal and leg muscles as they press against the veins. Inspirations of air also force the blood through the venous system, as do the movements of the intestines. If the leg muscles do not move for long periods of time, the blood collects in the lower part of the body and the amount available for the brain is decreased.

SYSTEMIC CIRCUITS. The circulatory system has been discussed so far as if the blood flowed through the body in a simple circular path. In fact, the blood can take one of several circuits through the body. Among these circuits are the coronary circuit through the arteries and veins of the heart; a circuit through the neck, head and brain; a circuit through the digestive organs; and the renal cir-

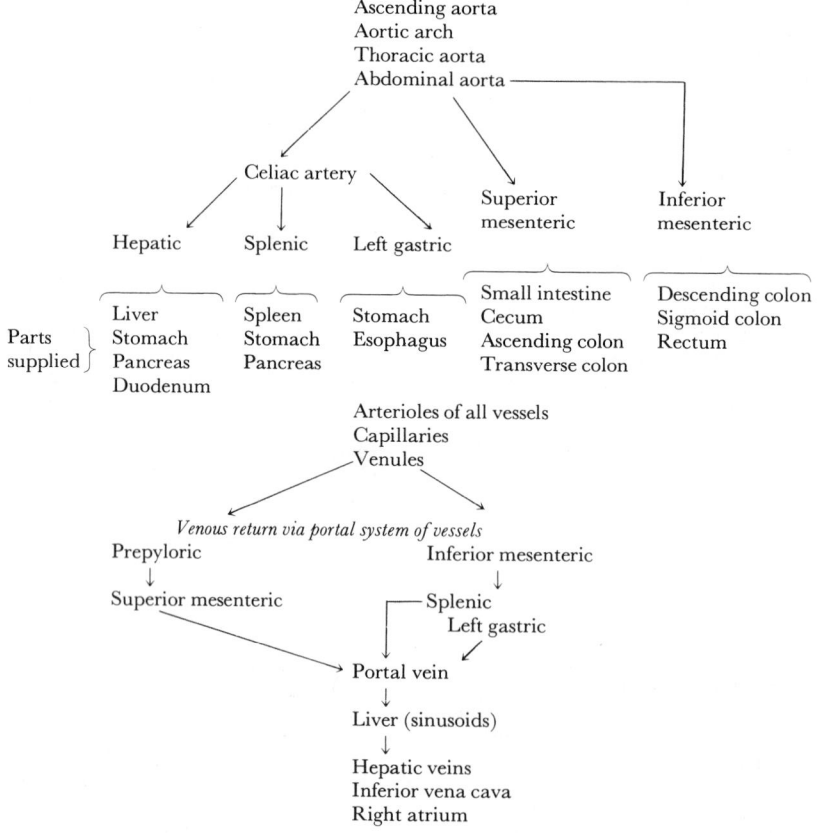

Portal circulation. (From King, B. G., and Showers, M. J.: Human Anatomy and Physiology. 5th ed. Philadelphia, W. B. Saunders Co., 1963.)

cuit through the kidneys. The importance of the renal circulation lies in the fact that the kidneys act as the cleansing filter of the circulatory system, removing a variety of products that have been cast off from the cells and body tissues. At any given time, about one-quarter of all the blood pumped through the body is passing through the renal circuit.

The most complex circuit (portal circulation) is that which flows through the digestive system, picking up proteins, carbohydrates, fats and chemicals from the intestines and delivering them to the tissues. Separate distributing arteries conduct the blood to the lower intestine, upper intestine, stomach, spleen and pancreas. The veins leading from these organs combine into the portal vein, which leads to the liver. Within the liver, the artery leading to the liver (the hepatic artery) and the portal vein subdivide themselves into a complex network of capillary-like vessels called sinusoids which bring the blood into closer contact with the cells of the liver. The liver cells withdraw glucose from the blood for storage as glycogen or release it as needed, and remove from the blood many harmful substances that might be toxic to body tissues. The blood leaving the liver flows to the inferior vena cava.

LYMPHATIC SYSTEM. The cells, chemicals and other components of the blood are suspended within the blood vessels in plasma. Similar fluid also fills the spaces between the tissue cells. Nutrients reaching the cells are carried there by this tissue fluid, and it also carries waste products from the cells to the capillaries. One function of the lymphatic system is to collect and return this fluid via the lymphatic vessels to the circulatory system. When this tissue fluid is within the lymphatic system, it is called lymph. In addition to draining off excess tissue fluid, the lymphatic capillaries also transport some waste products as well as dead blood cells, pathogenic organisms in case of infection and malignant cells from cancerous growths. From the lymphatic capillaries the lymph is carried into larger lymphatic vessels which contain one-way valves similar to those in the veins. Lymph nodes are interspersed among the lymph vessels and

filter their fluids. Eventually large lymph ducts (the thoracic duct and right lymphatic duct) empty into the right and left subclavian veins. The lymph is propelled by the same massaging action that causes the blood to circulate through the venous system. There are larger masses of lymphatic tissue called lymphatic organs, and among them are the SPLEEN, TONSILS, and THYMUS. These organs produce specialized leukocytes (lymphocytes) that help protect the body against infections.

CONTROL OF CIRCULATION. The organs and systems of the body vary greatly in the quantity of blood they require at different times. The needs of the brain are constant; the demands of the muscles are more varied. Heavy physical exertion may increase the rate of blood flow to the muscles eight times above the normal resting rate. In hot weather, a larger percentage of blood flows through the skin to cool the body. After every meal an extra supply of blood is required by the stomach to help digest and absorb the meal.

These changes in blood supply are accomplished automatically by the autonomic nervous system, which acts through the muscle fibers that surround the distributing arteries and arterioles. These muscle fibers either contract or relax according to the specific nerve signal transmitted to them by the medulla oblongata in the deepest part of the brain. As these muscle fibers contract or relax, they alter the diameter of the blood vessels and, therefore, the rate of blood flow. Certain chemicals, such as epinephrine, ephedrine, histamine and alcohol, as well as tobacco, can also affect the size of the blood vessels. These changes in the size of the blood vessels are entirely reflexive and the individual has no conscious control over them at all. Ordinarily, the autonomic nervous system maintains the muscles surrounding the arteries in a state of mild tension, which keeps the blood pressure at its normal level.

The brain requires a constant, unvarying supply of blood. Except for the presence of a special control system, this would be impossible to maintain, since every time a person moved or shifted posi-

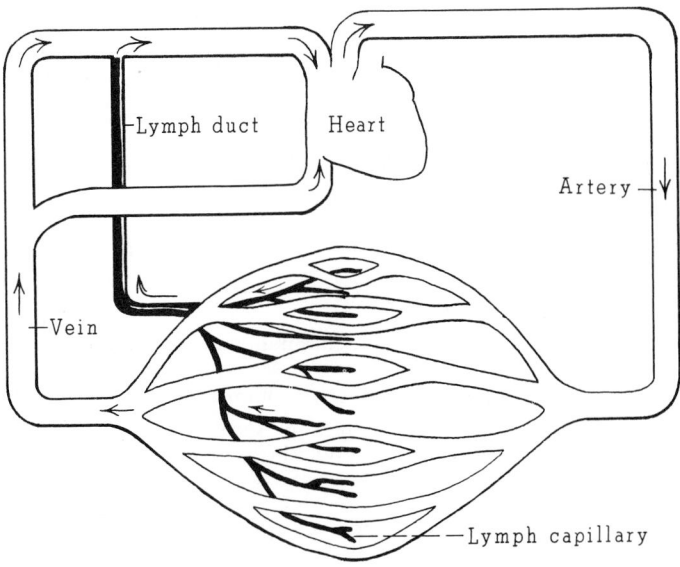

Diagram of lymphatic system, showing its relationship to the circulatory system. (From Jacob, S. W., and Francone, C. A.: Structure and Function in Man. 2nd ed. Philadelphia, W. B. Saunders Co., 1970.)

208

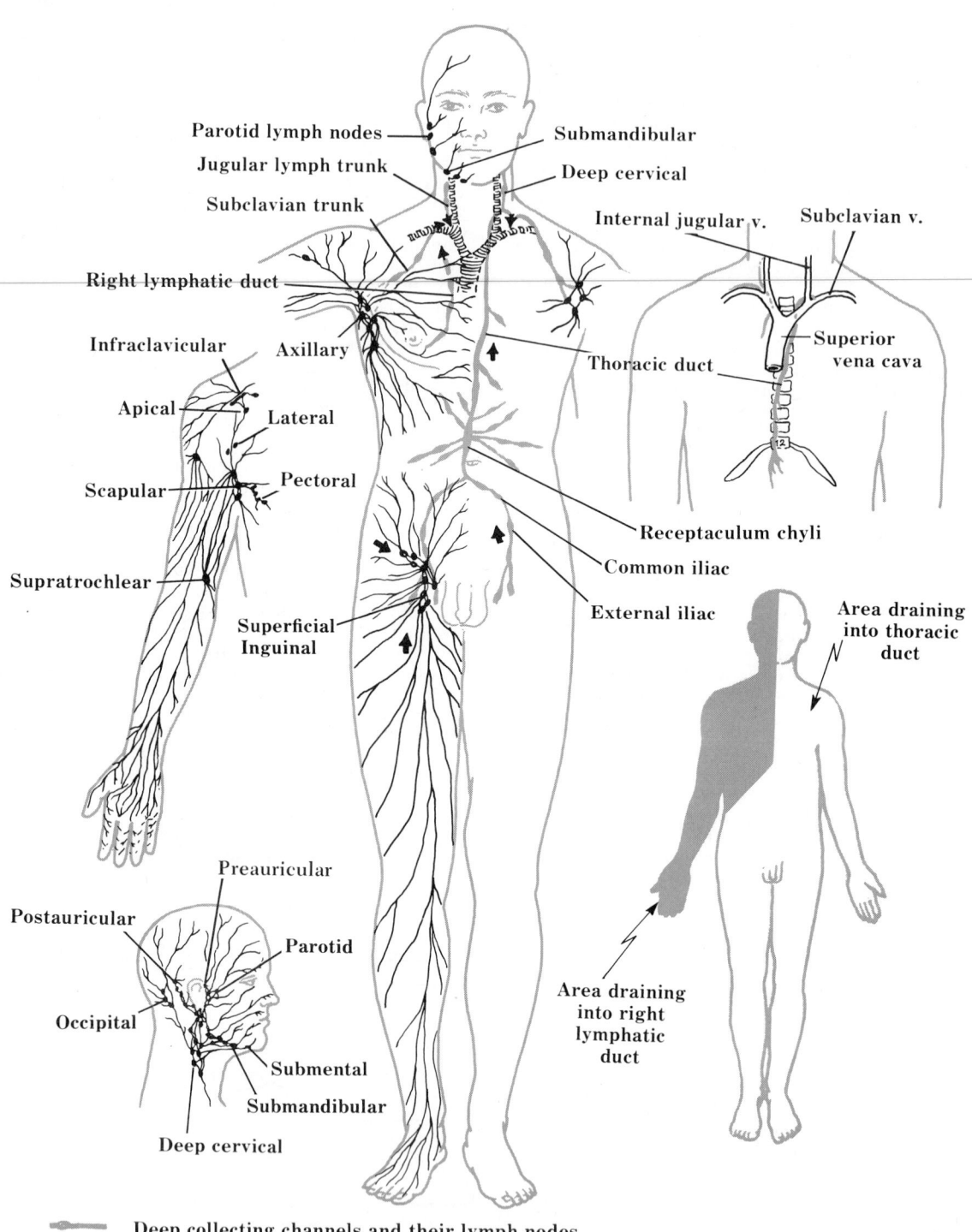

Deep collecting channels and their lymph nodes

Superficial collecting channels and their lymph nodes

Lymphatic system. (Redrawn from Jacob, S. W., and Francone, C. A.: Structure and Function in Man. 2nd ed. Philadelphia, W. B. Saunders Co., 1970.)

tion the quantity of blood flowing to the brain would change. The control system consists of the action of two nerves, one located in the aorta and the other in the carotid artery in the neck, which, acting together, register any changes in the blood pressure and cause the autonomic nervous system to change the rate of heartbeat and the size of the blood vessels to maintain the correct blood pressure.

circum- (ser'kum) word element [L.], *around.*

circumcision (ser"kum-sizh'un) surgical removal of the foreskin, or prepuce, of the penis. The operation is done to prevent phimosis, in which the foreskin is tightly wrapped around the tip of the glans and cannot be retracted with ease. This condition predisposes to infection and impedes the flow of urine. In the Jewish faith circumcision is a religious rite that must be performed on the eighth day after birth whenever possible.

Bleeding from the operative site is always a possibility even though the procedure is a relatively minor one. In addition to observing for bleeding, the raw area may be covered with a bland ointment and a small dressing until healing is complete. Some pediatricians prefer that no dressing be used and that the infant remain undiapered until healing takes place.

circumclusion (ser"kum-kloo'zhun) compression of an artery by a wire and pin.

circumduction (ser"kum-duk'shun) circular movement of a limb or of the eye.

circumflex (ser'kum-fleks) having a winding course.

circumpolarization (ser"kum-po"ler-ĭ-za'shun) the rotation of polarized light.

circumscribed (ser'kum-skrībd) bounded or limited; confined to a limited space.

circumstantiality (ser"kum-stan"she-al'ĭ-te) thinking or conversation characterized by unnecessary elaboration of trivial details.

cirrhonosus (sĭ-ron'o-sus) a fetal disease marked by a golden-yellow color of the pleura and peritoneum.

cirrhosis (sĭ-ro'sis) interstitial inflammation of an organ, particularly the liver. Cirrhosis is marked by degeneration of the liver cells and thickening of the surrounding tissue. adj., **cirrhot'ic.**

The person most likely to be struck by cirrhosis of the liver is a middle-aged male with a history of chronic alcoholism. It is thought that cirrhosis is caused primarily by severe malnutrition which often accompanies alcoholism, rather than by the alcohol itself. Cirrhosis may also stem from previous damage from toxins or infections.

SYMPTOMS AND TREATMENT. The symptoms of cirrhosis of the liver include fatigue, loss of weight, low resistance to infections and gastrointestinal disturbances. Ascites and jaundice are most often seen late in the course of cirrhosis. Increased pressure in the portal circulation may produce esophageal varicosities. Occasionally these varices may rupture and drain blood into the stomach. Spider angiomas (small bright red arterioles near the surface of the skin) frequently appear.

The treatment of cirrhosis is aimed at helping the liver rebuild and repair its damaged cells. It may include rest with moderate exercise, a high-protein

diet, administration of B vitamins and transfusions to replace blood lost. Since alcohol is damaging to the liver, the use of it is restricted.

NURSING CARE. Frequent, small feedings and protein and vitamin supplements are offered the patient to combat anorexia and assist the body in the repair of damaged tissues. Trays should be prepared attractively and served in a gracious manner. The patient will need much encouragement to eat his meals and supplemental feedings.

Observations for signs of bleeding are necessary because the liver no longer is able to produce normal amounts of prothrombin, which plays an important role in the clotting of blood. The patient may have hematemesis, tarry stools, bleeding gums, frequent and severe nosebleeds or bleeding under the skin. Care should be used in the brushing of teeth and the patient is instructed to avoid blowing his nose with force. The location of the site of bleeding should be noted and reported to the physician in charge.

Removal of fluid from the thoracic cavity (THORACENTESIS) or abdominal cavity (PARACENTESIS) may be necessary to relieve respiratory embarrassment or pressure on the abdominal organs caused by ascites. The character and amount of fluid removed are carefully observed and recorded.

Edema of the extremities demands constant vigilance against the breakdown of tissues and resulting decubitus ulcers. Frequent changes of position, skin care, periodic elevation of the extremities and passive exercises are required.

Intake and output are carefully measured and recorded. Diuretics may be given to assist in the elimination of excess fluid accumulating in the body.

Daily weighing is necessary to calculate the amount of fluid being retained or eliminated. The patient is weighed on the same scales and at the same time every day, preferably before breakfast.

During the terminal phase of his illness the patient must be protected from injury due to falls or attempted suicide. He has increasing weakness, lethargy and stupor. He may also suffer from mental changes with hallucinations and self-destructive tendencies.

atrophic c., cirrhosis marked by shrivelling and shrinkage in size of the liver.

biliary c., cirrhosis of the liver from chronic retention of bile.

fatty c., a form in which the liver cells become infiltrated with fat; seen commonly in acute alcoholism.

Laënnec's c., atrophic cirrhosis of the liver.

portal c., a degenerative and inflammatory disease of the liver leading to obstruction of the portal circulation.

cirsectomy (ser-sek'to-me) excision of a varicose vein.

cirsenchysis (ser-sen'kĭ-sis) therapeutic injection of a varicose vein.

cirsocele (ser'so-sēl) varicocele.

cirsodesis (ser-sod'ĕ-sis) ligation of a varicose vein.

cirsoid (ser'soid) resembling a varix.

cirsomphalos (ser-som'fah-los) a varicose state of the navel.

cirsotomy (ser-sot'o-me) incision of a varicosity.

cistern (sis'tern) a closed space serving as a reservoir for lymph or other body fluids, especially one of the enlarged subarachnoid spaces containing cerebrospinal fluid.

cisterna (sis-ter'nah), pl. *cister'nae* [L.] cistern.
 c. cerebellomedulla'ris, the enlarged subarachnoid space between the under surface of the cerebellum and the posterior surface of the medulla oblongata; called also cisterna magna.

cisternal (sis-ter'nal) pertaining to a cistern, especially the cisterna cerebellomedullaris.
 c. puncture, puncture of the cisterna cerebellomedullaris with a hollow needle inserted just below the occipital bone, to obtain a specimen of CEREBROSPINAL FLUID (see also SPINAL PUNCTURE).
 Preparation of the patient for this procedure should include a detailed explanation, because insertion of a needle so close to the brain may cause apprehension in the average layman. The physician may request that the back of the neck be shaved. The patient is positioned on his side with his head bent forward and held firmly by an attendant. Complications seldom occur, but the patient should be observed for signs of dyspnea or cyanosis during and immediately after the procedure. A cisternal puncture is often done in the out-patient clinic, and the patient is allowed to go home soon after it is completed.

cistron (sis'tron) a term used to designate a gene, when specified as a hereditary unit of function (identified by an experimental method called the cistrans test).

citrate (sit'rāt, si'trāt) a salt of citric acid.

citrated (sit'rāt-ed) treated with a salt of citric acid. Citrated blood is that treated with sodium citrate to prevent its coagulation.

citric acid (sit'rik) a crystalline acid from various fruits; used as a flavoring agent.
 c. a. cycle, tricarboxylic acid cycle.

citrinin (sit'ri-nin) a bacteriostatic derivative of the fungus *Penicillium citrinum.*

citrovorum factor (sit-rov'or-um) folinic acid, a factor necessary for the growth of *Leuconostoc citrovorum.*

citrulline (sit-rul'ēn) an amino acid.

citrullinuria (sit-rul"i-nu're-ah) the presence in the urine of large amounts of citrulline.

cittosis (si-to'sis) pica.

Cl chemical symbol, *chlorine.*

cl. centiliter.

clamp (klamp) a surgical device for compressing a part or structure.

clapotement (klah-pōt-maw') [Fr.] a splashing sound, as in succussion.

clarificant (klah-rif'i-kant) a substance that clears a liquid of turbidity.

Clark's rule (klarks) the dose of a drug for a child is obtained by multiplying the adult dose by the child's weight in pounds and dividing the result by 150.

clasmatocyte (klaz-mat'o-sīt) a macrophage.

class (klas) 1. a taxonomic category subordinate to a phylum and superior to an order. 2. a group of variables all of which show a value falling between certain limits.

clastic (klas'tik) undergoing or causing division.

clastothrix (klas'to-thriks) brittleness of the hair.

claudicant (klaw'di-kant) 1. pertaining to or characterized by claudication. 2. a patient with intermittent claudication.

claudication (klaw"di-ka'shun) limping or lameness.
 intermittent c., a complex of symptoms characterized by absence of pain or discomfort in a limb when at rest, the commencement of pain, tension and weakness after walking is begun, intensification of the condition until walking is impossible and the disappearance of symptoms after the limb has been at rest. It is associated with smoking, vascular spasm and atherosclerosis.
 venous c., intermittent claudication caused by venous stasis.

claustrophilia (klaws"tro-fil'e-ah) an abnormal desire to be in a closed room or space.

claustrophobia (klaws"tro-fo'be-ah) morbid fear of closed places.

claustrum (klaws'trum), pl. *claus'tra* [L.] a thin layer of gray matter on the lateral surface of the external capsule of the brain.

clavacin (klav'ah-sin) an antibiotic substance isolated from cultures of *Aspergillus clavatus,* but too toxic for clinical use.

Claviceps (klav'i-seps) a genus of parasitic fungi.

clavicle (klav'i-kl) an elongated, slender, curved bone lying horizontally at the root of the neck, in the upper part of the thorax; called also collarbone. adj., **clavic'ular.**

clavicotomy (klav"i-kot'o-me) cutting of the clavicle.

clavicula (klah-vik'u-lah), pl. *clavic'ulae* [L.] the clavicle.

claviformin (klav"i-for'min) an antibacterial substance derived from cultures of *Penicillium claviforme.*

clavus (kla'vus) a corn.
 c. hyster'icus, a sensation as if a nail were being driven into the head.

clawfoot (klaw'foot) atrophy and distortion of the foot.

clawhand (klaw'hand) atrophy and distortion of the hand, with flexion of the fingers; seen in cases of ulnar nerve injury, leprosy and syringomyelia.

clearance (klēr'ans) 1. the act of clearing; specifically, removal from the blood by an excretory organ of a particular substance, as removal of albumin, urea or certain dyes by the kidneys, or of rose bengal dye by the liver. 2. the space existing between opposed structures.

blood urea c., the volume of the blood cleared of urea per minute by renal elimination.

creatinine c., the volume of plasma cleared of creatinine in a unit of time by the kidney system.

inulin c., an expression of the renal efficiency in eliminating inulin from the blood, a measure of glomerular function.

urea c., blood urea clearance.

cleavage (klēv′ij) 1. division into distinct parts. 2. the early successive splitting of a fertilized ovum into smaller cells (blastomeres) by mitosis.

cleft (kleft) a fissure.

branchial c's, the clefts between the branchial arches of the embryo, formed by rupture of the membrane separating corresponding entodermal pouch and ectodermal groove.

c. lip, c. palate, congenital fissure, or split, of the lip (cleft lip) or of the roof of the mouth (cleft palate).

Cleft palate and cleft lip occur in about one birth per thousand and are sometimes associated with clubfoot (talipes) or other anatomic defects. They have no connection with mental retardation. Although poor health of the mother during pregnancy may have some effect on the development of her child, the old superstition that psychologic experiences of the pregnant mother can cause cleft palate and cleft lip has no scientific basis. However, it is true that parents who were born with cleft palate or cleft lip are somewhat more likely than other parents to have children with these defects.

Cleft palate and cleft lip result from failure of the two sides of the face to unite properly at an early stage of prenatal development. The defect may be limited to the outer flesh of the upper lip (the term harelip, suggesting the lip of a rabbit, is both inaccurate and unkind) or it may extend back through the midline of the upper jaw through the roof of the palate. Sometimes only the soft palate, located at the rear of the mouth, is involved.

The infant with a cleft palate is unable to suckle properly, because the opening between mouth and nose through the palate prevents suction. Feeding must be done by other means, with a dropper, a cup, a spoon or an obturator, a device inserted in the mouth to close the cleft while the baby is sucking. Cleft palate allows food to get into the nose, and it causes difficulty in chewing and swallowing. Later it will hinder speech, because consonants such as *g, b, d* and *f*, which are normally formed by pressure against the roof of the mouth, are distorted by resonance in the nasal cavity. The cleft may also prevent movements of the soft palate essential in clear speech.

TREATMENT. Treatment of cleft palate and cleft lip is by surgery, followed by measures to improve speech. A cleft palate should be reconstructed by plastic surgery when the child is about 18 months old, before he learns to talk. The corrective work usually requires only one operation. After surgery, the child often needs special training in speech to prevent his being handicapped and developing inferiority feelings.

Cleft lip usually can be corrected by surgery when the child reaches a weight of 12 to 15 lb., generally at the age of 2 to 3 months. Successful surgery often leaves only a thin scar and a greatly improved ability to form the *p, b* and *m* sounds.

A child born with a moderate case of cleft palate or cleft lip can look forward to a normal life—in appearance, speech and manner—if proper action is taken early. This means consulting and carefully following the advice of competent specialists in medicine, surgery, dentistry and speech.

The child should be patiently encouraged to overcome his handicap. He must not be pushed so hard as to become resentful or discouraged, nor should he be allowed to become too self-conscious or dependent. He needs opportunities to play normally with other children and to talk freely with adults. As he makes progress at a reasonable rate, his confidence will increase.

NURSING CARE. The main concerns during the preoperative period are maintenance of adequate nutrition, prevention of respiratory infections and speech therapy to prevent development of bad habits of speech.

Postoperative care must be aimed at prevention of trauma to or infection of the operative site. The child is not allowed to lie on his stomach until the incision is completely healed. Elbow restraints are used to keep the fingers and hands away from the mouth. The patient is usually fed with a special syringe with a rubber tip as long as he is on a liquid diet (about 7 to 10 days postoperatively). When he is given a soft diet care must be taken that the spoon or other eating utensils do not damage the suture line.

Mouth care is given frequently to keep the mouth clean and reduce the danger of infection. Dental caries often occurs in cleft palate and regular visits to the dentist are needed.

Tender loving care, always a part of pediatric nursing, is even more necessary when caring for these children. They must be reassured and kept quiet so that crying and restlessness do not undo the work done by the surgeon.

cleid(o)- (kli′do) word element [Gr.], *clavicle.*

cleidocranial (kli″do-kra′ne-al) pertaining to the clavicles and head.

c. dysostosis, a rare congenital condition in which there are defective ossification of the cranial bones and complete or partial absence of the clavicles, so that the shoulders are brought together in front.

cleidorrhexis (kli″do-rek′sis) fracture of a clavicle of the fetus in difficult labor.

cleidotomy (kli-dot′o-me) division of the clavicle of the fetus in difficult labor.

clemizole (klem′ĭ-zōl) a drug used as an antiallergic and antihistaminic.

climacteric (kli-mak′ter-ik, kli″mak-ter′ik) the combined phenomena accompanying cessation of the reproductive function in the female or diminution of testicular activity in the male.

climatotherapy (kli″mah-to-ther′ah-pe) treatment of disease by change of climate.

climax (kli′maks) the period of greatest intensity, as in the course of a disease.

clinic (klin′ik) 1. an establishment where patients are admitted for special study and treatment by a group of physicians practicing medicine together.

2. medical instruction based on observation of patients.

clinical (klin′ĭ-kl) pertaining to a clinic or to the bedside; pertaining to or founded on actual observation and treatment of patients, as distinguished from theoretical or experimental.

clinician (klĭ-nish′an) an expert clinical teacher or practitioner.

clinicogenetic (klin″ĭ-ko-jĕ-net′ik) pertaining to the clinical manifestations of a chromosomal (genetic) abnormality.

clinicopathologic (klin″ĭ-ko-path″o-loj′ik) relating to the clinical and pathologic manifestations of disease.

clinistix (klin′ĭ-stiks) trademark for an enzyme-impregnated strip of plastic used to test for sugar in the urine. The strip is dipped into the urine and results of positive or negative are indicated by the color of the strip. This test is not as accurate as the Clinitest or Benedict's test.

Clinitest (klin′ĭ-test) trademark for a reagent tablet used to test for the presence of sugar in the urine. Ten drops of water and 5 of urine are placed in a test tube. The tablet, which generates heat, is added and the solution is allowed to boil. Within a few moments the color of the solution is compared to a color chart similar to the one used for Benedict's test.

clinocephalism (kli″no-sef′ah-lizm) congenital flatness or concavity of the vertex of the head.

clinodactyly (kli″no-dak′til-e) permanent deviation or deflection of one or more fingers.

clinomania (kli″no-ma′ne-ah) a morbid inclination to remain lying down or to stay in bed.

clinometer (kli-nom′ĕ-ter) an instrument for measuring the paralysis of the ocular muscles as shown by torsion of the eyeballs.

cliseometer (klis″e-om′ĕ-ter) an instrument for measuring the angles between the long axis of the body and that of the pelvis.

Clistin (klis′tin) trademark for preparations of carbinoxamine maleate, an antihistamine.

clithrophobia (klith″ro-fo′be-ah) intense dread of being locked in.

clition (klit′e-on) the midpoint of the anterior border of the clivus.

clitoridectomy (klit″o-rĭ-dek′to-me) excision of the clitoris.

clitoriditis (klit″o-rĭ-di′tis) inflammation of the clitoris.

clitoridotomy (klit″o-rĭ-dot′o-me) incision of the clitoris.

clitoris (klit′o-ris) small, elongated, erectile body in the female, homologous with the penis in the male.

clitorism (klit′o-rizm) hypertrophy of the clitoris.

clitoritis (klit′o-ri′tis) inflammation of the clitoris.

clivus (kli′vus), pl. *cli′vi* [L.] a sloping surface, especially the surface of the posterior cranial fossa sloping downward from the pituitary fossa.

cloaca (klo-a′kah), pl. *cloa′cae* [L.] the common chamber in vertebrates below placental mammals into which fecal, urinary and reproductive elements pass before they are expelled from the body; such a structure also exists as a temporary feature in embryonic development of other species.

clone (klōn) 1. the asexual progeny of a single cell. 2. a strain of cells descended in culture from a single cell. adj., **clo′nal.**

clonic (klon′ik) pertaining to or characterized by clonus.

clonicity (klo-nis′ĭ-te) the condition of being clonic.

clonicotonic (klon″ĭ-ko-ton′ik) both clonic and tonic.

clonism (klon′izm) a succession of clonic spasms.

clonograph (klon′o-graf) an instrument for recording spasmodic movements.

clonorchiasis (klon″or-ki′ah-sis) infection with Clonorchis.

Clonorchis (klo-nor′kis) a genus of Asiatic liver flukes.

clonospasm (klon′o-spazm) clonic spasm.

clonus (klo′nus) spasm in which rigidity and relaxation succeed each other.
  ankle c., foot c., a series of convulsive movements of the ankle, induced by suddenly pushing up the foot while the leg is extended.
  toe c., rhythmic contraction of the great toe, induced by sudden passive extension of its first phalanx.
  wrist c., spasmodic contraction of the hand muscles, induced by forcibly bending the hand backward.

Clopane (klo′pān) trademark for preparations of cyclopentamine, a sympathomimetic drug used as a nasal decongestant and hypertensive.

Clostridium (klo-strid′e-um) a genus of Schizomycetes.
  C. botuli′num, the agent causing botulism in man.
  C. histolyt′icum, a species found in feces and soil.
  C. no′vyi, a species that is an important cause of gas gangrene.
  C. perfrin′gens, the most common causative agent of gas gangrene.
  C. tet′ani, a common inhabitant of soil and human and horse intestines, and the cause of TETANUS in man and domestic animals.

clostridium (klo-strid′e-um), pl. *clostrid′ia* [Gr.] an individual of the genus Clostridium.

clot (klot) a semisolidified mass, as of blood or lymph.

clotting (klot′ing) the formation of a jellylike substance over the ends or within the walls of a blood vessel, with resultant stoppage of the blood flow. This is one of the natural defense mechanisms of the body when injury occurs. A clot will usually form within 5 minutes after a blood vessel wall has been damaged. The exact process of clotting is not known; however, it is believed that the mechanism is triggered by the platelets, which disintegrate as they pass over rough places in the injured surface. As they disintegrate they release serotonin and thromboplastin. Serotonin causes constriction of the blood vessels and reduction of local blood pressure. Thromboplastin unites with calcium ions and other substances which promote the formation of fibrin. When examined under a microscope, a clot consists of a mesh of fine threads of fibrin in which are embedded erythrocytes and leukocytes and small amounts of fluid (serum).

Twelve factors considered essential to normal blood clotting have been described; they are designated by Roman numerals: *factor I*, a high-molecular-weight plasma protein that is converted to fibrin through the action of thrombin and that participates in stages 3 and 4 of blood clotting; called also fibrinogen. *factor II*, a glycoprotein present in the plasma that is converted into thrombin by extrinsic thromboplastin during the second stage of blood clotting; called also prothrombin. *factor III*, a material that has a number of sources in the body and is important in the formation of extrinsic thromboplastin; called also tissue thromboplastin. *factor IV*, an appellation that is, in the scheme of hemostasis, assigned to calcium, because of its requirement in the first, second and probably the third stages of blood clotting. *factor V*, a heat- and storage-labile material, present in plasma and not in serum, and functioning in the formation of intrinsic and extrinsic thromboplastins; called also accelerator globulin, accelerin and proaccelerin. *factor VI*, a factor previously called accelerin and thought to be an intermediate product of prothrombin conversion; it no longer is considered in the scheme of hemostasis, and hence it is assigned neither a name or a function at this time. *factor VII*, a heat- and storage-stable material, present in serum but not in plasma and participating only in the formation of extrinsic thromboplastin; called also prothrombinogen and serum prothrombin conversion accelerator, SPCA. *factor VIII*, a relatively storage-labile material present in plasma and not in serum, and participating only in the formation of extrinsic thromboplastin; a primary deficiency of this factor causes classic sex-linked hemophilia; called also antihemophilic factor (AHF) and antihemophilic globulin (AHG). *factor IX*, a relatively storage-stable substance, present in normal serum but not in plasma, that is involved in the generation of intrinsic thromboplastin; a deficiency of this factor results in a hemorrhagic syndrome called hemophilia B or Christmas disease which is similar to classical hemophilia A; called also plasma thromboplastin component, PTC. *factor X*, a heat-labile material with limited storage stability at room temperature, present in serum but not in plasma, that functions in the formation of both intrinsic and extrinsic thromboplastin; called also Stuart factor. *factor XI*, a stable factor, present in both serum and plasma, that together with factor XII forms a complex that activates factor IX in the formation of intrinsic thromboplastin; called also plasma thromboplastin antecedent, PTA. *factor XII*, a stable factor, present in plasma and serum, that is activated by contact with glass or other foreign substances and initiates the process of blood coagulation in vitro; its precise role during in vivo hemostasis remains unclear; called also Hageman factor. At least four platelet factors also exist that have a part in clotting.

It is possible for a clot to form within a blood vessel if the inner wall of the vessel has been

roughened by injury or disease. Clots may form in conditions such as arteriosclerosis, varicose veins and thrombophlebitis. An internal clot that remains at the place where it forms is called a thrombus; the general condition is called THROMBOSIS. If the clot (or pieces of it) breaks loose and flows through the blood vessels, it is called an embolus, and the condition is called EMBOLISM.

Clotting of the blood can be hastened by contact with injured tissue, by warming, by adding such coagulants as calcium, or by combination with thromboplastin and thrombin. The process can be retarded by cooling, by dilution, by adding oxalates and citrates or by administration of substances such as HEPARIN and Dicumarol, called ANTICOAGULANTS.

clubbing (klub′ing) proliferation of soft tissue about the terminal phalanges of fingers or toes, without osseous change.

clubfoot (klub′foot) a deformity in which the foot is twisted out of normal position. The medical term for this condition is talipes. The deformity is usually congenital but a few cases of clubfoot in older children may have been caused by injury or poliomyelitis. There are several types of clubfoot; the foot may be turned inward, outward, upward or downward. Sometimes a combination of these defects may be present.

There are several theories as to the cause of clubfoot. A familial tendency or arrested growth during fetal life may contribute to its development, or it may be caused by a defect in the ovum. It sometimes accompanies meningomyelocele as a result of paralysis. In mild clubfoot there are slight changes in the structure of the foot; more severe cases involve orthopedic deformities of both the foot and leg.

Treatment varies according to the severity of the deformity. Milder cases may be corrected with casts that are changed periodically, the foot being manipulated into position each time the cast is changed so that it gradually assumes normal position. A specially designed splint also may be used. It is made of two plates attached to shoes with a crossbar between the plates and special, set screws so that the angulation of the foot can be changed as necessary. More severe deformities require surgery of the tendons and bones, followed by the application of a cast to maintain proper position of the joint.

clubhand (klub′hand) deformity of the hand, resembling that of the foot in clubfoot.

clumping (klump′ing) aggregation of bacteria or other cells into irregular masses.

cluneal (kloo′ne-al) pertaining to the buttocks.

clunis (kloo′nis), pl. *clu′nes* [L.] buttock.

clysis (kli′sis) infusion of fluid into tissue or a body cavity, as an enema.

clyster (klis′ter) an enema.

C.M. [L.] *Chirur′giae Ma′gister* (Master in Surgery).

Cm chemical symbol, *curium.*

cm. centimeter.

cm.³ cubic centimeter.

C.M.A. Canadian Medical Association.

c./min. cycles per minute.

c. mm. cubic millimeter.

CN symbol, *cyanogen*.

C.N.A. Canadian Nurses' Association.

cnemial (ne'me-al) pertaining to the tibia, or shin.

C.N.M. Certified Nurse-Midwife.

C.N.S. central nervous system.

Co chemical symbol, *cobalt*.

coacervate (ko-as'er-vāt) a collection of less fully hydrated particles of a colloid system, with less solvent bound to them than they had before.

coacervation (ko-as"er-va'shun) the formation of coacervates in a colloid system.

coadaptation (ko"ad-ap-ta'shun) the mutual, correlated, adaptive changes in two interdependent organs.

coagglutination (ko"ah-gloo"tĭ-na'shun) agglutination by an antigen and the homologous antibody of the corpuscles of another animal.

coagglutinin (ko"ah-gloo'tĭ-nin) partial agglutinin.

coagulability (ko-ag"u-lah-bil'ĭ-te) the state of being capable of forming or of being formed into clots.

coagulant (ko-ag'u-lant) 1. causing coagulation. 2. an agent that causes coagulation.

coagulase (ko-ag'u-lās) an enzyme that accelerates the formation of blood clots, but is not involved in coagulation of blood in vivo.

coagulate (ko-ag'u-lāt) to form into a coagulum, or clot.

coagulation (ko-ag"u-la'shun) formation of a clot.
    c. factors, factors essential to normal blood clotting, whose absence, diminution or excess may lead to abnormality of the clotting; 12 factors, commonly designated by Roman numerals, have been described. (See also CLOTTING.)

coagulin (ko-ag'u-lin) 1. thromboplastin. 2. an antibody (precipitin) that coagulates its antigen.

coagulinoid (ko-ag'u-lin-oid") a coagulin whose activity has been destroyed by heat.

coagulometer (ko-ag"u-lom'ĕ-ter) an apparatus for determining clotting time of the blood.

coagulum (ko-ag'u-lum), pl. *coag'ula* [L.] a clot.

coal tar (kōl tar) a by-product obtained in destructive distillation of bituminous coal; used in ointment or solution in treatment of eczema.

coalescence (ko"ah-les'ens) a fusion or growing together.

coapt (ko'apt) to fit or bring together.

coaptation (ko"ap-ta'shun) a fitting together or adjustment of parts.

coarctate (ko-ark'tāt) to press close together, constrict.

coarctation (ko"ark-ta'shun) stricture or narrowing.
    c. of aorta, malformation characterized by deformity of the tunica media of the aorta, causing narrowing, usually severe, of the lumen of the vessel.

coarctotomy (ko"ark-tot'o-me) the cutting of a stricture.

coat (kōt) a layer of substance covering or enveloping another; in anatomic nomenclature called also tunica.
    buffy c., the thin yellowish layer of leukocytes overlying the packed erythrocytes in centrifuged blood.

cobalamin (ko-bal'ah-min) a cobalt-containing complex common to all members of the vitamin B_{12} group.

cobalt (ko'bawlt) a chemical element, atomic number 27, atomic weight 58.933, symbol Co. (See table of ELEMENTS.) RADIOISOTOPES of cobalt are used for implantation in the treatment of various forms of malignancy and also serve as the radioactive source in teletherapy machines.

cocaine (ko-kān', ko'kān) the active principle of the coca shrub, used as an anesthetic; applied topically or administered as a local or spinal anesthetic. Cocaine has limited use in its pure form but its derivatives are widely used. The drug must be administered with caution because of frequent idiosyncrasy even in small doses. Toxic effects include excitement, dizziness, headache, convulsions and hypotension. Barbiturates are sometimes given prior to the administration of cocaine to allay the side effects. If a reaction to cocaine does occur during its administration the drug is stopped immediately and barbiturates are given.

cocainism (ko'kān-izm) chronic poisoning due to prolonged use of cocaine.

cocainize (ko-kān'ĭz) to treat with cocaine.

cocarboxylase (ko"kar-bok'sĭ-lās) a coenzyme of carboxylase acting with the latter in splitting pyruvic acid.

cocarcinogenesis (ko-kar"sĭ-no-jen'ĕ-sis) the development of cancer only in preconditioned cells as a result of conditions favorable to its growth.

cocci (kok'si) plural of *coccus*.

Coccidia (kok-sid'e-ah) a group of sporozoa commonly parasitic in epithelial cells of the intestinal tract, including two genera, Eimeria and Isospora, sometimes found in domestic animals and man.

coccidial (kok-sid'e-al) pertaining to or caused by Coccidium.

Coccidioides (kok-sid"ĕ-oi'dēz) a genus of pathogenic fungi.
    C. immit'is, a species causing skin and lung lesions.

coccidioidin (kok-sid"e-oi'din) a sterile preparation from cultures of the organism used in a test for infection by *Coccidioides immitis.*

coccidioidomycosis (kok-sid″e-oi″do-mi-ko′sis) a fungal disease usually affecting the respiratory tract and caused by *Coccidioides immitis.* This fungus grows in hot, dry areas, especially in the southwestern United States, Mexico and parts of Central and South America. The disease is called also desert fever and San Joaquin Valley fever.

The spores are carried by the wind and enter the respiratory tract via the nose and mouth. After an incubation period of 7 to 21 days, symptoms appear that closely resemble those of influenza. There is extreme weakness, and pain and swelling of the joints resembling arthritis. The pulmonary symptoms and signs are similar to those of tuberculosis.

Treatment consists primarily of rest. Antibiotics may be given to prevent secondary bacterial infection. Amphotericin B has been used parenterally in treating the disease.

coccidioidosis (kok-sid″e-oi-do′sis) coccidioidomycosis.

coccidiosis (kok-sid″e-o′sis) infection by organisms of the group Coccidia.

Coccidium (kok-sid′e-um) a class of protozoans.

coccobacillus (kok″o-bah-sil′us) an oval bacterial cell intermediate between the coccus and bacillus forms.

coccobacteria (kok″o-bak-te′re-ah) spheroidal or rodlike bacteria.

coccogenous (kok-oj′ĕ-nus) produced by cocci.

coccoid (kok′oid) resembling a coccus.

cocculin (kok′u-lin) picrotoxin.

coccus (kok′us), pl. *cocci* [L.] a spherical bacterium belonging to the Micrococcaceae family and one of the three basic forms of bacteria, the other two being bacillus (rod-shaped) and spirillum (spiral-shaped). Almost all of the pathogenic cocci are either Staphylococci, which occur in clusters, or streptococci, which occur in short or long chains. Both staphylococci and streptococci are gram-positive and do not form spores.

The staphylococci are responsible for many serious infections, especially *Staphylococcus aureus,* which is the causative agent in boils, abscesses, osteomyelitis and a large variety of other infections. The staphylococcus has received much attention in recent years because of the ability of most strains to develop a resistance to antibiotics.

The most dangerous streptococci are those of the beta-hemolytic type. Various species of streptococci cause sore throat, scarlet fever, mastoiditis and septicemia.

coccyalgia, coccydynia (kok″se-al′je-ah) (kok″sĭ-din′e-ah) coccygodynia.

coccygeal (kok-sij′e-al) pertaining to or located in the region of the coccyx.

coccygectomy (kok″sĭ-jek′to-me) excision of the coccyx.

coccygeus (kok-sij′e-us) pertaining to the coccyx.

coccygodynia (kok″sĭ-go-din′e-ah) pain in the coccyx.

coccyx (kok′siks) the small bone caudad to the sacrum in man, formed by the union of four (sometimes five or three) rudimentary vertebrae, and forming the caudal extremity of the vertebral column; called also os coccygis.

cochineal (koch′ĭ-nēl) dried female insects of *Coccus cacti,* enclosing young larvae; used as a coloring agent or dye.

cochlea (kok′le-ah) a spiral cavity of the inner ear, shaped like a snail shell, that contains the organ of hearing. adj., **coch′lear.** The cochlea is filled with fluid and is connected with the middle ear by two membrane-covered openings, the oval window (fenestra vestibuli) and the round window (fenestra cochleae). Inside the cochlea is the organ of Corti, a structure of highly specialized cells that translate sound vibrations into nerve impulses. The cells of this organ have tiny hairlike strands (cilia) that protrude into the fluid of the cochlea.

Sound vibrations are relayed from the tympanic membrane (eardrum) by the bones of hearing in the middle ear to the oval window of the cochlea, where they set up corresponding vibrations in the fluid of the cochlea. These vibrations move the cilia of the organ of Corti, which then sends nerve impulses to the brain. (See also HEARING.)

cochleariform (kok″le-ar′ĭ-form) spoon-shaped.

cochleitis (kok″le-i′tis) inflammation of the cochlea.

cochleovestibular (kok″le-o-ves-tib′u-lar) pertaining to the cochlea and vestibule of the ear.

coconsciousness (ko-kon′shus-nes) consciousness secondary to the main stream of consciousness.

cocontraction (ko″kon-trak′shun) coordination of antagonistic muscles.

coctolabile (kok″to-la′bil) capable of being destroyed or altered by heating to the boiling point of water.

coctoprecipitin (kok″to-pre-sip′ĭ-tin) a precipitin produced by injecting a heated serum or other antigen.

coctostabile (kok″to-sta′bil) incapable of being altered by heating.

cod liver oil an oil pressed from the fresh liver of the cod and purified. It is one of the best-known natural sources of vitamin D, and a rich source of vitamin A. Because cod liver oil is more easily absorbed than other oils, it was formerly widely used as a nutrient and tonic, but it is rarely used today since more efficient sources are available. (See also VITAMIN.)

codeine (ko′dēn) an alkaloid obtained from opium or prepared from morphine by methylation; analgesic and antitussive.

c. phosphate, c. sulfate, preparations administered orally or parenterally for relief of pain.

codon (ko′don) the specific pattern of nucleotides (perhaps three) in the genetic material which corresponds to a particular amino acid in the genetic code.

coe- for words beginning thus, see also those beginning *ce-*.

coefficient (ko″ĕ-fish′ent) a number by which one value is to be multiplied in order to give another value, or a number that indicates the range of an effect produced under certain conditions.

c. of absorption, the volume of a gas absorbed by a unit volume of a liquid at 0° C. and a pressure of 760 mm. of mercury.

isotonic c., the quantity of salt that should be added to distilled water to prevent destruction of the erythrocytes when it is added to blood.

-coele (sēl) word element [Gr.], *cavity; space.*

coelenterate (se-len′ter-āt) 1. pertaining or belonging to Coelenterata, a phylum of invertebrates including jellyfish and other sea animals. 2. an individual member of the phylum Coelenterata.

coeloblastula (se″lo-blas′tu-lah) the common type of blastula, consisting of a hollow sphere composed of blastomeres.

coelom (se′lom) the body cavity, especially the cavity of a simple animal organism or the cavity between the somatic mesoderm and the splanchnic mesoderm in the developing embryo.

extraembryonic c., the cavity bordered by chorionic mesoderm and the mesoderm of the amnion and yolk sac.

coelosomy (se″lo-so′me) a developmental anomaly characterized by protrusion of the viscera from and their presence outside the body cavity.

coenzyme (ko-en′zīm) an organic molecule, usually containing phosphorus and some vitamins, sometimes separable from certain enzymes, which is required for the activation of an apoenzyme.

c. A, a substance essential for the metabolism of carbohydrates and fats and for the formation of acetylcholine. (See also PANTOTHENIC ACID.)

c. I, diphosphopyridine nucleotide.

c. II, triphosphopyridine nucleotide.

coeur (ker) [Fr.] heart.

c. en sabot (on să-bo′), a heart whose shape on a radiograph resembles that of a wooden shoe; noted in tetralogy of Fallot.

cofactor (ko′fak-tor) an element or principle whose presence is necessary for the functioning of another.

coferment (ko-fer′ment) coenzyme.

cognition (kog-nish′un) the processes involved in knowing.

cohesion (ko-he′zhun) the clinging together of separate particles in a single mass.

coil (koil) a winding structure or spiral; called also helix.

coilonychia (koi″lo-nik′e-ah) koilonychia.

coition (ko-ish′un) coitus.

coitophobia (ko″ĭ-to-fo′be-ah) morbid fear of coitus.

coitus (ko′ĭ-tus) sexual union by vagina between male and female; usually applied to the mating process in human beings.

c. incomple′tus, c. interrup′tus, coitus in which the penis is withdrawn from the vagina before ejaculation.

c. reserva′tus, coitus in which ejaculation of semen is intentionally suppressed.

colalgia (ko-lal′je-ah) pain in the colon.

colation (ko-la′shun) the process of straining or filtering.

colchicine (kol′chĭ-sēn) a poisonous alkaloid from *Colchicum autumnale;* used in treatment of gout and usually effective in terminating an attack of acute gout. Side effects include gastrointestinal symptoms and hypotension.

cold (kold) 1. an acute and highly contagious virus infection of the upper respiratory tract (see also COMMON COLD). 2. a relatively low temperature as compared with a normal temperature; the lack of heat. A total absence of heat is absolute zero, at which all molecular motion ceases.

A body temperature below 94° F. results in impairment of the heat-regulating center in the hypothalamus. As the temperature drops, sleepiness and coma develop, and as a result the central nervous system heat-control mechanism is depressed and shivering (a means of heat production) is prevented. FROSTBITE is a local freezing of a surface area of the body and results from exposure to extremely low temperatures. Circulatory disturbances and gangrene can result from frostbite.

Induced HYPOTHERMIA, in which the body temperature is deliberately lowered and maintained below 90° F., is sometimes used during heart and other types of surgery when it is necessary to stop the heart action for several minutes. This type of prolonged cooling does not have any seriously harmful effects on the body.

USE OF COLD APPLICATIONS

Effects. The primary effect of cold on the surface of the body is constriction of the blood vessels. Cold also causes contraction of the involuntary muscles of the skin. These actions result in a reduced blood supply to the skin and produce a marked pallor. If cold is prolonged there may be damage to the tissues because of the decreased blood supply.

Cold acts as a depressant to the activity of the cells and slows the heart action and pulse rate. By causing constriction of the blood vessels it may elevate the blood pressure. Intense cold numbs the sensory nerve endings so that impulses are not transmitted and sensations such as pain and taste are lost.

The secondary effects of cold are the opposite of its primary action. There is increased cell activity, dilatation of the blood vessels and increased sensitivity of the nerve endings. The outward appearance of the skin is a characteristic mottled blue or purple color, and there is stiffness and numbness of the affected part.

Purposes. Cold applications may be used to control bleeding or to check an inflammatory process. Application of cold may inhibit the swelling and relieve pain and loss of motion in an inflamed area; however, it will not reduce edema that is already present in the tissues. Because cold slows down activity of all living cells it may be used to check the growth of bacteria in a local infection.

Cold applications are used in the emergency treatment of burns because the cold reduces the loss of fluids from the blood vessels into the tissue spaces and thus controls edema.

Cool sponge baths, using cool water or alcohol, are often used to lower the body temperature when FEVER is present.

Methods. Cold is applied locally by the use of ice caps, ice collars and cold wet compresses. Ice caps are applied to the head for the relief of headache and treatment of fever, delirium and some types of head injury. An ice cap may also be used to check an inflammatory process within the pelvic or abdominal cavity, or to treat certain cardiac conditions. An ice cap usually is not left on for more than 1 hour and is used for less than an hour if the patient complains of cold or numbness or the area appears mottled. Unless otherwise ordered by the physician, ice caps and ice collars are always covered with a cotton cloth or towel before they are applied.

Ice collars are used to control bleeding and reduce swelling after tonsillectomy or other surgical conditions of the throat. They also may be applied to relieve nausea or to reduce discomfort from the passage of a nasogastric tube.

Cold compresses are most often applied to the eyes for relief of swelling and inflammation. They also may be used to relieve the symptoms of hemorrhoids.

coldsore (kold'sōr) a lesion caused by the virus of herpes simplex, usually on the lips, chin or cheeks.

colectomy (ko-lek'to-me) excision of the colon.

coleocystitis (ko″le-o-sis-ti'tis) inflammation of the vagina and bladder.

coleotomy (ko″le-ot'o-me) incision into the vagina.

colibacillemia (ko″lĭ-bas″ĭ-le'me-ah) the presence of *Escherichia coli* in the blood.

colibacillosis (ko″lĭ-bas″ĭ-lo'sis) infection with *Escherichia coli.*

colibacilluria (ko″lĭ-bas″ĭ-lu're-ah) the presence of *Escherichia coli* in the urine.

colibacillus (ko″le-bah-sil'us) *Escherichia coli.*

colic (kol'ik) 1. pertaining to the colon. 2. acute paroxysmal abdominal pain.

Colic usually refers to an attack of abdominal pain caused by spasmodic contractions of the intestine, most common during the first 3 months of life. The infant may pull up his arms and legs, cry loudly, turn red-faced and expel gas from the anus or belch it up from the stomach.

The exact cause of infant colic is not known but several factors may contribute to its occurrence. These include excessive swallowing of air, too rapid feeding or overfeeding, overexcitement and an anxious or easily disturbed mother. The infant can usually be relieved by being picked up, "bubbled" gently and given some warm water to drink. To relieve his tenseness he should be held and soothed with tender loving care. His condition is not serious and most infants gain weight and are healthy in spite of the colic.

biliary c., pain from abnormal contractions of the bile ducts, most often caused by gallstones.

lead c., acute abdominal pain caused by lead poisoning.

menstrual c., pain of menstruation.

renal c., intermittent and acute pain usually resulting from the presence of one or more calculi in the kidney or ureter. The pain begins in the kidney region and radiates forward and downward to envelop the abdomen, genitalia and legs. Other symptoms include nausea, vomiting, diaphoresis and a desire to urinate frequently.

colicoplegia (kol″ĭ-ko-ple'je-ah) combined colic and paralysis produced by lead poisoning.

coliform (kol'ĭ-form) resembling *Escherichia coli.*

coliplication (ko″lĭ-pli-ka'shun) coloplication.

colipuncture (ko″lĭ-pungk'tūr) colocentesis.

colipyuria (ko″lĭ-pi-u're-ah) pus in the urine due to infection with *Escherichia coli.*

colisepsis (ko″lĭ-sep'sis) infection with *Escherichia coli.*

colistimethate (ko-lis″tĭ-meth'āt) a colistin derivative used in the treatment of infections, particularly those of the urinary tract.

colistin (ko-lis'tin) an antibiotic substance produced by a microorganism in the soil, related chemically to polymyxin.

c. sulfate, a water-soluble salt of colistin, effective against several gram-negative bacilli, but not against Proteus.

colitis (ko-li'tis) inflammation of the colon. The most common form of colitis is mucous colitis, called also spastic colitis, irritable colon or functional bowel distress.

SYMPTOMS. In the early phase of mucous colitis, spasms occur in the lower portion of the bowel. They may be accompanied by cramp-like pain in the upper stomach. Frequently there is constipation, sometimes alternating with diarrhea. As the disturbance progresses, mucus is secreted more readily, and diarrhea becomes more likely.

CAUSES. The most common cause of mucous colitis is emotional stress or anxiety. This indicates that at least part of the treatment should be psychologic. The patient must learn to control his tension and anxiety so that they will not affect his physical well-being. Unwise eating habits, including too much roughage in the diet, and overdosing with laxatives can also cause some forms of colitis.

TREATMENT. Changes in diet and eating habits are recommended for the treatment of mucous colitis. The diet change depends on the symptoms. In most cases a bland diet with a minimum of roughage is advised. Food to which a patient has previously shown an intolerance should be totally excluded. Laxatives also should be excluded. Irritant substances such as strong seasonings, alcohol, coffee, tea and tobacco should be avoided. Meals should be serene, leisurely and as pleasant and attractive as possible. Proper exercise, a regular routine of daily living and the avoidance of emotional conflicts are all important. Mild sedatives and antispasmodic drugs may also be prescribed.

ulcerative c., a chronic ulceration in the colon producing diarrhea, loss of weight and sometimes anemia; it is less common and more serious than mucous colitis (see also ULCERATIVE COLITIS).

colitoxicosis (ko″li-tok″sĭ-ko'sis) intoxication caused by *Escherichia coli.*

colitoxin (ko″li-tok'sin) a toxin from *Escherichia coli.*

coliuria (ko″le-u're-ah) the presence of *Escherichia coli* in the urine.

collagen (kol'ah-jen) a scleroprotein present in connective tissue of the body adj., **collag'enous.**

c. **diseases,** a group of poorly understood diseases that cause deterioration of the connective tissues. Their cause is unknown, and the relationships among them are unclear. Apparently they are not infections. Widely varying symptoms often make early diagnosis difficult. These diseases are being diagnosed more often than in the past and are being studied intensively. The diseases are usually serious and may be fatal.

The four major forms of collagen diseases include systemic lupus erythematosus, periarteritis nodosa, scleroderma and dermatomyositis. In addition to these four diseases, rheumatoid arthritis and rheumatic fever are frequently held to belong to the group.

MECHANISM AND CAUSE. The connective tissues, found in every organ and every part of the body, consist mainly of cells and fibers embedded in matter called ground substance. The collagen diseases characteristically cause the ground substance itself to become fiber-like. This development in turn affects the organs of which the affected tissues are a part. Thus the symptoms may resemble diseases of these organs, whether heart, kidney, muscle, nerve or any other part of the body.

Medical research has discovered relatively little about these diseases but it is widely thought that they have an allergic basis. One view is that some other disease or a foreign substance causes the body to have a permanent or recurrent allergic reaction. Patients with mysterious fevers, painful joints and skin disorders are often suspected of having one of the collagen diseases. Some drugs also are suspected as being a source. Many patients are also subject to other well recognized allergic reactions.

collagenase (kol-laj'ĕ-nās) an enzyme that catalyzes the digestion of collagen.

collagenation (kol-laj″ĕ-na'shun) the appearance of collagen in developing cartilage.

collagenic (kol″ah-jen'ik) 1. producing collagen. 2. pertaining to collagen.

collagenoblast (kol-laj'ĕ-no-blast″) an immature collagen-producing cell.

collagenocyte (kol-laj'ĕ-no-sīt″) a mature collagen-producing cell.

collagenolysis (kol″ah-jĕ-nol'ĭ-sis) dissolution or digestion of collagen.

collagenosis (kol″ah-jĕ-no'sis) a disease characterized by areas of collagenous degeneration.

collapse (kŏ-laps') 1. to break down or flatten. 2. a state of extreme prostration.

c. **therapy,** collapse and immobilization of the lung in treatment of pulmonary disease; artificial pneumothorax.

collateral (kŏ-lat'er-al) 1. secondary or accessory. 2. a small side branch, as of a blood vessel or nerve.

collemia (kŏ-le'me-ah) a glutinous or viscid condition of the blood.

Colles' fracture (kol'ēz) a break in the lower end of the radius, the distal fragment being displaced backward.

C. **law,** a child affected with congenital syphilis, the mother showing no signs of the disease, will not infect the mother.

colliculectomy (kŏ-lik″u-lek'to-me) excision of the seminal colliculus.

colliculitis (kŏ-lik″u-li'tis) inflammation about the seminal colliculus.

colliculus (kŏ-lik'u-lus), pl. *collic'uli* [L.] a small elevation.

seminal c., a rounded projection on the floor of the prostatic portion of the urethra, on which are the opening of the prostatic utricle and, on either side of it, the orifices of the ejaculatory ducts; called also verumontanum.

collimation (kol″ĭ-ma'shun) in microscopy, the process of making light rays parallel; the adjustment of two or more optical axes with respect to each other.

colliquation (kol″ĭ-kwa'shun) liquefactive degeneration of tissue.

colliquative (kŏ-lik'wah-tiv) characterized by excessive liquid discharge, or by liquefaction of tissue.

collodiaphyseal (kol″o-di″ah-fiz'e-al) pertaining to the neck and shaft of a long bone, especially the femur.

collodion (kŏ-lo'de-on) pyroxylin dissolved in ether and alcohol.

flexible c., a mixture of collodion, camphor and castor oil, applied locally as a protectant.

salicylic acid c., flexible collodion containing salicylic acid, used topically as a keratolytic.

colloid (kol'oid) 1. gluelike. 2. a homogeneous, gelatinous material occurring in cells and tissues in a state of colloid degeneration. 3. a state of matter composed of single large molecules or groups of smaller molecules in a solid, liquid or gaseous state, dispersed (subdivided) in a continuous medium (disperse medium) which may also be solid, liquid or gas. Different types of colloids (colloid systems) are designated by their dispersed and dispersing phases. For example, if the dispersed phase is a solid and the dispersing phase a liquid, the system is called a sol, such as glue. Milk is an example of an emulsion, in which both phases are liquid, one an oil and one water. Colloids do not dissolve into true solutions and are not capable of passing through a semipermeable membrane, as in DIALYSIS. The physical opposite of a colloid is a crystalloid.

c. **bath,** a bath containing gelatin, bran, starch or similar substances, to relieve skin irritation and pruritus.

colloidal (kŏ-loi'dal) of the nature of a colloid.

c. **gold test,** a test of cerebrospinal fluid based on alterations in the albumin-globulin ratios that occur in certain disorders of the central nervous system. Normal spinal fluid, when diluted and added to a colloidal gold suspension, will not precipitate the colloidal gold. The extent of precipitation is indicative of various diseases such as multiple sclerosis, poliomyelitis and encephalitis. A positive reaction also occurs in the presence of neurosyphilis. The sample of spinal fluid must not contain blood because this will cause a false-positive reaction.

colloidin (kŏ-loi′din) a jelly-like principle produced in colloid degeneration.

colloidoclasia (kŏ-loi″do-kla′ze-ah) breaking up of the physical equilibrium of the colloid of the body, producing anaphylactic crises (colloidoclastic shock).

colloidopexy (ko-loi′do-pek″se) 1. metabolic fixation of colloids in the organism. 2. phagocytosis of small colloid particles.

colloma (kŏ-lo′mah) a colloid cancer; carcinoma whose degenerated substance has assumed glue-like character.

collonema (kol″o-ne′mah) myxoma.

collopexia (kol″o-pek′se-ah) fixation of the neck of the uterus.

collum (kol′um), pl. *col′la* [L.] the neck, or a neck-like part.
  c. distor′tum, torticollis.
  c. val′gum, coxa valga.

collutory (kol′u-to″re) mouthwash or gargle.

collyrium (kŏ-lir′e-um), pl. *collyr′ia* [L.] eyewash.

colo- (ko′lo) word element [Gr.], *colon.*

coloboma (kol″o-bo′mah) a developmental anomaly resulting from failure of closure of the embryonic ocular cleft, affecting the choroid, ciliary body, eyelid (palpebral coloboma, colobo′ma palpebra′le), iris (colobo′ma i′ridis), lens (colobo′ma len′tis), optic nerve or retina (colobo′ma ret′inae).

colocecostomy (ko″lo-se-kos′to-me) cecocolostomy.

colocentesis (ko″lo-sen-te′sis) surgical puncture of the colon.

coloclysis (ko-lok′li-sis) irrigation of the colon.

coloclyster (ko″lo-klis′ter) an enema introduced into the colon.

colocolic (ko″lo-ko′lik) pertaining to two separate portions of the colon.

colocolostomy (ko″lo-ko-los′to-me) anastomosis between two previously remote portions of the colon.

colocutaneous (ko″lo-ku-ta′ne-us) pertaining to the colon and skin, or communicating with the colon and the cutaneous surface of the body.

colocynth (kol′o-sinth) the dried pulp of the unripe but full-grown fruit of *Citrullus colocynthis;* hydragogue cathartic.

coloenteritis (ko″lo-en″ter-i′tis) enterocolitis.

colofixation (ko″lo-fik-sa′shun) fixation of the colon in cases of ptosis.

Cologel (kol′o-jel) trademark for a preparation of

methylcellulose, which acts as a mild laxative by increasing intestinal bulk.

coloileal (ko″lo-il′e-al) pertaining to or communicating with the colon and ileum.

colon (ko′lon) the part of the large intestine extending from the cecum to the rectum. adj., **colon′ic.** The colon is divided as follows: the ascending colon, which passes upward from the cecum to the lower edge of the liver where it bends and becomes the transverse colon. This section lies across the abdominal cavity from right to left, below the stomach, and then bends downward to become the descending colon. The descending colon extends downward along the left side of the abdomen. At the brim of the pelvis the colon extends in an S-shaped curve down to the sacrum where it becomes the rectum. The curved portion of the colon is called the sigmoid colon. (See also DIGESTIVE SYSTEM.)

colonitis (ko″lon-i′tis) inflammation of the colon; colitis.

colonometer (kol″o-nom′ĕ-ter) an instrument for counting colonies of bacteria.

colonopathy (ko″lon-op′ah-the) disease of the colon.

colonopexy (ko″lon-o-pek″se) sigmoidopexy.

colonorrhagia (ko″lon-o-ra′je-ah) hemorrhage from the colon.

colonorrhea (ko″lon-o-re′ah) a mucous discharge from the colon.

colonoscopy (ko″lon-os′ko-pe) endoscopic examination of the colon, frequently done with the instrument passed through the abdominal wall (transabdominal colonoscopy).

colony (kol′o-ne) a discrete group of organisms, as a collection of bacteria in a culture.

colopexy (kol′o-pek″se) sigmoidopexy.

coloplication (ko″lo-pli-ka′shun) the operation of taking a reef in the colon.

coloproctectomy (ko″lo-prok-tek′to-me) surgical removal of the colon and rectum.

coloproctitis (ko″lo-prok-ti′tis) inflammation of the colon and rectum.

coloproctostomy (ko″lo-prok-tos′to-me) anastomosis of the colon to the rectum.

coloptosis (ko″lop-to′sis) downward displacement of the colon.

colopuncture (ko′lo-pungk″tūr) colocentesis.

color (kul′er) 1. a property of a surface or substance due to absorption of certain light rays and reflection of others within the range of wavelengths (roughly 370 to 760 mμ) adequate to excite the retinal receptors. 2. radiant energy within the range of adequate chromatic stimuli of the retina, i.e., between the infrared and ultraviolet. 3. a sensory impression of one of the rainbow hues.
  c. blindness, inability to distinguish between certain colors. Genuine color blindness, a complete inability to see colors, is quite rare, affecting only

one person in 300,000. Generally the term describes some form of deficiency of color vision. The most common form is red-green confusion, which affects approximately 8 million people in the United States. There is no known cure for color deficiency.

Color vision is a function of the cones in the retina of the eye, which are stimulated by light and transmit impulses to the brain. It is now thought that there are three types of cones, each type stimulated by one of the primary colors in light (red, green and violet). Most cases of color deficiency affect either the red or green receptors, so that the two colors do not appear distinct from each other.

Color vision is usually tested with cards called pseudoisochromatic color plates. These have a letter, number or symbol printed in dots of one color in the midst of dots of gray or other colors. The normal person can see the symbol with no difficulty, but the person with color deficiency cannot distinguish it from the background.

Although color deficiency may occasionally result from injuries, diseases or certain drugs, most cases are hereditary. The deficiency is most often inherited by males through the mother, who carries the trait from her father although she is not color-deficient herself. In some cases, if the grandfather is color-deficient and the mother carries the trait, a daughter may inherit the disability. The ratio of men to women affected with inherited color deficiency is about 20 to 1.

c. index, an expression of the relative amount of hemoglobin contained in an erythrocyte compared with that of a normal individual of the patient's age and sex. The percentage of hemoglobin is divided by the percentage of erythrocytes.

Colorado tick fever a nonexanthematous febrile disease occurring in the Rocky Mountain regions of the United States where the tick vector of the causative virus is prevalent.

colorectitis (ko″lo-rek-ti′tis) inflammation of the colon and rectum.

colorectostomy (ko″lo-rek-tos′to-me) coloproctostomy.

colorectum (ko″lo-rek′tum) the distal 10 inches (25 cm.) of the bowel, including the distal portion of the colon and the rectum, regarded as a specific organ.

colorimeter (kul″er-im′ĕ-ter) an instrument for measuring color differences; especially one for measuring the color of the blood in order to determine the proportion of hemoglobin.

colorrhaphy (ko-lor′ah-fe) suture of the colon.

colosigmoidostomy (ko″lo-sig″moi-dos′to-me) the surgical creation of a new opening between the colon and sigmoid.

colostomy (ko-los′to-me) an artificial opening made on the surface of the abdomen for the purpose of evacuating the bowels and to act as a substitute for the rectum and anus. A colostomy is usually performed as a sequel to surgery in which the rectum has been removed and normal evacuation made impossible. The operation may also be required in occasional cases of ULCERATIVE COLITIS. A temporary colostomy may be done in certain cases

of abscess of the colon or intestinal obstruction.

A patient can soon learn to live with a colostomy and continue to lead a normal, active life for many years. Thousands of people living today have permanent colostomies that go completely unnoticed.

In general, the location of a colostomy depends on the site of the disorder. Most often the site is in the region of the descending colon, sigmoid flexure or rectum; in these cases, the operation is performed on the left side of the abdomen. If the trouble is in the ascending colon the operation will be on the right side, and if it is in the transverse colon, in the center.

NURSING CARE. Before the operation is performed, the physician will explain the type of surgery to be done and the need for such a procedure. The nurse should help the patient understand that a colostomy does not mean invalidism or permanent withdrawal from society. There should be written materials available for the patient to read. These can be obtained from the American Cancer Society, 219 East 42nd Street, New York, N.Y. 10017, free of charge and are written in an optimistic tone to help the patient adjust to his colostomy. Sometimes it helps the patient to talk with someone who has a colostomy and has learned to live a normal life with this handicap.

After surgery the patient should begin to care for his own colostomy as soon as he is able. While teaching the patient it is best to have an optimistic and encouraging attitude, helping him when necessary, but constantly encouraging him to become self-sufficient in handling the equipment needed. The equipment includes a 2-quart irrigating can or bag, rubber tubing, catheter, clamp and lubricating fluid. Other points to be considered include:

1. The colostomy should be irrigated at the same time every day. Later on, the irrigations may be necessary every 2 or 3 days. Some patients adjust very well and have spontaneous evacuations regularly without irrigations.

2. The length of time for complete evacuation varies from 15 minutes to 1 hour. The procedure is not completed until the bowel has been evacuated, and it is best not to hurry through the procedure.

3. The amount of solution depends on the individual patient and usually ranges from 1 pint to several quarts.

4. Irrigations and evacuation seem more normal if the patient is sitting on the toilet during the procedure.

5. Foods that are likely to cause diarrhea or lead to the formation of gas should be avoided. No special diet is required in the majority of cases and a normal well balanced diet is usually sufficient.

There are special colostomy bags that may be worn at all times to collect the intestinal contents. These may be worn in the early stages of adjustment to give the patient a sense of security. Colostomy bags should not be worn indefinitely, however, because they are a source of odor and do not give the patient complete freedom. The ultimate goal is complete control of the bowel movements so that only a small gauze square is needed over the opening to collect mucus that may leak from the colostomy.

colostrum (ko-los′trum) the first milk secreted by the female mammal before or after birth of the young.

colotomy (kŏ-lot′o-me) incision of the colon.

colotyphoid (ko″lo-ti′foid) typhoid fever with follicular ulceration of the colon.

colovaginal (ko″lo-vaj′ĭ-nal) pertaining to or communicating with the colon and vagina.

colovesical (ko″lo-ves′ĭ-kal) pertaining to or communicating with the colon and urinary bladder.

colp(o)- (kol′po) word element [Gr.], *vagina*.

colpalgia (kol-pal′je-ah) pain in the vagina.

colpatresia (kol″pah-tre′ze-ah) atresia of the vagina.

colpectasia (kol″pek-ta′ze-ah) dilatation of the vagina.

colpectomy (kol-pek′to-me) excision of the vagina.

colpeurysis (kol-pu′rĭ-sis) operative dilatation of the vagina.

colpitis (kol-pi′tis) inflammation of the vaginal mucosa.

colpocele (kol′po-sēl) vaginal hernia.

colpocleisis (kol″po-kli′sis) surgical closure of the vagina.

colpocystitis (kol″po-sis-ti′tis) inflammation of the vagina and bladder.

colpocystocele (kol″po-sis′to-sēl) protrusion of a fold of the vagina into the bladder.

colpocytogram (kol″po-si′to-gram) a differential listing of the cells observed in smears from the vaginal mucosa.

colpocytology (kol″po-si-tol′o-je) the quantitative and differential study of cells exfoliated from the epithelium of the vagina.

colpomicroscope (kol″po-mi′kro-skōp) an instrument for examining stained tissues of the cervix in situ.

colpomicroscopy (kol″po-mi-kros′ko-pe) microscopic examination of the stained tissues of the cervix in situ.

colpoperineoplasty (kol″po-per″ĭ-ne′o-plas″te) plastic repair of the vagina and perineum.

colpoperineorrhaphy (kol″po-per″ĭ-ne-or′ah-fe) suture of the vagina and perineum.

colpopexy (kol′po-pek″se) suturing of a relaxed vagina to the abdominal wall.

colpoplasty (kol′po-plas″te) plastic repair of the vagina.

colpoptosis (kol″pop-to′sis) prolapse of the vagina.

colporrhaphy (kol-por′ah-fe) suture of the vagina.

colporrhexis (kol″po-rek′sis) laceration of the vagina.

colposcope (kol′po-skōp) a speculum for examining the vagina.

colpospasm (kol′po-spazm) vaginal spasm.

colpostenosis (kol″po-stĕ-no′sis) narrowing of the vagina.

colpostenotomy (kol″po-stĕ-not′o-me) a cutting operation for stricture of the vagina.

colpotomy (kol-pot′o-me) incision of the vagina.

colpoxerosis (kol″po-ze-ro′sis) abnormal dryness of the vulva and vagina.

columbium (ko-lum′be-um) niobium.

columella (kol″u-mel′ah), pl. *columel′lae* [L.] a little column.
  c. na′si, the fleshy external termination of the septum of the nose.

column (kol′um) a supporting part.
  anterior c., a layer of white matter in either half of the spinal cord between the anterior horn and the anterior median fissure.
  gray c., the longitudinally oriented parts of the spinal cord in which the nerve cell bodies are found, comprising the gray matter of the spinal cord.
  lateral c., a layer of white matter in either half of the spinal cord between the posterior horn and nerve roots and the anterior horn and nerve roots.
  posterior c., a mass of white matter in the spinal cord on either side between the posterior horns and the posterior median fissure.
  vertebral c., the rigid structure in the midline of the back, composed of the vertebrae.

columning (kol′um-ing) support of the prolapsed uterus by means of tampons.

Coly-mycin (kol′e-mi″sin) trademark for preparations of colistimethate, an antibiotic.

colyone (ko′le-ōn) a substance formed in one organ which, when carried by the blood to another organ, decreases functional activity in the latter.

coma (ko′mah) a state of profound unconsciousness from which the patient cannot be aroused, even by powerful stimuli.
  diabetic c., the coma produced by severe diabetic acidosis (see also DIABETES MELLITUS).
  Kussmaul's c., coma with acetone in the urine from diabetes mellitus.

comatose (ko′mah-tōs) affected with coma.

combustion (kom-bus′chun) rapid oxidation with emission of heat.

comedo (kom′ĕ-do), pl. *comedo′nes*, a blackhead; an abnormal mass of keratin and sebum within the dilated orifice of a hair follicle (see also ACNE VULGARIS).

comedomastitis (kom″ĕ-do-mas-ti′tis) a condition characterized chiefly by dilatation of the collecting ducts of the mammary gland, with inflammation within and around the ducts.

comes (ko′mēz), pl. *com′ites* [L.] an accompanying structure, as an artery that accompanies a nerve trunk.

commensal (kŏ-men′sal) the organism or species that benefits by a symbiotic relationship with another organism or species without harming it.

commensalism (kŏ-men′sal-izm) the biologic association of two individuals or populations of different species, one of which is benefited and the other unaffected by the relationship.

comminution (kom″ĭ-nu′shun) a breaking into small fragments.

commissura (kom″ĭ-su′rah), pl. *commissu′rae* [L.] commissure.

commissure (kom′ĭ-shūr) a connecting band of tissue, e.g., at the junction of the upper and the lower lip, or connecting the cusps of the cardiac valves.

    anterior c., a cord of white fibers in front of the crura of the fornix of the cerebrum.

    middle c., a band of gray matter joining the optic thalami.

    posterior c., a white band joining the optic thalami posteriorly.

commissurorrhaphy (kom″ĭ-shūr-or′ah-fe) suture of connecting bands of a commissure, to lessen the size of the orifice.

commissurotomy (kom″ĭ-shūr-ot′o-me) splitting or incision at the junction of the connecting bands of a commissure, to increase the size of the orifice.

    mitral c., the breaking apart of the adherent leaves (commissure) of the mitral valve. This surgical procedure is indicated when the leaflets of the mitral valve have become scarred as a result of inflammation, usually as a complication of rheumatic fever. Normally, these leaflets of the valve open with each pulsation of the heart and allow blood to flow from the left atrium into the left ventricle. They then close as the ventricle fills again and thus prevent a backward flow of blood. Inflammation and scarring of these leaflets prevents their opening and closing as they should (mitral stenosis) and there is a resultant increase of pressure with the pulmonary artery and hypertrophy of the left ventricle.

    Commissurotomy may or may not involve open heart surgery. In one type of surgical procedure the surgeon feels rather than sees the diseased valve, and breaks apart the adhering leaflets with a finger or dilator. This closed cardiac surgery does not involve the use of the heart-lung machine because the heart is not emptied of blood and the heartbeat is not stopped.

    In an open-heart surgical procedure the surgeon can see the diseased valve and he can release the stenosed valve leaflets with his finger or with an instrument called a valvulotome. In this type of procedure the heart is emptied of blood and circulation of the patient's blood is maintained by a HEART-LUNG MACHINE.

    There usually is a dramatic relief of symptoms following mitral commissurotomy. In some cases, however, the valve is badly scarred or there are large deposits of calcium which prevent proper function of the valve and only partial relief can be obtained by surgery. Reoperation may be necessary in some cases when stenosis of the valve recurs.

common cold an acute and highly contagious virus infection of the upper respiratory tract; called also acute rhinitis. At least 20 identifiable viruses have been found to cause colds, and they may attack anyone with lowered resistance. Cold viruses are resistant to present antibiotics. Nor is there a really effective preventive vaccine as yet that will work against them in all situations for all people. Having a cold confers only a brief immunity.

    SYMPTOMS. All colds are not identical, because of different causative agents and individual reactions. Usually the common cold starts with a runny nose, sneezing, a stuffy feeling in the head, slight headache, watering of the eyes, general aching and listlessness, inability to concentrate and perhaps a slight fever. The affected membranes swell until the nasal passages are blocked. Often the inflammation spreads to the throat, causing sore throat and cough. The senses of smell and taste are blunted so that the patient hardly knows or cares what he is eating. He has no energy or ambition and just wants to lie down, as in fact he should.

    A cold usually begins to subside after several days. The nasal discharge lessens, the membranous swelling decreases and the patient is able to breathe through his nose again. The average cold lasts from 7 to 14 days.

    If at any stage the cold shows signs of getting worse—for example, if there are prolonged chills, noticeable fever (above 103° F.), aches in the chest, ears or face, shortness of breath, coughing up of blood-streaked or rust-colored mucus or persistent hoarseness—then a physician should be consulted.

    TREATMENT. To help avoid complications of all kinds, it is best to take a cold seriously from the beginning. Going to bed at the first signs will accomplish the dual purpose of speeding recovery and preventing the passing on of the cold to others. If it is not possible to stay in bed, extra hours of rest or sleep at night are important. During the "runny" stage, the patient should keep warm and avoid changing temperatures as much as possible. He should drink plenty of liquids and eat moderately of anything that appeals to him. The nose should be blown gently, to avoid forcing the infection into the sinuses and ears.

    Aspirin brings the quickest and safest relief. Antibiotics are *not* helpful for colds. They may be prescribed if complications occur. Among the complications that may accompany a cold is SINUSITIS, which occurs when the infection spreads and causes inflammation of the membranes of the paranasal sinuses. The infection may also affect the membranes of the middle ear.

    Other complications may occur if the infection enters the lower respiratory system, including laryngitis, bronchitis and pneumonia.

communicable disease (kŏ-mu′nĭ-kah-bl) a disease spread by direct contact with the infectious agents causing it. Modes of transmission include (1) direct contact with body excreta or discharges from an ulcer, open sore, etc.; (2) indirect contact with inanimate objects such as drinking glasses, toys, bedclothing, etc.; (3) vectors—flies, mosquitoes or other insects capable of spreading the disease.

    NURSING CARE. The patient with a communicable disease is isolated from others and confined to his room until he is no longer a source of infection (see also ISOLATION TECHNIQUE). All contaminated objects in the patient's immediate environment must be treated by disinfection or destroyed by burning so that the causative organisms are not carried to others. After each nursing procedure involving direct contact with the patient or contaminated objects, the nurse's hands are washed thoroughly with soap and running water for at least 1 full minute. The more prolonged the contact with an infected person and his surroundings, the more likely the chance for contamination. All persons concerned with the care of the patient should be familiar with the ways in which his specific disease can be spread.

compathy (kom'pah-the) sharing of emotional feelings with another person.

Compazine (kom'pah-zēn) trademark for preparations of prochlorperazine, a tranquilizer.

compensation (kom″pen-sa'shun) the counterbalancing of any defect of structure or function; a mental mechanism operating beyond conscious awareness by which an individual attempts to make up for real or fancied deficiencies.

complement (kom'plĕ-ment) a substance in normal blood serum that with specific amboceptor causes lysis of cells, destruction of bacteria and other phenomena.

   c.-fixation tests, tests that utilize antigen-antibody reaction and resulting hemolysis to determine the presence of various organisms in the blood. When complement is used up in this reaction it is said to be fixed. Examples of complement-fixation tests are the Wassermann and the Kolmer tests, both of which determine the presence of *Treponema pallidum* in the blood and are thus useful in the diagnosis of syphilis.

complex (kom'pleks) 1. a combination of various things, like or unlike. 2. a group of ideas that are part of the subconscious mental process and are associated with strong desires or emotional experiences. They usually are repressed and thus can give rise to morbid behavior characterized by utilization of escape mechanisms such as compensation or identification. 3. that portion of an electrocardiographic tracing that represents the systole of an atrium or ventricle.

   Electra c., a series of symptoms attributed to suppressed sexual desire of a daughter for her father, with hostility toward the mother.

   inferiority c., an abnormal feeling of inferiority, producing timidity or, as a compensation, exaggerated aggressiveness.

   Oedipus c., a series of symptoms attributed to suppressed sexual desire of a son for his mother, with hostility toward the father.

complexion (kom-plek'shun) the color and appearance of the skin of the face.

compliance (kom-pli'ans) the quality of yielding to pressure or force without disruption, or an expression of the measure of ability to do so, as an expression of the distensibility of an air- or fluid-filled organ, e.g., lung or urinary bladder, in terms of unit of volume per unit of pressure.

complication (kom″plĭ-ka'shun) a disease concurrent with another disease.

compos mentis (kom'pos men'tis) [L.] of sound mind.

compound (kom'pownd) 1. made up of diverse elements or ingredients. 2. in chemistry, a substance made up of two or more elements. The elements are united chemically, which means that each of the original elements loses its individual characteristics once it has combined with the other element(s). When elements combine they do so in definite proportions by weight; this is why the union of hydrogen and oxygen always produces water. Sugar, salt and vinegar are examples of compounds.

   Organic compounds are those containing carbon atoms; inorganic compounds are those that do not contain carbon atoms.

   acyclic c., aliphatic c., an organic compound that contains no ring structure of the atoms.

   cyclic c., a compound composed of several atoms linked together so as to form a ring.

   c. E, cortisone.

   c. F, cortisol.

   heterocyclic c., an organic compound that contains rings made up of more than one kind of atom.

compress (kom'pres) a square of gauze or similar dressing, for application of pressure or medication to a restricted area, or for local applications of heat or cold.

compression (kom-presh'un) the act of pressing upon or together; the state of being pressed together.

compulsion (kum-pul'shun) an overwhelming urge to perform an irrational act or ritual. adj., **compul'sive.**

   repetition c., the unconscious need to repeat earlier experiences, relationships or patterns of reaction.

conarium (ko-na're-um) the pineal gland.

conation (ko-na'shun) the conscious tendency to act.

conative (kon'ah-tiv) pertaining to the basic strivings of a person, as expressed in his behavior and actions.

concave (kon'kāv) rounded and somewhat depressed or hollowed out.

concavity (kon-kav'ĭ-te) a depression or hollowed surface.

concentration (kon″sen-tra'shun) 1. increase in strength by evaporation. 2. medicine that has been strengthened by evaporation of its nonactive parts. 3. the relative content of a contained or dissolved substance in a solution.

   hydrogen ion c., an expression of the degree of acidity or alkalinity (pH) of a solution.

   c. test, a test of renal function based on the patient's ability to concentrate urine.

conception (kon-sep'shun) 1. the union of male and female gametes, marking the beginning of a new organism. 2. an impression or idea.

conceptus (kon-sep'tus) the whole product of conception at any stage of development, from fertilization of the ovum to birth.

concha (kong'kah), pl. *con'chae* [L.] a shell-shaped structure.

   c. of auricle, the hollow of the auricle of the extended ear, bounded anteriorly by the tragus and posteriorly by the antihelix.

   nasal c., inferior, a bone forming the lower part of the lateral wall of the nasal cavity.

   nasal c., medial, the lower of two bony plates projecting from the inner wall of the ethmoidal labyrinth and separating the superior from the middle meatus of the nose.

   nasal c., superior, the upper of two bony plates projecting from the inner wall of the ethmoidal labyrinth and forming the upper boundary of the superior meatus of the nose.

   nasal c., supreme, a third thin bony plate occasionally found projecting from the inner wall of the ethmoidal labyrinth, above the two usually found.

   sphenoidal c., a thin curved plate of bone at the anterior and lower part of the body of the sphenoid bone, on either side, forming part of the roof of the nasal cavity.

conchitis   (kong-ki′tis) inflammation of a concha.

conchotomy   (kong-kot′o-me) incision of a concha.

conclination   (kon″kli-na′shun) inward rotation of the upper pole of the vertical meridian of each eye.

concordance   (kon-kor′dans) in genetics, the occurrence of a given trait in both members of a twin pair.

concrescence   (kon-kres′ens) a growing together of parts originally separate.

concretion   (kon-kre′shun) a hardened mass; calculus.

concussion   (kon-kush′un) a violent jar or shock, or the condition that results from such an injury.

   c. of the brain, vertigo, nausea, loss of consciousness and weak pulse from severe head injury. Breathing often is unusually rapid or slow. Outward evidence of the injury may include bleeding and contusions (bruises). When he regains consciousness the victim is likely to have severe headache, and he may have blurred vision. If severely injured, he may lapse into a coma.

   First Aid. The patient is kept lying down and quiet. He should be covered with a blanket or coat, and medical assistance should be obtained. Artificial respiration is given if breathing stops. Stimulants or drugs that may be depressants, e.g., pain relievers, should not be given; these drugs may mask the symptoms and make an accurate diagnosis difficult. (See also HEAD INJURY.)

condensation   (kon″den-sa′shun) 1. the act of rendering, or the process of becoming, more compact. 2. pathologic hardening of a part. 3. the unconscious union of concepts to produce a new idea or mental picture.

condenser   (kon-den′ser) 1. a vessel or apparatus for condensing gases or vapors. 2. a device for illuminating microscopic objects. 3. an apparatus for concentrating energy or matter.

conditioned reflex   (kon-dish′und) a reflex that does not occur naturally in the animal but that may be developed by regular association of some physiologic function with an unrelated outside event, such as ringing of a bell or flashing of a light.

condom   (kon′dum) a rubber sheath worn over the penis in coitus, to prevent impregnation or infection.

conductance   (kon-duk′tans) ability to conduct or transmit, as electricity or other energy or material; in studies of respiration, an expression of the amount of air reaching the alveoli per unit of time per unit of pressure, the reciprocal of resistance.

conduction   (kon-duk′shun) conveyance of energy, as of heat, sound or electricity.

   aerial c., air c., conduction of sound waves to the organ of hearing through the air.

bone c., conduction of sound waves to the inner ear through the bones of the skull.

conductivity   (kon″duk-tiv′ĭ-te) capacity for conduction.

condylarthrosis   (kon″dil-ar-thro′sis) an articulation in which a bony eminence is lodged in a joint cavity in an ellipsoid fashion.

condyle   (kon′dīl) a rounded eminence at the articular end of a bone.

condylectomy   (kon″dil-ek′to-me) excision of a condyle.

condylion   (kon-dil′e-on) the point at the lateral tip of the mandibular condyle.

condyloid   (kon′dĭ-loid) resembling a condyle.

condyloma   (kon″dĭ-lo′mah) an elevated wartlike lesion of the skin. adj., **condylo′matous.**

   c. acumina′tum, a papilloma of viral origin, sometimes occurring on skin or mucous surfaces of external genitalia.

   c. la′tum, a wide, flat, syphilitic condyloma with yellowish discharge.

condylotomy   (kon″dĭ-lot′o-me) transection of a condyle.

condylus   (kon′dĭ-lus), pl. *con′dyli* [L.] condyle.

cone   (kōn) a solid figure or body having a circular base and tapering to a point, especially one of the conelike structures of the retina, which, with the rods, form the light-sensitive elements of the retina. The cones make possible the perception of color.

   ether c., a cone-shaped device used over the face in administration of ether for anesthesia.

   c. of light, the triangular reflection of light seen on the tympanic membrane.

confabulation   (kon-fab″u-la′shun) the recitation of imaginary experiences to fill gaps in memory.

configuration   (kon-fig″u-ra′shun) the general form of a body. In chemisty, the arrangement in space of the atoms of a molecule. In gestalt psychology, an organized whole with interdependent parts so that the whole is more than the sum of its parts.

confinement   (kon-fīn′ment) restraint within a specific area; used especially to designate the termination of pregnancy with delivery of an infant.

conflict   (kon′flikt) a painful state of consciousness caused by presence of opposing impulses or desires and failure to resolve them, found to a certain extent in all persons.

confluence   (kon′floo-ens) a meeting of streams.

   c. of sinuses, the dilated point of confluence of the superior sagittal, straight, occipital and two transverse sinuses of the dura mater.

confusion   (kon-fu′zhun) disturbed orientation in regard to time, place or person, sometimes accompanied by disordered consciousness.

congener   (kon′jě-ner) something closely related to another thing, as a chemical compound closely related to another in composition and exerting similar or antagonistic effects.

congenital (kon-jen'ĭ-tal) present at and existing from the time of birth.

c. heart defect, a structural defect of the heart or great vessels or both, present at birth. Any number of defects may occur, singly or in combination. They result from improper development of the heart and blood vessels during the prenatal period. Between 30,000 and 40,000 children with one or more heart defects are born annually in the United States.

A fairly common defect is TETRALOGY OF FALLOT, so-called because it involves four major defects and was first described by Fallot. It can, in some instances, be corrected by surgery. Another defect, PATENT DUCTUS ARTERIOSUS, involves the persistent presence of a passage, the ductus arteriosus, between the aorta and pulmonary artery. Normally this passage closes at birth.

Ventricular septal defect is an opening between the ventricles, often described by laymen as a "hole in the heart." This defect results in a flow of blood directly from one ventricle to the other, resulting in a bypassing of the pulmonary circulation and producing varying degrees of cyanosis because of oxygen deficiency. Defective valves affecting the flow of blood to and from the heart may be associated.

A rarer congenital condition is transposition of the great vessels. In this defect the position of the chief blood vessels of the heart is reversed. The aorta rises from the right ventricle instead of the left, and the pulmonary artery emerges from the left ventricle rather than from the right. The result of this circulatory confusion is that oxygen-poor blood returning from the systemic circulation to the right side of the heart is pumped back into the general circulation instead of being transported to the lungs. Meanwhile, oxygen-rich blood flows aimlessly to and from the lungs. Transposition of the great vessels can sometimes be corrected by surgery.

Another congenital defect results when the foramen ovale, a window between the atria, fails to close completely after birth. This condition is called atrial septal defect. When an opening remains between the atria, some of the oxygen-rich blood from the left atrium passes into the right atrium and travels back to the lungs without being first transported through the body. Coarctation of the aorta results when a portion of the aorta is unusually narrow.

In many cases—depending on the severity of the defect and the physical condition of the patient—these congenital conditions can be treated by surgery. Some congenital defects are so minor that they do not significantly affect the action of the heart; these kinds of defects do not require surgery.

The cause of most congenital abnormalities is unknown. In a small number of cases, rubella (German measles) when contracted by the mother during the first 2 or 3 months of pregnancy can cause congenital defects in the baby.

congestion (kon-jes'chun) abnormal accumulation of blood in a part. adj., **conges'tiv.**

conglobation (kon"glo-ba'shun) the lumping together of particles in a mass.

conglutinant (kon-gloo'tĭ-nant) promoting union, as of the lips of a wound.

conglutination (kon-gloo"tĭ-na'shun) union or adherence of parts.

coniasis (ko-ni'ah-sis) the presence of dustlike concretions, as in the biliary tract.

coniofibrosis (ko"ne-o-fi-bro'sis) pneumoconiosis with connective tissue growth in the lungs.

coniosis (ko"ne-o'sis) a diseased state due to inhalation of dust.

coniotoxicosis (ko"ne-o-tok"sĭ-ko'sis) pneumoconiosis in which the irritant affects the tissues directly.

conization (ko"nĭ-za'shun) excision of a cone of tissue, as of the endocervical mucous membrane.

conjugata (kon"ju-ga'tah) the conjugate diameter of the pelvis.

conjugate (kon'ju-gāt) 1. joined or in pairs. 2. the conjugate diameter of the pelvis.

conjugation (kon"ju-ga'shun) the act of joining together. In biology, a method of reproduction in protozoa. In chemistry, the joining together of two compounds to produce another compound, such as the combination of a toxic product with some substance in the body to form a detoxified product which is then eliminated.

conjunctiva (kon"junk-ti'vah), pl. *conjuncti'vae* [L.] the delicate membrane lining the eyelids and covering the eyeball. adj., **conjuncti'val.**

conjunctivitis (kon-junk"tĭ-vi'tis) inflammation of the conjunctiva, the thin membrane that covers the eyeball and lines the eyelid. The disorder may be caused by bacteria or a virus, or by allergic, chemical or physical factors. Its infectious form (of bacterial or viral origin) is highly contagious. The type of conjunctivitis known as pinkeye is an example of a highly contagious conjunctivitis and must be handled with extreme care to prevent its spread.

gonorrheal c., an infectious disorder caused by the gonococcus, which is also the causative agent in gonorrhea.

inclusion c., conjunctivitis caused by a filterable virus and characterized by the presence of large basophilic inclusion bodies.

conjunctivoma (kon-junk"tĭ-vo'mah) a tumor of conjunctival tissue.

conjunctivoplasty (kon"junk-ti'vo-plas"te) plastic repair of the conjunctiva.

Conn's syndrome (konz) primary aldosteronism.

connective tissue (kŏ-nek'tiv) a fibrous type of body tissue with varied functions. The connective tissue system supports and connects internal organs, forms bones and the walls of blood vessels, attaches muscles to bones and replaces tissues of other types following injury.

Connective tissue consists mainly of long fibers embedded in noncellular matter, the ground substance. The density of these fibers and the presence or absence of certain chemicals make some connective tissues soft and rubbery and others hard and rigid. Compared with most other kinds of tissue, connective tissue has few cells. The fibers contain a protein called collagen, and the tissue for that reason is often called collagen tissue.

Collagen tissue can develop in any part of the

body, and the body uses this ability to help repair or replace damaged areas. Scar tissue is the most common form of this substitute. (See also COLLAGEN DISEASES.)

connexus (kō-nek'sus) a connection or connecting structure.

consanguinity (kon"sang-gwin'ĭ-te) blood relationship.

conscience (kon'shens) the moral, self-critical part of oneself; the conscious superego.

conscious (kon'shus) capable of responding to sensory stimuli and having subjective experiences.

consciousness (kon'shus-nes) responsiveness of the mind to impressions made by the senses.

consolidation (kon-sol"ĭ-da'shun) the process of becoming solidified, or more dense, as of a lung in pneumonia.

constellation (kon"stě-la'shun) a group of emotional ideas that have not become repressed.

constipation (kon"stĭ-pa'shun) ordinarily a condition in which the waste matter in the bowels is too hard to pass easily, or in which bowel movements are so infrequent that discomfort or uncomfortable symptoms result. Many people also use the term when referring to a sense of incomplete evacuation or when they feel they should have more frequent bowel movements. The frequency of bowel movements varies according to individual body make-up, type of intestine, eating habits, physical activity and custom.

CAUSES.   An organic cause of constipation can be a disease such as hypothyroidism. Or there may be a stricture or obstruction that prevents wastes from being passed through the intestines, as in the case of hernia, tumor or cancerous growth. Often constipation from such obstructions comes on suddenly.

SYMPTOMS.   Prolonged constipation, called obstipation, can cause such uncomfortable symptoms as nausea, heartburn, headache or distress in the rectum or intestines, which may last until the stool is passed. These symptoms are not due to the absorption of poisons from the waste material, as some people believe. Rather they are a reaction of the nerves when the rectum is distended by the matter it contains. This condition is uncomfortable rather than harmful.

PREVENTION AND TREATMENT.   Elimination is largely a matter of habit. Therefore it is desirable to establish a regular routine for it. Sensible living can also help to prevent or combat constipation. Emotional tension and strain can cause constipation. Therefore, it is important to avoid unnecessary tensions and worry, including concern over constipation itself.

When constipation does not respond to roughage added to the diet and an effort to improve bowel habits, an enema may be advisable, or a mild laxative such as petroleum and agar, aromatic cascara sagrada or milk of magnesia may be taken. Laxatives should be resorted to only after the bowels have been given a chance to function by themselves. The frequent and often unnecessary use of laxatives can be the cause of constipation, rather than its cure. Cathartics, such as castor oil, which are more powerful in their purgative action than laxatives, should never be used unless prescribed by a physician.

constitution (kon"stĭ-tu'shun) 1. the make-up or functional habit of the body. 2. the order in which the atoms of a molecule are joined together.

constitutional (kon"stĭ-tu'shun-al) affecting the whole body.

constriction (kon-strik'shun) a narrowing or compression.

constrictor (kon-strik'tor) that which causes constriction.

consultant (kon-sul'tant) a physician or surgeon whose opinion on diagnosis or treatment is sought by the physician originally attending a patient.

consultation (kon"sul-ta'shun) deliberation of two or more physicians about diagnosis or treatment in a particular case.

consumption (kon-sump'shun) 1. the act of consuming, or using up. 2. a wasting away of the body, applied especially to pulmonary tuberculosis.

contact (kon'takt) 1. mutual touching of two bodies. 2. the completion of an electric circuit. 3. a person who has been sufficiently near an infected person to have been exposed to the transfer of infectious material.

c. dermatitis, a skin rash marked by itching, swelling, blistering, oozing and scaling. It is caused by direct contact between the skin and a substance to which the person is allergic or sensitive. The rash usually occurs only on that area of the body that has come into contact with the irritating substance. The most common form of contact dermatitis is that caused by POISON IVY, OAK AND SUMAC. Other plants, too, sometimes cause an allergic reaction. Contact dermatitis may also be caused by industrial oils, medicines, cosmetics, perfumes, mouthwashes, deodorants, rubber, plastics, metals and clothing made of various materials and treated with certain preservatives and dyes. Some soaps, detergents and other cleansing products can cause a condition of the hands often referred to as "housewives' dermatitis" (or "dishpan hands"). (See also DERMATITIS.)

direct c., immediate c., contact of a healthy person with a diseased person, whereby a contagious disease may be communicated.

indirect c., contact of a healthy person with objects which may have been contaminated by an infected person.

c. lenses, corrective lenses that fit directly over the cornea of the eye, for correction of refractive errors. They do not actually touch the surface of the eye, but float on a thin layer of the fluid that naturally moistens the eyeball. Contact lenses are made of glass or plastic, and are invisible when in place. Their invisibility is one of their chief advantages. There are certain disadvantages to contact lenses. It takes time to become accustomed to wearing them, and even with practice most people cannot wear them for more than 6 or 8 hours at a time without irritation to the eyes. Since they must be molded to the exact shape of the patient's corneas, they are quite expensive.

mediate c., indirect contact.

contactant (kon-tak'tant) a substance that touches or may touch the surface of the body.

contactology (kon″tak-tol′o-je) the specialized field of knowledge related to the prescription and use of contact lenses.

contagion (kon-ta′jun) 1. the spread of disease from one person to another. 2. a disease which spreads from one person to another. 3. the living organism (germ or virus) by which disease is spread from one person to another.

contagiosity (kon-ta″je-os′ĭ-te) the quality of being contagious.

contagious (kon-ta′jus) readily transmitted by direct or indirect contact.

contagium (kon-ta′je-um) morbific matter that may spread disease.
  c. vi′vum, a living organism that causes disease.

contamination (kon-tam″ĭ-na′shun) the soiling or making inferior by contact or mixture.

content (kon′tent) that which is contained within a thing.
  latent c., the part of a dream that is hidden in the unconsciousness.
  manifest c., the part of a dream that is remembered after awakening.

continence (kon′tĭ-nens) the ability to exercise voluntary control over natural impulses, such as the urge to defecate or urinate. adj., **con′tinent.**

contra-aperture (kon″trah-ap′er-tūr) a second opening made in an abscess to facilitate the discharge of matter.

contraception (kon″trah-sep′shun) prevention of fertilization of the ovum and development of a new individual. Contraception may be achieved by several methods.
  RHYTHM METHOD. This is called the natural method since it uses no artificial means and is based on the natural cycle of ovulation in the female. The period of possible conception usually lasts from 2 days before ovulation through 1 day after it, or 3 days in all; during these days if conception is to be prevented the woman must abstain from coitus. The other days of the cycle constitute the so-called "safe period." In practice, however, the safe period is considered to be shorter, since ovulation generally occurs between the twelfth and sixteenth days of the cycle, so that any of these days must be counted as days of possible conception. (The first day of the cycle is the first day of menstruation.)
  To calculate the fertile period, it is necessary to keep an accurate record of menstrual cycles for 8 to 12 months. The length of the longest and shortest cycles must be carefully noted over this time.
  It is also possible to determine when ovulation takes place by daily readings of body temperature since the temperature is elevated after ovulation takes place.
  ORAL CONTRACEPTIVES. These are hormone-like products that duplicate the action of progesterone in women, preventing ovulation from taking place; popularly referred to as "the pill." A few patients experience some minor side effects, which are usually only temporary, such as nausea, a feeling of fullness or weight gain. Research on long-term side effects is incomplete.
  MECHANICAL AND CHEMICAL MEANS
  Condom and Cervical Diaphragm. The condom is a thin flexible sheath worn over the penis to prevent entry of spermatozoa into the vagina during coitus. The diaphragm is a soft rubber device shaped like a cup with a flexible spring forming the circular outer edge. It is inserted in the vagina in such a position that it covers the cervix uteri and prevents entry of spermatozoa. The diaphragm is used in conjunction with a spermicidal cream or jelly.
  Jellies, Creams and Foams. A number of contraceptive jellies, or gels, creams and aerosol foams are made to be used without any mechanical device. These are more powerful in their spermicidal effects than the creams and jellies made to be used with diaphragms. Doubt has been cast on their reliability and there have also been objections to them on esthetic grounds.
  INTRAUTERINE DEVICES. These consist of a ring, spiral, coil or loop that is permanently placed inside the uterine cavity. Although the mechanism is not completely understood, it is believed that these devices do not interfere with fertilization but rather in some way render implantation of the fertilized ovum impossible. The advantage of the intrauterine device is that once it has been inserted by the physician it can be left in place for as long as a year, after which it can be removed for a short period and then reinserted. (See also INTRAUTERINE CONTRACEPTIVE DEVICES.)
  ANTIZYGOTIC AGENTS. Experimental work is being carried on with agents that will inhibit the development of the ovum; to date the experiments have been confined to laboratory animals. Antispermatogenic agents, which would inhibit the development of sperm, are also being studied.

contraceptive (kon″trah-sep′tiv) 1. diminishing the likelihood of or preventing conception. 2. an agent that diminishes the likelihood of or prevents conception.

contractile (kon-trak′til) contracting under the proper stimulus.

contractility (kon″trak-til′ĭ-te) a capacity for movement, one of the fundamental properties of protoplasm; the ability to contract.

contraction (kon-trak′shun) a drawing together; a shortening or shrinkage.
  Braxton Hicks c's, painless contractions of the uterus during pregnancy, gradually increasing in frequency and intensity after the thirtieth week.
  carpopedal c., a kind of tetany in infants, with flexing of the fingers, toes, elbows and knees, and a general tendency to convulsions.
  Hicks c's, Braxton Hicks contractions.
  isometric c., contraction in which tension is developed, but length of the muscle is not changed.
  postural c., the state of muscular tension and contraction that just suffices to maintain the posture of the body.
  tetanic c., tonic c., sustained muscular contraction with alternating relaxation.
  Volkmann's c., Volkmann's contracture.

contracture (kon-trak′tūr) abnormal shortening of muscle tissue, rendering the muscle highly resistant to stretching. A contracture can lead to permanent disability. It can be caused by fibrosis of the tissues supporting the muscle or the joint, or by disorders of the muscle fibers themselves.

Improper support and positioning of joints affected by arthritis or injury, and inadequate exercising of joints in patients with paralysis can result in contractures. For example, a patient with arthritis or severe burns may assume a position most comfortable for him and will resist changing position because motion is painful. If the joints are allowed to remain in this position, the muscle fibers that normally provide motion will stretch or shorten to accommodate the position and eventually they will lose their ability to contract and relax.

In many cases contractures can be prevented by proper exercise (active or passive), and by adequate support of the joints to eliminate constant shortening or stretching of the muscles and surrounding tissues.

Dupuytren's c., a flexion deformity of the fingers or toes, due to shortening, thickening and fibrosis of the palmar or plantar fascia.

ischemic c., muscular contracture and degeneration due to interference with the circulation from pressure.

Volkmann's c., contraction of the fingers and sometimes of the wrist, with loss of power, after severe injury or improper use of a tourniquet or cast in the region of the elbow.

contrafissure (kon″trah-fish′er) a fracture in a part opposite the site of the blow.

contraindication (kon″trah-in″dĭ-ka′shun) a condition that forbids use of a particular treatment.

contralateral (kon″trah-lat′er-al) pertaining to or situated on the opposite side.

contrast medium (kon′trast) a radiopaque substance used in roentgenography to permit visualization of body structures.

contrecoup (kon″truh-koo′) [Fr.] injury produced at a site by a blow on the opposite side of the part or on a remote part.

control (kon-trōl′) 1. the governing or limitation of certain objects or events. 2. a standard against which experimental observations may be evaluated.

birth c., regulation of childbearing by measures designed to prevent conception.

contrusion (kon-troo′zhun) crowding of the teeth.

contuse (kon-tūz′) to bruise; to wound by beating.

contusion (kon-too′zhun) injury to tissues without breakage of skin; a bruise. In a contusion blood from the broken vessels accumulates in surrounding tissues, producing pain, swelling and tenderness. A discoloration appears as a result of blood seepage under the surface of the skin.

Most contusions heal without special treatment, but cold compresses may reduce bleeding, and thus reduce swelling and discoloration, and relieve pain. If a contusion is unusually severe, the injured part should be rested and slightly elevated. Later the application of heat may hasten the absorption of blood.

Serious complications may develop in some cases of contusion. Normally blood is drawn off from the bruised area in a few days, but there is possibility that blood clotted in the area will form a cyst or

calcify and require surgical treatment. The contusion may also be complicated by infection.

cerebral c., contusion of the brain following a HEAD INJURY. It may occur with extradural or subdural collections of blood, in which case the patient may be left with neurologic defects or EPILEPSY.

conus (ko′nus), pl. *co′ni* [L.] 1. a cone. 2. posterior staphyloma of the myopic eye.

c. arterio′sus, the anterosuperior portion of the right ventricle of the heart, at the entrance to the pulmonary trunk.

c. medulla′ris, the conical extremity of the spinal cord, at the level of the upper lumbar vertebrae.

convalescence (kon″vah-les′ens) the stage of recovery from an illness, operation or accidental injury.

convalescent (kon″vah-les′ent) 1. pertaining to or characterized by convalescence. 2. a patient who is recovering from a disease, operation or accidental injury.

convection (kon-vek′shun) the act of conveying or transmission, specifically transmission of heat in a liquid or gas by circulation of heated particles.

convergence (kon-ver′jens) a moving together, or inclination toward a common point; the coordinated movement of the two eyes toward fixation of the same near point. adj., **conver′gent.**

conversion (kon-ver′zhun) 1. the act of changing into something of different form or properties. 2. the transformation of emotions into physical manifestations. 3. manipulative correction of malposition of a fetal part during labor.

c. reaction, a type of mental mechanism that is unconsciously employed by an individual to solve a strong emotional conflict. In conversion reaction the patient "converts" his emotional distress into any of a wide variety of physical symptoms, none of which have any organic basis. Among the symptoms which may develop are deafness, blindness and paralysis of a limb. The symptom chosen by the patient can be related to his particular emotional conflict, and his reaction to the symptom appears to be one of indifference. This is not surprising when one realizes that the patient is using the symptom to obtain relief from a distressing conflict in his mind, and that such a symptom often provokes sympathy and a solicitous attitude from the person or persons involved in the conflict. Treatment of conversion reaction is aimed at helping the patient find more realistic ways of solving his emotional conflict.

convex (kon′veks) rounded and somewhat elevated.

convolution (kon″vo-lu′shun) an irregularity or elevation caused by the infolding of a structure upon itself.

convulsion (kun-vul′shun) involuntary spasm or contraction of muscles. In general there are three types of convulsions: clonic, in which opposing muscles contract and relax alternately, producing rhythmic movements; tonic, in which all the muscles tighten until the victim becomes rigid; and those that occur in jacksonian epilepsy, in which the muscular twitching begins in one area and spreads to another.

CAUSES. Convulsions may arise from any of a

number of changes in the chemical balance of the body. Insufficient amounts of sugar, calcium or various hormones in the blood may bring on seizures. Accumulation of waste products in the blood, such as occurs in uremia, or toxic conditions such as toxemia of pregnancy can produce convulsions. Disease or injury to the brain or central nervous system may also be severe enough to set off convulsions. Drug poisoning frequently produces convulsions. The seizures associated with EPILEPSY are a form of convulsion.

NURSING CARE. Prevention of injury to the patient is the first concern. If convulsions are likely, side rails should be applied to the bed and then padded with cotton blankets. The head of the bed should be covered with a folded blanket or pillow to avoid trauma to the head during the seizure. A padded tongue depressor is kept at the bedside at all times. This is used to place between the patient's teeth so that he will not bite his tongue or the inside of his mouth during the convulsion. No restraint should be used.

Observations before and during the convulsion should include: The time the convulsion began; whether the patient had any warning or specific symptoms (aura) just before the convulsion occurred, and the length of time it lasted; the type of convulsion and the area in which it began, and whether it was restricted to one part of the body or was generalized; whether the patient lost consciousness or was incontinent of urine or feces; the effects of the convulsion on the patient's pulse and respiration, and any other objective symptoms such as change in color or profuse perspiration.

convulsive (kon-vul′siv) of the nature of a convulsion.

Cooley's anemia (koo′lēz) thalassemia.

Coombs tests (koomz) laboratory tests that reveal certain antigen-antibody reactions; used in differentiating between various types of hemolytic anemias, for determining minor blood types, including the Rh factor, and for testing for anticipated ERYTHROBLASTOSIS FETALIS.

direct C. t., the test used to detect the presence of antibodies that may damage erythrocytes but will not cause visible agglutination. Clinically its most important use is in early diagnosis of erythroblastosis fetalis and autoimmune hemolytic anemias. It is used also in crossmatching blood for transfusions. Venous blood or blood from the umbilical cord may be used.

indirect C. t., a test for detecting incompatibility in transfusions when the recipient has a greater than normal risk of transfusion reaction. The test also can reveal the presence of anti-Rh antibodies in maternal blood during pregnancy. Either clotted blood or blood with an anticoagulant may be used.

coordination (ko-or″dī-na′shun) the harmonious functioning of interrelated organs and parts. Applied especially to the process of the motor apparatus of the brain which provides for the co-working of particular groups of muscles for the performance of definite adaptive useful responses.

copiopia (ko″pe-o′pe-ah) eyestrain.

copodyskinesia (ko″po-dis″kī-ne′ze-ah) difficulty of movement due to fatigue from habitual performance of a particular action.

copper (kop′er) a chemical element, atomic number 29, atomic weight 63.54, symbol Cu. (See table of ELEMENTS.) It is necessary for bone formation and for the formation of blood because it acts as a catalyst in the transformation of inorganic iron into hemoglobin. There is little danger of deficiency in ordinary diets because of relatively abundant supply and minute daily requirements.

c. sulfate, a compound used as an emetic and as a catalyst for iron when given in the treatment of anemia; serves also as an antidote in phosphorus poisoning.

coprecipitin (ko″pre-sip′ĭ-tin) a precipitin that acts on two or more organisms.

copremesis (kop-rem′ĕ-sis) the vomiting of fecal matter.

coprohematology (kop″ro-he″mah-tol′o-je) study of the blood content of the feces.

coprolalia (kop″ro-la′le-ah) the utterance of obscene words, especially words relating to feces.

coprolith (kop′ro-lith) a hard fecal concretion in the intestine.

coprology (kop-rol′o-je) the study of the feces.

coprophagia (kop″ro-fa′je-ah) eating of filth or feces.

coprophilia (kop″ro-fil′e-ah) a psychopathologic interest in filth, especially in feces and defecation.

coprophobia (kop″ro-fo′be-ah) fear of feces.

coproporphyria (kop″ro-por-fēr′e-ah) increased formation and excretion of coproporphyrin.

coproporphyrin (kop″ro-por′fĭ-rin) a prophyrin found in feces and urine.

coproporphyrinuria (kop″ro-por″fĭ-rĭ-nu′re-ah) the presence of coproporphyrin in the urine.

coprostasis (kop-ros′tah-sis) fecal impaction.

coprozoic (kop″ro-zo′ik) living in fecal matter.

copula (kop′u-lah) 1. any connecting part or structure. 2. amboceptor.

copulation (kop″u-la′shun) sexual union or coitus; usually applied to the mating process in lower animals.

cor (kor) [L.] heart.
c. bovi′num, a greatly enlarged heart, usually associated with aortic insufficiency.
c. pulmonale, a serious cardiac condition in which there is right ventricular heart failure due to increased pressure within the pulmonary artery. Acute cor pulmonale is an emergency situation arising from a sudden dilatation of the right ventricle as a result of pulmonary embolism. Chronic cor pulmonale develops gradually and is associated with chronic lung disorders such as pulmonary EMPHYSEMA, SILICOSIS and fibrosis of the lung following an infection. These conditions impair pulmonary circulation and thus create a "damming" effect on the blood flowing through the pulmonary artery. This in turn slows down the

flow of blood from the right ventricle, and the ventricle becomes hypertrophied and dilated.

SIGNS AND SYMPTOMS. Symptoms are similar to those of congestive heart failure from other causes: dyspnea, edema of the lower extremities, enlargement of the liver and distention of the veins in the neck. The hematocrit is increased as the body attempts to compensate for impaired circulation by producing more erythrocytes.

TREATMENT. Treatment is ultimately aimed at relief of the lung disorder causing the condition and relieving the pulmonary insufficiency. This includes the administration of bronchodilators and the use of a RESPIRATOR to reduce hypoxia and dyspnea. Severe polycythemia and hypervolemia may require phlebotomy to lower the blood volume and red cell count. The heart failure is treated with digitalis, diuretics, adequate rest and dietary measures. (See also HEART FAILURE.)

coracoid (kor'ah-koid) 1. like a crow's beak. 2. the coracoid process, a projection from the anterior the upper edge of the scapula.

Coramine (ko'rah-min) trademark for preparations of nikethamide, a central nervous system stimulant.

cord (kord) any long, cylindrical and flexible body or organ.
 spermatic c., the structure extending from the abdominal ring to the testis, comprising the pampiniform plexus, nerves, vas deferens, testicular artery and other vessels.
 spinal c., that part of the central nervous system lodged in the spinal canal, extending from the foramen magnum to about the level of the third lumbar vertebra.
 umbilical c., the structure connecting the fetus and placenta, and containing the channels through which fetal blood passes to and from the placenta (see also UMBILICAL CORD).
 vocal c's, the thyroarytenoid ligaments of the larynx, the superior pair being called the false, and the inferior pair the true, vocal cords.

cordal (kor'dal) pertaining to a cord; used specifically in referring to the vocal cords.

cordate (kor'dāt) heart-shaped.

cordectomy (kor-dek'to-me) excision of a cord, as of a vocal cord.

corditis (kor-di'tis) inflammation of the spermatic cord.

cordopexy (kor'do-pek"se) surgical fixation of a vocal cord.

cordotomy (kor-dot'o-me) chordotomy.

Cordran (kor'dran) trademark for preparations of flurandrenolone, a topical corticosteroid.

corectasis (kor-ek'tah-sis) morbid dilatation of the pupil.

corectome (ko-rek'tōm) a cutting instrument for iridectomy.

corectomy (ko-rek'to-me) iridectomy.

corectopia (kōr"ek-to'pe-ah) abnormal location of the pupil of the eye.

coredialysis (ko"re-di-al'ĭ-sis) creation of an artificial pupil by detaching the iris from the ciliary ligament.

corediastasis (ko"re-di-as'tah-sis) dilatation of the pupil.

corelysis (ko-rel'ĭ-sis) operative destruction of the pupil; especially detachment of adhesions of the iris to the cornea or lens.

coremorphosis (ko"re-mor-fo'sis) coreoplasty.

corenclisis (ko"ren-kli'sis) iridencleisis.

coreometer (ko"re-om'ě-ter) a device for measuring the pupil.

coreoplasty (ko're-o-plas"te) creation of an artificial pupil.

coretomy (ko-ret'o-me) iridotomy.

corium (ko're-um) the fibrous inner layer of the skin, the true skin, derived from the embryonic mesoderm, varying from 1/50 to 1/8 inch in thickness, well supplied with nerves and blood vessels and containing hair roots and sebaceous and sweat glands; on the palms and soles it bears ridges whose arrangement in whorls and loops is peculiar to the individual.

corn (korn) a circumscribed, conical, keratinous mass that causes severe pain by pressure on nerve endings in the corium. Corns are always caused by friction or pressure from poorly fitting shoes or hose. There are two kinds: the hard corn, usually located on the outside of the little toe or on the upper surfaces of the other toes; and the soft corn, a white, sodden mass usually found between the fourth and fifth toes.

cornea (kor'ne-ah) the clear, transparent anterior covering of the EYE. The cornea is subject to injury by foreign bodies in the eye, bacterial infection and viral infection, especially by the herpes simplex virus. The herpes zoster virus, which causes "shingles," can also infect the cornea. Prompt treatment of any corneal injury or infection is essential to avoid ulceration and loss of vision.

corneal (kor'ne-al) pertaining to the cornea.
 c. reflex, a reflex action of the eye resulting in automatic closing of the eyelid when the cornea is stimulated. The corneal reflex can be elicited in a normal person by gently touching the cornea with a wisp of cotton. Absence of the corneal reflex indicates deep coma or injury of one of the nerves carrying the reflex arc.

corneitis (kor"ne-i'tis) inflammation of the cornea.

corneo-iritis (kor"ne-o-i-ri'tis) inflammation of the cornea and iris.

corneosclera (kor"ne-o-skle'rah) the cornea and sclera regarded as one organ.

corneous (kor'ne-us) hornlike.

cornification (kor"nĭ-fĭ-ka'shun) the process of becoming horny.

cornified (kor'nĭ-fīd) converted into horny tissue.

cornu (kor'nu), pl. cor'nua [L.] 1. a hornlike excrescence or projection. 2. an anatomic structure that appears horn-shaped, especially in section.

c. ammo′nis, hippocampus.

c. sacra′le, either of two hook-shaped processes extending downward from the arch of the last sacral vertebra.

cornual (kor′nu-al) pertaining to a horn, especially to the horns of the spinal cord.

corona (kō-ro′nah), pl. *coro′nae* [L.] a crown; used in anatomic nomenclature to designate a crown-like eminence or encircling structure.

c. radia′ta, 1. the widely spread fibers radiating from the internal capsule to the various gyri of the cerebral hemisphere. 2. an investing layer of radially elongated follicle cells surrounding the zona pellucida of the ovum.

coronal (kŏ-ro′nal) pertaining to the crown of the head.

coronary (kor′o-na″re) encircling in the manner of a crown; a term applied to vessels, ligaments, etc.

c. arteries, two large arteries that branch from the ascending portion of the aorta and supply all of the heart muscle with blood.

c. occlusion, the occlusion, or closing off, of a coronary artery. It may occur when the artery is suddenly plugged by a blood clot developing within the vessel (coronary thrombosis), or it may result when mounting fatty deposits in the wall of the vessel finally clog the artery. Coronary occlusion and coronary thrombosis are commonly referred to as a "heart attack" because the situation is usually acute with severe symptoms resulting from damage to the heart muscle (myocardial infarction) and subsequent heart failure.

SYMPTOMS. There is a sudden painful pressure in the chest, occasionally radiating to the arms, throat or back and persisting for hours. There may be vomiting and nausea, which may cause the attack to be mistaken for acute indigestion. In many instances, the victim may be in a state of shock, with profuse perspiration, pallor and anxiety.

TREATMENT. Immediate care consists of combating shock and preventing further circulatory collapse. The victim should be kept lying down and all tight clothing should be loosened. Medical treatment usually includes administration of narcotics such as morphine sulfate and meperidine (Demerol) to relieve pain, and oxygen to relieve cyanosis and assist the heart in its efforts to circulate oxygenated blood through the body.

Absolute bed rest, anticoagulant drugs, dietary restrictions and administration of oxygen as necessary are included in the long-term care of the patient who has suffered a coronary occlusion. The extent of damage done to the myocardium determines the amount and type of activities the patient is allowed to resume after he has been discharged from the hospital. He must remain under the supervision of his physician for an indefinite period of time and should follow his physician's direction conscientiously so as to avoid repetition of an attack if at all possible.

NURSING CARE. During the acute phase of his illness the patient with a coronary occlusion must remain completely at rest. Most patients are restricted to bed, though some physicians may allow the patient to sit up in an armchair if he does not exert himself in any way and is lifted and carried from bed to chair. Whatever the patient's position, he must not be allowed to exert himself in any way

that will place a strain on his heart. As the damaged heart muscle heals he may gradually resume physical activity as directed by the physician. A complete and accurate record should be kept of the vital signs, and they should be taken at least every 4 hours or more frequently during the day, depending on the patient's condition in the earlier phase of the illness. An elevation of temperature often accompanies coronary occlusion because of the inflammation and necrosis produced in the heart muscle. Changes in the pulse and respiration should be reported immediately as they may indicate the development of complications. The patient is also observed for cyanosis, the development of edema, changes in blood pressure and changes in the cardiac rate or rhythm. The utilization of electronic monitoring equipment in coronary care units has aided in the early treatment and even prevention of the complications occurring in coronary occlusion.

c. sinus, a wide channel on the posterior surface of the heart which opens directly into the right atrium into which almost all of the veins of the heart drain.

c. thrombosis, formation of a clot in a coronary artery (see also CORONARY OCCLUSION).

coroner (kor′o-ner) an official of a local community who holds inquests concerning sudden, violent or unexplained deaths.

coroscopy (ko-ros′ko-pe) skiametry, the shadow test for determining the refractive powers of the eye.

corotomy (ko-rot′o-me) iridotomy.

corpulency (kor′pu-len″se) undue fatness; obesity.

corpus (kor′pus), pl. *cor′pora* [L.] body.

c. albi′cans, the mass of fibrous scar tissue replacing the corpus luteum.

cor′pora amyla′cea, starchlike masses in the prostate, neuroglia, etc.

c. callo′sum, an arched mass of white matter, situated at the bottom of the longitudinal fissure, and made up of transverse fibers connecting the cerebral hemispheres.

c. caverno′sum, either of the two columns of erectile tissue of the dorsum of the penis or clitoris.

c. fimbria′tum, a band of white matter bordering the lateral edge of the lower cornu of the lateral ventricle.

c. genicula′tum, one of a pair of tubercles on the lower part of the optic thalami.

c. hemorrhag′icum, 1. a blood clot in a corpus luteum. 2. the stage of a corpus luteum when it contains clotted blood.

c. lu′teum, a yellow mass formed in the graafian follicle after discharge of the ovum. (see also OVULATION).

cor′pora quadrigem′ina, four oval bodies behind the third ventricle of the cerebrum.

c. spongio′sum pe′nis, a column of erectile tissue surrounding the urethral portion of the penis.

c. stria′tum, a gray mass on the floor of either lateral ventricle.

corpuscle (kor′pusl) any small mass, organ or body. adj., **corpus′cular.**

blood c's, formed bodies in the blood.

colostrum c's, large rounded bodies in colostrum, containing droplets of fat and sometimes a nucleus.

Krause's c's, round bodies constituting nerve endings in the mucous membrane of the mouth, nose, eyes and genitalia.

malpighian c., the funnel-like structure constituting the beginning of the structural unit of the kidney (nephron) and comprising the malpighian capsule and its partially enclosed glomerulus.

Purkinje's c's, large, branched nerve cells composing the middle layer of the cortex of the cerebellum.

red blood c., erythrocyte.

white blood c., leukocyte.

correlation   (kor″ĕ-la′shun) in neurology, the union of afferent impulses within a nerve center to bring about an appropriate response.

correspondence   (kor″ĕ-spon′dens) the condition of being in agreement or conformity.

retinal c., the state concerned with the impingement of image-producing stimuli on the retinas of the two eyes.

corrosive   (kō-ro′siv) having a caustic and locally destructive effect.

Cortate   (kor′tāt) trademark for preparations of desoxycorticosterone acetate, a steroid.

Cort-dome   (kort′dōm) trademark for preparations of hydrocortisone, an adrenocortical steroid.

Cortef   (kor′tef) trademark for preparations of hydrocortisone, an adrenocortical steroid.

cortex   (kor′teks), pl. *cor′tices* [L.] an outer layer, as (1) the bark of the trunk or root of a tree, or (2) the outer layer of an organ or other structure, as distinguished from its inner substance. adj., **cor′tical.**

adrenal c., the thick, parenchymatous layer enclosing the medulla of the ADRENAL GLAND.

cerebellar c., the superficial gray matter of the cerebellum.

cerebral c., c. cer′ebri, the convoluted layer of gray matter covering each cerebral hemisphere (see also BRAIN).

renal c., the smooth-textured outer layer of the kidney composed mainly of glomeruli and secretory ducts, extending in columns between the pyramids constituting the renal medulla.

Corti's organ   (cor′tēz) the terminal acoustic apparatus within the scala media of the inner ear, including the rods of Corti and the auditory cells, with their supporting elements.

corticate   (kor′tĭ-kāt) having a cortex or bark.

corticectomy   (kor″tĭ-sek′to-me) excision of an area of cortex of an organ, as of a scar or microgyrus of the cerebral cortex in treatment of focal epilepsy.

corticifugal   (kor″tĭ-sif′u-gal) proceeding away from the cortex.

corticipetal   (kor″tĭ-sip′ĕ-tal) proceeding toward the cortex.

corticoadrenal   (kor″tĭ-ko-ad-re′nal) pertaining to the adrenal cortex.

corticoafferent   (kor″tĭ-ko-af′er-ent) conveying impulses toward the cerebral cortex; corticipetal.

corticoefferent, corticofugal (kor″tĭ-ko-ef′er-ent), (kor″tĭ-kof′u-gal) conveying impulses away from the cerebral cortex; corticifugal.

corticoid   (kor′tĭ-koid) a hormone of the adrenal cortex, or other natural or synthetic compound with similar activity.

corticopeduncular   (kor″tĭ-ko-pe-dung′ku-lar) pertaining to the cortex and peduncles of the brain.

corticopleuritis   (kor″tĭ-ko-ploo-ri′tis) inflammation of the cortical pleura.

corticospinal   (kor″tĭ-ko-spi′nal) pertaining to the cerebral cortex and spinal cord.

corticosteroid   (kor″tĭ-ko-ste′roid) any of the hormones elaborated by the cortex of the adrenal gland; called also adrenocortical hormone and adrenocorticosteroid. All the hormones are steroids having similar chemical structures, but they have quite different physiologic effects. Generally they are divided into GLUCOCORTICOIDS (cortisol or hydrocortisone, cortisone and corticosterone), MINERALOCORTICOIDS (aldosterone and desoxycorticosterone, and also corticosterone) and androgens.

At times of stress or emergency the adrenal cortex responds to a special alarm system which results in increased production of its hormones (alarm reaction). The corticosteroids help supply the body with emergency materials such as amino acids, fatty acids, glucose, sodium and water. These materials are used to provide energy, to increase resistance and aid in tissue repair and to maintain a normal fluid and electrolyte balance.

corticosterone   (kor″tĭ-ko-stēr′ōn) a hormone of the adrenal cortex; it is usually classified as a GLUCOCORTICOID, but it also has slight MINERALOCORTICOID activity.

corticosuprarenoma   (kor″tĭ-ko-su″prah-re-no′mah) a tumor derived from the adrenal cortex.

corticotrophic   (kor″tĭ-ko-trof′ik) adrenocorticotropic.

corticotrophin   (kor″tĭ-ko-tro′fin) corticotropin.

corticotropic   (kor″tĭ-ko-trop′ik) adrenocorticotropic.

corticotropin   (kor″tĭ-ko-tro′pin) 1. adrenocorticotropic hormone (see also ACTH). 2. a pharaceutical preparation derived from the anterior pituitary of mammals; used to stimulate adrenal cortical activity.

cortisol   (kor′tĭ-sol) a hormone from the adrenal cortex; the principal GLUCOCORTICOID. Called also 17-hydroxycorticosterone and, pharmaceutically, hydrocortisone.

cortisone   (kor′tĭ-sōn) a carbohydrate-regulating hormone from the adrenal cortex; one of the GLUCOCORTICOIDS. It can be extracted from animals and prepared synthetically from plants and is used in the treatment of adrenal deficiencies, for other disorders such as arthritis and rheumatic fever and in certain allergic conditions.

Cortogen   (kor′to-jen) trademark for preparations of cortisone.

Cortone (kor′tōn) trademark for preparations of cortisone.

Cortrophin (kor-tro′fin) trademark for preparations of corticotropin.

coruscation (kor″us-ka′shun) the sensation as of a flash of light before the eyes.

corybantism (kor″e-ban′tism) delirium with hallucinations.

Corynebacterium (ko-ri″ne-bak-te′re-um) a genus of Schizomycetes.
  C. diphthe′riae, the causative agent of diphtheria.
  C. pseudodiphtherit′icum, a nonpathogenic microorganism present in the upper respiratory tract.

coryza (ko-ri′zah) profuse discharge from the mucous membrane of the nose.
  allergic c., hay fever.

coryzavirus (ko-ri″zah-vi′rus) one of a group of viral agents isolated from patients with the common cold.

cosmetic (koz-met′ik) 1. improving the appearance. 2. an agent or substance used to improve the appearance.

cost(o)- (kos′to) word element [L.], *rib*.

costa (kos′tah), pl. *cos′tae* [L.] a rib. adj., **cos′tal.**

costectomy (kos-tek′to-me) excision of a rib.

costive (kos′tiv) 1. pertaining to, characterized by or producing constipation. 2. an agent that depresses intestinal motility.

costiveness (kos′tiv-nes) constipation.

costocervical (kos″to-ser′vĭ-kal) pertaining to the ribs and neck.

costochondral (kos″to-kon′dral) pertaining to a rib and its cartilage.

costoclavicular (kos″to-klah-vik′u-lar) pertaining to the ribs and clavicle.

costocoracoid (kos″to-kor′ah-koid) pertaining to the ribs and coracoid process.

costopneumopexy (kos″to-nu′mo-pek″se) fixation of the lung to a rib.

costosternal (kos″to-ster′nal) pertaining to the ribs and sternum.

costosternoplasty (kos″to-ster′no-plas″te) plastic repair of congenital chondrosternal depression, the sternum being straightened and supported with a segment of rib.

costotomy (kos-tot′o-me) transection of a rib.

costotransverse (kos″to-trans-vers′) lying between the ribs and the transverse processes of the vertebrae.

costovertebral (kos″to-ver′tĕ-bral) pertaining to a rib and a vertebra.

Cothera (ko-ther′ah) trademark for preparations of dimethoxanate hydrochloride, a cough medication.

co-twin (ko′twin) one of two individuals produced at the same gestation and born at the same time.

cotyledon (kot″ĭ-le′don) any subdivision of the uterine surface of the placenta.

couching (kowch′ing) displacement of the lens of the eye in cataract.

cough (kof) a sudden noisy expulsion of air from the lungs.
  dry c., cough without expectoration.
  productive c., cough attended with expectoration of material from the bronchi.
  reflex c., cough due to irritation of some remote organ.
  whooping c., pertussis, an infectious disease caused by *Bordetella pertussis*, characterized by coryza, bronchitis and a typical cough (see also WHOOPING COUGH).

coulomb (koo′lom) the unit of electrical quantity.

Coumadin (koo′mah-din) trademark for preparations of warfarin sodium, an anticoagulant.

coumarin (koo′mah-rin) colorless, prismatic crystals, $C_9H_6O_2$, used as a flavoring agent.

count (kownt) ascertainment of the number of individual units (e.g., blood corpuscles, cells) in a given series or quantity of solution.
  Addis c., a count of the cells in 10 cc. of urinary sediment as a means of calculating total urinary sediment in a 12-hour specimen.

counter (kown′ter) an apparatus for determining the number of units in any collection.
  Geiger c., Geiger-Müller c., a device for electrically determining the number of ionized particles emitted by a substance.
  scintillation c., a device for indicating the emission of ionizing particles, permitting determination of the concentration of radioisotopes in the body.

counterextension (kown″ter-eks-ten′shun) traction in a proximal direction coincident with traction in opposition to it.

counterirritant (kown″ter-ir′ĭ-tant) 1. producing counterirritation. 2. an agent that produces counterirritation.

counterirritation (kown″ter-ir″ĭ-ta′shun) superficial irritation intended to relieve some other irritation.

counteropening (kown″ter-o′pen-ing) a second opening, as in an abscess, made to facilitate drainage.

countertraction (kown′ter-trak″shun) traction opposed to another traction; used in reduction of fractures.

countertransference (kown″ter-trans-fer′ens) displacement of feelings and projection of needs and conflicts of the therapist onto the patient in psychotherapy.

coup (koo) [Fr.] stroke.
  c. de sabre (koo-duh-sahb), a linear, circumscribed lesion of scleroderma on the forehead or scalp, so called because of its resemblance to the scar of a saber wound.

coverglass (kuv′er-glas) a small plate of optical

glass of controlled thickness, used over material placed on a slide for microscopic study.

coverslip (kuv′er-slip) a small plate of plastic or other transparent substance used over material placed on a slide for microscopic study.

cowperitis (kow″per-i′tis) inflammation of the bulbourethral (Cowper's) glands, located in the urethral sphincter.

cowpox (kow′poks) a pustular eruption affecting cattle and related to smallpox in humans; called also vaccinia. Edward Jenner, in the 18th century, discovered that cowpox could be transmitted to humans who milked or tended cattle, and also noted that persons who contracted it in this way seldom contracted smallpox. This discovery led to vaccination against smallpox.

coxa (kok′sah), pl. *cox′ae* [L.] the hip, or hip joint.
c. pla′na, flattening of the head of the femur resulting from osteochondrosis of its epiphysis.
c. val′ga, deformity of the hip joint with increase in the angle of inclination between the neck and shaft of the femur.
c. va′ra, deformity of the hip joint with decrease in the angle of inclination between the neck and shaft of the femur.

coxalgia (kok-sal′je-ah) tuberculosis of the hip joint.

Coxiella (kok″se-el′ah) a genus of microorganisms of the order Rickettsiales.
C. burnet′ii, the causative agent of Q fever.

coxitis (kok-si′tis) inflammation of the hip joint.

coxodynia (kok″so-din′e-ah) pain in the hip.

coxofemoral (kok″so-fem′o-ral) pertaining to the hip and thigh.

coxotuberculosis (kok″so-tu-ber″ku-lo′sis) tuberculosis of the hip joint.

Coxsackie virus (kok-sak′e) one of a heterogeneous group of enteroviruses producing in man a disease resembling poliomyelitis, but without paralysis.
C. v. A disease, herpangina.

cozymase (ko-zi′mās) a coenzyme in yeast, muscle and blood serum.

c.p.m. counts per minute, an expression of the particles emitted after administration of a radioactive material such as the isotope iodine-131 (^{131}I).

Cr chemical symbol, *chromium.*

cradle (kra′dl) a frame for placing over the body of a patient, under the bed coverings, for application of heat or for protecting injured parts.
c. cap, an oily yellowish crust that sometimes appears on the scalp of nursing infants; also called milk crust (crusta lactea). The crust is caused by excessive secretion of the sebaceous glands in the scalp. Treatment consists of applications of oil or a bland ointment and frequent scalp shampoos until the crust is removed.
electric c., heat c., a frame with wiring for light bulbs, for applications of heat to the patient's body.

Craigia (kra′ge-ah) a genus of ameboid protozoa parasitic in the intestine and causing dysentery.

cramp (kramp) a painful spasmodic muscular contraction.
heat c., spasm accompanied by pain, weak pulse and dilated pupils; seen in workers in intense heat.
recumbency c's, cramping in the muscles of the legs and feet occurring while resting or during light sleep.
writers' c., spasm and neuralgia of the fingers, hand and forearm, due to excessive writing.

crani(o)- (kra′ne-o) word element [L.], *skull.*

cranial (kra′ne-al) pertaining to the cranium.
c. nerves, nerves that are attached to the brain and pass through the openings of the skull. There are 12 pairs of cranial nerves, symmetrically arranged so that they are distributed mainly to the structures of the head and neck. The one exception, the vagus nerve, extends beyond the head and carries among its fibers the motor fibers that go to the bronchi, stomach, gallbladder, small intestine and part of the large intestine. It also carries the fibers that control the release of secretions of the gastric glands and the pancreas, and inhibitory fibers to the heart.
Some of the cranial nerves are both sensory and motor; i.e., they control motion as well as conduct sensory impulses. Others are sensory or motor only.

CRANIAL NERVES (See also table of NERVES)		
I	Olfactory	Sensory
II	Optic	Sensory
III	Oculomotor	Mixed
IV	Trochlear	Mixed
V	Trigeminal	
	Ophthalmic	Sensory
	Maxillary	Sensory
	Mandibular	Mixed
VI	Abducens	Motor
VII	Facial	Mixed
VIII	Vestibulocochlear	
	Cochlear	Sensory
	Vestibular	Sensory
IX	Glossopharyngeal	Mixed
X	Vagus	Mixed
XI	Accessory	Motor
XII	Hypoglossal	Motor

craniectomy (kra″ne-ek′to-me) excision of a segment of the skull.

craniocele (kra′ne-o-sēl″) protrusion of part of the brain through the skull.

craniocerebral (kra″ne-o-ser′ĕ-bral) pertaining to the skull and brain.

cranioclasis (kra″ne-ok′lah-sis) crushing of the fetal skull in difficult labor.

cranioclast (kra′ne-o-klast″) an instrument for crushing the fetal skull in utero.

craniocleidodysostosis (kra″ne-o-kli″do-dis″os-to′sis) cleidocranial dysostosis.

craniodidymus (kra″ne-o-did′ĭ-mus) a fetal monster with two heads.

craniofacial (kra″ne-o-fa′shal) pertaining to the cranium and face.

craniograph (kra′ne-o-graf″) an instrument for outlining the skull.

craniology (kra″ne-ol′o-je) the scientific study of skulls.

craniomalacia (kra″ne-o-mah-la′she-ah) abnormal softness of the bones of the skull.

craniometer (kra″ne-om′ĕ-ter) an instrument for measuring the head.

craniometry (kra″ne-om′ĕ-tre) measurement of the skull and facial bones.

craniopagus (kra″ne-op′ah-gus) a double fetal monster joined at the head.

craniopharyngeal (kra″ne-o-fah-rin′je-al) pertaining to the cranium and pharynx.

craniopharyngioma (kra″ne-o-fah-rin″je-o′mah) a tumor arising from the remnants of the craniopharyngeal duct, an embryonic structure composed of the elongated Rathke's pouch joining the infundibulum of the embryonic pituitary gland.

cranioplasty (kra′ne-o-plas″te) plastic repair of the skull.

craniopuncture (kra′ne-o-pungk″tūr) exploratory puncture of the brain.

craniorachischisis (kra″ne-o-rah-kis′kĭ-sis) congenital fissure of the skull and vertebral column.

craniosacral (kra″ne-o-sa′kral) pertaining to the skull and sacrum.

cranioschisis (kra″ne-os′kĭ-sis) congenital fissure of the skull.

craniosclerosis (kra″ne-o-sklĕ-ro′sis) abnormal calcification and thickening of the cranial bones.

cranioscopy (kra″ne-os′ko-pe) diagnostic examination of the head.

craniospinal (kra″ne-o-spi′nal) pertaining to the skull and spine.

craniostenosis (kra″ne-o-stĕ-no′sis) narrowness of the skull due to premature closure of the cranial sutures.

craniostosis, craniosynostosis (kra″ne-os-to′-sis), (kra″ne-o-sin″os-to′sis) premature closure of the cranial sutures.

craniotabes (kra″ne-o-ta′bēz) reduction in mineralization of the skull, with abnormal softness of the bone and widening of the sutures and fontanels, occurring chiefly in rickets.

craniotome (kra′ne-o-tōm″) a cutting instrument used in craniotomy.

craniotomy (kra″ne-ot′o-me) opening of the skull, as for surgery on the brain or decompression of the fetal head in difficult labor.

craniotympanic (kra″ne-o-tim-pan′ik) pertaining to the skull and tympanum.

cranium (kra′ne-um), pl. *cra′nia* [L.] the skeleton of the head, exclusive of the mandible and facial bones.

crater (kra′ter) an excavated area with surrounding wall, such as is caused by ulceration.

craterization (kra″ter-ĭ-za′shun) excision of bone tissue to create a crater-like depression.

C-reactive protein test a nonspecific test for inflammation and necrosis; called also C.R.P. test. For reasons not clearly understood, inflammation and tissue breakdown give rise to the C-reactive protein, a substance that forms a precipitate with the C-polysaccharide of the pneumococcus. Blood from patients with inflammatory conditions or disorders accompanied by necrosis gives a positive result with the test, and it is therefore of some use in diagnosing or determining the progress of such disorders as rheumatoid arthritis, acute rheumatic fever, widespread malignancy and bacterial infections.

Creamalin (krēm′ah-lin) trademark for preparations of aluminum hydroxide gel, used as an antacid.

creatinase (kre-at′ĭ-nās) an enzyme that catalyzes the decomposition of creatine.

creatine (kre′ah-tin) a nonprotein substance synthesized in the body from three amino acids: arginine, glycine (aminoacetic acid) and methionine. Creatine readily combines with phosphate to form phosphocreatine, or creatine phosphate, which is present in muscle, where it serves as the storage form of high-energy phosphate necessary for muscle contraction.
  c. phosphokinase, an enzyme found mainly in muscle, heart and brain that catalyzes the transfer of the high-energy phosphate bond to and from creatine.

creatinemia (kre″ah-tĭ-ne′me-ah) excessive creatine in the blood.

creatinine (kre-at′ĭ-nin) a nitrogenous compound formed as a metabolic end product of creatine. It is formed in the muscle in relatively small amounts, passes into the blood and is excreted in the urine.
  A laboratory test for the creatinine level in the blood may be used as a measurement of kidney function. Since creatinine is normally produced in fairly constant amounts as a result of the breakdown of phosphocreatine and is excreted in the urine, an elevation in the creatinine level in the blood indicates a disturbance in kidney function. Normal range for the creatinine level is 0.6 to 1.3 mg. per 100 ml. of serum. The patient must be in a state of rest for the test, but fasting is not necessary. If the dyes Bromsulphalein and phenolsulfonphthalein have been given to the patient within the previous 24 hours, the creatine level may be elevated.

creatinuria (kre-at″ĭ-nu′re-ah) the presence of creatine in the urine.

creatorrhea (kre″ah-to-re′ah) the presence of muscle fibers in the feces.

creatotoxism (kre″ah-to-tok′sizm) acute gastroenteritis caused by bacterial toxins present in meat.

cremaster muscle (kre-mas′ter) the muscle that elevates the testis (see table of MUSCLES).

cremasteric (kre″mas-ter′ik) pertaining to the cremaster muscle.

crenated (kre′nāt-ed) having a notched or scalloped border; used to describe abnormal erythrocytes seen especially in hypertonic solutions.

crenation (kre-na′shun) the production of indentations in the surface of a cell, especially an erythrocyte, due to withdrawal of moisture from the cytoplasm, and giving it a notched appearance.

crenocyte (kre′no-sīt) a crenated erythrocyte.

creosote (kre′o-sōt) a mixture of phenols from wood tar; used as a disinfectant.

crepitant (krep′ĭ-tant) having a dry, crackling sound.

crepitation (krep″ĭ-ta′shun) a dry, crackling sound or sensation, such as that produced by the grating of the ends of a fractured bone.

crepitus (krep′ĭ-tus) 1. crepitation. 2. a crepitant rale.

crescent (kres′ent) a structure shaped like a new moon.
   Giannuzzi's c's, crescentic cell masses on the basement membrane of the acini of the glands that secrete mucus.
   sublingual c., the crescent-shaped area on the floor of the mouth, bounded by the lingual wall of the mandible and the base of the tongue.

cresol (kre′sol) a phenol from coal or wood tar; a preparation consisting of a mixture of isomeric cresol from coal tar or petroleum is used as a disinfectant.

cresomania (kres″o-ma′ne-ah) abnormal delusions of possessing great wealth.

crest (krest) a projection, or projecting structure or ridge, especially one surmounting a bone or its border.
   dental c., the maxillary ridge passing along the alveolar processes of the fetal maxillary bones.
   iliac c., the thickened, expanded upper border of the ilium.

cresylic acid (krĕ-sil′ik) cresol.

cretin (kre′tin) a patient exhibiting cretinism.

cretinism (kre′tĭ-nizm) arrested physical and mental development with dystrophy of bones and soft tissues, due to congenital lack of thyroid gland secretion from underfunctioning or absence of the gland. The child has a large head, short limbs, puffy eyes, a thick and protruding tongue, excessively dry skin, lack of coordination and mental retardation. The acquired or adult form of thyroid deficiency is MYXEDEMA.
   Administration of thyroid extract, which must be continued for life, can result in normal growth and mental development. If untreated, the child will become permanently dwarfed, probably mentally retarded and sterile.

cretinoid (kre′tĭ-noid) resembling a cretin.

cretinous (kre′tĭ-nus) affected with cretinism.

crevice (krev′is) a fissure.

gingival c., the space between the enamel of the neck of a tooth and the overlying unattached gingiva.

cribriform (krib′rĭ-form) perforated like a sieve.

cricoarytenoid (kri″ko-ar″ĭ-te′noid) pertaining to the cricoid and arytenoid cartilages.

cricoid (kri′koid) shaped like a signet ring.
   c. cartilage, a ringlike cartilage forming the lower and back part of the larynx.

cricoidectomy (kri″koi-dek′to-me) excision of the cricoid cartilage.

cricopharyngeal (kri″ko-fah-rin′je-al) pertaining to the cricoid cartilage and pharynx.

cricothyreotomy (kri″ko-thi″re-ot′o-me) incision through the cricoid and thyroid cartilages.

cricotomy (kri-kot′o-me) incision of the cricoid cartilage.

cricotracheotomy (kri″ko-tra″ke-ot′o-me) incision of the trachea through the cricoid cartilage.

Crigler-Najjar disease (krig′ler naj′er) a rare form of congenital familial nonhemolytic jaundice with kernicterus that results from defective bilirubin conjugation in the liver.

crinogenic (krin″o-jen′ik) causing secretion in a gland.

crisis (kri′sis) pl. *cri′ses* [L.] 1. the turning point of a disease. 2. a paroxysmal attack of pain, especially in tabes dorsalis.
   addisonian c., symptoms of fatigue, nausea and vomiting and weight loss accompanying an acute attack of Addison's disease.
   tabetic c., a painful paroxysm occurring in tabes dorsalis.
   thyroid c., thyrotoxic c., a sudden and dangerous increase of the symptoms of thyrotoxicosis.

crista (kris′tah) pl. *cris′tae* [L.] crest.
   cris′tae cu′tis, ridges of the skin produced by the projecting papillae of the corium on the palm of the hand and sole of the foot, producing a fingerprint and footprint characteristic of the individual; called also dermal ridges.
   c. gal′li, a thick triangular process projecting upward from the cribriform plate of the ethmoid bone.

C.R.N.A. Certified Registered Nurse Anesthetist.

Crocq's disease (kroks) acrocyanosis.

Crohn's disease (krōnz) inflammation of the terminal portion of the ileum; called also regional enteritis and regional ileitis.

cross (kros) a mating between organisms having different genes determining particular traits of inheritance.

crossbite (kros′bīt) a condition in which mandibular teeth are in buccal version to the maxillary teeth.

crossed eyes an eye condition in which both eyes cannot be focused on the same object at the same time; the result is that one eye focuses on the object, while the other eye is turned away from it. Called also squint or STRABISMUS.

crossing over (kros′ing o′ver) the exchange of

segments between homologous chromosomes, permitting new combinations of genes.

crossmatching (kros-mach'ing) a procedure vital in blood transfusions, testing for agglutination of donor erythrocytes by recipient's serum, and of recipient's red cells by donor serum.

crotamiton (kro"tah-mi'ton) a compound used in the treatment of scabies.

crotchet (kroch'et) a hook used in extracting the fetus after craniotomy.

croton oil (kro'ton) a cathartic used when rapid severe purgation is required. Because of its high toxicity and extreme irritant effect on the intestinal membranes, it has been deleted from the U.S.P. and replaced by equally effective but less dangerous drugs. It is administered by placing a few drops of the oil on a piece of bread or cube of sugar.

crotonism (kro'ton-izm) poisoning by croton oil.

croup (kroōp) a condition resulting from acute obstruction of the larynx caused by allergy, foreign body, infection or new growth, occurring chiefly in infants and children.

CHARACTERISTICS. Croup in itself is not a disease but a group of symptoms of varied origin with the following general characteristics: (1) obstruction of the upper respiratory tract, usually at the level of the larynx or just below it in the trachea; (2) hoarseness; (3) a cough, usually described as "barking"; and (4) a croaking sound, called stridor, during inspiration.

A typical attack of croup usually begins at night, and is often precipitated by exposure to cold air. The onset is sudden, with hoarse, "croupy" voice or cough, and what seems like difficult breathing. Spasms of choking that seem close to strangulation follow.

NURSING CARE. An atmosphere of high humidity is provided to liquefy the secretions and reduce the spasm of the laryngeal muscles. Warm, moist air may be provided by a vaporizer and croup tent. Cool, moist air is provided by special equipment such as a Croupette which cools the air and converts it into a fine mist. Cool air is preferred if the patient has a fever because the warm, moist air tends to elevate the body temperature. While providing an atmosphere of high humidity, it is important to keep the patient dry and comfortable and prevent chilling.

An emetic, such as syrup of ipecac, may be ordered to induce vomiting and thereby reduce laryngeal spasms. The child must have someone in attendance until the vomiting has stopped and there is no further danger of aspiration of the vomitus.

An attitude of calm does much to help the patient relax and also reassures the parents of the child. Although croup is very frightening, with a sudden onset and dramatic symptoms of asphyxia, it is rarely fatal and the prognosis is very good.

Observations include rate and character of respirations, color of the skin, degree of restlessness and anxiety and degree of prostration.

Crouzon's disease (kroo-zonz') craniofacial dysostosis.

crown (krown) the topmost part of an organ or structure; a crown-shaped structure, especially the exposed or enamel-covered part of a tooth.

artificial c., a metal, porcelain or plastic reproduction of a crown affixed to the remaining natural structure of a tooth.

crowning (krown'ing) the appearance of the fetal scalp at the vaginal orifice in childbirth.

C.R.P. C-reactive protein.

crucial (kroo'shal) 1. cross-shaped. 2. decisive.

cruciate (kroo'she-āt) shaped like a cross.

crucible (kroo'sĭ-bl) a laboratory vessel in which samples under study can be subjected to high temperatures.

cruciform (kroo'sĭ-form) cross-shaped.

cruor (kroo'or) a blood clot that contains erythrocytes.

crus (krus), pl. *cru'ra* [L.] a leg or leglike structure. adj., **cru'ral.**
c. cer'ebri, a structure comprising fiber tracts descending from the cerebral cortex to form the longitudinal fascicles of the pons.
c. of clitoris, the continuation of the corpus cavernosum of the clitoris diverging posteriorly to be attached to the pubic arch.
crura of diaphragm, two pillars that connect the diaphragm to the vertebral column.
crura of fornix, two flattened bands of white matter that unite to form the body of the fornix of the cerebrum.
c. of penis, the continuation of each corpus cavernosum of the penis, diverging posteriorly to be attached to the pubic arch.

crush syndrome (krush) the edema, oliguria and other symptoms of renal failure that follow crushing of a part, especially a large muscle mass.

crust (krust) the dried residue of exudate from an erosive or ulcerative skin lesion, or from the intact skin.

crusta (krus'tah), pl. *crus'tae* [L.] 1. any crust. 2. the part of the crus cerebri below the substantia nigra.

Crustacea (krus-ta'she-ah) a class of animals including the lobsters, crabs, shrimps, wood lice and water fleas.

crutches (kruch'ez) artificial supports, made of wood or metal, used by those who need aid in walking because of injury, disease or a birth defect.

TYPES. Crutches are made in different sizes suitable for persons of various heights. For the most part they are made of wood or tubular aluminum. The standard type is the tall crutch that fits under the armpits with double uprights and a small horizontal hand bar stretched between the uprights. The lower part is sometimes adjustable to allow for extensions. There always should be a rubber tip at the base, preferably a suction tip, to prevent slipping.

Gaining in popularity is the Lofstrand crutch, which consists of a single tube of aluminum surmounted by a metal cuff that fits around the forearm. The user supports his weight on a hand bar. He can release his hold on the handbar, as in grasping a handrail to climb stairs, without dropping the

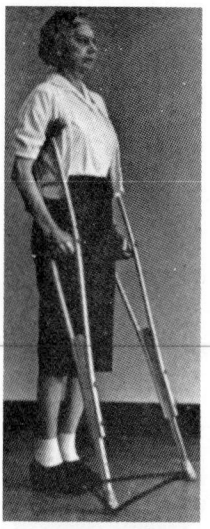

The four-point alternate gait is the slowest and safest crutch gait. It offers maximum balance and support because there are always three points of contact with the ground. From the left, it begins from the tripod position in which all gaits begin. The right crutch is brought forward, and then the left foot. The left crutch comes forward and then the right foot.

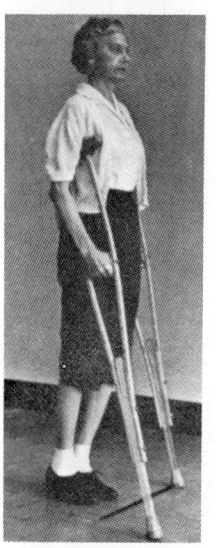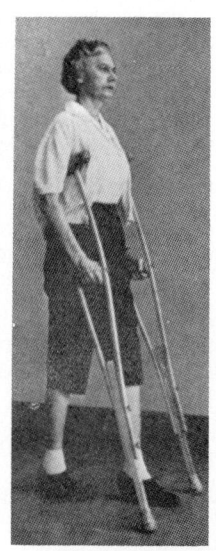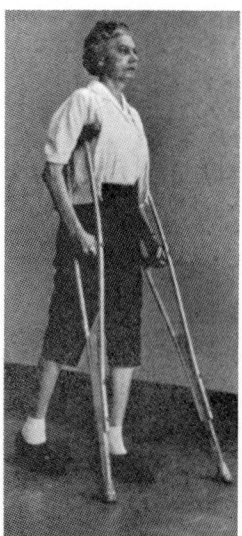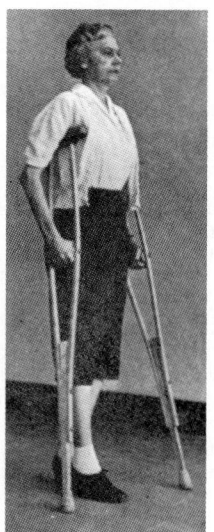

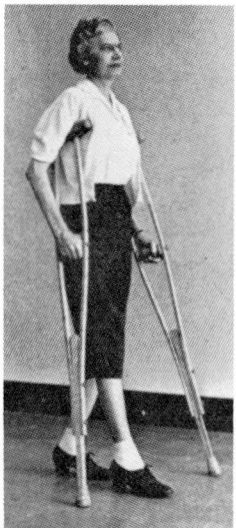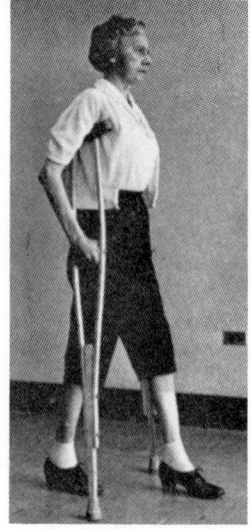

This three-point gait is used by patients who can bear some weight on the injured leg or foot. It begins from the tripod position. Then both crutches and the affected leg are brought forward at the same time. The patient must then rest lightly on the crutches while she moves the unaffected limb forward.

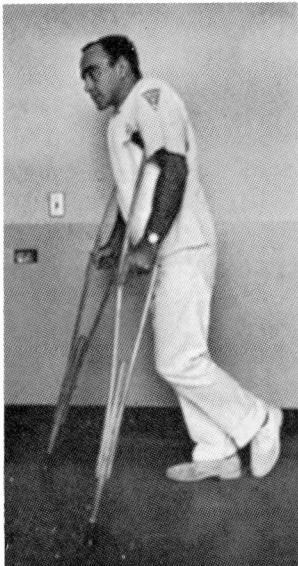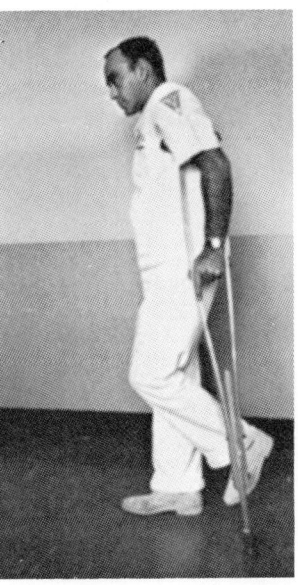

This three-point gait is used by patients who cannot bear any weight on the affected leg or foot. It begins from the tripod position. Both crutches are brought forward and the uninjured leg is brought forward through the crutches. The affected leg follows in a swinging movement because it is raised from the ground.

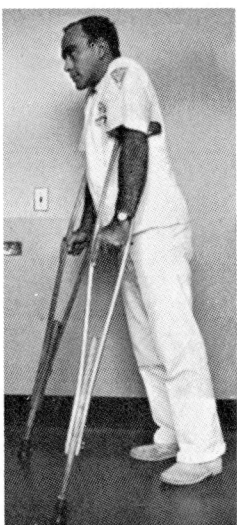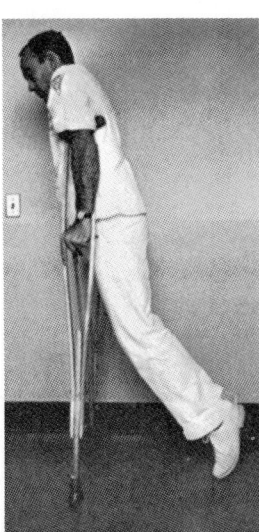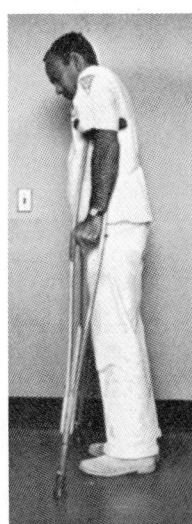

The swing-to gait is slower than the swing-through gait. From the tripod position, the patient places both crutches forward, either alternately or at the same time, and then swings his body ahead into a tripod position. The crutches and feet must never be even or the patient loses stability. In the drag-to gait, the patient slides his feet along the ground and does not raise them.

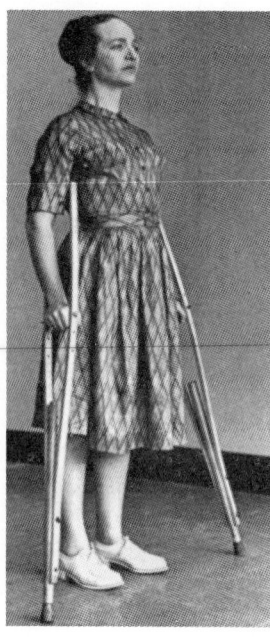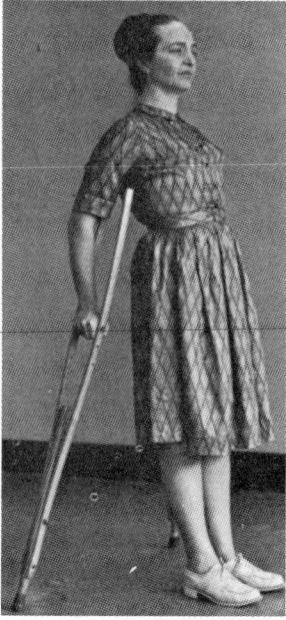

The swing-through gait is used mainly by paraplegics and severe arthritics who have good balance and muscle power in the arms and hands. From the tripod position, both crutches are brought forward, the patient bears down on the handpieces, lifts the body and swings it through the crutches into a reversed tripod position. To maintain balance in this gait, the pelvis moves first, then the shoulders and head.

crutch. A variation of the Lofstrand crutch is the Canadian elbow extensor crutch, which goes farther up the arm.

In walking with crutches, the means of locomotion is transferred from the legs to the arms. The muscles of the arms, shoulders, back and chest work together to manipulate the crutches. The kind of crutches used depends largely on the nature of the disability. In some cases, the legs may be partially able to function and bear some of the body's weight, so that there is less dependence on the crutches. In other cases leg BRACES may be needed to supplement the crutches.

GAITS. The user is taught one of several standard methods or gaits, according to his condition. Eventually he should be able to master at least two gaits: a fast one for making speed in the open, and a slow one for crowded places where the chief need is to maintain balance. A variety of gaits also helps to relieve fatigue because one set of muscles can rest while another works.

In describing a gait each foot and crutch is called a point, so that a two-point gait, for example, means that two points of the total of four are in contact with the ground during the performance of one step. A three-point gait may be used when one leg is stronger than the other, meaning that two crutches and the weaker leg hit the ground simultaneously while the next step is made by the stronger leg alone. There is also the so-called tripod gait, swinging gait and variations of them.

Cruveilhier's disease (kroo-vāl-yāz′) 1. simple ulcer of the stomach. 2. progressive myelopathic muscular atrophy.

cry(o)- (kri′o) word element [Gr.], *cold.*

cryalgesia (kri″al-je′ze-ah) pain on application of cold.

cryanesthesia (kri″an-es-the′ze-ah) loss of power of perceiving cold.

cryesthesia (kri″es-the′ze-ah) abnormal sensitiveness to cold.

crymophylactic (kri″mo-fi-lak′tik) resistant to cold.

crymotherapy (kri″mo-ther′ah-pe) cryotherapy.

cryobiology (kri″o-bi-ol′o-je) the science dealing with the effect of low temperatures on biological systems.

cryocardioplegia (kri″o-kar″de-o-ple′je-ah) cessation of contraction of the myocardium produced by application of cold during cardiac surgery.

cryocautery (kri″o-kaw′ter-e) cold cautery.

cryocrit (kri′o-krit) the percentage of the total volume of blood serum or plasma occupied by cryoprecipitates after centrifugation.

cryofibrinogen (kri″o-fi-brin′o-jen) a blood protein resembling fibrinogen that precipitates from plasma on cooling.

cryofibrinogenemia (kri″o-fi-brin″o-jĕ-ne′me-ah) the presence of cryofibrinogens in the blood.

cryogammaglobulin (kri″o-gam″ah-glob′u-lin) a gamma globulin readily precipitated from plasma on cooling.

cryogenic (kri″o-jen′ik) producing low temperatures.

cryoglobulin (kri″o-glob′u-lin) a serum globulin that precipitates, gels or crystallizes spontaneously at low temperatures.

cryoglobulinemia (kri″o-glob″u-lin-e′me-ah) the presence in the blood of cryoglobulins.

cryometer (kri-om′ĕ-ter) a thermometer for measuring very low temperature.

cryophilic (kri″o-fil′ik) preferring or growing best at low temperatures; psychrophilic.

cryoprecipitate (kri″o-pre-sip′ĭ-tāt) any precipitate that results from cooling.

cryoprotein (kri″o-pro′te-in) a blood protein that precipitates on cooling.

cryoscopy (kri-os′ko-pe) examination of fluids based on the principle that the freezing point of a solution varies according to the amount and nature of the solute.

cryostat (kri′o-stat) a device interposed in a cooling system by which temperature is automatically maintained between certain levels.

cryosurgery (kri″o-ser′jer-e) the destruction of tissue by application of extreme cold, as in the destruction of lesions in the thalamus for the treatment of Parkinson's disease and the treatment of certain malignant lesions of the skin and mucous membranes. The method has also been used successfully in some types of surgery of the eye, for example, in the removal of cataracts and the repair of retinal detachment.

cryotherapy (kri″o-ther′ah-pe) the therapeutic use of cold (see also HYPOTHERMIA).

cryotolerant (kri″o-tol′er-ant) able to withstand very low temperatures.

crypt (kript) a follicle or pit.
  anal c's, small recesses in the rectal mucosa, arranged circumferentially about the proximal margin of the anal canal and opening superiorly.
  c's of Lieberkühn, simple tubular glands opening on the surface of the intestinal mucous membrane.
  c's of tongue, deep, irregular invaginations from the surface of the lingual tonsil.
  tonsillar c's, the blind ends of the tonsillar fossulae on the palatine tonsils.

crypt(o)- (krip′to) word element [Gr.], *concealed; pertaining to a crypt.*

cryptectomy (krip-tek′to-me) excision or obliteration of a crypt.

cryptenamine (krip-ten′ah-mīn) a mixture of alkaloids from an extract of *Veratrum viride,* used to lower blood pressure.

cryptesthesia (krip″tes-the′ze-ah) subconscious perception of occurrences not ordinarily perceptible to the senses.

cryptitis (krip-ti′tis) inflammation of the mucous membrane of the anal crypts.

cryptocephalus (krip″to-sef′ah-lus) a fetal monster with an inconspicuous head.

cryptococcosis (krip″to-kok-o′sis) infection by fungi of the genus Cryptococcus.

Cryptococcus (krip″to-kok′us) a genus of fungi.
  C. capsula′tus, *Histoplasma capsulatum.*

C. neofor′mans, a species of yeastlike fungi of worldwide distribution, causing infection in man.

cryptodidymus (krip″to-did′ĭ-mus) a twin monster, one fetus being enclosed within the body of the other.

cryptoglioma (krip″to-gli-o′mah) one stage of glioma in which presence of the growth is masked.

cryptolith (krip′to-lith) a concretion in a crypt.

cryptomenorrhea (krip″to-men″o-re′ah) suppression of menstruation.

cryptomerorachischisis (krip″to-me″ro-rah-kis′-kĭ-sis) spina bifida occulta.

cryptomnesia (krip″tom-ne′ze-ah) the recall of events not recognized as part of one's conscious experience.

cryptophthalmos (krip″tof-thal′mos) congenital absence of the fissure between the eyelids, the eyeball being rudimentary or absent.

cryptopodia (krip″to-po′de-ah) swelling of the lower leg and foot, covering all but the sole of the foot.

cryptorchid (krip-tor′kid) a person with undescended testes.

cryptorchidectomy (krip″tor-kĭ-dek′to-me) excision of an undescended testis.

cryptorchidism, cryptorchism (krip-tor′kĭ-dizm), (krip-tor′kizm) retention of one or both of the testes in the abdominal cavity. As the unborn male child develops, the testes first appear in the abdomen at about the level of the kidney. They develop at this site, and in approximately the seventh month of fetal life start to descend to the upper part of the groin. From there they move into the inguinal canal and then, normally, into the scrotum. In its descent, a testis may sometimes be halted in the abdomen or within the canal, becoming an undescended testis.
  An improperly developed testis may never leave the abdomen, and it may not produce the hormones that cause secondary sex characters. A testis lodged in the canal may well produce these secondary sex characters, but cannot produce spermatozoa.
  Cases in which both testes fail to descend are most uncommon. Usually only one testis is involved and the other produces sufficient numbers of spermatozoa.
  TREATMENT. Often the undescended testis can be brought down into the scrotum by medical treatment with the gonadotropic hormone, and for physical and psychologic reasons this method is preferred.
  Frequently, however, surgery is required. The operation is not particularly serious and is usually successful. It is best performed when the patient is 5 to 7 years old, since operating at a later age may involve more risk to the cells that produce spermatozoa. The procedure is called an ORCHIOPEXY.

cryptorrhea (krip″to-re′ah) abnormal activity of an organ of internal secretion.

cryptoscope (krip′to-skōp) fluoroscope.

cryptotoxic (krip″to-tok′sik) having hidden toxic properties.

cryptoxanthin (krip″to-zan′thin) a pigment in egg yolk, green grass and yellow corn that can be converted in the body into vitamin A.

cryptozygous (krip″to-zi′gus) having the calvaria wider than the face, so that the zygomatic arches are concealed when the head is viewed from above.

crystal (kris′tal) a naturally produced angular solid of definite form.

crystallin (kris′tah-lin) globulin from the lens of the eye.

crystalline (kris′tah-lin) resembling a crystal in nature or clearness.
  c. lens, the transparent organ behind the pupil of the eye (see also LENS).

crystalloid (kris′tah-loid) 1. resembling a crystal. 2. a noncolloid substance. Crystalloids form true solutions and therefore are capable of passing through a semipermeable membrane, as in DIALYSIS. The physical opposite of a crystalloid is a colloid, which does not dissolve and does not form true solutions.

crystallophobia (kris″tah-lo-fo′be-ah) morbid fear of glass or glass objects.

crystalluria (kris″tah-lu′re-ah) the presence of crystals in the urine, causing irritation of the kidney.

crystalluridrosis (kris″tah-lu″rĭ-dro′sis) crystallization on the skin of urinary elements from the perspiration.

Crysticillin (kris″tĭ-sil′in) trademark for aqueous preparations of procaine penicillin G.

Crystodigin (kris″to-dij′in) trademark for preparations of crystalline digitoxin.

Crystoids (kris′toidz) trademark for anthelmintic pills of hexylresorcinol.

Cs chemical symbol, *cesium.*

C.S.F. cerebrospinal fluid.

C.S.M. cerebrospinal meningitis.

Cu chemical symbol, *copper* (L. *cuprum*).

cu. cubic.

cubitus (ku′bĭ-tus) the forearm. adj., **cu′bital.**

cuboid (ku′boid) resembling a cube; applied particularly to a bone of the foot.

cu. cm. cubic centimeter.

cuffing (kuf′ing) formation of a cufflike surrounding border, as of leukocytes about a blood vessel observed in certain infections.

cuirass (kwe-ras′) a covering for the chest.

cul-de-sac (kul-dĕ-sak′) [Fr.] a blind pouch.
  Douglas' c., a pouch between the anterior wall of the rectum and the posterior wall of the uterus.

culdocentesis (kul″do-sen-te′sis) transvaginal puncture of Douglas' cul-de-sac for aspiration of blood or pus.

culdoscope (kul′do-skōp) an endoscope used in culdoscopy.

culdoscopy (kul-dos′ko-pe) direct examination of the uterus and adnexa through an endoscope passed through the wall of the vagina posterior to the cervix.

Culex (ku′leks) a genus of mosquitoes, species of which transmit various disease-producing agents, e.g., microfilariae, sporozoa and viruses.

culicide (ku′lĭ-sīd) an agent that destroys mosquitoes.

Culicinae (ku-lĭ-si′ne) a tribe of mosquitoes, including the genera Aedes, Culex, Mansonia, Psorophora and others.

Cullen's sign (kul′enz) bluish discoloration around the umbilicus sometimes occurring in intraperitoneal hemorrhage, as following rupture of the uterine tube in ectopic pregnancy.

culmen (kul′men), pl. *kul′mina* [L.] the part of the cerebellum below the declivis.

cultivation (kul″tĭ-va′shun) the propagation of living organisms, applied especially to the growth of microorganisms or other cells in artificial media.

culture (kul′tūr) 1. the propagation of microorganisms or of living tissue cells in special media conducive to their growth. 2. a growth of microorganisms propagated on or in a medium. 3. the social heritage. adj., **cul′tural.**
  hanging-drop c., a culture in which the bacterium is inoculated into a drop of fluid on a coverglass.
  c. medium, any substance or preparation used for the cultivation of living cells.
  pure c., a culture of a single microorganism.
  smear c., a culture prepared by smearing the infective material across the surface of the culture medium.
  stab c., a bacterial culture into which the organisms are introduced by thrusting a needle deep into the medium.
  streak c., a bacterial culture in which the infectious material is implanted in streaks.
  tissue c., the cultivation of tissue cells in vitro.
  type c., a culture that is generally agreed to represent a particular species of microorganisms.

cu. mm. cubic millimeter.

cumulus (ku′mu-lus), pl. *cu′muli* [L.] a small elevation.
  c. ooph′orus, the hillock of cells where the young ovum is buried in the graafian follicle.

cuneate (ku′ne-āt) wedge-shaped.

cuneiform (ku-ne′ĭ-form) wedge-shaped; applied particularly to three bones of the foot.

cuneus (ku′ne-us), pl. *cu′nei* [L.] a wedge-shaped lobule on the medial aspect of the occipital lobe of the cerebrum.

cuniculus (ku-nik′u-lus), pl. *cunic′uli* [L.] a burrow in the skin made by the itch mite, *Sarcoptes scabiei.*

cup (kup) a depression or hollow.
  glaucomatous c., a depression of the optic disk due to persistently increased intraocular pressure, broader and deeper than a physiologic cup, and occurring first at the temporal side of the disk.

physiologic c., a slight depression sometimes observed in the optic disk.

cupola (ku'pŏ-lah) cupula.

cupping (kup'ing) formation of a depression in the normally flat optic disk.

cupric (ku'prik) pertaining to or containing divalent copper.
  c. sulfate, a blue crystalline powder used as an astringent and emetic.

cuprous (ku'prus) pertaining to or containing monovalent copper.

cuprum (ku'prum) [L.] copper (symbol Cu).

cupruresis (ku″proo-re'sis) the urinary excretion of copper.

cupula (ku'pu-lah), pl. *cu'pulae* [L.] a small, inverted cup or dome-shaped cap over a structure.

curare (koo-rah're) a South American arrow poison; used to produce muscle relaxation in shock therapy and surgical procedures.

cure (kūr) 1. a system of treatment. 2. eradication of disease.

curet (ku-ret') a spoon-shaped instrument for cleansing a diseased surface.

curettage (ku″rĕ-tahzh') [Fr.] the cleansing of a diseased surface with a curet.

curette (ku-ret') curet.

curettement (ku-ret'ment) curettage.

curie (ku're) a unit of radioactivity, defined as the quantity of any radioactive nuclide in which the number of disintegrations per second is 3.700×10^{10}; abbreviated Ci.

curiegram (ku'rĭ-gram) a photographic print made by radium emanation.

curie-hour (ku're-our″) a unit of dose equivalent to radioactive material disintegrating at the rate of 3.7×10^{10} atoms per second.

curietherapy (ku″re-ther'ah-pe) radium therapy.

curioscopy (ku″re-os'ko-pe) the detection and mapping of objects by means of the nuclear radiations coming from them.

curium (ku're-um) a chemical element, atomic number 96, atomic weight 247, symbol Cm. (See table of ELEMENTS.)

current (kur'ent) that which flows; electric transmission in a circuit.
  alternating c., a current that periodically flows in opposite directions.
  direct c., a current whose direction is always the same.

curtometer (ker-tom'ĕ-ter) an instrument for measuring curved surfaces.

curvature (ker'vah-tūr) a nonangular deviation from a straight course in a line or surface.
  greater c. of stomach, the left or lateral and inferior border of the stomach, marking the inferior junction of the anterior and posterior surfaces.
  lesser c. of stomach, the right or medial border of the stomach, marking the superior junction of the anterior and posterior surfaces.

  Pott's c., curvature of the vertebral column after Pott's disease.
  spinal c., abnormal deviation of the vertebral column, as in KYPHOSIS, lordosis and SCOLIOSIS.

curve (kerv) a line that is not straight, or that describes part of a circle, especially a line representing varying values in a graph.
  frequency c., a curve representing graphically the probabilities of different numbers of recurrences of an event.
  growth c., the curve obtained by plotting increase in size or numbers against the elapsed time.

Cushing's syndrome (koosh'ingz) a group of serious symptoms caused by overactivity of the cortices of the adrenal glands. This overactivity is commonly the result of an abnormal growth of the adrenal cortices, or it may be caused by a benign or malignant tumor of one of the adrenal glands. Very rarely the overactivity may be stimulated by a tumor of the pituitary gland or of an ovary.
  Symptoms of Cushing's syndrome include painful, fatty swellings on the body (the buffalo hump), moonlike fullness of the face, distention of the abdomen, impairment of sexual function, high blood pressure and general weakness. There may also be an unusual growth of body hair (hirsutism) and streaked purple markings on the body.
  Treatment for the disorder is surgical removal of part of the adrenal glands, if their abnormal growth is the cause, or removal of the tumor if that is the source of the condition. The syndrome is named for Dr. Harvey Cushing, the celebrated American brain surgeon and endocrinologist, who in 1932 was the first to describe it.

cusp (kusp) a pointed projection, such as on the crown of a tooth, or a segment of a cardiac valve.

cuspid (kus'pid) 1. the third tooth on either side from the midline in each jaw; called also canine tooth. 2. having one cusp.

cuspis (kus'pis), pl. *cus'pides* [L.] a cusp.

cutaneous (ku-ta'ne-us) pertaining to the skin.

cutdown (kut'down) creation of a small incised opening, especially in a vein (venous cutdown), to permit the passage of tubing to facilitate withdrawal of blood or transfusion of fluids.

cuticle (ku'tĭ-kl) 1. the outermost layer of the skin. 2. the flattened, elastic, keratinous rim of the posterior nail fold.

cutireaction (ku″tĭ-re-ak'shun) a response of the skin to application or introduction of an antigen.

cutis (ku'tis) the outer protective covering of the body; the skin.
  c. anseri'na, erection of the papillae of the skin, as from cold or shock; goose flesh.

cutitis (ku-ti'tis) dermatitis.

cutization (ku″tĭ-za'shun) conversion into skin.

cuvette (ku-vet') [Fr.] a glass container generally having well defined characteristics (dimensions, optical properties), to contain solutions or suspensions for study.

cwt. hundred weight.

cyan(o)- (si'ah-no) word element [Gr.], *blue*.

cyanate (si'ah-nāt) a salt of cyanic acid that contains the radical CNO.

cyanemia (si"ah-ne'me-ah) blueness of the blood.

cyanephidrosis (si"an-ef"ĭ-dro'sis) the excretion of bluish sweat.

cyanhemoglobin (si"an-he"mo-glo'bin) a compound formed by the action of hydrocyanic acid on hemoglobin, which gives the bright red color to blood.

cyanic acid (si-an'ik) a highly irritant compound, HOCN.

cyanide (si'ah-nīd) a binary compound of cyanogen. Some inorganic compounds, such as cyanide salts, potassium cyanide and sodium cyanide, are important in industry for extracting gold and silver from their ores and in electroplating. Other cyanide compounds are used in the manufacture of synthetic rubber and textiles. Cyanides are also used in pesticides.

Most cyanide compounds are deadly poisons. Treatment for cyanide poisoning varies according to the nature of the poison. In the case of swallowed poison like hydrocyanic acid, the poison itself will cause vomiting. If the victim is able to swallow, milk or water may be given. A large dose of hydrocyanic acid will cause almost instant death.

If a gas such as hydrogen cyanide has been inhaled, the victim should be taken into open air and given artificial respiration.

cyanmethemoglobin (si"an-met"he-mo-glo'bin) a crystalline, colored substance formed by the action of hydrocyanic acid on oxyhemoglobin at body temperature; used in measuring hemoglobin in the blood.

cyanmetmyoglobin (si"an-met-mi"o-glo'bin) a compound formed from metmyoglobin by addition of the cyanide ion to yield reduction to the ferrous state.

cyanocobalamin (si"ah-no-ko-bal'ah-min) a substance having hematopoietic activity apparently identical with that of the antianemia factor of liver; called also VITAMIN B$_{12}$ and extrinsic factor.

radioactive c., cyanocobalamin containing radioactive cobalt of mass number 57 or 60 used in diagnosis of pernicious anemia.

cyanoderma (si"ah-no-der'mah) blueness of the skin.

cyanogen (si-an'o-jen) a poisonous gas.

cyanomycosis (si"ah-no-mi-ko'sis) development of *Micrococcus pyocyaneus* in pus.

cyanopathy (si"ah-nop'ah-the) cyanosis.

cyanopia, cyanopsia (si"ah-no'pe-ah), (si-ah-nop'se-ah) a defect of vision in which objects appear tinged with blue.

cyanosed (si'ah-nōsd) affected with cyanosis.

cyanosis (si"ah-no'sis) a bluish discoloration of skin and mucous membranes due to excessive concentration of reduced hemoglobin in the blood. adj., **cyanot'ic.**

central c., severe generalized cyanosis with reduced oxygen saturation of arterial blood.

peripheral c., that due to an excessive amount of reduced hemoglobin in the venous blood as a result of extensive oxygen extraction at the capillary level.

cyasma (si-az'mah) pigmentation of the skin of pregnant women.

cybernetics (si"ber-net'iks) the science of communication and control in the animal and in the machine.

Cyclaine (si'klān) trademark for preparations of hexylcaine hydrochloride, a local anesthetic.

Cyclamycin (si'klah-mi"sin) trademark for preparations of triacetyloleandomycin, an antibiotic.

cyclandelate (si-klan'dĕ-lāt) a vasodilator for peripheral vascular disease.

cyclarthrosis (si"klar-thro'sis) a joint that permits rotation.

cycle (si'kl) a succession or recurring series of events.

carbon c., the steps by which carbon is extracted from the atmosphere, incorporated in the body of living organisms and ultimately returned to the air.

cardiac c., a complete cardiac movement, or heartbeat, including systole, diastole and the intervening pause.

citric acid c., tricarboxylic acid cycle.

estrous c., the sequence of changes in the reproductive organs of female mammals other than primates, culminating in the interval of heightened intensity of the sex urge known as estrus.

Krebs c., tricarboxylic acid cycle.

menstrual c., the period of the regularly recurring physiologic changes in the endometrium which culminate in its shedding (menstruation).

nitrogen c., the steps by which nitrogen is extracted from the nitrates of soil and water, incorporated as amino acids and proteins in the body of living organisms and ultimately reconverted to nitrates.

ovarian c., the sequence of physiologic changes in the ovary involved in ovulation.

sex c., sexual c., 1. the physiologic changes recurring regularly in the reproductive organs of female mammals when pregnancy does not supervene. 2. the period of sexual reproduction in an organism that also reproduces asexually.

tricarboxylic acid c., a series of biochemical reactions by which carbon chains of sugars, fatty acids and amino acids are metabolized to yield carbon dioxide, water and energy.

cyclectomy (si-klek'to-me) excision of a piece of the ciliary body.

cyclic (sik'lik) pertaining to or occurring in a cycle or cycles. The term is applied to chemical compounds that contain a ring of atoms in the nucleus.

cyclicotomy (si"klĭ-kot'o-me) division of the ciliary body.

cyclitis (si-kli'tis) inflammation of the ciliary body.

cyclizine (si'klĭ-zēn) an antihistamine and antinauseant to prevent motion sickness.

cyclobarbital (si"klo-bar'bĭ-tal) a short- to intermediate-acting barbiturate.

cycloceratitis (si″klo-ser″ah-ti′tis) cyclokeratitis.

cyclochoroiditis (si″klo-ko″roi-di′tis) inflammation of the ciliary body and choroid.

cyclodialysis (si″klo-di-al′ĭ-sis) creation of a communication between the anterior chamber of the eye and the suprachoroidal space, in glaucoma.

cyclodiathermy (si″klo-di″ah-ther′me) destruction of the ciliary body by diathermy.

cyclogram (si′klo-gram) a tracing of the visual field made with a cycloscope.

Cyclogyl (si′klo-jil) trademark for a preparation of cyclopentolate, an anticholinergic, cycloplegic-mydriatic drug.

cycloid (si′kloid) characterized by variations of mood from happiness to depression.

cyclokeratitis (si″klo-ker″ah-ti′tis) inflammation of the cornea and ciliary body.

cyclomethycaine (si″klo-meth′ĭ-kān) a compound used as a surface anesthetic.

cyclopentamine (si″klo-pen′tah-mēn) a sympathomimetic nasal decongestant and hypertensive.

cyclopentolate (si″klo-pen′to-lāt) an anticholinergic drug used to produce parasympathetic blockade and topically to the conjunctiva to dilate the pupil and paralyze accommodation.

cyclophoria (si″klo-fo′re-ah) tendency of the eyeball to rotate on its anteroposterior axis.

cyclophosphamide (si″klo-fos′fah-mīd) a white, crystalline powder used as an antineoplastic agent.

cyclopia (si-klo′pe-ah) a developmental anomaly characterized by a single orbital fossa, with the globe absent or rudimentary, apparently normal or duplicated.

cycloplegia (si″klo-ple′je-ah) paralysis of the ciliary structure of the eye.

cycloplegic (si″klo-ple′jik) 1. causing cycloplegia. 2. an agent that produces cycloplegia.

cyclopropane (si″klo-pro′pān) a powerful central nervous system depressant used as a general ANESTHETIC. The drug can be given in small doses and is particularly useful in anesthetizing elderly or poor-risk patients. This gas is highly explosive and requires special handling and precautions against sparks or flames which would result in an explosion.

Cyclops (si′klops) a genus of minute crustaceans, species of which act as hosts to certain intestinal parasites.

cyclops (si′klops) a fetal monster exhibiting cyclopia.

cycloscope (si′klo-skōp) a form of perimeter for mapping the visual fields.

cycloserine (si″klo-ser′ēn) a antibiotic substance elaborated by *Streptomyces orchidaceus* or *S. garyphalus*, used in treatment of urinary tract infections.

cyclosis (si-klo′sis) displacement of components in the protoplasm of a cell, without external deformation of the cell wall.

Cyclospasmol (si″klo-spaz′mol) trademark for preparations of cyclandelate, a peripheral vasodilator.

cyclothymia (si″klo-thi′me-ah) a condition characterized by alternating moods of elation and dejection. adj., **cyclothy′mic.**

cyclotomy (si-klot′o-me) incision of the ciliary muscle.

cyclotron (si′klo-tron) an apparatus for accelerating protons or deuterons to high energies by means of a constant magnet and an oscillating electric field.

cyclotropia (si″klo-tro′pe-ah) rotation of the eyeball on its anteroposterior axis.

cycrimine (si′krĭ-min) an agent used to produce parasympathetic blockade and in treatment of Parkinson's disease.

cyesiology (si-e″se-ol′o-je) scientific study of the phenomena of pregnancy.

cyesis (si-e′sis) pregnancy. adj., **cyet′ic.**

cylindroadenoma (sil″in-dro-ad″ĕ-no′mah) a degenerated adenoma containing cylindrical masses.

cylindroid (sil′in-droid) 1. shaped like a cylinder. 2. a mucous or spurious cast in urine.

cylindroma (sil″in-dro′mah) a malignant tumor, especially about the face.

cylindrosarcoma (sil″in-dro-sar-ko′mah) a tumor containing elements of cylindroma and sarcoma.

cylindruria (sil″in-droo′re-ah) the presence of cylindroids in the urine.

cyllosis (sĭ-lo′sis) clubfoot or other deformity of the foot.

cymbocephalic (sim″bo-sĕ-fal′ik) scaphocephalic.

cynanthropy (sin-an′thro-pe) a delusion in which the patient believes himself a dog.

cynophobia (sin″o-fo′be-ah) morbid fear of dogs.

cyogenic (si″o-jen′ik) producing pregnancy.

cyotrophy (si-ot′ro-fe) nutrition of the fetus.

cypridopathy (sip″rĭ-dop′ah-the) any venereal disease.

cypridophobia (sip″rĭ-do-fo′be-ah) morbid fear of acquiring venereal disease.

cyproheptadine (si″pro-hep′tah-dēn) a compound used as an antihistamine and antiserotonin.

cyrtometer (sir-tom′ĕ-ter) an instrument for determining the dimensions of curved surfaces.

cyst (sist) a sac or capsule containing a liquid or semisolid substance. Most cysts are harmless. Nevertheless they should be removed when possible because they occasionally may change into malignant growths, become infected or obstruct a gland. There are four main types of cysts: retention cysts, exudation cysts, embryonic cysts and parasitic cysts.

blue dome c., a benign retention cyst of the breast that shows a blue color.

branchial c., one formed from an incompletely closed branchial cleft (see also BRANCHIAL CYST).

chocolate c., one with dark, syrupy contents, resulting from a collection of brownish serum, as may occur in the ovary in ovarian endometriosis.

daughter c., a small cyst developed from the walls of a large cyst.

dermoid c., a cyst containing bone, hair, teeth, etc. (see also DERMOID CYST).

echinococcus c., hydatid cyst.

embryonic c., one developing from bits of embryonic tissue that have been overgrown by other tissues, or from developing organs that normally disappear before birth. An example is a BRANCHIAL CYST.

exudation c., a cyst formed by the slow seepage of fluid into a tissue, forming a pocket, or one developing in an existing cavity, such as a bursa.

hydatid c., the cyst stage of an embryonic tapeworm in which the cyst contains daughter cysts, each of which contains many scolices.

meibomian c., chalazion.

nabothian c., a cystic dilatation caused by inflammatory stenosis of the glands of the uterine cervix.

parasitic c., one forming around parasites (tapeworms, amebas, trichinae) that enter the body.

pilonidal c., a congenital lesion in the midline of the sacral region, overlying the junction of the sacrum and coccyx, lined with epithelium and producing hair, sebum and keratin.

retention c., a tumor-like accumulation of a secretion formed when the outlet of a secreting gland is obstructed. These cysts may develop in any of the secretory glands—the breast, pancreas, kidney, salivary or sebaceous glands and mucous membranes.

sebaceous c., a retention cyst of a sebaceous gland (see also SEBACEOUS CYST).

cyst(o)- (sis′to) word element [Gr.], cyst; bladder.

cystadenoma (sis-tad″ě-no′mah) cystoma blended with adenoma.

mucinous c., a multilocular tumor of the ovary, filled with a stringy mucoid material.

serous c., a cystic tumor of the ovary containing thin, clear yellow serum and some solid tissue.

cystalgia (sis-tal′je-ah) pain in the bladder.

cystectasia (sis″tek-ta′ze-ah) incision of the urethra and dilatation of the neck of the bladder for extraction of calculi.

cystectomy (sis-tek′to-me) 1. excision of a cyst. 2. excision of the urinary bladder.

cysteine (sis-te′in) an amino acid produced by acid hydrolysis of proteins, readily interconvertible with cystine.

cystencephalus (sis″ten-sef′ah-lus) a fetal monster with a brain like a membranous bag.

cystgastrostomy (sist″gas-tros′to-me) internal drainage of a pseudocyst of the pancreas into the stomach.

cystic (sis′tik) 1. pertaining to cysts. 2. relating to a bladder, especially the urinary bladder.

c. acid, an intermediate product in the oxidation of cysteine to taurine.

c. duct, the excretory duct of the gallbladder.

c. fibrosis, a hereditary condition marked by accumulation of excessively thick and tenacious mucus and abnormal secretion of sweat and saliva; called also cystic fibrosis of the pancreas, and mucoviscidosis. The disease is inherited as a mendelian recessive trait; both parents must be carriers. The cause of the disease is presumably the absence, insufficiency or abnormality of some essential hormone or enzyme.

EFFECTS. Symptoms and severity of cystic fibrosis vary widely. Although it is congenital, it may not manifest itself to any appreciable degree during the early weeks or months of life, or it may cause intestinal obstruction and perforation in the newborn. The chief cause of complications in cystic fibrosis is the extremely thick mucus produced. Normal mucus bathes and protects internal surfaces and transports chemicals produced in one organ through intricate small ducts for use in another organ. Normal mucus flows easily, carrying with it bacteria, dirt and wastes that will be eliminated from the body. The mucus of cystic fibrosis, in contrast, is highly adhesive. Bacteria and other matter stick to it, and it in turn clogs the lungs and usually interferes with the flow of digestive enzymes from the pancreas to the small intestine.

In the lungs, the mucus blocks the bronchioles, creating breathing difficulties. Infection develops, thereby increasing obstruction of the air passages. Air becomes trapped in the lungs (emphysema), and scattered small areas eventually collapse (patchy atelectasis). Repeated infections follow, inflaming and damaging lung tissue and leading to chronic lung disease. The organism that produces infection in cystic fibrosis is almost always a staphylococcus, but other organisms may be present in more severe cases.

When mucus prevents the pancreatic enzymes from reaching the duodenum (which occurs in approximately 80 per cent of cystic fibrosis patients), digestion is hindered. Fats especially are poorly digested and absorbed. The child may have a voracious appetite, yet fail to grow normally or gain weight. There may be marked signs of malnutrition. The outstanding symptom associated with pancreatic enzyme deficiency is frequent bulky, fatty and foul-smelling feces.

Between 5 and 10 per cent of cystic fibrosis babies are born with intestines obstructed by putty-like intestinal secretions (meconium ileus) and die unless the condition is diagnosed promptly and relieved by surgery within the first few days of life. Such relief does not protect the child against the other manifestations of cystic fibrosis, although these may not appear until later.

Because cysts and scar tissue on the pancreas were observed during autopsy when the disease was first being differentiated from other conditions, it was given the name cystic fibrosis of the pancreas. Although this term describes a secondary rather than primary characteristic, it has been retained.

DIAGNOSIS. Sweat in cystic fibrosis is excessively salty. Collapse of cystic fibrosis patients from salt loss during a heat wave led, in 1953, to recognition of the sweat abnormality. A sweat test, introduced the next year, remains the cornerstone of diagnosis of cystic fibrosis. If either the chloride or sodium content of the sweat is from three to five times higher than in normal children, there is a strong basis for suspecting cystic fibrosis. Supporting evidence can confirm the sweat test finding.

TREATMENT. Under careful supervision by a physician or physical therapist, parents are taught the principles of home treatment of cystic fibrosis. The child may be required to sleep regularly in a plastic mist tent, into which a dense fog is pumped to help liquefy mucus and check infection. Aerosol therapy is generally prescribed. Extracts of animal pancreas taken with meals, which should be high in protein and low in fat, compensate for pancreatic deficiency. Physical therapy involving POSTURAL DRAINAGE together with "clapping" and "vibrating" by the physical therapist or parent aids in loosening the mucus so that it can be coughed up and expectorated.

It is estimated that in the United States cystic fibrosis occurs once in every few thousand births. Caucasians appear more subject to it than Negroes, and among Orientals it seems to be rare.

NURSING CARE. Maintenance of the child's nutritional status may be difficult because of his tendency to cough and vomit frequently during feedings, and also because of difficulty in breathing. Small amounts of food, given slowly and at frequent intervals, are best for infants as well as for small children with cystic fibrosis.

Skin care is important, especially for infants and toddlers who are not yet toilet trained. The stools are likely to be copious and extremely irritating to the skin.

Frequent turning of the infant or bedridden child helps to prevent decubitus ulcers and lessens the danger of pneumonia, a constant threat to these children.

Prevention of infection is a most important aspect of the care of these children because of their extreme vulnerability to disorders of the respiratory tract.

Education of the parents must include the dietary regimen, use of the Croupette or aerosol therapy machine in the home, hygienic measures to prevent infections and the need for continuous medical follow-up and administration of medications prescribed for the child by the physician.

cysticercosis (sis″tĭ-ser-ko′sis) infection with cysticerci.

cysticercus (sis″tĭ-ser′kus), pl. *cysticer′ci* [Gr.] a larval form of tapeworm.

cystiform (sis′tĭ-form) resembling a cyst.

cystigerous (sis-tij′er-us) containing cysts.

cystine (sis′tēn, sis′tin) a naturally occurring amino acid, the chief sulfur-containing component of the protein molecule. It is sometimes found in the urine and in the kidneys in the form of minute hexagonal crystals, frequently forming cystine calculus in the bladder.

cystinemia (sis″tĭ-ne′me-ah) cystine in the blood.

cystinosis (sis″tĭ-no′sis) a congenital metabolic disturbance characterized by deposition of cystine throughout the reticuloendothelial system and in various organs, notably the kidneys.

cystinuria (sis″tĭ-nu′re-ah) excretion in the urine of excessive cystine as a result of a genetically determined error of renal transport.

cystistaxis (sis″tĭ-stak′sis) oozing of blood into the bladder.

cystitis (sis-ti′tis) inflammation of the bladder. The condition may result from an ascending infection coming from the exterior of the body by way of the urethra, or it may be caused by an infection descending from the kidney. A simple cystitis that does not involve the rest of the urinary tract is not as serious as the descending type in which the kidneys and ureters as well as the bladder are involved.

Often cystitis is not an isolated infection but is rather a result of some other physical condition. For example, urinary retention, calculi in the bladder, tumors or neurologic diseases impairing the normal function of the bladder may lead to cystitis.

SYMPTOMS AND TREATMENT. The most common symptoms of cystitis are dysuria, frequency and urgency of urination and in some cases hematuria. Chills and fever indicate involvement of the entire urinary tract and are not symptomatic of uncomplicated cystitis.

Treatment of acute cystitis consists of antibiotics, forcing of fluids, and bed rest. Hot sitz baths give some relief of the discomfort, and spasms of the bladder wall may respond to an antispasmodic drug such as hyoscyamine. Chronic cystitis is more difficult to cure and may require surgical dilatation of the urethra and antiseptic bladder instillations. In many cases removal of the underlying cause, such as chronic vaginal infection, relieves the cystitis.

cystitomy (sis-tit′o-me) incision of the capsule of the crystalline lens.

cystjejunostomy (sist″je-joo-nos′to-me) internal drainage of a pseudocyst of the pancreas into the jejunum.

cystocarcinoma (sis″to-kar″sĭ-no′mah) cystoma blended with carcinoma.

cystocele (sis′to-sēl) herniation of the urinary bladder into the vagina.

cystodynia (sis″to-din′e-ah) pain in the bladder.

cystoelytroplasty (sis″to-el′ĭ-tro-plas″te) surgical repair of a vesicovaginal fistula.

cystoepithelioma (sis″to-ep″ĭ-the″le-o′mah) cystoma blended with epithelioma.

cystofibroma (sis″to-fi-bro′mah) fibroma blended with cystoma.

cystogastrostomy (sis″to-gas-tros′to-me) surgical anastomosis of a pancreatic cyst to the stomach.

cystogram (sis′to-gram) the film obtained by cystography.
  voiding c., a radiogram of the urinary tract made while the patient is urinating.

cystography (sis-tog′rah-fe) roentgenography of the urinary bladder using a contrast medium, so that the outline of the organ can be seen clearly. This type of examination frequently is part of a complete x-ray study of the kidneys and ureters as well as the bladder. (See also PYELOGRAPHY.) It is useful in diagnosing tumors or other defects in the bladder wall, or calculi or other pathologic conditions of the bladder, especially when cystoscopy is impossible.

cystoid (sis′toid) resembling a cyst.

cystojejunostomy (sis″to-je-joo-nos′to-me) surgical anastomosis of a pancreatic cyst to the jejunum.

cystolith (sis'to-lith) a vesical calculus.

cystolithectomy (sis"to-lĭ-thek'to-me) removal of a vesical calculus.

cystolithiasis (sis"to-lĭ-thi'ah-sis) formation of vesical calculi.

cystolithic (sis"to-lith'ik) pertaining to a vesical calculus.

cystolithotomy (sis"to-lĭ-thot'o-me) incision of the urinary bladder with removal of calculus.

cystolutein (sis"to-lu'te-in) a yellow pigment from ovarian cysts.

cystoma (sis-to'mah) a cystic tumor.

cystometer (sis-tom'ĕ-ter) an apparatus for measuring the capacity of the bladder and the pressure reactions caused by injecting fluid into it.

cystometrogram (sis"to-met'ro-gram) the record obtained by cystometrography.

cystometrography (sis"to-mĕ-trog'rah-fe) the graphic recording of the pressure exerted at varying degrees of filling of the urinary bladder.

cystomorphous (sis"to-mor'fus) resembling a cyst or bladder.

cystomyxoadenoma (sis"to-mik"so-ad"ĕ-no'mah) cystomyxoma blended with adenoma.

cystomyxoma (sis"to-mik-so'mah) myxoma with cystic degeneration.

cystonephrosis (sis"to-nĕ-fro'sis) cystiform dilatation of the kidney.

cystopexy (sis'to-pek"se) fixation of the bladder to abdominal wall.

cystoplasty (sis'to-plas"te) plastic repair of the bladder.

cystoplegia (sis"to-ple'je-ah) paralysis of the bladder.

cystoproctoscopy (sis"to-prok-tos'to-me) surgical creation of a communication between the urinary bladder and the rectum.

cystoptosis (sis"top-to'sis) prolapse of the bladder into the urethra.

cystopyelitis (sis"to-pi"ĕ-li'tis) inflammation of the bladder and renal pelvis.

cystopyelonephritis (sis"to-pi"ĕ-lo-nĕ-fri'tis) inflammation of the bladder, renal pelvis and kidney.

cystorrhaphy (sis-tor'ah-fe) suture of the bladder.

cystorrhea (sis"to-re'ah) mucous discharge from the bladder.

cystosarcoma (sis"to-sar-ko'mah) sarcoma with contained cysts.

cystoschisis (sis-tos'kĭ-sis) fissure of the bladder.

cystoscope (sis'to-skōp) an endoscope especially designed for passing through the urethra into the bladder to permit inspection of the interior of that organ.

cystoscopy (sis-tos'ko-pe) examination of the bladder by means of a cystoscope, a hollow metal tube that is introduced into the urinary meatus and passed through the urethra and into the bladder. At the end of the cystoscope is an electric bulb that illuminates the bladder interior. By means of special lenses and mirrors the bladder mucosa is examined for inflammation, calculi or tumors.

A catheter can be passed through the cystoscope into the bladder or, if necessary, beyond, into the ureters and kidneys. In this way samples of urine can be obtained for diagnostic purposes. Also, radiopaque fluids can be injected into the bladder or ureters for x-rays of the urinary tract (see also PYELOGRAPHY).

cystostomy (sis-tos'to-me) the formation of an opening into the bladder.

cystotomy (sis-tot'o-me) incision of the bladder.

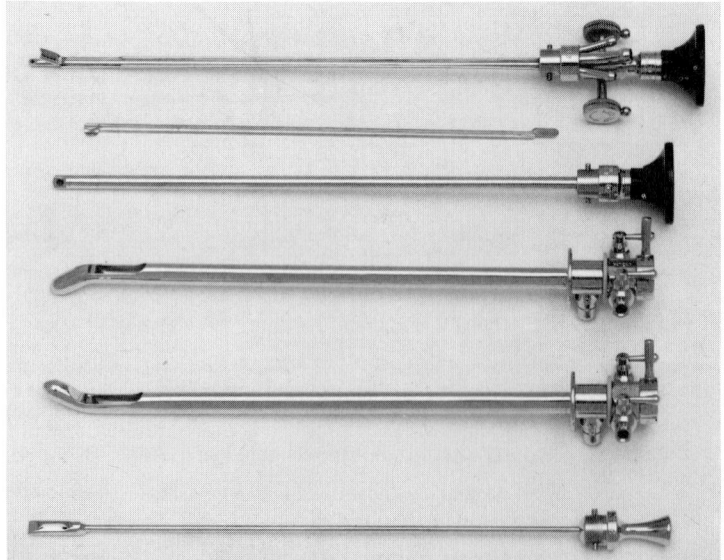

Cystoscope with lighting system. (Courtesy of American Cystoscope Makers, Inc.)

cystoureteritis (sis″to-u-re″ter-i′tis) inflammation involving the urinary bladder and ureters.

cystoureterogram (sis″to-u-re′ter-o-gram″) a roentgenogram of the bladder and ureter.

cystourethroscope (sis″to-u-re′thro-skōp″) an instrument for examining the posterior urethra and bladder.

cyt(o)- (si′to) word element [Gr.], *cell.*

-cyte (sīt) word element [Gr.], *mature cell.*

cythemolytic (si″them-o-lit′ik) pertaining to destruction of blood corpuscles.

cytoarchitectonic (si″to-ar″kī-tek-ton′ik) pertaining to the structural arrangement of cells.

cytobiology (si″to-bi-ol′o-je) the biology of cells.

cytoblast (si′to-blast) the cell nucleus.

cytocentrum (si″to-sen′trum) centrosome.

cytocerastic (si″to-sĕ-ras′tik) cytokerastic.

cytochemistry (si″to-kem′is-tre) the chemistry of cells.

cytochrome (si′to-krōm) a pigment universally present in aerobic cells; more than 20 such compounds, distinguishable by their absorption spectrums, have been studied.

cytochylema (si″to-ki-le′mah) the more fluid, finely granular substance of the cytoplasm of cells.

cytocide (si′to-sīd) an agent that destroys cells.

cytocinesia (si″to-si-ne′ze-ah) cytokinesis.

cytoclasis (si-tok′lah-sis) the destruction of cells. adj., **cytoclas′tic.**

cytoclesis (si″to-kle′sis) a form of energy, totally unrelated to electricity, light, heat or sound, that is generated by living tissues.

cytocyst (si′to-sist) a cyst enclosing a mass of merozoites.

cytodendrite (si″to-den′drīt) a dendrite given off from the cell itself, as distinguished from an axodendrite.

cytodiagnosis (si″to-di″ag-no′sis) diagnosis by examination of cells in body fluids.

cytodieresis (si″to-di-er′ĕ-sis) mitosis; indirect cell division.

cytodistal (si″to-dis′tal) remote from the cell of origin.

cytogene (si′to-jēn) a self-perpetuating cytoplasmic particle that traces origin to the genes of the nucleus.

cytogenesis (si″to-jen′ĕ-sis) development of the cell.

cytogenetic (si″to-jĕ-net′ik) pertaining to the cellular constituents concerned in heredity, i.e., chromosomes and genes.

cytogenetics (si″to-jĕ-net′iks) the science concerned with the cellular and molecular bases of heredity, variation, mutation, morphogenesis and evolution of organisms.

clinical c., the branch of cytogenetics concerned with relations between chromosomal abnormalities and pathologic conditions.

cytogenic (si″to-jen′ik) forming or producing cells.

cytoglycopenia (si″to-gli″ko-pe′ne-ah) deficient glucose content of the body or blood cells.

cytogony (si-tog′o-ne) cytogenic reproduction.

cytohistogenesis (si″to-his″to-jen′ĕ-sis) development of the structure of cells.

cytoid (si′toid) resembling a cell.

cytokalipenia (si″to-kal″ĭ-pe′ne-ah) a deficiency of potassium in the cells of the body.

cytokerastic (si″to-kĕ-ras′tik) pertaining to development of cells from a lower to a higher order.

cytokinesis (si″to-ki-ne′sis) division of the cytoplasm of a cell in the formation of daughter cells.

cytology (si-tol′o-je) the scientific study of cells.
exfoliative c., microscopic examination of cells desquamated from a body surface as a means of detecting malignant change.

cytolymph (si′to-limf) the more fluid, finely granular substance of the cytoplasm of cells; hyaloplasm.

cytolysin (si-tol′ĭ-sin) a lysin or antibody that produces disintegration of cells.

cytolysis (si-tol′ĭ-sis) the dissolution of cells.

cytomegalic inclusion disease (si″to-meg′ah-lik in-kloo′zhun) a disease, especially of newborns, due to infection with a cytomegalovirus, and characterized by hepatosplenomegaly and often by microcephaly and mental or motor retardation.

cytomegaloviruria (si″to-meg″ah-lo-vi-roo′re-ah) the presence in the urine of cytomegaloviruses.

cytomegalovirus (si″to-meg″ah-lo-vi′rus) one of a group of highly host-specific viruses infecting man, monkeys or rodents, producing unique large cells with inclusion bodies.

Cytomel (si′to-mel) trademark for a preparation of the sodium salt of liothyronine, a thyroid hormone preparation.

cytometaplasia (si″to-met″ah-pla′ze-ah) change in function or form of cells.

cytometer (si-tom′ĕ-ter) a device for counting cells.

cytometry (si-tom′ĕ-tre) the counting of blood cells.

cytomitome (si″to-mi′tōm) a fibril, or fibrillar network, of spongioplasm.

cytomorphology (si″to-mor-fol′o-je) the morphology of body cells.

cytomorphosis (si″to-mor-fo′sis) the changes through which cells pass in development.

cytomycosis (si″to-mi-ko′sis) a fatal disease marked by splenomegaly, irregular fever and leukopenia, caused by a fungus that attacks the phagocytic cells of the blood (the reticuloendothelial system); called also histoplasmosis.

cyton (si'ton) the cell body of a neuron.

cytopathic (si"to-path'ik) pertaining to or characterized by pathologic changes in cells.

cytopathogenesis (si"to-path"o-jen'ĕ-sis) production of pathologic changes in cells.

cytopathology (si"to-pah-thol'o-je) the study of cells in disease.

cytopenia (si"to-pe'ne-ah) deficiency in the cells of the blood.

cytophagy (si-tof'ah-je) absorption of cells by other cells.

cytophilic (si"to-fil'ik) having an affinity for cells.

cytophylaxis (si"to-fi-lak'sis) the protection of cells against cytolysis.

cytophysics (si"to-fiz'iks) the physics of cell activity.

cytophysiology (si"to-fiz"e-ol'o-je) the physiology of cells.

cytoplasm (si'to-plazm) the protoplasm of a cell surrounding the nucleus. adj., **cytoplas'mic.**

cytoscopy (si-tos'ko-pe) examination of cells.

cytosine (si'to-sēn) a pyrimidine base, one of the disintegration products of nucleic acid.

cytosome (si'to-sōm) the specific body of protoplasm in a particular cell.

cytospongium (si"to-spun'je-um) the spongioplasm of a cell.

cytostatic (si"to-stat'ik) 1. checking the growth and multiplication of cells. 2. an agent that suppresses the growth and multiplication of cells.

cytotaxis (si"to-tak'sis) the movement of a cell in response to stimulation by another cell.

cytotherapy (si"to-ther'ah-pe) treatment by use of animal cells.

cytothesis (si-toth'ĕ-sis) restitution of cells to their normal condition.

cytotoxic (si"to-tok'sik) having a deleterious effect upon cells.

cytotoxicosis (si"to-tok"sĭ-ko'sis) a toxic state of the cells.

cytotoxin (si"to-tok'sin) a toxin having a specific destructive effect on cells.

cytotrophoblast (si"to-trof'o-blast) the cellular (inner) layer of the trophoblast.

cytotropic (si"to-trop'ik) having an affinity for cells.

Cytoxan (si-tok'san) trademark for preparations of cyclophosphamide, an antineoplastic agent.

cytozyme (si'to-zīm) thromboplastin.

cytula (sit'u-lah) the impregnated ovum.

cyturia (sĭ-tu're-ah) presence of cells in the urine.

D

D chemical symbol, *deuterium*.

D- chemical prefix (written as small capital) that specifies that the substance corresponds in chemical configuration to the standard substance D-glyceraldehyde. Carbohydrates are named by this method to distinguish them by their chemical composition. The opposite prefix is L-.

d- prefix, *dextro-*.

dacry(o)- (dak're-o) word element [Gr.], *tears* (lacrimal apparatus of the eye).

dacryagogue (dak're-ah-gog") 1. causing a flow of tears. 2. an agent that provokes a flow of tears.

dacryoadenalgia (dak"re-o-ad"ĕ-nal'je-ah) pain in a lacrimal gland.

dacryoadenectomy (dak"re-o-ad"ĕ-nek'to-me) excision of a lacrimal gland.

dacryoadenitis (dak"re-o-ad"ĕ-ni'tis) inflammation of a lacrimal gland.

dacryoblennorrhea (dak"re-o-blen"o-re'ah) mucous flow from the lacrimal apparatus.

dacryocele (dak're-o-sēl") hernia of the lacrimal sac.

dacryocyst (dak're-o-sist") the lacrimal sac.

dacryocystalgia (dak"re-o-sis-tal'je-ah) pain in the lacrimal sac.

dacryocystectasia (dak"re-o-sis"tek-ta'ze-ah) dilatation of the lacrimal sac.

dacryocystectomy (dak"re-o-sis-tek'to-me) excision of the lacrimal sac.

dacryocystitis (dak"re-o-sis-ti'tis) inflammation of the lacrimal sac.

dacryocystoblennorrhea (dak"re-o-sis"to-blen"o-re'ah) mucous flow from the lacrimal sac.

dacryocystocele (dak"re-o-sis'to-sēl) protrusion of the lacrimal sac.

dacryocystoptosis (dak"re-o-sis"top-to'sis) prolapse of the lacrimal sac.

dacryocystorhinostenosis (dak"re-o-sis"to-ri"no-stĕ-no'sis) narrowing of the passage through which the tears enter the nose.

dacryocystorhinostomy (dak"re-o-sis"to-ri-nos'to-me) formation of an opening between the lacrimal sac and nasal cavity.

dacryocystorhinotomy (dak"re-o-sis"to-ri-not'o-me) passage of a probe through the lacrimal sac into the nasal cavity.

dacryocystostenosis (dak"re-o-sis"to-stĕ-no'sis) narrowing of the lacrimal sac.

dacryocystostomy (dak"re-o-sis-tos'to-me) incision of the lacrimal sac with drainage.

dacryocystotomy (dak"re-o-sis-tot'o-me) incision of the lacrimal sac.

dacryohemorrhea (dak"re-o-he"mo-re'ah) occurrence of a bloody discharge from the lacrimal glands.

dacryolith (dak're-o-lith") a calculus in a lacrimal gland or duct.

dacryoma (dak"re-o'mah) a tumor-like swelling due to obstruction of the lacrimal duct.

dacryon (dak're-on) the point where the lacrimal, frontal and upper maxillary bones meet.

dacryopyorrhea (dak"re-o-pi"o-re'ah) the discharge of tears mixed with pus.

dacryorrhea (dak"re-o-re'ah) excessive flow of tears.

dacryostenosis (dak"re-o-stĕ-no'sis) narrowing of a lacrimal passage or duct.

dacryosyrinx (dak"re-o-sir'inks) 1. lacrimal duct. 2. a lacrimal fistula. 3. a syringe for irrigating the lacrimal ducts.

Dactil (dak'til) trademark for preparations of piperidolate hydrochloride, an anticholinergic.

dactyl (dak'til) a digit.

dactyl(o)- (dak'tĭ-lo) word element [Gr.], *digit* (finger or toe).

dactylion (dak-til'e-on) webbing of the fingers or toes.

dactylitis (dak"tĭ-li'tis) inflammation of a finger or toe.

dactylography (dak"tĭ-log'rah-fe) the study of fingerprints.

dactylogryposis (dak"ti-lo-grĭ-po'sis) permanent flexion of the fingers.

dactylology (dak"tĭ-lol'o-je) communication by signs made with the fingers.

dactylolysis (dak"tĭ-lol'ĭ-sis) 1. surgical correction of webbing of the fingers or toes. 2. separation or loss of a finger or toe.

dactylomegaly (dak"tĭ-lo-meg'ah-le) large size of fingers and toes.

dactyloscopy (dak"tĭ-los'ko-pe) examination of fingerprints for identification.

dactylus (dak'tĭ-lus), pl. *dac'tyli* [L.] a dactyl, or digit.

Dakin's solution (da'kinz) an aqueous solution of chlorine compounds of sodium; germicide.

Dalton's law (dawl'tonz) the pressure exerted by a mixture of nonreacting gases is equal to the sum of the partial pressures of the separate components.

daltonism (dawl'ton-izm) red-green color blindness.

dam (dam) a sheet of latex rubber used to isolate teeth from the fluids of the mouth during dental treatments; used also in surgical procedures to isolate certain tissues or structures.

damp (damp) a noxious gas in a mine.
  black d., choke d., a gaseous mixture formed in a mine by the gradual absorption of the oxygen and the giving off of carbon dioxide by the coal.

damping (damp'ing) steady diminution of the amplitude of successive vibrations of an electric wave or current or sound wave.

D. and C. dilation and curettage.

dandruff (dan'druf) a scaly material from or on the scalp. The condition may spread unless checked and in rare cases may extend to the eyebrows, ears, nose and neck, causing a reddening of the skin in those areas. Called also SEBORRHEIC DERMATITIS.

Danilone (dan'ĭ-lōn) trademark for a preparation of phenindione, an anticoagulant.

danthron (dan'thron) a drug used as a laxative.

dapsone (dap'sōn) an antibacterial compound used in leprosy and tuberculosis.

Daranide (dar'ah-nīd) trademark for a preparation of dichlorphenamide, a carbonic anhydrase inhibitor.

Daraprim (dar'ah-prim) trademark for a preparation of pyrimethamine, an antimalarial drug.

Darbid (dar'bid) trademark for a preparation of isopropamide iodide, an anticholinergic.

Daricon (dar'ĭ-kon) trademark for a preparation of oxyphencyclimine hydrochloride, an anticholinergic.

Darier's disease (dar'e-āz) keratosis follicularis.

Darling's disease (dar'lingz) histoplasmosis.

Dartal (dar'tal) trademark for a preparation of thiopropazate dihydrochloride, a tranquilizer.

dartoid (dar'toid) resembling the dartos.

dartos (dar'tos) the contractile tissue under the skin of the scrotum; called also tunica dartos.

Darvon (dar'von) trademark for a preparation of dextropropoxyphene hydrochloride, an analgesic.

daturine (da-tu'rin) hyoscyamine.

DBI trademark for preparations of phenformin hydrochloride, an oral hypoglycemic drug.

D & C dilation and curettage.

D.D.S. Doctor of Dental Surgery.

DDT dichloro-diphenyl-trichloro-ethane, a powerful insect poison; used in dilution as a powder or in an oily solution as a spray.

deacidification (de″ah-sid″ĭ-fĭ-ka'shun) neutralization of acidity.

deactivation (de-ak″tĭ-va'shun) the process of rendering inactive.

deaf-mute (def'mūt) a person unable to hear or speak.

deafness (def'nes) impairment of HEARING. Total deafness is quite rate, but partial deafness is common; an estimated 15 million Americans suffer from some degree of deafness, and of these, perhaps 2.5 million are children whose defective hearing either is congenital (from birth) or developed before the age of 5.

CAUSES. The two major types of deafness are conductive deafness and sensorineural (nerve) deafness. In some cases both types may be present; this is called mixed deafness.

In conductive deafness sound vibrations are interrupted in the outer or middle ear before they reach the nerve endings of the inner ear. In the outer ear, a foreign body or an accumulation of cerumen (earwax) may block the external acoustic meatus. These cases generally can be cured by removal of the obstruction. In the middle ear, infections, often entering through a perforated tympanic membrane (eardrum) or the eustachian tube, may fill the chamber with fluid, hampering the passage of vibrations. The small bones of the middle ear (ossicles) may be damaged by injury or fixed in place by otosclerosis.

In sensorineural deafness, the outer and middle ear function normally, but damage to the nerve endings of the inner ear, the cochlear portion of the vestibulocochlear (eighth cranial) nerve or the hearing center in the brain causes either interruption or confusion of the sound messages. This damage may be caused by disease, head injury, tumor, excessively loud and sudden noise or continuous loud noise.

A great many cases of congenital deafness are caused by infectious diseases, especially viral infections, contracted by the mother during pregnancy. Of these, rubella (German measles) is the most common.

Impaired hearing or a predisposition to ear diseases may be inherited. The laws of heredity with respect to deafness, though not yet fully understood, are the subject of continuing research.

Two of the greatest contributing factors to deafness are pride and neglect. Many ear diseases that can be cured if treated early are allowed to lead to deafness because of these two factors. Symptoms such as ringing in the ears, a feeling of pressure in the ear or increasing hearing difficulty call for prompt medical consultation, if necessary with an ear specialist, or otologist.

TREATMENT. Medical science has made great progress in the treatment of conditions that are capable of causing deafness. Middle ear infections now yield to the antibiotics and sulfonamide drugs. The greatest progress, however, has been in the field of microsurgery. Special binocular microscopes and miniature surgical instruments have enabled the surgeon to operate freely in the small crowded chambers of the ear. Two examples of this type of microsurgery are TYMPANOPLASTY and STAPEDECTOMY. In a stapedectomy the stapes, or stirrup, is removed and replaced by a piece of stainless steel wire or plastic, which allows the chain of transmission of sound vibrations to function again. Tympanoplasty is useful in correcting other types of conductive deafness as well. If chronic ear infection or injury has destroyed one or more of the ossicles, they can be rebuilt or replaced. Through plastic surgery and grafting techniques, the skilled surgeon can rebuild the entire middle ear.

REHABILITATION.   There still remain many cases of deafness that cannot be improved by drugs or surgery. In particular, sensorineural deafness is not accessible to surgery because it involves parts deep in the inner ear or the brain itself.

For these patients, rehabilitation is required, with the aim of making the best use of what hearing remains. With proper training and the use of a suitable hearing aid where necessary, the deaf person can continue to lead a normal, useful life.

An important tool in rehabilitation is training in lip-reading. The patient is taught to use visual clues, such as the movements of the lips and tongue of the speaker, to supplement his hearing.

Another important tool is a correct HEARING AID. This should be selected with the help of an otologist, as different types of deafness require different instruments. Careful training in the use of the hearing aid also is necessary. After the silence of deafness, the patient may find it impossible at first to disregard the background noises that the instrument picks up. Also, some types of nerve deafness "scramble" sounds; training in the use of the hearing aid may enable the patient to distinguish among these sounds.

A third important component of rehabilitation is speech therapy. Since the deaf person is no longer able to hear his own voice, his speech often deteriorates. Proper training can help the patient prevent this deterioration, as well as correcting any speech defect that may already have developed.

DEAFNESS IN CHILDREN.   The problems of a child who is deaf from birth or shortly afterward are somewhat different from those of a person who loses his hearing during adult life. Since children learn to speak by imitating the sounds they hear, a child who cannot hear will be mute unless he is taught speech. This calls for special methods of teaching.

There are more than 350 schools and classes in the United States that specialize in teaching the partially and totally deaf child. These are located throughout the country, and many are publicly supported by taxes. There are also a number of summer camps that make it possible for the deaf child to continue his training throughout the year. Gallaudet College, in Washington, D.C., is the only college in the world devoted exclusively to educating the deaf. It is supported by the United States Government.

AGENCIES FOR THE DEAF.   The American Hearing Society is the best known of the organizations concerned with problems of the deaf. Located at 919 18th Street N.W., Washington, D.C. 20006, the society has affiliated agencies throughout the United States. The services offered by these branches include lip-reading classes, rehabilitation and hearing aid clinics. The American Speech and Hearing Association, 1001 Connecticut Avenue N.W., Washington, D.C. 20006, is a professional association of specialists in speech and hearing therapy. The Alexander Graham Bell Association for the Deaf, 1537 35th Street N.W., Washington, D.C. 20007, has one of the world's finest libraries on deafness, and functions as an information center on the subject. The Deafness Research Foundation, 366 Madison Avenue, New York, N.Y. 10017,

was founded several years ago to encourage medical research into the causes of deafness. Among the federal agencies concerned with questions of the deaf are the Children's Bureau of the Department of Health, Education and Welfare and the Office of Vocational Rehabilitation. The Veterans Administration offers assistance and rehabilitation to those whose hearing was injured during military service. Many states have agencies that deal with problems of the handicapped, including the deaf.

   cortical d., that due to disease of the cortical centers of the cerebrum.

   hysterical d., that which may appear or disappear in a hysterical patient without an organic cause being present.

deamidization (de-am″ĭ-dĭ-za′shun) liberation of the ammonia from an amide.

deaminase (de-am′ĭ-nās) an enzyme that promotes the removal of an amino group from a compound.

deamination (de-am″ĭ-na′shun) removal of the amino group, $-NH_2$, from a compound.

Deaner (de′ner) trademark for a preparation of deanol, a cerebral stimulant.

deanol acetaminobenzoate (de′ah-nol as″et-am″ĭ-no-ben′zo-āt) a drug used as a cerebral stimulant.

dearterialization (de″ar-te″re-al-ĭ-za′shun) 1. conversion of arterial into venous blood. 2. interruption of the supply of arterial (oxygenated) blood to an organ or part.

death (deth) the apparent extinction of life, as manifested by absence of heartbeat and respiration.

   black d., plague.

   cot d., crib d., the death, in its sleeping quarters, of an infant who had previously been apparently normal and well.

   neonatal d., death of an infant within 28 days after birth.

   d. rate, the number of deaths per stated number of persons (1000 or 10,000 or 100,000) in a certain region in a certain year.

debilitant (de-bil′ĭ-tant) 1. inducing weakness. 2. an agent that allays excitement.

debility (de-bil′ĭ-te) weakness.

débride (da-brēd′) [Fr.] to subject to removal of foreign matter and devitalized tissue.

débridement (da-brēd-maw′) [Fr.] removal of all foreign material and aseptic excision of all contaminated and devitalized tissues.

   enzymatic d., debridement of traumatized or diseased areas by use of proteolytic and fibrinolytic enzymes, such as streptodornase and streptokinase.

   surgical d., removal of foreign material and devitalized tissue by surgical excision.

debris (dĕ-bre′) accumulated fragments; rubbish. In dentistry, soft foreign matter loosely attached to the surface of a tooth.

deca- (dek′ah) 1. word element [Gr.], *ten;* also spelled *deka-.* 2. used in naming units of measurement to indicate a quantity 10 times the unit designated by the root with which it is combined, e.g., decagram.

decacurie (dek″ah-ku′re) a unit of radioactivity, being 10 curies.

Decadron (dek′ah-dron) trademark for preparations of dexamethasone, a corticosteroid.

decagram (dek′ah-gram) ten grams; 154.32 grains.

decalcification (de-kal″sĭ-fĭ-ka′shun) 1. removal of calcareous matter from tissues. 2. the loss of calcium salts from bone or teeth.

decalcify (de-kal′sĭ-fi) to deprive of calcium or its salts.

decaliter (dek′ah-le″ter) ten liters; 2.64 gallons.

decameter (dek′ah-me″ter) ten meters; 32.8 feet.

decannulation (de-kan″nu-la′shun) the removal of a cannula.

decanormal (dek″ah-nor′mal) of ten times normal strength.

decantation (de″kan-ta′shun) the pouring of a clear supernatant liquid from a sediment.

decapitation (de-kap″ĭ-ta′shun) removal of the head, as of the fetus in utero, or of a bone.

decapsulation (de-kap″su-la′shun) removal of a capsule.

decarboxylation (de″kar-bok″sĭ-la′shun) removal of the carboxyl group from a compound.

decay (de-ka′) 1. the gradual decomposition of dead organic matter. 2. the process or stage of decline; old age and its effects on mind and body.

decerebrate (de-ser′ĕ-brāt) functionally or anatomically deprived of influence of the brain (cerebrum).

decerebration (de-ser″ĕ-bra′shun) excision of the brain or interruption of its influence by transection of the spinal cord.

decholesterolization (de-ko-les″ter-ol-ĭ-za′shun) extraction of cholesterol from the system.

Decholin (de′ko-lin) trademark for preparations of dehydrocholic acid, a substance that hastens the flow of bile and the filling of the gallbladder. Because of its bitter taste on the tongue when injected into a vein, it is used to provide an end point for the measurement of the arm-tongue circulation time.

deci- (des′ĭ) word element [L.], *one-tenth;* used to indicate one-tenth of the unit designated by the root with which it is combined, e.g., decigram.

decibel (des′ĭ-bel) the unit of loudness of sound.

decidua (de-sid′u-ah) the membranous lining of the uterus shed after childbirth or at menstruation; called also the deciduous membrane. adj., **decid′ual.**
  basal d., d. basa′lis, that directly underlying the implanting ovum.
  capsular d., d. capsula′ris, that directly overlying the implanting ovum.

menstrual d., d. menstrua′lis, that which is shed at menstruation.
  parietal d., d. parieta′lis, true d., d. ve′ra, that lining the uterus elsewhere than at the site of the implanting ovum.

decidualitis (de-sid″u-al-i′tis) a bacterial disease leading to changes in the decidua.

deciduation (de-sid″u-a′shun) the shedding of the decidua.

deciduitis (de-sid″u-i′tis) inflammation of the decidua of pregnancy.

deciduoma (de-sid″u-o′mah) an intrauterine tumor derived from a retained decidua.
  d. malig′num, choriocarcinoma, a malignant tumor derived from retained decidua.

deciduomatosis (de-sid″u-o″mah-to′sis) excessive proliferation of decidual tissue in the nonpregnant state.

deciduosarcoma (de-sid″u-o-sar-ko′mah) chorioadenoma.

deciduous (de-sid′u-us) falling off; subject to being shed, as deciduous teeth.

decigram (des′ĭ-gram) one-tenth of a gram; 1.54 grains.

deciliter (des′ĭ-le″ter) one-tenth of a liter; 3.38 fluidounces.

decimeter (des′ĭ-me″ter) one-tenth of a meter; 3.9 inches.

decinormal (des″ĭ-nor′mal) of one-tenth normal strength.

decipara (des″ĭ-pah′rah) a woman who has had ten pregnancies that resulted in viable offspring; para X.

declination (dek″lĭ-na′shun) cyclophoria.

declivis (de-kli′vis) [L.] a slope or slanting surface.
  d. cerebel′li, the sloping posterior surface of the superior vermis of the cerebellum.

Declomycin (dek′lo-mi″sin) trademark for preparations of demethylchlortetracycline, an antibiotic.

décollement (da-kol-maw′) [Fr.] separation of an organ from adjoining tissue to which it normally adheres.

decolorizer (de-kul′or-iz″er) an agent that removes color, bleaches.

decompensation (de″kom-pen-sa′shun) inability of the heart to maintain adequate circulation; it is marked by dyspnea, venous engorgement, cyanosis and edema.

decomposition (de-kom″po-zish′un) dissolution, or chemical separation into component elements or simpler compounds.

decompression (de″kom-presh′un) return to normal environmental pressure after exposure to greatly increased pressure.
  cerebral d., removal of a flap of the skull and incision of the dura mater for the purpose of relieving intracranial pressure
  d. sickness, a disorder characterized by joint pains, respiratory manifestations, skin lesions and neurologic signs, occurring in aviators flying at

high altitudes and following rapid reduction of air pressure in a person's environment (see also BENDS).

decongestant (de″kon-jes′tant) 1. tending to reduce congestion or swelling. 2. an agent that reduces congestion or swelling, usually of the nasal membranes. Decongestants may be inhaled, taken as spray or nose drops or used orally in liquid or tablet form. The medication acts by reducing swelling of the nasal membranes and thus opening up the nasal passages. Among the leading medications used as decongestants are epinephrine, ephedrine and phenylephrine. Antihistamines, alone or in combination with decongestants, may also be effective.

A decongestant must be used several times a day to be helpful; but excessive use may cause headaches, dizziness or other disorders and sometimes the medicine itself may cause reactive nasal swelling.

decongestive (de″kon-jes′tiv) reducing congestion.

decontamination (de″kon-tam-ĭ-na′shun) the freeing of a person or an object of some contaminating substance such as war gas, radioactive material, etc.

decortication (de-kor″tĭ-ka′shun) removal of a cortex or of superficial substance.

decrepitation (de-krep″ĭ-ta′shun) crepitation.

decubitus (de-ku′bĭ-tus) 1. posture in bed. 2. the act of lying down. 3. a decubitus ulcer. adj., **decu′bital.**

Andral's d., lying on the unaffected side in the early stages of pleurisy.

dorsal d., lying on the back.

lateral d., lying on one side, designated right lateral decubitus when the subject lies on the right side and left lateral decubitus when he lies on the left side.

d. ulcer, due to local interference with the circulation; called also an ulceration, bedsore and pressure sore. The ulcer usually occurs over a bony prominence such as that of the sacrum, hip, heel, shoulder or elbow. Excessive or prolonged pressure produced by the weight of the body or limb is the primary cause. Factors that may contribute to the development of an ulcer include wrinkling or unevenness of the bedclothes, accumulation of perspiration and incontinence of urine or feces. The patients most likely to develop a decubitus ulcer are emaciated or diabetic patients, those confined to bed in traction or wearing a cast and those with generalized edema.

The prevention of a decubitus ulcer is far simpler than treatment and cure. Frequent changing of position of the patient who cannot move about in bed, thorough cleansing of the skin and gentle massage of the bony prominences to stimulate circulation are all important in avoiding pressure areas and ulcers. The use of sheepskin under the patient has been fairly successful in preventing pressure sores in patients confined to bed. Polyether urethan foam, a substance similar to foam rubber, can be used in large blocks as mattresses or in small squares with cut-out areas over the ulcer. These measures help relieve pressure and provide for increased circulation of blood to the affected area; they do not, however, replace such basic nursing care as frequent turning, cleanliness and massage of areas likely to develop decubitus ulcers.

Treatment of a decubitus ulcer is aimed at restoring circulation to the area as quickly and efficiently as possible, controlling secondary bacterial infection and initiating measures to promote healing. The patient should be positioned so that the ulcer and surrounding area are completely relieved of pressure. Exposure to sunlight, ultraviolet rays or heat lamp will aid in keeping the area dry and help promote healing. Medications in the form of liquid applications, ointments or powders are prescribed by the physician.

ventral d., lying on the ventral surface, or belly.

decussate (de-kus′āt) 1. to cross in the form of an X. 2. crossed like the letter X.

decussation (de″kus-sa′shun) 1. the position of one part crossing another, similar part. 2. the point of crossing; chiasm.

d. of pyramids, the crossing of the fibers of the pyramids of the medulla oblongata from one pyramid to the other.

dedifferentiation (de-dif″er-en″she-a′shun) regression from a more specialized or complex form to a simpler state.

deerfly (dēr′fli) a member of the genus Chrysops, an important vector of various organisms, e.g., *Pasteurella tularensis* and *Loa Loa.*

d. fever, tularemia.

defatted (de-fat′ed) deprived of fat.

defecation (def″ē-ka′shun) elimination of wastes and undigested food, as feces, from the rectum.

defect (de′fekt) a flaw, or imperfection.

filling d., an interruption in the contour of the inner surface of stomach or intestine revealed by roentgenography, indicating excess tissue or substance on or in the wall of the organ.

septal d., a defect in the cardiac septum resulting in an abnormal communication between opposite chambers of the heart.

defective (de-fek′tiv) 1. imperfect. 2. a person lacking in some physical, mental or moral quality.

defeminization (de-fem″ĭ-nĭ-za′shun) loss of normal secondary sex characters in the female.

defense (de-fens′) resistance to or protection from attack.

d. mechanism, a psychologic reaction or technique for protection against a stressful environmental situation or against anxiety.

deferens (def′er-ens) [L.] deferent.

deferent (def′er-ent) conducting or progressing away from a center or specific site of reference.

deferentectomy (def″er-en-tek′to-me) excision of a ductus deferens.

deferential (def″er-en′shal) pertaining to the ductus deferens.

defervescence (def″er-ves′ens) the decline of high temperature (fever) to normal.

defibrillation (de-fi″brĭ-la′shun) the stoppage of fibrillation of the heart.

defibrillator (de-fi′brĭ-la″tor) an apparatus that counteracts fibrillation by applying electric impulses to the heart; now used successfully in many cases of cardiac resuscitation.

defibrination (de-fi″bri-na′shun) the destruction or removal of fibrin, as from the blood.

deficiency (de-fish′en-se) a lack or shortage; a condition characterized by the presence of less than the normal or necessary supply or competence.
    d. disease, avitaminosis or other condition produced by dietary or metabolic deficiency; the term includes beriberi, scurvy, pellagra, etc.

deflection (de-flek′shun) a turning aside. In psychoanalysis, an unconscious diversion of ideas from conscious attention. In the electrocardiogram, a deviation of the curve from the isoelectric baseline, that is, any wave or complex.

defluxion (de-fluk′shun) a copious discharge or loss of any kind.

deformation (de″for-ma′shun) 1. deformity. 2. the process of deforming.

deformity (de-for′mĭ-te) distortion of any part or general disfigurement of the body.

defunctionalization (de-funk″shun-al-ĭ-za′shun) destruction of a function.

defundation (de″fun-da′shun) excision of the fundus of the uterus.

defurfuration (de-fer″fer-a′shun) the shedding of branlike scales from the skin.

deganglionate (de-gang′gle-ŏ-nāt″) to deprive of ganglia.

degenerate (de-jen′er-āt) 1. to change from a higher to a lower form. (de-jen′er-it) 2. characterized by degeneration. 3. a person whose moral or physical state is below the normal.

degeneration (de-jen″ĕ-ra′shun) deterioration; change from a higher to a lower form; especially change of tissue to a lower or less functionally active form. When there is chemical change of the tissue itself it is true degeneration; when the change consists in the deposit of abnormal matter in the tissues, it is infiltration.
    albuminoid d., albuminous d., cloudy swelling, an early stage of degenerative change characterized by swollen, parboiled-appearing tissues which may revert to normal.
    amyloid d., degeneration with deposit of lardacein in the tissues.
    caseous d., caseation.
    colloid d., degeneration with conversion into a gelatinous material.
    cystic d., degeneration with formation of cysts.
    fatty d., degeneration of tissue with abnormal accumulation of fat.
    fibroid d., degeneration into fibrous tissue.
    hepatolenticular d., a group of diseases characterized by degeneration of the liver cells and of the lenticular nucleus associated with increased absorption of copper; commonly called Wilson's disease.
    hyaline d., a regressive change in cells in which the cytoplasm takes on a homogeneous, glassy appearance.
    hydropic d., the appearance of vacuoles in the cytoplasm of cells in certain tissues in relatively mild infections and other conditions.
    lardaceous d., amyloid degeneration.
    lipoid d., a condition somewhat resembling fatty degeneration but in which the extraneous material is lipoid.
    mucoid d., degeneration with deposit of myelin and lecithin in the cells.
    mucous d., degeneration with accumulation of mucus in epithelial tissues.
    myxomatous d., degeneration with accumulation of mucus in connective tissues.
    wallerian d., degeneration of nerve fibers after separation from their nutritive centers.

deglutition (deg″loo-tish′un) the act of swallowing.

degradation (deg″rah-da′shun) conversion of a chemical compound to one less complex by splitting off one or more groups of atoms.

degustation (de″gus-ta′shun) the act or function of tasting.

dehiscence (de-his′ens) separation of edges previously joined; the formation of a fissure.
    wound d., separation of all the layers of an incision or wound.

dehumidifier (de″hu-mid′ĭ-fi″er) an apparatus for reducing the content of moisture in the atmosphere.

dehydrase (de-hi′drās) an enzyme that catalyzes the transference of water from a compound.

dehydration (de″hi-dra′shun) removal of water from the body or a tissue; or the condition that results from undue loss of water. Severe dehydration is a serious condition that may lead to fatal shock, acidosis and the accumulation of waste products in the body, as in UREMIA.
    Water accounts for more than half the body weight. Under normal conditions, a certain amount of fluid is lost daily. About 1.5 liters is removed by urination, and another 90 ml. is lost from the digestive tract in the feces. Through vaporization another liter is given off through the skin and lungs. To make up for these losses, about 2.5 liters of fluid must be taken into the body in food and fluids, and the cells contribute another 250 ml. through chemical activities.
    When the fluid intake is insufficient or the output is excessive, dehydration occurs.
    CAUSES. Abnormal dehydration may occur as a result of prolonged fever, diarrhea, acidosis and vomiting, and in severe injuries or surgical procedures in which there is loss of blood or body fluids. Dehydration is usually accompanied by a depletion of essential electrolytes dissolved in the body fluids. Without a normal supply of these fluids and electrolytes the body processes are impaired and eventual shock and death can occur.
    SYMPTOMS AND TREATMENT. The patient appears flushed and has dry skin and mucous membranes, cracked lips, loss of skin turgor and oliguria. Mental confusion and hypotension indicate a very severe dehydration.
    Treatment is aimed at replacement of fluids and specific electrolytes, and removal of the primary cause of dehydration.
    NURSING CARE. Accurate recording of fluid intake and fluid loss is essential. Special observations of profuse sweating, drainage from wounds or any

other visible loss of fluids are noted on the patient's chart. Daily weighing may be ordered to determine fluid loss or gain.

Intravenous administration of fluids must be done at the exact rate and in the amounts ordered. Rapid infusion of fluids to a dehydrated patient does not allow for proper diffusion into the tissues; thus, the vascular system is overloaded and added strain is placed on the heart.

dehydroandrosterone (de-hi″dro-an-dros′ter-ōn) an androgenic compound derived from male urine.

dehydrocholesterol (de-hi″dro-ko-les′ter-ol) a sterol found in the skin which, when properly irradiated, forms vitamin D.

activated 7-d., a compound used in prophylaxis and treatment of vitamin D deficiency.

dehydrocholic acid (de-hi″dro-ko′lik) a white, fluffy, bitter, odorless powder used to increase output of bile by the liver and the filling of the gallbladder. Preparations of this acid are used to aid the digestion of fats and increase absorption of fat-soluble vitamins. Drugs containing dehydrocholic acid are contraindicated in cases of biliary obstruction. Because of its bitter taste on the tongue when injected into a vein, it is used to provide an end point for the measurement of arm-tongue circulation time.

11-dehydrocorticosterone (de-hi″dro-kor″tĭ-ko-stēr′ōn) a steroid from the adrenal cortex that has a slight effect on protein and carbohydrate metabolism.

dehydrogenase (de-hi′dro-jen-ās″) an enzyme that catalyzes the transference of hydrogen ions.

glucose-6-phosphate d., an enzyme necessary for the oxidation of glucose-6-phosphate, an intermediate in carbohydrate metabolism. Hereditary deficiency of this enzyme in the erythrocytes is associated with a tendency toward hemolysis with certain antimalarial and sulfonamide drugs and fava beans (favism).

lactic d., an enzyme found in high concentrations in a number of tissues. It appears in the blood serum in elevated concentrations when these tissues are severely injured.

dehydrogenate (de-hi′dro-jen-āt″) 1. to remove hydrogen from. 2. a compound from which hydrogen has been removed.

de-iodination (de-i″o-din-a′shun) the loss or removal of iodine from a compound.

de-ionization (de-i″on-ī-za′shun) the removal of ions from a compound.

déjà vu (da′zhah voo′) [Fr.] an illusion that a new situation is a repetition of a previous experience.

dejecta (de-jek′tah) excrement.

dejection (de-jek′shun) 1. discharge of feces. 2. a mental state marked by depression and melancholy.

Dejerine's disease (deh″zher-ēnz′) hypertrophic interstitial neuropathy in infants.

Dejerine-Sottas disease (deh″zher-ēn′ sot′tahz) hypertrophic interstitial neuropathy.

delacrimation (de-lak″rĭ-ma′shun) excessive flow of tears.

delactation (de″lak-ta′shun) 1. weaning. 2. cessation of lactation.

Delalutin (del″ah-lu′tin) trademark for a preparation of hydroxyprogesterone caproate, used in the treatment of corpus luteum deficiency.

Delatestryl (del″ah-tes′tril) trademark for a preparation of testosterone enanthate, used in the treatment of hypogonadism.

deletion (de-le′shun) in genetics, loss from a chromosome of genetic material.

deligation (de″li-ga′shun) 1. ligation. 2. bandaging.

delinquent (de-ling′kwent) 1. lacking in some respect; characterized by antisocial, illegal or criminal behavior. 2. a person whose conduct is antisocial, illegal or criminal; applied to a minor exhibiting such conduct (juvenile delinquent).

deliquescence (del″ĭ-kwes′ens) the process of becoming liquid by absorption of water from the air.

delirium (dĕ-lēr′e-um) a disordered mental state with excitement and illusions. Almost any acute illness accompanied by very high fever can bring on delirium. Other causes are physical and mental shock, exhaustion, fear and anxiety, alcoholism, drug overdose and insulin shock.

NURSING CARE. The delirious patient must be protected from self-injury and carefully supervised so that accidental injury does not occur. The environment should be nonstimulating; the patient kept in a quiet secluded area free from noise, bright lights and other stimuli. When the delirium is prolonged, measures must be taken to ensure adequate fluid intake to combat dehydration, and proper attention must be given to elimination from the bladder and bowels. Medications such as sedatives or tranquilizing drugs may be ordered to relieve the symptoms.

d. tre′mens, delirium from the excessive, chronic use of alcoholic beverages. It may also occur in cases of addiction to narcotics. Delirium tremens (DT's) is a serious mental illness that is accompanied by illusions and vivid hallucinations, extreme restlessness, agitation, uncontrollable shaking and in general an increased body metabolism. The victim is extremely fearful and apprehensive because his illusions and hallucinations are very real to him.

TREATMENT AND NURSING CARE. The patient should be kept in a quiet, nonstimulating environment and approached in a calm, reassuring manner. He must be watched closely and protected from self-injury during the period of delirium and also when he is convalescing from his illness and is likely to feel great remorse and depression. He should be observed for signs of extreme fatigue, pneumonia or heart failure. Respiratory infections are quite common in these patients because of their weakened condition and inattention to personal hygiene.

The diet should be of high fluid intake and high in protein and carbohydrate content and low in fats. Dietary supplements usually include vitamin preparations, especially the B complex vitamins. If the patient is unable to cooperate by taking fluids and food by mouth, tube feeding and intravenous fluids may be necessary. Tranquilizing agents and sedatives are useful for therapy.

deliver (de-liv′er) 1. to aid in childbirth. 2. to remove, as a fetus, placenta or lens of the eye.

delivery (de-liv′er-e) 1. expulsion or extraction of the child at birth (see also LABOR). 2. removal of a part, as the placenta or lens.
   abdominal d., delivery of an infant through an incision made into the uterus through the abdominal wall (cesarean section).

Delta-cortef (del′tah-kor″tef) trademark for a preparation of prednisolone, a compound used as a glucocorticoid.

deltacortisone (del″tah-kor′tĭ-sōn) prednisone, a compound used as a glucocorticoid.

Deltalin (del′tah-lin) trademark for a preparation of synthetic vitamin D_2.

Deltasone (del′tah-sōn) trademark for a preparation of prednisone, a compound used as a glucocorticoid.

deltoid (del′toid) triangular.
   d. muscle, the muscular cap of the shoulder, an inverted triangle that abducts the arm. It is often used as a site for intramuscular injections.

deltoiditis (del″toi-di′tis) inflammation of the deltoid muscle.

Deltra (del′trah) trademark for a tablet containing prednisone, a compound used as a glucocorticoid.

delusion (de-lu′zhun) a false belief inconsistent with an individual's own knowledge and experience. adj., **delu′sional.**

Delvinal (del′vĭ-nal) trademark for preparations of vinbarbital, a short- to intermediate-acting barbiturate.

demecarium (dem″ĕ-ka′re-um) a compound used as a parasympathomimetic and to reduce intraocular pressure in glaucoma.

dementia (de-men′she-ah) progressive mental deterioration due to organic disease of the brain.
   paralytic d., d. paralyt′ica, a chronic disease of the brain characterized by degeneration of the cortical neurons and by progressive loss of mental and physical power, and resulting from antecedent syphilitic infection; called also general paresis.
   d. prae′cox, a term used for a large group of PSYCHOSES of psychogenic origin, often recognized during or shortly after adolescence but not infrequently in later maturity. The chief characteristics are disorientation, loss of contact with reality and splitting of the personality (schizophrenia). The types include the simple and the paranoid, and the forms known as hebephrenia and catatonia.
   senile d., a chronic brain disorder due to generalized atrophy of the brain, characterized by deterioration in intellectual functions.

Demerol (dem′er-ol) trademark for meperidine hydrochloride, a synthetic narcotic preparation.

demethylchlortetracycline (de-meth″il-klor″tet-rah-si′klēn) a broad-spectrum antibiotic produced by a mutant strain of *Streptomyces aureofaciens;* closely related to the other tetracyclines.

demilune (dem′ĭ-lūn) a crescent-shaped structure or cell.

demineralization (de-min″er-al-ĭ-za′shun) removal of mineral salts.

Demodex (dem′o-deks) a genus of mites parasitic within the hair follicles of the host, including the species *D. folliculo′rum* in man, and several other species in domestic and other animals.

demography (de-mog′rah-fe) the science dealing with social statistics, including questions of health, disease, births and mortality.

demorphinization (de-mor″fĭ-nĭ-za′shun) gradual withdrawal of morphine from one addicted to its use.

demucosation (de″mu-ko-za′shun) removal of mucous membrane.

demulcent (de-mul′sent) 1. soothing; bland. 2. a soothing mucilaginous medicine.

de Musset's sign (dĕ-mu-sāz′) rhythmic oscillation of the head caused by pulsations of the carotid arteries; a sign of aortic insufficiency.

demyelinate (de-mi′ĕ-lin-at″) to destroy or remove the myelin sheath of a nerve or nerves.

denarcotize (de-nar′ko-tīz) to deprive of narcotics or of narcotic properties.

denaturation (de-na″tūr-a′shun) the destruction of a substance, as the addition of methanol or acetone to alcohol to render it unfit for drinking.
   protein d., any nonproteolytic change in the chemistry, composition or structure of a native protein which causes it to lose some or all of its unique or specific characteristics.

dendraxon (den-drak′son) a nerve cell whose axon splits up into terminal filaments immediately after leaving the cell.

dendric (den′drik) pertaining to a dendrite.

dendriform (den′drĭ-form) tree-shaped.

dendrite (den′drīt) a long, branching protoplasmic process, such as the branches conducting impulses toward the body of a nerve cell.

dendritic (den-drit′ik) treelike in appearance or form.

dendroid (den′droid) branching like a tree.

dendron (den′dron) dendrite.

dendrophagocytosis (den″dro-fag″o-si-to′sis) the absorption by microglia cells of broken portions of astrocytes.

denervation (de″ner-va′shun) interruption of the nerve connection to an organ or part.

dengue (deng′e; Spanish, dan′ga) a painful, virus-caused disease that flourishes in tropical climates throughout the world. The virus that causes the disease is carried by the same species of mosquito that carries yellow fever, *Aedes aegypti.* Because of the intense pain in the bones, dengue is known also as "breakbone fever" and by other names based on the necessity of keeping the neck rigid, such as "dandy" and "giraffe." People who have had dengue are generally immunized against the disease for 5 years, and epidemics tend to recur at 5-year intervals. Occasional epidemics occur in the Gulf states of the United States.

SYMPTOMS. The symptoms of dengue begin within a week after the bite of the infected mosquito. The onset is marked by a severe headache and pain behind the eyes. Within hours the characteristic pain in the back and joints begins. Movement is difficult, and the temperature may rise as high as 106° F. A pink rash, congested eyeballs and a flushed face are outward symptoms. The disease usually has two stages of about 3 days and 2 days separated by a period of 24 hours in which the symptoms disappear, raising hopes of the end of the attack. The second stage is marked by the earlier symptoms and in addition a red rash appears on the elbows, knees and ankles, leading often to peeling skin. The total course of the disease is rarely more than 6 or 7 days. Although the sufferer is exhausted and less resistant to other diseases, dengue by itself is rarely fatal. Convalescence is slow.

TREATMENT AND PREVENTION. As there is no known remedy for dengue, the treatment is mainly palliative. An icecap to reduce the headache, analgesics to relieve the pain and a large intake of liquid are the basic essentials.

The best method of preventing dengue is by controlling the mosquito, and in some areas this has been successful. In areas lacking mosquito control, protective clothing should be worn outside and mosquito netting used indoors to reduce the risk of infection.

denidation (de″ni-da′shun) the disintegration and removal, during menstruation, of certain epthelial elements, potentially the nidus of an embryo.

Denis Browne splint (den′is brown) a splint for the correction of clubfoot, consisting of two metal footplates connected by a crossbar.

dens (dens), pl. *den′tes* [L.] a tooth or toothlike structure.

densimeter (den-sim′ĕ-ter) an apparatus for determining density or specific gravity.

densitometry (den″sĭ-tom′ĕ-tre) determination of variations in density by comparison with that of another material or with a certain standard.

density (den′sĭ-te) 1. the quality of being compact; the compactness of a substance. 2. the quantity of matter in a given space.

densography (den-sog′rah-fe) the measurement of the contrast densities in a roentgen negative.

dent(o)- (den′to) word element [L.], *tooth; toothlike.*

dentagra (den-tag′rah) 1. toothache. 2. a forceps or key for pulling teeth.

dental (den′tal) pertaining to the teeth.
  d. caries, tooth decay (see also CARIES).

dentalgia (den-tal′je-ah) toothache.

dentate (den′tāt) notched; tooth-shaped.

dentia (den′she-ah) 1. dentition. 2. a condition relating to development or eruption of the teeth.
  d. prae′cox, premature eruption of the teeth; presence of teeth in the mouth at birth.

d. tar′da, delayed eruption of the teeth, beyond the usual time for their appearance.

dentibuccal (den″tĭ-buk′al) pertaining to the cheek and teeth.

denticle (den′tĭ-kl) 1. a small toothlike process. 2. a distinct calcified mass within the pulp chamber or in the dentin of a tooth.

dentification (den″tĭ-fĭ-ka′shun) conversion into a toothlike structure.

dentifrice (den′tĭ-fris) a preparation for cleansing and polishing the teeth.

dentigerous (den-tij′er-us) containing or producing teeth.

dentilabial (den″tĭ-la′be-al) pertaining to the teeth and lips.

dentilingual (den″tĭ-ling′gwal) pertaining to the teeth and tongue.

dentimeter (den-tim′ĕ-ter) an instrument for measuring teeth.

dentin (den′tin) the chief substance of the teeth, forming the body, neck and roots, being covered by enamel on the exposed parts of the teeth and by cementum on the parts implanted in the jaws. adj., **den′tinal.**

dentinoblastoma (den″tĭ-no-blas-to′mah) a tumor of odontogenic origin, composed of round or spindle-shaped connective tissue cells, among which are islands of irregularly shaped masses of dentin.

dentinogenesis (den″tĭ-no-jen′ĕ-sis) the formation of dentin.
  d. imperfec′ta, imperfect formation of dentin, resulting in an unusual translucent or opalescent hue to the teeth.

dentinoma (den″tĭ-no′mah) an encapsulated tumor of the jaw, containing connective tissue and masses of dentin, with evidence of new dentin formation.

dentist (den′tist) a person licensed to practice dentistry.

dentistry (den′tis-tre) 1. that branch of the healing arts concerned with the teeth and associated structures of the oral cavity. 2. the work done by dentists, e.g., the creation of restorations, crowns and bridges, and surgical procedures performed in and about the oral cavity. 3. the practice of the dental profession collectively.
  operative d., dentistry concerned with restoration of parts of the teeth that are defective as a result of disease, trauma or abnormal development to a state of normal function, health and esthetics.
  preventive d., dentistry concerned with maintenance of a normal masticating mechanism by fortifying the structures of the oral cavity against damage and disease.
  prosthetic d., prosthodontics.

dentition (den-tish′un) the entire array of teeth in a jaw, consisting of natural teeth in position in the alveoli.
  deciduous d., the complement of teeth that erupt

first and are later succeeded by the permanent teeth.

mixed d., the complement of teeth in the jaws after eruption of some of the permanent teeth, but before all the deciduous teeth are shed.

permanent d., the complement of teeth that erupt after the deciduous teeth have been shed.

dentoalveolar (den″to-al-ve′o-lar) pertaining to a tooth and its alveolus.

dentoalveolitis (den″to-al″ve-o-li′tis) periodontitis.

dentulous (den′tu-lus) having natural teeth.

denture (den′tūr) a complement of teeth, either natural or artificial; ordinarily used to designate an artificial replacement for the natural teeth and adjacent tissues.

artificial d., an appliance worn in the mouth to replace missing natural teeth and associated structures.

complete d., an artificial denture replacing all the teeth of one jaw.

partial d., a removable or permanently attached appliance replacing one or more missing teeth in one jaw and receiving support and retention from underlying tissues and some or all of the remaining teeth.

denucleated (de-nu′kle-āt″ed) deprived of the nucleus.

denudation (de″nu-da′shun) the stripping or laying bare of any part.

denutrition (de″nu-trish′un) lack or failure of nutrition.

deobstruent (de-ob′stroo-ent) 1. removing obstructions. 2. a medicine that removes obstructions.

deodorant (deo-o′dor-ant) 1. destroying odors. 2. a deodorizing agent.

deorsum (de-or′sum) [L.] downward.

deorsumversion (de-or″sum-ver′zhun) the turning downward of a part, especially of the eyes.

deossification (de-os″ĭ-fĭ-ka′shun) loss or removal of the mineral elements of bone.

deoxidation (de-ok″sĭ-da′shun) deoxygenation, removal of oxygen from a chemical compound.

deoxy- (de-ok′se) a prefix used in naming chemical compounds, to designate a compound containing one less atom of oxygen than the reference substance. For words beginning thus, see also those beginning *desoxy-*.

deoxycholic acid (de-ok″sĭ-ko′lik) one of the bile acids, capable of forming soluble, diffusible complexes with fatty acids, and thereby allowing for their absorption in the small intestine.

deoxycorticosterone (de-ok″sĭ-kor′tĭ-ko-stēr′ōn) desoxycorticosterone.

deoxygenation (de-ok″sĭ-jē-na′shun) removal of oxygen.

deoxypentosenucleic acid (de-ok″sĭ-pen″tōs-nu-kle′ik) deoxyribonucleic acid.

deoxyribonuclease (de-ok″sĭ-ri″bo-nu′kle-ās) an enzyme that catalyzes the depolymerization of deoxyribonucleic acid (DNA).

deoxyribonucleic acid (de-ok″sĭ-ri″bo-nu-kle′ik) DNA; a nucleic acid that is a large complex molecule composed of phosphoric acid, a pentose (deoxyribose) and a mixture of purines and pyrimidines. DNA is the basic substance of GENES and carries the code of genetic information controlling development of the organism. DNA is a double molecule, capable of reproducing itself and also of producing ribonucleic acid (RNA), which in turn produces proteins. Since protein is the essential material of protoplasm, the importance of DNA in the vitality of the cell is obvious. The ability of DNA to reproduce itself explains how genes can reproduce again and again without changing their individual characteristics (See also HEREDITY).

deoxyribonucleoprotein (de-ok″sĭ-ri″bo-nu′kle-o-pro″te-in) a nucleoprotein in which the sugar is D-2-deoxyribose.

deoxyribose (de-ok″sĭ-ri′bōs) an aldopentose found in thymus nucleic acid.

dependence (de-pen′dens) the total psychophysical state of an addict in which the usual or increasing doses of the drug are required to prevent the onset of abstinence symptoms.

depersonalization (de-per″sun-al-ĭ-za′shun) a feeling of unreality or strangeness, related to one's self or to the external environment.

dephosphorylation (de-fos′for-ĭ-la′shun) removal of the phosphoryl, the trivalent PO group, from organic molecules.

depilate (dep′ĭ-lāt) to remove hair.

depilatory (de-pil′ah-tor″e) 1. removing hair. 2. an agent that removes the hair.

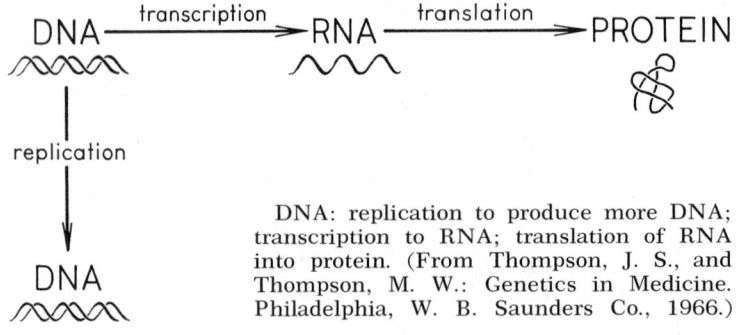

DNA: replication to produce more DNA; transcription to RNA; translation of RNA into protein. (From Thompson, J. S., and Thompson, M. W.: Genetics in Medicine. Philadelphia, W. B. Saunders Co., 1966.)

depolarization (de-po″lar-ĭ-za′shun) the abolition or disappearance of a difference in electrical charge.

depolymerization (de-pol″ĭ-mer-ĭ-za′shun) the conversion of a compound into one of smaller molecular weight and different physical properties without changing the percentage relations of the elements composing it.

deposit (de-poz′it) 1. sediment or dregs. 2. extraneous inorganic matter collected in the tissues or in an organ of the body.

Depo-testosterone (de″po-tes-tos′ter-ōn) trademark for a sustained-action preparation of testosterone.

depressant (de-pres′ant) 1. depressing or retarding. 2. an agent that retards any function, especially a drug that slows a function of the body or calms and quiets nervous excitement; a sedative. Among the best-known depressants are barbiturates. Alcohol is also a depressant, although its first effect is sometimes stimulating. (See also TRANQUILIZER).

depression (de-presh′un) 1. a hollow or fossa. 2. reduction of vital functional activity; in psychiatry, a morbid sadness or melancholy, distinguished from grief, which is realistic and proportionate to a personal loss. Depression may be symptomatic of a psychiatric disorder or it may constitute the principal manifestation of a neurosis or psychosis. adj., **depres′sive.**

Treatment of depression is often very difficult, requiring in most cases intensive psychotherapy to help the patient understand the underlying cause of his depression. Some form of shock therapy such as electric shock or insulin shock treatments is usually used in conjunction with the psychotherapy. Antidepressant drugs such as imipramine hydrochloride (Tofranil) and amitriptyline (Elavil) are often used in the treatment of depression. They are not true stimulants of the central nervous system, but they do alter the function of the reticular system in the midbrain and of the nuclei of the thalamus.

NURSING CARE. The severely depressed patient usually expresses three basic feelings associated with his mental state. These are physical inactivity and a lack of desire to socialize, feelings of worthlessness and loss of self-esteem and thoughts of self-injury or destruction. In planning the nursing care of the depressed patient one must always consider these attitudes and strive for some understanding as to why the patient behaves as he does. Although an optimistic approach should be used when helping the patient overcome his depression, the nurse must guard against excessive cheerfulness and attempts to "jolly" the patient into a better mood. Only by gradually gaining his attention and pointing out to him encouraging signs of his progress can she begin to help him in his early attempts to return to reality and socialize with others. As he progresses out of his depression the patient may become overdependent on the nurse and then later show signs of hostility toward her. She must, however, remain consistent in her relationship with him, demonstrating warmth and a sincere interest in him no matter what type of behavior he may exhibit.

The patient's physical inactivity will require attention to adequate nutrition, a normal balance of fluid intake and output, proper elimination and good skin care. He will need help in maintaining a pleasing personal appearance and good personal hygiene. At first it may be necessary for the nurse to initiate all such activities as bathing, dressing and even eating and drinking. As his condition improves the patient should take over responsibility for his personal care and grooming. If he is severely depressed he may be totally out of reach with reality and completely unresponsive to the nurse's presence. In such instances the nurse may be able to do little more than sit with the patient, letting him know by her presence that she is interested in his problem and that she does care enough to try to help him.

Constant vigilance must be maintained to prevent the depressed patient from injuring himself or committing suicide. Self-destructive behavior is a manifestation of the patient's feeling of worthlessness and loss of self-esteem. An awareness of the potential dangers in such a situation should help the nurse plan and provide a safe and congenial atmosphere. She should be alert to the early signs of a patient's intention to harm or destroy himself. Although physical restraint may eventually be necessary to control the patient, early recognition of the patient's deepening depression and appropriate measures to improve his mood will help eliminate the need for more drastic measures.

agitated d., depression with anxiety, as seen in involution melancholia.

anaclitic d., impairment of an infant's physical, social and intellectual development which sometimes follows a sudden separation from the mothering person.

congenital chrondrosternal d., a congenital deformity with a deep, funnel-shaped depression in the anterior chest wall.

emotional d., undue sadness or melancholy, due to no recognizable cause.

involutional d., depression sometimes accompanying menopause in women or decline in sexual or vocational activity in men.

reactive d., neurotic or psychotic depression due to environmental loss or stress.

situational d., reactive depression.

depressomotor (de-pres″o-mo′tor) diminishing motor action.

depressor (de-pres′or) that which depresses.
tongue d., an instrument for pressing down the tongue.

deradelphus (der″ah-del′fus) a twin monster with one neck and head.

deradenitis (der″ad-ĕ-ni′tis) inflammation of the glands of the neck.

deradenoncus (der″ad-ĕ-nong′kus) swelling of a gland of the neck.

derangement (de-rānj′ment) disorder.

Dercum's disease (der′kumz) adiposis dolorosa.

dereistic (de″re-is′tik) giving the imagination free play.

derencephalus (der″en-sef′ah-lus) a monster with no cranium, the cervical vertebrae containing the relics of a brain.

derepression (de″re-presh′un) in psychiatry, the coming back of ideas or impulses into conscious awareness that were earlier pushed from such awareness into the unconscious because they were personally intolerable.

deric (der'ik) pertaining to the ectoderm.

derivative (de-riv'ah-tiv) a chemical substance derived from another substance either directly or by modification or partial substitution.

derma (der'mah) corium.

dermabrasion (derm″ah-bra'shun) removal, by sandpaper or high-speed brush, of acne scars or nevi.

Dermacentor (der″mah-sen'tor) a genus of arthropods parasitic on various animals, and vectors of disease-producing microorganisms.

  D. anderso'ni, a species of tick common in the western United States, parasitic on numerous wild mammals, most domestic animals and man, and a vector of Rocky Mountain spotted fever, tularemia, Colorado tick fever and Q fever in the United States.

  D. varia'bilis, a tick parasitic on dogs and man, as well as many wild animals and most other domestic animals; a vector of spotted fever and tularemia.

dermadrome (der'mah-drōm) a complex of cutaneous symptoms commonly associated with an internal disorder.

dermal (der'mal) pertaining to the true skin, or corium.

Dermanyssus (der″mah-nis'us) a genus of mites parasitic on birds, sometimes affecting man.

dermatic (der-mat'ik) pertaining to the skin.

dermatitides (der″mah-tit'ĭ-dēz) inflammatory conditions of the skin considered collectively.

dermatitis (der″mah-ti'tis) inflammation of the skin. Dermatitis can result from various animal, vegetable and chemical substances, from heat or cold, from mechanical irritation, from certain forms of malnutrition or from infectious disease. In some cases, dermatitis may have a psychologic rather than a physical cause. The symptoms may include itching, redness, crustiness, blisters, watery discharges, fissures or other changes in the normal condition of the skin. The treatment of dermatitis varies greatly and is determined by the cause.

  TYPES OF DERMATITIS. One of the most common forms of the disorder, CONTACT DERMATITIS, results from contact of the skin with various substances. There are two types: allergic contact dermatitis and primary irritant dermatitis. Familiar examples of the allergic type are POISON IVY, OAK AND SUMAC, but many other substances may be the cause of an allergic reaction. These include rubber and plastics, industrial chemicals, cosmetics, clothing dyes, costume jewelry, some animals and plants, detergents, insecticides and paints.

  The second type of contact dermatitis is due to a direct irritating effect on the skin of certain chemical, physical or mechanical agents. In contrast to the allergic type, which affects only people who have a specific sensitivity, these agents cause dermatitis in everyone upon sufficient exposure. Acids, alkalis, petroleum products and mineral dusts are some of the chemical causes. A mild form

is the familiar "dishpan hands," resulting from contact with strong soaps and detergents.

  Such physical agents as excessive cold or heat may also cause inflammation of the skin. Prolonged exposure to extreme cold may result in CHILBLAINS or in FROSTBITE, and exposure to a hot sun may cause sunburn. When heat causes unusual sweating, miliaria (commonly called prickly heat) may result. All these familiar complaints are forms of dermatitis. Overexposure to x-rays is another factor which may cause skin inflammation. Mechanical agents, such as chafing, pressure or scratching, are other common causes of dermatitis. Pressure and friction resulting from ill fitting shoes cause corns and calluses, and pressure on bony parts of the body incurred in extended bed rest may cause decubitus ulcers.

  NURSING CARE. The patient with dermatitis frequently is uncomfortable, irritable and emotionally upset because of itching and the unsightly appearance produced by his condition. Efforts should be made to provide a quiet atmosphere that is conducive to rest, and to give the patient individual attention to help him feel acceptable to others.

  If large areas of the skin are involved there will be increased sensitivity to cold, making the patient more susceptible to chilling. Care must be used to protect the patient and the bed linen from dampness when wet compresses are prescribed.

  Bathing with ordinary soap and water is usually contraindicated and special colloid or medicated baths may be ordered to cleanse and soothe irritated or pruritic skin. After the bath the skin is dried by patting with a soft towel, *never* by rubbing. Scales, crusts and other exudates are *not* removed without specific orders from the physician. The skin should be handled gently, and great care used in changing the bedclothes or the patient's clothing. Lotions and alcohol routinely used in the hospital for back rubs or as skin fresheners must not be applied to the skin of these patients without written directions from the physician because they may aggravate the skin disorder.

  actinic d., d. actin'ica, dermatitis produced by exposure to rays of the sun or to ultraviolet radiation.

  atopic d., a skin condition occurring as a reaction to a substance to which the patient is sensitive.

  contact d., that due to direct contact with an allergen, usually accompanied by severe itching (see also CONTACT DERMATITIS).

  exfoliative d., dermatitis characterized by peeling of the skin and loss of hair; it may result from internal medication with such drugs as penicillin, quinine, sulfonamides, gold salts and iodides.

  infectious d., dermatitis caused by bacteria, fungi, viruses or other parasitic organisms.

  d. medicamento'sa, a skin eruption due to sensitivity to a drug that was ingested, inhaled or injected.

  pellagrous d., dryness and redness of the skin exposed to sunlight, characteristic symptoms of PELLAGRA.

  seborrheic d., d. seborrhe'ica, an inflammatory skin disease with yellowish, greasy scaling and usually itching (see also SEBORRHEIC DERMATITIS).

  d. venena'ta, contact dermatitis.

  x-ray d., skin inflammation due to exposure to x-rays.

dermatocellulitis (der″mah-to-sel″u-li'tis) inflammation of the skin and subcutaneous cellular tissue.

dermatocyst (der'mah-to-sist") a cyst of the skin.

dermatofibroma (der"mah-to-fi-bro'mah) a fibroma of the skin.

dermatofibrosarcoma (der"mah-to-fi"bro-sar-ko'-mah) a fibrosarcoma of the skin.

dermatogen (der-mat'o-jen) an antigen of any skin disease.

dermatogenic, dermatogenous (der"mah-to-jen'ik), (der"mah-toj'ĕ-nus) producing skin.

dermatoglyphics (der"mah-to-glif'iks) the study of the patterns of ridges of the skin of the fingers, palms, toes and soles, frequently found to be significant in genetic investigations.

dermatograph (der-mat'o-graf) 1. an instrument for marking the boundaries of the body. 2. a wheal made on the skin in dermographia.

dermatographia (der"mah-to-graf'e-ah) a condition in which persistent linear markings may be elicited by drawing a blunt instrument across the skin.

dermatoheteroplasty (der"mah-to-het'er-o-plas"te) grafting of skin taken from the body of another.

dermatoid (der'mah-toid) skinlike.

dermatology (der"mah-tol'o-je) that branch of medicine dealing with diseases of the skin.

dermatoma (der"mah-to'mah) an abnormal growth of skin tissue.

dermatome (der'mah-tōm) 1. the ventrolateral portion of an embryonic somite, which develops into the fibrous layer of the integument. 2. the cutaneous area developed from a single embryonic somite and receiving the greater part of its innervation from a single spinal nerve. 3. an instrument for excising areas of skin to be used for grafting.

dermatomegaly (der"mah-to-meg'ah-le) a condition in which the skin is larger than necessary to cover the body, so that it hangs in folds.

dermatomere (der'mah-to-mēr") any segment of the embryonic integument.

dermatomucosomyositis (der"mah-to-mu-ko"so-mi"o-si'tis) inflammation of the skin, mucous membrane and muscles.

dermatomycosis (der"mah-to-mi-ko'sis) a skin disease due to parasitic fungi.

dermatomyoma (der"mah-to-mi-o'mah) myoma involving the skin.

dermatomyositis (der"mah-to-mi"o-si'tis) an acute, subacute or chronic disease involving constant inflammation of the skin and muscles, leading to muscular decomposition and atrophy. It is included among the group of illnesses known as COLLAGEN DISEASES.
Among a variety of symptoms that point to the onset of the disease are fever, loss of weight, skin lesions and aching muscles. As the disease progresses there may be loss of the use of the arms and legs. Complications such as hardening may occur, similar to the changes seen in scleroderma. Occasionally steroids prove helpful in relieving symptoms, but the most beneficial treatment is physical therapy to maintain maximal use of the muscles.

dermatoneurosis (der"mah-to-nu-ro'sis) a neurogenic skin disorder.

dermatopathology (der"mah-to-pah-thol'o-je) pathology that is especially concerned with lesions of the skin.

dermatopathy (der"mah-top'ah-the) disease of the skin.

dermatophobia (der"ma-to-fo'be-ah) morbid dread of skin disease.

dermatophylaxis (der"mah-to-fi-lak'sis) protection against skin infection; protection of the skin against infection.

dermatophyte (der'mah-to-fīt") any one of a group of fungi that cause superficial infections of the skin, including Microsporum, Epidermophyton and Trichophyton.

dermatophytid (der"mah-tof'ĭ-tid) a secondary rash or eruption occurring in dermatomycosis.

dermatophytosis (der"mah-to-fi-to'sis) a superficial infection of the skin caused by a fungus.
d. furfura'cea, tinea versicolor.

dermatoplasty (der'mah-to-plas"te) plastic repair of the skin.

dermatosclerosis (der"mah-to-sklĕ-ro'sis) scleroderma.

dermatosis (der"mah-to'sis) any disorder of the skin.
precancerous d., any skin condition in which the lesions—warts, nevi or other excrescences—are likely to undergo malignant degeneration.
stasis d., skin disease marked by disturbances of the circulation and of lymphatic absorption.

dermatotherapy (der"mah-to-ther'ah-pe) treatment of skin diseases.

dermatotropic (der"mah-to-trop'ik) having a specific affinity for the skin.

dermis (der'mis) the true skin, or corium. adj., **der'mal, der'mic.**

dermoblast (der'mo-blast) the part of the mesoderm that develops into the true skin.

dermographia (der"mo-graf'e-ah) elicitation of a transient mark on the skin by stroking with a blunt-pointed instrument.

dermoid (der'moid) 1. skinlike. 2. a dermoid cyst.
d. cyst, a congenital cyst filled with sebaceous material and containing primary germ-cell layers and, perhaps, fetal remains. Upon removal the cysts are often found to contain hair, bone, teeth and cartilage. When these cysts occur in the ovary they may present no symptoms, but their long pedicles may cause twisting, resulting in acute abdominal pain. Treatment is surgical removal.

dermoidectomy (der"moi-dek'to-me) excision of a dermoid cyst.

dermolysis (der-mol'ĭ-sis) destruction of the skin.

dermomycosis (der"mo-mi-ko'sis) a skin disease produced by a fungus.

dermonecrotic (der"mo-nĕ-krot'ik) causing necrosis of the skin.

dermopathy (der-mop′ah-the) any skin disease.

dermophlebitis (der″mo-flĕ-bi′tis) inflammation of the veins of the skin.

dermophylaxis (der″mo-fi-lak′sis) the protective action of the skin against infections.

dermophyte (der′mo-fīt) a vegetable skin parasite.

dermoskeleton (der″mo-skel′ĕ-ton) the external and visible coverings of the body: skin, teeth, hair and nails.

dermosynovitis (der″mo-sin″o-vi′tis) malignant inflammation of the sole of the foot, with involvement of synovial sheaths.

dermotropic (der″mo-trop′ik) having a special affinity for epithelial surfaces of the body.

dermovascular (der″mo-vas′ku-lar) pertaining to the skin and blood vessels.

derodidymus (der″o-did′ĭ-mus) a fetal monster with one body, two necks and two heads.

Deronil (der′o-nil) trademark for a preparation of dexamethasone, a corticosteroid.

Descemet′s membrane (des-ĕ-māz′) the posterior lining membrane of the cornea.

descensus (de-sen′sus), pl. *descen′sus* [L.] downward displacement or prolapse.
   d. tes′tis, normal migration of the testis from its fetal position in the abdominal cavity to its location within the scrotum, usually during the last 3 months of gestation.
   d. u′teri, prolapse of the uterus.

desensitization (de-sen″sĭ-tĭ-za′shun) the abolition of sensitivity to a particular antigen.

desensitize (de-sen′sĭ-tīz) to render less sensitive.

desequestration (de″se-kwes-tra′shun) the release of sequestered material, e.g., release into the general circulation of blood previously withheld from it by physiologic or mechanical means.

deserpidine (de-ser′pĭ-dēn) a reserpine derivative used as a tranquilizer.

desert fever a fungal disease usually affecting the respiratory tract and lungs, although it may involve any or all of the body′s organs; called also San Joaquin Valley fever, desert rheumatism and COCCIDIOIDOMYCOSIS.

desiccant (des′ĭ-kant) promoting dryness.

desiccate (des′ĭ″kāt) to render thoroughly dry.

desiccation (des″ĭ-ka′shun) the act of drying.

desipramine hydrochloride (des-ip′rah-mēn) a compound used as an antidepressant for depression of psychogenic origin.

deslanoside (des-lan′o-sīd) a poisonous, white crystalline compound used as a cardiotonic and for controlling cardiac rhythm.

desmalgia (des-mal′je-ah) pain in a ligament.

desmectasia (des″mek-ta′ze-ah) the stretching of a ligament.

desmepithelium (des″mep-ĭ-the′le-um) the epithelium of the blood vessels, lymphatics and synovial membranes.

desmitis (des-mi′tis) inflammation of a ligament.

desmocranium (des″mo-kra′ne-um) the mass of dense mesenchyme enveloping the cranial end of the notochord at the fifth and sixth weeks, which is the earliest indication of the skull in the developing embryo.

desmocyte (des′mo-sīt) any supporting tissue cell.

desmodynia (des″mo-din′e-ah) pain in a ligament or ligaments.

desmoenzyme (des″mo-en′zīm) an enzyme that is bound to the protoplasm of a cell and that cannot be extracted by available methods.

desmography (des-mog′rah-fe) a description of ligaments.

desmoid (des′moid) 1. fibrous. 2. a hard or tough fibroma.

desmology (des-mol′o-je) the science of ligaments.

desmoma (des-mo′mah) fibroma.

desmoneoplasm (des″mo-ne′o-plazm) a connective tissue neoplasm.

desmopathy (des-mop′ah-the) any disease of the ligaments.

desmoplastic (des′mo-plas″tik) producing adhesions.

desoxy- (des-ok′se) for words beginning thus, see also those beginning *deoxy-*.

desoxycorticosterone (des-ok″sĭ-kor″tĭ-ko-stēr′-ōn) a hormone of the adrenal cortex very similar in structure to corticosterone. It is a MINERALOCORTICOID.
   d. acetate, a white crystalline powder used in the treatment of Addison′s disease.

desoxyephedrine (des-ok″se-ĕ-fed′rin) methamphetamine, an adrenergic and central nervous system stimulant.

Desoxyn (des-ok′sin) trademark for preparations of methamphetamine hydrochloride, an adrenergic and central nervous system stimulant.

desoxyphenobarbital (des-ok″sĭ-fe″no-bar′bĭ-tal) primidone, an anticonvulsant.

desquamation (des″kwah-ma′shun) shedding of material from a surface, as the shedding of cells from the skin or a mucous membrane. adj., **desquam′ative.**
   siliquose d., the shedding of dried vesicles from the skin.

detachment (de-tach′ment) the condition of being separated or set apart.
   d. of retina, retinal d., separation of the inner layers of the retina from the pigment layer, which remains attached to the choroid. The onset of symptoms may be gradual or sudden, depending on the cause, size and location of the area involved. The patient may see flashes of light and then days or weeks later notice cloudy vision or loss of central vision. Another common symptom is the sensation of spots or moving particles in the field of

vision. In severe retinal detachment there may be complete loss of vision.

The condition is treated surgically. Newer surgical procedures include the use of diathermy to seal the retinal break so that vitreous humor cannot leak between the retina and choroid. In some cases the vitreous is drained from the area in which it has accumulated so that the retina can be returned to its normal position. When sutures are used to hold the retina in place, the patient is confined to bed for 2 weeks postoperatively to avoid strain on the suture line. If one of the newer surgical techniques is used, the patient may be allowed out of bed the day after surgery but he must be warned to avoid vigorous movement of the head.

detergent (de-ter'jent) 1. cleansing. 2. a substance that combines the properties of wetting and emulsifying agents, facilitating removal of oil and dirt.

deterioration (de-tēr"e-o-ra'shun) 1. the process or state of growing worse. 2. disintegration or wearing away.

determination (de-ter"mĭ-na'shun) the establishment, during embryonic development, of the ultimate destiny of a particular region.

sex d., the process by which the sex of an organism is fixed, associated, in man, with the presence or absence of the Y chromosome.

determinism (de-ter'mĭ-nizm) the doctrine that the will is not free but is absolutely determined by psychic and physical conditions.

psychic d., the theory that mental processes are always determined by motives.

detoxicate (de-tok'sĭ-kāt) to deprive of toxic qualities.

detoxication, detoxification (de-tok"sĭ-ka'shun), (de-tok"sĭ-fĭ-ka'shun) the destruction of toxic properties of a substance, a major function of the liver.

detrition (de-trish'un) the wearing away, as of teeth, by friction.

detritus (de-tri'tus) particulate matter produced by or remaining after the wearing away or disintegration of a substance or tissue.

detruncation (de"trung-ka'shun) decapitation.

detubation (de"tu-ba'shun) the removal of a tube.

detumescence (de"tu-mes'ens) the subsidence of congestion and swelling.

deutan (du'tan) a person with anomalous color vision, marked by derangement or loss of the red-green sensory mechanism.

deuteranomalopia (du"ter-ah-nom"ah-lo'pe-ah) a variant of normal color vision with imperfect perception of the green hues.

deuteranope (du'ter-ah-nōp") a person exhibiting deuteranopia.

deuteranopia, deuteranopsia (du"ter-ah-no'pe-ah), (du"ter-ah-nop'se-ah) defective color vision, with retention of the sensory mechanism for two hues only—blue and yellow.

deuterate (du'ter-āt) to treat (combine) with deuterium (^{2}H).

deuterium (du-te're-um) the mass two isotope of hydrogen, symbol ^{2}H or D; it is available as a gas or heavy water (deuterium oxide) and is used as a tracer or indicator in studying fat and amino acid metabolism.

deuterohemophilia (du"ter-o-he"mo-fil'e-ah) a condition resembling hemophilia A (classic hemophilia).

deuteron (du'ter-on) the nucleus of the deuterium atom, considered to consist of one proton and one neutron.

deuteropathy (du"ter-op'ah-the) a disease that is secondary to another disease.

deutoplasm (du'to-plazm) the passive or inactive materials in protoplasm, especially reserve foodstuffs, such as yolk.

devascularization (de-vas"ku-lar-ĭ-za'shun) interruption of circulation of blood to a part due to obstruction or destruction of blood vessels supplying it.

Devegan (dev'ĕ-gan) trademark for a preparation of acetarsone, an antiprotozoan drug.

development (de-vel'up-ment) gradual growth or expansion, especially from a lower to a higher stage of complexity.

psychosexual d., development of the personality through the infantile and pregenital stages to sexual maturity.

developmental (de-vel"up-men'tal) pertaining to development.

d. anomaly, absence, deformity or excess of body parts as the result of faulty development of the embryo.

deviant (de've-ant) 1. varying from a determinable standard. 2. a person with characteristics varying from what is considered standard or normal.

color d., a person whose color perception varies from the norm.

deviation (de"ve-a'shun) a turning away from the regular standard or course. In ophthalmology, a tendency for the visual axes of the eye to fall out of alignment owing to muscular imbalance.

sexual d., sexual behavior that varies from that normally considered biologically or socially accepted (see also SEXUAL DEVIATION).

standard d., the measure of variability of any frequency curve.

devil's grip epidemic pleurodynia.

devisceration (de-vis"er-a'shun) removal of viscera.

devitalization (de-vi"tal-ĭ-za'shun) deprivation of vitality or life.

pulp d., destruction of vitality of the pulp of a tooth.

devolution (dev"o-lu'shun) the reverse of evolution; catabolic change.

dexamethasone (dek"sah-meth'ah-sōn) a glucocorticoid, used as an anti-inflammatory steroid with little salt-retaining action.

dexchlorpheniramine (deks″klōr-fen-i′rah-men) a pyridine derivative used as an antihistamine.

Dexedrine (dek′sĕ-drēn) trademark for preparations of dextroamphetamine, used in weight control and as a central nervous system stimulant.

Dexoval (dek′so-val) trademark for a preparation of methamphetamine, a central nervous system stimulant.

dexter (dek′ster) [L.] right; on the right side.

dextr(o)- (dek′stro) word element [L.], *right*.

dextrality (dek-stral′ĭ-te) the preferential use, in voluntary motor acts, of the right member of the major paired organs of the body, as the right eye, hand or foot.

dextran (dek′stran) a water-soluble, high-glucose polymer produced by the action of *Leuconostoc mesenteroides* on sucrose; used as a plasma substitute, for rapid expansion of the intravascular plasma volume.

dextrase (dek′strās) an enzyme that changes dextrose into lactic acid.

dextraural (dek-straw′ral) hearing better with the right ear.

dextrin (dek′strin) a carbohydrate formed during the hydrolysis of starch to sugar.

dextrinosis (dek″strĭ-no′sis) a condition characterized by accumulation in the tissues of an abnormal polysaccharide.
 limit d., a form of hepatic and muscle glycogen disease due to deficiency of debrancher enzyme.

dextrinuria (dek″strin-u′re-ah) presence of dextrin in the urine.

dextroamphetamine (dek″stro-am-fet′ah-mēn) the dextrorotatory isomer of amphetamine, having a more conspicuous stimulant effect on the central nervous system than racemic amphetamine in the same dosage; used to decrease appetite, as a respiratory stimulant, to stimulate peristalsis and to raise blood pressure.

dextrocardia (dek″stro-kar′de-ah) location of the heart in the right side of the thorax, the apex pointing to the right.
 mirror-image d., dextrocardia in which the right-to-left relation of the heart is reversed, venous blood passing through the chambers at the left, and arterial blood through the chambers at the right.

dextrocularity (dek″strok-u-lar′ĭ-te) dominance of the right eye.

dextromanual (dek″stro-man′u-al) right-handed.

dextromethorphan (dek″stro-meth′or-fan) a drug used as an antitussive.

dextropedal (dek-strop′ĕ-dal) right-footed.

dextrophobia (dek″stro-fo′be-ah) fear of objects on the right side of the body.

dextroposition (dek″stro-po-zish′un) displacement to the right.

dextropropoxyphene (dek″stro-pro-pok′sĭ-fēn) a drug used as an analgesic.

dextrorotation (dek″stro-ro-ta′shun) a turning to the right.

dextrorotatory (dek″stro-ro′tah-tor″e) turning the plane of polarization, or rays of light, to the right.

dextrose (dek′strōs) a sugar, called also glucose or grape sugar, containing six carbon atoms. Dextrose is considered one of the most important carbohydrates because it makes up 80 per cent of all simple sugar absorbed into the blood. It is present in the juice of many sweet fruits and in the blood of all animals. Through the process of metabolism, dextrose is used by the body to provide energy, or, in excess, it is converted into fat. The liver cells convert glucose into glycogen, so that it can be stored until needed. When the blood sugar drops below normal, there is increased production of epinephrine, which causes glycogen to be changed back into glucose and used for producing energy.
 Dextrose solutions are prepared commercially by the hydrolysis of disaccharides and polysaccharides. These solutions are available in strengths ranging from 5 to 50 per cent. A 5 per cent isotonic solution is the type most often given intravenously as a source of calories and also as a vehicle for water. When dehydration or other conditions call for the intravenous administration of fluids, plain water cannot be used because it would cause hemolysis (rupture of erythrocytes); therefore, an isotonic solution of dextrose and water is given. Highly concentrated solutions of dextrose are diuretic in action and may be used to reduce edema, particularly cerebral edema.

dextrosuria (dek″stro-su′re-ah) dextrose in the urine.

dextroversion (dek″stro-ver′zhun) location to the right; especially location of the heart to the right side of the chest, the apex pointing to the right, without change in relation of the chambers.

DFP diisopropyl fluorophosphate, a compound with anticholinesterase activity; a radioactive form containing radioactive phosphorus (^{32}P) has been used in studies of the various formed elements of the blood.

dg. decigram.

di- word element [Gr., L.], *two*.

diabetes (di″ah-be′tēz) inordinate and persistent increase in the urinary secretions; especially diabetes mellitus.
 bronze d., a primary disorder of iron metabolism, with deposits of iron-containing pigments in the body tissues, and often with pigmentation of the skin, diabetes mellitus and cirrhosis of the liver; called also hemochromatosis and iron storage disease.
 d. insip′idus, a metabolic disorder resulting from decreased activity of the posterior lobe of the pituitary gland. Reabsorption of water from the renal tubules is promoted by vasopressin, or antidiuretic hormone, a hormone from the posterior pituitary lobe. A deficiency of this hormone leads to the symptoms of diabetes insipidus which include excessive thirst and the passage of large amounts of urine with no excess of sugar. Treatment consists of administration of extracts of the posterior lobe of the pituitary gland or pure vasopressin.

d. melli′tus, a disorder of carbohydrate metabolism in which the ability to oxidize and utilize carbohydrates is lost as a result of disturbances in the normal insulin mechanism. A serious disruption of carbohydrate metabolism leads to abnormalities of protein and fat metabolism. The oxidation of fat is accelerated in diabetes, and thus there is an accumulation of the end products of fat metabolism in the blood and the development of the symptoms of ketosis, acidosis and coma.

Factors leading to disturbances in the normal insulin mechanism and the onset of diabetes mellitus include insufficient production of insulin from the beta cells of the islands of Langerhans in the pancreas, an increase in the insulin requirement by the tissue cells or a decrease in the effectiveness of insulin due to one or more insulin antagonists which can deactivate insulin. Any of these factors may produce the symptoms of diabetes mellitus.

Because the diabetic is unable to utilize the carbohydrates in his blood he is improperly nourished, no matter how much food he consumes. The accumulation of unused glucose leads to weakness, fatigue and a spilling over of sugar into the urine. The high level of sugar in the blood makes the untreated diabetic particularly susceptible to infection. In a prolonged severe diabetic condition, the raised fat and glucose level of the blood may cause damage to blood vessels and to tissues and organs containing blood vessels. The resulting poor circulation may be a factor leading to other complications such as gangrene of the hands or feet. The heart or kidneys may suffer damage, difficulty with vision may develop or the nervous system may be affected.

SYMPTOMS. Diabetes mellitus is characterized by elevated blood sugar (hyperglycemia), sugar in the urine (glycosuria), excessive urination (polyuria), increased thirst (polydipsia), increased appetite (polyphagia) and general weakness.

Although diabetes may develop in anyone, there are four groups of people who are most susceptible to the disorder: those who are obese (about 80 per cent of diabetics have a history of obesity), those who are over 40 years of age, women and those who have a history of diabetes in their families.

Diagnostic tests for diabetes mellitus include a urinalysis for sugar in the urine, and blood tests such as fasting blood sugar or the GLUCOSE TOLERANCE TEST, which indicates the ability of the body to utilize carbohydrates.

TREATMENT. Treatment of diabetes depends on the severity of the disease, the age of the patient and the symptoms exhibited. Primarily the disease is controlled by diet, exercise and the administration of INSULIN. Therapy is directed toward returning the carbohydrate metabolism as nearly as possible to normal. There is no cure for diabetes mellitus.

In the milder forms of diabetes which usually affect middle-aged or elderly persons who develop the disorder in later life, drugs that lower the blood sugar may be given orally. The oral hypoglycemic agents are not oral types of insulin; also they are not given as treatment for severe diabetes or diabetic acidosis. Examples of hypoglycemic agents include tolbutamide and chlorpropamide.

Diet. The diabetic diet usually consists basically of foods high in nutritive value and low in concentrated sweets. The exact type of diet is prescribed by the physician and must be followed precisely by the diabetic. This does not imply severe restriction of the diabetic's meals because most physicians prefer to give the patient an "exchange list" of foods which can be included, thereby providing a great variety for planning meals. The food-exchange lists prepared jointly by the American Diabetes Association, The American Dietetic Association and the Public Health Service are most often used. These lists are simple and easy to follow and can be obtained from The American Dietetic Association, 620 North Michigan Avenue, Chicago, Ill. 60611. The diet is explained to the patient by the physician, and detailed by the dietitian and nursing personnel. It should be stressed that all of the food must be eaten at the prescribed time, especially when insulin injections are given as part of the treatment.

FOOD EXCHANGE LISTS

List 1. *Milk Exchanges*

Carbohydrate – 12 gm., Protein 8 gm., Fat – 10 gm., Calories – 170

*Milk, whole – plain or homogenized	1 cup
Milk, evaporated	½ cup
*Milk, powdered	¼ cup
*Buttermilk	1 cup
*Milk, skim	1 cup

*Add 2 fat exchanges if fat free

List 2. *Vegetable Exchanges*

A. These vegetables may be used as desired in ordinary amounts. Carbohydrate, protein and fat negligible. Servings: raw unlimited; cooked ½–1 cup.

Asparagus	*Greens	Mushrooms
*Broccoli	Beets	Okra
*Brussels Sprouts	Chard	*Pepper
	Collard	Radishes
Cabbage	Dandelion	Rhubarb
Cauliflower	Kale	Sauerkraut
Celery	Mustard	String Beans,
*Chicory	Spinach	young
Cucumbers	Turnip	Summer
*Escarole		Squash
Eggplant		*Tomatoes
Lettuce		*Watercress

B. Restricted vegetables: 1 Serving = ½ cup = 100 grams. Carbohydrate – 7 gm., Protein – 2 gm., Calories – 35

Beets	Peas, green	*Squash, winter
*Carrots	*Pumpkin	Turnip
Onions	Rutabaga	

*High vitamin A value. Use one daily.

List 3. *Fruit Exchanges*

Carbohydrate – 10 gm., Calories – 40

Fresh, dried, cooked, canned, frozen without sugar

Apple	1 sm. 2″ diam.
Applesauce	½ cup
Apricots, fresh	2 medium
Apricots, dried	4 halves
Banana	½ small
Berries; Strawberries, Raspberries,	
Blackberries	1 cup
Blueberries	⅔ cup
Canteloupe	¼ (6″ diam.)
Cherries	10 large
Dates	2
Figs, fresh	2 large

FOOD EXCHANGE LISTS (*Continued*)

Figs, dried	1 small
Grapefruit	½ small
Grapefruit Juice	½ cup
Grapes	12
Grape Juice	¼ cup
Honeydew Melon	⅛ (7″ diam.)
Mango	½ small
Orange	1 small
Orange Juice	½ cup
Papaya	⅓ medium
Peach	1 medium
Pear	1 small
Pineapple	½ cup
Pineapple Juice	⅓ cup
Plums	2 medium
Prunes, dried	2 medium
Raisins	2 Tbsp.
Tangerine	1 large
Watermelon	1 cup

List 4. *Bread Exchanges*
Carbohydrate – 15 gm., Protein – 2 gm., Calories – 70

	Meas.
Bread	1 slice
Biscuit, Roll (2″ diam.)	1
Muffin (2″ diam.)	1
Cornbread (1½″ cube)	1
Flour	2½ Tbsp.
Cereal, cooked	½ cup
Cereal, dry (flake, puffed)	¾ cup
Rice, Grits, cooked	½ cup
Spaghetti, Noodles, etc.	
cooked	½ cup
Crackers,	
Graham (2½″ sq.)	2
Oyster	20 (½ cup)
Saltines (2″ sq.)	5
Soda (2½″ sq.)	3
Round, thin (1½″ diam.)	6 to 8
Vegetables	
Beans and Peas, dried,	
cooked (lima, navy, split pea,	
cowpeas, etc.)	½ cup
Baked Beans, no pork	¼ cup
Corn	⅓ cup
Parsnips	⅔ cup
Potatoes, white, baked, boiled	1 (2″ diam.)
Potatoes, white, mashed	½ cup
Potatoes, sweet, or Yams	¼ cup
Sponge Cake, plain (1½″ cube)	1
Ice Cream (Omit 2 fat	
exchanges)	½ cup

List 5. *Meat Exchanges*
Protein – 7 gm., Fat – 5 gm., Calories – 75

Meat and Poultry (med. fat)	1 oz.
(beef, lamb, pork, liver,	
chicken, etc.)	
Cold Cuts (4½″ sq., ⅛″ thick)	1 slice
Frankfurter (8 to 9/lb.)	1
Fish: Cod, Mackerel, etc.	1 oz.
Salmon, Tuna, Crab	¼ cup
Oysters, Shrimp, Clams	5 small
Sardines	3 med.
Cheese, cheddar, American	1 oz.
Cottage	¼ cup
Egg	1
Peanut Butter*	2 Tbsp.

*Limit use or adjust carbohydrate.

List 6. *Fat Exchanges*
Fat – 5 gm., Calories – 45

Butter or Margarine	1 tsp.
Bacon, crisp	1 slice
Cream, light, 20%	2 Tbsp.
Cream, heavy, 40%	1 Tbsp.
Cream Cheese	1 Tbsp.
French Dressing	1 Tbsp.
Mayonnaise	1 tsp.
Oil or Cooking Fat	1 tsp.
Nuts	6 small
Olives	5 small
Avocado	⅛ (4″ diam.)

Foods Allowed as Desired
Negligible Carbohydrate, Protein and Fat
Vegetables, List 2A

Coffee	Rhubarb
Tea	Mustard
Clear Broth	Pickle, sour
Bouillon	Pickle, dill –
	unsweetened
Gelatin, unsweetened	Saccharine
Rennet Tablets	Pepper
Cranberries	Spices
Lemon	Vinegar

Composition of Food Exchanges

LIST	FOOD	MEAS.	GM.	C	P	F	CAL.
1	Milk Exchanges	½ pint	240	12	8	10	170
2b	Vegetable Exch.	½ cup	100	7	2	—	35
3	Fruit Exch.	varies	—	10	—	—	40
4	Bread Exch.	varies	—	15	2	—	70
5	Meat Exchanges	1 oz.	30	—	7	5	75
6	Fat Exchanges	1 tsp.	5	—	—	5	45

From Meal Planning with Exchange Lists, prepared by Committees of the American Diabetes Association, Inc., and The American Dietetic Association in cooperation with the Chronic Disease Program, Public Health Service, Department of Health, Education and Welfare.

Composition of Food Exchanges

Diet Prescription

Carbohydrate	180 grams
Protein	80 grams
Fat	80 grams
Calories	1800

Foods for the Day

1 pint	Milk	List 1
any amount	Vegetable Exchanges	List 2A
1	Vegetable Exchange	List 2B
3	Fruit Exchanges	List 3
8	Bread Exchanges	List 4
7	Meat Exchanges	List 5
5	Fat Exchanges	List 6

EDUCATION OF THE PATIENT. The diabetic should be instructed in the nature of his disorder, the complications to be avoided and the role he must play in the control of his disease. If insulin injections are part of the treatment, instructions must include self-administration of insulin. When a diabetic cannot or will not give himself the injections, a member of the family is usually taught the procedure. The patient should also know how to test his urine for sugar and acetone. Recent developments have made the testing of urine a relatively simple procedure for the diabetic (see CLINITEST, CLINISTIX, ACETEST).

The patient is also given directions for the regulation of his diet, and is taught the effects of exercise on carbohydrate and fat metabolism and insulin supply, and the early warning signs of diabetic acidosis and INSULIN SHOCK. When signs of impending diabetic coma first appear the diabetic is told to administer insulin to himself. When insulin shock occurs, the patient is taught to consume some form of simple sugar such as sweetened orange juice, lumps of sugar or some candy. In both types of reaction the patient must call his physician immediately or go to a nearby hospital for emergency treatment. Special booklets written for the diabetic and useful in instruction of the patient and his family can be obtained from the American Diabetes Association or Eli Lilly & Co.

COMPLICATIONS. In general the complications of diabetes mellitus can be divided into emergency conditions and long-term disorders. The patient with severe diabetes who is taking insulin is particularly susceptible to the serious emergency situations of diabetic coma and insulin shock already mentioned. These disturbances in the normal glucose-insulin ratio in the blood can be brought about by dietary indiscretion, carelessness in the administration of insulin, infections and emotional or physical shocks.

Other complications developing over a period of time are believed to be caused by poor fat metabolism which results in atherosclerosis. The coronary arteries may be damaged, thereby producing heart disease, or atherosclerosis of peripheral arteries may cause poor circulation in the lower extremities. Retinal changes, sclerosis of the renal capillaries and nerve damage may also occur.

Because of poor circulation, a relatively high blood sugar level and decreased ability to repair damaged tissue, the diabetic may suffer serious complications from seemingly minor infections. Ulceration and gangrene, particularly of the lower extremities, are among these complications.

NURSING CARE. The care of the diabetic patient will depend to some degree on the severity of his disease, his age, his general physical condition and his ability to comprehend instructions and care for himself.

When the patient first learns he has diabetes he will need encouragement, moral support and specific instructions about his disease. The basic principles of good personal hygiene, cleanliness and prompt treatment of minor injuries or irritations of the skin must be stressed as important in the prevention of complications. Gangrene and possible loss of a lower limb can often be avoided by scrupulous foot care, including properly fitting shoes and stockings, correct trimming of the toenails and avoidance of injury to the feet and legs.

The hospitalized diabetic often requires frequent injections of insulin, and urinalyses for sugar and acetone. These procedures must be done accurately and at the specific times ordered by the physician so that a normal blood sugar can be maintained. The patient is observed carefully for signs of impending diabetic coma or insulin shock, and prompt action must be taken should either condition occur.

The meals of the diabetic are served at the exact times ordered and a record is kept of the amount and kinds of food and liquid accepted or refused by the patient.

diabetic (di″ah-bet′ik) 1. pertaining to or characterized by diabetes. 2. a person exhibiting diabetes.

brittle d., a patient with diabetes who spontaneously shows considerable oscillation between high and low levels of sugar in the blood.

diabetogenic (di″ah-bet″o-jen′ik) producing diabetes.

diabetogenous (di″ah-be-toj′ĕ-nus) caused by diabetes.

diabetometer (di″ah-be-tom′ĕ-ter) a polariscope for use in estimating the percentage of sugar in urine.

diabetophobia (di″ah-be″to-fo′be-ah) morbid fear of diabetes.

Diabinese (di-ab′ĭ-nēs) trademark for chlorpropamide, an oral hypoglycemic drug.

diabrotic (di″ah-brot′ik) 1. ulcerative; caustic. 2. a corrosive or escharotic substance.

diacele (di′ah-sēl) diacoele.

diacetate (di-as′ĕ-tāt) a salt of diacetic acid (acetoacetic acid).

diacetic acid (di″ah-se′tik) acetoacetic acid.

diacetylmorphine (di″ah-se″til-mor′fēn) heroin; a highly addictive narcotic derived from opium.

diacoele (di′ah-sēl) the third ventricle of the brain.

diacrisis (di-ak′rĭ-sis) 1. a disease characterized by change in the secretions. 2. a secretion or excretion. 3. diagnosis.

diacritical (di″ah-krit′ĭ-kal) diagnostic; pathognomonic.

diaderm (di′ah-derm) the two-layered embryo, consisting of ectoderm and entoderm.

SYMPTOMS OF DIABETIC COMA AND
INSULIN REACTION

DIABETIC COMA	INSULIN REACTION
Gradual onset, may be more rapid in active children	Sudden onset, begins abruptly
Skin hot and dry, face may be flushed	Perspiration, skin pale, cold and clammy
Deep, labored breathing	Shallow breathing
Nausea	Hunger
Drowsiness and lethargy	Mental confusion, strange behavior, nervousness
Fruity odor to breath	Double vision
Loss of consciousness	Loss of consciousness, convulsions (rarely)
Urine contains much sugar	There may be sugar in the urine, depending on the type of insulin and when it was taken
Blood sugar high	Blood sugar low

From Keane, C. B.: Essentials of Nursing. 2nd ed. Philadelphia, W. B. Saunders Co., 1969.

diadochokinesia   (di″ah-do″ko-ki-ne′ze-ah)   the function of arresting one motor impulse and substituting one that is diametrically opposite.

Diadol   (di′ah-dol)   trademark for a preparation of diallylbarbituric acid, an intermediate-acting sedative.

Diafen   (di′ah-fen)   trademark for a preparation of diphenylpyraline hydrochloride, an antihistamine.

Diagnex blue   (di′ag-neks)   trademark for a diagnostic agent for achlorhydria; it is a means of gastric analysis based on the fact that free hydrochloric acid releases a dye (Azure A) from a resin base. Once the dye is released it is absorbed from the intestinal tract and excreted in the urine. If no hydrochloric acid is present in the stomach the dye will not appear in the urine.

The test is valuable as a screening device to rule out achlorhydria, and is much less disturbing than other methods of gastric analysis, which require the passage of a stomach tube. It does not, however, give conclusive evidence sufficient for diagnosis of cases in which there is no secretion of hydrochloric acid.

Preparation of the patient requires that he be in a fasting state from the evening meal the night before the test is done. He may have water during this time. At 8 o'clock the morning of the test a urine specimen is obtained. Immediately afterward the patient is given a capsule containing caffeine that acts as a stimulant to gastric secretion. One hour later the dye resin is mixed with a glass of water and given to the patient. Another specimen of urine is collected 1 hour after the dye resin has been given. Absence of dye in the urine indicates absence of hydrochloric acid in the gastric secretions.

diagnose   (di′ag-nōs)   to identify or recognize a disease.

diagnosis   (di″ag-no′sis)   the art or method of identifying or recognizing a disease. adj., **diagnos′-tic.** Diagnosis is an important branch of medicine; it is also an important part of the daily routine of the general practitioner, as well as of that of every other physician. Difficult problems in diagnosis may require consultation with a specialist or admission to a hospital for special tests or perhaps for observation.

In making his diagnosis, a doctor follows a definite pattern of procedures. In some cases, he may be able to determine the nature of an illness without going through each of these steps; in others, all or almost all of the following procedures, questions and tests may be necessary.

In addition to questioning the patient regarding subjective symptoms that are evident only to the patient, the physician will also observe him for objective symptoms such as a rash, swelling or discoloration. He also obtains a medical history from the patient and inquires about his family history.

The physical examination includes inspection, palpation, percussion and auscuitation: looking, feeling and listening. By these means the physician is able to determine certain abnormalities in the body's structure and function. For viewing internal passages and organs he may employ various instruments such as the bronchoscope, speculum, cystoscope or proctoscope. With a fluoroscope he may examine structures deep inside the body. He may make an ELECTROCARDIOGRAM, or an ELECTROENCEPHALOGRAM.

Laboratory studies, including chemical studies, microscopic studies or physical tests on various secretions or samples of body tissues, may be used. Pathologic studies—examinations for structural and functional changes of tissues and organs—may constitute another part of the diagnostic procedure. The diagnosis may also be based on roentgenograms of parts of the patient's body. In some cases the physician may also wish to add consultative studies with medical specialists, such as neurologists or urologists. And in some instances a surgical exploration of the patient's body may be essential to a complete diagnosis.

clinical d., diagnosis based upon the symptoms shown by the patient.

differential d., the determination of which one of several diseases may be producing the symptoms.

physical d., diagnosis based on information obtained by inspection, palpation, percussion and auscultation.

diagnostician   (di″ag-nos-tish′an)   an expert in diagnosis.

diagraph   (di′ah-graf)   an instrument for recording outlines, as in craniometry.

diallylbarbituric acid   (di-al″il-bar″bĭ-tūr′ik)   an intermediate-acting sedative, its effect lasting from 18 to 24 hours.

dialysance   (di″ah-li′sans)   the minute rate of net exchange of solute molecules passing through a membrane in dialysis.

dialysate   (di-al′ĭ-sāt)   material obtained by dialysis.

dialysis   (di-al′ĭ-sis)   the diffusion of solute molecules through a semipermeable membrane, passing from the side of higher concentration to that of the lower; a method sometimes used in patients with defective renal function to remove from the blood elements that are normally excreted in the urine. Most membranes of the body's cells are semipermeable; that is, they allow the passage of certain smaller molecules of such crystalloids as glucose and urea, but prevent the passage of larger molecules of such colloids as plasma proteins and protoplasm.

Many body processes such as digestion, urine formation, respiration and distribution of nutrients and waste by the blood depend in part on dialysis. The principles of dialysis are utilized in the artificial KIDNEY and in PERITONEAL DIALYSIS.

extracorporeal d., dialysis by artificial kidney.

peritoneal d., dialysis through the peritoneum, the dialyzing solution being introduced into and removed from the peritoneal cavity, as either a continuous or an intermittent procedure (see also PERITONEAL DIALYSIS).

dialyzer   (di′ah-līz″er)   an apparatus for performing dialysis.

diameter   (di-am′ĕ-ter)   the length of a straight line passing through the center of a circle and connecting opposite points on its circumference; hence the distance between the two specified opposite points on the periphery of a structure such as the cranium or pelvis.

craniometric d's, imaginary lines connecting points on opposite surfaces of the cranium; the most important are: biparietal, that joining the parietal eminences; bitemporal, that joining the extremities of the coronal suture; occipitofrontal, that joining the root of the nose and the most prominent point of the occiput; occipitomental, that joining the external occipital protuberance and the chin; trachelobregmatic, that joining the anterior fontanel and the junction of the neck with the floor of the mouth.

pelvic d's, imaginary lines connecting opposite points of the pelvis; the most important are: anteroposterior (of inlet), that joining the sacrovertebral angle and the symphysis pubis; anteroposterior (of outlet), that joining the tip of the coccyx and the subpubic ligament; conjugate, the anteroposterior diameter of the inlet; diagonal conjugate, that joining the sacrovertebral angle and the subpubic ligament; external conjugate, that joining the depression above the spine of the first sacral vertebra and the middle of the upper border of the symphysis pubis; internal conjugate, that joining the sacral promontory and the upper edge of the symphysis pubis; true conjugate, that joining the sacrovertebral angle and the most prominent portion of the posterior aspect of the symphysis pubis; transverse (of inlet), that joining the two most widely separated points of the pelvic inlet; transverse (of outlet), that joining the ischial tuberosities.

diamide (di-am′id) a double amide.

diamine (di-am′in, di′ah-min) a double amine.

diaminuria (di-am″ĭ-nu′re-ah) diamines in the urine.

Diamox (di′ah-moks) trademark for preparations of acetazolamide, a diuretic.

diamthazole (di-am′thah-zōl) a drug used as an antifungal agent.

Dianabol (di-an′ah-bol) trademark for methandrostenolone, an anabolic hormone.

Diaparene (di-ap′ah-rēn) trademark for preparations of methylbenzethonium chloride, a local anti-infective used mainly in prevention of dermatitis in infants. Soap inhibits its action.

diapedesis (di″ah-pĕ-de′sis) the passage of blood corpuscles through intact vessel walls.

diaphane (di′ah-fān) the covering membrane of a cell.

diaphanometry (di″ah-fah-nom′ĕ-tre) measurement of the transparency of a liquid.

diaphanoscope (di″ah-fan′o-skōp) a device for examining body cavities by means of transmitted light.

diaphemetric (di″ah-fĕ-met′rik) pertaining to measurement of tactile sensibility.

diaphoresis (di″ah-fo-re′sis) profuse perspiration.

diaphoretic (di″ah-fo-ret′ik) 1. pertaining to, characterized by or promoting diaphoresis. 2. an agent that promotes diaphoresis.

diaphragm (di′ah-fram) 1. the strong, dome-shaped muscle separating the thoracic and abdominal cavities. On its sides, it is attached to the six lower ribs; at the front to the sternum; at the back to the spine. The esophagus, the aorta and vena cava and nerves pass through the diaphragm. When relaxed, the diaphragm is convex but it flattens as it contracts during inhalation, thereby enlarging the chest cavity and allowing for expansion of the lungs. (See also RESPIRATION.) 2. a thin septum dividing a cavity. 3. a disk with a fixed or flexible opening, mounted in relation to a lens, by which part of the light may be excluded from the area. 4. a contraceptive device of molded rubber or other soft plastic material, fitted over the cervix uteri to prevent entrance of spermatozoa. adj., **diaphragmat′ic.**

Bucky d., Bucky-Potter d., a device used in roentgenography to prevent scattered radiation from reaching the plate, thereby securing better contrast and definition.

pelvic d., the portion of the floor of the pelvis formed by the coccygeus muscles and the levator ani muscles, and their fascia.

urogenital d., the musculomembranous layer superficial to the pelvic diaphragm, extending between the ischiopubic rami.

diaphragmatocele (di″ah-frag-mat′o-sēl) diaphragmatic hernia.

diaphyseal (di″ah-fiz′e-al) pertaining to or affecting the shaft of a long bone (diaphysis).

diaphysectomy (di″ah-fĭ-zek′to-me) excision of part of a diaphysis.

diaphysial (di″ah-fiz′e-al) diaphyseal.

diaphysis (di-af′ĭ-sis) 1. the portion of a long bone between the ends or extremities, which are usually articular, and wider than the shaft; it consists of a tube of compact bone, enclosing the medullary cavity. Called also shaft. 2. the portion of a bone formed from a primary center of ossification.

diaplasis (di-ap′lah-sis) the setting of a fracture or reduction of a dislocation.

diapnoic (di″ap-no′ik) causing mild perspiration.

diapophysis (di″ah-pof′ĭ-sis) an upper transverse process of a vertebra.

diapyesis (di″ah-pi-e′sis) suppuration. adj., **diapyet′ic.**

diarrhea (di″ah-re′ah) rapid movement of fecal matter through the intestine resulting in poor absorption of water, nutritive elements and electrolytes and producing frequent, watery stools. adj., **diarrheic, diarrheal.** The major causes are local irritation of the intestinal mucosa by infectious or chemical agents (gastroenteritis), and emotional disorders which bring about increased peristalsis and increased secretion of mucus in the colon (psychogenic diarrhea or irritable colon).

In all types of diarrhea there is rapid evacuation of water and electrolytes resulting in a loss of these essential substances. Potassium supply especially is depleted by diarrhea, thus producing ACIDOSIS as well as DEHYDRATION.

SYMPTOMS. Diarrhea is accompanied by frequent and liquid bowel movements, abdominal cramps and general weakness. The stools often contain mucus and may be blood streaked. In chronic diarrhea the patient is likely to be anemic and suffering from malnutrition.

TREATMENT. Mild cases of diarrhea of short duration can be treated conservatively with a bland diet, increased intake of liquids and the administration of kaolin-pectin compounds to relieve the symptoms. Paregoric (camphorated tincture of opium) and other medicines are sometimes used to decrease peristalsis and relieve cramps.

More severe and chronic cases of diarrhea may be symptomatic of a wide variety of disorders including glandular disturbances, deficiency diseases, allergies and tumors of the intestinal tract. Since diarrhea is a symptom rather than a disease, extensive diagnostic procedures and laboratory tests may be necessary to determine the underlying cause. In the meantime symptomatic treatment must be instigated to relieve the dehydration, nutritional deficiencies and disturbances of acid-base balance produced by the loss of water, food elements and electrolytes in the stools. Liquids and semisolids may be given orally at frequent intervals if they can be tolerated by the patient. In cases in which vomiting accompanies the diarrhea or the stools occur with serious frequency, the fluids may be given intravenously. Antidiarrheal drugs such as paregoric are usually ordered in small doses to be given after each stool.

When diarrhea is psychogenic, psychotherapy may be used in conjunction with other methods of management.

NURSING CARE. The patient should be provided with an atmosphere conducive to rest and relaxation. Emotional factors must always be considered in cases of diarrhea, even though nervous tension may not always be the major cause of the disorder. The patient is likely to be embarrassed and inconvenienced by frequent trips to the bathroom or requests for the bedpan. The use of soap and warm water to cleanse the anal region after each bowel movement will help reduce local irritation and discomfort.

The number and character of each stool should be carefully noted and recorded on the patient's chart. Other observations include signs of dehydration and acidosis.

diarthric (di-ar'thrik) pertaining to or affecting two different joints; biarticular.

diarthrosis (di″ar-thro'sis), pl. *diarthro'ses* [Gr.] a specialized form of articulation in which there is more or less free movement, the union of the bony elements being surrounded by an articular capsule enclosing a cavity lined by synovial membrane; called also synovial joint.

d. rotato'ria, a joint characterized by mobility in a rotary direction.

diarticular (di″ar-tik'u-lar) pertaining to two joints.

diaschisis (di-as'ki-sis) loss of functional connection between various centers forming one of the cerebral mechanisms.

diascope (di'ah-skōp) a glass plate pressed against the skin to permit observation of changes produced in the underlying areas by the pressure.

diascopy (di-as'ko-pe) 1. examination by means of a diascope. 2. transillumination.

Diasone (di'ah-sōn) trademark for a preparation of sulfoxone, used in the treatment of leprosy.

diastalsis (di″ah-stal'sis) the forward movement of the bowel contents.

diastaltic (di″ah-stal'tik) 1. pertaining to diastalsis. 2. performed reflexly.

diastase (di'ah-stās) an enzyme that catalyzes the composition of cooked or uncooked starches to maltose.

diastasis (di-as'tah-sis) a separation; an interval in time or space, e.g., a short period of the cardiac cycle (dias'tasis cor'dis) just before contraction, or a separation between normally contiguous structures, as bones or muscles.

diastema (di″ah-ste'mah) a space or cleft.

diastematocrania (di″ah-stem″ah-to-kra'ne-ah) congenital longitudinal fissure of the cranium.

diastematomyelia (di″ah-stem″ah-to-mi-e'le-ah) abnormal division of the spinal cord by a bony spicule protruding from a vertebra or two.

diastematopyelia (di″ah-stem″ah-to-pi-e'le-ah) congenital median fissure of the pelvis.

diaster (di-as'ter) the double star figure in karyokinesis; called also amphiaster.

diastole (di-as'to-le) the phase of the cardiac cycle in which the heart relaxes between contractions; specifically, the period when the two ventricles are dilated by the blood flowing into them (see also BLOOD PRESSURE and HEART). adj., **diastol'ic.**

diataxia (di″ah-tak'se-ah) ataxia affecting both sides of the body.

diathermy (di'ah-ther″me) the use of high-frequency electric current for therapeutic or surgical purposes. The term is also applied to the apparatus employed. Heat is generated in the body tissues by their resistance to the passage of alternating electric current. In short-wave diathermy an oscillating current of very high frequency (10 million to 100 million cycles per second) is produced.

In medical diathermy, slight heat is applied to relax muscles, increase local blood supply and aid in the healing of tissues. In surgical diathermy, enough heat is generated so that the body cells in a particular area are coagulated and destroyed. This is done to remove warts and unwanted hair (electrolysis) and to cauterize tissues, as in the removal of minor growths on the cervix. Diathermy is also useful in stopping bleeding from small blood vessels during operations.

diathesis (di-ath'ĕ-sis) an unusual constitutional susceptibility or predisposition to a particular disease.

diatomic (di″ah-tom'ik) 1. containing two atoms. 2. bivalent.

diaxon (di-ak'son) a nerve cell with two axons.

diazo- (di-az'o) the group —N_2—.

dibasic (di-ba'sik) containing two replaceable hydrogen atoms, or furnishing two hydrogen ions.

Dibenzyline (di-ben'zĭ-lēn) trademark for a preparation of phenoxybenzamine hydrochloride, an adrenergic-blocking drug used as an antihypertensive and vasodilator.

Dibothriocephalus (di-both″re-o-sef′ah-lus) Diphyllobothrium.

dibucaine (di′bu-kān) a compound used as either a local or spinal anesthetic.

Dibuline (di′bu-lēn) trademark for a preparation of dibutoline sulfate.

dibutoline (di-bu′to-lēn) a compound used in parasympathetic blockade and as an antispasmodic.

dicephalous (di-sef′ah-lus) having two heads.

dicephalus (di-sef′ah-lus) a fetal monster with two heads.

dichlorisone (di-klōr′ĭ-sōn) a steroid used for topical antipruritic action.

dichlorphenamide (di″klōr-fen′ah-mīd) a compound used as a carbonic anhydrase inhibitor and to reduce intraocular pressure in glaucoma.

dichorial (di-ko′re-al) pertaining to or characterized by the presence of two chorions.

dichotomization (di-kot″ŏ-mĭ-za′shun) the process of dividing, or the state of being divided, into two parts.

dichotomy (di-kot′o-me) division into two parts.

dichroism (di′kro-izm) the showing of one color by reflected and of another by transmitted light.

dichromate (di-kro′māt) a salt containing the bivalent Cr_2O_7 radical.

dichromatic (di″kro-mat′ik) pertaining to or characterized by dichromatism.

dichromatism (di-kro′mah-tizm) 1. the quality of existing in or exhibiting two different colors. 2. dichromatopsia.

dichromatopsia (di″kro-mah-top′se-ah) a condition characterized by ability to perceive only two of the 160 colors discriminated by the normal eye.

dichromic (di-kro′mik) 1. showing only two colors. 2. containing two atoms of chromium.

dichromophilic (di″kro-mo-fil′ik) staining with both acid and basic dyes.

dichromophilism (di″kro-mof′ĭ-lizm) the quality of being dichromophilic.

Dick test (dik) a test for determination of susceptibility to scarlet fever.

dicliditis (dik″lĭ-di′tis) inflammation of a valve, especially a heart valve.

diclidotomy (dik″lĭ-dot′o-me) incision of a valve.

Dicodid (di-ko′did) trademark for preparations of dihydrocodeinone, an addictive analgesic and antitussive.

dicoelous (di-se′lus) 1. hollowed on each of two sides. 2. having two cavities.

dicophane (di′ko-fān) chlorophenothane, or DDT, an insecticide.

dicoria (di-ko′re-ah) double pupil.

dicoumarin (di-koo′mah-rin) Dicumarol; or BISHYDROXYCOUMARIN, an anticoagulant.

Dicrocoelium (dik″ro-se′le-um) a genus of flukes.
  D. dentrit′icum, a species of liver flukes that infest domestic animals and have been reported in man.

dicrotism (di′krŏ-tizm) the occurrence of two sphygmographic waves or elevations to one beat of the pulse. adj., **dicrot′ic.**

dictyoma (dik″te-o′mah) diktyoma.

Dicumarol (di-koo′mah-rol) trademark for a preparation of BISHYDROXYCOUMARIN, used as an anticoagulant in thrombotic states.

Dicurin (di-kur′in) trademark for a preparation of merethoxylline, a mercurial diuretic.

dicyclomine (di-si′klo-mēn) a compound used in parasympathetic blockade and as an antispasmodic.

didactylism (di-dak′til-izm) the presence of only two digits on a hand or foot.

didelphia (di-del′fe-ah) the condition characterized by the presence of a double uterus.

didymalgia (did″ĭ-mal′je-ah) pain in a testis.

didymitis (did″ĭ-mi′tis) inflammation of a testis.

didymous (did′ĭ-mus) occurring in pairs.

-didymus (did′ĭ-mus) word element [Gr.], *twin monster.*

diecious (di-e′shus) sexually distinct; having two sexes in separate individuals.

dielectrolysis (di″e-lek-trol′ĭ-sis) ionization and introduction of a drug into body tissues by passage of an electric current.

diencephalon (di″en-sef′ah-lon) 1. the posterior part of the forebrain, consisting of the hypothalamus, thalamus, metathalamus and epithalamus. 2. the posterior of the two brain vesicles formed by specialization of the prosencephalon in the developing embryo.

dienestrol (di″en-es′trol) a compound used as an estrogenic substance.

Dientamoeba (di-en″tah-me′bah) a genus of amebas commonly found in man.
  D. frag′ilis, a species frequently found in the appendix.

dieresis (di-er′ĕ-sis) 1. the division or separation of parts normally united. 2. mechanical separation of parts.

diet (di′et) 1. the total food consumed by an individual. 2. a prescription of food required or permitted to be eaten by a patient; called also therapeutic diet.
  acid-ash d., one of meat, fish, eggs and cereals with little fruit or vegetables and no cheese or milk.
  alkali-ash d., one of fruit, vegetables and milk with as little as possible of meat, fish, eggs and cereals.
  bland d., one that is free from any irritating or stimulating foods.
  elimination d., one for diagnosis of food allergy, based on omission of foods that might cause symptoms in the patient.

Types of Hospital Diets

	Clear Liquid Diet	Full Liquid Diet	Soft Diet	Regular–House General–Full
Characteristics	Temporary diet of clear liquids without residue; nonstimulating, nongas-forming, nonirritating	Foods liquid at room temperature or liquefying at body temperature	Normal diet modified in consistency to have no roughage. Liquids and semisolid food; easily digested	Practically all foods; simple, easy-to-digest foods, simply prepared, palatably seasoned
Adequacy	Inadequate: deficient in protein, minerals, vitamins and calories	Can be adequate with careful planning; adequacy depends on liquids used	Entirely adequate liberal diet	Adequate and well balanced
Use	Acute illness and infections. Postoperatively. Temporary food intolerance. To relieve thirst. Reduce colonic fecal matter 1 to 2 hour feeding intervals	Transition between clear liquid and soft diets. Postoperatively. Acute gastritis and infections. Febrile conditions. Intolerance for solid food 2 to 4 hour feeding intervals	Between full liquid and light or regular diet. Between acute illness and convalescence. Acute infections. Chewing difficulties. Gastrointestinal disorders. 3 meals with or without between-meal feedings	For uniformity and convenience in serving hospital patients. Ambulatory patients. Bed patients not requiring therapeutic diets
Foods	Water, tea, coffee, coffee substitutes. Fat-free broth. Carbonated beverages. Synthetic fruit juices. Ginger ale. Plain gelatin. Sugar	All liquids on clear liquid diet plus: All forms milk. Soups, strained. Fruit and vegetable juices. Eggnogs. Plain ice cream and sherbets. Junket and plain gelatin dishes. Soft custard. Cereal gruels	All liquids. Fine and strained cereals. Cooked tender or pureed vegetables. Cooked fruits without skins and seeds. Ripe bananas. Ground or minced meat, fish, poultry. Eggs and mild cheeses. Plain cake and puddings. Moderately seasoned foods	All basic foods
Modification	Liberal clear liquid diet includes: fruit juices, egg white, whole egg, thin gruels	Consistency for tube feedings: foods that will pass through tube easily	Low residue—no fiber. Bland—no chemical, thermal, physical stimulants. Cold soft—tonsillectomy. Mechanical soft—requiring no mastication. Light diet—intermediate between soft and regular. Note: Because of trend toward more liberal interpretation of diets and foods, soft diet may be combined with light diet in some hospitals	For a light or convalescent diet, fried foods, rich pastries, fat-rich foods, coarse vegetables, raw fruits may be omitted

From Keane, C. B.: Saunders Review for Practical Nurses. Philadelphia, W. B. Saunders Co., 1966.

high-calorie d., one that furnishes 4000 or more calories per day.

high-fat d., ketogenic diet.

high-protein d., one containing large amounts of protein, consisting largely of meats and vegetables.

hospital d., a routine diet plan provided in a hospital that includes general, soft and liquid diets and modifications of them to suit the needs of specific patients.

Karell d., a milk diet for nephritis and heart disease.

Kempner rice d., a special diet restricted to 10 oz. of rice daily, supplemented only by liberal quantities of sugar and fresh or preserved fruits, formerly used for hypertensive vascular disease and kidney disease.

ketogenic d., one containing large amounts of fat, with minimal amounts of protein and carbohydrate.

low-residue d., one with a minimum of cellulose and fiber and restriction of connective tissue found in certain cuts of meat. It is prescribed for irritations of the intestinal tract, after surgery of the large intestine, in partial intestinal obstruction or when limited bowel movements are desirable, as in colostomy patients. Called also low-fiber diet.

purine-free d., one omitting meat, fowl and fish, but using milk, eggs, cheese and vegetables.

Sippy d., a graduated diet for gastric ulcer.

dietetics (di″ĕ-tet′iks) the science of diet and nutrition.

diethazine (di-eth′ah-zēn) a compound used as an anticholinergic and in treatment of Parkinson's disease.

diethylcarbamazine (di-eth″il-kar-bam′ah-zēn) a compound used in combating filarial infections.

diethylpropion (di-eth″il-pro′pe-on) a compound used to curb appetite.

diethylstilbestrol (di-eth″il-stil-bes′trol) a synthetic estrogenic compound used in treating menopausal symptoms and vaginitis.

diethyltoluamide (di-eth″il-tol-u′ah-mīd) a compound used as an insect repellant.

dietitian (di″ĕ-tish′an) one skilled in the use of diet in health and disease.

dietotherapy (di″ĕ-to-ther′ah-pe) the scientific regulation of food in treating disease, especially important in patients with inborn errors of metabolism and various other metabolic diseases.

differentiation (dif″er-en″she-a′shun) the act or process of acquiring completely individual characteristics, such as occurs in the progressive diversification of cells and tissues in the embryo.

diffract (di-frakt′) to break up a ray of light into its component parts.

diffusate (di-fu′zāt) dialysate.

diffuse 1. (di-fūs′) not definitely limited or localized. 2. (di-fūz′) to pass through or to spread widely through a tissue or substance.

diffusion (di-fu′zhun) the continual movement and intermingling of molecules in liquids or gases. These movements are random and are caused by thermal agitation.

In the body fluids the molecules of water, gases and the ions of substances in solution are in constant motion. As each molecule moves about, it bounces off other molecules and loses some of its energy to each molecule it hits, but at the same time it gains energy from the molecules that collide with it.

The rate of diffusion is influenced by the size of the molecules; larger molecules move less rapidly, because they require more energy to move about. Molecules of a solution of higher concentration move more rapidly toward those of a solution of lesser concentration; in other words, *the rate of movement from higher to lower concentration is greater than the movement in the opposite direction.*

Other factors influencing the rate of diffusion from one substance to another are the size of the chamber in which the diffusion is taking place and the temperature within the chamber. *The rate of diffusion increases as the size of the chamber increases.* Molecular motion never ceases except at absolute zero; as the temperature increases so does the rate of motion of molecules. Thus, *the higher the temperature, the greater the molecular activity and, consequently, the greater the rate of diffusion.*

Many of the substances passing through the cell membrane are transported actively or passively by the process of diffusion. Without this constant motion of molecules there would be no exchange of nutrients and end products of cellular metabolism between the intracellular and extracellular fluid and the cell could not survive. The diffusion of water across cell membranes is called OSMOSIS. The diffusion of gases through the alveolar membrane is essential to respiration. The diffusion of nutrients through the intestinal membrane is essential to adequate nutrition of the body tissues.

digastric (di-gas′trik) having two bellies.

digenetic (di-jĕ-net′ik) having two stages of multiplication, one sexual in the mature forms, the other asexual in the larval stages.

digestant (di-jes′tant) 1. aiding digestion. 2. an agent capable of aiding digestion.

digestion (di-jes′chun) the conversion of materials into simpler compounds, physically or chemically, especially the breaking down of food into substances that can be absorbed into the blood and utilized by the body tissues. Digestion is accomplished by physically breaking down, churning, diluting and dissolving the food substances, and also by splitting them chemically into simpler compounds. Carbohydrates are eventually broken down to monosaccharides (simple sugars); proteins are broken down into amino acids; and fats are absorbed as fatty acids and glycerol (glycerin).

The digestive process takes place in the alimentary canal or DIGESTIVE SYSTEM. The salivary glands, liver, gallbladder and pancreas are located outside the alimentary canal, but they are considered accessory organs of digestion because their secretions provide essential enzymes.

gastric d., digestion by the action of gastric juice.

intestinal d., digestion by the action of intestinal juices.

lipolytic d., the splitting of fat into fatty acid and glycerin.

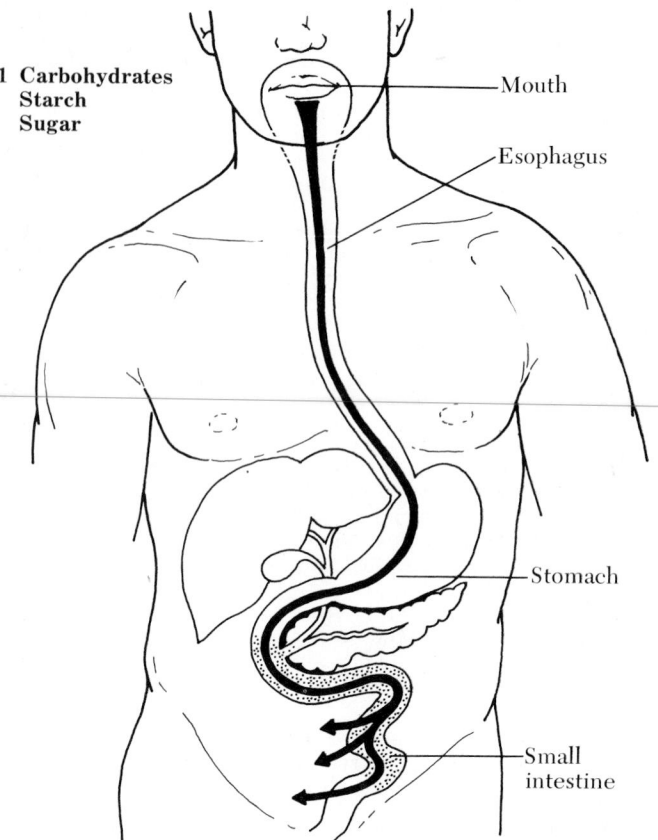

1 **Carbohydrates**
Starch
Sugar

Mouth

Esophagus

Stomach

Small intestine

Digestion.

1. *Carbohydrates* are digested in the mouth, where saliva converts some starch into sugar, and in the small intestine, where all starches and sugars are converted into monosaccharides, which are absorbed into the bloodstream from the small intestine.

2. *Fats* are digested principally in the small intestine. Broken down into fatty acids and glycerin by the intestinal and pancreatic juices, and emulsified by bile from the gallbladder, they are then absorbed through the intestinal walls.

3. *Protein* digestion begins in the stomach, where the gastric juice breaks them down into smaller molecules. Pancreatic and intestinal juices in the small intestine convert the proteins into amino acids, which are then absorbed from the intestine.

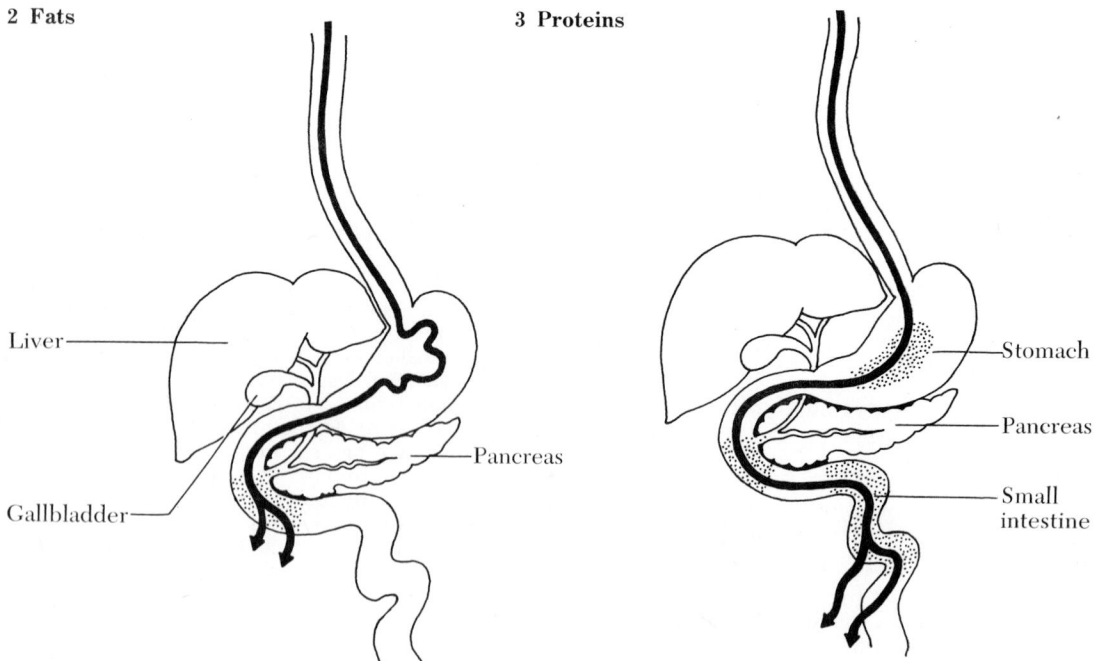

2 **Fats**

Liver

Gallbladder

Pancreas

3 **Proteins**

Stomach

Pancreas

Small intestine

pancreatic d., digestion by the action of pancreatic juice.

peptic d., gastric digestion.

primary d., digestion occurring in the gastrointestinal tract.

salivary d., digestion by the action of saliva.

secondary d., assimilation by body cells of nutritious material.

digestive (di-jes′tiv) pertaining to digestion.

d. system, the organs that have as their particular function the digestion of food. They include the mouth, teeth, tongue, pharynx, esophagus, stomach and intestines. The accessory organs of digestion, which contribute secretions important to digestion include the salivary glands, pancreas, liver and gallbladder.

MOUTH. The entrance to the alimentary canal is the MOUTH, where the teeth, tongue and jaws begin the process of digestion by mastication. Saliva is secreted into the mouth by three separate pairs of salivary glands located under the tongue, inside the lower jaw and in the cheek. Saliva softens and lubricates the food, dissolves some of it and begins the conversion of the starches into sugar by the action of ptyalin, the enzyme of the saliva. The saliva moistens the inside of the mouth, the tongue and the teeth, and rinses them after the food has departed on the next stage of its journey.

Four passageways meet at the back of the throat: the oral and nasal passages, the larynx and the esophagus. In the act of swallowing, the entrances to the nasal passages and the larynx are each sealed off momentarily by the soft palate and the epiglottis, so that the food can pass into the esophagus without straying into the respiratory tract.

STOMACH. Propelled by rhythmic muscular contractions called peristalsis, the food moves rapidly through the esophagus, past the cardiac sphincter—a circular muscle at the base of the esophagus—and into the STOMACH. Here the peristaltic motions are stronger and more frequent, occurring at the rate of three per minute, churning, liquefying and mixing the foods with the gastric juice. In the juice are the enzymes pepsin and lipase and, in infants, rennin; a secretion called mucin, which coats and protects the stomach lining; and hydrochloric acid. Together the pepsin and hydrochloric acid begin the splitting of the proteins in the food. The lipase in the stomach is a rather weak fat-splitting enzyme, able to act only on fats that are already emulsified, such as those in cream and the yoke of egg; more powerful lipase is available in the intestine, where most fats are digested.

The average adult stomach holds 1½ quarts. The stomach reaches its peak of digestive activity nearly 2 hours after a meal and may empty in 3 to 4½ hours; a heavy meal may take as long as 6 hours to pass into the small intestine.

SMALL INTESTINE. The food leaves the stomach in the form of *chyme,* a thick, liquid mixture. It passes through the pylorus, a sphincter muscle opening from the lower part of the stomach into the duodenum. This sphincter is closed most of the time, opening each time a peristaltic wave passes over it. The stomach is much wider than the rest of the canal and also has a J-shaped curve at its bottom, so that the passage of food through the pylorus is automatically slowed until the food is of the right consistency to flow through the narrow opening into the intestine.

The small intestine is about 20 feet long. The lining of the small intestine has deep folds and finger-like projections called villi that give it a surface of about 100 square feet through which the absorption of food can take place.

The duodenum, a C-shaped curve with a length of about 10 inches, is the first and widest part of the small intestine. Into it flows the pancreatic juice, with enzymes that break down starch, protein and fats. The common bile duct also empties into the duodenum. The bile emulsifies fats for the action of the fat-splitting enzymes.

Just below the duodenum is the jejunum, the longest portion of the small intestine, and beyond that is the ileum, the last and narrowest section of the small intestine. Along this whole length, carbohydrates, proteins and fats are broken down into sugars, amino acids, fatty acids and glycerin. The lining of the small intestine absorbs these nutrient compounds as rapidly as they are produced. The bulky and unusable parts of the diet pass into the large intestine.

LARGE INTESTINE. At the junction of the small and large intestines is the ileocecal valve, so called because it is at the end of the ileum and the beginning of the cecum. A small blind tube called the vermiform appendix is attached to the cecum. The longer part of the large intestine is called the colon and is divided into the ascending, transverse and descending colon, and the sigmoid flexure, an S-shaped bend at the distal end of the colon. The sigmoid colon empties into the rectum.

Along the 5½ feet or so of the large intestine, the liquid in the waste is gradually reabsorbed through the intestinal walls. Thus the waste is formed into fairly solid feces and pushed down into the rectum for eventual evacuation. This takes from 10 to 20 hours. The evacuation consists of bacteria, cells cast off from the intestines, some mucus and such indigestible substances as cellulose. The normal dark brown color of the stool is caused by bile pigments (see also FECES).

digit (dij′it) a finger or toe. adj., **dig′ital.**

Digitaline nativelle (dij″ĭ-tal′ēn na″tĭ-vel′) trademark for preparations of the crystalline pure glycoside of *Digitalis purpurea.*

Digitalis (dij″i-tal′is) a genus of herbs.

D. lana′ta, a Balkan species that yields digoxin and lanatoside.

D. purpu′rea, the foxglove, whose leaves furnish digitalis.

digitalis (dij″ĭ-tal′is) dried leaf of *Digitalis purpurea;* used as a cardiotonic agent. All drugs prepared from this digitalis leaf are members of the same group and principles of administration are the same. The drugs vary according to speed of action and potency. They may cause intoxication, symptoms of which include nausea, vomiting, visual disturbances and cardiac irregularity.

digitalism (dij′ĭ-tal-izm) the effect produced on the body by digitalis.

digitalization (dij″ĭ-tal-ĭ-za′shun) production of the physiologic effect of digitalis on the body.

digitation (dij″ĭ-ta′shun) 1. a finger-like process. 2. surgical creation of a functioning digit by making a cleft between two adjacent metacarpal bones, after amputation of the fingers.

digitonin (dij"ĭ-to'nin) a saponin from *Digitalis purpurea.*

digitoxin (dij"ĭ-tok'sin) a cardiotonic glycoside obtained from *Digitalis purpurea* and other species of the same genus; used in the treatment of congestive heart failure. It has a slowly developing action and slow elimination. Parenteral solutions should be diluted when given by vein.

diglossia (di-glos'e-ah) bifid tongue.

diglyceride (di-glis'er-īd) a glyceride containing two fatty acid molecules.

dignathus (dig-na'thus) a fetal monster with two lower jaws.

digoxin (dĭ-jok'sin) a cardiotonic glycoside obtained from the leaves of *Digitalis lanata;* used in the treatment of congestive heart failure. It has a relatively rapid action and rapid elimination.

dihydric (di-hi'drik) having two hydrogen atoms in each molecule.

dihydrocodeinone (di-hi"dro-ko'de-ĭ-nōn) an addictive synthetic analgesic and antitussive.

dihydroergotamine (di-hi"dro-er-got'ah-mēn) a product of the catalytic hydrogenation of ergotamine; used in the treatment of migraine.

dihydroestrin (di-hi"dro-es'trin) estradiol, an estrogen.

dihydrofolliculin (di-hi"dro-fŏ-lik'u-lin) estradiol, an estrogen.

dihydromorphinone hydrochloride (di-hi"dro-mor'fĭ-nōn) a white odorless powder used as a narcotic analgesic; called also hydromorphone hydrochloride.

dihydrostreptomycin (di-hi"dro-strep"to-mi'sin) a substance produced by the hydrogenation of streptomycin; used as an antibiotic, but with great care because of its ototoxicity.

dihydrotachysterol (di-hi"dro-tah-kis'ter-ol) a compound derived from ergosterol by irradiation; used to increase the blood calcium level.

dihydroxyaluminum aminoacetate (di"hi-drok"se-ah-lu'mĭ-num) an antacid compound.

dihydroxyfluorane (di"hi-drok"se-floo'o-rān) fluorescein.

dihydroxyphenylalanine (di"hi-drok"se-fen"il-al'ah-nēn) an amino acid produced by oxidation of tyrosine, and an intermediate product in the synthesis of both epinephrine and melanin. The levo form, called also L-dopa, is an experimental drug used in treating Parkinson's disease.

diiodohydroxyquin (di"i-o"do-hi-drok'se-kwin) an antiamebic and antitrichomonal.

diiodotyrosine (di"i-o"do-ti'ro-sēn) one of the thyroid hormones; an organic iodine-containing compound liberated from thyroglobulin by hydrolysis.

diktyoma (dik"te-o-'mah) a tumor of the ciliary epithelium.

dilaceration (di-las"er-a'shun) the rending asunder of a part or organ.

Dilantin (di-lan'tin) trademark for diphenylhydantoin, an anticonvulsant frequently used in the treatment of epilepsy.

dilatation (dil"ah-ta'shun) expansion, or the state of being expanded.
    d. of the heart, increase in the size of one or more of the cavities of the heart from weakness or relaxation.

dilation (di-la'shun) the process of expanding or enlarging.
    d. and curettage, expanding of the ostium uteri to permit scraping of the walls of the uterus; called also D & C.

dilator (di-la'tor) an instrument or agent, e.g., a muscle, that effects dilation.
    Bailey d., an instrument designed especially for use in dilating the aortic valve in cardiac surgery.

Dilaudid (di-law'did) trademark for preparations of dihydromorphinone hydrochloride, a narcotic analgesic.

Diloderm (di'lo-derm) trademark for preparations of dichlorisone acetate, an antipruritic.

diluent (dil'u-ent) 1. diluting. 2. an agent that dilutes or renders fluid.

dilution (di-lu'shun) 1. attenuation by admixture of a neutral agent. 2. an attenuated substance.

dimenhydrinate (di"men-hi'drĭ-nāt) an antihistaminic compound effective in relieving motion sickness and dizziness and nausea from other causes.

dimercaprol (di"mer-kap'rol) a colorless, liquid chelating agent used in the treatment of heavy metal poisoning; called also British antilewisite (BAL). The drug forms a relatively stable compound with arsenic, mercury and gold, thus protecting the vital enzyme systems of the cells against the effects of the metals. It is sometimes diluted with water and used to wash the stomach, some of the solution being permitted to remain in the stomach.
    Side effects include tachycardia, hypertension, nausea and vomiting, severe headaches and a sense of constriction of the chest. Barbiturates are usually ordered to relieve the symptoms, which should subside within an hour. The drug has a very disagreeable skunklike odor and should be handled carefully to avoid spilling.

Dimetane (di'mĕ-tān) trademark for preparations of brompheniramine, an antihistamine.

dimethisoquin (di"mĕ-thi'so-kwin) a compound used as a local anesthetic.

dimethoxanate (di-mĕ-thok'sĭ-nāt) a compound used as an antitussive.

dimethyl phthalate (di-meth'il thal'āt) a colorless oily liquid used as an insect repellent.

dimethyl sulfoxide (di-meth'il sul-fok'sīd) DMSO, a chemical with exceptional solvent properties that has been used experimentally in a variety of clinical conditions.

dimetria (di-me′tre-ah) double uterus.

dimorphism (di-mor′fizm) the quality of existing in two distinct forms. adj., **dimor′phous.**

dineuric (di-nu′rik) having two nerve cells.

diocoele (di′o-sēl) the cavity of the diencephalon; the third ventricle.

Dioctophyma (di-ok″to-fi′mah) a genus of nematode parasites.
   D. rena′le, a species found in the kidney in various carnivorous animals, and sometimes in man.

dioctyl calcium sulfosuccinate (di-ok′til kal′se-um sul″fo-suk′sĭ-nāt) a compound used as a fecal softener.

dioctyl sodium sulfosuccinate (di-ok′til so′de-um sul″fo-suk′sĭ-nāt) a compound used as a fecal softener and as a wetting agent.

Diodoquin (di″o-do′kwin) trademark for a preparation of diiodohydroxyquin, an antiamebic and antitrichomonal.

Diodrast (di′o-drast) trademark for a preparation of iodopyracet for injection, used for x-ray examination of the kidneys and urinary tract.

dioecious (di-e′shus) 1. having reproductive organs typical of only one sex in a single individual. 2. requiring two different hosts for completion of the life cycle.

Dioloxol (di″o-lok′sol) trademark for a preparation of mephenesin, a muscle relaxant.

diopter (di-op′ter) a unit adopted for calibration of lenses, being the reciprocal of the focal length when expressed in meters; symbol D.

dioptometry (di″op-tom′ĕ-tre) the measurement of ocular accommodation and refraction.

dioptrics (di-op′triks) the science of refracted light.

diovulatory (di-ov′u-lah-to″re) ordinarily discharging two ova in one ovarian cycle.

dioxide (di-ok′sīd) an oxide with two oxygen atoms.

dioxyline (di-ok′sĭ-lēn) a compound used as a vasodilator.

Dipaxin (di-pak′sin) trademark for a preparation of diphenadione, an anticoagulant.

dipeptidase (di-pep′tĭ-dās) an enzyme that attacks a dipeptide.

dipeptide (di-pep′tīd) a compound of two amino acids, containing a peptide group.

diperodon (di-per′o-don) a compound used as a surface anesthetic.

Dipetalonema (di-pet″ah-lo-ne′mah) a genus of nematode parasites of the superfamily Filarioidea; called also Acanthocheilonema.

diphallus (di-fal′us) a developmental anomaly characterized by duplication of the penis.

diphemanil methylsulfate (di-fe′mah-nil meth″-il-sul′fāt) an anticholinergic drug used generally for the same purposes as atropine or belladonna. It reduces pain, favors healing, diminishes gastric motility and reduces gastric acidity in peptic ulcer. Toxic symptoms are rare and include dry mouth, mydriasis and fever. The drug is contraindicated in patients with glaucoma.

diphenadione (di-fen″ah-di′ōn) a yellow crystalline compound used as an anticoagulant; it is one of the most potent and long acting of these drugs, and is effective in relatively small doses.

diphenhydramine (di″fen-hi′drah-min) a white crystalline powder; an antihistamine used in treatment of allergic disorders.

diphenoxylate (di″fen-ok′sĭ-lāt) a compound used to reduce intestinal motility.

diphenylhydantoin (di-fen″il-hi-dan′to-in) an anticonvulsant compound frequently used in the treatment of epilepsy.

diphenylpyraline (di-fen″il-pi′rah-lēn) a compound used as an antihistamine.

diphonia (di-fo′ne-ah) the production of two different voice tones in speaking.

diphosphopyridine nucleotide (di-fos″fo-pir′ĭ-dēn nu′kle-o-tīd″) a coenzyme widely distributed in nature and involved in many enzymatic reactions; called also coenzyme I.

diphtheria (dif-the′re-ah) a highly contagious childhood disease that generally affects the throat and, less frequently, the nose; caused by the bacillus *Corynebacterium diphtheriae*, it can be fatal if not treated promptly. Once one of the greatest childhood killers, diphtheria has now been almost conquered in the United States, although it is still widespread in many other countries. adj., **diphthe′rial, diphtherit′ic.**
   Diphtheria spreads in droplets of moisture from the mouth, nose or throat of an infected person. It may also be spread by handkerchiefs, towels, eating utensils or any other object used by an infected person or sprayed by his coughing or sneezing. It may also be transmitted by a healthy person who is nevertheless a carrier of the disease or by someone who is convalescing from diphtheria. The incubation period of the disease is generally between 2 and 5 days, sometimes longer. An infected person may continue to have the bacilli in his throat from 2 to 4 weeks after he has recovered from its effects.
   SYMPTOMS. The first symptoms of diphtheria usually include sore throat, fever, headache and nausea. Patches of grayish or dirty-yellowish membrane form in the throat, and gradually grow into one membrane. This membrane, combined with swelling of the throat, may interfere with swallowing or breathing. In severe cases, when other measures fail, a tracheostomy may be necessary to restore breathing.
   The diphtheria bacillus also produces a toxin that spreads throughout the body and may damage the heart and nerves permanently. Diagnosis of the disease can be verified by identifying the causative organisms from throat cultures.
   TREATMENT. Diphtheria antitoxin is administered to counteract the toxic reaction from the

bacillus. Prognosis depends on the severity of the infection and especially on how soon the antitoxin is given. Bed rest, antibiotics and general hygienic measures are used to combat the infection. Oxygen is administered as necessary to relieve dyspnea and cyanosis. Heart complications are usually more severe in adults; thus the convalescent period is extended for these patients. ISOLATION TECHNIQUE must be employed during the entire period that the patient is considered capable of spreading infection.

PREVENTION. Repeated exposure to the causative organisms may provide a natural immunity. Immunization, artificially induced through the administration of weakened toxins, should be begun between the sixth and eighth week of life. These injections usually are given in combination with pertussis (whooping cough) and tetanus immunizing agents (DPT injections), and are given 1 month apart in three separate injections.

diphtheroid (dif'thĕ-roid) 1. resembling diphtheria. 2. pseudodiphtheria.

diphthongia (dif-thon'je-ah) the utterance at the same time of two vocal sounds of the same pitch.

diphyllobothriasis (di-fil″o-both-ri'ah-sis) infection with Diphyllobothrium.

Diphyllobothrium (di-fil″o-both're-um) a genus of TAPEWORMS.
D. latum, fish tapeworm, a species of tapeworm found in man, dogs, cats and other fish-eating carnivorous animals.

diphyodont (dif'e-o-dont″) having two sets of teeth.

diplacusis (dip″lah-koo'sis) the perception of a single auditory stimulus as two separate sounds.

diplegia (di-ple'je-ah) paralysis of like parts on either side of the body. adj., **diple'gic.**

diplobacillus (dip″lo-bah-sil'us) a double bacillus.

diplobacterium (dip″lo-bak-te're-um) a double bacterium.

diploblastic (dip″lo-blas'tik) having two germ layers.

diplocardia (dip″lo-kar'de-ah) separation of the two halves of the heart.

diplococcemia (dip″lo-kok-se'me-ah) diplococci in the blood.

Diplococcus (dip″lo-kok'us) a genus of Schizomycetes.
D. pneumo'niae, pneumococcus, the commonest cause of lobar pneumonia, including some 80 serotypes distinguishable by the polysaccharide haptene of the capsular substance.

diplococcus (dip″lo-kok'us), pl. *diplococ'ci,* 1. an individual of the genus Diplococcus. 2. an organism consisting of a pair of cells.

diplocoria (dip″lo-ko're-ah) double pupil.

diploe (dip'lo-e) the spongy layer between the inner and outer compact layers of the bones covering the brain. adj., **diploet'ic, diplo'ic.**

diplogenesis (dip″lo-jen'ĕ-sis) duplication of a part.

diploid (dip'loid) having a pair of each chromosome characteristic of a species (2n or, in man, 46).

diploidy (dip'loi-de) the state of having two full sets of homologous chromosomes (2n).

diplomyelia (dip″lo-mi-e'le-ah) lengthwise fissure of the spinal cord.

diploneural (dip″lo-nu'ral) having a double nerve supply.

diplopia (di-plo'pe-ah) the perception of two images of a single object (double vision).
binocular d., perception of a separate image of a single object by each of the two eyes.
crossed d., horizontal diplopia in which the image perceived by the squinting eye is displaced to the opposite side of that perceived by the fixing eye.
direct d., horizontal diplopia in which the images bear the same lateral relation as the eyes to which they pertain.
horizontal d., diplopia in which the two images appear one beside the other.
vertical d., diplopia in which one image appears above the other in the same vertical plane.

diplosomia (dip″lo-so'me-ah) doubling of the body of a fetus.

diprosopus (di-pros'o-pus) a fetal monster with a double face.

diprotrizoate (di″pro-tri'zo-āt) a compound used as a contrast medium in roentgenography of the urinary tract.

dipsia (dip'se-ah) thirst.

dipsomania (dip″so-ma'ne-ah) an uncontrollable craving for alcoholic drink.

dipsotherapy (dip″so-ther'ah-pe) limitation of the amounts of fluids ingested.

dipygus (di-pi'gus) a fetal monster with a double pelvis.

dipylidiasis (dip″ĭ-lĭ-di'ah-sis) infection with Dipylidium.

Dipylidium (dip″ĭ-lid'e-um) a genus of tapeworms.
D. cani'num, the dog tapeworm, parasitic in dogs and cats and occasionally found in man.

dipyridamole (di″pi-rid'ah-mōl) a compound used to improve coronary circulation.

dipyrone (di'pi-rōn) a compound used as an analgesic and antipyretic.

director (di-rek'tor) a grooved instrument for guiding a knife or other surgical instrument.

Dirofilaria (di″ro-fi-la're-ah) a genus of nematode parasites of the superfamily Filarioidea.

dirofilariasis (di″ro-fil″ah-ri'ah-sis) infection with organisms of the genus Dirofilaria.

dis- (dis) word element [L.], *reversal* or *separation;* [Gr.], *duplication.*

disaccharide (di-sak'ah-rid, di-sak'ah-rīd) a sugar each molecule of which yields two molecules of monosaccharide on hydrolysis.

disarticulation (dis″ar-tik″u-la′shun) the separation of connecting bones at their site of articulation, as in amputation of an arm or leg.

disassimilation (dis″ah-sim″ĭ-la′shun) catabolic change.

disc (disk) disk.

discharge (dis-charj′) 1. a setting free, or liberation. 2. material or force set free, as electric energy, or an excretion or substance evacuated.

discission (dĭ-sizh′un) a cutting in two, or division, as of a soft cataract.

discitis (dis-ki′tis) inflammation of a disk, especially of an interarticular cartilage.

discogenic (dis″ko-jen′ik) caused by derangement of an intervertebral disk.

discography (dis-kog′rah-fe) diskography.

discoid (dis′koid) shaped like or resembling a disk.

discoplacenta (dis″ko-plah-sen′tah) a disk-shaped placenta.

discordance (dis-kor′dans) failure of occurrence of a given trait in one member of a twin pair.

discrete (dis-krēt′) made up of separated parts or characterized by lesions that do not become blended.

discus (dis′kus), pl. *dis′ci* [L.] disk.
 d. ooph′orus, d. ovig′erus, d. prolig′erus, cumulus oophorus.

disdiaclast (dis-di′ah-klast) a small, doubly refracting element found in the contractile substance of muscle.

disease (dĭ-zēz′) a definite morbid process having a characteristic train of symptoms. It may affect the whole body or any of its parts, and its etiology, pathology and prognosis may be known or unknown. For specific diseases, see under the specific name, as ADDISON'S DISEASE.
 autoimmune d., disease due to immunologic action of one's own cells or antibodies on components of the body.
 caloric d., any disease due to exposure to high temperature.
 collagen d's, a group of poorly understood diseases that cause deterioration of the connective tissues, including systemic lupus erythematosus, periarteritis nodosa, scleroderma, dermatomyositis and perhaps rheumatoid arthritis and rheumatic fever (see also COLLAGEN DISEASES).
 communicable d., a disease the causative agents of which may pass or be carried from one person to another directly or indirectly (see also COMMUNICABLE DISEASE).
 complicating d., one that occurs in the course of some other disease as a complication.
 constitutional d., one in which the whole body or an entire system of organs is affected.
 contagious d., communicable disease.
 deficiency d., a condition due to lack of some nutrient or other substance essential to well-being of the body.
 demyelinating d., a condition characterized by destruction of myelin.
 epizootic d., a disease that affects a large number of animals in some particular region within a short period of time.

 fifth venereal d., lymphogranuloma venereum.
 focal d., a localized disease.
 fourth d., Duke's disease.
 fourth venereal d., gangrenous balanitis.
 functional d., any disease that alters body functions but is not associated with any apparent organic lesion or change.
 genetotrophic d., a metabolic disease due to a genetically transmitted enzyme defect; called also inborn error of metabolism.
 hemorrhagic d., any one of a group of diseases marked by a tendency to hemorrhages from the membranes and into the tissues.
 idiopathic d., one that exists without any connection with any known cause.
 infectious d., one caused by some parasitic organism and transmitted from one person to another by transfer of the organism (see also COMMUNICABLE DISEASE).
 intercurrent d., a disease occurring during the course of another disease with which it has no connection.
 metabolic d., one caused by some defect in the chemical reactions of the cells of the body.
 occupational d., a disease arising from causes connected with the patient's occupation (see also OCCUPATIONAL DISEASES).
 periodic d., a condition characterized by regularly recurring intermittent episodes of fever, edema, arthralgia or gastric pain and vomiting, continuing for years in otherwise healthy persons.
 periodontal d., a disease process affecting the tissues about a tooth.
 secondary d., 1. a morbid condition subsequent to or a consequence of another disease. 2. a condition due to introduction of mature, immunologically competent cells into a host rendered capable of accepting them by heavy exposure to ionizing radiation.
 self-limited d., one that by its very nature runs a limited and definite course.
 septic d., one caused by putrefactive organisms within the body.
 sixth venereal d., lymphogranuloma venereum.
 specific d., one caused by a specific virus or poison.
 structural d., one accompanied by anatomic or histologic change in the tissues.
 systemic d., one affecting a number of tissues that perform a common function.
 third d., an infectious disease characterized by fever, lymphadenitis, conjunctivitis and a macular erythematous eruption of the trunk.
 venereal d., one acquired in sexual contact or coitus, including SYPHILIS, GONORRHEA, CHANCROID, LYMPHOGRANULOMA VENEREUM and GRANULOMA INGUINALE.

disengagement (dis″en-gāj′ment) liberation of the fetus, or part thereof, from the vaginal canal.

disequilibrium (dis″e-kwĭ-lib′re-um) unstable equilibrium.

disimmunize (dis-im′u-nīz) to cause an organism to lose its immunity.

disimpaction (dis″im-pak′shun) relief of the impacted portion of a fracture.

disinfect (dis″in-fekt′) to free from infection.

disinfectant (dis″in-fek′tant) 1. freeing from infection. 2. an agent that destroys infection-producing organisms. Heat and certain other physical agents such as live steam can be disinfectants, but in common usage the term is reserved for chemical substances such as mercury bichloride or phenol. Disinfectants are usually applied to inanimate objects since they are too strong to be used on living tissues. Chemical disinfectants are not always effective against spore-forming bacteria.

disinfection (dis″in-fek′shun) destruction of pathogenic germs or agents.
    concurrent d., disinfection of discharges and all infective matter through the course of a disease.
    terminal d., disinfection of a sick room and its contents at the termination of a disease.

disinfestation (dis″in-fes-ta′shun) the destruction of infesting insects, as lice.

disinsectization (dis″in-sek″tĭ-za′shun) removal of infesting insects.

disintegration (dis-in″tĕ-gra′shun) 1. the process of breaking up or decomposing. 2. disassimilation or catabolism.

Disipal (dis′ĭ-pal) trademark for a preparation of orphenadrine hydrochloride, a skeletal muscle relaxant.

disjunction (dis-junk′shun) the moving apart of chromosomes at anaphase of meiosis.

disk (disk) a flat, round structure or organ; often spelled disc in names of anatomic structures.
    articular d., a pad of fibrocartilage or dense fibrous tissue present in some synovial joints.
    Bowman's d., one of the segments making up a striated muscle fiber.
    embryonic d., the mass of cells of the developing fertilized ovum that gives rise to the new individual.

EVALUATION OF LIQUID GERMICIDES (BACTERIA ONLY)

COMPOUND	GENERAL USEFULNESS AS Disinfectants	Antiseptics	EFFECTIVENESS AGAINST TBC[1]	Spores	OTHER PROPERTIES
Mercurial compounds	None	Poor	None	None	Inact. by org. matter; bland
Phenolic compounds	Good	Poor	Good	Poor	Bad odor; irritating; not inact. by org. matter or soap; stable
Quaternary ammonium compounds ("Quats")	Good	Good	None	None	Neutr. by soap; rel. nontoxic; odorless; absorbed by gauze and fabrics
Chlorine compounds	Good[2]	Fair	Fair[2]	Fair[2]	Inact. by org. matter; corrosive
Iodine and iodophors	Good	Good	Good	Poor	Staining temporary; rel. nontoxic; corrosive
Alcohols	Good[3]	Very good[3]	Very good[3]	None	Volatile; strong conc. required; rapidly cidal; inact. by org. matter
Formaldehyde	Fair	None	Good[4]	Fair[4]	Toxic; irritating fumes
Glutaraldehyde	Good	None	Good	Good	Low protein coagulability; aqueous sol. useful for lens instruments and rubber articles; limited stability; corrodes carbon steel objects after 24 hours exposure
Combinations Iodine-alcohol	Fair	Very good	Very good	None	Stains fabrics
Formaldehyde-alcohol	Good[4]	None	Very good[4]	Good[4]	Toxic; irritating fumes; volatile

1. Tubercle bacillus
2. 4 to 5% conc.
3. 70 to 90% conc.
4. 5 to 8% formaldehyde (12 to 20% formalin)
From Evans, M. J.: Some contributions to prevention of infections. Nursing Clin. N. Amer., 3:641, 1968; modified from Spaulding, E. H.: J. Hosp. Res., 3:15, 1965.

intervertebral d., the layer of fibrocartilage between the bodies of adjoining vertebrae (see also slipped DISK).

intra-articular d., articular disk.

optic d., a circular area in the retina representing the termination of the optic nerve.

slipped d., the popular name for rupture of an intervertebral disk. The condition occurs most commonly in the lower back, occasionally in the neck and rarely in the upper portion of the spine.

Pads of cartilage and fiber enclosing a rubbery tissue known as the nucleus pulposus lie between the vertebrae. They act as cushions between the vertebrae, absorbing ordinary shocks and strains and shifting position to accommodate the various movements of the spine. Excessive strain may weaken the cartilage to the extent that the nucleus pulposus protrudes through it and forms a bulge. This bulge may push against the nerve roots in the spinal canal, causing pain.

CAUSES AND SYMPTOMS. Rupture, or herniation, of the disks may be caused by injury or by sudden straining with the spine in an unnatural position. The condition may come on gradually as a result of a progressive deterioration of the disks.

Symptoms depend upon the location and the extent to which the disk material has been pushed out. Most cases involve the disks between the fourth and fifth lumbar vertebrae or between the fifth lumbar vertebra and the sacrum. There is severe pain in the lower back and difficulty in walking. The sciatic nerve, which originates in the lower part of the spinal cord, is affected, with resulting pain at the back of the thigh and lower leg. A cough, sneeze or strain will send the pain along the course of the sciatic nerve to the calf or ankle.

When the disks of the cervical vertebrae are affected, severe pain in the back of the neck radiates down the arms to the fingers. Neck movements are restricted. Any neck motion, coughing, sneezing or straining will accentuate the pain.

DIAGNOSIS AND TREATMENT. Careful examination, including laboratory tests and x-ray examination, is necessary to distinguish the condition from other disturbances of the spine. The x-rays may reveal pathologic changes in the spine and narrowing of the space between the vertebrae.

Treatment for slipped disk varies according to the seriousness of the condition. Conservative treatment for a ruptured disk of the lower back consists of bed rest on a firm mattress over a bed board, local application of heat and the use of aspirin or other analgesics to relieve pain. Traction may be applied to the legs. In chronic cases the wearing of a surgical support may be helpful. Care must be taken to avoid aggravating the condition by excessive physical effort.

Cases of ruptured disk of the neck are treated in a similar manner with bed rest, heat, analgesics and traction. A collar may be worn to immobilize the neck when the patient is out of bed.

If the response to these measures is poor or if the condition becomes disabling, surgery may be necessary to relieve the pressure on the injured disk (see LAMINECTOMY).

NURSING CARE. The patient receiving conservative treatment for a slipped disk must always have his spine in good alignment so as to avoid pressure on the adjacent nerves. In addition to the firm mattress and bed boards he should be instructed in the proper method of turning himself by "log-rolling." To accomplish this the patient crosses his arms over his chest, flexes the knee opposite the side onto which he is to turn, and then rolls over in "one piece," being sure that his spine is not bent forward or twisted.

A footboard should be used to eliminate the weight of the bed clothes and also to prevent footdrop. A small bedpan is recommended for the patient's use so that he can roll onto it without discomfort. A folded towel or small pillow is placed under his lower back for support of the lumbar region. Measures must be taken to avoid constipation which is quite common and likely to cause increased pain as the patient strains to defecate. A nonconstipating diet may be sufficient; however, a mild laxative, such as one of the bulk laxatives, may also be necessary.

Heat, in the form of a heating pad or infrared lamp, often relieves the pain caused by muscle spasms. Care should be taken in the application of heat because of the danger of burning the patient who has a loss of sensory perception because of nerve damage caused by the slipped disk.

Most physicians prescribe a special corset to be worn by the patient whenever he is out of bed. The corset is designed to give proper support to the vertebral column and to relieve tension on the back muscles.

diskectomy (dis-kek'to-me) excision of an intervertebral disk.

diskiform (dis'kĭ-form) in the shape of a disk.

diskitis (dis-ki'tis) inflammation of a disk, especially of an intervertebral disk.

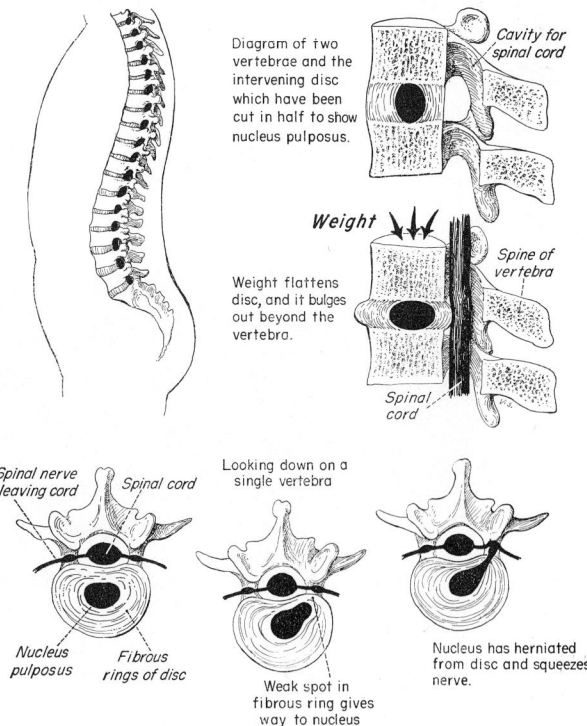

Slipped disk. (From Dowling, H. F., and Jones, T.: That the Patient May Know. Philadelphia, W. B. Saunders Co., 1959.)

diskography (dis-kog'rah-fe) roentgenography of the vertebral column after injection of radiopaque material into an intervertebral disk.

dislocation (dis"lo-ka'shun) displacement of a bone from a joint. The most common dislocations are those involving a finger, thumb or shoulder. Less common are those of the mandible, elbow, knee or hip. Symptoms include loss of motion, temporary paralysis of the involved joint, pain and swelling and sometimes shock.

A dislocation is usually caused by a blow or fall, although unusual physical effort may lead to this condition. Some dislocations, especially of the hip, are congenital, usually resulting from a faulty construction of the joint. Such a condition is best treated in infancy, with a cast and possibly surgery to correct the dislocation.

A dislocation should be treated as a fracture when first aid is administered. As soon as possible the dislocation is reduced by a surgeon. Traction, slight flexion, abduction and rotation will often reduce a dislocation. The affected joint is then immobilized to allow for healing of the torn ligaments, tendons and capsules. In some cases surgery may be necessary to stabilize the joint.

complete d., one in which the surfaces are entirely separated.

compound d., one in which the joint communicates with the outside air through a wound.

pathologic d., one due to disease of the joint or to paralysis of the muscles.

simple d., one in which there is no communication with the air through a wound.

dismemberment (dis-mem'ber-ment) amputation of an extremity, usually designating separation other than through a joint.

disodium edetate (di-so'de-um ed'ĕ-tāt) a chelating agent used specifically to remove calcium or lower blood calcium levels. It is used in the treatment of digitalis poisoning and in conditions in which there is hypercalcemia. Overuse may produce hypocalcemic tetany and osteoporosis.

disomus (di-so'mus) a double-bodied monster.

disorientation (dis-o"re-en-ta'shun) loss of recognition of time, place or persons.

dispensary (dis-pen'ser-e) a place for dispensation of free or low-cost medical treatment.

dispensatory (dis-pen'sah-tor"e) a book that describes medicines and their preparation and uses.

D. of the United States of America, a collection of monographs on unofficial drugs and drugs recognized by the Pharmacopeia of the United States, the Pharmacopoeia of Great Britain and the National Formulary, also on general tests, processes, reagents and solutions of the U.S.P. and N.F., as well as drugs used in veterinary medicine.

dispersate (dis'per-sāt) a suspension of finely divided particles of a substance.

disperse (dis-pers') 1. to scatter. 2. the particles suspended in a colloid solution.

dispersion (dis-per'zhun) a preparation in which particles of one material are incorporated throughout the substance of another.

displacement (dis-plās'ment) removal to an abnormal location or position; in psychology, unconscious transference of an emotion from its original object onto a more acceptable substitute.

disproportion (dis"pro-por'shun) abnormality of relation between two values or structures that are usually proportional.

cephalopelvic d., abnormally large size of the fetal skull in relation to the maternal pelvis, leading to difficulties in delivery.

dissect (dĭ-sekt', di-sekt') to perform dissection.

dissection (dĭ-sek'shun) 1. cutting up of an organism for study. 2. the separation of tissues, especially in surgical procedures.

blunt d., separation of tissues along natural lines of cleavage, by means of a blunt instrument or finger.

sharp d., separation of tissues by means of the sharp edge of a knife or scalpel, or with scissors.

dissector (dĭ-sek'tor) 1. one who dissects. 2. a handbook used as a guide for the act of dissecting.

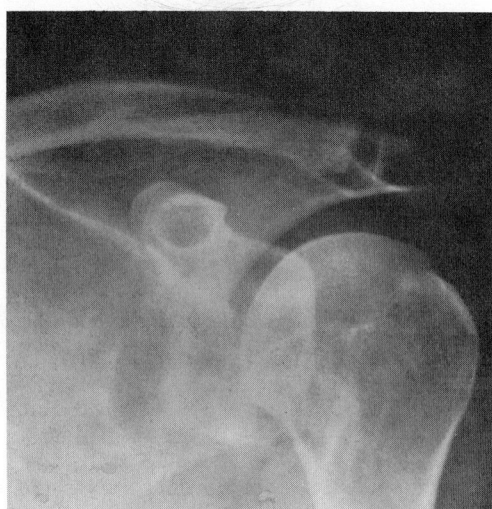
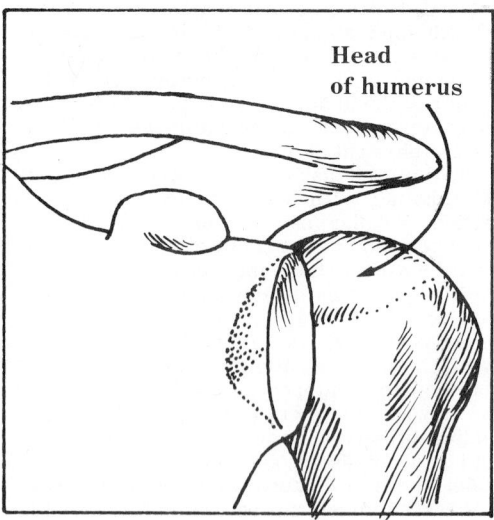

Shoulder dislocation.

disseminated   (dĭ-sem′ĭ-nāt″ed) scattered; distributed over a considerable area.

dissimilation   (dĭ-sim″ĭ-la′shun) disassimilation; catabolic change.

dissociation   (dĭ-so″se-a′shun) 1. separation into parts or elements. 2. a mental disorder in which ideas are split off from the personality and are buried in the unconscious.

dissolution   (dis″o-lu′shun) 1. death. 2. separation into component elements.

dissolve   (dĭ-zolv′) to liquefy by means of a solvent.

dissolvent   (dĭ-zol′vent) a solvent medium.

distad   (dis′tad) toward the distal part.

distal   (dis′tal) farthest from a point of reference, as from a center, a median line, the trunk, or the point of attachment or origin.

distance   (dis′tans) expression of the linear measurement of space separating two specified points.
   focal d., focal length.
   interocclusal d., the distance between the occluding surfaces of the maxillary and mandibular teeth with the mandible in physiologic rest position.
   interocular d., the distance between the eyes, usually used in reference to the interpupillary distance (the distance between the two pupils when the visual axes are parallel).
   target-skin d., the distance between the anode from which roentgen rays are reflected and the skin of the body surface interposed in their path.

distemper   (dis-tem′per) an acute, highly infectious viral disease in animals.

distention   (dis-ten′shun) the state of being distended, or stretched out; the act of distending.

distichia   (dis-tik′e-ah) the presence of a double row of eyelashes, causing irritation of the cornea.

distillate   (dis′tĭ-lāt) a product of distillation.

distillation   (dis″tĭ-la′shun) conversion of a liquid into vapors that are reconverted to liquid form, as a means of eliminating contaminants from the original solution.
   destructive d., distillation at a high temperature in the absence of air, as in the preparation of coal tar from coal.
   fractional d., separation of a mixture into a number of fractions, based on their different boiling points.

distobuccal   (dis″to-buk′al) pertaining to or formed by the distal and buccal surfaces of a tooth, or by the distal and buccal walls of a tooth cavity.

distoclusion   (dis″to-kloo′zhun) malrelation of the dental arches, with the lower jaw in a distal or posterior position in relation to the upper.

distomia   (di-sto′me-ah) the presence of two mouths.

distomiasis   (dis″to-mi′ah-sis) infection due to trematodes or flukes.

distortion   (dĭ-stor′shun) the state of being twisted out of shape or position; in psychiatry, the conversion of material offensive to the superego into acceptable form.

distraction   (dĭ-strak′shun) 1. diversion of attention. 2. separation of joint surfaces without rupture of their binding ligaments and without displacement.

distress   (dĭ-stres′) physical or mental anguish or suffering.

disulfiram   (di-sul′fĭ-ram) a compound that, when used in the presence of alcohol, produces distressing symptoms such as severe nausea and vomiting. It is a dangerous drug, should always be given under the supervision of a physician and is never given to a patient in a state of intoxication or without his full knowledge. Disulfiram acts as a blocking agent in the oxidation of alcohol, and stops the oxidation at the acetaldehyde stage, so that acetaldehyde accumulates in the body and produces nausea, vomiting, palpitation, dyspnea, lowered blood pressure and occasionally profound collapse.

dithiazanine   (di″thi-az′ah-nēn) a compound used as an anthelmintic.

diuresis   (di″u-re′sis) secretion of urine; often used to indicate increased function of the kidney.

diuretic   (di″u-ret′ik) 1. causing diuresis. 2. a substance that stimulates the flow of urine. Certain common substances such as tea, coffee and water act as diuretics. The diuretic drugs are prescribed chiefly to rid the body of excess fluid when it accumulates in tissues and causes swelling, a condition known as EDEMA. The mercurial diuretics reduce the reabsorption of water via the renal tubules and increase the amount of sodium excreted. They are given by injection only and are considered highly effective but have been supplanted by the newer oral compounds. Orally active diuretics such as the thiazides, ethacrynic acid and furosemide inhibit sodium and potassium reabsorption by the renal tubules, thereby increasing loss of fluid from the tissue. Acetazolamide (Diamox) is a diuretic that inhibits the reabsorption of sodium and bicarbonate. By increasing the loss of these salts from the body the diuretics cause an increase of excretion of body fluids as urine.

   Diuretic drugs are used chiefly in the treatment of edema resulting from conditions other than kidney disease since the abnormal kidney rarely responds to them. They are most useful in relieving edema accompanying congestive heart failure or diminished plasma proteins.

   NURSING CARE. For all patients receiving diuretic drugs, fluid intake and output should be totaled and recorded at least every 24 hours. Daily weights are also recorded. Symptoms of DEHYDRATION and overhydration should be reported immediately. Because of the danger of potassium depletion and sodium loss resulting from the action of some diuretic drugs, the patient may suffer from an acid-base imbalance. To avoid this, extra potassium is usually given with the thiazides, and frequent laboratory determinations of serum potassium, sodium, chloride and bicarbonate may be necessary.

Diuril   (di′u-ril) trademark for preparations of chlorothiazide, a diuretic.

diurnal   (di-er′nal) pertaining to or occurring during the daytime, or period of light.

divagation (di"vah-ga'shun) incoherent or wandering speech.

divalent (di-va'lent) having a valence of two.

divergence (di-ver'jens) a moving apart, or inclination away from a common point. adj., **diver'gent.**

diverticulectomy (di"ver-tik"u-lek'to-me) excision of a diverticulum.

diverticulitis (di"ver-tik"u-li'tis) inflammation of diverticula, small blind pouches that form in the lining and wall of the colon. Weakness of the muscles of the colon, sometimes produced by chronic constipation, leads to the formation of diverticula. Inflammation may occur as a result of collections of bacteria or other irritating agents trapped in the pouches.

Symptoms of diverticulitis include muscle spasms and cramplike pains in the abdomen, especially in the lower left quadrant. Diagnosis is confirmed by barium enema (see BARIUM TEST), in which the diverticula are clearly shown.

Treatment consists of bed rest, cleansing enemas, a bland or low-residue diet and drugs to reduce infection. In severe cases portions of the affected bowel may require surgical removal and a temporary colostomy.

diverticulogram (di"ver-tik'u-lo-gram") roentgenogram of a diverticulum.

diverticulosis (di"ver-tik"u-lo'sis) the presence of diverticula.

diverticulum (di"ver-tik'u-lum), pl. *divertic'ula* [L.] a blind pouch.

intestinal d., a pouch or sac formed by hernial protrusion of the mucous membrane through a defect in the muscular coat of the intestine.

Meckel's d., an occasional appendage of the ileum near the cecum; a relic of a fetal structure that connects the yolk sac with the intestinal cavity of the embryo.

pressure d., pulsion d., a sac or pouch formed by hernial protrusion of the mucous membrane through the muscular coat of the esophagus as a result of pressure from within.

traction d., a localized distortion, angulation or funnel-shaped bulging of the esophageal wall, due to adhesions resulting from external lesion.

division (dĭ-vizh'un) separation into parts.

cell d., the process by which cells reproduce.

direct cell d., amitosis.

indirect cell d., mitosis.

divulsion (dĭ-vul'shun) forcible separation of parts.

divulsor (dĭ-vul'ser) an instrument for forcible dilatation or separation of body parts.

Dix, (diks) Dorothea Lynde (1802–1887). American humanitarian. Born in Hampden, Maine, Miss Dix contributed to the establishment and improvement of many insane asylums and prisons in the United States, Europe and Japan, beginning with the establishment of the Boston Lunatic Asylum in 1839. During the Civil War she was appointed Superintendent of Female Nurses and organized the first nurse corps of the United States Army.

dizygotic (di"zi-got'ik) pertaining to or derived from two separate zygotes (fertilized ova); said of twins.

dizziness (diz'ĭ-nes) vertigo.

djenkolic acid (jen'kol-ik) an amino acid.

D.M.D. Doctor of Dental Medicine.

D.M.F. decayed, missing, filled (teeth): an index used in dental surveys.

DMSO dimethyl sulfoxide, a chemical with exceptional solvent properties that has been used experimentally in a variety of clinical conditions.

DNA deoxyribonucleic acid.

D.O. Doctor of Osteopathy.

D.O.A. dead on admission (arrival).

Dobell's solution (do-belz') a solution containing sodium borate; sodium bicarbonate, glycerin and phenol; a nonirritant wash for mucous membranes.

DOCA (do'kah) trademark for desoxycorticosterone, a mineralocorticoid.

Docibin (do'si-bin) trademark for a crystalline preparation of vitamin B_{12}.

dodecadactylon (do"dek-ah-dak'tĭ-lon) the duodenum.

dolich(o)- (dol'ĭ-ko) word element [Gr.], *long.*

dolichocephalic (dol"ĭ-ko-sĕ-fal'ik) having a cephalic index below 75; that is, long headed.

dolicomorphic (dol"ĭ-ko-mor'fik) having a long, thin, asthenic body type.

dolichopellic (dol"ĭ-ko-pel'ik) having a long oval pelvis.

dolichosigmoid (dol"ĭ-ko-sig'moid) an abnormally long sigmoid flexure.

dolichostenomelia (dol"ĭ-ko-ste"no-me'le-ah) extreme length and slenderness of the extremities, as in Marfan's syndrome.

Dolophine (do'lo-fēn) trademark for preparations of methadone, an analgesic.

dolor (do'lor) [L.] pain.

d. cap'itis, headache.

dolorific, dolorogenic (do"lor-if'ik) (do-lor"o-jen'-ik) producing pain.

domatophobia (dom"ah-to-fo'be-ah) fear of being in a house.

dominance (dom'ĭ-nans) 1. the supremacy, or superior manifestation, in a specific situation of one of two or more competitive or mutually antagonistic factors. 2. the appearance, in a heterozygote, of one of two mutually antagonistic parental characters.

dominant (dom'ĭ-nant) exerting a ruling or controlling influence.

d. gene, a gene that displaces its corresponding allele in the chain of inheritance; an example of a trait determined by a dominant gene is brown eye color (see also HEREDITY).

Donath-Landsteiner test (do'nath land'sti-ner) a test for paroxysmal hemoglobinuria based on the fact that the blood of patients with this disease contains isohemolysin and autohemolysin that unites with erythrocytes only at low temperatures (2 to 10° C.), hemolysis occurring only after warming with the complement to 37° C.

donor (do'ner) the person who furnishes blood or other body tissue to be transfused or grafted into the body of another.

   universal d., a donor whose blood cells are not agglutinated by the blood of any patient.

Donovan bodies (don'o-van) 1. *Donovania granulomatis.* 2. Leishman-Donovan bodies.

Donovania granulomatis (don-o-va'ne-ah gran-u-lo'mah-tis) a gram-negative, pleomorphic, rod-shaped microorganism that cannot be cultured on nonviable mediums, but grows in the yolk, yolk sac and amniotic fluid of the chick embryo. It is the causative organism of granuloma inguinale in man.

donovanosis (don"o-van-o'sis) granuloma inguinale.

dopa (do'pah) 3,4-dihydroxyphenylalanine, produced by oxidation of tyrosine, and an intermediate product in the synthesis of both epinephrine and melanin. The levo form, L-dopa, is an experimental drug used in treating Parkinson's disease.

dopamine (do'pah-mēn) a compound, hydroxytyramine, produced by the decarboxylation of dopa; an intermediate product in the synthesis of norepinephrine.

doraphobia (dor"ah-fo'be-ah) morbid dread of fur.

Dorbane (dor'bān) trademark for a preparation of danthron, a laxative.

Doriden (dor'ĭ-den) trademark for preparations of glutethimide, a central nervous system depressant.

dormifacient (dor"mĭ-fa'shent) conducive to sleep.

Dormison (dor'mĭ-son) trademark for a preparation of methylparafynol, a hypnotic.

dornase (dor'nās) deoxyribonuclease.

   pancreatic d., a stabilized preparation of deoxyribonuclease, prepared from beef pancreas; used as an aerosol to reduce tenacity of pulmonary secretions.

Dornavac (dor'nah-vak) trademark for a preparation of pancreatic dornase.

dors(o)- (dor'so) word element [L.], *the back; the dorsal aspect.*

Dorsacaine (dor'sah-kān) trademark for a preparation of benoxinate hydrochloride, a surface anesthetic for the eye.

dorsad (dor'sad) toward the back.

dorsal (dor'sal) directed toward or situated on the back surface; opposite the ventral.

dorsalis (dor-sa'lis) [L.] dorsal.

dorsiflexion (dor"sĭ-flek'shun) the act of bending a part backward.

dorsimeson (dor"sĭ-mes'on) the median lengthwise line of the back.

dorsocephalad (dor"so-sef'ah-lad) toward the back of the head.

dorsolateral (dor"so-lat'er-al) pertaining to the back and side.

dorsoventral (dor"so-ven'tral) 1. pertaining to the back and belly surfaces of a body. 2. passing from the back to the belly surface.

dorsum (dor'sum), pl. *dor'sa* [L.] the back; the posterior or superior surface of a body or body part, as of the foot or hand.

dosage (do'sij) the determination and regulation of doses.

dose (dōs) a portion of any therapeutic agent (drug or radiation) to be administered at one time.

   divided d., a relatively small dose repeated at short intervals.

   erythema d., that amount of roentgen rays which will cause a slight reddening of the skin.

   fatal d., lethal dose.

   infective d., I.D., that amount of pathogenic microorganisms which is sufficient to cause infection.

   infective d., median, $I.D._{.50}$, that amount of pathogenic microorganisms which will produce infection in 50 per cent of the test subjects.

   lethal d., L.D., that quantity of an agent which is sufficient to cause death.

   lethal d., median, $L.D._{.50}$, that which causes death of 50 per cent of the test subjects in 24 hours.

   lethal d., minimum, M.L.D., the amount of toxin that will just kill the experimental animal.

   maximum permissible d., M.P.D., that amount of radiation that is not expected to lead to bodily injury.

   skin d., the amount of radiation received on the surface of the skin.

dosimeter (do-sim'ĕ-ter) an instrument for measuring radiation dose.

dosimetry (do-sim'ĕ-tre) measurement of doses.

dossier (dos'e-a) the file containing the case history of a patient.

douche (doosh) [Fr.] a stream of water, gas or vapor directed against a part or into a cavity.

   vaginal d., irrigation of the vagina to cleanse the area, to apply medicated solutions to the vaginal mucosa and the cervix or to apply heat in order to relieve pain, inflammation and congestion. For the treatment to be effective the patient must be in the dorsal recumbent position with the hips level with the chest. Excessive pressure in administering the solution should be avoided so that the solution is not forced beyond the ostium uteri. Two commonly used solutions are saline and vinegar (30 ml. of vinegar to 1000 ml. of water, or about two tablespoonfuls of vinegar to a quart of water). The temperature of the solution should be 105° F.

Down's syndrome (downz) a congenital condition characterized by physical malformations and some degree of mental retardation. The disorder is also known as mongolism because the patient's facial characteristics resemble those of persons of the Mongolian race, and trisomy 21 because the disorder is concerned with a defect in the twenty-first chromosome.

The causes of Down's syndrome are not known. There is, however, a relatively high incidence of mongolism in children of mothers who are in the older childbearing age. A particular type of Down's syndrome that occurs in children of younger mothers seems to have a tendency to occur in certain families.

The term trisomy refers to the presence of three representative chromosomes in a cell instead of the usual pair. In Down's syndrome the twenty-first chromosome pair fails to separate when the germ cell (usually the ovum) is being formed. Thus the ovum contains 24 chromosomes, and when it is fertilized by a normal sperm carrying 23 chromosomes, the child is born with an extra chromosome (or a total of 47) per cell.

Although all of the physical characteristics of Down's syndrome are not found in a child suffering from this disorder, there usually is a combination of several of them so that diagnosis can be made without difficulty at birth. These characteristics include a small, flattened skull, a short, flat-bridged nose, wide-set eyes, epicanthus, a protruding tongue that is furrowed and lacks a central fissure, short, broad hands and feet with a wide gap between the first and second toes and a little finger that curves inward. The muscles are hypotonic and there is excessive mobility of the joints. The genitalia are often underdeveloped and congenital heart defects are not uncommon.

As the child grows older he remains below average in height and evidences some degree of mental retardation.

There is no cure for Down's syndrome. Depending on the level of intelligence, the child often can be helped to live productively. (See also MENTAL RETARDATION.)

doxylamine (dok″sil-am′ēn) a pyridine compound used as an antihistamine.

D.P. Doctor of Pharmacy.

D.P.H. Department of Public Health; Diplomate in Public Health; Doctor of Public Health.

DPT diphtheria, pertussis and tetanus; used in reference to triple-antigen immunization against these diseases.

Dr. Doctor.

dr. dram.

drachm (dram) dram.

dracunculiasis, dracunculosis (drah-kung″ku-li′ah-sis), (drah-kung″ku-lo′sis) infection by nematodes of the genus Dracunculus.

Dracunculus (drah-kung′ku-lus) a genus of nematode parasites.

D. medinen′sis, a species widely distributed in North America, Africa, the Near East, East Indies and India; frequently found in man.

draft (draft) a copious liquid potion or dose.

dragée (drah-zha′) [Fr.] a sugar-coated pill or medicated confection.

drain (drān) 1. to withdraw liquid gradually. 2. an appliance or substance that affords a channel of exit for discharge from a wound.

cigarette d., a drain made by surrounding a small strip of gauze with a protective covering of rubber, gutta-percha, etc.

Penrose d., a piece of small rubber tubing through which gauze has been pulled.

drainage (drān′ij) systematic withdrawal of fluids and discharges from a wound, sore or cavity.

postural d., therapeutic drainage in bronchiectasis, chronic bronchitis and lung abscess by placing the patient head downward so that the trachea will be inclined downward and below the affected area (see also POSTURAL DRAINAGE).

tidal d., drainage of the urinary bladder by an apparatus that alternately fills the bladder to a predetermined pressure and empties it by a combination of siphonage and gravity flow.

dram (dram) a unit of weight in the avoirdupois (27.344 grains, 1.77 grams) or apothecaries' (60 grains, 3.89 grams) system; symbol ℨ.

fluid d., a unit of liquid measure of the apothecaries' system, containing 60 minims, and equivalent to 3.697 ml. (See also Table of Weights and Measures in the Appendix.)

Dramamine (dram′ah-mēn) trademark for preparation of dimenhydrinate, an antihistamine effective against nausea and vomiting, especially in motion sickness.

drapetomania (drap″ĕ-to-ma′ne-ah) a morbid desire to run away.

drastic (dras′tik) 1. acting powerfully or thoroughly. 2. a violent purgative.

dream (drēm) a series of images occurring during SLEEP.

drepanocyte (drep′ah-no-sīt″) a sickle-shaped erythrocyte.

drepanocytosis (drep″ah-no-si-to′sis) occurrence of drepanocytes in the blood.

dressing (dres′ing) a bandage or other application for an external wound. A pressure dressing is used for maintaining constant pressure, as in the control of bleeding. A protective dressing is applied to shield a part from injury or from septic infection.

NURSING CARE. All dressings applied should be sterile and must be handled with care to avoid contamination of the wound. Before applying or changing a dressing, assemble all equipment, ointments, salves or other medications to be used. The wound is cleansed with a mild antiseptic each time a dressing is changed, unless otherwise directed by the physician. The hands are always washed with soap and running water immediately before changing dressings, even if sterile gloves are to be used.

A soiled dressing is removed by starting at the outer edges and releasing tape or other adhesive bandages, pulling *toward* the wound so as to avoid strain or damage to the healing tissues. This is done gently and slowly, and if there is dried exudate holding the dressing to the wound, sterile saline solution is applied until it loosens. All soiled dressings are placed in a paper bag, or wrapped in several thicknesses of newspaper. They are never left in the patient's room. They should be discarded in an incinerator or in a container provided for this purpose in the workroom.

If sterile technique is required for the changing of a dressing, sterile gloves are worn during the procedure. The first step is to open a sterile towel or wrapper and establish a sterile field from which to work. All principles of sterile technique must be observed when handling equipment. Containers of drugs to be applied are opened and the wrappings from dressings to be used are removed. After the equipment is ready and the soiled dressings are removed, the gloves are donned and the clean dressings applied.

Dressings may be held in place by a variety of tapes, bandages or binders. The type chosen will depend on the location of the wound and the tolerance of the patient's skin to different adhesives. Special straps called Montgomery straps or tapes are best when dressings must be changed frequently. If there is profuse drainage from the wound, absorbent pads may be applied and then covered with a moisture-proof dressing. After the procedure is completed all equipment is removed and the patient's unit is left in order. The hands should be washed immediately after leaving the patient's room or unit.

Drinalfa (drin-al'fah) trademark for preparations of methamphetamine hydrochloride, a central nervous system stimulant.

drip (drip) a slow, drop-by-drop instillation of a solution.
    Murphy d., slow instillation of fluid by rectum.

Drisdol (driz'dol) trademark for preparations of crystalline vitamin D.

drive (drīv) the force that activates human impulses.

Drolban (drol'ban) trademark for a preparation of dromostanolone propionate.

dromostanolone (dro″mo-stan'o-lōn) a steroid compound used as a palliative in advanced or metastatic carcinoma of the breast.

dromotropic (dro″mo-trop'ik) affecting conductivity of a nerve fiber.

dromotropism (dro-mot'ro-pizm) the quality or property of affecting the conductivity of a nerve fiber.

drop (drop) 1. a small spherical portion of liquid, which falls from the small opening in a pipet or medicine dropper; the quantity varies with the viscosity and specific gravity of the liquid, making use of this unit undesirable for medications requiring accurate measurement. 2. a descent or falling below the usual position.
    d. foot, paralysis of the anterior tibial muscles, causing the foot to drop or drag when walking.

droplet infection (drop'let) the transmission of microorganisms present in small drops of sputum expelled into the air by coughing, sneezing or speaking.

dropper (drop'er) a pipet or tube for dispensing liquids in drops.

dropsical (drop'sĭ-kal) affected with dropsy.

dropsy (drop'se) abnormal accumulation of serous fluid in a cavity or in the tissues; called also hydrops.
    d. of belly, ascites.

drowning (drown'ing) death from suffocation in water or other liquid. Drowning occurs because the liquid prevents breathing. The lungs of a drowned

person contain very little water or other liquid.

First-aid measures are begun as soon as the individual is rescued from the water. He should not be allowed to walk or remain standing if he has undergone a prolonged struggle to stay afloat because of the strain on his heart. Shock should be prevented by keeping the victim in a prone position with the head lower than the rest of the body. Blankets and other coverings are used only to prevent loss of body heat; the victim should not be kept overwarm. *No time should be lost in administering* ARTIFICIAL RESPIRATION *to anyone who has stopped breathing.* If the victim is unconscious but still breathing, he should be placed in a reclining position, preferably on his side. If the victim is not breathing and there is no evidence of a heartbeat, one person should administer artificial respiration while another carries out external CARDIAC MASSAGE.

Dr.P.H. Doctor of Public Health.

drug (drug) any medicinal substance.
    d. addiction, an acquired dependence upon narcotic or other drugs that stimulate or depress physiologic or mental activities. Drug addiction is a disease.

There is a difference in meaning between addiction and habituation. Addiction refers to the deep-seated dependence of the body's tissues upon a drug. With use, the body usually develops an increased tolerance, which creates the need for larger doses to gain the same effect. Habituation refers to the emotional dependence resulting from repeated use, but without the tendency to increase the dose.

The excessive use of drugs can result in deterioration of health and brain damage which can lead to paralysis or death. It is a habit generally repugnant to society and can involve the addict in serious legal complications. Although it is not a crime in the United States to be a drug addict, there are federal, state and local laws that forbid possession or sale of certain drugs not permitted in the United States and other laws regulating the distribution of authorized drugs.

REASONS FOR ADDICTION. Addiction can result from extensive exposure to drugs for the relief of pain, although this is not common. The majority of persons who become addicted do so because of psychologic or emotional needs to avoid facing deep personal problems. The use of drugs can create a false sense of well-being that temporarily, if inadequately, helps the user to escape from his problems. The use of drugs for this purpose only adds to a person's difficulties, because he is faced with additional problems of obtaining a supply of drugs through illegal sources. The main purpose in an addict's life frequently centers on how to obtain the money necessary to purchase more drugs for his addiction. Because of this, many addicts resort to criminal acts in their effort to maintain their addiction.

ADDICTIVE DRUGS. There are three main groups of drugs and medicines that are generally considered to be addictive: the opiates, the barbiturates and the amphetamines.

Opiates. The term opiates was first used in a federal law to describe the drugs derived from the poppy seed (opium). These include morphine, heroin and codeine. The word narcotics has been applied to the opiates because in heavy doses they produce stupor. Medically, many other stupor-producing drugs are often known as narcotics, but by federal law the term narcotics refers only to the opiates and synthetic drugs that have a similar effect and are addictive.

Barbiturates and Amphetamines. Of these two groups, barbiturates are frequently prescribed to produce calmness, sedation or sleep, depending upon the type and the strength of the dosage. When taken to excess and without the supervision of a physician, barbiturates can be fatal. They are also a frequent cause of death when taken with alcohol. Phenobarbital, amobarbital (Amytal), secobarbital (Seconal) and pentobarbital (Nembutal) are all barbiturates.

Amphetamines, or pep pills, are stimulants, in contrast to opiates and barbiturates, which are depressants. The best-known of the amphetamine group is Benzedrine.

Barbiturates are considered by most physicians as addictive; amphetamines, addictive to a lesser degree, are considered habit-forming. They are classified as such because abrupt withdrawal, particularly from barbiturates, can result in convulsions or serious side effects. Both are of a different nature from narcotic drugs and do not appeal to the narcotic addict because they are not as strong.

NONADDICTIVE DRUGS. It is important to remember that there is a difference between physiologic addiction and psychologic habituation. Whereas the addictive group of drugs is so known because of the body's physical dependence upon the drug, the body does not become dependent upon the nonaddictive group. However, most experts agree that people who use drugs to gain the effects that result will become psychologically dependent upon them. Because of the sensations derived from nonaddictive drugs, they can be just as dangerous, since they may become stepping-stones to the addictive drugs, particularly narcotics, as the user searches for stronger reactions. It is for this reason, completely aside from their adverse physical effects, that there is such concern for the seemingly mild effects young people gain from sniffing airplane glue. These first mild sensations can be the introduction that leads to a desire for stronger and for more dangerous drugs.

Among the major nonaddictive drugs, the best-known are marijuana (marihuana) and peyote. Marijuana, made from the dried leaves and flowering tops of the hemp plant (Cannabis), is commonly called "pot," "grass" or "tea." Hashish is a similar substance from the hemp plant. Both are no longer used as medicine and their importation into the United States is regulated by the Bureau of Narcotics, a branch of the Justice Department.

Peyote, a plant whose effects were discovered by the American Indians and used for their religious rites, grows in the southwest United States. Like marijuana, it produces hallucinations or dreamlike states. It is illegal throughout most of the country.

WITHDRAWAL AND TREATMENT. There are differences of opinion on the treatment methods of withdrawal from narcotic addiction. The most extreme method, often known as "cold turkey," is abrupt and uncomfortable. It is the natural process that occurs when no more drugs are taken. This method often occurs in jail when the addict is arrested for possessing drugs. In such instances, facilities are usually not available for gradual

withdrawal and the addict goes through abrupt withdrawal on his own.

If the narcotic addict's dosage has been mild, his withdrawal is equally mild and may include yawning, sneezing, watering eyes, perspiring and running nose. In the case of the heavy user, the symptoms become increasingly severe. These include severe cramps, vomiting, diarrhea and muscle spasms. Withdrawal in this manner lasts approximately 2 to 4 days. Since he cannot eat, an addict may lose 5 to 10 lb. during this period.

In the controlled withdrawal method, under the supervision of a physician a synthetic drug, such as methadone, is substituted for the narcotic, and the dosage is gradually decreased over a period of about 10 days.

HELP FOR THE ADDICT. Help available to the addict who wants to be cured of his addiction varies throughout the United States. The federal government maintains two Public Health Service hospitals, at Fort Worth, Tex., and Lexington, Ky., where treatment for addiction to opiates or habituation to marijuana or cocaine is given to volunteer applicants. These institutions are augmented by community and private facilities. The majority of addicts are found in metropolitan areas where drugs are more likely to be available and the addict is less noticeable.

In most of the major cities treatment is available in the larger hospitals, in many of which beds are available for controlled withdrawal. The amount of help or treatment available varies greatly. Some hospitals maintain a staff of psychiatrists, psychologists and social workers who offer the addict treatment for his psychologic addiction and help him to look realistically at some of the problems that drove him to drugs. Many of these treatment programs are known as "aftercare" because the addict returns regularly for additional care following his release from the hospital. For those addicts who are sent to prison, similar programs of individual and group treatment are offered to help him prepare for his return to the community.

The crucial period in the addict's adjustment following withdrawal is his attempt to find a place in community life. Job-hunting is difficult because he is often unable to explain his periods of unemployment and hospitalization. Many social service agencies offer treatment and support to these individuals during this period. It is often the difficulty in readjusting to community life that leads the addict to return to his previous habit of drug-taking.

PREVENTION. There is no need to break a narcotic habit if no habit has been formed. Therefore, the only sure method of prevention is never to start. Anyone with a desire to take drugs should consult his physician, who will probably be able to refer him for psychotherapy. A firm, unwavering "No!" is the only response that should be given to anyone offering any drug, whether it is heroin or a puff on a marijuana cigarette, unless the drug is prescribed by a physician for medical reasons.

drum (drum) the cavity of the middle ear, closed by the TYMPANIC MEMBRANE, to which the term "eardrum" is commonly applied.

drusen (droo'sen) 1. hyaline excrescences in the inner layer of the choroid of the eye. 2. rosettes of granules occurring in the lesions of actinomycosis.

Dubin-Johnson syndrome (doo'bin john'son) chronic idiopathic jaundice characterized by clinical exacerbations and remissions, and by the presence of a brown, coarsely granular pigment in the hepatic cells, which is pathognomonic of the condition.

Duchenne's disease (du-shenz′) 1. myelopathic muscular atrophy. 2. bulbar paralysis. 3. tabes dorsalis.

Duchenne-Aran disease (du-shen′ ar-ahn′) myelopathic muscular atrophy.

Ducubee (doo′ko-be) trademark for preparations of vitamin B_{12}.

duct (dukt) a canal or passage for fluids.
  alveolar d's, small passages connecting the respiratory bronchioles and the alveolar sacs.
  d. of Bartholin, the larger and longer of the sublingual ducts.
  bile d's, the passages for the conveyance of bile in and from the liver (see also BILE DUCTS).
  cochlear d., a spiral membranous tube in the body canal of the cochlea.
  common bile d., a duct formed by the union of the cystic and hepatic ducts.
  cystic d., the excretory duct of the gallbladder.
  efferent d., the duct that gives outlet to a glandular secretion.
  ejaculatory d., the channel formed by union of the excretory ducts of the testis and seminal vesicles, by which semen enters the urethra.
  endolymphatic d., a tubular process of the membranous labyrinth of the ear.
  excretory d., one through which the secretion is conveyed from a gland.
  hepatic d., the excretory duct of the liver, or one of its branches in the lobes of the liver.
  lacrimal d., the excretory duct of the lacrimal gland.
  lacrimonasal d., nasal duct.
  lactiferous d's, channels conveying the milk secreted by the lobes of the breast to and through the nipples.
  lymphatic d., left, thoracic duct.
  lymphatic d., right, a vessel draining lymph from the upper right side of the body, and joining the venous system at the junction of the right internal jugular and subclavian veins.
  mesonephric d., an embryonic duct of the mesonephros, which in the male becomes the ductus deferens and in the female is largely obliterated.
  müllerian d., either of the two ducts of the embryo that empty into the cloaca, in the female developing into the vagina, uterus and uterine tubes.
  nasal d., nasolacrimal d., the downward continuation of the lacrimal sac, opening on the lateral wall of the inferior meatus of the nose.
  pancreatic d., the main excretory duct of the pancreas, which usually unites with the common bile duct before entering the duodenum at the major duodenal papilla.
  parotid d., the duct by which the parotid glands empty into the mouth.
  prostatic d., any of the ducts conveying the prostatic secretion into the urethra.
  salivary d's, the ducts of the salivary glands.
  semicircular d's, the long ducts of the membranous labyrinth of the ear.
  seminal d's, the passages for conveyance of spermatozoa and semen.
  sublingual d's, the ducts of the sublingual salivary glands.
  tear d's, lacrimal ducts.

  thoracic d., a duct beginning in the receptaculum chyli and emptying into the venous system at the junction of the left subclavian and left internal jugular veins. It acts as a channel for the collection of lymph from the portions of the body below the diaphragm and from the left side of the body above the diaphragm.

ductile (duk′til) susceptible of being drawn out, as into a wire.

ductless (dukt′les) having no efferent duct.

ductule (duk′tūl) a minute duct.

ductulus (duk′tu-lus), pl. *duc′tuli* [L.] ductule.

ductus (duk′tus), pl. *duc′tus* [L.] duct.
  d. arterio′sus, a fetal blood vessel that joins the aorta and pulmonary artery.
  d. arterio′sus, patent, persistence of the fetal channel between the left pulmonary artery and aorta just distal to the left subclavian artery (see also PATENT DUCTUS ARTERIOSUS).
  d. def′erens, the excretory duct of the testis, which joins the excretory duct of the seminal vesicle to form the ejaculatory duct; called also vas deferens.
  d. veno′sus, a fetal vessel that connects the umbilical vein and the inferior vena cava.

Duke's disease (dūks) a mild contagious disease characterized by pharyngitis, lymphadenopathy and a generalized macular erythematous eruption.

Dulcolax (dul′ko-laks) trademark for preparations of bisacodyl, a laxative.

dullness (dul′nes) a quality of sound elicited by percussion, being short and high-pitched with little resonance.

dumb (dum) unable to speak.

dumping syndrome (dum′ping) a complex of symptoms, sometimes including diarrhea, occurring after ingestion of food by patients who have had partial gastrectomy (see also surgery of the STOMACH).

duodenal (du″o-de′nal) pertaining to the duodenum.
  d. ulcer, peptic ulcer of the duodenum (see also ULCER).

duodenectomy (du″o-dĕ-nek′to-me) excision of the duodenum.

duodenitis (du″o-dĕ-ni′tis) inflammation of the duodenum.

duodenocholedochotomy (du″o-de″no-ko-led″o-kot′o-me) incision of the duodenum and common bile duct.

duodenoduodenostomy (du″o-de″no-du″o-dĕ-nos′to-me) anastomosis of the two portions of a divided duodenum.

duodenoenterostomy (du″o-de″no-en″ter-os′to-me) anastomosis of the duodenum to some other part of the small intestine.

duodenohepatic (du″o-de″no-hĕ-pat′ik) pertaining to the duodenum and liver.

duodenoileostomy   (du″o-de″no-il″e-os′to-me) anastomosis of the duodenum to the ileum.

duodenojejunostomy   (du″o-de″no-je″joo-nos′to-me) anastomosis of the duodenum to the jejunum.

duodenorrhaphy   (du″o-dē-nor′ah-fe) suture of the duodenum.

duodenoscopy   (du″o-dē-nos′ko-pe) examination of the duodenum by an endoscope.

duodenostomy   (du″o-dě-nos′to-me) surgical formation of a permanent opening into the duodenum.

duodenotomy   (du″o-dě-not′o-me) incision of the duodenum.

duodenum   (du″o-de′num) the first or proximal portion of the small intestine; it is about 10 inches long. It plays an important role in digestion of food because both the common bile duct and the pancreatic duct empty into it. (See also DIGESTIVE SYSTEM.) It is subject to various disorders, the most common of which are peptic ULCER and obstruction due to dilatation of the intestine and stasis of the duodenal contents. The duodenum also may be the site of diverticula, fistulas and, rarely, tumors.

Duphaston   (du-fas′ton) trademark for a preparation of isopregnenone, a progestational agent.

duplication   (du-plĭ-ka′shun) in genetics, the presence of an extra portion of a gene or chromosome.

dupp   (dup) a syllable used to express the second sound heard at the apex of the heart in auscultation, shorter and higher pitched than the first sound (lubb).

Dupuytren's contracture   (du-pwe-trahnz′) a flexion deformity of the fingers or toes, due to shortening, thickening and fibrosis of the palmar or plantar fascia.

dura mater   (du′rah ma′ter) [L.] the outermost, toughest and most fibrous of the three membranes (meninges) covering the brain and spinal cord.

Duracillin   (du″rah-sil′in) trademark for preparations of crystalline procaine penicillin G.

dural   (du′ral) pertaining to the dura mater.

Durand-Nicolas-Favre disease   (du-ran′ ne-ko-lah fav′r) lymphogranuloma venereum.

duritis   (du-ri′tis) inflammation of the dura mater.

duroarachnitis   (du″ro-ar″ak-ni′tis) inflammation of the dura mater and arachnoid.

Duroziez's disease   (du-ro″ze-āz′) congenital mitral stenosis.

   D's sign, in aortic insufficiency, a murmur is heard on placing the stethoscope over the femoral artery.

D.V.M.   Doctor of Veterinary Medicine.

D.V.S.   Doctor of Veterinary Science; Doctor of Veterinary Surgery.

dwarf   (dwarf) an abnormally undersized person.

dwarfism   (dwar′fizm) underdevelopment of the body. Dwarfism may be the result of an abnormal development of the embryo, of nutritional or hormone deficiencies or of other diseases. The size of pygmies found in some parts of the world, such as the Philippines and equatorial Africa, is not the result of dwarfism; their small stature is a hereditary trait.

   A dwarf in adulthood may be as small as 2½ feet tall. The proportions of body to head and limbs may be normal or abnormal. The dwarf may also be deformed, and may suffer from mental retardation, depending on the cause of his condition.

   Achondroplasia is an abnormal development of the embryo that affects the growth of the bones. The patient's trunk is usually normal, but his head is unusually large and his arms and legs unusually small. Most fetuses with achondroplasia are stillborn. Those who reach adulthood do not suffer any lessening of their mental or sexual abilities, and may have unusual muscular strength. Achondroplasia does not significantly shorten the patient's life span.

   An infant who suffers from an insufficiency of thyroxine, a hormone secreted by the thyroid gland, may develop the symptoms of cretinism. These include an enlarged head, short limbs, puffy eyes, a thick and protruding tongue, very dry skin and lack of coordination. Cretinism can be treated by giving the patient an extract of thyroxine, and early treatment can result in normal growth and development. If the condition is not treated, however, the child will grow up dwarfed, mentally retarded and sexually sterile.

   Growth hormone, a hormone that plays a major role in the process of growth is produced in the pituitary gland. If this hormone is not produced in sufficient quantity, the patient's growth will be abnormally slight, although his head and limbs will be in normal proportion to his small torso. This condition has been treated experimentally with a special pituitary hormone that must be made from the pituitary glands of humans, although monkey hormones may be useful, too.

Dy   chemical symbol, *dysprosium.*

Dyclone   (di′klōn) trademark for preparations of dyclonine.

dyclonine   (di′klo-nēn) a compound used as a topical anesthetic.

dye   (di) a substance by which another material may be colored.

dynamic   (di-nam′ik) pertaining to strength or force.

dynamics   (di-nam′iks) 1. the scientific study of forces in action; a phase of mechanics. 2. the motivating or driving forces, physical or moral, in any field.

dynamograph   (di-nam′o-graf) an instrument for recording muscular power.

dynamometer   (di″nah-mom′ě-ter) an instrument for testing muscular power.

dynamoneure   (di-nam′o-nūr) a spinal neuron connected with the muscles.

dynamopathic   (di-nam″o-path′ik) affecting function; functional.

dyne   (dīn) the metric unit of force, being that amount which would, during each second, produce an acceleration of 1 cm. per second in a particle of 1 gram mass.

dyphilline (di-fil′lin) a theophylline compound used as a diuretic and as a bronchodilator and peripheral vasodilator.

dys- (dis) prefix [Gr], *bad; difficult.*

dysalbumose (dis-al′bu-mōs) an insoluble variety of albumose.

dysaphia (dis-a′fe-ah) impairment of the sense of touch.

dysarthria (dis-ar′thre-ah) difficulty in speaking because of impairment of the organs of speech or their innervation.

dysarthrosis (dis″ar-thro′sis) 1. deformity or malformation of a joint. 2. dysarthria.

dysaudia (dis-aw′de-ah) impaired hearing.

dysautonomia (dis″aw-to-no′me-ah) a familial condition marked by defective lacrimation, skin blotching, emotional instability, motor incoordination and hyporeflexia.

dysbarism (dis′bar-izm) a general term applied to any clinical syndrome caused by difference between the surrounding atmospheric pressure and the total gas pressure in the various tissues, fluids and cavities of the body, including such conditions as barosinusitis, barotitis media or expansion of gases in the hollow viscera.

dysbasia (dis-ba′ze-ah) impairment of the power of walking.

dysbulia (dis-bu′le-ah) weakness or perversion of the will.

dyscalculia (dis″kal-ku′le-ah) impairment of the ability to do mathematical problems because of brain injury or disease.

dyscephaly (dis-sef′ah-le) malformation of the cranium and bones of the face.

dyschiria (dis-ki′re-ah) loss of power to tell which side of the body has been touched.

dyscholia (dis-ko′le-ah) a disordered condition of the bile.

dyschondroplasia (dis″kon-dro-pla′ze-ah) a condition of abnormal growth of cartilage at the diaphyseal end of long bones with the formation of cartilaginous and bony tumors on the shafts of the long bones near the epiphyses.

dyschromatopsia (dis″kro-mah-top′se-ah) imperfect discrimination of colors.

dyschromia (dis-kro′me-ah) any disorder of the pigmentary layer of the skin.

dyschronism (dis-kro′nizm) disturbance of time sense.

dyscoria (dis-ko′re-ah) abnormality in shape of the pupil.

dyscorticism (dis-kor′tĭ-sizm) disordered functioning of the adrenal cortex.

dyscrasia (dis-kra′ze-ah) a morbid condition, usually referring to an imbalance of component elements. adj., **dyscrat′ic.**

blood d., an abnormal or pathologic condition of the blood.

dysdiadochokinesia (dis″di-ah-do″ko-ki-ne′ze-ah) derangement of the function of diadochokinesia.

dysdiemorrhysis (dis″di-ĕ-mor′ĭ-sis) retardation of the capillary circulation.

dysembryoma (dis″em-bre-o′mah) a tumor formed by maldevelopment of embryonic germ cells.

dysentery (dis′en-ter″e) a lower intestinal infection caused by bacteria, protozoa or virus, and associated with diarrhea and cramps. Dysentery is less prevalent today than in years past because of improved sanitary facilities throughout the world; it was formerly a common occurrence in crowded parts of the world and it particularly plagued army camps. It can be dangerous to infants, children, the elderly and others who are in a weakened condition.

In dysentery, there is an unusually fluid discharge of stool from the bowels, as well as fever, stomach cramps and spasms of involuntary straining to evacuate, with the passage of little feces. The stool is often mixed with pus and mucus and may be streaked with blood.

amebic d., a form common in tropical countries but also found in temperate areas, including the United States; caused by the protozoon *Entamoeba hystolytica.* It is usually less acute and violent than bacillary dysentery, but it frequently becomes chronic and causes unexplained attacks of diarrhea over a long period of time. It rarely causes death, but complications may result, including involvement of the liver, liver abscess and pulmonary abscess. Drugs used in treatment include emetine hydrochloride and chloroquine, among others.

bacillary d., the most common and violent form of the disease, caused by bacteria of the Shigella group.

Bacillary dysentery is most common in the tropics, the subtropics and the Orient. It can be fatal, especially among children. It can erupt anywhere where sanitation is poor and large groups of people, including carriers of the disease, are crowded together.

The disease is spread through the feces of carriers who have the bacteria in their intestines. They may be suffering from diarrhea or dysentery, or they may seem perfectly well and still carry the disease. It is transmitted by eating or drinking from anything contaminated with the bacteria from the feces of these carriers. Even touching something contaminated and then touching the mouth can cause infection. Flies also spread the disease.

Attacks of bacillary dysentery are always acute after the incubation period of a few days. Temperature may rise as high as 104° F., sometimes with symptoms of dehydration, shock and delirium. Bowel movements may be as many as 30 to 40 a day. Running its normal course, without special medicines, it is usually over within a few weeks from its outset, although an attack in a child may be more serious and last longer.

Antibiotics such as chlortetracycline (Aureomycin) and chloramphenicol are usually effective in relieving the symptoms and controlling bacillary dysentery in a day or two. They often completely cure it in that time. Sulfonamides, such as sulfa-diazine, are less effective because of the emergence of resistant strains of bacteria. With proper care, a violent attack may be over in a few days.

The greatest threat of dysentery is from dehydration. This condition is combated with intravenous administration of fluids and electrolytes lost in the watery stools.

Although the usual dysenteric illness may last a few weeks if not treated with special medicines, symptoms of intestinal ulceration, diarrhea and painful spasms in evacuating may in a few cases continue for a longer time.

viral d., a form caused by a virus. It is common in travelers who have eaten raw salads or fruit, or used contaminated tableware. With proper care, it should subside in 12 to 72 hours.

dyserethesia (dis″er-ĕ-the′ze-ah) impairment of sensibility.

dysergasia (dis″er-ga′ze-ah) a behavior disorder due to organic changes in the nervous system, with disorientation, hallucination and delirious reactions.

dysergia (dis-er′je-ah) motor incoordination due to nervous defect.

dysesthesia (dis″es-the′ze-ah) abnormality of sensation.

dysfunction (dis-fungk′shun) abnormal or imperfect functioning.

dysgalactia (dis″gah-lak′she-ah) disordered milk secretion.

dysgenesis (dis-jen′ĕ-sis) defective development; malformation.
　gonadal d., Turner's syndrome.

dysgenics (dis-jen′iks) the study of racial deterioration.

dysgenitalism (dis-jen′ĭ-tal-izm) abnormality of genital development.

dysgerminoma (dis-jer″mĭ-no′mah) a gonadal tumor derived from germinal epithelium that has not differentiated into cells of either male or female type.

dysgeusia (dis-gu′ze-ah) impairment of the sense of taste.

dysglandular (dis-glan′du-lar) marked by disorder of the glands of internal secretion.

dysglobulinemia (dis-glob″u-lin-e′me-ah) abnormality of the serum globulins.

dysglycemia (dis″gli-se′me-ah) any disorder of blood sugar metabolism.

dysgnathia (dis-na′the-ah) abnormality of the maxilla and mandible. adj., **dysgnath′ic.**

dysgnosia (dis-no′ze-ah) any abnormality of the intellect.

dysgonesis (dis″go-ne′sis) functional disorder of the reproductive organs.

dysgonic (dis-gon′ik) seeding badly; said of bacterial cultures that grow poorly.

dysgrammatism (dis-gram′ah-tizm) impairment of ability to speak grammatically because of brain injury or disease.

dysgraphia (dis-gra′fe-ah) loss or impairment of the ability to write because of brain injury or disease.

dyshematopoiesis (dis-hem″ah-to-poi-e′sis) defective blood formation.

dyshidrosis (dis″hĭ-dro′sis) an acute, recurrent, noninflammatory vesicular eruption limited to the palms and the soles; called also pompholyx.

dyshormonal (dis-hōr′mo-nal) due to disturbance of hormone secretion.

dyskaryosis (dis″kar-e-o′sis) abnormality of the nucleus of a cell. adj., **dyskaryot′ic.**

dyskeratosis (dis″ker-ah-to′sis) abnormal keratinization of the epidermis.

dyskinesia (dis-ki-ne′ze-ah) difficulty of movement.

dyslalia (dis-la′le-ah) difficulty in speaking due to deformity.

dyslexia (dis-lek′se-ah) impairment of ability to comprehend written language.

dyslipidosis (dis″lip-ĭ-do′sis) a localized or systemic disturbance of fat metabolism.

dyslogia (dis-lo′je-ah) impairment of the power of speaking and reasoning.

dysmasesis (dis″mah-se′sis) difficult mastication.

dysmelia (dis-me′le-ah) malformation of a limb or limbs due to disturbance in embryonic development.

dysmenorrhea (dis″men-ŏ-re′ah) painful menstruation, characterized by cramplike pains in the lower abdomen, and sometimes accompanied by headache, irritability, mental depression, malaise and fatigue. There are a variety of causes, but in many cases the factors involved may be extremely elusive. Relief can often be obtained by simple hygienic measures such as adequate rest, avoidance of constipation, moderate exercise, applications of moderate heat to the abdomen and removal of restricting clothing. Analgesics may be helpful. Hormone therapy may be required. Surgical procedures are rarely indicated unless a tumor or other demonstrable cause can be found.
　congestive d., that due to congestion of pelvic viscera.
　essential d., painful menstruation for which there is no demonstrable cause.
　inflammatory d., that due to inflammation.
　membranous d., severe dysmenorrhea with discharge of shreds of membrane.
　obstructive d., that due to mechanical obstruction to the discharge of menstrual fluid.

dysmetria (dis-me′tre-ah) inability to properly direct or limit motions.

dysmetropsia (dis″mĕ-trop′se-ah) a disturbance of visual appreciation of the size of objects.

dysmicrobialism (dis″mi-kro′be-al-izm″) disturbance of the normal balance of microorganisms, especially in the intestines.

dysmimia (dis-mim′e-ah) impairment of the power of expression by signs.

dysmnesia (dis-ne′ze-ah) disordered memory.

dysmorphophobia (dis″mor-fo-fo′be-ah) morbid dread of deformity.

dysmorphopsia (dis″mor-fop′se-ah) defective vision, with distortion of the shape of objects perceived.

dysmorphosis (dis″mor-fo′sis) malformation.

dysmyotonia (dis″mi-o-to′ne-ah) abnormal tonicity of muscle.

dysnomia (dis-no′me-ah) aphasia characterized by inability to correctly name certain things.

dysodontiasis (dis″o-don-ti′ah-sis) defective dentition.

dysontogenesis (dis″on-to-jen′ĕ-sis) defective embryonic development.

dysopia (dis-o′pe-ah) defective vision.

dysorexia (dis″o-rek′se-ah) impairment of the appetite.

dysosmia (dis-oz′me-ah) impairment of the sense of smell.

dysostosis (dis″os-to′sis) a condition due to defective ossification of fetal cartilages.
  cleidocranial d., a congenital condition in which there are defective ossification of the cranial bones and complete or partial absence of the clavicles, so that the shoulders are brought together in front.
  craniofacial d., deformity of the bones of the face and skull, attributed to premature fusion of the bones of the skull, a condition often having familial incidence.
  mandibulofacial d., a congenital condition with hypoplasia of facial bones, antimongoloid slant of palpebral fissures, deformity of ears, macrostomia and other abnormalities of face and jaw.
  metaphyseal d., a skeletal abnormality in which the epiphyses are normal or nearly so, and the metaphyseal tissues are replaced by masses of cartilage, producing interference with endochondral bone formation and expansion and thinning of the metaphyseal cortices.
  orodigitofacial d., anomalous development of the mouth and tongue, fingers, and frequently of the face, associated with a chromosomal abnormality.

dyspancreatism (dis-pan′kre-ah-tizm″) disorder of the pancreas.

dyspareunia (dis″pah-ru′ne-ah) painful coitus.

dyspepsia (dis-pep′se-ah) indigestion; difficulty of digestion. adj., **dyspep′tic.**
  acid d., dyspepsia with excessive formation of acid.
  atonic d., that due to deficient quantity or quality of the gastric juice, or to defective action of the gastric muscles.

dyspeptone (dis-pep′tōn) an insoluble peptone produced during digestion.

dysphagia (dis-fa′je-ah) difficulty in swallowing.

dysphasia (dis-fa′ze-ah) impairment of ability to understand and use the symbols of language, both spoken and written.

dysphemia (dis-fe′me-ah) stuttering or other speech disorder due to psychoneurosis.

dysphonia (dis-fo′ne-ah) difficulty in speaking. adj., **dysphon′ic.**

dysphoria (dis-fo′re-ah) disquiet; restlessness; malaise.

dysphoriant (dis-fo′re-ant) 1. producing dysphoria. 2. an agent that produces dysphoria.

dysphrasia (dis-fra′ze-ah) difficulty in speaking due to mental defect.

dyspigmentation (dis″pig-men-ta′shun) any abnormality of pigmentation.

dysplasia (dis-pla′ze-ah) an abnormality of development. adj., **dysplas′tic.**
  congenital alveolar d., idiopathic respiratory distress of the newborn.
  cretinoid d., a developmental abnormality characteristic of cretinism, consisting of retarded ossification and smallness of the internal and reproductive organs.
  fibrous d., localized overgrowth of fibrous tissue in bone, causing destructive resorption of cancellous and adjacent cortical bone, and sometimes distention and distortion of the contours of the affected bones; it may affect a single bone (monostotic fibrous dysplasia) or many bones (polyostotic fibrous dysplasia or Albright's syndrome).

dyspnea (disp-ne′ah) labored or difficult breathing. adj., **dyspne′ic.** Dyspnea is a symptom of a variety of disorders and is primarily an indication of inadequate ventilation, or of insufficient amounts of oxygen in the circulating blood.
  Physical exertion can produce dyspnea, as can hypoxia such as that experienced at high altitudes. Pathologic conditions that lead to dyspnea include: partial obstruction of the air passages, as in bronchitis, CROUP and ASTHMA; defects in the lungs or chest wall which restrict lung expansion; and heart diseases, such as congestive HEART FAILURE, which decrease the cardiac output.
  There are certain respiratory neuroses that are accompanied by dyspnea. The most common of these are HYPERVENTILATION, in which the patient breathes very rapidly, and a "sighing" type of respiration that follows a definite pattern of breathing at maximal depth and then breathing normally. These conditions can lead to respiratory ALKALOSIS because of a "blowing off" of carbon dioxide.
  cardiac d., difficult breathing due to heart disease.
  exertional d., dyspnea due to physical effort or exertion.
  orthostatic d., difficulty in breathing when in the erect position.
  paroxysmal d., respiratory distress occurring in attacks without apparent cause, usually during sleep at night.
  sighing d., a syndrome characterized by abnormally deep inspiration without significant alteration in the respiration rate and without wheezing.

dyspoiesis (dis″poi-e′sis) a disorder of formation, as of blood cells.

dysponderal (dis-pon′der-al) pertaining to disorder of weight, either obesity or underweight.

dyspragia (dis-pra′je-ah) the difficult performance of some function.

dyspraxia (dis-prak′se-ah) partial loss of ability to perform coordinated movements.

dysprosium (dis-pro′ze-um) a chemical element, atomic number 66, atomic weight 162.50, symbol Dy. (See table of ELEMENTS.)

dysproteinemia (dis-pro″te-in-e′me-ah) disorder of the protein content of the blood.

dysrhythmia (dis-rith′me-ah) disturbance of rhythm.
  cerebral d., electroencephalographic d., disturbance or irregularity in the rhythm of the brain waves.

dysspermia (dis-sper′me-ah) impairment of the semen.

dysstasia (dis-sta′ze-ah) difficulty in standing. adj., **dysstat′ic.**

dyssymbolia (dis″sim-bo′le-ah) inability to express thoughts in intelligent language.

dyssynergia (dis″sin-er′je-ah) muscular incoordination.

dyssystole (dis-sis′to-le) asystole; incomplete systole.

dystectia (dis-tek′she-ah) defective closure of the neural tube.

dysteleology (dis″te-le-ol′o-je) the science of rudimentary organs.

dysthermosia (dis″ther-mo′ze-ah) disturbance of heat production.

dysthymia (dis-thi′me-ah) mental distress.

dystimbria (dis-tim′bre-ah) defective resonance of the voice.

dystocia (dis-to′se-ah) difficult labor.
  fetal d., that due to malformation, abnormal position or size of fetus.

maternal d., that due to small or malformed pelvis of mother.
  placental d., difficult delivery of the placenta.

dystonia (dis-to′ne-ah) impairment of muscular tonus. adj., **dyston′ic.**

dystopia (dis-to′pe-ah) malposition; displacement. adj., **dystop′ic.**

dystrophia (dis-tro′fe-ah) [Gr.] dystrophy.
  d. adiposogenita′lis, adiposogenital dystrophy.
  d. epithelia′lis cor′neae, dystrophy of the corneal epithelium, with erosions.
  d. hypophysopri′va chron′ica, a condition caused by partial removal of the pituitary gland, marked by obesity, increased carbohydrate tolerance, hypothermia, hypoplasia of the gonads, retardation of skeletal growth and mental dullness.
  d. myoton′ica, a rare disease characterized by stiffness of the muscles followed in time by atrophy of the muscles of the neck and face, producing hatchet face or tapir mouth. The atrophy extends to the muscles of the trunk and extremities and is associated with cataract. Called also myotonia dystrophica.
  d. un′guium, alteration in texture and color of the nails, due to systemic or other disease.

dystrophoneurosis (dis-trof″o-nu-ro′sis) nervous disease due to malnutrition.

dystrophy (dis′tro-fe) faulty nutrition. adj., **dystroph′ic.**
  adiposogenital d., a condition associated with lesions of the hypothalamus and pituitary gland, marked by obesity and sexual infantilism; called also Fröhlich's syndrome.
  muscular d., progressive atrophy of the muscles with no discoverable lesion of the spinal cord (see also MUSCULAR DYSTROPHY).

dysuria (dis-u′re-ah) painful urination. adj., **dysu′ric.**

dysvitaminosis (dis″vi-tah-mĭ-no′sis) any disorder due to vitamin deficiency or excess.

dyszooamylia (dis-zo″o-ah-mi′le-ah) failure of the liver to store up glycogen.

dyszoospermia (dis″zo-o-sper′me-ah) a disorder of spermatozoa formation.

E

E. electromotive force, emmetropia, eye.

e. electron.

EACA epsilon-aminocaproic acid.

ear (ēr) the organ of hearing and of equilibrium. The ear is made up of the outer (external) ear, the middle ear and the inner (internal) ear.

The outer ear consists of the auricle, or pinna, and the external acoustic meatus. The auricle collects sound waves and directs them to the external acoustic meatus which conducts them to the tympanum (the cavity of the middle ear).

The tympanic membrane (eardrum) separates the outer ear from the middle ear. In the middle ear are the three ossicles, the malleus (hammer), incus (anvil) and stapes (stirrup), so called because of their resemblance to these objects. These three small bones form a chain across the middle ear from the tympanum to the oval window in the membrane separating the middle ear from the inner ear. The middle ear is connected to the nasopharynx by the eustachian tube, through which the air pressure on the inner side of the eardrum is equalized with the air pressure on its outside surface. The middle ear is also connected with the cells in the mastoid bone just behind the outer ear. Two muscles attached to the ossicles contract when loud noises strike the tympanic membrane, limiting its vibration and thus protecting it and the inner ear from damage.

In the inner ear (or labyrinth) is the cochlea, containing the nerves that transmit sound to the brain. The inner ear also contains the SEMICIRCULAR CANALS, which are essential to the sense of balance.

When a sound strikes the ear it causes the tympanic membrane to vibrate. The ossicles function as levers, amplifying the motion of the tympanic membrane, and passing the vibrations on to the cochlea. From there the vestibulocochlear (eighth cranial) nerve transmits the vibrations, translated into nerve impulses, to the auditory center in the brain. (See also HEARING.)

DISEASES OF THE EAR. Infections and inflammations of the ear include OTOMYCOSIS, a fungal infection of the outer ear; OTITIS MEDIA, an infection of the middle ear; and MASTOIDITIS, an infection of the mastoid cells. Deafness may result from infection or from other causes such as old age, injury to the ear or hereditary factors. Another cause of deafness is OTOSCLEROSIS. Disorders of equilibrium may be caused by imperfect functioning of the semicircular canals of the inner ear or from *labyrinthitis*, an inflammation of the inner ear. MENIÈRE'S DISEASE, believed to result from dilatation of the lymphatic channels in the cochlea, may also cause disturbances in balance.

SURGERY OF THE EAR. Surgical procedures on the ear usually are indicated when chronic infection has resulted in some destruction of the bones of the middle ear or mastoid. An exception is myrin-gotomy, incision of the tympanic membrane, which is sometimes necessary to relieve pressure behind the eardrum and allow for drainage from an inflammatory process in the middle ear. Surgical procedures involving plastic reconstruction of the small bones of the middle ear are extremely delicate and have been made possible by the development of special instruments and technical equipment. STAPEDECTOMY and TYMPANOPLASTY are examples of this type of surgery, which has done much to preserve hearing that would otherwise be lost as a result of infectious destruction or sclerosis of these bones.

NURSING CARE. Much can be done to prevent hearing loss resulting from destruction of the bones of the middle ear through education of the public in the danger of chronic ear infections. Otitis media is fairly common in infants and children and must be treated diligently by antibiotic therapy under the supervision of a physician. If infections of the middle ear are not treated properly, they tend to become chronic, often causing few or no symptoms until permanent damage has been done.

Nursing procedures used in the treatment of the ear include instillation of ear drops and IRRIGATIONS of the external ear. General principles of administration of ear drops include the following: Medications for the ear produce less discomfort if they are warmed slightly, but care must be taken that they are not overheated. When giving the drops it is important to avoid forcing air into the ear. The patient is instructed to turn his head so that it is tilted away from the affected side. After the ear drops are instilled the head is kept in a tilted position for a few minutes to prevent leakage of drops from the ear. Cotton is applied after instillation of the drops *only* when specifically ordered by the physician, as it may absorb the medication and prevent its reaching the area to be medicated. Before the ear drops are instilled the external acoustic meatus should be cleaned as necessary with a cotton-tipped applicator. To straighten the external acoustic meatus, one gently pulls the ear lobe upward and backward for adults, downward and backward for infants and small children.

Nursing care following surgery of the ear is aimed at prevention of infection and promoting the comfort of the patient. Since the ear is so close to the brain, it is extremely important to avoid introducing pathogenic organisms into the operative site. The external ear and surrounding skin must be kept scrupulously clean. If the patient's hair is long it should be braided or arranged so that it does not come in contact with the patient's ear and side of the face. Aseptic technique must be used in all nursing procedures immediately before and after surgery.

The patient should be instructed to avoid nose blowing, especially after surgery, when there is a possibility that such an action can alter pressure within the ear. Observation of the patient after surgery of the ear includes watching for signs of injury to the facial nerve. The patient will not be able to wrinkle his forehead, close his eye, pucker his lips or bare his teeth if the facial nerve has been damaged. This is often a temporary situation resulting from edema, and will subside as the edema is reduced. Some permanent damage may result, however, and signs of facial nerve damage should be reported to the surgeon. Vertigo is another common occurrence after surgery of the ear. It too is usually only temporary and will subside as the operative site heals. The situation does require special protective measures such as side rails, and support of the patient while he is up out of bed, so as to avoid falling and accidental injury.

Most surgeons prefer that the nurse not change dressings around the ear during the immediate postoperative period. Should excessive drainage require more dressings, these can be applied over the basic dressing. Any drainage should be noted and recorded and excessive drainage reported immediately to the surgeon.

cauliflower e., deformity caused by trauma to the ear.

earache (ēr′āk) pain in the ear; otalgia.

eardrum (ēr′drum) tympanic membrane.

earwax (ēr′waks) cerumen.

Eaton agent (e′ton a′jent) one of the pleuropneumonia-like organisms that cause primary atypical pneumonia.

ebonation (e″bo-na′shun) removal of loose pieces of bone from a wound.

Ebstein's anomaly (eb′stīnz) a malformation of the tricuspid valve, usually associated with an atrial septal defect.

ebullition (eb″u-lish′un) the state of boiling.

eburnation (e″ber-na′shun) conversion of bone into a hard, ivory-like mass.

eburneous (e-ber′ne-us) ivory-like.

ecaudate (e-kaw′dāt) tail-less.

ecbolic (ek-bol′ik) 1. stimulating the casting out of a material, as the secretion of a gland or the contents of the uterus. 2. an ecbolic agent.

eccentro-osteochondrodysplasia (ek-sen″tro-os″te-o-kon″dro-dis-pla′ze-ah) a condition in which ossification occurs from several centers instead of a single center, marked by dwarfing and bodily deformities.

eccentropiesis (ek-sen″tro-pi-e′sis) pressure from within outward.

ecchondroma, ecchondrosis (ek″kon-dro′mah), (ek″kon-dro′sis) a hyperplastic growth of cartilaginous tissue on the surface of a cartilage or projecting under the periosteum of a bone.

ecchymoma (ek″ĭ-mo′mah) swelling due to blood extravasation.

ecchymosis (ek″ĭ-mo′sis), pl. *ecchymo'ses* [Gr.] escape of blood into the tissues, producing a large and blotchy area of superficial discoloration (bruise). adj., **ecchymot'ic.**

eccrine (ek′rin) producing a fluid secretion without removing cytoplasm from the secreting cells.

eccrinology (ek″rĭ-nol′o-je) the study of secreting glands and secretions.

eccritic (ek-krit′ik) 1. promoting excretion. 2. an agent that promotes excretion.

eccyesis (ek″si-e′sis) ectopic pregnancy.

ecdemic (ek-dem′ik) brought into a region from without.

ECG electrocardiogram.

echinococcosis (e-ki″no-kok-o′sis) infection with the larval form of *Echinococcus granulosus* causing hydatid or echinococcus cysts.

Echinococcus (e-ki″no-kok′us) a genus of TAPEWORMS.

E. granulo′sus, a small tapeworm of dogs and wolves whose larvae may develop in mammals, forming hydatid cysts.

echinulate (e-kin′u-lāt) having small prickles or spines.

echoacousia (ek″o-ah-koo′ze-ah) subjective hearing of repetition of a sound after stimuli producing it have ceased.

echocardiogram (ek″o-kar′de-o-gram″) the record produced by echocardiography.

echocardiography (ek″o-kar″de-og′rah-fe) recording of the position and motion of the heart borders and valves by reflected echoes of ultrasonic waves transmitted through the chest wall.

echoencephalogram (ek″o-en-sef′ah-lo-gram″) the record produced by echoencephalography.

echoencephalography (ek″o-en-sef″ah-log′rah-fe) the mapping of intracranial structures by means of reflected echoes of ultrasound transmitted through the skull.

echolalia (ek″o-la′le-ah) automatic repetition by a patient of what is said to him.

echomimia (ek″o-mim′e-ah) purposeless repetition of the words of others.

echomotism (ek″o-mo′tizm) purposeless repetition of the movements of others.

echopraxis (ek″o-prak′sis) 1. the meaningless and purposeless repetition, on the part of a patient, of motions that have been started by the examining physician. 2. echomotism.

echothiophate (ek″o-thi′o-fāt) a compound used as a cholinesterase inhibitor and to reduce intraocular pressure in glaucoma.

echovirus (ek′o-vi″rus) a group of viruses, the name of which was derived from the first letters of the description "enteric cytopathogenic human orphan." At the time of the isolation of the viruses the diseases they caused were not known, hence the term "orphan," but it is now known that these viruses produce many different types of disease, including forms of meningitis, diarrhea and various respiratory diseases.

eclabium (ek-la′be-um) eversion of a lip.

eclampsia (e-klamp′se-ah) convulsive attacks of

peripheral origin; especially a toxemia of pregnancy marked by high blood pressure, albuminuria, convulsions and coma. Early prenatal care, including frequent blood pressure measurement and urinalysis, provides early detection of preeclampsia and adequate treatment to forestall the development of eclampsia.

TREATMENT. During the prenatal period efforts are made to limit the patient's weight gain to 8 ounces a week. Sodium intake is limited and diuretics may be administered. These same measures are used to treat preeclampsia. Hospitalization becomes necessary if the blood pressure continues to rise, weight gain cannot be controlled by the patient and cerebral, visual and gastrointestinal symptoms develop. The patient is placed on bed rest, her calorie and sodium intake is restricted and diuretics are administered. Medications that may be prescribed to control convulsive seizures include amobarbital (Amytal), chloral hydrate, paraldehyde and morphine sulfate. The patient who develops heart failure or pulmonary edema requires special medications and treatments to control these complications. If the eclampsia remains severe and progressive in spite of attempts to control it, and normal delivery of the infant is not expected within a reasonable period of time, the physician may decide to terminate the pregnancy.

NURSING CARE. The patient with mild eclampsia will need assistance and moral support in following the regime prescribed by her obstetrician. The nurse must explain to the patient the importance of following the doctor's orders, but she should avoid unduly frightening the patient. In severe eclampsia the patient is critically ill and the maternal and infant mortality rate is high. The patient is kept under constant observation and the temperature, pulse, respirations and blood pressure are recorded at least every hour. Intake and output are carefully measured. Because these patients are extremely restless and often confused, padded side rails must be kept in place and the head board padded with a pillow or folded blanket. To avoid precipitation of a convulsion or aggravation of the patient's restlessness, a quiet and nonstimulating environment must be provided. When a convulsion does occur the patient must be protected from injury (see CONVULSION). The nurse must be alert for signs of a precipitate delivery during a convulsion. Recovery from eclampsia usually is rapid and complete once delivery of the infant has taken place.

puerperal e., that occurring after or during childbirth.

uremic e., eclampsia due to uremia.

eclampsism (e-klamp'sizm) puerperal eclampsia without convulsive seizures.

eclamptogenic (e-klamp"to-jen'ik) causing eclampsia.

ecmnesia (ek-ne'ze-ah) forgetfulness of recent events with remembrance of more remote ones.

ecoid (e'koid) the colorless framework of an erythrocyte.

Ecolid (e'ko-lid) trademark for a preparation of chlorisondamine, an antihypertensive and ganglion-blocking agent.

ecology (e-kol'o-je) the scientific study of the interrelations of living organisms and their environment. adj., **ecolog'ic.**

ecomania (e"ko-ma'ne-ah) an attitude of mind that is dominating toward members of the family but humble toward those in authority.

ecosystem (e"ko-sis'tem) the fundamental unit in ecology, comprising the living organisms and the nonliving elements interacting in a certain defined area.

ecphylaxis (ek"fi-lak'sis) impotency of the antibodies or phylactic agents in the blood. adj., **ecphylac'tic.**

ecphyma (ek-fi'mah) an outgrowth or protuberance.

écraseur (a"krah-zer') [Fr.] an instrument with a loop of chain or wire for removing a part by enclosing and dividing it.

ecstrophy (ek'stro-fe) exstrophy; the turning inside out of an organ.

E.C.T. electroconvulsive therapy.

ect(o)- (ek'to) word element [Gr.], *external; outside.*

ectasia (ek-ta'ze-ah) expansion; dilatation. adj., **ectat'ic.**

ectental (ek-ten'tal) pertaining to the ectoderm and entoderm.

ecthyma (ek-thi'mah) an eruption of pustules with hard bases and areolae.

ectiris (ek-ti'ris) the retinal or external portion of the iris.

ectoantigen (ek"to-an'tĭ-jen) an antigen loosely attached to the outside of bacteria.

ectoblast (ek'to-blast) the ectoderm.

ectocardia (ek"to-kar'de-ah) displacement of the heart.

ectochoroidea (ek"to-ko-roi'de-ah) the outer layer of the choroid coat.

ectocinerea (ek"to-sĭ-ne're-ah) the cortical gray matter of the brain.

ectocolon (ek"to-ko'lon) dilatation of the colon.

ectocondyle (ek"to-kon'dīl) the external condyle of a bone.

ectocornea (ek"to-kor'ne-ah) the outer layer of the cornea.

ectocytic (ek"to-si'tik) outside the cell.

ectoderm (ek'to-derm) the outermost of the three primitive germ layers of the embryo; from it are derived the epidermis and epidermic tissues, such as the nails, hair and glands of the skin, the nervous system, external sense organs (eye, ear, etc.) and mucous membrane of the mouth and anus. adj., **ectoder'mal, ectoder'mic.**

ectodermosis (ek"to-der-mo'sis) a disorder involving tissues developed from the ectoderm.

ectoentad (ek"to-en'tad) from without inward.

ectoenzyme (ek"to-en'zīm) an extracellular enzyme.

ectogenous (ek-toj′ĕ-nus) originating outside the organism.

ectoglobular (ek″to-glob′u-lar) outside the blood corpuscles.

ectogony (ek-tog′o-ne) influence on the maternal organism by the developing zygote.

ectolysis (ek-tol′ĭ-sis) lysis or destruction of the ectoplasm.

ectomere (ek′to-mēr) one of the blastomeres taking part in formation of the ectoderm.

ectomesoblast (ek″to-mes′o-blast) the layer of cells not yet differentiated into ectoderm and mesoderm.

ectomorphy (ek′to-mor″fe) a type of body build in which tissues derived from the ectoderm predominate. There is relatively slight development of the visceral and body structures, and the body is linear and delicate.

-ectomy (ek′to-me) word element [Gr.], *excision; surgical removal.*

ectonuclear (ek″to-nu′kle-ar) outside the nucleus of a cell.

ectoparasite (ek″to-par′ah-sīt) a parasite attached to the outer surface or situated beneath the skin of the host. adj., **ectoparasit′ic.**

ectopia (ek-to′pe-ah) [L.] ectopy.
   e. cor′dis, location of the heart in an abnormal place, e.g., outside the chest wall or in the abdominal cavity.

ectopic (ek-top′ik) situated elsewhere than in the normal place.
   e. pregnancy, pregnancy in which the fertilized ovum becomes implanted outside the uterus. The ovum may rarely develop in the abdominal cavity, ovary or cervix uteri, but ectopic pregnancy is almost always found in one of the uterine (fallopian) tubes (see PREGNANCY). A spontaneous abortion may then occur, but more often the fetus will grow to a size large enough to burst the tube. This is an emergency situation requiring immediate treatment. The symptoms of a uterine tube ruptured by ectopic pregnancy are vaginal bleeding and a severe pain in one side of the abdomen. Prompt surgery is necessary to remove the damaged tube and the fetus, and to stop the bleeding. Fortunately, the removal of one tube usually leaves the other one intact, so that future pregnancy is possible.

ectoplasm (ek′to-plazm) the more peripheral layer of cytoplasm of a cell.

ectopy (ek′to-pe) displacement; abnormal situation.

ectoretina (ek″to-ret′ĭ-nah) the outermost layer of the retina.

ectoscopy (ek-tos′ko-pe) external inspection of an organ.

ectoskeleton (ek″to-skel′ĕ-ton) the dermoskeleton.

ectosteal (ek-tos′te-al) situated outside of a bone.

ectostosis (ek″to-sto′sis) ossification beginning underneath the perichondrium.

ectothrix (ek′to-thriks) a fungus that grows inside the shaft of a hair, but produces a conspicuous external sheath of spores.

ectozoon (ek″to-zo′on) an external animal parasite.

ectrodactyly (ek″tro-dak′tĭ-le) congenital absence of all or part of a digit.

ectromelia (ek″tro-me′le-ah) gross hypoplasia or aplasia of one or more long bones of one or more limbs.

ectromelus (ek-trom′ĕ-lus) a fetus with rudimentary arms and legs.

ectrometacarpia (ek″tro-met″ah-kar′pe-ah) gross hypoplasia or aplasia of a metacarpal bone.

ectrometatarsia (ek″tro-met″ah-tar′se-ah) gross hypoplasia or aplasia of a metatarsal bone.

ectrophalangia (ek″tro-fah-lan′je-ah) gross hypoplasia or aplasia of one or more phalanges of a finger or toe.

ectropion (ek-tro′pe-on) eversion or turning outward, as of the margin of an eyelid.

ectropionize (ek-tro′pe-ŏ-nīz″) to put into a state of eversion.

ectrosyndactyly (ek″tro-sin-dak′tĭ-le) absence of some of the digits with fusion of the existing ones.

ectylurea (ek″til-u-re′ah) a urea compound used to produce mild depression of the central nervous system.

ecuresis (ek″u-re′sis production of absolute dehydration of the body by excessive urinary excretion in relation to the intake of water.

eczema (ek′ze-mah) a skin rash characterized by itching, swelling, blistering, oozing and scaling of the skin.
   Eczema is a common allergic reaction in children but it also occurs in adults, usually in a more severe form. Childhood eczema often begins in infancy, the rash appearing on the face, neck and folds of elbows and knees. It may disappear by itself when the offending food is removed from the diet, or it may become more extensive and in some instances cover the entire surface of the body. Severe eczema can be complicated by skin infections.
   Childhood eczema may persist for several years or return after the child is older. A person who suffers eczema in childhood may develop some other allergic condition later, most commonly hay fever or asthma.
   CAUSE AND TREATMENT. Eczema is frequently caused by an allergic sensitivity to foods such as milk, fish or eggs or to dusts, pollens or similar substances that are inhaled. Allergic eczema is cured or controlled by some of the methods used for other allergic disorders (see ALLERGY).
   atopic e., eczema resulting from ingestion of or contact with a substance to which the individual is sensitive.
   e. bar′bae, eczema affecting the beard area of the face and neck.
   e. herpet′icum, a vesiculopustular eruption due to herpesvirus superimposed on areas of preexisting eczema.

e. hypertroph'icum, a form with permanent enlargement of the skin papillae.

solar e., an eczematous eruption on exposed areas of the body due to the burn-producing wavelengths of sunlight.

e. squamo'sum, eczema with adherent scales of epithelium.

stasis e., eczema of the legs, due to impeded circulation, with edema, pigmentation and ulceration.

e. vaccina'tum, a vesiculopapular eruption due to vaccinia virus, superimposed on preexisting eczema.

eczematous (ek-zem'ah-tus) of the nature of eczema.

edathamil (ĕ-dath'ah-mil) calcium disodium edetate, or EDTA, used in the treatment of metal poisoning.

edema (ĕ-de'mah) an abnormal accumulation of fluid in the intercellular spaces of the body. adj., **edem'atous.** Edema can be caused by a variety of factors, including hypoproteinemia in which a lowered concentration of plasma proteins decreases the osmotic pressure, thereby permitting passage of abnormal amounts of fluid out of the blood vessels and into the tissue spaces. Some other causes are poor lymphatic drainage, increased capillary permeability (as in inflammation) and congestive heart failure.

Local edema due to inflammation or poor drainage through the lymph vessels may be relieved by elevation of the part and application of cold to the area. Generalized edema is treated by the administration of DIURETICS, which increase the loss of certain salts and thereby increase removal of tissue fluids, which are eliminated as urine. Sodium, which enhances retention of fluid in the tissues, is restricted in the diet of patients with edema.

NURSING CARE. Edematous tissue breaks down quite readily because there is an interference with the normal exchange of nutrients and waste products within the tissue cells. Extreme care should be taken in handling edematous parts of the body, every effort should be made to keep the skin intact and it is necessary to change the patient's position frequently to avoid the development of decubitus ulcers.

In dependent edema it is helpful to elevate the lower extremities periodically and promote drainage of fluid via the lymph and blood vessels.

Severe edema accompanying an allergic reaction may prove fatal if the respiratory passages become occluded. An emergency tracheostomy set and equipment for the administration of epinephrine should be kept at the patient's bedside in the event acute respiratory embarrassment develops.

In all types of generalized edema the patient's intake and output are recorded at least every 24 hours. The physician may also request daily weighing of the patient so that fluid gain or loss can be determined. The patient should be weighed at the same time each day, preferably before breakfast, and using the same scales.

angioneurotic e., temporary edema suddenly appearing in areas of skin or mucous membrane, of allergic, neurotic or unknown origin.

cardiac e., edema due to heart disease with the resulting slowing of the peripheral blood flow and the rise in capillary pressure.

dependent e., edema affecting most severely the lowermost parts of the body.

e. neonato'rum, a disease of newborn infants marked by spreading edema with cold, livid skin.

pitting e., edema in which pressure for 30 seconds or so leaves a persistent depression in the tissues.

pulmonary e., an effusion of serous fluid into the air vesicles and interstitial tissue of the lungs.

purulent e., edema with purulent effusion.

edematogenic (ĕ-dem"ah-to-jen'ik) tending to produce or cause edema.

edentia (e-den'she-ah) absence of the teeth.

edentulous (e-den'tu-lus) without teeth.

edetate (ed'ĕ-tāt) calcium disodium edetate; disodium edetate.

edrophonium (ed"ro-fo'ne-um) an ammonium compound used as a parasympathomimetic, muscle stimulant, curare antagonist and diagnostic agent in myasthenia gravis.

EDTA calcium disodium edetate, used in the treatment of metal poisoning.

EEG electroencephalogram.

E.E.N.T. eye-ear-nose-throat.

effacement (ĕ-fās'ment) the obliteration of form or features; applied to the cervix uteri during labor when it is so changed that only the ostium uteri remains.

effect (ĕ-fekt') a condition or alteration produced by some agent or force.

additive e., an enhanced effect produced by the combined action of two agents, being greater than the sum of their separate effects.

cumulative e., a sudden marked effect after administration of a number of ineffective doses of a medication.

position e., in genetics, the changed effect produced by alteration of the relative positions of various genes on the chromosomes.

effectiveness (ĕ-fek'tive-nes) the ability to produce a specific result or to exert a specific measurable influence.

relative biologic e., an expression of the effectiveness of other types of radiation in comparison with that of 1 R of gamma or roentgen rays.

effector (ĕ-fek'tor) the organ that effects an organism's response to a stimulus.

effemination (ĕ-fem"ĭ-na'shun) development of feminine qualities in a male.

efferent (ef'er-ent) conducting or progressing away from a center or specific site of reference.

e. nerve, any nerve that carries impulses from the central nervous system toward the periphery (see also NEURON).

effleurage (ef"lu-rahzh') [Fr.] a centripetal stroking movement in massage.

efflorescence (ef"lo-res'ens) a rash or eruption; any skin lesion.

efflorescent (ef"lo-res'ent) becoming powdery by losing the water of crystallization.

effluvium (ĕ-floo've-um), pl. *efflu'via* [L.] 1. an outflowing or shedding, as of the hair. 2. an exhalation or emanation, especially one of noxious nature.

effortil (ef'or-til) an alcoholic compound used as a sympathomimetic and as a pressor agent.

effusion (ĕ-fu'zhun) 1. escape of a fluid into a part. 2. effused material.

egesta (e-jes'tah) the excretions or discharges from the body.

egestion (e-jes'chun) elimination from the body of waste products and residue of ingested nutrients.

egg (eg) an animal ovum, especially an ovum that is extruded from the maternal body before development of the embryo, and sometimes before fertilization.

ego (e'go) in psychoanalytic theory, one of the three major parts of the personality, the others being the ID and the SUPEREGO. The word ego is Latin for "I," that is, self or individual as distinguished from other persons. The ego is represented by certain mental mechanisms, such as perception and memory, and specific defense mechanisms that are used to adjust to the demands of primitive instinctual drives (the id) and the demands of the external world (superego). The ego may be considered the psychologic aspect of one's personality, the id comprising the physiologic aspects and the superego the social aspects. The ego controls and directs an individual's actions and seeks compromises between the id impulses, social and parental prohibitions and the pressures of reality.
    The word ego also is commonly used to express conceit or self-centeredness. This should not be confused with the psychiatric meaning described above.

egocentric (e"go-sen'trik) overly self-centered; having one's interest largely centered in or directed toward one's self.

egomania (e"go-ma'ne-ah) pathologic self-centeredness and selfishness.

egotropic (e"go-trop'ik) egocentric.

Ehrlich, (ār'lik) Paul (1854–1915). German bacteriologist. Born in Silesia of Jewish parents, he studied medicine and was early drawn to research on aniline dyes. Ehrlich did vast work on the problems of serology and immunity, and is known preeminently for his discovery of salvarsan or "606," an arsenical compound now called arsphenamine, which is a cure for syphilis. He differentiated the leukemias, classified the leukocytes, described polychromatophilia and is generally regarded the founder of hematology. In 1908 Ehrlich shared with Metchnikoff the Nobel prize for his work in immunology.

eidetic (i-det'ik) pertaining to or characterized by exact visualization of events or objects previously seen; a person having such an ability.

eidogen (i'do-jen) in embryology, a substance elaborated by a second-grade inductor, which is capable of modifying the form of an organ already induced.

eidoptometry (i"dop-tom'ĕ-tre) measurement of the acuteness of visual perception.

einsteinium (īn-sti'ne-um) a chemical element, atomic number 99, atomic weight 254, symbol Es. (See table of ELEMENTS.)

eisodic (i-sod'ik) afferent; centripetal.

ejaculatio (e-jak"u-la'she-o) [L.] ejaculation.
    e. prae'cox, ejaculation of the semen immediately after the beginning of the sexual act.

ejaculation (e-jak"u-la'shun) forcible, sudden expulsion; especially expulsion of semen from the male urethra, a reflex action that occurs as a result of sexual stimulation. adj., **ejac'ulatory.** The three components of semen are expelled in quick succession. First to emerge is a lubricating fluid produced by the bulbourethral glands in the penis. Next comes a fluid released into the urethral channel by the prostate; this fluid provides a neutral medium within which the sperm cells can swim. Lastly, the spermatic fluid, which has been stored in the seminal vesicles, is likewise injected into the urethral channel and ejaculated. (See also REPRODUCTION.)

ejecta (e-jek'tah) refuse cast off from the body.

EKG electrocardiogram.

EKY electrokymogram.

elastase (e-las'tās) a factor or enzyme capable of catalyzing the digestion of elastic tissue.

elastic (e-las'tik) susceptible of being stretched, compressed or distorted, and then tending to assume its original shape.
    e. cartilage, a substance that is more opaque, flexible and elastic than hyaline cartilage, and is further distinguished by its yellow color. The ground substance is penetrated in all directions by frequently branching fibers that give all of the reactions for elastin.
    e. tissue, connective tissue made up of yellow, elastic fibers, frequently massed into sheets.

elasticity (e"las-tis'ĭ-te) the ability of a material to undergo distortion and resume its original size and shape.

elastin (e-las'tin) a scleroprotein present in fibers of connective tissues, digestible by pepsin and trypsin, but not converted to gelatin in boiling water.

elastinase (e-las'tĭ-nās) an enzyme that dissolves elastic tissue.

elastofibroma (e-las"to-fi-bro'mah) a tumor consisting of both elastin and fibrous elements.

elastolysis (e"las-tol'ĭ-sis) the digestion of elastic substance or tissue. adj., **elastolyt'ic.**

elastoma (e"las-to'mah) a tumor of elastic tissue of the skin; pseudoxanthoma elasticum.

elastometer (e"las-tom'ĕ-ter) an instrument for measuring the elasticity of tissues.

elastomucin (e-las"to-mu'sin) a polysaccharide component of elastic tissue.

elastorrhexis (e-las"to-rek'sis) rupture of fibers composing elastic tissue.

elastosis (e"las-to'sis) degeneration of elastic tissue. adj., **elastot'ic.**

elation (e-la'shun) emotional excitement marked by acceleration of mental and bodily activity.

Elavil (el′ah-vil) trademark for preparations of amitriptyline, an antidepressant.

elbow (el′bo) the joint between the upper arm and the forearm. It joins the large bone of the upper arm, or humerus, with the two smaller bones of the lower arm, the radius and ulna.

Characteristics. The elbow is one of the body's more versatile joints, with a combined hinge and rotating action allowing the arm to bend and the hand to make a half turn. The flexibility of the elbow and shoulder joints together permits a nearly infinite variety of hand movements.

The action of the elbow is controlled primarily by the biceps and the triceps muscles. When the biceps contracts, the arm bends at the elbow. When the triceps contracts the arm straightens. In each action, the opposite muscle exerts a degree of opposing tension, moderating the movement so that it is smooth and even instead of sudden and jerky.

As in other joints, the ends of the bones meeting at the elbow have a smooth covering of cartilage, a tough rubbery substance that minimizes friction when the joint is moved. The elbow joint is lubricated with synovia. The bursa, a small sac of connective tissue, eases its movement. The bones forming the joint are held together by tough, fibrous ligaments.

The "funny bone" is not a bone but the ulnar nerve, a vulnerable and sensitive nerve that lies close to the surface near the point of the elbow. Hitting it causes a tingling pain or sensation that may be felt all the way to the fingers.

DISORDERS OF THE ELBOW. The elbows, like the knees, are continually exposed to bumps, twists and wrenches. A common injury of the elbow is a fracture of a bone near the joint. Another injury of the elbow is dislocation, in which the hinge joint is pulled apart by a violent twist or yank. Tendons and ligaments may be torn. In some cases, dislocation and fracture may occur together.

ARTHRITIS may affect the elbow and make it stiff or impossible to move. Special exercises, manipula-

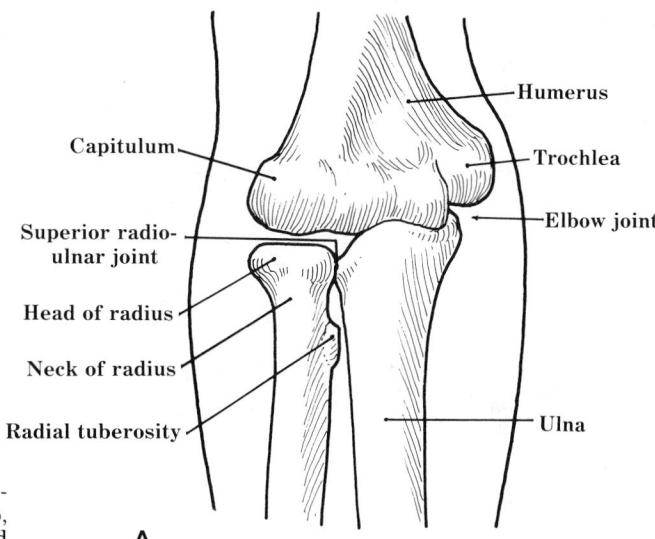

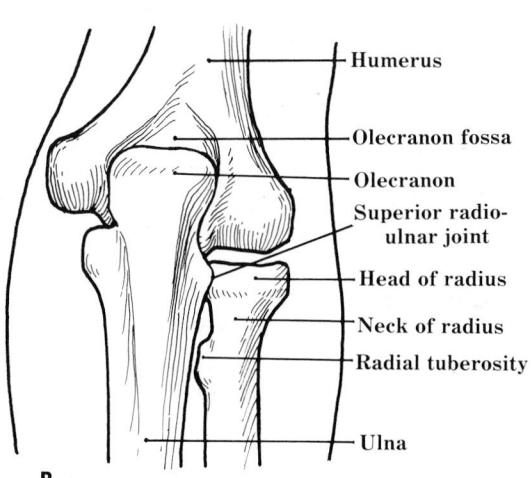

Elbow. *A*, Anterior view, right arm. *B*, Posterior view, right arm. (Redrawn from Jacob, S. W., and Francone, C. A.: Structure and Function in Man. 2nd ed. Philadelphia, W. B. Saunders Co., 1970.)

tion and heat therapy may be prescribed to help restore flexibility. BURSITIS can also cause pain in the elbow. It often results from excessive use of the joint. "Tennis elbow," which may affect people who never held a tennis racket, is a term often used for bursitis of the elbow but is more accurately a tendinitis, or inflammation of the tendons. Rest and heat therapy are usually effective in relieving the condition.

Electra complex (e-lek'trah) a series of symptoms attributed to suppressed sexual desire of a daughter for her father, with hostility toward the mother.

electric (e-lek'trik) of the nature of electricity.

e. shock, shock caused by electric current passing through the body. The longer the contact with electricity, the smaller the chance of survival. The victim's breathing may stop, and his body may appear stiff.

In giving first aid for electric shock, first the electric contact is broken as quickly as possible; this must be done with care to avoid exposure to the current. The rescuer, keeping in mind that water and metals are conductors of electricity, stands on a *dry* surface and does not touch the victim or electric wire with his bare hands.

The victim may have stopped breathing and appear to be paralyzed. In this case, ARTIFICIAL RESPIRATION is begun while someone else summons medical aid, and is continued until breathing is restored—which may be several hours.

Electroshock, or electroconvulsive, therapy is sometimes used therapeutically for mental illness, especially depression, although recent development of new medications has displaced its use in some cases (see also SHOCK THERAPY).

electrical (e-lek'trĭ-kal) pertaining to electricity.

electricity (e″lek-tris'ĭ-te) a form of energy generated by friction, induction or chemical means, which produces magnetic, chemical, thermal and radiant effects.

faradic e. 1. electricity produced by induction. 2. electricity in intermittent currents.

franklinic e., frictional e., static electricity.

galvanic e., electricity generated by chemical action. 2. electricity in uninterrupted currents.

induced e., electricity produced in a body by proximity to an electrified body.

magnetic e., electricity developed by means of a magnet.

static e., electricity generated by friction, or which does not move in currents.

voltaic e., galvanic electricity.

electroaffinity (e-lek″tro-ah-fin'ĭ-te) the tenacity with which the ions of an element hold their charges.

electroanalysis (e-lek″tro-ah-nal'ĭ-sis) chemical analysis by means of the electric current.

electrobiology (e-lek″tro-bi-ol'o-je) the science of the relations of electricity to living organisms.

electrobioscopy (e-lek″tro-bi-os'ko-pe) an electric test applied to determine whether life is present or not.

electrocardiogram (e-lek″tro-kar'de-o-gram″) the record produced by electrocardiography; a tracing representing the heart's electrical action derived by amplification of the minutely small electrical impulses normally generated by the heart. Called also ECG and EKG.

electrocardiograph (e-lek″tro-kar'de-o-graf″) the apparatus used in electrocardiography.

electrocardiography (e-lek″tro-kar″de-og'rah-fe) the graphic recording from the body surface of variation in electric potential produced by the heart. With the modern electrocardiograph, the current that accompanies the action of the heart is amplified 3000 times or more, and it moves a small, sensitively balanced lever in contact with moving paper. The pattern of heart waves that is traced on the paper indicates the heart's rhythm and other actions.

The normal electrocardiogram is composed of a P wave, Q, R and S waves known as the QRS COMPLEX, or QRS wave, and a T wave. The P wave occurs at the beginning of each contraction of the atria. The QRS wave occurs at the beginning of each contraction of the ventricles. The T wave seen in a normal electrocardiogram occurs as the ventricles recover electrically and prepare for the next contraction. There is a refractory period between these waves during which the muscle is inexcitable; this period is usually about 0.30 second.

The electric impulses in the heart muscle are picked up and conducted to the electrocardiograph by electrodes or leads connected to the body by small metal plates or other methods. The metal plates are moistened with a conductive paste and attached to the arms, legs and chest (cardiac area) of the patient.

Electrocardiography is a valuable diagnostic tool, used in some routine physical examinations and when a heart disorder occurs or is suspected. It helps diagnose the damage that may have been inflicted on the heart muscle by a coronary occlusion, the progress of rheumatic fever, the presence of abnormal rhythms or the effect of digitalis or other drugs. An electrocardiogram cannot always detect impending heart disease or all cardiovascular disorders. The readings are interpreted together with the results of other diagnostic tests.

electrocardiophonograph (e-lek″tro-kar″de-o-fo'-no-graf) an instrument for simultaneously recording the electric potentials and sounds produced by contraction of the heart.

electrocautery (e-lek″tro-kaw'ter-e) galvanocautery; cautery by a wire heated by galvanic electricity.

electrochemistry (e-lek″tro-kem'is-tre) the scientific study of electricity in relation to chemical reactions.

electrochromatography (e-lek″tro-kro″mah-tog' rah-fe) chromatography performed under the influence of an electric field.

electrocision (e-lek″tro-sizh'un) excision by electric current.

electrocoagulation (e-lek″tro-ko-ag″u-la'shun) coagulation of tissue by means of an electric current.

electrocontractility (e-lek″tro-kon″trak-til'ĭ-te) contractility to electric stimulation.

electroconvulsive therapy (e-lek″tro-kon-vul'-siv) electroshock therapy; the induction of convulsions by the passage of an electric current through the brain, as in the treatment of affective psychosis (see also SHOCK THERAPY).

electrocorticography (e-lek″tro-kor″tĭ-kog′rah-fe) electroencephalography with the electrodes applied directly to the cerebral cortex.

electrocortin (e-lek″tro-kor′tin) aldosterone.

electrode (e-lek′trōd) an electric conductor through which current enters or leaves a cell, apparatus or body.

   brush e., a wire brush connected with one of the poles of an electric battery; used for applying electricity to the body.

   calomel e., an electrode consisting of metallic mercury in contact with calomel and hydrochloric acid, used as a standard in the determination of hydrogen ion concentration because it develops a constant potential.

   depolarizing e., an electrode that has a resistance greater than that of the portion of the body enclosed in the circuit.

   hydrogen e., an electrode made by depositing platinum black on platinum and then allowing it to absorb hydrogen gas to saturation; used in determination of hydrogen ion concentration.

   indifferent e., a grounded electrode.

   spark ball e., an insulating handle having on one end a metallic ball; used in applying static sparks.

   therapeutic e., an electrode of carbon cored or filled with materials for medication.

electrodermography (e-lek″tro-der-mog′rah-fe) recording of the electrical resistance of the skin.

electrodesiccation (e-lek″tro-des″ĭ-ka′shun) dehydration of tissue by use of a monopolar current through a needle electrode.

electrodiagnosis (e-lek″tro-di″ag-no′sis) diagnosis by means of electricity.

electrodynamometer (e-lek″tro-di″nah-mom′ĕ-ter) an instrument used to measure the current of faradic electricity.

electroencephalogram (e-lek″tro-en-sef′ah-lo-gram″) the record produced by electroencephalography; a tracing of the electric impulses of the brain. Called also EEG.

electroencephalograph (e-lek″tro-en-sef′ah-lo-graf) the instrument used in electroencephalography.

electroencephalography (e-lek″tro-en-sef″ah-log′rah-fe) the recording of changes in electric potentials in various areas of the brain by means of electrodes placed on the scalp or on or in the brain itself, and connected to a vacuum tube radio amplifier, which amplifies the impulses more than a million times. The impulses are of sufficient magnitude to move an electromagnetic pen that records the brain waves.

The rate, height and length of the waves vary in different parts of the brain. Age and the degree of consciousness also cause the wave patterns to differ.

Electroencephalography is widely used in studying brain function and in tracing the connections between the parts of the central nervous system. It is particularly valuable in diagnosing epilepsy, brain tumor and other diseases of and injury to the brain.

An electroencephalogram is of little use in the study of those mental disorders and diseases that do not cause gross brain damage.

electrogastrography (e-lek″tro-gas-trog′rah-fe) the synchronous recording of the electrical and mechanical activity of the stomach.

electrohemostasis (e-lek″tro-he″mo-sta′sis) arrest of hemorrhage by electrocautery.

electrohysterography (e-lek″tro-his″ter-og′rah-fe) the recording of changes in electric potential associated with contractions of the uterine muscle.

electrokymogram (e-lek″tro-ki′mo-gram) the record produced by electrokymography.

electrokymography (e-lek″tro-ki-mog′rah-fe) the graphic recording of the movements of the heart or other moving organs as they appear on a fluoroscopic screen, by means of a photoelectric device.

electrology (e″lek-trol′o-je) scientific study of the nature, effects and uses of electricity.

electrolysis (e″lek-trol′ĭ-sis) 1. decomposition of a compound by means of electricity. 2. destruction of body tissue, as of hair roots, telangiectases, etc., by electricity.

electrolyte (e-lek′tro-līt) any compound that, when dissolved in water, separates into charged particles (ions) capable of conducting an electric current. Within the body, the electrolytes play an essential role in the workings of the cell, and in maintaining fluid balance and a normal acid-base balance.

The chief electrolyte ions are: sodium, a key regulator in water balance and also necessary to normal function of muscles and nerves; potassium, which is associated with acid-base balance and is one of the main constituents of cell protoplasm; and calcium, which plays an integral part in the clotting mechanism and is essential to normal muscle physiology. Magnesium and chloride also are considered to be vital electrolytes since they are essential to chemical changes necessary for normal body function.

Sodium and chloride are found in large amounts in the fluid outside the cell (extracellular fluid). Potassium, magnesium and phosphate are found in large amounts in the fluid inside the cell (intracellular fluid). The difference in electrolyte composition of these fluids causes an electric charge to develop across the cell membrane. This electric charge allows for many electrochemical reactions necessary for regulation of the functions of the cells: for example, transmission of nerve impulses, contraction of muscle tissue and secretion of glandular cells. Average electrolyte concentrations within each of the three major compartments of body fluids are given in the table.

electrolytic (e-lek″tro-lit′ik) pertaining to electrolysis or to an electrolyte.

electromagnet (e-lek″tro-mag′net) a piece of metal rendered temporarily magnetic by passage of electricity through a coil surrounding it.

electromagnetism (e-lek″tro-mag′nĕ-tizm) magnetism developed by an electric current.

AVERAGE ELECTROLYTE CONCENTRATIONS OF
THE BODY FLUIDS (mEq./L.)

	PLASMA	INTERSTITIAL FLUID	INTRA- CELLULAR FLUID
Cations			
Na$^+$ (Sodium)	142	147	15
K$^+$ (Potassium)	5	4	150
Ca^{++} (Calcium)	5	2.5	2
Mg^{++} (Magnesium)	2	1	27
	154	154.5	194
Anions			
Cl$^-$ (Chloride)	103	114	1
HCO$_3^-$ (Bicarbonate)	27	30	10
PO$_4^{--}$ (Phosphate)	2	2	100
SO$_4^{--}$ (Sulfate)	1	1	20
Organic acids	5	7.5	—
Proteinate	16	0	63
	154	154.5	194

From De Veber, G. A.: Fluid and electrolyte problems in
the postoperative period. Nursing Clin. N. Amer., *1*:275,
1966; modified from Weisberg, H. F.: Water, Electrolyte,
and Acid-Base Balance. 2nd ed. Baltimore, Md. 20202
U.S.A., The Williams & Wilkins Co., 1962.

electromassage (e-lek"tro-mah-sahzh') massage
combined with application of an electric current.

electrometer (e"lek-trom'ĕ-ter) an instrument for
measuring electricity.

electromotive force (e-lek"tro-mo'tiv) the force
that, by reason of differences in potential, causes a
flow of electricity from one place to another, giving
rise to an electric current.

electromyography (e-lek"tro-mi-og'rah-fe) the
recording of the electric potentials developed in
muscle.

electron (e-lek'tron) the unit of negative electricity. Electrons flowing in a conductor constitute
an electric current; when ejected from a radioactive substance, the beta particles; when revolving around the nucleus of an atom they determine
all of its physical and chemical properties except
mass and radioactivity, and are called the electron
cloud.

The number of electrons revolving around the
nucleus of an atom is equal to its atomic number.
An atom of oxygen, for instance, which has an
atomic number of 8, has eight electrons in orbit
around the nucleus in a manner similar to the

planets revolving around the sun in our solar
system.

Electrons greatly influence the behavior of an
atom toward other atoms. The combination of various ELEMENTS to form compounds is brought
about by the losing or gaining of electrons; the
process is sometimes called "sharing" of electrons. For example, the combination of the elements sodium and chlorine produce the compound
sodium chloride (table salt). This is accomplished
by the transfer of one electron from the outer orbit
of the sodium atom to the outer orbit of the chlorine
atom. This combining of elements by the loss or
gain of electrons is called electrovalence. After
the electron exchange, the atoms become charged
particles called ions.

electronarcosis (e-lek"tro-nar-ko'sis) narcosis
produced by passage of an electric current through
electrodes placed on the temples.

electronegative (e-lek"tro-neg'ah-tiv) 1. having
a negative charge or an excess of electrons. 2. able
to capture electrons.

electronic (e"lek-tron'ik) pertaining to or carrying
electrons.

electrophoresis (e-lek"tro-fo-re'sis) the movement of charged particles suspended in a liquid on
various media (e.g., paper, starch, agar), under the
influence of an applied electric field. The method is
used to analyze the plasma protein content in order
to diagnose certain diseases. adj., **electrophoret'ic.**

electrophorus (e"lek-trof'o-rus) a device for obtaining static electricity by means of friction.

electrophysiology (e-lek"tro-fiz"e-ol'o-je) observation of the effects of electricity upon the body in
health.

electroplexy (e-lek"tro-plek'se) electric shock.

electropneumatotherapy (e-lek"tro-nu"mah-to-
ther'ah-pe) treatment of voice weakness by air
forced electrically into the larynx.

electropositive (e-lek"tro-poz'ĭ-tiv) 1. having a
positive charge or a deficiency of electrons. 2. able
to give up electrons.

electropuncture (e-lek'tro-pungk"tūr) puncture
of tissues by electric needles.

electropyrexia (e-lek"tro-pi-rek'se-ah) production
of high body temperature by electric means.

electroradiometer (e-lek"tro-ra"de-om'ĕ-ter) an
electroscope for measuring radiant energy.

electroresection (e-lek"tro-re-sek'shun) resection
by electrocautery.

electroscission (e-lek"tro-sish'un) excision by
electricity.

electroscope (e-lek'tro-skōp) an instrument for detecting static electricity.

electroshock (e-lek'tro-shok) shock produced by
applying electric current to the brain (see also
SHOCK THERAPY).

electrosleep (e-lek'tro-slēp) sleep induced by
electrical stimulation of the brain.

electrostatics (e-lek"tro-stat'iks) the science of
static or frictional electricity.

electrostimulation (e-lek″tro-stim″u-la′shun) a form of electroshock treatment.

electrostriatogram (e-lek″tro-stri-a′to-gram) an electroencephalogram showing differences in electric potential recorded at various levels of the corpus striatum.

electrosurgery (e-lek″tro-ser′jer-e) the use of electricity in surgery.

electrosynthesis (e-lek″tro-sin′thĕ-sis) the formation of a compound under the influence of electricity.

electrotaxis (e-lek″tro-tak′sis) movement of organisms or cells in response to electric stimuli.

electrotherapy (e-lek″tro-ther′ah-pe) treatment of disease by electricity.

electrotonus (e″lek-trot′o-nus) the change effected in a nerve or muscle by passage of an electric current.

electrotropism (e″lek-trot′ro-pism) tropism in response to electric stimuli.

electrovalence (e-lek″tro-va′lens) the bond formed between two ions through the transfer of electrons.

electuary (e-lek′tu-a″re) a medicinal preparation consisting of a powdered drug made into a paste with honey or syrup.

eleidin (el-e′ĭ-din) a substance of peculiar nature, allied to keratin and protoplasm, found in the cells of the stratum lucidum of the skin.

element (el′ĕ-ment) 1. any one of the primary parts or constituents of a thing. 2. in chemistry, a simple substance that cannot be decomposed by ordinary chemical means; the basic "stuff" of which all matter is composed.

Chemical elements are made up of atoms. Each atom consists of a nucleus with a cloud of negatively charged particles (ELECTRONS) revolving around it. The two major components of the nucleus are protons and neutrons. The number of protons in the atoms of a particular element is always the same, and therefore the physical and chemical properties of the element are always the same. It is possible, however, for a chemical element to exist in several different forms, the difference depending on the number of neutrons in the nucleus of its atoms. Different forms of the same element are called isotopes.

There are at least 105 different chemical elements known. The table lists the elements, and the symbol, atomic weight and atomic number of each. The atomic number of an element is determined by the number of protons in the nucleus of an atom of the element. The mass number of an isotope is determined by the total number of neutrons and protons in the nucleus.

STABLE CHEMICAL ELEMENTS. A stable chemical element is one that contains an optimal ratio or range of ratios between the number of protons and neutrons in the nucleus. A stable element does not spontaneously transmute into another element and therefore does not give off radiations. The stable elements are those that have an atomic number below 84, except for a few, such as potassium and rubidium, which are weakly radioactive.

RADIOACTIVE CHEMICAL ELEMENTS. A radioactive chemical element does not contain an op-timal proton-to-neutron ratio in its atomic nuclei and therefore readily gives off nuclear particles until all nuclei have attained the optimal combination of protons and neutrons. The spontaneous releasing of its nuclear particles changes the radioactive atom into a new atom (transmutation).

As radioactive elements disintegrate and form new chemical elements a tremendous amount of energy is released. This emission of energy and nuclear particles is called RADIATION. The radiations may be electrically charged particles having size and mass, such as ALPHA PARTICLES and BETA PARTICLES, or they may be nonparticulate and contain no electrical charges, such as GAMMA RAYS. Most radioactive elements give off either alpha or beta particles and at the same time emit gamma radiation.

trace e., a chemical element present or needed in extremely small amount by plants and animals, such as manganese, copper, cobalt, zinc, iron.

transcalifornium e's, chemical elements with atomic numbers higher than 98.

transuranium e's, chemical elements with atomic numbers higher than 92, all of which have been produced artificially on earth by nuclear reactions and synthesis.

ele(o)- (el′e-o) word element [Gr.], *oil.*

eleoma (el″e-o′mah) a tumor caused by injection of oil into the tissues.

eleometer (el″e-om′ĕ-ter) an instrument for measuring the oil in a mixture.

eleopten (el″e-op′ten) the liquid part of a volatile oil.

eleotherapy (el″e-o-ther′ah-pe) therapeutic use of oil.

eleothorax (el″e-o-tho′raks) injection of oil into the pleural cavity.

elephantiasis (el″ĕ-fan-ti′ah-sis) massive subcutaneous edema, with accompanying thickening of the skin, the result of lymphatic obstruction. The disease derives its name from the symptoms, particularly swelling of the legs which makes them look like those of an elephant.

The condition is most often caused by a slender, threadlike parasite, the filarial worm, *Wuchereria bancrofti,* which enters the lymphatic system, causing an obstruction to drainage. The disease, sometimes called FILARIASIS, is transmitted by mosquitoes or flies which carry blood infected with filaria larvae. Elephantiasis is most often encountered in Central Africa, in some Pacific Islands and in other tropical and subtropical areas. It is rare or nonexistent in the temperate zone.

The first visible signs are inflammation of the lymph nodes, with temporary swelling in the affected area, red streaks along the leg or arm, pain and tenderness. Specific drugs are administered for destruction of the parasites; bandages and elevation of the affected area help relieve the swelling. Sanitary control to eliminate the carrier insects is the most effective approach to elimination of this disease.

elephantoid fever (el″ĕ-fan′toid) a recurrent acute febrile condition occurring with filariasis.

elimination (e-lim″ĭ-na′shun) discharge from the

TABLE OF CHEMICAL ELEMENTS

ELEMENT (DATE OF DISCOVERY)	SYMBOL	ATOMIC NUMBER	ATOMIC WEIGHT*	VALENCE	SP. GR. OR DENSITY (GRAMS/LITER)	DESCRIPTIVE COMMENT
Actinium (1899)	Ac	89	[227]	. . . .	10.07	radioactive element associated with uranium
Aluminum (1827)	Al	13	26.9815	3	2.6989	silvery-white metal, abundant in earth's crust, but not in free form
Americium (1944)	Am	95	[243]	3, 4, 5, 6	11.7	fourth transuranium element discovered
Antimony (prehistoric)	Sb	51	121.75	3, 5	6.691	exists in 4 allotropic forms
Argon (1894)	Ar	18	39.948	0?	1.7837 g./l.	colorless, odorless gas
Arsenic (1250)	As	33	74.9216	3, 5	5.73 / 4.73 / 1.97	(gray) semimetallic solid / (black) / (yellow)
Astatine (1940)	At	85	[210]	1, 3, 5, 7		radioactive halogen
Barium (1808)	Ba	56	137.34	2	3.5	silvery-white, alkaline earth metal
Berkelium (1949)	Bk	97	[247]	3, 4		fifth transuranium element discovered
Beryllium (1798)	Be	4	9.0122	2	1.848	light, steel-gray metal
Bismuth (1753)	Bi	83	208.980	3, 5	9.747	pinkish-white, crystalline, brittle metal
Boron (1808)	B	5	10.811	3	2.34, 2.37	crystalline or amorphous element, not occurring free in nature
Bromine (1826)	Br	35	79.909	1, 3, 5, 7	3.12 / 7.59 g./l.	mobile, reddish-brown liquid, volatilizing readily / red vapor with disagreeable odor
Cadmium (1817)	Cd	48	112.40	2	8.65	soft, bluish-white metal
Calcium (1808)	Ca	20	40.08	2	1.55	metallic element, forming more than 3 per cent of earth's crust
Californium (1950)	Cf	98	[249]	. . . .		sixth transuranium element discovered
Carbon (prehistoric)	C	6	12.01115	2, 3, 4	1.8–2.1 / 1.9–2.3 / 3.15–3.53	(amorphous) element widely distributed in nature / (graphite) / (diamond)
Cerium (1803)	Ce	58	140.12	3, 4	6.67–8.23	most abundant rare earth metal
Cesium (1860)	Cs	55	132.905	1	1.873	silvery-white, soft, alkaline metal
Chlorine (1774)	Cl	17	35.453	1, 3, 5, 7	3.214 g./l.	greenish-yellow gas of the halogen group
Chromium (1797)	Cr	24	51.996	2, 3, 6	7.18–7.20	steel-gray, lustrous, hard metal
Cobalt (1735)	Co	27	58.9332	2, 3	8.9	brittle, hard metal
Copper (prehistoric)	Cu	29	63.54	1, 2	8.96	reddish, lustrous, malleable metal
Curium (1944)	Cm	96	[247]	3	7	third transuranium element discovered
Dysprosium (1886)	Dy	66	162.50	3	8.536	rare earth metal with metallic bright silver luster

Element (date)	Symbol	Atomic Number	Atomic Weight	Valence	Sp. Gr. / Density	Description
Einsteinium (1952)	Es	99	[254]	......		seventh transuranium element discovered
Erbium (1843)	Er	68	167.26	3	9.051	soft, malleable rare earth metal
Europium (1896)	Eu	63	151.96	2, 3	5.259	lustrous, silvery-white rare earth metal
Fermium (1953)	Fm	100	[253]	......		eighth transuranium element discovered
Fluorine (1771)	F	9	18.9984	1	1.696 g./l.	pale yellow, corrosive gas of the halogen group
Francium (1939)	Fr	87	[223]	1		product of alpha disintegration of actinium
Gadolinium (1880)	Gd	64	157.25	3	7.8, 7.895	lustrous, silvery-white rare earth metal
Gallium (1875)	Ga	31	69.72	2, 3	5.907	beautiful, silvery-appearing metal
Germanium (1886)	Ge	32	72.59	2, 4	5.323	grayish-white, brittle metal
Gold (prehistoric)	Au	79	196.967	1, 3	19.32	malleable yellow metal
Hafnium (1923)	Hf	72	178.49	4	13.29	gray metal associated with zirconium
Hahnium (1970)	Ha	105	[260]			twelfth transuranium element discovered
Helium (1895)	He	2	4.0026	0	0.177 g./l.	inert gas
Holmium (1879)	Ho	67	164.930	3	8.803	relatively soft and malleable rare earth metal
Hydrogen (1766)	H	1	1.00797	1	0.08988 g./l.; 0.070	(gas) most abundant element in the universe; (liquid)
Indium (1863)	In	49	114.82	1, 2?, 3	7.31	soft, silvery-white metal
Iodine (1811)	I	53	126.9044	1, 3, 5, 7	4.93, 11.27 g./l.	grayish-black, lustrous solid or violet-blue gas
Iridium (1803)	Ir	77	192.2	3, 4	22.42	white, brittle metal of platinum family
Iron (prehistoric)	Fe	26	55.847	2, 3, 4, 6	7.874	fourth most abundant element in earth's crust
Krypton (1898)	Kr	36	83.80	0	3.733 g./l.	inert gas
Lanthanum (1839)	La	57	138.91	3	5.98-6.186	silvery-white, ductile, rare earth metal
Lawrencium (1961)	Lw	103	[257]	......		tenth transuranium element discovered
Lead (prehistoric)	Pb	82	207.19	2, 4	11.35	bluish-white, lustrous, malleable metal
Lithium (1817)	Li	3	6.939	1	0.534	lightest of all metals
Lutetium (1907)	Lu	71	174.97	3	9.872	rare earth metal
Magnesium (1808)	Mg	12	24.312	2	1.738	silvery-white metallic element; eighth in abundance in earth's crust
Manganese (1774)	Mn	25	54.9380	1, 2, 3, 4, 6, 7	7.21-7.44	exists in 4 allotropic forms
Mendelevium (1955)	Md	101	[256]	......		ninth transuranium element discovered
Mercury (prehistoric)	Hg	80	200.59	1, 2	13.546	heavy, silvery-white metal, liquid at ordinary temperatures
Molybdenum (1782)	Mo	42	95.94	2, 3, 4?, 5?, 6	10.22	silvery-white, very hard metal
Neodymium (1885)	Nd	60	144.24	3	6.80, 7.004	exists in 2 allotropic forms
Neon (1898)	Ne	10	20.183	0?	0.89990 g./l.	inert gas
Neptunium (1940)	Np	93	[237]	3, 4, 5, 6	18.0-20.45	first transuranium element discovered
Nickel (1751)	Ni	28	58.71	0, 1, 2, 3	8.902	silvery-white, malleable metal
Niobium (1801)	Nb	41	92.906	2, 3, 4?, 5	8.57	shiny white, soft, ductile metal
Nitrogen (1772)	N	7	14.0067	3, 5	1.2506 g./l.	colorless, odorless, inert element, making up 78 per cent of the air
Nobelium (?) (1958)	No	102	[253]	......		acceptance of this element considered premature
Osmium (1803)	Os	76	190.2	2, 3, 4, 8	22.57	bluish-white, hard metal of platinum family
Oxygen (1774)	O	8	15.9994	2	1.429 g./l.	colorless, odorless gas, third most abundant element in the universe

Table of Chemical Elements (*Continued*)

ELEMENT (DATE OF DISCOVERY)	SYMBOL	ATOMIC NUMBER	ATOMIC WEIGHT*	VALENCE	SP. GR. OR DENSITY (GRAMS/LITER)	DESCRIPTIVE COMMENT
Palladium (1803)	Pd	46	106.4	2, 3, 4	12.02	steel-white metal of the platinum family
Phosphorus (1669)	P	15	30.9738	3, 5	1.82 / 2.20 / 2.25–2.69	(white) waxy solid, transparent when pure / (red) / (black)
Platinum (1735)	Pt	78	195.09	1?, 2, 3, 4	21.45	silvery-white, malleable metal
Plutonium (1940)	Pu	94	[242]	3, 4, 5, 6	19.84	second transuranium element discovered
Polonium (1898)	Po	84	[210]	2, 4, 6	9.32	very rare natural element
Potassium (1807)	K	19	39.102	1	0.862	soft, silvery, alkali metal, seventh in abundance in earth's crust
Praseodymium (1885)	Pr	59	140.907	3, 4	6.782, 6.64	soft, silvery rare earth metal
Promethium (1941)	Pm	61	[147]	3		produced by irradiation of neodymium and praseodymium; identity established in 1945
Protactinium (1917)	Pa	91	[231]	4 or 5	15.37	bright lustrous metal
Radium (1898)	Ra	88	[226]	2	5(?)	brilliant white, radioactive metal
Radon (1900)	Rn	86	[222]	0	9.73 g./l.	heaviest known gas
Rhenium (1925)	Re	75	186.2	−1, 2, 3, 4, 5, 6, 7	21.02	silvery-white lustrous metal
Rhodium (1803)	Rh	45	102.905	−2, 3, 4, 5, 6, 7	12.41	silvery-white metal of platinum family
Rubidium (1861)	Rb	37	85.47	1, 2, 3, 4	1.532	soft, silvery-white, alkali metal
Ruthenium (1844)	Ru	44	101.07	0, 1, 2, 3, 4, 5, 6, 7, 8	12.41	hard white metal of platinum family
Rutherfordium (1969)	Rf	104	[261]			eleventh transuranium element discovered
Samarium (1879)	Sm	62	150.35	2, 3	7.536–7.40	bright silver lustrous metal
Scandium (1879)	Sc	21	44.956	3	2.992	soft, silvery-white metal
Selenium (1817)	Se	34	78.96	2, 4, 6	4.79, 4.28	exists in several allotropic forms
Silicon (1823)	Si	14	28.086	4	2.33	a relatively inert element, second in abundance in earth's crust
Silver (prehistoric)	Ag	47	107.870	1, 2	10.50	malleable, ductile metal with brilliant white luster
Sodium (1807)	Na	11	22.9898	1	0.971	most abundant of alkali metals, sixth in abundance in earth's crust
Strontium (1808)	Sr	38	87.62	2	2.54	exists in 3 allotropic forms
Sulfur (prehistoric)	S	16	32.064	2, 4, 6	1.957, 2.07	exists in several isotopic and many allotropic forms
Tantalum (1802)	Ta	73	180.948	2?, 3, 4?, 5	16.6	gray, heavy, very hard metal
Technetium (1937)	Tc	43	[99]	3?, 4, 6, 7	11.50	first element produced artificially
Tellurium (1782)	Te	52	127.60	2, 4, 6	6.24	silvery-white, lustrous element

Element (date)	Symbol	At. No.	At. Wt.	Valence	Sp. Gr.	Description
Terbium (1843)	Tb	65	158.924	3, 4	8.272	silvery-gray, malleable, ductile rare earth metal
Thallium (1861)	Tl	81	204.37	1, 3	11.85	very soft, malleable metal
Thorium (1828)	Th	90	232.038	4	11.66	silvery-white, lustrous metal
Thulium (1879)	Tm	69	168.934	2, 3		least abundant rare earth metal
Tin (prehistoric)	Sn	50	118.69	2, 4	5.75, 7.31	(gray) malleable metal existing in 2 or 3 allotropic forms, changing from white to gray on cooling and back to white on warming (white)
Titanium (1791)	Ti	22	47.90	2, 3, 4	4.54	lustrous white metal
Tungsten (1783)	W	74	183.85	2, 3, 4, 5, 6	19.3	steel-gray to tin-white metal
Uranium (1789)	U	92	238.03	3, 4, 5, 6	18.95	heavy, silvery-white metal
Vanadium (1801)	V	23	50.942	2, 3, 4, 5	6.11	bright, white metal
Xenon (1898)	Xe	54	131.30	0?	5.887 g./l.	one of the so-called rare or inert gases
Ytterbium (1878)	Yb	70	173.04	2, 3	6.977, 6.54	exists in 2 allotropic forms
Yttrium (1794)	Y	39	88.905	3	4.45	rare earth metal with silvery metallic luster
Zinc (1746)	Zn	30	65.37	2	7.133	bluish-white, lustrous metal, malleable at 100–150° C.
Zirconium (1789)	Zr	40	91.22	4	6.4	grayish-white, lustrous metal

*Figures in brackets represent mass number of most stable isotope.

TABLE OF ELEMENTS BY ATOMIC NUMBERS

1 hydrogen
2 helium
3 lithium
4 beryllium
5 boron
6 carbon
7 nitrogen
8 oxygen
9 fluorine
10 neon
11 sodium
12 magnesium
13 aluminum
14 silicon
15 phosphorus
16 sulfur
17 chlorine
18 argon
19 potassium
20 calcium
21 scandium
22 titanium
23 vanadium
24 chromium
25 manganese
26 iron
27 cobalt
28 nickel
29 copper
30 zinc
31 gallium
32 germanium
33 arsenic
34 selenium
35 bromine
36 krypton
37 rubidium
38 strontium
39 yttrium
40 zirconium
41 niobium
42 molybdenum
43 technetium
44 ruthenium
45 rhodium
46 palladium
47 silver
48 cadmium
49 indium
50 tin
51 antimony
52 tellurium
53 iodine
54 xenon
55 cesium
56 barium
57 lanthanum
58 cerium
59 praseodymium
60 neodymium
61 promethium
62 samarium
63 europium
64 gadolinium
65 terbium
66 dysprosium
67 holmium
68 erbium
69 thulium
70 ytterbium
71 lutetium
72 hafnium
73 tantalum
74 tungsten
75 rhenium
76 osmium
77 iridium
78 platinum
79 gold
80 mercury
81 thallium
82 lead
83 bismuth
84 polonium
85 astatine
86 radon
87 francium
88 radium
89 actinium
90 thorium
91 protactinium
92 uranium
93 neptunium
94 plutonium
95 americium
96 curium
97 berkelium
98 californium
99 einsteinium
100 fermium
101 mendelevium
102 [see nobelium]
103 lawrencium
104 rutherfordium
105 hahnium

body of indigestible materials and of waste products of body metabolism.

e. diet, one for diagnosing food allergy, based on omission of foods that might cause symptoms in the patient.

Elipten (e-lip'ten) trademark for a preparation of aminoglutethimide, an anticonvulsant.

elix. elixir.

elixir (e-lik'ser) a clear, sweetened, hydroalcoholic liquid for oral use.

Elkosin (el'ko-sin) trademark for preparations of sulfisomidine, a sulfonamide.

elliptocyte (e-lip'to-sīt) an elliptical erythrocyte.

elliptocytosis (e-lip"to-si-to'sis) a hereditary disorder in which the erythrocytes are largely elliptical and which is characterized by increased red cell destruction and anemia.

Elorine (el'o-rēn) trademark for a preparation of tricyclamol, an anticholinergic.

elution (e-loo'shun) separation of substances by extraction with a solvent.

elutriation (e-loo"tre-a'shun) purification of a substance by dissolving it in a solvent and pouring off the solution, thus separating it from the undissolved foreign material.

Em. emmetropia.

emaciation (e-ma"se-a'shun) a wasted, lean appearance due to extreme weight loss.

emailloid (e-ma'loid) a tumor developing from tooth enamel.

emanation (em"ah-na'shun) that which is given off, such as a gaseous disintegration product given off from radioactive substances.

radium e., radon.

emanotherapy (em"ah-no-ther'ah-pe) treatment by means of emanations, such as radium emanation, or radon.

emasculation (e-mas"ku-la'shun) removal of the penis or testes.

embalming (em-bahm'ing) treatment of a dead body to retard decomposition.

embedding (em-bed'ing) fixation of tissue in a firm medium before cutting microscopic sections.

embolalia (em"bo-la'le-ah) insertion of meaningless words in a spoken sentence.

embolectomy (em"bo-lek'to-me) removal of an embolus through an incision in the blood vessel wall.

embolic (em-bol'ik) pertaining to embolism or an embolus.

embolism (em'bo-lizm) the transfer of a mass or object within the vascular system from its point of origin or entrance to a distant site, causing obstruction to the flow of blood. The obstructing material (embolus) is most often a blood clot, but may be a fat globule, air bubble, piece of tissue or clump of bacteria.

SYMPTOMS. The symptoms of an embolism usually do not appear until the embolus lodges within a blood vessel and suddenly obstructs the blood flow. Emboli usually lodge at divisions of an artery where the vessel narrows. The signs of obstruction appear almost immediately with severe pain at the site. If the embolus lodges in an extremity the area becomes pale, numb and cold to the touch. Fainting, nausea and vomiting and eventually severe shock may occur. Unless the obstruction is relieved, gangrene of the adjacent tissues served by the affected vessel develops.

TREATMENT. Whenever possible the embolism is treated medically with vasodilating drugs and applications of warmth to improve collateral circulation and to dilate the blood vessels. Surgical treatment of an embolism consists of an embolectomy in which the affected blood vessel is incised and the embolus removed. When this is difficult, sympathectomy may be beneficial.

NURSING CARE. Since an embolus often arises from a thrombus that has broken away from a vessel wall and entered the general circulation, it is extremely important to use care in moving postoperative patients or those confined to bed over a long period of time. Although frequent changing of position and early ambulation are necessary to the prevention of thrombosis, sudden and extreme movements should be avoided. Under no circumstances should the legs be massaged to relieve "muscle cramps," especially when the pain is located in the calf and the patient has not been up and about; pain in the calf may be symptomatic of a thrombosis.

The introduction of air into the blood vessels or tissues can occur through careless handling of equipment being used for intravenous therapy or when air bubbles in syringes are not eliminated before parenteral injections.

cerebral e., embolism of a cerebral artery, one of the three main causes of CEREBRAL VASCULAR ACCIDENT (stroke).

pulmonary e., obstruction of the pulmonary artery or one of its branches by an embolus. The embolus usually is a blood clot swept into circulation from a large peripheral vein—particularly one in the leg or pelvis. Plugging of a large pulmonary vessel can cause sudden death. Symptoms include sudden onset of chest pain, a cough productive of bright red sputum, tachycardia and rapid, shallow respirations. Treatment usually consists of administration of oxygen, morphine sulfate to relieve pain and anticoagulant drugs to aid in removal of the clot.

embolophrasia (em"bo-lo-fra'ze-ah) insertion of meaningless phrases in a spoken sentence.

embolus (em'bo-lus), pl. *em'boli* [Gr.] a mass of undissolved material, usually part or all of a thrombus, carried in the bloodstream and frequently causing obstruction of a vessel (EMBOLISM).

saddle e., one situated astride the bifurcation of a large artery, sometimes blocking both branches.

embrocation (em"bro-ka'shun) a liniment or medicine for external application.

embryectomy (em"bre-ek'to-me) excision of an extrauterine embryo or fetus.

embryo (em'bre-o) a new organism in the earliest stage of development; the human young from the time of fertilization of the ovum until the beginning of the third month. After the second month the unborn baby is usually referred to as the fetus. adj., **embry'onal, embryon'ic.**

Immediately after fertilization takes place cell division begins and progresses at a rapid rate. At approximately 4 weeks the cell mass becomes a recognizable embryo from 7 to 10 mm. long with rudimentary organs. The beginnings of the eyes, ears and extremities can be seen. By the end of the second month the embryo has grown to a length of 2 to 2.5 cm., and the head is the most prominent part because of the rapid development of the brain; the sex can be distinguished at this stage.

At the time of fertilization the ovum contains the potential beginnings of a human being. As cell division takes place the cells of the blastoderm (embryonic disk) gradually form three layers from which all the body structures develop. The ectoderm (outer layer) gives rise to the epidermis of the skin and its appendages, and to the nervous system. The mesoderm (middle layer) develops into muscle, connective tissue, the circulatory organs, circulating lymph and blood cells, endothelial tissues within the closed vessels and cavities and the epithelium portion of the urogenital system. From the entoderm (internal layer) are derived those portions not arising from the ectoderm, the liver, pancreas and the lungs.

embryocardia (em″bre-o-kar′de-ah) a state in which the heart tones resemble the tic-tac ones of fetal life, indicating severe heart disease.

embryoctony (em″bre-ok′to-ne) destruction of the fetus in utero.

embryography (em″bre-og′rah-fe) description of the embryo.

embryology (em″bre-ol′o-je) the science of the development of embryos. adj., **embryolog′ic.**

embryoma (em″bre-o′mah) a tumor containing embryonic elements.

embryonization (em-bre″o-nĭ-za′shun) return of a tissue to embryonic form.

embryonoid (em′bre-ŏ-noid″) resembling an embryo.

embryopathy (em″bre-op′ah-the) disordered embryonic development with consequent congenital anomalies.

rubella e., congenital deformities in an infant due to rubella (German measles) in the mother during early pregnancy.

embryoplastic (em′bre-o-plas″tik) pertaining to formation of an embryo.

embryotocia (em″bre-o-to′se-ah) abortion.

embryotomy (em″bre-ot′o-me) dismemberment of the fetus in difficult labor in which a normal delivery is impossible.

embryotoxon (em″bre-o-tok′son) congenital opacity of the margin of the cornea.

embryotroph (em′bre-o-trōf″) the nutritive material utilized by the early embryo.

embryotrophy (em″bre-ot′ro-fe) nourishment of the early embryo.

embryulcus (em″bre-ul′kus) a hooked instrument for extracting a dead fetus from the uterus.

emedullate (e-med′u-lāt) to deprive of marrow.

emergent (e-mer′jent) 1. coming out from a cavity or other part. 2. coming on suddenly.

emesis (em′ĕ-sis) the act of vomiting.

emetic (e-met′ik) 1. causing vomiting. 2. an agent that causes vomiting. A strong solution of salt (1 tablespoon to 1 cup of water), mustard water (1 tablespoon to 1 cup of water) and powdered ipecac or ipecac syrup are examples of emetics.

Emetics should not be used when lye or other strong alkalis or acids have been swallowed, since vomiting may rupture the already weakened walls of the esophagus. Among the acids and alkalis for which emetics should not be used are sodium hydroxide (caustic soda), potassium hydroxide (caustic potash) and carbolic acid. Emetics should be avoided also when kerosene, gasoline, nail polish remover or lacquer thinner has been swallowed, since vomiting of these substances may draw them into the lungs.

tartar e., antimony potassium tartrate, used in parasitic infections.

emetine (em′ĕ-tēn) an alkaloid derived from ipecac or produced synthetically.

e. hydrochloride, a white or slightly yellowish crystalline compound used in the treatment of amebiasis.

emetocathartic (em″ĕ-to-kah-thar′tik) both emetic and cathartic.

E.M.F. electromotive force.

-emia (e′me-ah) word element [Gr.], *condition of the blood.*

eminence (em′ĭ-nens) a projection or prominence.

eminentia (em″ĭ-nen′she-ah), pl. *eminen′tiae* [L.] eminence.

emissary (em′ĭ-sār″e) affording an outlet, as the veins exiting from the skull to drain blood from the venous sinuses of the dura mater.

emission (e-mish′un) discharge, especially of semen.

nocturnal e., involuntary discharge of semen during sleep.

Emivan (em′ĭ-van) trademark for preparations of ethamivan, a respiratory stimulant.

emmenagogue (ĕ-men′ah-gog) 1. promoting menstruation. 2. a drug that promotes the menstrual flow.

emmenia (ĕ-me′ne-ah) menstruation. adj., **emmen′ic.**

emmenology (em″ĕ-nol′o-je) sum of what is known about menstruation.

emmetrope (em′ĕ-trōp) a person with normal vision.

emmetropia (em″ĕ-tro′pe-ah) the ideal optical condition, parallel rays coming to a focus on the retina. adj., **emmetrop′ic.**

emollient (e-mol′yent) 1. soothing and softening, as an emollient bath given for various skin disorders. 2. a soothing medication, administered to reduce itching and pain, thereby promoting healing.

emotion (e-mo′shun) a feeling or state of mental

excitement that is usually accompanied by physical changes in the body. adj., **emotional**. The physical form of emotion may be outward and evident to others, as in crying, laughing, blushing or a variety of facial expressions. However, emotion is not always reflected in one's appearance and actions even though psychic changes are taking place. Joy, grief, fear and anger are examples of emotions.

empathize (em'pah-thīz) to comprehend intellectually the feelings of another.

empathy (em'pah-the) intellectual understanding of something in another person which is foreign to one's self. adj., **empath'ic**.

emphlysis (em'flĭ-sis) a vesicular eruption.

emphractic (em-frak'tik) 1. clogging or obstructive. 2. an agent that closes the pores of the skin.

emphysema (em″fĭ-se'mah, em″fĭ-ze'mah) abnormal presence of air or gas in body tissues. The term is generally used to designate chronic pulmonary emphysema, a lung disorder in which the terminal bronchioles become plugged with mucus. Eventually there is a loss of elasticity in the lung tissue too so that inspired air becomes trapped in the lungs, making breathing difficult, especially during the expiratory phase.

bullous e., emphysema in which bullae form in areas of lung tissue so that these areas do not contribute to respiration.

chronic pulmonary e., emphysema of the lungs that develops slowly over a period of years and in some persons may gradually lead to serious disability. It is found most frequently in men over 40.

In many cases, it occurs as a result of prolonged respiratory difficulties, such as chronic bronchial ASTHMA, BRONCHITIS or TUBERCULOSIS, that have caused partial obstruction of the smaller divisions of the bronchi.

Chronic emphysema may also occur without serious preceding respiratory problems. Some authorities suggest that a defect in the elastic tissue of the lungs may make certain persons susceptible to the disease. It is found with some frequency in aged persons whose lungs have lost their natural elasticity.

Chronic emphysema of the lungs kills over 10,000 Americans a year, and the number of deaths has been increasing sharply. The reasons for this are not fully known. As with other respiratory ailments, however, one factor may be the increasing pollution of the air that accompanies urbanization, industrialization and the growing number of automobiles. Another reason may be the increase in tobacco smoking. Although there is no proof that smoking actually causes emphysema, there is a higher proportion of smokers who inhale or smoke heavily among emphysema sufferers than among the general population. It is known that the continuance of smoking seriously aggravates the disease.

SYMPTOMS AND TREATMENT. As the lungs become less efficient, breathing becomes more difficult for chronic emphysema sufferers. There is often a persistent cough that is moist and wheezing in nature. The patient often develops a barrel-shaped chest and has an anxious facial expression. Cardiac complications, especially enlargement and dilatation of the right ventricle with resultant right heart failure, may develop from pulmonary emphysema.

Treatment is aimed at correction of the deficiency in pulmonary ventilation as much as possible. Bronchodilators are administered to enlarge the bronchioles and provide an adequate airway. Expectorants and liquefying agents are given to aid in the removal of mucus and other materials obstructing the bronchioles. POSTURAL DRAINAGE may also be prescribed to clear the bronchial passages by inducing the gravitational flow of sputum. Special breathing exercises and the use of a respirator that employs the principle of intermittent positive pressure breathing (IPPB) are helpful in increasing the volume of air the patient is able to exhale. Antibiotics and corticosteroids may be helpful.

familial e., emphysema occurring in different members of a family and considered to be due to a familial predisposition to the disease.

interlobular e., air between the lobes of the lung.

interstitial e., pulmonary emphysema due to destruction of the walls of the alveoli.

interstitial e., spontaneous, presence of air in the interstitial tissues of the lungs after spontaneous rupture of the alveoli.

intestinal e., a condition marked by accumulation of gas under the tunica serosa of the intestine.

lobar e., emphysema involving less than all the lobes of the affected lung.

lobar e., infantile, a condition characterized by overinflation, commonly affecting one of the upper lobes and causing respiratory distress in early life, usually necessitating lobectomy; called also congenital lobar emphysema.

subcutaneous e., air or gas in the connective tissues under the skin.

surgical e., subcutaneous emphysema following operation.

unilateral e., a condition in which an entire lung is overinflated and does not empty on expiration.

vesicular e., pulmonary emphysema due to dilatation of the alveoli.

emphysematous (em″fĭ-sem'ah-tus) of the nature of or affected with emphysema.

empiricism (em-pir'ĭ-sizm) skill or knowledge from mere experience. adj., **empir'ic**.

Empirin (em'pĭ-rin) trademark for tablets containing acetylsalicylic acid, acetophenetidin and caffeine, used as an analgesic. One form of Empirin contains codeine and requires a prescription.

emporiatrics (em-po″re-at'riks) that branch of medicine particularly concerned with health problems of travelers about the world.

emprosthotonos (em″pros-thot'o-nos) tetanic forward flexure of the body.

emptysis (emp-ti'sis) expectoration, especially of blood.

empyema (em″pi-e'mah) the presence of pus in a body cavity, particularly the presence of a purulent exudate within the pleural cavity (pyothorax). It occurs as an occasional complication of pleurisy or some other respiratory disease. Symptoms include dyspnea, coughing, chest pain on one side, malaise and fever. Thoracentesis may be done to confirm the diagnosis and determine the specific causative organism. The condition is treated with antibiotics, rest and sedative cough mixtures.

empyesis (em″pi-e'sis) a pustular eruption.

empyocele (em-pi′o-sēl) a purulent tumor of the scrotum.

emul. emulsion.

emulgent (e-mul′jent) draining out.

emulsifier (e-mul″sĭ-fi′er) a substance used to make an emulsion.

emulsion (e-mul′shun) a liquid that contains droplets of another liquid with which it will not mix and in which it will not dissolve. An emulsion is an example of a colloid system in which both phases are liquid. Margarine, cold cream and various medicated ointments are emulsions. In some emulsions the suspended particles tend to join together and settle out; hence the container must be shaken each time the emulsion is used.

emulsoid (e-mul′soid) a colloid system in which there is a mutual attraction between the two phases.

emulsum (e-mul′sum) [L.] emulsion.

emunctory (e-mungk′to-re) 1. excretory or cleansing. 2. an excretory organ.

emylcamate (e-mil′kah-māt) a compound used as a tranquilizer.

enamel (e-nam′el) the calcified tissue of ectodermal origin covering the crown of a tooth.

mottled e., defective enamel, with a chalky white appearance or brownish stain, caused by excessive amounts of fluorine in drinking water during the period of enamel calcification.

e. organ, a process of epithelium forming a cap over a dental papilla and developing into the enamel.

enanthem (en-an′them) an eruption upon a mucous surface. adj., **enanthem′atous.**

enanthesis (en″an-the′sis) a skin eruption from an internal disease.

enanthrope (en′an-thrōp) a source of disease within the body.

enantiomorph (en-an′te-o-morf″) one of a pair of isomeric substances, the molecular structures of which are mirror opposites of each other.

enantiopathy (en-an″te-op′ah-the) 1. any disease antagonistic to another. 2. the curing of one disease by inducing an antagonistic disease.

enarthritis (en″ar-thri′tis) inflammation of an enarthrosis.

enarthrosis (en″ar-thro′sis) a joint in which the rounded head of one bone fits in a cuplike depression in another, permitting motion in any direction; called also ball-and-socket joint.

encapsulation (en-kap″su-la′shun) enclosure within a capsule.

encelialgia (en″se-le-al′je-ah) pain in an abdominal organ.

encephal(o)- (en-sef′ah-lo) word element [Gr.], *brain.*

encephalalgia (en″sef-ah-lal′je-ah) cephalalgia; pain in the head; headache.

encephalasthenia (en″sef-al-as-the′ne-ah) lack of brain power.

encephalatrophy (en″sef-ah-lat′ro-fe) atrophy of the brain.

encephalic (en″sĕ-fal′ik) pertaining to the brain.

encephalin (en-sef′ah-lin) a nitrogenous glycoside said to be obtained from the brain.

encephalitis (en″sef-ah-li′tis) inflammation of the brain and its coverings (the meninges), producing persistent drowsiness, delirium and, rarely, coma. adj., **encephalit′ic.**

There are several different forms of encephalitis, a few of which are occasionally epidemic in limited areas of the United States. The epidemic forms are caused by a virus transmitted to man by the bite of mosquitoes and ticks. The condition can also occur as a rare complication of some other virus disease, and it is occasionally produced by contact with a toxic substance, such as lead.

Encephalitis is known also as sleeping sickness. There are no specific drugs for this condition. Treatment and nursing care are aimed at relief of symptoms and prevention of complications.

acute disseminated e., postinfection encephalitis.

cortical e., inflammation involving only the cortex of the brain.

Economo's e., epidemic e., a viral disease of obscure pathology, occurring epidemically.

equine e., equine encephalomyelitis.

hemorrhagic e., e. hemorrha′gica, inflammation of the brain with hemorrhagic exudate.

herpes e., a viral disease resembling equine encephalomyelitis.

e. hyperplas′tica, acute nonsuppurating encephalitis.

infantile e., inflammation of the brain in children following infections, injury, etc., and causing the cerebral palsies of children.

Japanese B e., a form of epidemic encephalitis of varying severity occurring in Japan and other Pacific islands, China, Manchuria, U.S.S.R. and probably much of the Far East.

lead e., encephalitis with cerebral edema due to lead poisoning.

lethargic e., a form of epidemic encephalitis characterized by increasing languor, apathy and drowsiness.

e. neonato′rum, encephalitis of the newborn.

e. periaxia′lis, massive inflammation of the white matter of the cerebral hemispheres, beginning in the occipital lobes and characterized by early disappearance of the myelin; the disease occurs mostly in children and young subjects and begins with blindness.

postinfection e., an acute disease of the central nervous system seen in patients convalescing from infectious diseases.

postvaccinal e., acute encephalitis sometimes occurring after vaccination.

Russian spring-summer e., a form of epidemic encephalitis acquired in forests from infected ticks, but also transmitted in other ways, as by ingestion of the flesh of infected mammals or birds, or milk of infected goats. It ranges in severity from mild to fatal cases, with degenerative changes in organs other than those of the nervous system.

St. Louis e., a viral disease observed first in 1932 in Illinois. It occurs during the late summer and early fall, and is similar to western equine encephalomyelitis.

encephalocele (en-sef′ah-lo-sēl″) local herniation of neural tissue through a defect in the skull.

encephalocystocele (en-sef"ah-lo-sis'to-sēl) hernial protrusion of the brain distended by fluid.

encephalodialysis (en-sef"ah-lo-di-al'ĭ-sis) softening of the brain.

encephalogram (en-sef'ah-lo-gram") the film obtained by encephalography.

encephalography (en-sef"ah-log'rah-fe) radiography of the brain.

encephaloid (en-sef'ah-loid) 1. resembling the brain or brain substance. 2. encephaloma.

encephalolith (en-sef'ah-lo-lith") a brain calculus.

encephalology (en-sef"ah-lol'o-je) scientific study of the encephalon.

encephaloma (en-sef"ah-lo'mah) encephaloid cancer; a malignant growth of brainlike texture.

encephalomalacia (en-sef"ah-lo-mah-la'she-ah) abnormal softening of the brain.

encephalomeningitis (en-sef"ah-lo-men"in-ji'-tis) meningoencephalitis; inflammation of the brain and its membranes.

encephalomeningocele (en-sef"ah-lo-mě-ning'-go-sěl) protrusion of the brain and meninges through the skull.

encephalomeningopathy (en-sef"ah-lo-men"in-gop'ah-the) disease involving the brain and meninges.

encephalomere (en-sef'ah-lo-mēr") one of the segments making up the embryonic brain.

encephalometer (en"sef-ah-lom'ě-ter) an instrument for measuring the skull.

encephalomyelitis (en-sef"ah-lo-mi"ě-li'tis) inflammation of the brain and spinal cord.
    acute disseminated e., postinfection encephalitis.
    benign myalgic e., a disease, usually occurring in epidemics, characterized by headache, fever, myalgia, muscular weakness and emotional lability.
    equine e., eastern, a viral disease similar to western equine encephalomyelitis, but occurring principally in the Atlantic and Gulf Coast states.
    equine e., Venezuelan, a viral disease of horses and mules; the infection in man resembles influenza, with little or no indication of nervous system involvement.
    equine e., western, a viral disease of horses and mules, communicable to man, occurring chiefly as a meningoencephalitis, with little involvement of the medulla oblongata or spinal cords; observed in the United States chiefly west of the Mississippi River.
    granulomatous e., a disease marked by granulomas and necrosis of the walls of the cerebral and spinal ventricles.
    postvaccinal e., inflammation of the brain and spinal cord following vaccination or infection with vaccinia virus.

encephalomyeloneuropathy (en-sef"ah-lo-mi"-ě-lo-nu-rop'ah-the) disease involving the brain, spinal cord and nerves.

encephalomyelopathy (en-sef"ah-lo-mi"ě-lop'ah-the) disease involving the brain and spinal cord.

encephalomyeloradiculitis (en-sef"ah-lo-mi"ě-lo-rah-dik"u-li'tis) inflammation of the brain, spinal cord and spinal nerve roots.

encephalomyeloradiculopathy (en-sef"ah-lo-mi"ě-lo-rah-dik"u-lop'ah-the) disease involving the brain, spinal cord and spinal nerve roots.

encephalomyocarditis (en-sef"ah-lo-mi"o-kar-di'-tis) a disease of virus origin, characterized by lesions in the central nervous system and by degenerative and inflammatory changes in skeletal and cardiac muscle.

encephalon (en-sef'ah-lon) the brain; with the spinal cord (medulla spinalis) constituting the central nervous system.

encephalopathy (en-sef"ah-lop'ah-the) any disorder of the brain.
    boxer's e., a syndrome of prize fighters due to cumulative punishment absorbed in the boxing ring, characterized by slowing of mental functions, bouts of confusion and scattered memory loss.
    lead e., brain disease caused by lead poisoning.
    progressive subcortical e., a familial disease of unknown origin, characterized by headache, dysphasia, weakness of the arms and legs and visual failure progressing to blindness.

encephalopuncture (en-sef"ah-lo-pungk'tūr) puncture into the brain substance.

encephalopyosis (en-sef"ah-lo-pi-o'sis) a purulent condition in the brain.

encephalorrhagia (en-sef"ah-lo-ra'je-ah) cerebral hemorrhage.

encephalosclerosis (en-sef"ah-lo-sklě-ro'sis) hardening of the brain.

encephalosis (en"sef-ah-lo'sis) any organic brain disease.

encephalotomy (en"sef-ah-lot'o-me) incision of the fetal head in difficult labor.

enchondroma (en"kon-dro'mah) a hyperplastic growth of cartilaginous tissue remaining in the interior of a cartilage or bone.

enchondromatosis (en-kon"dro-mah-to'sis) a condition characterized by hamartomatous proliferation of cartilage cells within the metaphysis of several bones, causing thinning of the overlying cortex and distortion of the growth in length.

enchondrosarcoma (en-kon"dro-sar-ko'mah) sarcoma containing cartilaginous tissue.

enchondrosis (en"kon-dro'sis) hyperplastic growth within a cartilage or bone.

enchylema (en"ki-le'mah) the more fluid, finely granular substance of the cytoplasm of cells, called also hyaloplasm.

enclave (en'klāv) tissue detached from its normal connection and enclosed within another organ.

enclitic (en-klit'ik) having the planes of the fetal head inclined to those of the maternal pelvis.

encopresis (en"ko-pre'sis) incontinence of feces not due to organic defect or illness.

encranial (en-kra'ne-al) situated within the cranium.

encyesis (en″si-e′sis) normal uterine pregnancy.

encyst (en-sist′) to enclose in a sac or cyst.

end(o)- (en′do) word element [Gr.], *within; inward.*

endadelphos (end″ah-del′fos) a monster fetus in which a parasitic twin is enclosed within the body of another.

Endamoeba (en″dah-me′bah) a genus of amebas parasitic in the intestines of invertebrates, distinguishable from Entamoeba by the characteristics of the nucleus.

endangium (en-dan′je-um) the membrane that lines blood vessels.

endaortitis (en″da-or-ti′tis) inflammation of the membrane lining the aorta.
    bacterial e., the presence of bacterial vegetations on the endothelial surface of the aorta.

endarterectomy (en″dar-ter-ek′to-me) excision of thickened areas of the innermost coat of an artery.

endarteritis (en″dar-ter-i′tis) inflammation of the innermost coat of an artery.
    e. oblit′erans, a form in which the lumen of the vessel becomes obliterated.

endarteropathy (en″dar-ter-op′ah-the) noninflammatory disorder of the innermost coat of an artery.

end-artery (end-ar′ter-e) an artery that does not anastomose with other arteries.

end-brain (end′brān) telencephalon.

end-bud (end′bud) 1. an ovoid or spheroid body located at the termination of a nerve fiber, and dispersed in skin, mucous membranes, muscles, joints and connective tissue of the internal organs. 2. tail bud.

end-bulb (end′bulb) end-bud (1).

endemic (en-dem′ik) 1. present in a community at all times, but occurring in only small numbers of cases. 2. a disease of low morbidity that is constantly present in a human community.

endemiology (en-de″me-ol′o-je) the science dealing with all the factors relating to occurrence of endemic disease.

endemoepidemic (en″de-mo-ep″ĭ-dem′ik) endemic, but occasionally becoming epidemic.

endergonic (en″der-gon′ik) characterized or accompanied by the absorption of energy; requiring the input of free energy.

endermic (en-der′mik) administered through the skin.

endermosis (en″der-mo′sis) 1. administration of medicines by absorption through the skin. 2. herpetic affection of mucous membranes.

enderon (en′der-on) the deeper part of the skin or mucous membrane.

endoaneurysmorrhaphy (en″do-an″u-riz-mor′-ah-fe) opening of an aneurysmal sac and suture of the orifices.

endoangiitis (en″do-an″je-i′tis) inflammation of the intima of blood vessels.

endoantitoxin (en″do-an″tĭ-tok′sin) an antitoxin contained within a cell.

endoappendicitis (en″do-ah-pen″dĭ-si′tis) inflammation of mucous membrane of the vermiform appendix.

endoarteritis (en″do-ar″ter-i′tis) endarteritis.

endoblast (en′do-blast) the cell nucleus.

endobronchitis (en″do-brong-ki′tis) inflammation of the lining membrane of the bronchi.

endocardial (en″do-kar′de-al) 1. situated or occurring within the heart. 2. pertaining to the endocardium.

endocarditis (en″do-kar-di′tis) inflammation of the inner lining of the heart, usually involving the heart valves. Bacterial endocarditis is an acute or subacute, febrile, systemic disease characterized by bacterial infection of the heart valves or irregular areas on the endocardium, with formation of bacteria-laden vegetations on these areas. Intensive chemotherapy with antibiotic drugs has done much to reduce the seriousness of this disease.
    acute bacterial e., a rapidly progressing endocarditis that usually is a part of an acute septicemia due to a variety of bacteria.
    rheumatic e., cardiac involvement in rheumatic fever.
    subacute bacterial e., a protracted form of endocarditis caused by various bacteria, usually in association with *Streptococcus viridans.*
    syphilitic e., endocarditis resulting from extension of syphilitic infection from the aorta.
    vegetative e., verrucous e., nonbacterial endocarditis with formation of shreds of fibrin on the ulcerated valves; frequently found in cases of systemic lupus erythematosus.

endocardium (en″do-kar′de-um) the membrane lining the chambers of the heart and covering the cusps of the various valves.

endocervicitis (en″do-ser″vĭ-si′tis) inflammation of the mucous membrane of the cervix uteri.

endocervix (en″do-ser′viks) 1. the mucous membrane lining the canal of the cervix uteri. 2. the region of the opening of the cervix uteri into the uterine cavity.

endochondral (en″do-kon′dral) situated, formed or occurring within cartilage.

endochorion (en″do-ko′re-on) the inner chorionic layer.

endochrome (en′do-krōm) the coloring matter within a cell.

endocolitis (en″do-ko-li′tis) inflammation of the mucous membrane of the colon.

endocolpitis (en″do-kol-pi′tis) inflammation of vaginal mucous membrane.

endocomplement (en″do-kom′plĕ-ment) a complement contained within the erythrocyte as distinguished from that contained in the serum.

endocorpuscular (en″do-kor-pus′ku-lar) contained within a corpuscle.

endocranial (en″do-kra′ne-al) within the cranium.

endocranitis (en″do-kra-ni′tis) inflammation of endocranium.

endocranium (en″do-kra′ne-um) the dura mater lining the cranium.

endocrine (en′do-krin) 1. secreting internally. 2. pertaining to internal secretions.

  e. glands, glands that regulate body activity by special secretions, the hormones, which are delivered directly into the blood. Each of the glands within the endocrine system has one or more specific functions, but they all are dependent upon the other glands in the system for maintenance of a normal hormonal balance in the body.

  The PITUITARY GLAND (hypophysis cerebri), which is about the size of a pea, lies at the base of the brain and is called the master gland because it regulates the functions of other endocrine glands. It also has some vital functions of its own, such as controlling the body's growth through the growth hormone (somatotropin).

  Some pituitary hormones that directly affect other glands in the endocrine system are: thyro-tropic hormone (thyroid-stimulating hormone, TSH), which stimulates the thyroid gland; adreno-corticotropic hormone (ACTH), which affects the cortex of the adrenal gland; and the gonadotropic hormones (FSH, LH and LTH), which have a role in the development and proper functioning of the gonads.

  The THYROID GLAND is situated in the neck, its two lateral lobes lying on either side of the larynx. It secretes the hormone thyroxine, which controls the metabolic rate. The PARATHYROID GLANDS are located behind the thyroid and are embedded in its capsule. There are two pairs of parathyroid glands; their secretion, parathyroid hormone, regulates the blood calcium and phosphorus levels.

  Small groups of specialized cells, scattered throughout the pancreas, are known as the islands of Langerhans. They secrete the hormone insulin, which is necessary for proper utilization of carbohydrates.

  The ADRENAL GLANDS, one atop each kidney, are each two glands in one, being made up of two parts, the cortex and medulla, with separate hormonal secretions. There are at least 26 hormones produced by the adrenal glands, including epinephrine,

FUNCTIONS OF ENDOCRINE GLANDS

GLAND	HORMONE	ACTION OF HORMONE
PITUITARY		
Anterior lobe	Thyrotropic hormone	Stimulates thyroid gland
	Somatotropic hormone	Stimulates growth
	Gonadotropic hormones (LH, FSH, LTH)	Affect growth, maturity and functioning of primary and secondary sex organs
	Adrenocorticotropic hormone (ACTH)	Stimulates cortex of adrenal glands
Posterior lobe	Antidiuretic hormone	Decreases production of urine
	Oxytocic principle	Stimulates uterine contractions
THYROID	Thyroxine Triiodothyronine	Stimulates metabolism (catabolic phase)
PARATHYROID	Parathyroid hormone	Regulates blood calcium level
ADRENAL		
Cortex	Hormones divided into three main groups:	
	Glucocorticoids	Tend to increase amount of sugar in blood
	Mineralocorticoids	Tend to increase amount of blood sodium and decrease amount of potassium in blood
	Androgens (male hormones)	Govern certain secondary sex characteristics All corticoids important for defense against stress or injury to body tissues
Medulla	Epinephrine (Adrenaline); "fight or flight" hormone	Elevates blood pressure; converts glycogen to glucose when needed by muscles for energy; increases heartbeat rate; dilates bronchioles
OVARIES	Estrone and progesterone	Stimulate development of secondary sex characteristics Effect repair of endometrium after menstruation
TESTES	Testosterone	Essential for normal functioning of male reproductive organs Stimulates development of male secondary sex characteristics
ISLANDS OF LANGERHANS OF PANCREAS	Insulin	Promotes metabolism of carbohydrates

From Keane, C. B.: Saunders Review for Practical Nurses. Philadelphia, W. B. Saunders Co., 1966.

corticosterone and aldosterone. They are vital to the protection of the body during stress and danger, and to the adaptation of the body to changes in its environment.

The GONADS, or sex glands, consist of the TESTES in the male and the OVARIES in the female. Besides producing sperm and ova, respectively, they manufacture the androgens and estrogens, hormones responsible for the special characteristics of the male and female, respectively.

The PINEAL GLAND and the THYMUS are also sometimes included as endocrine glands, although the exact function of each is unknown.

endocrinism (en-dok'rĭ-nizm) endocrinopathy.

endocrinology (en″do-krĭ-nol'o-je) study of the glands of internal secretion.

endocrinopathy (en″do-krĭ-nop'ah-the) a disorder of the internal secretions.

endocrinosis (en″do-krĭ-no'sis) dysfunction of an endocrine gland.

endocrinotherapy (en″do-kri″no-ther'ah-pe) treatment of disease by the administration of endocrine preparations.

endocrinotropic (en″do-kri-no-trop'ik) having an affinity for the endocrine glands.

endocrinous, endocritic (en-dok'rĭ-nus), (en″do-krit'ik) pertaining to internal secretions.

endocystitis (en″do-sis-ti'tis) inflammation of the bladder mucosa.

endoderm (en'do-derm) entoderm.

Endodermophyton (en″do-der-mof'ĭ-ton) the former name of a genus of fungi causing skin infections; now called Trichophyton.

endodontics (en″do-don'tiks) the branch of dentistry concerned with the etiology, prevention, diagnosis and treatment of conditions that affect the dental pulp and apical periodontal tissues.

endodontitis (en″do-don-ti'tis) inflammation of the dental pulp.

endodontium (en″do-don'she-um) dental pulp.

endoenteritis (en″do-en″tĕ-ri'tis) inflammation of the intestinal mucosa.

endoenzyme (en″do-en'zīm) an intracellular enzyme; an enzyme that is retained in a cell and does not normally diffuse out of the cell into the surrounding medium.

endogain (en'do-gān) the primary gain of emotional illness, which operates on a deeply unconscious level in its initiation.

endogamy (en-dog'ah-me) 1. fertilization by union of separate cells having the same chromatin ancestry. 2. restriction of marriage to persons within the same community. adj., **endog'amous.**

endogastrectomy (en″do-gas-trek'to-me) excision of the gastric mucosa.

endogastritis (en″do-gas-tri'tis) inflammation of the gastric mucosa.

endogenous (en-doj'ĕ-nus) produced within or caused by factors within the organism.

endoglobular (en″do-glob'u-lar) within the blood corpuscles.

endointoxication (en″do-in-tok″sĭ-ka'shun) poisoning by an endogenous toxin.

endolabyrinthitis (en″do-lab″ĭ-rin-thi'tis) inflammation of the membranous labyrinth of the ear.

endolaryngeal (en″do-lah-rin'je-al) situated on or occurring within the larynx.

Endolimax (en″do-li'maks) a genus of amebas found in the colon of man, other mammals, birds, amphibians and cockroaches.

endolumbar (en″do-lum'bar) within the lumbar portion of the spinal cord.

endolymph (en'do-limf) fluid within the membranous labyrinth of the ear.

endolysin (en-dol'ĭ-sin) a lysin existing in a leukocyte and acting directly on bacteria.

endolysis (en-dol'ĭ-sis) dissolution of the cytoplasm of a cell.

endomastoiditis (en″do-mas″toi-di'tis) inflammation of the interior of the mastoid antrum and cells.

endometriosis (en″do-me″tre-o'sis) a condition in which tissue more or less perfectly resembling the uterine mucous membrane occurs aberrantly in various locations in the pelvic cavity. The condition may be characterized by pelvic pain, abnormal uterine or rectal bleeding, dysmenorrhea and symptoms of pressure within the pelvic cavity. Sterility and dyspareunia also may be present.

Treatment is based on the age of the patient and the extent of the endometrial growth. In young married women exogenous hormone therapy is employed, and, whenever feasible, the patient is encouraged to become pregnant since interruption of menstruation is thought to retard the progress of the disease. In older women and in cases of extensive growth, surgical treatment involving complete hysterectomy is indicated. X-ray therapy in doses large enough to produce destruction of the reproductive organs is sometimes employed when there is definite evidence of advanced endometriosis and surgery is contraindicated or refused.

endometritis (en″do-me-tri'tis) inflammation of the endometrium.
　puerperal e., endometritis following childbirth.

endometrium (en″do-me'tre-um) the mucous membrane lining the uterus. adj., **endome'trial.**

endomitosis (en″do-mi-to'sis) mitosis taking place without dissolution of the nuclear membrane, resulting in doubling of the number of chromosomes within the nucleus.

endomixis (en″do-mik'sis) mingling of nuclear and cytoplasmic substance of a cell.

endomorphy (en'do-mor″fe) a type of body build in which tissues derived from the entoderm predominate. There is relative preponderance of soft roundness throughout the body, with large digestive viscera and accumulations of fat, the body usually presenting large trunk and thighs and tapering extremities.

endomyocarditis (en″do-mi″o-kar-di′tis) inflammation of the endocardium and myocardium.

endomysium (en″do-mis′e-um) the sheath of delicate reticular fibrils that surrounds each muscle fiber.

endoneuritis (en″do-nu-ri′tis) inflammation of the endoneurium.

endoneurium (en″do-nu′re-um) connective tissue between the fibers of a fascicle of a nerve.

endoparasite (en″do-par′ah-sīt) a parasite that lives within the body of the host. adj., **endoparasit′-ic.**

endopelvic (en″do-pel′vik) within the pelvis.

endopeptidase (en″do-pep′tĭ-dās) a peptidase capable of acting on any peptide linkage in a peptide chain.

endopericarditis (en″do-per″ĭ-kar-di′tis) inflammation of the endocardium and pericardium.

endoperimyocarditis (en″do-per″ĭ-mi″o-kar-di′-tis) inflammation of the endocardium, pericardium and myocardium.

endoperitonitis (en″do-per″ĭ-to-ni′tis) inflammation of the serous lining of the peritoneal cavity.

endophlebitis (en″do-flĕ-bi′tis) inflammation of the intima of a vein.

endophthalmitis (en″dof-thal-mi′tis) inflammation of the internal structures of the eye.

endophytic (en″do-fit′ik) growing inward; proliferating internally.

endoplasm (en′do-plazm) the more centrally located cytoplasm of a cell.

endoplast (en′do-plast) the nucleus of a cell.

endoreduplication (en″do-re-du″plĭ-ka′shun) reproduction of elements within the nucleus of a cell not followed by chromosome movements and cytoplasmic division.

end-organ (end′or-gan) any terminal structure of a nerve.

endorhinitis (en″do-ri-ni′tis) inflammation of the mucous membrane of the nasal passages.

endosalpingitis (en″do-sal″pin-ji′tis) inflammation of the lining membrane of the oviduct (uterine tube).

endosalpingoma (en″do-sal″ping-go′mah) an epithelial tumor of the oviduct (uterine tube).

endosalpinx (en″do-sal′pinks) the mucous membrane lining the oviduct (uterine tube).

endoscope (en′do-skōp) an instrument used for direct visual inspection of hollow organs or body cavities. Specially designed endoscopes are used for such examinations as BRONCHOSCOPY, CYSTOSCOPY, GASTROSCOPY and PROCTOSCOPY.

Although the design of an endoscope may vary according to its specific use, all endoscopes have similar working elements. The viewing part (scope) may be a hollow metal or fiber tube fitted with a lens system that permits viewing in a variety of directions. The endoscope also has a light source, power cord and power source. Accessories that might be used with an endoscope for diagnostic or therapeutic purposes include suction tip, tubes and suction pump; forceps for removal of biopsy tissue or a foreign body; and electrode tip for cauterization.

endoscopy (en-dos′ko-pe) visual examination of interior structures of the body with an endoscope. adj., **endoscop′ic.**

endosepsis (en″do-sep′sis) septicemia originating from causes inside the body.

endosite (en′do-sīt) an internal parasite.

endoskeleton (en″do-skel′ĕ-ton) the framework of hard structures, embedded in and supporting the soft tissues of the body of higher animals, derived principally from the mesoderm.

endosmosis (en″dos-mo′sis) inward osmosis; inward passage of liquid through a membrane, by which one fluid passes through a septum into a cavity that contains fluid of a different density.

endosome (en′do-sōm) a body thought to consist of deoxyribonucleic acid, observed in the vesicular nucleus of certain cells.

endosteal (en-dos′te-al) occurring inside a bone.

endosteitis (en-dos″te-i′tis) inflammation of the endosteum.

endosteoma (en-dos″te-o′mah) a tumor in the medullary cavity of a bone.

endosteum (en-dos′te-um) the lining membrane of a hollow bone.

endostoma (en″dos-to′mah) a bony tumor within a bone.

endothelioangiitis (en″do-the″le-o-an″je-i′tis) a condition resembling lupus erythematosus, attended by fever, arthritis, pericarditis and angiitis.

endotheliocyte (en″do-the′le-o-sīt″) a large mononuclear phagocytic cell of the blood and tissues.

endotheliocytosis (en″do-the″le-o-si-to′sis) abnormal increase of endotheliocytes.

endotheliolysin (en″do-the″le-ol′ĭ-sin) an antibody that causes the dissolution of endothelial cells.

endothelioma (en″do-the″le-o′mah) an endothelial tumor.

endotheliotoxin (en″do-the″le-o-tok′sin) a toxin that destroys endothelium.

endothelium (en″do-the′le-um), pl. *endothe′lia* [Gr.] the layer of epithelial cells that lines the cavities of the heart and of the blood and lymph vessels, and the serous cavities of the body. adj., **endothe′lial.**

endothermal, endothermic (en″do-ther′mal), (en″do-ther′mik) 1. characterized by the absorption of heat. 2. pertaining to endothermy.

endothermy (en′do-ther″me) production of heat in the tissues by the resistance they offer to the passage of the high-frequency current.

endothoracic (en″do-tho-ras′ik) within the thorax; situated internal to the ribs.

endothrix (en'do-thriks) a fungus whose growth is confined chiefly within the shaft of a hair, without formation of conspicuous external spores.

endotoxic (en"do-tok'sik) retaining its toxin within itself; said of certain bacteria.

endotoxicosis (en"do-tok"sĭ-ko'sis) poisoning by an endotoxin.

endotoxin (en"do-tok'sin) a heat-stable toxin present in the bacterial cell but not in cell-free filtrates of cultures of intact bacteria. They are found primarily in enteric bacilli, in which they are identical with the O antigen, but are also found in certain of the gram-negative cocci and in Pasteurella and Brucella species. The endotoxins are pyrogenic and increase capillary permeability, the activity being substantially the same regardless of the species of bacteria from which they are derived.

endotoxoid (en"do-tok'soid) a toxoid prepared from an endotoxin.

endotracheal (en"do-tra'ke-al) within the trachea.

endotracheitis (en"do-tra"ke-i-'tis) inflammation of the mucous membrane of the trachea.

endovasculitis (en"do-vas"ku-li'tis) inflammation of the intima of a blood vessel.

endovenous (en"do-ve'nus) within a vein.

endoxan (en-dok'san) cyclophosphamide, an antineoplastic agent.

end-plate (end'plāt) a flattened terminal discoid expansion at the ending of a motor nerve fiber upon a muscle fiber.

Endrate (en'drāt) trademark for disodium edetate, a chelating agent used to lower blood calcium levels.

enema (en'ĕ-mah) 1. introduction of fluid into the rectum. 2. a solution introduced into the rectum to promote evacuation of feces or as a means of ad-

ministering nutrient or medicinal substances, anesthetics or opaque material in roentgen examination of the lower intestinal tract (see also BARIUM TEST). Unless otherwise ordered, the solution is warmed to 105° F., the patient is placed in Sims's left lateral position and the rectal tube is inserted. The container of fluid is usually held 18 inches above the buttocks.

energy (en'er-je) power that may be translated into motion, overcoming resistance or effecting physical change; the ability to do work. Energy assumes several forms: it may be thermal (in the form of heat), electrical, mechanical, chemical, radiant or kinetic. In doing work, the energy is changed from one form to another or to several forms. In these changes some of the energy is "lost" in the sense that it cannot be recaptured and used again. Usually there is loss in the form of heat, which escapes or is dissipated unused. All energy changes give off a certain amount of the energy as heat.

All activities of the body require energy, and all needs are met by the consumption of food containing energy in chemical form. The human diet comprises three main sources of energy: carbohydrates, proteins and fats. Of these three, carbohydrates most readily provide the kind of energy needed to activate muscles. Proteins work to build and restore body tissues. The body transforms chemical energy derived from food by the process of METABOLISM, an activity that takes place in the individual cell. Molecules of the food substances providing energy pass through the cell wall. Inside the cell, chemical reactions occur that produce the new forms of energy and yield by-products such as water and waste materials.

enervation (en"er-va'shun) 1. lack of nervous energy. 2. removal of a nerve or a section of a nerve.

enflagellation (en-flaj"ĕ-la'shun) the formation of flagella.

ENEMAS

TYPE	PREPARATION	PURPOSES
Magnesium, glycerin, and water (one, two, three)	Mix 1 oz. magnesium sulfate, 2 oz. glycerin and 3 oz. hot water.	To increase intestinal fluids thereby causing pressure and stimulating peristalsis; glycerin acts as lubricant
Milk and molasses	Mix 180 ml. milk with 180. ml. molasses	Carminative: To relieve distention caused by flatus; to stimulate peristalsis
Oil retention	120 ml. mineral oil or glycerin, heated to 100° F.	To soften feces
Saline	1 tsp. salt to 1 pt. water	To relieve constipation or cleanse the rectal area, especially for removal of mucus
Soapsuds (S.S.)	30 ml. pure castile soap to 500 ml. water	Cleansing of rectal area; soap acts as an irritant to intestinal lining, stimulates peristalsis
Sodium bicarbonate	Add 1 tsp. sodium bicarbonate (baking soda) to 500 ml. water	To soothe mucous membranes and neutralize gastrointestinal acids

engagement (en-gāj'ment) the entrance of the fetal head or presenting part into the superior pelvic strait.

engastrius (en-gas'tre-us) a double fetal monster in which one fetus is contained within the abdomen of the other.

engorgement (en-gorj'ment) excessive fullness of any organ or passage.

engram (en'gram) a lasting mark or trace. The term is applied to the definite and permanent trace left by a stimulus in the protoplasm of a tissue. In psychology, it is the lasting trace left in the psyche by anything that has been experienced psychically; a latent memory picture.

engraphia (en-gra'fe-ah) the production by stimuli of definite traces (engrams) on the protoplasm, which, with repetition, induce a habit that persists after the stimuli have ceased.

enhematospore (en-hem'ah-to-spōr") a spore of the malarial parasite found in the blood.

enhexymal (en-hek'sĭ-mal) hexobarbital, an ultra-short acting barbiturate.

enkatarrhaphy (en"kah-tar'ah-fe) suturing together of the sides of tissues alongside a structure, burying it.

enomania (e"no-ma'ne-ah) 1. periodic craving for strong drink. 2. delirium tremens.

enophthalmos (en"of-thal'mos) abnormal recession of the eyeballs in the orbit.

enostosis (en"os-to'sis) a bony growth in the hollow of a bone.

ensiform (en'sĭ-form) sword-shaped.
  e. cartilage, the xiphoid process.

ensomphalus (en-som'fah-lus) a double monster with bodies partially united.

enstrophe (en'stro-fe) inversion; a turning inward.

E.N.T. ear, nose and throat.

entad (en'tad) toward a center; inwardly.

ental (en'tal) inner; central.

Entamoeba (en"tah-me'bah) a genus of amebas parasitic in the intestines of vertebrates.
  E. co'li, a nonpathogenic form found in the intestinal tract of man.
  E. histolyt'ica, a species causing AMEBIC DYSENTERY and abscess of the liver.
  E. tropica'lis, *Entamoeba histolytica.*

entasia (en-ta'ze-ah) a constrictive spasm.

enter(o)- (en'ter-o) word element [Gr.] *intestines.*

enteradenitis (en"ter-ad"ĕ-ni'tis) inflammation of the intestinal glands.

enteral (en'ter-al) within the intestine.

enteramine (en"ter-am'ēn) serotonin.

enterectomy (en"ter-ek'to-me) excision of a portion of the intestine.

enterelcosis (en"ter-el-ko'sis) ulceration of the intestine.

enteric (en-ter'ik) pertaining to the intestine.
  e.-coated, a trade term designating a special coating applied to tablets or capsules which prevents release and absorption of their contents until they reach the intestines.
  e. fever, typhoid fever.

enteritis (en"tĕ-ri'tis) inflammation of the intestine; a general condition that can be produced by a variety of causes. Bacteria and certain viruses may irritate the intestinal tract and produce symptoms of abdominal pain, nausea, vomiting and diarrhea. Similar effects may result from poisonous foods such as mushrooms and berries, or from a harmful chemical present in food or drink. Enteritis may also be the consequence of overeating, alcoholic excesses or emotional tension.
  Rest and bland diet are generally prescribed. In cases of bacterial infection antibiotics may be helpful. Severe dehydration, which may accompany enteritis, is treated with replacement of lost fluids and electrolytes.
  choleriform e., an acute cholera-like diarrheal disease with a high fatality rate prevalent in epidemic and endemic forms in the Western Pacific area since 1938.
  e. cys'tica chron'ica, a form marked by cystic dilatations of the intestinal glands, due to closure of their openings.
  e. gra'vis, an often fatal disease characterized by severe abdominal pain, nausea, vomiting and bloody diarrhea, with mucosal necrosis and hemorrhage and edema of the submucosa, most prominent in the jejunum and proximal ileum.
  membranous e., mucous e., mucous colitis.
  e. necrot'icans, an inflammation of the intestines due to *Clostridium perfringens* and characterized by necrosis.
  e. nodula'ris, enteritis with enlargement of the lymph nodes.
  phlegmonous e., a condition with symptoms resembling those of peritonitis and secondary to other intestinal diseases, e.g., chronic obstruction, strangulated hernia, carcinoma.
  e. polypo'sa, enteritis marked by polypoid growths in the intestine, due to proliferation of the connective tissue.
  regional e., inflammation of the terminal portion of the ileum; called also regional ileitis and Crohn's disease.

enteroanastomosis (en"ter-o-ah-nas"to-mo'sis) enteroenterostomy.

enteroantigen (en"ter-o-an'tĭ-jen) an antigen derived from feces.

Enterobacteriaceae (en"ter-o-bak-te"re-a'se-e) a family of Schizomycetes occurring as plant or animal parasites.

enterobiliary (en"ter-o-bil'e-a"re) pertaining to the intestines and the bile passages.

Enterobius (en"ter-o'be-us) a genus of nematode worms.
  E. vermicula'ris, the seatworm or pinworm, a small white worm parasitic in the upper part of the large intestine. (See also WORMS.)

enterocele (en'ter-o-sēl") intestinal hernia.

enterocentesis (en"ter-o-sen-te'sis) surgical puncture of the intestine.

enterocholecystostomy (en″ter-o-ko″le-sis-tos′-to-me) surgical creation of an opening from the gallbladder to the small intestine.

enterocholecystotomy (en″ter-o-ko″le-sis-tot′o-me) incision of the gallbladder and intestine.

enterocinesia (en″ter-o-si-ne′se-ah) peristalsis.

enteroclysis (en″ter-ok′lǐ-sis) the injection of liquids into the intestine.

enterococcus (en″ter-o-kok′us) a streptococcus of the human intestine.

enterocoele (en′ter-o-sēl″) the abdominal cavity.

enterocolectomy (en″ter-o-ko-lek′to-me) resection of part of the small intestine and colon.

enterocolitis (en″ter-o-ko-li′tis) inflammation of the small intestine and colon.
 hemorrhagic e., inflammation of the small intestine and colon, characterized by hemorrhagic breakdown of the intestinal mucosa, with inflammatory cell infiltration.
 pseudomembranous e., an acute, superficial necrosis of the mucosa of the small intestine and colon, characterized by the passage of shreds or casts of the bowel wall.

enterocolostomy (en″ter-o-ko-los′to-me) anastomosis of the small intestine to the colon.

enterocrinin (en″ter-ok′rǐ-nin) a hormone from animal intestines that stimulates the glands of the small intestine.

enterocutaneous (en″ter-o-ku-ta′ne-us) pertaining to or communicating with the intestine and the skin, or surface of the body.

enterocyst (en′ter-o-sist″) a cyst proceeding from subperitoneal tissue.

enterocystocele (en″ter-o-sis′to-sēl) hernia of the bladder and intestine.

enterocystoma (en″ter-o-sis-to′mah) cystic tumor of the intestine.

enterodynia (en″ter-o-din′e-ah) pain in the intestine.

enteroenterostomy (en″ter-o-en″ter-os′to-me) anastomosis between two normally remote parts of the intestine.

enteroepiplocele (en″ter-o-e-pip′lo-sēl) hernia of the intestine and omentum.

enterogastritis (en″ter-o-gas-tri′tis) inflammation of the small intestine and stomach.

enterogastrone (en″ter-o-gas′trōn) a hormone of the duodenum that mediates the humoral inhibition of gastric secretion and motility produced by ingestion of fat.

enterogenous (en″ter-oj′ĕ-nus) arising within the intestine.

enterogram (en′ter-o-gram″) an instrumental tracing of the movements of the intestine.

enterohepatitis (en″ter-o-hep″ah-ti′tis) inflammation of the intestine and liver.

enterohepatopexy (en″ter-o-hep″ah-to-pek′se) fixation to the liver of a seromuscular flap of a defunctionalized loop of the proximal small intestine.

enterohydrocele (en″ter-o-hi′dro-sēl) hernia with hydrocele.

enterokinase (en″ter-o-ki′nās) an enzyme present in intestinal juice that catalyzes the conversion of trypsinogen to trypsin.

enterolith (en′ter-o-lith″) a calculus in the intestine.

enterolysis (en″ter-ol′ĭ-sis) surgical separation of intestinal adhesions.

enteromegaly (en″ter-o-meg′ah-le) enlargement of the intestines.

enteromycosis (en″ter-o-mi-ko′sis) fungal disease of the intestine.

enteron (en′ter-on) the intestine.

enteroneuritis (en″ter-o-nu-ri′tis) inflammation of the nerves of the intestine.

enteronitis (en″ter-o-ni′tis) inflammation of the small intestine; enteritis.

enteroparesis (en″ter-o-par′ĕ-sis) relaxation and dilatation of the intestine.

enteropathy (en″ter-op′ah-the) a disease of the intestine.

enteropexy (en′ter-o-pek″se) surgical fixation of the intestine.

enteroplasty (en′ter-o-plas″te) plastic repair of the intestine.

enteroplegia (en″ter-o-ple′je-ah) paralysis of the intestine.

enteroptosis (en″ter-op-to′sis) abnormal downward displacement of the intestines.

enterorrhagia (en″ter-o-ra′je-ah) intestinal hemorrhage.

enterorrhaphy (en″ter-or′ah-fe) suture of the intestine.

enterorrhexis (en″ter-o-rek′sis) rupture of the intestine.

enteroscope (en′ter-o-skōp″) an instrument for inspecting the inside of the intestine.

enterosepsis (en″ter-o-sep′sis) intestinal sepsis due to putrefaction of the contents of the intestines.

enterosorption (en″ter-o-sorp′shun) accumulation of a substance in the bowel by virtue of its passage from the circulating blood.

enterospasm (en′ter-o-spazm″) intestinal colic.

enterostasis (en″ter-o-sta′sis) intestinal stasis.

enterostenosis (en″ter-o-stě-no′sis) narrowing or stricture of the intestine.

enterostomy (en″ter-os′to-me) the artificial formation of a permanent opening into the intestine through the abdominal wall (see also COLOSTOMY).

enterotomy (en″ter-ot′o-me) incision of the intestine.

enterotoxin (en″ter-o-tok′sin) 1. a toxin specific for the cells of the intestinal mucosa. 2. a toxin arising in the intestine. 3. an exotoxin that is protein in nature and relatively heat-stable, produced by staphylococci and causing food poisoning.

enterotoxism (en″ter-o-tok′sizm) absorption of toxins from the intestine.

enterotropic (en″ter-o-trop′ik) affecting the intestines.

enterovaginal (en″ter-o-vaj′ĭ-nal) pertaining to or communicating with the intestine and the vagina, as an enterovaginal fistula.

enterovesical (en″ter-o-ves′ĭ-kal) pertaining to or communicating with the intestine and urinary bladder.

Entero-vioform (en″ter-o-vi′o-form) trademark for a preparation of iodochlorhydroxyquin, used largely for treatment of trichomoniasis and amebiasis.

enterovirus (en″ter-o-vi′rus) one of a group of morphologically similar viruses infecting the gastrointestinal tract and discharged in the excreta, including the poliovirus, Coxsackie virus and echovirus.

enterozoon (en″ter-o-zo′on) an animal parasite in the intestines.

entoblast (en′to-blast) the entoderm.

entocele (en′to-sēl) an internal hernia.

entochondrostosis (en″to-kon″dros-to′sis) the development of bone within cartilage.

entochoroidea (en″to-ko-roi′de-ah) the inner layer of the choroid of the eye.

entocineria (en″to-sĭ-ne′re-ah) the internal gray matter of the brain or spinal cord.

entocyte (en′to-sīt) the cell contents.

entoderm (en′to-derm) the innermost of the three primitive germ layers of the embryo; from it are derived the epithelium of the pharynx, respiratory tract (except the nose), digestive tract, bladder and urethra. adj., **entoder′mal, entoder′mic.**

entoectad (en″to-ek′tad) from within outward.

entomere (en′to-mēr) a blastomere normally destined to become entoderm.

entomion (en-to′me-on) the tip of the posteroinferior, or mastoid, angle of the parietal bone.

entomology (en″to-mol′o-je) that branch of biology concerned with the study of insects.
    medical e., that concerned with insects that cause disease or serve as vectors of microorganisms that cause disease in man.

entomophobia (en″to-mo-fo′be-ah) morbid dread of insects, mites, ticks, etc.

entopic (en-top′ik) occurring in the proper place.

entoptic (en-top′tik) originating within the eye.

entoptoscopy (en″top-tos′ko-pe) inspection of the interior of the eye.

entoretina (en″to-ret′ĭ-nah) the nervous or inner layer of the retina.

entotic (en-tot′ik) originating within the ear.

entozoon (en″to-zo′on) an internal animal parasite. adj., **entozo′ic.**

entropion (en-tro′pe-on) inversion, or the turning inward, as of the margin of an eyelid.
    e. u′veae, inversion of the margin of the pupil.

enucleation (e-nu″kle-a′shun) removal of an organ or other mass intact from its supporting tissues, as of the eyeball from the orbit.

enuresis (en″u-re′sis) inability to control urination, especially at night during sleep; bed-wetting. adj., **enuret′ic.** It occurs most often in children who are very sound sleepers or who have small bladder capacity. In many cases enuresis is due to emotional rather than physical causes. If it persists after the age of 6, a physical or emotional disorder is likely to be present.

environment (en-vi′ron-ment) the sum total of all the conditions and elements that make up the surroundings of an individual.

Enzactin (en-zak′tin) trademark for preparations of triacetin, a topical antifungal agent.

enzygotic (en″zi-got′ik) developed from one zygote.

enzyme (en′zīm) a substance, usually protein in nature, that initiates and accelerates a chemical reaction. adj., **enzymat′ic.** The substance acted upon by an enzyme is called a substrate. In an enzymatic reaction a portion of one substrate is transferred to another substrate or metabolized. Each enzyme is specific for a certain type of substrate and may catalyze the reaction in either direction.
    Enzymes are essential for a number of the life processes and are responsible for functions such as digestion, maintenance of acid-base balance and energy utilization.
    The digestive enzymes are divided into three groups: the amylases, or starch splitters; the lipases, or fat splitters; and the proteases, which split proteins.
    Enzymes are sensitive to changes in acidity and alkalinity and can act as toxins. If obstruction of the pancreatic duct causes powerful digestive enzymes of the pancreas to be retained and made active in that organ, acute symptoms can occur. A slowing up of the enzymatic action can also cause serious illness or death.
    It is thought that improper functioning of enzymes causes some nerve disorders. There has been a growing recognition of a number of hereditary diseases caused by defective enzyme systems. Phenylketonuria (PKU), for example, is caused by the inherited inability of the body to convert the amino acid phenylalanine into tyrosine.
    By a number of biochemical tests performed in clinical laboratories the activity levels of many enzymes in body fluids (e.g., serum) can be determined, and variations from previously normal levels can help the physician in diagnosing and following the course of a disease, e.g., myocardial infarction and pancreatitis.
    activating e., one that activates a given amino acid by attaching it to the corresponding transfer ribonucleic acid.
    adaptive e., induced enzyme.
    amylolytic e., one that catalyzes the conversion of starch into sugar.
    brancher e., an enzyme that acts on glucose

residues in starch, and is important in the formation of glycogen.

clotting e., coagulating e., one that catalyzes the conversion of soluble into insoluble proteins.

constitutive e., one produced by a microorganism regardless of the presence or absence of the specific substrate acted upon.

deamidizing e., one that splits up the amino acids into ammonia compounds.

debrancher e., an enzyme that acts on glucose residues of the glycogen molecule, and is important in glycogenolysis; deficiency of this enzyme results in a condition known as limit dextrinosis.

decarbolizing e., one that splits carbon dioxide from organic acids.

digestive e., a substance that catalyzes the process of digestion.

glycolytic e., one that catalyzes the oxidation of sugar.

induced e., one whose production requires or is stimulated by a specific small molecule, the inducer, which is the substrate of the enzyme or a compound structurally related to it.

lipolytic e., one that catalyzes the decomposition of fat.

mucolytic e., one that catalyzes the depolymerization of mucopolysaccharides.

peptolytic e., one that catalyzes the decomposition of peptone.

proteolytic e., one that catalyzes the hydrolysis of proteins and protein split products to peptone.

redox e., one that catalyzes oxidation-reduction reactions.

steatolytic e., one that splits up fat.

sucroclastic e., one that decomposes sugar.

transferring e., one that catalyzes the transference of various radicals between molecules.

uricolytic e., one that metabolizes uric acid into urea.

Warburg's respiratory e., a protein existing in many tissues and serving as an important factor in tissue respiration.

yellow e's, a number of substances that have been isolated from various organs and tissues and that take part in oxidations and reductions in the body; all contain riboflavin in their prosthetic groups.

enzymolysis (en″zi-mol′ĭ-sis) disintegration induced by an enzyme.

enzymosis (en″zi-mo′sis) fermentation induced by an enzyme.

enzymuria (en″zi-mu′re-ah) the presence of enzymes in the urine.

eonism (e′o-nizm) the wearing of feminine clothing or the adoption of feminine habits and sexual behavior by a male.

eosin (e′o-sin) a coloring matter used as a dye in preparing various specimens, especially plasma samples, for microscopic study.

eosinopenia (e″o-sin″o-pe′ne-ah) deficiency of eosinophils in the blood.

eosinophil (e″o-sin′o-fil) 1. an element readily stainable by eosin. 2. a medium-sized leukocyte, with a two- or three-lobed nucleus and cytoplasm containing large granules that stain bright red, normally constituting 1 to 2 per cent of the leukocytes in the blood.

eosinophilia (e″o-sin″o-fil′e-ah) 1. affinity for

eosin. 2. an excess in the number of eosinophils, seen frequently in allergic states. adj., **eosinophil′ic.**

tropical e., a disease characterized by anorexia, malaise, cough, leukocytosis and an increase in eosinophils.

eosinophilic (e″o-sin″o-fil′ik) staining readily with eosin.

epaxial (ep-ak′se-al) situated above the axis.

epencephalon (ep″en-sef′ah-lon) the embryonic structure from which arise the pons and cerebellum.

ependyma (ĕ-pen′dĭ-mah) the membrane lining the cerebral ventricles and the central canal of the spine. adj., **epen′dymal.**

ephebiatrics (e-fe″be-at′riks) the branch of medicine that deals especially with the diagnosis and treatment of diseases and problems peculiar to youth (18 to 25 years).

ephebic (ĕ-fe′bik) pertaining to puberty.

ephebogenesis (ef″e-bo-jen′ĕ-sis) the bodily changes occurring at puberty.

ephebogenic (ef″e-bo-jen′ik) leading to the changes associated with puberty.

ephebology (ef″e-bol′o-je) the study of puberty.

ephedrine (ĕ-fed′rin, ef′ĕ-drin) an alkaloid obtained from the shrub *Ephedra equisetina* or produced synthetically; used, in the form of ephedrine hydrochloride or ephedrine sulfate, as a sympathomimetic, as a pressor substance, to relieve bronchial spasm and as a central nervous system stimulant. It may be administered orally, topically, intramuscularly or intravenously.

ephelis (ĕ-fe′lis), pl. *ephel′ides* [Gr.] a freckle.

ephidrosis (ef″ĭ-dro′sis) profuse perspiration.

Ephynal (ef′ĭ-nal) trademark for a preparation of vitamin E.

epi- (ep′ĭ) word element [Gr.], *upon.*

epiblepharon (ep″ĭ-blef′ah-ron) a condition in which a fold of the skin stretches along the border of the lower eyelid and presses against the eyeball.

epibulbar (ep″ĭ-bul′bar) situated upon the eyeball.

epicanthus (ep″ĭ-kan′thus) a vertical fold of skin on either side of the nose, sometimes covering the inner canthus; a normal characteristic in persons of certain races, but anomalous in others.

epicardia (ep″ĭ-kar′de-ah) the lower portion of the esophagus, extending from the esophageal hiatus to the cardia, the upper orifice of the stomach.

epicardiectomy (ep″ĭ-kar′de-ek′to-me) an operation by which the heart is supplied with a collateral circulation from the pericardium.

epicardium (ep″ĭ-kar′de-um) the layer of the pericardium that is in contact with the heart.

epicele (ep′ĭ-sēl) the fourth ventricle of the brain.

epichorion (ep″ĭ-ko′re-on) the portion of uterine mucosa enclosing the fertilized ovum.

epicondyle (ep″ĭ-kon′dīl) an eminence or projection above the condyle of a bone.

epicranium (ep″ĭ-kra′ne-um) the structures collectively that cover the skull.

epicritic (ep″ĭ-krit′ik) determining accurately; said of cutaneous nerve fibers, that are sensitive to fine variations of touch or temperature.

epicystotomy (ep″ĭ-sis-tot′o-me) cystotomy by the suprapubic method.

epicyte (ep′ĭ-sīt) the wall or envelope of a cell.

epidemic (ep″ĭ-dem′ik) 1. occurring in a great number of cases in a community at the same time. 2. the simultaneous occurrence in a community of a great many cases of a specific disease.

epidemiology (ep″ĭ-de″me-ol′o-je) the scientific study of factors that influence the frequency and distribution of infectious diseases in man.

epidermal (ep″ĭ-der′mal) 1. any material originating from animal epidermis (hairs, scales, feathers) that may cause allergy in hypersensitive persons. 2. epidermic.

epidermis (ep″ĭ-der′mis) the outermost, nonvascular layer of the skin, derived from the embryonic ectoderm, varying in thickness from 1/200 to 1/20 inch, and composed of four layers: the desquamating horny layer, replaced by growth from below; the clear layer; the granular layer, a transition state between the innermost, the malpighian, layer and the outer two. adj., **epider′mic.**

epidermitis (ep″ĭ-der-mi′tis) inflammation of the epidermis.

epidermodysplasia (ep″ĭ-der″mo-dis-pla′ze-ah) faulty development of the epidermis.
   e. verrucifor′mis, an inherited dysplasia of the upper layers of the epidermis.

epidermoid (ep″ĭ-der′moid) 1. resembling the epidermis. 2. a brain tumor formed by inclusion of epidermal cells.

epidermoidoma (ep″ĭ-der″moi-do′mah) a usually benign tumor developing in the scalp, in the diploic space or between the dura mater and the inner table of the skull.

epidermolysis (ep″ĭ-der-mol′ĭ-sis) 1. looseness of the skin. 2. a condition in which the outer skin peels away from its underlying structures.
   e. bullo′sa, a variety with formation of deep-seated bullae that appear after irritation.

epidermoma (ep″ĭ-der-mo′mah) an outgrowth on the skin.

epidermomycosis (ep″ĭ-der″mo-mi-ko′sis) any dermatitis caused by fungi or yeasts.

epidermophytid (ep″ĭ-der-mof′ĭ-tid) a skin eruption occurring as an allergic response to Epidermophyton.

epidermophytin (ep″ĭ-der-mof′ĭ-tin) a vaccine for epidermophytosis prepared from cultures of Epidermophyton.

Epidermophyton (ep″ĭ-der-mof′ĭ-ton) a genus of fungi. *E. flocco′sum* attacks both skin and nails and is one of the causative organisms of tinea cruris, tinea pedis (athlete's foot) and tinea unguium.

epidermophytosis (ep″ĭ-der″mo-fi-to′sis) infection by the fungus Epidermophyton.

epidiascope (ep″ĭ-di′ah-skōp) an instrument for projecting the images of opaque bodies upon a screen.

epididymectomy (ep″ĭ-did″ĭ-mek′to-me) excision of the epididymis.

epididymis (ep″ĭ-did′ĭ-mis), pl. *epididym′ides* [Gr.] an elongated, cordlike structure along the posterior border of the testis in the ducts of which the sperm are stored. adj., **epidid′ymal.**

epididymitis (ep″ĭ-did″ĭ-mi′tis) inflammation of the epididymis. Nonspecific epididymitis may result from an infection in the urinary tract, especially in the prostate. Rarely it may be traced to an infection elsewhere in the body. Tuberculosis, mumps and gonorrhea may be complicated by epididymitis. Symptoms include sudden severe pain in the testes followed by scrotal swelling and tenderness. Treatment is usually with antibiotics, rest in bed and avoidance of alcoholic beverages, spiced foods, sexual excitement and physical exercise until all symptoms have disappeared.

epididymodeferentectomy (ep″ĭ-did″ĭ-mo-def″-er-en-tek′to-me) excision of the epididymis and vas deferens.

epididymo-orchitis (ep″ĭ-did″ĭ-mo-or-ki′tis) inflammation of the epididymis and testis.

epididymotomy (ep″ĭ-did″ĭ-mot′o-me) incision of the epididymis.

epididymovasostomy (ep″ĭ-did″ĭ-mo-vas-os′to-me) anastomosis of the epididymis to the vas deferens.

epidural (ep″ĭ-du′ral) external to the dura mater.

epifolliculitis (ep″ĭ-fŏ-lik″u-li′tis) inflammation of the hair follicles.

epigain (ep″ĭ-gān) the unconscious portion of the secondary external advantage to be derived from an emotional illness.

epigaster (ep″ĭ-gas′ter) hindgut; the embryonic structure from which the large intestine is formed.

epigastrium (ep″ĭ-gas′tre-um) the upper abdominal region, overlying the stomach. adj., **epigas′-tric.**

epigenesis (ep″ĭ-jen′ĕ-sis) development from simpler to more complex forms through division and progressive differentiation of the component cells.

epigenetics (ep″ĭ-jĕ-net′iks) the science concerned with the causal analysis of development.

epiglottis (ep″ĭ-glot′is) a leaflike flap of cartilage between the back of the tongue and the entrance to the larynx and trachea. The muscular action of swallowing closes the opening to the trachea by placing the larynx against the epiglottis. This prevents food and drink from entering the larynx and trachea, directing it instead into the esophagus.

epilation (ep″ĭ-la′shun) removal of hair.

epilatory (e-pil'ah-tor"e) 1. pertaining to removal of hair. 2. an agent for removing hair.

epilemma (ep"ĭ-lem'ah) the sheath of a terminal nerve fiber.

epilepsy (ep'ĭ-lep"se) a disorder of the nervous system in which the major symptom is a convulsive seizure, which is the result of a temporary disturbance of the brain impulses. It is sometimes called cerebral dysrhythmia, meaning a disturbance of the brain's normal rhythm. There are an estimated 1,860,000 persons with epilepsy in the United States, making it the most common organic disorder of the nervous system.

Brain damage or mental deterioration occurs in only a very small percentage of certain types of epilepsy, or in cases that have been grossly neglected over a long period of years.

SYMPTOMS. Epilepsy is characterized by momentary or prolonged loss of consciousness and involuntary convulsive movements. In minor seizures, or petit mal, the loss of consciousness lasts only a few seconds. Although there is often twitching about the eyes or mouth, the victim remains seated or standing and appears to have had no more than a lapse of attention or a moment of absentmindedness. Petit mal occurs most frequently in children.

In major seizures, or grand mal, the victim falls to the floor unconscious, often with foaming at the mouth, biting and violent shaking of the limbs. The patient may hurt himself during such a seizure. Fortunately, epileptics frequently experience a warning called the aura, such as ringing in the ears, spots before the eyes or tingling in the fingers, before an attack. This may give them time to lie down and avoid falls.

In the third type of seizure, psychomotor epilepsy, there is a very brief clouding of consciousness with some repeated meaningless movement, such as clapping of hands. It is followed by brief periods of forgetfulness. Another type, focal epilepsy, is characterized by seizures that are predominantly one-sided or local, or present localized features.

All three types of seizures last from a few seconds to a few minutes. The frequency of seizures may vary from one a year or so to several a day. The term epilepsy equivalent refers to any disturbance, mental or physical, that may take the place of an epileptic seizure.

CAUSES. Acquired epilepsy, called also symptomatic epilepsy, has a physical cause, such as brain tumor, injury to the brain at birth or a wound or blow to the head. These injuries irritate the brain and set off abnormal electrical discharge. In a small percentage of cases, this form of epilepsy may be cured by surgery to remove the tumor or repair the injury.

In jacksonian epilepsy, the specific portion of the brain controlling certain muscles may be diseased or irritated. The convulsions start in a specific group of muscles, such as those in the hand or leg, and progress to involve other muscles. They may, in some cases, develop into a complete grand mal attack, with loss of consciousness.

Idiopathic epilepsy is the most common type, and usually manifests itself early in life. Eighty per cent of victims have their first seizures before the age of 18. This type of epilepsy does not seem to be inherited, although there is evidence that a predisposition to it may run in families. The cause is still unknown.

TREATMENT. Anticonvulsant drugs are very helpful in the treatment of epilepsy. These include phenobarbital, diphenylhydantoin (Dilantin), trimethadione (Tridione) and others. The patient must take these drugs as ordered by the physician so that seizures can be controlled effectively. Although the anticonvulsants do not cure epilepsy, they can usually prevent the disabling effects of the disease, so that the patient can hold a responsible position and lead practically a normal life with few restrictions.

The Epilepsy Foundation of America, 733 15th Street, Washington, D.C. 20005, supplies information on all aspects of epilepsy, and can refer victims of epilepsy to specialists and clinics in their locality.

NURSING CARE. Because of ignorance and superstition, there is still some stigma attached to epilepsy. Nurses need to do their part in counteracting this through educational efforts. The patient and his family, as well as the general public, should become familiar with all aspects of this disorder. The patient must understand the importance of taking the prescribed drugs as ordered by his physician. Specific nursing measures to be taken during an epileptic seizure are identical to those for any patient having a seizure and can be found under CONVULSION.

epileptic (ep"ĭ-lep'tik) 1. pertaining to epilepsy. 2. a person subject to attacks of epilepsy.

epileptogenic (ep"ĭ-lep"to-jen'ik) causing an epileptic seizure.

epileptoid (ep"ĭ-lep'toid) 1. resembling epilepsy or its manifestations. 2. occurring in severe or sudden paroxysms.

epileptology (ep"ĭ-lep-tol'o-je) the study of epilepsy.

epimenorrhagia (ep"ĭ-men"o-ra'je-ah) abnormally profuse menstruation.

epimenorrhea (ep"ĭ-men"o-re'ah) abnormally frequent menstruation.

epimer (ep'ĭ-mer) one of two or more isomers which differ only in the position of one carbon atom.

epimere (ep'ĭ-mēr) one of the dorsal portions of the fusing myotomes in embryonic development, forming muscles innervated by the dorsal rami of the spinal nerves.

epimerite (ep"ĭ-mer'īt) an organ of protozoa by which they attach themselves to epithelial cells.

epimicroscope (ep"ĭ-mi'kro-skōp) a microscope in which the specimen is illuminated by light passing through a condenser built around the objective.

epimorphosis (ep"ĭ-mor-fo'sis) the regeneration of a piece of an organism by proliferation at the cut surface.

epimysium (ep"ĭ-mis'e-um) the outer fibrous sheath about a striated muscle.

epinephrectomy (ep"ĭ-ne-frek'to-me) adrenalectomy.

epinephrine (ep"ĭ-nef'rin) a hormone produced by the medulla, or inner core, of the ADRENAL

GLANDS; called also Adrenaline. Its function is to aid in the regulation of the sympathetic branch of the AUTONOMIC NERVOUS SYSTEM. At times when a person is highly stimulated, as by fear, anger or some challenging situation, extra amounts of epinephrine are released into the bloodstream, preparing the body for energetic action. The arteries are contracted and blood pressure rises; heartbeat speeds up and so does breathing; the rate at which the blood will clot is increased, and so is the rate of oxygen consumption by the body. Simultaneously, extra sugar is released into the blood from its storage place in the liver for quick conversion into energy. The person has a suddenly increased feeling of muscular strength and aggressiveness.

Some disorders of the adrenal glands, such as Addison's disease, reduce the output of epinephrine below normal. By contrast, excessive activity of the adrenals often seen in highly emotional persons, tends to produce tenseness, palpitation, high blood pressure, perhaps diarrhea and overaggressiveness. Certain adrenal tumors result in the production of too much epinephrine. Removal of the tumor relieves symptoms.

Epinephrine can be administered parenterally, topically or by inhalation, and acts as a vasoconstrictor, antispasmodic and sympathomimetic. It is used as an emergency heart stimulant and to relieve symptoms in allergic conditions such as urticaria (hives) and asthma. It is the most effective drug for counteracting the lethal effects of anaphylactic shock.

epinephritis (ep″i-ně-fri′tis) inflammation of an adrenal gland.

epineural (ep″i-nu′ral) situated upon a neural arch.

epineurium (ep″i-nu′re-um) the sheath of a nerve.

epinosis (ep″i-no′sis) a psychic or imaginary state of illness secondary to an original illness.

epionychium (ep″e-o-nik′e-um) situated on or above the ear.

epiphora (e-pif′o-rah) overflow of tears from obstruction of the lacrimal duct.

epiphysiolysis (ep″i-fiz″e-ol′i-sis) separation of the epiphysis from the diaphysis of a bone.

epiphysis (e-pif′i-sis), pl. *epiph′yses* [Gr.] 1. the end of a long bone, usually wider than the shaft, and either entirely cartilaginous or separated from the shaft by a cartilaginous disk. 2. part of a bone formed from a secondary center of ossification, commonly found at the ends of long bones, on the margins of flat bones and at tubercles and processes; during the period of growth epiphyses are separated from the main portion of the bone by cartilage. 3. the pineal gland. (*epiphysis cere′bri*). adj., **epiphys′eal.**

epiphysitis (e-pif″i-si′tis) inflammation of the cartilage joining the epiphysis to a shaft.

epipial (ep″i-pi′al) situated upon the pia mater.

epiplocele (e-pip′lo-sēl) omental hernia.

epiploenterocele (ep″i-plo-en′ter-o-sēl″) hernia containing intestine and omentum.

epiplomerocele (ep″i-plo-me′ro-sēl) femoral hernia containing omentum.

epiplomphalocele (ep″i-plom-fal′o-sēl) umbilical hernia containing omentum.

epiploon (e-pip′lo-on), pl. *epip′loa* [Gr.] the greater omentum. adj., **epiplo′ic.**

episclera (ep″i-skle′rah) the loose connective tissue forming the external surface of the sclera.

episcleritis (ep″i-skle-ri′tis) inflammation of the outer layers of the sclera.

episioclisia (e-piz″e-o-kli′se-ah) surgical closure of the vulva.

episioperineoplasty (e-piz″e-o-per″i-ne′o-plas″te) plastic repair of the vulva and perineum.

episioperineorrhaphy (e-piz″e-o-per″i-ne-or′ah-fe) suture of the vulva and perineum.

episioplasty (e-piz′e-o-plas″te) plastic repair of the vulva.

episiorrhaphy (e-piz″e-or′ah-fe) suture of the vulva.

episiostenosis (e-piz″e-o-stě-no′sis) narrowing of the vulva.

episiotomy (e-piz″e-ot′o-me) incision of the vulva, most often done during the second stage of labor to avoid lacerations of the perineum as the infant is delivered.

episome (ep′i-sōm) a block of genetic material capable of existing in the cell in two alternate forms, one replicating autonomously in the cytoplasm and the other replicating as part of the chromosome.

epispadias (ep″i-spa′de-as) a congenital malformation with absence of the upper wall of the urethra, occurring in both sexes, but more commonly in the male, the urethral opening being located anywhere on the dorsum of the penis. adj., **epispa′diac.**

epispastic (ep″i-spas′tik) vesicant; blistering.

episplenitis (ep″i-sple-ni′tis) inflammation of the capsule of the spleen.

epistaxis (ep″i-stak′sis) hemorrhage from the nose; nosebleed. A minor nosebleed may be caused by a blow on the nose, irritation from foreign bodies or vigorous nose-blowing during a cold. Sometimes it occurs in connection with menstruation. If bleeding persists in spite of the following first-aid measures, medical attention is advisable.

The victim should sit up with the head tilted back. The soft portion of the nose is grasped firmly between the thumb and forefinger. If this does not stop the bleeding, small wads of cotton or gauze are gently inserted into the nose and then the nostrils are pressed firmly together again. This often helps a clot to form. If a clot fails to form, cold compresses are applied about the nose, the lips and the back of the neck. If the bleeding still persists, cauterization of the blood vessel may be necessary.

Sometimes nosebleed has serious underlying causes. Arteriosclerosis is a possible cause in the elderly. Polyps and other fleshy growths in the nose, food allergy, hypertension, vitamin deficiencies or any disease producing a bleeding tendency may produce nosebleed. Nosebleeds in children are sometimes a sign of rheumatic fever. If the nose bleeds often or profusely or if the bleeding is difficult to stop, a physician should be consulted.

Bleeding from the nose that does not originate in the nose itself is a serious indication that some damage has been done internally, either by injury or disease. Medical attention is necessary to trace the bleeding to its source. The blood probably originates in the stomach, the lungs, within the skull or in passages related to these parts.

episternal (ep″ĭ-ster′nal) 1. situated upon the sternum. 2. pertaining to the episternum.

episternum (ep″ĭ-ster′num) the manubrium, or upper piece of the sternum.

epitendineum (ep″ĭ-ten-din′e-um) the fibrous sheath covering a tendon.

epithalamus (ep″ĭ-thal′ah-mus) the pineal gland and adjacent structures of the forebrain.

epithelialization (ep″ĭ-the″le-al-ĭ-za′shun) the covering of a denuded area with epithelium; conversion into epithelium.

epitheliitis (ep″ĭ-the″le-i′tis) inflammation of the epithelium.

epithelioblastoma (ep″ĭ-the″le-o-blas-to′mah) a tumor made up of cells of epithelial origin.

epithelioid (ep″ĭ-the′le-oid) resembling epithelium.

epitheliolysin (ep″ĭ-the″le-ol′ĭ-sin) an antibody that causes dissolution of epithelial cells.

epitheliolysis (ep″ĭ-the″le-ol′ĭ-sis) destruction of epithelial tissue.

epithelioma (ep″ĭ-the″le-o′mah) a malignant tumor largely of epithelial cells. adj., **epithelio′-matous.**

e. adenoi′des cys′ticum, a rare form of basal cell carcinoma, appearing as heaped-up lesions on the skin, especially of the face.

epitheliosis (ep″ĭ-the″le-o′sis) proliferation of conjunctival epithelium, forming trachoma-like granules.

epitheliotropic (ep″ĭ-the″le-o-trop′ik) having a special affinity for epithelial cells.

epithelium (ep″ĭ-the′le-um), pl. *epithe′lia* [Gr.] the covering of internal and external surfaces of the body, including the lining of vessels and other small cavities. It consists of cells joined by small amounts of cementing substances. Epithelium is classified into types on the basis of the number of layers deep and the shape of the superficial cells. adj., **epithe′lial.**

ciliated e., epithelium having motile, hairlike processes on its free surface.

columnar e., epithelium whose cells are of much greater height than width.

cuboidal e., epithelium whose cells are of approximately the same height and width, and appear square in transverse section.

germinal e., a layer of cells between the primitive mesentery and each mesonephros which becomes the epithelial covering of the gonad and perhaps gives rise to the germ cells.

glandular e., that composed of secreting cells.

pavement e., a variety composed of flattened cells in layers.

pigmented e., that made up of cells containing melanin or other pigment.

sense e., epithelium containing end-organs receiving stimuli of sensation.

squamous e., epithelium whose cells are thin and platelike.

stratified e., epithelium made up of cells arranged in two or more layers.

transitional e., a type characteristically found lining hollow organs, such as the urinary bladder, that are subject to great mechanical change due to contraction and distention, originally thought to represent a transition between stratified squamous and columnar epithelium.

epithelization (ep″ĭ-the″lĭ-za′shun) the formation of skin over a denuded area or wound.

epitonic (ep″ĭ-ton′ik) abnormally tense and tonic.

epitrichium (ep″ĭ-trik′e-um) the superficial layer of the epidermis of the embryo and fetus.

epitrochlea (ep″ĭ-trok′le-ah) the inner condyle of the humerus.

epituberculosis (ep″ĭ-tu-ber″ku-lo′sis) a condition resembling tuberculosis, but not caused by *Mycobacterium tuberculosis.*

epiturbinate (ep″ĭ-tur′bĭ-nāt) the soft tissue covering the nasal concha (turbinate bone).

epitympanum (ep″ĭ-tim′pah-num) the upper part of the tympanum.

epizoon (ep″ĭ-zo′on), pl. *epizo′a* [Gr.] an external animal parasite. adj., **epizo′ic.**

epizootic (ep″ĭ-zo-ot′ik) 1. occurring in a great number of cases in an animal community at the same time. 2. the simultaneous occurrence in an animal community of a great many cases of a specific disease.

eponychium (ep″o-nik′e-um) 1. an extension of the horny layers of the skin over the nail. 2. the horny embryonic membrane from which the nail is developed.

eponym (ep′o-nim) the name of a person used to designate a disease, organ or other entity, e.g., Hodgkin's disease, Cowper's gland, Schick test. adj., **eponym′ic.**

epoophoron (ep″o-of′o-ron) a vestigial structure associated with the ovary.

epoxytropine tropate (e-pok″se-tro′pēn tro′pāt) methscopolamine, used in parasympathetic blockade.

Eprolin (ep′ro-lin) trademark for a preparation of vitamin E.

epsilon-aminocaproic acid (ep′sĭ-lon am″ĭ-no-kah-pro′ik) a synthetic amino acid that is a potent inhibitor of fibrinolysis, plasminogen activator and plasmin.

Epsom salt (ep′sum) white crystalline salt, magnesium sulfate, formerly much used as a cathartic, but little used today.

epulis (ep-u′lis), pl. *epu′lides* [Gr.] a fibrous tumor of the gingiva.

epulosis (ep″u-lo′sis) a scarring over.

Equanil (ek′wah-nil) trademark for preparations of meprobamate, a tranquilizer.

equation (e-kwa′zhun) an expression of equality.
   Henderson-Hasselbalch e., a formula for calculating the pH of a buffer solution such as blood plasma, pH = pK′ + log $\frac{(BA)}{(HA)}$; (HA) is the concentration of a weak acid; (BA) the concentration of a weak salt of this acid; pK′ the buffer system.

equilibration (e″kwĭ-lĭ-bra′shun) the achievement of a balance between opposing elements or forces.

equilibrium (e″kwĭ-lib′re-um) a state of balance between opposing forces or influences. In the body, equilibrium may be chemical or physical. A state of chemical equilibrium is reached when the body tissues contain the proper proportions of various salts and water. Physical equilibrium, such as the state of balance required for walking, standing or sitting, is achieved by a very complex interplay of opposing sets of muscles. The labyrinth of the inner ear contains the semicircular canals, or organs of balance, and relays to the brain information about the body's position and also the direction of body motions.
   dynamic e., the condition of balance between varying, shifting and opposing forces that is characteristic of living processes.

equine (e′kwīn) pertaining to, characteristic of or derived from the horse.

equinophobia (e-kwi″no-fo′be-ah) morbid fear of horses.

equinovarus (e-kwi″no-va′rus) talipes equinovarus; inward flexion of the foot.

equipotentiality (e″kwĭ-po-ten″she-al′ĭ-te) the quality or state of having similar and equal power; the capacity for developing in the same way and to the same extent.

equivalent (e-kwiv′ah-lent) 1. of equal force, power or value. 2. the unvarying quantity of one body necessary to replace a fixed weight of another body.
   epilepsy e., any disturbance, mental or physical, that may take the place of an epileptic seizure.
   Joule's e., the energy expended in raising the temperature of one unit weight of water one degree.

Er chemical symbol, *erbium.*

erasion (e-ra′zhun) abrasion or scraping.

Erb-Goldflam disease (erb gōlt′flahm) myasthenia gravis.

erbium (er′be-um) a chemical element, atomic number 68, atomic weight 167.26, symbol Er. (See table of ELEMENTS.)

erectile (e-rek′tīl) capable of erection.

erection (e-rek′shun) the process of becoming upright and turgid; applied especially to the swelling and rigidity that occur in the penis as a result of sexual or other types of stimulation. Impulses received by the nervous system stimulate a flow of blood from the arteries leading to the penis, where the erectile tissue fills with blood, and the penis becomes firm and erect. Erection makes possible the transmission of semen into the body of the female (see REPRODUCTION). Erection can also occur to some extent in the clitoris and the nipples of the female.

erector (e-rek′ror) [L.] that which erects, particularly a muscle that holds up or raises a part.

eremophobia (er″ĕ-mo-fo′be-ah) morbid fear of being alone.

erepsin (e-rep′sĭn) a proteolytic enzyme of the intestinal juice.

erethin (er′ĕ-thin) the poisonous principle of tuberculin.

erethism (er′ĕ-thizm) excessive irritability or sensitivity to stimulation.

erethisophrenia (er″ĕ-thiz″o-fre′ne-ah) exaggerated mental excitability.

erg (erg) a unit of work or energy, equivalent to 2.4×10^{-8} gram (small) calories, or to 0.624×10^{12} electron volts.

ergasia (er-ga′ze-ah) 1. a hypothetical substance that stimulates the activity of body cells. 2. the total of an individual's functions and behavior.

ergasiomania (er-ga″se-o-ma′ne-ah) a morbid desire to be continually at work.

ergasiophobia (er-ga″se-o-fo′be-ah) morbid fear of overexertion.

ergasthenia (er″gas-the′ne-ah) debility from overwork.

ergastic (er-gas′tik) having potential energy.

ergocalciferol (er″go-kal-sif′er-ol) a white, odorless, crystalline compound; an oil-soluble, antirachitic vitamin.

ergocardiography (er″go-kar″de-og′rah-fe) the recording of moment-to-moment electromotive forces of the heart while the subject is engaging in muscular activity.

ergograph (er′go-graf) an instrument for measuring work done in muscular action.

ergonovine (er″go-no′vin) an ergot alkaloid used as an oxytocic and to relieve migraine.

ergophobia (er″go-fo′be-ah) morbid dread of work.

ergophore (er′go-fōr) the group of atoms in a molecule that brings about the specific activity of the substance.

ergoplasm (er′go-plazm) the specific kinetic or motor substance of a cell; functional protoplasm; called also kinoplasm.

ergosterol (er-gos′ter-ol) a sterol occurring in animal and plant tissues which on ultraviolet irradiation becomes a potent antirachitic substance, vitamin D_2.

ergot (er′got) a dried product made from the fungus *Claviceps purpurea,* which affects the rye plant. Ergot is used as an oxytocic and smooth muscle stimulant. It can also cause poisoning if incorporated in bread made from rye flour.

ergotamine (er-got'ah-min) an alkaloid derived from ergot, used as an oxytocic and in treatment of migraine.

ergotherapy (er″go-ther'ah-pe) treatment by physical exertion.

ergotism (er'go-tizm) chronic poisoning produced by ingestion of ergot.

Ergotrate (er'go-trāt) trademark for preparations of ergonovine, an oxytocic.

erogenous (ĕ-roj'ĕ-nus) causing sexual excitement.
  e. zones, portions of the body stimulation of which produces sexual response, e.g., the oral, anal and genital orifices and the nipples.

erosio (e-ro'ze-o) [L.] erosion.
  e. intergita'lis blastomycet'ica, a fungus infection causing maceration between the fingers.

erosion (e-ro'zhun) an eating or gnawing away; a kind of ulceration; in dentistry, the wasting away or loss of substance of a tooth by a chemical process that does not involve known bacterial action. adj., **ero'sive.**
  cervical e., ulceration of the endocervix and of the vaginal portion of the cervix, due to chemical irritation.

erotic (ĕ-rot'ik) pertaining to love or to sexual energy.

eroticism, erotism (e-rot'ĭ-sizm), (er'o-tizm) the expression of one's instinctual energy or drive, often used in special reference to the sex drive.
  anal e., fixation of psychosexual feelings at the anal phase of personality development; thought to lead to certain personality traits and to obsessive-compulsive disorders.
  genital e., achievement and maintenance of libido at the genital phase of psychosexual development, permitting acceptance of normal adult relationships and responsibilities.
  oral e., fixation of psychosexual feelings at the oral phase of personality development; thought to lead to passive, dependent character traits and sometimes to obesity and alcoholism.

erotize (er'o-tīz) to endow with erotic meaning or significance.

erotogenic (ĕ-ro″to-jen'ik) arousing sexual desire.

erotomania (ĕ-ro″to-ma'ne-ah) morbidly exaggerated sexual behavior.

erotophobia (ĕ-ro″to-fo'be-ah) morbid dread of sexual love.

errhine (er'īn) causing sneezing and secretion from the nose.

Ertron (er'tron) trademark for preparations of vitamin D₂.

eructation (e″ruk-ta'shun) the oral ejection of gas or air from the stomach.

eruption (e-rup'shun) emergence from beneath a surface, as of teeth through the gingivae or of lesions on the skin; applied also to various skin lesions not due to external injury. adj., **erup'tive.**
  creeping e., an eruption due to the larva of a fly or to a helminth; called also larva migrans.
  Kaposi's varicelliform e., a vesiculopustular eruption of viral origin, superimposed upon preexisting eczema.

erysipelas (er″ĭ-sip'ĕ-las) a febrile disease characterized by inflammation and redness of the skin and subcutaneous tissues, and due to Group A hemolytic streptococci.
  The visible symptoms of erysipelas, a form of cellulitis, are round or oval patches on the skin that promptly enlarge and spread, becoming swollen, tender and red. The affected skin is hot to the touch, and, occasionally, the adjacent skin blisters. Headache, vomiting, fever and sometimes complete prostration can occur. Sulfonamide compounds or antibiotics are used in the treatment. Care must be taken to avoid spreading the disease to other areas of the body.
  swine e., a rather unusual form of the disease that primarily affects domestic animals, particularly swine, but also other species including fish and shellfish. It may be transmitted to human beings through abrasive contact with either sick or healthy animals, or through skin injuries caused by articles that have been in contact with the animals. It is caused by a relatively harmless bacillus, *Erysipelothrix insidiosa*, and is characterized by bluish red swellings, usually on the hands. Called also erysipeloid.

erysipelatous (er″ĭ-sĭ-pel'ah-tus) of the nature of erysipelas.

erysipeloid (er″ĭ-sip'ĕ-loid) swine erysipelas.

Erysipelothrix (er″ĭ-sip'ĕ-lo-thriks″) a genus of Schizomycetes containing a single species.
  E. insidio'sa, a species of microorganisms occurring as gram-positive rods and filaments, the causative organism of swine erysipelas, or erysipeloid, and also infecting sheep, turkeys and rats; called also *E. rhusiopath'iae.* An erythematous-edematous lesion, commonly on the hand, resulting from contact with infected meat, hides or bones, represents the usual type of infection in man.

erythema (er″ĭ-the'mah) congestive or exudative redness of the skin caused by engorgement of the capillaries in the lower layers of the skin. It occurs with any skin injury, infection or inflammation.
  e. ab ig'ne, persistent erythema and pigmentation from long-continued exposure to excessive heat without burning.
  e. margina'tum, a type of erythema multiforme in which the reddened areas are disk-shaped, with elevated edges.
  e. mi'grans, geographic tongue.
  e. multifor'me, a disease state with highly polymorphic skin lesions, including macular papules, vesicles and bullae.
  toxic e., e. tox'icum, a generalized erythematous eruption due to administration of a drug or to bacterial toxins or other toxic substances.

erythematous (er″ĭ-them'ah-tus) of the nature of erythema.

erythr(o)- (ĕ-rith'ro) word element [Gr.], *red.*

erythrasma (er″ĭ-thraz'mah) a chronic infection of the skin, marked by development of red or brownish patches on the inner side of the thigh, on the scrotum and in the axilla.
  Baerensprung's e., tinea cruris affecting the thighs.

erythredema polyneuropathy (ĕ-rith″rĕ-de'mah pol'ĭ-nu-rop'ah-the) a condition occurring in infants, marked by swollen, bluish red hands and feet and disordered digestion, followed by multiple arthritis and muscular weakness; called also acrodynia.

erythremia (er"ĭ-thre'me-ah) polycythemia, a disease due to an excess of erythrocytes. adj., **erythrem'ic.**

erythrism (ĕ-rith'rizm) redness of the hair and beard. adj., **erythris'tic.**

erythrityl tetranitrate (ĕ-rith'rĭ-til tĕ"trah-ni'-trāt) a synthetic vasodilator.

erythroblast (ĕ-rith'ro-blast) an immature cell from which an erythrocyte, or red blood corpuscle, develops. adj., **erythroblas'tic.**

   basophilic e., a cell with a slightly clumped nuclear chromatin and basophilic cytoplasm without hemoglobin, which follows the pronormoblast developmentally.

   polychromatophilic e., a cell of the stage following the basophilic erythroblast, in which there is increased chromatin clumping and the earliest appearance of pink cytoplasmic hemoglobin.

erythroblastemia (ĕ-rith"ro-blas-te'me-ah) the presence in the peripheral blood of abnormally large numbers of nucleated red cells.

erythroblastoma (ĕ-rith"ro-blas-to'mah) a tumor arising from erythroblasts.

erythroblastomatosis (ĕ-rith"ro-blas"to-mah-to'-sis) a condition marked by the formation of erythroblastomas.

erythroblastopenia (ĕ-rith"ro-blas"to-pe'ne-ah) abnormal deficiency of erythroblasts.

erythroblastosis (ĕ-rith"ro-blas-to'sis) the presence of erythroblasts in the circulating blood.

   e. feta'lis, e. neonator'um, a blood dyscrasia of the newborn characterized by agglutination and hemolysis of erythrocytes and usually due to incompatibility between the infant's blood and the mother's. In most cases the fetus has Rh-positive blood and its mother has Rh-negative blood (see RH FACTOR). Called also hemolytic disease of the newborn.

   In Rh incompatibility the mother builds up immune bodies against the cells of the fetus; these bodies pass through the placenta, entering the fetal circulation. They then proceed to destroy the fetal erythrocytes very rapidly. In order to compensate for this rapid destruction of red blood cells, there is an ever increasing effort of the fetus to avoid anemia and death results in the release of very immature red blood cells (erythroblasts). Thus an extremely high percentage of the fetal erythrocytes are erythroblasts, and the condition is called erythroblastosis.

   SYMPTOMS. If the fetus survives under these circumstances, it is jaundiced and usually anemic at birth. The immune bodies from the mother's blood usually circulate in the baby's blood for 1 to 2 months after birth, continuing their destruction of red blood cells unless an exchange transfusion is done.

   Other symptoms depend on the number of red cells destroyed and the amount of damage done to other tissues of the body such as the brain and central nervous system.

   TREATMENT. The usual treatment for erythro-

blastosis fetalis is exchange transfusion in which the infant's blood is replaced with Rh-negative blood. The average amount used for transfusion of this kind is 400 ml. This measure stops the destruction of the infant's red cells, and gradually the Rh-negative blood is replaced with the baby's own blood. In about 6 weeks the immune bodies left over from the mother's blood have been destroyed and are no longer a menace to the baby.

   Recent developments in the management of erythroblastosis include AMNIOCENTESIS and intrauterine fetal TRANSFUSION. The former is puncture of the amniotic sac through the maternal abdomen and is done for the purpose of obtaining a sample of AMNIOTIC FLUID for analysis. This allows for determination of concentration of bilirubin pigments and protein in the amniotic fluid; a high concentration indicates excessive destruction of fetal erythrocytes. If there is a mild hemolysis the mother is watched closely and allowed to deliver at term. In more severe cases induced labor and premature delivery are usually advised so that further destruction of erythrocytes will not take place and an exchange transfusion can be performed as soon as possible. For cases of very severe hemolysis it has been recommended that an intrauterine transfusion be administered to the fetus. This is a very delicate procedure, not without risks, and advised only if the mother's past history and the present evidence indicate that the infant would not survive or would suffer damage from erythroblastosis. Both amniocentesis and intrauterine transfusion are hazardous procedures that should be performed only by trained personnel in well equipped medical centers.

erythrochloropia (ĕ-rith"ro-klo-ro'pe-ah) visual recognition of only red and green, not blue and yellow.

erythrochromia (ĕ-rith"ro-kro'me-ah) hemorrhagic, red pigmentation of the cerebrospinal fluid.

erythroclasis (er"ĭ-throk'lah-sis) fragmentation of the red blood corpuscles. adj., **erythroclas'tic.**

erythrocuprein (ĕ-rith"ro-koo'prin) a copperprotein compound contained in erythrocytes.

erythrocyanosis (ĕ-rith"ro-si"ah-no'sis) bluish or red discoloration of skin, with swelling, burning and itching.

erythrocyte (ĕ-rith'ro-sīt) a red blood cell, or corpuscle. adj., **erythrocyt'ic.** The erythrocytes are biconcave disks that have no nuclei and are about 7.7 microns in diameter. The cell when mature consists mainly of hemoglobin and a supporting framework called the stroma. Erythrocyte formation (erythropoiesis) takes place in the red bone marrow in the adult, and in the liver, spleen and bone marrow of the fetus. Erythrocyte formation requires an ample supply of certain dietary elements such as iron, cobalt and copper, amino acids and certain vitamins.

   The functions of erythrocytes include transportation of oxygen and carbon dioxide. They also are important in the maintenance of a normal acid-base balance, and, since they help determine the viscosity of the blood, they also influence its specific gravity.

   The average life span of a red blood cell is 120 days. Since they are subjected to much wear and tear in circulation they become more fragile and eventually are removed by cells of the reticuloendothelial system, particularly in liver, bone marrow and spleen. In spite of this constant destruction and production of red cells, the body maintains a fairly constant number of erythrocytes: between 4 and 5 million per cu. mm. of blood in women and 5 to 6 million per cu. mm. in men. A decreased number of erythrocytes constitutes one form of ANEMIA.

Red blood cells are destroyed whenever they are exposed to solutions that are not isotonic to blood plasma. If the erythrocyte is placed in a solution that is more dilute than plasma (distilled water for example) the cell will swell until osmotic pressure bursts the cell membrane. If the erythrocyte is placed in a solution more concentrated than plasma, the cell will lose water and shrivel or crenate. It is for this reason that solutions to be given intravenously must be isotonic to plasma.

e. sedimentation rate, an expression of the extent of settling of erythrocytes in a vertical column of blood per unit of time (see also SEDIMENTATION RATE).

erythrocythemia (ĕ-rith″ro-si-the′me-ah) increase in the number of erythrocytes in the blood.

erythrocytin (ĕ-rith″ro-si′tin) a substance in red cells thought to function in the first stage of blood clotting.

erythrocytolysis (ĕ-rith″ro-si-tol′ĭ-sis) dissolution of erythrocytes.

erythrocytometer (ĕ-rith″ro-si-tom′ĕ-ter) a device for measuring or counting erythrocytes.

erythrocyto-opsonin (ĕ-rith″ro-si″to-op-so′nin) an opsonin that acts on erythrocytes.

erythrocytorrhexis (ĕ-rith″ro-si″to-rek′sis) a morphologic change in erythrocytes, consisting in the escape from the cells of round, shining granules and splitting off of particles; called also plasmorrhexis.

erythrocytosis (ĕ-rith″ro-si-to′sis) increase in the number of erythrocytes as a result of a known stimulus; secondary polycythemia.

stress e., a relative polycythemia observed in anxiety-prone persons.

erythroderma (ĕ-rith″ro-der′mah) abnormal redness of the skin over widespread areas of the body.

atopic e., a chronic, diffuse dermatitis occurring in allergic infants.

congenital ichthyosiform e., a generalized hereditary dermatitis with scaling.

e. desquamati′vum, severe seborrheic dermatitis, leading to desquamation of skin and exposure of corium.

lymphoblastic e., a condition marked by chronic redness of the skin, associated with absolute leukocytosis, with relative increase in the lymphocytes.

lymphomatous e., widespread redness of the skin associated with lymphoma.

maculopapular e., a reddish eruption composed of maculae and papules.

psoriatic e., a generalized psoriasis, showing the chemical characteristics of exfoliative dermatitis.

squamous e., an eruption of scaly groups of papules.

erythrogenesis (ĕ-rith″ro-jen′ĕ-sis) the production of erythrocyte s.

e. imperfec′ta, congenital hypoplastic anemia.

erythrogenic (ĕ-rith″ro-jen′ik) 1. producing erythrocytes. 2. producing or causing a rash.

erythrogonium (ĕ-rith-ro-go′ne-um) a very immature erythroblast.

erythroid (er′ĭ-throid) of a red color.

erythrokinetics (ĕ-rith″ro-ki-net′iks) the quantitative, dynamic study of in-vivo production and destruction of erythrocytes.

erythroleukemia (ĕ-rith″ro-lu-ke′me-ah) a malignant blood dyscrasia with atypical erythroblasts and myeloblasts in the peripheral blood.

erythroleukosis (ĕ-rith″ro-lu-ko′sis) excessive formation of both erythrocytes and leukocytes in the blood.

erythrolysin (er″ĭ-throl′ĭ-sin) a substance capable of causing erythrocytolysis.

erythrolysis (er″ĭ-throl′ĭ-sis) erythrocytolysis; dissolution of erythrocytes.

erythromania (ĕ-rith″ro-ma′ne-ah) uncontrollable blushing.

erythromelalgia (ĕ-rith″ro-mel-al′je-ah) neuritis marked by burning pain and redness of the extremities.

erythromelia (ĕ-rith″ro-me′le-ah) progressive redness of the skin on the extensor surfaces of the legs and arms.

erythromycin (ĕ-rith″ro-mi′sin) an antibiotic obtained from *Streptomyces erythreus*. It is effective against a wide variety of organisms, including gram-negative and gram-positive bacteria and many rickettsial and viral infectious agents. It may be administered orally or parenterally.

erythron (er′ĭ-thron) the circulating erythrocytes and the erythrocyte-forming tissues of the body.

erythroneocytosis (ĕ-rith″ro-ne″o-si-to′sis) the presence of immature erythrocytes in the blood.

erythropenia (ĕ-rith″ro-pe′ne-ah) deficiency in the number of erythrocytes.

erythrophage (ĕ-rith′ro-fāj) a phagocyte that absorbs blood pigments and destroys erythrocytes.

erythrophil (ĕ-rith′ro-fil) an element that stains easily with red.

erythrophilous (er″ĭ-throf′ĭ-lus) easily staining red.

erythrophobia (ĕ-rith″ro-fo′be-ah) 1. morbid flushing. 2. morbid aversion to red.

erythrophthisis (ĕ-rith″ro-thi′sis) a condition characterized by severe impairment of the restorative power of the erythrocyte-forming tissues.

erythroplasia (ĕ-rith″ro-pla′ze-ah) a condition of mucous membrane characterized by erythematous papular lesions.

e. of Queyrat, a condition characterized by an erythematous papular lesion on the glans penis or prepuce.

erythropoiesis (ĕ-rith″ro-poi-e′sis) the formation of erythrocytes. adj., **erythropoiet′ic**.

erythropoietin (ĕ-rith″ro-poi′ĕ-tin) a factor in the plasma that stimulates the production of red cells.

erythroprecipitin (ĕ-rith″ro-pre-sip′ĭ-tin) a precipitin specific for erythrocytes.

erythroprosopalgia (ĕ-rith″ro-pros″o-pal′je-ah) a nervous disorder marked by redness and pain in the face.

erythropsia (er″ĭ-throp′se-ah) a defect of vision in which objects appear tinged with red.

erythropsin (er″ĭ-throp′sin) rhodopsin, the visual purple.

erythrosis (er″ĭ-thro′sis) reddish discoloration of the skin and mucous membranes.

erythrotoxin (ĕ-rith″ro-tok′sin) a toxin acting on erythrocytes.

erythruria (er″ĭ-throo′re-ah) excretion of red urine.

Es chemical symbol, *einsteinium.*

eschar (es′kar) a slough produced by burning or by a corrosive application.

escharotic (es-kah-rot′ik) 1. capable of producing an eschar; corrosive. 2. a corrosive or caustic agent.

Escherichia (esh″ĕ-rik′e-ah) a genus of Schizomycetes occasionally pathogenic for man.
 E. coli, a species of organisms constituting the greater part of the intestinal flora of man and other animals; called also colon bacillus. Pathogenic strains are the cause of many cases of urinary tract infections and of epidemic diarrheal diseases, especially in children.

eschrolalia (es″kro-la′le-ah) coprolalia; the use of foul language.

escutcheon (es-kuch′an) the pattern of distribution of the pubic hair.

eserine (es′er-ēn) physostigmine, a cholinesterase inhibitor.

Esidrix (es′ĭ-driks) trademark for a preparation of hydrochlorothiazide, a diuretic and antihypertensive.

-esis (e′sis) word element [Gr.], *state; condition.*

Eskabarb (es′kah-barb) trademark for a preparation of phenobarbital, a hypnotic and sedative.

Eskadiazine (es″kah-di′ah-zēn) trademark for a preparation of sulfadiazine, an antibacterial agent.

Esmarch bandage (es′mark) a rubber bandage used to render an operative area bloodless before operation.

eso- (es′o) word element [Gr.], *within.*

esoethmoiditis (es″o-eth″moi-di′tis) inflammation of the ethmoid sinuses.

esogastritis (es″o-gas-tri′tis) inflammation of the gastric mucosa.

esophageal (e-sof″ah-je′al) pertaining to the esophagus.

esophagectasia (e-sof″ah-jek-ta′ze-ah) dilatation of the esophagus.

esophagectomy (e-sof″ah-jek′to-me) excision of the esophagus.

esophagism (e-sof′ah-jism) spasm of the esophagus.

esophagitis (e-sof″ah-ji′tis) inflammation of the ESOPHAGUS.
 peptic e., inflammation of the esophagus due to a reflux of acid and pepsin from the stomach.

esophagobronchial (e-sof″ah-go-brong′ke-al) pertaining to or communicating with the esophagus and a bronchus.

esophagocele (e-sof′ah-go-sēl″) esophageal hernia.

esophagoduodenostomy (e-sof″ah-go-du″o-dĕ-nos′to-me) anastomosis of the esophagus to the duodenum.

esophagodynia (e-sof″ah-go-din′e-ah) pain in the esophagus.

esophagoenterostomy (e-sof″ah-go-en″ter-os′-to-me) creation of an opening between the esophagus and a part of the intestine.

esophagoesophagostomy (e-sof″ah-go-e-sof″ah-gos′to-me) anastomosis between two normally remote parts of the esophagus.

esophagogastrectomy (e-sof″ah-go-gas-trek′to-me) excision of the esophagus and stomach.

esophagogastroanastomosis (e-sof″ah-go-gas″-tro-ah-nas″to-mo′sis) esophagogastrostomy.

esophagogastroplasty (e-sof″ah-go-gas′tro-plas″te) plastic repair of the esophagus and stomach.

esophagogastroscopy (e-sof″ah-go-gas-tros′ko-pe) endoscopic inspection of the esophagus and stomach.

esophagogastrostomy (e-sof″ah-go-gas-tros′to-me) anastomosis of the esophagus to the stomach.

esophagography (e-sof″ah-gog′rah-fe) roentgenography of the esophagus.

esophagojejunoplasty (e-sof″ah-go-je-joo′no-plas″te) restoration of the esophagus with a segment of jejunum.

esophagojejunostomy (e-sof″ah-go-je″joo-nos′to-me) anastomosis of the esophagus to the jejunum.

esophagolaryngectomy (e-sof″ah-go-lar″in-jek′-to-me) excision of the upper cervical esophagus and larynx.

esophagomalacia (e-sof″ah-go-mah-la′she-ah) softening of the walls of the esophagus.

esophagometer (e-sof″ah-gom′ĕ-ter) an instrument for measuring the esophagus.

esophagomyotomy (e-sof″ah-go-mi-ot′o-me) incision through the muscular coat of the esophagus.

esophagoplasty (e-sof′ah-go-plas″te) plastic repair of the esophagus.

esophagoplication (e-sof″ah-go-pli-ka′shun) infolding of the wall of an esophageal pouch.

esophagoptosis (e-sof"ah-gop-to'sis) prolapse of the esophagus.

esophagorespiratory (e-sof"ah-go-re-spi'rah-to"-re) pertaining to or communicating with the esophagus and respiratory tract (trachea or a bronchus).

esophagoscope (e-sof'ah-go-skōp") an endoscope for examination of the esophagus.

esophagoscopy (e-sof"ah-gos'ko-pe) direct visual examination of the esophagus with an esophagoscope. Esophagoscopy usually is done as a diagnostic procedure for the purpose of locating and inspecting a disorder of the esophagus. After the esophagoscope has been inserted it is possible to obtain samples of tissue for microscopic study. In some instances the esophagoscope can be used to remove a foreign object that has become lodged in the esophagus.

NURSING CARE. Food and liquids are withheld for at least 6 hours prior to the procedure so that the stomach will be empty and there will be no regurgitation during the procedure. An operative permit should be signed before this examination is done. Sedatives are usually given about an hour before the procedure to relax the patient and help him cooperate with the physician. Although the procedure is not painful, it is uncomfortable and difficult for the patient. The throat is anesthetized with a local anesthetic such as cocaine or tetracaine (Pontocaine) to depress the gag reflex and reduce local reaction to the passage of the instrument. Since there may be some toxic reaction to the local anesthetic the patient should be observed carefully for dyspnea, excitement, dizziness or headache and an emergency tray containing barbiturates should be readily available.

The patient is placed on his back with his head and shoulders extending over the edge of the treatment table. The patient's head is supported by an attendant and if it seems likely that he will move about he is restrained. This is necessary because a sudden movement might cause perforation of the esophagus.

Food and fluids are withheld for several hours after the procedure is completed, and the patient is instructed not to take anything by mouth until the gag reflex has returned. This is necessary because there is danger of aspiration as long as the gag reflex is depressed. Hoarseness and a sore throat usually remain for a few days after the examination.

esophagostenosis (e-sof"ah-go-stĕ-no'sis) stricture of the esophagus.

esophagostomy (e-sof"ah-gos'to-me) the creation of an artificial opening into the esophagus.

esophagotomy (e-sof"ah-got'o-me) incision of the esophagus.

esophagotracheal (e-sof"ah-go-tra'ke-al) pertaining to or communicating with the esophagus and trachea.

esophagus (e-sof'ah-gus) the hollow muscular tube extending from the pharynx to the stomach, consisting of an outer fibrous coat, a muscular layer, a submucous layer and an inner mucous membrane. The junction between the stomach and esophagus is closed by a muscular ring known as the cardiac sphincter, which opens to allow the passage of food into the stomach. In an adult the esophagus is usually 10 to 12 inches long. (See also DIGESTIVE SYSTEM.)

Disorders of the esophagus often involve either an obstruction or a reflux (backward flow) of food and gastric juices. Foreign bodies, accidentally swallowed and lodged in the esophageal passage, can obstruct the flow of foods and fluids, as can malignant or benign tumors. The term ACHALASIA is used to describe a particular disturbance in motility which leads to obstruction at the level of the cardiac sphincter.

Esophagitis, inflammation of the mucous membrane lining the esophagus, may occur in conjunction with gastroenteritis, or as a result of a backward flow of the gastric contents upward into the esophagus. The symptoms of hiatus hernia are due in large part to this type of reflux. Hiatus hernia is a protrusion of the stomach, colon or other intestinal organs through the esophageal hiatus, a narrow opening in the diaphragm through which the esophagus normally passes. When the herniation occurs the normal downward passage of food is interrupted.

Esophageal varices are varicose veins of the esophagus and occur most often as a result of obstruction in the portal circulation, especially in portal hypertension. These varices are potentially dangerous since they tend to rupture easily and may result in serious hemorrhage.

Visual examination of the interior lining of the esophagus is accomplished by ESOPHAGOSCOPY.

esosphenoiditis (es"o-sfe"noi-di'tis) osteomyelitis of the sphenoid bone.

esotropia (es"o-tro'pe-ah) deviation of a visual axis toward that of the other eye when fusion is a possibility.

E.S.P. extrasensory perception.

E.S.R. erythrocyte sedimentation rate.

essence (es'ens) 1. the distinctive or individual principle of anything. 2. a mixture of alcohol with a volatile oil.

essential (ĕ-sen'shal) 1. constituting the necessary or inherent part of a thing. 2. idiopathic; self-existing; having no obvious external exciting cause.

E.S.T. electroshock therapy.

ester (es'ter) a compound formed from an alcohol and an acid by removal of water.

esterase (es'ter-ās) an enzyme that catalyzes the hydrolysis of esters.

esterification (es-ter"i-fi-ka'shun) conversion of an acid into an ester by combination with an alcohol and removal of a molecule of water.

esterolysis (es"ter-ol'i-sis) the hydrolysis of an ester into its alcohol and acid. adj., **esterolyt'ic.**

esthematology (es"them-ah-tol'o-je) esthesiology.

esthesioblast (es-the'ze-o-blast") ganglioblast, an embryonic cell of the spinal ganglia.

esthesiology (es-the"ze-ol'o-je) the scientific study or description of the sense organs and sensations.

esthesiomania (es-the"ze-o-ma'ne-ah) mental disorder with perverted moral sense.

esthesiometer   (es-the″ze-om′ĕ-ter) an instrument for measuring tactile sensibility.

esthesioneurosis (es-the″ze-o-nu-ro′sis) disease of the sensory nerves.

esthesiophysiology (es-the″ze-o-fiz″e-ol′o-je) the physiology of sensation and sense organs.

esthesioscopy (es-the″ze-os′ko-pe) marking on the skin of areas in which pain is felt.

estheticokinetic   (es-thet″ĭ-ko-ki-net′ik) both sensory and motor.

estradiol (es″trah-di′ol, es-tra′de-ol) an estrogenic compound available as **e. benzoate**, used for parenteral injection; **e. dipropionate**, which is absorbed more slowly; or **e. valerate**, a form used for oral administration.

estrin (es′trin) an estrogenic hormone.

estrinization   (es″trin-ĭ-za′shun) production of the cellular changes in the vaginal epithelium characteristic of estrus.

estrogen (es′tro-jen) 1. an estrus-producing substance. 2. a general name for the principal female sex hormones. These hormones are manufactured in the ovaries and, though each has a slightly different function, they are closely related and are usually referred to collectively as estrogen.
   Estrogen is responsible for development of the reproductive organs and secondary sex characters of the female. The production of natural estrogen is intensified during ovulation, pregnancy and menstruation.
   Synthetic preparations of estrogens may be used therapeutically in the relief of menopausal symptoms and in the treatment of prostatic cancer and breast cancer. They are also used to suppress lactation in women following delivery. In some cases they are helpful in relieving vaginitis.

estrogenic   (es″tro-jen′ik) producing estrus.

estrone (es′trōn) an estrogenic steroid isolated from the urine of pregnant animals.

estrous   (es′trus) having the characteristics of estrus.

estruation (es″troo-a′shun) the state of being in estrus.

Estrugenone (es″troo-jen′ōn) trademark for a preparation of estrone.

estrum (es′trum) any form of recurrent excitement.

estrus (es′trus) 1. the recurrent period of sexual excitement in adult female mammals. 2. the cycle of changes in the reproductive organs produced as a result of ovarian hormonal activity. adj., **es′trual.**

e.s.u. electrostatic unit.

Etamon (et′ah-mon) trademark for a solution of tetraethylammonium (chloride), a ganglionic blocking agent.

ethacrynic acid (eth″ah-krin′ik) a powerful diuretic used orally or parenterally, and effective in promoting sodium and chloride excretion.

ethamivan (ĕ-tham′ĭ-van) a compound used as a respiratory stimulant and to hasten recovery from general anesthesia.

ethanol (eth′ah-nol) the major ingredient of alcoholic beverages; called also ethyl alcohol and grain alcohol.

ethaverine (eth″ah-ver′ēn) a compound used as a relaxant for vascular smooth muscle.

ethchlorvynol (eth-klōr′vĭ-nol) a hypnotic and sedative compound.

ethene (eth′ēn) ethylene.

ether (e′ther) 1. the subtle fluid believed to fill all space. 2. a colorless, transparent, volatile liquid, used by inhalation to produce general ANESTHESIA; called also ethyl ether.
   nitrofurfuryl methyl e., a compound used as a topical fungicide and sporicide for skin infections.
   vinyl e., a clear liquid anesthetic compound used by inhalation to produce general anesthesia.

ethereal (e-the′re-al) 1. pertaining to, prepared with, containing or resembling ether. 2. vanishing; unstable; delicate.

etherization   (e″ther-ĭ-za′shun) induction of anesthesia by means of ether.

ethinamate (ĕ-thin′ah-māt) a compound used as a hypnotic.

ethinyl trichloride (eth′ĭ-nil) trichloroethylene, an anesthetic.

ethisterone (ĕ-this′ter-ōn) a progestational steroid.

ethmocarditis (eth″mo-kar-di′tis) inflammation of the connective tissue of the heart.

ethmoid (eth′moid) sievelike; cribriform.
   e. bone, the sievelike bone that forms a roof for the nasal fossae and part of the floor of the anterior cranial fossa.

ethmoidal (eth-moi′dal) pertaining to the ethmoid bone.

ethmoidectomy (eth″moi-dek′to-me) excision of the ethmoid bone.

ethmoiditis (eth″moi-di′tis) inflammation of the ethmoid bone.

ethmoidotomy (eth″moi-dot′o-me) incision of the ethmoid bone.

ethnic (eth′nik) pertaining to the races of mankind.

ethnobiology   (eth″no-bi-ol′o-je) the scientific study of physical characteristics of different races of mankind.

ethnology (eth-nol′o-je) the science dealing with comparison and analytical study of the human races.

ethoheptazine (eth″o-hep′tah-zēn) a compound used as an analgesic.

ethohexadiol (eth″o-heks-a′de-ol) a compound used as an insect repellant.

ethology (e-thol′o-je) the scientific study of animal behavior.

ethopropazine (eth"o-pro'pah-zēn) a phenothiazine compound used to produce parasympathetic blockade and to reduce tremors in Parkinson's disease.

ethosuximide (eth"o-suk'sǐ-mīd) a compound used as an anticonvulsant in treatment of petit mal epilepsy.

ethotoin (e-tho'to-in) a compound used as an anticonvulsant in grand mal epilepsy.

ethoxazene (eth-ok'sah-zēn) a compound used to relieve pain associated with chronic urinary tract infections.

ethoxzolamide (eth"ok-zol'ah-mīd) a diuretic of the carbonic anhydrase inhibitor type, used mainly in edema, glaucoma and epilepsy.

ethyl (eth'il) the common alcohol radical, C_2H_5.
  e. acetate, a transparent, colorless liquid used as a flavoring agent.
  e. alcohol, alcohol, the major ingredient of alcoholic beverages; called also ethanol and grain alcohol.
  e. aminobenzoate, a white, crystalline substance used as a topical anesthetic.
  e. biscoumacetate, a white, odorless, bitter, crystalline solid used as an anticoagulant.
  e. bromide, a colorless, volatile liquid having anesthetic properties.
  e. carbamate, urethan.
  e. chloride, a colorless, volatile liquid used as a general and a topical anesthetic.
  e. oxide, a transparent, colorless liquid used as a solvent.
  e. phenylephrine, effortil.
  e. vanillin, fine white or slightly yellowish crystals used as a flavoring agent.

ethylene (eth'ǐ-lēn) a colorless, highly flammable gas with a slightly sweet taste and odor, used for inducing general ANESTHESIA.

ethylenediamine (eth'ǐ-lēn-di"ah-mēn) a volatile, colorless liquid with an ammonia odor that is used as a solvent and in organic synthesis.

ethylmorphine hydrochloride (eth"il-mor'fēn) a white or faintly yellow microcrystalline powder; used as a narcotic and antitussive.

ethylnorepinephrine (eth"il-nor-ep"ǐ-nef'rin) a compound used as a sympathomimetic and in treatment of bronchial asthma; called also ethylnoradrenaline and ethylnorsuprarenin.

ethylstibamine (eth"il-stib'ah-mēn) a synthetic antimony compound used in treatment of cutaneous leishmaniasis.

ethynylestradiol (eth"ǐ-nil-es"trah-di'ol) a derivative of estradiol used for oral administration.

etiology (e"te-ol'o-je) the science dealing with causes of disease. adj., **etiolog'ic.**

etioporphyrin (e"te-o-por'fǐ-rin) a porphyrin obtained from hematoporphyrin.

Eu chemical symbol, *europium.*

eu- (u) word element [Gr.], *normal; good; well; easy.*

Eubacteriales (u"bak-te"re-a'lēz) an order of Schizomycetes comprising the true bacteria.

Eubacterium (u"bak-te're-um) a genus of Schizomycetes found in the intestinal tract as parasites and as saprophytes in soil and water.

eubiotics (u"bi-ot'iks) the science of healthy living.

eubolism (u'bo-lizm) a condition of normal metabolism.

eucalyptol (u"kah-lip'tol) a colorless liquid obtained from eucalyptus oil and other sources; used as an expectorant and flavoring agent.

eucalyptus oil (u"kah-lip'tus) a volatile oil from fresh leaf of species of Eucalyptus; used as a flavoring agent.

eucatropine (u-kat'ro-pēn) a compound used as a mydriatic.

euchlorhydria (u"klōr-hi'dre-ah) the presence of the normal amount of acid in the gastric juice.

eucholia (u-ko'le-ah) normal condition of the bile.

euchromatin (u-kro'mah-tin) the gene-bearing fraction of chromatin, composed of deoxyribonucleic acid (DNA) with higher proteins of the globulin type.

eucrasia (u-kra'ze-ah) the proper balance of different factors constituting a healthy state.

eudiemorrhysis (u"di-ě-mor'ǐ-sis) the normal flow of blood through the capillaries.

eudiometer (u"de-om'ě-ter) an instrument for measuring and analyzing gases.

eudipsia (u-dip'se-ah) ordinary, normal thirst.

euergasia (u"er-ga'ze-ah) normal mental functioning.

euesthesia (u"es-the'ze-ah) a normal state of the senses.

eugamy (u'gah-me) the union of gametes each of which contains the proper complement of chromosomes.

eugenics (u-jen'iks) the scientific study and practice of principles that will improve the hereditary qualities of future generations.
  negative e., that concerned with prevention of reproduction by individuals having inferior or undesirable traits.
  positive e., that concerned with promotion of optimal mating and reproduction by individuals having desirable or superior traits.

eugenol (u'jě-nol) a phenol from clove oil and other sources, used as a dental analgesic.

euglobulin (u-glob'u-lin) one of a class of globulins characterized by being insoluble in water but soluble in saline solutions.

euglycemia (u"gli-se'me-ah) a normal level of glucose in the blood.

eugonic (u-gon'ik) growing luxuriantly; said of bacteria.

eukaryosis (u"kar-e-o'sis) the state of having a true nucleus.

eukinesia (u″ki-ne′ze-ah) normal or proper motor function or activity. adj., **eukinet′ic.**

Eulenburg's disease (oil′en-burgz) myotonia congenita.

eumetria (u-me′tre-ah) a normal condition of nerve impulse, so that a voluntary movement just reaches the intended goal; the proper range of movement.

eunuch (u′nuk) a castrated male.

eunuchoid (u′nŭ-koid) 1. resembling a eunuch. 2. a person who resembles a eunuch.

eupancreatism (u-pan′kre-ah-tizm″) normal functioning of the pancreas.

eupepsia (u-pep′se-ah) good digestion. adj., **eupep′tic.**

euphoretic (u″fo-ret′ik) 1. pertaining to or characterized by euphoria. 2. an agent that produces euphoria.

euphoria (u-fo′re-ah) a subjectively pleasant feeling of well-being, marked by confidence and assurance. adj., **euphor′ic.**

euphoriant (u-for′e-ant) 1. conducive to a feeling of well-being. 2. an agent that is conducive to a feeling of well-being.

eupiesis (u″pi-e′sis) normal pressure. adj., **eupiet′ic.**

euplastic (u-plas′tik) forming sound tissues.

euploidy (u′ploi-de) the state of having a balanced set or sets of chromosomes, in any number.

eupnea (ūp-ne′ah) normal respiration. adj., **eupne′ic.**

eupraxia (u-prak′se-ah) intactness of reproduction of coordinated movements. adj., **euprac′tic.**

eupyrexia (u-pi-rek′se-ah) a slight fever in the early stage of an infection.

Eurax (u′raks) trademark for preparations of crotamiton, used in the treatment of scabies.

eurhythmia (u-rith′me-ah) regularity of the pulse.

europium (u-ro′pe-um) a chemical element, atomic number 63, atomic weight 151.96, symbol Eu. (See table of ELEMENTS.)

Eurotium (u-ro′she-um) a genus of fungi or molds.

eury- (u′re) word element [Gr.], *wide; broad.*

eurycephalic (u″rĭ-sĕ-fal′ik) having a wide head.

euryon (u′re-on) a point on either parietal bone marking either end of the greatest transverse diameter of the skull.

euscope (u′skōp) a device for projecting the image of a microscopic field upon a screen.

eusitia (u-sish′e-ah) normal appetite.

eustachian tube (u-sta′ke-an) a narrow channel that connects the tympanum with the nasopharynx. The eustachian tube serves to equalize pressure on either side of the tympanic membrane (eardrum). In children this tube is wider and shorter than in adults, and thus children are especially prone to infections of the middle ear that originate in the pharynx and travel through the tube.

euthanasia (u″thah-na′ze-ah) 1. an easy death. 2. the painless induction of death in a patient with an incurable disease or condition; called also mercy killing.

euthenics (u-then′iks) the science of race improvement by regulation of environment.

euthermy (u-ther′me) the state of being tolerant of a wide range of temperature. adj., **euther′mic.**

euthyroid (u-thi′roid) characterized by normal activity (secretion) of the thyroid gland.

eutocia (u-to′she-ah) natural or normal parturition.

Eutrombicula (u″trom-bik′u-lah) a genus of mites. **E. alfreddugè′si,** *Trombicula alfreddugèsi,* the chigger.

eutrophia (u-tro′fe-ah) a state of normal nutrition.

evacuant (e-vak′u-ant) 1. promoting evacuation. 2. an agent that promotes evacuation.

evacuation (e-vak″u-a′shun) 1. removal, especially the removal of any material from the body by discharge through a natural or artificial passage. 2. material discharged from the body, especially the discharge from the bowels.

evagination (e-vaj″ĭ-na′shun) protrusion of a part or organ.

Evans blue (ev′anz) an odorless green, bluish green or brown powder dye, used as a diagnostic aid in estimation of blood volume. The dye is injected into the bloodstream and after a sufficient period of time samples of the blood are taken to determine the degree of dilution of the dye.

eventration (e″ven-tra′shun) 1. protrusion of abdominal viscera. 2. removal of abdominal viscera. **e. of the diaphragm,** elevation of the diaphragm into the thoracic cavity.

eversion (e-ver′zhun) a turning outward.

Evipal (e′vĭ-pal) trademark for a preparation of hexobarbital, an ultra-short-acting barbiturate.

evisceration (e-vis″er-a′shun) removal of the viscera or the internal contents of a body, as removal of the contents of the eyeball.

evolution (ev″o-lu′shun) a process of development in which an organ or organism becomes more and more complex by the differentiation of its parts; a continuous and progressive change according to certain laws and by means of resident forces. **convergent e.,** the development, in animals that are only distantly related, of similar structures in adaptation to similar environment. **organic e.,** the evolution of living things; the theory that organisms now living have developed by gradual modifications from simpler organisms.

evulsion (e-vul′shun) forcible tearing away of a part.

ex (eks)[L.] preposition, *out; away from.*

exacerbation (eg-zas″er-ba′shun) increase in severity.

exacrinous (eks-ak′rĭ-nus) pertaining to external secretion of a gland.

examination (eg-zam″ĭ-na′shun) inspection and investigation of a patient as a means of diagnosing disease.

physical e., examination of the bodily state of a patient by ordinary physical means, as inspection, palpation, percussion and auscultation.

exanthem (eg-zan′them) an eruption or rash on the skin.

e. sub′itum, an acute viral disease of infants, with fever and a macular or maculopapular eruption (see also ROSEOLA INFANTUM).

exanthema (eg″zan-the′mah), pl. *exanthem′ata* [Gr.] exanthem.

exanthematous (eg″zan-them′ah-tus) characterized by an eruption or rash.

exanthrope (ek′zan-thrōp) a source of disease outside the body.

exarteritis (eks″ar-ter-i′tis) inflammation of the outer arterial coat.

exarticulation (eks″ar-tik″u-la′shun) amputation at a joint.

excavation (eks″kah-va′shun) 1. the act of hollowing out. 2. a hollowed-out space, or pouchlike cavity.

atrophic e., cupping of the optic disk, due to atrophy of the optic nerve fibers.

excavator (eks′kah-va″tor) a scoop or gouge for surgeons' use.

excentric (ek-sen′trik) out of, or away from, a center.

excerebration (ek″ser-ĕ-bra′shun) removal of the brain.

excipient (ek-sip′e-ent) a gummy or syrupy material in which an active ingredient (powder) is incorporated to be made into pills.

excise (ek-sīz′) to remove by cutting.

excision (ek-sizh′un) removal by cutting out or off, often applied to surgical removal of an entire organ or body structure.

excitability (ek-sīt″ah-bil′ĭ-te) readiness to respond to a stimulus; irritability.

excitant (ek-sīt′ant) a medicine that arouses functional activity.

excitation (ek″si-ta′shun) stimulation or irritation.

direct e., stimulation of a muscle by means of an electrode on the muscle substance.

indirect e., stimulation of a muscle through stimulation of its nerve.

excitomotor (ek-si″to-mo′tor) arousing muscular activity.

excitonutrient (ek-si″to-nu′tre-ent) stimulating nutrition.

excitor (ek-si′tor) a nerve that stimulates a part to greater activity.

excitosecretory (ek-si″to-se-kre′to-re) producing increased secretion.

excitovascular (ek-si″to-vas′ku-lar) causing vascular changes.

exclave (eks′klāv) a detached part of an organ.

exclusion (ek-skloo′zhun) surgical isolation of a part, as of a segment of intestine, without removal from the body.

excoriation (ek″sko-re-a′shun) any superficial loss of substance, such as that produced on the skin by scratching.

excrement (ek′skrĕ-ment) excreted or fecal matter.

excrementitious (ek″skrĕ-men-tish′us) pertaining to excrement.

excrescence (ek-skres′ens) an abnormal outgrowth.

excreta (ek-skre′tah) waste material excreted or eliminated from the body, including FECES, URINE and PERSPIRATION. Mucus and carbon dioxide also can be considered excreta. The organs of excretion are the intestinal tract, kidneys, lungs and skin.

excrete (ek-skrēt′) to separate and eliminate useless matter.

excretion (ek-skre′shun) the elimination of waste products from the body. Ordinarily, what is meant by excretion is the evacuation of feces. Technically, excretion can refer to the expulsion of any matter, whether from a single cell or from the entire body, or to the matter excreted. adj., **ex′cretory.**

excursion (ek-skur′zhun) a range of movement regularly repeated in performance of a function, e.g., excursion of the jaws in mastication. adj., **excur′sive.**

excystation (ek″sis-ta′shun) escape or removal from a cyst.

exercise (ek′ser-sīz) performance of physical exertion for improvement of health or correction of physical deformity.

active e., motion imparted to a part by voluntary contraction and relaxation of its controlling muscles.

active resistive e., motion voluntarily imparted to a part against resistance.

muscle-setting e., static exercise.

passive e., motion imparted to a part by another person or outside force, without voluntary participation by the patient.

range of motion e's, exercises designed to keep the joints mobile and functioning normally.

static e., active contraction and relaxation of a muscle or group of muscles without producing motion of a joint that it ordinarily mobilizes.

exeresis (ek-ser′ĕ-sis) removal of a nerve, vessel or other part or organ.

exergonic (ek″ser-gon′ik) accompanied by the release of free energy.

exfoliation (eks-fo″le-a′shun) separation of fragments of dead bone or of skin in scales.

exhalation (eks″hah-la′shun) 1. the expulsion of air or other vapor from the lungs. 2. escape in the form of vapor. 3. vapor escaping from a body or substance.

exhaustion (eg-zos′chun) loss of ability to react or to function because of continued stimulation or activity.

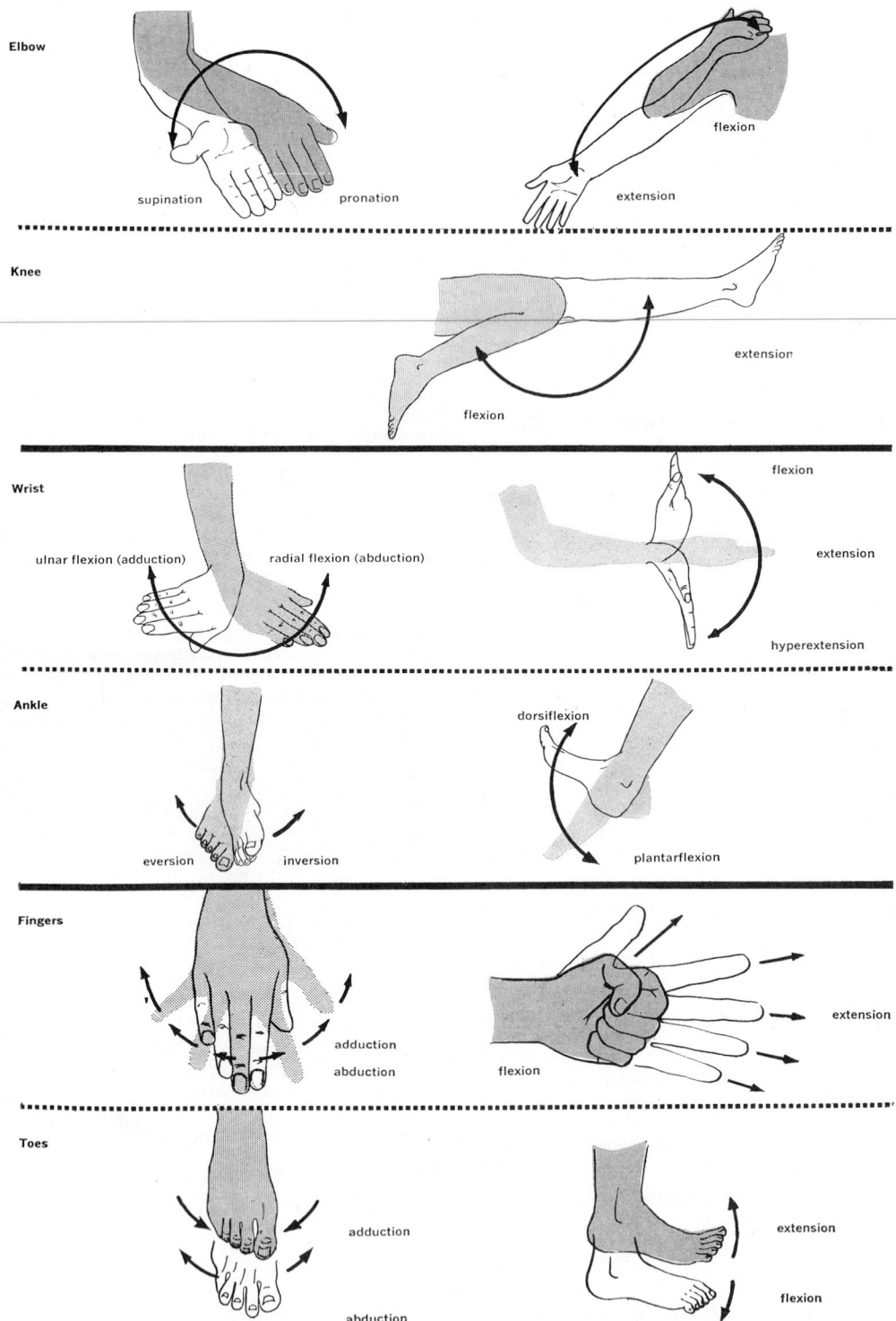

Ranges of motion. All exercises can be performed from the supine position in bed except hyperextension of the spine, hips and shoulders and flexion of the knees, for which the person must lie prone or on his side. (From Kelly, M. M.: Exercises for bedfast patients. Amer. J. Nursing, *66*:2209, 1966.)

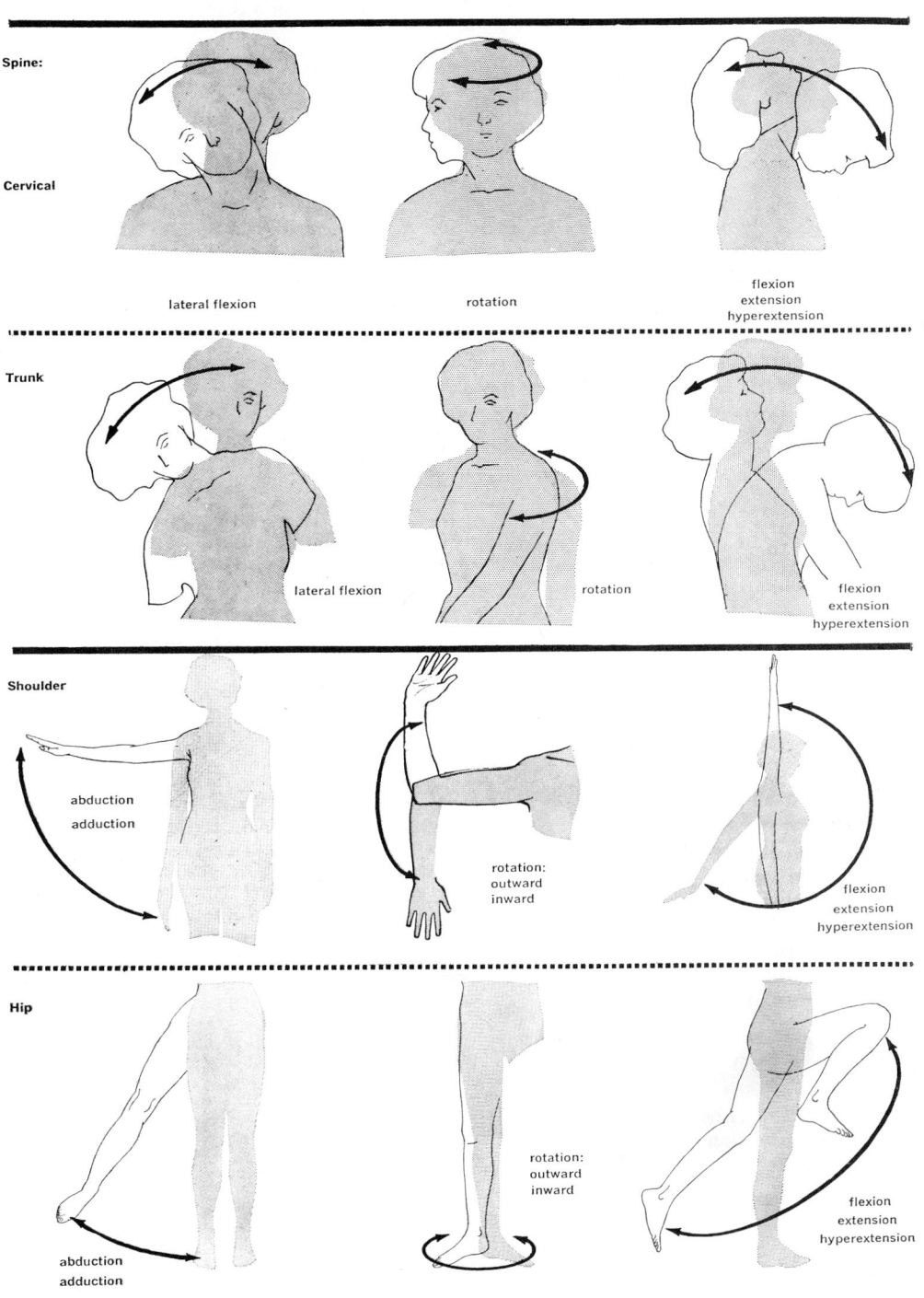

Spine:

Cervical

lateral flexion   rotation   flexion
extension
hyperextension

Trunk

lateral flexion   rotation   flexion
extension
hyperextension

Shoulder

abduction
adduction

rotation:
outward
inward

flexion
extension
hyperextension

Hip

abduction
adduction

rotation:
outward
inward

flexion
extension
hyperextension

heat e., a condition caused by exposure to excessive heat (see also HEAT EXHAUSTION).

exhibitionism (ek″sĭ-bish′ĕ-nizm) an abnormal tendency to make a display of one's self, in its severest form leading to exposure of the genitalia. It is more common in men than in women, and in adults it is difficult to correct. It may be resorted to by an individual who is unable for physical or psychologic reasons to gain sexual gratification by normal means. A common cause is a feeling of sexual inadequacy; for this the exposure is a compensation. Exhibitionism may also be a form of masochism in which a feeling of guilt drives the person to behavior for which he knows he will be punished. Psychotherapy is necessary to deal with this type of sexual deviation.

exhibitionist (ek″sĭ-bish′ĕ-nist) a person who indulges in exhibitionism.

exo- (ek′so) word element [Gr.], *outside of; outward.*

exobiology (ek″so-bi-ol′o-je) the science concerned with study of life on planets other than the earth.

exocardia (ek″so-kar′de-ah) abnormal position of the heart.

exocardial (ek″so-kar′de-al) 1. situated outside the heart. 2. pertaining to exocardia.

exocolitis (ek″so-ko-li′tis) inflammation of the outer coat of the colon.

exocrine (ek′so-krin) secreting externally.

exocrinology (ek″so-krĭ-nol′o-je) the study of substances secreted externally by individuals which effect integration of a group of organisms.

exodeviation (ek″so-de″ve-a′shun) a turning outward.

exodontics (ek″so-don′tiks) that branch of dentistry dealing with extraction of teeth.

exoenzyme (ek″so-en′zīm) an enzyme that acts outside the cell that secretes it.

exoerythrocytic (ek″so-ĕ-rith″ro-sit′ik) occurring or situated outside the red blood cells (erythrocytes), a term applied to a stage in the development of certain malarial parasites that takes place in tissue cells instead of in erythrocytes.

exogamy (ek-sog′ah-me) 1. fertilization by union of elements derived from different cells. 2. heterosexuality.

exogastritis (ek″so-gas-tri′tis) inflammation of the external coat of the stomach.

exogenous (ek-soj′ĕ-nus) originating outside or caused by factors outside the organism.

exometritis (ek″so-me-tri′tis) inflammation of the outer surface of the uterus.

exomphalos (ek-som′fah-lus) undue prominence of the navel.

exopathic (ek″so-path′ik) originating outside the body.

exopeptidase (ek″so-pep′tĭ-dās) a proteolytic enzyme whose action is limited to terminal peptide linkages.

exophthalmia, exophthalmos (ek″sof-thal′me-ah), (ek″sof-thal′mos) abnormal protrusion of the eye. adj., **exophthal′mic.** It results in a marked stare and is usually due to an overactive thyroid gland. Occasionally the condition is caused by an infection of the eye or a tumor behind the eye.

exophylaxis (ek″so-fi-lak′sis) protective against disease from the outside. adj., **exophylac′tic.**

exophytic (ek″so-fit′ik) growing outward; proliferating externally or on the surface of an organ or other structure.

exoplasm (ek′so-plazm) the peripheral part of the protoplasm of a cell.

exorbitism (ek-sor′bĭ-tizm) protrusion of the eyeball.

exormia (ek-sor′me-ah) a papular skin eruption.

exoserosis (ek″so-se-ro′sis) an oozing of serum or exudate.

exoskeleton (ek″so-skel′ĕ-ton) an external hard framework that supports and protects the soft tissues of lower animals, derived from the ectoderm. In vertebrates the term is sometimes applied to structures produced by the epidermis, as hair, nails, hoofs, teeth, etc.

exosmosis (ek″sos-mo′sis) osmosis or diffusion from within outward.

exostosis (ek″sos-to′sis), pl. *exosto′ses* [Gr.] a benign new growth protruding from the outer contour of bones and characteristically capped by growing cartilage.
   e. mul′tiplex cartilagin′ea, dyschondroplasia.

exothermal, exothermic (ek″so-ther′mal) (ek″so-ther′mik) marked by the evolution of heat; liberating heat.

exotoxin (ek″so-tok′sin) a toxic substance formed by bacteria that is found outside the bacterial cell, or free in the culture medium. adj., **exotox′ic.** Exotoxins are heat labile, and protein in nature. They are detoxified with retention of antigenicity by treatment with formaldehyde, and are the most poisonous substances known to man. Bacteria of the genus Clostridium are the most frequent producers of exotoxins, and diphtheria, botulism and tetanus are all caused by such toxins.

exotropia (ek″so-tro′pe-ah) deviation of a visual axis away from that of the other eye when fusion is a possibility; called also divergent strabismus and walleye.

expander (ek-span′der) an agent that increases volume or bulk.
   plasma volume e., a solution given instead of blood transfusion, to increase the volume of fluid circulating in the blood vessels.

expectorant (ek-spek′to-rant) 1. promoting expectoration. 2. an agent that promotes expectoration.
   liquefying e., an expectorant that promotes the ejection of mucus from the respiratory tract by decreasing the viscosity of that already present.

expectoration (ek-spek″to-ra′shun) the ejection

of sputum and other materials from the air passages.

experiment (ek-sper'ĭ-ment) a procedure undertaken to discover or demonstrate some fact or general truth. adj., **experimen'tal.**

 check e., crucial experiment.

 control e., one made under standard conditions, to test the correctness of other observations.

 crucial e., one so designed and prepared for by previous work that it will settle some point.

expiration (ek"spĭ-ra'shun) the expulsion of air or other vapor from the lungs. adj., **expi'ratory.**

expire (ek-spīr') 1. to breathe out. 2. to die.

explant 1. (eks-plant') to take from the body and place in an artificial medium for growth. 2. (eks'plant) material taken from the body and grown in an artificial medium.

expression (eks-presh'un) 1. the act of squeezing out. 2. the process of making manifest, especially the revelation of emotions on the face.

expressivity (eks"pres-siv'ĭ-te) the extent to which a heritable trait is manifested by an individual carrying the principal gene or genes conditioning it.

expulsive (eks-pul'siv) tending to expel or extrude.

exsanguination (eks-sang"gwĭ-na'shun) 1. forcible expulsion of blood from a part. 2. the state of being deprived of blood.

exsection (ek-sek'shun) an excision or cutting out.

exsiccosis (ek"sĭ-ko'sis) the state of an organism depleted of its necessary fluid intake.

exsorption (ek-sorp'shun) outward movement of material through a membrane.

exstrophy (ek'stro-fe) the turning inside out of an organ.

 e. of the bladder, a congenital malformation in which, from deficiency of the abdominal wall and bladder, the latter organ appears to be turned inside out, having the internal surface of the posterior wall showing through the opening in the anterior wall.

exsufflation (ek"suf-fla'shun) the act of exhausting the air content of a cavity, especially the lungs, by artificial or mechanical means.

exsufflator (ek"suf-fla'tor) an apparatus that, by the sudden production of negative pressure, can reproduce in the bronchial tree the effects of a natural, vigorous cough.

ext. external; extract.

extender (ek-sten'der) something that increases dimension in space or duration in time.

 plasma volume e., plasma volume expander.

extension (ek-sten'shun) 1. an increase in measurement or duration. 2. the straightening of a flexed limb.

 Buck's e., extension of fractured leg by weights, the foot of the bed being raised so that the body makes counterextension.

 Codivilla's e., extension for fractures made by a weight pulling on a nail passed through the lower end of the bone.

extensor (ek-sten'sor) [L.] that which extends, especially a muscle that extends a joint.

 e. surface, the aspect of a joint of a limb (such as the knee or elbow) toward which the movement of extension is directed.

exteriorization (ek-stēr"e-or-ĭ-za'shun) the process of bringing an interior body structure temporarily outside the body; in psychiatry, the turning of interests and drives outwardly into work, recreation and social pursuits.

extern (ek'stern) 1. a physician belonging to the staff of a hospital, but attending only during the day. 2. one of the hospital staff who attends to the outpatient department.

externalization (ek-ster"nah-lĭ-za'shun) a mental mechanism operating outside of and beyond conscious awareness in which the emotion of an internal conflict is directed outwardly.

externus (ek-ster'nus) external; in official anatomic nomenclature, designating a structure farther from the center of an organ or cavity.

exteroception (ek"ster-o-sep'shun) the perception of stimuli originating outside or at a distance from the body.

exteroceptive (ek"ster-o-sep'tiv) receiving impulses from the ectodermal covering or exterior of the body.

exteroceptor (ek"ster-o-sep'tor) a receptor organ that responds to stimuli arising outside the body.

exterofective (ek"ster-o-fek'tiv) responding to external stimuli; a term applied to the cerebrospinal nervous system.

exterogestate (ek"ster-o-jes'tāt) 1. developing outside the uterus, but still requiring complete care to meet all physical needs. 2. an infant during the period of exterior gestation, that is, from the time of its emergence from the uterus until it creeps, or about the age of 9 months.

extima (ek'stĭ-mah) the outermost coat of a blood vessel; the adventitia.

extirpation (ek"ster-pa'shun) complete removal; eradication.

extra- (ek'strah) word element [L.], *outside; beyond the scope of; in addition.*

extra-articular (ek"strah-ar-tik'u-lar) outside a joint.

extracapsular (ek"strah-kap'su-lar) outside a capsule.

extracellular (ek"strah-sel'u-lar) outside a cell or cells.

extracerebral (ek"strah-ser'ĕ-bral) outside the cerebrum.

extracorporeal (ek"strah-kor-po're-al) outside the body.

 e. circulation, the circulation of blood outside of the body, as through an artificial kidney for removal of substances usually excreted in the urine, or through a heart-lung apparatus for carbon dioxide-oxygen exchange. Extracorporeal circulation through the heart-lung machine has come into relatively common use in open-heart surgery.

extract (ek'strakt) a concentrated preparation of a vegetable or animal drug.

    allergenic e., an extract of the protein of any substance to which a person may be sensitive.

    liver e., a brownish, somewhat hygroscopic powder prepared from mammalian livers; used as a hematopoietic.

    malt e., a product containing dextrin, maltose, a small amount of glucose and amylolytic enzymes; used as a nutritive and emulsifying agent.

    ox bile e., a brown or brownish or greenish yellow powder with a characteristic odor and bitter taste; used as a choleretic.

    parathyroid e., a preparation of the active principles of parathyroid glands.

    thyroid e., a pharmaceutical substance derived from the thyroid glands of certain animals and used in the treatment of hypothyroidism.

extraction (ek-strak'shun) 1. the act of removing or pulling out. 2. the separation of a constituent from a compound or mixture by use of a suitable volatile solvent.

    breech e., extraction of an infant from the uterus in cases of breech presentation.

    flap e., removal of a cataract by making a flap in the cornea.

extractive (ek-strak'tiv) a substance separated by extraction.

extractor (ek-strak'tor) an instrument for removing bullets, etc.

extradural (ek"strah-du'ral) outside the dura mater.

extraembryonic (ek"strah-em"bre-on'ik) not occurring as a part of the embryo proper; applied specifically to the fetal membranes.

extramarginal (ek"strah-mar'ji-nal) below the limit of consciousness.

extramastoiditis (ek"strah-mas"toi-di'tis) inflammation of tissues adjoining the mastoid process.

extrasensory perception (ek"strah-sen'so-re) awareness gained otherwise than through the usual physical senses.

extrasystole (ek"strah-sis'to-le) a cardiac contraction caused by an impulse arising outside the sinoatrial node and occurring earlier than expected in the dominant or usual rhythm.

    atrial e., an extrasystole in which the stimulus is thought to arise in the atrium elsewhere than at the sinoatrial node.

    atrioventricular e., one in which the stimulus is supposed to arise in the atrioventricular node.

    interpolated e., a contraction taking place between two normal heartbeats.

    nodal e., atrioventricular extrasystole.

    retrograde e., a premature ventricular contraction, due to transmission of the stimulus backward over the bundle of His.

    ventricular e., one in which the stimulus is thought to arise in the ventricular portion of the bundle of His.

extrauterine (ek"strah-u'ter-in) outside the uterus

    e. pregnancy, ectopic pregnancy.

extravasation (ek-strav"ah-za'shun) escape of fluid from its proper vessel into the tissues.

extravascular (ek"strah-vas'ku-lar) outside a vessel.

extraversion (ek"strah-ver'zhun) extroversion.

extravert (ek'strah-vert) extrovert.

extremitas (ek-strem'ĭ-tas), pl. *extremita'tes* [L.] extremity.

extremity (ek-strem'ĭ-te) 1. a termination of an elongated or pointed structure. 2. a limb of the body.

extrinsic (ek-strin'sik) of external origin.

    e. factor, a constituent of food that combines with intrinsic factor to produce blood formation; called also vitamin B_{12} and cyanocobalamin.

extroversion (ek"stro-ver'zhun) direction of one's energy and interests toward external environmental and social phenomena.

extrovert (ek'stro-vert) a person whose interest is turned outward.

extrude (ek-strood') to force out, or to occupy a position distal to that normally occupied.

extrusion (ek-stroo'zhun) 1. a pushing out. 2. in dentistry, the condition of a tooth pushed too far forward from the line of occlusion.

extubation (eks"tu-ba'shun) removal of a tube.

exudate (eks'u-dāt) material that has escaped from blood vessels and been deposited in tissues or on tissue surfaces, usually as a result of inflammation.

exudation (eks"u-da'shun) 1. the escape of fluid, cells or cellular debris from blood vessels and deposition in or on the tissue. 2. exudate. adj., exu'dative.

exumbilication (eks"um-bil"ĭ-ka'shun) protrusion of the umbilicus.

exuvia (ek-su've-ah), pl. *exu'viae* [L.] something that is shed; slough.

eye (i) the organ of vision. In the embryo the eye develops as a direct extension of the brain, and thus is a very delicate organ. To protect the eye the bones of the skull are shaped so that an orbital cavity protects the dorsal aspect of each eyeball. In addition, the conjunctival sac covers the front of the eyeball and lines the upper and lower eyelids. Tears from the lacrimal duct constantly wash the eye to remove foreign objects, and the lids and eyelashes aid in protecting the front of the eye.

    Structure. The eyeball has three coats. The cornea is the clear transparent layer on the front of the eyeball. It is a continuation of the sclera (the white of the eye), the tough outer coat that helps protect the delicate mechanism of the eye. The choroid is the middle layer and contains blood vessels. The third layer, the retina, contains rods and cones, which are specialized cells that are sensitive to light. Behind the cornea and in front of the lens is the iris, the circular pigmented band around the pupil. The iris works much like the

Ching.

Please pool
about . 40 sera
for me - I need
it ~~today~~ for the Wed.
Seminar.

Thanks

Carol

Also I would like about
10 tubes of lipemic serum.

diaphragm in a camera, widening or narrowing the pupil to adjust to different light conditions.

FUNCTION. The refraction or bending of light rays so that they focus on the retina and can thus be transmitted to the optic nerve is accomplished by three structures: the aqueous humor, a watery substance between the cornea and lens; the lens, a crystalline structure just behind the iris; and the vitreous humor, a jelly-like substance filling the space between the lens and the retina. Unlike the lens of a camera, the lens of the eye focuses by a process called accommodation. This means that when the eye sees something in the distance, muscles pull the lens, stretching it until it is thin and almost flat, so that the light rays are only slightly bent as they pass through it. When the object is close, the muscles relax and the elastic lens becomes thicker, bending the light rays and focusing them on the retina.

Because the eye must function under many different circumstances, there are two different sets of nerve cells in the retina, the cone-shaped and the rod-shaped cells. They cover the full range of adaptation to light, the cones being sensitive in bright light, and the rods in dim light. The cones are responsible for color vision. It is now believed that there are three types of cones, each containing a substance that reacts to light of a different color — one set for red, one for green and the third for violet. These are the primary colors in light, which, when mixed together, give white. White light stimulates all three sets of color cells; any other color stimulates one or two. Lack of a set of color cells causes COLOR BLINDNESS, which usually affects either the red or the green cells.

The optic nerve, which transmits the nerve impulses from the retina to the visual center of the brain, contains nerve fibers from the many nerve cells in the retina. The small spot where it leaves the retina does not have any light-sensitive cells, and is called the blind spot.

The eyes are situated in the front of the head in such a way that human beings have stereoscopic vision, the ability to judge distances. Because the eyes are set apart, each eye sees farther around an object on its own side than does the other. The brain superimposes the two slightly different images and judges distances from the composite image. (See also VISION.)

DISORDERS OF THE EYE. If the eyeball is too short or too long, the lens focuses the image not on the retina, but behind or in front of it. The former condition is called hyperopia, or farsightedness, and the latter myopia, or nearsightedness. An irregularity in the curvature of the cornea or lens can cause the impaired vision of ASTIGMATISM.

STRABISMUS, or crossed eyes, is usually caused by weakness in some of the muscles that control movement of the eyeball.

CONJUNCTIVITIS is an inflammation of the membrane that covers the front of the eyeball and lines the eyelids.

When small pieces of the retina become detached from the underlying layers, the result is DETACHMENT OF THE RETINA. Repair by surgery can usually prevent blindness produced by retinal detachment.

PRESBYOPIA (usually taking the form of hyperopia) occurs in older persons and develops as the lens loses its elasticity with the passing years. Correction is easily made with properly prescribed eyeglasses.

The three major disorders causing blindness in the United States are CATARACT, GLAUCOMA and TRACHOMA.

Foreign bodies in the eyes are common occurrences. Cinders, grit or other foreign bodies are best removed by lifting the eyelid by the lashes. The foreign body will usually remain on the surface of the lid, and can easily be removed. Particles embedded in the eyeball must be removed by a physician.

Eyestrain is fatigue of the eyes caused by improper use, uncorrected defects in the vision or an eye disorder. Symptoms may include aching or pains in the eyes, or a hot, scratchy feeling in the eyelids. Headache, blurring or dimness of vision and sometimes dizziness or nausea may also occur.

eyeball (i'bawl) the ball or globe of the eye.

eyebrow (i'brow) the hairy ridge above the eye; supercilium.

eyecup (i'kup) a small vessel for application of cleansing or medicated solution to the exposed area of the eyeball.

eyeglass (i'glas) a lens for aiding the sight.

eyeground (i'grownd) the fundus of the eye.

eyelash (i'lash) one of the hairs growing on the edge of an eyelid.

eyelid (i'lid) either of two movable folds (upper and lower) protecting the anterior surface of the eyeball.

eyepiece (i'pēs) the lens or system of lenses of a microscope nearest the eye of the observer when the instrument is in use.

eyestrain (i'strān) eye fatigue caused by overuse of the eye or by an uncorrected defect in focus of the eye.

F

F chemical symbol, *fluorine*.

F. Fahrenheit, French (catheter size).

F₁ first filial generation, a term used in genetics.

F₂ second filial generation, a term used in genetics.

fabella (fah-bel′ah), pl. *fabel′lae* [L.] a sesamoid fibrocartilage in the gastrocnemius muscle.

fabism (fa′bizm) favism.

Fabry's syndrome (fah-brēz′) a genetically transmitted disorder characterized by remittent attacks of fever, lightning pains and burning dysesthesias of the extremities, proteinuria and hematuria, and cutaneous lesions.

face (fās) the anterior aspect of the head.
    moon f., the peculiar rounded face resulting from excess of adrenocortical hormones or corticosteroids.

facet (fas′et) a small, nearly plane area on a bone or other hard surface.

facetectomy (fas″ĕ-tek′to-me) excision of a facet of a bone.

faci(o)- (fa′she-o) word element [L.], *face*.

facial (fa′shal) pertaining to the face.
    f. nerve, the seventh cranial nerve; its motor fibers supply the muscles of facial expression. These are a complex group of cutaneous muscles that move the eyebrows, skin of the forehead, corners of the mouth and other parts of the face concerned with frowning, smiling, achieving a look of surprise or any of the many and varied expressions of emotion. The sensory fibers of the facial nerve provide a sense of taste in the forward two-thirds of the tongue, and also supply the submaxillary, sublingual and lacrimal glands for secretion.
    Irritation of the facial nerve can produce a paralysis known as BELL'S PALSY. Usually the paralysis involves only one side of the face with a resulting distortion of facial expression, inability to close the mouth on one side and difficulty in closing the eye on the affected side.

facies (fa′she-ēz), pl. *fa′cies* [L.] 1. a specific surface, e.g., the anterior aspect of the head, or face. 2. the expression or appearance of the face.
    adenoid f., the stupid expression, with open mouth, in children with adenoid growths.
    f. hepat′ica, a thin face with sunken eyeballs, sallow complexion and yellow conjunctivae, characteristic of certain chronic liver disorders.
    f. hippocrat′ica, a drawn, pinched and livid appearance indicative of approaching death.
    f. leonti′na, a lion-like appearance seen in certain cases of leprosy.

facilitation (fah-sil″ĭ-ta′shun) hastening or assistance of a natural process; specifically, the effect produced in nerve tissue by the passage of an impulse. The resistance is diminished so that second application of the stimulus evokes the reaction more easily.

faciobrachial (fa″she-o-bra′ke-al) pertaining to the face and arm.

faciocephalalgia (fa″she-o-sef″al-al′je-ah) pertaining to the face and arm.

faciocervical (fa″she-o-ser′vĭ-kal) pertaining to the face and neck.

faciolingual (fa″she-o-ling′gwal) pertaining to the face and tongue.

facioplasty (fa′she-o-plas″te) plastic surgery of the face.

facioplegia (fa″she-o-ple′je-ah) facial paralysis.

facioscapulohumeral (fa″she-o-skap″u-lo-hu′mer-al) pertaining to the face, scapula and arm.

F.A.C.O.G. Fellow of the American College of Obstetricians and Gynecologists.

F.A.C.P. Fellow of American College of Physicians.

F.A.C.S. Fellow of American College of Surgeons.

F.A.C.S.M. Fellow of the American College of Sports Medicine.

factitial (fak-tish′al) produced by artificial means.

factitious (fak-tish′us) artificial; not natural.

factor (fak′tor) an agent or element that contributes to the production of a result.
    accelerator f., factor V, one of the CLOTTING factors.
    antianemia f., an element essential for the maturation of erythrocytes and the prevention of anemia.
    antihemophilic f., AHF, clotting factor VIII, deficiency of which causes classic sex-linked hemophilia. It is available in a preparation for preventive and therapeutic use. Called also antihemophilic globulin.
    antihemorrhagic f., vitamin K.
    antipernicious anemia f., cyanocobalamin.
    antirachitic f., vitamin D.
    antiscorbutic f., ascorbic acid.
    antisterility f., vitamin E.
    citrovorum f., folinic acid, a factor necessary for the growth of *Leuconostoc citrovorum*.
    clotting f's, coagulation f's, factors essential to normal blood clotting, whose absence, diminution or excess may lead to abnormality of the clotting; 12 factors, commonly designated by Roman numerals, have been described (see also CLOTTING).
    extrinsic f., a constituent of food that combines with intrinsic factor to produce blood formation; called also vitamin B₁₂ and cyanocobalamin.

Hageman f., factor XII, one of the CLOTTING factors.

intrinsic f., a mucoprotein, normally found in gastric juice, that is necessary for the absorption and assimilation of cyanocobalamin (extrinsic factor) contained in food. It is essential for the production of the antianemia factor and is absent in PERNICIOUS ANEMIA.

multiple f's, two or more independent pairs of genes that affect the same character in the same way and in an additive fashion.

plasma converting f., factor V, one of the CLOTTING factors.

platelet f's, factors important in hemostasis that are contained in or attached to the platelets.

Rh f., Rhesus f., an antigen found in some 25 different serologically distinct types in about 85 per cent of the Caucasian population (see also RH FACTOR).

rheumatoid f., a protein of high molecular weight in the serum of most patients with rheumatoid arthritis, detectable by serologic tests.

spreading f., hyaluronidase.

Stuart f., factor X, one of the CLOTTING factors.

facultative (fak′ul-ta″tiv) capable of adaptation to different conditions.

f. anaerobe, a microorganism that can live either with or without oxygen.

faculty (fak′ul-te) a normal power or function, especially of the mind.

fae- for words beginning thus, see those beginning *fe-*.

Fahr. Fahrenheit.

Fahr-Volhard disease (far fōl′hart) malignant nephrosclerosis.

Fahrenheit thermometer (far′en-hīt) a thermometer on which the freezing point of water is at 32 and the normal boiling point of water at 212 degrees (212° F.)

failure (fāl′yer) inability to perform or to function properly.

heart f., inability of the heart to expel blood from the ventricles (see also HEART).

left ventricular f., inadequate ability of the left ventricle to pump sufficient blood to the systemic circulation.

right ventricular f., inability of the right ventricle to expel an adequate amount of blood, with subsequent venous engorgement and sequelae.

fainting (fānt′ing) sudden loss of consciousness resulting frequently from an insufficient supply of blood to the brain; syncope. This may be due to a nervous reaction stemming from such causes as fear, hunger, pain or any emotional or physical shock. Although fainting may be considered a very mild form of shock, it is not as serious and usually is not accompanied by the rapid, weak pulse and cold, clammy skin characteristic of true shock. The person who is about to faint should be made to lie down with the legs somewhat elevated, and collar and clothing loosened. If this is not feasible, he should lower his head between his knees for about 5 minutes.

If a person has lost consciousness, he should be kept lying down with the feet and legs slightly elevated. Tight clothing should be loosened. Smelling salts (ammonium carbonate) or aromatic spirits of ammonia may be held under the victim's nose

until he revives. Prolonged loss of consciousness indicates a condition more serious than simple fainting and should be treated by a physician.

falcial (fal′shal) pertaining to the falx cerebri.

falciform (fal′sī-form) sickle-shaped.

f. ligament, a sickle-shaped sagittal fold of peritoneum that helps to attach the liver to the diaphragm and separates the right and left lobes of the liver.

falcula (fal′ku-lah) the falx cerebelli.

falcular (fal′ku-lar) sickle-shaped.

fallopian tube (fah-lo′pe-an) uterine tube.

Fallot's tetralogy (fal-ōz′ tĕ-tral′o-je) a combination of congenital cardiac defects, namely, pulmonary stenosis, ventricular septal defects, dextroposition of the aorta, so that it overrides the interventricular septum and receives venous as well as arterial blood, and right ventricular hypertrophy (see also TETRALOGY OF FALLOT).

fallout (fawl′owt) the settling of radioactive fission products from the atmosphere after explosion of an atomic or thermonuclear bomb.

falx (falks), pl. *fal′ces* [L.] a sickle-shaped structure.

f. cerebel′li, a small fold of dura mater in the posterior cranial fossa.

f. cer′ebri, a sickle-shaped fold of dura mater in the longitudinal fissure that separates the two cerebral hemispheres.

F.A.M.A. Fellow of American Medical Association.

familial (fah-mil′e-al) occurring in or affecting members of the same family.

family (fam′ĭ-le) 1. a group descended from a common ancestor. 2. a taxonomic category subordinate to an order (or suborder) and superior to a tribe (or subfamily); names of families end typically in *-aceae* (plants) or *-idae* (animals).

Fanconi's disease (fan-kōn′ez) congenital aplastic anemia of childhood with musculoskeletal defects.

F's syndrome, a familial, slowly progressive kidney disease, with progressive degeneration of the renal parenchyma and metabolic disorders.

Fannia (fan′e-ah) a genus of flies whose larvae have caused both intestinal and urinary infestation in man.

fantasy (fan′tah-se) an imagined series of events (see also PHANTASY).

far. faradic; pertaining to faradic electricity.

farad (far′ad) the unit of electric capacity; capacity to hold 1 coulomb with a potential of 1 volt.

faradic electricity (fah-rad′ik) 1. electricity produced by induction. 2. electricity in intermittent currents.

faradism (far′ah-dizm) 1. faradization. 2. faradic electricity.

faradization (far″ah-dī-za′shun) therapeutic use of faradic electricity.

farsightedness (far-sīt'ed-nes) a condition in which vision for distant objects is better than for near objects; called also HYPEROPIA.

fascia (fash'e-ah), pl. *fas'ciae* [L.] a band or sheet of tissue investing and connecting muscles. adj., **fas'cial.**

  aponeurotic f., deep f., a dense, firm, fibrous membrane investing the trunk and limbs and giving off sheaths to the various muscles.

  extrapleural f., a prolongation of the endothoracic fascia, important as possibly modifying the auscultatory sounds at the apex of the lung.

  f. la'ta, the external investing fascia of the thigh.

  Scarpa's f., part of the deep layer of superficial abdominal fascia crossing the inguinal ligament.

  superficial f., the thin tough membrane covering the muscles and lying immediately under the skin.

  thyrolaryngeal f., the fascia covering the thyroid gland and attached to the cricoid cartilage.

  transverse f., part of the inner investing layer of the abdominal wall.

fascicle (fas'ĭ-kl) a small bundle or cluster, especially of nerve or muscle fibers.

fascicular (fah-sik'u-lar) clustered together; pertaining to or arranged in bundles or clusters.

fasciculation (fah-sik″u-la'shun) spontaneous contractions of a number of muscle fibers supplied by a single motor nerve filament.

fasciculus (fah-sik'u-lus), pl. *fascic'uli* [L.] fascicle.

fasciectomy (fas″e-ek'to-me) excision of fascia.

fasciitis (fas″e-i'tis) inflammation of a fascia.

  nodular f., proliferative f., a benign, reactive proliferation of fibroblasts in the subcutaneous tissues and commonly associated with the deep fascia.

  pseudosarcomatous f., a benign soft tissue tumor occurring subcutaneously and sometimes arising from deep muscle and fascia.

fasciodesis (fas″e-od'ĕ-sis) suture of a fascia to skeletal attachment.

Fasciola (fah-si'o-lah) a genus of flukes, parasitic worms.

  F. hepat'ica, a species parasitic in the liver and bile ducts of herbivorous mammals and found also in man; usually known as the liver fluke.

fasciola (fah-si'o-lah), pl. *fasci'olae* [L.] 1. a small band or striplike structure. 2. a small bandage. 3. a fluke of the genus Fasciola.

fascioliasis (fas″e-o-li'ah-sis) infection of the body with Fasciola.

fasciolopsiasis (fas″e-o-lop-si'ah-sis) infection with Fasciolopsis.

Fasciolopsis (fas″e-o-lop'sis) a genus of trematodes or flukes, parasitic worms.

  F. bus'ki, a species of flukes parasitic in the intestines.

fascioplasty (fas'e-o-plas″te) plastic repair of a fascia.

fasciorrhaphy (fas″e-or'ah-fe) suture of a fascia.

fasciotomy (fas″e-ot'o-me) incision of a fascia.

fast (fast) immovable, or unchangeable; resistant to the action of a specific drug or to staining.

fastigium (fas-tij'e-um) the highest point.

fat (fat) 1. the adipose or fatty tissue of the body. 2. an oily substance consisting of glycerin (a form of alcohol called also glycerol) and a group of fatty acids, chiefly palmitic, stearic and oleic acids, combined as glycerin esters. Fats consist of carbon, hydrogen and oxygen in various chemical combinations. They occur in most foods, especially in meats and dairy products. Fats may be solid, such as butter, or liquid, such as olive oil.

The fat-soluble vitamins, A, D and K, are found in fats. Between 15 and 35 per cent of the average human diet is fat, and about 95 per cent of the fat we eat is absorbed and utilized or stored in the body. In addition, fat is produced by the body from carbohydrates and some from proteins. Fat accounts for some 15 per cent of the average person's body weight.

Digestion of fat is accomplished in the intestines. The products of fat digestion are absorbed through the intestinal walls and distributed by the blood to various storage regions in the body. Some fat is used for tissue building but most of it is stored for future energy needs. These reserves are continuously being converted into carbohydrates for the body's work, and are continuously being replaced by new reserves.

When the intake of food exceeds the energy needs of the body, the food stored as fat accumulates in layers under the skin. Such fat layers provide insulation for the body against low temperatures. The insulating effect is due to the fact that there are few blood vessels in fatty tissue, and hence the heat of circulating blood is lost slowly from the body.

OBESITY. Although people vary in their tendency to put on fat, OBESITY is almost invariably the result of eating more than one needs. Obesity is a definite hazard to health. It places an unnatural burden on the heart and for this reason is a common cause of coronary occlusion (heart attack). DIABETES MELLITUS and ARTERIOSCLEROSIS are major and serious diseases invited by obesity.

SATURATED AND UNSATURATED FATS. Fats are composed of fatty acids in various combinations with glycerin. These fatty acids (and the fats they form) can be classified as saturated or unsaturated. The molecules of saturated fatty acids are constructed with single bonds between the carbon and hydrogen atoms so that they contain all the hydrogen possible; i.e., they are "saturated" with hydrogen. Unsaturated fatty acids contain double bonds so that they can take on more hydrogen under certain conditions. All of the common unsaturated fatty acids are liquid at room temperature. Through the process of hydrogenation, hydrogen can be incorporated into certain unsaturated fatty acids so that they are converted into solid fats for cooking purposes. Margarine is an example of the hydrogenation of unsaturated fatty acids into a solid substance.

Recent research has indicated that the unsaturated fats (called also polyunsaturates) are less likely than saturated fats to be used by the body in ways injurious to health. The theory supporting this claim is that the body's normal supply of cholesterol and its concentration in serum are increased by saturated fats, which are found mainly in animal fats, such as meat, butter and eggs. The unsaturated fats, found in large quantities in vegetable oils such as corn oil and safflower oil, are thought to help reduce the amount of cholesterol in the blood. Some researchers hold that eating foods rich in cholesterol itself, such as the animal fats, will also increase the amount of cholesterol in the blood.

Although the body's own normal production of cholesterol is essential to the functioning of body systems, it is known that the formation of fatty deposits in the arteries, a condition called *atherosclerosis,* can impede the flow of blood and cause damage to the coronary arteries of the heart and other arteries. Cholesterol is recognized as an important factor in these conditions, although its exact contribution is still not clear (see also CHOLESTEROL).

fatal (fa′tal) causing death; deadly; mortal.

fatigability (fat″ĭ-gah-bil′ĭ-te) easy susceptibility to fatigue.

fatigue (fah-tēg′) a state of increased discomfort and decreased efficiency resulting from prolonged exertion; a generalized feeling of tiredness or exhaustion. Fatigue is a normal reaction to intense physical exertion, emotional strain or lack of rest. It is the body's way of saying that one ought to slow down, relax and get more rest and sleep. Fatigue that is not relieved by rest may have a more serious origin. It may be a symptom of generally poor physical condition, of specific disease or of severe emotional stress.

Poor living habits, including improper diet, lack of sleep and insufficient fresh air and exercise, are a common cause of fatigue. Often, however, fatigue signals an oncoming illness. Fatigue is associated with a wide variety of diseases, including tuberculosis, anemia, thyroid disorders, heart ailments, diabetes mellitus and cancer.

Sometimes fatigue is psychologic in origin. Tiredness and a loss of interest in one's work may actually result from boredom with the daily routine. If one is certain that there is nothing wrong physically, steps should be taken to vary the daily round, to seek new and more active ways to spend leisure time, perhaps to revive old interests that have been neglected.

Sometimes the demands made upon a person's nervous system are excessive and nervous exhaustion, or nervous prostration, occurs. This state of abnormal fatigue is usually brought on by the inability to cope emotionally with long periods of trouble. Insomnia combines with deep discouragement, and the person is mentally and physically exhausted. The resulting symptoms are sometimes grouped together under the descriptive term, neurasthenia, or nerve weakness. They include poor memory, irritability, aches and pains, lack of appetite, heart palpitations and dizziness. Occasionally, because of his emotional state, the person has difficulty with a particular organ and may suffer from an imaginary ailment. A cardiac neurosis, in which the individual is convinced he has heart disease is fairly common. The combat fatigue suffered by soldiers in battle is a type of neurosis.

fatty (fat′e) pertaining to fat.

f. acid, an organic compound of carbon, hydrogen and oxygen that combines with glycerin to form fat. All fats are esters of fatty acids and glycerin, the fatty acids accounting for 90 per cent of the molecule of most natural fats. Fatty acids may be satu-

rated or unsaturated, depending on their content of hydrogen. Saturated fatty acids contain all the hydrogen atoms possible in the molecule. They are solid at room temperature and are the components of the common animal fats, such as butter and lard. Unsaturated fatty acids contain one or more free bonds which allow for taking on more hydrogen atoms under certain conditions; in other words, they are not "saturated" with hydrogen atoms. The unsaturated fatty acids are liquid at room temperature and are found in oils such as olive oil and linseed oil.

From a nutritional standpoint, some fatty acids are essential for proper growth and metabolism, and a deficiency of these fatty acids can lead to eczema and other skin disorders. Such deficiencies are rare, however, because the fatty acids occur in abundance in many foods, such as butter, whole milk, egg yolk, nuts and vegetables.

f. degeneration, degeneration of tissue with abnormal accumulation of fat.

fauces (faw′sēz) the passage from the mouth to the pharynx.

faucitis (faw-si′tis) inflammation of the fauces.

faveolate (fah-ve′o-lāt) honeycombed.

faveolus (fah-ve′o-lus) a small pit or depression.

favism (fa′vizm) an acute hemolytic anemia caused by ingestion of fava beans or inhalation of the pollen of the plant, occurring in certain individuals as a result of a genetic abnormality with a deficiency in an enzyme, glucose-6-phosphate dehydrogenase, in the erythrocytes.

favus (fa′vus) a type of tinea capitis, with formation of prominent honeycomb-like masses, due to *Trichophyton schoenleini.*

F-Cortef (ef-kor′tef) trademark for a preparation of fludrocortisone, a synthetic corticoid.

F.D. fatal (lethal) dose; focal distance (focal length).

F.D.$_{50}$ median fatal (lethal) dose.

F.D.A. Food and Drug Administration.

Fe chemical symbol, *iron* (L. *ferrum.*)

febricide (feb′rĭ-sīd) 1. destroying fever. 2. an agent that destroys fever.

febrifacient (feb″rĭ-fa′shent) producing fever.

febrifuge (feb′rĭ-fūj) a remedy that dispels fever.

febrile (feb′ril) pertaining to fever; feverish.

febriphobia (feb″rĭ-fo′be-ah) morbid fear of fever.

fecal (fe′kal) pertaining to or of the nature of feces.

fecalith (fe′kah-lith) an intestinal concretion composed of fecal material.

fecaloid (fe′kal-oid) resembling feces.

fecaloma (fe″kal-o′mah) a tumor-like accumulation of feces in the rectum.

fecaluria (fe″kal-u′re-ah) the presence of fecal matter in the urine.

feces (fe′sēz) body waste discharged from the intestine; also called stool, excreta or excrement. The feces are formed in the colon and pass down into the rectum by the process of peristalsis. When the rectum is sufficiently distended, nerve endings in its wall signal a need for evacuation, which is made possible by a voluntary relaxation of the sphincter muscles around the outer part of the anus.

The frequency of bowel movements varies according to the individual body make-up, type of intestine, eating habits, physical activity and custom. Although one bowel movement a day is the average, a movement every 2 or 3 days may be considered normal. A balanced diet and an established routine can promote regular bowel movements.

CHARACTERISTICS. Normally the stool is soft and formed and brownish in color. An abnormality in color, odor or consistency usually indicates a disorder of the intestinal tract or of the accessory organs of the digestive system. Black, tarry stools may indicate intestinal bleeding, especially in the upper portion of the tract. Some drugs, such as those containing iron or bismuth, can produce tarry stools. Bright red blood in the feces can indicate a wide variety of disorders ranging from HEMORRHOIDS to a malignancy of the rectum. Clay-colored stools result from an absence or deficiency of BILE in the intestinal tract, and indicate obstruction of the biliary tract or decreased production of bile by the liver. Greenish-colored feces often accompany diarrhea, especially in infants, and may be caused by growth of certain bacteria.

Bulky, fatty stools, having a foul odor, are characteristic of CYSTIC FIBROSIS. Other causes of fatty feces include GALLBLADDER disease, pancreatic disorders, SPRUE and excessive intake of fat in the diet. Feces containing large amounts of mucus often occur in COLITIS and other irritations of the intestinal tract.

The stool of a newborn, full-term infant is called meconium. It is a dark greenish brown color, smooth and semisolid in consistency.

DISINFECTION. In many types of communicable diseases it is necessary to decontaminate the feces before they are flushed into the sewage system. Chlorinated lime, Lysol or formalin may be used for this purpose. The contents of the bedpan used by the patient should be thoroughly covered with the disinfectant and allowed to stand for several hours. The contents are then disposed of in a hopper or commode, and the bedpan is rinsed and sterilized, preferably with live steam or by autoclave.

OBSERVATIONS. Because the characteristics of the feces can be of help in the diagnosis of various diseases, it is important to inspect the stool for color, consistency, odor and number of stools per day. Abnormalities should be noted on the patient's chart or reported to the physician.

SPECIMENS. A sample of the feces (stool specimen) may be required as a diagnostic aid. The specimen should be collected in a sterile bedpan and transferred into a sterile container, using a wooden spatula or tongue blade for this purpose. In order for certain types of intestinal parasites to be discovered in the feces, the specimen must be fresh and kept warm until examined in the laboratory. Microorganisms that may be detected include the typhoid and paratyphoid bacilli, the anthrax bacilli and *Entomoeba histolytica*, which causes AMEBIC DYSENTERY.

Specimens of the feces may be examined for occult (hidden) blood. This test is indicated when intestinal bleeding is suspected but the stools do not appear to contain blood when examined by gross inspection.

feculent (fek′u-lent) having sediment.

fecundation (fe″kun-da′shun) fertilization; impregnation.

fecundity (fe-kun′dĭ-te) the ability to produce offspring frequently and in large numbers.

feeblemindedness (fe″bl-mīnd′ed-nes) mental deficiency from arrested mental development.

feedback (fēd′bak) the return of some of the output of a system as input.

feeding (fēd′ing) the taking or giving of food.
  artificial f., feeding of a baby with food other than mother's milk.
  breast f., the feeding of an infant at the breast (see also BREAST FEEDING).
  extrabuccal f., administration of food other than through the mouth.
  forced f., administration of food by force to those who cannot or will not receive it.
  intravenous f., administration of nutrient fluids through a vein (see also INTRAVENOUS INFUSION).
  tube f., feeding of liquids and semisolid foods through a nasogastric tube (see also TUBE FEEDING).

Feer's disease (fārz) acrodynia.

Fehling's solution (fa′lingz) (1) 34.66 Gm. cupric sulfate in water to make 500 cc.; (2) 173 Gm. crystallized potassium and sodium tartrate and 50 gm. sodium hydroxide in water to make 500 cc.; mix equal volumes of (1) and (2) at time of use.

fellatio (fĕ-la′she-o) oral stimulation or manipulation of the penis.

felon (fel′on) a purulent infection involving the pulp of the distal phalanx of a finger.

feltwork (felt′werk) a complex of closely interwoven fibers, as of nerve fibers.

female (fe′măl) an individual of the sex that produces ova or bears young.

feminism (fem′ĭ-nizm) the possession of female characteristics, usually referring to the presence of such characteristics in the male.

feminization (fem″ĭ-nĭ-za′shun) the development of female characteristics.
  testicular f., a condition in which the subject is phenotypically female, but lacks nuclear sex chromatin and is of XY chromosomal sex.

femoral (fem′o-ral) pertaining to the femur or to the thigh.
  f. artery, the chief artery of the thigh (see table of ARTERIES).
  f. nerve, the largest branch of the lumbar plexus (see table of NERVES).
  f. vein, the chief vein of the thigh (see table of VEINS).

femorocele (fem′o-ro-sēl″) femoral hernia.

femorotibial (fem″o-ro″tib′e-al) pertaining to the femur and tibia.

femur (fe′mur), pl. *fem′ora* [L.] the thigh bone, extending from the pelvis to the knee; the longest and strongest bone in the body. Its proximal end articulates with the acetabulum, a cup-like cavity in the pelvic girdle. The greater and lesser trochanters are the two processes (prominences) at the proximal end of the femur.

fenestra (fĕ-nes′trah), pl. *fenes′trae* [L.] a small opening or window.
   f. coch′leae, a small, round, membrane-filled opening between the middle ear and internal ear; called also round window.
   f. vestib′uli, a small, oval opening between the middle ear and inner ear into which the foot of the stapes fits; called also oval window.

fenestrate (fen′es-trāt) to pierce with one or more openings.

fenestration (fen″es-tra′shun) 1. the act of perforating or condition of being perforated. 2. the surgical creation of a new opening in the labyrinth of the ear for the restoration of hearing in cases of otosclerosis.
   aortopulmonary f., a congenital anomaly consisting of a communication between the aorta and the pulmonary artery just above the semilunar valves.

Feosol (fe′o-sol) trademark for preparations of ferrous sulfate, an iron preparation.

Fergon (fer′gon) trademark for preparations of ferrous gluconate, an iron preparation.

ferment (fer′ment) a substance that causes fermentation.

fermentation (fer″men-ta′shun) the decomposition of an organic substance into simpler compounds through the agency of an enzyme.

fermentogen (fer-men′to-jen) a substance that may be converted into a ferment.

fermentum (fer-men′tum) [L.] yeast.

fermium (fer′me-um) a chemical element, atomic number 100, atomic weight 253, symbol Fm. (See table of ELEMENTS.)

ferric (fer′ik) containing iron in its trivalent form and yielding trivalent ions in aqueous solution.
   f. ammonium citrate, an iron preparation sometimes used in treatment of anemia.
   f. ammonium tartrate, a compound used orally in iron deficiency anemia.
   f. chloride, $FeCl_3$, sometimes used as an astringent for skin disorders and as a styptic.
   f. subsulfate solution, a solution of iron used undiluted as a styptic.

ferricyanide (fer″ĭ-si′ah-nīd) a compound containing the trivalent $Fe(CN)_6$ radical.

ferritin (fer′ĭ-tin) the iron-apoferritin complex, which is one of the forms in which iron is stored in the body.

ferrocholinate (fer″o-ko′lin-āt) a compound of ferric chloride and choline dihydrogen citrate, used as a hematinic.

ferrocyanide (fer″o-si′ah-nīd) a compound containing the tetravalent $Fe(CN)_6$ radical.

ferrokinetics (fer″o-ki-net′iks) the scientific study of the turnover or rate of change of iron in the body.

Ferrolip (fer′o-lip) trademark for preparations of ferrocholinate, a hematinic.

ferrotherapy (fer″o-ther′ah-pe) therapeutic use of iron and iron compounds.

ferrous (fer′us) containing iron in its divalent form and yielding divalent ions in aqueous solution.
   f. carbonate, a hematinic useful in treatment of iron deficiency anemia but extremely irritating to the gastric and intestinal mucosa.
   f. fumarate, an iron preparation used in treatment of iron deficiency anemia.
   f. gluconate, a hematinic that is less irritating to the gastrointestinal tract than ferrous sulfate and generally used as a substitute when ferrous sulfate cannot be tolerated.
   f. iodide, an iron preparation in syrup form given in treatment of iron deficiency anemia.
   f. sulfate, a hematinic used in treatment of iron deficiency anemia. It is believed to be less irritating than equivalent amounts of ferric salts and is more effective.
   All iron preparations should be administered after meals, never on an empty stomach. The patient should be warned that the drugs cause stools to turn dark green or black. Overdosage may cause severe systemic reactions.

ferrum (fer′um) [L.] iron (symbol Fe).

fertility (fer-til′ĭ-te) the ability to beget or conceive children. Many factors, including poor diet, general ill health and emotional stress, may lessen fertility. Sterility, or a complete inability to conceive children, is fairly rare. Most childless couples can be helped to have children with medical assistance in determining and correcting the conditions which lessen their fertility.
   Impotence in the male is inability to maintain an erection or to achieve orgasm, making coitus impossible. It has no direct relationship with fertility, except that in preventing completion of the sexual act it also prevents conception. An impotent man may be very fertile, because his testes produce many sperm cells, while one who is virile may suffer from decreased fertility. A great many cases of impotence are the result of emotional disturbances, and can often be successfully treated.
   FERTILITY IN WOMEN. Any disturbance of the endocrine glands may lessen fertility. These glands influence every stage of the sexual cycle, from the maturing of the ovum in the ovary to its implantation in the uterus. Thus, an imbalance in the endocrine system may affect fertility in several different ways. The ovum may fail to mature, or may be sterile, or the fertilized ovum may not come to rest properly in the uterus. Many types of endocrine disturbance can now be corrected by administration of hormones.
   Any deformation of the reproductive organs may affect fertility. In a few cases, the uterus may be undeveloped. More common, however, is retroverted uterus, which was thought for some years to be a cause of infertility. In those cases in which the retroverted uterus does contribute to infertility, exercises or a mechanical support may often be sufficient to correct the condition.

If the uterine tubes are blocked, the ovum and sperm will be prevented from uniting. This condition can be detected by passing a gas such as carbon dioxide into the uterus under controlled pressure. The gas goes into the tubes and, if the tubes are open, escapes into the abdomen, from which it is harmlessly discharged. In some cases, it is thought that the gas may unblock stopped-up tubes, as well as detect them. Similar information is obtained by instilling a radiopaque material into the uterus and tubes and obtaining x-rays. In the rare instances in which a portion of the tube is completely blocked, surgery may be advised. As long as one tube and one ovary continue to function normally, however, the woman continues to be fertile to some degree, even if the tube and the ovary are on opposite sides of the uterus.

Painful intercourse (dyspareunia) may result in infertility by diminishing the frequency of intercourse. This is an abnormal condition and should have medical attention. Pain during intercourse may be a result of a malfunction of the glands that lubricate the vagina. Often the difficulty is psychologic in origin, the result of sexual fears or inhibitions. Most serious of this type of condition is vaginismus, in which the muscles in the vagina contract, blocking the entry of the penis and making intercourse impossible.

Among other conditions that can cause infertility or sterility in women is salpingitis, an inflammation of the uterine tubes, a principal complication of gonorrhea, although it may also result from tuberculosis and other infections. Eventually the tubes become closed at both ends and pus accumulates within them, a condition known as pyosalpinx. Another cause of sterility is chronic cervicitis, resulting in production of mucus harmful to the migration of the sperm into the uterus.

Proper nutrition may be an important factor in fertility. A healthy diet is a necessary part of any treatment designed to remedy infertility. Vitamin supplements are occasionally suggested.

Weight control is another factor in treatment for infertility, since both overweight and underweight women are found to have less than normal fertility.

Emotional stress may directly or indirectly lessen fertility. Repressed hostilities or fears of pregnancy may cause muscle spasms which reduce the chance of pregnancy. Although the effects of emotional factors are still somewhat mysterious, it appears that these factors may affect fertility in other ways as well. Often a couple adopt a child after giving up hope, and unexpectedly have a child of their own shortly afterward, possibly because of the decrease in anxiety. In many cases, psychologic counseling is an important part of treatment for infertility, particularly if the doctor can find no organic reason for it.

FERTILITY IN MEN. At one time, a couple's inability to have children was almost always ascribed to infertility in the wife. It is now recognized that in about 40 per cent of all childless couples, the husband is lacking in fertility. This is not related to virility, which is the ability to perform intercourse, but to the quantity and vitality of the sperm cells in the sexual emission. There is no disturbance of the sexual act. The only way of discovering low fertility in the male is by laboratory examination of the semen.

To determine the fertility of the male, the physician examines a sample of the semen under the microscope. Infertility may result from too few sperm cells, or from a high proportion of malformed cells, or from a low level of vitality of the sperm. Also, an obstruction in the passages from the testes may block or prevent the exit of the sperm.

Treatment for male infertility varies with the cause of the infertility. In some cases, increased rest and a better diet may be sufficient to raise the level of effective sperm cells. When several factors are involved, medical treatment or psychotherapy may be necessary. In a few cases, the man may be wholly sterile, as may happen as a result of mumps suffered in adolescence or adulthood. Gonorrhea and tuberculosis may also cause sterility.

fertilization (fer″tĭ-lĭ-za′shun) in human reproduction, the process by which the male's sperm unites with the female's ovum. By this event, also called conception, a new life is created and the sex and other biologic traits of the new individual are determined. These traits are determined by the combined genes and chromosomes that exist in the sperm and ovum.

After injection into the vagina, the sperm cells—millions of them—make use of their whiplike tails to swim through the cervix toward the uterus. Most are destroyed along the way by secretions in the vagina, but some reach the uterus and a few may enter the UTERINE TUBES. A very small number may survive as long as 48 hours. If during this period only one sperm succeeds in entering a uterine tube and meeting there an ovum ready to be fertilized, conception can occur. This event is possible only during a period of about 4 days of the month. After the sperm lodges in the ovum, the tail disappears, but the head unites with the ovum to form the embryo. (See also REPRODUCTION.)

fertilizin (fer″tĭ-li′zin) a substance of the plasma membrane and gelatinous coat of the ovum; thought to bind the spermatozoon to the ovum and also to be concerned with its engulfment by the ovum.

fervescence (fer-ves′ens) increase of fever or body temperature.

festinant (fes′tĭ-nant) hastening; rapidly accelerating.

festination (fes″tĭ-na′shun) a gait in which quicker and quicker steps are taken.

fetal (fe′tal) pertaining to a fetus.
  f. circulation, the circulation of blood through the body of the fetus and to and from the placenta through the umbilical cord. Oxygenated blood from the placenta is carried to the embryo by the umbilical vein. The blood from the embryo is returned to the placenta by two umbilical arteries. Oxygenation of the fetal blood and disposal of its waste products is carried on through the placenta. When the lungs begin to function at birth some of the fetal vessels, such as the ductus arteriosus, and the fetal passages, such as the foramen ovale, begin to fall into disuse. This is a gradual process of fibrosis that takes place in the period after birth.

fetalization (fe″tal-ĭ-za′shun) retention in the adult of characters that at an earlier stage of evolution were only infantile and were rapidly lost as the organism attained maturity.

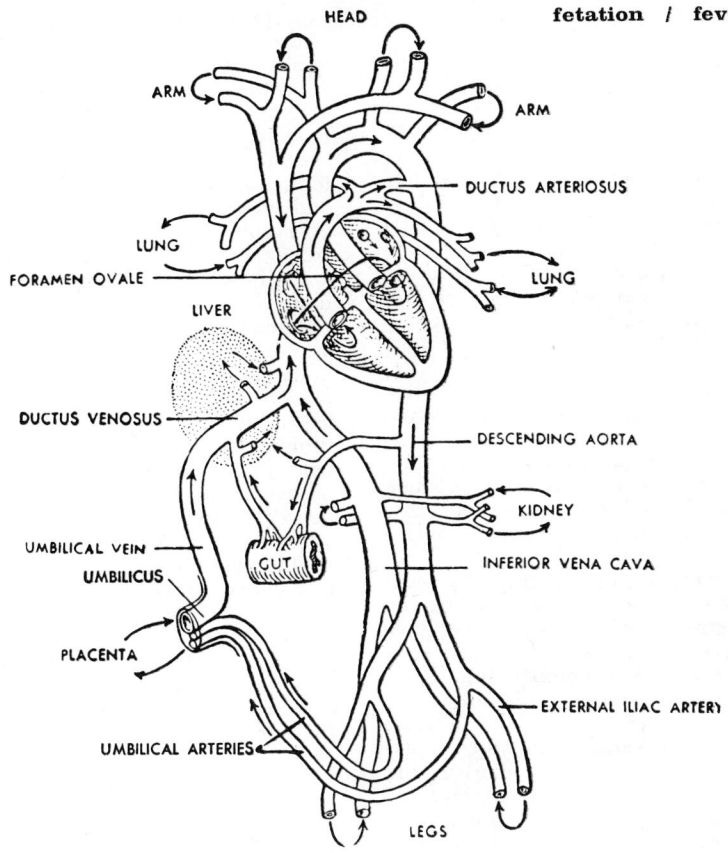

Fetal circulation. (From King, B. G., and Showers, M. J.: Human Anatomy and Physiology. 6th ed. Philadelphia, W. B. Saunders Co., 1969.)

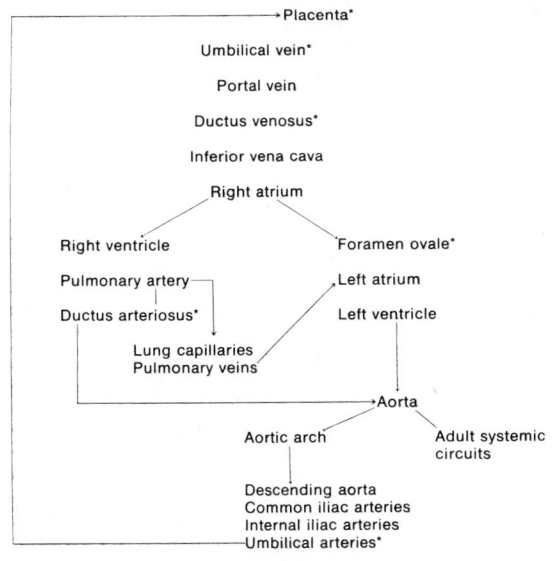

*Cease function at birth or shortly after.

fetation (fe-ta'shun) 1. development of the fetus. 2. pregnancy.

feticide (fēt'ĭ-sīd) the killing of a fetus in utero.

fetid (fet'id) having a rank, disagreeable smell.

fetish (fet'ish, fe'tish) an object or act to which special significance is attributed, e.g., an object, body part or maneuver charged with special erotic interest.

fetography (fe-tog'rah-fe) roentgenography of the fetus in utero.

fetometry (fe-tom'ĕ-tre) measurement of the fetus or of the fetal head.

fetoplacental (fe″to-plah-sen'tal) pertaining to the fetus and placenta.

fetor (fe'tor) stench or offensive odor.
  f. o'ris, halitosis.

fetus (fe'tus) [L.] the developing young in the uterus; applied especially to the human young from the seventh to ninth week of gestation until birth; before that time it is known as an EMBRYO. adj., fe'tal.
  calcified f., lithopedion; a stony or petrified fetus.
  f. in fe'tu, a teratoma within the body of an infant produced by separate growth of cells split off from the developing embryo.
  mummified f., a dried-up and shriveled fetus.
  f. papyra'ceus, a fetus flattened by being pressed against the uterine wall by a living twin.
  parasitic f., an incomplete minor fetus attached to a larger, more completely developed fetus, or autosite.

fever (fe'ver) 1. an abnormally high body temperature; pyrexia. 2. any disease characterized by marked increase of temperature, acceleration of the pulse, increased tissue destruction and delirium.

Fever is a warning that there is some disturbance of normal bodily processes. While the physiologic mechanism of fever is not fully understood, it is an indication that the temperature-regulating mechanisms of the body are out of order, and the body's delicate balance between the rate of producing heat and the rate of dissipating it is upset. This is thought to be due to chemical reactions resulting from disease.

Fever is almost always present in infectious diseases, and usually accompanies seriously infected cuts, burns and other wounds. Abnormalities in the brain that affect the hypothalamus, where the heat-regulating center is located, can produce fever. Some drugs, as well as the hormone thyroxine, can cause an elevation of the body temperature.

Some medical scientists consider fever a protective device of the body because certain pathogenic organisms are destroyed when the temperature rises well above normal. It is also believed that the increased metabolic rate accompanying fever allows the cells to increase their production of immune substances that defend the body against bacterial invasion. Fever brings discomfort, weakness or fatigue and sometimes pain, causing the patient to rest and in this way conserving his energy for battle against the disease. Sometimes fever itself is destructive, as in SUNSTROKE. Prolonged or very high fever usually must be controlled.

NORMAL AND ABNORMAL TEMPERATURE. Although fever is defined as an abnormal temperature increase, it is not always easy to determine when an increase in temperature is abnormal. This is especially true of the lower temperature readings. If the temperature is 100° F. by mouth or 101° F. or above by rectum, fever is almost decidedly present. However, a mouth temperature of 99° F. may or may not indicate fever even though the reading is above the manufacturer's 98.6° F. arrow on the thermometer scale. This arrow indicates normal temperature on the basis of a statistical average, and is by no means the normal temperature for everyone. Normal temperature varies somewhat from person to person. Also, in each person there are slight temperature variations throughout the day.

Since it is sometimes important to judge whether or not fever is present by interpreting readings under the 100° F. mark, it is recommended that a person determine his own particular normal, or basal, temperature. This is done by averaging a number of readings taken over a period of time. Once the basal temperature is determined, it can be assumed that when there is an increase of a degree or two above that figure (and in all cases when the reading is over 100° F.), fever is present.

There are a few exceptions to this rule. Children often have a slightly raised temperature after lively activity, and adults have a considerably raised temperature while engaged in strenuous sports. This rise is of course temporary and disappears with rest. During and soon after emotional excitement there may also be a rise in temperature. In women there is a slight increase in temperature at the time of ovulation.

EFFECTS OF FEVER. The feverish person feels weak. Often there is a sensation of soreness in muscles and bones, and there may also be chills, headache, thirst, loss of appetite, constipation, a coated tongue and dry skin. In children a sudden onset of high fever may bring on CONVULSIONS and DELIRIUM although the illness itself may not be serious.

In fever the pulse rate is likely to increase at the rate of about eight to ten beats per minute for each degree of temperature rise. The metabolic rate—the speed of chemical reactions in the body—also increases.

TREATMENT. The treatment of fever includes detection and elimination of the primary cause whenever possible, and the relief of symptoms. Fluids are given orally or intravenously as necessary to prevent dehydration. Frequent, small feedings of high-calorie, high-protein liquids are recommended to combat fatigue and the debility brought about by an increased metabolic rate. Vitamin supplements may be prescribed in prolonged, low-grade fevers.

Antipyretic drugs such as aspirin and sodium salicylate are used when the body temperature rises to a dangerous level. In cases of extreme fever, as in sunstroke, it is sometimes advisable to cool the patient quickly in a bath of cold water. Other measures to reduce body temperature are discussed under Nursing Care.

NURSING CARE. The feverish patient's temperature, pulse and respiration should be taken and recorded at least every 4 hours, and more frequently if the temperature rises above 102° F. or if the patient has chills or signs of delirium. The shivering accompanying a fever is a reaction of the body to the cold of its environment. The patient feels cold because his body temperature is much higher in relation to the surrounding air than it normally is. In response to the stimulus of cold the muscles begin a rhythmic contraction in an effort

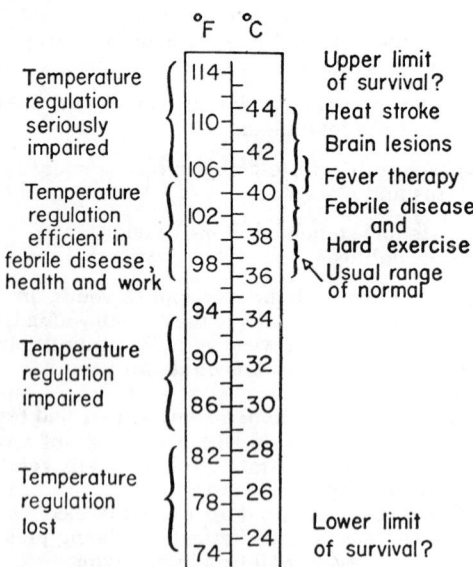

Body temperatures under different conditions. (From DuBois, E. F.: Fever and the Regulation of Body Temperature. Springfield, Ill., Charles C Thomas, 1948.)

to produce more heat. When this occurs warmth should be provided the patient in the form of extra blankets and the application of a hot water bottle filled with warm, *not hot,* water. At the same time efforts should be made to bring the body temperature down to the normal range if the physician has left a written order to this effect. Because fever is considered beneficial in some cases, it is important to know the wishes of the physician in regard to the use of nursing measures to reduce fever.

Sponging alternate parts of the body and extremities with cool water or a mixture of alcohol and water is an effective means of reducing fever. The purpose of the sponging is to increase evaporation of moisture and thereby increase heat loss from the body surface. The part being sponged should be left exposed to the air until it is almost dry, and then lightly covered while another part of the body is being sponged. Alcohol is often used with the cool bath water because it evaporates more quickly than water. An ice cap or cold compress to the forehead helps to reduce the fever and relieve headache and delirium. In some instances the physician may order a cool water enema.

During the sponging procedure the patient's temperatue is taken every 30 minutes. A sudden reduction in temperature is not desirable, and should the patient's temperature appear to be dropping too quickly the sponge bath is discontinued. After the procedure is completed the bed linens and patient's gown should be changed as necessary to leave him dry and comfortable.

A prolonged or extremely high fever is likely to produce severe dehydration. For this reason the patient is observed for symptoms of fluid depletion, the fluid intake and output are measured and recorded and the urine is observed for color and concentration. If delirium or convulsions are likely to accompany the fever, side rails should be applied to the bed and someone should be in constant attendance to prevent the patient from injuring himself.

For specific types of fevers, see the eponymic or descriptive name; as TYPHOID FEVER.

f. blister, an itching or stinging sore (called also coldsore) on the skin or mucous membrane, due to a virus infection. It is most commonly seen on the lip or mouth. The medical name for this eruption is herpes febrilis, or herpes simplex.

childbed f., puerperal fever.

continuous f., persistently elevated body temperature, showing no or little variation and never falling to normal during any 24-hour period.

induced f., fever brought on artificially, as by diathermy or by the injection of malarial organisms.

intermittent f., elevated body temperature showing fluctuation each day, with periods when it falls to normal or below normal values.

Murchison-Pel-Ebstein f., a type observed in some patients with Hodgkin's disease, characterized by irregular episodes of pyrexia of several days' duration, with intervening periods in which the temperature is normal.

periodic f., a hereditary condition characterized by repetitive febrile episodes and anatomic disturbances, occurring in precise or irregular cycles of days, weeks or months.

puerperal f., an infectious disease of childbirth (see also PUERPERAL FEVER).

recurrent f., relapsing f., elevated body temperature for one or several days, alternating with similar periods of normal or subnormal temperature;

an acute infectious disease due to a species of Borrelia (see also RELAPSING FEVER).

remittent f., elevated body temperature showing fluctuation each day, but never falling to normal.

fiber (fi′ber) an elongated threadlike structure of organic tissue.

A f's, myelinated somatic afferent and efferent nerve fibers conducting at speeds of 5 to 120 meters per second.

adrenergic f's, nerve fibers that liberate epinephrine-like substances at the time of passage of nerve impulses across a synapse.

arciform f., arcuate f., a bow-shaped fiber crossing the anterior aspect of the medulla oblongata.

axial f., the axon of a nerve fiber.

B f's, myelinated efferent preganglionic fibers of autonomic nerves, conducting at 3 to 15 meters per second.

C f's, nonmyelinated fibers of the autonomic nervous system, conducting at a velocity of 0.6 to 2.3 meters per second.

collagenous f., a soft, flexible, white fiber that is the most characteristic constituent of all types of connective tissues.

Corti's f's, Corti's rods.

dark f's, muscle fibers rich in sarcoplasm and having a dark appearance.

gray f's, nonmedullated fibers found largely in the sympathetic nerves.

lattice f., reticular fiber.

light f's, muscle fibers poor in sarcoplasm and more transparent than dark fibers.

medullated f's, grayish white nerve fibers whose axons are sheathed in myelin.

motor f's, nerve fibers transmitting motor impulses only.

muscle f., a unit of structure of muscle, made up of the coalesced protoplasm of a varying number of cells, and containing contractile fibrils.

nerve f., a slender process of a neuron, especially the prolonged axon that conducts nerve impulses.

nonmedullated f's, nerve fibers that lack the myelin sheath.

osteogenetic f's, osteogenic f's, precollagenous fibers formed by osteoclasts and becoming the fibrous component of bone matrix.

postganglionic f's, nerve fibers passing to involuntary muscle and gland cells, the cell bodies of which lie in the autonomic ganglia.

preganglionic f's, nerve fibers passing to the autonomic ganglia, the cell bodies of which lie in the brain or spinal cord.

projection f's, bundles of axon fibers that connect the cerebral cortex with the brain stem.

Purkinje's f's, beaded muscular fibers forming a network in the subendocardial tissue of the ventricles of the heart. They are thought to be concerned in the conduction of stimuli from the atria to the ventricles.

radicular f's, fibers in the roots of the spinal nerves.

reticular f., one of the connective tissue fibers, staining with silver, forming the reticular framework of lymphoid and myeloid tissue, and occurring in interstitial tissue of glandular organs, the papillary layer of the skin and elsewhere.

Rolando's f's, the external arcuate fibers of the medulla oblongata.

Sharpey's f's, those that pass from the periosteum and embed in the periosteal lamellae.

spindle f's, achromatic filaments extending between the poles of a dividing cell and making a spindle-shaped configuration.

T f., a fiber given off at right angles from the axon of a unipolar ganglion cell.

fiberscope (fi'ber-skōp) a flexible instrument for direct visual examination of the interior of hollow organs or body cavities, constructed of fibers having special optical properties.

fibr(o)- (fi'bro) word element [L.], fiber; fibrous.

fibra (fi'brah), pl. fi'brae [L.] fiber.

fibralbumin (fi″bral-bu'min) globulin.

fibremia (fi-bre'me-ah) the presence of fibrin in the blood.

fibril (fi'bril) a minute fiber or filament. adj., fibril'lar.

fibrillation (fi″brĭ-la'shun) 1. a transitory muscular contraction resulting from spontaneous activation of single muscle cells or fibers. 2. the quality of being made up of fibrils.

atrial f., auricular f., a cardiac arrhythmia characterized by extremely rapid, irregular atrial impulses, ineffectual atrial contractions and irregular, rapid ventricular beats.

ventricular f., a cardiac arrhythmia characterized by rapid, irregular and ineffective twitchings of the ventricles. Ventricular fibrillation is a frequent cause of CARDIAC ARREST. An apparatus called a defibrillator sometimes is used to alleviate fibrillation. The defibrillator delivers an electric shock to the heart muscle, depolarizing the muscle and ending the irregular contractions. The heart is then able to resume normal, regular contractions.

fibrilloceptor (fi-bril'o-sep″tor) a receptor at the terminal of a neurofibril that receives the stimuli.

fibrillolysis (fi″bril-ol'ĭ-sis) the dissolution of fibrils.

fibrin (fi'brin) an insoluble protein that is essential to clotting of blood, formed from fibrinogen by action of thrombin (see also CLOTTING).

fibrination (fi″brĭ-na'shun) excess of fibrin in the blood.

fibrinemia (fi″brĭ-ne'me-ah) the presence of fibrin in the blood.

fibrinocellular (fi″brĭ-no-sel'u-lar) made up of fibrin and cells.

fibrinogen (fi-brin'o-jen) a high-molecular-weight protein in the blood plasma that by the action of thrombin is converted into fibrin; called also clotting factor I. In the clotting mechanism, fibrin threads form a meshwork for the basis of a blood clot. Most of the fibrinogen in the circulating blood is formed in the liver. Normal quantities of fibrinogen in the plasma vary from 100 to 700 mg. per 100 ml. of plasma. (See also CLOTTING.)
Commercial preparations of human fibrinogen are used to restore blood fibrinogen levels to normal after extensive surgery, or to treat diseases and hemorrhagic conditions that are complicated by AFIBRINOGENEMIA.

fibrinogenemia (fi-brin″o-jĕ-ne'me-ah) the presence of an excessive amount of fibrinogen in the blood.

fibrinogenolysis (fi-brin″o-jĕ-nol'ĭ-sis) dissolution or inactivation of fibrinogen in the blood.

fibrinogenopenia (fi-brin″o-jen″o-pe'ne-ah) decreased fibrinogen in the blood.

fibrinoid (fi'brĭ-noid) a homogeneous, eosinophilic, relatively acellular refractile substance with some of the staining properties of fibrin.

fibrinokinase (fi″brĭ-no-ki'nās) a nonwater-soluble plasminogen activator derived from animal tissues.

fibrinolysin (fi″brĭ-nol'ĭ-sin) any enzyme that catalyzes the digestion of fibrin.

fibrinolysis (fi″brĭ-nol'ĭ-sis) the splitting up or dissolution of fibrin. adj., fibrinolyt'ic.

fibrinopenia (fi″brĭ-no-pe'ne-ah) deficiency of fibrin in the blood.

fibrinopeptide (fi″brĭ-no-pep'tīd) a substance split off from fibrinogen, during blood clotting, by the action of thrombin.

fibrinorrhea (fi″brĭ-no-re'ah) a profuse discharge containing fibrin.

f. plas'tica, membranous dysmenorrhea.

fibrinoscopy (fi″brĭ-nos'ko-pe) the diagnosis of disease by artificial digestion and examination of the fibers or fibrinous matter of the sputum, blood, effusions, etc.

fibrinosis (fi″brĭ-no'sis) excess of fibrin in the blood.

fibrinous (fi'brĭ-nus) of the nature of fibrin.

fibrinuria (fi″brĭ-nu're-ah) discharge of fibrin in the urine.

fibroadenia (fi″bro-ah-de'ne-ah) fibroid degeneration of gland tissue.

fibroadenoma (fi″bro-ad″ĕ-no'mah) adenoma containing fibrous elements.

fibroadipose (fi″bro-ad'ĭ-pōs) both fibrous and fatty.

fibroangioma (fi″bro-an″je-o'mah) an angioma containing fibrous elements.

fibroareolar (fi″bro-ah-re'o-lar) both fibrous and areolar.

fibroblast (fi'bro-blast) an immature fiber-producing cell capable of differentiating into a chondroblast, collagenoblast or osteoblast.

fibroblastoma (fi″bro-blas-to'mah) a tumor arising from connective tissue cells.

fibrocalcific (fi″bro-kal-sif'ik) pertaining to or characterized by partially calcified fibrous tissue.

fibrocarcinoma (fi″bro-kar″sĭ-no'mah) carcinoma containing fibrous elements.

fibrocartilage (fi″bro-kar′tĭ-lij) cartilage made up of parallel, thick, compact collagenous bundles, separated by narrow clefts containing the typical cartilage cells.

fibrochondritis (fi″bro-kon-dri′tis) inflammation of fibrocartilage.

fibrochondroma (fi″bro-kon-dro′mah) chondroma containing fibrous elements.

fibrocystic (fi″bro-sis′tik) characterized by an overgrowth of fibrous tissue and the development of cystic spaces.
   f. disease of pancreas, cystic fibrosis.

fibrocystoma (fi″bro-sis-to′mah) cystoma containing fibrous elements.

fibrocyte (fi′bro-sīt) a cell that produces fibrous tissue; called also fibroblast.

fibrocytogenesis (fi″bro-si″to-jen′ĕ-sis) development of connective tissue fibrils.

fibroelastic (fi″bro-e-las′tik) both fibrous and elastic.

fibroelastosis (fi″bro-e″las-to′sis) overgrowth of fibroelastic elements.
   endocardial f., a condition characterized by left ventricular hypertrophy, conversion of the endo-cardium into a thick fibroelastic coat and reduction in ventricular capacity.

fibroenchondroma (fi″bro-en″kon-dro′mah) en-chondroma containing fibrous elements.

fibroglioma (fi″bro-gli-o′mah) glioma containing fibrous elements.

fibroid (fi′broid) 1. resembling fiber or a fibrous structure. 2. fibroma.
   f. tumor, a common benign tumor of the uterus properly designated as myoma of the UTERUS.

fibroidectomy (fi″broi-dek′to-me) excision of a uterine myoma.

fibrolipoma (fi″bro-lĭ-po′mah) a lipoma contain-ing fibrous elements.

fibroma (fi-bro′mah) a tumor composed mainly of fibrous or fully developed connective tissue.
   chondromyxoid f. of bone, a benign neoplasm ap-parently derived from cartilage-forming connective tissue.
   f. myxomatodes, myxofibroma; myxoma blended with fibroma.
   nonosteogenic f., a degenerative and proliferative lesion of the medullary and cortical tissues of bone.
   odontogenic f., a benign tumor of the jaw arising from the embryonic portion of the tooth germ, the dental papilla or dental follicle, or later from the periodontium.

fibromatosis (fi″bro-mah-to′sis) a condition char-acterized by the presence of numerous fibromas.
   f. gingi′vae, a diffuse fibroma of the gingivae and palate, manifested as a dense, smooth or nodu-lar overgrowth of the tissues.

fibromatous (fi-bro′mah-tus) of the nature of fibroma.

fibromembranous (fi″bro-mem′brah-nus) both fibrous and membranous.

fibromuscular (fi″bro-mus′ku-lar) both fibrous and muscular.

fibromyectomy (fi″bro-mi-ek′to-me) excision of a fibromyoma.

fibromyitis (fi″bro-mi-i′tis) inflammation of muscle with fibrous degeneration.

fibromyoma (fi″bro-mi-o′mah) a myoma contain-ing fibrous elements.

fibromyomectomy (fi″bro-mi″o-mek′to-me) exci-sion of a fibromyoma.

fibromyositis (fi″bro-mi″o-si′tis) inflammation of fibromuscular tissue.

fibromyxoma (fi″bro-mik-so′mah) a myxoma con-taining fibrous elements.

fibromyxosarcoma (fi″bro-mik″so-sar-ko′mah) a sarcoma containing fibrous and mucous elements.

fibroneuroma (fi″bro-nu-ro′mah) a neuroma con-taining fibrous elements.

fibropapilloma (fi″bro-pap″ĭ-lo′mah) a papilloma containing fibrous tissue.

fibropericarditis (fi″bro-per″ĭ-kar-di′tis) fibrous pericarditis.

fibroplasia (fi″bro-pla′ze-ah) the formation of fibrous tissue, as in the healing of a wound. adj., **fibroplas′tic.**
   retrolental f., a condition characterized by the presence of opaque tissue behind the lens, leading to detachment of the retina and arrest of growth of the eye, generally attributed to use of high con-centrations of oxygen in the care of premature infants.

fibroplastin (fi″bro-plas′tin) paraglobulin.

fibrosarcoma (fi″bro-sar-ko′mah) a sarcoma containing fibrous elements.
   odontogenic f., a malignant tumor of the jaws, originating from one of the mesenchymal compo-nents of the tooth or tooth germ.

fibroserous (fi″bro-se′rus) composed of both fibrous and serous elements.

fibrosis (fi-bro′sis) formation of fibrous tissue; fibroid degeneration. adj., **fibrot′ic.**
   cystic f., overgrowth of fibrous tissue in an organ, with development of cystic spaces.
   cystic f. of pancreas, a generalized hereditary disorder with widespread dysfunction of exocrine glands, chronic pulmonary disease, pancreatic deficiency, high levels of electrolytes in sweat and sometimes biliary cirrhosis. (See also CYSTIC FIBROSIS.)
   mediastinal f., development of whitish, hard fi-brous tissue in the upper portion of the mediasti-num, sometimes obstructing the air passages and large blood vessels.
   periureteral f., progressive development of fibrous tissue spreading from the great midline vessels and causing strangulation of one or both ureters.
   postfibrinous f., that occurring in tissues in which fibrin has been deposited.
   proliferative f., that in which the fibrous elements

continue to proliferate after the original causative factor has ceased to operate.

pulmonary f., interstitial, diffuse, progressive fibrosis of the walls of pulmonary alveoli, leading to deficient aeration of the blood, dyspnea, cyanosis and cor pulmonale.

f. u'teri, a morbid condition characterized by overgrowth of the smooth muscle and increase in the collagenous fibrous tissue of the uterus, producing a thickened, coarse, tough myometrium.

fibrositis (fi″bro-si'tis) inflammatory hyperplasia of the white fibrous tissue, especially of the muscle sheaths and fascial layers of the locomotor system, causing pain and stiffness; called also muscular rheumatism.

fibrous (fi'brus) composed of fibers.

f. dysplasia, localized overgrowth of fibrous tissue in bone, causing destructive resorption of cancellous and adjacent cortical bone, and sometimes distention and distortion of contours of the affected bones; it may affect a single bone (monostotic fibrous dysplasia) or many bones (polyostotic fibrous dysplasia, or Albright's syndrome).

fibula (fib'u-lah) the lateral and smaller of the two bones of the leg.

F.I.C.S. Fellow of the International College of Surgeons.

field (fēld) a limited area, such as the area of a slide visible through the lens system of a microscope.

auditory f., the area within which stimuli will produce the sensation of sound.

high-power f., the area of a slide visible under the high magnification system of a microscope.

low-power f., the area of a slide visible under the low magnification system of a microscope.

morphogenetic f., an embryonic region out of which definite structures normally develop.

visual f., the area within which stimuli will produce the sensation of sight with the eye in a straight-ahead position.

filaceous (fi-la'shus) composed of filaments.

filament (fil'ah-ment) a delicate fiber or thread.

filamentous (fil″ah-men'tus) composed of long, threadlike structures.

Filaria (fi-la're-ah) a name formerly given a genus of nematode parasitic worms.

F. bancrof'ti, *Wuchereria bancrofti.*

F. lo'a, *Loa loa.*

F. medinen'sis, *Dracunculus medinensis.*

filaria (fi-la're-ah), pl. *fila'riae* [L.] a slender, threadlike worm, especially one of a series formerly included in the genus Filaria. adj., **fila'rial.**

filariasis (fil″ah-ri'ah-sis) an infectious tropical disease caused by parasitic nematode worms formerly included in the genus Filaria. The organism causing the most common form of filariasis is *Wuchereria bancrofti.* Most often encountered in central Africa, the southwest Pacific and eastern Asia, the disease also occurs in the West Indies and in tropical South and Central America. It is transmitted by the Culex mosquito or by mites or flies. The larvae invade lymphoid tissues and then grow to adult worms an inch or two long. The resulting obstruction of the lymphatic circulation causes swelling, inflammation and pain. Repeated infections over many years, with impaired circulation and formation of excess connective tissue, may cause enlargement of the affected part, usually the arm, leg or scrotum. In cases of extreme enlargement, known as ELEPHANTIASIS, the affected part may grow to two or three times its normal size.

The larvae can be killed by treatment with diethylcarbamazine, but there is as yet no effective way of treating the adult worms. Edema of the legs can be reduced by rest and by the use of pressure bandages. The prognosis is favorable for all but the most severe cases.

filaricide (fi-lār'ĭ-sīd) an agent that destroys filariae.

Filarioidea (fi-la″re-oi'de-ah) a superfamily of nematode parasites, the adults of which are long, threadlike worms found in lymph nodes, other tissues and body cavities, and the larvae of which (microfilariae) are found in the blood.

filiform (fil'ĭ-form, fi'lĭ-form) threadlike.

filipuncture (fil'ĭ-pungk″tūr) insertion of a wire or thread into an aneurysm.

fillet (fil'et) 1. a loop, as of cord or tape, for making traction. 2. a loop-shaped structure, such as a band of nerve fibers in the brain.

olivary f., the nerve fascicle surrounding an olivary body.

film (film) 1. a thin layer or coating. 2. a thin sheet of material (e.g., gelatin, cellulose acetate) specially treated for use in photography or radiography; used also to designate the sheet after exposure to the energy to which it is sensitive.

bite-wing f., an x-ray film for radiography of oral structures, with a protruding tab to be held between the upper and lower teeth.

gelatin f., absorbable, a sterile, nonantigenic, absorbable, water-insoluble coating used as an aid in surgical closure and repair of defects in the dura mater and pleura.

spot f., a radiograph of a small anatomic area obtained (1) by rapid exposure during fluoroscopy to provide a permanent record of a transiently observed abnormality, or (2) by limitation of radiation passing through the area to improve definition and detail of the image produced.

x-ray f., film sensitized to roentgen (x) rays, either before or after exposure.

filopressure (fi″lo-presh'ur) compression of a blood vessel by a thread.

filter (fil'ter) a device for eliminating certain elements, as (1) particles of certain size from a solution, or (2) rays of certain wavelength from a stream of radiant energy.

Berkefeld's f., one composed of diatomaceous earth, impermeable to ordinary bacteria.

Kitasato's f., an unglazed porcelain cylinder through which liquids are drawn by suction.

Pasteur-Chamberland f., a hollow column of unglazed porcelain through which liquids are forced by pressure.

Wood's f., a screen permitting passage of ultraviolet rays and absorbing rays of visible light.

filterable, filtrable (fil'ter-ah-bl), (fil'trah-bl) capable of passing through the pores of a filter;

said of viruses that will pass through a filter that will not permit the passage of larger microorganisms.

filtrate (fil'trāt) a liquor that passed through a filter.

glomerular f., the fluid that passes from the blood through the glomeruli of the kidney and is excreted as urine.

filtration (fil-tra'shun) passage through a filter or through a material that prevents passage of certain molecules.

filtratometer (fil"trah-tom'ĕ-ter) an instrument for measuring gastric filtrates.

filum (fi'lum), pl. *fi'la* [L.] a threadlike structure.

f. termina'le, the slender fibrous strand anchoring the spinal cord to the coccyx.

fimbria (fim'bre-ah), pl. *fim'briae* [L.] an elongated process such as one of the components making up a fringe, or a structure resembling such a component.

f. hippocam'pi, the band of white matter along the median edge of the ventricular surface of the hippocampus.

fimbriae of uterine tube, the numerous divergent fringelike processes on the distal part of the infundibulum of the uterine tube.

fimbriate (fim'bre-āt) fringed.

finger (fing'ger) one of the five digits of the hand.

clubbed f., enlargement of the distal phalanx of a finger.

hammer f., mallet f., permanent flexion of the distal phalanx of a finger.

webbed f's, fingers abnormally joined by strands of tissue at their base.

first aid (ferst ād) emergency care and treatment of an injured person before complete medical and surgical treatment can be secured.

fish-skin disease ichthyosis.

fish-slime disease septicemia from puncture wound by a fish spine.

Fishberg concentration test (fish'berg) a laboratory test used to determine the ability of the kidneys to concentrate urine. Samples of urine are collected and tested for specific gravity. The patient is allowed no food or water from the evening meal the night before the test until after completion of the test. A specimen of urine is collected at 10:00 A.M. and another at 11:00 A.M. Normal concentration is indicated by a specific gravity of 1.020.

fission (fish'un) division into parts; segmentation.

binary f., the halving of the nucleus and then the cytoplasm of the cell, as in protozoa.

nuclear f., disintegration of a heavy atomic nucleus into smaller nuclei.

fissiparous (fĭ-sip'ah-rus) propagated by fission.

fissula (fis'u-lah), pl. *fis'sulae* [L.] a small cleft.

fissura (fis-ur'rah), pl. *fissu'rae* [L.] fissure.

fissure (fish'er) a narrow slit or cleft, especially one of the deeper or more constant furrows separating the gyri of the brain.

abdominal f., a congenital cleft in the abdominal wall.

anal f., a painful lineal ulcer at the margin of the anus.

anterior median f., a longitudinal furrow along the midline of the ventral surface of the spinal cord, extending nearly one-third of the anteroposterior diameter.

f. of Bichat, the transverse fissure between the fornix and the upper surface of the cerebellum.

branchial f., branchial cleft.

callosomarginal f., one on the median surface of each cerebral hemisphere midway between the corpus callosum and the margin of the surface.

central f., fissure of Rolando.

collateral f., a longitudinal fissure on the inferior surface of the cerebral hemisphere between the fusiform gyrus and the hippocampal gyrus.

Henle's f's, spaces filled with connective tissue between the muscular fibers of the heart.

hippocampal f., one from the splenium to the tip of the temporal lobe.

interparietal f., one between the parietal convolutions of the brain.

longitudinal f., the deep fissure between the cerebral hemispheres.

maxillary f., a groove on the maxilla for the maxillary process of the palatine bone.

occipital f., a deep fissure between the parietal and occipital lobes of the cerebrum.

palpebral f., the slit or opening between the eyelids.

portal f., the transverse fissure of the liver.

posterior median f., a shallow vertical groove on the posterior surface of the spinal cord in the median plane.

precentral f., one parallel to the fissure of Rolando and anterior to it.

presylvian f., the anterior branch of the fissure of Sylvius.

f. of Rolando, a groove running obliquely across the superolateral surface of the cerebral hemisphere, separating the frontal from the parietal lobe.

f. of Sylvius, one that separates the anterior and middle lobes of the cerebrum.

transverse f., 1. the fissure crossing transversely the under surface of the right lobe of the liver. 2. the horseshoe-shaped fissure from the descending cornu of the cerebrum on one side to that on the other.

Wernicke's f., one separating the parietal and temporal lobes from the occipital lobe.

zygal f., a cerebral fissure consisting of two branches connected by a stem.

fistula (fis'tu-lah) any abnormal, tubelike passage within body tissue. Some fistulas are created surgically, for diagnostic or therapeutic purposes; others occur as a result of injury or as congenital abnormalities. Among the many kinds of fistulas, the anal type (fistula in ano) is one of the most common. This generally develops as a result of a break, or fissure, in the wall of the anal canal or rectum, or an abscess here. Treatment is by surgery. In women, difficult labor in childbirth may result in the formation of a vesicovaginal fistula between the bladder and the vagina, with resulting leakage of urine into the vagina. In the vesicointestinal fistula, there is leakage of urine from the bladder into the intestine. In rectovaginal fistula, feces escape through the wall of the anal canal or rectum into the vagina. The latter condition, formerly a serious hazard of childbirth, is now rare; also, like other kinds of fistulas, it can be corrected by surgery.

With the types of fistulas described here, typical symptoms are pain in the affected region and an abnormal discharge through the skin near the anus or through the vagina. Fistulas at different places of the body may be caused by tuberculosis, actinomycosis (a fungus infection), the presence of diverticula or some other serious disease, and the fistula itself may be a site of infection and discomfort.

arteriovenous f., a fistula between an artery and a vein.

blind f., one open at one end only, opening on the skin (external blind fistula) or on a mucous surface (internal blind fistula).

branchial f., an unclosed branchial cleft.

complete f., one extending from the skin to an internal body cavity.

craniosinus f., one between the cerebral space and one of the sinuses, permitting escape of cerebrospinal fluid into the nose.

Eck's f., an artificial communication made between the portal vein and the vena cava.

fecal f., a colonic fistula opening on the external surface of the body and discharging feces.

gastric f., an abnormal passage communicating with the stomach; often applied to an artificially created opening, through the abdominal wall, into the stomach.

horseshoe f., a semicircular fistulous tract about the anus.

incomplete f., blind fistula.

pulmonary arteriovenous f., congenital, a congenital anomalous communication between the pulmonary arterial and venous systems, allowing unoxygenated blood to enter the systemic circulation.

umbilical f., an abnormal passage communicating with the gut or the urachus at the umbilicaus.

fistulectomy (fis″tu-lek′to-me) excision of a fistula.

fistulization (fis″tu-li̅-za′shun) surgical creation of an opening from the body surface to an internal organ or passage.

fistulotomy (fis″tu-lot′o-me) incision of a fistula.

fistulous (fis′tu-lus) of the nature of a fistula.

fixation (fik-sa′shun) 1. the act or operation of holding, suturing or fastening in a fixed position. 2. the condition of being held in a fixed position. 3. in psychiatry, the cessation of the development of personality at a stage short of complete maturity. 4. in microscopy, the hardening and preserving for microscopic examination of fresh tissue or microorganisms by heating or by immersion in a hardening solution.

f. of complement, addition of another serum containing an antibody and the corresponding antigen to a hemolytic serum, making the complement incapable of producing hemolysis (see also COMPLEMENT FIXATION TESTS).

skeletal f., immobilization of the ends of a fractured bone by metal wires or plates applied directly to the bone (internal skeletal fixation) or on the body surface (external skeletal fixation).

fixative (fik′sah-tiv) an agent for hardening and preserving specimens for histologic study.

flaccid (flak′sid) weak, soft and flabby; applied especially to muscles.

flagellate (flaj′ĕ-lāt) an organism of the subphylum Mastigophora, having one or more flagella.

flagelliform (flah-jel′ĭ-form) shaped like a flagellum or lash.

flagellosis (flaj″ĕ-lo′sis) infection with a flagellate protozoan.

flagellum (flah-jel′um), pl. *flagel'la* [L.] a filamentous, cytoplasmic projection from a cell, such as is characteristic of protozoa of the subphylum Mastigophora. The flagellum is an organ of locomotion for the organism.

Flagyl (flaj′il) trademark for a preparation of metronidazole, a trichomonacide.

Flajani's disease (flah-jan′ēz) exophthalmic goiter.

flame (flām) 1. the luminous, irregular appearance usually accompanying combustion, or an appearance resembling it. 2. to render sterile by exposure to a flame.

flank (flangk) the side of the body between the ribs and ilium.

flap (flap) a portion of superficial tissue (skin with subcutaneous tissue, cornea, etc.) partially detached from underlying tissue; used in repair of defects in remote parts of the body, as in plastic surgery.

island f., a segment of skin and subcutaneous tissue, with a pedicle made up of only the nutrient vessels.

jump f., a graft cut from the abdomen and attached to a flap of the same size on the forearm. The forearm flap is transferred later to some other part of the body.

musculocutaneous f., a flap containing skin and muscle.

skin f., a thin flap containing little subcutaneous tissue.

sliding f., a flap carried to its new position by sliding.

flare (flār) an area of redness on the skin around an infective lesion or around the point of application of an irritant.

flask (flask) a laboratory vessel, usually of glass and with a constricted neck.

flatfoot (flat′foot) absence of the normal arch of the sole of the foot.

flatness (flat′nes) a quality of sound elicited by percussion, being short and high-pitched.

flatulence (flat′u-lens) excessive formation of gases in the stomach or intestine. adj., **flat′ulent.**

flatus (fla′tus) gas or air in the stomach or intestine.

flatworm (flat′werm) an individual organism of the phylum Platyhelminthes (see also WORMS).

flav(o)- (fla′vo) word element [L.], *yellow.*

flavedo (flah-ve′do) yellowness, as of the skin.

flavism (fla′vizm) yellowness of the hair.

flavone (fla′vōn) a substance, $C_{15}H_{10}O_2$, the basis of several yellow dyes.

flavonoid (fla′vo-noid) one of a group of substances resembling vitamin P having antihemorrhagic properties.

flavonol (fla′vo-nol) a yellow, crystalline substance, a hydroxyl derivative of flavone.

flaxseed (flak′sēd) linseed; used in laxatives and as an emollient.

fl. dr. fluid dram.

flea (fle) a small, wingless insect with mouthparts of the piercing-sucking type, ectoparasitic on birds and mammals; fleas act as vectors of such diseases as plague, tularemia and brucellosis.

Fleming (flem′ing) Sir Alexander (1881–1955). Scottish bacteriologist and discoverer of penicillin. He was born at Lochfield in Scotland and served as a captain in the army medical corps during World War I. The first result of his search for an antibacterial substance that would not be toxic to human tissue was the discovery of lysozyme, but his ephochal discovery was of penicillin in 1938. In 1943 he was made fellow of the Royal Society, was knighted and given the John Scott medal in 1944 and was awarded the Nobel prize in 1945.

flesh (flesh) soft tissue of plant or animal organisms; muscular tissue of animals.
　goose f., cutis anserina; erection of the papillae of the skin, as from cold or shock.
　proud f., soft, edematous, unhealthy-looking granulation tissue.

fletcherism (flech′er-izm) thorough mastication of food.

flex (fleks) to bend or put in a state of flexion.

flexibilitas (flek″sĭ-bil′ĭ-tas) [L.] flexibility.
　f. ce′rea, passive retention by the body or limbs of any position in which they are placed.

flexibility (flek″sĭ-bil′ĭ-te) the state of being unusually pliant.
　waxy f., flexibilitas cerea.

flexion (flek′shun) the act of bending; decreasing of the angle at the joint between two bones.

flexor (flek′sor) that which flexes, especially a muscle that flexes a joint.
　f. surface, the aspect of a joint of a limb on the side toward which the movement of flexion is directed.

flexura (flek-shu′rah), pl. *flexu′rae* [L.] flexure.

flexure (flek′sher) a bend or fold; a curve.
　caudal f., the bend at the tail end of the embryo.
　cephalic f., a sharp bend at the level of the midbrain of an early vertebrate embryo.
　cervical f., a gentle curvature in the early vertebrate embryo, in the region of the future neck.
　colic f., left, the angular junction of the transverse and descending colon.
　colic f., right, the angular junction of the ascending and transverse colon.
　dorsal f., a flexure in the mid-dorsal region of the embryo.
　duodenojejunal f., the bend at the junction of duodenum and jejunum.
　hepatic f., the bend at the junction of the ascending and transverse colon.
　lumbar f., the ventral curvature in the lumbar region of the back.

　mesencephalic f., a bend in the neural tube of the embryo at the level of the mesencephalon, or midbrain.
　pontine f., a flexure of the hindbrain in the embryo.
　sacral f., caudal flexure.
　sigmoid f., the bend at the junction of descending colon and rectum.
　splenic f., left colic flexure.

flint disease (flint) chalicosis.

floating kidney a condition in which the kidney does not remain fixed in its normal position. NEPHROPTOSIS refers to a dropping of the kidney from its normal position. Surgical correction, by nephropexy, is necessary when the condition interferes with normal kidney function.

floccillation (flok″sĭ-la′shun) carphology; picking at the bedclothes by a delirious patient.

flocculation (flok″u-la′shun) a colloid phenomenon in which the disperse phase separates in discrete, usually visible, particles rather than in a continuous mass, as in coagulation.

flocculent (flok′u-lent) containing downy or flaky shreds.

flocculoreaction (flok″u-lo-re-ak′shun) a serum reaction characterized by flocculation.

flocculus (flok′u-lus), pl. *floc′uli* [L.] a small tuft or mass, as of wool or other fibrous material. adj., **floc′cular.**

flora (flo′rah) the collective plant organisms of a given locality.
　intestinal f., the bacteria normally residing within the lumen of the intestine.

florantyrone (flo-ran′ti-rōn) a butyric acid compound used as a hydrocholeretic.

Floraquin (flōr′ah-kwin) trademark for a preparation of diiodohydroxyquin, an antiamebic and antitrichomonal.

Florinef (flōr′ĭ-nef) trademark for preparations of fludrocortisone, a synthetic corticoid.

Floropryl (flōr′o-pril) trademark for preparations of isoflurophate, an anticholinesterase inhibitor and a miotic used in glaucoma.

fl. oz. fluid ounce.

flu (floo) a common term for INFLUENZA, a virus disease that is highly contagious and may be serious if not treated promptly.

fluctuation (fluk″tu-a′shun) a wavelike motion or alteration of condition or position.

fludrocortisone (floo″dro-kor′tĭ-sōn) a synthetic corticoid with effects similar to those of hydrocortisone and desoxycorticosterone.

fluid (floo′id) 1. a material that flows readily in the natural state; a liquid or gas. 2. composed of elements that yield to pressure without disruption of the mass. 3. one of the ultimate states of matter, being composed of molecules that can move about within limits, permitting change in the shape of the mass without disruption of the substance.

allantoic f., the fluid contained within the allantois.

amniotic f., the fluid within the amnion that bathes the developing fetus (see also AMNIOTIC FLUID).

body f's, the fluids within the body; normally they make up about 57 per cent of the total body weight; although obesity may decrease the percentage to as low as 45 per cent.

Although the body fluids are continually in motion, moving in and out of the cells, tissue spaces and vascular system, physiologists consider them to be "compartmentalized." Fluid within the cell membrane is called intracellular fluid and comprises about two-thirds of the total body fluids. The remaining one-third is outside the cell and is called extracellular fluid. The extracellular fluid can be further divided into tissue fluid (interstitial fluid), blood plasma (intravascular fluid), cerebrospinal fluid, fluid in the eye (intraocular fluid) and fluid of the gastrointestinal tract.

Intracellular fluid serves as a medium for the basic materials needed by the cells for growth, repair and carrying on their various functions. Extracellular fluid is mainly concerned with transporting substances from one part of the body to another; for example, it carries the nutrients and chemicals needed by the cells for metabolism and also the waste products of cell metabolism. Through the process of DIFFUSION there is a continual interchange between intracellular and extracellular fluid and between the fluid in the blood vessels and tissue spaces. Extracellular fluid is carried by the circulatory system and the lymphatic system, and is essential to the transportation of such substances as glucose from the intestinal tract to the cells, waste products from the cells to the kidneys and lungs and urea from the liver to the kidney.

The ELECTROLYTE composition of intracellular fluid differs from that of extracellular fluid. Intracellular fluid contains large amounts of potassium, magnesium and phosphates. Extracellular fluid contains large amounts of sodium, chloride and

bicarbonate ions. The difference in electrolyte composition is important in maintaining an electrical charge across the cell membrane. This charge is necessary for the transmission of nerve impulses, for muscle contraction and for glandular secretions.

It is obvious that the maintenance of adequate body fluids and a normal balance between intracellular and extracellular fluids is essential to the life of the cell and to the health and well-being of the individual. Disturbances in this balance can produce EDEMA, DEHYDRATION, SHOCK, UREMIA and other serious or even fatal disorders. (See also INTRAVENOUS INFUSION.)

cerebrospinal f., the fluid contained within the ventricles of the brain, the subarachnoid space and the central canal of the spinal cord (see also CEREBROSPINAL FLUID).

f. dram, a unit of liquid measure of the apothecaries' system, containing 60 minims, and equivalent to 3.697 ml.

f. ounce, a unit of liquid measure of the apothecaries' system, being 8 fluid drams, or the equivalent of 29.57 ml.

spinal f., the fluid within the spinal canal.

subarachnoid f., cerebrospinal fluid.

synovial f., synovia.

fluidextract (floo"id-ek'strakt) a liquid preparation of a vegetable drug, containing alcohol as a solvent or preservative, or both, each milliliter of which contains the therapeutic constituents of 1 Gm. of the standard drug it represents.

fluidrachm (floo'ĭ-dram) fluid dram.

fluke (flook) an organism of the class Trematoda (phylum Platyhelminthes), characterized by a body that is usually flat and often leaflike. These parasitic trematode worms can infect the blood, liver, intestines and lungs. SCHISTOMIASIS is an infection of the body with flukes of the genus Schistosoma, the so-called blood flukes.

flumen (floo'men), pl. *flu'mina* [L.] a stream.

flu'mina pilo'rum, the lines along which the hairs of the body are arranged.

flumethiazide (floo"mě-thi'ah-zīd) a sulfonamide compound used as a diuretic and antihypertensive.

fluocinolone acetonide (floo"o-sin'o-lōn ah-set'-o-nīd) a steroid compound with anti-inflammatory action used for topical application to skin lesions.

fluohydrisone (floo"o-hi'drĭ-sōn) fludrocortisone, a synthetic corticoid.

fluohydrocortisone (floo"o-hi"dro-kor'tĭ-sōn) fludrocortisone, a synthetic corticoid.

fluorescein (floo"o-res'e-in) an orange-red powder used in manufacture of various dyes.

sodium f., a compound used in solution applied topically to the eye to detect injury to the cornea.

fluorescence (floo"o-res'ens) the emission of radiation, especially that from the visible spectrum, as a result of exposure to and absorption of radiation from another source.

fluoridation (floo"or-ĭ-da'shun) the addition of a fluoride, a chemical salt containing fluorine, to drinking water. This has been found to reduce the occurrence of dental caries in children by about one-half.

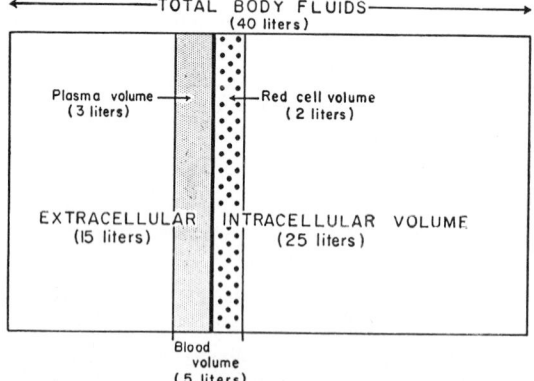

Diagrammatic representation of the body fluids, showing the extracellular fluid volume, intracellular fluid volume, blood volume and total body fluids. (From Guyton, A. C.: Textbook of Medical Physiology. 4th ed. Philadelphia, W. B. Saunders Co., 1971.)

Minute traces of fluoride are found in almost all food, but the quantity apparently is too small to meet the requirements of the body in building tooth enamel that resists cavities. Drinking water containing one part fluoride to one million parts of water does meet this need. It has been found to reduce tooth decay in children by as much as 40 to 60 per cent. Since few natural water supplies contain the necessary amount of fluoride, it usually must be added if protection against tooth decay is desired. Recent evidence suggests that the fluoridation of water has little direct effect in reducing tooth decay in adults. But children raised on fluoridated water develop a resistance to tooth decay that carries over into their adult lives.

In spite of all the evidence in favor of fluoridation, some communities have hesitated to add the chemical to their water. Where this is true, it is possible to obtain other means of fluoride protection. Dentists may apply fluoride solutions directly to a child's teeth, beginning as soon as the first teeth appear, and repeat this treatment every 3 or 4 years until the child is 13. This has been found to reduce caries by about 40 per cent.

Fluoridated water can be bought by the bottle or prepared at home, but both methods require special care and are far more costly to the individual than is the fluoridation of a public water supply. The dentist or physician may prescribe sodium fluoride drops to be added to milk, water or juice. The use of these drops must be carefully supervised, since a slight excess of fluoride causes mottling of teeth and since, like most medicines, fluoride in large amounts is a poison. A dentifrice containing fluoride may also prove effective. The physician or dentist should be consulted before any fluoride preparation is used.

fluoride (floo'ō-rīd) any binary compound of fluorine.

fluoridization (floo″or-ĭ-dĭ-za′shun) fluoridation.

fluorimetry (floo″or-im′ĕ-tre) determination of the spectral range of fluorescence of a substance in solution.

fluorination (floo″or-ĭ-na′shun) 1. treatment with fluorine. 2. fluoridation.

fluorine (floo′or-ēn) a chemical element, atomic number 9, atomic weight 18.998, symbol F. (See table of ELEMENTS).

fluorography (floo″or-og′rah-fe) photography of the image revealed on a fluorescent screen; called also fluororoentgenography.

fluorometholone (floor″o-meth′o-lōn) a compound used as a glucocorticoid with anti-inflammatory effects on the skin.

fluorophosphate (floo″or-o-fos′fāt) an organic compound containing fluorine and phosphorus.

fluororoentgenography (floo″or-o-rent″gen-og′-rah-fe) the photographic recording of fluoroscopic images on small films, using a fast lens; used in mass roentgenography of the chest. Called also fluorography and photofluorography.

fluoroscope (floo′or-o-skōp″) an instrument for visual observation of the deep structures of the body by means of x-ray. The patient is put into position so that the part to be viewed is placed between an x-ray tube and a fluorescent screen. X-rays from the tube pass through the body and project the bones and organs as shadowy images on the screen. Examination by this method is called fluoroscopy.

The advantage of the fluoroscope is that the action of joints, organs and entire systems of the body can be observed directly. The use of radiopaque media aids in this process. (See also BARIUM TEST.)

fluoroscopy (floo″or-os′ko-pe) examination by means of the fluoroscope

fluorosis (floo″o-ro′sis) a condition due to ingestion of excessive amounts of fluorine.
   dental f., a mottled discoloration of the enamel of the teeth occurring in chronic endemic fluorosis.
   endemic f., chronic, a condition due to long-continued ingestion of excessive amounts of fluorine.

Fluothane (floo′o-thān) trademark for a preparation of halothane, a general anesthetic.

fluoxymesterone (floo-ok″se-mes′ter-ōn) a compound used as an anabolic androgen in palliative treatment of certain cancers.

fluphenazine (floo-fen′ah-zēn) a compound used as a tranquilizer and antiemetic.

fluprednisolone (floo″pred-nis′o-lōn) a compound used as an anti-inflammatory corticosteroid in treatment of joint disease and allergic disturbances.

flurandrenolone (floor″an-dren′o-lōn) a corticosteroid applied locally to skin lesions.

flush (flush) redness of the face and neck.
   hectic f., the peculiar flush of the face in wasting disease.
   malar f., hectic flush over the cheekbone in pulmonary tuberculosis.

flutter (flut′er) a tremulous, generally ineffective movement.
   atrial f., rapid heart action with the atria contracting regularly at a rate of 250 to 350 per minute.
   impure f., a form in which the atrial rhythm is irregular.
   mediastinal f., mobility of the mediastinum, each inspiration of the healthy lung drawing the mediastinum toward itself.
   pure f., a form in which the atrial rhythm is regular.
   ventricular f., a possible transition stage between ventricular tachycardia and ventricular fibrillation, the electrocardiogram showing rapid, uniform and virtually regular oscillations, 250 or more per minute.

flux (fluks) 1. an excessive discharge. 2. matter discharged.
   bloody f., dysentery.

fly (fli) a two-winged insect that is often the vector of organisms causing disease.

Fm chemical symbol, *fermium.*

focus (fo′kus), pl. *fo′ci* [L.] 1. the point of convergence of light rays or sound waves. 2. chief center of a morbid process. adj., **fo′cal.**
   epileptogenic f., the area of the cerebral cortex

responsible for causing epileptic seizures, as revealed in the encephalogram.

foe- for words beginning thus, see those beginning *fe-*.

fog (fog) a colloid system in which the dispersion medium is a gas and the disperse particles are liquid.

fogging (fog'ing) dimming of the vision by use of appropriate lenses before the eyes, as a means of relaxing accommodation.

fold (fōld) a doubling or reflection of a body structure.
   amniotic f., the folded edge of the amnion where it rises over and finally encloses the embryo.
   aryepiglottic f's, aryepiglottidean f's, folds of mucous membrane extending between the arytenoid cartilage and the epiglottis.
   costocolic f., a fold of peritoneum from the diaphragm to the left colic flexure.
   Douglas's semilunar f., the lower part of the posterior wall of the sheath of the rectus muscle of the abdomen.
   gluteal f., the crease separating the buttocks from the thigh.
   head f., a fold of blastoderm at the cephalic end of the developing embryo.
   nail f., the fold of connective tissue embracing the base and sides of the nail of a finger or toe.
   neural f., one of the paired folds lying on either side of the neural plate that form the neural tube.
   tail f., a fold in the early embryo, ensheathing the hindgut.
   vestigial f., a pericardial fold over the root of the left lung.
   vocal f., a fold of mucous membrane in the larynx, forming the inferior boundary of the ventricle of the larynx, the vocal muscle being situated deep to it; called also true vocal cord.

folic acid (fo'lik) one of the B-group vitamins. Folic acid is necessary to the proper formation of blood in the body, and a deficiency of this vitamin typically produces anemia. Green vegetables and liver are major sources of folic acid in the diet. Folic acid deficiency may result from the inability of the body to utilize the vitamin.
   f. a. antagonist, a compound, such as aminopterin, that neutralizes the action of folic acid, thus producing a folic acid deficiency; used particularly in treatment of leukemias and Hodgkin's disease.

folie (fo-le') [Fr.] psychosis.
   f. à deux (ah duh') the occurrence of psychosis simultaneously in two closely associated persons.
   f. circulaire (ser"ku-lār') the circular form of manic-depressive psychosis.
   f. du doute (du doot) persistent obsessive doubting, vacillation and indecision.
   f. du pourquoi (du poor-kwah') psychopathologic constant questioning.
   f. gémellaire (zha"mĕ-lār') psychosis occurring simultaneously in twins.
   f. musculaire (mus"ku-lār') severe chorea.
   f. raisonnante (rez"un-ahnt') the delusional form of any psychosis.

folinic acid (fo-lin'ik) a factor in crude liver, yeast extracts and other biological material; called also citrovorum factor.

folium (fo'le-um), pl. *fo'lia* [L.] a leaflike structure, especially one of the leaflike subdivisions of the cerebellar cortex.

follicle (fol'ĭ-kl) a sac or pouchlike depression or cavity. adj., **follic'ular.**
   atretic f., a graafian follicle that has involuted.
   dental f., the structure within the substance of the jaws enclosing a tooth before its eruption.
   gastric f's, lymphoid masses in the gastric mucosa.
   graafian f., an ovarian follicle in which an ovum matures, before its rupture containing an eccentric cavity filled with fluid (see also GRAAFIAN FOLLICLE).
   hair f., a pouchlike depression in the skin in which a hair develops from the matrix at its base and grows to emerge from its opening on the body surface.
   lymphatic f., a small collection of lymphoid tissue in the mucous membrane of the gastrointestinal tract.
   ovarian f., the ovum and its encasing cells, at any stage of its development.
   primordial f., an ovarian follicle consisting of an ovum enclosed by a single layer of cells.
   sebaceous f., a sebaceous gland of the skin.
   thyroid f's, discrete cystlike units filled with a colloid substance, constituting the lobules of the thyroid gland.
   vesicular f., a graafian follicle before rupture and discharge of the ovum.

follicle-stimulating hormone one of the gonadotropic hormones of the anterior lobe of the PITUITARY GLAND that stimulates the growth and maturation of graafian follicles in the ovary, and stimulates spermatogenesis in the male.

folliclis (fol'ĭ-klis) papulonecrotic tuberculid with lesions on the hands.

folliculin (fŏ-lik'u-lin) estrone.

folliculitis (fŏ-lik"u-li'tis) inflammation of the hair follicles at their openings in the skin. An example of folliculitis is sycosis barbae, called also barber's itch, which affects the follicles of the beard.
   Folliculitis is caused by staphylococci. It is marked by pustules in the hair follicles, intense itching and pain when the hairs are touched or moved as in shaving. The disease can be stubborn and last for months or even years. Occasionally it leads to skin abscess. The condition is treated with antibiotics locally or systemically.
   keloid f., infection of hair follicles of the back of the neck and scalp, occurring chiefly in men, producing large, irregular keloid plaques and scarring.

folliculoma (fŏ-lik"u-lo'mah) an ovarian tumor derived from epithelium of the graafian follicles.

folliculus (fŏ-lik'u-lus), pl. *follic'uli* [L.] follicle.

Follutein (fŏ-lu'te-in) trademark for a preparation of chorionic gonadotropin.

Folvite (fōl'vīt) trademark for preparations of folic acid.

fomentation (fo"men-ta'shun) a warm, moist application.

fomes (fo'mēz), pl. *fo'mites* [L.] an inanimate

object or material on which disease-producing agents may be conveyed.

fontanel (fon″tah-nel′) a soft spot in the skull of a young infant. Actually there are two soft spots close together, representing gaps in the bone structure which will be filled in by bone during the normal process of growth. The anterior fontanel is diamond shaped and lies at the junction of the frontal and parietal bones. This fontanel usually fills in and closes between the eighth and fifteenth months of life. The posterior fontanel lies at the junction of the occipital and parietal bones, is triangular in shape and usually closes by the third or fourth month of life. Though these "soft spots" may appear very vulnerable, they may be touched gently without harm. Care should be exercised that they be protected from strong pressure or direct injury.

food (fo͞od) anything which, when taken into the body, serves to nourish or build up the tissues or to supply heat.

f. poisoning, a condition caused by food that is contaminated with bacteria or chemicals, or by poisonous berries, contaminated shellfish or poisonous mushrooms. Food poisoning usually causes inflammation of the gastrointestinal tract (gastroenteritis). This may occur quite suddenly, soon after the poisonous food has been eaten. The symptoms are acute, and include tenderness, pain or cramps in the abdomen, nausea, vomiting, diarrhea, weakness and dizziness. In mushroom poisoning, there may be dimness of vision and symptoms resembling those of alcoholic intoxication.

Food poisoning is often falsely attributed to ptomaines, substances that are formed when protein foods "spoil," or decompose. Because ptomaines produce toxic reactions when injected into experimental animals, "ptomaine poisoning" was formerly believed to be responsible for food-poisoning symptoms in human beings. It is now known that the human digestive system is well able to cope with these substances. Although they should be avoided, spoiled foods are not necessarily harmful. When they are, it is because foods in the process of decomposition frequently harbor disease-causing bacteria.

Bacterial food poisoning may be staphylococcal in origin or it may result from other microorganisms, as in BOTULISM or salmonella infections.

Staphylococcal poisoning is the most common form of food poisoning in the United States. If a food handler is afflicted with a staphylococcal infection, or if he is a carrier, one of the rare persons who carries the disease without suffering infection, he may pass the bacteria on to food. In some foods, the bacteria will multiply very quickly, especially if the food is not refrigerated. Staphylococci are toxin-producing bacteria which do not harm the body directly but produce poisonous substances in the body, causing disease symptoms. The symptoms of staphylococcal poisoning result from the effects of the toxins which have built up in the staphylococci-harboring food. The condition does not spread throughout the body and is not contagious.

Custard-filled pastry is the food most liable to contain staphylococci. Other susceptible foods are cream, milk, cheddar cheese, potato salad, many kinds of sauces and processed meats, especially ham. These foods should always be purchased from reliable dealers and be kept refrigerated.

Staphylococcal poisoning is characterized by a sudden, sometimes violent onset of nausea, vomiting and weakness. There may be severe diarrhea. It is rarely serious, except for young children, the elderly and persons who are weakened by other illness. Symptoms may appear as soon as a half hour or as late as 4 hours after the contaminated food is eaten.

There are a number of poisonous berries and over 80 kinds of poisonous mushrooms. Every year people die or become seriously ill because they have decided that one of these looks good enough to eat. Children are frequently tempted by poisonous holly berries or the berries that grow on privet (the shrub often used for hedges). Adults often place their faith in some incorrect notion, such as the old superstition that you can tell mushrooms from toadstools by cooking a silver coin with them; the coin is supposed to tarnish if the variety is poisonous. These mistaken notions cause a number of deaths every year. Although it is possible to learn to identify poisonous mushrooms and berries, it is much wiser to play safe. Children should be trained not to eat things they find in the woods or fields.

Mushroom poisoning causes a sudden reduction in the concentration of sugar in the blood. There may be convulsions, severe abdominal pain, intense thirst, nausea, vomiting and diarrhea. Symptoms appear 6 to 15 hours after eating.

Mussels and clams may grow in beds contaminated by the typhoid bacillus (*Salmonella typhi*) and other germs. Mussels, clams and certain other shellfish are dangerous during some seasons of the year. They become poisonous as a result of feeding on microorganisms that appear in the ocean during the warm months, particularly in the Pacific. Shellfish poisoning is characterized by paralysis of the respiratory tract. The symptoms vary. There may be trembling about the lips or loss of power in the muscles of the neck. Symptoms develop within 5 to 30 minutes after eating.

FIRST AID FOR FOOD POISONING

1. Give the patient weak tea and, when he can tolerate them, soft foods.

2. Keep the patient warm and apply heat to the abdomen by means of an electric pad or hot water bottle.

3. The patient should be seen by a physician as soon as possible.

Botulism and Poisoning from Mushrooms, Berries or Shellfish. If the patient has difficulty seeing, swallowing or breathing; or if his eyes are sunken; or if his breath has a sweet, fruity odor, his condition is serious and a physician should be called immediately.

Food and Drug Administration an agency of the Department of Health, Education and Welfare whose principal purpose is to enforce the Federal Food, Drug and Cosmetic Act. The agency insures that foods for sale in the United States are safe, pure and wholesome; that drugs and therapeutic devices are safe and effective; that cosmetics are harmless; and that all these products are correctly labeled and packaged. The F.D.A. is also responsible for enforcing the federal act that requires informative labels on any household product that is toxic, corrosive, irritant, inflammable or generates pressure through decomposition or heat.

If a product in interstate commerce is proved to

be faulty, the F.D.A. is authorized to bring court action or seize the adulterated or incorrectly labeled merchandise and to prosecute the responsible person or company.

foodstuff (fōōd′stuf) any nutrient material taken in by a living organism for production of energy or building of tissue.

foot (foot) the terminal part of the leg.

athlete's f., a fungus infection of the skin of the foot (see also ATHLETE'S FOOT).

drop f., paralysis of the anterior tibial muscle, causing the foot to drop or drag during walking.

immersion f., a morbid condition occurring in persons in water for considerable periods.

Madura f., maduromycosis of the foot.

march f., painful swelling of the foot, usually with fracture of a metatarsal bone.

trench f., a morbid condition resulting from inaction and prolonged exposure to cold and moisture.

footboard (foot′bōrd) a device placed at the foot of the bed and situated so that the feet rest firmly against it and are at right angles to the legs. It is used to relieve the weight of the bedclothes and to maintain proper positioning of the feet while a patient is confined to bed. Its purpose is to prevent the development of footdrop. It also helps maintain good posture because it prevents the patient from slipping down in bed.

A footboard can be made from wood or improvised from a cardboard box. When the patient is a child and immobilization of the foot, as well as correct positioning, is desired, rubber-soled tennis shoes can be nailed to the footboard and the child's feet laced into the shoes.

foot-candle (foot-kan′dl) a unit of illumination, the amount of light at 1 foot from a standard candle; it is 1 lumen per foot.

footdrop (foot′drop) dropping of the foot from paralysis of the anterior muscles of the leg.

footplate (foot′plāt) the flat portion of the stapes.

foot-pound (foot′pownd) the amount of energy necessary to raise 1 pound of mass a distance of 1 foot.

foramen (fo-ra′men), pl. *foram′ina* [L.] a natural opening or passage; used as a general term in anatomic nomenclature to designate such a passage, especially on or into a bone.

apical f., the foramen at the end of the root of a tooth.

auditory f., external, the external acoustic meatus.

auditory f., internal, the passage for the auditory (vestibulocochlear) and facial nerves in the pars petrosa of the temporal bone.

Bichat's f., a canal from the subarachnoid space to the third ventricle.

f. cae′cum, cecal f., 1. the foramen between the frontal bone and the crista galli. 2. a canal over the root and dorsum of the tongue. 3. one in the mucous membrane of the posterior wall of the pharynx.

condyloid f., anterior, the passage in the occipital bone for the hypoglossal nerve.

condyloid f., posterior, a fossa behind either occipital condyle.

epiploic f., an opening connecting the two sacs of the peritoneum, situated below and behind the porta hepatis.

interventricular f., a passage from the third to the lateral ventricle of the brain.

intervertebral f., anterior, a passage for spinal nerves and vessels between the laminae of adjacent vertebrae.

intervertebral f., posterior, a space between the articular processes of adjacent vertebrae.

jugular f., a space made by the jugular notches of the temporal and occipital bones.

f. mag′num, a large opening in the anterior inferior part of the occipital bone, between the cranial cavity and spinal canal.

mastoid f., a small hole behind the mastoid process.

f. of Monro, interventricular foramen.

obturator f., the large opening between the pubic bone and the ischium.

optic f., a passage for the optic nerve and ophthalmic artery at the apex of the orbit.

f. ova′le, 1. the septal opening in the fetal heart that provides a communication between the atria. The opening closes at birth; failure to close results in atrial septal defect (see also CONGENITAL HEART DEFECT). 2. an aperture in the great wing of the sphenoid for vessels and nerves.

palatine f., anterior, an orifice in the anterior part of the roof of the mouth for a nerve and artery.

f. rotun′dum, a round opening in the great wing of the sphenoid for the superior maxillary nerve.

sacral foramina, anterior, eight passages on the pelvic surface of the sacrum for the anterior branches of the sacral nerves.

sacral foramina, posterior, eight passages on the dorsal surface of the sacrum for the posterior branches of the sacral nerves.

sphenopalatine f., a space between the orbital and sphenoidal processes of the palatine bone.

f. spino′sum, a hole in the great wing of the sphenoid for the middle meningeal artery.

supraorbital f., a notch of the frontal bone for the supraorbital vessels and nerve.

Thebesius's foramina, the orifices of the smallest cardiac veins (thebesian veins) in the right atrium.

vertebral f., the large opening in a vertebra formed by its body and its arch.

f. of Vesalius, an opening at the inner side of the foramen ovale of the sphenoid.

Weitbrecht's f., a foramen in the capsule of the shoulder joint.

f. of Winslow, epiploic foramen.

force (fōrs) energy or power; that which originates or arrests motion or other activity.

catabolic f., energy derived from the metabolism of food.

electromotive f., the force that, by reason of differences in potential, causes a flow of electricity from one place to another, giving rise to an electric current.

nerve f., nervous f., 1. the ability of nerve tissue to conduct stimuli. 2. in psychiatry, the amount of nervous capital or stamina a person possesses.

reserve f., energy above that required for normal functioning. In the heart it is the power that will take care of the additional circulatory burden imposed by bodily exertion.

forceps (fōr′seps), pl. *for′cipes* [L.] a two-pronged instrument for grasping or seizing.

alligator f., strong toothed forceps having a double clamp.

bayonet f., a forceps whose blades are offset from the axis of the handles.

capsule f., a forceps for removing the lens capsule in cataract.

Chamberlen f., the original form of obstetric forceps.

clamp f., a forceps-like clamp with an automatic lock, for compressing arteries.

dressing f., forceps with scissor-like handles for grasping lint, drainage tubes, etc., in dressing wounds.

obstetric f., forceps for making traction on the fetus in difficult labor.

rongeur f., a forceps designed for use in cutting bone.

Fordyce's disease (fōr′dĭs-ez) a congenital condition characterized by minute yellowish white papules on the oral mucosa.

forearm (fōr′arm) the part of the arm between the elbow and wrist.

forebrain (fōr′brān) the portion of the brain developed from the anterior of the three primary brain vesicles in the early embryo, and comprising the diencephalon and telencephalon; called also prosencephalon.

foreconscious (fōr′kon-shus) preconscious; material not ordinarily in consciousness, but subject to voluntary recall.

forefinger (fōr′fing-ger) the first or index finger.

forefoot (fōr′foot) the front part of the foot, comprising the toes and metatarsal region.

foregut (fōr′gut) the embryonic organ from which the pharynx, esophagus, stomach and part of the small intestine are derived.

forehead (fōr′ed) the part of the head above the eyes; the anterior portion of the cranium.

foreskin (fōr′skin) prepuce; a loose fold of skin that covers the glans penis. It is a continuation of the loose skin that covers the entire penis and scrotum.

formaldehyde (fōr-mal′dĕ-hīd) a gaseous compound with strongly disinfectant properties. It is used in solution for disinfection of excreta and utensils and also in the preparation of toxoids from toxins.

formalin (fōr′mah-lin) a 40 per cent solution of gaseous formaldehyde.

formatio (fōr-ma′she-o), pl. *formatio′nes* [L.] formation.

formation (fōr-ma′shun) 1. the giving or taking of form. 2. a structure or definite shape.

reaction f., a mental mechanism by which one assumes an attitude that is the reverse of, and a substitute for, a repressed antisocial impulse.

formic acid (fōr′mik) a colorless, pungent liquid from the secretion of ants, nettles, etc.

formication (fōr″mĭ-ka′shun) a sensation as if ants were creeping on the body.

formiciasis (fōr″mĭ-si′ah-sis) a morbid condition caused by ant bites.

formilase (fōr′mĭ-lās) an enzyme that changes acetic acid into formic acid.

formiminoglutamic acid (fōrm-im″ĭ-no-glootam′ik) a product in the metabolism of histidine, the appearance of which in urine is used as a test of folic acid deficiency.

formol (fōr′mol) formaldehyde solution.

formula (fōr′mu-lah), pl. *for′mulae, for′mulas* [L.] 1. an expression, using numbers or symbols, of the composition of, or of directions for preparing, a compound, such as a medicine, or of a procedure to follow to obtain a desired result, or of a single concept. 2. a milk mixture for feeding an infant, composed of milk and other ingredients—usually sugar and water—in proportions prescribed by the pediatrician (see also INFANT).

chemical f., a combination of chemical symbols representing the elements and the number of their atoms in a molecule of a chemical compound.

empirical f., a chemical formula that expresses the proportions of the elements composing the molecule.

graphic f., structural formula.

molecular f., a chemical formula expressing the number of atoms of each element of which the molecule is composed.

official f., one officially established by a pharmacopeia or other recognized authority.

rational f., structural formula.

spatial f., stereochemical f., a chemical formula giving the numbers of atoms of each element present in a molecule of a substance, which atom is linked to which, the types of linkages involved and the relative positions of the atoms in space.

structural f., a chemical formula showing the spatial arrangement of the atoms and the linkage of every atom.

formulary (fōr′mu-ler″e) a collection of formulae.

National F., a book published at regular intervals under supervision of the Council of the American Pharmaceutical Association, establishing official standards for certain drugs.

fornix (fōr′niks), pl. *for′nices* [L.] an archlike structure or the vaultlike space created by such a structure.

Forthane (fōr′thān) trademark for a preparation of methylhexaneamine, used for relief of nasal congestion.

fossa (fos′ah), pl. *fos′sae* [L.] a pit or depression; applied to numerous depressions in various tissues of the body where they come in contact with or articulate with other structures.

amygdaloid f., the depression in which the tonsil is lodged.

cerebral f., any of the depressions on the floor of the cranial cavity.

condyloid f., either of two pits on the lateral portion of the occipital bone.

coronoid f., a depression in the humerus for the coronoid process of the ulna.

cranial f., any one of the three hollows in the base of the cranium for the lobes of the brain.

digastric f., a groove on the inner aspect of the mastoid process.

glenoid f., mandibular fossa.

hypogastric f., a depression on the interior surface of the anterior abdominal wall, between the hypogastric folds.

iliac f., a large, smooth, concave area occupying much of the inner surface of the ala of the ilium, especially anteriorly. From it arises the iliac muscle.

interpeduncular f., a depression on the inferior surface of the midbrain, between the two cerebral peduncles, the floor of which is the posterior perforated substance.

ischiorectal f., a triangular space between the rectum and the tuberosity of the ischium.

mandibular f., a prominent depression in the inferior surface of the pars squamosa of the temporal bone at the base of the zygomatic process, in which the condyle of the mandible rests; called also glenoid fossa.

nasal f., the portion of the nasal cavity anterior to the middle meatus.

navicular f., f. navicula'ris, 1. a cavity behind the vaginal aperture. 2. an expansion of the urethra in the glans penis. 3. the fossa between the helix and antihelix. 4. a depression on the internal pterygoid process of the sphenoid bone.

f. ova'lis, a fossa in the right atrium of the heart; the remains of the fetal foramen ovale.

ovarian f., a shallow pouch on the posterior surface of the broad ligament of the uterus in which the ovary is located.

pituitary f., the depression in the sphenoid that lodges the pituitary gland.

sigmoid f., the curved fossa on the mastoid process.

subarcuate f., a depression in the posterior inner surface of the pars petrosa of the temporal bone.

subpyramidal f., a depression on the internal wall of the middle ear.

subsigmoid f., a fossa between the mesentery of the sigmoid flexure and that of the descending colon.

supraspinous f., a depression above the spine of the scapula.

f. tempora'lis, the area on the side of the cranium outlined posteriorly and superiorly by the temporal lines, anteriorly by the frontal and zygomatic bones and laterally by the zygomatic arch.

tibiofemoral f., a space between the articular surfaces of the tibia and femur.

fossette (fŏ-set') 1. a small depression. 2. a small, deep corneal ulcer.

fossula (fos'u-lah), pl. *fos'ulae* [L.] a small fossa.

Fothergill's disease (foth'er-gilz) tic douloureux.

foulage (foo-lahzh') [Fr.] kneading and pressing of the muscles in massage.

fourchette (foor-shet') [Fr.] the posterior junction of the labia minora.

fovea (fo've-ah), pl. *fo'veae* [L.] a small pit or depression.

f. centra'lis ret'inae, a tiny pit in the center of the macula lutea, composed of slim, elongated cones; it is the area of clearest vision, because here the layers of the retina are spread aside, permitting light to fall directly on the cones.

foveate (fo've-āt) pitted.

foveation (fo"ve-a'shun) formation of pits on a surface, as on the skin.

foveola (fo-ve'o-lah), pl. *fove'olae* [L.] a minute pit or depression.

Fowler's position (fow'lerz) the head of the patient's bed is raised 18 to 20 inches above the level.

Fowler's solution (fow'lerz) potassium arsenite solution, used as a hematinic and in certain skin lesions.

Fox-Fordyce disease (foks for'dīs) a condition of unknown causation characterized by plugging of the pores of the apocrine sweat glands and vesiculation of the epidermis.

foxglove (foks'gluv) digitalis.

F.P. freezing point.

F.R. flocculoreaction.

Fr chemical symbol, *francium.*

fracture (frak'tūr) a break in the continuity of bone. It may be caused by trauma, by twisting due to muscle spasm or indirect loss of leverage or by disease that results in decalcification of the bone.

TREATMENT. Immediate first aid consists in splinting the bone. No attempt should be made to set the bone; it should be splinted "as it lies"; i.e., it should be supported in such a way that the injured part will remain steady and will resist jarring if the victim is moved.

A fracture is treated by reduction, which means that the broken ends are pulled into alignment and the continuity of the bone is established so that healing can take place and the bone is "made whole" again. Closed reduction is performed by manual manipulation of the fractured bone so that the fragments are brought into proper alignment; no surgical incision is made. Open reduction is done only when it is necessary to débride and cleanse the area, as in an open fracture. A fracture may also require internal fixation with pins, nails, metal plates or screws to stabilize the alignment.

Once reduction is accomplished the bone is immobilized by application of a CAST or by an apparatus exerting TRACTION on the distal end of the bone.

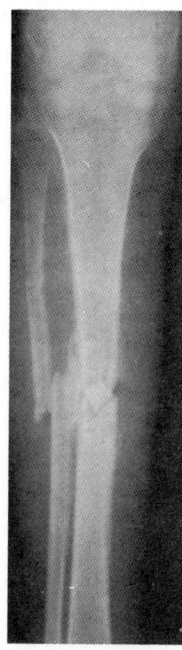

X-ray film of a fracture of the tibia and fibula. (From Meschan, I.: Roentgen Signs in Clinical Practice. Philadelphia, W. B. Saunders Co., 1966.)

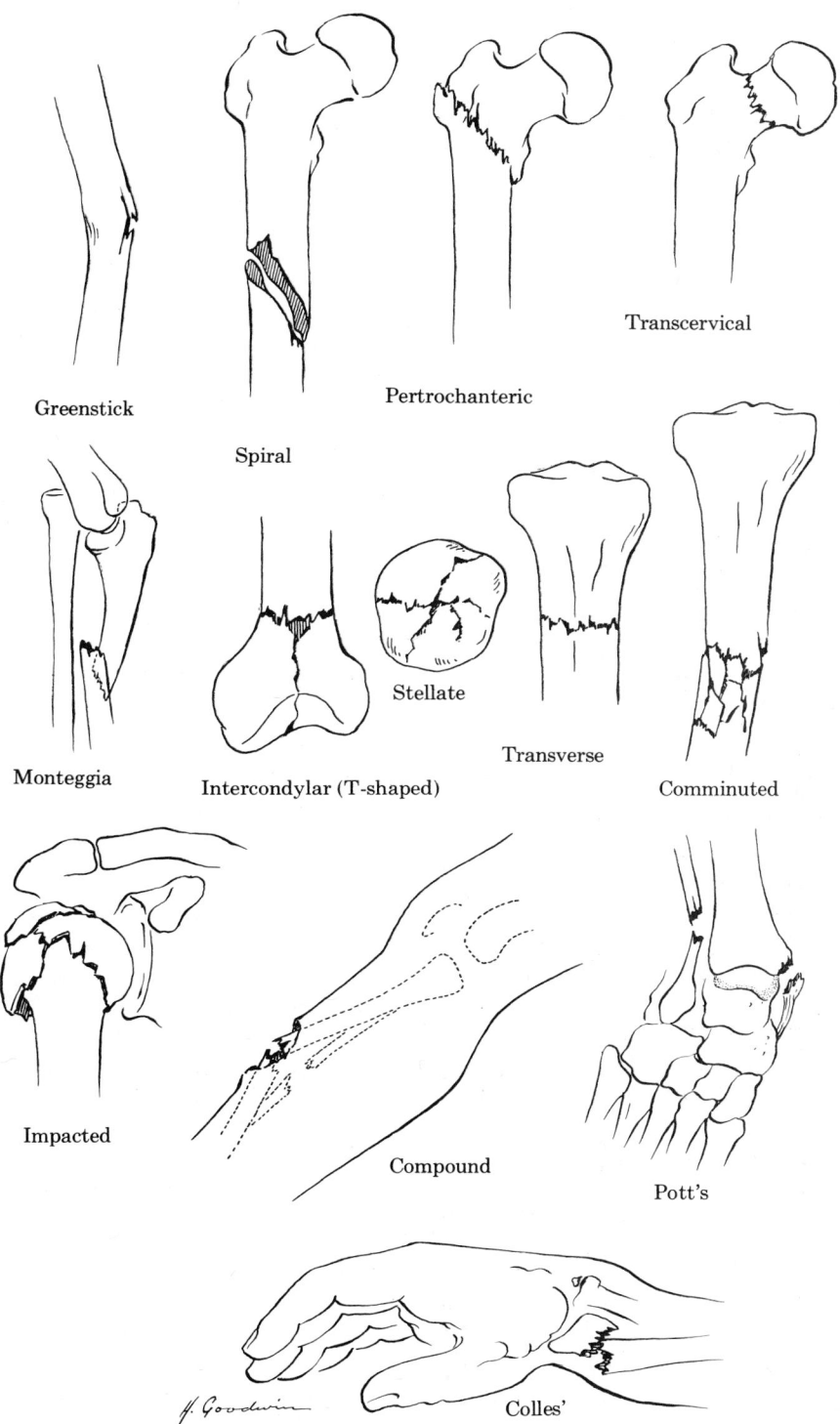

Types of fractures. (From Dorland's Illustrated Medical Dictionary. 24th ed. Philadelphia, W. B. Saunders Co., 1965.)

avulsion f., separation of a small fragment of bone cortex at the site of attachment of a ligament.

Barton's f., one involving only a small portion of the articular surface of the distal end of the radius.

Bennett's f., a longitudinal fracture of the first metacarpal bone, complicated by subluxation.

capillary f., one that appears on a roentgenogram as a fine, hairlike line, the segments of bone not being separated; sometimes seen in fractures of the skull.

chip f., avulsion fracture.

closed f., one in which there is no wound on the body surface communicating with the break in the bone.

Colles' f., a break in the lower end of the radius, the distal fragment being displaced backward.

Colles' f., reversed, one in the lower end of the radius, the distal fragment being displaced anteriorly.

comminuted f., one in which two or more communicating breaks divide the bone into more than two fragments.

complete f., one involving the entire cross section of the bone.

compound f., open fracture.

compression f., disruption of the normal continuity and structure of a bone resulting from unusual and excessive compressive force.

depressed f., one in which the fragment of bone is forced beneath the line of its normal contour.

double f., one in which the bone is divided by two noncommunicating lines of fracture.

Dupuytren's f., Pott's fracture.

Duverney's f., fracture of the ilium just below the anterior inferior spine.

fissure f., one extending longitudinally along the shaft of a long bone.

greenstick f., an incomplete fracture of a long bone, with a longitudinal split of the shaft.

impacted f., fracture in which one fragment is firmly driven into the other.

incomplete f., one that does not involve the complete cross section of the bone.

interperiosteal f., greenstick fracture.

intrauterine f., fracture of a fetal bone incurred in utero.

lead pipe f., buckling of the cortex on one side of the shaft of a long bone.

Monteggia's f., one in the proximal half of the shaft of the ulna, with dislocation of the head of the radius.

open f., one in which a wound through the adjacent or overlying soft tissues communicates with the site of the break.

pathologic f., one occurring in diseased bone with only slight or no trauma.

pertrochanteric f., fracture of the femur passing through the greater trochanter.

ping-pong f., fracture of the skull with the bone fragment depressed below the normal level of the surface.

Pott's f., fracture of lower part of fibula with serious injury of the lower tibial articulation.

simple f., closed fracture.

Smith's f., Colles' fracture, reversed.

spiral f., a fracture twisting around the shaft of a bone.

spontaneous f., pathologic fracture.

sprain f., avulsion fracture.

Stieda's f., a fracture of the internal condyle of the femur sometimes causing hypertrophy of the condyle.

transcervical f., one through the neck of the femur.

trophic f., one due to a trophic disturbance.

fracture-dislocation (frak′tūr-dis″lo-ka′shun) a fracture of a bone near a joint, also involving dislocation.

frae- for words beginning thus, see those beginning *fre-*.

fragilitas (frah-jil′ĭ-tas) [L.] fragility.

    f. crin′ium, fragility of the hair, with resultant longitudinal splitting of the shaft.

    f. os′sium congen′ita, osteogenesis imperfecta.

fragility (frah-jil′ĭ-te) susceptibility or lack of resistance to influences capable of causing disruption of continuity or integrity.

    f. of blood, erythrocyte fragility.

    capillary f., abnormal susceptibility of capillary walls to rupture.

    erythrocyte f., susceptibility of erythrocytes to hemolysis when subjected to mechanical trauma (mechanical fragility) or when exposed to increasingly hypotonic saline solutions (osmotic fragility). A test of erythrocyte osmotic fragility is used in diagnosing hemolytic anemia.

fragilocyte (frah-jil′o-sīt) an erythrocyte abnormally sensitive to hypotonic salt solution.

fragilocytosis (frah-jil″o-si-to′sis) the presence of fragilocytes in the blood.

fragmentation (frag″men-ta′shun) division into small pieces.

frambesia (fram-be′ze-ah) yaws.

frambesioma (fram-be″ze-o′mah) the primary lesion of frambesia, consisting of a large single projecting nodule.

frame (frām) a rigid supporting structure.

    Balkan f., an apparatus for continuous extension in treatment of fractures of the femur, consisting of an overhead bar, with pulleys attached, by which the leg is supported in a sling.

    Bradford f., a rectangular structure of gas pipe across which are stretched two strips of canvas, used for patients with fractures or disease of the hip or spine.

    quadriplegic standing f., a device for supporting in the upright position a patient whose four limbs are paralyzed.

    spectacle f., a device for holding lenses before the eyes.

    Stryker f., an apparatus similar to the Bradford frame, used for patients with fractures and injuries to the spinal cord (see also STRYKER FRAME).

Francis' disease (fran′siz) tularemia.

francium (fran′se-um) a chemical element, atomic number 87, atomic weight 223, symbol Fr. (See table of ELEMENTS.)

franklinization (frank″li-ni-za′shun) therapeutic use of static electricity.

F.R.C.P. Fellow of the Royal College of Physicians.

F.R.C.S. Fellow of the Royal College of Surgeons.

freckle (frek′l) a pigmented spot on the skin due

to accumulation of melanin resulting from exposure to sunlight.

cold f., lentigo.

freezing point (fre′zing) the temperature at which a liquid begins to freeze; for water, 0° C., or 32° F.

Frei's disease (frīz) lymphogranuloma venereum.

F's test, intracutaneous injection of antigen derived from infected chick embryos, used in the diagnosis of lymphogranuloma venereum.

Freiberg's disease (fri′bergz) osteochondritis of a metatarsal head, usually the head of the second or third metatarsal bones.

Frejka splint (fra′kah) one used for securing abduction of the heads of the femurs in congenital dislocation of the hip.

fremitus (frem′i-tus) a thrill or vibration, especially one perceptible on palpation or auscultation.

tactile f., a vibration or thrill of the chest wall in speaking, perceived on palpation.

tussive f., a thrill felt on chest while the patient coughs.

vocal f., a vibration or thrill of the chest wall in speaking, perceived on auscultation.

French scale (french) a scale used for denoting size of catheters, sounds and other tubular instruments, each unit being roughly equivalent to 0.33 mm. in diameter.

frenectomy (fre-nek′to-me) excision of a frenum (frenulum).

frenotomy (fre-not′o-me) the cutting of a frenum (frenulum).

frenulum (fren′u-lum), pl. *fren′ula* [L.] a small fold of integument or mucous membrane that limits the movements of an organ or part.

f. of clitoris, a fold on the urethral surface of the clitoris, formed by the anterior junction of the labia minora.

f. labio′rum puden′di, fourchette.

f. lin′guae, the midline fold connecting the under surface of the tongue and floor of the mouth.

f. of prepuce of penis, a fold of thin integument from the inferior angle of the exterior urethral orifice to the inner sheath of the prepuce.

frenum (fre′num), pl. *fre′na* [L.] a restraining structure; frenulum.

frequency (fre′kwen-se) 1. in statistics, the number of occurrences of a determinable entity per unit of time or population. 2. the number of vibrations made by a particle or ray in 1 second; in electricity, the rate of oscillation or alternation in an alternating current; the number of complete cycles produced by an alternating current generator per second.

Freud (froid) Sigmund (1856–1939). Clinical neurologist and founder of psychoanalysis. Born in Freiberg in Moravia, and educated at the University of Vienna, he studied in Paris in 1885 under the neurologist J. M. Charcot, who encouraged him to investigate hysteria from a psychologic point of view. Freud stressed the existence of an unconscious that exerts a dynamic influence on consciousness, and was led to develop his method of "free association" in order to discover these buried memories. He emphasized the role of sexuality in the development of neurotic conditions, and

published *Interpretation of Dreams* (1900), *Psychopathology of Everyday Life* (1901) and many more works. He was also director of the *International Journal of Psychology.* Fleeing the Nazi regime in Vienna in 1938, he died in London.

freudian (froi′de-an) pertaining to Sigmund Freud and his doctrines that certain nervous disorders are caused by the existence of unconscious sexual and other drives, and that they can be cured by bringing these repressions into conciousness by PSYCHOANALYSIS.

friable (fri′ah-bl) broken easily into small pieces.

friction (frik′shun) the act of rubbing.

Fried's rule (frēds) the dose of a drug for an infant less than 2 years old is obtained by multiplying the child's age in months by the adult dose and dividing the result by 150.

Friedländer's disease (frēd′len-derz) endarteritis obliterans.

Friedman's test (frēd′manz) a test for pregnancy, based on the effects on ovaries of a mature, nonpregnant female rabbit, produced by injection of the patient's urine (see also PREGNANCY TESTS).

Friedreich's ataxia (frēd′rīks) an inherited disease, usually beginning in childhood or youth, with sclerosis of the dorsal and lateral columns of the spinal cord. It is attended by ataxia, speech impairment, lateral curvature of the vertebral column and peculiar swaying and irregular movements, with paralysis of the muscles, especially of the lower extremities.

F's disease, 1. paramyoclonus multiplex. 2. Friedreich's ataxia.

frigidity (frĭ-jid′ĭ-te) partial or complete inability of the female to be aroused sexually or to achieve orgasm.

frigorific (frig″o-rif′ik) producing coldness.

Fröhlich's syndrome (fra′liks) a condition associated with lesions of the hypothalamus and pituitary gland, marked by obesity and sexual infantilism; called also adiposogenital dystrophy. It is treated with pituitary extract.

frolement (frōl-maw′) [Fr.] 1. a rustling sound heard in pericardial disease. 2. a brushing movement in massage.

frons (fronz) [L.] the forehead.

frontad (frun′tad) toward a front, or frontal aspect.

frontal (frun′tal) pertaining to the upper, anterior part of the head, or forehead.

f. bone, the unpaired bone constituting the anterior part of the skull.

f. lobe, the anterior portion of the cerebral cortex.

frontalis (fron-ta′lis) [L.] frontal.

frost (frost) a deposit resembling frozen dew or vapor.

urea f., the appearance on the skin of salt crystals left by evaporation of the sweat in uremia.

frostbite (frost′bīt) injury to tissues due to exposure to cold. Usually the first areas of the body to freeze are the nose, ears, fingers and toes. The flesh feels cold to the touch, and the frozen parts become pale and feel numb. There may also be some prickly or itchy sensation. A person suffering from frostbite may feel no warning pain.

In mild cases of frostbite proper treatment can rather quickly restore normal circulation of blood. In more serious cases the area may become painfully inflamed, and blistering may follow. Especially severe frostbite can cause death of the injured tissues and gangrene may result.

TREATMENT. The frozen parts should be gradually and gently rewarmed. Hot water bottles or other applications of heat are contraindicated, as is rubbing or massaging, which may further damage the injured tissues. Cool or lukewarm water may be used to rewarm the frozen parts. If water is not available the part may be rewarmed by covering it with warm clothing or by placing it in contact with any other part of the body that is warm. Contrary to a common theory, frostbite should *never* be treated by rubbing the affected area with snow or by the application of snow or ice.

frottage (fro-tahzh′) [Fr.] a rubbing movement in massage.

frozen section (fro′zen) a specimen of tissue that has been quick-frozen, cut by microtome and stained immediately for rapid diagnosis of possible malignant lesions. A specimen processed in this manner is not satisfactory for detailed study of the cells, but it is valuable because it is quick and gives the surgeon immediate information regarding the malignancy of a piece of tissue.

fructose (fruk′tōs) a colorless or white crystalline sugar; called also levulose and fruit sugar. It is used in solution as a fluid and nutrient replenisher.

fructosuria (fruk″to-su′re-ah) fructose in the urine.

frustration (frus-tra′shun) the feeling aroused by the blocking of sought gratifications and satisfactions, ordinarily by forces outside one's self.

FSH follicle-stimulating hormone.

Fuadin (fu′ah-din) trademark for a preparation of stibophen, used in schistosomal and leishmanial infections.

fuchsin (fook′sin) a dark red dye with germicidal properties.
  acid f., a compound used in preparation of a staining solution.
  basic f., a compound used in preparation of an antifungal solution.

-fugal (fu′gal) word element [L.], *driving away; fleeing from; repelling.*

fugue (fūg) transitory abnormal behavior marked by aimless wandering and some alteration of consciousness, usually but not always followed by amnesia.

fulguration (ful″gu-ra′shun) treatment by electric sparks.

fulminate (ful′mĭ-nāt) to occur suddenly with great intensity. adj., **ful′minant.**

Fulvicin (ful′vĭ-sin) trademark for a preparation of griseofulvin, an antibiotic used specifically for treatment of fungus infections of the skin.

fumagillin (fu″mah-jil′in) an antibiotic elaborated by strains of *Aspergillus fumigatus;* used as an amebicide.

fumigation (fu″mĭ-ga′shun) exposure to disinfecting fumes.

Fumiron (fūm′i-ron) trademark for a preparation of ferrous fumarate, used in treatment of iron deficiency anemia.

function (fungk′shun) the special, normal or proper action of any part or organ.

functional (fungk′shun-al) pertaining to or fulfilling a function.
  f. disease, a disease without a discoverable lesion or organic cause.

fundament (fun′dah-ment) 1. a base or foundation upon which something rests. 2. the anus and parts adjacent to it.

fundectomy (fun-dek′to-me) excision of the fundus of an organ, as of the stomach or uterus.

fundiform (fun′dĭ-form) shaped like a loop or sling.

fundoplication (fun″do-pli-ka′shun) mobilization of the lower end of the esophagus and plication of the fundus of the stomach up around it, in the treatment of reflux esophagitis.

fundus (fun′dus), pl. *fun′di* [L.] the bottom or base of anything; used in anatomic nomenclature as a general term to designate the bottom or base of an organ, or the part of a hollow organ farthest from its mouth. adj., **fun′dal, fun′dic.**
  f. of bladder, the base or posterior surface of the urinary bladder.
  f. of eye, the back portion of the interior of the eyeball, visible through the pupil by use of the ophthalmoscope.
  f. of gallbladder, the rounded end of the gallbladder, remote from its opening into the cystic ducts.
  f. of stomach, the part of the stomach to the left and above the level of the opening between the stomach and esophagus.
  f. tym′pani, the floor of the cavity of the middle ear.
  f. u′teri, f. of uterus, the part of the uterus above the orifices of the uterine tubes.

fundusectomy (fun″dŭ-sek′to-me) excision of the fundus of the stomach.

fungal (fun′gal) pertaining to or caused by a fungus.

fungate (fun′gāt) to grow in fungus-like masses.

fungemia (fun-je′me-ah) the presence of fungi in the bloodstream.

fungi (fun′ji) [L.] plural of *fungus.*

fungicide (fun′jĭ-sīd) an agent that destroys fungi. adj., **fungici′dal.**

fungicidin (fun″jĭ-si′din) nystatin, an antifungal antibiotic.

fungiform (fun′jĭ-form) shaped like a fungus or mushroom.

fungistasis (fun″jĭ-sta′sis) inhibition of the growth of fungi. adj., **fungistat′ic.**

fungistat (fun′jĭ-stat) a substance that checks the growth of fungi.

fungitoxic (fun″jĭ-tok′sik) exerting a toxic effect upon fungi.

Fungizone (fun′jĭ-zōn) trademark for a preparation of amphotericin B, an antibiotic used for systemic fungus infections.

fungoid (fun′goid) resembling a fungus.
   chignon f., a nodular growth on the hair.

fungosity (fun-gos′ĭ-te) a fungoid growth or excrescence.

fungous (fun′gus) of the nature of a fungus.

fungus (fun′gus), pl. *fun′ji* [L.] any vegetable organism of the class to which mushrooms and molds belong. Fungi are present in the soil, air and water, but only a few species can cause disease. Among the fungus diseases (mycoses) are HISTO-PLASMOSIS, COCCIDIOIDOMYCOSIS (desert fever), RINGWORM, ATHLETE'S FOOT, and THRUSH. Although the fungus diseases develop slowly, are difficult to diagnose and are resistant to treatment, they are rarely fatal.

funicle (fu′nĭ-kl) funiculus.

funiculitis (fu-nik″u-li′tis) 1. inflammation of the spermatic cord. 2. inflammation of that portion of a spinal nerve root which lies within the intervertebral canal.

funiculus (fu-nik′u-lus), pl. *funic′uli* [L.] a cordlike structure or part, especially one of the large bundles of nerve tracts making up the white matter of the spinal cord. adj., **funic′ular.**
   anterior f., f. ante′rior, the ventral mass of fibers on either side of the spinal cord, between the anterior median fissure and the anterolateral sulcus.
   lateral f., f. latera′lis, the lateral mass of fibers on either side of the spinal cord, between the anterolateral and posterolateral sulci.
   posterior f., f. poste′rior, the posterior mass of fibers on either side of the spinal cord, between the posterolateral and posterior median sulci.
   f. spermat′icus, the spermatic cord.

funiform (fu′nĭ-form) resembling a rope or cord.

funnel chest (fun′el) a deformity of the front of the chest wall, characterized by a funnel-shaped depression with its apex over the lower end of the sternum; called also PECTUS EXCAVATUM.

Furacin (fu′rah-sin) trademark for preparations of nitrofurazone, an antibacterial agent.

Furadantin (fūr″ah-dan′tin) trademark for preparations of nitrofurantoin, an antibacterial used in urinary tract infections.

furazolidone (fu″rah-zol′ĭ-dōn) a yellow, odorless, crystalline powder; used as a local antibacterial and antiprotozoan.

furcal (fur′kal) forked.

furfuraceous (fur″fu-ra′shus) like dandruff or bran.

furosemide (fur-o′sĕ-mīd) a compound used as an oral diuretic.

Furoxone (fur-ok′sōn) trademark for preparations of furazolidone, a local antibacterial and antiprotozoan.

furrow (fur′o) a groove or trench.
   atrioventricular f., the transverse groove marking off the atria of the heart from the ventricles.
   digital f., any one of the transverse lines on the palmar surface of a finger.
   gluteal f., the furrow that separates the buttocks.

furuncle (fu′rung-kl) a focal suppurative inflammation of the skin and subcutaneous tissues, enclosing a central slough or "core"; called also BOIL. It is caused by bacteria, which enter through the hair follicles or sweat glands, and its formation is favored by constitutional or digestive derangement and local irritation.

furunculosis (fu-rung″ku-lo′sis) the occurrence of a number of furuncles.

furunculous (fu-rung′ku-lus) of the nature of a furuncle.

fuscin (fus′in) a brown pigment of the retinal epithelium.

fusiform (fu′zĭ-form) spindle-shaped.

fusion (fu′zhun) the combining or blending of distinct bodies into one, as (1) the fusion into a single image of the separate impressions received by the two eyes, or (2) the surgical process of making a formerly movable structure (joint) immovable.
   diaphyseal-epiphyseal f., operative establishment of bony union between the epiphysis and diaphysis of a bone, to arrest growth in length of the bone.
   nerve f., nerve anastomosis done to induce regeneration for resupplying empty tracts of a nerve with new growth of fibers.
   spinal f., surgical fixation of the joint of two or more vertebrae.

Fusobacterium (fu″zo-bak-te′re-um) a genus of Schizomycetes occurring in the mouth and large intestine.
   F. plau′ti-vincen′ti, a microorganism found in necrotizing ulcerative gingivitis (trench mouth).

fusocellular (fu″zo-sel′u-lar) having spindle-shaped cells.

fusospirillosis (fu″zo-spi″rĭ-lo′sis) Vincent's angina, or trench mouth.

fusospirochetal (fu″zo-spi″ro-ke′tal) caused by fusiform bacilli and spirochetes.

fusospirochetosis (fu″zo-spi″ro-ke-to′sis) Vincent's angina, or trench mouth.

fusus (fu′sus), pl. *fu′si* [L.] 1. a spindle-shaped structure. 2. a minute air vesicle in a hair shaft.

G

G. gram.

Ga chemical symbol, *gallium.*

gadolinium (gad″o-lin′e-um) a chemical element, atomic number 64, atomic weight 157.25, symbol Gd. (See table of ELEMENTS.)

gag (gag) 1. a surgical device for holding the mouth open. 2. to retch, or strive to vomit.
  g. reflex, elevation of the soft palate and retching elicited by touching the back of the tongue or the wall of the pharynx.

Gaisböck's disease (gīz′bekz) polycythemia hypertonica; polycythemia without spleen enlargement, but with hypertrophy of the heart and increased blood pressure.

gait (gāt) the manner of progression in walking.
  ataxic g., a gait in which the foot is raised high, the sole striking the ground at once and suddenly.
  cerebellar g., a staggering walk indicative of cerebellar disease.
  spastic g., a gait in which the legs are held together and move in a stiff manner, the toes seeming to drag and catch.
  steppage g., one in which the toes are strongly lifted and the heel reaches the ground first.
  tabetic g., ataxic gait.

galactacrasia (gah-lak″tah-kra′ze-ah) an abnormal state of mother's milk.

galactagogue (gah-lak′tah-gog) 1. increasing the flow of milk. 2. an agent that increases the flow of milk.

galactan (gah-lak′tan) a carbohydrate that yields galactose upon hydrolysis.

galactase (gah-lak′tās) a proteolytic enzyme that hydrolyzes caseinogen in the stomach.

galactemia (gal″ak-te′me-ah) the presence of milk in the blood.

galactic (gah-lak′tik) pertaining to milk.

galactidrosis (gah-lak″tĭ-dro′sis) the sweating of a milky fluid.

galactin (gah-lak′tin) a basic principle found in milk; called also prolactin.

galactoblast (gah-lak′to-blast) a colostrum corpuscle in the gland acini.

galactocele (gah-lak′to-sēl) 1. a milk-containing tumor of the mammary gland. 2. a hydrocele filled with milky fluid.

galactoma (gal″ak-to′mah) galactocele (1).

galactophorous (gal″ak-tof′o-rus) conveying milk.

galactophygous (gal″ak-tof′ĭ-gus) arresting the flow of milk.

galactoplania (gah-lak″to-pla′ne-ah) secretion of milk in some abnormal part.

galactopoietic (gah-lak″to-poi-et′ik) concerned in production of milk.

galactopyra (gah-lak″to-pi′rah) milk fever.

galactorrhea (gah-lak″to-re′ah) excessive secretion by the mammary gland.

galactoschesis (gal″ak-tos′kĕ-sis) suppression of milk secretion.

galactoscope (gah-lak′to-skōp) a device showing the proportion of cream in milk; called also lactoscope.

galactose (gah-lak′tōs) a monosaccharide derived from lactose.
  g. tolerance test, a laboratory test done to determine the liver's ability to convert the sugar galactose into glycogen. Two methods may be used. The oral method requires about 5 hours to complete, and the intravenous method, which is more accurate, requires about 2 hours. With the oral method, elimination of more than 3 Gm. of galactose in the urine during a 5-hour period indicates liver damage. With the intravenous method, all galactose should have been eliminated from the blood 45 minutes after its injection.

galactosemia (gah-lak″to-se′me-ah) a genetically determined biochemical disorder in which there is a lack of the enzyme necessary for proper metabolism of galactose. Normally the sugar derived from lactose in milk is changed by enzymatic action into glucose. In galactosemia the enzyme galactose-1-phosphate uridyl transferase is absent. This means that normal conversion of galactose to glucose does not take place and the galactose accumulates in the tissues and blood.
  The disorder becomes manifest soon after birth and is characterized by feeding problems, vomiting and diarrhea, abdominal distention, enlargement of the liver, mental retardation and elevated blood and urine galactose levels. Cataracts also may develop.
  The disorder can be detected by a sensitivity test so that early diagnosis and treatment are possible. If the disease is detected early, before there is damage to the central nervous system, the symptoms of the disorder can be prevented.
  Treatment consists of exclusion from the diet of milk and all foods containing galactose or lactose. Milk substitutes are used and the diet is planned to substitute necessary nutrients normally obtained from products containing lactose or galactose.

galactosis (gal″ak-to′sis) the formation of milk.

galactostasis (gal″ak-tos′tah-sis) 1. cessation of milk secretion. 2. abnormal collection of milk.

galactosuria (gah-lak″to-su′re-ah) galactose in the urine.

galactotherapy (gah-lak″to-ther′ah-pe) treatment of a nursing infant by medication given the mother.

galactotoxin (gah-lak″to-tok′sin) a poison produced in milk by growth of a microorganism.

galactotrophy (gal″ak-tot′ro-fe) feeding with milk.

galactozymase (gah-lak″to-zi′mās) a starch-liquefying enzyme.

galacturia (gal″ak-tu′re-ah) chyluria; the discharge of urine with a milky appearance.

galea (ga′le-ah), pl. *ga′leae* [L.] a helmet-like structure.

    g. aponeurot′ica, the aponeurotic structure of the scalp, connecting the frontal and occipital bellies of the occipitofrontal muscle.

Galen (ga′len) [Claudius Galenus] (A.D. 130–200). The celebrated Greek physician to the Roman Emperor Marcus Aurelius. Although he did not dissect the human cadaver, he made many valuable anatomic and physiologic observations on animals (and applied many of them inaccurately to man), and his writings on these and other subjects were extensive. His influence on medicine was profound for many centuries—his teleology ("nature does nothing in vain") being particularly attractive to the medieval mind, although it was stultifying as regards advances in medical thought and practice.

galenicals, galenics (gah-len′ĭ-kals), (gah-len′-iks) medicines prepared according to the formulae of Galen. The term is now used to denote standard preparations containing one or several organic ingredients, as contrasted with pure chemical substances.

galeophobia (ga″le-o-fo′be-ah) morbid fear of cats; ailurophobia.

gall (gawl) the bile.

gallamine triethiodide (gal′ah-min tri″eth-i′o-dīd) a compound used to relax skeletal muscles.

gallbladder (gawl′blad-er) a small saclike organ located below the liver. It serves as a storage place for bile. The gallbladder may be subject to such disorders as inflammation and the formation of GALLSTONES.

Acute inflammation of the gallbladder (CHOLE-CYSTITIS) causes severe pain and tenderness in the right upper abdomen, accompanied by fever, nausea, prostration and sometimes jaundice. If the inflammation does not subside quickly, the gallbladder must be removed before it becomes gangrenous and ruptures.

Chronic inflammation of the gallbladder may cause habitual indigestion, accompanied by flatulence and nausea. The indigestion is most evident after heavy meals or meals of fatty foods. There also may be repeated attacks of pain in the right upper abdomen; these may be very brief or may last as long as several hours. Gallstones are often present. The condition may respond to conservative treatment with diet and medications or it may require surgical removal of the gallbladder, especially if there are gallstones.

Diagnosis of disorders of the gallbladder is aided by CHOLECYSTOGRAPHY; x-ray films are made after a contrast medium has been administered so that the gallbladder and bile ducts are clearly silhouetted. Studies may be done to determine the presence of gallstones or obstructions to the flow of bile in the biliary tract.

SURGERY OF THE GALLBLADDER. The two surgical procedures most commonly performed on the gallbladder are cholecystectomy and cholecystostomy. In cholecystectomy the gallbladder is removed; in cholecystostomy an incision is made into the gallbladder for the purpose of drainage. Surgical procedures involving the common bile duct are sometimes done in the treatment of various disorders of the gallbladder and biliary tract and may entail a surgical incision into the common bile duct (choledochotomy) which is usually done for removal of gallstones (choledocholithotomy).

Nursing Care. During the preoperative period the patient usually receives a thorough physical

GALACTOSEMIA: FOOD PLAN FOR ALL THE FAMILY MEMBERS

| | Servings During One Day | | |
Food Group	Preschool	School Age	Adults
Milk (Nutramigen for child with galactosemia)[1]	3 to 4 cups	4 or more cups	2 cups
Fruits[2] and vegetables[3]	4 or more small servings	4 or more	4 or more
Meats, fish, eggs, poultry[4]	2 or more small servings	2 or more	2 or more
Breads and cereals (milk free for child with galactosemia)	4 or more	4 or more	4 or more

From "Parent's Guide for the Galactose-free Diet," published by the California State Department of Health, 2151 Berkeley Way, Berkeley, California.

[1]If Nutramigen is not drunk in these amounts, calcium and vitamin D should be given as supplements.

[2]Include every day a serving of one of these: citrus, tomato, melon, strawberries, broccoli, raw cabbage, green peppers.

[3]Include a deep yellow or dark green, leafy vegetable at least every other day. Omit beets, peas and Lima beans for the child with galactosemia.

[4]Nuts, peanuts and peanut butter are also included in this group.

examination as well as specific tests for liver function and x-ray studies of the gallbladder and bile ducts. Since nausea and flatulence are common occurrences in these patients both before and after surgery, a nasogastric tube is usually inserted prior to surgery.

When the patient returns from the operating room a careful check should be made for drainage tubes, which may have been inserted during surgery. Most drains are devised so that bile and serous fluid from the operative site drain directly onto the dressings applied over the wound. Other drains or tubes, such as the T tube or Y tube, should be opened immediately and attached to a drainage apparatus so that the bile is collected in a bottle and can be measured periodically. In either case dressings over the wound are checked frequently for signs of hemorrhage or abnormalities in the drainage. When bile leakage is excessive the dressings will need frequent reinforcing and the outer layers will require frequent changing to keep the patient dry and comfortable and to avoid irritation of the skin around the incision.

It is especially important to observe the patient for signs of jaundice, bile pigment in the urine and light-colored stools during the postoperative period. Any of these conditions may indicate improper drainage of bile from the gallbladder and resultant accumulation of bile pigments in the blood. If the patient complains of severe abdominal pain before or after removal of drains or tubes, this situation should be reported to the physician at once.

Galli Mainini test (gal'e mi-ne'ne) a test for pregnancy; sperm are found in the urine of male frogs 1 to 4 hours after injection of urine from a pregnant woman (see also PREGNANCY TESTS).

gallium (gal'e-um) a chemical element, atomic number 31, atomic weight 69.72, symbol Ga. (See table of ELEMENTS.)

gallon (gal'on) a unit of liquid measure (4 quarts, or 3.785 liters).

gallstone (gawl'stōn) a stonelike mass, called a calculus, that forms in the gallbladder. The presence of gallstones is known medically as cholelithiasis. Their cause is unknown, although there is evidence of a connection between gallstones and obesity. They are most common in women after pregnancy, and in men and women past 35.

Gallstones may be present for years without causing trouble. The usual symptoms, however, are vague discomfort and pain in the upper abdomen. There may be indigestion and nausea, especially after eating fatty foods. X-rays will generally reveal the presence of gallstones, either directly or by use of a dye introduced into the gallbladder (CHOLECYSTOGRAPHY).

The most common complication of gallstones occurs when one of the stones escapes from the gallbladder and travels along the common bile duct, where it may lodge, blocking the flow of bile to the intestine and causing obstructive jaundice. This condition should be corrected by surgery before the liver is damaged.

When a gallstone travels through or obstructs a bile duct it can cause severe biliary colic, probably the most severe pain that can be experienced. The pain is located in the upper right quadrant of the abdomen, and radiates through to the scapula. Morphine is usually not given to relieve the pain because it increases spasm of the biliary sphincters. Other drugs such as papaverine hydrochloride and atropine may be given to promote relaxation and thereby relieve the pain. Treatment may also include insertion of a nasogastric tube for the purpose of gastric suction to relieve distention in the upper gastrointestinal tract.

Surgery is the preferred method of treatment and is performed as soon as the patient is able to withstand it. In most cases the gallbladder is removed and a tube is inserted to establish drainage of bile that has been dammed up by the stone. (See also surgery of the GALLBLADDER.)

Galton's law (gawl'tonz) each parent contributes, on an average, one-fourth, or $(0.5)^2$, of an individual's heritage, each grandparent one-sixteenth, or $(0.5)^4$, and so on, the occupier of each ancestral place in the nth degree contributing $(0.5)^{2n}$ of the heritage.

galvanic current (gal-van'ik) a steady direct electric current.

galvanism (gal'vah-nizm) uninterrupted electric current.

galvanization (gal"vah-nĭ-za'shun) treatment by galvanism.

galvanocautery (gal"vah-no-kaw'ter-e) cautery by a wire heated by galvanic electricity.

galvanocontractility (gal"vah-no-kon"trak-til'ĭ-te) contractility on stimulation by galvanic current.

galvanofaradization (gal"vah-no-far"ah-dī-za'-shun) the application of continuous and interrupted currents together.

galvanogustometer (gal"vah-no-gus-tom'ĕ-ter) an apparatus for clinical determination of taste thresholds by use of a galvanic current.

galvanometer (gal"vah-nom'ĕ-ter) an instrument for measuring galvanic electricity.
  string g., an apparatus for detecting very minute electric currents, consisting of a delicate thread of silvered quartz or platinum stretched between poles of a strong magnet.

galvanopalpation (gal"vah-no-pal-pa'shun) testing of nerves of the skin by means of galvanic electricity.

galvanoscope (gal-van'o-skōp) an instrument that shows the presence of galvanic electricity.

galvanosurgery (gal"vah-no-ser'jer-e) surgical application of galvanism.

galvanotaxis (gal"vah-no-tak'sis) 1. orientation of an organism in response to the influence of an electric current. 2. arrangement of a living organism in a fluid medium in relation to the direction of flow of the medium.

galvanotherapy (gal"vah-no-ther'ah-pe) treatment by means of uninterrupted electric current.

galvanothermy (gal"vah-no-ther'me) heating by galvanic electricity.

galvanotonus (gal"vah-not'o-nus) tonic response to galvanism.

galvanotropism (gal"vah-not'ro-pizm) movements in organs of animals and plants under the influence of an electric current.

gamete (gam′ēt) 1. one of two cells, male and female, whose union is necessary in sexual reproduction to initiate the development of a new individual. 2. the complete sexual form of malarial plasmodium as found in the anopheles mosquito. adj., **gamet′ic.**

gametocide (gam′ĕ-to-sīd″) an agent that destroys malarial gametes.

gametocyte (gah-met′o-sīt) the sexual plasmodial cell in malarial blood that produces gametes in the insect host.

gametogenesis (gam″ĕ-to-jen′ĕ-sis) the formation or production of gametes.

gametology (gam″ĕ-tol′o-je) the study of gametes.

gamma (gam′ah) the third letter of the Greek alphabet, γ; used in names of chemical compounds to distinguish one of three or more isomers or to indicate the position of substituting atoms or groups.
 g. globulin, a plasma protein developed in the lymphoid tissues and reticuloendothelial system in response to invasion by harmful agents such as bacteria, viruses and toxins. There are three types of plasma proteins: albumin, globulins and fibrinogen. Fibrinogen and albumin are manufactured by the liver; fibrinogen plays a vital role in the process of clotting. Gamma globulins are specific protein molecules that react chemically with the invading agent and are capable of destroying it; thus they play an important role in providing IMMUNITY. Almost all ANTIBODIES produced in defense of the body are gamma globulin molecules.
 Commercial preparations of gamma globulin are derived from blood serum and are used for prevention, modification and treatment of various infectious diseases. This type of gamma globulin, which is an immune serum, contains almost all the known antibodies circulating in the blood. It provides a passive immunity, usually for about 6 weeks. Certain specific types of gamma globulin may be used to raise the body's resistance to measles, mumps and poliomyelitis.
 The production of gamma globulin may be increased in the body by the invasion of harmful microorganisms. An abnormal amount of gamma globulin in the blood, a condition known as hypergammaglobulinemia, may be indicative of a chronic infection or certain malignant blood diseases.
 There is also a rare condition, AGAMMAGLOBULINEMIA, in which the body is unable to produce gamma globulin; patients suffering from this condition are extremely susceptible to infection and must be given frequent injections of gamma globulin serum.
 g. rays, electromagnetic emissions from radioactive substances. Gamma rays are similar to and have the same general properties as x-rays, except that they are produced through the disintegration of certain radioactive elements.
 Radium, uranium and thorium are examples of radioactive metals that emit three types of rays: alpha, beta and gamma rays. Of these three forms of radiation, the gamma rays are the most penetrating and therefore are sometimes used in the treatment of deep-seated malignancies (see also RADIOTHERAPY).

gamma benzene hexachloride (gam′ah ben′zēn

hek″sah-klōr′īd) lindane, used to treat scabies and pediculosis.

gammacism (gam′ah-sizm) imperfect utterance of *g* and *k* sounds.

gammaglobulinopathy (gam″ah-glob″u-lin-op′-ah-the) abnormality of the gamma globulins in the blood.

gammagram (gam′ah-gram) 1. a graphic record of the gamma rays emitted by an object or substance. 2. a radiogram produced by use of gamma rays as the radiant energy.

gammagraphic (gam″ah-graf′ik) pertaining to the recording of gamma rays in the study of organs after the administration of radioactive isotopes.

gamma-pipradol (gam″ah-pip′rah-dol) azacyclonol, a tranquilizer.

gammopathy (gah-mop′ah-the) gammaglobulinopathy.

Gamna's disease (gam′naz) splenomegaly with thickening of the splenic capsule and the presence of small brownish areas (Gamna nodules), iron-containing pigment being deposited in the splenic pulp.

gamogenesis (gam″o-jen′ĕ-sis) sexual reproduction.

gamogony (gam-og′o-ne) the development of merozoites into male and female gametes, which later fuse to form a zygote.

gamophobia (gam″o-fo′be-ah) morbid fear of marriage.

gampsodactylia (gamp″so-dak-til′e-ah) clawlike deformity of the toes.

gangli(o)- (gang′gle-o) word element [Gr.], *ganglion.*

ganglial (gang′gle-al) pertaining to a ganglion.

gangliasthenia (gang″gle-as-the′ne-ah) asthenia due to disease of a ganglion.

gangliated (gang′gle-āt″ed) provided with ganglia.

gangliectomy (gang″gle-ek′to-me) excision of a ganglion.

gangliform (gang′glī-form) resembling a ganglion.

gangliitis (gang″gle-i′tis) inflammation of a ganglion.

ganglioblast (gang′gle-o-blast″) an embryonic cell of the spinal ganglia.

gangliocyte (gang′gle-o-sīt″) a ganglion cell.

gangliocytoma (gang″gle-o-si-to′mah) a tumor containing ganglion cells.

ganglioform (gang′gle-o-form″) gangliform.

ganglioglioma (gang″gle-o-gli-o′mah) a glioma containing ganglion cells.

ganglioglioneuroma (gang″gle-o-gli″o-nu-ro′-mah) a nerve tumor containing ganglion cells, glia cells and nerve fibers.

gangliolytic (gang″gle-o-lit′ik) ganglioplegic.

ganglioma (gang″gle-o′mah) tumor of the lymphatic ganglia.

ganglion (gang′gle-on), pl. *gan′glia, ganglions* [Gr.] 1. a knot or knotlike mass; used in anatomic nomenclature as a general term to designate a group of nerve cell bodies located outside the central nervous system. The parasympathetic ganglia are located in, on or near the organs being innervated. The sympathetic ganglia are arranged in a chainlike fashion on either side of the spinal cord. 2. a form of cystic tumor occurring on an aponeurosis or tendon, as in the wrist.

Arnold's g., auricular g., one situated below the foramen ovale, sending nerves to the muscles of the tympanic membrane and palate; called also otic ganglion.

autonomic ganglia, aggregations of cell bodies of neurons of the autonomic nervous system.

basal ganglia, masses of gray matter centrally embedded with the thalamus in the cerebral hemisphere, comprising the corpus striatum (caudate and lentiform nucleï), amygdaloid body and claustrum. Sometimes the thalamus is considered as part of the basal ganglia; the tuber cinereum, corpora geniculata bodies and even the corpora quadrigemina have also been included. Called also basal nuclei.

cardiac g., a ganglion of the superficial cardiac plexus under the arch of the aorta.

carotid g., a ganglion in the lower part of the cavernous sinus.

carotid g., inferior, one in the lower part of the carotid canal.

carotid g., superior, one in the upper part of the carotid canal.

celiac ganglia, two large masses, one on either side of the midline, near the adrenal glands, which with the nerve fibers uniting them form the solar plexus.

cephalic ganglia, the ciliary, otic, pterygopalatine and submaxillary ganglia, all mainly of the sympathetic system.

cerebral g., thalamus.

cerebrospinal ganglia, those associated with the cranial and spinal nerves.

cervical g., inferior, a ganglion between the transverse process of the lowest cervical vertebra and the neck of the first rib.

cervical g., middle, a ganglion adjacent to the fifth cervical vertebra.

cervical g., superior, a ganglion opposite the second and third cervical vertebrae.

cervicothoracic g., a ganglion on the sympathetic trunk anterior to the lowest cervical or first thoracic vertebra. It is formed by a union of the seventh and eighth cervical and first thoracic ganglia. Called also stellate ganglion.

cervicouterine g., one near the cervix uteri.

ciliary g., a ganglion in the posterior part of the orbit.

coccygeal g., glomus coccygeum.

Corti's g., spiral ganglion.

dorsal root g., spinal ganglion.

false g., an enlargement on a nerve that does not have a true ganglionic structure.

Frankenhäuser's g., cervicouterine ganglion.

gasserian g., trigeminal ganglion.

geniculate g., a ganglion on the facial nerve in the aqueduct of Fallopius.

g. im′par, the ganglion commonly found in front of the coccyx, where the sympathetic trunks of the two sides unite.

jugular g., a node on (1) the root of the vagus nerve or (2) the glossopharyngeal nerve, both in the jugular foramen.

lenticular g., ciliary ganglion.

Ludwig's g., a ganglion near the right atrium of the heart.

lumbar ganglia, four or five pairs of ganglia on either side behind the abdominal aorta.

lymphatic g., any lymph node.

ophthalmic g., orbital g., ciliary ganglion.

otic g., a parasympathetic ganglion next to the medial surface of the mandibular division of the trigeminal nerve, just inferior to the foramen ovale, sending nerves to the muscles of the tympanic membrane and palate.

parasympathetic ganglia, aggregations of cell bodies of neurons of the parasympathetic nervous system.

petrous g., a ganglion on the glossopharyngeal nerve at the lower border of the petrous bone.

pterygopalatine g., a parasympathetic ganglion in a fossa in the sphenoid bone, formed by postganglionic cell bodies that synapse with preganglionic fibers from the fascial nerve via the nerve of the pterygopalatine canal. Called also sphenopalatine ganglion.

sacral ganglia, four or five pairs of ganglia on the ventral face of the sacrum.

Scarpas's g., vestibular ganglion.

sensory g., a name sometimes applied to the collective masses of nerve cell bodies in the brain subserving the function of sensation.

simple g., a cystic tumor in a tendon sheath.

sphenopalatine g., pterygopalatine ganglion.

spinal ganglia, ganglia on the posterior root of each spinal nerve.

spiral g., ganglia between the plates of the spiral lamina, sending filaments to the organ of Corti.

stellate g., cervicothoracic ganglion.

submandibular g., submaxillary g., a ganglion located superior to the deep part of the submandibular gland, on the lateral surface of the hypoglossus muscle; it receives a parasympathetic root from the lingual nerve, and a sympathetic root derived from the plexus on the facial artery.

suprarenal g., a ganglion at the junction of the great splanchnic nerves.

sympathetic ganglia, aggregations of cell bodies of neurons of the sympathetic nervous system.

thoracic ganglia, the ganglia on the thoracic portion of the sympathetic trunk, usually about ten on either side.

trigeminal g., a ganglion on the sensory root of the fifth cranial nerve, situated in a cleft within the dura mater (trigeminal cave) on the anterior part of the pars petrosa of the temporal bone, and giving off the ophthalmic and maxillary and part of the mandibular nerve. Called also gasserian ganglion and ganglion semilunare.

tympanic g., a ganglion on the tympanic branch of the glossopharyngeal nerve.

vestibular g., a ganglion on the vestibular part of the vestibulocochlear nerve near the external acoustic meatus.

Walther's g., glomus coccygeum.

Wrisberg's g., cardiac ganglion.

ganglionectomy (gang″gle-o-nek′to-me) excision of a ganglion.

ganglioneure (gang′gle-o-nūr″) any cell of a nerve ganglion.

ganglioneuroma (gang″gle-o-nu-ro′mah) a tumor made up of ganglion cells.

ganglionic (gang″gle-on′ik) pertaining to a ganglion.

   g. blockade, inhibition by drugs of nerve impulse transmission at autonomic ganglionic synapses.

ganglionitis (gang″gle-o-ni′tis) inflammation of a ganglion.

ganglionostomy (gang″gle-o-nos′to-me) surgical creation of an opening into a cystic tumor on a tendon sheath or aponeurosis.

ganglioplegic (gang″gle-o-ple′jik) 1. blocking transmission of impulses through the sympathetic and parasympathetic ganglia. 2. an agent that blocks impulses through the sympathetic and parasympathetic ganglia.

gangrene (gang′grēn) the death and putrefaction of body tissue, caused by stoppage of circulation to an area, often as a result of infection or injury. adj., **gang′grenous.** Although it usually affects the extremities, gangrene sometimes may involve the internal organs. Symptoms depend on the site and include fever, pain, darkening of the skin and an unpleasant odor. If the condition involves an internal organ, it is generally attended by pain and collapse. Treatment includes correcting the causes, and is frequently successful with modern medications and surgery.

   Types of Gangrene. The three major types of gangrene are moist, dry and gas gangrene. Moist and dry gangrene result from loss of blood circulation due to various causes; gas gangrene occurs in wounds infected by species of Clostridium that break down tissue by gas production and by toxins.

   Moist gangrene is caused by sudden stoppage of blood, resulting from burning by heat or acid, severe freezing, physical accident that destroys the tissue, a tourniquet that has been left on too long or a clot or other embolism. At first, tissue affected by moist gangrene has the color of a bad bruise, is swollen and often blistered. The gangrene is likely to spread with great speed. Toxins are formed in the affected tissues and absorbed.

   Dry gangrene occurs gradually and results from slow reduction of the blood flow in the arteries. It occurs only in the extremities, and can occur with arteriosclerosis, in old age or in advanced stages of diabetes mellitus. buerger's disease can also sometimes cause dry gangrene. Symptoms include gradual shrinking of the tissue which becomes cold and lacking in pulse, and turns first brown and then black. Usually a line of demarcation is formed where the gangrene stops owing to the fact that the tissue above this line continues to receive an adequate supply of blood.

   Internal Gangrene. In strangulated hernia, a loop of intestine is caught in the bulge and its blood supply is cut off; gangrene may occur in that section of tissue. In acute appendicitis, areas of gangrene may occur in the walls of the appendix with consequent rupture through a gangrenous area. In severe cases of cholecystitis, which is usually associated with gallstones, gangrene may develop where the stones compress the mucous membrane. Thrombosis of the mesenteric artery may result in gangrene. Gangrene can be a rare complication of lung abscess in pneumonia; a symptom is brown sputum with a foul smell.

   Prevention. To prevent gangrene in an open wound, the wound should be kept as clean as possible. If a tourniquet is applied, it must be loosened

for about 1 minute in every 10 minutes to keep fresh blood in the tissue. Burned skin requires careful and antiseptic handling. Frostbite is especially dangerous, for the freezing impedes circulation and skin becomes tender and easily broken.

Gantrisin (gan′tri-sin) trademark for preparations of sulfisoxazole, an antibacterial sulfonamide.

gargle (gar′gl) 1. a solution for rinsing the mouth and throat. 2. to rinse the mouth and throat by holding a solution in the open mouth and agitating it by expulsion of air from the lungs.

gargoylism (gar′goil-izm) a hereditary condition with large head, grotesque facies, thickening of lips, nostrils and ears, deformed limbs and claw-like hands, associated with Hurler's syndrome.

gas (gas) one of the four ultimate states of matter, being composed of widely scattered molecules that are freely movable; an aeriform fluid without independent shape or volume. adj., **gas′eous.**

   coal g., a gas produced by the destructive distillation of coal and used for domestic cooking. It is poisonous because it contains carbon monoxide.

   g. gangrene, a condition often resulting from dirty, lacerated wounds in which the muscles and subcutaneous tissue become filled with gas and a serosanguineous exudate. It is due to species of Clostridium that break down tissue by gas production and by toxins.

   laughing g., nitrous oxide.

   marsh g., methane.

   mustard g., a vesicant gas employed in war. It produces blistering and subsequent sloughing of the skin with involvement of the eyes and respiratory tract. Death results from bronchopneumonia; called also dichlorodiethylsulfide.

   g. pains, pains caused by distention of the stomach or intestines by accumulations of air or other gases. The presence of gas is indicated by the distention of the abdomen and by belching or the discharge of gas by rectum. Gas-forming foods include highly flavored vegetables such as onions, cabbage and turnips, and members of the bean family. Melons and raw apples are gas-forming fruits. Seasonings and other chemical irritants are also likely to produce gas in the intestinal tract.

   sewer g., the mixture of gases and vapors from a sewer; often dangerous from the contained materials resulting from the decay of organic matter.

   tear g., a gas that produces severe lacrimation by irritating the conjunctivae.

gaster (gas′ter) [Gr.] stomach.

gasterangiemphraxis (gas″ter-an″je-em-frak′-sis) obstruction of blood vessels of the stomach.

Gasterophilus (gas″ter-of′ĭ-lus) a genus of flies, the horse bot flies, the larvae of which develop in the gastrointestinal tract of horses and may sometimes infect man.

gastr(o)- (gas′tro) word element [Gr.], *stomach.*

gastradenitis (gas″trad-ĕ-ni′tis) inflammation of the gastric glands.

gastralgia (gas-tral′je-ah) pain in the stomach.

gastramine (gas′trah-min) betazole, a substance used to stimulate gastric secretion.

gastraneuria (gas″trah-nu′re-ah) defective nervous tone of the stomach.

gastrasthenia (gas"tras-the'ne-ah) a weak state of the stomach.

gastratrophia (gas"trah-tro'fe-ah) atrophy of the stomach.

gastrectasia (gas"trek-ta'ze-ah) dilatation of the stomach.

gastrectomy (gas-trek'to-me) excision of the stomach (total gastrectomy) or of a portion of it (partial or subtotal gastrectomy). Indications for surgical removal of part or all of the stomach include malignant tumors and gastric ULCER that does not respond to medical management or is complicated by perforation or hemorrhage. (See also surgery of the STOMACH.)

gastric (gas'trik) pertaining to the stomach.

g. analysis, analysis of the stomach contents by microscopy and tests to determine the amount of acid present. The tests performed are of value in diagnosing peptic ulcer, cancer of the stomach and pernicious anemia. They include tests for free and total acid, for occult blood and for lactic acid. Hyperacidity frequently is associated with benign ulcers; free acid is decreased in malignant tumors. Achlorhydria, or total absence of free hydrochloric acid, is characteristic of untreated pernicious anemia.

Procedures for a gastric analysis vary according to the type of test meal or stimulating substance given to increase the flow of gastric juices. Alcohol, caffeine or histamine may be used as a stimulant. All gastric analyses require that the patient be in a fasting state, that he refrain from smoking and that he remain calm and undisturbed prior to withdrawal of the stomach's contents. Measures must be taken to make the passage of the stomach tube as easy as possible for the patient under the circumstances. Once the stomach tube is in place specimens are obtained at varying intervals, depending on the stimulant administered.

One type of gastric analysis does not require the passage of a stomach tube. This is the DIAGNEX BLUE TEST, sometimes called a "tubeless gastric analysis." This test determines free hydrochloric acid by qualitative means; though it is of value as a screening device, it cannot be used as conclusive evidence in those cases in which hydrochloric acid is not excreted.

g. juice, the secretion of glands in the walls of the stomach for use in digestion. Its essential ingredients are pepsin, an enzyme that breaks down proteins in food, and hydrochloric acid, which destroys bacteria and is of assistance in the digestive process.

At the sight and smell of food, the stomach increases its output of gastric juice. When the food reaches the stomach, it is thoroughly mixed with the juice, the breakdown of the proteins is begun and the food then passes on to the duodenum for the next stage of digestion.

Normally the hydrochloric acid in gastric juice does not irritate or injure the delicate stomach tissues. However, in certain persons the stomach produces too much gastric juice, especially between meals when it is not needed, and the gastric secretions presumably erode the stomach lining, producing a peptic ULCER, and also hinder its healing once an ulcer has formed.

g. ulcer, an ulcer of the inner wall of the stomach. It is one of the two most common types of peptic ulcer, the other type being duodenal ulcer. (See also ULCER.)

gastricism (gas'trĭ-sizm) gastric disorder.

gastricsin (gas-trik'sin) a proteolytic enzyme isolated from gastric juices, differing from pepsin in molecular weight and in amino acid content.

gastrin (gas'trin) a hormone in extracts of pyloric mucosa that stimulates secretion by the gastric glands.

gastritis (gas-tri'tis) inflammation of the lining of the stomach. Gastritis is one of the most common stomach disorders, and occurs in acute, chronic and toxic forms.

acute g., severe gastritis caused by food poisoning, overeating, excessive intake of alcoholic beverages or bacterial or viral infection, and often accompanied by enteritis. The outstanding symptom of acute gastritis is abdominal pain. There is a feeling of distention, with loss of appetite, nausea and headache. There may be a slight fever and vomiting.

The substance causing the irritation can often be identified and it should of course be avoided. A bland diet of liquids and easily digested food should be followed for 2 or 3 days. Simply prepared solid foods in small quantities can then be added.

chronic g., an inflammation of the stomach that may occur repeatedly or continue over a period of time. Pain, especially after eating, and symptoms associated with indigestion occur in chronic gastritis. Among its possible causes are vitamin deficiencies, abnormalities of the gastric juice, ulcers, hiatus hernia, excessive use of alcohol, chronic emotional tension or a combination of any of these factors.

Chronic gastritis is treated with a bland diet. Food should be taken frequently, in small amounts. Antacids may also be used in moderation to minimize stomach acidity. A tranquilizer or mild sedative may help relieve tension and thus speed the healing process.

toxic g., gastritis resulting from ingestion of a corrosive substance such as a strong acid or poison. There is acute burning and cramping stomach pain, accompanied by diarrhea and vomiting. The vomitus may be bloody. The victim may collapse.

This condition is an emergency and immediate measures must be taken to prevent serious damage to the tissues of the stomach. First-aid measures are begun at once to flush out and neutralize the poison. If the poison is an acid, the victim is given plenty of milk, or, if milk is not available, water or a tablespoonful of milk of magnesia in a cup of water. If the poison is an alkali, milk is also the best antidote, although water or any fruit juice may be substituted.

gastroanastomosis (gas"tro-ah-nas"to-mo'sis) gastrogastrostomy.

gastroblennorrhea (gas"tro-blen"o-re'ah) excessive secretion of mucus in the stomach.

gastrobrosis (gas"tro-bro'sis) perforation of the stomach.

gastrocele (gas'tro-sēl) hernia of the stomach.

gastrocolic (gas"tro-kol'ik) pertaining to the stomach and colon.

gastrocolitis (gas"tro-ko-li'tis) inflammation of the stomach and colon.

gastrocoloptosis (gas"tro-ko"lop-to'sis) downward displacement of the stomach and colon.

gastrocolostomy (gas"tro-ko-los'to-me) anastomosis of the stomach to the colon.

gastrocolotomy (gas"tro-ko-lot'o-me) incision of the stomach and colon.

gastrodiaphany (gas"tro-di-af'ah-ne) exploration of the stomach by means of an electric lamp passed down the esophagus.

gastrodidymus (gas"tro-did'ĭ-mus) symmetrical conjoined twins joined in the abdominal region.

Gastrodiscoides (gas"tro-dis-koi'dēz) a genus of trematodes parasitic in the intestinal tract.

gastroduodenal (gas"tro-du"o-de'nal) pertaining to the stomach and duodenum.

gastroduodenectomy (gas"tro-du"o-dĕ-nek'to-me) excision of the stomach and duodenum.

gastroduodenitis (gas"tro-du"o-dĕ-ni'tis) inflammation of the stomach and duodenum.

gastroduodenostomy (gas"tro-du"o-dĕ-nos'to-me) anastomosis of the stomach to a normally remote part of the duodenum.

gastrodynia (gas"tro-din'e-ah) pain in the stomach.

gastroenteralgia (gas"tro-en"ter-al'je-ah) pain in the stomach and intestines.

gastroenteric (gas"tro-en-ter'ik) pertaining to the stomach and intestines.

gastroenteritis (gas"tro-en"tĕ-ri'tis) inflammation of the lining of the stomach and intestines. Psychologic causes of gastroenteritis include fear, anger and other forms of emotional upset. Allergic reactions to certain foods can cause gastroenteritis, as can irritation by excessive use of alcohol. Severe gastroenteritis, with such symptoms as headache, nausea, vomiting, weakness, diarrhea and gas pains, may result from various infectious and contagious diseases, such as typhoid fever, influenza and food poisoning.

gastroenteroanastomosis (gas"tro-en"ter-o-ah-nas"to-mo'sis) anastomosis of the stomach to the intestine.

gastroenterocolitis (gas"tro-en"ter-o-ko-li'tis) inflammation of the stomach, small intestine and colon.

gastroenterologist (gas"tro-en"ter-ol'o-jist) a specialist in gastroenterology.

gastroenterology (gas"tro-en"ter-ol'o-je) study of diseases of the stomach and intestine.

gastroenteropathy (gas"tro-en"ter-op'ah-the) any disease of the stomach and intestine.

gastroenteroptosis (gas"tro-en"ter-op-to'sis) downward displacement of the stomach and intestines.

gastroenterostomy (gas"tro-en"ter-os'to-me) anastomosis of the stomach to the intestine.

gastroenterotomy (gas"tro-en"ter-ot'o-me) incision of the stomach and intestine.

gastroesophagitis (gas"tro-e-sof"ah-ji'tis) inflammation of the stomach and esophagus.

gastroesophagostomy (gas"tro-e-sof"ah-gos'to-me) anastomosis between the stomach and esophagus.

gastrogastrostomy (gas"tro-gas-tros'to-me) surgical creation of an anastomosis between the pyloric and cardiac ends of the stomach, performed for hourglass contraction of the stomach, a condition in which the organ contracts at the middle.

gastrogavage (gas"tro-gah-vahzh') artificial feeding through a tube passed into the stomach.

gastrogenic (gas"tro-jen'ik) originating in the stomach.

gastrograph (gas'tro-graf) an instrument for registering motions of the stomach.

gastrohepatic (gas"tro-hĕ-pat'ik) pertaining to the stomach and liver.

gastrohepatitis (gas"tro-hep"ah-ti'tis) inflammation of the stomach and liver.

gastrohydrorrhea (gas"tro-hi"dro-re'ah) secretion of a watery fluid by the stomach.

gastrohyperneuria (gas"tro-hi"per-nu're-ah) excessive activity of the stomach nerves.

gastrohyponeuria (gas"tro-hi"po-nu're-ah) defective activity of the stomach nerves.

gastroileac (gas"tro-il'e-ak) pertaining to the stomach and ileum.

gastroileitis (gas"tro-il"e-i'tis) inflammation of the stomach and ileum.

gastroileostomy (gas"tro-il"e-os'to-me) anastomosis of the stomach to the ileum.

gastrointestinal (gas"tro-in-tes'tĭ-nal) pertaining to the stomach and intestine.
    g. series, G.I. series, an examination of the upper gastrointestinal tract using barium as the contrast medium for a series of x-ray films. Called also a barium meal (see BARIUM TEST).
    g. tract, the stomach and intestines; the portion of the digestive tract from the cardia to the anus (see also DIGESTIVE SYSTEM).

gastrojejunocolic (gas"tro-je-joo"no-kol'ik) pertaining to the stomach, jejunum and colon.

gastrojejunostomy (gas"tro-je-joo-nos'to-me) anastomosis of the stomach to the jejunum.

gastrolienal (gas"tro-li-e'nal) pertaining to the stomach and spleen.

gastrolith (gas'tro-lith) a calculus in the stomach.

gastrolithiasis (gas"tro-lĭ-thi'ah-sis) formation of gastroliths.

gastrology (gas-trol'o-je) study of the stomach and its diseases.

gastrolysis (gas-trol'ĭ-sis) freeing of the stomach from adhesions.

gastromalacia (gas"tro-mah-la'she-ah) softening of the wall of the stomach.

gastromegaly   (gas"tro-meg'ah-le) enlargement of the stomach.

gastromycosis   (gas"tro-mi-ko'sis) fungus infection of the stomach.

gastromyxorrhea   (gas"tro-mik"so-re'ah) excessive secretion of mucus by the stomach.

gastronephritis   (gas"tro-nĕ-fri'tis) inflammation of the stomach and kidney.

gastropancreatitis   (gas"tro-pan"kre-ah-ti'tis) inflammation of the stomach and pancreas.

gastroparalysis   (gas"tro-pah-ral'ĭ-sis) paralysis of the stomach.

gastropathy   (gas-trop'ah-the) any disease of the stomach.

Gastrophilus   (gas-trof'ĭ-lus) Gasterophilus.

gastrophrenic   (gas"tro-fren'ik) pertaining to the stomach and diaphragm.

gastroplasty   (gas'tro-plas"te) plastic repair of the stomach.

gastroplegia   (gas'tro-ple'je-ah) gastroparalysis.

gastroplication   (gas"tro-pli-ka'shun) plication of the stomach wall.

gastroptosis   (gas"trop-to'sis) downward displacement of the stomach.

gastroptyxis   (gas"tro-tik'sis) an operation for reducing a dilated stomach.

gastropulmonary   (gas"tro-pul'mo-ner"e) pertaining to the stomach and lungs.

gastropylorectomy   (gas"tro-pi"lo-rek'to-me) excision of the pyloric part of the stomach.

gastropyloric   (gas"tro-pi-lor'ik) pertaining to the stomach and pylorus.

gastrorrhagia   (gas"tro-ra'je-ah) hemorrhage from the stomach.

gastrorrhaphy   (gas-tror'ah-fe) suture of the stomach.

gastrorrhea   (gas"tro-re'ah) excessive secretion by the glands of the stomach.

gastrorrhexis   (gas"tro-rek'sis) rupture of the stomach.

gastroschisis   (gas-tros'kĭ-sis) a congenital fissure of the abdominal cavity.

gastroscope   (gas'tro-skōp) an endoscope especially designed for passage into the stomach to permit examination of its interior. The gastroscope is a hollow, cylindrical tube fitted with special lenses and lights. The newer types of gastroscope are made of glass fiber (fiberscope) which is more flexible. Each glass fiber reflects light and creates a mirror effect, making it possible to "go around corners," and facilitating visualization of the curvature of the stomach.

gastroscopy   (gas-tros'ko-pe) inspection of the interior of the stomach with a gastroscope.

NURSING CARE.   For 6 to 8 hours prior to the examination the patient is not allowed to take any food or liquids by mouth. The stomach should be empty during the procedure to facilitate inspection of its lining and to avoid vomiting and aspiration of liquids into the lungs.

A sedative, usually a barbiturate, and an analgesic such as meperidine (Demerol) are given 30 minutes

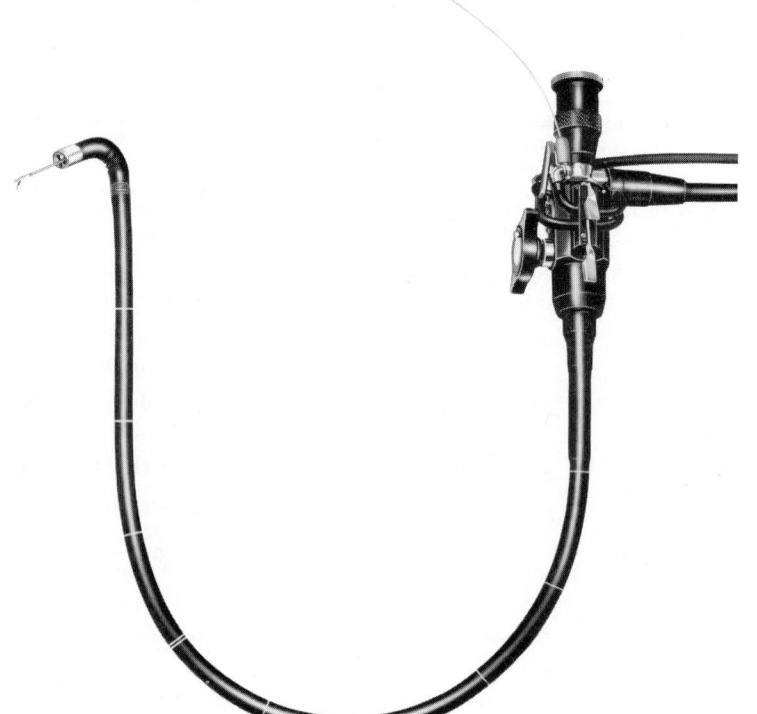

Fiber optic gastroscope. (Courtesy of American Cystoscope Makers, Inc.)

to 1 hour before the examination. The patient is awake during the procedure, which is not painful but is uncomfortable and exhausting. The sedatives help relieve apprehension and fear so that the patient can be more cooperative during the examination.

A local anesthetic such as cocaine or tetracaine (Pontocaine) is sprayed on the posterior pharynx to depress the gag reflex and reduce local reaction to the passage of the gastroscope. The patient is watched for toxic reaction to these drugs, and an emergency tray containing barbiturates must be readily available.

For passage of the conventional metal gastroscope the patient should be lying on his back. He may sit on the side of the bed or lie on his side facing the physician if a fiberscope is passed. If it seems likely that the patient will not be able to lie still he should be restrained, as there is danger that a sudden movement may cause the endoscope to perforate the esophagus or stomach.

After the procedure is completed the patient should be provided with rest and an opportunity to sleep. Foods and liquids are withheld until the gag reflex returns (usually about 4 hours).

gastrosis (gas-tro′sis) any disease of the stomach.

gastrospasm (gas′tro-spazm) spasm of the stomach.

gastrosplenic (gas″tro-splen′ik) pertaining to the stomach and spleen.

gastrostaxis (gas″tro-stak′sis) oozing of blood from the stomach.

gastrostenosis (gas″tro-stĕ-no′sis) abnormal constriction of the stomach.

gastrostogavage (gas-tros″to-gah-vahzh′) feeding through a gastric fistula.

gastrostolavage (gas-tros″to-lah-vahzh′) washing of the stomach through a gastric fistula.

gastrostoma (gas-tros′to-mah) a gastric fistula.

gastrostomy (gas-tros′to-me) the creation of an opening into the stomach. This procedure is done to provide for the administration of food and liquids when stricture of the esophagus or other conditions make swallowing impossible.

NURSING CARE. The patient who is to undergo this type of surgery usually has been ill for some time. He often has nutritional deficiencies brought on by a steadily increasing difficulty in swallowing. Sometimes the patient is a small child who has accidentally swallowed lye or some other caustic substance, or he may be an adult who has taken a corrosive poison in an attempted suicide. Some elderly patients with obstructive carcinoma of the esophagus or throat may also require gastrostomy.

A primary consideration in the care of these patients is the patient's acceptance of the gastrostomy as a substitute for eating. There are many social and emotional factors associated with eating and sharing a meal with others. The nursing staff must be sensitive to the problems the patient will encounter in his adjustment to the changes a gastrostomy may bring to his life. Whenever possible the patient should be taught to feed himself and care for his gastrostomy. It is important that he have privacy while doing this and that he be encouraged to ask questions and seek assistance from the nursing staff.

The skin around the opening must be protected from irritation by the gastric juices, which may leak from the opening and act as a corrosive on the skin. In some cases the gastrostomy tube can be removed after each feeding. A device called the Barnes-Redo prosthesis is available for use by patients with a permanent gastrostomy. This device is designed so that a cap can be fitted over a nylon tube permanently installed in the opening. When food or liquids are to be given the cap is unscrewed and a catheter is passed into the nylon tube. After feeding is completed the catheter is removed and the cap is screwed tightly over the nylon tube.

Feedings for a gastrostomy patient are gradually increased according to his tolerance. At first, water and glucose are given at regular intervals. If there is no leakage and the patient has no difficulty with these liquids, other liquids and puréed foods are gradually added until a full meal can be tolerated.

In order to stimulate gastric secretions and aid digestion, the patient should see, smell and taste small amounts of food before each feeding. It is recommended that he be allowed to chew small bits of food even though he cannot swallow them. This allows for proper stimulation of the gums and teeth and helps promote the health of the mouth and teeth.

Feedings should be warmed before they are given through the tube. Although commercially prepared liquid feedings are more convenient, they often cause diarrhea and are not as nutritionally adequate as regular meals. The foods to be given through the tube should be cooked until they are soft and then puréed in an electric blender. They can be diluted with the water in which they have been cooked, so that no vitamins are lost. The hospital or clinic dietician usually must work very closely with the patient and his family, instructing them in the planning and preparation of the patient's meals and offering suggestions for a variety of foods that will provide a well balanced diet.

gastrosuccorrhea (gas″tro-suk″o-re′ah) continuous secretion of gastric juice.

gastrotherapy (gas″tro-ther′ah-pe) 1. treatment of stomach diseases. 2. treatment of pernicious anemia with extract of gastric mucosa.

gastrothoracopagus (gas″tro-thor″ah-kop′ah-gus) symmetrical conjoined twins joined at the abdomen and thorax.

gastrotomy (gas-trot′o-me) incision of the stomach.

gastrotonometer (gas″tro-to-nom′ĕ-ter) an instrument for measuring intragastric pressure.

gastrotrachelotomy (gas″tro-tra″kĕ-lot′o-me) cesarean section with a transverse incision across the cervix.

gastrotropic (gas″tro-trop′ik) having affinity for the stomach.

gastrotympanites (gas″tro-tim″pah-ni′tēz) tympanitic distention of the stomach.

gastrula (gas′troo-lah) an embryo in the stage following the blastula stage, consisting of two layers of cells, the ectoderm and entoderm, enclosing a central cavity or archenteron.

gastrulation (gas″troo-la′shun) the formation of a gastrula.

Gatch bed (gach) a bed fitted with a jointed back rest and knee rest by which the patient can be raised to a sitting position and kept so.

gatophobia (gat″o-fo′be-ah) morbid dread of cats; ailurophobia.

Gaucher's disease (go-shāz′) a familial disorder characterized by splenomegaly, skin pigmentation, scleral pinguiculae and presence of distinctive cells (Gaucher's cells) in the liver, spleen and bone marrow. In the infantile form it results in delayed development and early death.

gauntlet (gawnt′let) a bandage covering hand and fingers like a glove.

gauze (gawz) white cotton cloth of plain weave of varying closeness.
  absorbent g., white cotton cloth of various thread counts and weights, supplied in various lengths and widths and in different forms (rolls or folds).
  petrolatum g., a sterile material produced by saturation of sterile absorbent gauze with sterile white petrolatum.

gavage (gah-vahzh′) [Fr.] feeding by a tube passed into the stomach; called also TUBE FEEDING.

g. cal. gram calorie (small calorie).

Gd chemical symbol, *gadolinium.*

Ge chemical symbol, *germanium.*

Gee's disease (gēz) celiac disease; called also Gee-Herter disease, Gee-Herter-Heubner disease, Gee-Thayson disease.

Geiger counter, Geiger-Müller counter (gi′ger), (gi′ger mil′er) a device for electrically determining the number of ionized particles emitted by a substance; used as a means of determining the presence of radioactivity.

gel (jel) a colloid that is firm in consistency, although containing much liquid; a colloid in a gelatinous form.

gelatin (jel′ah-tin) a substance obtained by partial hydrolysis of collagen derived from skin, white connective tissue and bones of animals; used as a vehicle for various drugs or in manufacture of capsules, and suggested for intravenous use as a plasma substitute. In absorbable sponge form it is used as a hemostatic agent.

gelatinase (jĕ-lat′ĭ-nās) an enzyme that liquefies gelatin.

gelatinize (jĕ-lat′ĭ-nīz) to convert into a jelly.

gelatinoid (jĕ-lat′ĭ-noid) resembling gelatin.

gelatinolytic (jĕ-lat″ĭ-no-lit′ik) splitting up gelatin.

gelatinous (jĕ-lat′ĭ-nus) like jelly or gelatin.

gelation (jĕ-la′shun) conversion of a sol into a gel.

Gelfilm (jel′film) trademark for absorbable gelatin film, used as a hemostatic agent.

Gelfoam (jel′fōm) trademark for preparations of absorbable gelatin sponge, used as a hemostatic agent.

gelose (jel′ōs) agar.

gelosis (je-lo′sis) a hard, swollen lump.

gemellology (jem″el-ol′o-je) the scientific study of twins and twinning.

geminate (jem′ĭ-nāt) paired; in twos.

geminus (jem′ĭ-nus), pl. *gem′ini* [L.] a twin. **gem′ini aequa′les,** monozygotic twins.

gemmangioma (jem″an-je-o′mah) a vascular tumor composed of embryonal cells.

gemmation (jĕ-ma′shun) development of a new organism from a protuberance on the body of the parent, a form of asexual reproduction; called also budding.

gemmule (jem′ūl) 1. a reproductive bud; the immediate product of gemmation. 2. any one of the many little excrescences upon the protoplasmic process of a nerve cell.

Gemonil (jem′o-nil) trademark for a preparation of metharbital, an anticonvulsant barbiturate.

-gen (jen) word element [Gr.], *an agent that produces.*

genal (je′nal) pertaining to the cheek.

gender (jen′der) the category (male, female, intersex) to which an individual is assigned on the basis of sex.

gene (jēn) one of the units of heredity arranged in linear fashion along a chromosome. Genes make up segments of the complex DEOXYRIBONUCLEIC ACID (DNA) molecule that controls cellular reproduction and function. There are thousands of genes in the chromosomes of each cell nucleus; they play an important role in heredity because they control the individual physical, biochemical and physiologic traits inherited by offspring from their parents. Through the genetic code of DNA they also control the day-to-day functions and reproduction of all cells in the body. For example, the genes control the synthesis of structural proteins and also the enzymes that regulate various chemical reactions that take place in a cell.
  The gene is capable of replication. When a cell multiplies by mitosis each daughter cell carries a set of genes that is an exact replica of that of the parent cell. This characteristic of replication explains how genes can carry hereditary traits through successive generations without change.
  allelic g's, genes situated at corresponding loci in a pair of chromosomes.
  complementary g's, two independent pairs of genes, neither of which will produce its effect in the absence of the other.
  dominant g., one that produces an effect in the organism regardless of the state of the corresponding allele.
  lethal g., one whose presence brings about the death of the organism or permits survival only under certain conditions.
  mutant g., one that has undergone a detectable mutation.
  nonstructural g's, units of a chromosome that are not concerned with formation of templates for messenger RNA (ribonucleic acid); the operator and regulator genes.

operator g., one that controls, through interaction with a repressor, the activity of adjacent structural genes.

recessive g., one that produces an effect in the organism only when it is transmitted by both parents.

regulator g., a segment of a chromosome that directs the synthesis of a repressor.

repressor g., one that controls formation of a repressor.

sex-linked g., one that is carried on or linked to a sex chromosome (X or Y).

structural g., one that forms templates for messenger RNA and is thereby responsible for the amino acid sequence of specific polypeptides.

supplementary g's, two independent pairs of genes that interact in such a way that one dominant will produce its effect even in the absence of the other, but the second requires the presence of the first to be effective.

genera (jen'er-ah) [L.] plural of *genus.*

generation (jen″ĕ-ra'shun) 1. the process of reproduction. 2. a class composed of all individuals removed by the same number of successive ancestors from a common predecessor, or occupying positions on the same level in a genealogical (pedigree) chart.

alternate g., reproduction by alternate asexual and sexual means in an animal or plant species.

asexual g., production of a new organism not originating from union of gametes.

direct g., asexual generation.

filial g., first, the offspring of the first mating in a particular genetic experiment; designated F_1.

filial g., second, offspring resulting from mating of two individuals of the first filial generation in a particular genetic experiment; designated F_2.

parental g., the two individuals first mating in a particular genetic study.

sexual g., production of a new organism from the zygote formed by the union of gametes.

spontaneous g., the alleged development of living organisms from lifeless matter; abiogenesis.

generative (jen'ĕ-ra″tiv) pertaining to reproduction.

generic (jĕ-ner'ik) 1. pertaining to a genus. 2. distinctive.

genesiology (jĕ-ne″ze-ol'o-je) the science of generation.

genesis (jen'ĕ-sis) creation; origination; used as a word termination joined to an element indicating the thing created, e.g., carcinogenesis.

genetic (jĕ-net'ik) pertaining to or carried by a gene or genes; hereditary.

g. code, the system by which information is transferred from genetic material to proteins, the pattern of nucleotides in the nucleic acids being thought to determine each amino acid in the chain making up each protein.

geneticist (jĕ-net'ĭ-sist) a student of genetics.

genetics (jĕ-net'iks) the branch of biology dealing with the phenomena of heredity and the laws governing it.

biochemical g., the science concerned with the chemical and physical nature of genes and the mechanism by which they control the development and maintenance of the organism.

The field of biochemical genetics is relatively new and recently it has become the study of the cause of many specific diseases that are now known to be inherited. These diseases include those resulting from the improper synthesis of hemoglobins and protein, such as sickle cell anemia and thalassemia, both of which are hereditary anemias; inborn errors of metabolism, such as PHENYLKETONURIA and GALACTOSEMIA, in which lack of or alteration of a specific enzyme prohibits proper metabolism of carbohydrates, proteins or fats and thus produces pathologic symptoms; and genetically determined variations in response to certain drugs, for example, isoniazid.

clinical g., the study of the possible genetic factors influencing the occurrence of a pathologic condition. In addition to the diseases mentioned under biochemical genetics, other aspects of clinical genetics include the study of chromosomal aberrations, such as those that cause mental retardation and DOWN'S SYNDROME (mongolism), and immunogenetics, or the genetic aspects of antigens, antibodies and their reactions, which has particular significance in the area of TRANSPLANTATION of body organs.

genetopathy (jen″ĕ-top'ah-the) any disease affecting the reproductive function.

genetotrophic (jĕ-net″o-trōf'ik) pertaining to genetics and nutrition; relating to problems of nutrition that are hereditary in nature, or transmitted through the genes.

genetous (jen'ĕ-tus) dating from fetal life.

genial (je'ne-al) pertaining to the chin.

genic (jen'ik) pertaining to genes.

-genic (jen'ik) word element [Gr.], *giving rise to; causing.*

genicular (jĕ-nik'u-lar) pertaining to the knee.

geniculate (jĕ-nik'u-lāt) bent like a knee.

geniculum (jĕ-nik'u-lum), pl. *genic'ula* [L.] a little knee; used in anatomic nomenclature to designate a sharp kneelike bend in a small structure or organ.

genioplasty (je'ne-o-plas″te) plastic surgery of the chin.

genital (jen'ĭ-tal) pertaining to reproduction.

genitalia (jen″ĭ-ta'le-ah) the reproductive organs; called also the genitals. (See also REPRODUCTIVE ORGANS.)

The internal female reproductive organs consist of the ovaries, uterine tubes, uterus and vagina. The external genitalia, referred to collectively as the vulva, consist of the mons pubis, labia majora, labia minora, clitoris, vestibule of the vagina, vulvovaginal glands and the bulb of the vestibule.

The male genitalia consist of the testes, seminiferous (semen-carrying) tubules, epididymides, ductus deferentes, ejaculatory ducts, seminal vesicles, prostate, bulbourethral glands and glans penis.

genitaloid (jen'ĭ-tal-oid″) pertaining to the primordial germ cells, before future sexuality is distinguishable.

genito- (jen'ĭ-to) word element [L.] relating to the organs of reproduction.

genitofemoral (jen″ĭ-to-fem'o-ral) pertaining to the reproductive organs and thigh.

genitoplasty (jen'ĭ-to-plas″te) plastic surgery on the reproductive organs.

genitourinary system (jen″ĭ-to-u'rĭ-ner″e) the organs of reproduction, together with the organs concerned with production and excretion of urine; called also urogenital system. (See also REPRODUCTIVE ORGANS, KIDNEY, URETER, BLADDER and URETHRA.)

genoblast (jen'o-blast) 1. the nucleus of the impregnated ovum. 2. a mature germ cell.

genodermatosis (je″no-der″mah-to'sis) a genetically determined disease or malformation that involves the skin.

genome (je'nōm) the complete set of hereditary factors contained in the haploid set of chromosomes. adj., **genom'ic.**

genoneme (jen'o-nēm) the axial thread of a chromosome in which lie the genes.

genotype (je'no-tīp) the hereditary constitution of an organism. adj., **genotyp'ic.**

-genous (jen'us) word element [Gr.], *arising or resulting from; produced by.*

gentian (jen'shan) the dried roots of *Gentiana lutea;* used as a bitter tonic.
  g. violet, a faintly odorous compound used as a dye and in medicine as an anthelmintic and anti-infective; called also methylrosaniline chloride.

gentianophilous (jen″shan-of'ĭ-lus) staining readily with gentian violet.

gentianophobous (jen″shan-of'ŏ-bus) not staining with gentian violet.

gentiavern (jen'shah-vern) gentian violet.

genu (je'nu), pl. *gen'ua* [L.] the knee.
  g. extror'sum, bowleg.
  g. intror'sum, knock-knee.
  g. recurva'tum, hyperextensibility of the knee joint.
  g. val'gum, knock-knee.
  g. va'rum, bowleg.

genus (je'nus), pl. *gen'era* [L.] a taxonomic category (taxon) subordinate to a tribe (or subtribe) and superior to a species (or subgenus).

genyplasty (jen'ĭ-plas″te) plastic surgery of the cheek.

geobiology (je″o-bi-ol'o-je) the biology of terrestrial life.

geode (je'ōd) a dilated lymph space.

geomedicine (je″o-med'ĭ-sin) the branch of medicine dealing with the influence of climatic and environmental conditions on health.

geophagism, geophagy (je-of'ah-jizm), (je-of'ah-je) the eating of earth (soil) or clay.

geotaxis (je″o-tak'sis) geotropism.

geotrichosis (je″o-trĭ-ko'sis) infection with fungus of the genus Geotrichum.

Geotrichum (je-ot'rĭ-kum) a genus of fungi sometimes found in lesions in the lungs.

geotropism (je-ot'ro-pizm) a growth curvature occurring in response to the stimulation of gravity.

gephyrophobia (je-fi″ro-fo'be-ah) fear of walking on a bridge or other structure near the water.

geratic (jĕ-rat'ik) pertaining to old age.

geratology, gereology (jer″ah-tol'o-je), (jer″e-ol'o-je) the science dealing with old age.

geriatrics (jer″e-at'riks) the branch of medicine devoted to the medical problems and care of elderly persons. It is related to the science of gerontology, which is the study of the aging process in all its aspects, social as well as biologic. Geriatrics grows increasingly important as modern medicine and a rising standard of living lengthen life expectancy and increase the proportion of aged persons in society.

  An important part of geriatrics is concerned with helping older persons to live happy and satisfying lives. Geriatric specialists encourage their patients to follow useful and interesting pursuits and to adopt a sound mental attitude toward aging itself. The prevention of disease is also important in geriatrics, and stress is placed on suitable exercise, rest and nutrition, and on maintenance of proper body weight. Regular and thorough medical examinations are another essential factor in the control of illness.

  There are few illnesses, if any, that affect only elderly persons. Certain disorders, however, tend to be characteristic problems of advancing age. These include decline of vision and hearing and deterioration of the teeth. The wear and tear of living may also produce increasing stiffness and other disorders of the joints, and the bones may become somewhat brittle and tend to break more easily.

  Among the diseases that often affect older persons are arteriosclerosis and heart disease. Other disorders that may often occur in the aged are hernia, cataract, enlargement of the prostate in men, cancer and prolapse of the rectum or uterus. Advances in modern surgery have made it possible to treat these conditions in elderly patients with excellent results.

  In geriatrics, increasing emphasis is also being given to the older person's psychologic welfare—his social contacts, economic security, interest in living, work opportunities after retirement and a continuing sense of belonging to society. Geriatrics recognizes that health of mind is essential to the health of the body.

germ (jerm) 1. a pathogenic microorganism. 2. living substance capable of developing into an organ, part or organism as a whole; a primordium.
  wheat g., the embryo of wheat, which contains tocopherol, thiamine, riboflavin and other vitamins.

German measles (jer'man me'zelz) a contagious virus disease, most common in children between the ages of 3 and 12 years; called also RUBELLA or 3-day measles. The disease is usually mild in children, but it has been found to cause various developmental abnormalities in fetuses of mothers who contract it during pregnancy.

germanium (jer-ma′ne-um) a chemical element, atomic number 32, atomic weight 72.59, symbol Ge. (See table of ELEMENTS.)

germicidal (jer″mĭ-si′dal) destructive to pathogenic microorganisms.

germicide (jer′mĭ-sīd) an agent that destroys pathogenic microorganisms.

germinal (jer′mĭ-nal) pertaining to a germ.

germination (jer″mĭ-na′shun) the beginning of development of a plant embryo.

germinative (jer′mĭ-na″tiv) germinal.

gerocomia (jer″o-ko′me-ah) the hygiene of the elderly.

geroderma, gerodermia (jer″o-der′mah), (jer″o-der′me-ah) wrinkling and thickening of the skin, like that of old age.

gerodontics (jer″o-don′tiks) dentistry dealing with the dental problems of older people.

gerodontology (jer″o-don-tol′o-je) study of the dentition and dental problems in the aged and aging.

geromarasmus (jer″o-mah-raz′mus) the emaciation of old age.

geromorphism (jer″o-mor′fizm) premature old age.

gerontal (jĕ-ron′tal) pertaining to old age.

gerontology (jer″on-tol′o-je) the study of old age, its phenomena, diseases, etc.

gerontopia (jer″on-to′pe-ah) the improved sight of old age.

gerontotherapeutics (je-ron″to-ther″ah-pu′tiks) the science of retarding and preventing the development of many of the aspects of senescence.

gerontoxon (jer″on-tok′son) arcus senilis.

gestagen (jes′tah-jen) a hormone with progestational activity.

gestaltism (gĕ-stawl′tizm) the theory in psychology that the objects of mind, as immediately presented to direct experience, come as complete unanalyzable wholes or forms (Gestalten) that cannot be split up into parts.

gestation (jes-ta′shun) the development of the new individual within the uterus, from conception to birth.
    abdominal g., development of the fertilized ovum in the abdominal cavity.
    ectopic g., development of the fertilized ovum outside the uterus; ectopic pregnancy.
    g. period, the duration of pregnancy, in the human female about 266 days.

gestosis (jes-to′sis) any toxemic manifestation in pregnancy.

geumaphobia (gu″mah-fo′be-ah) abnormal fear of tastes or flavors.

GFR glomerular filtration rate.

G.I. gastrointestinal; globin (zinc) insulin.

giantism (ji′an-tizm) gigantism.

Giardia (je-ar′de-ah) a genus of flagellate protozoa parasitic in many species of vertebrates.
    G. intestina′lis, G. lam′blia, a species parasitic in the intestines of man.

giardiasis (je″ar-di′ah-sis) infection with Giardia.

gibbosity (gĭ-bos′ĭ-te) the condition of being humped.

gibbous (gib′us) humped; protuberant.

gibbus (gib′us) a hump.

Gibraltar fever (jĭ-brawl′ter) brucellosis.

Gierke's disease (gēr′kez) a disease characterized by abnormal storage of glycogen in children; marked by enlargement of the liver and hypoglycemia and lack of response to epinephrine's glycogen-mobilizing effect. An enzyme deficiency is responsible for the abnormal glycogen metabolism. Called also glycogenosis and glycogen storage disease.

giga- (gi′gah) word element [Gr.], *huge;* used in naming units of measurement to designate an amount 10^9 (one billion) times the size of the unit to which it is joined, e.g., gigameter (10^9 meters); symbol G.

gigantism (ji-gan′tizm, ji′gan-tizm) abnormal overgrowth of the body or a part. Generally applied to a rare abnormality of the PITUITARY GLAND that causes excessive growth in a child so that he becomes an unusually tall adult. If the abnormality is extreme, he may reach a height of 8 feet or more, although the body proportions usually are normal.
    The condition is brought on by overproduction of growth hormone occurring before the growing ends of bone have closed. The opposite condition, DWARFISM, is caused by underproduction of the same hormone. (Overproduction of growth hormone in adults causes ACROMEGALY.) Gigantism can be corrected only by early diagnosis in childhood and removal by surgery of part of the pituitary gland or by x-ray treatment.

gigantocyte (ji-gan′to-sīt) a very large erythrocyte.

gigantosoma (ji-gan″to-so′mah) gigantism.

Gilbert's disease (zhēl-bārz′) constitutional hyperbilirubinemia.

Gilford-Hutchinson disease (gil′ford-huch′in-sun) progeria.

Gilles de la Tourette's disease (zhēl″dĕ-lah-toor-etz′) motor incoordination with echolalia and coprolalia.

gingiva (jin-ji′vah), pl. *gingi′vae* [L.] the fleshy structure covering the tooth-bearing border of the jaw; the gum. adj., **gingi′val.**
    alveolar g., the portion overlying the alveolar process and firmly attached to it.
    areolar g., the portion attached to the alveolar process by loose areolar connective tissue.
    buccal g., the portion that is applied to the buccal surfaces of the posterior teeth.
    cemental g., the portion attached to cementum of a tooth, but lying crownward of the alveolar process.

free g., the portion covering part of the crowns of the teeth, but not attached to them.

labial g., the portion that is applied to the labial surfaces of the teeth.

lingual g., the portion that is applied to the lingual surfaces of the teeth.

marginal g., free gingiva.

gingivalgia (jin″ji-val′je-ah) neuralgia of the gingiva.

gingivectomy (jin″ji-vek′to-me) surgical excision of all loose infected and diseased gingival tissue to eradicate periodontal infection and reduce the depth of the gingival sulcus.

gingivitis (jin″ji-vi′tis) a general term for inflammation of the gums, of which bleeding is one of the primary symptoms. Other symptoms include swelling, redness, pain and difficulty in chewing. There are numerous causes for this condition, and it can lead to a more serious disorder, pyorrhea alveolaris or periodontitis.

One of the most common causes of gingivitis is the accumulation of food particles in the crevices between the gums and the teeth. Other causes are general poor health, irregular teeth, badly fitting fillings or dentures that irritate the gums and infections such as Vincent's angina, or TRENCH MOUTH.

Gingivitis is best prevented by correct brushing of the teeth and proper gum care. A good diet containing the necessary minerals and vitamins is also important. Vitamin deficiencies and anemia and other blood dyscrasias are often accompanied by gingivitis.

gingivo- (jin′ji-vo) word element [L.], *gingival.*

gingivoglossitis (jin″ji-vo-glŏ-si′tis) inflammation of the gingiva and tongue.

gingivolabial (jin″ji-vo-la′be-al) pertaining to the gingiva and lips.

gingivoplasty (jin′ji-vo-plas″te) surgical remodeling of the gingiva.

gingivosis (jin″ji-vo′sis) a chronic, diffuse inflammation of the gums, with desquamation of papillary epithelium and mucous membrane.

gingivostomatitis (jin″ji-vo-sto″mah-ti′tis) inflammation of the gingiva and oral mucosa.

herpetic g., an infection of the gingiva and oral mucosa by herpesvirus, characterized by fever, redness and swelling, without necrosis of the gingival papillae or margins.

ginglymus (jing′gli-mus) a joint that allows movement in but one plane, forward and backward like a door hinge; called also hinge joint.

girdle (ger′dl) an encircling or confining structure.

pectoral g., shoulder girdle.

pelvic g., the encircling bony structure supporting the lower limbs.

shoulder g., thoracic g., the encircling bony structure supporting the upper limbs.

Gitaligin (ji-tal′i-jin) trademark for a preparation of amorphous gitalin, a cardiotonic.

gitalin (jit′ah-lin) a glycoside of digitalis.

amorphous g., a glycosidal constituent of the leaves of *Digitalis purpurea;* used as a cardiotonic.

glabella (glah-bel′ah) space between the eyebrows.

glabrous (gla′brus) smooth.

gladiolus (glah-di′o-lus) the main portion of the sternum.

glairy (glār′e) resembling white of an egg.

gland (gland) an organ that secretes a specific substance. Glands are divided into two main groups, endocrine and exocrine.

The ENDOCRINE GLANDS, or ductless glands, discharge their secretions directly into the blood; they include the adrenal, pituitary, thyroid and parathyroid glands, the islands of Langerhans in the pancreas, the gonads, the thymus and the pineal gland.

The exocrine glands, which discharge through ducts opening on an external or internal surface, include the salivary, sebaceous and sweat glands, the liver, the gastric glands, the pancreas, the intestinal, mammary and lacrimal glands and the prostate.

The organs sometimes called lymph glands are more accurately called lymph nodes; they are not glands in the usual sense.

acinar g., acinous g., one made up of several oval or spherical sacs (acini).

adrenal g., a triangular structure above either kidney, an endocrine gland consisting of cortex and medulla, the latter secreting epinephrine and the cortex secreting hormones affecting growth and the gonads (see also ADRENAL GLAND).

albuminous g's, certain glands of the digestive tract secreting a watery fluid.

apocrine g., one whose discharged secretion contains part of the secreting cells.

axillary g's, lymph nodes situated in the axilla.

Bartholin g's, vulvovaginal glands, two minute glands, one on each side of the vagina, their ducts opening on the vulva (see also BARTHOLIN GLANDS).

Bowman's g's, tubular glands in the olfactory mucosa.

bronchial g's, lymph nodes at the root of a bronchus.

Brunner's g's, glands in the duodenum secreting intestinal juice.

bulbocavernous g's, bulbourethral g's, two glands embedded in the substance of the sphincter of the male urethra, posterior to the membranous part of the urethra; their secretion lubricates the urethra; called also Cowper's glands.

cardiac g's, those of the cardiac extremity of the stomach.

carotid g's, carotid bodies.

celiac g's, lymph nodes anterior to the abdominal aorta.

ceruminous g's, glands that secrete cerumen.

choroid g., the choroid plexus, regarded as the secretor of the cerebrospinal fluid.

circumanal g's, specialized sweat and sebaceous glands around the anus.

Cobelli's g's, glands in the mucous membrane of the esophagus.

coccygeal g., a vascular body near the tip of the coccyx.

compound g., one with branching ducts.

conglobate g., a lymph node.

conglomerate g., compound gland.

Cowper's g's, 1. bulbourethral glands. 2. Bartholin, or vulvovaginal glands.

dental g., one of the white areas on the mucous membrane of the jaw over the point of emergence of the tooth.

duodenal g's, Brunner's glands.

Ebner's g's, mucous glands of the tongue.

eccrine g., one that produces a simple fluid secretion without admixture of cell plasm or cell contents.

enterochromaffin g., a type found in the mucosa of the intestines, characterized by the presence in the cell protoplasm of granules that stain with chromium salts and are impregnable with silver.

Fränkel's g's, minute glands that open below the edge of the vocal cord.

fundic g's, very numerous, tubular glands in the mucosa of the fundus and body of the stomach that secrete the gastric juice.

gastric g's, the secreting glands of the stomach, including the fundic, cardiac and pyloric glands.

Gay g's, highly developed sweat glands.

genal g's, glands in the submucous tissue of the cheek.

glossopalatine g's, mucous glands at the posterior end of the smaller sublingual glands.

hair g., the sebaceous gland of a hair follicle.

haversian g's, folds on synovial surfaces regarded as secretors of synovia.

hematopoietic g's, glands that take a part in formation of the blood elements.

hemolymph g's, glands containing blood sinuses occurring along with the lymph nodes.

holocrine g., one whose discharged secretion contains the entire secreting cells.

interscapular g., a mass of lymphoid tissue in the neck and scapular region in the embryo.

intestinal g's, straight tubular glands in the mucous membrane of the intestines, opening, in the small intestine, between the bases of the villi, and containing argentaffin cells.

jugular g., a lymph node behind the clavicular insertion of the sternocleidomastoid muscle.

Krause's g's, mucous glands in the middle portion of the conjunctiva.

lacrimal g's, the glands that secrete tears.

g's of Lieberkühn, intestinal glands.

Littre's g's, acinar glands in the spongy portion of the urethra.

mammary g., the milk-secreting organ of female mammals, existing also in a rudimentary state in the male (see also BREAST).

meibomian g's, sebaceous glands between the cartilage and conjunctiva of the eyelids.

merocrine g., one whose discharged secretion contains no part of the secreting cells.

Moll's g's, small glands at the edges of the eyelids.

Montgomery's g's, sebaceous glands in the mammary areola.

mucous g's, glands that secrete mucus.

parathyroid g's, small bodies in the region of the thyroid glands, developed from the entoderm of the brachial clefts, numbering one to four, commonly two; they are concerned with the metabolism of calcium and phosphorus (see also PARATHYROID GLANDS).

parotid g., the large salivary gland in front of the ear (see also PAROTID GLAND).

peptic g's, a set of mucous glands on the mucous membrane of the stomach, believed to secrete the gastric juice.

pilous g., the sebaceous gland of a hair follicle.

pineal g., a small, conelike, glandular body in the brain whose role in the human is largely unknown (see also PINEAL GLAND).

pituitary g., an epithelial body of dual origin, resting on the sphenoid bone and connected to the brain by a stalk; it consists of two lobes, the anterior lobe, secreting several important hormones that regulate the proper functioning of the other endocrine glands, and the posterior lobe, whose cells are sites of storage for a pressor and an oxytocic principle. Called also hypophysis cerebri. (See also PITUITARY GLAND.)

prostate g., prostate.

pyloric g's, the pepsin-secreting glands of the stomach situated near the pylorus.

salivary g., any gland that secretes saliva, as the parotid, submaxillary or sublingual (see also SALIVARY GLANDS).

sebaceous g., one of the tiny glands of the skin that secrete an oily material (sebum) into the hair follicles.

sentinel g., an enlarged lymph node, considered to be pathognomonic of some pathologic condition elsewhere.

sex g's, gonads.

Skene's g's, two mucous glands just within the meatus of the female urethra; called also paraurethral ducts.

solitary g's, isolated lymphoid nodules in the mucosa of the large and small intestines.

sublingual g., a salivary gland on either side under the tongue.

submandibular g., submaxillary g., a salivary gland on the inner side of each ramus of the lower jaw.

sudoriparous g's, sweat glands.

suprarenal g., adrenal gland.

sweat g., one of the glands distributed over the entire body surface which promote cooling of the body by evaporation of the secretion (see also SWEAT GLAND).

target g., one specifically affected by a pituitary hormone.

thymus g., thymus.

thyroid g., an endocrine gland concerned with metabolism, situated in the neck at the level of the fifth to seventh cervical vertebrae, and serving an important function in regulating body metabolism (see also THYROID GLAND).

tubular g., one without an excretory duct, the terminal portion being a straight tubule that opens directly on an epithelial surface.

Tyson's g's, small sebaceous glands on the corona of the penis and of the labia majora and minora.

vulvovaginal g's, two minute glands, one on either side of the vagina, their ducts opening on the vulva (see also BARTHOLIN GLANDS).

Waldeyer's g's, glands in the attached edge of the eyelid.

Weber's g's, the tubular mucous glands of the tongue.

glanders (glan'derz) a disease of horses communicable to man, and caused by the glanders bacillus, *Actinobacillus mallei*. It is marked by a purulent inflammation of mucous membranes and an eruption of nodules on the skin which coalesce and break down, forming deep ulcers, which may end in necrosis of cartilage and bones. Called also equinia.

glandilemma (glan″di-lem′ah) the capsule or outer envelope of a gland.

glandula (glan′du-lah), pl. *glan′dulae* [L.] gland.

glandular (glan′du-lar) pertaining to or of the nature of a gland.

g. fever, disease characterized by changes in the leukocytes, occurring most commonly in children and young adults; called also infectious MONO-NUCLEOSIS.

glandule (glan′dūl) a small gland.

glans (glanz), pl. *glan′des* [L.] a small, rounded mass or glandlike body.

g. clitor′idis, the distal end of the clitoris.

g. pe′nis, the cap-shaped expansion of the corpus spongiosum at the end of the penis.

Glanzmann's disease (glanz′manz) thrombasthenia.

glass-blower's disease an infection with enlargement of the parotid gland occurring in glassblowers.

glasses (glas′ez) lenses arranged in a frame holding them in the proper position before the eyes, as an aid to vision.

bifocal g., those having two segments that give the proper correction for near and for far vision.

trifocal g., lenses that have three different refracting powers, one for distant, one for intermediate and one for near vision.

glaucarubin (glaw″kah-ru′bin) a crystalline glycoside obtained from the fruit of *Simaruba glauca*; used as an amebicide.

glaucoma (glaw-ko′mah) a disease of the eye characterized by increased intraocular pressure resulting in damage to the retina and the optic nerve and eventually to blindness if it is not treated successfully. adj., **glauco′matous.** Glaucoma is responsible for almost half of all cases of adult blindness, and strikes more than 2 per cent of all those over 40 years of age in the United States. It rarely occurs in anyone under 40. There is evidence that it is much more common in patients with diabetes mellitus. The cause is unknown, but proper treatment, given early enough, can halt its disabling effects.

The normal eye is filled with aqueous humor in an amount carefully regulated to maintain the shape of the eyeball. In glaucoma, the balance of this fluid is disturbed; fluid is formed more rapidly than it leaves the eye, and pressure builds up. The increased pressure damages the retina and disturbs the vision, for example, by the loss of side vision. If not relieved by proper treatment, the pressure will eventually damage the optic nerve, interrupting the flow of impulses and causing blindness.

There are two principal forms of glaucoma. The acute form may cause a sudden dimming of the vision, often with severe pain in the eye. Chronic glaucoma, which is more common, does not usually cause pain, and affects the vision very gradually. The patient frequently does not notice the effects of chronic glaucoma until after he has already suffered some loss of vision.

SYMPTOMS AND DIAGNOSIS. The symptoms of glaucoma are loss of side vision, so that the patient seems to be "looking down a rifle barrel," blurred or fogged vision and the appearance of colored rings or halos around bright objects. These symptoms do not necessarily indicate glaucoma, but anyone over 40 who experiences any of them should consult an ophthalmologist immediately.

Glaucoma is diagnosed with the help of a tono-meter, which measures the pressure inside the eyeball.

TREATMENT. Treatment for glaucoma varies with the type and severity of the case. If it is detected early, it can generally be treated satisfactorily with miotics and other drugs that help reduce the pressure inside the eye. In some advanced cases, relatively simple surgery may be necessary to provide the fluid with a new outflow channel.

The effects of untreated glaucoma cannot be remedied. If the condition is neglected until partial or total blindness sets in, the retina and optic nerve cannot be repaired to restore sight.

gleet (glēt) chronic gonorrheal urethritis.

Glénard's disease (gla-narz′) splanchnoptosis.

glenoid (gle′noid) resembling a pit or socket.

g. cavity, the cavity in the head of the scapula for articulation with the humerus.

g. fossa, a depression in the temporal bone where the condyle of the lower jaw rests; called also mandibular fossa.

glia (gli′ah) neuroglia; the supporting structure of the brain and spinal cord, composed of specialized cells and their processes.

gliacyte (gli′ah-sīt) a cell of the neuroglia.

gliadin (gli′ah-din) a tough protein from wheat gluten.

glial (gli′al) pertaining to glia or neuroglia.

glioblastoma (gli″o-blas-to′mah) glioma.

gliococcus (gli″o-kok′us) a micrococcus forming gelatinous matter.

gliocyte (gli′o-sīt) gliacyte.

gliocytoma (gli″o-si-to′mah) a tumor composed of cells.

gliogenous (gli-oj′ĕ-nus) produced or formed by neuroglia.

glioma (gli-o′mah) a tumor composed of neuroglia in any of its stages of development.

g. ret′inae, a tumor of the retina resembling glioma.

gliomatosis (gli″o-mah-to′sis) overdevelopment of the neuroglia in the spinal cord.

gliomatous (gli-o′mah-tus) of the nature of glioma.

gliosarcoma (gli″o-sar-ko′mah) glioma combined with sarcoma.

gliosis (gli-o′sis) excessive development of neuroglia tissue.

gliosome (gli′o-sōm) a small granule seen in glia cells.

Glisson's capsule (glis′unz) a sheath of connective tissue enclosing the hepatic artery, hepatic duct and portal vein.

G's disease, rickets.

globin (glo′bin) the protein constituent of hemoglobin; also any member of a group of proteins similar to the typical globin.

globinometer (glo″bĭ-nom′ĕ-ter) an instrument for determining the proportion of oxyhemoglobin in the blood.

globule (glob′ūl) a small spherical mass, especially an erythrocyte. adj., **glob′ular.**

globulimeter (glob″u-lim′ĕ-ter) an instrument for estimating the number of erythrocytes in a given quantity of blood.

globulin (glob′u-lin) a type of simple animal protein found in body fluids and cells. The plasma proteins are divided into three main types: fibrinogen, globulins and albumin. Globulins are further divided into three groups: alpha, beta and gammà globulins. The alpha and beta globulins perform various functions in the circulation, such as transporting other proteins to various parts of the body, combining with other substances so they can be transported and chemically reacting with other substances. The GAMMA GLOBULINS are essential to the establishment of immunity because nearly all ANTIBODIES are gamma globulin molecules.

   accelerator g., a substance present in plasma, but not in serum, that functions in the formation of intrinsic and extrinsic thromboplastin; called also clotting factor V.

   antihemophilic g., AHG, a sterile preparation containing a fraction of normal human plasma of unknown composition which shortens the coagulation time of shed hemophilic blood; called also clotting factor VIII.

   antilymphocyte g., ALG, a substance used as an immunosuppressive agent in organ transplantation, usually in combination with immunosuppressive drugs; it is a derivative of antilymphocyte serum.

   immune serum g., a serum globulin that has been modified in response to infection or to injection of certain materials and contains antibodies to the antigens eliciting their production; used as a passive immunizing agent against measles or tetanus and in prophylaxis or treatment of whooping cough.

globulinemia (glob″u-lin-e′me-ah) globulin in the blood.

globulinuria (glob″u-lin-u′re-ah) globulin in the urine.

globulolysis (glob″u-lol′ĭ-sis) destruction of erythrocytes. adj., **globulolyt′ic.**

globulose (glob′u-lōs) a product of the digestion of globulins.

globus (glo′bus), pl. *glo′bi* [L.] 1. a sphere or ball; a large spherical mass. 2. a subjective sensation as of a lump or mass.

   g. hyster′icus, the subjective sensation of a lump in the throat.

   g. pal′lidus, the smaller and more medial part of the lentiform nucleus.

glomangioma (glo-man″je-o′mah) an extremely painful, small, firm, rounded, red-blue tumor, usually occurring in the distal portion of a finger or toe, in the skin or in deeper tissues.

glomectomy (glo-mek′to-me) excision of a glomus.

glomerulitis (glo-mer″u-li′tis) inflammation of the glomeruli of the kidney.

glomerulonephritis (glo-mer″u-lo-nĕ-fri′tis) a variety of nephritis characterized by inflammation of the capillary loops in the glomeruli of the kidney. It occurs in acute, subacute and chronic forms and is usually secondary to an infection, especially with the hemolytic streptococcus.

glomerulopathy (glo-mer″u-lop′ah-the) a noninflammatory disease of the kidney glomeruli.

   diabetic g., intercapillary glomerulosclerosis.

glomerulosclerosis (glo-mer″u-lo-sklĕ-ro′sis) arteriolar nephrosclerosis.

   intercapillary g., Kimmelstiel-Wilson syndrome, a degenerative complication of diabetes mellitus, manifested as albuminuria, edema, hypertension, renal insufficiency and retinopathy.

glomerulus (glo-mer′u-lus), pl. *glomer′uli* [L.] a small convoluted mass of capillaries, especially a network of vascular tufts encased in the malpighian capsule of the kidney. adj., **glomer′ulan.**

   The glomerulus is an integral part of the NEPHRON, the basic unit of the KIDNEY. Each nephron is capable of forming urine by itself, and each kidney has approximately a million nephrons. The specific function of each glomerulus is to bring blood (and the waste products it carries) to the nephron. As the blood flows through the glomerulus, about one-fifth of the plasma passes through the glomerular membrane, collects in the malpighian capsule and then flows through the renal tubules. Much of this fluid passes back into the blood via the small capillaries around the tubules (peritubular capillaries). The continuous filtration of fluid from the glomeruli and its reabsorption into the peritubular capillaries is made possible by a high pressure in the glomerular capillary bed and a low pressure in the peritubular bed.

   Any disease of the glomeruli, such as acute or chronic glomerulonephritis, must be considered serious because it interferes with the basic functions of the kidneys, that is, filtration of liquids and excretion of certain end products of metabolism and excess sodium, potassium and chloride ions that may accumulate in the blood.

glomoid (glo′moid) resembling a glomus.

glomus (glo′mus), pl. *glom′era* [L.] a small body composed primarily of fine arterioles connecting directly with veins, and having a rich nerve supply.

   g. carot′icum, carotid body.

   g. choroi′deum, an enlargement of the choroid plexus of the lateral ventricle.

   coccygeal g., g. coccyg′eum, a collection of arteriovenous anastomoses formed, close to the tip of the coccyx, by the median sacral artery.

gloss(o)- (gloss′o) word element [Gr.], *tongue.*

glossal (glos′al) pertaining to the tongue.

glossalgia (glŏ-sal′je-ah) pain in the tongue.

glossectomy (glŏ-sek′to-me) excision of the tongue.

Glossina (glŏ-si′nah) a genus of biting flies, including the tsetse; important as vectors of trypanosomes.

   G. palpa′lis, the species that transmits the trypanosomes causing sleeping sickness.

glossitis (glŏ-si′tis) inflammation of the tongue.

   rhomboid g., median, a congenital anomaly of the tongue, with a flat or slightly raised reddish patch or plaque on the dorsal surface.

glossocele (glos′o-sēl) swelling and protrusion of the tongue.

glossodynia (glos″o-din′e-ah) pain in the tongue.

glossograph (glos′o-graf) an apparatus for registering tongue movements in speech.

glossolalia (glos″o-la′le-ah) unintelligible speech.

glossology (glŏ-sol′o-je) 1. the sum of knowledge regarding the tongue. 2. a treatise on nomenclature.

glossolysis (glŏ-sol′ĭ-sis) paralysis of the tongue.

glossopathy (glŏ-sop′ah-the) disease of the tongue.

glossopharyngeal (glos″o-fah-rin′je-al) pertaining to the tongue and pharynx.
  g. nerve, the ninth cranial nerve; it supplies the carotid sinus, mucous membrane and muscles of the pharynx, soft palate and posterior third of the tongue, and the taste buds in the posterior third of the tongue. By serving the carotid sinus, the glossopharyngeal nerve provides for reflex control of the heart. It is also responsible for the swallowing reflex, for stimulating secretions of the parotid glands and for the sense of taste in the posterior third of the tongue.

glossoplasty (glos′o-plas′te) plastic surgery of the tongue.

glossoplegia (glos″o-ple′je-ah) paralysis of the tongue.

glossorrhaphy (glŏ-sōr′ah-fe) suture of the tongue.

glossospasm (glos′o-spazm) spasm of the tongue.

glossotomy (glŏ-sot′o-me) incision of the tongue.

glossotrichia (glos″o-trik′e-ah) hairy tongue.

glottic (glot′ik) pertaining to the glottis or tongue.

glottis (glot′is), pl. *glot′tides* [Gr.] the vocal apparatus of the larynx, consisting of the true vocal cords (vocal folds) and the opening between them.

glottitis (glŏ-ti′tis) glossitis.

glottology (glŏ-tol′o-je) glossology.

gluc(o)- (gloo′ko) word element [Gr.], *sweetness; glucose.* See also words beginning *glyco-.*

glucagon (gloo′kah-gon) a secretion of the pancreas that increases the concentration of sugar in the blood. The commercial preparation, glucagon hydrochloride, is used to relieve hypoglycemic coma from any cause, especially hyperinsulinism.

glucase (gloo′kas) an enzyme from plants changing starch into dextrose.

glucide (gloo′sid) a term denoting carbohydrates and glycosides.

glucinium (gloo-sin′e-um) beryllium.

glucocorticoid (gloo″ko-kor′tĭ-koid) any of the hormones of the adrenal cortex having a gluconeogenesis-increasing effect, i.e., cortisol (hydrocortisone), cortisone and corticosterone. These hormones influence protein, fat and carbohydrate metabolism. They promote mobilization of fat from fat stores and transport of amino acids into the extracellular compartment. By increasing the concentration of amino acids in the blood the gluco-

corticoids provide the liver with the chemical needed to convert proteins and fats into glucose (gluconeogenesis). The amino acids in the blood are also used by the body in times of stress to repair cellular damage and to build tissue resistance to trauma (see also ALARM REACTION). The various glucocorticoids are used therapeutically for their anti-inflammatory effects.

glucogenic (gloo″ko-jen′ik) producing sugar.

glocohemia (gloo″ko-he′me-ah) sugar in the blood.

glucokinetic (gloo″ko-ki-net′ik) activating sugar so as to maintain the sugar level of the body.

glucokinin (gloo″ko-kin′in) a substance obtained from vegetable tissues that produces hyperglycemia when injected into animals.

gluconate (gloo′ko-nāt) a salt of gluconic acid.
  ferrous g., a compound used in the treatment of iron deficiency anemia.

gluconeogenesis (gloo″ko-ne″o-jen′ĕ-sis) the formation of sugar by the liver from noncarbohydrate molecules.

gluconic acid (gloo-kon′ik) an intermediate product formed in the biosynthesis of pentoses.

glucophore (gloo′ko-fōr) the group of atoms in a molecule that gives the compound a sweet taste.

glucoprotein (gloo″ko-pro′te-in) glycoprotein.

glucosamine (gloo″ko-sam′in) a derivative of glycoprotein obtained from mucin and chitin by hydrolysis.

glucosan (gloo′ko-san) a polysaccharide of indefinite composition, yielding chiefly glucose on hydrolysis.

glucose (gloo′kōs) a simple sugar, called also DEXTROSE; the principal monosaccharide in human blood and body fluids.
  liquid g., a product obtained by incomplete hydrolysis of starch, consisting chiefly of dextrose with dextrins, maltose and water.
  g.-1-phosphate, an intermediate in carbohydrate metabolism.
  g.-6-phosphate, an intermediate in carbohydrate metabolism.
  g. tolerance test, a test to determine a person's response to a specific amount of glucose. It is often used to detect abnormalities of carbohydrate metabolism such as occur in diabetes mellitus, hypoglycemia and liver and adrenocortical dysfunction.
  There are two types of glucose tolerance tests. In the standard test, which is used most often, the patient is given a single dose of 100 Gm. of glucose, and blood and urine specimens are collected periodically for up to 6 hours. The Exton and Rose test is also useful for the diagnosis of diabetes mellitus and is completed in 1 hour.
  In the standard test the patient must be in a fasting state when the test is begun, and a blood sample is taken for measurement of fasting glucose before the test dose is given. Glucose is given dissolved in water and flavored with lemon juice, or commercial preparations in the form of a carbonated drink or gelatin, which are more palatable and provide exactly 100 Gm. of glucose, may be used.
  One-half hour after the glucose is ingested a blood sample and urine specimen are obtained. The specimens are collected at hourly intervals for the

next 4 or 5 hours as indicated. Each specimen must be labeled with the exact time it was collected. The patient may be allowed to drink water during the testing period but he may not drink anything else or eat or smoke until the test is completed.

Usually the patient experiences some weakness and perspires excessively, and he may faint during the test. These are normal reactions to a fall in the blood glucose level as insulin is secreted in response to the presence of glucose.

In both the standard test and in the Exton and Rose test the patient is usually fed a high-carbohydrate diet for 3 days before the test. In the Exton and Rose test the patient is given 50 Gm. of glucose, and blood and urine samples are obtained 30 minutes later. Immediately after these specimens are collected he is given a second dose of 50 Gm. of glucose. Half an hour later specimens of blood and urine are obtained.

NORMAL VALUES. *Standard test* (results given in milligrams per 100 ml. of blood): fasting—80 mg.; 30 min.—150 mg.; 60 min.—135 mg.; 2 hours —100 mg.; 2½ hours—80 mg. *Exton and Rose test* (results given in milligrams per 100 ml. of blood): Fasting—80 mg., urine neg.; 30 min.—150 mg., urine neg.; 1 hour—160 mg., urine neg.

glucoside (gloo'ko-sīd) a vegetable principle (glycoside) decomposable into glucose and another substance.

glucosin (gloo'ko-sin) a base derived from glucose by the action of ammonia.

glucosulfone (gloo″ko-sul'fōn) a compound derived from dapsone.
g. sodium, a compound used in treatment of leprosy.

glucosuria (gloo″ko-su're-ah) abnormally high sugar content.

glucurolactone (gloo″ku-ro-lak'tōn) a compound used in treatment of arthritis, neuritis and fibrositis.

glucuronic acid (gloo″ku-ron'ik) a compound found in various animal and plant tissues.

glucuronidase (gloo″ku-ron'ĭ-dās) an enzyme that splits compounds of glucuronic acid.

glucuronolactone (gloo″ku-ro″no-lak'tōn) glucurolactone.

glutamic acid (gloo-tam'ik) a crystalline dibasic compound, an important amino acid, but not essential to growth.
g. a. hydrochloride, a compound used as a gastric acidifier.

glutamic oxaloacetic transaminase (gloo-tam'ik ok″sah-lo-ah-se'tik trans-am'ĭ-nās) GOT, an enzyme normally present in serum and various tissues, especially the heart and liver; it is released into the serum as a result of tissue injury and is present in increased concentration in myocardial infarction or acute damage to liver cells.

glutamic pyruvic transaminase (gloo-tam'ik pi-roo'vik trans-am'ĭ-nās) GPT, an enzyme present in the body, especially the liver, observed in higher concentration in the serum of patients with acute damage to liver cells.

glutamine (gloo'tah-min) a nitrogen compound occurring in body tissues and having a part in the production of ammonia by the kidney.

Glutan H-C-L (gloo'tan āch-se-el) trademark for capsules containing glutamic acid hydrochloride, a gastric acidifier.

glutaraldehyde (gloo″tahr-al'dĕ-hīd) a compound used as a disinfectant and as a tissue fixative for light and electron microscopy because of its preservation of fine structural detail and localization of enzyme activity.

glutathione (gloo″tah-thi'ōn) a compound in animal and plant tissues that acts as a carrier of oxygen.
oxidized g., the precursor of reduced glutathione.
reduced g., a tripeptide present in red blood cells, deficiency of which probably predisposes erythrocytes to the oxidant and hemolytic effects of certain drugs.

gluteal (gloo'te-al) pertaining to the buttocks.
g. muscles, three muscles, the greatest; middle and least, that extend, abduct and rotate the thigh; called also gluteus maximus, medius and minimus muscles. (See also table of MUSCLES.)
g. nerves, nerves that innervate the gluteal muscles (see also table of NERVES).

glutelin (gloo'tĕ-lin) a simple protein from the seeds of cereals.

gluten (gloo'ten) the protein of wheat and other grains that gives dough its tough elastic character; avoidance of this substance will alleviate sprue and celiac disease in certain persons.

glutethimide (gloo-teth'ĭ-mīd) a compound used as a central nervous system depressant.

glutin (gloo'tin) a viscid constituent found in cereal proteins and collagen.

glutinous (gloo'tĭ-nus) adhesive; sticky.

glutitis (gloo-ti'tis) inflammation of the buttock.

glycase (gli'kās) an enzyme that converts maltose and maltodextrin into dextrose.

glycemia (gli-se'me-ah) sugar in the blood.

glyceric acid (glĭ-ser'ik) an intermediate product in the transformation in the body of carbohydrate to lactic acid formed by oxidation of glycerin.

glyceride (glis'er-īd) an organic acid ester of glycerin, designated, according to the number of ester linkages, as a mono-, di- or triglyceride.

glycerin (glis'er-in) a clear, colorless, syrupy liquid, used as an emollient and as a solvent for drugs; a product, along with fatty acids, of the hydrolysis of ingested fats.

glycerite (glis'er-īt) a preparation of a medicinal substance in glycerin.

glycerol (glis'er-ol) glycerin.

glycerophosphate (glis″er-o-fos'fāt) a combination of a base with glycerin and phosphoric acid.

glyceryl (glis'er-il) the radical of glycerin.
g. monostearate, a white, waxlike solid, used in cosmetic creams.
g. triacetate, triacetin, a topical antifungal agent.
g. trinitrate, a colorless or yellowish, oily liquid; a vasodilator used principally in ANGINA PECTORIS; called also nitroglycerin.

glycine (gli′sēn) a colorless crystalline powder derivable from many proteins; used as a dietary supplement. Called also aminoacetic acid and glycocoll.

glycobiarsol (gli″ko-bi-ar′sol) an odorless, slightly colored amorphous powder, used in amebiasis.

glycocholic acid (gli″ko-ko′lik) a combination of glycine and cholic acid present in bile.

glycoclastic (gli″ko-klas′tik) breaking up sugars.

glycocoll (gli′ko-kol) glycine.

glycogen (gli′ko-jen) a polysaccharide that is the chief carbohydrate storage material in animals. adj., **glycogen′ic.** It is formed by and largely stored in the liver, being depolymerized to glucose and liberated as needed. Called also animal starch.
   g. disease, g. storage disease, glycogenosis.

glycogenase (gli′ko-jě-nās″) an enzyme that splits glycogen into dextrin and maltose.

glycogenesis (gli″ko-jen′ě-sis) production of glycogen.

glycogenolysis (gli″ko-jě-nol′ĭ-sis) the splitting up of glycogen into dextrose.

glycogenosis (gli″ko-jě-no′sis) a disease characterized by abnormal storage of glycogen in children; marked by enlargement of the liver, hypoglycemia and lack of response to epinephrine's glycogen-mobilizing effect. An enzyme deficiency is responsible for the abnormal glycogen metabolism. Called also glycogen storage disease, von Gierke's disease, etc.

glycogeusia (gli″ko-gu′se-ah) a sweet taste in the mouth.

glycohemia (gli″ko-he′me-ah) sugar in the blood.

glycol (gli′kol) any one of a group of aliphatic dihydric alcohols, having marked hygroscopic properties and useful as solvents and plasticizers.

glycolic acid (gli-kol′ik) an intermediate product in the transformation in the body of serine to glycine.

glycolipid (gli″ko-lip′id) a compound of an alcohol, fatty acids and a carbohydrate.

glycolysis (gli-kol′ĭ-sis) the breaking down of sugars into simpler compounds. adj., **glycolyt′ic.**

glyconeogenesis (gli″ko-ne″o-jen′ě-sis) the formation of carbohydrates from molecules that are not themselves carbohydrates.

glyconucleoprotein (gli″ko-nu″kle-o-pro′te-in) a nucleoprotein having the carbohydrate group largely developed.

glycopenia (gli″ko-pe′ne-ah) abnormally low blood sugar; hypoglycemia.

glycopexis (gli″ko-pek′sis) fixation or storing of sugar.

glycophilia (gli″ko-fil′e-ah) a condition in which a small amount of glucose produces hyperglycemia.

glycoprotein (gli″ko-pro′te-in) a protein combined with a carbohydrate, but not containing phosphoric acid, purines or pyrimidines.

glycoptyalism (gli″ko-ti′ah-lizm) glucose in the saliva.

glycopyrrolate (gli″ko-pir′o-lāt) a compound used to produce parasympathetic blockade and to reduce gastric acid secretion and hypermotility.

glycorachia (gli″ko-ra′ke-ah) sugar in the cerebrospinal fluid.

glycoregulation (gli″ko-reg″u-la′shun) the control of sugar metabolism.

glycorrhea (gli″ko-re′ah) any sugary discharge from the body.

glycosamine (gli″ko-sam′in) glucosamine.

glycosecretory (gli″ko-se-kre′to-re) concerned in secretion of glycogen.

glycosemia (gli″ko-se′me-ah) glucose in the blood.

glycosialia (gli″ko-si-a′le-ah) sugar in the saliva.

glycosialorrhea (gli″ko-si″ah-lo-re′ah) excessive flow of saliva containing sugar.

glycoside (gli″ko-sīd) a compound containing a carbohydrate molecule, especially such a compound occurring in plants.
   cardiac g., any one of a group of glycosides occurring in certain plants (such as Digitalis) that have a characteristic action on the heart.

glycosine (gli-ko′sin) 1. a principle that sometimes unites with urea in the kidneys, forming uric acid. 2. an extract from the pancreas.

glycosometer (gli″ko-som′ě-ter) an instrument for determining the proportion of sugar in urine.

glycostatic (gli″ko-stat′ik) tending to maintain a constant sugar level.

glycosuria (gli″ko-su′re-ah) abnormally high sugar content in the urine.
   renal g., glycosuria due to an abnormally low threshold of the kidney for glucose.

glycotaxis (gli″ko-tak′sis) metabolic distribution of glucose to body tissues.

glycotropic (gli″ko-trop′ik) having an affinity for sugar; causing hyperglycemia.

glycuresis (gli″ku-re′sis) the normal increase in the glucose content of the urine that follows an ordinary carbohydrate meal.

glycylglycine (glis″il-glis′in) the simplest polypeptide.

glycyltryptophan (glis″il-trip′to-fan) a dipeptide used as a test for cancer of the stomach.

glycyrrhiza (glis″ĭ-ri′zah) dried roots of *Glycyrrhiza glabra,* or licorice; used in various pharmaceutical preparations.

glyoxylic acid (gli″ok-sil′ik) a compound formed in the oxidative deamination of glycine.

Glytheonate (gli-the′o-nāt) trademark for a preparation of theophylline sodium glycinate, a smooth muscle relaxant and diuretic.

Gm., gm. gram.

gnath(o)- (na′tho) word element [Gr.], *jaw.*

gnathitis (nah-thi′tis) inflammation of the jaw.

gnathocephalus (na″tho-sef′ah-lus) a headless fetal monster with jaws.

gnathodynamometer (na″tho-di″nah-mom′ĕ-ter) an instrument for measuring the force exerted in closing the jaws.

gnathology (nah-thol′o-je) the science dealing with the masticatory apparatus as a whole.

gnathoplasty (na′tho-plas″te) plastic repair of the jaw.

gnathoschisis (nah-thos′kĭ-sis) congenital cleft of the upper jaw.

gnosia (no′se-ah) the faculty of perceiving and recognizing. adj., **gnos′tic.**

goiter (goi′ter) enlargement of the thyroid gland, causing a swelling in the front part of the neck. adj., **goit′rous.** Simple endemic goiter is usually caused by lack of iodine in the diet. Although the administration of iodine will not cure simple goiter, it will prevent it or stop an existing goiter from enlarging. If there is evidence of pressure against the throat, or the possibility of a malignancy, the goiter may be removed surgically.

Exophthalmic, or toxic, goiter (known also as Graves' disease) is accompanied by excessive concentrations of thyroid hormones in the blood, which produce the symptoms of HYPERTHYROIDISM. There is protrusion of the eyeballs (exophthalmos) and there may be other ocular changes. Treatment of this type of goiter may include surgical removal of the thyroid or medical management with administration of iodine compounds and other antithyroid drugs. Depending on the age and sex of the patient, therapeutic doses of radioactive iodine may also be used.

    aberrant g., goiter of an accessory thyroid gland.

    adenomatous g., enlargement caused by adenoma of the thyroid gland.

    Basedow g., exophthalmic goiter.

    colloid g., a large, soft thyroid gland with distended spaces filled with colloid.

    cystic g., one with cysts formed by mucoid or colloid degeneration.

    fibrous g., goiter in which the capsule and the stroma of the thyroid gland are hyperplastic.

    follicular g., parenchymatous goiter.

    intrathoracic g., goiter situated in the thoracic cavity.

    nodular g., thyroid enlargement with circumscribed nodules within the gland.

    papillomatous g., adenomatous goiter.

    parenchymatous g., goiter marked by increase in follicles and proliferation of epithelium.

    perivascular g., goiter growing around a blood vessel.

    retrovascular g., goiter with a process or processes behind an important blood vessel.

    substernal g., goiter situated below the sternum.

    suffocative g., one that causes dyspnea by pressure.

    toxic g., exophthalmic goiter.

    vascular g., enlargement of the thyroid due chiefly to dilatation of the blood vessels.

goitrogen (goi′tro-jen) a goiter-producing agent.

goitrogenicity (goi″tro-jĕ-nis′ĭ-te) the tendency to produce goiter.

goitrogenous (goi-troj′ĕ-nus) producing goiter.

gold (gōld) a chemical element, atomic number

79, atomic weight 196.967, symbol Au. (See table of ELEMENTS.) Gold and many of its compounds are used in medicine, especially in treating rheumatoid arthritis. Gold salts are among the most toxic of therapeutic agents and must be given only under strict medical supervision. Toxic reactions may vary from mild to severe kidney or liver damage and blood dyscrasias.

    radioactive g., a RADIOISOTOPE of gold; used in treating certain types of cancer.

    g. sodium thiomalate, an odorless, fine, white to yellowish powder with a metallic taste; used in treatment of rheumatoid arthritis and nondisseminated lupus erythematosus.

    g. sodium thiosulfate, used in treatment of rheumatoid arthritis.

    g. thioglucose, aurothioglucose, used in treating rheumatoid arthritis.

Goldflam's disease (gōlt′flahmz) myasthenia gravis; called also Goldflam-Erb disease.

Goldschieder's disease (gōld′shi-derz) epidermolysis bullosa.

Golgi apparatus (gol′je) a complex of membranes and vesicles in a cell, seen in stained preparations as an irregular network of blackened canals or solid strands; thought to play an important role in cellular activities, especially those dealing with secretion.

gomphiasis (gom-fi′ah-sis) looseness of the teeth.

gomphosis (gom-fo′sis) an articulation in which a spike of bone fits into a bony socket.

gonad (go′nad, gon′ad) a sex gland, the OVARY in the female and the TESTIS in the male. adj., **gonad′al, gonad′ial.** The ovary produces the ovum and the testis produces the spermatozoon. In addition, the gonads secrete hormones that influence the development of the reproductive organs at puberty, and they control other physical traits that differentiate men from women, such as pitch of the voice, body form and size (the secondary sex characters). The hormones produced by the ovary include ESTROGEN and PROGESTERONE. The principal hormone produced by the testis is called TESTOSTERONE.

gonadectomy (go″nah-dek′to-me) removal of a gonad.

gonadogenesis (go-nad″o-jen′ĕ-sis) development of the gonads in the embryo.

gonadokinetic (go-nad″o-ki-net′ik) stimulating activity of the gonads.

gonadopathy (go″nah-dop′ah-the) disease of the gonads.

gonadotherapy (go-nad″o-ther′ah-pe) treatment with gonadal hormones.

gonadotrophic (go-nad″o-trōf′ik) gonadotropic.

gonadotrophin (go-nad″o-trōf′in) gonadotropin.

gonadotropic (go-nad″o-trop′ik) having a stimulating effect upon the gonads.

    g. hormone, one that affects the gonads, especially the anterior pituitary hormone that has this effect.

gonadotropin (go-nad″o-trōp′in) a substance that has a stimulating effect upon the gonads, especially the hormone secreted by the anterior pituitary.

chorionic g., such a substance found in human pregnancy urine; used in treatment of underdevelopment of the gonads (see also CHORIONIC GONADOTROPIN).

gonadotropism (go″nah-dot′ro-pizm) dominance of the gonads in the endocrine constitution.

gonaduct (go′nah-dukt) a tubular channel for passage of ova or spermatozoa.

gonagra (go-nag′rah) gouty seizure of the knee.

gonalgia (go-nal′je-ah) pain in the knee.

gonangiectomy (go-nan″je-ek′to-me) excision of the vas deferens.

gonarthritis (gon″ar-thri′tis) inflammation of the knee joint.

gonarthrocace (gon″ar-throk′ah-se) tuberculous arthritis of the knee joint.

gonarthrotomy (gon″ar-throt′o-me) incision into the knee joint.

gonecystis (gon″ĕ-sis′tis) a seminal vesicle.

gonecystitis (gon″ĕ-sis-ti′tis) inflammation of a seminal vesicle.

gonecystolith (gon″ĕ-sis′to-lith) a concretion in a seminal vesicle.

gonecystopyosis (gon″ĕ-sis″to-pi-o′sis) suppuration of a seminal vesicle.

gonepoiesis (gon″ĕ-poi-e′sis) formation of the semen.

gonidium (go-nid′e-um), pl. *gonid′ia* [Gr.] a spore that is not born free, but is formed in a case or receptacle.

goniometer (go″ne-om′ĕ-ter) an instrument for measuring angles.
  finger g., one for measuring the limits of flexion and extension of the joints between the phalanges of the fingers.

gonion (go′ne-on), pl. *go′nia* [Gr.] the most inferior, posterior and lateral point on the angle of the mandible.

goniopuncture (go″ne-o-pungk′tūr) insertion of a knife blade through clear cornea, just within the limbus, across the anterior chamber of the eye and through the opposite corneoscleral wall, in treatment of glaucoma.

gonioscope (go′ne-o-skōp″) an instrument for examination of the angle of the anterior chamber of the eye.

gonioscopy (go″ne-os′ko-pe) examination of the angle of the anterior chamber of the eye.

goniotomy (go″ne-ot′o-me) an operation for glaucoma; it consists in opening Schlemm's canal under direct vision.

gonococcemia (gon″o-kok-se′me-ah) gonococci in the blood.

gonococcide (gon″o-kok′sīd) an agent destructive to gonococci.

gonococcus (gon″o-kok′us), pl. *gonococ′ci* [L.] the causative organism of gonorrhea, *Neisseria gonorrhoeae.* adj., **gonococ′cal.**

gonocyte (gon′o-sīt) the primitive reproductive cell of the embryo.

gonophore (gon′o-fōr) an accessory reproductive organ.

gonorrhea (gon″o-re′ah) a highly contagious bacterial infection of the genitourinary system. adj., **gonorrhe′al.** It is the most common venereal disease.
  CAUSE. Gonorrhea is caused by the bacterial organism *Neisseria gonorrhoeae,* or gonococcus. Characteristically, the gonococcus attacks the mucous membranes of the genital and urinary organs, producing inflammation and pus. In adults the disease is almost always contracted by coitus with an infected person.
  Occasionally the gonococci may attack the membranes of the eye, resulting in blindness if untreated. This is not common in adults. The eyes of babies, however, may be infected at birth during passage through the birth canal of an infected mother. The condition that results is called ophthalmia neonatorum, and in the past it was a major cause of blindness in babies. Today it is routine, and required by law in some states, for all newborn infants to receive eye drops (penicillin or silver nitrate) at birth as a protection against gonorrheal infection.
  SYMPTOMS. The first symptoms of gonorrhea usually appear within a week after exposure to the gonococcus, but they may take as long as 3 weeks to develop. In men the inflammation generally causes a painful burning sensation during urination, and the infected penis discharges a whitish fluid, or pus. If the condition remains untreated, the discharge increases and continues for 2 or 3 months. As the infection spreads to other membranes, complications such as inflammation of the prostate and the testes may result and may cause sterility.
  A woman infected with gonorrhea may feel no pain and notice no early symptoms. She may, however, experience pain in the lower abdomen, with or without a burning sensation during urination or a whitish discharge from the vagina. If the infection is allowed to reach other organs of her reproductive system, the ovaries and the uterine tubes may become inflamed and sterility may result.
  If uncontrolled, the gonococcal infection may continue to spread and affect other parts of the body such as the bladder, kidneys and rectum. The disease can also cause inflammation of the joints, resulting in painful arthritis. As the infection spreads it can lead to meningitis or to peritonitis, and may even cause death if the gonococci enter the blood and lodge in the valves of the heart, causing endocarditis.
  DIAGNOSIS AND TREATMENT. Diagnosis is confirmed by the presence of gonococci in the discharge from the penis or vagina or in fluid from any affected area. Gonorrhea can be cured with comparative speed, particularly in its early stages. Penicillin and other antibiotics, as well as the sulfonamide drugs, are effective in treatment. The drug of choice is usually penicillin, administered in a single dose of the long-acting form, which provides concentrations of the drug in the blood for several weeks. The patient cannot be considered cured until cultures taken from the discharge are

NURSING CARE. The greatest danger in caring for these patients is contamination of the eyes and a resulting gonorrheal conjunctivitis. Special care must be taken with bed linens, urinals and bed-pans since these can be grossly contaminated with vaginal or urethral discharge. While administering nursing care the nurse's hands should be covered with rubber gloves and then washed thoroughly for a full minute after the gloves are removed. It is best to wear a protective gown such as that worn during isolation technique whenever personal care is given the patient. Although gonorrhea is contracted by coitus, the gonococci can infect the eyes or an open wound or break in the skin.

gonycampsis (gon″ĭ-kamp′sis) curvature of the knee.

gonycrotesis (gon″ĭ-kro-te′sis) knock-knee.

gonyocele (gon′e-o-sel″) synovitis of the knee.

gonyoncus (gon″e-ong′kus) tumor of the knee.

Goodell's sign (good′elz) if the cervix uteri is soft as one's lip, the woman is pregnant; if it is as hard as one's nose, she is not.

GOT glutamic oxaloacetic transaminase, an enzyme found in many body cells.

gouge (gowj) an instrument for cutting bone.

goundou (gōōn′doo) osteogenic periostitis of the nose, thought to be a sequel of yaws.

gout (gowt) a disease in which uric acid appears in excessive quantities in the blood and may be deposited in the joints and other tissues. During an acute attack of gout there is swelling, inflammation and extreme pain in a joint, frequently that of the big toe. After several years of attacks, the chronic form of the disease may set in, permanently damaging and deforming joints and destroying cells of the kidney. About 95 per cent of all cases occur in men and the first attack rarely occurs before the age of 30.

CAUSES. The causes of gout are not fully understood. It is a disorder of the metabolism of purines. These nitrogenous substances are found in high-protein foods and the net product of their metabolism is uric acid. For unknown reasons, the uric acid, normally expelled in the urine, is retained in the blood in excess amounts. Uric acid crystals are deposited in the joints and in cartilage, where they form lumps called tophi. The uric acid crystals also predispose to the formation of calculi in the kidney (kidney stones) and lead to permanent damage of the kidney cells.

ACUTE GOUT. The acute form of gout usually strikes without warning. The affected joint, which in 70 per cent of cases is that of the big toe, becomes swollen, inflamed and very painful. The first attack may follow an operation, infection or minor irritation such as tight shoes, or it may have no apparent cause. The patient may have a headache or fever, and often cannot walk because of the pain.

Without treatment, acute attacks of gout usually last a few days or weeks. The symptoms then disappear completely until the next attack. As the disease progresses, the attacks tend to last longer and the intervals between attacks become shorter.

Treatment. An acute attack of gout can be treated successfully with any of several medicines.

Colchicine has long been used to treat gout. In most cases, colchicine relieves the pain and swelling in 72 hours or less, although it does not affect the high concentration of uric acid. In very severe attacks, or for patients who are not helped by colchicine, phenylbutazone or oxyphenbutazone may be used instead. Corticotropin or the cortisones may be combined with one of these medicines. A relatively new medication, indomethacin, has also been effective in acute cases.

The patient should be kept in bed, with the affected joint protected, throughout the attack and for 24 hours after it subsides. Walking too soon after the attack may set off another one.

CHRONIC GOUT. After a number of acute attacks of gout, the patient who goes without medical treatment may develop the symptoms of chronic gout. This seldom occurs less than 10 years after the first acute attack.

The joints affected by chronic gout degenerate in the same way as joints affected by RHEUMATOID ARTHRITIS, and they may eventually lose their ability to move. In 10 to 20 per cent of those with chronic gout, damage to the renal tubules occurs as the result of the formation of kidney stones.

Treatment. Chronic gout is treated with probenecid or other medicines which promote the urinary excretion of uric acid. Other treatment may also be necessary if the kidney is involved. Sometimes surgery to remove the tophi and correct deformities may be helpful.

MANAGEMENT BETWEEN ATTACKS. If acute gout is recognized at an early stage and treated correctly, the development of the chronic form can generally be prevented.

Since uric acid is the end product of purine metabolism, the patient is usually put on a diet limiting the amount of foods of a high purine content, such as sweetbreads, kidney, liver, sardines, anchovies and meat extracts and gravies. He also should keep his weight within normal limits and is instructed to increase his daily intake of liquids to encourage the production of urine. Medications such as probenecid, which prevents the retention of uric acid in the body and the formation of tophi, may be prescribed. Another drug, allopurinol, which prevents the formation of uric acid by blocking an enzyme step, has been used successfully in the long-term treatment of gout.

G.P. general paresis; general practitioner.

GPT glutamic pyruvic transaminase, an enzyme derived mainly from the liver cells.

gr. grain.

graafian follicle (graf′e-an) a small sac, embedded in the OVARY, that encloses an ovum. At puberty each ovary has a large number of immature follicles, each of which contains an undeveloped egg cell. These structures are called primordial, or primitive, graafian follicles. About every 28 days between puberty and the onset of menopause, one of these follicles develops to maturity, or ripens.

As the follicle ripens, it increases in size. The ovum within becomes larger, the follicular wall becomes thicker, and fluid collects in the follicle and surrounds the egg. The follicle also secretes estradiol, the hormone that prepares the endometrium to receive a fertilized egg. As the follicle matures, it moves to the surface of the ovary and forms a projection. When fully mature, the graafian follicle breaks open and releases the ovum, which passes into the UTERINE TUBES. This release of the ovum is called OVULATION; it occurs midway in the menstrual cycle, generally about 14 days after the commencement of the menstrual flow.

The released ovum travels down the tube to the uterus, a process that takes about 3 days. Meanwhile, the empty graafian follicle in the ovary becomes filled with cells containing a' yellow substance, the corpus luteum, or yellow body. The corpus luteum secretes progesterone, a hormone that causes further change in the endometrium, allowing it to provide a good milieu in which a fertilized ovum can grow through the stages of gestation to become a fetus.

gracile (gras′il) slender; delicate.

gradatim (gra-da′tim) [L.] by degrees; gradually.

gradient (gra′de-ent) rate of increase or decrease of a variable value, or its representative curve.

graduate (grad′u-āt) 1. a cylindrical or tapered laboratory vessel, usually of glass, with a scale showing the capacity in milliliters or fluid ounces. 2. person who has received an academic or professional degree.

graduated (grad′u-āt″ed) marked by a succession of lines; progressing by regularly marked intervals or degrees.

graft (graft) a fragment of skin or other body tissue for transplantation.

   autodermic g., autoepidermic g., a skin graft taken from the patient's own body.

   autologous g., a graft taken from another area of the patient's own body; an autograft.

   avascular g., a graft of tissue in which not even transient vascularization is achieved.

   bone g., a piece of bone used to take the place of a removed bone or bony defect.

   cable g., a nerve graft made up of several sections of nerve in the manner of a cable.

   cutis g., skin from which epidermis and subcutaneous fat have been removed, used instead of fascia in various plastic procedures.

   delayed g., a graft or flap of skin that is sutured back into its bed and subsequently shifted.

   dermic g., a graft composed of a bit of derma or corium.

   epidermic g., a piece of epidermis implanted on a raw surface.

   fascia g., a graft of tissue taken from the external investing fascia of the leg (fascia lata).

   fascicular g., a nerve graft in which bundles of nerve fibers are approximated and sutured separately.

   free g., a graft of tissue completely freed from its bed.

   full-thickness g., a skin graft consisting of the full thickness of the skin.

   heterodermic g., a skin graft taken from a person other than the patient.

   heterologous g., a graft of tissue derived from an individual of a different species, or of synthetic or nonorganic material; a heterograft.

   homologous g., a graft of tissue obtained from the body of another animal of the same species but with a genotype differing from that of the recipient; a homograft.

   isologous g., a graft of tissue obtained from the body of another individual of the same genotype as the recipient; an isograft.

   lamellar g., replacement of the superficial layers of an opaque cornea by a thin layer of clear cornea from a donor eye.

   Ollier-Thiersch g., a very thin graft including

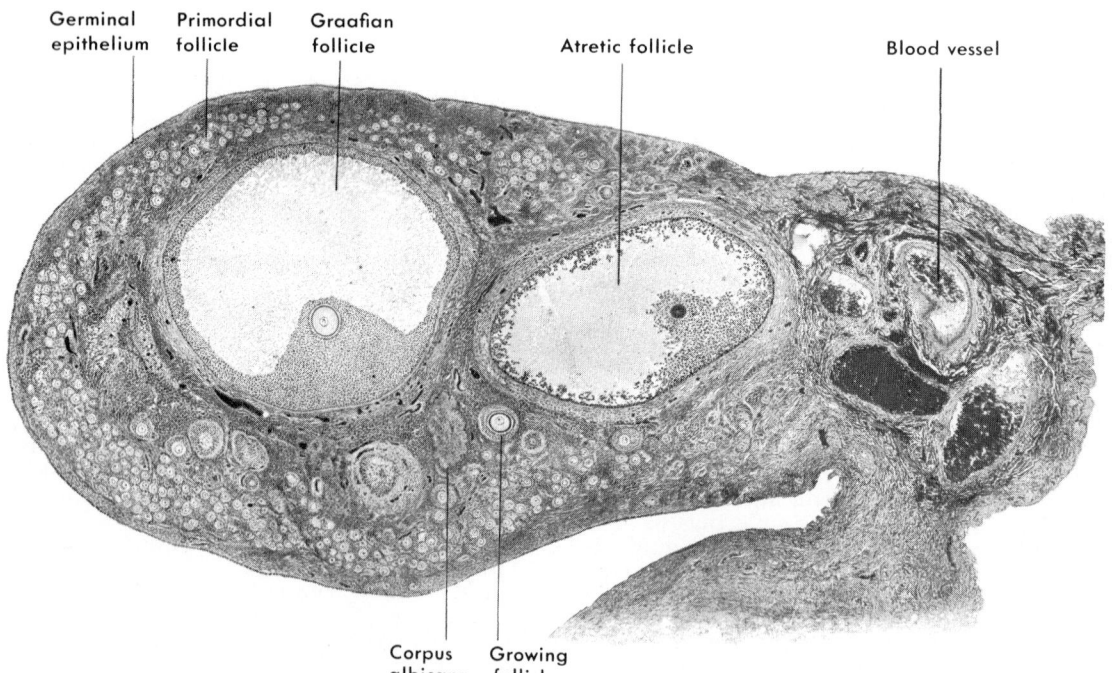

Germinal epithelium   Primordial follicle   Graafian follicle   Atretic follicle   Blood vessel

Corpus albicans   Growing follicle

Retouched photomicrograph of transection of ovary of *Macacus rhesus*. (From Bloom, W., and Fawcett, D. W.: A Textbook of Histology. 9th ed. Philadelphia, W. B. Saunders Co., 1968.)

the epidermis and nearly always some of the derma.

omental g's, strips of omentum to cover the line of enterorrhaphy.

pedicle g., one consisting of the full thickness of the skin and the subcutaneous tissue attached by a pedicle.

penetrating g., a full-thickness corneal transplant.

periosteal g., a piece of periosteum to cover a denuded bone.

pinch g., a piece of skin graft about ¼ inch in diameter, obtained by elevating the skin with a needle and slicing it off with a knife.

postmortem g., tissue taken from a body after death and stored under proper conditions, to be used later in a patient requiring a graft of such tissue (skin, cornea, etc.).

skin g., a bit of skin implanted to replace a lost part of the integument.

Thiersch g., Ollier-Thiersch graft.

thyroid g., a piece of thyroid tissue implanted in the body as a remedy for myxedema.

grafting (graf'ting) transplantation of skin or other tissue from another part of the body or from another person to serve as replacement for damaged or missing tissue. The purpose may be to encourage healing, to improve function, to act as a safeguard against infection, to improve appearance or, more recently, to replace a diseased body organ.

Grafting of skin is most common, but other tissues can be grafted, such as bone, cartilage, muscle, fat, blood vessels, nerves and certain body organs. Usually, grafts are either autologous — that is, taken from the same individual — or homologous, taken from another individual. The autologous graft (autograft) is the most commonly used and the most successful. A graft from an identical twin or from an individual closely related genetically is an isologous graft, or isograft, and a graft in which the donor and recipient are of different species is a heterologous graft, or heterograft.

SKIN GRAFTING.   The most important function of skin grafting is to promote the healing of large surfaces that have been burned or wounded, or that have become ulcerated or cancerous.

The skin to be grafted is cut usually from the chest, thigh or abdomen, from the lower part of the neck or from behind the ear. It may be removed in very thin strips or as a thin layer of superficial skin, and it must be placed in its new location without delay. If delay is unavoidable, it is placed in a saline solution or refrigerated.

In this kind of so-called free graft, in which the skin is cut entirely away from the body before transplantation, the skin is sewed into place and a pressure dressing is applied or a tissue glue is used. The skin must then depend for its nourishment on the surrounding tissue in the new location.

If a large thick area of skin containing much underlying tissue is to be moved, it is usually done by means of a pedicle graft — that is, the skin is not completely removed but is left partially attached to the body so that it continues to receive nourishment from its original site while it is beginning to grow in its new site. For example, an injured hand that needs the transplant may be strapped against the abdominal wall to receive a pedicle graft of skin from the abdomen. (See also PLASTIC SURGERY.)

OTHER GRAFTS.   Eye surgeons have developed one of the most dramatic and useful grafting procedures, called keratoplasty, in which part or all of

a diseased cornea that has become opaque is removed and replaced by healthy corneal tissue from an eye bank.

Cartilage and bone are other tissue that can be successfully transplanted from one individual to another. Cartilage lends itself particularly well to various shapes and is widely used in reconstructive surgery. Bone grafts are sometimes used instead of metal plates in operations to repair fractures. They are also used to replace diseased bone.

Transplanting of an entire organ from one person to another has been attempted, as well as transplants from animal to human. There has been promise of success in some instances of kidney transplants, especially when the donor and recipient have been identical twins (see TRANSPLANTATION). The major problem in this procedure is the rejection phenomena. Heart transplants have also now been performed in humans. Surgical and scientific ingenuity are now tending toward the construction of artificial organs, substituting for the heart, kidney or other organs (see ARTIFICIAL ORGAN). Arteries of plastic tubing have already been used in surgical procedures.

Graham's law (gra'amz) the rate of diffusion of a gas through porous membranes varies inversely with the square root of its density.

grain (grān) 1. the seed of cereal plants. 2. a unit of weight in the avoirdupois or apothecaries' system, being the equivalent of 64.8 milligrams; abbreviated gr. (See also Table of Weights and Measures in the Appendix.)

gram (gram) the basic unit of mass (weight) of the metric system, being the equivalent of 15.432 grains; abbreviated G., Gm. or gm. (See also Table of Weights and Measures in the Appendix.)

-gram (gram) word element [Gr.], *written; recorded.*

Gram's stain (gramz) a stain for bacteria, used as one means of identifying unknown bacterial organisms.

gramicidin (gram″ĭ-si'din) an antibacterial substance produced by the growth of *Bacillus brevis,* one of the two principal components of tyrothricin; called also gramicidin D.

gram-molecule (gram-mol'ĕ-kūl) a quantity in grams equal to the molecular weight of the substance.

gram-negative (gram-neg'ah-tiv) not staining with Gram's stain, a primary characteristic of certain microorganisms.

gram-positive (gram-poz'ĭ-tiv) staining with Gram's stain, a primary characteristic of certain microorganisms.

grand mal (grahn mahl) [Fr.] a major epileptic seizure attended by loss of consciousness and convulsive movements, as distinguished from petit mal, a minor seizure (see also EPILEPSY).

granular (gran'u-lar) made up of granules or grains.

granulatio (gran″u-la'she-o), pl. *granulatio'nes* [L.] a granular mass.

granulation (gran″u-la′shun) 1. a small rounded mass. 2. the production of small rounded masses, as in the healing of a wound of soft tissue.

exuberant g's, excessive proliferation of granulation tissue in the healing of a wound.

g. tissue, material formed in repair of wounds of soft tissue, consisting of connective tissue cells and ingrowing young vessels. It ultimately forms cicatrix.

granule (gran′ūl) 1. a small rounded body. 2. a medicinal pellet.

agminated g's, small protoplasmic particles occurring in the blood, supposed to be disintegrated blood corpuscles.

albuminous g's, granules seen in the cytoplasm of many normal cells, which disappear on the addition of acetic acid, but are not affected by ether or chloroform.

aleuronoid g's, colorless myeloid colloidal bodies found in the base of pigment cells.

alpha g's, coarse, highly refractive, eosinophil granules of leukocytes, composed of albuminous matter.

amphophil g's, beta granules.

azur g's, azurophil g's, granules that stain easily with azure dyes; they are coarse, reddish granules and are seen in many lymphocytes.

Babes-Ernst g's, metachromatic granules.

basophil g's, granules staining with basic dyes.

beta g's, presecretion granules found in the pituitary gland and islands of Langerhans of the pancreas.

carbohydrate g's, particles of carbohydrate matter in body fluids in the course of being assimilated.

chromatic g's, chromophilic g's, Nissl bodies.

cone g's, the nuclei of the visual cells in the outer nuclear layer of the retina which are connected with the cones.

delta g's, fine basophil granules in the lymphocytes.

eosinophil g's, those staining with eosin.

epsilon g's, neutrophil granules.

fuchsinophil g's, those staining with fuchsin.

gamma g's, basophil granules found in the blood, bone marrow and tissues.

Grawitz's g's, minute granules seen in the erythrocytes in lead poisoning.

hyperchromatin g's, azur granules.

iodophil g's, granules staining brown with iodine, seen in polymorphonuclear leukocytes in various acute infectious diseases.

juxtaglomerular g's, osmophilic secretory granules present in the juxtaglomerular cells, closely resembling zymogen granules.

Kolliker's interstitial g's, granules seen in the sarcoplasm of muscle fibers.

metachromatic g's, deeply staining masses irregular in size and number seen in the protoplasm of various bacteria.

Much's g's, granules and rods found in tuberculous sputum which do not stain by the usual processes for acid-fast bacilli but do stain with Gram's stain.

Neusser's g's, basophil granules seen about the nuclei of leukocytes.

neutrophil g's, neutrophilic granules from the protoplasm of polymorphonuclear leukocytes.

Nissl's g's, Nissl bodies.

oxyphil g's, alpha granules.

pigment g's, small masses of coloring matter in pigment cells.

Plehn's g's, basophil granules in the conjugating form of malarial parasite.

protein g's, minute particles of various proteins, some anabolic and others catabolic.

rod g's, the nuclei of the visual cells in the outer nuclear layer of the retina which are connected with the rods.

Schüffner's g's, coarse red granules in parasitized erythrocytes in tertian malarial staining with polychrome methylene blue.

Schule's g's, Plehn's granules.

seminal g's, the small granular bodies in the semen.

thread g's, mitochondria.

zymogen g's, granules in the cells of the salivary glands.

granulitis (gran″u-li′tis) miliary tuberculosis.

granuloadipose (gran″u-lo-ad′ĭ-pōs) containing granules of fat.

granuloblast (gran′u-lo-blast″) an immature granulocyte.

granulocyte (gran′u-lo-sīt″) any cell containing granules, especially a leukocyte containing neutrophil, basophil or eosinophil granules in its cytoplasm.

band-form g., a stage in the development of the granular leukocyte in which the nuclear indentation is more than half the width of the hypothetical round nucleus, and its opposite ends become approximately parallel for an appreciable distance.

granulocytemia (gran″u-lo-si-te′me-ah) an excess of granulocytes in the blood.

granulocytopenia (gran″u-lo-si″to-pe′ne-ah) deficiency of granulocytes in the blood.

primary g., agranulocytosis.

granulocytopoiesis (gran″u-lo-si″to-poi-e′sis) the production of granulocytes.

granulocytosis (gran″u-lo-si-to′sis) granulocytemia.

granulofilocyte (gran″u-lo-fil′o-sīt) a reticulocyte.

granuloma (gran″u-lo′mah) a circumscribed mass consisting mainly of histiocytes, occurring in reaction to the presence of a living agent (infectious granuloma) or a foreign body, or sometimes idiopathically.

benign g. of thyroid, chronic inflammation of the thyroid gland, converting it into a bulky tumor that later becomes extremely hard.

coccidioidal g., the secondary, progressive, chronic (granulomatous) stage of coccidioidomycosis.

dental g., a proliferating mass of chronic inflammatory tissue contained within an extension of the periodontium of a tooth.

eosinophilic g., a type of xanthomatosis characterized by the presence of rarefactions or cysts in one or more bones and sometimes associated with eosinophilia.

g. fissura′tum, a firm, whitish, fissured, fibrotic granuloma of the gum and buccal mucosa, occurring in the fold between the jaw and cheek.

foreign body g., a localized histiocytic reaction to a foreign body in the tissue.

g. inguina′le, a venereal disease that is associated with uncleanliness and is caused by the microorganism *Donovania granulomatis*, sometimes, called *Donovan body*. Although granuloma inguinale is generally considered to be a venereal disease, there is no absolute proof that it is transmitted by sexual contact. It is possible that natural resistance to the disease is very high, so that only a few of the persons exposed are affected.

Generally, 10 days to 3 months elapse after exposure before the first symptoms appear. Small painless ulcers that bleed easily may occur first. Swelling in the groin may then follow. A new ulcer or ulcers may appear as the old one heals, so that granuloma inguinale may eventually cover the reproductive organs, buttocks and lower abdomen. The extensive sores give off a foul odor. As persons who have the disease seem to develop little immunity to it, granuloma inguinale may be present for many years.

In recent years, both streptomycin and tetracyclines have been successfully employed to treat the disease. Excellent results have been obtained with triacetyloleandomycin. There is no known preventive for granuloma inguinale, although the disease is rare where sanitary living conditions prevail.

g. ir'idis, a nonmalignant and highly vascular growth of the iris.

lipoid g., a granuloma containing lipoid cells.

lipophagic g., a granuloma attended by the loss of subcutaneous fat.

Majocchi's g., a condition characterized by the development of nodules at the borders of indistinct scaling patches of the lower half of the lower leg, due to *Trichophyton rubrum* infection.

malignant g., g. malig'num, Hodgkin's disease.

paracoccidioidal g., South American blastomycosis.

peripheral giant cell reparative g., a pedunculated or sessile lesion apparently arising from periodontium or mucoperiosteum, and usually due to trauma.

g. pyogen'icum, septic g., a fungating pedunculated growth in which the granulations consist of masses of pyogenic organisms.

swimming pool g., a papular lesion at the site of a swimming pool injury, caused by an organism related to the tubercle bacillus (*Mycobacterium tuberculosis*), which tends to heal spontaneously in a few months or years.

g. telangiectat'icum, a form characterized by numerous dilated blood vessels.

g. trop'icum, yaws.

ulcerating g. of the pudenda, venereal g., g. vene'reum, granuloma inguinale.

granulomatosis (gran″u-lo″mah-to′sis) the formation of multiple granulomas.

g. siderot'ica, Gamna's disease.

Wegener's g., a progressive disease, with granulomatous lesions of the respiratory tract, focal necrotizing arteriolitis with mainly glomerular renal involvement, and, finally, widespread inflammation of all organs of the body.

granulomatous (gran″u-lo′mah-tus) composed of granulomas.

granulomere (gran′u-lo-mēr″) the center portion of a platelet in a dry, stained blood smear, apparently filled with fine, purplish red granules, thought possibly to be due to an artifact.

granulopenia (gran″u-lo-pe′ne-ah) decreased number of granulocytes in the blood.

granulopexis (gran″u-lo-pek′sis) the fixation of granules.

granuloplastic (gran′u-lo-plas″tik) forming granules.

granulopoiesis (gran″u-lo-poi-e′sis) the formation and development of granulocytes.

granulopotent (gran″u-lo-po′tent) able to form granules.

granulosa cell tumor (gran″u-lo′sah) an ovarian tumor originating in the solid mass of cells (granulosa cells) that surrounds the ovum in a developing graafian follicle. It is associated with excessive production of estrogen, inducing endometrial hyperplasia with menorrhagia. Called also folliculoma and oophoroma.

granulosarcoma (gran″u-lo-sar-ko′mah) mycosis fungoides.

granulose (gran′u-lōs) the more soluble portion of starch.

granulosis (gran″u-lo′sis) the formation of granules.

g. ru'bra na'si, a red granular eruption of the skin of the nose.

granulotherapy (gran″u-lo-ther′ah-pe) treatment by stimulating production of leukocytes.

granum (gra′num) [L.] grain.

graph (graf) a diagram showing relationship between different variable factors.

graphorrhea (graf″o-re′ah) the writing of a meaningless flow or words.

graphospasm (graf′o-spazm) writer's cramp.

-graphy (graf′e) word element [Gr.], *making of a graphic record.* adj., **graph'ic.**

grattage (grah-tahzh′) [Fr.] removal of granulations or follicles by scraping.

gravedo (grah-ve′do) coryza, or nasal catarrh.

gravel (grav′el) calculus occurring in small particles.

Graves' disease (grāvz) exophthalmic goiter.

gravid (grav′id) pregnant; containing developing young.

gravida (grav′ĭ-dah) a pregnant woman.

g. I, primigravida.

g. II, secundigravida.

g. III, tertigravida.

gravidocardiac (grav″ĭ-do-kar′de-ak) pertaining to heart disease in pregnancy.

gravidopuerperal (grav″ĭ-do-pu-er′per-al) pertaining to or occurring during pregnancy and the puerperium.

gravimetric (grav″ĭ-met′rik) pertaining to measurement by weight.

gravity (grav′ĭ-te) weight; tendency toward the center of the earth.

specific g., the weight of a substance compared with that of another taken as a standard (see also SPECIFIC GRAVITY).

gray matter gray areas of the nervous system, so called because the nerve fibers in these areas are not enveloped in a white fatty material called the MYELIN sheath. These fibers are described as unmyelinated, or nonmedullated. White matter is the term used to describe the tissues composed of myelinated, or medullated, fibers.

The bodies of the nerve cells are centered in the gray matter. The cerebral cortex is composed of gray matter and there are some deep-seated masses of gray matter within the cerebellum. In the spinal cord there is a central core of gray matter surrounded by white matter. On a cross section of the spinal cord the gray matter follows the general pattern of the letter H.

green (grēn) 1. the color of grass or of an emerald. 2. a green dye.

benzaldehyde g., malachite green.

indocyanine g., a dye used in tests of cardiovascular function.

malachite g., a dye used as a stain for bacteria and as an antiseptic for wounds.

Paris g., an emerald green compound of copper and arsenic, used as an insecticide on plants.

Greenfield's disease (grēn'fēldz) late infantile metachromatic leukoencephalopathy.

grenz rays (grenz) very soft electromagnetic radiation of wavelengths 1 to 5 angstroms.

grid (grid) 1. a grating. 2. a chart with horizontal and vertical lines for plotting curves.

baby g., a direct-reading chart on infant growth.

Wetzel g., a direct-reading chart for evaluating physical fitness in terms of body build, developmental level and basal metabolism.

grip (grip) 1. influenza. 2. a grasping or clasping.

devil's g., epidemic pleurodynia.

grippe (grip) influenza.

griseofulvin (gris"e-o-ful'vin) antibiotic used orally for treatment of fungal infections of the skin, nails and scalp. Treatment usually must be prolonged and patient must be watched for signs of leukopenia, which often occurs when drug is administered over a long period of time.

groin (groin) the junction of abdomen and thigh.

groove (groōv) a narrow, linear hollow or depression.

branchial g., an external furrow lined with ectoderm, occurring in the embryo between two branchial arches.

Harrison's g., one on the thorax, caused by contraction of the diaphragm, seen in children who have had rickets.

medullary g., neural g., that formed by beginning invagination of the neural plate to form the neural tube.

ground substance (ground) the basic homogeneous material of a tissue or organ, in which the specific components occur.

group (groōp) a collection of similar units or of closely related entities, such as a number of different atoms that act as a unit when entering or leaving chemical combination (a radical), or a particular combination of atoms in a molecule responsible for a characteristic (e.g., taste, odor) of the compound.

acetyl g., the radical, CH_3CO.

alcohol g., an organic radical consisting of one atom each of carbon and oxygen with three atoms of hydrogen (primary alcohol group), with two atoms of hydrogen (secondary alcohol group), or with only one atom of hydrogen (tertiary alcohol group).

alkyl g., an organic radical produced by loss of one hydrogen atom from an aliphatic hydrocarbon.

amino g., the radical, NH_2.

azo g., the divalent radical, $-N=N-$.

blood g's, categories into which blood can be classified on the basis of agglutinogens (see also BLOOD TYPES).

carbonyl g., a functional group consisting of carbon joined to oxygen with a double bond, two carbon electrons remaining unpaired (C:O).

carboxyl g., a carbonyl group united with a hydroxyl group, one electron of the carbon remaining unpaired (COOH).

coli-aerogenes g., a group of microorganisms including *Escherichia coli, Aerobacter aerogenes* and a variety of intermediate forms; called also coliform bacilli or coliform bacteria.

colon-typhoid-dysentery g., a group of gram-negative bacteria more or less resembling *Escherichia coli.*

hydroxyl g., the univalent radical, OH.

methyl g., the organic radical, $-CH_3$.

nitro g., the monovalent radical, $-NO_2$.

nitroso g., the monovalent radical, $-N=O$.

peptide g., the bivalent radical, $-CO.NH-$, formed by reaction between the amino and carboxyl groups of adjacent amino acids.

prosthetic g., the nonamino acid portion of a protein molecule.

saccharide g., a combination of carbon, hydrogen and oxygen atoms in a hypothetical molecule, $C_6H_{10}O_5$, the number of which in the compound determines the specific name of the polysaccharide.

zymophore g., zymophore.

grouping (groōp'ing) arrangement or classification in groups.

antigenic structural g., haptene.

g. of blood, classification of blood according to the blood group to which it belongs.

haptenic g., haptene.

growing pains (gro'ing) rheumatic-type pains in the arms or legs of children, once believed to be caused by the growing process. It is now recognized that growth does not cause pain and that these pains can be a symptom of many different disorders.

growth (grōth) 1. the progressive development of a living thing, especially the process by which the body reaches its point of complete physical development. 2. an abnormal formation of tissue, such as a tumor.

HUMAN GROWTH. Human growth from infancy to maturity involves great changes in body size and appearance, including the development of the sexual characteristics. The growth process is not a steady one: at some times growth occurs rapidly, at others slowly. Individual patterns of growth vary widely because of differences in heredity and environment. Children tend to have physiques similar to those of their parents or of earlier forebears; however, environment may modify this tendency. Living conditions, including nutrition and hygiene, have considerable influence on growth.

Glands and Growth. The regulators of growth are the ENDOCRINE GLANDS, which are themselves subject to hereditary influence. The PITUITARY GLAND secretes growth hormone, which controls general body growth, particularly the growth of the skeleton, and also influences METABOLISM.

In addition to influencing growth directly, the pituitary has a central role in regulating the other endocrine glands. These other glands in turn control many body functions, and they secrete the various hormones that directly regulate metabolism.

Variations in Growth Rates. The growth of different individuals varies a great deal. It should be remembered that the rate of growth we call "normal" is really only an average rate. There is a wide range of growth rates, almost all of them quite normal. Of the children of a given sex and age, only about two-thirds will have physical measurements that fall close to the average.

Periods of Rapid Growth. Children in general have two periods of noticeably rapid growth. One occurs after birth, the other near puberty. In the first year of life the average baby grows about 50 per cent in height and about triples his weight. Thereafter his development proceeds more slowly until he reaches the rapid growth associated with puberty, which generally takes place between the ninth and thirteenth years in girls and between the eleventh and fifteenth years in boys.

During the pubertal period of rapid growth the sexual differences become evident. The girl begins to assume the characteristics of a woman's physique, with full breasts, rounded hips and soft deposits of fatty tissue, and she begins menstruation. The boy likewise undergoes changes associated with masculinity: enlargement of the testes, broadening of shoulders and deepening of the voice. In both sexes the appearance of pubic hair accompanies these developments. The average girl may attain her adult size by the age of 17, the average boy by 18 or 19.

GROWTH DISORDERS. Disorders in growth are usually traceable to excess or shortage of pituitary secretions, and may arise from hereditary defects or from glandular abnormalities. Abnormally large secretions of growth hormone can produce GIGANTISM. Failure of the pituitary gland to develop sufficiently or to secrete adequate amounts of growth hormone may result in DWARFISM. In adulthood, overproduction of growth hormone may lead to ACROMEGALY, a disorder characterized by abnormal growth of the hands and feet and coarse thickening of the facial features. In certain cases, such hormonal imbalance or deficiency may be relieved by surgery or by giving hormone substitutes. These growth disorders are uncommon, however.

g. hormone, a substance secreted by the anterior lobe of the PITUITARY GLAND that directly influences protein, carbohydrate and lipid metabolism and controls the rate of skeletal and visceral growth.

grumous (groo'mus) lumpy or clotted.

grutum (groo'tum) milium.

GSH reduced glutathione.

G6PD glucose-6-phosphate dehydrogenase.

GSSG oxidized glutathione.

g.u. genitourinary.

guanase (gwan'ās) an enzyme found in the thymus, adrenal glands and pancreas.

guanethidine (gwan-eth'i-den) an adrenergic-blocking agent, used as an antihypertensive.

guanidoacetic acid (gwan"ĭ-do-ah-se'tik) an intermediate product in the synthesis of creatine.

guanine (gwan'ēn) a purine that is an essential component of nucleic acids.

guaranine (gwah-rah'nin) caffeine.

Guillain-Barré syndrome (ge-yan"bar-ra') a syndrome described in encephalitis of virus origin consisting of absence of fever, pain or tenderness in the muscles, motor weakness, abolition of tendon reflexes and great increase in the protein in the cerebrospinal fluid without corresponding increase in cells; called also radiculoneuritis.

guillotine (gil'o-tēn) a surgical instrument with a movable blade that slides in the grooves of a rigid frame, used for removing tonsils.

Gull's disease (gulz) atrophy of the thyroid gland with myxedema.

Gull-Sutton disease (gul sut'on) generalized arteriosclerosis.

gullet (gul'et) the passage to the stomach.

gum (gum) 1. a mucilaginous excretion of various plants. 2. gingiva.

gumma (gum'ah) a soft, gummy tumor in tertiary syphilis.

gummatous (gum'ah-tus) of the nature of gumma.

gummy (gum'e) resembling gum or gumma.

gustation (gus-ta'shun) the sense of taste. adj., gus'tatory.

gustometer (gus-tom'ēter) an instrument used in the quantitative determination of taste thresholds.

gustometry (gus-tom'ĕ-tre) measurement of acuity of the sense of taste.

gut (gut) 1. the bowel or intestine. 2. catgut.

gutta (gut'ah), pl. *gut'tae* [L.] drop.
  g. rosa'cea, acne rosacea.
  g. sere'na, amaurosis.

gutta-percha (gut"ah-per'chah) the coagulated latex of a number of tropical trees of the family *Sapotaceae*, resembling rubber and used in medicine and surgery for mechanical purposes.

guttat. [L.] *gutta'tim* (drop by drop).

guttate (gut'āt) resembling a drop.

guttatim (gŭ-ta'tim) drop by drop.

guttering (gut'er-ing) cutting of a gutter-like excision in bone.

guttural (gut'er-al) pertaining to the throat.

gymnobacterium (jim"no-bak-te're-um) a microorganism that has no flagella.

gymnocyte (jim'no-sīt) a cell with no cell wall.

gymnophobia (jim"no-fo'be-ah) morbid fear of the naked body.

gymnospore (jim'no-spōr) a spore without an envelope.

gynaeco- for words beginning thus, see those beginning *gyneco-*.

gynandrism (jĭ-nan'drizm) a mixture of female and male characteristics in the male.

gynandroblastoma (jĭ-nan"dro-blas-to'mah) a tumor containing elements of both male and female germ cells.

gynandroid (jĭ-nan'droid) a female with masculine characteristics.

gynandromorph (jĭ-nan'dro-morf) an organism exhibiting gynandromorphism.

gynandromorphism (jĭ-nan"dro-mor'fizm) the presence of chromosomes of both sexes in different tissues of the body, producing a mosaic of male and female sex characteristics.

gynecic (jĭ-ne'sik) pertaining to women.

gynecogenic (jin"ĕ-ko-jen'ik) producing female characteristics or reactions.

gynecography (jin"ĕ-kog'rah-fe) roentgenography of the female reproductive organs.

gynecoid (jin'ĕ-koid) woman-like.

gynecologist (jin"ĕ-kol'o-jist) a specialist in gynecology.

gynecology (jin"ĕ-kol'o-je) the branch of medicine dealing with diseases of the reproductive organs in women. adj., **gynecolog'ic.**

gynecomania (jin"ĕ-ko-ma'ne-ah) satyriasis.

gynecomastia (jin"ĕ-co-mas'te-ah) overdevelopment of mammary glands in the male.

gynecopathy (jin"ĕ-kop'ah-the) disease peculiar to women.

gynephobia (jin"ĕ-fo'be-ah) morbid aversion to women.

Gynergen (jin'er-jen) trademark for ergotamine tartrate, an oxytocic used also to treat migraine.

gyniatrics (jin"e-at'riks) the treatment of diseases of women.

gynomerogon (jin"o-mer'o-gon) an organism produced by gynomerogony and containing only the maternal set of chromosomes.

gynomerogony (jin"o-mer-og'o-ne) development of a portion of a fertilized ovum containing only the female pronucleus.

gynopathic (jin"o-path'ik) pertaining to disease of women.

gynoplastics (jin'o-plas"tiks) plastic surgery of female genitalia.

gypsum (jip'sum) calcium sulfate.

gyration (ji-ra'shun) revolution about a fixed center.

gyre (jīr) gyrus.

gyrectomy (ji-rek'to-me) excision or resection of a cerebral gyrus, or a portion of the cerebral cortex.

Gyrencephala (ji"ren-sef'ah-lah) a group of higher mammals having a brain marked by gyri.

gyroma (ji-ro'mah) a tumor of the ovary, consisting of a convoluted, highly refracting mass.

gyrospasm (ji'ro-spazm) rotatory spasm of the head.

gyrotrope (ji'ro-trōp) rheotrope, an instrument for reversing an electric current.

gyrus (ji'rus), pl. *gy'ri* [L.] one of the many convolutions of the surface of the brain caused by infolding of the cortex (gy'ri cere'bri), separated by fissures or sulci.

  angular g., one continuous anteriorly with the supramarginal gyrus.
  annectent g., any one of four gyri connecting the occipital and parietotemporal lobes.
  Broca's g., inferior frontal gyrus of the left hemisphere.
  central g., anterior, one on the frontal lobe.
  central g., posterior, one on the parietal lobe.
  cingulate g., g. cin'guli, one embracing the entire upper surface of the corpus callosum and continuous with the gyrus hippocampi.
  frontal g., any of the three (inferior, middle and superior) gyri of the frontal lobe.
  fusiform g., one connecting the temporal and occipital lobes.
  hippocampal g., g. hippocam'pi, one on the inferior surface of each cerebral hemisphere, lying between the hippocampal and collateral fissures; called also parahippocampal gyrus.
  infracalcarine g., one on the under surface of the temporal lobe.
  lingual g., median occipitotemporal gyrus.
  marginal g., one in the frontal lobe bordering on the callosomarginal fissure.
  occipital g., any of the three (superior, middle and inferior) gyri of the occipital lobe.
  occipitotemporal g., lateral, fusiform gyrus.
  occipitotemporal g., median, one on the tentorial surface of the temporal lobe, continuous anteriorly with the hippocampal gyrus and ending posteriorly in the occipital lobe.
  orbital gyri, irregular gyri on the orbital surface of the frontal lobe.
  parahippocampal g., hippocampal gyrus.
  parietal g., ascending, one between the fissure of Rolando, the interparietal fissure and the fissure of Sylvius.
  parietal g., superior, the superomedial border of the parietal lobe.
  quadrate g., precuneus.
  g. rec'tus, a cerebral convolution on the orbital aspect of the frontal lobe.
  Retzius' g., sagittal g., a large gyrus of the brain running parallel with the sagittal sutura of the skull.
  subcollateral g., fusiform gyrus.
  g. supracallo'sus, a rudimentary gyrus on the upper surface of the corpus callosum.
  supramarginal g., that part of the inferior parietal convolution which curves around the upper end of the fissure of Sylvius.
  temporal g., any gyrus of the temporal lobe, including inferior, middle, superior and transverse gyri (the anterior transverse temporal gyrus represents the cortical center for hearing).
  g. transiti'vus, annectant gyrus.
  uncinate g., hippocampal gyrus.

H

H chemical symbol, *hydrogen.*

H. [L.] *ho'ra* (hour).

H⁺ symbol, *hydrogen ion.*

Ha chemical symbol, *hahnium.*

habena (hah-be'nah) the peduncle of the pineal gland.

habenula (hah-ben'u-lah), pl. *haben'ulae* [L.] 1. any frenulum, especially one of a series of structures in the cochlea. 2. a triangular area in the dorsomedial aspect of the thalamus rostral to the pineal gland.

habit (hab'it) 1. an action that has become automatic or characteristic by repetition. 2. predisposition; bodily temperament.

habituation (hah-bit″u-a'shun) acquired tolerance from repeated use or exposure to a specific stimulus or substance; applied to a condition due to repeated consumption of a drug, with a desire to continue its use, but with little or no tendency to increase the dose. (See also DRUG ADDICTION.)

habitus (hab'ĭ-tus) [L.] habit; body conformation.
  h. enteroptot'icus, the body conformation seen in enteroptosis, marked by a long, narrow abdomen.
  h. phthis'icus, a body conformation predisposing to pulmonary tuberculosis, marked by pallor, emaciation, poor muscular development and small bones.

hachement (ahsh-maw') [Fr.] a hacking or chopping stroke in massage.

hae- for words beginning thus, see also those beginning *he-.*

Haemadipsa (he″mah-dip'sah) a genus of leeches.

Haemaphysalis (hem″ah-fis'ah-lis) a genus of ticks, several species of which are important as vectors of disease.

Haemophilus (he-mof'ĭ-lus) a genus of Schizomycetes.
  H. aegyp'tius, an organism related to *H. influenzae,* and the cause of acute contagious conjunctivitis.
  H. ducrey'i, the causative agent of chancroid.
  H. influen'zae, a species that produces an upper respiratory infection and a serious form of meningitis, especially in infants.
  H. vagina'lis, a hemophilic bacterium associated, possibly causally, with human vaginitis.

hafnium (haf'ne-um) a chemical element, atomic number 72, atomic weight 178.49, symbol Hf. (See table of ELEMENTS.)

Hageman factor (hāg'ē-man) clotting factor XII.

hahnium (hah'ne-um) a chemical element, atomic

number 105, atomic weight 260, symbol Ha. (See table of ELEMENTS.)

Hailey-Hailey disease (ha'le-ha'le) benign chronic familial pemphigus.

hair (hār) a threadlike structure, especially the specialized epidermal structure developing from a papilla sunk in the corium, produced only by mammals and characteristic of that group of animals.
  auditory h's, hairlike attachments of the epithelial cells of the inner ear.
  beaded h., hair marked with alternate swellings and constrictions; seen in monilethrix.
  h. bulb, the bulbous expansion at the lower end of a hair root.
  burrowing h., one that grows horizontally in the skin.
  club h., a hair whose root is surrounded by a bulbous enlargement composed of keratinized cells, preliminary to normal loss of the hair from the follicle.
  h. follicle, a pouchlike depression in the skin in which a hair develops from the matrix at its base and grows to emerge from its opening on the body surface.
  Frey's h's, stiff hairs mounted in a handle; used for testing the sensitiveness of pressure points of the skin.
  ingrown h., one that has curved and reentered the skin.
  lanugo h., the fine hair on the body of the fetus.
  pubic h., the hair on the external genitalia; called also pubes.
  resting h., one that has ceased growing, but has not yet been shed from the follicles.

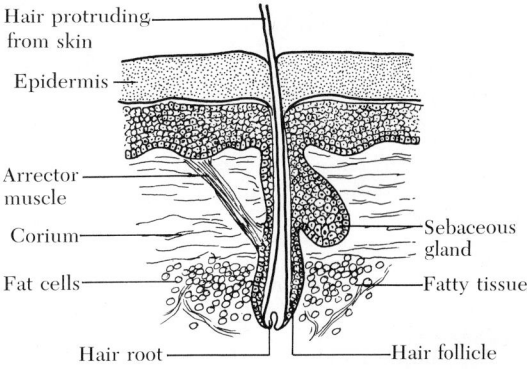

Structure of a hair. The follicle is the protective casing of the hair root. The action of the arrector muscle causes so-called goose flesh (cutis anserina) when the skin is cold.

ringed h., a condition in which a hair appears to be marked by alternating bands of white.

sensory h's, hairlike projections on the surface of sensory epithelial cells.

tactile h's, hairs sensitive to touch.

taste h's, short hairlike processes projecting freely into the lumen of the pit of a taste bud from the peripheral ends of the taste cells.

terminal h., the coarse hair on various areas of the body during adult years.

hairball (hār′bawl) a concretion of hair sometimes found in the stomach or intestines of man or other animals.

halation (hah-la′shun) indistinctness of the visual image by illumination from the same direction as the object.

halazone (hal′ah-zōn) a white, crystalline powder used as a disinfectant for water supplies.

Haldrone (hal′drōn) trademark for a preparation of paramethasone acetate, a corticosteroid.

half-life (haf′līf) the time in which the radioactivity usually associated with a particular isotope is reduced by half through radioactive decay.

halibut liver oil (hal′ĭ-but) a fixed oil from fresh or suitably preserved livers of halibut species; used as a source of vitamin A.

halide (hal′īd) a compound of a halogen with an element or radical.

halisteresis (hah-lis″ter-e′sis) deficiency of mineral salts in a part, as in bone.

halitosis (hal″ĭ-to′sis) offensive odor of the breath.

halitous (hal′ĭ-tus) covered with vapor or moisture.

halitus (hal′ĭ-tus) an expired breath.

Hallervorden-Spatz syndrome (hal′er-for″den spatz) a fatal, familial condition of unknown origin, characterized by neurologic symptoms and intellectual impairment.

Hallopeau's disease (al-o-pōz′) lichen sclerosus et atrophicus.

hallucination (hah-lu″sĭ-na′shun) a sensory impression (sight, touch, sound, smell or taste) that has no basis in external stimulation. Hallucinations can have psychologic causes, as in mental illness, or they can result from drugs, alcohol, organic illnesses, such as brain tumor or senility, or exhaustion. When hallucinations have a psychologic origin, they usually represent a disguised form of a repressed conflict.

auditory h., a hallucination of hearing; the most common type.

gustatory h., a hallucination of taste.

haptic h., tactile hallucination.

hypnagogic h., a hallucination occurring between sleeping and awakening.

olfactory h., a hallucination of smell.

tactile h., a hallucination of touch.

visual h., a hallucination of sight.

hallucinogen (hah-lu′sĭ-no-jen″) an agent capable of producing hallucinations or false sensory perceptions. adj., **hallucinogen′ic.** Drugs that have hallucinogenic properties include mescaline, LSD (lysergic acid diethylamide) and psilocybin. Certain mushrooms and seeds and cactus button (peyote) are also hallucinogenic. The experiences brought about by the use of hallucinogens involve a more acute "awareness" of one's environment and a distorted response to visual, auditory and tactile stimuli. They can also cause a person to exhibit behavior that is symptomatic of a psychotic state of mind.

Hallucinogenic drugs have been used experimentally in research on mental illness; their value in determining brain function and the mechanisms of mental illness is yet to be proved. Abuse of the hallucinogenic compounds by persons who have obtained them through illicit channels, or taken them in medically unsupervised or socially unacceptable settings, has led to the regulation of their distribution by the Food and Drug Administration. Indiscriminate use of these compounds can bring on psychotic states and may result in permanent harm to the psyche.

hallucinogenesis (hah-lu″sĭ-no-jen′ĕ-sis) the production of hallucinations.

hallucinosis (hah-lu″sĭ-no′sis) the experiencing of hallucinations.

acute h., alcoholic h., alcoholic psychosis marked by auditory hallucinations and delusions of persecution.

hallux (hal′uks) the great toe.

h. doloro′sa, a painful disease of the great toe, usually associated with flatfoot.

h. flex′us, a bent great toe.

h. mal′leus, hammer toe affecting the great toe.

h. rig′idus, painful stiffness of the first metatarsophalangeal joint due to degenerative arthritis.

h. val′gus, angulation of the great toe toward the other toes of the foot.

h. va′rus, angulation of the great toe away from the other toes of the foot.

halmatogenesis (hal″mah-to-jen′ĕ-sis) a sudden alteration of type from one generation to another.

halo (ha′lo) a circular structure, such as a luminous circle seen surrounding an object or light.

Fick's h., a colored circle appearing around a light, experienced by wearers of contact lenses.

h. glaucomato′sus, glaucomatous h., a narrow light zone surrounding the optic disk in glaucoma.

senile h., a zone of variable width around the optic disk, due to exposure of various elements of the choroid as a result of senile atrophy of the pigmented epithelium.

halogen (hal′o-jen) an element of a closely related chemical family, all of which form similar (saltlike) compounds in combination with sodium. The halogens are bromine, chlorine, fluorine and iodine.

halometer (hah-lom′ĕ-ter) an instrument for estimating the size of erythrocytes by measuring the diffraction halos they produce.

halophilic (hal″o-fil′ik) pertaining to or characterized by an affinity for salt; requiring a high concentration of salt for optimal growth.

Halotestin (hal″o-tes′tin) trademark for a preparation of fluoxymesterone, an androgen used in the palliative treatment of certain cancers.

halothane (hal′o-thān) a colorless, mobile, non-flammable, heavy liquid used by inhalation to produce ANESTHESIA.

hamarthritis (ham″ar-thri′tis) arthritis of all the joints.

hamartia (ham-ar′she-ah) a defect of tissue combination in development.

hamartoblastoma (ham-ar″to-blas-to′mah) a specific tumor of embryonic tissue.

hamartoma (ham″ar-to′mah) an overgrowth of tissue of the types commonly present in an organ, but not existing in the usual arrangement.
vascular h., hemangioma.

hamartomatosis (ham″ar-to″mah-to′sis) the presence of multiple hamartomas.

hamartomatous (ham″ar-to′mah-tus) pertaining to a disturbance in growth of a tissue in which the cells of a circumscribed area outstrip those of the surrounding areas.

hamartoplasia (ham″ar-to-pla′ze-ah) overdevelopment of tissue in response to trauma.

Hamman's disease (ham′anz) spontaneous interstitial emphysema of the lungs.

Hamman-Rich syndrome (ham′an rich) diffuse interstitial pulmonary fibrosis.

hammer (ham′er) the malleus, the largest of the three bones of the ear.
h. toe, a condition in which the proximal phalanx of the toe—most often that of the second toe—is extended and the second and distal phalanges are flexed, causing a clawlike appearance.

hamstring (ham′string) a tendon that laterally bounds the depression in the posterior region of the knee (popliteal space).
inner h's, the tendons of the gracilis, sartorius and two other muscles of the leg.
outer h., the tendon of the biceps muscle of the thigh.

hamulus (ham′u-lus), pl. ham′uli [L.] any hook-shaped process.

hand (hand) the terminal part of an arm, or of the upper (anterior) extremity of a primate.
ape h., one with the thumb permanently extended.
drop h., wristdrop.
obstetrician's h., the contraction of the hand in tetany; the hand is flexed at the wrist, the fingers at the metacarpophalangeal joints but extended at the interphalangeal joints, the thumb being strongly flexed into the palm.
writing h., in Parkinson's disease, assumption of the position by which a pen is commonly held.

hand-foot-and-mouth disease a mild, highly infectious virus disease of children, with vesicular lesions in the mouth and on the hands and feet.

Hand-Schüller-Christian disease (hand shil′er kris′chan) a chronic disorder of the reticuloendothelial system that is found principally in children and young adults; called also Schüller-Christian disease, Hand's disease and chronic idiopathic xanthomatosis.
The three classic symptoms of the syndrome are softened areas of the skull and other flat, membran-

ous bones, exophthalmos and diabetes insipidus. However, all three symptoms are rarely found in one patient. Otitis frequently accompanies the disease. Skin lesions resembling those of seborrheic dermatitis may appear, as may xanthomas.
There is no specific treatment. X-ray therapy is sometimes helpful in treating specific local lesions and corticosteroids have been used with success in some cases. Complete recovery does occur, but about 40 per cent of the cases terminate fatally.

H and E hematoxylin and eosin (stain).

handedness (hand′ed-nes) the preferential use of the hand of one side in all voluntary motor acts.

handicap (han′de-kap) any physical or mental defect or characteristic that prevents a person from taking part freely in the activities appropriate for his age. A handicap may be the result of an accident or a disease, or it may be congenital. It may be obvious—blindness, paralysis or disfiguring scars—or unnoticeable—a heart defect, slight mental retardation or a chronic disease, such as hemophilia.

hangnail (hang′nāl) a shred of epidermis at one side of a nail. Hangnail is prevented by gently pushing the cuticle instead of cutting it, and it is treated by clipping off the shred of skin and applying antiseptic to the area to prevent infection.

Hanot's disease (an-ōz′) biliary cirrhosis.

Hansen's bacillus (han′sunz) *Mycobacterium leprae*, the causative agent of leprosy.
H's disease, leprosy.

hapalonychia (hap″ah-lo-nik′e-ah) abnormal softening of the nails.

haphalgesia (haf″al-je′ze-ah) pain on touching objects.

haphephobia (haf″ĕ-fo′be-ah) morbid fear of contact.

haploid (hap′loid) having half the number of chromosomes characteristically found in the somatic cells of an organism; typical of the gametes of a species whose union restores the diploid number.

haploidy (hap′loi-de) the state of having only one member of each pair of homologous chromosomes.

hapten, haptene (hap′ten), (hap′tēn) the portion of an antigenic molecule or complex that determines its immunologic specificity. adj., **hapten′ic.**

haptic (hap′tik) tactile.

haptics (hap′tiks) the science of the sense of touch.

haptoglobin (hap″to-glo′bin) a serum alpha-2 globulin glycoprotein that binds free hemoglobin; different types, genetically determined, are distinguished electrophoretically.

haptophore (hap′to-fōr) the specific group of atoms in a toxin molecule by which it attaches itself to another molecule; it is capable of neutralizing antitoxin and of acting as an antigen to stimulate specific antitoxin production by body cells.

harelip (hār′lip) congenitally cleft lip (see also CLEFT LIP).

Harmonyl (har′mo-nil) trademark for preparations of deserpidine, a tranquilizer.

Harrison antinarcotic act (har′ĭ-sun) a federal law, enacted March 1, 1915, that regulates the possession, sale, purchase and prescription of opium and coca and all their preparations, natural and synthetic derivatives and salts. These include the drugs cocaine, morphine, codeine and papaverine. Laws patterned after the Harrison antinarcotic act in some states prohibit the possession or sale of derivatives of barbituric acid except under proper licenses, so that they may not be dispensed without a prescription.

Hartmann's solution (hart′manz) a solution containing sodium chloride, sodium lactate and phosphates of calcium and potassium; used parenterally in acidosis and alkalosis.

Hartnup disease (hart′nup) a genetically determined disorder of tryptophan transport, with pellagra-like skin lesions, transient cerebellar ataxia, constant renal aminoaciduria and other biochemical abnormalities.

harvest fever a form of spirochetosis affecting harvest workers.

Harvey (har′ve) William (1578–1657). English physician and physiologist. Born at Folkestone in Kent, he attended the universities of Cambridge and Padua, and announced in 1628 his discovery of the circulation of blood, which was a model of accurate experimentation and inductive proof, and the first application of quantitative demonstration in any biologic investigation. His *De generatione animalium* is important in the history of embryology, for in it Harvey rejected the doctrine of preformation of the fetus and stated that almost all animals, and man himself, are produced from eggs.

Hashimoto's disease (hash″ĭ-mo′tōz) a progressive disease of the thyroid gland with degeneration of its epithelial elements and replacement by lymphoid and fibrous tissue; called also struma lymphomatosis.

hashish (hash-ēsh′) the stalks and leaves of the hemp plant, Cannabis, with narcotic properties similar to those of marijuana.

haustration (hos-tra′shun) 1. the formation of a haustrum. 2. a haustrum.

haustrum (hos′trum), pl. *haus′tra* [L.] one of the pouches of the colon, produced by collection of circular muscle fibers at 1 or 2 cm. distances, and responsible for the sacculated appearance.

Haverhill fever (ha′ver-il) a form of RATBITE FEVER, an acute febrile disease caused by *Streptobacillus moniliformis,* transmitted by the bite of an infected rat, and characterized by an erythematous eruption and more or less generalized arthritis, with adenitis, headache and vomiting; first described in Haverhill, Mass., in 1926.

haversian canal (ha-ver′shan) one of the anastomosing channels of the haversian system in compact bone, containing blood and lymph vessels, nerves and marrow.

h. system, a haversian canal and its concentrically arranged lamellae, constituting the basic unit of structure in compact bone (osteon).

hay fever an allergy characterized by sneezing itchy and watery eyes, running nose and burning palate and throat.

Like all allergies, hay fever is caused by sensitivity to certain substances—most commonly pollens and the spores of molds. Pollen is the fertilizing element of flowering plants. It is a fine dust, easily airborne, that enters the body by inhalation. Ragweed pollen is a particular nuisance to persons subject to hay fever. Mold is a fungus that grows on animal and vegetable matter. The spores of molds are dustlike reproductive units that are also present in the air we breathe.

The amount of pollen in the air varies with the season and geographic area. East of the Rocky Mountains, the peak of the regional hay fever season occurs between mid-August and mid-September, when the air is heavy with the pollen of the ragweed plant. An appreciable number of hay fever sufferers are also reactive to the spring pollens from grasses and trees. Mold-bearing plants such as wheat, barley and corn are prevalent in the agricultural areas of the Midwest, and attacks of hay fever caused by mold spores are common there as these crops ripen.

Hay fever deserves to be recognized as more than a mere nuisance. By causing lack of sleep and loss of appetite, it can lower the body's resistance to disease. It can cause inflammation of the ears, sinuses, throat and bronchi. A number of hay fever sufferers develop ASTHMA.

Hay fever can be relieved, although not cured, by antihistamines and sympathomimetic drugs such as ephedrine and phenylpropanolamine hydrochloride. Sedatives may be prescribed for nervous or tense persons. A series of preventive injections (desensitization) may be recommended in advance of the hay fever season. This consists of administering controlled and gradually increasing amounts of the offending substance in order to develop a certain amount of immunity. In some cases it may be helpful to avoid part of the hay fever season by taking a vacation in an area that is relatively free of the annoying pollen. Air conditioning may also help give relief by filtering much of the pollen from the air. (See also ALLERGY.)

Hb hemoglobin.

HCl hydrochloric acid.

H disease Hartnup disease.

H & E hematoxylin and eosin (stain).

He chemical symbol, *helium.*

head (hed) the anterior or superior part of a structure or organism, in vertebrates containing the brain and the organs of special sense.

articular h., an eminence on a bone by which it articulates with another bone.

h. injury, traumatic injury to the head resulting from a fall or violent blow. Such an injury may be open or closed and may involve a brain concussion, skull fracture or contusions of the brain. All head injuries are potentially dangerous because there may be a slow leakage of blood from damaged blood vessels into the brain, or the formation of a blood clot which gradually increases pressure against brain tissue (subdural or extradural hematoma). These conditions may not present symptoms for several days or months after the head injury.

TREATMENT. The patient with a head injury is treated conservatively at first unless an open fracture of the skull demands surgical débridement, or a large hematoma requires immediate relief of increasing intracranial pressure. The physician usually limits the amount of sedative or analgesic drugs allowed the patient as these may mask developing symptoms. The patient is kept in bed in a quiet, nonstimulating environment. Adequate nutrition is provided by INTRAVENOUS INFUSIONS if he is unconscious and unable to swallow. If unconsciousness is prolonged, the physician may order TUBE FEEDING.

NURSING CARE. Observation of the patient is extremely important in determining the extent of injury. Any one of the following symptoms should be reported to the physician: (1) changes in the patient's blood pressure, pulse or respiration rate, especially slowing of the pulse with a rising blood pressure; (2) extreme restlessness or excitability following a period of comparative calm; (3) deepening stupor or loss of consciousness; (4) headache that increases in intensity; (5) vomiting, especially persistent, projectile vomiting; (6) unequal size of the pupils; (7) leakage of cerebrospinal fluid (clear yellow or pink-tinged) from the nose or ear; (8) inability to move one or more extremity.

Patients who are unconscious must be watched closely for respiratory difficulty or inability to swallow. If the patient cannot swallow, his head must be turned to the side and his mouth and trachea suctioned as necessary to prevent aspiration of mucus into the lungs. A TRACHEOSTOMY set and RESPIRATOR should be readily at hand in case severe respiratory embarrassment occurs.

Side rails are applied and the head board of the bed is padded with pillows or a blanket if the patient is delirious or if convulsions are anticipated. An accurate record of the patient's intake and output is kept and the patient is observed for signs of retention of urine, incontinence or abdominal distention.

nerve h., the optic disk.

headache (hed′āk) a pain or ache in the head. One of the most common ailments of man, it is a symptom rather than a disorder in itself. It accompanies many diseases and conditions, including emotional distress. (See also MIGRAINE.)

Although recurring headache may be an early sign of serious organic disease relatively few headaches are caused by disease-induced structural changes. Most result from vasodilation of blood vessels in tissues surrounding the brain, or from tension in the neck and scalp muscles.

Treatment of headache varies according to its severity and its tendency to recur. A mild transient headache can be relieved by the administration of an analgesic such as aspirin; however, aspirin and other drugs should not be taken habitually. It is best to determine the primary cause of the headache. A tranquilizer may be useful when stress and tension are shown to be responsible for recurring headaches. If the cause is found to be a vascular disturbance, the physician may prescribe vasoconstricting drugs such as ergotamine or ergotamine plus caffeine.

healing (hēl′ing) the restoration of structure and function of injured or diseased tissues. The healing processes include blood clotting, tissue mending, scarring and bone healing.

INFLAMMATION. When an injury occurs, the body's first-aid mechanisms automatically begin to operate. The blood vessels in the neighborhood of the injury dilate to provide an increased blood supply. At the same time the pores in the thin walls of the capillaries also widen, letting more plasma than usual flow through to the injured tissues. The immediate result is twofold: the increased flow of blood and plasma brings the body's repair materials to the spot in large quantities, and the increase in

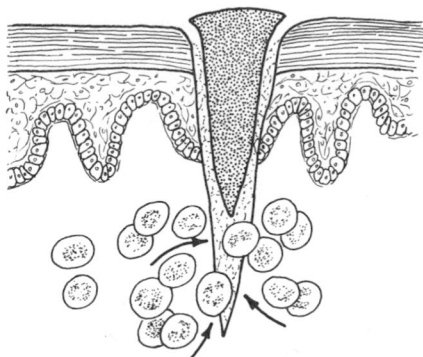

Formation of a blood clot in a wound

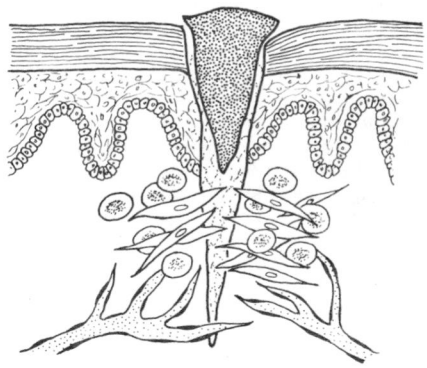

Fibroblasts repair wound, clot shrinks

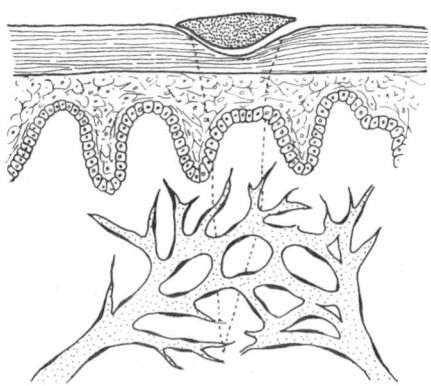

Normal blood supply returns to healing wound

Wound healing.

fluid at the spot distends tissues, presses on nerves and raises the local temperature. This whole process is called inflammation. It is one of the body's protective devices. Inflammation causes pain, which impairs the function of the injured part.

BLOOD CLOTTING. If the skin is broken and there is bleeding, another mechanism, blood CLOTTING, goes into operation at the site of the injury. Twelve essential clotting substances, or factors, have been recognized. Of the four chief ones, only three are ordinarily present in the blood; the fourth is locked in the tissues. Not until tissue is damaged, and the fourth substance is liberated, is the blood clotting, or coagulating, mechanism put to work.

In the BLOOD there are fragments of protoplasm known as platelets. Even though no more than a few drops of blood may flow from a cut, platelets by the tens of thousands come in contact with the rough edge of injured tissue, and they disintegrate. Thus they liberate thromboplastin, the fourth substance essential for clotting, at the spot where it is needed. The thromboplastin acts upon one of the constituents of the blood, prothombin, and in the presence of calcium, also a normal constituent of the blood, the prothrombin changes to a similar but active material, thrombin. Now the newly formed thrombin reacts with another chemical in the blood, fibrinogen, to form fibrin. This substance, the end product of the series of chemical reactions, is insoluble and spongelike and has the property of being able to contract. It forms a network of threads that enmesh the erythrocytes; it pulls them together, as it contracts, into a tough mass called a clot, which acts like a cork to stop up the opening.

The platelets help to stop the flow of blood in two additional ways. They release a chemical that stimulates the muscle walls of nearby blood vessels to contract, narrowing the channels along which blood is flowing to the cut and also narrowing the cut end that needs to be plugged. And the platelets themselves, being sticky, act as a natural adhesive, helping to seal up the cut. They are both chemical and mechanical agents.

THE MENDING PROCESS. The same materials that arrest bleeding prepare the site for mending. The fibrin threads contract and pull together the edges of the wound under the natural adhesive patch of the clot, and the repair cells go to work. These repair cells are a variety of connective tissue, long and spindle-shaped, with fibrous branches; they bind the edges of the wound neatly together. This done, their work is ended; their remnants and the remnants of cells damaged in the injury are cleared away by scavenger cells (phagocytes), cellular sanitation squads that keep all kinds of microscopic debris from cluttering the body tissues.

SCAR. When a cut is relatively clean and small, the edges of tissue are brought together in a neat seam and there is no visible evidence of the repair. The repair cells have acted as basting stitches, and they are disposed of when the tissues themselves effect a permanent juncture with their own cells. A clean, dry surgical incision in which there is practically no loss of tissue heals in much the same way.

When a wound is extensive, with uneven edges, the repair cells are unable to pull the edges together. Instead, they build a bridge across the gap. These cells of connective tissue, the fibroblasts, are not skin and cannot change into skin. They harden into tough, contracting, white scar tissue (granulation tissue).

In the type of wound just described, the physician stitiches the edges of the damaged tissues together, giving the body the conditions under which it can do its own repair work. But when so much tissue has been lost that the wound must be left open or gaping, as in an abscess or ulcer, this cannot be done, and the fibroblasts must fill in the wound from the depth and sides before it can be covered over. In addition to being unsightly, the scars from extensive wounds may interfere with nerves, blood vessels and muscles. In such cases, PLASTIC SURGERY may be necessary or advisable to restore function or for cosmetic reasons.

BONE HEALING. When a bone is broken, the healing process works on similar principles; but the task requires different material, as strong as the original bone and capable of hardening rapidly. The first repair cells bind the broken ends of bone together, and along these bonds, the osteoblasts, bone-forming cells, begin at once to grow. Callus, a tough binding material, holds the break firm until the new bone is properly hardened, and eventually it also turns into true bone. When the task is done, bone-scavenger cells (osteoclasts) clear away excess repair cells and trim the mended area to nearly its original size. When the break is jagged and the ends are out of alignment, the body's repair mechanisms fill in with their mending materials, but often not adequately. The physician helps the natural process by setting the fracture and giving the body the necessary start for a good bone repair job.

There are various factors that favorably influence the healing process. The chief ones are youth (healing is slow in elderly people), rest of the injured part, adequate nutrition, with plency of protein and vitamins, and warmth.

h. by first intention, union of accurately coapted edges of a wound, with an irreducible minimum of granulation tissue.

h. by second intention, union by adhesion of granulating surfaces.

h. by third intention, union by filling of the wound with granulations.

health   (helth) a state of physical, mental and social well-being.

public h., the field of medicine that is concerned with safeguarding and improving the physical, mental and social well-being of the community as a whole.

healthy   (helth′e) pertaining to, characterized by or promoting health.

hearing   (hēr′ing) the sense by which sounds are perceived, by conversion of sound waves into nerves impulses, which are then interpreted by the brain. The organ of hearing is the EAR, which is divided into three sections, the outer, middle and inner ear. Each plays a special role in hearing. Connecting the middle ear with the nasopharynx is the eustachian tube, through which air enters to equalize the pressure on both sides of the TYMPANIC MEMBRANE (eardrum).

The function of the outer ear is to collect the sound waves and direct them into the external acoustic meatus and toward the eardrum.

In the middle ear are three tiny bones, the malleus (hammer), incus (anvil) and stapes (stirrup), called collectively the ossicles. The malleus is attached to the tympanic membrane, and the stapes connects with the COCHLEA in the inner ear.

The cochlea, named for a snail shell, which it closely resembles, is a tube coiled in two and a half turns. Deep inside its fluid-filled convolutions, which are further complicated by dividing membranes, is the organ of Corti, containing the nerve endings of hearing which convert sound into impulses for the vestibulocochlear nerve to carry to the brain.

HOW THE EAR WORKS.   When sound waves strike the tympanic membrane, they start it vibrating. Most of the sound waves simply bounce off; what remains may be a very tiny vibration of the drum. To be useful, the ear must be able to record very light sound, and yet survive a violent sound such as a thunderclap.

The problem of protecting the tympanic membrane is handled by two tiny muscles that damp the vibrations in the eardrum and ossicles. The main problem, that of hearing, is solved by the ear's transmitting chain of membrane-ossicles-cochlea, a mechanical transformer that converts the large-amplitude sound waves striking the drum into smaller, more concentrated vibrations.

The ossicles act as a series of levers, each one amplifying the minute movement of the eardrum as it passes it along. By the time the stirrup taps the window of the cochlea, it has 22 times the pressure of the original vibration. The thin oval window membrane vibrates in turn, setting the fluid in the cochlea in motion along its spiral course. The constricted channel of the cochlea multiplies the pressure still further, until the original vibrations reach the nerve ends in the form of powerful sideways motions rubbing against the sensitive hairlike cells of the organ of Corti. The vibrations are transformed into impulses that pass along the vestibulocochlear nerve to the brain, and the waves of pressure in the cochlea are released by way of another membrane-covered window, the round window, at the other end of the cochlea.

It is still not certain how the organ of Corti transforms the vibrations into nerve impulses. There are two major theories. One, the Helmholtz theory, points out that the organ of Corti is shaped much like a piano or harp, with long strands at one end and short ones at the other. Perhaps these strands vibrate sympathetically, each strand for a different note, just as the strings of a harp or piano will vibrate when another instrument is played nearby. The second theory, the telephone theory,

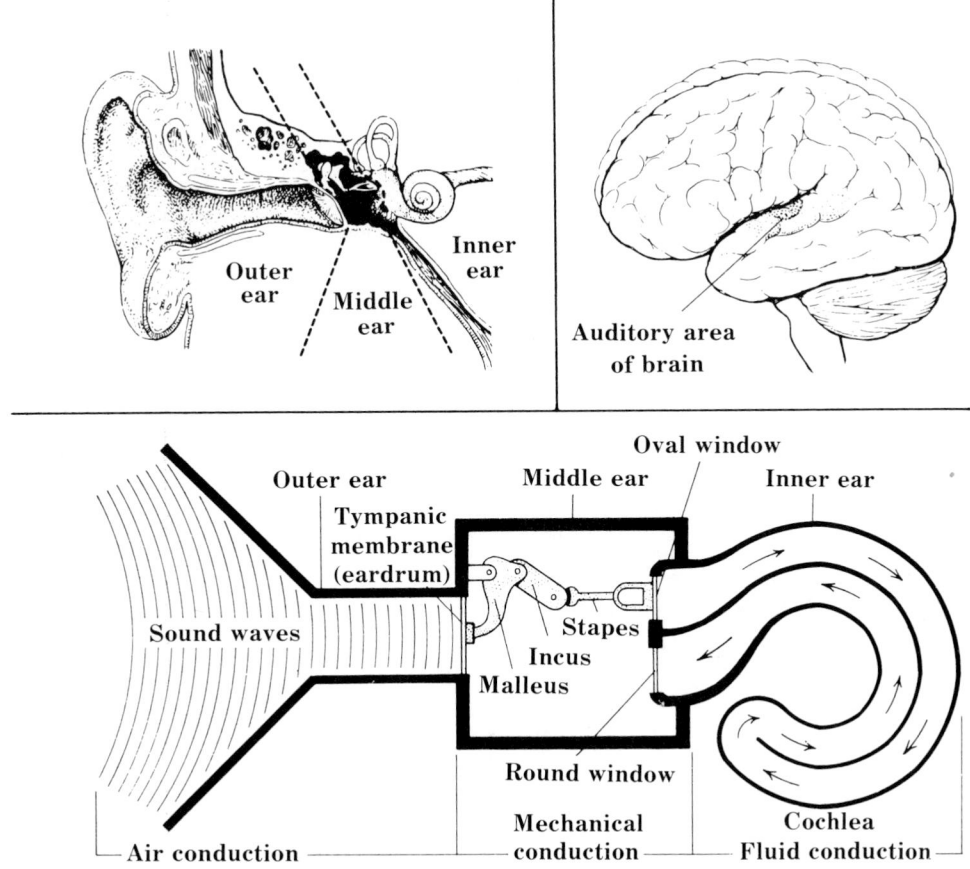

As sound is conducted from the external ear to the inner ear, the sound waves undergo considerable transformation. The tympanic membrane (eardrum), ossicles and cochlea act as a mechanical transformer to concentrate the sound waves so that they can be picked up by nerve endings in the inner ear and transmitted to the brain.

holds that the frequency of notes is transmitted to the brain by nerve impulses of the same frequency. This is the principle on which the telephone is based.

There are technical objections to both theories. It is possible that the organ of Corti operates on both principles—for example, like the telephone for low notes and according to the Helmholtz theory for high notes, with the two systems overlapping in the middle range, where the ear is more sensitive.

Whatever system the ear uses, it is a remarkably versatile organ. The human ear can distinguish more than 1500 separate musical tones, can recognize thousands of different sounds and can hear clearly from the softest whisper to the roar of a factory or a battleship's guns.

h. aid, an instrument to amplify sounds for the hard of hearing. There are two types of electronic hearing aids: the air-conduction type, which is worn in the external acoustic meatus, and the bone-conduction type, which is worn in back of the ear over the mastoid process.

Those who have conductive deafness can often use any one of the better aids with good results. Patients with OTOSCLEROSIS will probably need the bone-conduction type of instrument. Those with sensorineural deafness, caused by injury to the vestibulocochlear nerve, and mixed deafness may have more trouble selecting a suitable hearing aid, and may get less satisfactory results.

Those wearing a hearing aid for the first time should have special training in its proper use. A hearing aid picks up and amplifies all the sounds in the vicinity. Often a person whose hearing has declined gradually will have lost the facility to ignore background noises. When he first tries a hearing aid, his ears will be assaulted by the sounds of passing cars, of doors slamming, of telephones ringing. Training in how to filter out these noises and concentrate on the essential is necessary if the person is to get good results from his hearing aid. For best results, this should be combined with lessons in lip-reading.

The National Association of Hearing and Speech Agencies, 919 18th Street, N.W., Washington, D.C. 20006, has affiliates throughout the United States that offer many services to those with hearing difficulties.

heart   (hart) a hollow muscular organ lying slightly to the left of the midline of the chest. The heart serves as a pump controlling the blood flow in two circuits, the pulmonary and the systemic (see also CIRCULATORY SYSTEM).

DIVISIONS OF THE HEART.   The septum, a thick muscular wall, divides the heart into right and left halves. Each half is again divided into upper and lower quarters or chambers. The lower chambers are called ventricles; the upper chambers are called atria. The right side of the heart, consisting of the right atrium and right ventricle, sends blood into the pulmonary circuit. The left side, consisting of the left atrium and left ventricle, sends blood into the systemic circuit.

VALVES OF THE HEART.   Between the right atrium and right ventricle is the tricuspid valve. Similarly, the left atrium and left ventricle are connected by the mitral, or bicuspid, valve. In addition to the valves between the atrium and ventricle on each side of the heart, there are valves at the blood's exit points: the pulmonary valve opening from the right ventricle into the pulmonary artery, and the aortic valve opening from the left ventricle into the aorta. These valves, both within the heart and leading out of it, open and shut in such a way as to keep the blood flowing in one direction through the heart's two separate pairs of chambers: from atrium to ventricle and out through its appropriate artery.

LAYERS OF THE HEART.   The heart wall is composed of three layers of tissues. Its chambers are lined by a delicate membrane, the endocardium. The thick muscular wall essential to normal pumping action of the heart is called the myocardium. The thin but sturdy membranous sac surrounding the exterior of the heart is called the pericardium.

THE HEART'S PACEMAKER.   The heart is made up of special muscle tissue, capable of continuous rhythmic contraction without tiring. The impulse that starts the heartbeat has its origin in an area

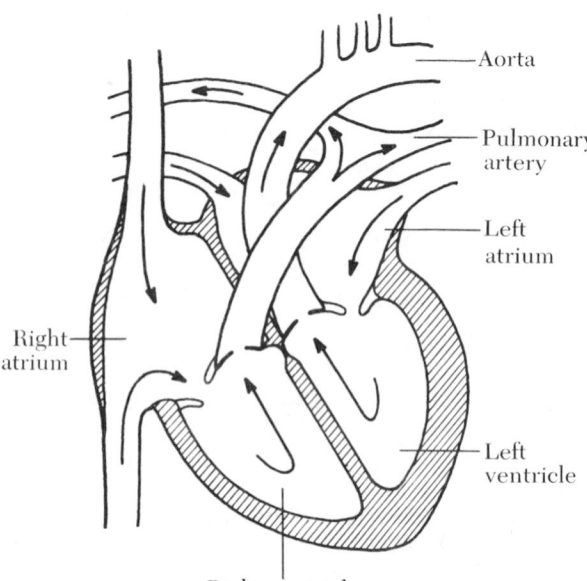

Aorta

Pulmonary artery

Left atrium

Right atrium

Left ventricle

Right ventricle

Blood enters the right atrium from the body and then passes into the right ventricle, where it is pumped into the lungs. It returns from the lungs into the left atrium. It enters the left ventricle and then is pumped to the body via the aorta.

of the right atrium called the sinoatrial node; it is this special tissue that acts as a pacemaker for the heart. It transmits the impulse in a fraction of a second through the atria to another group of similarly sensitive fibers called the atrioventricular node, which conducts the stimulus into the ventricular walls, resulting in contraction of the ventricles. (See also PACEMAKER.)

PUMPING ACTION. Although the right and left sides of the heart serve two separate branches of the circulation, each with its distinct function, they are coordinated so that the heart efficiently serves both sides with a single pumping action. The valve action on both sides is also coordinated with the two phases of the pumping action. Thus during diastole, the relaxation phase, oxygen-poor blood returning from the systemic circulation and accumulated in the right atrium pours into the right ventricle. At the same time, the oxygen-rich blood that has accumulated in the left atrium returning from the pulmonary circulation pours into the left ventricle. The walls of both atria contract to press blood into the relaxed ventricles. In the next contraction phase (systole) the valve between the atrium and ventricle on each side closes, and the muscular walls contract the ventricles and force the blood through the pulmonary artery and the aorta. At the end of the contraction the pulmonary and aortic valves snap shut, preventing any backward surge of the blood into the ventricles. The diastole follows, the ventricles again filling with the flow from their separate atria, and the cycle is repeated.

DISORDERS OF THE HEART. The heart is subject to a variety of disorders. Among them are CONGENITAL HEART DEFECTS, which begin or exist at the time of birth. Disorders of this nature may interfere with the flow of the blood from the heart to the lungs. TETRALOGY OF FALLOT and PATENT DUCTUS ARTERIOSUS are examples of congenital heart defects.

In syphilitic heart disease, there is damage to the aorta or the aortic valve, interfering with the proper functioning of the valve, so that the blood may flow backward into the heart as well as forward from the ventricle.

Another heart ailment is rheumatic heart disease, associated with RHEUMATIC FEVER. The disease can injure the endocardium, the valves or the muscle fibers. The valves may lose their original efficiency, so that passage of the blood is hindered.

Coronary insufficiency is a condition in which the coronary arteries are unable to transport an adequate supply of oxygenated blood to nourish the heart muscle itself. One form of coronary insufficiency, ANGINA PECTORIS, may be precipitated by hampered circulation of the blood caused by arteriosclerotic narrowing of the coronary artery, combined with a stepped-up demand for oxygen during exercise or some other form of exertion.

A "heart attack" is the common description for the condition in which the formation of a blood clot within a coronary artery may shut off, or occlude, the blood flow to a section of the heart muscle. This is called CORONARY OCCLUSION or THROMBOSIS, and can damage or cause permanent injury to the affected area of myocardium.

HEART FAILURE is the inability of the heart to perform its function of pumping sufficient blood to assure a normal flow through the circulation. The heart is unable to pump out the blood returned to it from the veins. In the condition known as congestive heart failure, one or more chambers of the heart do not empty adequately during contraction of the heart muscle. This results in shortness of breath, edema and abnormal retention of sodium and water in body tissues.

Cardiac arrhythmias are disturbances in the normal rate and rhythm of the heartbeat. Electrical impulses that affect the rate and rhythm of the heartbeat are generated in the heart's pacemaker— the sinoatrial node—and distributed to the heart muscle by the heart's conduction system. The sinoatrial node is subject to the influence of the autonomic nervous system and it also responds to chemical changes in the blood and to certain drugs. Tissue necrosis such as that following myocardial infarction or resulting from arteriosclerotic coronary artery disease also can block the passage of electrical impulses. When there is a disturbance in any part of the heart's conduction system or electric generating function the patient may experience a heartbeat that is speeded up (tachycardia) or slowed down (bradycardia). The various forms of arrhythmia are sinus arrhythmia, extrasystole, heart block, atrial fibrillation, atrial flutter and paroxysmal tachycardia.

HEART SURGERY. Many heart disorders can be corrected by surgery of the heart. Since the 1950's, special techniques in heart surgery have become possible, primarily because of several new developments. One was the introduction of antibiotics to aid in controlling infection. Another was the technique of induced HYPOTHERMIA which allows for removal of the body's supply of oxygenated blood for as long as 8 to 10 minutes without causing damage to body tissues. Thus hypothermia permits surgeons to drain the heart in order to repair defects.

A third development was the invention of the HEART-LUNG MACHINE, or pump-oxygenator. This machine, when connected to the patient's circulatory system, relieves the heart and lungs of their tasks of pumping and oxygenating blood, by providing for extracorporeal circulation.

Among the severe congenital defects which in many cases may be treated surgically are patent ductus arteriosus, coarctation of the aorta and atrial and ventricular septal defect. Another congenital (sometimes acquired) heart defect that may be treated surgically is pulmonary stenosis.

Acquired heart defects that may in certain cases be treated by surgery include stenosis, or narrowing of the mitral or aortic valves, constrictive pericarditis and aneurysm of the aorta or of the heart wall itself.

Nursing Care. Prior to surgery the patient is given instructions in coughing and deep breathing so that he can perform these procedures after surgery. They are necessary to provide complete expansion of the lungs and to prevent pulmonary complications postoperatively. He is also told what to expect postoperatively; for example, he can expect a tight feeling in his chest, there may be a tube inserted in the chest cavity, and his blood pressure, pulse and respiration rate will be taken and recorded frequently. To allay his fears of choking or suffocating and to familiarize him with some of the machinery that may be used after surgery, some physicians wish to have the patient acquainted with the suction machine and the respirator, which are kept available in case of need.

During the preoperative period it is important to observe the patient carefully so as to become familiar with his individual characteristics, such as rate and volume of pulse, depth and rate of respiration, tolerance to physical activity and tolerance to pain or discomfort. Later, these preoperative observations are used as a basis for comparison with the patient's postoperative condition.

Preparation of the patient's unit for postoperative care should include assembling a suction apparatus for removing mucus from the mouth and throat, poles for holding infusion bottles and equipment for taking and recording blood pressure. An oxygen tank may be set up and if a mucolytic agent such as Alevaire is to be administered, this equipment should also be on hand. To avoid delay in an emergency, a cardiac arrest tray containing scalpel, hemostats and rib spreaders should be readily available in the event CARDIAC MASSAGE is necessary. One should also be prepared for assisting with a THORACENTESIS should the accumulation of fluid in the chest require this procedure. If hypothermia has been used during surgery, it will be necessary to have equipment available for keeping the body at lowered temperatures and also for applying external heat when hypothermia is discontinued.

Immediately after surgery the radial pulse, respiration and blood pressure are observed for character and rate as often as every 5 minutes until they become stabilized. Use of monitoring intruments allows for continued observation of these variables. Any change in blood pressure, variance in the volume or rhythm of pulse or respiratory changes must be reported at once. Generalized cyanosis is reported to the physician, as is blanching or mottling of the lower extremities, which may indicate the presence of an embolism. Surgical dressings are checked carefully and at frequent intervals for signs of hemorrhage or restriction of chest expansion. All drainage tubes, such as urinary catheter or nasogastric tube, must be attached to the proper apparatus for drainage. The amount and type of drainage obtained is carefully observed and recorded. The chest catheter is attached to closed drainage or to chest suction apparatus (see THORACIC SURGERY). After the patient has recovered from anesthesia he usually is put in Fowler's position. The surgeon may allow him to lie on his back or on the operative side.

Maintenance of a patent airway is most important in these patients because retention of secretions in the respiratory tract is common. Coughing is encouraged. In some cases suctioning, bronchoscopy or tracheostomy may be required to open the airway and remove mucous plugs and secretions. Oxygen is administered as needed. Positioning of the patient should be done only according to the specific wishes of the surgeon since improper positioning may produce thrombosis or other complications in certain types of surgery.

heart block a condition in which the atria and ventricles of the heart contract independently, causing interference in the rate or regularity of the heartbeat.

When isolated impulses from the atria fail to reach the ventricles, heartbeats are missed and the block is called incomplete. When no impulses reach the ventricles from the atria the heart block is complete, with the result that the atria and the ventricles beat at separate rates. In this case the beats remain regular but the rate of the ventricular beats is greatly slowed down.

Heart block can occur with various forms of heart disease, and as a result of excessive dosage of digitalis. A particularly severe instance of heart block can be complicated by the Stokes-Adams disease, in which a sudden attack of unconsciousness results from the slowed heartbeat. It may be accompanied by convulsions.

The treatment for heart block caused by digitalis overdosage is to stop the medication temporarily and give reduced amounts thereafter. When heart block results from a form of heart disease, treatment is given for the underlying cause. An artificial PACEMAKER may be used in the treatment of complete heart block and Stokes-Adams disease.

arborization h. b., a form in which there is interference with the fine terminal Purkinje fibers.

atrioventricular h. b., a form in which the blocking is at the atrioventricular junction.

bundle-branch h. b., a form of heart block in which the two ventricles contract independently of each other.

complete h. b., a condition in which the functional relation between the parts of the bundle of His is destroyed by a lesion, so that the atria and ventricles act independently of each other.

interventricular h. b., bundle-branch heart block.

sinoatrial h. b., a form in which the blocking is located between the atria and the mouths of the great veins and coronary sinus.

heart failure inability of the heart to perform its proper function of expelling blood from the ventricles.

backward h. f., heart failure produced by passive engorgement of the venous system.

congestive h. f., a condition resulting from cardiac output inadequate for physiologic needs, with shortness of breath, edema and abnormal retention of sodium and water in body tissues.

TREATMENT. Treatment for heart failure includes rest to reduce the oxygen requirements of the body, medications such as digitalis to strengthen the heart action and diuretics to control the edema, along with dietary measures.

NURSING CARE. The patient with acute congestive failure is usually placed on complete bed rest with severe limitation of activities as long as the symptoms of edema, dyspnea, ascites and venous engorgement are present. He must be fed, bathed, dressed and otherwise cared for as though he could not lift a finger to help himself. For some patients this is extremely difficult and depressing. Care should be taken not to give the patient the impression that he is causing any difficulties for those assigned to his care.

In addition to measuring the patient's intake and output it is usually necessary to record his weight daily. This information is used as a guide to the response to medication and treatment and the amount of fluid being retained in the tissues.

Oxygen is administered as needed to relieve dyspnea and cyanosis. The position of the patient in bed may also help relieve these symptoms. If the patient tires easily while sitting up in Fowler's position, he may rest more comfortably if he is allowed to lay his arms and head on an overbed table that has been padded with pillows (orthopneic position). Since edematous tissue breaks down more readily and is thus more susceptible to ulceration than normal tissue, routine skin care is extremely important.

Dietary restrictions, such as limiting the intake of sodium to reduce edema, should be explained thoroughly to the patient and his family. If fluids by mouth also are restricted, care should be taken to regulate the amount taken at any given period so that the total amount allowed is evenly distributed over a 24-hour period.

Chronic congestive failure does not always require hospitalization. Medications such as digitalis and a diuretic are used to control the condition and may keep the patient free of symptoms unless complications develop.

forward h. f., diminution in the amount of blood propelled in a forward direction by the heart.

left ventricular h. f., failure of the left ventricle to maintain a normal output of blood. Since the left ventricle does not empty completely, it cannot accept blood returning from the lungs via the pulmonary veins. The pulmonary veins become engorged and fluid seeps out through the veins and collects in the pleural cavity. Pulmonary edema and pleural effusion result. In many cases heart failure begins on the left side and eventually involves both sides of the heart.

right ventricular h. f., failure of proper functioning of the right ventricle, with subsequent engorgement of the systemic veins, producing swelling of the legs, enlargement of the liver and ascites.

total h. f., a condition due to weakening of the myocardium as a whole, with engorgement of the neck veins and liver, and edema of the legs.

unilateral h. f., inadequate output of blood involving only one side of the heart.

heart-lung machine a mechanical device that temporarily takes over the functions of the heart and lungs; called also a pump-oxygenator. It is used as an aid to surgery.

The "heart" of the machine is a pump that draws blood from the patient's vessels before it reaches the heart. The blood is routed through a "lung" chamber (usually made of plastic), where it receives oxygen. The oxygenated blood is then returned to the patient's vessels and pumped through his circulatory system. This method of circulating the blood outside the patient's body is known as extracorporeal circulation.

heart murmur any sound in the heart region other than normal heart sounds (see also MURMUR). A murmur may be caused by several different factors, including changes in the valves of the heart or blood leaking through a disease-scarred valve that does not close properly.

RHEUMATIC FEVER is a common cause of heart murmur. A murmur may also indicate other types of heart disease. In many cases, however, the murmur may be of the innocent or "functional" type, which does not indicate any heart damage at all and causes no trouble. Such murmurs vary from time to time, and often go away completely.

heart rate the number of contractions of the cardiac ventricles per unit of time.

heart sounds the sounds heard on the surface of the chest in the heart region. They are amplified by and heard more distinctly through a stethoscope. These sounds are caused by the vibrations of the normal cardiac cycle. They may be produced by muscular action, valvular actions, motion of the heart and blood as it passes through the heart.

The first heart sound is heard as a firm but not sharp "lubb" sound. It consists of four components: a low-frequency, indistinct vibration caused by ventricular contraction; a louder sound of higher frequency caused by closure of the mitral and tricuspid valves; a vibration caused by opening of the semilunar valves and early ejection of blood from the ventricles; and a low-pitched vibration produced by rapid ejection.

The second heart sound is shorter and higher pitched than the first, is heard as a "dupp" and is produced by closure of the aortic and pulmonary valves.

The third heart sound is very faint and is caused by blood rushing into the ventricles. It can be heard in most normal persons between the ages of 10 and 20 years.

The fourth heart sound is rarely audible in a normal heart but can be demonstrated on graphic records. It is short and of low frequency and intensity, and is caused by atrial contraction. The vibrations arise from atrial muscle and from blood flow into, and distention of, the ventricles.

ABNORMALITIES IN HEART SOUNDS. Failure of the heart muscle to contract is characterized by a gallop or triple rhythm. Accentuation of the third heart sound (protodiastolic gallop) is caused by the filling of a large flabby ventricle with blood under high venous pressure. A presystolic gallop is an accentuated fourth heart sound and is also caused by blood filling a dilated and inert ventricle. Merging of the third and fourth heart sounds is called a mesodiastolic or summation gallop. A very rare abnormality in which four heart sounds are heard distinctly is called a "locomotive" rhythm.

Extracorporeal circulation, illustrating flow of blood from the body and return. The coronary arteries are filled, but no blood enters the cardiac chambers (except coronary venous return). (From Storer, E. H., Pate, J. W., and Sherman, R. T.: The Science of Surgery. New York, McGraw-Hill Book Co., 1964.)

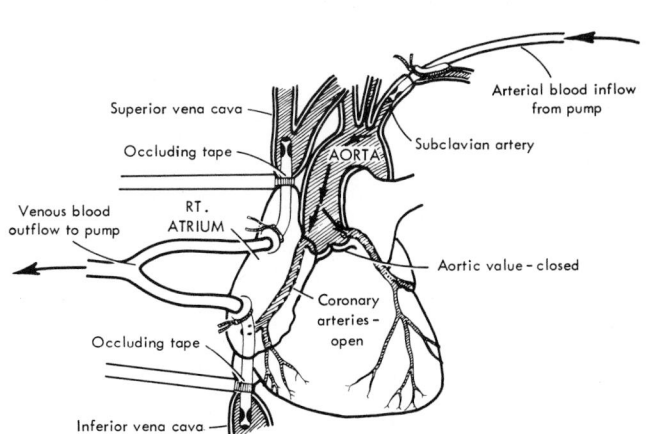

Superior vena cava

Occluding tape

Venous blood outflow to pump

RT. ATRIUM

Occluding tape

Inferior vena cava

AORTA

Arterial blood inflow from pump

Subclavian artery

Aortic value – closed

Coronary arteries – open

HEART MURMURS are sounds other than the normal heart sounds emanating from the heart region. They are often heard as blowing or hissing sounds as blood leaks through diseased and malfunctioning valves.

heartbeat (hart′bēt) the cycle of contraction of the heart muscle, during which the chambers of the heart contract. The beat begins with a rhythmic impulse in the sinoatrial node, which serves as a pacemaker for the heart. (See also HEART.)

heartburn (hart′burn) a burning sensation in the esophagus, or below the sternum in the region of the heart. It is one of the common symptoms of indigestion.

Heartburn often occurs when there is distention of a part of the esophagus, particularly the lower part. This may happen when the stomach regurgitates part of its contents, forcing them upward into the esophagus. Since this matter is acid, it acts as an irritant, producing discomfort or pain.

Excessive acidity (hyperacidity) is thought to be a cause of heartburn, occurring when the stomach secretes an excessive amount of hydrochloric acid. Recent evidence, however, indicates that hyperacidity in itself may not be the actual cause, and that heartburn results from excessive gastric secretions only when there is improper eating or emotional disturbance.

There is no doubt that emotional disturbance, excitement and nervous tension are frequent causes of heartburn. The functions of the stomach, both those of motion and secretion, are controlled by the VAGUS NERVE, one of the cranial nerves. Emotional stress can stimulate this nerve, which in turn starts the churning of the stomach and the flow of the various gastric juices; it can also cause contraction and spasm of the pylorus. If some of the stomach contents are displaced into the esophagus during this nervous activity, heartburn may result.

Treatment of heartburn is aimed at determining its underlying cause. Antacids may be used to relieve the symptoms but they will not cure heartburn and should not be used indiscriminately.

HEAT human erythrocyte agglutination test.

heat (hēt) energy that raises the temperature of a body or material substance; also, the rise of the temperature itself. Heat is a form of kinetic energy, associated with molecular motion, and generated in various ways, including combustion, friction, chemical action and radiation. The total absence of heat is absolute zero, at which all molecular activity ceases.

BODY HEAT. *Heat Production.* Body heat is the by-product of the metabolic processes of the body. The hormones thyroxine and epinephrine increase metabolism and consequently increase body heat. Muscular activity also produces body heat. At complete rest (basal metabolism) the amount of heat produced from muscular activity may be as low as 25 per cent of the total body heat. During exercise or shivering the percentage may rise to 60 per cent.

Body temperature is regulated by the thermostatic center in the HYPOTHALAMUS. A body temperature above the normal range is called FEVER.

Heat Loss. Loss of body heat occurs in three ways: by radiation (heat waves), by conduction to air or objects in contact with the body and by evaporation of perspiration. Some body heat is lost in expiration of air and in elimination of urine and feces.

APPLICATIONS OF EXTERNAL HEAT. *Purposes.* Local applications of heat may be used to provide warmth and promote comfort, rest and relaxation. Heat is also applied locally to promote suppuration and drainage from an infected area by hastening the inflammatory process; to relieve congestion and swelling by dilating the blood vessels, thereby increasing circulation; and to improve repair of diseased or injured tissues by increasing local metabolism.

Effects. Factors that determine the physiologic action of heat include the type of heat used, length of time it is applied, age and general condition of the patient and area of body surface to which the heat is applied. Moist heat is more penetrating than dry heat. Prolonged applications of heat produce an increase in skin secretions, resulting in a softening of the skin and a lowering of its resistance. Extreme heat produces constriction of the blood vessels; moderate heat produces vascular dilation. Repeated applications of heat will result in an increased tolerance to heat so that the individual may be burned without his being aware of it. Elderly persons and infants are more susceptible to burns from high temperatures.

Heat applied to an infected area can localize the infection; for this reason, external heat should not be applied to the abdomen when appendicitis is suspected because it may lead to rupture of the inflamed appendix.

Methods. Heat may be applied in the form of hot water bottles, electric or chemical heating pads, heat lamps or an electric light bulb with a heat cradle.

1. Basal metabolism

2. Muscular activity
— Shivering —

3. Thyroxine effect on cells

4. Sympathetic effect on cells

5. Temperature effect on cells

1. Radiation

2. Evaporation
—Convection—

3. Conduction
—Convection—

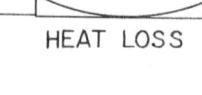

HEAT PRODUCTION   HEAT LOSS

Balance of heat production versus heat loss. (From Guyton, A. C.: Textbook of Medical Physiology. 4th ed. Philadelphia, W. B. Saunders Co., 1971.)

Hot water bottles should be filled with water not exceeding 125° F., and should be about half full; the air is expelled before the bottle is sealed. The hot water bottle is covered with a flannel or cotton covering before it is applied and this covering should remain dry at all times, unless the hot water bottle is used over moist dressings to keep them warm. The hot water bottle should be refilled at least every 2 hours.

Electric heating pads are never used over wet dressings or in other areas where moisture may come in contact with the electricity. Those used in hospitals should have an automatic control and the thermostat should be turned to low or medium.

Chemical heating pads, such as the Hydrocollator Pack, require the addition of hot water to the pad so that a heat-producing chemical reaction will take place. These pads are heavier than electric heating pads and hot water bottles but even so the patient should not be allowed to lie on the pad because a serious burn may result. The pad should be supported over the patient so that its weight does not cause discomfort. It provides moist heat for a prolonged period of time, and one must always be aware of the danger of burning the patient. Most chemical heating pads require at least 12 thicknesses of towelling between the pad and the patient.

Heat lamps may generate heat through ultraviolet or infrared radiation. Ultraviolet rays are more penetrating than infrared rays. Moderate radiation from ultraviolet rays produces local vasodilation and stimulates growth of tissue cells. It must be used with caution because of the danger of producing deep burns.

Infrared rays provide surface heat but penetrate to a depth of only 10 mm. Prolonged and intense application can lead to burning and blistering of the skin. Before being exposed to infrared rays, the skin should be cleansed and all ointments or other medicinal preparations removed.

The heat cradle employs an ordinary bed cradle to support the top bed covers and an electric light bulb to generate heat. This type of apparatus is often used for patients with circulatory disturbances of the extremities.

Uses. Local applications of heat are used for a variety of disorders. Perineal lacerations and surgical incisions heal more readily when dry heat is applied. Circulatory disturbances of the extremities, and the ulcers they sometimes cause, are amenable to applications of heat. Moderate heat is used to relax the muscles and reduce spasm that often accompanies muscle strain.

Heat, applied by boiling, autoclaving, flaming or burning, is a commonly used physical antiseptic.

h. exhaustion, a disorder resulting from overexposure to heat or to the sun; called also heat prostration. Long exposure to extreme heat or too much activity under a hot sun causes excessive sweating, which removes large quantities of salt and fluid from the body. When the amount of salt and fluid in the body falls too far below normal, heat exhaustion may result.

SYMPTOMS. The early symptoms of heat exhaustion are headache and a feeling of weakness and dizziness, usually accompanied by nausea and vomiting. There may also be cramps in the muscles of the arms, legs or abdomen. These first symptoms are similar to the early signs of SUNSTROKE, or heat stroke, but the disorders are not the same and should be treated differently. In heat exhaustion, the person turns pale and perspires profusely. His skin is cool and moist, his pulse and breathing are rapid. His body temperature remains at a normal level or slightly below or above. He may seem confused and may find it difficult to coordinate his body movements. Ordinarily he remains conscious.

TREATMENT. In cases of heat exhaustion, a physician should be called and the victim should lie quietly in a cool place. He should be given half a teaspoonful of salt dissolved in tomato juice or in half a glass of water every 15 minutes for 2 hours if he tolerates it. After he has taken the salt, hot tea or coffee may be given.

If the condition is accompanied by cramps, the pain may be relieved by gentle massage of the painful area or by firm hand pressure. In cases of severe heat exhaustion and cramps, it may be necessary to keep the victim at rest in bed for a day or more.

PREVENTION. Heat exhaustion and other heat disorders may be prevented by avoiding long exposure to sun or heat. When the weather is very hot, or when working in an extremely hot place, it is essential to drink plenty of water. Salt tablets should be taken if the stomach tolerates them, or a half to one teaspoonful of salt can be added to each quart of drinking water. Regular breaks from work are necessary, and in the event of weakness or dizziness, the victim should stop working at once and rest in a cool place.

latent h., the heat that a body may absorb without changing its temperature.

molecular h., the product of the molecular weight of a substance multiplied by its specific heat.

prickly h., h. rash, miliaria; inflammation of the skin, due to retention of sweat, occurring during hot, humid weather.

sensible h., the heat that, when absorbed by a body, produces a rise in temperature.

specific h., the number of calories required to raise the temperature of 1 Gm. of a particular substance one degree centigrade.

h. stroke, sunstroke.

hebephrenia (heb″ĕ-fre′ne-ah) a clinical form of schizophrenia coming on soon after the onset of puberty and marked by rapid deterioration, hallucinations, absurd delusions, senseless laughter and silly mannerisms (see also PSYCHOSIS). adj., **hebephren′ic.**

Heberden's disease (he′ber-denz) rheumatoid arthritis.

H's nodes, small, hard nodules, formed usually at the distal interphalangeal joints of the fingers in osteoarthritis.

hebetic (hĕ-bet-′ik) pertaining to puberty.

hebetude (heb′ĕ-tūd) mental dullness.

heboidophrenia (hĕ-boi″do-fre′ne-ah) schizophrenia marked by simple dementia.

hebosteotomy, hebotomy (he-bos″te-ot′o-me), (he-bot′o-me) pubiotomy.

hecatomeric (hek″ah-to-mer′ik) having processes that divide in two, one going to each side of the spinal cord; said of certain neurons.

hecto- (hek′to) word element [Fr.], *hundred;* used in naming units of measurement to designate an amount 100 times (10^2) the size of the unit to which it is joined, e.g., hectoliter (100 liters).

hectogram   (hek′to-gram) one hundred grams; 3.53 ounces.

hectoliter (hek′to-le″ter) one hundred liters; 26.42 gallons.

hectometer (hek′to-me″ter) one hundred meters; 109.36 yards.

hedonism   (he′don-izm) excessive devotion to pleasure.

Hedulin (hed′u-lin) trademark for a preparation of phenindione, an anticoagulant.

heel (hēl) the hindmost part of the foot; by extension, a part comparable to the heel of the foot, or the hindmost portion of an elongate structure.
    Thomas h., a shoe correction consisting of a heel ½ inch longer and ⅙ to ⅛ inch higher on the inside; used to bring the heel of the foot into varus and to prevent depression in the region of the head of the talus.

Heerfordt's disease (hār′forts) uveoparotid fever.

Hegar's sign (ha′garz) compressibility of the cervix, owing to softening of the isthmus of the uterus in early pregnancy.

Heine-Medin disease (hi′nĕ-ma′din) poliomyelitis.

HeLa cells (he′lah) cells of the first continuously cultured carcinoma strain, descended from a human cervical carcinoma; used in the study of life processes, including viruses, at the cell level.

helcoid (hel′koid) like an ulcer.

helcology   (hel-kol′o-je) the science of ulcers.

helcoplasty (hel′ko-plas″te) plastic surgery of ulcers.

helcosis (hel-ko′sis) the formation of an ulcer.

Heleidae (hĕ-le′ĭ-de) a family of flies, species of which suck the blood of man and may serve as vectors of disease.

heli(o)- (he′le-o) word element [Gr.], *sun.*

helianthin (he″le-an′thin) an orange-yellow aniline dye used as a pH indicator.

helicine (hel′ĭ-sin) spiral.

helicoid (hel′ĭ-koid) coiled; spiral.

helicopodia   (hel″ĭ-ko-po′de-ah)   a   peculiar dragging gait of certain paralyses.

helicotrema (hel″ĭ-ko-tre′mah) the passage that connects the scala tympani and the scala vestibuli at the apex of the cochlea.

heliophobia (he″le-o-fo′be-ah) morbid fear of sunlight.

heliotaxis (he″le-o-tak′sis) the motile response of an organism to the stimulus of light.

heliotherapy (he″le-o-ther′ah-pe) treatment of disease by exposing the body to the sun's rays; therapeutic use of the sun bath.

heliotropism   (he″li-ot′ro-pizm) the tendency of an organism to orient itself in relation to the stimulus of light.

helium (he′le-um) a chemical element, atomic number 2, atomic weight 4.003, symbol He. (See table of ELEMENTS.)

helix (he′liks) 1. a coiled structure. 2. the superior and posterior free margin of the pinna of the ear.
    Watson-Crick h., a representation of the structure of deoxyribonucleic acid (DNA), consisting of two coiled chains, each of which contains information completely specifying the other chain.

Hellin's law (hel′inz) one in about 80 pregnancies ends in the birth of twins; one in about 6400, of triplets; one in about 512,000, of quadruplets.

helminth (hel′minth) a worm or wormlike parasitic organism.

helminthagogue (hel-min′thah-gog) vermifuge; an agent that expels worms or intestinal animal parasites.

helminthemesis (hel″min-them′ĕ-sis) the vomiting of worms.

helminthiasis   (hel″min-thi′ah-sis) a morbid state due to infection with worms.

helminthicide   (hel-min′thĭ-sīd) vermicide, an agent that destroys worms or intestinal animal parasites.

helminthology   (hel″min-thol′o-je) the scientific study of worms.

helminthoma (hel″min-tho′mah) a tumor caused by a parasitic worm.

heloma (he-lo′mah) a corn.
    h. du′rum, hard corn, the usual type occurring over joints of the toes.
    h. mol′le, a soft corn.

helotomy (he-lot′o-me) excision of a corn or callus.

hemabarometer (hem″ah-bah-rom′ĕ-ter) an instrument for ascertaining the specific gravity of blood.

hemachrome (he′mah-krōm, hem′ah-krōm) the red coloring matter of blood.

hemacyanin (he″mah-si′ah-nin) hematocyanin.

hemacyte (he′mah-sīt) hemocyte; a blood corpuscle.

hemacytometer (he″mah-si-tom′ĕ-ter) an instrument used in counting blood cells, commonly applied to a combination of counting chambers with coverglasses and pipets for erythrocytes and leukocytes, all meeting established specifications.

hemacytozoon (he″mah-si″to-zo′on) hemocytozoon.

hemad (he′mad) toward the hemal or ventral side.

hemadynamometer (he″mah-di″nah-mom′ĕ-ter) an instrument for measuring blood pressure; hemodynamometer.

hemadynamometry (he″mah-di″nah-mom′ĕ-tre) measurement of blood pressure.

hemafacient   (he″mah-fa′shent)   1.   producing

blood; hematopoietic. 2. an agent that induces the production of blood.

hemagglutination (he″mah-gloo″tĭ-na′shun) agglutination of erythrocytes.

hemagglutinin (he″mah-gloo′tĭ-nin) an antibody that causes agglutination of erythrocytes.

cold h., one that acts only at temperatures near 4° C.

warm h., one that acts only at temperatures near 37° C.

hemagogue (he′mah-gog) promoting the discharge of blood from the body.

hemal (he′mal) pertaining to blood or blood vessels.

hemanalysis (he″mah-nal′ĭ-sis) analysis of the blood.

hemangiectasis (he-man″je-ek′tah-sis) dilatation of blood vessels.

hemangioblast (he-man′je-o-blast″) a mesodermal cell that gives rise to both vascular endothelium and hemocytoblasts.

hemangioblastoma (he-man″je-o-blas-to′mah) a capillary hemangioma of the brain consisting of proliferated blood vessel cells or angioblasts.

hemangioendothelioblastoma (he-man″je-o-en″do-the″le-o-blas-to′mah) a tumor of mesenchymal origin of which the cells tend to form endothelial cells and line blood vessels.

hemangioendothelioma (he-man″je-o-en″do-the″le-o′mah) a true neoplasm consisting predominantly of masses of endothelial cells growing in and about vascular channels.

hemangioma (he-man″je-o′mah) a benign tumor made up of newly formed blood vessels, clustered together. Hemangioma may be present at birth in various parts of the body, including the liver and bones. In the majority of cases, however, it appears as a network of small blood-filled capillaries near the surface of the skin, forming a reddish or purplish birthmark. These marks are not malignant.

Types of hemangiomas include "strawberry" or "raspberry" marks, port-wine stains and cavernous hemangiomas; the latter is a less common type in which the birthmark has a soft, spongy consistency. With the exception of port-wine stains, superficial hemangiomas often disappear of their own accord as the person grows older. Cavernous hemangiomas should be treated early, since the lesions tend to grow and there is the possibility of severe hemorrhage should the lesion be injured and start to bleed. Treatment is by irradiation, injection of a sclerosing agent or surgery.

hemangiopericyte (he-man″je-o-per′ĭ-sīt) pericyte.

hemangiopericytoma (he-man″je-o-per″ĭ-si-to′mah) a tumor composed of spindled cells with a rich vascular network, which apparently arises from pericytes.

hemangiosarcoma (he-man″je-o-sar-ko′mah) a malignant tumor of vascular tissue; called also angiosarcoma.

hemaphein (hem″ah-fe′in) a brown coloring matter of the blood and urine.

hemapoiesis (hem″ah-poi-e′sis) hematopoiesis.

hemapophysis (hem″ah-pof′ĭ-sis) a costal cartilage.

hemarthros, hemarthrosis (hem-ar′thros), (hem″ar-thro′sis) blood in a joint cavity.

hemase (hem′ās) an enzyme found in the blood.

hemasthenosis (hem″as-thĕ-no′sis) defective state or defective circulation of the blood.

hemat(o)- (hem′ah-to) word element [Gr.], *blood.* See also words beginning *hem-* and *hemo-.*

hematachometer (hem″ah-tah-kom′ĕ-ter) an instrument for measuring the speed of blood currents; hemotachometer.

hemataerometer (hem″at-a″er-om′ĕ-ter) an instrument for measuring gases in the blood.

hematein (hem″ah-te′in) a compound occurring in reddish brown plates with a metallic luster; the coloring principle of hematoxylin.

hematemesis (hem″ah-tem′ĕ-sis) the vomiting of blood. The appearance of the vomitus depends on the amount and character of the gastric contents at the time blood is vomited and on the length of time the blood has been in the stomach. Gastric acids change bright red blood to a brownish color and the vomitus is often described as "coffee-ground" color. Bright red blood in the vomitus indicates a fresh hemorrhage and little contact of the blood with gastric juices.

The most common causes of hematemesis are peptic ulcer, gastritis, esophageal lesions or varices and cancer of the stomach. Benign tumors, traumatic postoperative bleeding and swallowed blood from points in the nose, mouth and throat can also produce hematemesis.

hematencephalon (hem″at-en-sef′ah-lon) effusion of blood in the brain.

hematherapy (hem″ah-ther′ah-pe) treatment of disease by administration of blood; hemotherapy.

hemathermous (hem″ah-ther′mus) warm-blooded; hematothermal.

hematic (he-mat′ik) pertaining to the blood.

hematidrosis (hem″ah-tĭ-dro′sis) excretion of bloody sweat.

hematimeter (hem″ah-tim′ĕ-ter) device for counting blood corpuscles; a hemacytometer.

hematin (hem′ah-tin) heme.

hematinemia (hem″ah-tĭ-ne′me-ah) the presence of heme (hematin) in the blood.

hematinic (hem″ah-tin′ik) an agent that increases the amount of hemoglobin in the circulating blood, for example, iron preparations, liver extract, whole blood, and the B complex vitamins.

hematinometer (hem″ah-tĭ-nom′ĕ-ter) an instrument for measuring the hemoglobin of the blood; hemoglobinometer.

hematobilia (hem″ah-to-bil′e-ah) bleeding into the biliary passages.

hematobium (hem″ah-to'be-um) an organism living in the blood.

hematoblast (hem'ah-to-blast″) a cell that develops into an erythrocyte.

hematocele (hem'ah-to-sēl″) an effusion of blood into a cavity, especially into the tunica vaginalis testis.

hematocelia (hem″ah-to-se'le-ah) effusion of blood into the peritoneal cavity.

hematochezia (hem″ah-to-ke'ze-ah) blood in the feces.

hematochromatosis (hem″ah-to-kro″mah-to'sis) staining of tissues with blood pigment.

hematochyluria (hem″ah-to-ki-lu're-ah) blood and chyle in the urine.

hematocolpometra (hem″ah-to-kol″po-me'trah) progressive accumulation of menstrual blood in the vagina and uterus.

hematocolpos (hem″ah-to-kol'pos) accumulation of blood in the vagina.

hematocrit (he-mat'o-krit) the volume percentage of erythrocytes in whole blood. The hematocrit (which means, literally, "to separate blood") is determined by centrifuging a blood sample to separate the cellular elements from the plasma; the results of the test indicate the ratio of cell volume to plasma volume and are expressed as milliliters of packed cells per 100 ml. of blood, or in volumes per 100 ml. Normal range is 45 to 50 volumes per 100 ml. for males, and 40 to 45 volumes per 100 ml. for females. The hematocrit, in conjunction with other hematologic tests, provides information about the size, functioning capacity and number of erythrocytes.

hematocryal (hem″ah-to-kri'al) cold-blooded.

hematocrystallin (hem″ah-to-kris'tah-lin) hemoglobin.

hematocyanin (hem″ah-to-si'ah-nin) a chromoprotein occurring in the blood of mollusks and arthropods. It is a blue respiratory pigment and contains 0.17 to 0.38 per cent of copper.

hematocyst (hem'ah-to-sist″) effusion of blood in the bladder or in a cyst.

hematocytopenia (hem″ah-to-si″to-pe'ne-ah) decrease in the cellular elements of the blood.

hematocytosis (hem″ah-to-si-to'sis) increase in the cellular elements of the blood.

hematocyturia (hem″ah-to-si-tu're-ah) blood corpuscles in the urine.

hematodialysis (hem″ah-to-di-al'ĭ-sis) hemodialysis.

hematogen (hem'ah-to-jen″) any blood-producing substance.

hematogenesis (hem″ah-to-jen'ĕ-sis) the formation of blood.

hematogenic (hem″ah-to-jen'ik) 1. hematopoietic. 2. hematogenous.

hematogenous (hem″ah-toj'ĕ-nus) produced by or derived from the blood; disseminated through the bloodstream or by the circulation.

hematoid (hem'ah-toid) like blood.

hematoidin (hem″ah-toi'din) a crystalline pigment lacking iron, generally found where blood has extravasated into the tissues.

hematologist (he″mah-tol'o-jist) a specialist in hematology.

hematology (he″mah-tol'o-je) the science dealing with study of the blood. adj., **hematolog'ic.**

hematolymphangioma (hem″ah-to-lim-fan″je-o'mah) a tumor composed of blood and lymph vessels.

hematolysis (hem″ah-tol'ĭ-sis) hemolysis.

hematoma (he″mah-to'mah) a tumor-like mass produced by coagulation of extravasated blood in a tissue or cavity. Contusions (bruises) and black eyes are familiar forms of hematoma that are seldom serious. Hematomas can occur almost anywhere on the body; they are almost always present with a fracture and are especially serious when they occur inside the skull, where they may produce local pressure on the brain. In minor injuries the blood is absorbed unless infection develops.

CRANIAL HEMATOMA. The two most common kinds of cranial hematomas are extradural (epidural) and subdural. The word dural refers to the dura mater. Extradural hematoma occurs above the dura mater, between it and the skull. It is most often caused by a heavy blow to the head that damages the upper surface of the dura mater. Blood seeps into the surrounding tissue, forming a tumor-like mass or hematoma. Since the skull is rigid, the hematoma presses inward against the brain. If the pressure continues, the brain can be affected. An extradural hematoma can involve rupture of an artery, with hemorrhage, causing severe pressure that can be quickly fatal.

Subdural hematoma occurs beneath the dura mater, between the tough casing and the more delicate membranes covering the tissue of the brain, the pia-arachnoid. This kind of injury is more often caused by the head's striking an immovable object, such as the floor, than by a blow from a moving object. There may be no severe head injury or fracture. A blow to the head can cause the brain to move violently, tearing blood vessels and forming a swelling that may include fluid from the brain tissue. A chronic subdural hematoma may remain and increase in size.

Symptoms. The most common symptoms of extradural hematoma occur within a few hours after injury. There can be a sudden or gradual loss of consciousness, partial or full paralysis on the side opposite the injury and dilation of the pupil of the eye on the same side as the injury.

The symptoms of chronic subdural hematoma are similar to those of a brain tumor, and may come and go. Diagnosis is difficult, particularly in older people. There may be subtle personality changes, or the patient may become confused, weak in various parts of the body, vague and drowsy.

Subdural hematoma may occasionally occur in babies as a result of birth injury. Unless the injury is discovered and treated at an early stage, the child's mental and physical development may be retarded, and spastic paralysis can occur. Early surgery is usually successful in preventing permanent symptoms and disabilities.

Treatment. Prompt surgery is the only treatment for extradural hematoma. The clotted blood is removed by a combination of suction and irrigation methods through openings made in the skull, and the bleeding is controlled. The same surgery is used for subdural hematomas.

SEPTAL HEMATOMA. Injury to the nose sometimes causes hematoma of the nasal septum. Its symptoms include nasal obstruction and headache. The condition may be treated by incision and drainage or may clear up spontaneously in a few weeks. If the hematoma becomes infected, an abscess may result, requiring drainage and treatment with antibiotics.

hematomediastinum (hem″ah-to-me″de-ah-sti′-num) effusion of blood in the mediastinum.

hematometra (hem″ah-to-me′trah) progressive accumulation of menstrual blood in the uterus.

hematometry (he″mah-tom′ĕ-tre) measurement of hemoglobin and various cells of the blood.

hematomphalocele (hem″at-om-fal′o-sēl) umbilical hernia containing blood.

hematomphalus (hem″at-om′fah-lus) 1. hematomphalocele. 2. blue discoloration around the navel in ruptured ectopic pregnancy.

hematomycosis (hem″ah-to-mi-ko′sis) the presence of a fungus in the blood.

hematomyelia (hem″ah-to-mi-e′le-ah) hemorrhage into the gray matter of the spinal cord.

hematomyelitis (hem″ah-to-mi″ĕ-li′tis) acute myelitis with bloody effusion.

hematomyelopore (hem″ah-to-mi′ĕ-lo-pōr″) formation of canals in the spinal cord due to hemorrhage.

hematonephrosis (hem″ah-to-nĕ-fro′sis) the presence of blood in the renal pelvis.

hematopathology (hem″ah-to-pah-thol′o-je) the study of diseases of the blood; hemopathology.

hematophagous (hem″ah-tof′ah-gus) subsisting on blood.

hematophilia (hem″ah-to-fil′e-ah) hemophilia.

hematophyte (hem′ah-to-fīt″) any vegetative microorganism or species living in the blood.

hematopneic (hem″ah-top-ne′ik) pertaining to oxygenation of the blood.

hematopoiesis (hem″ah-to-poi-e′sis) production of blood or of its constituent elements, usually taking place in the bone marrow. adj., **hematopoiet′-ic.**

extramedullary h., the formation of and development of blood cells outside the bone marrow, as in the spleen, liver and lymph nodes.

hematoporphyria (hem″ah-to-por-fēr′e-ah) a constitutional state marked by abnormal quantity of porphyrin (uroporphyrin and coproporphyrin) in the tissues and secreted in the urine, pigmentation of the face (and later of the bones), sensitivity of the skin to light, vomiting and intestinal disturbance; called also PORPHYRIA.

hematoporphyrin (hem″ah-to-por′fĭ-rin) an iron-free derivative of heme, a product of the decomposition of hemoglobin.

hematoporphyrinemia (hem″ah-to-por″fĭ-rĭ-ne′-me-ah) hematoporphyrin in the blood.

hematoporphyrinism (hem″ah-to-por′fĭ-rin-izm″) a condition marked by hematoporphyrinemia and sensitivity to sunlight.

hematoporphyrinuria (hem″ah-to-por″fĭ-rĭ-nu′-re-ah) hematoporphyrin in the urine.

hematorhachis (hem″ah-tor′ah-kis) hemorrhage into or beneath the meninges of the spinal cord.

hematorrhea (hem″ah-to-re′ah) copious hemorrhage.

hematosalpinx (hem″ah-to-sal′pinks) an accumulation of blood in the uterine tube.

hematoscheocele (hem″ah-tos′ke-o-sēl″) hematoma of the scrotum.

hematoscope (hem′ah-to-skōp″) a device used in examining thin layers of blood.

hematoscopy (hem″ah-tos′ko-pe) the inspection of blood.

hematosepsis (hem″ah-to-sep′sis) septicemia; the presence of bacteria or their toxins in the blood.

hematospectroscopy (hem″ah-to-spek-tros′ko-pe) spectroscopic examination of blood.

hematospermatocele (hem″ah-to-sper-mat′o-sēl) a spermatocele containing blood.

hematospermia (hem″ah-to-sper′me-ah) blood in the semen.

hematosteon (hem″ah-tos′te-on) hemorrhage into the medullary cavity of a bone.

hematothermal (hem″ah-to-ther′mal) warm-blooded.

hematotoxic (hem″ah-to-tok′sik) 1. pertaining to hematotoxicosis. 2. poisonous to the blood and hematopoietic system.

hematotoxicosis (hem″ah-to-tok″sĭ-ko′sis) toxic damage to the blood-forming organs.

hematotrachelos (hem″ah-to-trah-ke′los) distention of the cervix uteri with blood, because of atresia of the ostium uteri or the vagina.

hematotropic (hem″ah-to-trop′ik) having a special affinity for the blood or erythrocytes.

hematoxylin (hem″ah-tok′sĭ-lin) an acid coloring matter obtained from the wood of a tree (*Haematoxylon campechianum*); used as a stain for histologic specimens.

hematozoon (hem″ah-to-zo′on) any animal microorganism or species living in the blood.

hematuresis (hem″ah-tu-re′sis) hematuria.

hematuria (hem″ah-tu′re-ah) the discharge of blood in the urine. The urine may be slightly blood tinged, grossly bloody or a smoky brown color.

Hematuria is symptomatic of disease or injury to a part of the urinary system. Tumors of the bladder, cystitis, urethritis and small kidney stones passing along the ureter can cause blood in the urine. Vascular diseases and some types of kidney disorders produce hematuria. Traumatic injury to the kidney is usually but not always accompanied by hematuria.

Nursing Care. When hematuria is suspected because of the outward appearance of the urine, a specimen should be saved and sent to the laboratory for microscopic analysis. An accurate record of the patient's intake and output is kept and the characteristics of the urine should be noted on the patient's chart. If hematuria occurs suddenly and unexpectedly this should be reported immediately to the physician in charge.

heme (hēm) the nonprotein, insoluble, iron protoporphyrin constituent of hemoglobin, of various other respiratory pigments and of many cells, both animal and vegetable. It is an iron compound of protoporphyrin and so constitutes the pigment portion or protein-free part of the hemoglobin molecule. Formerly called hematin.

hemeralopia (hem″er-al-o′pe-ah) day blindness; defective vision in a bright light.

hemi- (hem′ĭ) word element [Gr.], *half.*

hemiacardius (hem″e-ah-kar′de-us) an unequal twin in which the heart is rudimentary.

hemiachromatopsia (hem″e-ah-kro″mah-top′se-ah) loss of the normal perception of color in half of the visual field.

hemiamyosthenia (hem″e-ah-mi″os-the′ne-ah) lack of muscular power on one side of the body.

hemianacusia (hem″e-an″ah-koo′ze-ah) loss of hearing in one ear.

hemianalgesia (hem″e-an″al-je′ze-ah) analgesia on one side of the body.

hemianencephaly (hem″e-an″en-sef′ah-le) congenital absence of one side of the brain.

hemianesthesia (hem″e-an″es-the′ze-ah) anesthesia of one side of the body.

hemianopia, hemianopsia (hem″e-ah-no′pe-ah), (hem″e-ah-nop′se-ah) defective vision or blindness in half of the visual field; usually applied to bilateral defects caused by a single lesion.

hemianosmia (hem″e-an-oz′me-ah) absence of the sense of smell in one nostril.

hemiapraxia (hem″e-ah-prak′se-ah) inability to perform coordinated movements on one side of the body.

hemiataxia (hem″e-ah-tak′se-ah) ataxia on one side of the body.

hemiatrophy (hem″e-at′ro-fe) atrophy of one side of the body.

hemiballismus (hem″ĭ-bah-liz′mus) violent motor restlessness of half of the body, most marked in the upper extremity.

hemic (he′mik, hem′ik) pertaining to blood.

hemicardia (hem″ĭ-kar′de-ah) the presence of only one side of a four-chambered heart.

hemicellulose (hem″ĭ-sel′u-lōs) a cellular plant material that is more soluble than cellulose.

hemicephalia (hem″ĭ-sĕ-fa′le-ah) congenital absence of one side of the skull.

hemicephalus (hem″ĭ-sef′ah-lus) a monster with one cerebral hemisphere.

hemichromatopsia (hem″ĭ-kro″mah-top′se-ah) defective perception of color in half of the visual field.

hemicolectomy (hem″ĭ-ko-lek′to-me) excision of approximately half of the colon.

hemicorporectomy (hem″ĭ-kor″po-rek′to-me) surgical removal of the lower part of the body, including the bony pelvis, external genitalia and the lower part of the rectum and anus.

hemicrania (hem″ĭ-kra′ne-ah) 1. headache on one side of the head. 2. a developmental anomaly with absence of half of the cranium.

hemicraniosis (hem″ĭ-kra″ne-o′sis) hyperostosis of one side of the cranium and face.

hemidiaphoresis (hem″ĭ-di″ah-fo-re′sis) sweating of one side of the body.

hemidysesthesia (hem″ĭ-dis″es-the′ze-ah) a disorder of sensation affecting only one side of the body.

hemidystrophy (hem″ĭ-dis′tro-fe) unequal development of the two sides of the body.

hemiectromelia (hem″e-ek″tro-me′le-ah) a developmental anomaly with imperfect limbs on one side of the body.

hemiepilepsy (hem″e-ep′ĭ-lep″se) epilepsy of one side of the body.

hemifacial hem″ĭ-fa′shal) affecting one side of the face.

hemigastrectomy (hem″ĭ-gas-trek′to-me) excision of half of the stomach.

hemigeusia (hem″ĭ-gu′ze-ah) absence of the sense of taste on one side of the tongue.

hemiglossectomy (hem″ĭ-glŏ-sek′to-me) excision of part of the tongue.

hemiglossitis (hem″ĭ-glŏ-si′tis) inflammation of half of the tongue

hemignathia (hem″ĭ-na′the-ah) a developmental anomaly characterized by partial or complete lack of the lower jaw on one side.

hemihidrosis (hem″ĭ-hĭ-dro′sis) sweating on one side of the body.

hemihypalgesia (hem″ĭ-hi″pal-je′ze-ah) diminished sensitivity to pain on one side of the body.

hemihyperesthesia (hem″ĭ-hi″per-es-the′ze-ah) increased sensitivity of one side of the body.

hemihyperhidrosis (hem″ĭ-hi″per-hĭ-dro′sis) excessive perspiration on one side of the body.

hemihyperplasia (hem″ĭ-hi″per-pla′ze-ah) overdevelopment of one side of the body or of half of an organ or part.

hemihypertonia (hem″ĭ-hi″per-to′ne-ah) increased tonicity of muscles on one side of the body.

hemihypertrophy (hem″ĭ-hi-per′tro-fe) overgrowth of one side of the body.

hemihypesthesia (hem″ĭ-hi″pes-the′ze-ah) diminished sensitivity on one side of the body.

hemihypoplasia (hem″ĭ-hi″po-pla′ze-ah) underdevelopment of one side of the body or of half of an organ or part.

hemihypotonia (hem″ĭ-hi″po-to′ne-ah) diminished tonicity of one side of the body.

hemilaminectomy (hem″ĭ-lam″ĭ-nek′to-me) excision of part of a vertebral lamina.

hemilaryngectomy (hem″ĭ-lar″in-jek′to-me) excision of part of the larynx.

hemilateral (hem″ĭ-lat′er-al) affecting one side of the body only.

hemilesion (hem″ĭ-le′zhun) a lesion on one side of the spinal cord.

hemimelia (hem″ĭ-me′le-ah) a developmental anomaly characterized by absence of all or part of the distal half of a limb.

heminephrectomy (hem″ĭ-ne-frek′to-me) excision of part (half) of a kidney.

hemiopia (hem″e-o′pe-ah) hemianopia.

hemipagus (hem-ip′ah-gus) twin fetuses joined at the thorax.

hemiparalysis (hem″ĭ-pah-ral′ĭ-sis) paralysis of one side of the body.

hemiparanesthesia (hem″ĭ-par″an-es-the′ze-ah) anesthesia of the lower half of one side.

hemiparaplegia (hem″ĭ-par″ah-ple′je-ah) paralysis of the lower half of one side.

hemiparesis (hem″ĭ-par′ĕ-sis) paralysis affecting one side of the body.

hemiparesthesia (hem″ĭ-par″es-the′ze-ah) perverted sensation on one side.

hemipeptone (hem″ĭ-pep′tōn) a form of peptone obtained from pepsin digestion.

hemiplegia (hem″ĭ-ple′je-ah) paralysis of one side of the body; usually caused by a brain lesion, such as a tumor, or by a cerebral vascular accident. The paralysis occurs on the side opposite the brain disorder. This is explained by the fact that motor axons from the cerebral cortex enter the medulla oblongata and form two well defined bands known as the pyramidal tracts. The majority of the fibers in these tracts cross to the opposite side; therefore damage to the right hemisphere of the brain affects motor control of the left half of the body. (See also CEREBRAL VASCULAR ACCIDENT for symptoms and nursing care of the patient with hemiplegia.)

hemiprostatectomy (hem″ĭ-pros″tah-tek′to-me) excision of half of the prostate.

Hemiptera (hem-ip′ter-ah) an order of arthropods (class Insecta) characterized usually by the presence of two pairs of wings; including some 30,000 species, known as the true bugs, and characterized by having mouth parts adapted to piercing or sucking.

hemipyocyanin (hem″ĭ-pi″o-si′ah-nin) an antibiotic produced by the growth of *Pseudomonas aeruginosa,* which is active against certain fungi.

hemirachischisis (hem″ĭ-rah-kis′kĭ-sis) fissure of the vertebral column without prolapse of the spinal cord.

hemisacralization (hem″ĭ-sa″kral-ĭ-za′shun) fusion of the fifth lumbar vertebra to the first segment of the sacrum on only one side.

hemisection (hem″ĭ-sek′shun) division into two parts.

hemispasm (hem′ĭ-spazm) spasm affecting only one side.

hemisphere (hem′ĭ-sfēr) half of a spherical or roughly spherical structure or organ.
  cerebral h., one of the paired structures constituting the largest part of the brain, consisting of the extensive cerebral cortex, corpus striatum and rhinencephalon, and containing the lateral ventricle.
  dominant h., that cerebral hemisphere which is more concerned than the other in the integration of sensations and the control of many functions.

hemispherium (hem″ĭ-sfe′re-um), pl. *hemisphe′-ria* [L.] hemisphere.

hemisystole (hem″ĭ-sis′to-le) absence of contraction of the left ventricle after every other contraction of the atrium.

hemithorax (hem″ĭ-tho′raks) one side of the chest; the cavity lateral to the mediastinum.

hemithyroidectomy (hem″ĭ-thi″roi-dek′to-me) excision of one lobe of the thyroid.

hemivagotony (hem″ĭ-va-got′o-ne) irritability of the vagus nerve on one side.

hemivertebra (hem″ĭ-ver′tĕ-brah) 1. either lateral half of a vertebra. 2. a developmental anomaly in which only half of a vertebra is present.

hemizygosity (hem″ĭ-zi-gos′ĭ-te) the state of having only one of a pair of alleles transmitting a specific character. adj., **hemizy′gous.**

hemizygote (hem″ĭ-zi′got) an individual exhibiting hemizygosity.

hemo- (he′mo) word element [Gr.], *blood.* See also words beginning *hem-* and *hemato-*.

hemoalkalimeter (he′mo-al″kah-lim′ĕ-ter) an apparatus for estimating the alkalinity of the blood.

hemobilia (he″mo-bil′e-ah) hematobilia.

hemobilinuria (he″mo-bil″ĭ-nu′re-ah) blood cells and bile pigments in the urine.

hemocatheresis (he″mo-kah-ther′ĕ-sis) the destruction of erythrocytes.

hemochorial (he″mo-ko′re-al) denoting a type of

placenta in which maternal blood comes in direct contact with the chorion.

hemochromatosis (he″mo-kro″mah-to′sis) a disorder of iron metabolism with excess deposition of iron in the tissues, skin pigmentation, cirrhosis of the liver and decreased carbohydrate tolerance. Called also bronze diabetes and iron storage disease.

hemochrome (he′mo-krōm) an oxygen-carrying pigment of the blood.

hemochromogen (he″mo-kro′mo-jen) a compound formed by the combination of heme with a nitrogenous compound.

hemochromometer (he″mo-kro-mom′ĕ-ter) an instrument for making color tests of the blood.

hemochromoprotein (he″mo-kro″mo-pro′te-in) a colored, conjugated protein with respiratory functions, found in the blood of animals.

hemocidal (he″mo-si′dal) destroying blood cells.

hemoclasis (he-mok′lah-sis) destruction of erythrocytes.

hemoconcentration (he″mo-kon″sen-tra′shun) increase in the proportion of formed elements in the blood.

hemocrystallin (he″mo-kris′tah-lin) hemoglobin.

hemoculture (he″mo-kul′tūr) a bacteriologic culture of the blood.

hemocuprein (he″mo-koo′prin) a copper and protein compound isolated from erythrocytes.

hemocyanin (he″mo-si′ah-nin) hematocyanin.

hemocyte (he′mo-sīt) a blood corpuscle.

hemocytoblast (he″mo-si′to-blast) a primitive cell from which all blood corpuscles develop.

hemocytoblastoma (he″mo-si″to-blas-to′mah) a tumor containing undifferentiated blood cells.

hemocytocatheresis (he″mo-si″to-kah-ther′ĕ-sis) destruction of erythrocytes.

hemocytogenesis (he″mo-si″to-jen′ĕ-sis) formation of blood cells.

hemocytology (he″mo-si-tol′o-je) the study of blood cells.

hemocytolysis (he″mo-si-tol′ĭ-sis) hemolysis.

hemocytometer (he″mo-si-tom′ĕ-ter) hemacytometer.

hemocytophagy (he″mo-si-tof′ah-je) ingestion and destruction of blood cells by the histiocytes of the reticuloendothelial system.

hemocytopoiesis (he″mo-si″to-poi-e′sis) formation of blood cells, hematopoiesis.

hemocytotripsis (he″mo-si″to-trip′sis) disintegration of blood cells by pressure.

hemocytozoon (he″mo-si″to-zo′on) a parasitic animal microorganism inhabiting blood cells.

hemodiagnosis (he″mo-di″ag-no′sis) diagnosis by examination of the blood.

hemodialysis (he″mo-di-al′ĭ-sis) removal of certain elements from the blood by virtue of difference in rates of their diffusion through a semipermeable membrane while the blood is being circulated outside the body. (See also KIDNEY.)

hemodialyzer (he″mo-di′ah-līz″er) an apparatus for performing hemodialysis.

hemodiastase (he″mo-di′as-tās) an enzyme found in the blood.

hemodilution (he″mo-di-lu′shun) increase in the fluid content of blood, resulting in diminution of the proportion of formed elements.

hemodipsia (he″mo-dip′se-ah) a desire to drink blood to assuage thirst.

hemodromometer (he″mo-dro-mom′ĕ-ter) an instrument for measuring the speed of the blood current.

hemodynamics (he″mo-di-nam′iks) the study of the movements of the blood.

hemodynamometer (he″mo-di″nah-mom′ĕ-ter) an instrument for measuring blood pressure.

hemoendothelial (he″mo-en-do-the′le-al) denoting a type of placenta in which maternal blood comes in contact with the endothelium of chorionic vessels.

hemoferrum (he″mo-fer′um) oxyhemoglobin.

hemoflagellate (he″mo-flaj′ĕ-lāt) a flagellate protozoan parasitic in the blood.

hemofuscin (he″mo-fus′in) brown coloring matter of the blood.

hemogenesis (he″mo-jen′ĕ-sis) the formation of blood; hematogenesis.

hemogenic (he″mo-jen′ik) pertaining to production of blood.

hemoglobin (he″mo-glo′bin) the oxygen-carrying pigment of the blood, the principal protein in the erythrocyte; it makes up approximately 33 per cent of the cell and averages between 14 and 16 Gm. per 100 ml. of whole blood. The pigment in hemoglobin gives blood its red color.

Hemoglobin is a chromoprotein, that is, a protein combined with a colored compound. The protein is globin; the pigment is heme, which is red. When erythrocytes are broken down, degradation of hemoglobin releases the pigment bilirubin which is converted into pigments responsible for the characteristic color of bile. Heme is a complex molecule containing iron.

Hemoglobin has the property of combining chemically with certain gases to form various substances; one of the most important is oxyhemoglobin, formed by the combination of oxygen and hemoglobin. This function of hemoglobin is important in respiration because it provides a means of transporting oxygen from the lungs to the tissues. The oxygen combined with hemoglobin in arterial blood is responsible for its bright red color; venous blood has a darker color because of its lower oxygen content.

Hemoglobin also combines readily with carbon monoxide; this is what happens in carbon monoxide poisoning.

Hemoglobin has been classified according to

various types. For example, adult hemoglobin, fetal hemoglobin and hemoglobin in sickle cell anemia are called hemoglobin A, F and S, respectively. Hemoglobins C, D, E, F, I and J are found in persons with certain blood abnormalities.

Hemoglobin determinations are often used as aids in diagnosing different types of anemias. The amount of hemoglobin may be expressed in grams per 100 ml. of blood or in percentages of normalcy. A value as low as 80 per cent may be considered within the normal range. The results reported in grams are considered more accurate. The normal range expressed in these terms is 14.5 to 16.0 Gm. per 100 ml. of blood for men, and 13.0 to 15.5 Gm. per 100 ml. of blood for women.

h. C disease, a hereditary condition in Negroes characterized by a third type of adult hemoglobin, distinguishable from hemoglobin A and hemoglobin S.

hemoglobinated (he″mo-glo′bin-āt″ed) filled with or containing hemoglobin.

hemoglobinemia (he″mo-glo″bĭ-ne′me-ah) abnormal presence of hemoglobin in the blood plasma.

hemoglobinolysis (he″mo-glo″bĭ-nol′ĭ-sis) the splitting up of hemoglobin.

hemoglobinometer (he″mo-glo″bĭ-nom′ĕ-ter) a laboratory instrument for colorimetric determination of the hemoglobin content of the blood.

hemoglobinorrhea (he″mo-glo″bĭ-no-re′ah) escape of hemoglobin from the erythrocytes.

hemoglobinous (he″mo-glo′bĭ-nus) containing hemoglobin.

hemoglobinuria (he″mo-glo″bĭ-nu′re-ah) the presence of hemoglobin in the urine. adj., **hemoglobinu′ric.**

epidemic h., hemoglobinuria of young infants, with cyanosis, jaundice, etc.

intermittent h., paroxysmal hemoglobinuria.

malarial h., blackwater fever.

paroxysmal h., that occurring episodically, after exertion (march hemoglobinuria) or idiopathically, with hemolytic anemia, leukopenia and possible thrombocytopenia (nocturnal paroxysmal hemoglobinuria).

paroxysmal cold h., sudden passage of hemoglobin in the urine following exposure to cold.

toxic h., that which is consequent upon the ingestion of various poisons.

hemogram (he′mo-gram) a graphic representation of the differential blood count.

hemoid (he′moid) resembling blood.

hemokinesis (he″mo-ki-ne′sis) augmentation of the flow of blood in the body.

hemolith (he′mo-lith) a concretion in the walls of a blood vessel.

hemolymph (he′mo-limf) 1. blood and lymph. 2. nutrient fluid or blood of certain invertebrates.

hemolymphangioma (he″mo-lim-fan″je-o′mah) hematolymphangioma.

hemolysate (he-mol′ĭ-sāt) the product resulting from hemolysis.

hemolysin (he-mol′ĭ-sin) a substance that liberates hemoglobin from erythrocytes.

hemolysis (he-mol′ĭ-sis) rupture of erythrocytes with release of hemoglobin into the plasma.

Some microbes form substances called hemolysins that have the specific action of destroying red blood corpuscles; the beta-hemolytic streptococcus is an example.

Intravenous administration of a hypotonic solution or plain distilled water will cause the red cells to fill with fluid until their membranes rupture and the cells are destroyed.

In a transfusion reaction or in ERYTHROBLASTOSIS FETALIS, incompatibility causes the red blood cells to clump together. The agglutinated cells become trapped in the smaller vessels and eventually disintegrate, releasing hemoglobin into the plasma. Kidney damage may result as the hemoglobin crystallizes and obstructs the renal tubules, producing renal shutdown and uremia.

Snake venoms and certain vegetable poisons, e.g., mushrooms, may cause hemolysis. A great variety of chemical agents can lead to destruction of erythrocytes if there is exposure to a sufficiently high concentration of the substance. These chemical hemolytics include arsenic, lead, benzene, acetanilid, nitrites and potassium chlorate.

hemolytic (he″mo-lit′ik) pertaining to, characterized by or producing hemolysis.

h. anemia, anemia caused by the increased destruction of erythrocytes. It may result from Rh incompatibility (see RH FACTOR and ERYTHROBLASTOSIS FETALIS); from mismatched blood transfusions; from industrial poisons such as benzene, trinitrotoluene (TNT) or aniline; and from hypersensitivity to certain antibiotics and tranquilizers. Hemolytic anemia may also appear in the course of other diseases such as widespread cancer, leukemia, Hodgkin's disease, acute alcoholism and liver diseases. In addition to the usual symptoms of anemia, the patient may exhibit JAUNDICE.

Severe hemolytic anemia may be very quickly fatal. Victims of it must be hospitalized immediately so that transfusions can be given and other treatment begun. If the cause of the condition can be located, and if it can be successfully treated, there is a good chance of recovery. In some cases, surgery to remove the SPLEEN may bring about great improvement. (See also ANEMIA for nursing care.)

h. disease of newborn, a condition marked by excessive blood destruction in newborn infants; caused by transplacental transfer of antibodies produced by the mother in response to passage of incompatible blood from the fetal to the maternal circulation and usually the result of incompatibility of the Rh factor. (See also ERYTHROBLASTOSIS FETALIS.)

h. jaundice, a rare, chronic and generally hereditary disease characterized by periods of excessive hemolysis due to abnormal fragility of the erythrocytes, which are small and spheroidal. It is accompanied by enlargement of the spleen and by jaundice. The hereditary or congenital form is known as congenital family icterus and familial acholuric jaundice; the acquired form is known as acquired hemolytic jaundice.

hemolytopoietic (he″mo-lit″o-poi-et′ik) pertaining to destruction and formation of blood cells.

hemomediastinum (he″mo-me″de-ah-sti′num) hematomediastinum.

hemometer (he-mom′ĕ-ter) hemoglobinometer.

hemometra (he″mo-me′trah) hematometra.

hemonephrosis (he″mo-nĕ-fro′sis) effused blood in the renal pelvis; hematonephrosis.

hemopathology (he″mo-pah-thol′o-je) the study of diseases of the blood.

hemopathy (he-mop′ah-the) disease of the blood. adj., **hemopath′ic.**

hemoperfusion (he″mo-per-fu′zhun) continuous circulation of blood outside the body through a material, such as charcoal, for removal of injurious factors from the bloodstream.

hemopericardium (he″mo-per″ĭ-kar′de-um) effused blood in the pericardial cavity.

hemoperitoneum (he″mo-per″ĭ-to-ne′um) effused blood in the peritoneal cavity.

hemopexin (he″mo-pek′sin) an enzyme that coagulates blood.

hemopexis he″mo-pek′sis) coagulation of blood.

hemophagocyte (he″mo-fag′o-sīt) a cell that destroys blood corpuscles.

hemophil (he′mo-fil) 1. thriving on blood. 2. a microorganism that grows best in media containing hemoglobin.

hemophilia (he″mo-fil′e-ah) a condition characterized by impaired coagulability of the blood, and a strong tendency to bleed. The classic disease is hereditary, and limited to males, being transmitted always through the female to the second generation, but many similar conditions attributable to the absence of different factors from the blood are now recognized.

SYMPTOMS. In addition to excessive bleeding from minor wounds, a hemophiliac may be subject to spontaneous hemorrhages under the skin and in the gums, gastrointestinal tract, joints and muscles. Hemarthrosis may cause the joints to stiffen and may result in permanent crippling if it is permitted to go untreated.

TREATMENT. General treatment is directed toward raising the level of clotting factor VIII (AHF, or antihemophilic factor) in the patient's blood. Serious occurrences of bleeding require transfusion of fresh whole blood or of blood plasma to replace lost blood and to increase temporarily the clotting power of the hemophiliac. The patient must learn to avoid trauma and to obtain prompt medical attention for any bleeding, no matter how slight it may seem. Before any surgery or dental treatment the patient must be given an infusion of special plasma. Also, arrangements should be made for blood donors so that there will be sufficient blood available for transfusion if it is needed. Whenever these patients must receive injections, a small needle is used, pressure is applied at the site after the needle is withdrawn and the area should be inspected frequently for bleeding until the danger of hemorrhage is past.

h. A, a hereditary hemophilic state transmitted by the female to the male as a sex-linked recessive abnormality, and due to absence of a specific clotting factor.

h. B, a hereditary hemorrhagic diathesis due to lack of clotting factor IX, transmitted by the female to the male as a sex-linked recessive abnormality; called also Christmas disease.

h. C, a hemorrhagic diathesis transmitted as an autosomal dominant and due to a lack of clotting factor XI.

h. calcipri′va, a bleeding tendency due to deficiency of calcium in the blood.

classic h., hemophilia. A.

hereditary h., a bleeding tendency due to a genetically determined deficiency of some factor in the blood.

vascular h., angiohemophilia.

hemophiliac (he″mo-fil′e-ak) 1. a person affected with hemophilia. 2. pertaining to hemophilia.

hemophilic (he″mo-fil′ik) 1. pertaining to hemophilia. 2. living or growing especially well in blood.

hemophilioid (he″mo-fil′e-oid) resembling classic hemophilia clinically, but not due to the same deficiency in the blood.

Hemophilus (he-mof′ĭ-lus) a genus name formerly given a taxon of microorganisms growing best (or only) in the presence of hemoglobin.

H. parapertus′sis, *Bordetella parapertussis.*

H. pertus′sis, *Bordetella pertussis.*

hemophobia (he″mo-fo′be-ah) fear of blood.

hemophoric (he″mo-for′ik) conveying blood.

hemophthalmia (he″mof-thal′me-ah) extravasation of blood inside the eye.

hemopleura (he″mo-ploo′rah) hemothorax.

hemopneumopericardium (he″mo-nu″mo-per″ĭ-kar′de-um) effused blood and air in the pericardium.

hemopneumothorax (he″mo-nu″mo-tho′raks) hemothorax and pneumothorax together.

hemopoiesis (he″mo-poi-e′sis) hematopoiesis.

hemoprotein (he″mo-pro′te-in) a conjugated protein whose nonprotein portion is heme.

hemoptysis (he-mop′tĭ-sis) coughing and spitting of blood as a result of bleeding from any part of the respiratory tract. In true hemoptysis the sputum is bright red and frothy with air bubbles; it must not be confused with the dark red or black color of hematemesis.

Although recent developments in drug therapy have reduced the incidence of serious bleeding in tuberculous patients, tuberculosis remains a common cause of hemoptysis. Other causes may be bronchiectasis, lung abscess or malignancy. In acute pneumonia the sputum may be bright red or it may contain old blood, which gives it a characteristic rusty appearance. Vascular disorders such as congestive heart failure, pulmonary infarction and aortic aneurysm can also cause hemoptysis.

Treatment is aimed at the primary cause of the symptom. The patient with severe hemorrhage is more likely to die from drowning in his own blood than from blood loss. Emergency measures for severe hemoptysis include application of an ice pack to the neck and chest, administration of a sedative and absolute bed rest with the head of the bed elevated slightly. The patient may be given codeine to depress the cough reflex, and he should be instructed to cough with the glottis open, without straining.

hemorrhage (hem'ŏ-rij) the escape of blood from a ruptured vessel. Hemorrhage can be external, internal or into the skin or other tissues. Blood from an artery is bright red in color and comes in spurts; that from a vein is dark red and comes in a steady flow.

SYMPTOMS. Aside from the obvious flow of blood from a wound or body orifice, massive hemorrhage can be detected by other signs such as restlessness, cold and clammy skin, thirst, increased and thready pulse, rapid and shallow respirations and a drop in blood pressure. If the hemorrhage continues unchecked, the patient may complain of visual disturbances, ringing in the ears or extreme weakness.

FIRST AID
From Severe Wound

1. Apply direct pressure on the wound with a thick compress of gauze or any other available clean cloth. If necessary, use bare hands or fingers.

2. When bleeding has been controlled, bind the compress firmly in place with strips of cloth.

3. If direct pressure does not control bleeding, apply digital pressure at the appropriate pressure point.

Internal Bleeding

1. Following injury, blood flowing from the mouth, nose or ears may indicate fracture of the skull or serious internal injury. Do *not* move the patient. Summon medical help immediately.

2. Until help arrives, the patient should be covered with a blanket or coat. If possible, keep the head and chest a little lower than the body and elevate the legs.

Further treatment consists of measures to stop the flow of blood, to combat shock and circulatory collapse and to replace lost blood by transfusion.

capillary h., oozing from minute vessels.

cerebral h., a hemorrhage into the cerebrum or occurring within the cranium; one of the three main causes of CEREBRAL VASCULAR ACCIDENT (stroke).

concealed h., internal hemorrhage.

fibrinolytic h., that due to abnormalities in the fibrinolytic system and not dependent on hypofibrinogenemia.

internal h., that in which the extravasated blood remains within the body.

petechial h., subcutaneous hemorrhage occurring in minute spots.

postpartum h., that which follows soon after labor.

primary h., that which soon follows an injury.

secondary h., that which follows an injury after a considerable lapse of time.

hemorrhagenic (hem"o-rah-jen'ik) causing hemorrhage.

hemorrhagic (hem"o-raj'ik) pertaining to or characterized by hemorrhage.

h. disease of newborn, a self-limited hemorrhagic disorder of the first days of life, caused by a marked deficiency of blood clotting factors II and VII, and most probably involving also factors IX and X.

epidemic h. fever, an acute infectious disease characterized by fever, purpura, peripheral vascular collapse and acute renal failure, caused by a filterable agent thought to be transmitted to man by mites or chiggers.

hemorrhea (hem"o-re'ah) hematorrhea.

hemorrheology (he"mo-re-ol'o-je) the scientific study of the deformation and flow properties of cellular and plasmatic components of blood in macroscopic, microscopic and submicroscopic dimensions, and the rheologic properties of vessel structure with which the blood comes in direct contact.

hemorrhoid (hem'ŏ-roid) an enlarged vein in the mucous membrane inside or just outside the rectum that causes pain, itching, discomfort and bleeding.

Hemorrhoids (called also piles) are usually caused by straining to evacuate hard, dry stools. They sometimes occur in pregnancy because of pressure on the veins from the enlarged uterus. They may result from pressure on the veins caused by a disorder of the liver or the heart or may by symptomatic of a tumor or growth that causes pressure against the veins.

Temporary relief from hemorrhoids can usually be obtained by cold compresses, sitz baths or an analgesic ointment. Treatment of the condition is surgical removal of the hemorrhoids by ligation and excision (HEMORRHOIDECTOMY).

external h., one distal to the pectinate line.

internal h., one originating above the pectinate line and covered by mucous membrane.

prolapsed h., an internal hemorrhoid that has descended below the pectinate line and protruded outside the anal sphincter.

strangulated h., an internal hemorrhoid that has prolapsed sufficiently and for long enough time for its blood supply to become occluded by the constricting action of the anal sphincter.

hemorrhoidectomy (hem"ŏ-roi-dek'to-me) surgical excision of hemorrhoids. Although the operation is considered minor and dressings may not be needed, the patient may experience much discomfort and require analgesic drugs and frequent nursing measures to relieve discomfort.

NURSING CARE. Postoperatively the patient must be watched for signs of hemorrhage, an uncommon occurrence but one that can develop quickly. The patient may be placed on his abdomen to relieve pressure on the operative site, or he may lie on his back with a rubber air ring under the buttocks for support. Warm sitz baths are usually begun the day after surgery to relieve discomfort. Compresses of witch hazel or some other astringent agent may be applied to reduce swelling and promote healing.

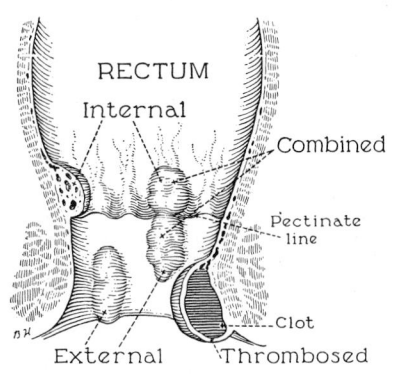

Types of hemorrhoids.

Difficulty in evacuating often occurs during the immediate postoperative period. Sitz baths are quite helpful in relieving this situation.

hemosiderin (he″mo-sid′er-in) an insoluble form of storage iron, visible microscopically both with and without the use of special stains.

hemosiderosis (he″mo-sid″ĕ-ro′sis) a focal or general increase in tissue iron stores without associated tissue damage.

hemosozic (he″mo-so′zik) preventing destruction of blood corpuscles.

hemospasia (he″mo-spa′ze-ah) withdrawal of blood.

hemospermia (he″mo-sper′me-ah) hematospermia.

hemostasis (he″mo-sta′sis) arrest of the escape of blood by either natural (clot formation or vessel spasm) or artificial (compression or ligation) means. adj., **hemostat′ic.**

hemostat (he′mo-stat) an agent (instrument or drug) used to check the escape of blood.

hemostyptic (he″mo-stip′tik) chemically hemostatic.

hemotachometer (he″mo-tah-kom′ĕ-ter) an instrument for measuring the speed of the blood flow.

hemotherapy (he″mo-ther′ah-pe) the use of blood in treating disease.

hemothorax (he″mo-tho′raks) collection of blood in the pleural cavity.

hemotoxic (he″mo-tok′sik) pertaining to or producing toxic destruction of blood cells.

hemotoxin (he″mo-tok′sin) an exotoxin characterized by hemolytic activity.

hemotroph (he′mo-trōf) nutritive material from the circulating blood of the maternal body, utilized by the early embryo.

henbane (hen′bān) hyoscyamus.

Henle's loop (hen′lēz) the U-shaped loop of the uriniferous tubule of the kidney.

Henry's law (hen′rēz) the solubility of a gas in a liquid solution is proportionate to the partial pressure of the gas.

hepar (he′par) [L.] liver.

heparin (hep′ah-rin) a mucopolysaccharide acid occurring in tissues, but most abundantly in the liver, or a mixture of active principles from the livers or lungs of domestic animals, which renders the blood incoagulable; used in the prevention and treatment of thrombosis, in postoperative pulmonary embolism and frostbite and in repair of vascular injury. Heparin is an ANTICOAGULANT and a patient receiving this drug must be watched for signs of spontaneous bleeding.

heparinize (hep′er-ĭ-nīz″) to treat with heparin in order to increase the clotting time of the blood.

hepat(o)- (hep′ah-to) word element [Gr.], *liver.*

hepatalgia (hep″ah-tal′je-ah) pain in the liver.

hepatatrophia (hep″ah-tah-tro′fe-ah) atrophy of the liver.

hepatectomize (hep″ah-tek′to-mīz) to deprive of the liver by surgical removal.

hepatectomy (hep″ah-tek′to-me) surgical excision of liver tissue.

hepatic (hĕ-pat′ik) pertaining to the liver.
  h. duct, the excretory duct of the liver, or one of its branches in the lobes of the liver.

hepatic(o)- (hĕ-pat′ĭ-ko) word element [Gr.], *hepatic duct.*

hepaticoduodenostomy (hĕ-pat″ĭ-ko-du″o-dĕ-nos′to-me) anastomosis of the hepatic duct to the duodenum.

hepaticoenterostomy (hĕ-pat″ĭ-ko-en″ter-os′to-me) anastomosis of the hepatic duct to the intestine (duodenum or jejunum).

hepaticogastrostomy (hĕ-pat″ĭ-ko-gas-tros′to-me) anastomosis of the hepatic duct to the stomach.

hepaticojejunostomy (hĕ-pat″ĭ-ko-je″joo-nos′to-me) anastomosis of the hepatic duct to the jejunum.

hepaticolithotomy (hĕ-pat″ĭ-ko-lĭ-thot′o-me) incision of the hepatic duct with removal of calculi.

hepaticolithotripsy (hĕ-pat″ĭ-ko-lith′o-trip″se) crushing of a calculus in the hepatic duct.

hepaticostomy (hĕ-pat″ĭ-kos′to-me) fistulization of the hepatic duct.

hepaticotomy (hĕ-pat″ĭ-kot′o-me) incision of the hepatic duct.

hepatin (hep′ah-tin) glycogen.

hepatitis (hep″ah-ti′tis) inflammation of the liver. It may be secondary to other disorders such as AMEBIC DYSENTERY, CIRRHOSIS or infectious MONONUCLEOSIS, it may be drug induced or it may be a viral infection (infectious hepatitis). The virus can be transmitted by the fecal oral route through contaminated foods or liquids. In serum hepatitis the virus is present in the serum of a blood donor and is transmitted by administration of infected blood or blood products. Improved sterilization techniques for disinfecting needles, syringes, intravenous equipment and other articles that might be contaminated with the virus, and the use of disposable equipment, have largely erased this source of infection.

SYMPTOMS. The symptoms of hepatitis include loss of appetite, nausea, fever, local tenderness in the region of the liver and enlargement of the liver. As the disease progresses, jaundice becomes evident and there is rapid loss of weight and strength.

TREATMENT. Bed rest is prescribed and continued until the patient is free of symptoms. During the convalescent period physical activities are limited, sometimes for as long as 2 to 3 months, to prevent permanent damage to the liver. The diet is planned to provide an adequate intake of protein to repair damaged tissue cells, and a high intake of carbohydrates, which are thought to have a protective effect on the liver cells. There are no specific drugs used in the treatment of hepatitis.

NURSING CARE. The patient with infectious hepatitis is isolated during the acute phase of the disease (see ISOLATION TECHNIQUE). Special care must be used in the handling of all articles and equipment contaminated by bodily excretions from the patient. The patient must be encouraged to rest as much as possible and to eat all of the meals and between-meal feedings offered to him. If nausea or other conditions interfere with the adequate intake of the prescribed diet, the situation should be reported to the physician so that supplemental feedings may be administered intravenously.

homologous serum h., serum hepatitis.

infectious h., a subacute disease due to a virus, with liver enlargement, fever, gastrointestinal distress, headache, anorexia and jaundice.

serum h., a virus infection transmitted by inadequately sterilized syringes and needles and by administration of infectious blood, plasma or blood products.

transfusion h., serum hepatitis.

hepatization (hep″ah-tĭ-za′shun) conversion of the air-containing lung into solid tissue, resembling that of the liver, occurring in lobar pneumonia.

gray h., a late stage, in which the exudate of fibrin and pus produces a gray color.

red h., the early stage, when the tissue is red because of the extravasated erythrocytes.

hepatocele (hep′ah-to-sēl″) hernia of the liver.

hepatocellular (hep″ah-to-sel′u-lar) pertaining to or affecting liver cells.

hepatocirrhosis (hep″ah-to-sĭ-ro′sis) cirrhosis of the liver.

hepatocolic (hep″ah-to-kol′ik) pertaining to the liver and colon.

hepatocuprein (hep″ah-to-koo′prin) a copper-containing compound present in liver tissue.

hepatocystic (hep″ah-to-sis′tik) pertaining to the liver and gallbladder.

hepatodynia (hep″ah-to-din′e-ah) pain in the liver.

hepatogenic (hep″ah-to-jen′ik) giving rise to or forming liver tissue.

hepatogenous (hep″ah-toj′ě-nus) originating in or caused by the liver.

hepatogram (hep′ah-to-gram″) 1. a tracing of the liver pulse in the sphygmogram. 2. a roentgenogram of the liver.

hepatography (hep″ah-tog′rah-fe) 1. a treatise on the liver. 2. roentgenography of the liver.

hepatolenticular degeneration (hep″ah-to-len-tik′u-lar) a group of diseases characterized by degeneration of the liver cells and of the lenticular nucleus associated with increased absorption of copper; commonly called Wilson's disease.

hepatolienography (hep″ah-to-li″ě-nog′rah-fe) roentgenography of the liver and spleen.

hepatolith (hep′ah-to-lith″) a calculus in the liver.

hepatolithectomy (hep″ah-to-lĭ-thek′to-me) excision of a calculus from the liver.

hepatolithiasis (hep″ah-to-lĭ-thi′ah-sis) formation of calculi in the liver or gallbladder.

hepatology (hep″ah-tol′o-je) the scientific study of the liver and its diseases.

hepatolysin (hep″ah-tol′ĭ-sin) a substance destructive to liver cells.

hepatolysis (hep″ah-tol′ĭ-sis) destruction of the liver cells.

hepatoma (hep″ah-to′mah) a tumor of the liver.

hepatomalacia (hep″ah-to-mah-la′she-ah) softening of the liver.

hepatomegaly (hep″ah-to-meg′ah-le) enlargement of the liver.

hepatomelanosis (hep″ah-to-mel″ah-no′sis) melanosis of the liver.

hepatometry (hep″ah-tom′ě-tre) determination of the size of the liver.

hepatomphalocele (hep″ah-tom′fah-lo-sēl″) omphalocele with liver also in the membranous sac outside the abdomen.

hepatonephric (hep″ah-to-nef′rik) pertaining to the liver and kidney.

hepatopathy (hep″ah-top′ah-the) any disease of the liver.

hepatopexy (hep′ah-to-pek″se) fixation of the displaced liver to the abdominal wall.

hepatopleural (hep″ah-to-ploo′ral) pertaining to the liver and pleura.

hepatoptosis (hep″ah-to-to′sis) downward displacement of the liver.

hepatopulmonary (hep″ah-to-pul′mo-ner″e) pertaining to the liver and lungs.

hepatorenal (hep″ah-to-re′nal) pertaining to the liver and kidneys.

hepatorrhaphy (hep″ah-tor′ah-fe) suture of the liver.

hepatorrhexis (hep″ah-to-rek′sis) rupture of the liver.

hepatoscopy (hep″ah-tos′ko-pe) examination of the liver.

hepatosis (hep″ah-to′sis) any functional disorder of the liver.

serous h., veno-occlusive disease of the liver.

hepatosolenotropic (hep″ah-to-so-le″no-trop′ik) having an affinity for or exerting a specific effect on the cholangioles and interlobular ducts of the liver.

hepatosplenography (hep″ah-to-sple-nog′rah-fe) roentgenography of the liver and spleen.

hepatosplenomegaly (hep″ah-to-sple″no-meg′ah-le) enlargement of the liver and spleen.

hepatotherapy (hep″ah-to-ther′ah-pe) administration of liver or liver extract.

hepatotomy (hep″ah-tot′o-me) incision of the liver.

hepatotoxemia (hep″ah-to-tok-se′me-ah) septicemia originating in the liver.

hepatotoxicity (hep″ah-to-tok-sis′ĭ-te) the property of exerting a deleterious effect upon the liver cells.

hepatotoxin (hep″ah-to-tok′sin) a toxin that destroys liver cells.

hepatotropic (hep″ah-to-trop′ik) having a special affinity for the liver.

hepta- (hep′tah) word element [Gr.], *seven.*

heptabarbital (hep″tah-bar′bĭ-tal) a short- to intermediate-acting barbiturate.

heptachromic (hep″tah-kro′mik) 1. pertaining to or exhibiting seven colors. 2. having vision for all seven colors of the spectrum.

heptad (hep′tad) an element with a valence of seven.

heptapeptide (hep″tah-pep′tīd) a polypeptide containing seven amino acids.

heptaploidy (hep′tah-ploi″de) the state of having seven sets of chromosomes.

heptose (hep′tōs) a sugar whose molecule contains seven carbon atoms.

heptosuria (hep″to-su′re-ah) heptose in the urine.

hereditary (hĕ-red′ĭ-ter″e) transmissible or transmitted from parent to offspring; genetically determined.

heredity (hĕ-red′ĭ-te) the transmission of traits from parents to offspring. The hereditary material is contained in the ovum and sperm, so that the child's heredity is determined at the moment of conception.

CHROMOSOMES AND GENES. Inside the nucleus of each germ cell are structures called *chromosomes.* A chromosome is composed of DEOXYRIBONUCLEIC ACID (DNA) on a framework of protein. Genes are segments of the DNA molecule; there are thousands of GENES in each cell. Each gene carries a specific hereditary trait. These traits are physical, biochemical and physiologic. Thus genes affect not only the physical appearance of an individual but also his physiologic makeup, his tendency to develop certain diseases and the daily activities of all the cells of his body.

The human ovum contains 23 chromosomes. The sperm also contains 23 chromosomes, and aside from the pair determining the sex, each one is similar in shape and size to one in the ovum. When the sperm penetrates the ovum, the fertilized ovum thus contains 23 pairs of chromosomes, or 46 chromosomes in all.

The fertilized ovum then begins to reproduce itself by dividing (mitosis). The original cell divides and forms two cells, each of these divides and forms a total of four cells and so on until a many-celled embryo begins to take form.

In the process of cell division, the chromosomes in the nucleus have the ability to make duplicates of themselves. They do not split in two, but instead each one produces another chromosome exactly like itself. When the two cells are formed from one, the chromosomes are divided so that each cell contains the same number and kind of chromosomes as the original. For this reason, all the cells in the developing embryo and in the human body, except the ovum and sperm, contain identical sets of 46 chromosomes.

The ovum and the sperm are formed by a special process of cell division (meiosis) in which each sperm or ovum receives only one member of each chromosome pair. If this were not true, and sperm or ova contained the full complement of 46 chromosomes, the cells of the offspring would have 92 chromosomes, their offspring would have 184 and so on. As it is, the amount of hereditary material in the body cells remains constant from generation to generation.

In the formation of the germ cells, it is a matter of chance which member of each pair of chromosomes goes to a given ovum or sperm. It is also purely a matter of chance which sperm fertilizes an ovum. Incredible as it seems, there are, all in all, about 70 trillion possible combinations of chromosomes that a child can inherit.

INHERITED TRAITS. Although many of the details of human heredity are not known, in general we can say that the child receives a set of genes from his parents. These genes, or hereditary determinants, develop into characteristics which reflect those of his parents, grandparents and other ancestors. Before birth these inherited traits are influenced by conditions within the mother's body. After birth they are shaped in various ways by environmental influences such as diet, training and education.

Some specific aspects of human heredity are well understood, for example, the inheritance of eye color. Remember that one member of a chromosome pair is contributed by one parent and the other by the other parent. A gene in one chromosome acts on the same trait as a gene in the same position on the other chromosome.

It has been found that one gene may be more powerful in its influence than the other gene that acts on the same trait. The more powerful gene is then said to be dominant, and the other gene is said to be recessive. A gene that produces blue eyes, for example, is recessive to a gene that produces brown eyes.

SEX DETERMINATION. Of the 23 pairs of chromosomes in each of the body cells, one pair is distinctly different from the others. The members of this pair are the sex chromosomes, and they determine the sex of offspring. In the female, they look alike and are termed X chromosomes. But in the male, one sex chromosome is an X chromosome and the other is a smaller, Y chromosome. Thus each egg cell produced by the male contains either an X or a Y chromosome. If a sperm containing a Y chromosome fertilizes an egg, the child will be male. If the sperm has an X chromosome, the child will be female.

SEX-LINKED TRAITS. Certain hereditary traits are known as sex-linked because they are carried on the X chromosome. Color blindness is an example. This condition, in which colors appear as varying shades of gray, is rare in females but appears in about 8 per cent of the male population. The genes for color vision are located on the X chromosomes, and the gene for normal vision is dominant to that for color blindness. A female having one gene for normal vision on one X chromosome and one for color blindness on the other will have normal vision, since the color blindness gene is recessive. A male, however, having only one X chromosome, will be color blind if that chromosome has the recessive gene, since there is no corresponding dominant gene to suppress it.

It is possible for a female to be color blind, if she has two of the recessive genes, but it is quite rare that these two genes come together in one person.

Another characteristic associated with sex is baldness. The gene for baldness is dominant in males and recessive in females. Thus a male need have only one gene for baldness for the trait to be expressed, but a female must have two.

HEREDITARY DISEASES. Hereditary diseases should be distinguished from congenital birth defects. A congenital defect is one that the infant is born with, such as a cleft lip, a birthmark or congenital syphilis, but the defect can arise during conception or pregnancy and not be related to heredity. Hereditary diseases, on the other hand, are passed from generation to generation by genes. Some diseases, such as cystic fibrosis, are transmitted by recessive genes.

Classic *hemophilia* is a hereditary disease transmitted by a sex-linked gene. A recessive gene carried on the X chromosome is responsible for it, and it is transmitted in the same way as color blindness. In the extremely rare case of a female carrying two recessive genes for the trait, the victim usually dies at the onset of menstruation.

Medical scientists believe that although certain diseases are not inherited directly, the tendency to contract them may be inherited. Epilepsy, for example, occurs more frequently in some families than in others. The tendency to develop allergy, asthma and bronchitis also seems to run in families. Whether these conditions actually develop in a person with such a tendency depends on environmental circumstances. Strong evidence indicates that nearsightedness, farsightedness and night blindness have a hereditary basis.

Certain mental disorders are known to be hereditary. It has been discovered in recent years that there is an abnormality in the chromosomes in children afflicted with DOWN'S SYNDROME (mongolism). This condition is classified as a trisomy, which refers to the state of having an extra chromosome per cell. Inborn errors of metabolism such as PHENYLKETONURIA and GALACTOSEMIA are inherited.

ROLE OF MUTATION. Mutation is the term used for a spontaneous change in a chromosome or gene. Normally chromosomes duplicate themselves exactly during cell division. Occasionally, however, the new cells contain an altered gene or chromosome. If the mutation occurs in an ovum or sperm involved in reproduction, the new trait will be expressed in the offspring.

Many mutations are so minor that they have no visible effect. A mutation that is very harmful will usually result in the death of the fetus and spontaneous abortion. Occasionally a mutation is beneficial. Favorable mutations gradually tend to spread through a population. The accumulation of mutations over millions of years has contributed to evolution.

heredofamilial (her″ĕ-do-fah-mil′e-al) hereditary in certain families.

heredopathia (her″ĕ-do-path′e-ah) any inherited pathologic condition.

hermaphrodism (her-maf′ro-dizm) hermaphroditism.

hermaphrodite (her-maf′ro-dīt) an individual

whose body contains tissue of both male and female gonads. The ovaries and testes may be present as separate organs, or ovarian and testicular tissue may be combined in the same organ (ovotestis). In human beings this is a rare and abnormal condition.

hermaphroditism (her-maf′ro-di-tizm″) the presence of both ovarian and testicular tissue in the same individual, a rare condition in human beings. Hermaphroditism is not to be confused with pseudohermaphroditism, in which an individual with only one kind of gonad possesses reproductive organs that reflect some characteristics of the opposite sex, owing to improper balance of male and female hormones or other endocrine disorder.

   bilateral h., that in which gonadal tissue typical of both sexes occurs on each side of the body.

   false h., pseudohermaphroditism.

   lateral h., presence of gonadal tissue typical of one sex on one side of the body and tissue typical of the other sex on the opposite side.

   protandrous h., that in which the male organs develop first, and those typical of the female sex develop later.

   protogynous h., that in which the female gonads function first, the sexual role later being reversed.

   synchronous h., that in which the gonads of both sexes are functional at the same time.

   true h., coexistence in the same person of both ovarian and testicular tissue, with somatic characters typical of both sexes.

hermetic (her-met′ik) impervious to the air.

hernia (her′ne-ah) the abnormal protrusion of part of an organ through the structures normally containing it. adj., **her′nial.** In this condition, a weak spot or other abnormal opening in a body wall permits part of the organ to bulge through. A hernia may develop in various parts of the body; it occurs most commonly in the region of the abdomen.

A layman's term for hernia is rupture. The word rupture is misleading, because it suggests tearing and nothing is torn in a hernia. A hernia is either acquired or congenital.

Although various supports and trusses can be tried in an effort to contain the hernia, the best treatment of this condition is surgical repair of the weakness in the muscle wall through which the hernia protrudes. This procedure is called HERNIORRHAPHY.

   h. cer′ebri, protrusion of brain substance through the skull.

   crural h., femoral hernia.

   cystic h., cystocele.

   diaphragmatic h., protrusion of some of the contents of the abdomen through an opening in the diaphragm into the chest cavity. The condition may be congenital or acquired, in some cases as a result of a severe injury. Hiatal hernia is one type of diaphragmatic hernia.

Symptoms, which are noted especially when the stomach is full after a meal, include heartburn, indigestion, difficulty in breathing and pain that may in some instances extend to the neck and arms. Some cases require surgical treatment. In less severe cases, treatment includes small meals of bland, easily digested food, moderate exercise and sleeping with the upper part of the body in a raised position.

esophageal h., hiatal hernia.

fat h., hernial protrusion of peritoneal fat through the abdominal wall.

femoral h., protrusion of a loop of intestine into the femoral canal, a tubular passageway that carries nerves and blood vessels to the thigh; this type occurs more often in women than in men.

hiatal h., hiatus h., protrusion of a structure, often a portion of the stomach, through the esophageal hiatus of the diaphragm.

Holthouse's h., hernia that is both femoral and inguinal.

incarcerated h., one that cannot be readily reduced, but without obstruction or strangulation; sometimes applied to an irreducible hernia with intestinal obstruction but no strangulation.

incisional h., hernia after operation at the site of the surgical incision, owing to improper healing or to excessive strain on the healing tissue; such strain may be caused by excessive muscular effort, such as that involved in lifting or severe coughing, or by obesity, which creates additional pressure on the weakened area.

inguinal h., hernia occurring in the groin, or inguen, where the abdominal folds of flesh meet the thighs. It is often the result of increased pressure within the abdomen, whether due to lifting, coughing, straining or accident. Inguinal hernia accounts for about 75 per cent of all hernias.

A sac formed from the peritoneum and containing a portion of the intestine or omentum, or both, pushes either directly outward through the weakest point in the abdominal wall (direct hernia) or downward at an angle into the inguinal canal (indirect hernia). Indirect inguinal hernia (the common form) occurs more often in males because it follows the tract that develops when the testes descend into the scrotum before birth, and the hernia itself may descend into the scrotum. In the female, the hernia follows the course of the round ligament of the uterus.

Inguinal hernia begins usually as a small breakthrough. It may be hardly noticeable, appearing as a soft lump under the skin, no larger than a marble, and there may be little pain. As time passes, the pressure of the contents of the abdomen against the weak abdominal wall may increase the size of the opening and, accordingly, the size of the lump formed by the hernia. In the early stages, an inguinal hernia is usually reducible—it can be pushed gently back into its normal place.

strangulated h., one that is tighly constricted. As any hernia progresses and bulges out through the weak point in its containing wall, the opening in the wall tends to close behind it, forming a narrow neck. If this neck is pinched tight enough to cut off the blood supply, the hernia will quickly swell and become strangulated. This is a very dangerous condition that can appear suddenly and requires immediate medical attention. Unless the blood supply is restored promptly, gangrene can set in and may cause death.

If a hernia suddenly grows larger, becomes tense and will not go back into place, and there is pain and nausea, the hernia is strangulated. Occasionally, especially in the elderly, there is no pain or tenderness when a hernia is strangulated.

umbilical h., protrusion of part of the intestine at the umbilicus, occurring most frequently in infants (see also UMBILICAL HERNIA).

ventral h., incisional hernia.

herniation (her″ne-a′shun) abnormal protrusion of an organ or other body structure through a defect or natural opening in a covering membrane, muscle or bone.

h. of nucleus pulposus, rupture or prolapse of the nucleus pulposus into the spinal canal, or against the spinal cord (see also slipped DISK).

hernioid (her′ne-oid) resembling hernia.

herniology (her″ne-ol′o-je) the study of hernia.

hernioplasty (her′ne-o-plas″te) surgical repair of hernia, with reconstruction of the abdominal wall.

herniorrhaphy (her″ne-or′ah-fe) surgical repair of HERNIA, with suture of the abdominal wall. When the weakened area is very large, hernioplasty is done and some type of strong synthetic material is sewn over the defect to reinforce the area.

Nursing care is similar to that for any type of abdominal surgery. The patient is protected from respiratory infections which may cause coughing and undue strain on the suture line. Ambulation is usually not restricted and the physician instructs the patient in activities he may resume when discharged from the hospital.

heroin (her′o-in) a highly addictive narcotic derived from opium; also called diacetylmorphine. Its sale is prohibited in the United States and in many other countries of the world. Because of its potency, it is the most popular drug of the addict, and is used by the great majority of confirmed addicts.

heroinism (her′o-in-izm″) addiction to the use of heroin.

herpangina (her″pan-ji′nah) a febrile viral disease of children marked by vesicular or ulcerated lesions on the fauces or soft palate.

herpes (her′pēz) an inflammatory viral skin disease marked by clusters of small vesicles. adj., **herpet′ic.**

h. febri′lis, eruption of skin lesions characteristic of herpes simplex, as a concomitant of fever, commonly occurring about the lips or nose; called also fever blister and coldsore.

h. gestatio′nis, a herpes peculiar to pregnant women.

h. i′ris, a form seen in rings on the hands and feet.

h. sim′plex, an acute infectious virus disease characterized by groups of watery blisters on the skin and mucous membranes, such as around the lips or nose (coldsores) or on the mucous surface of the genitalia. It often accompanies fever (herpes febrilis, fever blisters). Treatment is neither specific nor very satisfactory. Tincture of benzoin and camphorated lip ice may help dry the lesions. In some cases smallpox vaccination reduces the occurrence of the lesions.

When the virus of herpes simplex infects the eye it may cause keratoconjunctivitis and, if untreated, corneal ulceration.

h. zoster, an acute virus disease characterized by inflammation of spinal ganglia and by a vesicular eruption along the area of distribution of a sensory nerve, caused by the virus of chickenpox; called also shingles and zoster.

The disease may appear in persons who have been exposed to chickenpox, and it sometimes accompanies other diseases such as pneumonia, tuberculosis and lymphoma or is triggered by trauma or injection of certain drugs. In some cases it appears without any apparent reason for activation.

Treatment is symptomatic and is aimed at relieving the pain and itching of the blisters. Local applications of calamine lotion or other lotions to dry the blisters may help. Herpes zoster is a very exhausting disease, especially for elderly people, because the constant itching and pain are difficult to control, even with systemic analgesics in some cases.

Herpes zoster affecting the eye causes severe conjunctivitis and possible ulceration and scarring of the cornea if not treated successfully.

herpesvirus (her″pēz-vi′rus) the viral agent causing herpes simplex.

herpetiform (her-pet′ĭ-form) resembling herpes.

heter(o)- (het′er-o) word element [Gr.], *other; dissimilar.*

heteradelphus (het″er-ah-del′fus) a twin monster with one fetus more developed than the other.

heteradenia (het″er-ah-de′ne-ah) an abnormality of gland tissue.

heterecious (het″er-e′shus) requiring different hosts in different stages of development; a characteristic of certain parasites.

heteresthesia (het″er-es-the′ze-ah) variation of cutaneous sensibility on adjoining areas.

heteroagglutination (het″er-o-ah-gloo″tĭ-na′-shun) heterohemagglutination.

heteroantibody (het″er-o-an″tĭ-bod′e) an antibody combining with antigens originating from a species foreign to the antibody producer.

heteroantigen (het″er-o-an′tĭ-jen) an antigen originating from a species foreign to the antibody producer.

heteroautoplasty (het″er-o-aw′to-plas″te) surgical transfer of tissue from one part of the body to another.

heteroblastic (het″er-o-blas′tik) originating in a different kind of tissue.

heterocephalus (het″er-o-sef′ah-lus) a fetal monster with two unequal heads.

heterochromatin (het″er-o-kro′mah-tin) material of the chromosomes that remains condensed and deeply staining during interphase, considered metabolically inert.

heterochromatosis, heterochromia (het″er-o-kro″mah-to′sis), (het″er-o-kro′me-ah) diversity of color in a part normally of one color.

h. i′ridis, difference in color of the iris in the two eyes, or in different areas in the same iris.

heterochronia (het″er-o-kro′ne-ah) irregularity in time; occurrence at abnormal times.

heterochronic (het″er-o-kron′ik) 1. pertaining to or characterized by heterochronia. 2. existing for different periods of time; showing a difference in ages.

heterochthonous (het″er-ok′tho-nus) originating in an area other than that in which it is found.

heterocyclic (het″er-o-si′klik) having or pertaining to a closed chain or ring formation that includes atoms of different elements.

heterodermic (het″er-o-der′mik) performed with skin from another individual.

heterodont (het′er-o-dont″) having teeth of different shapes, as molars, incisors, etc.

heterodromous (het″er-od′ro-mus) moving or acting in other than the usual or forward direction.

heteroerotism (het″er-o-er′o-tizm) sexual feeling directed toward another person.

heterogamety (het″er-o-gam′ĕ-te) production by an individual of one sex (as the human male) of unlike gametes with respect to the sex chromosomes.

heterogamy (het″er-og′ah-me) the conjugation of gametes differing in size and structure, to form the zygote from which the new organism develops.

heterogeneity (het″er-o-jĕ-ne′ĭ-te) the state of being heterogeneous.

heterogeneous (het″er-o-je′ne-us) not of uniform composition, quality or structure.

heterogenesis (het″er-o-jen′ĕ-sìs) 1. alternation of generation. 2. asexual generation. 3. the development of a living thing from some other kind of living thing, as a virus from a cell.

heterogenote (het′er-o-je″nōt) a cell that has an additional genetic fragment, different from its intact genotype; usually resulting from transduction.

heterogenous (het″er-oj′ĕ-nus) of other origin; not originating in the body.

heterogony (het″er-og′o-ne) heterogenesis.

heterograft (het′er-o-graft″) a graft of tissue obtained from an animal of a species other than that of the recipient.

heterography (het″er-og′rah-fe) writing of other than the intended words.

heterohemagglutination (het″er-o-he″mah-gloo″tĭ-na′shun) agglutination of erythrocytes by a hemagglutinin derived from an individual of a different species.

heterohemagglutinin (het″er-o-he″mah-gloo′tĭ-nin) a hemagglutinin that agglutinates erythrocytes of organisms of other species.

heterohemolysin (het″er-o-he-mol′ĭ-sin) a hemolysin that destroys erythrocytes of animals of other species than that of the animal in which it is formed.

heteroinoculation (het″er-o-ĭ-nok″u-la′shun) inoculation from one individual to another.

heterokinesis (het″er-o-ki-ne′sis) the differential distribution of the sex chromosomes in the developing gametes of a heterogametic organism.

heterolalia (het″er-o-la′le-ah) utterance of inappropriate or meaningless words instead of those intended.

heterolateral (het″er-o-lat′er-al) relating to the opposite side.

heterologous (het″er-ol′o-gus) 1. made up of tissue not normal to the part. 2. derived from an individual of a different species or one having a different genetic constitution.

heterolysin (het″er-ol′ĭ-sin) heterohemolysin.

heterolysis (het″er-ol′ĭ-sis) destruction of blood cells of an animal by serum from another species.

heteromeric (het″er-o-mer′ik) sending processes through one of the commissures to the white matter of the opposite side of the spinal cord.

heterometaplasia (het″er-o-met″ah-pla′ze-ah) formation of tissue foreign to the part where it is formed.

heteromorphosis (het″er-o-mor-fo′sis) the development, in regeneration, of an organ or structure different from the one that was lost.

heteromorphous (het″er-o-mor′fus) of abnormal shape or structure.

heteronomous (het″er-on′ŏ-mus) subject to different laws; in biology, subject to different laws of growth or specialized along different lines.

hetero-osteoplasty (het″er-o-os′te-o-plas″te) osteoplasty with bone taken from another individual.

heteropagus (het″er-op′ah-gus) a conjoined twin monster consisting of inequally developed components.

heteropathy (het″er-op′ah-the) abnormal or morbid sensibility to stimuli.

heterophany (het″er-of′ah-ne) a difference in manifestations of the same condition.

heterophasia, heterophemia (het″er-o-fa′ze-ah), (het″er-o-fe′me-ah) the utterance of words other than those intended by the speaker.

heterophil (het″er-o-fil″) 1. a finely granular polymorphonuclear leukocyte represented by neutrophils in man, but characterized in other mammals by granules that have variable sizes and staining characteristics. 2. heterophilic.

heterophilic (het″er-o-fil′ik) 1. having affinity for other antigens or antibodies besides the one for which it is specific. 2. staining with a type of stain other than the usual one.

heterophonia (het″er-o-fo′ne-ah) any abnormality of the voice.

heterophoria (het″er-o-fo′re-ah) deviation of the visual axis of one eye when the other eye is covered and fusion is prevented.

heterophthalmia (het″er-of-thal′me-ah) difference in the direction of the axes, or in the color, of the two eyes.

heteroplasia (het″er-o-pla′ze-ah) replacement of normal by abnormal tissues.

heteroplasty (het′er-o-plas″te) plastic repair with tissue derived from an individual of a different species or with synthetic or nonorganic material.

heteroploid (het′er-o-ploid″) 1. characterized by heteroploidy. 2. an individual or cell with an abnormal number of chromosomes.

heteroploidy (het′er-o-plo″de) the state of having an abnormal number of chromosomes.

heteropsia (het″er-op′se-ah) unequal vision in the two eyes.

heteropyknosis (het″er-o-pik-no′sis) 1. the quality of showing variations in density throughout. 2. a state of differential condensation observed in different chromosomes, or in different regions of the same chromosome; it may be attenuated (negative heteropyknosis) or accentuated (positive heteropyknosis).

heterosexual (het″er-o-seks′u-al) pertaining to the opposite sex; directed toward a person of the opposite sex.

heterosexuality (het″er-o-seks″u-al′ĭ-te) attraction to persons of the opposite sex.

heterosis (het″er-o′sis) the existence, in the first generation of a hybrid, of greater vigor than is shown by either parent.

heterostimulation (het″er-o-stim″u-la′shun) stimulation of an animal with antigenic material originating from foreign species.

heterotaxia (het″er-o-tak′se-ah) abnormal position of viscera.

heterotherm (het′er-o-therm″) an organism that exhibits different temperatures at different times or under different conditions.

heterothermy (het′er-o-ther″me) exhibition of widely different body temperatures at different times or under different conditions. adj., **heterother′mic.**

heterotonia (het″er-o-to′ne-ah) a state characterized by variations in tension or tone.

heterotopia (het″er-o-to′pe-ah) displacement or misplacement of parts. adj., **heterotop′ic.**

heterotoxin (het″er-o-tok′sin) a toxin formed outside the body.

heterotransplant (het″er-o-trans′plant) tissue taken from one individual and transplanted into one of a different species.

heterotrichosis (het″er-o-trĭ-ko′sis) growth of hairs of different colors on the body.

heterotroph (het′er-o-trōf″) a heterotrophic organism.

heterotrophic (het″er-o-trof′ik) not self-sustaining; requiring complex organic substances (growth factors) for nutrition.

heterotropia (het″er-o-tro′pe-ah) deviation of the visual axis of one eye when the other eye is fixing, with the result that single binocular vision is prevented.

heterotypic (het″er-o-tip′ik) pertaining to, characteristic of or belonging to a different type.

heteroxenous (het″er-ok′sĕ-nus) requiring more than one host to complete the life cycle.

heterozygosity (het″er-o-zi-gos′ĭ-te) the state of

having different alleles in regard to a given character. adj., **heterozy'gous.**

heterozygote (het″er-o-zi′gōt) an individual exhibiting heterozygosity.

HETP hexaethyltetraphosphate, a suggested agent for treating myasthenia gravis.

Hetrazan (het′rah-zan) trademark for preparations of diethylcarbamazine, a compound used in combating filarial infections.

Heubner-Herter disease (hoib′ner her′ter) celiac disease.

heuristic (hu-ris′tik) encouraging or promoting investigation; conducive to discovery.

hex(a) (hek′sah) word element [Gr.], *six.*

hexabasic (hek″sah-ba′sik) having six atoms replaceable by a base.

Hexa-betalin (hek″sah-ba′tah-lin) trademark for preparations of pyridoxine hydrochloride, vitamin B₆.

hexachlorophene (hek″sah-klo′ro-fēn) a crystalline compound used for its detergent and germicidal properties.

hexachromic (hek″sah-kro′mik) 1. pertaining to or exhibiting six colors. 2. able to distinguish only six of the seven colors of the spectrum.

hexad (hek′sad) 1. a group or combination of six similar or related entities. 2. an element with a valence of six.

hexadimethrine (hek″sah-di-meth′rēn) a compound used to neutralize the anticoagulant action of heparin.

hexaethyltetraphosphate (hek″sah-eth″il-tet″-rah-fos′fat) a powerful anticholinesterase that has been tried in the treatment of myasthenia gravis.

hexamethonium (hek″sah-mĕ-tho′ne-um) an ammonium compound used as a ganglion-blocking agent and antihypertensive.

hexamine (hek′sah-min) methenamine, a urinary antiseptic.

hexaploidy (hek′sah-ploi″de) the state of having six sets of chromosomes (6n).

hexatomic (hek″sah-tom′ik) containing six replaceable atoms.

hexavalent (hek″sah-va′lent) having a valence of six.

Hexavibex (hek″sah-vi′beks) trademark for a preparation of pyridoxine hydrochloride, vitamin B₆.

hexavitamin (hek″sah-vi′tah-min) a preparation of vitamin A, vitamin D, ascorbic acid, thiamine hydrochloride, riboflavin and niacinamide.

hexestrol (hek-ses′trol) a compound used as an estrogenic substance.

hexethal (hek′sĕ-thal) a short- to intermediate-acting barbiturate.

hexetidine (hek-set′ĭ-dēn) a compound used as an antibacterial, antifungal and antitrichomonal agent.

hexobarbital (hek″so-bar′bĭ-tal) an ultra-short-acting barbiturate.
h. sodium, an agent used intravenously to produce general anesthesia.

hexobarbitone (hek″so-bar′bĭ-tōn) hexobarbital.

hexocyclium (hek″so-si′kle-um) a compound used as an anticholinergic and antispasmodic.

hexokinase (hek″so-ki′nās) an enzyme that catalyzes the transfer of a high-energy phosphate group of a donor to D-glucose, producing D-glucose-6-phosphate.

hexosamine (hek′sōs-am″in) a nitrogenous sugar in which an amino group replaces a hydroxyl group.

hexose (hek′sōs) a monosaccharide containing six carbon atoms in a molecule.

hexosephosphate (hek″sōs-fos′fāt) an ester of glucose with phosphoric acid that aids in the absorption of sugars and is important in carbohydrate metabolism.

hexuronic acid (hek″su-ron′ik) ascorbic acid.

hexylcaine (hek′sil-kān) a compound used as a local anesthetic.

hexylresorcinol (hek″sil-rĕ-zor′sĭ-nol) a compound used as an anthelmintic.

HF Hageman factor, or clotting factor XII.

Hf chemical symbol, *hafnium.*

Hg chemical symbol, *mercury* (L. *hydrargyrum*).

Hgb. hemoglobin.

hiatus (hi-a′tus), pl. *hia′tus* [L.] a gap, cleft or opening. adj., **hia′tal.**
aortic h., h. aor′ticus, the aortic opening in the diaphragm.
esophageal h., h. esophage′us, the opening in the diaphragm for the passage of the esophagus and the vagus nerves.
h. hernia, protrusion of any structure through the esophageal hiatus of the diaphragm.

hibernation (hi″ber-na′shun) the dormant state in which certain animals pass the winter.
artificial h., a state of reduced metabolism, muscle relaxation and a twilight sleep resembling narcosis, produced by controlled inhibition of the sympathetic nervous system and causing attenuation of the homeostatic reactions of the organism.

hibernoma (hi″ber-no′mah) a rare tumor made up of large polyhedral cells with a coarsely granular cytoplasm, occurring on the back or around the hips.

hiccough, hiccup (hik′up) spasmodic involuntary contraction of the diaphragm that results in uncontrolled breathing in of air; called also singultus. The peculiar noise of hiccups is produced by the attempt to inhale while the air passages are partially closed.
Hiccups may be due to a variety of causes, such as rapid eating or irritation in the digestive system or the respiratory system, or of the diaphragm muscle itself. Hiccups sometimes occur as a complication following some kinds of surgery, and in serious diseases such as uremia and epidemic

encephalitis. They may also have emotional causes. Hiccups are serious only when they persist for a long time; usually they stop after a few minutes.

Standard home remedies for hiccups include holding the breath, swallowing sugar or a bread crust, pulling the tongue forward, applications of cold to the back of the neck, simply sipping water slowly and breathing into a paper bag. The paper bag device has the effect of cutting off the normal exchange of air with the surrounding atmosphere. The air in the bag, after a few breaths, will have an increasingly high carbon dioxide content, and so will the air in the lungs, and finally the blood. As a consequence, the automatic respiratory centers in the brain call for stronger and deeper breathing to get rid of the carbon dioxide. This frequently makes the contractions of the diaphragm more regular and eliminates the hiccups.

In extreme cases of prolonged hiccups sedative drugs or tranquilizers may be necessary.

hidr(o)- (hid′ro) word element [Gr.], *sweat.*

hidradenitis (hi″drad-ĕ-ni′tis) inflammation of the sweat glands.

h. suppurati′va, a severe, chronic, recurrent suppurative infection of the apocrine sweat glands.

hidradenoma (hi″drad-ĕ-no′mah) adenoma of the sweat glands; called also syringocystadenoma.

hidrocystoma (hid″ro-sis-to′mah) a retention cyst of a sweat gland.

hidropoiesis (hid″ro-poi-e′sis) the formation of sweat.

hidrorrhea (hid″ro-re′ah) profuse perspiration.

hidrosadenitis (hi″dros-ad″ĕ-ni′tis) inflammation of the sweat glands.

hidroschesis (hĭ-dros′kĕ-sis) suppression of perspiration.

hidrosis (hĭ-dro′sis) 1. sweating. 2. disease of the sweat glands. adj., **hidrot′ic.**

hieralgia (hi″er-al′je-ah) pain in the sacrum.

hierolisthesis (hi″er-o-lis-the′sis) displacement of the sacrum.

high blood pressure a disorder of the circulatory system marked by excessive pressure of the blood against the walls of the arteries (see also HYPERTENSION).

hilitis (hi-li′tis) inflammation of a hilus.

hilum (hi′lum) hilus.

hilus (hi′lus), p., *hi′li* [L.] a depression or pit on an organ, giving entrance and exit to vessels and nerves. adj., **hi′lar.**

hindbrain (hīnd′brān) the portion of the brain developed from the most caudal of the three primary brain vesicles of the early embryo, comprising the metencephalon and myelencephalon.

hindfoot (hīnd′foot) the posterior portion of the foot, comprising the region of the talus and calcaneus.

hindgut (hīnd′gut) a pocket formed beneath the caudal portion of the developing embryo, which develops into the distal portion of the small intestine, the colon and the rectum.

Hinton test (hin′ton) a serologic test for syphilis.

hip (hip) the region of the body at the articulation of the femur and the hip at the base of the lower trunk. These bones meet at the hip joint.

At each hip joint, the smooth, rounded head of the femur fits into the deeply recessed socket (the acetabulum) in the hip bone, which comprises the ilium, ischium and pubis. The joint is covered by a tough, flexible protective capsule and is heavily reinforced by strong ligaments that stretch across the joint.

As in most joints, the ends of the bones, where they meet at the hip joint, are covered with a layer of cartilage that reduces friction and absorbs shock. The synovial membrane lines the socket and lubricates the joint with synovia. Cushioning is provided by small fluid-filled sacs, or bursae.

FRACTURE AND DISLOCATION. The hip is much more susceptible to fracture than to dislocation. The hip joint is very stable and possesses great strength; severe injury is necessary to dislocate it and it will often fracture first. Hip fractures usually involve the neck or the base of the neck of the femur. A fracture usually causes the leg to appear shortened, with the foot pointing outward; usually the victim is unable to raise his leg and there is pain, swelling and discoloration around the joint. The diagnosis is confirmed by x-ray examination.

A wrench of considerable force, such as may occur in an automobile accident, in skiing or in football, may dislocate the hip. Dislocation usually tears the capsule and ligaments that bind the joint together, and fragments may be torn from the rim of the hip socket.

First-aid measures are the same for a fractured or dislocated hip. In either case the injured person will probably not be able to lift his heel while lying on his back. If the victim must be moved, his legs should be gently brought together and tied at the thigh and ankle; the uninjured leg is used as a splint. If possible, a stretcher should be improvised for carrying him.

CONGENITAL DISLOCATION. Congenital dislocation of the hip occurs more frequently in females than in males. It may not be evident until the child starts to walk, when it causes limping or waddling. It is important that the condition be recognized before the child does much walking on the weakened joint. Early treatment can cure the condition, but neglect for a year or two may make reconstruction of the hip joint necessary.

OTHER HIP DISORDERS. Like most joints, the hip may be affected by ARTHRITIS and by BURSITIS, or inflammation of the bursae.

A condition known as slipped capital femoral epiphysis occasionally occurs in growing children. The epiphysis is a cartilaginous disk found at the heads of long bones throughout the body; it is the site at which bone growth takes place and it becomes permanently united to the bone only when growth has finished. There is an epiphyseal line at the top of the femur where the head of the bone joins its neck. Injury to the femur of a child, or its subjection to unusual pressure, may cause the epiphysis to slip out of alignment. This produces shortening of the leg, limitation of movement of the hip and pain. If the condition is diagnosed early enough it may be corrected with splints and plaster casts.

Hippel's disease (hip′elz) angiomatosis of the retina.

hippocampus (hip″o-kam′pus), pl. *hippocam′pi* [L.] a curved structure on the floor of the inferior horn of the lateral ventricle.

h. ma′jor, hippocampus.

h. mi′nor, a white elevation on the floor of the posterior horn of the lateral ventricle, called also calcar avis.

Hippocrates (hĭ-pok′rah-tēz) (late 5th century B.C.). "Father of Medicine." Son of a priest-physician, he was born on the island of Cos. By stressing that there is a natural cause for disease he did much to dissociate the care of the sick from the influence of magic and superstition. His carefully kept records of treatment and solicitous observation of the ill provided a foundation for clinical medicine in the case report; and by reporting also unsuccessful methods of treatment he anticipated the modern scientific attitude. The way for the professional nurse was prepared by his emphasis on the importance of skilled bedside care, and his bedside example demonstrated the value of clinical instruction. A moral code for medicine has been established by his ideals of ethical conduct and practice as embodied in the Oath.

"I swear by Apollo the physician, by Æsculapius, Hygeia, and Panacea, and I take to witness all the gods, all the goddesses, to keep according to my ability and my judgment the following Oath:

"To consider dear to me as my parents him who taught me this art; to live in common with him and if necessary to share my goods with him; to look upon his children as my own brothers, to teach them this art if they so desire without fee or written promise; to impart to my sons and the sons of the master who taught me and the disciples who have enrolled themselves and have agreed to the rules of the profession, but to these alone, the precepts and the instruction. I will prescribe regimen for the good of my patients according to my ability and my judgment and never do harm to anyone. To please no one will I prescribe a deadly drug, nor give advice which may cause his death. Nor will I give a woman a pessary to procure abortion. But I will preserve the purity of my life and my art. I will not cut for stone, even for patients in whom the disease is manifest; I will leave this operation for practitioners (specialists in this art). In every house where I come I will enter only for the good of my patients, keeping myself far from all intentional ill-doing and all seduction, and especially from the pleasures of love with women or with men, be they free or slaves. All that may come to my knowledge in the exercise of my profession or outside my profession or in daily commerce with men, which ought not to be spread abroad, I will keep secret and will never reveal. If I keep this oath faithfully, may I enjoy my life and practice my art, respected by all men and in all times; but if I swerve from it or violate it, may the reverse be my lot."

hippuria (hĭ-pu′re-ah) excess of hippuric acid in urine.

hippuric acid (hĭ-pu′rik) a compound formed by conjugation of benzoic acid and glycine.

hippus (hip′us) abnormal exaggeration of the rhythmic contraction and dilation of the pupil, independent of changes in illumination or in fixation of the eyes.

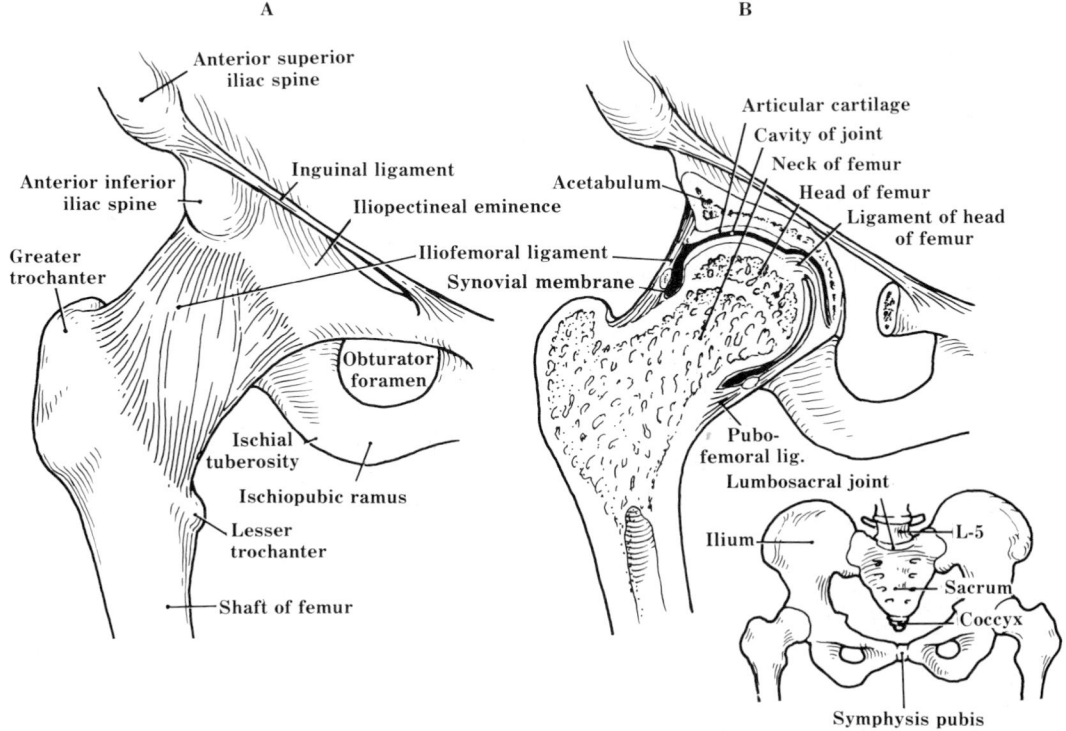

Hip joint. (Redrawn from Jacob, S. W., and Francone, C. A.: Structure and Function in Man, 2nd ed. Philadelphia, W. B. Saunders Co., 1970.)

hircus (her'kus), pl. *hir'ci* [L.] 1. the hair growing in the axilla. 2. tragus.

Hirschsprung's disease (hirsh'sproongz) massive enlargement of the colon, resulting from obstruction caused by an aganglionic segment of intestine; called also aganglionic megacolon.

hirsute (her'sūt) shaggy; hairy.

hirsuties, hirsutism (her-su'she-ēz), (her'sūt-izm) abnormal growth of hair.

hirudicide (hĭ-roo'dĭ-sīd) an agent that is destructive to leeches.

hirudin (hĭ-roo'din) the active principle of the buccal secretion of leeches.

His's bundle (his'ez) a muscular band connecting the atria with the ventricles of the heart; called also atrioventricular bundle.
   H's disease, trench fever; called also His-Werner disease.

Histadyl (his'tah-dil) trademark for preparations of methapyrilene, an antihistamine.

Histalog (his'tah-log) trademark for a preparation of betazole, an analogue of histamine, used as a substitute for histamine in gastric analysis.

histaminase (his-tam'ĭ-nās) an enzyme that inactivates histamine.

histamine (his'tah-min) a substance produced by the breakdown of histidine, a common amino acid derived from protein that occurs naturally in the body. Histamine is found in all tissues of the body.
   Although histamine was discovered in 1909, its role is still not fully understood. Histamine normally functions as a stimulant to the production of gastric juice. It also dilates the small blood vessels, as part of the regular adaptation of the body to changing inner and exterior conditions. An excess of histamine can dilate blood vessels to the extent that extravasation occurs. This appears as the reddening and swelling known as inflammation. Continued extravasation causes edema.
   In certain people, histamine may also bring on a severe form of headache, known medically as histaminic cephalalgia. It usually occurs during sleep, and is caused by release of histamine into the system. It is treated by desensitizing the patient to histamine.
   An excess of histamine apparently is released when the body comes in contact with certain substances to which it is sensitive. This excess histamine is believed to be the final cause of hay fever, urticaria (hives) and most other allergies, as well as certain stomach upsets and some headaches. It is possible that histamine also causes vomiting, diarrhea and muscular spasm, since these reactions are seen in animals injected with histamine. The fact that a person suffering from shock has large amounts of histamine in the blood suggests that histamine also plays a role in this condition, but its presence may be an incidental side effect.
   Substances that block some of the effects of histamine, the ANTIHISTAMINES, have proved useful in preventing some types of vomiting, and they are the main medications for relieving allergies.
   h. phosphate, a compound used in tests of gastric function and to reduce sensitivity to histamine.

histaminemia (his"tah-min-e'me-ah) histamine in the blood.

histaminia (his"tah-min'e-ah) shock produced by histamine.

histenzyme (his-ten'zĭm) an enzyme from the kidney that catalyzes the splitting of hippuric acid into benzoic acid and glycine.

histidine (his'tĭ-din) a naturally occurring amino acid, essential for optimal growth of infants.
   h. monohydrochloride, small, colorless crystals, used in treatment of ulceration of the intestines.

histidinemia (his"tĭ-dĭ-ne'me-ah) excessive histidine in the blood.

histioblast (his'te-o-blast") an immature histiocyte.

histioblastoma (his"te-o-blas-to'mah) reticuloendothelioma.

histiocyte (his'te-o-sīt" a large phagocytic tissue cell of the reticuloendothelial system.

histiocytoma (his"te-o-si-to'mah) a tumor containing histiocytes.

histiocytomatosis (his"te-o-si-to"mah-to'sis) any general disorder of the reticuloendothelial system.

histiocytosis (his"te-o-si-to'sis) a condition marked by the abnormal appearance of histiocytes in the blood.
   lipid h., Niemann-Pick disease.
   h. X, a generic term embracing eosinophilic granuloma, Letterer-Siwe disease and Hand-Schüller-Christian disease.

histiogenic (his"te-o-jen'ik) formed by the tissues.

histioid (his'te-oid) histoid.

histio-irritative (his"te-o-ir'ĭ-ta"tiv) irritative to tissue.

histoblast (his'to-blast) a tissue-forming cell.

histochemistry (his"to-kem'is-tre) that branch of histology that deals with the staining and description of chemical components in cells and in the intercellular materials of tissues.

histochromatosis (his"to-kro"mah-to'sis) a general term for affections of the reticuloendothelial system.

histoclastic (his"to-klas'tik) breaking down tissue.

histocompatibility (his"to-kom-pat"ĭ-bil'ĭ-te) the quality of a cellular or tissue graft enabling it to be accepted and functional when transplanted to another organism.

histodiagnosis (his"to-di"ag-no'sis) diagnosis by microscopic examination of the tissues.

histodialysis (his"to-di-al'ĭ-sis) disintegration or breaking down of tissue.

histogenesis (his"to-jen'ĕ-sis) differentiation of cells into the specialized tissues forming the various organs and parts of the body.

histogram (his'to-gram) a graph in which values found in a statistical study are represented by lines or symbols placed horizontally or vertically, to indicate frequency distribution.

histography (his-tog'rah-fe) description of the tissues.

histohematin (his″to-hem′ah-tin) one of a group of red tissue pigments; called also cytochrome.

histohematogenous (his″to-hem″ah-toj′ĕ-nus) formed from tissues and blood.

histohypoxia (his″to-hi-pok′se-ah) abnormally diminished concentration of oxygen in the tissues.

histoid (his′toid) developed from one tissue.

histoincompatibility (his″to-in″kom-pat″ĭ-bil′ĭ-te) the quality of a cellular or tissue graft preventing its acceptance or functioning when transplanted to another organism.

histokinesis (his″to-ki-ne′sis) movement in the tissues of the body.

histology (his-tol′o-je) microscopic study of the form and structure of the various tissues making up living organisms. adj., **histolog′ic.**
   normal h., the science of healthy tissues.
   pathologic h., the science of diseased tissues.

histolysis (his-tol′ĭ-sis) breaking down of tissues.

histoma (his-to′mah) any tissue tumor.

histone (his′tōn) a simple protein, soluble in water and insoluble in dilute ammonia, found combined as salts with acidic substances, such as nucleic acids or heme, in animal tissues.

histonomy (his-ton′o-me) the scientific study of tissues based on the translation into biologic terms of quantitative laws derived from histologic measurement.

histonuria (his″to-nu′re-ah) histone in the urine.

histopathology (his″to-pah-thol′o-je) pathologic histology.

histophysiology (his″to-fiz″e-ol′o-je) physiology of the minute elements of tissues.

Histoplasma (his″to-plaz′mah) a genus of fungi.
   H. capsula′tum, a species of pathogenic fungus that may cause infection (histoplasmosis) in man.

histoplasmin (his″to-plaz′min) a preparation of growth products of *Histoplasma capsulatum,* injected intracutaneously as a test for histoplasmosis.

histoplasmosis (his″to-plaz-mo′sis) a systemic fungal disease caused by inhalation of dust contaminated by *Histoplasma capsulatum*. Histoplasmosis is a disease of the rural Midwest, but it has been seen in most sections of the United States, including urban areas. It is not transmitted from one person to another. The disease begins in the lungs and may spread to other organs. Many cases of asymptomatic infection are believed to occur. The first symptoms resemble those of influenza, including fever and extreme fatigue. On x-ray the lungs may resemble tuberculous lungs.
   The specific drug used in the treatment of histoplasmosis is amphotericin B, an antifungal antibiotic. In extreme cases surgery may be necessary to remove the affected portions of the lung.

historrhexis (his″to-rek′sis) the breaking up of tissue.

histoteliosis (his″to-tēl″e-o′sis) the final differentiation of cells whose fate has already been determined irreversibly.

histotherapy (his″to-ther′ah-pe) treatment by administration of animal tissues.

histothrombin (his″to-throm′bin) thrombin derived from connective tissue.

histotome (his′to-tōm) a cutting instrument used in microtomy.

histotomy (his-tot′o-me) dissection of tissues; microtomy.

histotoxic (his″to-tok′sik) poisonous to tissue.

histotribe (his′to-trīb) an instrument for crushing tissues to secure hemostasis.

histotroph (his′to-trōf) an amorphous nutritive material derived from maternal tissue other than the blood, utilized by the early embryo.

histotrophic (his″to-trof′ik) encouraging formation of tissue.

histotropic (his″to-trop′ik) having affinity for tissue cells.

histrionism (his′tre-o-nizm″) a morbid or hysterical adoption of an exaggerated manner and gestures. adj., **histrion′ic.**

hives (hīvz) a vascular reaction characterized by sudden outbreaks of itching and burning swellings on the skin; called also URTICARIA.

HNO₂ nitrous acid.

HNO_2 nitrous acid.

HNO_3 nitric acid.

Ho chemical symbol, *holmium.*

H_2O water.

H_2O_2 hydrogen peroxide.

hoarseness (hōrs′nes) a rough quality of the voice.

Hodgkin's disease (hoj′kinz) a painless, progressive and fatal condition characterized by pruritus and enlargement of the lymph nodes, spleen and lymphoid tissue generally, which often begins in the neck and spreads through the body. Although Hodgkin's disease can occur at any age, it affects primarily those between the ages of 20 and 40 and is almost twice as frequent among men as among women. Called also malignant granuloma and lymphogranuloma.
   SYMPTOMS. The first sign of the disease is often swelling of the lymph nodes, usually those of the neck, armpit or groin, but sometimes those lying deep within the chest or abdomen. Severe itching is often an early sign of the disorder.
   As Hodgkin's disease progresses, it is usually marked by sweating, weakness, fever and loss of weight and appetite. It spreads through the lymphatic system, involving other lymph nodes elsewhere in the body as well as the spleen, liver and bone marrow. The lymph nodes and the spleen and liver may swell, and by obstructing other organs may cause coughing, breathlessness or enlargement of the abdomen. The patient often becomes anemic, and because of blood changes the body becomes less able to combat infections.

Patients are classified according to stages of development of the malignancy. In stage I only one localized lymph region is affected; in stage II two or three adjacent regions are involved as well as the original site, and the patient may or may not experience symptoms of a generalized disease; in stage III two or more distant lymphatic regions have been invaded by the malignancy.

The course of Hodgkin's disease varies considerably. In some cases the progression may be very slow, with periods of remission and exacerbations. In others the disease spreads rapidly and death occurs within months.

DIAGNOSIS AND TREATMENT. The presence of Hodgkin's disease is definitely established by lymph node biopsy.

Treatment is by large doses of radiation, often in conjunction with chemotherapy. The drugs used include mechlorethamine hydrochloride (nitrogen mustard), thio-tepa and chlorambucil. These drugs are toxic; if a side effect such as bone marrow depression occurs, it may be necessary to change to another drug.

If treatment is begun early in the progress of the disease, there usually is a remission of symptoms and the patient's life is greatly prolonged. If untreated, Hodgkin's disease may be fatal within 3 years.

hodoneuromere (ho″do-nu′ro-mēr) a segment of the embryonic trunk with its pair of nerves and their branches.

Hoffmann's sign (hof′manz) a sudden nipping of the nail of the index, middle or ring finger produces flexion of the terminal phalanx of the thumb and of the second and third phalanx of some other finger; called also digital reflex.

holandric (hol-an′drik) inherited exclusively through the male descent; transmitted through genes located on the Y chromosome.

holarthritis (hol″ar-thri′tis) inflammation of all the joints.

holergasia (hol″er-ga′ze-ah) a psychiatric disorder involving the entire personality.

holistic (ho-lis′tik) pertaining to totality, or to the whole.

holmium (hol′me-um) a chemical element, atomic number 67, atomic weight 164.930, symbol Ho. (See table of ELEMENTS.)

holoacardius (hol″o-ah-kar′de-us) an unequal twin in which the heart is entirely absent.

holoblastic (hol″o-blas′tik) undergoing cleavage in which the entire ovum participates; completely dividing.

Holocaine (ho′lo-kān) trademark for a preparation of phenacaine, a local anesthetic.

holocrine (hol′o-krin) wholly secretory: noting that type of glandular secretion in which the entire secreting cell, along with its accumulated secretion, forms the secreted matter of the gland, as in the sebaceous glands; cf. apocrine and merocrine.

holodiastolic (hol″o-di″ah-stol′ik) pertaining to the entire diastole.

holoendemic (hol″o-en-dem′ik) affecting practically all the residents of a particular region.

holoenzyme (hol″o-en′zīm) an active substance formed by combination of a coenzyme and an apoenzyme.

hologynic (hol″o-jin′ik) inherited exclusively through the female descent; transmitted through genes located on attached X chromosomes.

holophytic (hol″o-fit′ik) resembling a plant in every respect.

holorachischisis (hol″o-rah-kis′kĭ-sis) fissure of the entire vertebral column with prolapse of the spinal cord.

holosystolic (hol″o-sis-tol′ik) pertaining to the entire systole.

holotetanus (hol″o-tet′ah-nus) general tetanus.

holotonia (hol″o-to′ne-ah) muscular spasm of the whole body.

holozoic (hol″o-zo′ik) resembling an animal in every respect.

homaluria (hom″ah-lu′re-ah) production and excretion of urine at a normal, even rate.

Homan's sign (ho′manz) discomfort behind the knee on forced dorsiflexion of the foot; a sign of thrombosis in the leg.

homatropine (ho-mat′ro-pin) an alkaloid obtained by the condensation of tropine and mandelic acid; used to produce parasympathetic blockade and as a mydriatric.
   h. hydrobromide, a compound used topically in the eye as a cycloplegic and mydriatic.
   h. methylbromide, a parasympatholytic compound used in the treatment of gastrointestinal spasm and hyperchlorhydria.

homeo- (ho′me-o) word element [Gr.], *similar; same; unchanging.*

homeokinesis (ho″me-o-ki-ne′sis) the reception of identical amounts and kinds of chromatin by the daughter cells in meiosis.

homeomorphous (ho″me-o-mor′fus) of like form and structure.

homeo-osmosis (ho″me-o-oz-mo′sis) the maintenance by a cell, tissue, organ or organism of its fluid milieu at relatively constant and stable osmotic pressure (or tonicity), independent of the tonicity of the surrounding medium.

homeopathy (ho″me-op′ah-the) a system of therapeutics founded by Samuel Hahnemann (1755–1843) in which diseases are treated by drugs that are capable of producing in healthy persons symptoms like those of the disease to be treated, the drug being administered in minute doses.

homeoplasia (ho″me-o-pla′ze-ah) formation of new tissue like that adjacent to it.

homeostasis (ho″me-o-sta′sis) a tendency to uniformity or stability in the normal body states of the organism. adj., **homeostat′ic.**

homeotherapy (ho″me-o-ther′ah-pe) treatment with a substance similar to the causative agent of the disease.

homeothermal (ho″me-o-ther′mal) homoio-thermic.

homeotransplant (ho″me-o-trans′plant) homo-transplant.

homeotypical (ho″me-o-tip′ĭ-kal) resembling the normal or usual type.

homergy (hom′er-je) normal metabolism.

homicide (hom′ĭ-sīd) the taking of the life of another person.

homo- (ho′mo) word element [Gr.], *same; similar.*

homoarterenol (ho″mo-ar″tĕ-re′nol) nordefrin, a sympathomimetic agent.

homocerebrin (ho″mo-ser′ĕ-brin) a principle obtainable from brain substance.

homochrome (ho′mo-krōm) taking the same color as the stain.

homodromous (ho-mod′ro-mus) moving or acting in the same or in the usual direction.

homogametic (ho″mo-gah-met′ik) having only one kind of gamete with respect to the sex chromosomes.

homogenate (ho-moj′ĕ-nāt) material obtained by homogenization.

homogeneity (ho″mo-jĕ-ne′ĭ-te) the state of being homogeneous.

homogeneous (ho″mo-je′ne-us) of uniform quality, composition or structure.

homogenesis (ho″mo-jen′ĕ-sis) reproduction by the same process in each generation.

homogenic (ho″mo-jen′ik) homozygous.

homogenicity (ho″mo-jĕ-nis′ĭ-te) homogeneity.

homogenize (ho-moj′ĕ-nīz) to convert into material that is of uniform quality or consistency throughout.

homogentistic acid (ho″mo-jen-tis′ik) 2,5-dihydroxyphenyl acetic acid, an intermediate product in the metabolism of tyrosine and phenylalanine, excreted in urine in an inborn error of metabolism (PHENYLKETONURIA).

homoglandular (ho″mo-glan′du-lar) pertaining to the same gland.

homograft (ho′mo-graft) a graft of tissue from another animal of the same species, but having a different genotype.

homohemotherapy (ho″mo-he″mo-ther′ah-pe) treatment by injection of blood from another individual of the same species.

homoiopodal (ho″moi-op′ŏ-dal) having processes of one kind only, as nerve cells.

homoiotherm (ho-moi′o-therm) an animal that exhibits homoiothermy; a so-called warm-blooded animal.

homoiothermy (ho-moi′o-ther″me) maintenance of a constant body temperature despite variation in environmental temperature. adj., **homoiother′-mic.**

homolateral (ho″mo-lat′er-al) ipsilateral; pertaining to or situated on the same side.

homologous (ho-mol′ŏ-gus) 1. corresponding in structure, position and origin to another organ. 2. derived from an animal of the same species but of different genotype, as a homograft.

homologue (hom′ŏ-log) any homologous organ or part.

homology (ho-mol′ŏ-je) the state of being homologous.

homolysin (ho-mol′ĭ-sin) isohemolysin.

homonomous (ho-mon′ŏ-mus) subject to the same laws; in biology, subject to the same laws of growth or developed along the same line.

homonymous (ho-mon′ĭ-mus) having the same or corresponding sound or name.

homophilic (ho″mo-fil′ik) acting only with a specific antigen.

homoplastic (ho″mo-plas′tik) denoting a transplantation or grafting of tissue taken from another individual of the same species.

homoplasty (ho′mo-plas″te) 1. operative replacement of lost parts or tissues by similar parts from another individual of the same species. 2. similarity between organs or their parts not due to common ancestry.

homorganic (hom″or-gan′ik) produced by the same or by homologous organs.

homosexual (ho″mo-seks′u-al) 1. sexually attracted by persons of the same sex. 2. an individual sexually attracted by persons of the same sex.

homosexuality (ho″mo-seks″u-al′ĭ-te) sexual attraction toward persons of the same sex. It is found in both men and women.

During a child's emotional development, his sexual energies are directed at various times toward those of his own sex and toward those of the opposite sex. As he becomes mature, these energies focus on the opposite sex, but traces of the earlier attitudes usually remain. As a result, occasional homosexual feelings or dreams may occur. Homosexual experiences also may occur in a normal person who is put in an unusual situation, such as continued isolation from members of the opposite sex. He usually returns eventually to normal relationships. These isolated experiences should not be confused with homosexuality as a continued, preferred sexual outlet. This is considered a personality disorder, and indicates a need for psychiatric treatment.

There are a number of theories to explain homosexuality, but most of them agree on the basic pattern. During early childhood, the child normally tends to identify with the parent of the same sex. A girl wants to be like, and replace, her mother; a boy, his father. If for some reason the child identifies too strongly with the parent of the opposite sex, he may be oriented at an early age in the direction of homosexuality. The child may also be driven in the direction of homosexuality by a feeling of inadequacy or a fear of the opposite sex.

homostimulant (ho″mo-stim′u-lant) stimulating the organ from which it is derived.

homotherm (ho′mo-therm) homoiotherm.

homotopic (ho″mo-top′ik) occurring at the same place upon the body.

homotransplant (ho″mo-trans′plant) tissue taken from one individual and transplanted into another of the same species.

homotype (ho′mo-tīp) a part or object similar to another, but oppositely oriented.

homozygosis (ho″mo-zi-go′sis) the formation of a zygote by the union of gametes of similar genetic constitution.

homozygosity (ho″mo-zi-gos′ĭ-te) the state of having identical alleles in regard to a given character or to all characters. adj., **homozy′gous.**

homozygote (ho″mo-zi′gōt) an individual exhibiting homozygosity.

homunculus (ho-mung′ku-lus) a dwarf without deformity or disproportion of parts.

hookworm (hook′werm) a parasitic roundworm, found mostly in the southeastern part of the United States, that enters the human body through the skin and migrates to the intestines where it attaches itself to the intestinal wall and sucks blood from it for nourishment. Once fairly common, hookworm disease is now largely confined to poor, rural areas where modern sanitation is lacking.

The kind of hookworm most common in the United States and Central America is *Necator americanus,* which literally means "American killer." This hookworm is about half an inch long, with sharp hooklike teeth and a muscular gullet used in sucking blood. The female, slightly larger than the male, can lay more than 10,000 eggs a day, any one of which can hatch into a larva and invade the human body. Another common hookworm is *Ancylostoma duodenale.*

The larval hookworms enter the body by burrowing through the skin, usually that of the sole of the foot. The first sign of the disease may appear on the skin as small eruptions that develop into pus-filled blisters; this condition is sometimes called "ground itch."

Meanwhile the hookworms enter blood vessels and are carried by the blood into the lungs. They leave the lungs, propel themselves up the trachea, are swallowed and washed through the stomach and end up in the intestines. Here, if left alone, they will make a permanent home, using their host's body as a source of nourishment.

By the time they reach the intestines, about 6 weeks after they enter the body as larvae, the worms are full-grown adults. Each worm now attaches itself by its hooked teeth to the intestinal wall, where it sucks its host's blood by contraction and expansion of its gullet. If large numbers of worms are present, they can cause considerable loss of blood and severe anemia. The symptoms include pallor and loss of energy; the appetite may increase.

The thousands of eggs laid every day by each female worm pass out of the body in the stool, in which they can easily be seen. If the stool is not properly disposed of, the larvae that hatch from the eggs may infect other persons.

TREATMENT AND PREVENTION. A nutritious, high-protein diet supplemented by iron is given to relieve anemia and improve the health. Specific drugs include hexylresorcinol, tetrachloroethylene and chenopodium oil. When left untreated, hookworm can cause not only anemia but also bronchial inflammation and, occasionally, stunting of growth, retardation of mental development and even death.

Hookworm infection can be prevented by installation of sanitary toilets or, if that is not possible, by disposal of human feces in deep holes so that the soil with which the human foot comes in contact is not contaminated. Shoes should be worn out of doors to protect the feet from infection.

hordeolum (hōr-de′o-lum) inflammation of a gland of the eyelid; called also STY.

horismascope (ho-ris′mah-skōp) an instrument for examining the urine for albumin.

horismology (hōr″iz-mol′o-je) the science dealing with the definition of terms.

horizocardia (hŏ-ri″zo-kar′de-ah) horizontal position of the heart.

horizon (hŏ-ri′zon) a specific anatomic stage of embryonic development, of which 23 have been defined, beginning with the unicellular fertilized egg and ending 7 to 9 weeks later, with the beginning of the fetal stage.

hormesis (hōr-me′sis) stimulation by a subinhibitory concentration of a toxic substance.

Hormodendrum (hōr″mo-den′drum) a genus of fungi. The species *H. pedrosoi* and *H. compactum* are causes of chromoblastomycosis.

hormonagogue (hōr-mōn′ah-gog) an agent that increases the production of hormones.

hormone (hōr′mon) a glandular secretion produced in the body and dispatched through the bloodstream. adj., **hormo′nal.** Hormones act as chemical messengers to body organs, stimulating certain life processes and retarding others. Growth, reproduction, sexual attributes and even mental conditions and personality traits are dependent on hormones.

Hormones are produced by various organs and body tissues, but mainly by the ENDOCRINE GLANDS, such as the pituitary, thyroid and gonads (testes and ovaries). Each gland apparently manufactures several kinds of hormones; the adrenal glands alone produce more than 25 varieties. The total number of hormones is still unknown, but each has its unique function and its own chemical formula. After a hormone is discharged by its parent gland into the capillaries or the lymph, it may travel a circuitous path through the bloodstream to exert influence on cells, tissues and organs (target organs) far removed from its site of origin.

One of the best-known hormones is insulin, a protein substance manufactured by the islands of Langerhans in the pancreas that is important in carbohydrate metabolism. Other important hormones are THYROXINE, an iodine-carrying amino acid produced by the thyroid gland; CORTISONE, a member of the steroid family from the adrenal glands; and the sex hormones, ESTROGEN from the ovaries and ANDROGEN from the testes.

Certain hormone substances can now be synthesized in the laboratory for treatment of human disease. Animal hormones can also be used, as endocrine hormones are to some extent interchangeable among species. Extracts from the pancreas of cattle, for example, enabled diabetes sufferers to live normal lives even before the chemistry of insulin was fully understood.

We now know that any significant imbalance in the kind and number of hormones produced by the glands must be corrected if the body and mind are to function properly. Extreme imbalances account for such forms of abnormal development as DWARFISM and CRETINISM. Hormonal imbalance can also cause changes in personality such as excessive excitability, lethargy or fatigue. Thanks to modern endocrinology, hormone and glandular disorders are yielding more and more to the physician's treatment.

adaptive h., one that is secreted during adaptation to unusual circumstances.

adrenocortical h., one of the steroids produced by the adrenal cortex (see also CORTICOSTEROID).

adrenocorticotropic h., a hormone elaborated by the anterior lobe of the pituitary gland that stimulates the action of the adrenal cortex (see also ACTH).

adrenomedullary h's, substances secreted by the adrenal medulla, including epinephrine and norepinephrine.

androgenic h's, the masculinizing hormones, androsterone and testosterone.

antidiuretic h., ADH, one from the posterior lobe of the PITUITARY GLAND that suppresses the secretion of urine; vasopressin.

A.P.L. h., chorionic gonadotropin.

chromaffin h., epinephrine.

corpus luteum h., progesterone.

cortical h., corticosteroid.

estrogenic h., one that produces estrus in female mammals.

follicle-stimulating h., a hormone of the anterior lobe of the pituitary gland that stimulates follicular growth in the ovary and spermatogenesis in the testis.

gonadotropic h., one that has an influence on the gonads.

growth h., a substance that stimulates growth, especially a secretion of the anterior lobe of the PITUITARY GLAND that directly influences protein, carbohydrate and lipid metabolism and controls the rate of skeletal and visceral growth.

interstitial cell-stimulating h., luteinizing hormone.

lactation h., lactogenic h., a hormone of the anterior pituitary that regulates lactation.

luteinizing h., a hormone of the anterior pituitary concerned in production of corpora lutea in the ovary and secretion of testosterone by the interstitial cells of the testis; called also interstitial cell-stimulating hormone.

luteotropic h., lactogenic hormone.

melanocyte-stimulating h., MSH, a substance from the anterior pituitary that influences the formation or deposition of melanin in the body.

parathyroid h., a substance secreted by the parathyroid glands that influences calcium and phosphorus metabolism and bone formation.

placental h., an estrogenic hormone derived from the placenta.

progestational h's, substances, including PROGESTERONE, that are concerned mainly with preparing the endometrium for nidation of the fertilized ovum if conception has occurred.

sex h's, hormones having estrogenic (female sex

hormones) or androgenic (male sex hormones) activity.

somatotrophic h., somatotropic h., growth hormone.

thyrotropic h., a hormone of the anterior lobe of the pituitary gland that exerts a stimulating influence on the thyroid gland; called also thyrotropin and thyroid-stimulating hormone (TSH).

hormonology (hōr″mo-nol′o-je) the science of hormones; clinical endocrinology.

hormonopoiesis (hōr-mo″no-poi-e′sis) the production of hormones.

hormonoprivia (hōr-mo″no-priv′e-ah) a morbid condition resulting from a lack of hormones; it may be the result of hyposecretion or of surgical removal of an endocrine gland.

hormonotherapy (hōr-mo″no-ther′ah-pe) treatment by the use of hormones.

horn (hōrn) a pointed projection such as the paired processes on the head of various animals, or other structure resembling them in shape.

anterior h. of spinal cord, the horn-shaped structure seen in transverse section of the spinal cord, formed by the anterior column of the cord.

cicatricial h., a hard, dry outgrowth from a cicatrix, commonly scaly and rarely osseous.

h. of clitoris, an occasional formation of a horny mass under the prepuce of the clitoris.

posterior h. of spinal cord, the horn-shaped structure seen in transverse section of the spinal cord, formed by the posterior column of the cord.

sebaceous h., a hard outgrowth of the contents of a sebaceous cyst.

warty h., a hard, pointed outgrowth of a wart.

Horner's syndrome (hōr′nerz) sinking in of the eyeball, ptosis of the upper eyelid, slight elevation of the lower lid, constriction of the pupil, narrowing of the palpebral fissure and anhidrosis caused by paralysis of the cervical sympathetic nerve supply.

horopter (hōr-op′ter) the sum of all points seen in binocular vision with the eyes fixed.

host (hōst) 1. an animal or plant that harbors and provides sustenance for another organism. 2. the recipient of an organ or other tissue derived from another organism.

accidental h., one that accidentally harbors an organism that is not ordinarily parasitic in the particular species.

alternate h., intermediary host.

definitive h., final h., the organism in which a parasite passes its adult and sexual existence.

intermediary h., intermediate h., the organism in which a parasite passes its larval or nonsexual existence.

h. of predilection, the host preferred by a parasite.

primary h., definitive host.

reservoir h., one that becomes infected by a pathogenic parasite and may serve as the source from which the parasite is transmitted to other animals.

secondary h., intermediary host.

transfer h., one that is used until the appropriate definitive host is reached, but is not necessary to completion of the life cycle of the parasite.

housemaid's knee a swelling at the front of the knee, caused by enlargement of a bursa in front of the patella (kneecap), with accumulation of fluid within it.

The condition is so called because it was formerly supposed to be common among domestic workers who injured the knee by frequent kneeling.

The knee swells, is tender to the touch and hurts when bent; if the bursa continues to be aggravated, these symptoms become acute. The injury may result in BURSITIS. Infection is possible if the knee is cut or scratched.

The condition can be treated by withdrawal of the fluid with a hollow needle and syringe. Sometimes the bursa must be removed altogether to prevent a chronic or recurrent condition.

Howell-Jolly bodies (how'el zho-le') small, round or oval bodies seen in erythrocytes when stains are added to fresh blood and found in various anemias and leukemias and after splenectomy.

Hp haptoglobin, a serum protein that binds free hemoglobin.

HPO hyperbaric (high-pressure) oxygenation.

hr. hour.

HSA human serum albumin.

5-HT serotonin (5-hydroxytryptamine).

ht. height.

Huhner test (hoon'er) determination of the number and condition of spermatozoa in mucus aspirated from the canal of the cervix uteri within 2 hours after coitus.

hum (hum) a low, steady, prolonged sound.
 venous h., a continuous steady sound heard over the larger veins.

Humatin (hu'mah-tin) trademark for preparations of paromomycin sulfate, an antibiotic.

humectant (hu-mek'tant) 1. moistening. 2. a diluent medicine.

humectation (hu″mek-ta'shun) the act of moistening.

humeral (hu'mer-al) of or pertaining to the humerus.

humeroradial (hu″mer-o-ra'de-al) pertaining to the humerus and radius.

humerus (hu'mer-us) the bone of the upper arm, extending from shoulder to elbow. It consists of a shaft and two enlarged extremities. The proximal end has a smooth round head that articulates with the scapula to form the shoulder joint. Just below the head are two rounded processes called the greater and lesser tubercles. Just below the tubercles is the "surgical neck," so named because of its liability to fracture. The distal end of the humerus has two articulating surfaces: the trochlea, which articulates with the ulna, and the capitulum, which articulates with the radius.

humidifier (hu-mid'ĭ-fi″er) an apparatus for controlling humidity by adding moisture to the air.

humidity (hu-mid'ĭ-te) the degree of moisture in the air.

humor (hu'mor), pl. *humo'res, humors* [L.] any fluid or semifluid in the body. adj., **hu'moral.**
 aqueous h., the fluid produced in the eye and filling the spaces (anterior and posterior chambers) in front of the lens and its attachments.
 crystalline h., the crystalline lens.
 ocular h., any one of the humors of the eye—aqueous, crystalline or vitreous.
 vitreous h., the fluid portion of the vitreous body; often used to designate the entire gelatinous mass.

humoralism (hu'mor-al-izm″) the obsolete doctrine that all diseases arise from some change of the humors.

Humorsol (hu'mor-sol) trademark for a solution of demecarium bromide, used in the treatment of glaucoma.

hunchback (hunch'bak) a rounded deformity, or hump, of the back, or a person with such a deformity. The condition is called also KYPHOSIS and is the result of an abnormal backward curvature of the spine.

hunger (hung'ger) a craving, as for food.
 air h., dyspnea affecting both inspiration and expiration.

Hunter (hun'ter) John (1728–1793). "Founder of scientific surgery." Born in England, he learned dissection from his brother William and then acquired extensive knowledge of gunshot wounds in the army, of which he was later appointed surgeon-general. Upon retiring from the army, he practiced surgery and lectured on anatomy and surgery. His merit rests with the sound pathologic reasons upon which his surgical procedures were based. Hunter was also the first to study teeth scientifically. In 1783 he was elected a member of the Royal Society of Medicine and of the Royal Academy of Surgery at Paris.

Huntington's chorea (hunt'ing-tunz) a rare hereditary disease of the brain characterized by quick involuntary movements, speech disturbances and mental deterioration due to degenerative changes in the cerebral cortex and basal ganglia; called also chronic or hereditary chorea.

The disease appears in adulthood, usually between the ages of 30 and 45, and the patient's condition deteriorates over a period of 15 years or so, progressing to total incapacitation and death. There is no treatment as yet that is successful in curing this disorder. Sedatives and tranquilizers may be used to relieve the symptoms.

Hurler's syndrome (hoor'lerz) a hereditary disorder of mucopolysaccharide metabolism, characterized by abnormal elimination of mucopolysaccharides and by typical craniofacial changes (gargoylism).

Hutchinson's disease (huch'in-sunz) progeria.

HVL half-value layer.

hyalin (hi'ah-lin) a translucent albuminoid substance obtainable from the products of amyloid degeneration.

hyaline (hi'ah-līn) glassy; pellucid.
 h. cartilage, cartilage with a glassy, translucent appearance, the matrix and embedded collagenous fibers having the same index of refraction.
 h. membrane disease, a disorder of the alveoli and respiratory passages that results in inadequate

expansion of the lungs. Infants with this disease do not secrete adequate quantities of a substance called surfactant, which is secreted by the epithelium of the alveoli and decreases the surface tension of the fluids lining the alveoli and bronchioles. When the surface tension is kept low, air can pass through the fluids and into the alveoli. If the surface tension is not decreased by adequate supplies of surfactant, the alveoli cannot fill with air and there is partial or complete collapse of the lung (atelectasis). Thus the infant with hyaline membrane disease suffers from respiratory embarrassment with severe DYSPNEA and cyanosis.

The cause of hyaline membrane disease is not known, but it seldom occurs in full-term infants, and may develop in infants whose mothers are diabetic or in infants delivered by cesarean section.

There is no cure for hyaline membrane disease. The infant is given oxygen as needed and usually is fed through a stomach tube to avoid aspiration of liquids into the lungs. As a safeguard against pneumonia, which frequently accompanies this disease, antibiotics may be prescribed. Infants who are able to survive the first few days usually recover very quickly.

hyalinization (hi″ah-lin″ĭ-za′shun) conversion into a substance resembling glass.

hyalinosis (hi″ah-lĭ-no′sis) hyaline degeneration.

hyalinuria (hi″ah-lĭ-nu′re-ah) hyalin in the urine.

hyalitis (hi″ah-li′tis) inflammation of the vitreous body.
    asteroid h., hyalitis marked by spherical or star-shaped bodies in the vitreous.
    h. puncta′ta, a form marked by small opacities.
    h. suppurati′va, purulent inflammation of the vitreous humor of the eye.

hyaloenchondroma (hi″ah-lo-en″kon-dro′mah) a chondroma of hyaline cartilage.

hyalogen (hi-al′o-jen) an albuminous substance occurring in cartilage, vitreous humor, etc., and convertible into hyalin.

hyaloid (hi′ah-loid) pellucid; like glass.

hyaloiditis (hi″ah-loi-di′tis) hyalitis.

hyalomere (hi′ah-lo-mēr″) the pale, homogeneous portion of a blood platelet, possibly an artifact.

Hyalomma (hi″ah-lom′ah) a genus of ticks occurring only in Africa, Asia and Europe; ectoparasites of animals and man, they may transmit disease and cause serious injury by their bite.

hyalomucoid (hi″ah-lo-mu′koid) the mucoid of the vitreous body.

hyalonyxis (hi″ah-lo-nik′sis) the act of puncturing the vitreous body.

hyalophagia (hi″ah-lo-fa′je-ah) the eating of glass.

hyalophobia (hi″ah-lo-fo′be-ah) fear of glass.

hyaloplasm (hi′ah-lo-plazm″) 1. the fluid portion of the cytoplasm of a cell, in which the other elements are dispersed. 2. the conducting medium of the axon.
    nuclear h., karyolymph.

hyaloserositis (hi″ah-lo-se″ro-si′tis) inflammation of serous membranes marked by conversion of the serous exudate into a pearly coating.

hyalosome (hi-al′o-sōm) a structure resembling the nucleolus of a cell, but staining only slightly.

hyaluronic acid (hi″ah-lu-ron′ik) a sulfate-free polysaccharide in the vitreous humor, synovia, skin, umbilical cord, tumors and hemolytic streptococci.

hyaluronidase (hi″ah-lu-ron′ĭ-dās) an enzyme that acts on hyaluronic acid, the "cement material" of connective tissues. When hyaluronidase is mixed with fluids administered subcutaneously, absorption is more rapid and less uncomfortable. This is especially valuable when large amounts of fluid must be given by hypodermoclysis instead of intravenously. The drug should be dissolved just before it is used and usually is injected with the first portion of the fluid to be given. Hyaluronidase should not be given in areas where there is infection. Since it hastens absorption, it must be given with caution when administered with toxic drugs, as the toxic reaction can occur very rapidly.

Hyazyme (hi′ah-zīm) trademark for a preparation of hyaluronidase for injection.

hybrid (hi′brid) an offspring of parents of different species.

hydantoin (hi-dan′to-in) a crystalline base derivable from allantoin.

hydatid (hi′dah-tid) a cystlike structure; applied especially to the cyst stage of an embryonic tapeworm of the genus Echinococcus in which the cyst contains daughter cysts, each of which contains many scolices.
    h. disease, infection due to larval forms of certain tapeworms (Echinococcus) and characterized by the development of expanding cysts.
    h. mole, a mole formed by the proliferation of the chorionic villi, resulting in a mass of cysts that resembles a bunch of grapes.
    h. of Morgagni, a cystlike remnant of the müllerian duct attached to a testis or to the oviduct.
    sessile h., the hydatid of Morgagni connected with a testis.
    stalked h., the hydatid of Morgagni connected with an oviduct.

hydatidiform (hi″dah-tid′ĭ-form) resembling a hydatid.

hydatidocele (hi″dah-tid′o-sēl) a tumor of the scrotum containing hydatids.

hydatidoma (hi″dah-tĭ-do′mah) a tumor containing hydatids.

hydatidosis (hi″dah-tĭ-do′sis) infection with hydatids.

hydatidostomy (hi″dah-tĭ-dos′to-me) incision and drainage of a hydatid cyst.

hydatiduria (hi″dah-tĭ-du′re-ah) excretion of hydatid cysts in the urine.

Hyde's disease (hīdz) prurigo nodularis.

Hydeltra (hi-del′trah) trademark for preparations

of prednisolone, a compound used as a gluco-corticoid.

hydr(o)- (hi′dro) word element [Gr.], *hydrogen; water.*

hydracetin (hi-dras′ĕ-tin) acetylphenylhydrazine, an erythrocyte depressant.

hydraeroperitoneum (hi-dra″er-o-per″ĭ-to-ne′-um) water and gas in the peritoneal cavity.

hydragogue (hi′drah-gog) 1. increasing the fluid content of the feces. 2. a purgative that causes evacuation of watery stools.

hydralazine hydrochloride (hi-dral′ah-zēn) an antihypertensive and vasodilator; used in periph-eral vascular disease, essential and early malig-nant hypertension, thrombophlebitis and other conditions in which dilation of the blood vessels of the extremities is desired.

The drug may be administered orally, intramus-cularly or intravenously. Dosage is adjusted to the individual patient's response. The blood pressure should be checked frequently, especially during parenteral administration of the drug. Side effects are rare with therapeutic doses but the drug must be administered with caution to patients with coronary artery disease, advanced kidney damage and existing or incipient cerebral vascular acci-dent.

hydramnios (hi-dram′ne-os) excess of amniotic fluid.

hydranencephaly (hi″dran-en-sef′ah-le) absence of the cerebral hemispheres, their normal site being occupied by fluid.

hydrargyria (hi″drar-jir′e-ah) chronic poisoning from mercury.

hydrargyrum (hi-drar′jĭ-rum) [L.] mercury (symbol Hg).

hydrarthrosis (hi″drar-thro′sis) an accumulation of watery fluid in the cavity of a joint.

hydrate (hi′drāt) 1. a compound of hydroxyl with a radical. 2. a salt or other compound that contains water. 3. to combine with water.

hydraulics (hi-draw′liks) the science of liquids in motion.

hydrazine (hi′drah-zin) 1. a gaseous diamine. 2. any one of its substitution derivatives.

hydremia (hi-dre′me-ah) excess of water in the blood.

hydrencephalocele (hi″dren-sef′ah-lo-sēl″) her-nial protrusion of brain tissue containing a cavity communicating with the cerebral ventricles.

hydrencephalus, hydrencephaly (hi″dren-sef′-ah-lus), (hi″dren-sef′ah-le) hydrocephalus.

hydriatrist (hi″dre-at′rist) a specialist in hydro-therapy.

hydroa (hi-dro′ah) a skin disease with vesicular patches.

hydroappendix (hi″dro-ah-pen′diks) distention of the vermiform appendix with watery fluid.

hydrobilirubin (hi″dro-bil″ĭ-roo′bin) a bile pig-ment.

hydrocalycosis (hi″dro-kal″ĭ-ko′sis) distention of a single calix of the kidney with accumulated urine.

hydrocarbon (hi″dro-kar′bon) an organic com-pound that contains carbon and hydrogen only.
  alicyclic h., one that has cyclic structure and ali-phatic properties.
  aliphatic h., a compound in which the carbons are attached in a chain with no ring form.
  aromatic h., one that has cyclic structure and a closed conjugated system of double bonds.
  saturated h., one that has the maximum number of hydrogen atoms for a given carbon structure.
  unsaturated h., an aliphatic or alicyclic hydro-carbon that has less than the maximum number of hydrogen atoms for a given carbon structure.

hydrocele (hi′dro-sēl) a painless swelling of the scrotum caused by a collection of fluid between the tunica vaginalis testis, the outermost covering of the testes. It can be removed by withdrawing the fluid by tapping through the outer layer of tissue, or by cutting away the outer layer of tissue. The latter operation makes it impossible for the hydrocele to recur.

hydrocelectomy (hi″dro-se-lek′to-me) excision of a hydrocele.

hydrocenosis (hi″dro-se-no′sis) removal of drop-sical fluid.

hydrocephalocele (hi″dro-sef′ah-lo-sēl″) hydren-cephalocele.

hydrocephaloid (hi″dro-sef′ah-loid) resembling hydrocephalus.
  h. disease, a condition resembling hydrocephalus, but with depressed fontanels, following severe diarrhea.

hydrocephalus (hi″dro-sef′ah-lus) a condition characterized by enlargement of the cranium caused by abnormal accumulation of fluid; called also water on the brain. adj., **hydrocephal′ic.** Al-though hydrocephalus occurs occasionally in adults it is usually associated with a congenital defect in infants. When the regular flow or absorption of the CEREBROSPINAL FLUID is impaired by a congenital malformation of the internal skull, the fluid accu-mulates in the brain and enlarges the ventricles.

There is no known effective treatment for hydro-cephalus other than surgery. The procedures most often used employ the shunt technique, so called because it shunts the fluid away from the cranial cavity and into the jugular vein, where it is ab-sorbed into the bloodstream. The shunt technique is not the final answer to all problems of hydro-cephalus, and research continues on possible alter-native methods.

NURSING CARE. The child with hydrocephalus requires frequent changing of position of the head as well as of the body. Decubitus ulcers (pressure sores) on the head are a constant threat because of the weight and size of the head and the child's inability to move it. The child should be picked up and held frequently, especially during feeding periods. Care must be taken that the head is well supported while the child is being held.

hydrochlorate (hi″dro-klo′rāt) a salt of hydro-chloric acid.

hydrochloric acid (hi″dro-klōr′ik) HCl, a normal constituent of gastric juice in man and other animals. The absence of free hydrochloric acid in the stomach, called achlorhydria, may be found with chronic gastritis, gastric carcinoma, pernicious anemia, pellagra and alcoholism. This condition is also referred to as gastric anacidity.

Hyperacidity of the gastric juice is often associated with emotional stress and tension and is believed to be a factor in the development of peptic ULCER.

Dilute hydrochloric acid may be administered to aid digestion in achlorhydria. The preparation should be given well diluted and the patient is instructed to take the solution through a straw to avoid damage to the teeth. It is administered 30 minutes before each meal.

hydrochlorothiazide (hi″dro-klōr″o-thi′ah-zīd) a white, crystalline compound used as a diuretic and antihypertensive agent.

hydrocholecystis (hi″dro-ko″le-sis′tis) distention of gallbladder with watery fluid.

hydrocholeretic (hi″dro-ko″ler-et′ik) 1. pertaining to an increased output by the liver of bile of low specific gravity. 2. an agent that stimulates an increased output of bile of low specific gravity.

hydrocirsocele (hi″dro-sir′so-sēl) hydrocele with variocele.

hydrocodone (hi″dro-ko′dōn) dihydrocodeinone, an antitussive.

hydrocolloid (hi″dro-kol′oid) a colloid in which water is the dispersion medium.

hydrocolpos (hi″dro-kol′pos) collection of watery fluid in the vagina.

hydrocortamate (hi″dro-kor′tah-māt) a compound used in treatment of dermatoses.

hydrocortisone (hi″dro-kor′tĭ-sōn) the pharmaceutical term for cortisol, a corticosteroid used for its anti-inflammatory action.

Hydrocortone (hi″dro-kor′tōn) trademark for preparations of hydrocortisone, a corticosteroid.

hydrocyanic acid (hi″dro-si-an′ik) a volatile liquid that is extremely poisonous because it checks the oxidation process in protoplasm.

hydrocyst (hi′dro-sist) a cyst with watery contents.

hydrocystoma (hi″dro-sis-to′mah) hidrocystoma.

hydrodipsia (hi″dro-dip′se-ah) thirst for water.

Hydrodiuril (hi″dro-di′u-ril) trademark for a preparation of hydrochlorothiazide, a diuretic and antihypertensive.

hydrogel (hi′dro-jel) a gel that contains water.

hydrogen (hi′dro-jen) a chemical element, atomic number 1, atomic weight 1.00797, symbol H. (See table of ELEMENTS.)
   h. dioxide, hydrogen peroxide.
   heavy h., hydrogen having double the mass of ordinary hydrogen.
   h. ion concentration, the degree of concentration of hydrogen ions (the acid element) in a solution, used to indicate or express the reaction of that solution. Its symbol is pH.
   h. monoxide, water, H_2O.

h. peroxide, H_2O_2, used in solution as an antibacterial agent. A 3 per cent solution foams on touching skin or mucous membrane and appears to have a mechanical cleansing action.
   h. sulfide, an ill-smelling, colorless, poisonous gas, H_2S; much used as a chemical reagent. Called also hydrosulfuric acid.

hydrogenate (hi′dro-jen-āt″) to cause to combine with hydrogen.

hydrogymnastics (hi″dro-jim-nas′tiks) exercise performed under water.

hydrohymenitis (hi″dro-hi″men-i′tis) inflammation of a serous membrane.

hydrokinesitherapy (hi″dro-ki-ne″sĭ-ther′ah-pe) treatment by underwater exercise.

hydrokinetic (hi″dro-ki-net′ik) relating to movement of water or other fluid, as in a whirlpool bath.

hydrokinetics (hi″dro-ki-net′iks) the science dealing with fluids in motion.

hydrolase (hi′dro-lās) an enzyme that catalyzes the hydrolysis of a compound.

hydrology (hi-drol′o-je) the study of water and its uses.

Hydrolose (hi′dro-lōs) trademark for a preparation of methylcellulose, a laxative.

hydrolymph (hi′dro-limf) the thin blood of certain animals.

hydrolysate (hi-drol′ĭ-zat) a compound produced by hydrolysis.
   protein h., a mixture of amino acids prepared by splitting a protein with acid, alkali or enzyme. Such preparations provide the nutritive equivalent of the original material in the form of its constituent amino acids and are used in special diets or for patients unable to take the ordinary food proteins.

hydrolysis (hi-drol′ĭ-sis) the cleavage of a compound by the addition of water, the hydroxyl group being incorporated in one fragment and the hydrogen atom in the other. adj., **hydrolyt′ic.**

hydrolyst (hi′dro-list) an agent that promotes hydrolysis.

hydroma (hi-dro′mah) hygroma.

hydromeningitis (hi″dro-men″in-ji′tis) 1. meningitis with serous effusion. 2. inflammation of Descemet's membrane.

hydromeningocele (hi″dro-mĕ-ning′go-sēl) protrusion of the meninges, containing fluid, through a defect in the skull or vertebral column.

hydrometer (hi-drom′ĕ-ter) an instrument for determining the specific gravity of a fluid.

hydrometra (hi″dro-me′trah) collection of watery fluid in the uterus.

hydrometrocolpos (hi″dro-me″tro-kol′pos) collection of watery fluid in the uterus and vagina.

hydrometry (hi-drom′ĕ-tre) measurement of specific gravity with a hydrometer.

hydromicrocephaly (hi″dro-mi″kro-sef′ah-le)

smallness of the head with an abnormal amount of cerebrospinal fluid.

hydromorphone (hi″dro-mor′fōn) a hydrogenated ketone of morphine; used as an analgesic.

   h. hydrochloride, a crystalline compound used as a narcotic analgesic.

hydromphalus (hi-drom′fah-lus) a cystic accumulation of watery fluid at the umbilicus.

hydromyelia (hi″dro-mi-e′le-ah) dilatation of the central canal of the spinal cord with an abnormal accumulation of fluid.

hydromyelomeningocele   (hi″dro-mi″ĕ-lo-mĕ-ning′go-sēl) a defect of the spine marked by protrusion of the membranes and tissue of the spinal cord, forming a fluid-filled sac.

hydromyoma (hi″dro-mi-o′mah) a cystic myoma containing fluid.

hydronephrosis (hi″dro-nĕ-fro′sis) distention of the renal pelvis and calices with urine; if it is allowed to progress, the functioning units of the kidney are destroyed. The collecting tubules dilate and the muscular walls of the renal pelvis and calices stretch, are replaced by fibrous tissue and eventually form a large, fluid-filled, functionless sac.

   The cause of hydronephrosis is obstruction or atrophy of the urinary tract. Mechanical obstruction may result from ureteral tumors, calculi, NEPHROPTOSIS, benign or malignant hyperplasia of the prostate or carcinoma of the bladder, urethra or glans penis. Inflammatory obstruction is the outcome of a urinary tract infection that produces edema and narrowing of the ureters or urethra. Rarely there occurs during pregnancy a loss of muscle tone in the urinary tract. The atony is thought to be induced by placental hormones.

   SYMPTOMS. The patient usually complains of recurrent attacks of pain in the kidney region. The pain may be described as dull and nagging or sharp. Examination of the urine often reveals the presence of pus and blood; there is fever if infection develops. If both kidneys are involved, uremia develops as the functional units of the kidneys are destroyed.

   Diagnosis is established by extensive urologic examination with detailed PYELOGRAPHY, which usually reveals the cause of the obstruction and accumulation of fluid in the pelvis.

   TREATMENT. The urinary tract must be drained by whatever means necessary; this may involve a simple dilatation of the ureter or urethra or it may require surgery of the affected kidney. When urinary tract infection is present as a cause or result of the hydronephrosis, urinary antiseptics and antibiotics are administered until the urine becomes sterile.

hydropericarditis (hi″dro-per″ĭ-kar-di′tis) pericarditis with watery effusion.

hydropericardium (hi″dro-per″ĭ-kar′de-um) excessive amount of serous fluid in the pericardial cavity.

hydroperinephrosis (hi″dro-per″ĭ-nĕ-fro′sis) collection of watery fluid around the kidney.

hydroperitoneum (hi″dro-per″ĭ-to-ne′um) collection of watery fluid in the peritoneal cavity.

hydrophilia (hi″dro-fil′e-ah) the property of absorbing water. adj., **hydrophil′ic.**

hydrophobia (hi″dro-fo′be-ah) rabies.

hydrophysometra (hi″dro-fi″so-me′trah) collection of fluid and gas in the uterus.

hydropic (hi-drop′ik) affected with dropsy, or hydrops.

hydroplasmia (hi″dro-plaz′me-ah) dilution of the blood plasma.

hydropneumatosis (hi″dro-nu″mah-to′sis) collection of fluid and gas in the tissues.

hydropneumopericardium (hi″dro-nu″mo-per″ĭ-kar′de-um) fluid and gas in the pericardium.

hydropneumoperitoneum (hi″dro-nu″mo-per″ĭ-to-ne′um) fluid and gas in the peritoneal cavity.

hydropneumothorax (hi″dro-nu″mo-tho′raks) the presence of both noninflammatory fluid and air or gas within the pleural cavity.

hydroposia (hi″dro-po′ze-ah) the drinking of water.

hydropotherapy (hi″dro-po-ther′ah-pe) therapeutic injection of ascitic fluid.

hydrops (hy′drops) [L.] abnormal accumulation of serous fluid in the tissues or in a body cavity; called also dropsy.

   fetal h., h. feta′lis, accumulation of fluid in the entire body of the newborn infant, in hemolytic disease due to antibodies present in the blood of the Rh-negative mother.

hydropyonephrosis (hi″dro-pi″o-nĕ-fro′sis) urine and pus in the kidney and its pelvis.

hydrorheostat (hi″dro-re′o-stat) a rheostat in which water furnishes resistance.

hydrorrhea (hi″dro-re′ah) a watery discharge.

   h. gravida′rum, watery discharge from the gravid uterus.

hydrosalpinx (hi″dro-sal′pinks) accumulation of watery fluid in a uterine tube.

hydroscheocele (hi-dros′ke-o-sēl″) a scrotal hernia containing fluid.

hydroscope (hi′dro-skōp) an instrument for detecting the presence of water.

hydrosis (hi-dro′sis) hidrosis.

hydrosol (hi′dro-sol) a colloid in which the dispersion medium is a liquid.

hydrostabile (hi″dro-sta′bil) tending to maintain constant weight under diet restrictions or in gastrointestinal disease.

hydrostat (hi′dro-stat) a device for regulating the height of a fluid in a column or reservoir.

hydrostatic (hi″dro-stat′ik) pertaining to a liquid in a state of equilibrium.

hydrostatics (hi″dro-stat′iks) the science of equilibrium of fluids.

hydrosudotherapy (hi″dro-su″do-ther′ah-pe) hydrotherapy with induction of perspiration.

hydrosulfuric acid (hi″dro-sul-fu′rik) hydrogen sulfide.

hydrosyringomyelia (hi″dro-sĭ-ring″go-mi-e′le-ah) distention of the central canal of the spinal cord, with the formation of cavities and degeneration.

hydrotaxis (hi″dro-tak′sis) an orientation movement of motile organisms or cells in response to the influence of water or moisture.

hydrotherapy (hi″dro-ther′ah-pe) use of water in any form, either externally or internally, in treatment of disease.

hydrothermic (hi″dro-ther′mik) relating to the temperature effects of water, as in hot baths.

hydrothionemia (hi″dro-thi″o-ne′me-ah) hydrogen sulfide in the blood.

hydrothionuria (hi″dro-thi″o-nu′re-ah) hydrogen sulfide in the urine.

hydrothorax (hi″dro-tho′raks) the presence of noninflammatory serous fluid within the pleural cavity.

hydrotropism (hi-drot′ro-pizm) a growth response of a nonmotile organism to the presence of water or moisture.

hydrotympanum (hi″dro-tim′pah-num) watery fluid in the middle ear.

hydroureter (hi″dro-u-re′ter) distention of the ureter with fluid.

hydrous (hi′drus) containing water.

hydrovarium (hi″dro-va′re-um) watery fluid in an ovary.

hydroxide (hi-drok′sīd) any compound of hydroxyl with another radical.

hydroxy- (hi-drok′se) a prefix in chemical terms indicating presence of the univalent radical OH.

hydroxyacetanilide (hi-drok″se-as″ĕ-tan′ĭ-lid) acetaminophen, an analgesic.

hydroxyamphetamine (hi-drok″se-am-fet′ah-mēn) a compound used as a sympathomimetic nasal decongestant, pressor and mydriatic.

hydroxyapatite (hi-drok″se-ap′ah-tīt) a compound that is probably the main inorganic constituent of bone and teeth.

hydroxybenzene (hi-drok″sĭ-ben′zēn) phenol.

hydroxybutyric acid (hi-drok″sĭ-bu-tir′ik) oxybutyric acid.

hydroxychloroquine (hi-drok″sĭ-klo′ro-kwin) a compound used as a suppressant for lupus erythematosus and against malaria.

hydroxycorticosterone (hi-drok″sĭ-kor″tĭ-ko-stēr′on) cortisol, a corticosteroid.

hydroxydione (hi-drok″sĭ-di′ōn) a compound used to produce basal anesthesia.

hydroxyl (hi-drok′sil) the univalent radical OH.

hydroxylysine (hi-drok″sĭ-li′sēn) a naturally occurring amino acid.

hydroxyprogesterone (hi-drok″sĭ-pro-jes′ter-ōn) a long-acting progesterone used in treatment of corpus luteum deficiency.

hydroxyproline (hi-drok″sĭ-pro′lēn) a naturally occurring amino acid.

hydroxystilbamidine (hi-drok″sĭ-stil-bam′ĭ-dēn) a compound used in treatment of leishmaniasis and blastomycosis.

hydroxytetracycline (hi-drok″sĭ-tĕ″trah-si′klēn) oxytetracycline, an antibiotic.

hydroxytryptamine (hi-drok″sĭ-trip′tah-mēn) serotonin.

hydroxyzine (hi-drok′sĭ-zēn) a compound used as a tranquilizer.

hydruria (hi-droo′re-ah) excretion of urine of low specific gravity.

hygeiophrontis (hi″je-o-fron′tis) anxious concern about one's own health; suggested to supplant hypochondriasis.

hygiene (hi′jēn) 1. the science of health and its preservation. 2. a condition or practice, such as cleanliness, that is conducive to preservation of health. adj., **hygien′ic.**
  mental h., the science dealing with development of healthy mental and emotional reactions and habits.
  oral h., the proper care of the mouth and teeth.
  social h., the science dealing with prevention and cure of venereal disease.

hygienics (hi″je-en′iks) a system of principles for promoting health.

hygienist (hi′je-en″ist) a specialist in hygiene.
  dental h., an auxiliary member of the dental profession, trained in the art of removing calcareous deposits and stains from surfaces of teeth and in providing additional services and information on prevention of oral disease.

hygro- (hi′gro) word element [Gr.], *moisture.*

hygroma (hi-gro′mah) an accumulation of fluid in a sac, cyst or bursa. adj., **hygrom′atous.**
  cystic h., h. cys′ticum, an endothelium-lined, fluid-containing lesion of lymphatic origin, encountered most often in infants and children and occurring in various regions of the body, most commonly in the posterior triangle of the neck, behind the sternocleidomastoid muscle (hygroma colli cysticum).
  Fleischmann's h., enlargement of a bursa in the floor of the mouth, to the outer side of the genioglossus muscle.

hygrometer (hi-grom′ĕ-ter) an instrument for measuring atmospheric moisture.

hygroscope (hi′gro-skōp) an instrument for showing variation in atmospheric moisture.

hygroscopic (hi″gro-skop′ik) readily absorbing moisture.

hygrostomia (hi″gro-sto′me-ah) excessive secretion of saliva.

Hygroton (hi′gro-ton) trademark for a preparation of chlorthalidone, a diuretic.

hyl(o)- (hi'lo) word element [Gr.], *matter (material; substance).*

hyle (hi'le) the primitive substance from which all matter is derived.

hylotropy (hi-lot'ro-pe) the ability of a substance to change from one physical form to another, e.g., solid to liquid, liquid to gas, without change in chemical composition.

hymen (hi'men) the membranous fold partly closing the vaginal orifice.

hymenectomy (hi"men-ek'to-me) excision of a membrane, especially of the hymen.

hymenitis (hi"men-i'tis) inflammation of the hymen.

hymenolepiasis (hi"men-o-lep-i'ah-sis) infection due to organisms of species of Hymenolepis.

Hymenolepis (hi"men-ol'ĕ-pis) a genus of TAPEWORMS; three species, *H. diminu'ta, H. lanceola'ta* and *H. na'na,* have been found in man.

hymenology (hi"men-ol'o-je) the science of the membranes.

hymenotomy (hi"men-ot'o-me) incision of the hymen.

hyoepiglottidean (hi"o-ep"ĭ-glŏ-tid'e-an) pertaining to the hyoid bone and epiglottis.

hyoglossal (hi"o-glos'al) pertaining to the hyoid bone and tongue.

hyoid (hi'oid) shaped like Greek letter upsilon (*v*).
  h. bone, a horseshoe-shaped bone situated at the base of the tongue, just below the thyroid cartilage.

hyoscine (hi'o-sin) scopolamine.

hyoscyamine (hi"o-si'ah-mēn) an alkaloid usually obtained from species of the plant Hyoscyamus or other genera of the family Solanaceae.
  h. sulfate, a salt used as a parasympatholytic.

hyoscyamus (hi"o-si'ah-mus) the dried leaf of *Hyoscyamus niger;* used in tincture or extract to produce parasympathetic blockade.

hypacusia (hi"pah-ku'ze-ah) diminished acuteness of the sense of hearing.

hypalbuminosis (hi"pal-bu"mĭ-no'sis) deficiency of albumins in blood.

hypalgesia (hi"pal-je'ze-ah) diminished sensibility to pain.

hypamnios (hi-pam'ne-os) deficiency of amniotic fluid.

hypanakinesia (hi"pan-ah-ki-ne'se-ah) defective motor (muscular) activity, as of the stomach.

hypaxial (hi-pak'se-al) beneath the axis of the vertebral column.

hyper- (hi'per) word element [Gr.], *abnormally increased; excessive.*

hyperacid (hi"per-as'id) abnormally or exessively acid.

hyperacidity (hi"per-ah-sid'ĭ-te) excessive acidity.

hyperactivity (hi"per-ak-tiv'ĭ-te) excessive activity.

hyperacusia (hi"per-ah-ku'ze-ah) abnormal acuteness of the sense of hearing.

hyperacute (hi"per-ah-kūt') extremely acute.

hyperadenosis (hy"per-ad"ĕ-no'sis) enlargement of glands.

hyperadiposis (hi"per-ad"ĭ-po'sis) extreme fatness.

hyperadrenalemia (hi"per-ah-dre"nah-le'me-ah) increased amount of adrenal secretion in the blood.

hyperadrenalism, hyperadrenia (hi"per-ah-dren'al-izm), (hi"per-ah-dre'ne-ah) overactivity of the adrenal glands.

hyperadrenocorticalism, hyperadrenocorticism (hi"per-ah-dre"no-kor'tĭ-kal-izm"), (hi"per-ah-dre"no-kor'tĭ-sizm) hypersecretion of the adrenal cortex; CUSHING'S SYNDROME.

hyperaffectivity (hi"per-ah"fek-tiv'ĭ-te) abnormally increased sensibility to mild superficial stimuli; abnormally heightened emotional reactivity.

hyperalbuminemia (hi"per-al-bu"mĭ-ne'me-ah) excessive albumin content of the blood.

hyperaldosteronemia (hi"per-al-dos'ter-o-ne'me-ah) excess of aldosterone in the blood.

hyperaldosteronism (hi"per-al-dos'ter-ōn-izm") aldosteronism.

hyperaldosteronuria (hi"per-al-dos'ter-o-nu're-ah) excess of aldosterone in the urine.

hyperalgesia (hi"per-al-je'ze-ah) excessive sensitiveness to pain.

hyperalkalinity (hi"per-al"kah-lin'ĭ-te) excessive alkalinity.

hyperammoniemia (hi"per-ah-mo"ne-e'me-ah) excess of ammonia in the blood.

hyperammoniuria (hi"per-ah-mo"ne-u're-ah) excess of ammonia in the urine.

hyperanakinesia (hi"per-an"ah-ki-ne'ze-ah) excessive motor activity.
  h. ventric'uli, excessive motor activity of the stomach.

hyperandrogenism (hi"per-an'dro-jen-izm") excessive secretion of androgens.

hyperaphia (hi"per-a'fe-ah) abnormal acuteness of the sense of touch.

hyperazotemia (hi"per-az"o-te'me-ah) excess of nitrogenous matter in the blood.

hyperazoturia (hi"per-az"o-tu're-ah) excess of nitrogenous matter in the urine.

hyperbaria (hi"per-bār'e-ah) disorder due to exposure to extremely high atmospheric pressure.

hyperbaric (hi"per-bār'ik) characterized by greater than normal pressure or weight; applied to gases under greater than atmospheric pressure, or to a solution of greater specific gravity than another taken as a standard of reference.
  h. oxygenation, exposure to oxygen under condi-

tions of greatly increased pressure; abbreviated HPO, for high-pressure oxygenation. This treatment is given to patients who, for various reasons, need more oxygen than they can take in by breathing while in the ordinary atmosphere, or even in an oxygen tent.

The patient is placed in a sealed enclosure, called a hyperbaric chamber. Compressed air is introduced to raise the atmospheric pressure to several times normal. At the same time the patient is given pure oxygen through a face mask. The increase in atmospheric pressure forces enough air into the patient so that the pressure within his body equals the pressure outside. Thus all his tissues become flooded with more than the usual supply of oxygen. While the patient is in the chamber, pressure changes are controlled with extreme care to avoid injury to his lungs or other tissues.

USE OF HYPERBARIC OXYGENATION. This form of treatment may be administered in many types of disorders in which oxygen supply is deficient. If, because of injury or disease, the lungs or heart are unable to maintain good circulation, the increase in oxygen can temporarily compensate for the reduction in circulation. If injury or disease has caused the breaking or blocking of arteries, an extra supply of oxygen in the vessels that are still functioning will help.

Hyperbaric oxygenation has been used with apparent success in some cases of heart surgery and other operations during which a forced supply of oxygen to the patient is vital. During such operations, the surgeon and his assistants must work within the chamber. Since the high pressure could cause the physical and mental disturbances of BENDS, as sometimes happens with deep-sea divers, it must be carefully controlled. All persons must be decompressed after leaving the chamber.

Patients suffering from tetanus and gas gangrene, infections caused by bacteria that are resistant to antibiotics but vulnerable to oxygen, are helped by hyperbaric oxygenation. The technique is apparently also useful in radiotherapy for cancer. When full of oxygen, cancer cells seem more vulnerable to radiation.

Carbon monoxide poisoning can be treated by hyperbaric oxygenation. Carbon monoxide molecules, displacing the oxygen in the erythrocytes,

usually cause asphyxiation, but hyperbaric oxygenation can often keep the patient alive until the carbon monoxide has been eliminated from his system.

hyperbilirubinemia (hi″per-bil″i-roo″bĭ-ne′me-ah) excess of bilirubin in the blood.

hyperbrachycephalic (hi″per-brak″e-sĕ-fal′ik) having a cephalic index of 85.5 or more.

hyperbulia (hi″per-bu′le-ah) excessive willfulness.

hypercalcemia (hi″per-kal-se′me-ah) excess of calcium in the blood.
   idiopathic h., a condition of infants, associated with vitamin D intoxication, characterized by elevated serum calcium levels, increased density of the skeleton, mental deterioration and nephrocalcinosis.

hypercalciuria (hi″per-kal″se-u′re-ah) excess of calcium in the urine.

hypercapnia, hypercarbia (hi″per-kap′ne-ah), (hi″per-kar′be-ah) excess of carbon dioxide in the blood.

hypercatabolism (hi″per-kah-tab′o-lizm) abnormally increased catabolism.

hypercatharsis (hi″per-kah-thar′sis) excessive purgation.

hypercellularity (hi″per-sel″u-lar′ĭ-te) abnormal increase in the number of cells present, as in bone marrow.

hypercenesthesia (hi″per-sen″es-the′ze-ah) an exaggerated feeling of well-being.

hyperchloremia (hi″per-klo-re′me-ah) excess of chlorides in the blood.

hyperchlorhydria (hi″per-klōr-hi′dre-ah) excess of HYDROCHLORIC ACID in the gastric juice.

hypercholesteremia, hypercholesterolemia (hi″per-ko-les″ter-e′me-ah), (hi″per-ko-les″ter-ol-e′me-ah) excess of cholesterol in the blood.

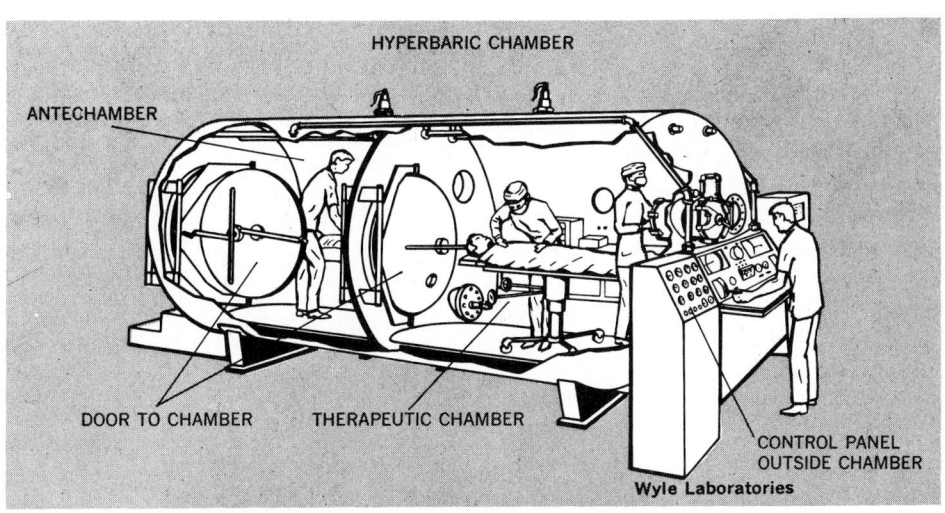

Hyperbaric chamber. (Courtesy of Wyle Laboratories.)

hypercholia (hi″per-ko′le-ah) excessive secretion of bile.

hyperchromatism (hi″per-kro′mah-tizm) excessive pigmentation; especially a form of degeneration of a cell nucleus in which it becomes filled with particles of pigment, or chromatin.

hyperchromatosis (hi″per-kro″mah-to′sis) 1. increased staining capacity. 2. hyperchromatism.

hyperchromemia (hi″per-kro-me′me-ah) a high color index of the blood.

hyperchromia (hi″per-kro′me-ah) 1. hyperchromatism. 2. abnormal increase in the hemoglobin content of the erythrocytes. adj., **hyperchro′mic.**

hyperchylia (hi″per-ki′le-ah) excessive secretion of gastric juice.

hyperchylomicronemia (hi″per-ki″lo-mi″kro-ne′-me-ah) the presence in the blood of an excessive number of particles of fat (chylomicrons).

hypercinesia (hi″per-si-ne′ze-ah) hyperkinesia.

hypercoagulability (hi″per-ko-ag″u-lah-bil′i-te) abnormally increased coagulability of the blood.

hypercorticism (hi″per-kor′ti-sizm) hyperadrenocorticism.

hypercrine (hi′per-krin) due to endocrine hyperfunction.

hypercrinism (hi″per-krin′izm) excessive secretion of an endocrine gland.

hypercryalgesia, hypercryesthesia (hi″per-kri″al-je′ze-ah), (hi″per-kri″es-the′ze-ah) excessive sensitiveness to cold.

hypercupriuria (hi″per-ku″pre-u′re-ah) excess of copper in the blood.

hypercyanotic (hi″per-si″ah-not′ik) extremely cyanotic.

hypercyesis (hi″per-si-e′sis) superfetation.

hypercythemia (hi″per-si-the′me-ah) excess of erythrocytes.

hypercytosis (hi″per-si-to′sis) a condition characterized by an abnormally increased number of cells, especially of leukocytes.

hyperdactylia (hi″per-dak-til′e-ah) the presence of supernumerary digits on the hand or foot.

hyperdiastole (hi″per-di-as′to-le) excessive cardiac diastole.

hyperdicrotic (hi″per-di-krot′ik) markedly dicrotic.

hyperdiploidy (hi″per-dip′loi-de) the state of having more than the diploid number of chromosomes (>2n).

hyperdipsia (hi″per-dip′se-ah) intense thirst of relatively brief duration.

hyperdistention (hi″per-dis-ten′shun) excessive distention.

hyperdiuresis (hi″per-di″u-re′sis) excessive secretion of urine.

hyperdontia (hi″per-don′she-ah) a condition characterized by the presence of supernumerary teeth.

hyperdynamia (hi″per-di-na′me-ah) excessive muscular activity.

hypereccrisia (hi″per-ĕ-kriz′e-ah) excessive excretion.

hyperelectrolytemia (hi″per-e-elek″tro-li-te′-me-ah) abnormally increased electrolyte content of the blood.

hyperemesis (hi″per-em′ĕ-sis) excessive vomiting.
  h. gravida′rum, excessive and pernicious vomiting of pregnancy, usually in the first trimester. The condition is more serious than simple MORNING SICKNESS, which is a common discomfort during the first 3 months of pregnancy. The exact cause of hyperemesis gravidarum is not known; however, psychologic factors are thought to play an important role in its development and control.
  SYMPTOMS. The patient complains of uncontrollable nausea, persistent retching and vomiting, inability to take any food by mouth and exhaustion due to restlessness and lack of sleep. As the condition persists the patient becomes severely dehydrated, develops a fever and may show signs of peripheral nerve involvement and jaundice. The urine may contain blood, bile, albumin and ketone bodies as starvation develops. Although hyperemesis gravidarum is rarely fatal, these latter symptoms indicate a grave illness that demands prompt treatment.
  TREATMENT. The physical symptoms of the patient are relieved by intravenous administration of fluids and nutrients and mild sedation to promote rest and relaxation. There is some controversy as to the value of psychotherapy; however, it is generally agreed that the patient will need help in overcoming emotional problems and nervous tension if they contribute to the occurrence of the disorder.
  Dietary treatment may include limiting the intake of liquids, eating a snack of crackers or dry toast before arising and avoiding excessive fat in the diet.
  NURSING CARE. The hospitalized patient should be placed in a quiet, well ventilated room that is free from odors or sights that may cause nausea. She should be encouraged to talk about her fears and anxieties if she indicates a desire to do so. The nursing staff should be alert to signs of depression or fears of pregnancy, labor or the responsibilities of motherhood. Recovery is much more likely if the patient is able to vocalize her fears and seek aid in solving the mental conflicts that may be an underlying cause of her illness. Those who care for her should be sympathetic, optimistic and reassuring in discussing her condition with her.
  h. lacten′tium, the vomiting of nursing babies.

hyperemia (hi″per-e′me-ah) excess of blood in a part.
  active h., arterial h., that due to local or general relaxation of arterioles.
  leptomeningeal h., congestion of the pia-arachnoid.
  passive h., that due to obstruction to flow of blood from the area.
  reactive h., that due to increase in blood flow after its temporary interruption.
  venous h., passive hyperemia.

hyperemotivity (hi″per-e″mo-tiv′i-te) hyperaffectivity.

hyperencephalus (hi″per-en-sef′ah-lus) a monster fetus with the brain exposed.

hyperendocrinism (hi″per-en-dok′rĭ-nizm) excess of any internal secretion.

hypereosinophilia (hi″per-e″o-sin″o-fil′e-ah) excess of eosinophils in the blood.

hyperephidrosis (hi″per-ef″ĭ-dro′sis) excessive sweating.

hyperepinephrinemia (hi″per-ep″ĭ-nef″rĭ-ne′me-ah) excessive epinephrine in the blood.

hypererethism (hi″per-er′ĕ-thizm) extreme irritability.

hyperergasia, hyperergy (hi″per-er-ga′ze-ah), (hi″per-er′je) increased capacity to react to a specific stimulus.

hypererythrocythemia (hi″per-ĕ-rith″ro-si-the′-me-ah) excess of erythrocytes in the blood; hypercythemia.

hyperesthesia (hi″per-es-the′ze-ah) a state of abnormally increased sensitivity to stimuli.

hyperestrinemia (hi″per-es″trĭ-ne′me-ah) excessive estrin in the blood.

hyperestrinism (hi″per-es′trin-izm) excessive secretion of estrin, characterized by functional uterine bleeding.

hyperestrogenemia (hi″per-es″tro-jĕ-ne′me-ah) excessive estrogen in the blood.

hyperestrogenism (hi″per-es′tro-jen-izm″) excessive secretion of estrogen.

hyperextension (hi″per-ek-sten′shun) excessive extension of a limb or part.

hyperferremia, hyperferricemia (hi″per-fĕ-re′-me-ah), (hi″per-fer″ĭ-se′me-ah) excess of iron in the blood.

hyperfunction (hi″per-fungk′shun) excessive functioning of a part or organ.

hypergalactia (hi″per-gah-lak′she-ah) excessive secretion of milk.

hypergammaglobulinemia (hi″per-gam″ah-glob″u-lin-e′me-ah) increased gamma globulins in the blood.

hypergenesis (hi″per-jen′ĕ-sis) excessive development.

hypergenitalism (hi″per-jen′ĭ-tal-izm″) hypergonadism.

hypergeusesthesia, hypergeusia (hi″per-gu″-zes-the′ze-ah), (hi″per-gu′ze-ah) abnormal acuteness of the sense of taste.

hypergigantosoma (hi″per-ji-gan″to-so′mah) excessive size of the body.

hyperglandular (hi″per-glan′du-lar) marked by excessive glandular activity.

hyperglobulia (hi″per-glo-bu′le-ah) excess of erythrocytes; erythrocytosis.

hyperglobulinemia (hi″per-glob″u-lin-e′me-ah) excess of globulin in the blood.

hyperglycemia (hi″per-gli-se′me-ah) excess of glucose in the blood. adj., **hyperglyce′mic.**

hyperglyceridemia (hi″per-glis″er-ĭ-de′me-ah) excess of glycerides in the blood.

hyperglycinemia (hi″per-gli″sĭ-ne′me-ah) excessive glycine in the blood.

hyperglycistia (hi″per-gli-sis′te-ah) excess of sugar in the tissues.

hyperglycogenolysis (hi″per-gli″ko-jĕ-nol′ĭ-sis) excessive splitting up of glycogen in the body.

hyperglycoplasmia (hi″per-gli″ko-plaz′me-ah) excessive sugar in the blood plasma.

hyperglycorachia (hi″per-gli″ko-ra′ke-ah) excessive sugar in the cerebrospinal fluid.

hyperglycosemia (hi″per-gli″ko-se′me-ah) hyperglycemia.

hyperglycosuria (hi″per-gli″ko-su′re-ah) excessive glycosuria.

hypergnosia (hi″per-no′se-ah) a paranoic condition marked by distortion of perception with a tendency to project psychic conflicts to the environment.

hypergonadism (hi″per-go′nad-izm) abnormally increased functional activity of the gonads, with excessive growth and precocious sexual development.

hyperhedonia (hi″per-he-do′ne-ah) morbid increase of enjoyment.

hyperhidrosis (hi″per-hĭ-dro′sis) abnormally increased secretion of sweat.

hyperhormonism (hi″per-hōr′mōn-izm) excessive hormone secretion.

hyperhydration (hi″per-hi-dra′shun) abnormally increased water content of the body.

hyperidrosis (hi″per-ĭ-dro′sis) hyperhidrosis.

hyperinosemia (hi″per-in″o-se′me-ah) excess of fibrin in the blood.

hyperinsulinism (hi″per-in′su-lin-izm″) 1. excessive secretion of insulin by the pancreas, resulting in hypoglycemia. 2. insulin shock from overdosage of insulin.

hyperinvolution (hi″per-in″vo-lu′shun) excessive involution.

hyperisotonic (hi″per-i″so-ton′ik) noting a serum containing more salt than is necessary to preserve the erythrocytes.

hyperkalemia (hi″per-kah-le′me-ah) excess of potassium in the blood. adj., **hyperkale′mic.**

hyperkeratinization (hi″per-ker″ah-tin-ĭ-za′-shun) excessive development of keratin in the epidermis.

hyperkeratosis (hi″per-ker″ah-to′sis) 1. hypertrophy of the cornea. 2. thickening of the stratum corneum of the skin.

hyperketonemia (hi″per-ke″to-ne′me-ah) increased concentration of ketone bodies in the blood.

hyperketonuria (hi″per-ke″to-nu′re-ah) excessive ketone in the urine.

hyperketosis (hi″per-ke-to′sis) excessive formation of ketone.

hyperkinemia (hi″per-ki-ne′me-ah) abnormally high cardiac output.

hyperkinesia (hi″per-ki-ne′ze-ah) abnormally increased motor function or activity.

hyperlactation (hi″per-lak-ta′shun) lactation in greater than normal amount or for a longer than normal period.

hyperlecithinemia (hi″per-les″ĭ-thin-e′me-ah) excessive lecithin in the blood.

hyperleukocytosis (hi″per-lu″ko-si-to′sis) excess of leukocytes in the blood.

hyperlipemia (hi″per-li-pe′me-ah) excess of lipids in the blood.

hyperlipoproteinemia (hi″per-lip″o-pro″te-ine′me-ah) excess of lipoproteins in the blood.

hyperliposis (hi″per-lĭ-po′sis) excess of fat in the blood serum or tissues.

hyperlithuria (hi″per-lĭ-thu′re-ah) excess of uric (lithic) acid in the urine.

hypermastia (hi″per-mas′te-ah) 1. excessive size of mammary glands. 2. the presence of one or more supernumerary mammary glands; polymastia.

hypermegasoma (hi″per-meg″ah-so′mah) excessive bodily development.

hypermelanotic (hi″per-mel″ah-not′ik) characterized by an excessive deposit of melanin.

hypermenorrhea (hi″per-men″o-re′ah) excessive uterine bleeding occurring at regular intervals, the period of flow being of usual duration.

hypermetabolism (hi″per-mĕ-tab′o-lizm) increased metabolism.
  extrathyroidal m., abnormally elevated basal metabolism unassociated with thyroid disease.

hypermetaplasia (hi″per-met″ah-pla′ze-ah) excessive metaplasia.

hypermetria (hi″per-me′tre-ah) excessive range of movement.

hypermetrope (hi″per-met′rōp) hyperope.

hypermetropia (hi″per-mĕ-tro′pe-ah) farsightedness; hyperopia.

hypermnesia (hi″perm-ne′ze-ah) excessive crowding or unusual clarity of memory images.

hypermodal (hi″per-mo′dal) in statistics, relating to the values or items located to the right of the mode in a variations curve.

hypermorph (hi′per-morf) 1. a person who is tall, but of low sitting height. 2. in genetics, a hypermorphic mutant gene, i.e., one exaggerating or increasing normal activity.

hypermotility (hi″per-mo-til′ĭ-te) excessive or abnormally increased motility.

hypermyotonia (hi″per-mi″o-to′ne-ah) excessive muscular tonicity.

hypermyotrophy (hi″per-mi-ot′ro-fe) excessive development of muscular tissue.

hypernatremia (hi″per-na-tre′me-ah) excess of sodium in the blood.

hypernephroma (hi″per-nĕ-fro′mah) a tumor of the kidney whose cells resemble those from the adrenal cortex.

hypernitremia (hi″per-ni-tre′me-ah) excess of nitrogen in the blood.

hypernoia (hi″per-noi′ah) excessive mental activity.

hypernormal (hi″per-nor′mal) in excess of what is normal.

hypernormocytosis (hi″per-nor″mo-si-to′sis) excessive proportion of neutrophils in the blood.

hypernutrition (hi″per-nu-trish′un) overfeeding and its ill effects.

hyperonychia (hi″per-o-nik′e-ah) hypertrophy of the nails.

hyperope (hi′per-ōp) a person with hyperopia.

hyperopia (hi″per-o′pe-ah) farsightedness; a visual defect in which parallel light rays reaching the eye come to focus behind the retina, vision being better for distant objects than for near. (See also VISION.)
  Most children are born with some degree of farsightedness. As the child grows the condition decreases and usually disappears by the age of 8 years. If the child is excessively farsighted, however, the constant effort to focus may cause headaches and fatigue.
  The eyeglasses used to correct hyperopia are convex; that is, they bend the light rays toward the center, helping the lens of the eye to focus them on the retina.

hyperorchidism (hi″per-or′kĭ-dizm) abnormally increased functional activity of the testes.

hyperorexia (hi″per-o-rek′se-ah) excessive appetite.

hyperosmia (hi″per-oz′me-ah) abnormal acuteness of the sense of smell.

hyperosmolarity (hi″per-oz″mo-lar′ĭ-te) abnormally increased osmotic concentration of a solution.

hyperostosis (hi″per-os-to′sis) excessive growth of bony tissue.
  h. fronta′lis intern′a, a new formation of bone tissue protruding in patches on the internal surface of the cranial bones in the frontal region.
  infantile cortical h., a disease of young infants characterized by soft tissue swellings over the affected bones, fever and irritability, and marked by periods of remission and exacerbation.

hyperovaria (hi″per-o-va′re-ah) excessive ovarian activity.

hyperoxaluria (hi″per-ok″sah-lu′re-ah) excess of oxalate in the urine.

primary h., a genetic disorder characterized by urinary excretion of oxalate, with nephrolithiasis, nephrocalcinosis and often a generalized deposit of calcium oxalate.

hyperoxemia (hi″per-ok-se′me-ah) excessive acidity of the blood.

hyperoxia (hi″per-ok′se-ah) an abnormally increased supply or concentration of oxygen.

hyperpancreorrhea (hi″per-pan″kre-o-re′ah) excessive secretion from the pancreas.

hyperparasite (hi″per-par′ah-sīt) an individual or species parasitic on an organism that is itself parasitic upon a third species of organism.

hyperparathyroidism (hi″per-par″ah-thi′roi-dizm) abnormally increased activity of the parathyroid glands, causing loss of calcium from the bones and excessive secretion of calcium and phosphorus by the kidney. Among the symptoms are kidney stones, back pain, joint pains, thirst, nausea and vomiting. The condition also makes bones more subject to fracture.

About 90 per cent of cases of primary hyperparathyroidism are caused by a benign tumor. Secondary hyperparathyroidism is usually associated with abnormal growth of the parathyroid glands. It is most commonly found in chronic kidney disease, but is also found in childhood rickets and osteomalacia.

If a parathyroid tumor is present, it is removed surgically. If there is abnormal growth of all of the parathyroids, three of the glands and part of the fourth must be removed surgically.

The outlook for the patient is directly related to the extent of kidney damage. Damaged bones, despite deformity, fracture and cysts, will heal completely if the tumor is removed. Once significant kidney damage has occurred, however, it may continue to progress.

hyperpepsinemia (hi″per-pep″sĭ-ne′me-ah) abnormally high level of pepsin in the blood.

hyperpepsinia (hi″per-pep-sin′e-ah) excessive secretion of pepsin in the stomach.

hyperpepsinuria (hi″per-pep″sĭ-nu′re-ah) abnormally high level of pepsin in the urine.

hyperphalangism (hi″per-fal′an-jizm) the presence of a supernumerary phalanx on a finger or toe.

hyperphasia (hi″per-fa′ze-ah) excessive talkativeness.

hyperphonesis (hi″per-fo-ne′sis) intensification of the sound in auscultation or percussion.

hyperphosphatasia (hi″per-fos″fah-ta′ze-ah) excess of phosphatase in the body.

hyperphosphatemia (hi″per-fos″fah-te′me-ah) an excess of phosphates in the blood.

hyperphosphaturia (hi″per-fos″fah-tu′re-ah) an excess of phosphates in the urine.

hyperphrenia (hi″per-fre′ne-ah) 1. extreme mental excitement. 2. accelerated mental activity.

hyperpiesis (hi″per-pi-e′sis) abnormally high pressure, in particular, high blood pressure.

hyperpituitarism (hi″per-pĭ-tu′ĭ-tar-izm″) a

condition due to pathologically increased activity of the PITUITARY GLAND.

hyperplasia (hi″per-pla′ze-ah) increase in volume of a tissue or organ caused by the formation and growth of new cells. adj., **hyperplas′tic.**

hyperplasmia (hi″per-plaz′me-ah) 1. excess in the proportion of blood plasma to corpuscles. 2. increase in size of erythrocytes through absorption of plasma.

hyperplasminemia (hi″per-plaz″mĭ-ne′me-ah) excess of plasmin in the circulating blood.

hyperploidy (hi″per-ploi″de) the state of having more than the typical number of chromosomes in unbalanced sets.

hyperpnea (hi″perp-ne′ah) abnormal increase in depth and rate of respiration.

hyperponesis (hi″per-po-ne′sis) a feeling of being unduly weighed down by one's duties and responsibilities.

hyperporosis (hi″per-po-ro′sis) excessive callus formation.

hyperposia (hi″per-po′ze-ah) abnormally increased ingestion of fluids for relatively brief periods.

hyperpotassemia (hi″per-pot″ah-se′me-ah) hyperkalemia; excess of potassium in the blood.

hyperpragic (hi″per-praj′ik) characterized by excessive activity.

hyperpraxia (hi″per-prak′se-ah) abnormal activity; restlessness.

hyperprolinemia (hi″per-pro″lĭ-ne′me-ah) excessive proline in the blood.

hyperprosexia (hi″per-pro-sek′se-ah) occupation of the mind by one idea to the exclusion of all others.

hyperproteinemia (hi″per-pro″te-ĭ-ne′me-ah) excess of protein in the blood.

hyperproteinuria (hi″per-pro″te-ĭ-nu′re-ah) excess of protein in the urine.

hyperproteosis (hi″per-pro″te-o′sis) excess of protein in the diet.

hyperpselaphesia (hi″perp-sel″ah-fe′ze-ah) increased tactile sensitiveness.

hyperpsychosis (hi″per-si-ko′sis) exaggeration of the function of thought.

hyperptyalism (hi″per-ti′ah-lizm) abnormally increased secretion of saliva.

hyperpyrexia (hi″per-pi-rek′se-ah) excessively high fever.

hyperreactor (hi″per-re-ak′tor) an individual showing greater than normal response to a stimulus.

hyperreflexia (hi″per-re-flek′se-ah) exaggeration of reflexes.

hyperresonance (hi″per-rez′o-nans) a sound elicited by percussion, of pitch lying between that of resonance and tympany.

hypersalemia (hi″per-sah-le′me-ah) abnormally increased content of salt in the blood.

hypersalivation (hi″per-sal″ĭ-va-shun) hyperptyalism.

hypersecretion (hi″per-se-kre′shun) excessive secretion.

hypersegmentation (hi″per-seg″men-ta′shun) the appearance of being divided into multiple segments or lobes.

hypersensibility (hi″per-sen″sĭ-bil′ĭ-te) exaggerated sensibility.

hypersensitivity (hi″per-sen″sĭ-tiv′ĭ-te) a state of altered reactivity in which the body reacts to a foreign agent more strongly than normal; anaphylaxis and allergy are forms of hypersensitivity.

hypersensitization (hi″per-sen″sĭ-tĭ-za′shun) creation of an abnormally sensitive condition.

hypersialosis (hi″per-si″ah-lo′sis) excessive secretion of the salivary glands; hyperptyalism.

hypersomnia (hi″per-som′ne-ah) pathologically excessive sleep.

hypersphyxia (hi″per-sfik′se-ah) increased activity of the circulation with increased blood pressure.

hypersplenism (hi″per-splen′izm) a morbid state resulting from hyperfunctioning of the spleen.

hypersthenia (hi″per-sthe′ne-ah) increased strength or tonicity.

hypersthenuria (hi″per-sthĕ-nu′re-ah) excretion of urine of abnormally high molecular concentration.

hypersystole (hi″per-sis′to-le) abnormal exaggeration of the systole.

hypertelorism (hi″per-te′lo-rizm) abnormally increased distance between two organs or parts.

   ocular h., orbital h., increase in the interocular distance, often associated with cleidocranial or craniofacial dysostosis and sometimes with mental deficiency.

hypertensin (hy″per-ten′sin) angiotensin, a vasoconstrictor substance in the blood.

hypertensinogen (hi″per-ten-sin′o-jen) a globulin in the blood that is acted on by renin to produce hypertension (angiotensin).

hypertension (hi″per-ten′shun) excessive pressure of the blood against the arterial walls; usually restricted to the condition in which the resting systolic pressure is consistently greater than 160 mm. of mercury, the diastolic pressure is over 90 mm. of mercury, and the individual complains of the symptoms of hypertension; called also high blood pressure.

   In a large percentage of cases, the causes of hypertension cannot be determined. Such cases are called essential (or idiopathic) hypertension. The others can be traced to definite diseases such as kidney disorders, tumors of the adrenal glands, Cushing's syndrome or coarctation of the aorta.

Mild cases of hypertension may not present any symptoms for years and the patient may not know that he has high blood pressure. When symptoms do appear they may include headache, fatigue, weakness, shortness of breath and failing vision. High blood pressure is rarely a direct cause of death. It is more often an indication that there is something wrong, either physically or emotionally, that must be corrected; it tends to weaken other systems of the body so that they may fail and cause serious illness. About 15 per cent of the deaths in patients with hypertension are caused by cerebral vascular accident (stroke), and 65 per cent are caused by heart disease.

Malignant hypertension occurs most often in persons in their twenties or thirties and differs from other types of hypertension in that it progresses very rapidly and may prove fatal if not treated immediatly after symptoms develop, before damage is done to the blood vessels. Especially affected are the blood vessels in the eye. The kidneys or heart may fail, or the cerebral blood vessels may rupture, resulting in a cerebral vascular accident. With proper care under a physician's continuous supervision, malignant hypertension can be kept under control for years.

Treatment of hypertension consists of rest as indicated to lower the blood pressure to within safe limits, sedatives to relieve tension and promote rest and antihypertensive drugs, which lower the blood pressure. Examples of these drugs are rauwolfia serpentina, reserpine and hydralazine hydrochloride.

Restricting the intake of sodium may be necessary if edema is present, and since obesity tends to increase the blood pressure, a reducing diet may be prescribed. If emotional tensions are the cause of hypertension, psychotherapy may be desirable.

   portal h., abnormally increased pressure in the portal circulation.

hypertensive (hi″per-ten′siv) 1. characterized by or causing increased tension or pressure, as abnormally high blood pressure. 2. a person with abnormally high blood pressure.

hypertensor (hi″per-ten′sor) a substance that raises the blood pressure.

hypertetraploidy (hi″per-tĕ′trah-ploi″de) the state of having more than the tetraploid number of chromosomes in unbalanced sets ($4n + x$).

hyperthecosis (hi″per-the-ko′sis) hyperplasia and excessive luteinization of the cells of the inner stromal layer of the ovary.

hyperthelia (hi″per-the′le-ah) the presence of supernumerary nipples.

hyperthermalgesia (hi″per-ther″mal-je′ze-ah) abnormal sensitiveness to heat.

hyperthermesthesia (hi″per-therm″es-the′ze-ah) increased sensibility for heat.

hyperthermia, hyperthermy (hi″per-ther′me-ah), (hi″per-ther′me) greatly increased temperature.

hyperthrombinemia (hi″per-throm″bĭ-ne′me-ah) excess of thrombin in the blood.

hyperthrombocytemia (hi″per-throm″bo-si-te′-me-ah) excess of platelets in the blood.

hyperthymia (hi″per-thi′me-ah) excessive emotionalism.

hyperthymism (hi″per-thi′mizm) excessive thymus activity.

hyperthyroidism (hi″per-thi′roi-dizm) excessive functional activity of the THYROID GLAND. The condition is called also thyrotoxicosis, and is often accompanied by GOITER. Symptoms include profuse sweating, dislike of heat, palpitation, insomnia, nervousness and excitability. The basal metabolic rate is increased. Sometimes there is diarrhea. There may also be bulging of the eyes, in which case the condition may be referred to as exophthalmic goiter, or Graves' disease.

TREATMENT. Medical treatment includes drugs that inhibit the production of thyroxine (antithyroid drugs). Preparations of iodine, such as Lugol's solution, and radioactive iodine are widely used, as are thiourea and its derivatives. In addition to these drugs the patient is placed on a regimen of rest and freedom from emotional excitement in an effort to lower the metabolic rate. A diet high in caloric and vitamin content is prescribed to compensate for weight loss and high energy output.

NURSING CARE. The environment of the patient should be as quiet and conducive to relaxation as possible. Emotional outbursts are not uncommon in these patients and they should be handled calmly and without retaliation because the patient cannot control them. Nursing personnel and visitors should avoid conversations or activities that might disturb the patient or excite him emotionally.

Patients receiving radioactive iodine therapeutically are usually isolated until the drug is completely eliminated from the body. Radioactive iodine is excreted by the kidneys and circulates in the blood; thus, precautions are necessary with the handling of needles and syringes used for the patient, and with bedpans or specimen bottles used for collecting urine. If the patient receives small amounts of radioactive iodine he is usually allowed to go home immediately after taking the medication and no special precautions are necessary. All patients must, however, be observed for signs of thyroid crisis, due to radiation-induced thyroiditis, after administration of the drug. Another complication of treatment with radioactive iodine is underactivity of the gland and development of the symptoms of MYXEDEMA.

Patients receiving preparations of iodine should be observed for signs of toxicity. These include a metallic taste in the mouth and sore gums. All iodine preparations are given through a straw to avoid discoloration of the teeth.

hypertonia (hi″per-to′ne-ah) abnormally increased tonicity or strength.
h. oc′uli, high intraocular pressure.

hypertonic (hi″per-ton′ik) 1. pertaining to or characterized by an increased tonicity or tension. 2. having an osmotic pressure greater than that of the solution with which it is compared.

hypertonicity (hi″per-to-nis′ĭ-te) the state or quality of being hypertonic.

hypertoxicity (hi″per-tok-sis′ĭ-te) an exaggerated or increased toxic quality.

hypertrichiasis, hypertrichosis (hi″per-trĭ-ki′-ah-sis), (hi″per-trĭ-ko′sis) excessive hairiness, which may be generalized or local, as on the pinna of the ear in males, a trait thought to be transmitted on the Y chromosome.

hypertriploidy (hi″per-trip′loi-de) the state of having more than the triploid number of chromosomes in unbalanced sets $(3n + x)$.

hypertrophy (hi-per′tro-fe) increase in volume of a tissue or organ produced entirely by enlargement of existing cells. adj., **hypertroph′ic.**
ventricular h., hypertrophy of the myocardium of a ventricle, causing undue deviation of the axis of the electrocardiogram.

hypertropia (hi″per-tro′pe-ah) upward deviation of the visual axis of one eye when the other eye is fixing.

hyperuresis (hi″per-u-re′sis) polyuria; excessive excretion of urine.

hyperuricemia (hi″per-u″rĭ-se′me-ah) an excess of uric acid in the blood.

hypervascular (hi″per-vas′ku-lar) extremely vascular.

hypervegetative (hi″per-vej′ĕ-ta″tiv) denoting a constitutional body type in which the visceral, nutritional functions predominate.

hypervenosity (hi″per-ve-nos′ĭ-te) excessive development of veins.

hyperventilation (hi″per-ven″tĭ-la′shun) 1. increase of air in the lungs above the normal amount. 2. abnormally prolonged and deep breathing, usually associated with acute anxiety or emotional tension. It is most commonly seen in nervous, anxious females who have other functional disturbances related to emotional problems. A transient, respiratory ALKALOSIS commonly results from hyperventilation. More prolonged hyperventilation may be caused by disorders of the central nervous system, or by drugs, such as high concentrations of salicylate, that increase sensitivity of the respiratory centers.

Symptoms of hyperventilation include "faintness" or impaired consciousness without actual loss of consciousness. At the outset the patient may have felt a tightness of the chest, a sensation of smothering and some degree of apprehension. Other symptoms may be related to the heart and digestive tract; for example, palpitation or pounding of the heart, fullness in the throat and pain over the stomach region. In prolonged attacks the patient may exhibit tetany with muscular spasm of the hands and feet.

Immediate treatment consists of having the patient rebreathe in a paper bag, to replace the carbon dioxide he has been "blowing off" during hyperventilation. He may need to be convinced that there is nothing serious wrong with him in the organic sense and that he can control the "attack" by using the paper bag for rebreathing. Treatment of the underlying emotional disturbance is recommended.

hyperviscosity (hi″per-vis-kos′ĭ-te) excessive viscosity.

hypervitaminosis (hi″per-vi″tah-mĭ-no′sis) a condition produced by ingestion of excessive amounts of vitamins.

hypervolemia (hi″per-vo-le′me-ah) abnormal increase in the volume of circulating fluid (plasma) in the body.

hypesthesia (hi″pes-the′ze-ah) abnormally diminished sensitiveness; hypoesthesia.

hypha (hi′fah), pl. *hy′phae* [L.] a filament composing the mycelium of a fungus.

hyphedonia (hīp″he-do′ne-ah) diminution of power of enjoyment.

hyphema (hi-fe′mah) hemorrhage into the anterior chamber of the eye.

hyphemia (hi-fe′me-ah) oligemia, or deficiency of blood.

hyphidrosis (hīp″hĭ-dro′sis) too scanty perspiration.

Hyphomycetes (hi″fo-mi-se′tēz) a genus of fungi including the molds, etc.

hypinosis (hip″ĭ-no′sis) diminished fibrin in the blood; hypoinosemia.

hypisotonic (hīp″i-so-ton′ik) less than isotonic; hypoisotonic.

hypn(o)- (hip′no) word element [Gr.], *sleep; hypnosis.*

hypnagogic (hip″nah-goj′ik) 1. producing sleep. 2. occurring during sleep.

hypnagogue (hip′nah-gog) 1. producing sleep. 2. an agent that produces sleep.

hypnalgia (hip-nal′je-ah) pain during sleep.

hypnoanalysis (hip″no-ah-nal′ĭ-sis) psychoanalysis with use of hypnosis to help uncover unconscious material.

hypnoanesthesia (hip″no-an″es-the′ze-ah) reduction of sensitivity to pain by hypnosis.

hypnodontics (hip″no-don′tiks) the application of hypnosis and controlled suggestion in the practice of dentistry.

hypnogenetic, hypnogenic (hip″no-jĕ-net′ik), (hip″no-jen′ik) causing or producing sleep.

hypnoid (hip′noid) resembling hypnosis.

hypnoidization (hip″noi-dĭ-za′shun) the production of light hypnosis.

hypnolepsy (hip′no-lep″se) abnormal sleepiness.

hypnology (hip-nol′o-je) the scientific study of sleep or of hypnotism.

hypnonarcosis (hip″no-nar-ko′sis) light hypnosis combined with narcosis.

hypnosis (hip-no′sis) an artifically induced passive state in which there is increased amenability and responsiveness to suggestions and commands. In hypnosis, a drowsy phase is followed by a sleep that is light or deep, depending on the cooperation of the sleeper. Although this sleep seems normal, a part of the sleeper remains aware of the outside world and of the wishes of the hypnotist.
STATE OF HYPNOSIS. The nature of hypnosis and the way it works are still largely unknown. One widely accepted theory is that the person's ego—that is, the part of his mind that consciously restrains his instincts—is temporarily weakened under hypnosis at his own wish. How deeply he responds depends on many psychologic and biologic factors. The ability to respond to hypnosis varies from person to person; it tends to increase after successive experiences.

It is not true that a hypnotized person will do absolutely anything he is asked. Most subjects, for instance, will not respond to any suggestions they would consider immoral or illegal if they were awake.

USE OF HYPNOSIS. A common medical use of hypnosis is in treating mental illness. Historically, Sigmund Freud developed his theory of the unconscious as a result of his experiments with a hypnotized patient. Out of this theory came some of the techniques of PSYCHOANALYSIS. By lessening the mind's unconscious defenses, hypnosis can make some patients able to recall and even reexperience important childhood events that have long been forgotten or repressed by the conscious mind.

In certain cases when the use of anesthetics is not advisable, hypnosis has been used successfully during dental treatment, setting of fractures and childbirth, usually in addition to pain-killing medicines.

Hypnosis should be used only for medical purposes, under the supervision of a physician or psychiatrist. It should never be used for the purpose of entertainment.

hypnotherapy (hip″no-ther′ah-pe) treatment by hypnotism or by inducing sleep.

hypnotic (hip-not′ik) 1. pertaining to hypnosis or sleep. 2. an agent that induces sleep.

hypnotism (hip′no-tizm) the induction of hypnosis.

hypnotize (hip′no-tīz) to put into a condition of hypnosis.

hypnotoxin (hip″no-tok′sin) a hypothetical toxin that is supposed to accumulate during the waking hours until it is sufficient to inhibit the activity of the cortical cells and induce sleep.

hypo (hi′po) 1. a colloquial abbreviation of hypodermic. 2. sodium thiosulfate, used as a photographic fixing agent.

hypo- (hi′po) word element [Gr.], *abnormally decreased; deficient.*

hypoacidity (hi″po-ah-sid′ĭ-te) decreased acidity.

hypoadenia (hi″po-ah-de′ne-ah) diminished glandular activity.

hypoadrenalism (hi″po-ah-dren′al-izm) deficiency of adrenal activity.

hypoadrenocorticism (hi″po-ah-dre″no-kor′tĭ-sizm) diminished activity of the adrenal cortex; Addison's disease.

hypoaffectivity (hi″po-ah″fek-tiv′ĭ-te) abnormally diminished sensitivity to superficial stimuli; abnormally decreased emotional reactivity.

hypoalbuminemia (hi″po-al-bu″mĭ-ne′me-ah) diminished albumin in the blood.

hypoaldosteronemia (hi″po-al-dos′ter-o-ne′me-ah) abnormally low level of aldosterone in the blood.

hypoaldosteronism (hi″po-al-dos′ter-ōn-izm″) deficiency of aldosterone in the body.

hypoaldosteronuria (hi″po-al-dos′ter-o-nu′re-ah) abnormally low level of aldosterone in the urine.

hypoalimentation (hi″po-al″ĭ-men-ta′shun) insufficient nourishment.

hypoalkalinity (hi″po-al″kah-lin′ĭ-te) the state of being less alkaline than normal. adj., **hypoal′kaline.**

hypoazoturia (hi″po-az″o-tu′re-ah) diminished nitrogenous material in the urine.

hypobaric (hi″po-bār′ik) characterized by less than normal pressure or weight; applied to gases under less than atmospheric pressure, or to solutions of lower specific gravity than another taken as a standard of reference.

hypobaropathy (hi″po-bār-op′ah-the) decompression sickness (see BENDS).

hypoblast (hi′po-blast) the entoderm.

hypobulia (hi″po-bu′le-ah) abnormal feebleness of will.

hypocalcemia (hi″po-kal-se′me-ah) diminished calcium in the blood.

hypocalcia (hi″po-kal′se-ah) deficiency of calcium.

hypocalciuria (hi″po-kal″se-u′re-ah) an abnormally diminished amount of calcium in the urine.

hypocapnia, hypocarbia (hi″po-kap′ne-ah), (hi″-po-kar′be-ah) diminished carbon dioxide in the blood.

hypocatalasemia (hi″po-kat″ah-la-se′me-ah) diminished content of catalase in the blood.

hypocatalasia (hi″po-kat″ah-la′ze-ah) reduced level of catalase in all or most of the body tissues, due to a genetic defect.

hypocellularity (hi″po-sel″u-lar′ĭ-te) abnormal decrease in the number of cells present, as in bone marrow.

hypochloremia (hi″po-klo-re′me-ah) diminished chlorides in the blood.

hypochlorhydria (hi″po-klōr-hi′dre-ah) deficiency of hydrochloric acid in the gastric juice.

hypochlorization (hi″po-klōr″ĭ-za′shun) diminution of sodium chloride in the diet.

hypochlorous acid (hi″po-klōr′us) an unstable compound used as a disinfectant and bleaching agent.

hypochloruria (hi″po-klo-ru′re-ah) diminished chloride content in the urine.

hypocholesteremia, hypocholesterolemia (hi″-po-ko-les″ter-e′me-ah), (hi″po-ko-les″ter-ol-e′me-ah) low level of cholesterol in the blood.

hypochondria (hi″po-kon′dre-ah) hypochondriasis.

hypochondriac (hi″po-kon′dre-ak) 1. pertaining to the hypochondrium. 2. a person affected with hypochondriasis.

hypochondriasis (hi″po-kon-dri′ah-sis) abnormal concern about one's health. The hypochondriac exaggerates trivial symptoms and often believes that he is suffering from some serious ailment.
　　True hypochondriasis is a type of neurosis caused by an unresolved conflict in the patient's unconscious mind. His fears are usually related to a specific organ, such as the heart, eyes or lungs. This organ often has a deep symbolic connection with the inner conflict causing the neurosis. In many cases, the relationship between the patient's mind and the organ on which his fears center is so strong that he develops real symptoms, even though there is no physical disorder to explain them.
　　The treatment of hypochondria is usually difficult and of long duration. Psychotherapy is the most effective means of dealing with this disorder.

hypochondrium (hi″po-kon′dre-um) the abdominal region on either side, just below the thorax.

hypochromatism (hi″po-kro′mah-tizm) abnormally deficient pigmentation; especially deficiency of chromatin in a cell nucleus.

hypochromatosis (hi″po-kro″mah-to′sis) the gradual fading and disappearance of the nucleus (the chromatin) of a cell.

hypochromemia (hi″po-kro-me′me-ah) abnormally low color index of the blood.

hypochromia (hi″po-kro′me-ah) 1. hypochromatism. 2. decrease of hemoglobin in the erythrocytes so that they are abnormally pale. adj., **hypochro′mic.**

hypochromotrichia (hi″po-kro″mo-trik′e-ah) abnormally reduced pigmentation of the hair.

hypochromy (hi″po-kro′me) increase in the intensity of absorption of light.

hypochylia (hi″po-ki′le-ah) deficient secretion of gastric juice.

hypocinesia (hi″po-si-ne′ze-ah) hypokinesia.

hypocitremia (hi″po-sĭ-tre′me-ah) abnormally low content of citric acid in the blood.

hypocitruria (hi″po-sĭ-tru′re-ah) excretion of urine containing an abnormally small amount of citric acid.

hypocoagulability (hi″po-ko-ag″u-lah-bil′ĭ-te) abnormally decreased coagulability of the blood.

hypocondylar (hi″po-kon′dĭ-lar) below a condyle.

hypocorticism (hi″po-kor′tĭ-sizm) hypoadrenocorticism.

hypocrinism (hi″po-krin′izm) deficient secretion of an endocrine gland.

hypocupremia (hi″po-ku-pre′me-ah) abnormally diminished concentration of copper in the blood.

hypocyclosis (hi″po-si-klo′sis) insufficient accommodation in the eye.

hypocythemia (hi″po-si-the′me-ah) deficiency in the number of erythrocytes in the blood.

hypocytosis (hi″po-si-to′sis) hypoleukocytosis; deficiency of leukocytes in the blood.

hypodactylia (hi″po-dak-til′e-ah) less than the usual number of digits on the hand or foot.

hypodermic (hi″po-der′mik) 1. beneath the skin;

injected into subcutaneous tissues. 2. a hypodermic, or subcutaneous, injection.

hypodermoclysis (hi″po-der-mok′lĭ-sis) the introduction, into the subcutaneous tissues, of fluids, especially physiologic sodium chloride solution, in large quantity. The most common sites for insertion of the needles for hypodermoclysis are the anterior aspect of the thighs and the loose tissue below each breast. This method of introducing fluids into the body is contraindicated in cases of edema, and it may be complicated by abscess formation, puncture of a large blood vessel and necrosis and sloughing of the tissues due to poor absorption. For these reasons the intravenous method of fluid therapy usually is preferred to hypodermoclysis.

hypodiaphragmatic (hi″po-di″ah-frag-mat′ik) below the diaphragm.

hypodiploidy (hi″po-dip′loi-de) the state of having less than the diploid number of chromosomes (<2n).

hypodipsia (hi″po-dip′se-ah) abnormally diminished thirst.

hypodynamia (hi″po-di-na′me-ah) abnormally diminished power.

hypoeccrisia (hi″po-ē-kriz′e-ah) diminished excretion.

hypoelectrolytemia (hi″po-e-lek″tro-li-te′me-ah) abnormally decreased electrolyte content of the blood.

hypoemotivity (hi″po-e″mo-tiv′ĭ-te) hypoaffectivity.

hypoendocrinism (hi″po-en-dok′rĭ-nizm) abnormally decreased activity of an organ of internal secretion.

hypoeosinophilia (hi″po-e″o-sin″o-fil′e-ah) decrease of the eosinophils of the blood; eosinopenia.

hypoergasia (hi″po-er-ga′ze-ah) abnormally decreased functional activity.

hypoergia (hi″po-er′je-ah) 1. hypoergasia. 2. hyposensitivity to allergens.

hypoergic (hi″po-er′jik) 1. less energetic than normal. 2. pertaining to or characterized by hypoergy.

hypoergy (hi″po-er′je) abnormally diminished reactivity.

hypoesthesia (hi″po-es-the′ze-ah) a state of abnormally decreased sensitivity to stimuli.

hypoevolutism (hi″po-e-vol′u-tizm) abnormally retarded development.

hypoferremia (hi″po-fĕ-re′me-ah) deficiency of iron in the blood.

hypofibrinogenemia (hi″po-fi-brin″o-jĕ-ne′me-ah) deficiency of fibrinogen in the blood.

hypofunction (hi″po-fungk′shun) diminished functioning of a part or organ.

hypogammaglobulinemia (hi″po-gam″ah-glob″-u-lin-e′me-ah) an abnormally low level of gamma globulin in the blood (see also AGAMMAGLOBULINEMIA).

acquired h., hypogammaglobulinemia that becomes manifest after early childhood; the condition may be primary (that is, without discoverable underlying cause) or secondary (that is, associated with such conditions as multiple myeloma, lymphoma and chronic lymphoid leukemia, in which there is failure of gamma globulin synthesis).

congenital h., hypogammaglobulinemia in which the manifestations of immunologic inadequacy appear shortly after birth.

hypogastric (hi″po-gas′trik) pertaining to the hypogastrium.

hypogastrium (hi″po-gas′tre-um) the lowest middle abdominal region.

hypogenesis (hi″po-jen′ĕ-sis) defective development.

hypogenitalism (hi″po-jen′ĭ-tal-izm″) lack of sexual development because of deficient activity of the gonads; hypogonadism.

hypogeusesthesia, hypogeusia (hi″po-gu″zes-the′ze-ah), (hi″po-gu′ze-ah) abnormally diminished acuteness of the sense of taste.

hypoglandular (hi″po-glan′du-lar) marked by decreased glandular (hormonal) activity.

hypoglobulia (hi″po-glo-bu′le-ah) decrease of erythrocytes.

hypoglossal (hi″po-glos′al) beneath the tongue.
h. nerve, the twelfth cranial nerve; it provides motion for the muscles of the tongue.

hypoglottis (hi″po-glot′is) 1. the under side of the tongue. 2. a cystic tumor beneath the tongue.

hypoglycemia (hi″po-gli-se′me-ah) an abnormally low level of sugar (glucose) in the blood. The condition may result from an excessive rate of removal of glucose from the blood or from decreased secretion of glucose into the blood. Overproduction of insulin from the islands of Langerhans or an overdose of exogenous insulin can lead to increased utilization of glucose, so that glucose is removed from the blood at an accelerated rate. Some large tumors of the retroperitoneal area and tumors of the islands of Langerhans can increase the production of insulin and result in rapid removal of glucose from the blood. Because the liver is the source of most of the glucose entering the blood while a person is fasting, damage to the liver cells can result in impaired ability to convert glycogen into glucose. If secretion of the adrenocortical hormones, especially the GLUCOCORTICOIDS, is deficient, the protein precursors of glucose are not available and the blood glucose level drops as the liver's glycogen supply is depleted.

SYMPTOMS. Hypoglycemia may be tolerated by normal persons for brief periods of time without symptoms; however, if the blood sugar level remains very low for a prolonged period of time, symptoms of cerebral dysfunction develop. These include mental confusion, hallucinations, convulsions and eventually deep coma as the nervous system is deprived of the glucose needed for its normal metabolic activities. Other symptoms are a result of a greatly increased secretion of epinephrine, a normal response to hypoglycemia. The patient then experiences increased pulse rate, tachycardia, a rise in blood pressure, sweating and anxiety. (See also INSULIN SHOCK.)

TREATMENT. An acute episode of hypoglycemia

demands emergency treatment with intravenous injections of glucose. If the patient can swallow and no facilities for intravenous therapy are available, sugar, candy, sweetened fruit juice or honey may be given by mouth.

Specific treatment depends on the primary cause of hypoglycemia. If hyperinsulinism is due to a tumor or hyperplasia of the islands of Langerhans, surgical intervention is necessary to remove this cause of hypoglycemia. The large sarcomas of the retroperitoneal or mediastinal areas that cause hyperinsulinism also must be treated surgically.

When the cause of hypoglycemia is an endocrine or liver disease that results in decreased secretion of glucose, treatment includes dietary changes that are aimed at avoiding extremes in blood glucose level and maintaining an adequate level of glucose in the blood at all times. The diet is high in protein and fat and low in carbohydrate content and is given in frequent, small feedings during the day and before retiring. This regimen avoids extreme fluctuations in blood glucose concentration by restricting carbohydrate intake, and supplies adequate precursors of glycogen through the protein intake.

Drugs that may be administered to help control the symptoms of hypoglycemia include atropine and belladonna, and such corticosteroids as cortisol.

hypoglycemic (hi″po-gli-se′mik) pertaining to, characterized by or producing hypoglycemia.

h. drugs, drugs that lower the blood sugar level. The hormone INSULIN lowers the blood sugar by increasing the metabolism of sugar. Some synthetic hypoglycemic agents such as chlorpropamide and tolbutamide are used in the treatment of older diabetics. Since their usefulness is restricted to patients who have some functioning cells in the islands of Langerhans, they are not recommended for those suffering from juvenile and ketotic types of diabetes mellitus.

hypoglycogenolysis (hi″po-gli″ko-jĕ-nol′ĭ-sis) defective splitting up of glycogen in the body.

hypoglycorachia (hi″po-gli″ko-ra′ke-ah) abnormally low sugar content in the cerebrospinal fluid.

hypogonadism (hi″po-go′nad-izm) decreased functional activity of the gonads, with retardation of growth and sexual development.

hypohidrosis (hi″po-hĭ-dro′sis) abnormally diminished secretion of sweat.

hypohypnotic (hi″po-hip-not′ik) marked by light sleep or hypnosis.

hypoimmunity (hi″po-ĭ-mu′nĭ-te) lowered or diminished immunity.

hypoinosemia (hi″po-in″o-se′me-ah) diminished fibrin in the blood.

hypoinsulinism (hi″po-in′su-lin-izm″) deficient secretion of insulin.

hypoisotonic (hi″po-i″so-ton′ik) less than isotonic; said of a solution having a lesser osmotic power than another.

hypokalemia (hi″po-kah-le′me-ah) deficiency of potassium in the blood. adj., **hypokale′mic.**

hypokinemia (hi″po-ki-ne′me-ah) abnormally low cardiac output.

hypokinesia (hi″po-ki-ne′ze-ah abnormally diminished motor function or activity.

hypolarynx (hi″po-lar′inks) the part of the larynx below the glottis.

hypolemmal (hi″po-lem′al) located beneath a sheath, as the end-plates of motor nerves under the sarcolemma of muscle.

hypoleukocytosis (hi″po-lu″ko-si-to′sis) deficiency of leukocytes in the blood.

hypoleydigism (hi″po-li′dig-izm) abnormally diminished functional activity of Leydig's cells.

hypomania (hi″po-ma′ne-ah) mania of a mild type.

hypomastia (hi″po-mas′te-ah) abnormal smallness of mammary glands.

hypomelancholia (hi″po-mel″an-ko′le-ah) melancholia with slight mental disorder.

hypomenorrhea (hi″po-men″o-re′ah) uterine bleeding of less than the normal amount occurring at regular intervals, the period of flow being of the same or less than usual duration.

hypomere (hi′po-mēr) 1. one of the ventrolateral portions of the fusing myotomes in embryonic development, forming muscles innervated by the ventral rami of the spinal nerves. 2. the lateral plate of mesoderm that develops into the walls of the body cavity.

hypometabolism (hi″po-mĕ-tab′o-lizm) decreased metabolism.

hypometria (hi″po-me′tre-ah) diminished range of movement.

hypomineralization (hi″po-min″er-al-ĭ-za′shun) abnormal decrease in mineral elements in the blood.

hypomnesia (hi″pom-ne′ze-ah) defective memory.

hypomorph (hi′po-morf) 1. a person short in standing height. 2. in genetics, a hypomorphic mutant gene, i.e., showing only a slight reduction of its effectiveness.

hypomotility (hi″po-mo-til′ĭ-te) deficient power of movement in any part.

hypomyotonia (hi″po-mi″o-to′ne-ah) deficient muscular tonicity.

hypomyxia (hi″po-mik′se-ah) decreased secretion of mucus.

hyponatremia (hi″po-na-tre′me-ah) deficiency of sodium in the blood.

hyponoia (hi″po-noi′ah) sluggish mental activity.

hyponychium (hi″po-nik′e-um) the thickened epidermis beneath the free distal end of the nail of a digit.

hypo-orchidism (hi″po-or′kĭ-dizm) defective endocrine activity of the testes.

hypo-ovaria (hi″po-o-va′re-ah) deficient ovarian activity.

hypopancreatism (hi″po-pan′kre-ah-tizm″) diminished activity of the pancreas.

hypoparathyroidism (hi″po-par″ah-thi′roi-dizm) a disorder caused by underproduction of the parathyroid hormone. It most often occurs as a result of accidental removal of, or damage to, one or all of the parathyroids during thyroid surgery. Insufficiency of parathyroid hormone causes lowering of the calcium content of the blood and may result in TETANY, of which the most obvious sign is spasm of the muscles, especially those of the fingers and toes.

Treatment consists of raising the lowered calcium content of the blood. There are various forms in which calcium can be administered, and calcium injections will bring immediate improvement. However, if there is complete absence of parathyroid function the patient will have to continue to take oral preparations of calcium indefinitely. Transplantation of parathyroid glands has been attempted as substitution therapy.

hypopepsinia (hi″po-pep-sin′e-ah) deficiency in pepsin secretion of the stomach.

hypophalangism (hi″po-fal′an-jizm) absence of a phalanx on a finger or toe.

hypophamine (hi-pof′ah-min) the active principle of the posterior lobe of the pituitary gland.
alpha h., oxytocin.
beta h., vasopressin.

hypopharynx (hi″po-far′ingks) the lower part of the pharynx.

hypophonesis (hi″po-fo-ne′sis) diminution of the sound in auscultation or percussion.

hypophosphatasia (hi″po-fos″fah-ta′ze-ah) deficiency of alkaline phosphatase in the body.

hypophosphatemia (hi″po-fos″fah-te′me-ah) deficiency of phosphates in the blood.

hypophrenia (hi″po-fre′ne-ah) feeblemindedness.

hypophrenic (hi″po-fren′ik) 1. below the diaphragm. 2. feebleminded.

hypophrenium (hi″po-fre′ne-um) the peritoneal space between the diaphragm and the transverse colon.

hypophrenosis (hi″po-fre-no′sis) feeblemindedness.

hypophysectomy (hi-pof″ĭ-sek′to-me) excision of the hypophysis cerebri, or pituitary gland.

hypophysin (hi-pof′ĭ-sin) secretion from the hypophysis cerebri.

hypophysioprivic (hi″po-fiz″e-o-priv′ik) due to deficiency of the internal secretion of the hypophysis cerebri.

hypophysis (hi-pof′ĭ-sis), pl. *hypoph′yses* [Gr.] any process or outgrowth, especially the hypophysis cerebri. adj., **hypophys′eal.**
h. cer′ebri, an epithelial body at the base of the brain, attached by a stalk to the hypothalamus; called also PITUITARY GLAND. It is composed of two main lobes, the anterior lobe (adenohypophysis, anterior pituitary), secreting several important hormones that regulate the proper functioning of the other endocrine glands, and the posterior lobe (neurohypophysis, posterior pituitary), which releases a pressor and an oxytocic principle.
h. sic′ca, posterior pituitary.

hypophysitis (hi-pof″ĭ-si′tis) inflammation of the hypophysis cerebri.

hypophysoma (hi-pof″ĭ-so′mah) a tumor of the hypophysis cerebri.

hypopiesis (hi″po-pi-e′sis) abnormally low pressure, in particular, low blood pressure.

hypopigmentation (hi″po-pig″men-ta′shun) abnormally decreased pigmentation.

hypopituitarism (hi″po-pĭ-tu′ĭ-tar-izm″) a condition due to pathologically diminished activity of the pituitary gland due to pressure from basophil adenoma and marked by excessive deposit of fat and the persistence or acquirement of adolescent characteristics.

hypoplasia, hypoplasty (hi″po-pla′ze-ah), (hi′po-plas″te) incomplete development of an organ or tissue. adj., **hypoplas′tic.**

hypopnea (hi-pop′ne-ah) abnormal decrease in depth and rate of respiration.

hypoporosis (hi″po-po-ro′sis) deficient callus formation.

hypoposia (hi″po-po′ze-ah) abnormally diminished ingestion of fluids.

hypopotassemia (hi″po-pot″ah-se′me-ah) hypokalemia; deficiency of potassium in the blood.

hypopraxia (hi″po-prak′se-ah) abnormally diminished activity.

hypoprosody (hi″po-pros′o-de) diminution of the normal variation of stress, pitch and rhythm of speech.

hypoproteinemia (hi″po-pro″te-ĭ-ne′me-ah) deficiency of protein in the blood.

hypoprothrombinemia (hi″po-pro-throm″bĭ-ne′-me-ah) deficiency of prothrombin in the blood.

hypopselaphesia (hi″pop-sel″ah-fe′ze-ah) dullness of tactile sensitiveness.

hypopsychosis (hi″po-si-ko′sis) diminution of the function of thought.

hypoptyalism (hi″po-ti′ah-lizm) abnormally decreased secretion of saliva.

hypopyon (hi-po′pe-on) pus in the anterior chamber of the eye.

hyporeactor (hi″po-re-ak′tor) an individual showing less than normal response to a stimulus.

hyporeflexia (hi″po-re-flek′se-ah) diminution or weakening of reflexes.

hyposalemia (hi″po-sah-le′me-ah) diminution of salt in the blood.

hyposalivation (hi″po-sal″ĭ-va′shun) hypoptyalism.

hyposarca (hi″po-sar′kah) anasarca; accumulation of great amounts of fluid in all the body tissues.

hyposecretion (hi″po-se-kre′shun) diminished secretion.

hyposensitivity (hi″po-sen″sĭ-tiv′ĭ-te) 1. abnormally decreased sensitivity. 2. the specific or general ability to react to a specific allergen reduced by repeated and gradually increasing doses of the offending substance.

hyposensitization (hi″po-sen″sĭ-tĭ-za′shun) reduction of sensitivity to a particular antigen, by appropriate treatment.

hyposmia (hi-poz′me-ah) diminished acuteness of the sense of smell.

hyposmolarity (hi-poz″mo-lar′ĭ-te) abnormally decreased osmotic concentration of a solution.

hyposomnia (hi″po-som′ne-ah) pathologically diminished sleep.

hypospadias (hi″po-spa′de-as) a developmental anomaly in the male in which the urethra opens on the under side of the penis or on the perineum.
   female h., a developmental anomaly in the female in which the urethra opens into the vagina.

hyposphyxia (hi″po-sfik′se-ah) decreased activity of the circulation, with lowered blood pressure.

hypostasis (hi-pos′tah-sis) 1. deposit or sediment. 2. formation of a deposit. adj., **hypostat′ic.**

hyposteatolysis (hi″po-ste″ah-tol′ĭ-sis) inadequate hydrolysis of fats during digestion.

hyposthenia (hi″pos-the′ne-ah) diminished strength or tonicity.

hyposthenuria (hi″pos-thĕ-nu′re-ah) excretion of urine of abnormally low molecular concentration.

hypostomia (hi″po-sto′me-ah) a developmental anomaly characterized by abnormal smallness of the mouth, the slit being vertical instead of horizontal.

hypostypsis (hi″po-stip′sis) moderate astringency.

hyposulfite (hi″po-sul′fit) sodium thiosulfate.

hyposynergia (hi″po-sĭ-ner′je-ah) defective coordination.

hyposystole (hi″po-sis′to-le) abnormal diminution of the systole.

hypotelorism (hi″po-te′lo-rizm) abnormally decreased distance between two organs or parts.
   ocular h., orbital h., abnormal decrease in the intraocular distance.

hypotension (hi″po-ten′shun) diminished tension; lowered blood pressure. A consistently low blood pressure with a systolic pressure less than 100 mm. of mercury is no cause for concern. In fact, low blood pressure often is associated with long life and an old age free of illness. An extremely low blood pressure is occasionally a symptom of a serious condition. In shock there is a disproportion between the blood volume and the capacity of the circulatory system, resulting in greatly reduced blood pressure.
   Hypotension may be associated with Addison's disease and inadequate thyroid function, but in both cases the primary disease produces so many other symptoms that the hypotension is considered comparatively unimportant.

   orthostatic h., postural h., a form of low blood pressure that occurs on assumption of the erect position or on prolonged standing.

hypotensive (hi″po-ten′siv) 1. characterized by or causing diminished tension or pressure, as abnormally low blood pressure. 2. a person with abnormally low blood pressure.

hypotensor (hi″po-ten′sor) a substance that lowers the blood pressure.

hypotetraploidy (hi″po-tĕ′trah-ploi″de) the state of having fewer than the tetraploid number of chromosomes in unbalanced sets $(4n - x)$.

hypothalamotomy (hi″po-thal″ah-mot′o-me) production of lesions in the posterolateral part of the hypothalamus, in treatment of psychotic disorders.

hypothalamus (hi″po-thal′ah-mus) a portion of the brain, lying beneath the thalamus at the base of the cerebrum, and forming the floor and part of the walls of the third ventricle.
   Some cells in the hypothalamus control heat production and others control heat loss; thus the hypothalamus is said to contain the temperature-regulating center of the body. It also contains the mechanism for regulating functional activity of the posterior lobe of the PITUITARY GLAND, and the secretory activity of the anterior lobe of the pituitary. Because of its influence in the production of pituitary hormones, the hypothalamus indirectly plays an important role in the regulation of fat and carbohydrate metabolism, in body fluid balance and electrolyte content and in internal secretion of other endocrine glands.
   The hypothalamus is a coordinating center for the autonomic nervous system and therefore influences many involuntary actions such as gastrointestinal motility and secretion, sweating, changes in arterial pressure and urinary output. Behaviorial functions associated with the hypothalamus include sleep, wakefulness, alertness and reactions to pain and pleasure.

hypothenar (hi-poth′ĕ-nar) the ridge on the palm along the bases of the fingers and the medial side.

hypothermia, hypothermy (hi″po-ther′me-ah), hi″po-ther′me) low temperature. adj., **hypother′mal, hypother′mic,** Hypothermia may be symptomatic of a disease or disorder of the temperature-regulating mechanism of the body, or it may be induced for certain surgical procedures or as a therapeutic measure.
   induced h., deliberate reduction of the temperature of all or part of the body; sometimes used as an adjunct to anesthesia in surgical procedures involving a limb, and as a protective measure in cardiac and neurologic surgery. The hypothermia may be continued only for the duration of the operation or it may be prolonged for as long as 5 days, depending on the reason for its use.
   LOCAL HYPOTHERMIA. This is a type of refrigeration anesthesia restricted to a part of the body, such as a limb. It usually is used to produce surgical anesthesia immediately before amputation. The advantages of this type of anesthesia include minimal risk of shock, lowering of cell metabolism and elimination of the need for inhalation anesthesia in patients who are poor surgical risks.
   The part to be anesthetized is packed in ice or

wrapped in a special refrigeration unit consisting of coiled tubes. Tourniquets are applied to the limb to inhibit circulation and avoid general chilling of the patient. The limb is chilled for 3 to 5 hours before amputation.

GENERAL HYPOTHERMIA. Generalized lowering of the body temperature decreases the metabolism of tissues and thereby the need for oxygen; it is used in various surgical procedures, especially on the heart. The body temperature is maintained between 89° F. (32° C.) and 78° F. (26° C.).

To induce general hypothermia, the patient may be immersed in ice water, packed in crushed ice or ice packs or wrapped in a cooling blanket containing coils through which cold water and alcohol are circulated. The fastest method for achieving hypothermia is extracorporeal cooling of the blood; the patient's blood is removed through a cannula inserted in a large vessel, circulated through refrigerated coils and returned via another cannulated vessel.

Rewarming the patient is accomplished simply by removing the ice packs or cooling blankets and allowing the temperature to rise gradually and naturally. In most cases regular blankets are used to maintain body warmth. External heat in the form of hot water bottles or warm tub baths, if used at all, must be applied with extreme caution to avoid burning the patient.

NURSING CARE. During hypothermia and the rewarming process the patient's temperature, pulse, respiration and blood pressure must be checked frequently. Special electronic thermometers are often used so that the body temperature can be monitored at all times. In prolonged hypothermia, cardiac irregularities or respiratory difficulties may develop quickly; the patient must be watched constantly for changes in the vital signs, and any changes must be reported immediately. The skin also should be observed for signs of developing decubitus ulcers, edema or marked discoloration.

The patient should be turned every 2 hours, with special attention to proper positioning and good body alignment. Decreased secretion of saliva and mouth-breathing demand frequent mouth care. The eyes may need to be irrigated frequently and covered with compresses moistened with physiologic saline solution if the corneal reflex is diminished and eye secretions are reduced.

Intake and output are measured and recorded. An indwelling catheter is inserted prior to induction of hypothermia and is left in place until normal body temperature is established. This is necessary because urinary output is diminished during hypothermia. Fluids are given intravenously and the oral intake of food and liquids is prohibited because of depression of the gag reflex.

Shivering during prolonged hypothermia must be avoided as it tends to elevate the body temperature and increase metabolic needs, thereby defeating the purpose of hypothermia. Chlorpromazine may be ordered as a precaution against shivering.

During the rewarming process the patient must be observed for signs of increased tendency to bleed and of gastric distention; these are common complications. After the body temperature returns to normal and becomes stabilized the patient is allowed to progress to a normal diet and physical activities.

symptomatic h., pathologic reduction of body temperature as a result of decreased heat production or increased heat loss. Hypothyroidism, severe blood loss with circulatory failure, and damage to the heat-producing cells of the hypothalamus can lead to decreased heat production. Prolonged exposure to cold, overdosage of antipyretic drugs, such as aspirin, and profuse sweating (diaphoresis) are some causes of increased heat loss and resultant hypothermia.

hypothrombinemia   (hi″po-throm″bĭ-ne′me-ah) diminution of thrombin in the blood, resulting in a tendency to bleeding.

hypothymia   (hi″po-thi′me-ah) abnormally diminished emotionalism.

hypothymism   (hi″po-thi′mizm) diminished thymus activity.

hypothyroidism   (hi″po-thi′roi-dizm) deficiency of THYROID GLAND activity, with underproduction of thyroxine, or the condition resulting from it. adj., **hypothy′roid.** In its severe form it is called MYXEDEMA and is characterized by physical and mental sluggishness, obesity, loss of hair, enlargement of the tongue and thickening of the skin. In children the condition is known as CRETINISM.

hypotonia   (hi″po-to′ne-ah) abnormally decreased tonicity or strength.

hypotonic   (hi″po-ton′ik) 1. having an abnormally reduced tonicity or tension. 2. having an osmotic pressure lower than that of the solution with which it is compared.

hypotoxicity   (hi″po-tok-sis′ĭ-te) abnormally reduced toxic quality.

hypotransferrinemia   (hi″po-trans-fer″ĭ-ne′me-ah) deficiency of transferrin in the blood.

hypotrichosis   (hi″po-trĭ-ko′sis) congenital absence of body hair, which may be partial or complete.

hypotriploidy   (hi″po-trip′loi-de) the state of having fewer than the triploid number of chromosomes in unbalanced sets ($3n - x$).

hypotrophy   (hi-pot′ro-fe) 1. bacterial nutrition in which the organism is nourished by its host's nutrition. 2. abiotrophy.

hypotropia   (hi″po-tro′pe-ah) downward deviation of the visual axis of one eye while the other is fixing.

hypotympanotomy   (hi″po-tim″pah-not′o-me) surgical opening of the hypotympanum.

hypotympanum   (hi″po-tim′pah-num) the lower part of the cavity of the middle ear, in the temporal bone.

hypouremia   (hi″po-u-re′me-ah) an abnormally low level of urea in the blood.

hypouresis   (hi″po-u-re′sis) oliguria; diminished excretion of urine.

hypovaria   (hi″po-va′re-ah) hypo-ovaria; deficient ovarian activity.

hypovegetative   (hi″po-vej′ĕ-ta″tiv) denoting a constitutional body type in which somatic systems predominate in contrast to visceral organs.

hypovenosity (hi"po-ve-nos'ĭ-te) incomplete development of veins.

hypoventilation (hi"po-ven"tĭ-la'shun) decrease of air in the lungs below the normal amount.

hypovitaminosis (hi"po-vi"tah-mĭ-no'sis) a condition produced by lack of an essential vitamin.

hypovolemia (hi"po-vo-le'me-ah) abnormally decreased volume of circulating fluid (plasma) in the body.

hypoxemia (hi"pok-se'me-ah) deficient oxygenation of the blood.

hypoxia (hi-pok'se-ah) a broad term meaning diminished availability of oxygen to the body tissues. adj., **hypox'ic.** Its causes are many and varied. There may be a deficiency of oxygen in the atmosphere, as in ALTITUDE SICKNESS, or a pulmonary disorder that interferes with adequate ventilation of the lungs. Anemia or circulatory deficiencies can lead to inadequate transport and delivery of oxygen to the tissues. Finally, edema or other abnormal conditions of the tissues themselves may impair the exchange of oxygen and carbon dioxide between the capillaries and the tissues.

SYMPTOMS. Signs and symptoms of hypoxia vary according to its cause. Generally they include dyspnea, rapid pulse, syncope and mental disturbances such as delirium or euphoria. Cyanosis is not always present and in some cases is not evident until the hypoxia is far advanced. The localized pain of ANGINA PECTORIS due to hypoxia occurs because of impaired oxygenation of the myocardium. Discoloration of the skin and eventual ulceration that sometimes accompany varicose veins are a result of hypoxia of the involved tissues.

TREATMENT. The treatment of hypoxia depends on the primary cause. Administration of oxygen by inhalation may be useful in some cases and of no help in others. For example, in situations in which there is difficulty with the transport of oxygen from the lungs to other parts of the body, increasing the intake of oxygen will do little to correct the problem of distribution. In some vascular diseases the administration of vasodilators may help increase circulation, hence oxygen supply, to the tissues.

hyps(o)- (hip'so) word element [Gr.], *height.*

hypsarhythmia (hip"sah-rith'me-ah) a term for an electroencephalographic abnormality sometimes observed in infants, with random high-voltage slow waves and spikes arising from multiple foci and spreading to all cortical areas; the disorder is characterized by spasms or quivering spells, and is commonly associated with mental retardation.

hypsokinesis (hip"so-ki-ne'sis) a backward swaying or falling in erect posture, seen in paralysis agitans and other neurologic disorders.

hypsophobia (hip"so-fo'be-ah) fear of great heights.

hypsotherapy (hip"so-ther'ah-pe) therapeutic use of high altitudes.

hyster(o)- (his'ter-o) word element [Gr.], *uterus.*

hysteralgia (his"tĕ-ral'je-ah) pain in the uterus.

hysterectomy (his"tĕ-reck'to-me) surgical removal of the UTERUS.

hysteresis (his-tĕ-re'sis) the failure of coincidence of two associated phenomena, such as that exhibited in the differing temperatures of gelation and of liquefaction of a reversible colloid.

hystereurynter (his"ter-u-rin'ter) an instrument for dilating the ostium uteri.

hystereurysis (his"ter-u'rĭ-sis) dilation of the ostium uteri.

hysteria (his-te're-ah) a form of psychoneurosis in which the individual converts anxiety created by emotional conflict into physical symptoms that have no organic basis; called also conversion reaction or conversion hysteria. The term hysteria is also used to describe a state of tension or excitement in which there is a temporary loss of control over the emotions. adj., **hyster'ical.**

The patient with conversion hysteria is mentally ill. He converts his mental distress into physical symptoms in an effort to escape severe emotional conflict. The physical symptoms may include blindness, deafness, mutism or paralysis of an arm or leg. In most cases the symptom can be related to some aspect of the conflict. For example, a college student interested in creative writing, but majoring in music because her parents want her to, may attempt to solve the problem by developing a loss of hearing. She then has an excuse for not continuing with the study of music and can at the same time satisfy her own desires without openly defying her parents. The patient who employs such methods is unaware that he is using the physical symptom to solve his emotional problem. Treatment is by PSYCHOTHERAPY in which the patient is helped to resolve the emotional conflict in a more normal manner.

The milder form of hysteria that is characterized by such symptoms as crying, pointless laughter, shouting, aimless walking about or a temper tantrum usually results from an incident in which a person is pushed beyond his normal endurance. It might be provoked by danger, severe fright or the reception of bad news.

hysteritis (his"tĕ-ri'tis) inflammation of the uterus.

hysterocatalepsy (his"ter-o-kat'ah-lep"se) hysteria with cataleptic symptoms.

hysterocele (his'ter-o-sēl") hernia of the uterus.

hysterocleisis (his"ter-o-kli'sis) surgical closure of the ostium uteri.

hysterocolpectomy (his"ter-o-kol-pek'to-me) hysterectomy with excision of the vagina.

hysterodynia (his"ter-o-din'e-ah) pain in the uterus.

hysteroepilepsy (his"ter-o-ep'ĭ-lep"se) severe hysteria with epileptic convulsions.

hysterogenic (his"ter-o-jen'ik) causing hysterical phenomena or symptoms.

hysterography (his"tĕ-rog'rah-fe) roentgenography of the uterus.

hysteroid (his"ter-oid) resembling hysteria.

hysterolith (his'ter-o-lith") a uterine calculus.

hysterology (his"tĕ-rol'o-je) study of the uterus.

hysterolysis (his"tĕ-rol'ĭ-sis) freeing of the uterus from adhesions.

hysteromania (his"ter-o-ma'ne-ah) 1. hysterical mania. 2. nymphomania.

hysterometer (his"tĕ-rom'ĕ-ter) an instrument for measuring the uterus.

hysterometry (his"tĕ-rom'ĕ-tre) measurement of the uterus.

hysteromyoma (his"ter-o-mi-o'mah) myoma of the uterus.

hysteromyomectomy (his"ter-o-mi"o-mek'to-me) local excision of a myoma of the uterus.

hysteromyotomy (his"ter-o-mi-ot'o-me) incision of the uterus for removal of a solid tumor.

hysteroneurosis (his"ter-o-nu-ro'sis) nervous disease due to a uterine lesion.

hystero-oophorectomy (his"ter-o-o"of-o-rek'to-me) excision of the uterus and ovaries.

hysteropathy (his"tĕ-rop'ah-the) any uterine disease.

hysteropexy (his'ter-o-pek"se) fixation of the uterus by surgery.

hysteropia (his"tĕ-ro'pe-ah) a hysterical disorder of vision.

hysteroptosis (his"ter-op-to'sis) prolapse of the uterus.

hysterorrhaphy (his"tĕ-ror'ah-fe) 1. suture of the uterus. 2. hysteropexy.

hysterorrhexis (his"ter-o-rek'sis) rupture of the uterus.

hysterosalpingectomy (his"ter-o-sal"pin-jek'to-me) excision of the uterus and uterine tubes.

hysterosalpingography (his"ter-o-sal"ping-gog'-rah-fe) roentgenography of the uterus and uterine tubes.

hysterosalpingo-oophorectomy (his"ter-o-sal-ping"go-o"of-o-rek'to-me) excision of the uterus, uterine tubes and ovaries.

hysterosalpingostomy (his"ter-o-sal"ping-gos'-to-me) anastomosis of a uterine tube of the uterus.

hysteroscope (his'ter-o-skōp") an endoscope used in direct visual examination of the canal of the uterine cervix and the cavity of the uterus.

hysterospasm (his'ter-o-spazm") spasm of the uterus.

hysterotomy (his"tĕ-rot'o-me) incision of the uterus.

hysterotrachelorrhaphy (his"ter-o-tra"kĕ-lor'-ah-fe) suture of the uterus and uterine cervix.

hysterotrachelotomy (his"ter-o-tra"kĕ-lot'o-me) incision of the uterus and uterine cervix.

hysterotraumatism (his"ter-o-traw'mah-tizm) hysterical symptoms following injury.

hysterotubography (his"ter-o-tu-bog'rah-fe) hysterosalpingography.

Hytakerol (hi-tak'er-ol) trademark for preparations of dihydrotachysterol, used to increase the blood calcium level.

hyzone (hi'zōn) an unstable triatomic form of hydrogen, H_3.

I

I chemical symbol, *iodine.*

-ia (e′ah) word element, *state; condition; disease.*

ianthinopsia (i-an″thĭ-nop′se-ah) a perversion of color vision in which objects are seen as violet.

-iasis (i′ah-sis) word element [Gr.], *condition of.*

iateria (i″ah-te′re-ah) therapeutics.

iatr(o)- (i-at′ro) word element [Gr.], *medicine; physician.*

iatric (i-at′rik) pertaining to medicine or to a physician.

iatrochemistry (i-at″ro-kem′is-tre) the name of a school of medicine of the 17th century, which espoused the theory that all phenomena of life and disease were based on chemical action.

iatrogenic (i-at″ro-jen′ik) resulting from an attitude or activity of a physician. An iatrogenic disorder is one produced inadvertently as a result of treatment by a physician for some other disorder.

iatrology (i″ah-trol′o-je) the science of medicine.

iatrophysics (i-at″ro-fiz′iks) treatment of disease by physical or mechanical means.

I.C.D. intrauterine contraceptive device.

Iceland disease benign myalgic encephalomyelitis.

ichor (i′kor) a watery discharge from wounds or sores. adj., **i′chorous.**

ichorrhea (i″ko-re′ah) copious discharge of ichor.

ichthammol (ik-tham′ol) an ammoniated coal tar product, used in ointment form for certain skin diseases.

ichthyismus (ik″the-iz′mus) disease caused by eating rancid or poisonous fish.

ichthyoacanthotoxin (ik″the-o-ah-kan″tho-tok′-sin) the toxin secreted by venomous fishes.

ichthyohemotoxin (ik″the-o-he″mo-tok′sin) a toxic substance found in the blood of certain fishes.

ichthyoid (ik′the-oid) fishlike.

ichthyootoxin (ik″the-o-″o-tok′sin) a toxic substance derived from the roe of certain fishes.

ichthyosarcotoxin (ik″the-o-sar″ko-tok′sin) a toxin found in the flesh of poisonous fishes.

ichthyosis (ik″the-o′sis) dryness, roughness and scaliness of the skin, resulting from failure of shedding of the keratin produced by the skin cells. adj., **ichthyot′ic.**
    i. follicula′ris, keratosis follicularis.
    i. hys′trix, a variety with dry, warty knobs.
    i. seba′cea, seborrhea.

ichthyotoxicology (ik″the-o-tok″sĭ-kol′o-je) the science of poisons derived from certain fish, their cause, detection and effects, and treatment of conditions produced by them.

ichthyotoxin (ik″the-o-tok′sin) a toxin derived from fish.

I.C.N. International Council of Nurses.

I.C.S. International College of Surgeons.

ICSH interstitial cell-stimulating hormone (luteinizing hormone).

ictal (ik′tal) pertaining to, characterized by or caused by a sudden attack, such as an acute epileptic seizure.

icteric (ik-ter′ik) pertaining to or affected with jaundice.
    i. index, a rough determination of the concentration of bilirubin in the serum; it is indicative of liver function. The color intensity of the serum is measured and reported in units. Preparation of the patient includes fasting because chyle can render the sample of blood unsatisfactory. Normal range for the icteric index is 4 to 8 units.

icterogenic (ik″ter-o-jen′ik) causing jaundice.

icterohepatitis (ik″ter-o-hep″ah-ti′tis) inflammation of the liver with marked jaundice.

icteroid (ik′ter-oid) resembling jaundice.

icterus (ik′ter-us) jaundice.
    congenital family i., hereditary or congenital hemolytic jaundice.
    cythemolytic i., icterus due to excessive formation of bile from destruction of erythrocytes.
    i. gra′vis, acute yellow atrophy of the liver.
    i. neonato′rum, jaundice in newborn infants.

ictus (ik′tus) a stroke, blow or sudden attack.

I.D. infective dose.

I.D.₅₀ median infective dose.

id (id) 1. a freudian term used to describe that part of the personality which harbors the unconscious, instinctive impulses that lead to immediate gratification of primitive needs such as hunger, the need for air, the need to move about and relieve body tension and the need to eliminate. Id impulses are physiologic and body processes, as opposed to the EGO and SUPEREGO, which are psychologic and social processes. The id is dominated by the pleasure principle and some gratification of the id impulses is necessary for survival of a person's personality. 2. a skin eruption occurring as an allergic reaction to an agent causing primary lesions elsewhere.

-id (id) word element [Gr.], indicating a skin condition occurring secondarily to a primary infection.

467

-ide (īd) suffix indicating a binary compound.

idea (i-de′ah) a mental impression or conception.

autochthonous i., a strange idea that comes into the mind in some unaccountable way, but is not a hallucination.

compulsive i., an idea that persists despite reason and will and that drives one to action, usually inappropriate.

dominant i., an impression that controls or colors every action and thought.

fixed i., an impression that stays in the mind and cannot be changed by reason.

i. of reference, an idea that the words and actions of others refer to one's self.

ideal (i-de′al) a pattern or concept of perfection.

ego i., an ideal of perfection developed in childhood through identification with a loved person.

idealization (i-de″ah-lī-za′shun) 1. a mental mechanism by which an object or person is unconsciously overvalued and emotionally aggrandized. 2. concentration upon and exaggeration of the liked attributes of a person. 3. the conscious or partly conscious process of building a person, principle or system into a standard of excellence.

ideation (i″de-a′shun) clear mental presentation of an object.

idee fixe (e-da′ fēks′) a psychopathologically fixed idea or belief, of a delusional nature.

identification (i-den″tĭ-fĭ-ka′shun) a mental mechanism by which an individual unconsciously takes as his own the characteristics, postures, achievements or other identifying traits of other persons or groups. Identification plays a major role in the development of the SUPEREGO and of awareness and acceptance of the standards and rules accepted by society. However, as a person matures emotionally, his own self-identity should become clearer as he relates more to his own personal achievements and less to the accomplishments and successes of others with whom he identifies.

Identification is not to be confused with imitation, which is a conscious process. It should be pointed out also that overuse of identification as a defense mechanism denies one the opportunity of enjoying the benefits and self-satisfaction derived from his own accomplishments.

ideogenetic (i″de-o-jĕ-net′ik) induced by or related to vague sense impressions rather than organized images.

ideogenous (i″de-oj′ĕ-nus) aroused by an idea or thought.

ideology (i″de-ol′o-je, id″e-ol′o-je) 1. the science of the development of ideas. 2. the body of ideas characteristic of an individual or of a social unit.

ideomotion (i″de-o-mo′shun) muscular action induced by mental energy.

ideophrenia (i″de-o-fre′ne-ah) a morbid mental state characterized by perversion of ideas.

idio- (id′e-o) word element [Gr.], *self; peculiar to a substance or organism itself.*

idiocy (id′e-o-se) mental deficiency so severe as to render the patient incapable of guarding against common physical dangers, the mental age being less than 2 years.

amaurotic familial i., a familial condition characterized by subnormal mentality and blindness, due to a defect of lipid metabolism (see also AMAUROTIC FAMILIAL IDIOCY).

mongolian i., a term formerly used for marked mental deficiency associated with Down's syndrome.

idioglossia (id″e-o-glos′e-ah) speech characterized by imprecise pronunciation of letters, creating virtually a new language peculiar to the individual.

idiometritis (id″e-o-me-tri′tis) inflammation of the uterine muscle.

idiopathic (id″e-o-path′ik) self-originated; occurring without known cause.

idiopathy (id″e-op′ah-the) a morbid state arising without known cause.

idioplasm (id′e-o-plasm″) the self-reproducing portion of a cell; germ plasm.

idiosome (id′e-o-sōm″) 1. an ultimate element of living matter. 2. the centrosome of a spermatocyte, together with the surrounding Golgi apparatus and mitochondria.

idiosyncrasy (id″e-o-sing′krah-se) 1. a habit or quality of body or mind peculiar to any individual. 2. an abnormal susceptibility to some drug, protein or other agent that is peculiar to the individual.

idiot (id′e-ot) a mentally defective person of the lowest order of intellectual potential (mental age less than 2 years).

mongolian i., a term formerly applied to a patient with Down's syndrome and severe mental retardation.

i.-savant, a person of subnormal intelligence who has a particular mental faculty developed to a high degree, e.g., mathematic ability, memory.

idiotrophic (id″e-o-trof′ik) capable of selecting its own nourishment.

idioventricular (id″e-o-ven-trik′u-lar) pertaining to the cardiac ventricle alone.

idoxuridine (ī″doks-u′rĭ-dēn) an antiviral used specifically for the treatment of herpes simplex (dendritic) keratitis.

Ig immunoglobulin.

ignipuncture (ig″nĭ-pungk′tūr) therapeutic puncture with hot needles.

ignis (ig′nis) [L.] fire.

i. sa′cer, 1. ergotism. 2. herpes zoster.

ile(o)- (il′e-o) word element [L.], *ileum.*

ileac, ileal (il′e-ak), (il′e-al) pertaining to the ileum.

ileectomy (il″e-ek′to-me) excision of the ileum.

ileitis (il″e-i′tis) inflammation of the ileum, or lower portion of the small intestine. It may result from infection, obstruction, severe irritation or faulty absorption of material through the intestinal walls.

A specific type of inflammation of unknown cause involving the small and large intestines is known as regional ileitis, regional enteritis or Crohn's disease.

The advanced stage is marked by hardening, thickening and ulceration of parts of the bowel lining. An obstruction may cause the development of a fistula.

A common symptom of ileitis is pain in the lower right quadrant of the abdomen or around the umbilicus. Other symptoms include loss of appetite, loss of weight, anemia and diarrhea, which may alternate with periods of constipation. Treatment may require medication to remove any source of infection, special diet or surgery if there is obstruction.

ileocecal (il″e-o-se′kal) pertaining to the ileum and cecum.
  i. valve, the valve guarding the opening between the ileum and the cecum.

ileocecostomy (il″e-o-se-kos′to-me) anastomosis of the ileum to the cecum.

ileocolic (il″e-o-kol′ik) pertaining to the ileum and colon.

ileocolitis (il″e-o-ko-li′tis) inflammation of the ileum and colon.
  i. ulcero′sa chron′ica, chronic ileocolitis with fever, rapid pulse, anemia, diarrhea and right iliac pain.

ileocolostomy (il″e-o-ko-los′to-me) anastomosis of the ileum to the colon.

ileocolotomy (il″e-o-ko-lot′o-me) incision of the ileum and colon.

ileocystostomy (il″e-o-sis-tos′to-me) use of an isolated segment of ileum to create a passage from the urinary bladder to an opening in the abdominal wall.

ileoileostomy (il″e-o-il″e-os′to-me) anastomosis between two parts of the ileum.

ileorectal (il″e-o-rek′tal) pertaining to or communicating with the ileum and rectum.

ileorrhaphy (il″e-or′ah-fe) suture of the ileum.

ileosigmoidostomy (il″e-o-sig″moi-dos′to-me) anastomosis of the ileum to the sigmoid colon.

ileostomy (il″e-os′to-me) surgical creation of an opening into the ileum.

ileotomy (il″e-ot′o-me) incision of the ileum.

Iletin (il′ĕ-tin) trademark for preparations of insulin.

ileum (il′e-um) the distal portion of the small intestine, ending at the cecum.
  duplex i., congenital duplication of the ileum.

ileus (il′e-us) intestinal obstruction, especially failure of peristalsis. The condition frequently accompanies peritonitis and usually results from disturbances in neural stimulation of the bowel. It also may occur in many painful conditions involving the thoracolumbar region, for example, the colicky pains of GALLSTONES or KIDNEY stones and spinal injuries.
  SYMPTOMS. The principal symptoms of ileus are abdominal pain and distention, vomiting (the vomitus may contain fecal material) and constipation. If the intestinal obstruction is not relieved, the circulation in the wall of the intestine is impaired and the patient appears extremely ill with symptoms of shock and dehydration.

TREATMENT. Distention of the abdomen is relieved by decompression, which involves INTUBATION with a long, balloon-tipped tube (e.g., MILLER-ABBOTT TUBE) that extends to the site of the obstruction, and use of constant suction. Because of the disruption in absorption of fluids and nutrients from the intestinal tract, fluids, electrolytes and glucose are given intravenously. Surgical intervention to remove the cause of ileus is usually necessary when the obstruction is complete or the bowel is likely to become gangrenous. The type of surgical procedure will depend on the condition of the bowel and the cause of the obstruction. In some cases ileostomy or COLOSTOMY, either temporary or permanent, may be necessary. (See also INTESTINAL OBSTRUCTION.)
  adynamic i., ileus resulting from inhibition of bowel motility, which may be produced by numerous causes, most frequently peritonitis.
  dynamic i., spastic ileus.
  mechanical i., obstruction of the intestines resulting from mechanical causes.
  meconium i., ileus in the newborn due to blocking of the bowel with thick meconium.
  paralytic i., adynamic ileus.
  spastic i., obstruction of the bowel resulting from persisting contracture of the intestinal musculature.
  i. subpar′ta, ileus due to pressure of the gravid uterus on the pelvic colon.

ili(o)- (il′e-o) word element [L.], *ilium.*

iliac (il′e-ak) pertaining to the ilium.

iliadelphus (il″e-ah-del′fus) a twin monster joined at the pelvis; iliopagus.

Ilidar (il′ĭ-dar) trademark for a preparation of azapetine, used for sympathetic blockade and to dilate peripheral blood vessels.

iliofemoral (il″e-o-fem′o-ral) pertaining to the ilium and femur.

ilio-inguinal (il″e-o-ing′gwĭ-nal) pertaining to the iliac and inguinal regions.

iliolumbar (il″e-o-lum′bar) pertaining to the iliac and lumbar regions.

iliopagus (il″e-op′ah-gus) symmetrical conjoined twins united in the iliac region.

iliopectineal (il″e-o-pek-tin′e-al) pertaining to the ilium and pubes.

ilium (il′e-um), pl. *il′ia* [L.] the lateral, flaring portion of the hip bone.

illumination (ĭ-lu″mĭ-na′shun) the lighting up of a part, cavity, organ or object for inspection.

illuminator (ĭ-lu′mĭ-na″tor) the source of light for viewing an object.

illusion (ĭ-lu′zhun) a mental impression derived from misinterpretation of an actual sensory stimulus.

Ilotycin (i″lo-ti′sin) trademark for preparations of erythromycin, an antibiotic.

I.M. intramuscularly.

I.M.A. Industrial Medical Association.

image (im′ij) a picture or concept with more or less likeness to an objective reality.

body i., a three-dimensional concept of one's self, recorded in the cortex by the perception of ever changing postures of the body, and constantly changing with them.

mirror i., 1. the image of light made visible by the reflecting surface of the cornea and lens when illuminated through the slit lamp. 2. an image with right and left relations reversed, as in the reflection of an object in a mirror.

motor i., the organized cerebral model of the possible movements of the body.

imago (ĭ-ma′go) 1. the adult or definitive form of an insect. 2. in psychoanalysis, a childhood memory or fantasy of a loved person that persists in adult life.

imbalance (im-bal′ans) lack of balance; especially lack of balance between muscles, as in insufficiency of ocular muscles.

autonomic i., disturbance of the involuntary nervous system.

sympathetic i., vagotonia.

vasomotor i., autonomic imbalance.

imbecile (im′bĕ-sil) a mentally defective person of the second lowest order of intellectual potential (mental age between 3 and 7 years), usually requiring custodial and complete protective care.

imbecility (im″bĕ-sil′ĭ-te) mental deficiency sufficient to render the patient incapable of managing himself or his own affairs, the mental age being between 3 and 7 years.

imbibition (im″bĭ-bish′un) absorption of a liquid.

imbricated (im′brĭ-kāt″ed) overlapping like shingles.

imidazole (im″id-az′ōl) iminazole.

imide (im′īd) any compound containing the bivalent group, > NH.

iminazole (im″in-az′ōl) a radical occurring in histidine.

imipramine (ĭ-mip′rah-mēn) a compound used as an antidepressant in psychoses, neuroses and nonpsychotic disorders in which there is depressed emotional tone.

immature (im″ah-tūr) unripe or not fully developed.

immersion (ĭ-mer′zhun) 1. the plunging of a body into a liquid. 2. the use of the microscope with the object and object glass both covered with a liquid.

immiscible (ĭ-mis′ĭ-bl) incapable of being mixed.

immobilization (ĭ-mo″bĭ-lĭ-za′shun) the rendering of a part incapable of being moved.

immune (ĭ-mūn′) not susceptible to a particular disease.

i. reaction, the response of an organism to elements recognized as nonself, with production of plasmocytes, lymphocytes and antibodies, leading to ultimate rejection of the foreign material.

immunifacient (ĭ-mu″nĭ-fa′shent) producing immunity.

immunity (ĭ-mu-nĭ′-te) resistance of the body to the effects of a harmful agent, such as pathogenic microorganisms or their toxins. Immunity occurs as a result of the antigen-antibody reaction that takes place whenever a foreign agent or its product enters the bloodstream. (See also ANTIBODY and ANTIGEN). Immune substances that aid in the body's defense against disease include lysins, which have a dissolving action; antitoxins, which neutralize poisons produced by the microorganisms; agglutinins, which clump the microorganisms together, enabling bacteria-destroying cells in the blood to destroy many at one time; and opsonins, which sensitize the bacteria so that they may be more easily engulfed by the phagocytes. These immune substances are believed to be produced by certain cells in lymphoid tissue.

acquired i., that which results from antibodies not normally present in the blood; called also induced immunity.

active i., immunity produced by natural or artificial stimulation so that the body produces its own antibodies. It may be produced by an attack of the specific disease or by introduction of vaccines or toxoids by injections.

cellular i., acquired immunity (usually to an infectious agent) in which the role of phagocytic cells is predominant.

humoral i., acquired immunity in which the role of circulating antibody is predominant.

infection i., resistance to infection by reason of an already existing infection by the same or a homologous organism.

natural i., an innate resistance to disease due to the presence of antibodies occurring normally in the blood.

passive i., a state of nonsusceptibility to certain microorganisms produced by injection of ready-made antibodies present in immune serum (antiserum) or gamma globulin.

immunization (im″u-nĭ-za′shun) the process of rendering a subject immune, or of becoming immune. Called also inoculation and vaccination; the word vaccine originally referred to the substance used to immunize against smallpox, the first immunization developed. Now, however, the term is used for any preparation used in active immunization.

active i., inoculation, usually by injection, with a specific antigen to promote antibody formation in the body. The antigenic substance may be in one of four forms: (1) dead disease bacteria, as in typhoid immunization; (2) dead viruses, as in the Salk poliomyelitis injection; (3) live attenuated virus, e.g., smallpox vaccine and Sabin polio vaccine (taken orally); and (4) toxoids, altered forms of toxins produced by bacteria, as in immunization against tetanus and diphtheria.

Since active immunization induces the body to produce its own antibodies and to go on producing them, protection against disease will last several years, in some cases for life.

passive i., transient immunization produced by the introduction into the system of serum (antiserum) or antitoxin that already contains antibodies. The person immunized is protected only as long as these antibodies remain in his blood and are active—usually from 4 to 6 weeks.

immunochemistry (im″u-no-kem′is-tre) study of the chemistry of immunity.

immunoelectrophoresis (im″u-no-e-lek″tro-fo-re′sis) a method of distinguishing proteins and

mobility and antigenic specificities.

immunogenetics (im″u-no-jĕ-net′iks) the scientific study of the interrelations of immune reactions and genetic constitution.

immunogenic (im″u-no-jen′ik) producing immunity.

immunogenicity (im″u-no-jĕ-nis′ĭ-te) the ability of a substance to induce specific resistance.

immunoglobulin (im″u-no-glob′u-lin) serum globulin having antibody activity. Most of the antibody activity apparently resides in the gamma fraction of globulin. Immunoglobulins can be divided into at least three molecular species by electrophoretic and other methods. A system of nomenclature for these various immunoglobulins has been proposed, whereby Ig (or γ) means immunoglobulin, and the individual types are designated IgG (γG), IgM (γM) and IgA (γA). Preliminary studies show, for example, that patients with severe staphylococcal infections of the eye have low serum IgM levels, as compared with other Ig levels.

immunology (im″u-nol′o-je) the scientific study of immunity.

immunopolysaccharide (im″u-no-pol″e-sak′ah-rīd) a polysaccharide that is responsible for the immunologic specificity of a microorganism.

immunosuppression (im″u-no-sŭ-presh′un) inhibition of the formation of antibodies to antigens that may be present; used in transplantation procedures to prevent rejection of the transplanted organ or tissue. adj., **immunosuppres′sive.**

immunotherapy (im″u-no-ther′ah-pe) treatment by production of immunity.

immunotoxin (im″u-no-tok′sin) an antitoxin.

immunotransfusion (im″u-no-trans-fu′zhun) transfusion of blood from a donor previously immunized by vaccine prepared from the patient's serum or of blood from a person recently recovered from the same disease.

impaction (im-pak′shun) the condition of being wedged in firmly.

  fecal i., a collection of hardened feces in the rectum or sigmoid.

impar (im′par) not even; unequal; unpaired.

impedance (im-pe′dans) obstruction or opposition to passage or flow, as of an electric current or other form of energy.

  acoustic i., an expression of the opposition to passage of sound waves, being the product of the density of a substance and the velocity of sound in it.

Active Immunization Schedule for Infants

Age	Preparation	Dose
2 months	Triple antigen (DPT)	0.5 cc.[a]
3 months	Triple antigen (DPT)	
4 months	Triple antigen (DPT)	
2 months	Trivalent poliovaccine (Sabin)	2 cc. by mouth[b]
4 months	Trivalent poliovaccine (Sabin)	
6 months	Trivalent poliovaccine (Sabin)	
9 months	Smallpox vaccine	Multiple pressure technique over deltoid or triceps muscle
12 months	Measles vaccine	0.5 cc.[c]

[a]Diphtheria toxoid, approximately 20 Lf units per cc.: pertussis, 12 N.I.H. units per 1.5 cc.: tetanus toxoid, approximately 20 Lf units per cc. For all vaccines the manufacturer's directions regarding volume of dose and site of inoculation should be followed.

[b]Live, attenuated poliovaccine (Sabin) should not be fed from June through October.

[c]Live, attenuated measles vaccine may be administered safely without simultaneous administration of gamma globulin (0.01 cc. per lb. at different site with different syringe), but giving gamma globulin will reduce the reaction to the live measles vaccine. The "further attenuated measles vaccine" (Schwarz strain) may be used without the simultaneous administration of gamma globulin.

Rubella vaccine and mumps vaccine are usually given during the second year of life.

Schedule of Recall or Booster Immunizations for Children

Age	Preparation	Dose
15 months	1. Triple antigen (DPT)	0.5 cc.
	2. Trivalent poliovaccine (Sabin)	2 cc. by mouth[a]
4 years	Triple antigen (DPT)	0.25–0.5 cc.
6 years	Smallpox vaccine	Multiple pressure technique
8 years	Diphtheria-tetanus toxoid (standard)	0.1 cc.[b]
12 years and every 4 years	Diphtheria-tetanus toxoid (adult)	0.5 cc.[c]
	Smallpox vaccine	Multiple pressure technique

[a]One feeding of trivalent poliovaccine (Sabin) is recommended for booster dose. The need for further booster doses of poliovaccine (Sabin) has not been established.

[b]Standard diphtheria-tetanus toxoid not recommended for children over 10 years of age without preliminary Schick test and toxoid sensitivity test. It contains diphtheria toxoid, approximately 20 Lf units per cc., and tetanus toxoid, 20 Lf units per cc.

[c]Adult type of diphtheria-tetanus toxoid contains 1 to 2 Lf units of diphtheria toxoid and 7.5 to 10 Lf units of tetanus toxoid per dose (0.5 cc.) and may be used without preliminary Schick and diphtheria toxoid sensitivity tests.

From Active immunization for common infectious diseases. Nursing Clin. N. Amer., *1*:347, 1966.

imperforate (im-per'fo-rāt) not open; abnormally closed.

impermeable (im-per'me-ah-bl) not permitting passage, as for fluid.

impetigo (im"pĕ-ti'go) a skin disease characterized by pustules and caused by streptococci, often in association with staphylococci. The disease occurs most frequently in children, especially in very young infants because of their low resistance. It is spread by direct contact with the moist discharges of the lesions. If not properly treated, it can be serious or even fatal to newborn infants.
Treatment consists of cleansing the lesions with soap and water and then wiping the surrounding skin with alcohol. Care should be taken to avoid spreading the infection and the patient should be isolated. The lesions should be kept dry and open to the air as much as possible. Local applications of an antibiotic ointment may clear up the lesions; however, systemic administration of antibiotics usually is recommended.

implant (im-plant') 1. to insert or graft. 2. (im'-plant) material inserted or grafted into the body, or a small container holding radon or radium, for internal application of its radiation.

implantation (im"plan-ta'shun) 1. embedding of a material within the tissues, as of medication, or of a device such as an artificial pacemaker, or of the fertilized ovum in the uterine lining. 2. the insertion of a part or tissue such as skin, nerve or tendon in a new site in the body.

impotence (im'po-tens) partial or complete inability of the male to perform the sexual act or to achieve orgasm.

impregnation (im"preg-na'shun) 1. fertilization of the ovum. 2. saturation.

impressio (im-pres'e-o), pl. *impressio'nes* [L.] impression (1).

impression (im-presh'un) 1. an indentation or dent. 2. a negative copy or counterpart of some object made by bringing into contact with the object, with varying degrees of pressure, some plastic material that later becomes solidified. 3. an effect on the mind or senses produced by external objects.

impulse (im'puls) 1. an instinctive urge. 2. a sudden pushing force.
cardiac i., the impulse or beat of the heart at the fifth intercostal space at the left side of the sternum.
nerve i., the impulse or activity propagated along nerve fibers.

impulsion (im-pul'shun) a state characterized by an instinctive urge to commit an unlawful or socially unacceptable act.

In chemical symbol, *indium.*

inactivation (in-ak"tĭ-va'shun) destruction of activity, as of a serum by the action of heat or other means.

inalimental (in"al-ĭ-men'tal) not nutritious.

inanition (in"ah-nish'un) the physical condition that results from complete lack of food; starvation.

inappetence (in-ap'ĕ-tens) lack of appetite or desire.

inarticulate (in"ar-tik'u-lāt) 1. without definite articulations. 2. incapable of articulate speech.

inassimilable (in"ah-sim'ĭ-lah-bl) not susceptible of being utilized as nutriment.

inborn (in'born) formed or implanted during fetal life.

inbreeding (in'brēd-ing) the mating of closely related individuals or of individuals having closely similar genetic constitutions.

incarceration (in-kar"sĕ-ra'shun) abnormal confinement or constriction.

incest (in'sest) culturally prohibited sexual activity between persons of close blood relationship.

incidence (in'sĭ-dens) the rate at which a certain event occurs, as the number of new cases of a specific disease occurring during a certain period.

incineration (in-sin"ĕ-ra'shun) the act of burning to ashes.

incisal (in-si'zal) cutting.

incision (in-sizh'un) 1. a cut or wound. 2. the act of cutting.

incisive (in-si'siv) 1. having the power or quality of cutting; sharp. 2. pertaining to the incisor teeth.

incisor (in-si'zor) any one of the four front teeth of either jaw.

incisure (in-si'zher) a cut, notch or incision.

inclination (in"klĭ-na'shun) a sloping or leaning; the angle of deviation from a particular line or plane of reference.
i. of the pelvis, the angle between the axis of the body and that of the pelvis.

inclusion (in-kloo'zhun) 1. enclosure within something else. 2. anything that is enclosed.
i. bodies, round, oval or irregular-shaped bodies occurring in the protoplasm or nuclei of cells of the body, as in disease caused by filterable virus infection such as rabies, smallpox, herpes.
cell i., a usually lifeless, often temporary, constituent in the cytoplasm of a cell.
i. conjunctivitis, an inflammatory condition of the conjunctiva, caused by a filterable virus and characterized by the presence of large basophilic inclusion bodies.

incoagulability (in"ko-ag"u-lah-bil'ĭ-te) the state of being incapable of coagulation.

incompatible (in"kom-pat'ĭ-bl) not suited for harmonious coexistence or simultaneous administration; not to be combined in the same preparation or taken concomitantly.

incompetent (in-kom'pĕ-tent) 1. not able to function properly. 2. not responsible for actions, usually because of severe emotional disorder.

incontinence (in-kon'tĭ-nens) inability to refrain from yielding to normal impulses, as the urge to defecate or urinate.
Fecal incontinence may result from disorders of the nervous system or weakening of the anal sphincters in elderly persons. Anal or rectal surgery

and anal tears resulting from childbirth also may impair control.

Urinary incontinence has many possible causes. Stress, anger or anxiety can increase the urge to urinate. Incontinence sometimes occurs after surgery or in connection with irritation of the urinary tract by inflammation or injury. In some instances incontinence is due to an obstruction that prevents normal emptying of the urinary bladder, resulting in constant dribbling of the overflow. An uncontrolled flow can result from spasm of the bladder, or from the development of a fistula between the bladder and urethra, vagina or rectum. Damage to the spinal cord or brain by injury or disease also hinders bladder control.

NURSING CARE. Both physical and emotional problems usually are involved in cases of incontinence. Although solutions to these problems may appear impossible, an attitude of optimism and patience is essential if the patient is to be helped. All nursing measures are aimed at keeping the patient dry, clean, odorless and as comfortable as possible. Regularity in eating, a definite routine for elimination, frequent offering of the bedpan and prompt response to the patient's request for a bedpan can do much to help him learn control. Waterproof materials and specially designed receptacles for collecting waste are useful in preventing irritation to the skin and reducing the unpleasant odors that arise from incontinence.

stress i., involuntary escape of urine due to strain on the orifice of the bladder, as in coughing or sneezing.

incoordination (in″ko-or″dī-na′shun) lack of normal adjustment of muscular motions; failure to work harmoniously.

incorporation (in-kor″po-ra′shun) 1. thorough mixing of a substance with another. 2. in psychiatry, a primitive mental mechanism whereby a person unconsciously and symbolically takes within himself another person, parts of another person, or other significant nonmaterial elements.

increment (in′krĕ-ment) increase or augmentative growth; the amount by which a value or quantity is increased.

incretion (in-kre′shun) an internal secretion.

incrustation (in″krus-ta′shun) 1. the formation of a crust. 2. a crust or scab.

incubate (in′ku-bāt) 1. to provide proper conditions for growth and development, as to maintain optimal temperature for the growth of bacteria. 2. material that has been incubated.

incubation (in″ku-ba′shun) the induction of development, especially of pathogenic organisms within the body, or in a special medium.

i. period, the interval of time required for development; especially the time between invasion of the body by a pathogenic organism and appearance of the first symptoms of disease. Incubation periods vary from a few days to several months, depending on the causative organism and type of disease.

incubator (in′ku-ba″ter) an apparatus for main-

INCUBATION PERIODS OF COMMUNICABLE DISEASES

Usually about 0–7 days

DISEASE	INCUBATION PERIOD AVG.	RANGE	ISOLATION	IMMUNIZATION
Anthrax	1–4	(1–7)	"Clean" technique	
Bacillary dysentery	2–4	(1–7)	Till stool negative	
Chancroid	3–5	(1–12)	From sexual contact	
Cholera	3	(1–5)	Till stool negative (quarantine)	
Dengue	5–6	(3–15)	Screen	
Diphtheria	2–5		Till nose and throat negative	Toxoid/antitoxin
Epidemic diarrhea of newborn	6–7	(2–21)	Yes (quarantine)	
Erysipelas	0–2		"Clean" technique	
Food poisoning				
Staphylococcus	2–4	(1–6) hr.		
Salmonella	12	(6–48) hr.	From food handling	Antitoxin
Botulinus	18–24	(2–48) hr.		
Gonorrhea	3–5	(1–14)	From sexual contact and children	
Impetigo contagiosa	5		From child contacts	
Infectious keratoconjunctivitis	5–7			
Influenza	1–3		Acute stage	Formalin-virus
Meningitis, meningococcic	7	(2–10)	24 hr., if treated	
Paratyphoid	1–10		Till stool and urine negative	Vaccine
Plague	3–6		Till well	Formalin-vaccine
Pneumonia, bacterial	1–3		Respiratory precautions	
Puerperal infection	1–3		Till well	
Relapsing fever (tick)	3–6	(2–12)		
Rocky Mountain spotted fever	3–10			Yolk-sac vaccine
Scabies	1–2		From school	
Scarlet fever	2–5		Respiratory precautions	
Tularemia	3	(1–10)		
Yellow fever	3–6		Screen	Modified-virus

taining optimal conditions (temperature, humidity, etc.,) for growth and development, especially one used in the early care of premature infants. The primary purpose of the incubator is to surround the infant with some of the environmental conditions normally provided in the uterus and necessary until he reaches approximately the level of development of a full-term infant.

The temperature within the incubator is regulated so that the infant's temperature is maintained between 96° and 98° F. (35.5° to 36.5° C.). Humidity is kept at 50 to 60 per cent unless there is respiratory difficulty, in which case the humidity may be raised as high as 85 to 100 per cent. Oxygen is added in concentrations not exceeding 30 to 40 per cent only as long as the infant is cyanotic because of the danger of retrolental fibroplasia with high concentrations of oxygen.

incubus (in'ku-bus) 1. nightmare. 2. a heavy mental burden.

incudal (ing'ku-dal) pertaining to the incus.

incudectomy (ing"ku-dek'to-me) excision of the incus.

incudiform (ing-ku'dĭ-form) anvil-shaped.

incudomalleal (ing"ku-do-mal'e-al) pertaining to the incus and malleus.

incudostapedial (ing"ku-do-stah-pe'de-al) pertaining to the incus and stapes.

incurable (in-kūr'ah-bl) 1. not susceptible of being cured. 2. a person with a disease that cannot be cured.

incus (ing'kus) the middle of the three ossicles of the ear; called also anvil.

Indecidua (in"de-sid'u-ah) a division of the class Mammalia, including the mammals without a decidua.

index (in'deks) 1. the second digit of the hand, or

INCUBATION PERIODS OF COMMUNICABLE DISEASES (*Continued*)

Usually about 7–14 days

DISEASE	INCUBATION PERIOD AVG.	RANGE	ISOLATION	IMMUNIZATION
Coccidioidomycosis	10–15	(7–21)	Till sputum negative	
Equine encephalitis	5–15			
Infectious mononucleosis	11	(7–15)	Respiratory precautions	
Leptospirosis	9–10	(4–19)		
Lymphocytic choriomeningitis	8–13			
Measles	9–14		Till 5 days after rash	Immune globulin
Pertussis	5–9	(2–21)	From school and susceptibles	Vaccine
Poliomyelitis	7–14	(3–35)	First 2 weeks	Vaccine
Primary atypical pneumonia	11	(7–21)	Respiratory precautions	
Psittacosis	6–15		Till afebrile	
Relapsing fever (louse)	7	(5–12)	To delouse	
Scrub typhus	7–10	(7–14)		
Smallpox	12	(7–21)	Till scabs off (quarantine)	Vaccinia
Trichinosis	9	(2–28)		
Typhoid fever	7–14	(3–38)	Till stool and urine negative	Vaccine
Typhus fever	12	(6–15)	To delouse (quarantine)	Vaccine

Usually over 14 days

DISEASE	INCUBATION PERIOD AVG.	RANGE	ISOLATION	IMMUNIZATION
Amebic dysentery	21–28	(8–90)	From food handling	
Brucellosis	14	(6–30+)		
Chickenpox	14	(12–21)	Till skin clear	
German measles	16–18	(10–21)	First week	
Granuloma inguinale	10–90		From sexual contact	
Hepatitis, infectious	25	(15–35)	Stool disinfection for 3 weeks	Immune globulin
Hepatitis, serum	80–100	(60–180)		
Lymphogranuloma venereum	7–28		From sexual contact	
Malaria	10–17	(to 35+)	Screen	
Mumps	18	(12–26)	Till glands down	
Q fever	14–21			Vaccine
Rabies	14–42	(10–180)	Aseptic technique	Attenuated vaccine
Rickettsialpox	10–24			
Syphilis	21	(10–90)	From sexual contact and children	
Tetanus	4–21			Toxoid
Tuberculosis	Variable		"Open" cases	BCG vaccine
Yaws	30–90		Desirable till treated	

From The SK&F Pocket Book of Medical Tables. 15th ed. Philadelphia, Smith Kline & French Laboratories, 1966.

the forefinger. 2. the numerical ratio of measurement of any part in comparison with a fixed standard.

alveolar i., the degree of prominence of the jaws.

centromeric i., the ratio of the length of the shorter arm of a mitotic chromosome to the total length of the chromosome.

cephalic i., 100 times the maximal breadth of the skull divided by its maximal length.

cerebral i., the ratio of the greatest transverse to the greatest anteroposterior diameter of the cranial cavity.

color i., the relative amount of hemoglobin in an erythrocyte compared with that of a normal individual of the same age and sex. The percentage of hemoglobin is divided by the percentage of erythrocytes.

hand i., 100 times the breadth of the hand divided by the length of the hand.

hemolytic i., a formula for calculating increased erythrocyte destruction.

icteric i., the ratio of bilirubin in the blood (see also ICTERIC INDEX).

length-breadth i., cephalic index.

length-height i., vertical index.

leukopenic i., any variation from the normal leukocyte count after ingestion of food to which a patient is allergic.

mitotic i., an expression of the number of mitoses found in a stated number of cells.

nasal i., 100 times the width of the nose, divided by its length.

opsonic i., the resisting power of the blood against bacilli, as compared with the normal.

orbital i. (of Broca), 100 times the height of the opening of the orbit divided by its width.

pelvic i., 100 times the anteroposterior diameter of the pelvis divided by the maximal width across the inlet.

phagocytic i., the average number of bacteria ingested per leukocyte of the patient's blood.

refraction i., refractive i., the refracting power of any substance compared with that of air.

sacral i., 100 times the breadth of the sacrum divided by the length.

thoracic i., the ratio of the anteroposterior diameter of the thorax to the transverse diameter.

ventilation i., the ratio of the residual volume of the lung to total lung capacity.

vertical i., 100 times the height of the skull divided by its length.

vital i., the ratio of births to deaths within a given time in a population.

volume i., the index indicating the size of the erythrocytes as compared to the normal.

indican (in'dĭ-kan) 1. a substance formed by decomposition of tryptophan in the intestines and found in the urine. 2. a yellow indoxyl glycoside from indigo plants.

indicator (in'dĭ-ka″ter) a substance that makes manifest a condition of a solution (acid: alkaline), or the end point of a reaction.

indigestible (in″dĭ-jes'tĭ-bl) not susceptible of digestion.

indigestion (in″dĭ-jes'chun) failure of digestive function; dyspepsia. Among the symptoms of indigestion are heartburn, nausea, flatulence, cramps, a disagreeable taste in the mouth, belching and sometimes vomiting or diarrhea. Ordinary indigestion can result from eating too much or too fast; from eating when tense, tired or emotionally up-

set; from food that is too fatty or spicy; and from heavy fried food or food that has been badly cooked or processed.

Indigestion and its symptoms may also accompany other disorders such as allergy, migraine, influenza, typhoid fever, food poisoning, peptic ulcer, inflammation of the gallbladder (chronic cholecystitis), appendicitis and coronary occlusion ("heart attack").

indigitation (in-dij″ĭ-ta'shun) intussusception.

indigo (in'dĭ-go) a blue dyeing material from plants and also made synthetically.

indigotindisulfonate (in″dĭ-go″tin-di-sul'fo-nāt) a dye used in tests for measurement of kidney function.

indium (in'de-um) a chemical element, atomic number 49, atomic weight 114. 82, symbol In. (See table of ELEMENTS.)

individuation (in″dĭ-vid″u-a'shun) 1. the process of developing individual characteristics. 2. differential regional activity in the embryo occurring in response to organizer influence.

indocyanine green (in″do-si'ah-nēn) a dye used in tests of cardiovascular function.

indole (in'dōl) a compound formed during the putrefaction of proteins, which contributes to the characteristic odor of feces.

indomethacin (in″do-meth'ah-sin) a compound used as an anti-inflammatory, analgesic and antipyretic agent.

indoxyl (in-dok'sil) an oily substance found in urine.

induction (in-duk'shun) the process or act of inducing, or causing to occur, especially (1) the specific morphogenetic effect of a chemical stimulus transmitted from one part of the embryo to another, bringing about the orderly development of the various organs and body structures, or (2) the generation of electric phenomena in a body by influence of an electrified body near it.

inductor (in-duk'tor) a tissue elaborating a chemical substance that acts to determine the growth and differentiation of embryonic parts.

inductotherm (in-duk'to-therm) an apparatus for producing high body temperature by electric induction.

inductothermy (in-duk'to-ther″me) production of artificial fever by the inductotherm.

indulin (in'du-lin) a coal tar dye used as a histologic stain.

indurated (in'du-rāt″ed) hardened; abnormally hard.

induration (in″du-ra'shun) the quality of being hard; the process of hardening; an abnormally hard spot. adj., **indura'tive.**

black i., hardening and pigmentation of the lung, as in anthracosis.

brown i., 1. a deposit of altered blood pigment in the lung in pneumonia. 2. marked increase of the connective tissue of the lung and excessive pigmentation, due to long-continued congestion from valvular heart disease, or to anthracosis.

  cyanotic i., hardening of an organ from chronic venous congestion.

  granular i., cirrhosis.

  gray i., induration of lung tissue in or after pneumonia, without pigmentation.

  red i., interstitial pneumonia in which the lung is red and congested.

inebriant   (ĭ-ne′bre-ant) an intoxicating agent.

inelastic   (in″e-las′tik) lacking elasticity.

inemia   (in-e′me-ah) fibrin in the blood.

inert   (in-ert′) inactive.

inertia   (in-er′she-ah) [L.] inactivity.

  colonic i., absence of efficient contraction of the muscular coat of the colon, leading to distention of the organ and constipation.

  i. u′teri, uterine i., absence of effectual contraction of the muscular wall of the uterus, leading to prolonged labor.

in extremis   (in ek-stre′mis) [L.] at the point of death.

infancy   (in′fan-se) the first 2 years of life.

infant   (in′fant) a young child from birth to 2 years of age.

  NEEDS OF THE INFANT.   Emotional and physical needs include love and security, a sense of trust, warmth and comfort, feeding and sucking pleasure.

  GROWTH AND DEVELOPMENT.   Development is a continuous process, and each child progresses at his own rate. There is a developmental sequence, which means that the changes leading to maturity are specific and orderly. The various types of growth and development and the accompanying changes in appearance and behavior are interrelated; that is, physical, emotional, social and spiritual developments affect one another in the progress toward maturity.

  Development of muscular control proceeds from the head downward (cephalocaudal development). The infant controls the head first and gradually acquires the ability to control the neck, then the arms and finally the legs and feet. Control begins near the body and progresses outward to the arms and hands and the legs and feet. Movements are general and random at first, beginning with use of the larger muscles and progressing to specific smaller muscles, such as those needed to handle small objects.

  Factors that influence growth and development are: hereditary traits, sex, environment, nationality and race and physical makeup.

  INFANT CARE.   A plan of care should be designed within the framework of the natural rhythms of a normal infant. The plan should be sensible, taking into account the family's needs as well as the needs of the infant.

  Bathing.   A sponge bath is usually advised during the first 2 weeks of life. After that, the tub bath provides not only cleanliness but also an opportunity for exercise as the infant kicks and splashes in the water. There is no definite time at which the bath should be given, but it is best to plan the bath before a feeding.

  The room should be warm (about 75 to 80° F.) and free from drafts. The temperature of the bath water should be about 90 to 100° F., or comfortably warm to the inner arm. The scalp should be washed with soap and water once or twice a week, or daily if the baby has CRADLE CAP. Special attention should be given to the folds and creases of the arms, legs and genitalia. A lotion may be applied after the bath but it usually is not necessary; talcum, if used at all, should be applied sparingly to avoid caking and accumulations in the folds of the skin which may harbor bacteria.

  Clothing.   The infant's garments should be loose so that he can move about freely. He should be kept comfortably warm, but not overheated because this leads to prickly heat. The number of gowns, shirts, diapers or other articles of clothing needed will depend on laundry facilities and the taste and wishes of the family. Diapers require special laundering to remove all traces of soap and stains and to destroy bacteria. Ideally, diapers should be boiled for 5 minutes in soapy water and then washed and rinsed thoroughly, with several rinses to remove the soap. If possible they should be hung outdoors to dry.

  Fresh Air.   A daily outing for fresh air and sunshine is recommended if the temperature is above freezing and if there is no strong wind. Sunburn, overheating and glare in the infant's eyes should be avoided.

  Sleep.   The average infant spends a large part of his time sleeping. Needs of individual infants vary, but at 3 months most infants sleep about 16 hours out of the 24. This length of time will gradually decrease as he grows older.

  ARTIFICIAL FEEDING.   The advantages and disadvantages of breast feeding as opposed to artificial feeding are discussed under BREAST FEEDING. In artificial feeding the infant is fed from a bottle until he learns to drink from a cup. A formula prescribed by the pediatrician is given; when the baby is about 2 to 4 weeks of age, cereal and pureed foods are added to the diet. Vitamins A, D and C (usually in the form of orange juice) are given every day. At about 4 months boiled egg yolk may be given and soup may also be tried. When an infant is first given solid foods he may make a sucking action with his tongue and then push the food out of his mouth. This does not indicate a dislike for the taste; the infant is simply learning how to handle solid foods in his mouth. At 5 months custards and simple puddings may be given for variety. At 6 months a variety of food can be offered and the infant may be weaned from the breast or bottle to a cup. By 12 months the infant should be able to handle most simple foods but his interest in eating may dwindle as he begins to notice other things that distract his attention.

  Preparation of Formula.   The type of milk and sugar to be used in the formula depends on the pediatrician's orders and the infant's tolerance. Evaporated milk, condensed milk, homogenized milk or dried milk can be used. The sugar included in the formula may be sucrose (cane sugar), dextrose or a mixture of dextrose and maltose. There are several proprietary milk products available; some are said to closely resemble breast milk in composition. They have the advantages of convenience, sterility and compactness and usually require only the addition of boiled water for preparation.

  Generally there are two methods for sterilizing the formula: the terminal method and the aseptic method. In the terminal method the formula is prepared and poured into bottles and filled bottles are sterilized by heat. In the aseptic method the form-

Average Achievement Levels of Infants, 1 Month to 1 Year

1 Month

Physical
  Weight: 8 pounds. Gains about 5 to 7 ounces weekly during first 6 months of life.
  Height: Gains approximately 1 inch a month for the first 6 months.
  Pulse: 120–150
  Respirations: 30–60
Motor Control
  Head sags when supported. May lift head from time to time when he is held against his mother's shoulder
  Makes crawling movements when prone on a flat surface
  Lifts head intermittently, though unsteadily, when in prone position. Cervical curve begins to develop as the infant learns to hold his head erect
  Can turn his head to the side when prone
  Can push with feet against a hard surface to move himself forward
  Has "dance" reflex when held upright with feet touching the bed or examining table.
  Shows a well developed tonic neck reflex (head turned to one side, the arm extended on the same side and the other arm flexed to his shoulder)
  Holds hands in fists. Does not reach with hands. Can grasp an object placed in his hand, but drops it immediately
Vision
  Stares indefinitely at his surroundings and apparently notices faces and bright objects, but only if they are in his line of vision. Activity diminishes when he regards a human face
  Can follow an object to the midline of vision
Vocalization and Socialization
  Utters small throaty sounds
  Smiles indefinitely
  Shows a vague and indirect regard of faces and bright objects
  Cries when hungry or uncomfortable

2 Months

Physical
  Posterior fontanel closed
Motor Control
  Can hold head erect in midposition. Can lift head and chest a short distance above bed or table when lying on his abdomen
  Tonic neck and Moro reflexes are fading
  Can turn from side to back
  Can hold a rattle for a brief time
Vision
  Can follow a moving light or object with his eyes
Vocalization and Socialization
  Shows a "social smile" in response to another's smile. This is the beginning of social behavior. It may not appear until the third month
  Has learned that by crying he will get attention. His crying becomes differentiated; the sound of his crying varies with the reason for crying, e.g. hunger, sleepiness or pain
  Pays attention to the speaking voice

3 Months

Physical
  Weight: 12–13 pounds
Motor Control
  Holds his hands up in front of him and stares at them
  Plays with hands and fingers
  Reaches for shiny objects but misses them
  Can carry hand or object to mouth at will
  Holds head erect and steady. Raises chest, usually supported on forearms
  Has lost the walking or dancing reflex
  Grasping reflex has weakened
  Sits, back rounded, knees flexed when supported
Vision
  Shows binocular coordination (vertical and horizontal vision) when an object is moved from right to left and up and down in front of his face
  Turns eyes to an object in his marginal field of vision
  Voluntarily winks at objects which threaten his eyes
Vocalization and Socialization
  Laughs aloud and shows pleasure in making sounds
  Cries less
  Smiles in response to mother's face

AVERAGE ACHIEVEMENT LEVELS OF INFANTS, 1 MONTH TO 1 YEAR (*Continued*)

4 MONTHS

Physical
  Weight: Between 13 and 14 pounds
  Drools between 3 and 4 months of age. This indicates the appearance of saliva. He does not know how to swallow saliva, which therefore runs from his mouth
Motor Control
  Symmetrical body postures predominate
  Holds head steady when in sitting position
  Lifts head and shoulders at a 90-degree angle when on abdomen and looks around
  Tries to roll over. Can turn from back to side
  Thumb apposition in grasping occurs between third and fourth months
  Holds hands predominantly open. Activates arms at sight of preferred toy
  Sits with adequate support and enjoys being propped up
  Tonic neck reflex has disappeared
  Sustains portion of own weight
Vision
  Recognizes familiar objects
  Stares at rattle placed in his hand and takes it to his mouth
  Follows moving objects well. Even the most difficult types of eye movements are present
  Arms are activated on sight of dangling toy
Vocalization and Socialization
  Laughs aloud and smiles in response to smiles of others
  Initiates social play by smiling
  Vocalizes socially; i.e. he coos and gurgles when talked to
  He does not cry when scolded. He is very "talkative"
  "Talking" and crying follow each other quickly
  Shows evidence of wanting social attention and of increasing interest in other members of the family
  Enjoys having people with him

5 MONTHS

Physical
  Weight: Twice the birth weight (15–16 pounds)
Motor Control
  Sits with slight support. Holds back straight when pulled to sitting position
  Can use thumb in partial apposition to fingers more skillfully
  Can balance head well
  Reaches for objects which are beyond his grasp. Grasps objects independently of direct stimulation of the palm of the hand (partial grasp). Grasps with the whole hand. Accepts an object handed to him
  Has completely lost the Moro reflex
Vocalization and Socialization
  Vocalizes his displeasure when a desired object is taken from him

6 MONTHS

Physical
  Gains about 3 to 5 ounces weekly during the second 6 months of life
  Grows about ½ inch a month
  May be teething
Motor Control
  Sits momentarily without support if placed in a favorable leaning position
  Grasps with simultaneous flexion of fingers
  Retains transient hold on 2 blocks, one in either hand
  Pulls himself up to a sitting position
  Completely turns over from stomach to stomach with rest periods during the complete turn. This ability is important in protecting him from falling out of bed
  Springs up and down when sitting
  Bangs with object held in his hand, rattle or spoon
  Hitches. Hitching is locomotion backward when in a sitting position. Movement of the body is aided by use of his arms and hands. This ability is usually present by the sixth month
Vocalization and Socialization
  Babbles from the third to the eighth month
  Vocalizes several well defined syllables. Actively vocalizes pleasure with crowing or cooing. Babbling is not linked with specific objects, people or situations
  Cries easily on slight provocation (change of position or withdrawal of a toy)
  Thrashes arms and legs when frustrated
  Begins to recognize strangers (fifth to sixth month)

AVERAGE ACHIEVEMENT LEVELS OF INFANTS, 1 MONTH TO 1 YEAR (*Continued*)

7 MONTHS

Motor Control
When lying down, lifts head as if he were trying to sit up
Sits briefly, leaning forward on his hands. Control of trunk is more advanced
Plays with his feet and puts them in his mouth
Bounces actively when held in a standing position
Can approach a toy and grasp it with one hand
Can transfer a toy from one hand to the other with varying degrees of success
Rolls more easily from back to stomach
Vocalization and Socialization
Vocalizes his eagerness
Vocalizes "m-m-m" when crying
Makes polysyllabic vowel sounds
Emotional development, 7 to 8 months: Shows fear of strangers
Emotional instability shown by easy and quick changes from crying to laughing

8 MONTHS

Motor Control
Sits alone steadily
Complete thumb apposition
Hand-eye coordination is perfected to the point that random reaching and grasping no longer persist
Vocalization and Socialization
Greets strangers with coy or bashful behavior, turning away, hanging his head, crying or even screaming, and refuses to
play with strangers or even accept toys from them
Shows nervousness with strangers
Emotional development: "Eight months' anxiety," to be distinguished from anaclitic depression, occurs between the
sixth and eighth months as a result of the child's increased capacity for discriminating between friend and stranger
Affection or love of family group appears
Emotional instability still shown by easy changes from laughing to crying
Stretches arm to loved adult as in invitation to come

9 MONTHS

Motor Control
Shows good coordination and sits alone
Holds his bottle with good hand-mouth coordination. Can put the nipple in and out of his mouth at will
Preference for the use of one hand is marked
Crawls instead of hitching. Crawling may be seen as early as the fourth month; the average age is about nine months.
In crawling the infant is prone, his abdomen touching the floor, his head and shoulders supported with the weight
borne on the elbows. The body is pulled along by the movement of the arms while the legs drag. The leg movements
may resemble swimming or kicking movements
Creeps. This is a more advanced type of locomotion than crawling. The trunk is carried above the floor, but parallel to it.
The infant uses both his hands and knees in propelling himself forward. Not all infants follow this pattern of hitching,
crawling and creeping. Different children stress different means of locomotion and may even skip a stage. (This is
particularly likely if an infant is sick or for some other reason is unable to practice moving about)
Raises himself to a sitting position. Requires help to pull self to feet
Vocalization and Socialization
Shows the beginning of imitative expression. Sounds stand for things to him. Says "Da-da" or some such expression
Responds to adult anger. Cries when scolded.

10 MONTHS

Motor Control
Sits steadily for an indefinite time. Does not enjoy lying down unless he is sleepy
Makes early stepping movements when held
Pulls himself to his feet, holding to the crib rail or similar support. (This is a good time to begin use of the play pen or
yard)
Creeps and cruises about very well. (Cruising is walking sideways while holding on to a supporting object with both
hands)
Can pick up objects fairly well and pokes them with his fingers
Feeds himself a cracker or some such food which he can hold in his hand
Is able crudely to release a toy
Can bring his hands together
Vocalization and Socialization
Says one or two words and imitates an adult's inflection
Pays attention to his name
Plays simple games as bye-bye and pat-a-cake (motor control is such that he can bring his hands together) and peek-a-boo

ula and bottles are sterilized separately and then the bottles are filled and capped under aseptic conditions.

Enough formula for 24 hours should be prepared at one time and poured into 8-oz. bottles. The bottles of formula are kept refrigerated until one is needed for feeding; it is then reheated to a tepid temperature. (Recent evidence, however, shows that infants tolerate cold formula as well as that which has been warmed.) Any formula left in the bottle after feeding should be poured out and the bottle and nipple immediately rinsed with cold water to remove the milk.

Feeding the Infant. The infant should be picked up and held during the feeding. This provides him with physical contact that conveys a sense of warmth and security, and also avoids the dangers of strangulation or aspiration of the formula and prevents the possibility of the infant sucking air from a half-empty bottle. He should be positioned so that his head and shoulders are elevated and well supported.

The opening in the nipple may be a cross-cut or a group of small holes. The nipple should be firm and the opening small enough so that some sucking effort is required and the formula is not taken too rapidly.

During the feeding the infant's position should be changed so that he can eliminate bubbles of air that may have accumulated in his stomach. The position for "burping" or "bubbling" the infant is not important as long as his head and shoulders are higher than the rest of his body. He may be turned on his abdomen for burping. Holding the infant in a sitting position in one's lap is less likely to contaminate the infant than is the shoulder method. After the feeding is completed the infant should be placed in bed on his side or abdomen to facilitate removal of air from the stomach and reduce the danger of aspiration if he regurgitates some of the formula.

floppy i., one exhibiting severe generalized hypotonia.

immature i., one weighing between 17 oz. and $2\frac{1}{5}$ lb. (500 to 999 Gm.) at birth, with little chance of survival.

mature i., one weighing $5\frac{1}{2}$ lb. (2500 Gm.) or more at birth, with optimal chance of survival.

newborn i., the human young during the first 2 to 4 weeks after birth.

postmature i., one having an accurate history of a prolonged gestation period and weighing more than 9 lb. (4082 Gm.) at birth.

premature i., one weighing between $2\frac{1}{2}$ and $5\frac{1}{2}$ lb. (1000 to 2499 Gm.) at birth, with poor to good chance of survival (see also PREMATURE INFANT).

infantile (in'fan-tīl) relating to the stage of infancy; having features or traits characteristic of early childhood.

i. paralysis, poliomyelitis.

infantilism (in-fan'tĭ-lizm) persistence of the characters of childhood in adult life, marked by mental retardation, underdevelopment of the reproductive organs and often, but not always, smallness of stature.

infarct (in'farkt) a localized area of ischemic

AVERAGE ACHIEVEMENT LEVELS OF INFANTS, 1 MONTH TO 1 YEAR (*Continued*)

11 MONTHS

Motor Control
   Stands erect with the help of his mother's hand or supporting himself by holding on to some object as the side of his play yard

12 MONTHS

Physical
   Weight: Three times his birth weight (21–22 pounds)
   Height: 29 inches
   Head and chest are equal in circumference
   Has 6 teeth
   Pulse: 100–140 per minute.
   Respirations: 20–40 per minute
Motor Control
   Stands for a moment alone, or possibly longer
   Walks with help. Cruises, walking sideways around chairs or from chair to chair, holding on with one hand
   Lumbar curve and the compensating dorsal curve develop as he learns to walk
   Can sit down from standing position without help
   Holds a crayon adaptively to make a stroke and can mark on a piece of paper
   Can pick up small bits of food and transfer them to his mouth. Can drink from a cup and eat from a spoon, but requires help. He likes to eat with his fingers
   Cooperates in dressing; e.g. he can put his arm through a sleeve. Can take off his socks
Vocalization and Socialization
   Can say 2 words besides "Mama" and "Dada"
   Slow vocabulary growth, as a rule, owing to his interest in walking
   Knows his own name
   Uses expressive jargon. Communicates with himself and those around him
   Inhibits simple acts on command. Recognizes the meaning of "No, no"
   Shows jealousy, affection, anger and other emotions. He may cry for affection. He loves an audience, and will repeat a performance which brings a response. Crying is more often associated with irritation or frustration than it formerly was. Stiffens in resistance
   Loves rhythms
   Still egocentric, concerned only with himself

From Marlow, D. R.: Textbook of Pediatric Nursing. 3rd ed. Philadelphia, W. B. Saunders Co., 1969.

necrosis produced by occlusion of the arterial supply or the venous drainage of the part.

anemic i., one due to interruption of flow of arterial blood to the area.

bone i., an area of bone tissue that has become necrotic as a result of loss of its arterial blood supply.

hemorrhagic i., that due to interruption of drainage of venous blood from the area.

pale i., anemic infarct.

red i., hemorrhagic infarct.

septic i., one in which the tissues have been invaded by pathogenic organisms.

white i., anemic infarct.

infarction (in-fark'shun) the development or presence of an infarct.

cardiac i., myocardial infarction.

cerebral i., an ischemic condition of the brain, causing a persistent focal neurologic deficit in the area affected.

intestinal i., occlusion of an artery or arteriole in the wall of the intestine, resulting in the formation of an area of coagulation necrosis.

myocardial i., formation of an infarct in the heart muscle, due to interruption of the blood supply to the area (see also CORONARY OCCLUSION).

pulmonary i., infiltration of an airless area of lung with blood cells, due to obstruction of the pulmonary artery or one of its branches by an embolus or thrombus.

infection (in-fek'shun) 1. a morbid state caused by multiplication of pathogenic microorganisms within the body. 2. the invasion of an organism by any pathogenic (or nonpathogenic) organisms such as bacteria, viruses, protozoa, helminths and fungi.

Several factors are necessary to the development of an infection. The microorganisms must enter the body in sufficient numbers and they must be virulent, or capable of destroying healthy tissues. The host must be susceptible to the disease. If the host has developed immunity to the disease, either by having had the disease or by having undergone immunization, he will not be affected by the microorganisms. Some persons have greater natural resistance to infections than others. Finally, the disease must be transmitted through the proper route.

The body responds to the invasion by the formation of ANTIBODIES and by a series of physiologic changes known as INFLAMMATION.

Infection may be transmitted by direct contact, by indirect contact or by vectors. Direct contact may be with body excreta such as urine, feces or mucus, or with drainage from an open sore, ulcer or wound. Indirect contact refers to transmission via inanimate objects such as bed linens, bedpans, drinking glasses or eating utensils. Vectors are flies, mosquitoes or other insects capable of harboring and spreading the infectious agent.

air-borne i., infection by agents transmitted through the air.

cross i., infection transmitted between patients infected with different pathogenic microorganisms.

droplet i., infection by microorganisms present in droplets of sputum expelled into the air during talking or by coughing or sneezing.

dust-borne i., infection by agents that have become affixed to particles of dust and are transmitted by that means.

ectogenous i., infection due to organisms that have gained entrance to the body from outside, as through surgical or accidental wounds, or a natural orifice.

endogenous i., a morbid state produced by organisms normally present in the body.

focal i., the presence of microorganisms in circumscribed colonies, but causing general symptoms.

germinal i., transmission of infection to the child by means of the ovum or sperm of the parent.

latent i., persistence in the body of microorganisms that have ceased to multiply.

mixed i., infection with more than one kind of organism at the same time.

secondary i., infection by a bacterium following an infection by a bacterium of another kind.

septic i., septicemia.

terminal i., an acute infection occurring near the end of a disease and causing death.

water-borne i., infection by microorganisms transmitted in water.

infectious (in-fek'shus) liable to be communicated by infection.

i. disease, one caused by some parasitic organism and transmitted from one person to another by transfer of the organism (see also COMMUNICABLE DISEASE).

infective (in-fek'tiv) of the nature of an infection; infectious.

inferior (in-fēr'e-or) situated below, or directed downward; in official anatomic nomenclature, used in reference to the lower surface of an organ or other structure.

infertility (in″fer-til'ĭ-te) absence of ability to produce offspring. adj., **infer'tile.**

infestation (in″fes-ta'shun) invasion of the body by arthropods, including insects, mites and ticks.

infiltrate (in-fil'trāt) 1. to penetrate the interstices of a tissue or substance. 2. material deposited by infiltration.

infiltration (in″fil-tra'shun) the deposit or diffusion in tissue of substances not normal to it.

adipose i., fatty infiltration.

calcareous i., deposit of lime and earthy salts in the tissues.

cellular i., infiltration of tissues with round cells.

fatty i., the abnormal accumulation of fat within healthy cells as the result of a systemic metabolic derangement.

urinous i., the extravasation of urine into a tissue.

waxy i., deposition of amyloid.

infirmary (in-fir'mah-re) a place for the care of ill patients.

inflammation (in″flah-ma'shun) a tissue response to injury or destruction of the cells. adj., **inflam'matory.** The injury may be caused by a physical blow, or by exposure to an excessive amount of radiation from sunlight, x-rays or an ultraviolet lamp; or it may be caused by corrosive chemicals, burns, extreme heat or cold or foreign objects. Inflammation is also the usual response to a bacterial infection.

The physiologic changes that take place during the inflammatory process include vascular dilatation, leukocytosis and fluid exudation. The vascular changes occur at the site of the injury to the tissues. There is automatic dilatation of the capillaries and arterioles so that a greater supply of blood is brought to the area. The speed of circulation is decreased with the result that leukocytes leave the blood vessels and enter the tissue spaces. The vascular changes are responsible for the redness that accompanies inflammation.

Leukocytosis means an increase in the number of white blood cells. The injured tissues release chemicals that attract these leukocytes to the site of injury. There they ingest, or surround and destroy, the cause of the inflammation.

Body fluids also collect at the site. This increase of fluids is called exudation. The exudate brings immune bodies (antibodies) and special enzymes, and also helps in the removal of dead bacteria, destroyed tissue cells and blood cells.

The four classic symptoms of inflammation are redness (rubor), swelling (tumor), heat (calor), and pain (dolor). Loss of function of the part may also occur.

TREATMENT. Treatment of inflammation depends on the cause. Heat can sometimes be applied to an inflammation to promote the circulation of blood through the area. On the other hand application of cold initially may reduce swelling and thus reduce pain. If the inflammation results from a wound, the wound should be cleaned and painted with a mild antiseptic.

The treatment of advanced or widespread conditions of inflammation is intended to destroy the bacteria, increase the patient's resistance to any possible infection and eliminate from the body any toxins formed by the bacteria. Treatment therefore consists of medicines such as the sulfonamides and antibiotics, vitamins to help increase the patient's resistance to infection and antitoxins to help eliminate any toxins. Surgery may be required to remove foreign bodies, drain pus and otherwise promote healing.

acute i., a tissue response usually of sudden onset and accompanied by the cardinal signs of heat, redness, swelling, pain and loss of function.

catarrhal i., a condition characterized by outpouring of large amounts of mucinous secretion, occurring only in tissues capable of secreting mucus.

chronic i., prolonged and persistent inflammation.

exudative i., a tissue response ordinarily of short duration, characterized by vascular congestion and exudation of fluids and leukocytes.

fibrinous i., a tissue response characterized by outpouring of large amounts of fibrinogen and precipitation of masses of fibrin.

granulomatous i., a tissue response, usually chronic, attended by formation of granulomas.

interstitial i., inflammation affecting primarily the materials between the essential structural elements.

parenchymatous i., inflammation affecting chiefly the essential structural elements.

productive i., one attended by a new growth of connective tissue.

pseudomembranous i., a response characterized by formation on a mucosal surface of a false membrane composed of precipitated fibrin, necrotic epithelium and inflammatory leukocytes.

reactive i., one occurring around a foreign body or a focus of degeneration.

serous i., inflammation marked by outpouring of watery, low-protein fluid derived from blood serum or secretions of serosal mesothelial cells.

simple i., one without pus or other specific inflammatory product.

specific i., one due to a particular microorganism.

subacute i., a condition intermediate between chronic and acute inflammation, exhibiting some of the characteristics of each.

suppurative i., that characterized by production of large amounts of pus or purulent exudate.

toxic i., one due to a poison.

traumatic i., one that follows a wound or injury.

ulcerative i., that in which necrosis on or near the surface leads to loss of tissue and creation of a local defect (ulcer).

inflation (in-fla′shun) distention with air, gas or fluid.

influenza (in″floo-en′zah) an acute infectious epidemic disease caused by a filterable virus. adj., **influen′zal.** Four main types of the virus have been recognized, arbitrarily labeled by researchers as types A, B, C and D, and sometimes subdivided, as into A_1 and A_2. The A_2 virus is a comparatively new strain that first emerged in 1957. The disease it produces is often called Asian flu.

SYMPTOMS. Influenza has a brief incubation period. The symptoms appear suddenly and though the virus enters the respiratory tract it soon affects the entire body. The symptoms include fever, chills, headache, sore throat, cough, gastrointestinal disturbances, muscular pain and neuralgia.

TREATMENT. There is no drug that will cure influenza. An antibiotic may be prescribed to ward off complications of secondary bacterial infections such as pneumonia and bronchitis. Bed rest, increasing the intake of fluids, and aspirin to relieve aches and discomfort and help control fever are prescribed.

PREVENTION. A vaccine is available, although it does not always provide complete immunity against all forms of influenza viruses that may be present. The vaccine is strongly advised for people over 65, pregnant women and all who have chronic heart, lung or kidney disease. Other precautions include avoiding contact with others who have influenza, avoiding crowded places when there is a local epidemic and observing good personal hygiene to increase the body's resistance.

infra-axillary (in″frah-ak′sĭ-ler″e) below the axilla.

infraclavicular (in″frah-klah-vik′u-lar) below the clavicle.

infracostal (in″frah-kos′tal) below a rib.

infrahyoid (in″frah-hi′oid) below the hyoid bone.

inframaxillary (in″frah-mak′sĭ-ler″e) below the jaw.

infranuclear (in″frah-nu′kle-ar) below the nucleus.

infraorbital (in″frah-or′bĭ-tal) beneath the orbit.

infrapatellar (in″frah-pah-tel′ar) beneath the patella.

infrapsychic (in″frah-si′kik) below the psychic level; automatic.

infrared (in″frah-red′) beyond the red end of the visible spectrum.

i. rays, a form of electromagnetic radiation beyond the red end of the visible spectrum and therefore not visible to man. They are capable of penetrating body tissues to a depth of 10 mm. Sources of infrared rays include heat lamps, hot water bottles, steam radiators and incandescent light bulbs.

Infrared rays are used therapeutically to promote muscle relaxation, to speed up the inflammatory process and to increase circulation to a part of the body. (See also HEAT.)

infrascapular (in″frah-skap′u-lar) beneath the scapula.

infrasonic (in″frah-son′ik) below the frequency range of the waves normally perceived as sound by the human ear.

infraspinous (in″frah-spi′nus) beneath the spine of the scapula.

infrasternal (in″frah-ster′nal) beneath the sternum.

infraversion (in″frah-ver′zhun) 1. downward deviation of the eye. 2. shortness of a tooth in relation to the place of occlusion.

infundibuliform (in″fun-dib′u-lĭ-form) shaped like a funnel.

infundibulum (in″fun-dib′u-lum), pl. *infundib′-ula* [L.] any funnel-shaped passage, in particular the conus arteriosus, the anterosuperior portion of the right ventricle of the heart. adj., **infundib′ular.**
 ethmoidal i., 1. a passage connecting the nasal cavity with the anterior ethmoidal cells and frontal sinus. 2. a sinuous passage connecting the middle meatus of the nose with the anterior ethmoidal cells and often with the frontal sinus.
 i. of hypothalamus, a hollow, funnel-shaped mass in the brain, extending to the posterior lobe of the pituitary gland.
 i. of uterine tube, the distal, funnel-shaped portion of the uterine tube.

infusion (in-fu′zhun) 1. steeping of a substance in water to obtain its soluble principles. 2. a solution obtained by steeping a substance in water. 3. the introduction of a solution into a vein by gravity. (See also INTRAVENOUS INFUSION.) Note—An *infusion* flows in by gravity, an *injection* is forced in by a syringe, an *instillation* is dropped in, an *insufflation* is blown in and an *infection* slips in unnoticed.

ingesta (in-jes′tah) material taken into the body by mouth.

ingestant (in-jes′tant) a substance that is or may be taken into the body by mouth or through the digestive system.

ingestion (in-jes′chun) the taking of nutrient material into the digestive tract of the body.

ingravescent (in″grah-ves′ent) gradually becoming more severe.

ingrown nail (in′grōn) overlapping of the anterior corners of a nail by the flesh of the digit, causing pain, inflammation and possible infection. The condition occurs most frequently in the great toe, and is often caused by pressure from tight-fitting shoes. Another common cause is improper cutting of the toenails, which should be cut straight across or with a curved toenail scissors so that the sides are a little longer than the middle.

inguen (ing′gwen), pl. *in′guina* [L.] the groin.

inguinal (ing′gwĭ-nal) pertaining to the groin.
 i. hernia, hernia occurring in the groin; protrusion of intestine or omentum, or both, either directly through a weak point in the abdominal wall (direct inguinal hernia) or downward into the inguinal canal (indirect inguinal hernia). (See also HERNIA.)

INH trademark for preparations of isoniazid, used in treatment of tuberculosis.

inhalant (in-ha′lant) a gaseous substance that is or may be taken into the body by way of the nose and trachea (through the respiratory system).

inhalation (in″hah-la′shun) the drawing of air or other vapor into the lungs.

inhaler (in-ha′ler) an instrument for administering a medicated vapor.

inheritance (in-her′ĭ-tans) 1. the acquisition of characters or qualities by transmission from parent to offspring. 2. that which is transmitted from parent to offspring.
 criss-cross i., inheritance by offspring of characters from the parent of the opposite sex.
 holandric i., inheritance by all the males, but not by the females.
 maternal i., the transmission of characters that are dependent on peculiarities of the egg cytoplasm produced, in turn, by nuclear genes.
 monofactorial i., the acquisition of a characteristic or quality whose transmission depends on a single gene.
 multifactorial i., the acquisition of a characteristic or quality whose manifestation is subject to modification by a number of genes.

inhibition (in″ĭ-bish′un, in″hĭ-bish′un) the imposition of restraint or arrest of a process.
 competetive i., prevention of the action of an effector substance or agent by another substance or agent that enters into combination with the element on which the effector substance acts or which is essential to its action.

inhibitor (in-hib′ĭ-tor) a substance or agent that depresses the activity of another substance or agent, particularly a substance that checks the action of an enzyme or a tissue organizer, or the growth of microorganisms.

inion (in′e-on) the external occipital protuberance.

iniopagus (in″e-op′ah-gus) a twin monster joined at the occiput.

initis (ĭ-ni′tis) inflammation of muscular substance.

injected (in-jek′ted) 1. filled by injection. 2. congested.

injection (in-jek′shun) 1. introduction of a fluid substance into the body, usually by means of a syringe or other device connected to a hollow needle. 2. the solution so administered.
 Immunizing substances, or inoculations, are generally given by injection. When a patient is unconscious, injection may be the only means of administering medication, and in some cases nourishment. Some medicines cannot be given by mouth because chemical action of the digestive juices would change or reduce their effectiveness,

or because they would be removed from the body too quickly to have any effect. Certain potent medicines must be injected because they would irritate body tissues if administered any other way. Occasionally a medication is injected so that it will act more quickly.

In addition to the most common types of injections described below, injections are sometimes made into arteries, bone marrow, the spine, the sternum, the pleural space of the chest region, the peritoneal cavity and the joint spaces. In sudden heart failure, heart-stimulating drugs may be injected directly into the heart (intracardiac injection).

NURSING CARE. When drawing the drug to be administered into the syringe, the tip, plunger and inside of the barrel of the syringe must not be contaminated. The shaft of the needle should be covered with a plastic cover to avoid contamination after the drug has been drawn into the syringe. The site of injection is cleansed with an antiseptic. After the needle is inserted, the plunger is drawn back; if blood returns in the syringe in an intramuscular or subcutaneous injection, the needle is in a blood vessel and must be withdrawn and inserted in another site.

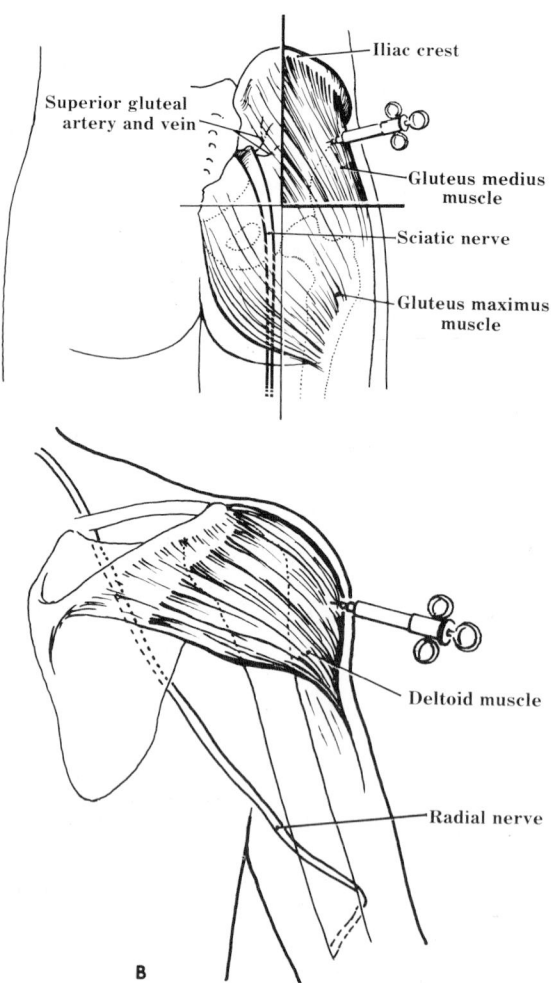

Intramuscular injection.

hypodermic i., subcutaneous injection.

intracutaneous i., intradermal i., injection of small amounts of material into the substance of the skin. This method is used in diagnostic procedures and in administration of regional anesthetics, as well as in treatment procedures. In certain allergy tests the allergen is injected intradermally. These injections are given in an area where the skin and hair are sparse, usually on the inner part of the forearm. A 25-gauge needle, 3/8 or 1/2 inch long, is recommended. The needle is inserted at a 10- to 15-degree angle to the skin.

intramuscular i., injection into the substance of the muscles, usually those of the upper arm, thigh or buttock. Intramuscular injections are given when the substance is to be absorbed quickly. They should be given with extreme care, especially in the buttock, because the sciatic nerve may be injured or a large blood vessel may be entered if the injection is not made correctly into the upper, outer quadrant of the buttock. The deltoid muscle at the shoulder is also used, but less commonly than the gluteus muscle of the buttock; care must be taken to insert the needle in the center, 2 cm. below the acromion.

The needle should be at least 1½ inches long so that the liquid is injected deep into the muscle tissue. The gauge of the needle depends on the viscosity of the fluid being injected. As a general rule, not more than 5 ml. is given in an intramuscular injection. The needle is inserted at a 90-degree angle to the skin. When the gluteus maximus muscle is the site chosen for the injection, the patient should be in a prone position with the toes turned in if possible. This position relaxes the muscle and makes the injection less painful.

intravenous i., an injection made into a vein. Intravenous injections are used when rapid absorption is called for, when fluid cannot be taken by mouth or when the substance to be administered is too irritating to be injected into the skin or muscles. In certain diagnostic tests and x-ray examinations a drug or dye may be administered intravenously. Blood transfusions also are given by this route. (See also INTRAVENOUS INFUSION.)

The needle used is usually 20 or 22 gauge, about 1½ inches long. Extreme care must be taken not to give an overdose in the injection; any medication or dye given by vein acts very rapidly, and there is little time for emergency procedures in case of error.

subcutaneous i., injection made into the subcutaneous tissues. Although usually fluid medications are injected, occasionally solid materials, such as steroid hormones, are administered subcutaneously in small, slowly absorbed pellets to prolong their effect. Subcutaneous injections may be given wherever there is subcutaneous tissue, usually in the upper, outer arm or thigh. A 25-gauge needle 3/4 inch long is usually used, and the amount injected should not exceed 2 ml. The needle is held at a 45-degree angle to the skin.

injury (in'jur-e) a specific impairment of body structure or function caused by an outside agent or force, which may be physical, chemical or psychic.

inlay (in'la) 1. a graft that is inserted into the substance of an organ or other body structure. 2. in dentistry, a filling first made to correspond with the form of a dental cavity and then cemented into the cavity.

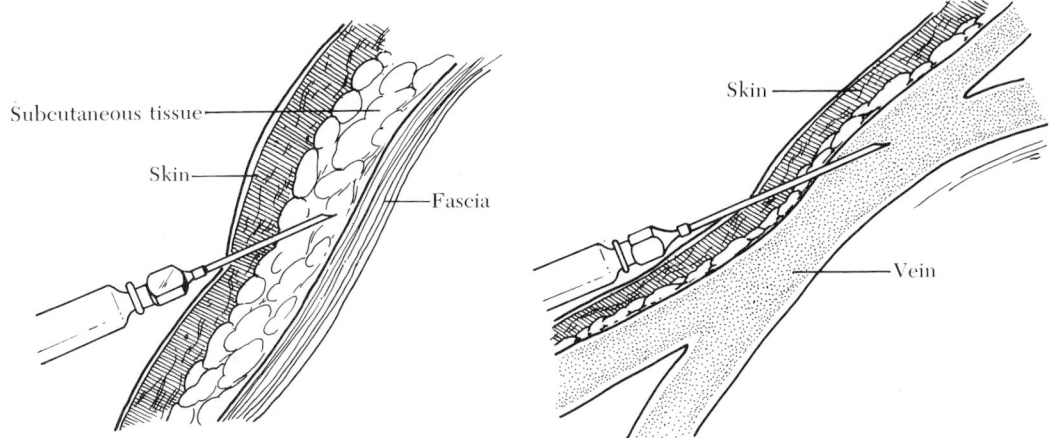

Left: subcutaneous, or hypodermic, injection, in which fluid medicines are introduced into the body through a hypodermic needle that pierces only the skin and the tissue beneath it. Right: intravenous injection, in which the needle is inserted into a vein. Only occasionally are injections made into arteries.

inlet (in'let) a means or route of entrance.
  pelvic i., the upper limit of the pelvic cavity.

innate (ĭ-nāt', in'āt) inborn; hereditary; congenital.

innervation (in"er-va'shun) the distribution or supply of nerves to a part.

innidiation (ĭ-nid"e-a'shun) development of cells in a part to which they have been carried.

innocent (in'o-sent) not harmful or malignant.

innocuous (ĭ-nok'u-us) not hurtful.

innominate (ĭ-nom'ĭ-nāt) nameless or unnamed.
  i. artery, brachiocephalic trunk, the first branch of the arch of the aorta.
  i. bone, the hip bone.
  i. veins, the brachiocephalic veins, which unite to form the superior vena cava.

inochondritis (in"o-kon-dri'tis) inflammation of a fibrocartilage.

inochondroma (in"o-kon-dro'mah) fibrochondroma; chondroma containing fibrous elements.

inoculability (ĭ-nok"u-lah-bil'ĭ-te) the state of being inoculable.

inoculable (ĭ-nok'u-lah-bl) 1. transmissible by inoculation. 2. not immune against a transmissible disease.

inoculation (ĭ-nok"u-la'shun) 1. introduction of pathogenic microorganisms into the body to stimulate the production of antibodies and immunity. 2. introduction of infectious material into culture medium in an effort to produce growth of the causative organism.

inoculum (ĭ-nok'u-lum) material used in inoculation.

inocystoma (in"o-sis-to'mah) a fibrous tumor with cystic degeneration.

inocyte (in'o-sīt) a cell of fibrous tissue.

inogenesis (in"o-jen'ĕ-sis) the formation of fibrous tissue.

inogenous (in-oj'ĕ-nus) produced from or forming tissue.

inoperable (in-op'er-ah-bl) not susceptible of being cured by surgery.

inorganic (in"or-gan'ik) 1. having no organs. 2. not of organic origin.
  i. acid, an acid containing no carbon atoms.
  i. chemistry, that branch of chemistry which deals with compounds that do not contain carbon.

inosclerosis (in"o-sklĕ-ro'sis) fibrous induration.

inosemia (in"o-se'me-ah) excess of fibrin in the blood.

inosinic acid (in"o-sin'ik) the parent compound of all purines.

inositol (in-o'sĭ-tol) a compound found in many plants, microorganisms and animal tissues, capable of facilitating removal of fats from the liver; it is a vitamin of the B complex.

inosituria (in"o-si-tu're-ah) inositol in the urine.

inotropic (in'o-trop"ik) affecting the force of muscular contractions.

in ovo (in o'vo) [L.] in the egg, especially in a chick embryo.

inquest (in'kwest) inquiry before a coroner into the manner of a death.

insalubrious (in"sah-lu'bre-us) injurious to health.

insane (in-sān) mentally deranged.

insanity (in-san'ĭ-te) severe mental disorder that may make a person irresponsible, unreasonable and unable to function normally in society. His thoughts and actions are distinctly different from accepted patterns of behavior.
  The term is a legal rather than a medical one, and includes different kinds of mental illness, such as SCHIZOPHRENIA and affective PSYCHOSIS. A person who is judged insane by a court is not held legally responsible for his actions and may have to be institutionalized.

inscriptio (in-skrip'she-o), pl. *inscriptio'nes* [L.] inscription.
   i. tendin'ea, a fibrous band traversing the belly of a muscle and dividing it into two parts.

inscription (in-skrip'shun) a writing, mark or line; that part of a prescription giving the name, size or strength, and quantity of the agent, or the name and amount of each of the ingredients to be combined.

insect (in'sekt) an individual of the class Insecta.
   i. bites and stings, injuries caused by the mouth parts and venom of insects and of certain related creatures, known as arachnids—spiders, scorpions, ticks—but popularly classified with insects. Bites and stings can be the cause of much discomfort. Usually there is no real danger although a local infection can develop from scratching. Some insects, however, establish themselves on the skin as parasites, others inject poison and still others transmit disease. A knowledge of first-aid measures for bites and stings can do much to relieve discomfort, to prevent infection and, in some cases, even to save a life.

FIRST AID FOR INSECT BITES AND STINGS
   Stings of Bees, Wasps, Hornets, Yellow Jackets
   1. For bee sting, scrape stinger out with fingernail or remove with tweezers, holding tweezers flat against skin to avoid squeezing more venom into wound.
   2. To relieve itching, apply (a) paste of sodium bicarbonate (baking soda) and water, or (b) compress moistened with ammonia water, or (c) calamine lotion.
   In Case of Allergic Reaction to Bee or Wasp Stings
   1. Call a physician immediately.
   2. If the sting is on a limb, apply a constricting bandage above the sting as follows: Use a wide, strong piece of cloth; tie a half knot; place a stick over it and tie a full knot.
   3. Twist the stick to tighten the bandage but do not make it so tight that it causes a throbbing sensation.
   4. Loosen for 1 minute every 10 minutes.
   5. Apply ice or cold compresses.
   6. Remove stinger.
   7. Do not give the person alcohol or allow him to walk to the doctor or to the hospital.
   Chigger Bites
   1. If exposed to chiggers, wash body with soap and water as soon as possible.
   2. Apply denatured alcohol or sulfur ointment to the skin.
   3. Apply ice water, or bathe affected parts with a solution of sodium bicarbonate (baking soda) and water, ammonia water or an alcohol solution, to relieve skin irritation.
   Ticks
   1. To remove ticks, dab kerosene, gasoline or some kind of oil on skin where ticks are embedded. If ticks do not drop off in half an hour, remove them carefully with tweezers or in some other way, being careful not to use bare hands.
   2. Wash the bite and paint with antiseptic.
   Stings of Poisonous Scorpions, Spiders, Centipedes
   1. Call a physician immediately.
   2. Have patient lie down.
   3. If sting is on a limb, apply a constricting ban-

dage above the sting as follows: Use a wide, strong piece of cloth; tie a half knot; place a stick over it and tie a full knot.
   4. Twist the stick to tighten the bandage but do not make it so tight that it causes a throbbing sensation.
   5. Loosen for 1 minute every 10 minutes.
   6. Apply ice to the sting.
   7. Do not give the person alcohol or allow him to walk to the doctor or to the hospital.

Insecta (in-sek'tah) a class of animals (phylum Arthropoda) characterized by division of the body into three distinct regions: head, thorax and abdomen.

insecticide (in-sek'tĭ-sīd) an agent that kills insects.

Insectivora (in"sek-tiv'o-rah) an order of small, terrestrial and nocturnal mammals that feed on insects.

insectivore (in-sek'tĭ-vōr) an individual of the order Insectivora.

insemination (in-sem"ĭ-na'shun) introduction of sperm into the female reproductive tract for the purpose of fertilization.
   artificial i., instrumental introduction of semen into the female genital tract.

insenescence (in"sĕ-nes'ens) the process of growing old.

insensible (in-sen'sĭ-bl) 1. devoid of sensibility or consciousness. 2. not perceptible to the senses.

insertion (in-ser'shun) attachment, as the site of attachment of a skeletal muscle on the bone that is moved when the muscle contracts.
   velamentous i., attachment of the umbilical cord to the fetal membranes.

insidious (in-sid'e-us) coming on in a stealthy manner.

insight (in'sīt) in psychiatry, recognition of the abnormality of one's own emotional reactions or motives.

in situ (in si'tu) [L.] in its normal place; confined to the site of origin.

insoluble (in-sol'u-bl) not susceptible of being dissolved.

insomnia (in-som'ne-ah) sleeplessness; an inability to fall asleep easily or to remain asleep throughout the night. The frequency of persistent insomnia is high.
   The causes of insomnia may be physical or psychologic or, most often, a combination of both. Some persons are more sensitive to conditions around them than others, and may be kept awake by slight noises, light or sharing their bed. Beverages that contain caffeine, such as coffee, tea and cola drinks, keep some people awake. A heavy meal shortly before bedtime may prevent sleep. Drinking large quantities of fluids may cause an uncomfortable feeling of distention of the bladder.
   The type of bedding may be a cause of insomnia. Changing to a firmer or softer mattress, doing without a pillow or making other changes in the bedding may help. Those who are bothered by the weight of blankets may sleep better under lightweight blankets, or with a device that supports the bedclothes at the foot of the bed.

Personal problems and worries about job, finances or family matters may cause wakefulness, and the inability to sleep disappears when the problems are solved. More difficult to deal with are the deeper psychologic problems such as anxiety, irrational fears and tensions or frequent nightmares that produce resistance to sleep.

insorption (in-sorp'shun) movement of a substance into the blood, especially from the gastrointestinal tract into the circulating blood.

inspection (in-spek'shun) visual examination for detection of features or qualities perceptible to the eye.

inspersion (in-sper'zhun) sprinkling, as with powder.

inspiration (in"spī-ra'shun) the drawing of air into the lungs. adj., **inspi'ratory.**

inspissated (in-spis'āt-ed) thickened; made less fluid.

instability (in"stah-bil'ĭ-te) the quality of being unsteady or changeable.

   emotional i., the quality of being too changeable in feeling tone.

instillation (in"stĭ-la'shun) the dropping of liquid into a cavity, as into the eye.

instinct (in'stinkt) an innate tendency to a certain action or mode of behavior. adj., **instinc'tive.**

   death i., an unconscious drive toward dissolution and death.

   herd i., the tendency to adopt the standards of thought and action of a group.

instrumentarium (in"stroo-men-ta're-um) the equipment or instruments required for any particular operation or purpose; the physical adjuncts with which a physician combats disease.

insufficiency (in"sŭ-fish'en-se) inability to perform properly an allotted function.

   aortic i., inadequacy of the aortic valve, permitting blood to flow back into the left ventricle of the heart.

   cardiac i., inability of the heart to perform its function properly.

   coronary i., decrease in flow of blood through the coronary blood vessels.

   ileocecal i., inability of the ileocecal valve to prevent backflow of contents from the cecum into the ileum.

   pulmonary i., 1. insufficiency of the pulmonary valve. 2. inability of the lungs to allow for adequate gas exchange, marked by hypoxia and hypercapnia.

   valvular i., failure of a cardiac valve to close perfectly, so that blood passes back through the orifice; named, according to the valve affected, aortic, mitral, pulmonary or tricuspid.

insufflation (in"sŭ-fla'shun) the blowing of a powder, vapor or gas into a cavity.

   perirenal i., injection of air around the kidney for roentgen examination of the adrenal glands.

   tubal i., insufflation of air or gas through the uterus into the uterine tubes as a test of their patency.

insufflator (in'sŭ-fla"tor) an instrument for blowing gas or powder into a cavity.

insula (in'su-lah), pl. *in'sulae* [L.] a triangular area of the cerebral cortex that forms the floor of the lateral cerebral fossa.

insulation (in"sŭ-la'shun) 1. the surrounding of a space or body with material designed to prevent the entrance or escape of radiant energy. 2. interposition of a nonconductor to prevent the communication of electricity to other bodies.

insulin (in'su-lin) the active antidiabetic principle secreted by the islands of Langerhans, in the pancreas. This hormone regulates the rate at which the body utilizes carbohydrates; various preparations of it are used in the treatment of DIABETES MELLITUS.

Types of insulin vary in the rapidity of action and the duration of effectiveness. Regular insulin is effective almost immediately after injection and reaches its peak of action within 2 hours. It is used most often in diabetic emergencies and in regulating dosage for a patient when diabetes is first diagnosed. Crystalline insulin is made of zinc-insulin crystals and is usually given to patients who are allergic to regular insulin. Other types of insulin developed in recent years contain substances that prolong the action of insulin. Protamine zinc insulin (PZI), isophane insulin (NPH), globin zinc insulin and insulin lente are examples of long-acting preparations of insulin.

ADMINISTRATION OF INSULIN. Protamine zinc, isophane and lente insulin are all cloudy and milky in appearance and must be thoroughly mixed by gently rolling the bottle between the palms before the drug is withdrawn from the ampule. Vigorous shaking is avoided because it produces air bubbles that may alter the dosage measured in the syringe.

Insulin is measured in units, and is available in varying strengths, for example, U40, U80 and

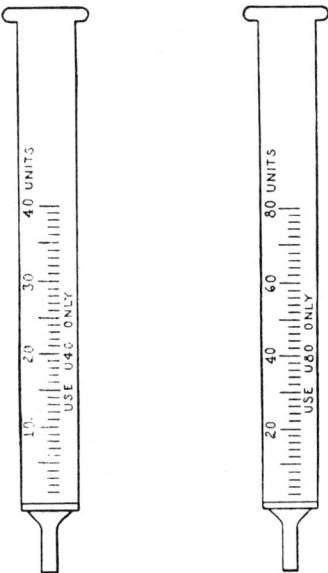

Insulin syringes. The markings on the U40 syringe are red, and on the U80, green. (From Wilder, R. M.: A Primer for Diabetic Patients. 9th ed. Philadelphia, W. B. Saunders Co., 1950.)

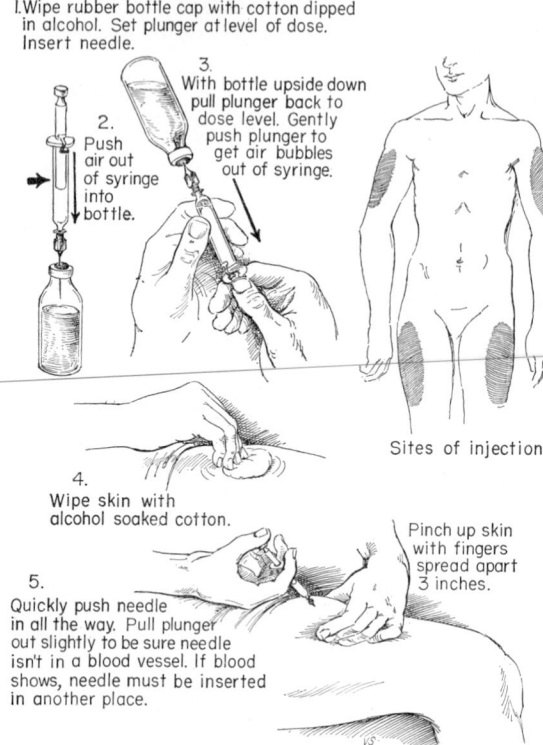

1. Wipe rubber bottle cap with cotton dipped in alcohol. Set plunger at level of dose. Insert needle.

2. Push air out of syringe into bottle.

3. With bottle upside down pull plunger back to dose level. Gently push plunger to get air bubbles out of syringe.

Sites of injection

4. Wipe skin with alcohol soaked cotton.

Pinch up skin with fingers spread apart 3 inches.

5. Quickly push needle in all the way. Pull plunger out slightly to be sure needle isn't in a blood vessel. If blood shows, needle must be inserted in another place.

Injection of insulin. (From Dowling, H. F., and Jones, T.: That the Patient May Know. Philadelphia, W. B. Saunders Co., 1959.)

U100. The term U40 means that there are 40 units per milliliter of insulin. When measuring the drug in an insulin syringe one must *be careful to use the calibrations on the syringe that correspond with the strength of insulin being used.* If the insulin is marked U80, then the measurements on the syringe must be for U80 insulin. Some insulin syringes have calibrations for U40 insulin on one side and for U80 insulin on the other. Others have calibrations for U40 or U80 or U100 only.

Insulin is injected deep into the subcutaneous tissue of the upper arm or thigh. Because of the frequency with which the injections are given, the sites should be rotated to avoid the formation of excessive amounts of scar tissue and to provide ample time for healing before the site is used again. The anterior surface of the abdomen may also be used as a site of injection.

HYPOGLYCEMIA and INSULIN SHOCK result when the level of insulin in the body is too high, because of overdose, failure to eat a full meal at the expected time, more than the usual amount of exercise, an emotional or physical upset or some change in the body chemistry, as in infection, surgical operation, etc.

i. shock, a condition of circulatory insufficiency caused by an overdose of insulin or decreased food intake with the usual dose. Insulin shock is an ever present danger against which those who take insulin for diabetes mellitus must learn to protect themselves.

SYMPTOMS. The first reaction to an overdose of insulin is usually tremors, cold sweating and ex-treme hunger. The symptoms may differ in some cases, and can include nausea, dizziness, headache and marked drowsiness. If the urine is tested at this time, it will show no sugar or a trace at most. The blood sugar content likewise is drastically lowered. The patient suddenly becomes weaker and has a quickened pulse and perhaps muscular spasms, such emotional reactions as excessive laughing or crying and convulsions.

The ultimate stage of insulin shock is unconsciousness. This is a serious emergency requiring the services of a physician. Death seldom occurs, but an undue delay can result in permanent harm.

In the past, insulin shock, produced intentionally, was sometimes used in treatment of schizophrenia.

TREATMENT. Insulin shock occurs most often when meals are delayed or irregular, and sometimes after unusual physical exertion. Diabetics should recognize the symptoms of insulin shock and immediately take some form of sugar at the first sign of such an attack, either sugar by the lump or spoonful, or a glass of orange juice with sugar added. (See also DIABETES MELLITUS.)

First Aid for Insulin Shock

1. If the person is conscious, immediately give him sugar or a food rich in sugar, such as candy or orange juice.

2. If the patient is semiconscious or unconscious, don't force food or liquid. Call a physician, or take the patient to a hospital.

insulinemia (in″su-lin-e′me-ah) insulin in the blood.

insulinogenic (in″su-lin″o-jen′ik) caused by insulin.

insulinoid (in′su-lin-oid″) resembling insulin.

insulitis (in″su-li′tis) cellular infiltration of the islands of Langerhans, possibly in response to invasion by an infectious agent.

insuloma (in″su-lo′mah) adenoma of the islands of Langerhans of the pancreas.

insulopathic (in″su-lo-path′ik) pertaining to abnormal insulin secretion.

insusceptibility (in″su-sep″ti-bil′i-te) the state of being unaffected or uninfluenced.

intake (in′tāk) substance taken into the body by ingestion or parenterally, usually expressed quantitatively, as the amount of fluid or caloric intake.

integration (in″tĕ-gra′shun) assimilation into a common body or activity to achieve a common purpose.

biological i., the acquisition of functional coordination during embryonic development through humoral and nervous influences.

DIFFERENCES BETWEEN INSULIN SHOCK AND DIABETIC ACIDOSIS

	INSULIN SHOCK	DIABETIC ACIDOSIS
Cause	Too much insulin	Too little insulin
Symptoms		
Onset	Sudden	Gradual
Breathing	Shallow	Noisy and deep
Skin	Moist	Dry
Hunger, thirst	Extreme hunger	Extreme thirst
Urine	Little or no sugar	Much sugar
Treatment	Sugar is eaten	Insulin is injected

primary i., recognition by a child that his body is a unit apart from the environment.

secondary i., sublimation of the separate elements of the early sexual instinct into the mature psychosexual personality.

integument (in-teg′u-ment) the natural covering of the body; the skin. adj., **integumen′tary.**

integumentum (in-teg″u-men′tum) [L.] integument.

in tela (in te′lah) [L.] in tissue; relating especially to stained histologic preparations.

intellect (in′tĕ-lekt) the mind, thinking faculty or understanding.

intelligence (in-tel′ĭ-jens) a general term for the practical functioning of the mind. It is basically a combination of reasoning, memory, imagination and judgment. Each of these faculties relies upon the others.

The brain may store up many memories, but they are useful only when brought to surface consciousness at the right time and in the right connection. Imagination is the faculty of associating several memories—they may be of facts, images or sensations—to produce another fact or image. In general, the more efficiently the brain combines memories in an orderly fashion, the greater the intelligence. Imagination, however, must be governed by reason and judgment. Reason is the ability to draw logical conclusions by relating memories and observations. Judgment relies on experience to choose between different forms of reasoning. All these factors are controlled by the cerebral cortex (see also BRAIN).

In speaking of general intelligence, authorities often distinguish between a number of different kinds of basic mental ability. One of these is verbal aptitude, the ability to understand the meaning of words and to use them effectively in writing or speaking. Another is skill with numbers, the ability to add, subtract, multiply and divide and to use these skills in problems. The capacity to work with spatial relationships, that is, with visualizing how objects take up space, is still another (for example, how two triangles can fit together to make a square). Perception, memory and reasoning may also be considered different basic abilities. Often a person is more proficient in some of these areas than he is in others. Commonly, for example, a child may excel in using words but have some difficulty with arithmetic, or the opposite may be true.

In the United States, schoolgirls often achieve verbal skills more quickly than boys, while boys are often more skillful in spatial relations and number work. As a person grows older and as his interests and needs develop and change, his aptitudes may change as well.

These abilities are the ones that are usually examined by intelligence tests. There are others, however, that may be as important or more important. Determination and perseverance make intelligence effective and useful. Artistic talent, such as proficiency in art or music, and creativity, the ability to use thought and imagination to produce original ideas, are difficult to measure but are certainly part of intelligence.

i. quotient, I.Q., a numerical expression of intellectual capacity obtained by multiplying the mental age of the subject, ascertained by testing, by 100 and dividing by his chronologic age.

intensimeter (in″ten-sim′ĕ-ter) a device for measuring intensity of roentgen rays.

intention (in-ten′shun) the union of the edges of a wound in HEALING.

inter- (in′ter) word element [L.], *between.*

interarticular (in″ter-ar-tik′u-lar) between articulating surfaces.

interatrial (in″ter-a′tre-al) between the atria of the heart.

interbrain (in′ter-brān) diencephalon.

intercadence (in″ter-ka′dens) occurrence of an occasional extra beat between two pulse beats.

intercalary (in-ter′kah-ler″e) inserted between; interposed.

intercellular (in″ter-sel′u-lar) between the cells.

intercentral (in″ter-sen′tral) between, or connecting, nerve centers.

interchondral (in″ter-kon′dral) between cartilages.

intercilium (in″ter-sil′e-um) the space between the eyebrows.

interclavicular (in″ter-klah-vik′u-lar) between the clavicles.

intercondylar (in″ter-kon′dĭ-lar) between two condyles.

intercostal (in″ter-kos′tal) between two ribs.

intercostalis (in″ter-kos-ta′lis), pl. *intercosta′les* [L.] intercostal.

intercourse (in′ter-kōrs) interchange or communication between individuals.
  sexual i., coitus.

intercricothyrotomy (in″ter-kri″ko-thi-rot′o-me) incision of the larynx through the lower part of the fibroelastic membrane of the larynx (cricothyroid membrane); inferior laryngotomy.

intercurrent (in″ter-kur′ent) occurring during the course of, as a disease occurring during the course of an already existing disease.

interdigital (in″ter-dij′ĭ-tal) between two digits (fingers or toes).

interdigitation (in″ter-dij″ĭ-ta′shun) 1. an interlocking of parts by finger-like processes. 2. one of a set of finger-like processes.

interface (in′ter-fās) in chemistry, the surface of separation or boundary between two phases of a heterogeneous system.

interfascicular (in″ter-fah-sik′u-lar) between adjacent fascicles.

interfemoral (in″ter-fem′o-ral) between the thighs.

interferon (in″ter-fēr′on) a protein produced by interaction of animal cells and viruses that is capable of inhibiting virus multiplication.

interfibrillary (in″ter-fib′rĭ-lār″e) between fibrils.

interfilar (in″ter-fi′lar) between the fibrils of a reticulum.

interganglionic (in″ter-gang″gle-on′ik) between ganglia.

intergenic (in″ter-jen′ik) occurring between two genes.

interictal (in″ter-ik′tal) occurring between attacks or paroxysms.

interlobar (in″ter-lo′bar) between lobes.

interlobitis (in″ter-lo-bi′tis) inflammation of the pleura between lobes of the lung.

interlobular (in″ter-lob′u-lar) between lobules.

intermaxillary (in″ter-mak′sĭ-ler″e) between the maxillae.

intermedius (in″ter-me′de-us) [L.] intermediate.

intermeningeal (in″ter-mĕ-nin′je-al) between the meninges.

intermitotic (in″ter-mi-tot′ik) between successive mitoses.

intermural (in″ter-mu′ral) between the walls of an organ or organs.

intermuscular (in″ter-mus′ku-lar) between muscles.

intern (in′tern) a medical graduate serving and residing in a hospital preparatory to being licensed to practice medicine.

internal (in-ter′nal) situated or occurring within or on the inside.

internalization (in-ter″nal-ĭ-za′shun) a mental mechanism whereby certain external attributes, attitudes or standards are unconsciously taken within oneself.

internatal (in″ter-na′tal) between the nates, or buttocks.

interneuron (in″ter-nu′ron) a neuron between the primary afferent neuron and the final motor neuron.

internist (in-ter′nist) a specialist in diseases of the internal organs.

internship (in′tern-ship) the position of an intern in a hospital, or the term of service.

internuclear (in″ter-nu′kle-ar) between nuclei.

internuncial (in″ter-nun′shal) transmitting impulses between two different parts.

internus (in-ter′nus) [L.] internal.

interoceptive (in″ter-o-sep′tiv) receiving impulses from the viscera, or from the interior of the body.

interoceptor (in″ter-o-sep′tor) a sensory nerve terminal located in and transmitting impulses from the viscera.

interofective (in″ter-o-fek′tiv) affecting the interior of the organism—a term applied to the autonomic nervous system.

interogestate (in″ter-o-jes′tāt) 1. developing with-in the uterus. 2. an infant developing within the uterus or during the period of interior gestation.

interoinferiorly (in″ter-o-in-fēr′e-or-le) inwardly and downwardly.

interolivary (in″ter-ol′ĭ-ver″e) between the olivary bodies.

interorbital (in″ter-or′bĭ-tal) between the orbits.

interosseous (in″ter-os′e-us) between two bones.

interosseus (in″ter-os′e-us), pl. *interos′sei* [L.] an interosseous muscle.

interpalpebral (in″ter-pal′pĕ-bral) between the eyelids.

interparietal (in″ter-pah-ri′ĕ-tal) between the parietal bones.

interparoxysmal (in″ter-par″ok-siz′mal) between paroxysms.

interphalangeal (in″ter-fah-lan′je-al) situated between two contiguous phalanges.

interphase (in′ter-fāz) the stage in the life of a cell before it begins to divide mitotically, or between the first and second divisions in meiosis.

interplant (in′ter-plant) an embryonic part isolated by transference to an indifferent environment provided by another embryo.

interpolation (in-ter″po-la′shun) 1. surgical transplantation of tissue. 2. the determination of intermediate values in a series on the basis of observed values.

interproximal (in″ter-prok′sĭ-mal) between two adjoining surfaces.

interpubic (in″ter-pu′bik) between the pubic bones.

interpupillary (in″ter-pu′pĭ-ler″e) between the pupils.

interscapular (in″ter-skap′u-lar) between the scapulae.

intersex (in′ter-seks) 1. intersexuality. 2. an individual showing one or more contradictions of the morphologic criteria of sex.
  female i., one who has only female gonadal tissue and shows sex chromatin in the somatic cells.
  male i., one who has only male gonadal tissue and shows no sex chromatin in the somatic cells.
  true i., one who has both male and female gonadal tissue; the chromatin test may be either positive or negative in result.

intersexuality (in″ter-seks″u-al′ĭ-te) a blending of the characters of both sexes.

interspinalis (in″ter-spi-na′lis), pl. *interspina′les* [L.] between spines of the vertebrae.

interstice (in-ter′stis) an interval, space or gap in a tissue or structure.

interstitial (in″ter-stish′al) pertaining to or situated in the intervals in a tissue or structure.
  i. cell-stimulating hormone, luteinizing hormone.
  i. cells of testis, cells located in the seminiferous tubules that furnish the internal secretion of the testis; called also Leydig cells.

i. fluid, that portion of the body fluid outside the cells and plasma volume; the extracellular fluid minus the plasma volume.

intertransverse (in″ter-trans-vers′) situated between or connecting the transverse processes of the vertebrae.

intertrigo (in″ter-tri′go) a skin irritation caused by friction between two moist, adjacent skin surfaces. Symptoms include burning, itching, moistness, redness and cracking of the skin. The condition is frequently accompanied by bacterial or fungal infection. It is most likely to occur in obese persons, and particularly in those with diabetes mellitus. Intertrigo is most prevalent in hot and humid regions.

In treatment of intertrigo, the opposing body surfaces should be thoroughly cleansed and dried, and then sprinkled with talcum powder containing zinc oxide. Sometimes gauze strips between the adjacent skin surfaces will keep the area dry and exposed to air.

intertubular (in″ter-tu′bu-lar) between tubules.

interureteral, interureteric (in″ter-u-re′ter-al), (in″ter-u″re-ter′ik) between the ureters.

intervaginal (in″ter-vaj′ĭ-nal) between sheaths.

interval (in′ter-val) the space between two objects or parts; the lapse of time between two events.
cardioarterial i., the time between the apex beat and arterial pulsation.
lucid i., a period of full possession of the faculties between periods of mental disturbance.
postsphygmic i., the time between the beginning of dilation of the ventricles of the heart and the opening of the atrioventricular valves.
presphygmic i., the time between the beginning of contraction of the ventricles of the heart and the opening of the arterial valves.
QRST i., the ventricular complex of the ELECTRO-CARDIOGRAM.

intervalvular (in″ter-val′vu-lar) between valves.

intervascular (in″ter-vas′ku-lar) between blood vessels.

interventricular (in″ter-ven-trik′u-lar) between the ventricles of the heart.

intervertebral (in″ter-ver′tĕ-bral) between two vertebrae.
i. disk, the layer of fibrocartilage between the bodies of adjoining vertebrae (see also DISK).

intervillous (in″ter-vil′us) situated between or among villi.

intestinal (in-tes′tĭ-nal) pertaining to the intestine.
i. flu, a popular term for what may be any one of several disorders of the stomach and intestinal tract. The symptoms are nausea, diarrhea, abdominal cramps and fever.
During the acute stage all foods should be avoided. Carbonated soft drinks such as ginger ale or cola can be taken in moderation to relieve the nausea. Cola is also useful in offsetting the effects of the diarrhea.
When the symptoms subside, the diet should at first be confined to liquids and soft, bland foods. Milk and dairy products, butter and fats generally, fruits and greens should be avoided completely until the patient is free of all symptoms. If the symptoms persist a physician should be consulted.
i. obstruction, impairment, arrest or reversal of the normal flow of intestinal contents. Causes may be mechanical or neural or both. Some of the more common causes are HERNIA, ADHESIONS of the peritoneum, VOLVULUS, INTUSSUSCEPTION, malignant or benign tumor, congenital defect or local inflammation. Failure of peristalsis (adynamic ILEUS) is frequently associated with PERITONITIS; it also may occur with GALLSTONES, renal colic or a spinal injury.
SYMPTOMS. The most characteristic symptoms are abdominal pain, vomiting and distention. The symptoms may be mild at first and in its early stages the condition can be confused with less serious disorders of the intestinal tract. Under no circumstances should the patient be given a laxative or purgative because it will aggravate the situation. If the obstruction continues the patient suffers from dehydration and shock because of inadequate absorption of fluids, electrolytes and nutrients from the intestinal tract. If the bowel becomes strangulated and circulation to the bowel wall is obstructed, the patient shows signs of peritonitis with extreme tenderness and rigidity of the abdomen.
TREATMENT. The basic steps of treatment are decompression of the intestine, replacement of fluids and electrolytes and removal of the cause of the obstruction.
Decompression is accomplished by INTUBATION with a special tube (usually the MILLER-ABBOTT TUBE) that is designed to reach past the pyloric sphincter and into the intestine. Constant suction is then applied to remove accumulations of gas and liquids.
Fluids, sodium chloride and glucose are administered intravenously at a specific rate as ordered by the physician. Transfusions of whole blood plasma may be given as necessary to restore normal blood values.
Surgical removal of the cause of obstruction is usually necessary in cases of complete obstruction. If there is no evidence of strangulation of the bowel, the surgeon may choose to postpone surgery until dehydration and shock have been overcome and a normal electrolyte balance is restored. The type of surgical procedure performed depends on the cause of the obstruction and whether or not the intestine is gangrenous. In some cases a COLOSTOMY may be necessary before the damaged portion of the bowel is removed. A surgical incision into the cecum with insertion of a drainage tube (cecostomy) may be done when intestinal intubation is not successful in relieving distention.
NURSING CARE. Observations of the patient with intestinal obstruction include location and character of abdominal pain, degree of distention and occurrence or absence of bowel movements or passing of flatus. Should defecation occur a specimen is saved for examination and laboratory analysis. If there is vomiting, the amount and special characteristics of the vomitus should be noted and recorded. In severe cases of obstruction of the small bowel the vomitus may contain fecal material because of the reversal of peristalsis and forcing of the intestinal contents backward into the stomach.
Foods and fluids by mouth are restricted. If a Miller-Abbott tube has been inserted it should be irrigated as necessary to keep the lumen open so that intestinal decompression by suction siphonage

is achieved. Frequent mouth care is necessary to relieve the dryness and foul taste that accompanies intestinal obstruction and vomiting.

Urinary output is measured and recorded because there is a possibility that pressure on the bladder will produce urinary retention. In some cases catheterization may be necessary.

Preoperative Care. If conservative measures fail to relieve the obstruction, or if the bowel has become strangulated, surgery is indicated. Before the operation the surgeon may order a low enema. The entire abdomen is shaved. Suction siphonage is continued and the intestinal tube is left in place when the patient goes to the operating room.

Postoperative Care. Routine postoperative care of the patient with abdominal surgery is indicated. Specific nursing measures depend on the type of surgical procedure done. Suction siphonage is usually continued until peristalsis resumes. The passing of flatus or feces should be noted on the patient's chart because it indicates a return of normal peristaltic movements of the bowel. In some cases a cecostomy tube or rectal tube is inserted during surgery; the tube is attached to a drainage bottle and the amount and type of material collected in the bottle are recorded. If there is evidence that the tube has become obstructed the surgeon should be notified, because he may wish to order saline irrigations to keep the tube open and draining freely. The skin around the site of insertion of a cecostomy tube should be protected with gauze impregnated with petrolatum. The area must be washed frequently to avoid erosion of the skin by intestinal contents leaking around the tube.

See also COLOSTOMY for nursing care after that procedure.

i. tract, the small and large intestines in continuity. The long, coiled tube of the intestine is the part of the digestive system where most of the digestion of food takes place.

The small intestine has three parts: the duodenum (connected to the stomach), the jejunum and the ileum. The small intestine is small only in diameter; in length it is about 20 feet.

The large intestine, just below the ileum of the small intestine, is about 5½ feet long. It is made up of the cecum (to which the appendix is attached), the colon (comprising the ascending, transverse and descending colon and the sigmoid) and the rectum.

The digestion of food is completed in the small intestine. The digested food is absorbed through the walls of the small intestine into the blood (see also DIGESTIVE SYSTEM).

Indigestible parts of the food pass into the large intestine. Here the liquid from the wastes is gradually absorbed back into the body through the intestinal walls. The waste itself is formed into fairly solid feces and pushed down into the rectum for evacuation.

Among the disorders of the intestinal tract are the disturbances of function, such as DIARRHEA, CONSTIPATION and COLITIS; the organic diseases, ULCERATIVE COLITIS, APPENDICITIS and ILEITIS; and communicable diseases, such as DYSENTERY. Colitis is characterized by constipation, sometimes alternating with diarrhea. Ulcerative colitis is a disorder in which ulcers may appear in the wall of the large intestine. Ileitis is a disorder of the ileum or small intestine. A symptom of both is diarrhea.

Dysentery, which is characterized by diarrhea, is the result of infection by bacteria, viruses or various parasites.

intestine (in-tes′tin) the membranous tube extending from the pylorus of the stomach to the anus, consisting of the small intestine and large intestine (see also INTESTINAL TRACT).

intestinum (in″tes-ti′num), pl. *intesti′na* [L.] intestine.

intima (in′ti-mah) the innermost coat of a blood vessel; called also tunica intima.

intima-pia (in″ti-mah-pi′ah) the combined intima of blood vessels and pia mater surrounding the arteries of the brain.

intimectomy (in″ti-mek′to-me) endarterectomy; excision of thickened areas of the innermost coat of an artery.

intimitis (in″ti-mi′tis) endarteritis; inflammation of the innermost coat of an artery.

Intocostrin (in″to-kos′trin) trademark for a preparation of chondodendron tomentosum extract, a curare derivative used as a strong muscle relaxant.

intorsion (in-tor′shun) tilting of the upper part of the vertical meridian of the eye toward the midline of the face.

intoxication (in-tok″si-ka′shun) poisoning; in popular usage, the term means drunkenness produced by alcoholic beverages.

Intoxication in the sense of poisoning can be caused by carbon monoxide, lead or other toxic agents. Some medications can be poisonous in excessive doses. Intoxication can also occur in persons who have an allergy to medications such as penicillin, to various serums and to other substances. Any type of drug addiction is medically recognized as a state of intoxication. In addition to those mentioned there are the commonly recognized types of poisoning, such as those caused by chemicals and food contaminants.

Acid intoxication and alkaline intoxication are acidosis and alkalosis, respectively, of a severe grade.

Intoxication in the sense of drunkenness occurs when the concentration of alcohol in the blood reaches about one-tenth of 1 per cent. (See also ALCOHOLISM.)

intra- (in′trah) word element [L.], *inside of; within.*

intra-abdominal (in″trah-ab-dom′i-nal) within the abdomen.

intra-arterial (in″trah-ar-te′re-al) within an artery.

intra-articular (in″trah-ar-tik′u-lar) within a joint.

intracapsular (in″trah-kap′su-lar) within a capsule.

intracardiac (in″trah-kar′de-ak) within the heart.

intracartilaginous (in″trah-kar″ti-laj′i-nus) within a cartilage.

intracellular (in″trah-sel′u-lar) within a cell or cells.

intracervical (in″trah-ser′vĭ-kal) within the canal of the cervix uteri.

intracranial (in″trah-kra′ne-al) within the cranium.

intracutaneous (in″trah-ku-ta′ne-us) within the substance of the skin.
   i. injection, an injection made into the substance of the skin (see also intracutaneous INJECTION).

intracystic (in″trah-sis′tik) within the bladder or a cyst.

intrad (in′trad) inwardly.

intradermal (in″trah-der′mal) within the substance of the skin.
   i. injection, an injection made into the substance of the skin (see also intradermal INJECTION).

intraduodenal (in″trah-du″o-de′nal) within the duodenum.

intradural (in″trah-du′ral) within the dura mater.

intraerythrocytic (in″trah-ĕ-rith″ro-sit′ik) occurring or situated inside erythrocytes.

intrafebrile (in″trah-feb′ril) occurring in the febrile stage.

intragastric (in″trah-gas′trik) within the stomach.

intragenic (in″trah-jen′ik) within a gene.

intralesional (in″trah-le′zhun-al) within a localized lesion.

intralocular (in″trah-lok′u-lar) within the loculi of a structure.

intralumbar (in″trah-lum′bar) within the lumbar portion of the spinal cord.

intraluminal (in″trah-lu′mĭ-nal) within the lumen of a tubular structure.

intramastoiditis (in″trah-mas″toi-di′tis) inflammation of the antrum and cells of the mastoid process.

intramural (in″trah-mu′ral) within the walls of an organ.

intramuscular (in″trah-mus′ku-lar) within the muscular substance.
   i. injection, an injection made into the muscular substance (see also intramuscular INJECTION).

intraocular (in″trah-ok′u-lar) within the eye.

intraoperative (in″trah-op′er-a″tiv) performed or occurring during a surgical operation.

intraparietal (in″trah-pah-ri′ĕ-tal) in the substance of a wall.

intrapartum (in″trah-par′tum) occurring during childbirth or during delivery.

intraperitoneal (in″trah-per″ĭ-to-ne′al) within the peritoneal cavity.

intrapleural (in″trah-ploo′ral) within the pleura.

intrapsychic (in″trah-si′kik) taking place within the mind.

intrapulmonary (in″trah-pul′mo-ner″e) within the substance of the lung.

intraspinal (in″trah-spi′nal) within the substance of the spinal cord.

intrasternal (in″trah-ster′nal) within the sternum.

intrathoracic (in″trah-tho-ras′ik) within the thorax.

intratracheal (in″trah-tra′ke-al) endotracheal.

intratympanic (in″trah-tim-pan′ik) within the tympanum.

intrauterine (in″trah-u′ter-in) within the uterus.
   i. contraceptive device, I.U.D., a mechanical device inserted into the uterine cavity for the purpose of contraception. These devices are made of stainless steel, nylon or polyethylene and are manufactured in various sizes and shapes. Examples include the Hall-Stone ring, Lippes loop, Brinberg bow and Margulies coil. Their exact effect is not known but it is believed that they increase mobility of the ovum through the uterine tube and interfere with implantation of the fertilized ovum.
   Intrauterine devices must be inserted by a gynecologist and the patient is usually instructed to have yearly follow-up examinations. Contraindications to insertion include recent pelvic infection, suspected pregnancy, cervical stenosis, myoma of the uterus and abnormal uterine bleeding. They are not recommended for women who have never been pregnant because of the severe pain and bleeding that they produce in the majority of these patients.

intravasation (in-trav″ah-za′shun) entrance of abnormal material into vessels.

intravascular (in″trah-vas′ku-lar) within a vessel or vessels.

intravenous (in″trah-ve′nus) within a vein.
   i. infusion, administration of fluids through a vein; called also venoclysis and intravenous feeding. This method of feeding is used most often when a patient is suffering from severe dehydration and is unable to drink fluids because he is unconscious, recovering from an operation, unable to swallow normally or vomiting persistently. Medications are also given directly into the veins when necessary (see also intravenous INJECTION).
   The fluid to be infused is prescribed by the physician; it consists of sterile solution, usually with a small amount of sodium chloride or glucose or both. In some circumstances, such as after surgery, vitamins and antibiotics may be given in the fluid. Rubber or plastic tubing conducts the fluid from its glass container to an intravenous needle or small-gauge catheter. The flow of fluid is regulated by a control clip on the tubing close to the container, and there is a glass or plastic drip regulator in the line through which the rate at which the fluid is flowing from the container can be observed. The container is hung upside down 2 to 3 feet above the bed and the needle is inserted into a vein in the lower part of the patient's arm or leg. The needle is held in place by a piece of adhesive. After the slight prick when the needle is first inserted, the patient feels no pain or discomfort beyond the necessity of having his arm immobilized.
   When the control clip is first opened, the number of drops per minute flowing from the container is

counted at the drip regulator. The rate of flow is set according to the physician's instructions.

Another method of administering fluids is under the skin (subcutaneous infusion, or clysis); it is useful with children, whose veins may be too small to pierce. Subcutaneous infusion may also be resorted to when it is difficult to insert a needle into a vein.

NURSING CARE. Before the intravenous infusion is begun the patient's arm or leg is immobilized in a comfortable position, preferably with a special board designed for this purpose. The tape, gauze or canvas straps used to hold the limb stationary are applied snugly, but not so tight as to impede circulation. The label of each container of fluid or medication is very carefully checked against the physician's orders before it is connected to the infusion apparatus.

While the solution is being given the apparatus is checked frequently to see that the solution is passing through the drip regulator at the prescribed rate per minute. The area where the needle or catheter enters the vein should be watched for signs of swelling. If swelling occurs, or if the patient complains of severe pain in the area, the flow of solution is reduced to a minimum immediately and the physician is consulted. Both these signs may indicate infiltration of the fluid into the surrounding tissues. The needle is not removed until the infusion is completed or until a new site is chosen for venipuncture and continuation of the infusion.

Following completion of the venoclysis the tubing is clamped off and the needle or catheter is withdrawn. The site is covered immediately with a small gauze square or cotton ball and slight pressure is applied until bleeding stops. A small sterile bandage should be placed over the site to prevent infection.

The amount and type of solution, time the infusion was started and completed and any untoward reaction of the patient are recorded on the patient's chart.

intraventricular (in″trah-ven-trik′u-lar) within a ventricle.

intravital (in″trah-vi′tal) occuring during life.

intra vitam (in′trah vi′tam) [L.] during life.

intrinsic (in-trin′sik) of internal origin; innate.

i. factor, a mucoprotein, normally found in gastric juice, which is necessary for the assimilation and absorption of cyanocobalamin (extrinsic factor vitamin B_{12}) contained in food, an essential for the production of the antianemia factor. It is absent in PERNICIOUS ANEMIA.

introitus (in-tro′ĭ-tus), pl. *intro′itus* [L.] the entrance to a cavity or space.

introjection (in″tro-jek′shun) mental identification with another person or object.

intromission (in″tro-mish′un) the entrance of one part or object into another.

introspection (in″tro-spek′shun) contemplation or observation of one's own thoughts and feelings; self-analysis.

introsusception (in″tro-sŭ-sep′shun) intussusception.

introversion (in″tro-ver′zhun) 1. a turning inside out. 2. direction of one's energy and interests toward one's self and the inner world of experience.

introvert (in′tro-vert) a person whose interests are turned inward upon himself.

intubation (in″tu-ba′shun) insertion of a tube. The purpose of intubation varies with the location and type of tube inserted; generally the procedure is done to allow for drainage, to maintain an open airway or for the administration of anesthetics or oxygen.

Intubation into the stomach or intestine is done to remove gastric or intestinal contents for the relief or prevention of distention, or to obtain a specimen for analysis. A rubber or plastic nasogastric tube is introduced through the nose and into the stomach. The stomach tube is shorter than the Miller-Abbott tube, which is balloon-tipped and is designed to pass through the stomach and into the intestine. The tubes usually are attached to a suction apparatus so that gas and liquids can be removed. A nasogastric tube also may be inserted for the purpose of providing nourishment (see also TUBE FEEDING).

A tube may be inserted in the common bile duct to allow for drainage of bile from the ducts that drain the liver after surgery on the gallbladder or the common bile duct.

Tracheal intubation can be achieved by the insertion of an endotracheal tube into the trachea via the nose or mouth. A rubber, plastic or metal AIRWAY may be used to administer anesthetics or to remove mucus or other secretions obstructing the air passages and to keep the tongue forward until gag reflex returns. TRACHEOSTOMY is also a form of tracheal intubation.

Oxygen is sometimes administered by way of a nasal catheter (oropharyngeal insufflation). This method is usually considered less effective than an oxygen mask or tent.

intuition (in″tu-ish′un) instinctive knowledge; awareness not gained through the use of conscious reasoning.

intumescence (in″tu-mes′ens) a normal or abnormal enlargement or swelling, such as the enlargement of the spinal cord in the cervical or lumbar region.

intussusception (in″tŭ-sŭ-sep′shun) telescoping of one part of the intestine into an adjoining section, causing INTESTINAL OBSTRUCTION.

Intussusception is a rather rare disorder. Most cases occur in children during the first year of life, and some cases occur in the second year, but very few thereafter. The condition may be caused by a growth in the intestine or by any condition that causes the intestine to contract strongly. Frequently there is no obvious cause. The child seems healthy, yet paroxysms of abdominal pain begin, with vomiting and restlessness. Within 12 to 24 hours bloody mucus is passed by rectum. On the second day a high fever may appear. Death can occur within 2 to 4 days after the onset unless the condition is remedied by surgery.

The diagnosis may be confirmed by BARIUM TEST in the form of a barium enema. This examination will frequently reduce the intussusception and in some cases will completely correct the telescoping of the intestine. Treatment by surgery may be advised and ordinarily gives a permanent cure.

intussusceptum (in″tŭ-sŭ-sep′tum) a portion of intestine that has telescoped into another part.

intussuscipiens (in″tŭ-sŭ-sip′e-ens) the portion of the intestine containing the intussusceptum.

inulin (in′u-lin) a starchlike substance found in some plants, which on hydrolysis yields fructose. It is used as a measure of glomerular function in tests of renal function.

inunction (in-ungk′shun) 1. the rubbing of the skin with an ointment. 2. an ointment to be applied to the skin.

in utero (in u′ter-o) [L.] in the uterus; before delivery or birth.

invagination (in-vaj″ĭ-na′shun) the telescoping of an organ in the manner of a pouch.

Inversine (in-ver′sēn) trademark for a preparation of mecamylamine, used in ganglionic blockade and as an antihypertensive.

inversion (in-ver′zhun) 1. a turning inward, or other reversal of normal relationship of a part. 2. in genetics, the reunion of the middle segment in reverse position after breakage of a chromosome at two points.
   carbohydrate i., hydrolysis of the complex carbohydrates to simple sugars.

invert (in′vert) an individual who has adopted the attitudes and behavior of the opposite sex, manifested by overt homosexuality, trans-sexualism or transvestism.

invertase (in-ver′tās) invertin.

invertebrate (in-ver′tĕ-brāt) 1. having no vertebral column. 2. an animal organism that has no vertebral column.

invertin (in-ver′tin) an enzyme that converts cane sugar into invert sugar.

investment (in-vest′ment) a covering or outer layer of a structure of the body.

inveterate (in-vet′er-it) confirmed and chronic; difficult to cure.

in vitro (in vit′ro) [L.] in glass; referring to studies performed under artificial conditions in the laboratory on tissues removed from a living organism.

in vivo (in vi′vo) [L.] in life; referring to studies performed on tissues and organs not removed from the living organism.

involucrum (in″vo-lu′krum), pl. *involu′cra* [L.] a covering or sheath, such as contains the sequestrum of a necrosed bone.

involuntary (in-vol′un-tār″e) performed independently of the will

involution (in″vo-lu′shun) 1. a rolling or turning inward. 2. retrograde change of the entire body or in a particular organ, as the retrogression of the uterus after expulsion of the fetus. 3. the regressive changes occurring in the body in old age.

Io chemical symbol, *ionium.*

Iodamoeba (i-o″dah-me′bah) a genus of amebas, including I. *buetsch′lii,* parasitic in man, and I. *su′is,* found in pigs.

iodide (i′o-dīd) a binary compound of iodine.

iodination (i″o-dĭ-na′shun) the incorporation or addition of iodine in a compound.

iodine (i′o-dīn) a chemical element, atomic number 53, atomic weight 126.904, symbol I. (See table of ELEMENTS.) Salts of iodine and tincture of iodine were once used as antiseptics. Iodine is a strong poison, however, and has largely been replaced by other antiseptics that are less irritating to the tissues and equally effective. Since iodine salts are opaque to x-rays, they can be combined with other compounds and used as contrast media in diagnostic x-ray examinations of the gallbladder and kidneys.
   protein-bound i., iodine firmly bound to protein in the blood plasma. The determination of protein-bound iodine content is a test of thyroid function (see also PROTEIN-BOUND IODINE TEST). Iodine makes up 65 per cent of thyroxine, a hormone produced by the thyroid gland.
   radioactive i., a RADIOISOTOPE of the element, which emits gamma rays; called also radioiodine. It is often used as a tracer in the diagnosis of thyroid gland disorders. Larger doses are used therapeutically in HYPERTHYROIDISM and exophthalmic GOITER.

iodinophilous (i″o-din-of′ĭ-lus) easily stainable with iodine.

iodipamide (i″o-dip′ah-mīd) a compound used as a radiopaque medium in cholecystography.

iodism (i′o-dizm) ill health due to injudicious use of the iodides.

iodoalphionic acid (i″o-do-al″fe-on′ik) a white or yellowish compound used as a contrast medium in cholecystography.

iodobrassid (i-o″do-bras′id) a compound used in iodide therapy and as a radiopaque medium.

iodochlorhydroxyquin (i″o-do-klōr″hi-drok′sĭ-kwin) a spongy, brownish yellow powder, containing 40 to 41.5 per cent of iodine and 11.9 to 12.2 per cent of chlorine; used in treating amebiasis and trichomoniasis.

iododerma (i″o-do-der′mah) skin eruption from use of iodides.

iodoform (i-o′do-form) a greenish yellow powder or lustrous crystals, about 96 per cent iodine; used as a local antibacterial.

iodoglobulin (i″o-do-glob′u-lin) an iodine-containing globulin (protein).

iodomethamate (i-o″do-meth′ah-māt) an acid compound used as a radiopaque medium for urography.

iodophilia (i″o-do-fil′e-ah) a condition in which potassium iodide staining produces brown discoloration of particles in the leukocytes; it indicates the presence of toxemia or severe anemia.

iodophthalein (i″o-do-thal′ēn) an iodine-containing compound.
   i. sodium, a compound used as a radiopaque medium in cholecystography.

iodopyracet (i-o″do-pi′rah-set) a compound used as a radiopaque medium for urography.

iodotherapy (i″o-do-ther′ah-pe) use of iodine and iodides as remedies.

iodum (i-o′dum) [L.] iodine.

ion (i′on) an atom or group of atoms carrying an electric charge and forming one of the elements of an ELECTROLYTE. adj., **ion′ic.**
   dipolar i., one that is charged both positively and negatively.
   hydrogen i., the positively charged hydrogen atom (H^+), which is the positive ion of all acids.
   hydroxyl i., the negatively charged group, OH^-, present to excess in alkaline solutions.

ion-exchange resin a high-molecular-weight, insoluble polymer of simple organic compounds with the ability to exchange its attached ions for other ions in the surrounding solution. They are classified as cation- or anion-exchange resins, depending on which ions the resin exchanges. Cation-exchange resins are used to restrict sodium absorption in edematous states; anion-exchange resins are used as antacids in the treatment of ulcers.

ionium (i-o′ne-um) a radioactive isotope of thorium, which is transformed into radium; symbol, Io.

ionization (i″on-ĭ-za′shun) the breaking up of molecules into their component ions.
   i. chamber, an enclosure containing two or more electrodes between which an electric current may be passed when the enclosed gas is ionized by radiation; used for determining the intensity of x-rays and other rays.

ionogen (i-on′o-jen) a substance that may be ionized.

ionometer (i″o-nom′ĕ-ter) an instrument for measuring the intensity or quantity of x-rays.

ionotherapy, iontophoresis (i″o-no-ther′ah-pe), (i-on″to-fo-re′sis) the introduction of ions into the body by an electric current, for therapeutic purposes.

iopanoic acid (i″o-pah-no′ik) a cream-colored powder used as an opaque medium in cholecystography.

iophendylate (i″o-fen′dĭ-lāt) a compound used as a radiopaque medium for roentgenography of the spine and of the biliary tract.

iophenoxic acid (i″o-fen-oks′ik) a compound used as a radiopaque medium for cholecystography.

iophobia (i″o-fo′be-ah) morbid fear of poisons.

iothiouracil (i″o-thi″o-u′rah-sil) a compound used in preparation for thyroidectomy and in treatment of hyperthyroidism.

ipecac (ip′ĕ-kak) the dried rhizome and roots of *Cephaelis ipecacuanha* or *Cephaelis acuminata;* used as an emetic or expectorant.

ipomea (i″po-me′ah) the dried root of *Ipomaea orizabensis;* used as a cathartic.

IPPB intermittent positive pressure breathing, a principle used in the operation of certain types of RESPIRATORS.

Ipral (ip′ral) trademark for preparations of probarbital, an intermediate-acting barbiturate.

iproniazid (i″pro-ni′ah-zid) a compound used as an antidepressant, antituberculotic and antihypertensive.

ipsi- (ip′se) word element [L.], *same; self.*

ipsilateral (ip″sĭ-lat′er-al) pertaining to or situated on the same side.

I.Q. intelligence quotient (see also INTELLIGENCE).

Ir chemical symbol, *iridium.*

Ircon (ir′kon) trademark for a preparation of ferrous fumarate, used in iron deficiency anemia.

iridal (i′rĭ-dal) pertaining to the iris.

iridalgia (i″rĭ-dal′je-ah) pain in the iris.

iridauxesis (ir″id-awk-se′sis) thickening of the iris.

iridectasis (ir″ĭ-dek′tah-sis) dilatation of the iris, or pupil of the eye.

iridectomesodialysis (ir″ĭ-dek″to-me″so-di-al′ĭ-sis) excision and separation of adhesions around the inner edge of the iris to form an artificial pupil.

iridectomy (ir″ĭ-dek′to-me) excision of part of the iris.

iridectopia (ir″id-ek-to′pe-ah) displacement of the iris of the eye.

iridemia (ir″ĭ-de′me-ah) hemorrhage from the iris.

iridencleisis (ir″ĭ-den-kli′sis) formation of an artificial pupil by strangulation of a slip of the iris in a corneal incision.

irideremia (ir″ĭ-der-e′me-ah) absence of the iris.

iridesis (i-rid′ĕ-sis) formation of artificial iris.

iridic (i-rid′ik) pertaining to the iris.

iridium (ĭ-rid′e-um, ī-rid′e-um) a chemical element, atomic number 77, atomic weight 192.2, symbol Ir. (See table of ELEMENTS.)

iridoavulsion (ir″ĭ-do-ah-vul′shun) tearing away of the iris.

iridocapsulitis (ir″ĭ-do-kap″su-li′tis) inflammation of the iris and lens capsule.

iridocele (i-rid′o-sēl) hernial protrusion of a slip of the iris.

iridochoroiditis (ir″ĭ-do-ko″roi-di′tis) inflammation of the iris and choroid.

iridocoloboma (ir″ĭ-do-kol″o-bo′mah) fissure of the iris.

iridoconstrictor (ir″ĭ-do-kon-strik′tor) a muscle element or an agent that acts to constrict the pupil of the eye.

iridocyclectomy (ir″ĭ-do-si-klek′to-me) excision of the iris and ciliary body.

iridocyclitis (ir″ĭ-do-si-kli′tis) inflammation of the iris and ciliary body.

iridocyclochoroiditis (ir″ĭ-do-si″klo-ko″roi-di'tis) inflammation of the iris, ciliary body and choroid.

iridocystectomy (ir″ĭ-do-sis-tek'to-me) a plastic operation on the iris.

iridodesis (ir″ĭ-dod'ĕ-sis) formation of an artificial pupil by ligating the iris.

iridodialysis (ir″ĭ-do-di-al'ĭ-sis) separation or loosening of the iris from its attachments, as in the surgical creation of a new pupil (coredialysis).

iridodilator (ir″ĭ-do-di-la'tor) a muscle element or an agent that acts to dilate the pupil of the eye.

iridodonesis (ir″ĭ-do-do-ne'sis) abnormal tremulousness of the iris on movement of the eye, seen in subluxation of the lens.

iridokeratitis (ir″ĭ-do-ker″ah-ti'tis) inflammation of the iris and cornea.

iridokinesis (ir″ĭ-do-ki-ne'sis) contraction and expansion of the iris.

iridoleptynsis (ir″ĭ-do-lep-tin'sis) thinning of the iris.

iridology (ir″ĭ-dol'o-je) the study of the iris as associated with disease.

iridolysis (ir″ĭ-dol'ĭ-sis) surgical release of adhesions of the iris.

iridomalacia (ir″ĭ-do-mah-la'she-ah) softening of the iris.

iridomesodialysis (ir″ĭ-do-me″so-di-al'ĭ-sis) loosening of adhesions around the inner edge of the iris.

iridomotor (ir″ĭ-do-mo'tor) pertaining to movements of the iris.

iridoncus (ir″ĭ-dong'kus) tumor of the iris.

iridoparalysis (ir″ĭ-do-pah-ral'ĭ-sis) paralysis of the pupil.

iridoperiphakitis (ir″ĭ-do-per″ĭ-fah-ki'tis) inflammation of the lens capsule.

iridoplegia (ir″ĭ-do-ple'je-ah) paralysis of the sphincter of the iris, with lack of contraction or dilation of the pupil.

iridoptosis (ir″ĭ-dop-to'sis) prolapse of the iris.

iridorhexis (ir″ĭ-do-rek'sis) 1. rupture of iris. 2. tearing away of iris.

iridosclerotomy (ir″ĭ-do-sklĕ-rot'o-me) puncture of the sclera and of the edge of the iris.

iridosteresis (ir″ĭ-do-stĕ-re'sis) removal of all or part of the iris.

iridotasis (ir″ĭ-dot'ah-sis) stretching of the iris in treatment of glaucoma.

iridotomy (ir″ĭ-dot'o-me) incision of the iris.

iris (i'ris) the circular pigmented membrane behind the cornea, perforated by the pupil; the most anterior portion of the vascular tunic of the eye, it is made up of a flat bar of circular muscular fibers surrounding the pupil, a thin layer of plain muscle fibers by which the pupil is dilated and, posteriorly, of two layers of pigmented epithelial cells.

iritis (i-ri'tis) inflammation of the iris. The condition may be acute, occurring suddenly with pronounced symptoms, or chronic, with less severe but longer-lasting symptoms.

CAUSE.   The cause of iritis is often obscure. Frequently the condition is associated with rheumatic diseases, particularly rheumatoid arthritis, and with diabetes mellitus, syphilis, diseased teeth, tonsillitis and other infections. It may also be caused by injury.

SYMPTOMS.   Iritis is characterized by severe pain, usually radiating to the forehead and becoming worse at night. The eye is usually red and the pupil contracts and may be irregular in shape; there is extreme sensitivity to light, together with blurring of vision and tenderness of the eyeball. The iris becomes swollen and discolored. If not treated promptly, iritis can be dangerous because of scarring and adhesions that may cause impaired vision and possibly blindness.

TREATMENT.   Caring for iritis calls for treatment of the underlying cause and then dilation of the pupil with atropine drops to prevent scarring or adhesions. Certain steroid drugs may be used to reduce the inflammation quickly. Warm compresses may also help to lessen the inflammation and pain. A protective covering allows the eye to rest.

With proper treatment, acute iritis usually clears up fairly quickly, although it may recur. For permanent relief, elimination or control of the underlying cause is necessary.

iritoectomy (ir″ĭ-to-ek'to-me) excision of part of the iris.

iritomy (i-rit'o-me) iridotomy.

irium (ir'e-um) sodium lauryl sulfate.

iron (i'ern) a chemical element, atomic number 26, atomic weight 55.847, symbol Fe. (See table of ELEMENTS.) Iron is chiefly important to the human body because it is the main constituent of hemoglobin, and a constant although small intake of iron in food is needed to replace erythrocytes that are destroyed in the body processes.

Most iron reaches the body in food, where it occurs naturally in the form of iron compounds. These are converted for use in the body by the action of the hydrochloric acid produced in the stomach. This acid separates the iron from the food and combines with it in a form that is readily assimilable by the body. Vitamin C enhances the absorption of food iron. The administration of alkalis hampers iron absorption.

IRON DEFICIENCIES.   The amount of new iron needed every day by the adult body is about 15 mg. A child needs a bit more in proportion to his weight. Although these amounts are very small, iron deficiencies may cause serious disorders.

The most common form of anemia results from iron deficiency. A great loss of blood, such as may result from bleeding ulcers, hemorrhoids or injury, may cause a deficiency of iron. Women who lose much blood in menstruation may have to supplement their diet with iron-rich food. Iron deficiency sometimes occurs in pregnancy as a result of increased demands on the mother's blood. Iron deficiency may also occur in infants, since milk contains little iron. Although babies are born with an extra supply of hemoglobin, by the age of 2 or 3 months they need iron-rich food to supplement milk.

Iron preparations, such as ferrous sulfate, may be

necessary in treatment of iron deficiency anemia; they should be administered after meals, never on an empty stomach. The patient should be warned that the drugs cause stools to turn dark green or black. Overdosage may cause severe systemic reactions.

FOOD SOURCES OF IRON. Liver is the richest source of iron, containing enough in 6 oz. for a whole day's supply for an adult. Other iron-rich foods include lean meat, oysters, kidney beans, whole-wheat bread, kale, spinach, egg yolk, turnip tops, beet greens, carrots, apricots and raisins.

i. lung, a type of RESPIRATOR that provides controlled, automatic breathing for a patient whose respiratory muscles are paralyzed; called also Drinker respirator.

radioactive i., a RADIOISOTOPE of iron; used in studies of hemoglobin formation and breakdown.

i. storage disease, hemochromatosis.

Ironate (i'ron-āt) trademark for a preparation of ferrous sulfate, used in iron deficiency anemia.

Irosul (i'ro-sul) trademark for preparations of ferrous sulfate, used in iron deficiency anemia.

irotomy (i-rot'o-me) iridotomy.

irradiate (ĭ-ra'de-āt) to treat with radiant energy.

irradiation (ĭ-ra"de-a'shun) the passage of penetrating rays, such as x-rays, gamma rays, ultraviolet rays or infrared rays, through any object or substance; exposure to RADIATION.

There are many kinds of rays, all traveling at the speed of light. Every living thing is subject to some irradiation by cosmic rays, ultraviolet rays in sunlight and other natural radiation in the environment. Such radiation is usually slight and harmless. In large amounts, certain kinds of radiation – those rays with a greater frequency and producing more energy – cause direct harm to living cells.

USES. Irradiation of certain foods, including milk, kills harmful bacteria and prevents spoilage. X-ray photography is used in industrial research and in diagnosis of disorders within the body.

Radiation therapy usually refers to treatment by x-rays and gamma rays. X-rays are produced by bombarding a tungsten target with high-speed electrons in a vacuum tube; gamma rays are emitted by radium and other radioactive substances, including RADIOISOTOPES of iodine, gold, phosphorus and cobalt. X-rays may be employed to kill organisms causing skin diseases, for example, or to destroy the abnormal cells that form tumors. Gonads, blood cells and cancer cells are especially sensitive to radiation, particularly to x-rays and gamma rays. These rays are used principally for the treatment of cancer, and the radiotherapist attempts to destroy diseased cells without producing other ill effects.

Other rays are also used medically. Infrared rays produce a radiant heat used for the treatment of sprains and bursitis; tissues such as muscles and joints are relaxed and soothed by the penetration of these rays. Ultraviolet rays are used in sun lamps to treat skin diseases such as acne and psoriasis.

PROTECTION AGAINST HARMFUL EFFECTS. Excessive radiation can cause RADIATION SICKNESS in the person exposed; sterility or genetic mutations in offspring are other possible results of excessive exposure to radiation. Hence the great danger from the blasts of atomic explosives and from the radioactive materials (fallout) scattered by these blasts.

The harmful effects of radiation are determined by both the degree of exposure and the type of radiation. Prevention must take into account time, distance and shielding of both areas and people. Persons who are employed in nuclear power plants or other places where radioactive materials are accumulated must be properly shielded, and should wear or carry a dosimeter on which the amount of radiation received is recorded. Proper shielding is necessary also for radiologists, nurses and others who spend much time near radiation emitted from either machinery or materials. (See also RADIATION PROTECTION.)

Since radiation effects, such as those of x-rays, build up in the body, a person should not be exposed to any more radiation during his lifetime than is necessary, and all radiation therapy must be under the control of a competent medical practitioner. In many states, all radiation-producing equipment must be registered.

Radiologists reduce harmful effects by limiting the field of exposure, by means of fast films, filters and other technical devices. This shortens measurably the length of exposure of patients receiving medical and dental x-rays.

irrigation (ir"ĭ-ga'shun) washing of a body cavity or wound by a stream of water or other fluid.

GENERAL PRINCIPLES. A steady, gentle stream is used in irrigation. The pressure should be sufficient to reach the desired area, but not enough to force the fluid beyond the area to be irrigated. The greater the height of the container of solution, the greater will be the pressure exerted by the stream of solution. Return flow of solution must always be allowed for. Directions about the type of solution to be used, the strength desired and correct temperature should be followed carefully. Aseptic technique must be observed if sterile irrigation is ordered.

BLADDER. The purpose is to cleanse the bladder or to apply medication to the bladder lining. Aseptic technique must be used. The amount and type of solution will be ordered by the physician. A syringe and basin are used for single irrigations; other apparatus may be used for continuous or intermittent irrigations.

EAR. The stream is kept flowing steadily but with very low pressure; excessive pressure is painful and may spread infection to the middle ear. The patient usually is seated for this procedure, but he may lie on his side, with the ear to be irrigated uppermost while the solution is entering the ear. The head is turned to allow for return flow. The output flow of solution must never be obstructed.

EYE (CONJUNCTIVAL SAC). The patient's head is turned to the side so that the eye to be irrigated is lower than the other eye. The solution is allowed to run over the eyelids to cleanse them and to accustom the patient to the flow of the solution. The flow of solution is directed from the inner to outer corner of the eye. The eyelids are separated by exerting pressure on the facial bones, not on the eyeball.

PERINEUM. The purpose of the procedure is to cleanse the vulva. The type of solution is specified by the physician. Flow of the solution is from front to back. The patient is instructed to wipe from the front to back to avoid contamination from the anal region.

THROAT (ORAL PHARYNX). This type of irrigation reaches a more extensive area than does gargling. The temperature of the solution may be slightly higher than for other irrigations because the mouth and throat are more accustomed to hot liquids. The patient may be more comfortable sitting, with his head bent forward slightly. The patient is instructed to hold his breath while the solution is flowing.

irritability (ir″ĭ-tah-bil′ĭ-te) 1. ability of an organism or a specific tissue to react to the environment. 2. the state of being abnormally responsive to slight stimuli or unduly sensitive.

    muscular i., the normal contractile quality of muscle.

    nervous i., the ability of a nerve to transmit impulses.

    tactile i., responsiveness to stimulation arising from touching an object.

irritable (ir′ĭ-tah-bl) 1. capable of reacting to a stimulus. 2. abnormally sensitive to stimuli.

irritant (ir′ĭ-tant) 1. causing irritation. 2. an agent that causes irritation.

irritation (ir″ĭ-ta′shun) 1. the act of stimulating. 2. a state of overexcitation and undue sensitiveness.

ischemia (is-ke′me-ah) deficiency of blood in a part, due to functional constriction or actual obstruction of a blood vessel. adj., **ische′mic.**

    myocardial i., deficiency of blood supply to the heart muscle, due to obstruction or constriction of the coronary arteries.

ischi(o)- (is′ke-o) word element [Gr.], *ischium,* referring to the inferior portion of the hip bone.

ischiadic, ischial, ischiatic (is″ke-ad′ik), (is′ke-al), (is″ke-at′ik) pertaining to the ischium, the inferior portion of the hip bone.

ischidrosis (is″kĭ-dro′sis) suppression of secretion of sweat.

ischiobulbar (is″ke-o-bul′bar) pertaining to the ischium and the bulb of the urethra.

ischiocele (is′ke-o-sēl″) hernia at the sacrosciatic notch.

ischiodidymus (is″ke-o-did′ĭ-mus) conjoined twins united at the pelvis.

ischiodynia (is″ke-o-din′e-ah) pain in the ischium.

ischiofemoral (is″ke-o-fem′o-ral) pertaining to the ischium and femur.

ischiofibular (is″ke-o-fib′u-lar) pertaining to the ischium and fibula.

ischiohebotomy (is″ke-o-he-bot′o-me) ischiopubiotomy.

ischioneuralgia (is″ke-o-nu-ral′je-ah) sciatica.

ischiopagus (is″ke-op′ah-gus) a twin fetal monster united at the pelvis, the axes of the bodies forming a straight line.

ischiopubic (is″ke-o-pu′bik) pertaining to the ischium and pubes.

ischiopubiotomy (is″ke-o-pu″be-ot′o-me) transection of the bar of bone constituting the lower margin of the obturator foramen and formed by the conjoined rami of the ischium and pubis.

ischiorectal (is″ke-o-rek′tal) pertaining to the ischium and rectum.

ischium (is′ke-um) the inferior, dorsal portion of the hip bone.

ischo- (is′ko) word element [Gr.], *suppression; deficiency.*

ischochymia (is″ko-ki′me-ah) suppression of gastric digestion.

ischomenia (is″ko-me′ne-ah) suppression of the menstrual flow.

ischuria (is-ku′re-ah) retention or suppression of the urine.

iseikonia (i″si-ko′ne-ah) equality in size of the two retinal images.

island (i′land) an isolated mass of tissue.

    blood i., a group of cells in the mesoderm of the early embryo, from which the blood vessels and blood corpuscles are later derived.

    i's of Langerhans, masses in the pancreas composed of cells smaller than the ordinary cells. They produce the hormone insulin and their degeneration is one of the causes of DIABETES MELLITUS.

    i. of Reil, an isolated part of the cerebral cortex in the fissure of Sylvius.

islet (i′let) an island.

    i's of Langerhans, islands of Langerhans.

Ismelin (is′me-lin) trademark for a preparation of guanethidine, an antihypertensive.

iso- (i′so) word element [Gr.], *equal.*

isoagglutinin (i″so-ah-gloo′tĭ-nin) an agglutinin acting on cells of animals of the same species as that from which it is derived, an isohemagglutinin.

isoamyl nitrite (i″so-am′il ni′trīt) amyl nitrite, a vasodilator.

isoanaphylaxis (i″so-an″ah-fi-lak′sis) anaphylaxis produced by serum from an individual of the same species.

isoantibody (i″so-an′tĭ-bod″e) an antibody combining with an antigen present in tissues of some, but not all, individuals of the same species as the antibody producer.

isoantigen (i″so-an′tĭ-jen) an antigen present in tissues of some, but not all, individuals of the same species as the antibody producer.

isobar (i′so-bahr) 1. one of several nuclides having the same number of nucleons, but different combinations of protons and neutrons, i.e., the same mass number, but different atomic numbers. 2. a series of points on a map or chart that when connected depict a line of constant atmospheric pressure.

isobornyl thiocyanoacetate (i″so-bor′nil thi″o-si″ah-no-as′ĕ-tāt) a compound used as a pediculicide.

isocaloric (i″so-kah-lo′rik) providing the same number of calories.

isocarboxazid (i″so-kar-bok′sah-zid) a compound used as an antidepressant and to reduce pain of angina pectoris.

isocellular (i″so-sel′u-lar) made up of identical cells.

isochromatic (i″so-kro-mat′ik) of the same color throughout.

isochromatophil (i″so-kro-mat′o-fil) staining alike with the same stain.

isochromosome (i″so-kro′mo-sōm) a chromosome whose two arms are exact duplicates.

isochronic, isochronous (i″so-kron′ik), (i-sok′ro-nus) 1. passing through the same phases at the same time. 2. performed in the same period of time.

isocoria (i″so-ko′re-ah) equality of size of the pupils of the two eyes.

isocortex (i″so-kor′teks) that portion of the cerebral cortex made up of layers developing between the sixth and eighth fetal months.

isocytolysin (i″so-si-tol′ĭ-sin) a cytolysin acting on cells of animals of the same species as that from which it is derived.

isocytosis (i″so-si-to′sis) equality in size of cells, especially erythrocytes.

isodactylism (i″so-dak′tĭ-lizm) relatively even length of the fingers.

isodiametric (i″so-di″ah-met′rik) measuring the same in all diameters.

isodontic (i″so-don′tik) having all the teeth alike.

isoelectric (i″so-e-lek′trik) showing no variation of electric potential.

isoenergetic (i″so-en″er-jet′ik) exhibiting equal energy.

isoenzyme (i″so-en′zīm) one of the many forms of a protein catalyst, differing chemically, physically and/or immunologically.

isoflurophate (i″so-floo′ro-fāt) a compound used as an anticholinesterase inhibitor and as a miotic in glaucoma.

isogamety (i″so-gam′ĕ-te) production by an individual of one sex of gametes identical with respect to the sex chromosome.

isogamy (i-sog′ah-me) the conjugation of gametes identical in size and structure to form the zygote from which the new organism develops.

isogeneic (i″so-jĕ-ne′ik) having the same genetic constitution.

isogeneric (i″so-jĕ-ner′ik) of the same kind; belonging to the same species.

isogenesis (i″so-jen′ĕ-sis) identity in development.

isograft (i′so-graft) a graft of tissue from a donor of the same genotype as the recipient.

isohemagglutination (i″so-he″mah-gloo″tĭ-na′-shun) agglutination of erythrocytes caused by a hemagglutinin from another individual of the same species.

isohemagglutinin (i″so-he″mah-gloo′tĭ-nin) a hemagglutinin that agglutinates the erythrocytes of other individuals of the same species.

isohemolysin (i″so-he-mol′ĭ-sin) a hemolysin acting on the blood of animals of the same species as that from which it is derived.

isohemolysis (i″so-he-mol′ĭ-sis) hemolysis of blood corpuscles of an animal produced by serum from another animal of the same species.

isohypercytosis (i″so-hi″per-si-to′sis) increase of leukocytes with normal proportions of neutrophils.

isohypocytosis (i″so-hi″po-si-to′sis) decrease of leukocytes with normal proportion of neutrophils.

isoimmunization (i″so-im″u-nĭ-za′shun) development of antibodies in response to antigens from individuals of the same species.

isolate (i′so-lāt) 1. to separate from others, or set apart. 2. a group of individuals prevented by geographic, genetic, ecologic or social barriers from interbreeding with others of their kind.

isolateral (i″so-lat′er-al) 1. equilateral. 2. ipsilateral.

isolation (i″so-la′shun) the act of separating or setting apart, or state of being set apart, e.g., the segregation of patients with a communicable disease or, in psychology, failure to connect behavior with its motives, or contradictory attitudes and behavior with each other.

i. technique, special precautionary measures and procedures used in the care of a patient with a communicable disease. The patient is isolated from others and confined to a designated area until he is no longer a source of infection. All objects that have been contaminated by infectious agents must be disinfected or destroyed (preferably by burning) to prevent the spread of infection.

Disinfection may be concurrent or terminal. Concurrent disinfection refers to immediate destruction of the infectious agents as they leave the body, or after they have contaminated linen, eating utensils, hospital equipment or other objects that have come in contact with the patient or his excreta. Concurrent disinfection is a continuous process in the daily care of the patient.

Terminal disinfection refers to destruction of pathogenic microorganisms remaining in the patient's environment after he is no longer considered to be a source of infection.

GENERAL PRINCIPLES OF NURSING CARE. Pathogenic microorganisms enter and leave the human body in a number of ways, for example, through the respiratory tract, intestinal tract, skin and mucous membranes. All persons concerned with the care of a patient with a communicable disease should be thoroughly familiar with the ways in which the specific disease may be spread. (For modes of transmission, see COMMUNICABLE DISEASE).

The more prolonged the contact with an infected person and his surroundings, the more likely the chance for contamination. Specific measures must be taken to avoid contracting the illness or spreading it to others.

The factors most important in preventing spread of a communicable disease are proper disinfecting technique and conscientious handwashing. The hands are used for many nursing tasks and are therefore most likely to be excellent sources of infection if they are not washed properly after each contact with the patient.

The spread of microorganisms can be kept at a minimum if it is always kept in mind that one must touch only "clean" to "clean" and "contaminated" to "contaminated." Once a clean article comes in contact with a contaminated article, both must be considered contaminated. In this context the word "clean" does not mean unsoiled; it means that an object is free from the organisms causing the patient's illness. Unsoiled linen, for example, might be contaminated with infectious agents and therefore could not be considered clean.

While carrying out the multitude of special procedures and precautionary measures necessary in isolation technique, one must not forget their psychologic impact on the patient. He should be told the reason for the precautions with special emphasis on concern for his well-being as well as for the protection of others. Unless he is very seriously ill some provision should be made for diversional activities that will help relieve the loneliness and boredom that result from isolation from other human beings.

Visitors must be limited to a very few persons and they should be instructed in the ways in which the patient's disease can be spread and the precautions necessary to prevent infection of others. If the patient is a child and his parents are allowed to stay with him, they should wear gowns, masks, and head coverings while they are in the patient's unit. Toys, books and other items brought into the unit for the child's amusement must be of the type that can be thoroughly disinfected; otherwise it will be necessary to dispose of them when he is no longer ill.

SETTING UP THE ISOLATION UNIT. Specific steps in setting up the unit will depend on hospital policy and the patient's disease. When the patient is being cared for in the home it is necessary to improvise with the facilities available. Ideally the patient should be in a room with an adjoining bath, both rooms being considered as the unit and as contaminated areas. When a bathroom is available, there is running water for handwashing and for obtaining and disposing of bath water. When running water is not available in the unit, basins and a pitcher are needed for proper handwashing.

If the patient has not entered the unit before it is set up, upholstered furniture, rugs and other articles that would be difficult or impossible to disinfect should be removed. The usual items included in a hospital unit such as wash basin, water pitcher and glass, soap and soap dish, bedpan and urinal are kept in their usual places, cleansed daily and disinfected terminally. Supplies of extra linen and isolation gowns and masks are kept in an area away from the immediate surroundings of the patient. Paper or plastic bags are used to line the inside of the wastebasket in the patient's room and also the container for discarded paper towels. Small paper bags are used at the bedside for disposal of paper tissues used by the patient. Most hospitals use large, sturdy paper bags for contaminated linen; however, some may use laundry bags marked "isolation." The linen is given special handling and often is autoclaved before laundering so that all microorganisms are destroyed. In the home the linen should be soaked in a disinfectant before laundering.

Hospital equipment such as thermometer tray, stethoscope and sphygmomanometer are kept in the patient's unit for his individual use and are disinfected terminally. Disposable needles and syringes, intravenous equipment, catheters and drainage tubes are discarded in a lined container set aside for this purpose.

Rubber gloves, catheter trays and other equipment that is not disposable must be soaked in Lysol solution for 30 minutes before it is cleaned, dried and returned to the hospital supply room.

The patient's bathroom should contain antibacterial soap, paper towels, a nail brush and Lysol or other disinfectant for soaking articles. If the patient's excreta is to be disinfected before it is flushed into the sewage system, chlorinated lime or Lysol may be used for this purpose (see also FECES).

SPECIFIC NURSING PROCEDURES. *Handwashing.* Proper washing of the hands is necessary each time the patient receives care, or the nurse realizes that her hands are grossly contaminated. Running water is much preferred to the use of a basin and pitcher of water. When running water is not available a second person must assist by pouring water from a pitcher over the hands of the person washing her hands.

Friction between the hands during the handwashing is very important in removal of microorganisms from the lines and crevices in the skin. A clean nail brush is used to clean beneath the fingernails. The wrists and arms usually can be considered uncontaminated; therefore the hands are kept below the level of the elbows during the handwashing procedure. If bar soap is used, it is kept in the hands during the entire procedure until the hands are rinsed for the last time. The hands should be washed for one full minute.

When foot pedals are not used to control the flow of water, the faucet handles are to be considered contaminated and a paper towel must be used to turn off the water after the hands have been cleaned.

Gown Technique. A gown is worn whenever one enters the isolation unit and is removed when one leaves. A hat rack or other device is placed inside the patient's unit and is used to hold a gown that has been worn, and is therefore contaminated on the outside, but is not soiled and can be worn again. The outside of the gown is contaminated and so the gown is hung with the contaminated side out. The inside of the gown and the neck band are considered clean because they are not touched by the hands after they have been contaminated. When donning the gown the nurse removes it from the hook by grasping the inside of the neckband. She then slides her arms into the sleeves, keeping her hand inside one sleeve as she adjusts the other. The back edges of the gown are brought together away from the body and then folded over and tied.

When removing the gown the back ties are loosened first. The cuff of the left sleeve is pulled over the hand, and with the left hand inside the sleeve the right sleeve is pulled down over the right hand. The gown is then shrugged off the shoulders and the hands removed from the sleeves. If the gown is to be discarded it is rolled with the inside out. If it is to be worn again it is hung on the hook with the contaminated side to the outside. Immediately after the gown is removed the hands must be washed.

Face Mask. The mask is worn to protect the nurse from contamination by droplet infection. Sneezing or coughing by the patient may release infectious organisms from his respiratory tract. A mask should fit snugly and cover both the nose and mouth. It should not be worn for more than 1 hour at a time. If it is necessary to stay in the patient's immediate environment for a longer period than this, the mask is discarded and replaced by a fresh one.

Gloves. Gloves are worn if there are dressings to be changed, or if there is the possibility of gross contamination of the hands from excreta. The gloves are removed by grasping the cuff on the outside and turning the glove wrong side out. The ungloved hand is then slipped under the cuff of the other glove so that it is removed by turning it wrong side out. The gloves are then placed in a basin of Lysol solution or other disinfectant and soaked for 30 minutes. The hands are washed immediately after removal of the gloves.

Cap. Most hospitals use a disposable cap to be worn over the hair during care of the patient in isolation. A clean cap is worn each time one enters the patient's unit and is discarded before leaving the unit. When removing the cap, care must be taken to avoid contamination of the hands if they have already been washed.

Feeding the Patient. Disposable plates, cups and food trays are preferred. The meal can be prepared in the kitchen and brought to the patient's unit. Silverware is usually kept in the patient's unit, washed after use and wrapped in a paper towel until it is needed again. Uneaten food is wrapped in a paper bag or newspaper and placed in a lined container. If a bathroom is available, some of the food may be flushed down the toilet. Milk and other liquids can be disposed of in the same manner.

Transporting the Patient to Other Departments. In rare instances it may be necessary to take the patient to another part of the hospital, for example, to the operating room, x-ray department or diagnostic clinic. The patient must be dressed in an isolation gown, mask and cap. The stretcher or wheel chair is covered with a clean sheet. If the patient is able to walk, the wheel chair or stretcher is rolled to the door of the room. If he cannot walk to the door, newspapers are placed on the floor of the unit (which must always be considered grossly contaminated) and the wheel chair or stretcher is rolled to the bedside. Immediately before transporting the patient to another area, the department should be called and warned that the patient is coming so that adequate preparations can be made.

On return of the patient to the unit, his gown, mask and cap are removed and placed in the proper container. The sheet on the stretcher or wheel chair also is removed and placed in the container for contaminated linen. The wheelchair or stretcher is washed with Lysol solution and returned to its proper place.

TERMINAL DISINFECTION. If the patient is to continue to stay in the hospital and the isolation is discontinued, he should be given a bath and shampoo, dressed in clean clothes and placed in a clean room while disinfection is carried out. If he is to be discharged, the bath, shampoo and change of clothes are done immediately before he leaves the hospital and he is placed in another room until he is discharged.

All equipment must be decontaminated or wrapped and prepared for discard before it is removed from the unit. A special technique called "fogging" is used in some hospitals when decontamination is desired, although the National Communicable Disease Center does not recognize it as an effective method of decontamination. If fogging is done, the unit is prepared by opening all drawers and closet doors so that as many areas as possible can be exposed to the disinfecting mist. The bed is stripped of linen and rolled up so the springs are exposed. Equipment such as suction machines is left in the room after it has been thoroughly washed. The room is kept closed for a specified period of time and then arranged as necessary for the admission of another patient.

In the home the furniture in the room is washed with Lysol solution and the windows are opened so that the room is exposed to fresh air for several hours. The mattress and bed covers should be exposed to direct sunlight for 8 hours if possible.

isolecithal (i″so-les′ĭ-thal) having a small amount of yolk evenly distributed throughout the cytoplasm of the ovum.

isoleucine (i″so-lu′sēn) a naturally occurring amino acid, one of those essential for human metabolism.

isologous (i-sol′o-gus) characterized by an identical genotype.

isolysis (i-sol′ĭ-sis) isohemolysis.

isomer (i′so-mer) one of two or more nuclides having the same mass number and atomic number, but existing in the excited state with a higher energy and other properties differing from those of the ground state nuclide.

isomerase (i-som′er-ās) an enzyme that catalyzes the process of isomerization, such as the interconversion of aldoses and ketoses.

isomerism (i-som′ĕ-rizm) the existence of two or more compounds (isomers) having the same number and kinds of atoms in the molecule, and the same molecular weight, but differing in arrangement of the atoms. adj., **isomer′ic.**

isomerization (i-som″ĕ-rĭ-za′shun) the process whereby any isomer is converted into another, usually requiring special conditions of temperature, pressure or catalysts.

isometheptene (i″so-meth′ep-tēn) a compound used as a sympathomimetic and antispasmodic.

isometric (i″so-met′rik) maintaining, or pertaining to, the same measure, or length.

isometropia (i″so-mĕ-tro′pe-ah) equality in refraction of the two eyes.

isomorphism (i″so-mor′fizm) identity in form; in genetics, referring to genotypes of polyploid organisms that produce similar gametes even though containing genes in different combinations on homologous chromosomes.

isoniazid (i″so-ni′ah-zid) an antibacterial compound used in treatment of tuberculosis.

isonicotinoylhydrazine (i″so-nik″o-tin″o-il-hi′-drah-zēn) isoniazid.

isopathy (i-sop′ah-the) treatment by administering the agent producing the disease.

isopepsin (i″so-pep′sin) pepsin changed by heat.

isophoria (i″so-fo′re-ah) correspondence of the visual axes of the two eyes.

Isophrin (i′so-frin) trademark for a preparation of phenylephrine, a local vasoconstrictor.

isoplastic (i′so-plas″tik) taken from an animal of the same species.

isoprecipitin (i″so-pre-sip′ĭ-tin) a precipitin acting on serum of animals of the same species as that from which it is derived.

isopregnenone (i″so-preg′ne-nōn) a compound used as a progestational agent and as a test of pregnancy.

isoprenaline (i″so-pren′ah-lēn) isoproterenol.

isopropamide (i″so-pro′pah-mīd) a compound used in parasympathetic blockade and as an antispasmodic.

isopropanol (i″so-pro′pah-nol) isopropyl alcohol, a transparent, volatile, colorless liquid used as a rubbing compound.

isopropyl meprobamate (i″so-pro′pil mě-pro′bah-māt) carisoprodol, a muscle relaxant.

isoproterenol (i″so-pro″tě-re′nol) an odorless, white, crystalline powder used as a sympathomimetic, cardiac stimulant and antispasmodic, and in relief of bronchospasm.

isopter (i-sop′ter) a curve representing areas of equal visual acuity in the field of vision.

isopyknosis (i″so-pik-no′sis) 1. the quality of showing uniform density throughout. 2. uniformity of condensation observed in comparison of different chromosomes or in different areas of the same chromosome.

Isordil (i′sor-dil) trademark for preparations of isosorbide dinitrate, a coronary vasodilator.

isorrhea (i″so-re′ah) a steady equilibrium between the intake and output, by the body, of water and/or solutes.

isosexual (i″so-seks′u-al) pertaining to or characteristic of the same sex.

isosmotic (i″soz-mot′ik) having the same osmotic pressure.

isosorbide dinitrate (i″so-sor′bīd di-ni′trāt) a compound used as a coronary vasodilator in treatment of coronary insufficiency.

Isospora (i-sos′po-rah) a genus of coccidia, including *I. belti*, which causes a coccidial diarrhea in man, and *I. hom′inis*, a nonpathogenic species sometimes temporarily present in the small intestine of man.

isospore (i′so-spōr) a spore that develops directly into an adult.

isosthenuria (i″sos-thě-nu′re-ah) maintenance of a constant osmolality of the urine, regardless of changes in osmotic pressure of the blood.

isostimulation (i″so-stim″u-la′shun) stimulation of an animal with antigenic material from other animals of the same species.

isotherapy (i″so-ther′ah-pe) isopathy.

isotherm (i′so-therm) a line on a map or chart depicting the boundaries of an area in which the temperature is the same.

isothermal (i″so-ther′mal) having the same temperature.

isothiazine (i″so-thi′ah-zēn) ethopropazine, a drug used in Parkinson's disease.

isothipendyl (i″so-thi′pen-dil) a compound used as an antihistamine.

isotone (i′so-tōn) one of several nuclides having the same number of neutrons, but differing in number of protons in their nuclei.

isotonic (i″so-ton′ik) of the same tonicity or strength; of a solution, having the same osmotic pressure as the solution being compared with it.

isotope (i′so-tōp) a chemical element having the same atomic number as another (i.e., the same number of nuclear protons), but having a different atomic mass (i.e., a different number of nuclear neutrons); now usually indicated by the conventional chemical symbol with the atomic mass number in the left superscript position, as ^{14}C.
    radioactive i., one transmuted into another element with emission of radiations. These isotopes occur naturally or may be produced by bombardment of a common chemical element with high-velocity particles. (See also RADIOISOTOPE.)
    stable i., one that does not transmute into another element with emission of radiations.

isotopology (i″so-to-pol′o-je) the scientific study of isotopes and of their uses and applications.

isotropic (i″so-trop′ik) transmitting light equally in all directions.

isotropy (i-sot′ro-pe) the quality or condition of being isotropic.

isotypical (i″so-tip′ĭ-kal) belonging to the same type.

isoxsuprine (i-sok′su-prēn) a compound used as a vasodilator and uterine relaxant.

isozyme (i′so-zīm) isoenzyme.

issue (ish′ū) a suppurating sore, made and kept open by inserting an irritant substance.

isthmectomy (is-mek′to-me) excision of an isthmus, especially of the isthmus of the thyroid.

isthmitis (is-mi′tis) inflammation of the isthmus faucium.

isthmoparalysis, isthmoplegia (is″mo-pah-ral′ĭ-sis), (is″mo-ple′je-ah) paralysis of the isthmus faucium.

isthmospasm (is′mo-spazm) spasm of an isthmus.

isthmus (is′mus) a narrow strip of tissue or narrow passage connecting two larger parts. adj., **isth′mian.**
    i. of eustachian tube, the narrowest part of the eustachian tube.
    i. fau′cium, the passage between the mouth and fauces.
    i. rhombenceph′ali, that part of the embryonic hindbrain comprising the anterior medullary velum, the superior cerebellar peduncles and uppermost part of the fourth ventricle.
    i. of thyroid, the band of tissue joining the lobes of the thyroid.
    i. of uterine tube, the narrower, thicker-walled portion of the uterine tube closest to the uterus.

i. of uterus, the constricted part of the uterus between the cervix and the body of the uterus.

Isuprel (i'su-prel) trademark for a preparation of isoproterenol, a sympathomimetic bronchodilator.

isuria (i-su're-ah) excretion of urine at a uniform rate.

itch (ich) 1. a skin disease attended with itching. 2. scabies.

barber's i., infection and irritation of the hair follicles of the beard region (see also SYCOSIS BARBAE).

dhobie i., a contact dermatitis in India, caused by marking fluid used by native washermen (dhobie).

grain i., itching dermatitis due to a mite parasitic on various plants, which bites human beings who come in close contact with the host plants.

grocers' i., an eczema of the hands said to be sometimes due to a sugar mite.

ground i., an itching eruption caused by the presence of larval forms of certain roundworms.

seven-year i., scabies.

swimmers' i., schistosome dermatitis.

washerman's i., dhobie itch.

water i., schistosome dermatitis.

itching (ich'ing) a teasing irritation of the skin, arousing the desire to scratch.

iteroparity (it″er-o-par′ĭ-te) the state, in an individual organism, of reproducing repeatedly, or more than once in a lifetime.

-itides (it′ĭ-dēz) plural of *-itis*.

-itis (i′tis) word element, *inflammation.*

ITP idiopathic thrombocytopenic purpura.

Itrumil (it′roo-mil) trademark for a preparation of iothiouracil, a drug that depresses thyroid activity.

I.U. International unit.

IUCD intrauterine contraceptive device.

IUD intrauterine contraceptive device.

I.V. intravenously.

I.V.T. intravenous transfusion.

Ixodes (ik-so′dēz) a genus of ticks that become parasitic on man and animals.

ixodiasis (ik″so-di′ah-sis) fever caused by bites of ticks of the genus Ixodes.

ixodic (ik-sod′ik) pertaining to, or caused by, ticks.

J

J symbol, *Joule's equivalent.*

jacket (jak'et) an encasement or covering for the trunk, especially the thorax.

 plaster-of-paris j., a casing of plaster of paris enveloping the body, for the purpose of giving support or correcting deformities (see also CAST).

 Sayre's j., a plaster-of-paris jacket used as a support for the vertebral column.

 strait j., a contrivance for restraining the arms of a violently disturbed person.

jacksonian epilepsy (jak-so'ne-an) a progression of involuntary clonic movement or sensation, with retention of consciousness.

jactitation (jak″tĭ-ta'shun) restless tossing to and fro in acute illness.

Jaksch's disease (yaksh) infantile pseudoleukemia.

janiceps (jan'ĭ-seps) a fetal monster with one head and two opposite faces.

jaundice (jawn'dis) yellowness of skin and eyes caused by excess of BILE pigment. It is usually first noticeable in the eyes, although it may come on so gradually that it is not immediately noticed by those in daily contact with the jaundiced person.

 Jaundice is not a disease. It is a symptom of one of a number of different diseases and disorders of the LIVER, GALLBLADDER and blood. One such disorder is the presence of a gallstone in the common bile duct, which carries bile from the liver to the intestine. This may obstruct the flow of bile, causing it to accumulate and enter the bloodstream. The obstruction of bile flow may cause bile to enter the urine, making it dark in color, and also decrease the bile in the stool, making it light and clay-colored. This condition requires surgery to remove the gallstone before it causes serious liver injury.

 Jaundice may also be a symptom of infectious (viral) HEPATITIS. This very infectious disease may result in damage to the liver if not treated.

 Certain diseases of the blood, such as hemolytic anemia, increase the amount of yellow pigment in the bile, causing jaundice.

 The pigment causing jaundice is called BILIRUBIN. It is derived from hemoglobin that is released when erythrocytes are hemolyzed and therefore is constantly being formed and introduced into the blood as worn-out or defective erythrocytes are destroyed by the body. Normally the liver cells absorb the bilirubin and secrete it along with other bile constituents. If the liver is diseased, or if the flow of bile is obstructed, or if destruction of erythrocytes is excessive, the bilirubin accumulates in the blood and eventually will produce jaundice. A diagnostic test for determination of the level of bilirubin in the blood, called the van den Bergh test, is of value in detecting elevated bilirubin levels at the earliest stages before jaundice appears, when liver disease or hemolytic anemia is suspected.

 acholuric j., jaundice without bile pigments in urine or with only minute quantities of them.

 acute infectious j., infectious hepatitis.

 catarrhal j., infectious hepatitis.

 hemolytic j., a rare, chronic and generally hereditary disease characterized by periods of excessive hemolysis due to abnormal fragility of the erythrocytes, which are small and spheroidal. It is accompanied by enlargement of the spleen and by jaundice. The hereditary or congenital form is known as congenital family icterus, and familial acholuric jaundice; the acquired form is known as acquired hemolytic jaundice.

 hemorrhagic j., leptospiral jaundice.

 hepatocellular j., jaundice caused by injury to or disease of the liver cells.

 homologous serum j., human serum j., serum hepatitis.

 infectious j., infective j., 1. infectious hepatitis. 2. leptospiral jaundice.

 leptospiral j., an acute infectious disease characterized by nephritis, jaundice, fever, muscular pain and enlargement of the liver and spleen, and caused by a spirochete, *Leptospira icterohaemorrhagiae.* The symptoms last from 10 days to 2 weeks and recovery is usually uneventful. Called also Weil's disease.

 obstructive j., that due to an impediment to the flow of bile from the liver to the duodenum.

 physiologic j., mild icterus neonatorum during the first few days after birth.

jaw (jaw) one of the two opposing rigid structures of the mouth of vertebrates, for seizing prey, for biting or for masticating food.

 lumpy j., actinomycosis.

jaw-winking (jaw-wingk'ing) elevation of a congenitally ptotic eyelid when the mouth is opened, giving the appearance of constant winking.

jejunectomy (je″joo-nek'to-me) excision of the jejunum.

jejunitis (je″joo-ni'tis) inflammation of the jejunum.

jejunocecostomy (je-joo″no-se-kos'to-me) anastomosis of the jejunum to the cecum.

jejunocolostomy (je-joo″no-ko-los'to-me) anastomosis of the jejunum to the colon.

jejunoileitis (je-joo″no-il″e-i'tis) inflammation of the jejunum and ileum.

jejunoileostomy (je-joo″no-il″e-os'to-me) anastomosis of the jejunum to the ileum.

jejunojejunostomy (je-joo″no-je″joo-nos'to-me) surgical creation of an anastomosis between two portions of the jejunum.

jejunorrhaphy (je″joo-nor'ah-fe) suture of the jejunum.

jejunostomy (je″joo-nos′to-me) surgical creation of a permanent opening through the abdominal wall to the jejunum.

jejunotomy (je″joo-not′o-me) incision of the jejunum.

jejunum (je-joo′num) the second portion of the small intestine, between the duodenum and the ileum. adj., **jeju′nal.**

jelly (jel′e) an elastic, homogeneous mass.
　cardiac j., a jelly present between the endothelium and myocardium of the embryonic heart that transforms into the connective tissue of the endocardium.
　contraceptive j., a nongreasy jelly used in the vagina for prevention of conception.
　petroleum j., a soft, semisolid substance prepared from petroleum, used as a basis for ointments; petrolatum.
　Wharton's j., the substance of the umbilical cord.

Jenner (jen′er) Edward (1749–1823). English physician. Born at Berkeley, Gloucestershire, he discovered the principle of smallpox vaccination in 1796. By experimental demonstration, Jenner turned a local country tradition that dairymaids who had contracted cowpox did not acquire smallpox into a permanent working principle in science.

jennerian (jĕ-ne′re-an) relating to Edward Jenner, who developed vaccination.

jerk (jerk) a spasmodic muscular movement.
　ankle j., plantar extension of the foot elicited by a tap on the Achilles tendon, preferably while the patient kneels on a bed or chair, the feet hanging free over the edge; called also Achilles reflex and triceps surae reflex.
　biceps j., biceps reflex.
　elbow j., involuntary flexion of the elbow on striking the tendon of the biceps or triceps muscle.

　jaw j., jaw-jerk reflex.
　knee j., contraction of the quadriceps muscle and extension of the leg elicited by tapping the patellar ligament when the leg hangs loosely flexed at a right angle (see also KNEE JERK).
　tendon j., tendon reflex.

joint (joint) the junction of two or more bones of the body. The primary function of a joint is to provide motion and flexibility to the human frame.

Some joints are immovable, such as certain fixed joints where segments of bone are fused together in the skull. Other joints, such as those between the vertebrae, have extremely limited motion. However, most joints allow considerable motion.

Many joints have an extremely complex internal structure. They are composed not merely of ends of bones but also of ligaments, which are tough whitish fibers binding the bones together; cartilage, which is connective tissue covering and cushioning the bone ends; the articular capsule, a fibrous tissue that encloses the ends of the bones; the synovial membrane, which lines the capsule and secretes a lubricating fluid (synovia); and sometimes bursae, which are fluid-filled sacs that cushion the movements of muscles and tendons.

Joints are classified by variations in structure that make different kinds of movement possible. The movable joints are usually subdivided into hinge, pivot, gliding, ball-and-socket, condyloid and saddle joints.

DISEASES AND DISORDERS. Joints are often subject to great stress in day-to-day living; likewise they are exposed daily to injuries of all kinds because of their prominent location on the body. Wrenches and SPRAINS are fairly common. DISLOCATIONS are only slightly less frequent and they may be the aftermath of disease as well as accident.

Joints are also subject to inflammation. The two most prevalent types are OSTEOARTHRITIS, a degenerative joint disorder common to elderly people, and RHEUMATOID ARTHRITIS, which may occur in even the very young and the cause of which is largely unknown. BURSITIS is inflammation of one or more bursae. It may cause pain and partial or

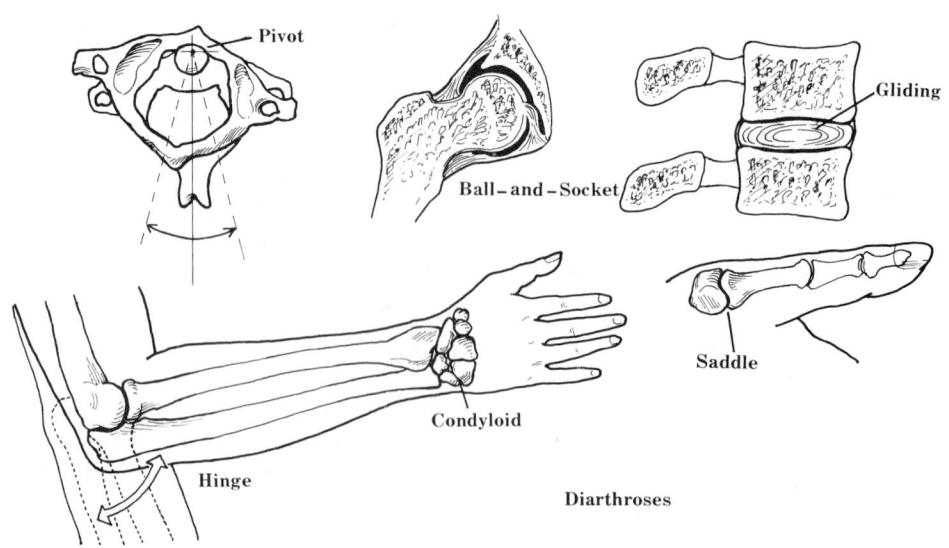

Joints.

complete immobility of the adjacent joint; it may be either acute or chronic. Synovitis, painful inflammation of the lining of the synovial membrane, may be caused either by external injury or by disease, for example, pneumonia, rheumatism or syphilis. ANKYLOSIS is immobility and solidification of a joint.

arthrodial j., gliding joint.

ball-and-socket j., a synovial joint in which the rounded or spheroidal surface of one bone moves within a cup-shaped depression on another bone, allowing greater freedom of movement than any other type of joint.

cartilaginous j., one in which the bones are united by cartilage, providing slight flexible movement; it includes symphysis and synchondrosis.

condyloid j., one in which an ovoid head of one bone moves in an elliptical cavity of another, permitting all movements except axial rotation. Such a joint is found at the wrist, connecting the radius and carpal bones, and at the base of the index finger.

diarthrodial j., synovial joint.

fibrous j., one in which the bones are connected by fibrous tissue and no or very little motion is possible; it includes suture, syndesmosis and gomphosis.

gliding j., a synovial joint in which the opposed surfaces are flat or only slightly curved, so that the bones slide against each other in a simple and limited way. The intervertebral joints are gliding joints, and many of the small bones of the wrist and ankle meet in gliding joints. Called also arthrodial joint and plane joint.

hinge j., a synovial joint that allows movement in only one plane, foreward and backward. Examples are the elbow and the interphalangeal joints of the fingers. The jaw is primarily a hinge joint but it can also move somewhat from side to side. The knee and ankle joints are hinge joints that also allow some rotary movement. Called also ginglymus.

pivot j., a joint that allows only rotary movement; an example is the joint between the first and second cervical vertebrae (the atlas and axis).

plane j., gliding joint.

saddle j., a joint whose movement resembles that of a rider on horseback, who can shift in several directions at will; there is a saddle joint at the base of the thumb, so that the thumb is more flexible and complex than the other fingers, and more difficult to treat if injured.

synarthrodial j., fibrous joint.

synovial j., a specialized form of articulation permitting more or less free movement, the union of the bony elements being surrounded by an articular capsule enclosing a cavity lined by synovial membrane. Called also diarthrosis.

joule (jōol) a unit of work energy, i.e., the work done in moving a body a distance of 1 meter against a force of 1 newton, or the energy expended by a current of 1 ampere flowing for 1 second through a resistance of 1 ohm.

jugal (joo'gal) pertaining to the cheek or zygomatic (cheek) bone.

jugale (joo-ga'le) the point at the angle of the zygomatic bone.

jugular (jug'u-lar) pertaining to the neck.
j. veins, large veins that return blood to the heart from the head and neck.

Each side of the neck has two sets of jugular veins, external and internal. The external jugular carries blood from the face, neck and scalp and has two branches, posterior and anterior. The internal jugular vein receives blood from the brain, the deeper tissues of the neck and the interior of the skull. The external jugular vein empties into the subclavian vein, and the internal jugular vein joins it to form the brachiocephalic vein, which carries the blood to the superior vena cava, where it continues to the heart.

If one of these veins is severed, rapid loss of blood will result and air bubbles may enter the circulatory system unless preventive measures are taken. If such an accident should occur, a compress should be applied to the wound with pressure. Under no circumstance is a tourniquet used.

jugum (joo'gum), pl. *ju'ga* [L.] a depression or ridge connecting two structures.
j. pe'nis, a forceps for compressing the penis.

juice (jōos) any fluid from animal or plant tissue.
gastric j., the secretion of glands in the wall of the stomach (see also GASTRIC JUICE).
intestinal j., the liquid secretion of glands in the intestinal lining.
pancreatic j., the enzyme-containing fluid secreted by the pancreas and conducted through its ducts to the duodenum.

junction (jungk'shun) the place of meeting or coming together.
myoneural j., the point of junction of a nerve fiber with the muscle that it innervates.
sclerocorneal j., the line of union of the sclera and cornea.

junctura (jungk-tu'rah), pl. *junctu'rae* [L.] a junction or joint.

jurisprudence (joor"is-proo'dens) the science of the law.
medical j., the science of the law as applied to the practice of medicine.

juvantia (joo-van'she-ah) adjuvant and palliative medicines.

juvenile (ju've-nīl) pertaining to youth or childhood; young or immature.

juxta-articular (juks"tah-ar-tik'u-lar) in the region of a joint.

juxtaglomerular (juks"tah-glo-mer'u-lar) near to or adjoining a glomerulus of the kidney.

juxtapyloric (juks"tah-pi-lor'ik) near the pylorus.

juxtaspinal (juks"tah-spi'nal) near the vertebral column.

K

K chemical symbol, *potassium* (L. *kalium*).

K., Ka cathode.

Kahler's disease (kah'lerz) multiple myeloma.

Kahn test (kahn) a serologic test for the diagnosis of syphilis.

kainophobia (ki″no-fo′be-ah) morbid fear of new things.

kak- for words beginning thus, see also those beginning *cac-*.

kakidrosis (kak″ĭ-dro′sis) excretion of foul-smelling perspiration.

kakosmia (kak-oz′me-ah) an offensive odor.

kala-azar (kah″lah-ah-zar′) a fatal epidemic fever of tropical Asia, resembling malaria, caused by *Leishmania donovani*, a protozoan parasite. The sandfly is the vector.
SYMPTOMS. Symptoms are usually vague, resembling those of incipient pulmonary tuberculosis. The disease is often confused with malaria. There may be fever, chills, malaise, cough, anorexia and loss of weight. The Leishmania organisms multiply in the cells of the reticuloendothelial system, eventually causing hyperplasia of the cells, especially those of the liver and spleen. Diagnosis is confirmed by demonstration of the parasite.
TREATMENT. The drug of choice is *ethylstibamine*. In some cases that are resistant to this drug, other compounds must be tried.
Bed rest is prescribed for patients debilitated by anemia. A decrease in white cell count (leukopenia) often accompanies the disease, and therefore the patient's resistance to secondary infections is lowered. In some cases transfusion may be necessary to bring blood values back to normal. The patient is given a well balanced diet and liberal amounts of fluids. Special mouth care and attention to the skin are necessary to avoid complications.

kalemia, kaliemia (kah-le′me-ah), (ka″le-e′me-ah) the presence of potassium in the blood.

kaligenous (kah-lij′ĕ-nus) producing potash.

kaliopenia (ka-″le-o-pe′ne-ah) deficiency of potassium in the body.

kalium (ka′le-um) [L.] potassium (symbol K).

kaliuresis (ka″le-u-re′sis) excretion of potassium in the urine.

kaliuretic (ka″le-u-ret′ik) 1. pertaining to or promoting kaliuresis. 2. an agent that promotes kaliuresis.

kallidin (kal′ĭ-din) bradykinin; a type of kinin liberated by the action of kallikrein on a globulin of blood plasma.

kallikrein (kal″ĭ-kre′in) a type of enzyme present in pancreas, saliva, urine, blood plasma, etc., which liberates kallidin (bradykinin) from a globulin of blood plasma and hence has vasodilator and whealing actions.

kallikreinogen (kal″ĭ-kri′no-jen) the inactive precursor of kallikrein which is normally present in blood.

kanamycin (kan″ah-mi′sin) a broad-spectrum antibiotic derived from *Streptomyces kanamyceticus.*

kansasiin (kan-sas′e-in) a product prepared from *Mycobacterium kansasii*, comparable to tuberculin, used in a cutaneous test of hypersensitivity.

Kantrex (kan′treks) trademark for preparations of kanamycin, an antibiotic.

kaolin (ka′o-lin) native hydrated aluminum silicate, powdered and freed from gritty particles by elutriation; used as an adsorbent in diarrhea.

kaolinosis (ka″o-lin-o′sis) pneumoconiosis from inhaling particles of kaolin.

Kaposi's disease (kap′o-sēz) 1. xeroderma pigmentosum. 2. Kaposi's varicelliform eruption. 3. Kaposi's sarcoma.
K's **sarcoma,** multiple soft, bluish nodules of the skin with hemorrhages, which may become neoplastic.
K's **varicelliform eruption,** a vesiculopustular skin disorder of viral origin, superimposed upon a pre-existing eczema.

Kappadione (kap″ah-di′ōn) trademark for preparations of menadiol sodium diphosphate, used to promote the formation of prothrombin.

karyo- (kar′e-o) word element [Gr.], *nucleus.*

karyoblast (kar′e-o-blast″) a cell at the beginning of the erythrocytic series.

karyochromatophil (kar″e-o-kro-mat′o-fil) 1. having a stainable nucleus. 2. a cell with an easily staining nucleus.

karyochrome (kar′e-o-krōm″) a nerve cell with an easily staining nucleus.

karyoclasis (kar″e-ok′lah-sis) the breaking down of a cell nucleus.

karyocyte (kar′e-o-sīt″) 1. a nucleated cell. 2. an early normoblast.

karyogamy (kar″e-og′ah-me) cell conjugation with union of nuclei.

karyogenesis (kar″e-o-jen′ĕ-sis) the formation of a cell nucleus.

karyokinesis (kar″e-o-ki-ne′sis) division of the nucleus of a cell in the formation of daughter cells.

karyolymph (kar′e-o-limf″) the fluid portion of

the nucleus of a cell, in which the other elements are dispersed.

karyolysis (kar″e-ol′ĭ-sis) the dissolution of the nucleus of a cell.

karyomegaly (kar″e-o-meg′ah-le) abnormal enlargement of the nucleus of a cell, not caused by polyploidy.

karyomere (kar′e-o-mēr″) 1. chromomere (1). 2. a vesicle containing only a small portion of the typical nucleus, usually after abnormal mitosis.

karyomitome (kar″e-om′ĭ-tōm) the nuclear chromatin network.

karyomitosis (kar″e-o-mi-to′sis) mitosis.

karyomorphism (kar″e-o-mor′fizm) the shape of a cell nucleus.

karyon (kar′e-on) the nucleus of a cell.

karyophage (kar′e-o-fāj″) an intracellular sporozoon.

karyoplasm (kar′e-o-plazm″) the protoplasm of a cell contained within the nuclear membrane; called also nucleoplasm.

karyopyknosis (kar″e-o-pik-no′sis) shrinkage of a cell nucleus, with condensation of the chromatin.

karyorrhexis (kar″e-o-rek′sis) fragmentation of the nucleus of a cell.

karyosome (kar′e-o-sōm″) a spherical mass of chromatin in the cell nucleus.

karyostasis (kar″e-os′tah-sis) the so-called resting stage of the nucleus between mitotic divisions.

karyotheca (kar″e-o-the′kah) the nuclear membrane.

karyotype (kar′e-o-tīp″) the chromosomal elements typical of a cell, arranged according to the Denver classification and drawn in their true proportions, based on the average of measurements determined in a number of cells (see also CHROMOSOME).

kat(a)- (kat′ah) word element [Gr.], *down; against*. See also words beginning *cat(a)-*.

katathermometer (kat″ah-ther-mom′ĕ-ter) a thermometer for showing decrease in temperature.

kelis (ke′lis) 1. keloid. 2. morphea.

keloid (ke′loid) a scarlike growth that rises above the skin surface, and is rounded, hard, shiny and white, or sometimes pink. A keloid is a benign tumor that has its origin usually in a scar from surgery or a burn or other injury. Keloids are generally considered harmless and noncancerous, although they may produce contractures. Ordinarily they cause no trouble beyond an occasional itching sensation.

Surgical removal is not usually effective because it results in a high rate of recurrence. However, radium and x-ray therapy often are of substantial help, provided care is taken not to destroy the surrounding healthy tissue.

keloidosis (ke″loi-do′sis) a condition marked by the formation of keloids.

keloma (ke-lo′ma) a keloid.

keloplasty (ke′lo-plas″te) any plastic operation on a scar.

kelotomy (ke-lot′o-me) relief of hernial strangulation by cutting.

Kemadrin (kem′ah-drin) trademark for a preparation of tricyclamol, an anticholinergic.

Kempner rice diet (kemp′ner) a special diet restricted to 10 oz. of rice daily, supplemented only by liberal quantities of sugar and fresh or preserved fruits, formerly used for hypertensive vascular disease and kidney disease.

Kenacort (ken′ah-kort) trademark for preparations of triamcinolone, a corticosteroid.

Kenalog (ken′ah-log) trademark for preparations of triamcinolone acetonide, a corticosteroid.

Kenny treatment (ken′e) treatment of poliomyelitis by wrapping the patient in woolen cloths wrung out of hot water and reeducating muscles by passive exercises after pain has subsided.

keno- (ken′o) word element [Gr.], *empty*.

kenophobia (ke″no-fo′be-ah) morbid dread of large open spaces.

kenotoxin (ke″no-tok′sin) a toxin produced by muscular contraction.

kerasin (ker′ah-sin) a cerebroside containing lignoceric acid.

kerat(o)- (ker′ah-to) word element [Gr.], *horny tissue; cornea*.

keratalgia (ker″ah-tal′je-ah) pain in the cornea.

keratectasia (ker″ah-tek-ta′ze-ah) protrusion of the cornea.

keratectomy (ker″ah-tek′to-me) excision of a portion of the cornea.

keratiasis (ker″ah-ti′ah-sis) the presence of horny warts on the skin.

keratic (kĕ-rat′ik) pertaining to horn; horny.

keratin (ker′ah-tin) a scleroprotein that is the principal constituent of epidermis, hair, nails, horny tissues and the organic matrix of the enamel of the teeth. Its solution is sometimes used in coating pills when the latter are desired to pass through the stomach unchanged.

keratinization (ker″ah-tin″ĭ-za′shun) formation of microscopic fibrils of keratin in the keratinocytes.

keratinocyte (kĕ-rat′ĭ-no-sīt″) the cell of the epidermis that synthesizes keratin, known in its successive stages in the various layers of the skin as basal cell, prickle cell and granular cell.

keratinous (kĕ-rat′ĭ-nus) composed of keratin.

keratitis (ker″ah-ti′tis) inflammation of the cornea. Keratitis may be deep, when the infection causing it is carried in the blood or spreads to the cornea from other parts of the eye, or superficial, caused by bacteria or virus infection or by allergic reaction. Microorganisms causing the inflammation can be introduced into the cornea during the removal of foreign bodies from the eye. All infections of the eye are potentially serious because opaque fibrous tissue or scar tissue may form on the cornea during the healing process and cause partial or total loss of vision.

CAUSES. There are several kinds of keratitis. Dendritic keratitis is a viral form caused by the herpes simplex virus; it usually affects only one eye. A bacterial form, acute serpiginous keratitis, may result from infection by pneumococci, streptococci or staphylococci. Some kinds of keratitis — dendritic keratitis, for example — may follow symptoms of upper respiratory tract infection, such as fever.

Burns of the cornea, such as those produced by chemicals or ultraviolet rays, also give rise to a form of keratitis. In trachoma, a contagious disease of the conjunctiva, the eyes become inflamed, and small, gritty particles develop on the cornea. Herpetic keratitis may accompany herpes zoster.

Interstitial keratitis is often caused by congenital syphilis, although occasionally it may also result from acquired syphilis. When caused by congenital syphilis, the disease usually appears when the child is between the ages of 5 and 15. In rare cases, interstitial keratitis may also stem from tuberculosis or rheumatic infection in other parts of the body.

SYMPTOMS. Symptoms vary somewhat among the different forms of keratitis, but pain, which may be severe, and inability to tolerate light (photophobia) are usual. There may also be considerable effusion of tears and a conjunctival discharge.

TREATMENT. Antibiotics are the usual treatment for keratitis caused by an infectious organism. Cortisone is used for other forms, but may be dangerous in some patients. A new compound, idoxuridine, has given promising results in dendritic keratitis. In cases of syphilitic interstitial keratitis, the syphilis is treated. Congenital interstitial keratitis can be prevented if syphilis is detected early in pregnancy by means of blood tests, and the mother is treated.

keratoacanthoma (ker″ah-to-ak″an-tho′mah) a rapidly growing papular lesion with a superficial crater filled with a keratin plug, usually on the face.

keratocele (ker′ah-to-sēl″) hernial protrusion of the innermost layer of the cornea.

keratocentesis (ker″ah-to-sen-te′sis) puncture of the cornea.

keratoconjunctivitis (ker″ah-to-kon-junk″tĭ-vi′-tis) inflammation of the cornea and conjunctiva.

epidemic k., an acute viral infection of the eye, with systemic symptoms and occurring in epidemics.

k. sic′ca, a condition marked by hyperemia of the conjunctiva, thickening and drying of the corneal epithelium and itching and burning of the eye.

keratoconus (ker″ah-to-ko′nus) conical protrusion of the central part of the cornea, resulting in an irregular astigmatism.

keratocyte (ker′ah-to-sīt″) one of the flattened connective tissue cells between the lamellae of fibrous tissue composing the cornea, with branch-

ing processes that intercommunicate with those of other cells.

keratoderma (ker″ah-to-der′mah) hypertrophy of the stratum corneum of the skin.

k. blennorha′gica, a symptom complex characterized by peculiar crusted, hornlike lesions on hands and feet and sometimes elsewhere.

k. climacter′icum, endocrine k., circumscribed hyperkeratosis of palms and soles, occurring in menopausal women.

keratodermatitis (ker″ah-to-der″mah-ti′tis) inflammation of the skin associated with hypertrophy of the stratum corneum.

keratodermia (ker″ah-to-der′me-ah) keratoderma.

keratogenous (ker″ah-toj′ĕ-nus) producing horny tissue, or keratin.

keratoglobus (ker″ah-to-glo′bus) prominent globular protrusion of the cornea.

keratohelcosis (ker″ah-to-hel-ko′sis) ulceration of the cornea.

keratoid (ker′ah-toid) resembling horn; hornlike.

keratoiditis (ker″ah-toi-di′tis) keratitis.

keratoiridoscope (ker″ah-to-i-rid′o-skōp) a compound microscope for examining the eye.

keratoiritis (ker″ah-to-i-ri′tis) inflammation of the cornea and iris.

keratoleptynsis (ker″ah-to-lep-tin′sis) removal of the anterior thickness of the cornea and covering the denuded area with conjunctiva.

keratoleukoma (ker″ah-to-lu-ko′mah) white opacity of the cornea.

keratolysis (ker″ah-tol′ĭ-sis) separation of the stratum corneum of the epidermis.

keratolytic (ker″ah-to-lit′ik) 1. pertaining to or promoting keratolysis. 2. an agent that promotes keratolysis.

keratoma (ker″ah-to′mah) any growth of horny tissue.

keratomalacia (ker″ah-to-mah-la′she-ah) softening of cornea.

keratome (ker′ah-tōm) a knife for incising the cornea.

keratometer (ker″ah-tom′ĕ-ter) an instrument for measuring the curves of the cornea.

keratometry (ker″ah-tom′ĕ-tre) measurement of corneal curves.

keratomycosis (ker″ah-to-mi-ko′sis) fungus disease of the cornea.

keratonosis (ker″ah-to-no′sis) any disease of the horny structure of the epidermis.

keratonyxis (ker″ah-to-nik′sis) puncture of the cornea.

keratopathy (ker″ah-top′ah-the) noninflammatory disease of the cornea.

band k., a condition characterized by an abnormal circumcorneal band.

keratoplasty (ker'ah-to-plas"te) plastic surgery of the cornea.

   optic k., transplantation of corneal material to replace scar tissue that interferes with vision.

   tectonic k., transplantation of corneal material to replace tissue that has been lost.

keratoprotein (ker"ah-to-pro'te-in) the protein of the horny tissues of the body, such as the hair, nails and epidermis.

keratorhexis (ker"ah-to-rek'sis) rupture of the cornea.

keratoscleritis (ker"ah-to-sklĕ-ri'tis) inflammation of cornea and sclera.

keratoscope (ker'ah-to-skōp") an instrument for examining the cornea.

keratosis (ker"ah-to'sis) formation of horny growth or tissue. adj., **keratot'ic.**

   k. follicula'ris, a rare hereditary condition manifested by areas of crusting, verrucous papular growths, usually occurring symmetrically on the trunk, axillae, neck, face, scalp and retroauricular areas.

   k. palma'ris et planta'ris, a disease marked by thickening of the skin of the palms and soles.

   k. pharynge'us, horny projections from the tonsils and pharyngeal walls.

   k. pila'ris, formation of a hard elevation around each hair follicle.

   k. puncta'ta, keratosis occurring as small spots or points.

   seborrheic k., k. seborrhe'ica, formation of a small, sharply marginated, yellowish or brownish lesion, covered by a thin, greasy scale.

   k. seni'lis, a harsh, dry state of the skin in old age.

keratotomy (ker"ah-tot'o-me) incision of the cornea.

keraunophobia (kĕ-raw"no-fo'be-ah) morbid dread of lightning.

kerectomy (kĕ-rek'to-me) removal of a part of the cornea.

kerion (ke're-on) a pustular disease of the scalp.

kernicterus (ker-nik'ter-us) a condition in the newborn marked by severe neural symptoms, associated with high levels of bilirubin in the blood.

Kernig's sign (ker'nigz) in the dorsal decubitus position the patient can easily and completely extend the leg; in the sitting posture or when lying with the thigh flexed upon the abdomen the leg cannot be completely extended; it is a sign of meningeal irritation.

keto- (ke'to) word element denoting the possession of the carbonyl group ($>C:O$).

keto acids (ke'to) compounds containing the groups CO (carbonyl) and COOH (carboxyl).

ketogenesis (ke"to-jen'ĕ-sis) the production of ketones (ketone bodies).

ketogenic (ke"to-jen'ik) conducive to the production of ketones (ketone bodies).

   k. diet, one containing large amounts of fat, with minimal amounts of protein and carbohydrate; used sometimes in the treatment of epilepsy.

ketolysis (ke-tol'ĭ-sis) the splitting up of ketone bodies.

ketone (ke'tōn) a chemical compound characterized by the presence of the bivalent carbonyl group ($>C:O$).

   k. bodies, substances synthesized by the liver as a step in the combustion of fats; they are beta-oxybutyric acid, acetoacetic acid and acetone. Called also acetone bodies.

   Initially, the combustion of fatty acids produces ketones, which eventually are broken down into carbon dioxide and water by the liver and other tissues of the body. Under abnormal conditions, such as uncontrolled DIABETES MELLITUS, starvation or the intake of a diet composed almost entirely of fat, the breakdown of fatty acids may be halted at the ketone stage, causing increasing levels of ketone bodies in the blood. This condition is called KETOSIS and is directly related to improper utilization or inadequate supplies of carbohydrates, which are necessary for proper combustion of fats.

ketonemia (ke"to-ne'me-ah) the presence of ketone bodies in the blood.

ketonuria (ke"to-nu're-ah) the presence of excessive amounts of ketone bodies in the urine.

ketose (ke'tōs) a sugar that contains the ketone radical ($>C:O$).

ketosis (ke"to'sis) the accumulation of large quantities of ketone bodies in the body tissues and fluids. adj., **ketot'ic.** Ketosis is the result of incomplete combustion of fatty acids, which in turn is the result of improper utilization of, or lack of availability of, carbohydrates. When carbohydrates cannot be used as the source of energy, the body draws on its supply of fats. Deficiency of carbohydrates triggers several hormonal responses and greatly increases the removal of fatty acids from fatty tissues. As a result, large quantities of fatty acids must be oxidized, more in fact than the body cells can handle; thus their oxidation is incomplete and ketones accumulate in the blood and tissues.

   Ketosis may result in severe ACIDOSIS because the ketone bodies beta-oxybutyric acid and acetoacetic acid decrease the blood pH and, more important, because when the keto acids are excreted in the urine they take with them large quantities of sodium. The result is a depletion of the alkaline part of the body's buffer system, so that the acid-base balance is upset in favor of acidosis.

   Ketosis occurs in uncontrolled DIABETES MELLITUS because carbohydrates are not properly utilized, and in starvation because carbohydrates simply are not available for utilization. Ketosis is sometimes produced intentionally in the treatment of epilepsy by means of the ketogenic diet, which contains large amounts of fat and little carbohydrate and protein.

   The patient with ketosis often has a sweet or "fruity" odor to his breath. This is produced by acetone, a ketone body that is highly volatile and is blown off in small amounts with air expired from the lungs. Although ketosis can give rise to acidosis, acidosis can occur without any corresponding ketosis.

ketosteroid (ke"to-ste'roid) a steroid that contains the ketone radical ($>C:O$).

   17-k., a steroid with a ketone radical on the seventeenth carbon atom; normally found in human urine and occurring in excessive amounts in certain pathologic conditions.

ketosuria (ke"to-su're-ah) ketose in the urine.

kev kilo (1000) electron volts (3.82×10^{-17} gram (small) calories, or 1.6×10^{-9} ergs).

kg. kilogram.

kg.-m. kilogram-meter.

kidney (kid'ne) one of two glandular organs, almost bean-shaped, located in the lumbar region, that secrete urine. Their function is to regulate the content of water and other substances in the blood, and to remove from the blood various wastes. PHYSIOLOGY. In an average adult each kidney is about 4 inches long, 2 inches wide and 1 inch thick, and weighs 4 to 6 oz. In this small area the kidney contains over a million microscopic filtering units, the NEPHRONS. Blood arrives at the kidney by way of the renal artery, and is distributed through arterioles into many millions of capillaries which lead into the nephrons. Fluids and dissolved salts in the blood pass through the walls of the capillaries and are collected within the central capsule of each nephron, the malpighian capsule. The glomerulus, a tuft of capillaries within the capsule, acts as a semipermeable membrane permitting a protein-free ultrafiltrate of plasma to pass through. This filtrate is forced into hairpin-shaped collecting channels in the nephrons, called tubules. Capillaries in the walls of the tubules reabsorb the water and the salts required by the body and deliver them to a system of small kidney veins which, in turn, carry them into the renal vein and return them to the general circulation. Excess water and other waste materials remain in the tubules as urine. The urine contains, besides water, a quantity of urea, uric acid, yellow pigments, amino acids and trace metals. The urine moves through a system of ducts into a collecting funnel (renal pelvis) in each kidney, whence it is led into the two ureters.

KIDNEY
(partly in hemisection)

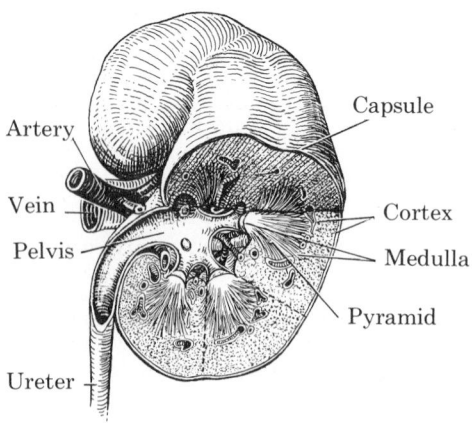

Artery

Capsule

Vein

Pelvis

Cortex

Medulla

Pyramid

Ureter

Kidney. (From Dorland's Illustrated Medical Dictionary. 24th ed. Philadelphia, W. B. Saunders Co., 1965.)

Filtering Capacity. About 1½ quarts (1500 cc.) of urine are excreted daily by the average adult. The efficiency of the normal kidney is one of the most remarkable aspects of the body. It has a filtering capacity of a quart of blood per minute—that is, 15 gallons per hour, or 360 gallons per day. Ordinarily it draws off from the blood about 180 quarts of fluid daily, and returns usually 98 to 99 per cent of the water plus the useful dissolved salts, according to the body's changing needs.

Maintaining Salt and Water Balance. The development of kidneys was an essential step in the evolution of species that could live in fresh water and eventually on dry land. The kidneys still preserve a salt-water environment inside the body, maintaining the proper balance between the salts (ELECTROLYTES) and water. If the water becomes excessive, salt will continue to be returned to the blood while more of the water is excreted in the urine. The opposite happens if there is an excess of salts. Similarly, the kidneys regulate the amount of potassium in the blood. These functions of the kidneys are controlled by hormones.

Maintaining Acid-Base Balance. The kidneys help control the body's acidity by converting some of the amino acids into ammonia, an alkaline chemical. The kidneys also manufacture enzymes that aid in this conversion.

DISORDERS OF THE KIDNEYS. Disorders of the kidney include inflammation, infection, obstruction, structural defects, injuries, calculus formation and tumors.

PYELITIS is an inflammation of the renal pelvis. When the inflammation reaches deeper portions of the kidneys, it is called pyelonephritis.

NEPHRITIS is widespread inflammation of the kidney, usually affecting the inner mesh of capillaries (glomeruli). It appears to be caused in certain cases by an allergic reaction to certain varieties of streptococci. NEPHROSIS (called also the nephrotic syndrome) is a noninflammatory condition in which the kidneys lose their control over the water content of the blood, producing widespread edema.

When the kidneys are so badly damaged that they can no longer remove urea and other waste products from the blood, a condition called UREMIA develops. It has many causes, such as severe trauma to the kidney, nephritis, chronic pyelonephritis, hypertension, severe gout, renal calculi with infection, overdose of vitamin D and diabetes mellitus.

Kidney infection is potentially serious. Many disorders can be completely cured if treated early. Unchecked infection can destroy the organs and lead to uremia. Failure of both kidneys may result in death, because no other organ can eliminate waste products of the blood. Fortunately, one kidney or even less than half a kidney is capable of performing the task of purification. Hence a diseased kidney can be removed, and the other will carry on the function. If both must be removed—a rare circumstance—or if both are destroyed by disease, the only hope is the use of an artifical kidney. Recently attempts have been made to transplant a kidney from one person to another, with some success.

Antibiotics and other medicines are prescribed for many kidney diseases caused by infection. In a kidney disorder stemming from such diseases as tuberculosis or diabetes mellitus, the underlying disease must also be treated. The kidneys are also subject to cancer.

The formation of kidney stones or calculi, may occur as a result of a metabolic disorder or from the excess concentration of a substance such as calcium in the blood. The salts in solution in the urine may also crystallize around small fragments of matter.

Structural defects in kidneys may be congenital or acquired. A kidney may be displaced, fused, malformed or totally absent. Floating kidney, or NEPHROPTOSIS, is a condition in which the kidney is displaced, usually to a position somewhat lower than normal. This condition may be corrected by a surgical procedure called NEPHROPEXY.

SURGERY OF THE KIDNEY. Surgical removal of the kidney is called nephrectomy, and is done when the kidney is unable to function because of severe disease or injury. Fortunately, one kidney or even less than half a kidney is capable of performing the necessary task of eliminating waste products of the blood.

When obstruction prevents an adequate flow of urine from the kidney, nephrostomy may be performed. This procedure involves a surgical incision into the pelvis of the kidney and usually includes the insertion of a tube or catheter so that drainage can be established. Removal of large kidney stones may entail a "splitting" of the kidney; that is, an incision is made from one end of the kidney to the other. Removal of a calculus from the pelvis of the kidney is known as a pyelolithotomy. If the stone is located in the upper ureter it is removed by a procedure known as a ureterolithotomy. This operation involves an abdominal incision but the kidney is not incised.

Nursing Care. The site of the incision for surgery of the kidney creates special nursing problems. The incision is referred to as a flank incision and, because it is directly below the diaphragm, deep breathing, coughing and other measures necessary to prevent pulmonary complications are extremely painful and difficult for the patient. Narcotic drugs that relieve pain are usually ordered to be given every 4 hours so that coughing and deep breathing can be done. In addition to these measures, the patient should be turned from side to side and encouraged to get out of bed as soon as ordered by the physician.

If a nephrostomy tube has been inserted, care must be taken that it does not kink while the patient is lying in bed. When he moves about there should be enough slack in the connecting tubes so that there is no tension exerted on the nephrostomy tube. It should be remembered that any type of CATHETER or drainage tube inserted during surgery of the kidney or ureters has been left in place for the purpose of drainage. Those responsible for the postoperative care of the patient must constantly be alert to the possibility of obstruction of catheters or tubes, or their accidental removal. In either case the surgeon should be notified immediately so that steps can be taken to reestablish drainage and prevent serious damage to the kidney.

In most cases when a nephrectomy has been done, a Penrose drain is left in place to facilitate removal of serous material collecting in the space left by the kidney. There will, of course, be no urine in this drainage. It may be blood tinged at first, but should not continue to be bright red in color; if it does, it may indicate hemorrhage and should be reported immediately. The amount, color, consistency and odor of drainage should be noted and recorded on the patient's chart. Dressings may be changed or reinforced as necessary to keep the patient dry and comfortable. A sterile safety pin may be attached to the end of the drain to keep it in place. The drain must not be compressed by the weight of the patient's body. Small pillows are used to support the area around the drain when the patient is lying on the operative side.

Abdominal distention frequently occurs after renal surgery. Fluids by mouth should be given slowly at first until there is evidence that peristalsis is normal. Warm fluids are preferred to iced drinks. Citrus fruit juices and milk are usually contraindicated. A rectal tube and medications to stimulate peristalsis are often ordered to facilitate the passage of flatus.

Hemorrhage is likely to occur after kidney surgery, especially when the highly vascular parenchyma has been incised. The times at which hemorrhage is most likely to occur are the day of surgery and 8 to 12 days after surgery when there is sloughing of tissue during the healing process. Dressings should be observed frequently and any undue drainage of bright red blood must be reported immediately.

amyloid k., one affected with amyloid degeneration.

artificial k., a device used as a substitute for nonfunctioning kidneys to remove endogenous metabolites from the blood, or as an emergency measure to remove exogenous poisons such as bromides or barbiturates. Originally the artificial kidney was used only as a temporary substitute until the kidneys could recover and resume normal function. With the development of a new type of cannula that is a semipermanent appliance in the patient's arm, it is now possible to treat patients with chronic renal failure.

There are several types of artificial kidneys available but all require the same basic components and all employ the principle of a semipermeable membrane through which dialysis takes place. The artificial kidney utilizes a cellophane membrane, the patient's blood and a wash or dialyzing solution. The blood usually is removed from the brachial or radial artery and continuously recirculated through the dialyzing tube, which is immersed in the dialyzing solution. This solution is of lower concentration than the patient's blood, and so the solutes in the blood pass through the membrane into the dialyzing solution, until an equilibrium is achieved. Thus are waste products or toxins, or both, removed from the patient's blood.

Artificial kidney: schematic drawing showing the tips of the cannula within the vein and artery. (From Fellows, B. J.: The role of the nurse in a chronic dialysis unit. Nursing Clin. N. Amer., *1*:577, 1966.)

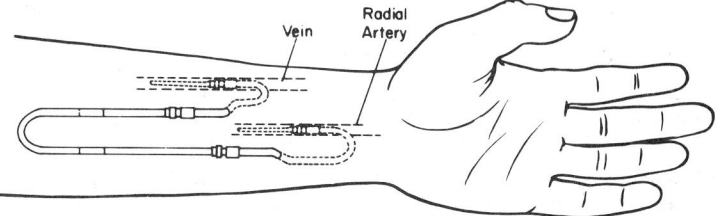

This procedure is sometimes called hemodialysis because the dialysis takes place between the patient's blood and the dialyzing solution. Another method is PERITONEAL DIALYSIS, in which the dialyzing membrane is the membrane lining the peritoneal cavity, and the dialyzing solution is introduced into the peritoneal cavity.

Patients treated by the artificial kidney are given heparin before treatment is begun so that there will be no clotting of blood during the procedure. In peritoneal dialysis no anticoagulation is necessary.

cicatricial k., a shriveled, irregular and scarred kidney due to suppurative pyelonephritis.

cirrhotic k., contracted k., granular kidney.

fatty k., one affected with fatty degeneration.

floating k., one that is loosened and displaced (see also NEPHROPTOSIS).

fused k., a single anomalous organ developed as a result of fusion of the renal primordia.

granular k., one affected with chronic interstitial inflammation.

horseshoe k., an anomalous organ resulting from fusion of the corresponding poles of the renal primordia.

lump k., a solid, irregularly lobed organ of bizarre shape resulting from fusion of the kidney primordia in the embryo.

medullary sponge k., a large, smooth kidney with dilated collecting tubules.

polycystic k., a congenital condition of nodular (cystic) enlargement, usually involving both kidneys.

small white k., an atrophied and degenerated state of the kidney following chronic interstitial nephritis.

sponge k., medullary sponge kidney.

wandering k., floating kidney.

waxy k., amyloid kidney.

Kienböck's disease (kēn'beks) chronic osteitis of the lunate bone.

kilo- (kil'o) word element [Gr.], *one thousand;* used in naming units of measurement to designate an amount 10^3 times the size of the unit to which it is joined.

kilogram (kil'o-gram) a unit of mass (weight) of the metric system, 1000 grams; equivalent to 15,432 grains, or 2.205 pounds (avoirdupois) or 2.679 pounds (apothecaries' weight); abbreviated kg.

kilogram-meter (kil'o-gram-me"ter) a unit of work, representing the energy required to raise 1 kg. of weight 1 meter vertically against gravitational force.

kiloliter (kil'o-le"ter) one thousand liters; 264 gallons.

kilometer (kil'o-me"ter) one thousand meters; five-eighths of a mile.

kilounit (kil"o-u'nit) a quantity equivalent to one thousand (10^3) units.

kilovolt (kil'o-volt) one thousand volts.

Kimmelstiel-Wilson syndrome (kim'el-stēl wil'son) intercapillary glomerulosclerosis, with diabetes mellitus, nephrosis and gross albuminuria.

kinanesthesia (kin"an-es-the'ze-ah) loss of the power of perceiving sensations of movement.

kinase (ki'nās) 1. an enzyme that catalyzes the transfer of a high-energy group of a donor to an acceptor. 2. an enzyme that activates a zymogen.

kine- (kin'e) word element [Gr.], *movement.* See also words beginning *cine-.*

kinematics (kin"ĕ-mat'iks) that phase of mechanics which deals with the possible motions of a material body.

kinematograph (kin"ĕ-mat'o-graf) an instrument for showing pictures of objects in motion.

kinemia (ki-ne'me-ah) cardiac output.

kineplasty (kin'ĕ-plas"te) plastic amputation; amputation in which the stump is so formed as to be utilized for motor purposes.

kinergety (kin-er'jĕ-te) the capacity for kinetic energy.

kinesalgia (kin"ĕ-sal'je-ah) pain on muscular exertion.

kinescope (kin'ĕ-skōp) an instrument for ascertaining ocular refraction.

kinesi(o)- (ki-ne'se-o) word element [Gr.], *movement.*

kinesia (ki-ne'ze-ah) motion sickness.

kinesialgia (ki-ne"se-al'je-ah) kinesalgia.

kinesiatrics (ki-ne"se-at'riks) kinesitherapy.

kinesimeter (kin"ĕ-sim'ĕ-ter) instrument for quantitative measurement of motions.

kinesiology (ki-ne"se-ol'o-je) scientific study of movement of body parts.

-kinesis (ki-ne'sis) word element [Gr.], *movement.*

kinesitherapy (ki-ne"sĭ-ther'ah-pe) treatment of disease by movements.

kinesthesia (kin"es-the'ze-ah) the sense by which one is aware of position and movement of various body parts. adj., **kinesthet'ic.**

kinesthesiometer (kin"es-the"ze-om'ĕ-ter) an apparatus for testing kinesthesia.

kinesthesis (kin"es-the'sis) kinesthesia.

kinetia (ki-ne'te-ah) kinetosis.

kinetic (ki-net'ik) pertaining to or producing motion.

kineticist (ki-net'i-sist) a specialist in kinetics.

kinetics (ki-net'iks) the scientific study of the turnover, or rate of change, of a specific factor in the body, commonly expressed as units of amount per unit time.

chemical k., the scientific study of the rates at which chemical reactions occur.

kinetocardiogram (ki-ne"to-kar'de-o-gram") the record produced by kinetocardiography.

kinetocardiography (ki-ne"to-kar"de-og'rah-fe) graphic recording of the slow vibrations of the chest wall in the region of the heart, representing the absolute motion at a given point on the chest.

kinetochore (ki-ne'to-kōr) a clear region where the arms of a chromosome meet.

kinetogenic (ki-ne″to-jen′ik) causing or producing movement.

kinetoplasm (ki-ne′to-plazm) the most highly contractile portion of the cytoplasm of a cell; the energy plasm; the term is applied to the chromatophilic elements in the nervous tissue.

kinetosis (ki″ne-to′sis) any disorder due to unaccustomed motion.

kinetotherapy (ki-ne″to-ther′ah-pe) kinesitherapy.

kingdom (king′dum) one of the three major categories into which natural objects are usually classified: the animal (including all animals), plant (including all plants) and mineral (including all substance and objects without life).

kinin (ki′nin) an endogenous peptide that acts on blood vessels, smooth muscles and nociceptive nerve endings, such as bradykinin.
  venom k., a peptide found in the venom of insects.

kink (kingk) a bend or twist.
  ileal k., Lane's k., obstruction of the terminal portion of the small intestine.

kinocilium (ki″no-sil′e-um), pl. *kinocil′ia,* a motile, protoplasmic filament on the free surface of a cell.

kinoplasm (ki′no-plazm) the specific kinetic or motor substance of a cell; functional protoplasm. Called also ergoplasm.

kinotoxin (ki″no-tok′sin) a toxin produced as a result of fatigue.

kiotomy (ki-ot′o-me) excision of the vulva.

Kirschner wire (kērsh′ner) a steel wire for skeletal transfixion of fractured bones and for obtaining skeletal traction in fractures. It is inserted through the soft parts and the bone and held tight in a clamp.

kl. kiloliter.

Klebs-Löffler bacillus (klebz lef′ler) the diphtheria bacillus, *Corynebacterium diphtheriae.*

Klebsiella (kleb″se-el′ah) a genus of Schizomycetes frequently found in the respiratory or intestinal tract in man.
  K. friedlan′deri, K. pneumo′niae, an organism occurring in patients with lobar pneumonia and other infections of the respiratory tract.

kleptomania (klep″to-ma′ne-ah) an abnormal, uncontrollable desire to steal. This should not be confused with the stage children naturally go through before they understand the concept of ownership. Repeated stealing by an older child may be done simply for the sake of adventure, or it may be an indication of emotional disturbance.
  In an adult, the uncontrollable impulse to steal arises from a serious psychologic problem, or neurosis. Since the impulse is an irrational one rooted in subconscious needs of which the person who steals is not aware, he often does not actually covet the object he steals. Sometimes the impulse is expressed by ostensibly borrowing an object and not returning it.

Kline test (klīn) a serologic test performed for the diagnosis of syphilis.

Klinefelter's syndrome (klīn fel-terz) a condition characterized by the presence of small testes, with fibrosis and hyalinization of seminiferous tubules, without involvement of the interstitial cells of the testes, and by increase in urinary gonadotropins; associated with an abnormality of the sex chromosomes.

Klippel-Feil disease (klī-pel′ fīl) arthritic general pseudoparalysis.

knee (ne) a complex hinge joint, one of the largest joints of the body, and one that sustains great pressure. The knee is formed by the head of the tibia, the lower end of the femur and the patella, or kneecap. The bones are joined by ligaments, and the patella is secured to the adjacent bones by powerful tendons. The fibula is attached at the side of the knee to the tibia. Crescent-shaped pads of cartilage lying on top of the tibia cushion it from the femur and form the gliding surfaces of the joint in motion.
  Further cushioning is supplied by bursae, which are located around the main joint, between it and the patella and on the outside of the patella. A cap-

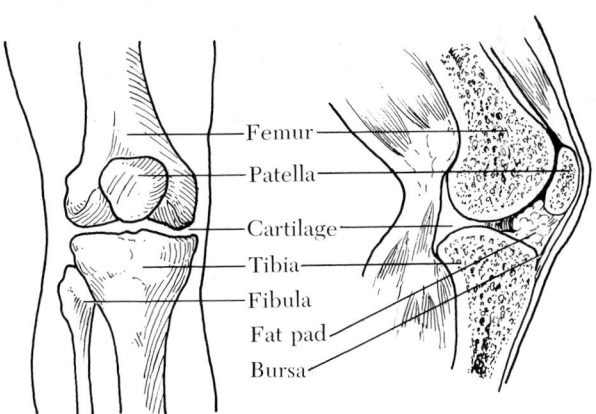

Femur
Patella
Cartilage
Tibia
Fibula
Fat pad
Bursa

Left: knee joint, front view. Right: knee joint, flexed, in profile.

sule of ligaments binds the whole assembly to-gether. The capsule is lined with synovial mem-brane, which secretes a lubricating fluid (synovia) that makes possible a smooth, gliding motion.

DISORDERS OF THE KNEE. Twists and wrenches of the knee may result from a blow or from pres-sure. If the injury is followed by swelling and sore-ness, rest and heat are usually helpful. An elastic bandage may be helpful to bolster the knee against further stress and strain. If symptoms are severe or persistent, they should be reported to a physician.

HOUSEMAID'S KNEE results from frequent kneel-ing on hard surfaces, causing injury to the front of the knee and inflammation of the bursa in front of the patella.

Water on the knee is an excessive accumulation of synovia within the knee joint. The condition may follow a knee injury or result from an infec-tion or acute arthritis. The patella is raised or "floats" on the accumulated fluid, and there is general swelling around the knee. In most cases, the effusion subsides if the joint is rested.

The knee is subject to many joint inflammations that come under the general heading of ARTHRITIS. When the knee is severely inflamed, the patient is confined to bed, and the knee is bound and splinted to rest the joint.

The knee is subject to bone and joint injuries, including DISLOCATION, SPRAIN and FRACTURE. A fractured patella without wide separation of the parts is often treated by immobilization of the leg for several weeks with a cast or splint, so that the parts can grow together. The surgeon extracts with a needle or syringe the excess blood or fluid that has accumulated in the knee. If the injury is a complicated one, with wide separation of the parts, the parts may be bound together surgically with fine steel wire or similar material. Torn soft tissues are sewed together, and the knee is immobilized in a plaster cast for 4 or 5 weeks.

Trick knee is a colloquial term referring to a knee that is highly susceptible to injury and that may constantly or intermittently give trouble. It often occurs in athletes, who initially suffer a twist or blow that is sufficiently violent to tear ligaments or to weaken or displace other internal components of the knee. Thereafter, under the stress of athletic competition, the knee may unexpectedly give way or "lock." Upon manipulation the knee often snaps back to normal position. Wearing an elastic bandage during strenuous activity may help keep such a weakened knee in position.

Another condition that interferes with free knee movement may be caused by loose fragments in the knee resulting from tuberculosis of the bone, arthritis or inflammation of the synovial membrane that lines the knee joint.

KNOCK-KNEE, an inward curving of the knees, is usually caused by irregular bone growth or by weak ligaments; formerly rickets was a common cause.

k. jerk, a kick reflex produced by a light tap or blow on the patellar ligament. To test this reflex, the lower part of the leg is allowed to hang relaxed, usually by crossing the legs at the knees. The physi-cian taps the ligament below the patella with a small rubber hammer. The normal reaction is con-traction of the quadriceps muscle, causing involun-tary extension of the lower leg. Called also patellar reflex and quadriceps reflex.

The knee jerk is a stretch reflex; striking the patellar ligament stretches the quadriceps muscle at the front of the thigh and causes it to contract. Two nerves are involved: one receives the stimulus and transmits the impulse to the spinal cord, and the other, a motor nerve, receives the impulse and relays it to the quadriceps muscle.

Inadequate response to the knee jerk test may mean that the reflex mechanism involved is in some way impaired. In some people the knee jerk is normally so light that it is nearly imperceptible, and the physician makes other tests to check the reflex mechanism.

knock-knee (nok'ne) a childhood deformity, de-veloping gradually, in which the knees rub to-gether or "knock" in walking and the ankles are far apart; called also genu valgum. At one time, knock-knee and bowleg were common symptoms of rickets. Knock-knee is now more often caused by an irregularity in the growth of the leg bones, some-times stemming from injury to the bone ends at the knee, or by weak ligaments. The weight of the body, which is not supported properly, turns the knees in and the weak lower legs buckle until the ankles are spread far apart.

Knock-knee in young children varies in serious-ness. Milder cases frequently disappear after early childhood as bones, ligaments and muscles strengthen and coordination improves. More seri-ous cases can often be corrected by strengthening exercises and by proper manipulation of the joints. Sometimes braces are used to ensure the proper alignment of growing legs.

In a very young child, knock-knee involves only the soft bone ends where the bone grows. If allowed to continue for a number of years, the condition can lead to abnormal developments in body structure. The sooner corrective measures are taken, the more effective the treatment is likely to be.

knot (not) a knoblike structure or an entangle-ment, as of two ends of a thread or suture.

surgeon's k., surgical k., a knot in which the thread is passed twice through the same loop.

knuckle (nuk'l) the dorsal aspect of any inter-phalangeal joint, or any similarly bent structure.

Köbner's disease (keb'nerz) epidermolysis bullo-sa.

Koch's law (kōks) in order for a given organism to be established as the cause of a given disease, the following conditions must be fulfilled: (1) the microorganism is present in every case of the dis-ease; (2) it is to be cultivated in pure culture; (3) inoculation of such culture must produce the dis-ease in susceptible animals; (4) it must be obtained from such animals, and again grown in a pure cul-ture. Called also Koch's postulates.

Köhler's disease (ka'lerz) osteochondrosis of the navicular bone.

K's second disease, osteochondritis of a meta-tarsal head, usually of the head of the second or third metatarsal bone.

koilo- (koi'lo) word element [Gr.], *hollowed; de-pressed.*

koilonychia (koi"lo-nik'e-ah) a disorder of the nails, which are abnormally thin and concave from side to side, with the edges turned up.

koilorrhachic (koi"lo-rak'ik) having a vertebral

column in which the lumbar curvature is anteriorly concave.

koilosternia (koi″lo-ster′ne-ah) pectus excavatum (funnel chest).

koinotropic (koi″no-trop′ik) having a well balanced personality with a normal social outlook.

Kolmer test (kōl′mer) a complement-fixation technique used in the diagnosis of syphilis or other infections.

kolp- for words beginning thus, see those beginning *colp-*.

Konakion (kon″ah-ki′on) trademark for a preparation of vitamin K, used in prevention and treatment of hypoprothrombinemia.

konometer (ko-nom′ĕ-ter) an apparatus for counting the dust particles in the air.

Koplik's spots (kop′liks) small, irregular, bright red spots on the buccal and lingual mucosa, with a minute bluish white speck in the center of each, that are pathognomonic of beginning measles.

Korsakoff's syndrome (kor-sak′ofs) a mental disorder associated with chronic alcoholism and caused in part by vitamin B$_1$ (thiamine) deficiency; called also Korsakoff's psychosis. Characteristics include disturbances of orientation, memory defect, susceptibility to external stimulation and suggestion and hallucinations. There is irreversible brain damage; confinement to an institution is a frequent outcome of this condition.

Kr chemical symbol, *krypton*.

Krabbe's disease (krab′ēz) diffuse infantile familial cerebral sclerosis, a variety of demyelinating encephalopathy.

Kraepelin's classification (kra′pa-linz) a classification of manic-depressive and schizophrenic groups of mental disease.

kraurosis (kraw-ro′sis) a dried, shriveled condition.
  k. vul′vae, shriveling and dryness of the vulva.

krebiozen (krĕ-bi′o-zen) a substance alleged to be capable of curing cancer.

Krebs cycle (krebz) tricarboxylic acid cycle.

kreotoxism (kre″o-tok′sizm) poisoning by meat.

Krukenberg's tumor (kroo′ken-bergz) a type of carcinoma of the ovary, usually metastatic from cancer of the gastrointestinal tract.

krypton (krip′ton) a chemical element, atomic number 36, atomic weight 83.80, symbol Kr. (See table of ELEMENTS.)

Kuf's disease (kōōfs) a late juvenile form of amaurotic familial idiocy.

Kümmel's disease (kim′elz) a form of spondylitis of unknown origin or occurring at a great interval after the injury causing it, with collapse of the vertebra and thinning of the intervertebral disks.

kuru (koo′roo) a chronic, progressive disorder involving the central nervous system, observed in natives of a region of the Australian Trust Territory of New Guinea.

Kussmaul disease (koos′mowl) an inflammatory disease of the coats of the small and medium-sized arteries of the body with inflammatory changes around the vessels and marked symptoms of systemic infection; called periarteritis nodosa, polyarteritis nodosa and panarteritis.
  K. respiration, difficult breathing occurring in paroxysms, and often preceding diabetic coma; called also air hunger.

kv. kilovolt.

kvp. kilovolt peak (the maximal amount of voltage that an x-ray machine is using).

kwashiorkor (kwash″e-or′kor) a disease of infants and young children that is due primarily to protein deficiency. The condition occurs soon after weaning and is characterized by edema, "pot belly," pigmentation changes of skin and hair and impaired growth and development.

Kwell (kwel) trademark for preparations of lindane, a compound used to treat scabies and pediculosis.

Kyasanur Forest disease (kyah′sah-nor for′est) a highly fatal virus disease of monkeys in the Kyasanur Forest of India, communicable to man.

kyestein (ki-es′te-in) an albuminoid that floats on decomposing urine.

kymatism (ki′mah-tizm) myokymia; quivering of muscles.

kymogram (ki′mo-gram) the graphic record (tracing or film) produced by the kymograph.

kymograph (ki′mo-graf) an instrument for recording variations or undulations, arterial or other.

kymoscope (ki′mo-skōp) a device used in observing the blood current.

Kynex (ki′neks) trademark for preparations of sulfamethoxypyridazine, an antibacterial used in urinary tract and other infections.

kynocephalus (ki″no-sef′ah-lus) a monster with a head like that of a dog.

kynurenine (kin″u-re′nin) a metabolite of tryptophan found in the urine of normal mammals.

kyogenic (ki″o-jen′ik) producing pregnancy.

kyphos (ki′fos) the hump in the spine in kyphosis.

kyphoscoliosis (ki″fo-sko″le-o′sis) backward and lateral curvature of the spine, such as that seen in vertebral osteochondrosis (Scheuermann's disease).

kyphosis (ki-fo′sis) abnormally increased convexity in the curvature of the thoracic spine as viewed from the side; called also hunchback. adj., **kyphot′ic.** The condition may be the result of an acquired disease, an injury or a congenital disorder or disease. It never develops from poor posture.
  This spinal deformity usually is caused by vertebral tuberculosis (POTT'S DISEASE), or by some other destructive inflammation of the vertebrae (spondylitis). Kyphosis sometimes occurs with certain forms of poliomyelitis and with diseases

that cause bone destruction, as happens in osteitis deformans (Paget's disease). An injury, such as a fracture of the spine, treated improperly or not at all, may also result in hunchback. There are some rare cases of kyphosis caused by congenital deformities and diseases. One example, achondroplasia, or fetal rickets, is a congenital bone disorder that affects growth and bone formation.

There are no specific symptoms of kyphosis besides back pain and increasing immobility of the spine. Symptoms vary with the cause, and any back pain or injury should be investigated.

kyrtorrhachic (kir″to-rak′ik) having a vertebral column in which the lumbar curvature is anteriorly convex.

kyto- for words beginning thus, see those beginning *cyto-*.

L

L. *left; length; liter; lumbar.*

L- chemical prefix (written as small capital) that specifies that the substance corresponds in chemical configuration to the standard substance L-glyceraldehyde. Carbohydrates are named by this method to distinguish them by their chemical composition. The opposite prefix is D-.

l- prefix, *levo-*.

L₀ Ehrlich's symbol for a toxin-antitoxin mixture that is completely neutralized and will not kill an animal.

L+ Ehrlich's symbol for a toxin-antitoxin mixture that contains one fatal dose in excess and will kill the experimental animal.

L & A light and accommodation reflexes of the pupils.

La chemical symbol, *lanthanum.*

labia (la'be-ah) [L.] plural of *labium.*

labial (la'be-al) pertaining to a lip, or labium.

labialism (la'be-ah-lizm″) defective speech with use of labial sounds.

labile (la'bil) 1. gliding; moving from point to point over the surface; unstable. 2. chemically unstable.

lability (lah-bil'ĭ-te) the quality of being labile. In psychiatry, emotional instability; a tendency to show alternating states of gaiety and somberness.

labioglossolaryngeal (la″be-o-glos″-o-lah-rin'-je-al) pertaining to the lips, tongue and larynx.

labioglossopharyngeal (la″be-o-glos″o-fah-rin'-je-al) pertaining to the lips, tongue and pharynx.

labiograph (la'be-o-graf″) an instrument for registering movements of the lips in speaking.

labioincisal (la″be-o-in-si'zal) pertaining to or formed by the labial and incisal surfaces of a tooth.

labiology (la″be-ol'o-je) the study of the movements of the lips in speaking or singing.

labiomancy (la'be-o-man″se) lip-reading.

labiomental (la″be-o-men'tal) pertaining to the lips and chin.

labiopalatine (la″be-o-pal'ah-tīn) pertaining to the lips and palate.

labioplasty (la'be-o-plas″te) plastic repair of a lip; cheiloplasty.

labium (la'be-um), pl. *la'bia* [L.] a border or edge; a lip.

l. ma'jus (pl. *la'bia majo'ra*), the hairy fold of skin on either side of the vulva.
l. mi'nus (pl. *la'bia mino'ra*), the small fold of skin on either side, between the labia majora and the opening of the vagina.

labor (la'bor) the function of the female organism by which the product of conception is expelled from the uterus through the vagina to the outside world. The process of labor takes place in three stages: (1) opening or dilation of the cervix uteri; (2) passage of the fetus through the birth canal, or vagina; and (3) separation and expulsion of the placenta.
Labor is believed to be triggered by the release of oxytocin after a fall in the levels of other hormones. Normally at the end of pregnancy oxytocin, which is stored in the posterior lobe of the pituitary gland, is released and stimulates contraction of the uterine muscles.
FIRST STAGE OF LABOR. The beginning of labor is usually indicated by one or more of the following signs: (1) Show: passage from the vagina of small quantities of blood-tinged mucus. (2) Breaking the "bag of waters": normal rupture of membranes that is indicated by a gush or slow leakage of amniotic fluid from the vagina. (3) Labor pains.
The first two of these signs are almost always unmistakable. Labor pains, however, can be confusing. True labor pains are regularly, or rhythmically, spaced, and are accompanied by contractions of the uterus. At first the pain may be only slight; like a cramp, it increases to a peak before fading away. It also seems to start in the small of the back but after a time moves around to the front of the body. The pains are regularly spaced with a pain-free period between. The contractions of the uterus can be felt if the hand is placed on the abdomen.
As labor progresses, the intervals between the contractions of the uterine muscle become shorter and the contractions become more intense. Sometimes the membranes rupture before labor contractions begin.
This first stage of childbirth is known as the dilation period. The uterus is like a large rubber bottle with a half-inch-long neck that is almost closed. Its narrow opening, the cervical canal, must be stretched to a diameter of about 4 inches to make room for the passage of the baby. As the uterine muscles contract, the cervix gradually dilates. This period usually lasts from 8 to 10 hours, but it can be longer or much shorter.
SECOND STAGE OF LABOR. This second period, called the expulsion stage, usually lasts about an hour and a half for the first child, and half an hour for subsequent children. After the cervix is fully dilated, the baby must be pushed through and out of the vagina. The mother helps during this process by holding her breath and bearing down.
THIRD STAGE OF LABOR. In this final stage the placenta detaches itself from the uterine wall and

is expelled. The process takes about 15 minutes, and is painless.

NURSING CARE. Once labor has begun the patient should have someone in constant attendance. She will derive much emotional support from one who is warm, kind and understanding, and displays a genuine interest in her welfare and that of her infant. It is best to have the same person care for her through the entire labor and birth process.

During labor the strength, frequency and duration of contractions are noted and recorded. It is expected that the contractions will increase in all three characteristics, but a sudden change in any one should be reported to the physician immediately. The rate, regularity and volume of the fetal heart tones are checked and recorded periodically. Some apprehensive patients may be helped by allowing them to listen to the infant's heartbeat.

Food and fluids are withheld during active labor, but thirst may cause some discomfort and may be lessened by allowing the patient to moisten her lips with a gauze sponge dipped in ice water. Frequent bathing of the face with a cool washcloth often helps relieve the flushed feeling brought about by the actual hard work being done by the mother. Frequent changing of the patient's gown and the quilted pad protecting the bed linens may be necessary to keep her clean, dry and comfortable.

If hospital policy allows the husband to remain with his wife during labor, he should be instructed in ways in which he can help his wife and at the same time feel that he is making some contribution in this very important event in their lives. He may wish to participate in keeping a record of the contractions or he might appreciate the opportunity to listen to the fetal heart tones occasionally. If the patient feels that sacral support during each contraction helps mitigate the pain, the husband can be shown how to do this. Both husband and wife should be informed of the progress being made during labor so they can feel that something is being accomplished by their efforts.

The mother should be instructed to relax between contractions so as to conserve her strength. She should not bear down until the cervix is dilated, since this effort will only serve to exhaust her and may cause lacerations of the cervix. After the cervix is fully dilated she can speed the birth process by holding her breath and contracting her abdominal muscles. Controlled breathing exercises learned in classes for expectant parents promote relaxation and aid labor.

Although serious complications rarely develop during labor, they can occur and must be watched for. Observations to report immediately include hyperactivity of the fetus; vaginal bleeding in excess of a heavy show; a rapid and irregular pulse and drop in blood pressure; sudden rise in blood pressure; headache, visual disturbances, extreme restlessness or rapidly developing edema. A sudden cessation of contractions or a contraction that does not relax may indicate a serious disturbance in the labor process. The appearance of meconium in the vaginal discharge may indicate fetal distress unless the infant is in a breech position.

artificial l., induced labor.

dry l., that in which the bag of waters ruptures before contraction of the uterus begins.

false l., Braxton Hicks contractions.

induced l., that which is brought on by extraneous means, e.g., by the use of drugs that cause uterine contractions.

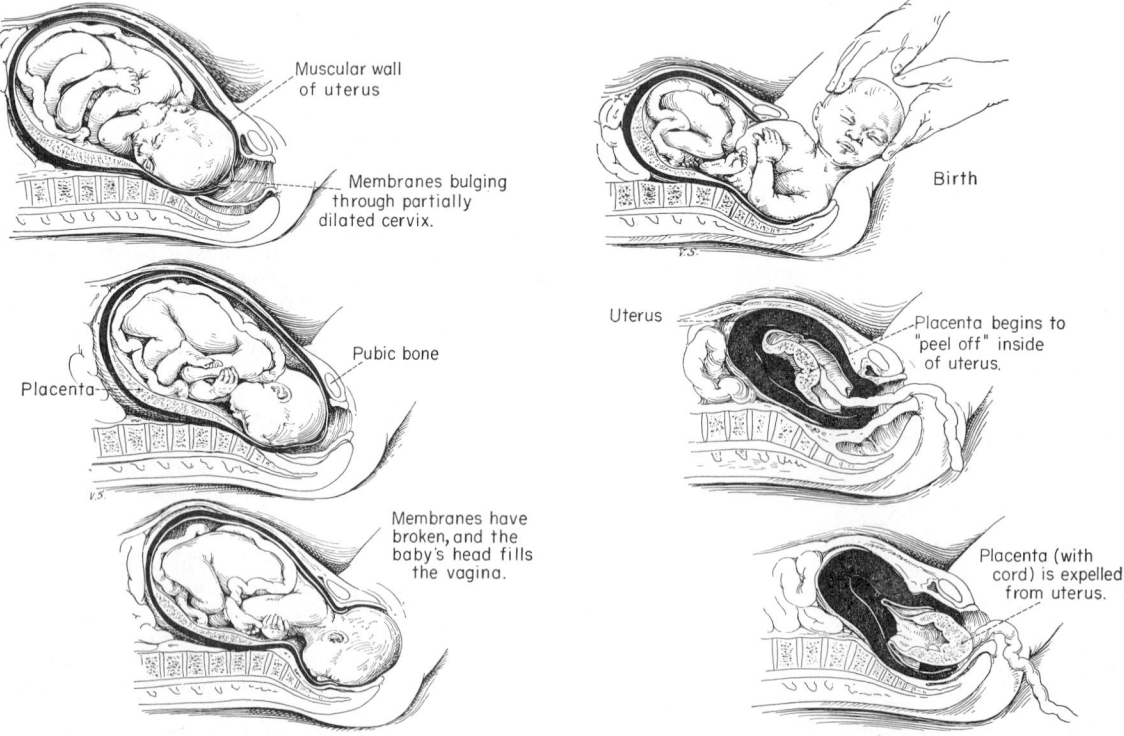

Childbirth. (From Dowling, H. F., and Jones, T.: That the Patient May Know. Philadelphia, W. B. Saunders Co., 1959.)

instrumental l., delivery facilitated by use of instruments, particularly forceps.

missed l., retention of the dead fetus in utero after the normal time of delivery.

precipitate l., delivery accomplished with undue speed.

premature l., expulsion of a viable infant before the normal end of gestation; usually applied to interruption of pregnancy between the twenty-eighth and thirty-seventh weeks.

spontaneous l., delivery occurring without artificial aid.

laboratory (lab'o-rah-tor"e) a place for making tests or doing experimental work.

labrum (la'brum), pl. *la'bra* [L.] an edge, rim or lip.

labyrinth (lab'ĭ-rinth) a system of intercommunicating cavities or canals, such as that constituting the inner ear, which is made up of the vestibule, cochlea and SEMICIRCULAR CANALS. adj., **labyrin'thine.** The cochlea is concerned with hearing, and the vestibule and semicircular canals with equilibrium (sense of balance).

The bony portion of the labyrinth (osseous labyrinth) is composed of a series of canals tunneled out of the temporal bone. Inside the osseous labyrinth is the membranous labyrinth, which conforms to the general shape of the osseous labyrinth but is much smaller. A fluid called perilymph fills the space between the osseous and membranous labyrinths. Fluid inside the membranous labyrinth is called endolymph. These fluids play an important role in the transmission of sound waves and the maintenance of body balance.

Disorders of the inner ear, such as labyrinthitis and MENIÈRE'S DISEASE, are characterized by episodes of dizziness, ringing in the ears and hearing loss.

ethmoidal l., either of the paired lateral masses of the ethmoid bone, consisting of numerous thin-walled cellular cavities, the ethmoidal cells.

labyrinthectomy (lab"ĭ-rin-thek'to-me) excision of the labyrinth.

labyrinthitis (lab"ĭ-rin-thi'tis) inflammation of the labyrinth.

labyrinthotomy (lab"ĭ-rin-thot'o-me) incision of the labyrinth.

lac (lak), pl. *lac'ta* [L.] milk.

laceration (las"ĕ-ra'shun) a wound produced by the tearing of body tissue, as distinguished from a cut or incision.

External lacerations may be small or large and may be caused in many ways. Some common causes of lacerations are a blow from a blunt instrument, a fall against a rough surface and an accident with machinery.

A laceration may be a ragged tear with many tag ends of skin or a torn flap of skin and flesh. Although the bleeding may be less than that caused by a cut, the danger of infection may be greater. In a laceration there is likely to be more damage to surrounding tissue, with a greater area exposed.

Because of the danger of infection, cleaning the laceration is the first and most important step in treatment. If the wound is not extensive or deep, the cleaning is simply done with soap and water. The wound is then covered with dry sterile gauze. If parts of the wound are deep, medical attention

should be sought and immunity against tetanus established.

Lacerations within the body occur when an organ is compressed or moved out of place by an external or internal force. This kind of laceration may result from a blow that does not penetrate the skin. Surgical repair is usually necessary for internal lacerations.

lacertus (lah-ser'tus), pl. *lacer'ti* [L.] a name given certain fibrous attachments of muscles.

lachry- for words beginning thus, see those beginning *lacri-*.

lacrimal (lak'rĭ-mal) pertaining to tears.

l. apparatus, a group of organs concerned with the production and drainage of tears; it is a protective device that helps keep the eye moist and free of dust and other irritating particles.

The lacrimal gland, which secretes tears, lies over the upper, outer corner of the eye; its excretory ducts branch downward toward the eyeball. A constant stream of tears washes down over the front of the eye and is drained off through two small openings located in the inner corner of the eye. Through these openings the tears pass into the lacrimal duct, then through the lacrimal sac into the nasolacrimal duct and finally into the nasal cavity.

lacrimase (lak'rĭ-mās) an enzyme from the lacrimal secretion.

lacrimation (lak"rĭ-ma'shun) secretion and discharge of tears.

lacrimonasal (lak"rĭ-mo-na'zal) pertaining to the lacrimal sac and nose.

lacrimotomy (lak"rĭ-mot'o-me) incision of the lacrimal gland, duct or sac.

lactacidase (lak-tas'ĭ-dās) the enzyme of lactic acid bacteria.

lactacidemia (lak-tas"ĭ-de'me-ah) lactic acid in the blood.

lactaciduria (lak-tas"ĭ-du're-ah) lactic acid in the urine.

lactagogue (lak'tah-gog) an agent that promotes the flow of milk; galactagogue.

lactalase (lak'tah-lās) an enzyme that changes dextrose into lactic acid.

lactalbumin (lak"tal-bu'min) the albumin from milk.

lactase (lak'tās) an enzyme that catalyzes the conversion of lactose into glucose and galactose.

lactate (lak'tāt) a salt of lactic acid.

lactation (lak-ta'shun) the secretion of milk by the breasts. The word is also used to describe the period of weeks or months during which a child is nursed.

Lactation is thought to be brought about by action of progesterone and estrogen and specific pituitary hormones, such as lactogenic hormone (prolactin). Lactation does not begin until at least 3 days after the birth of the baby. Before that, and immediately after birth, the breast secretes colostrum, a fluid containing substances valuable to the baby until milk is formed.

lacteal (lak'te-al) 1. pertaining to milk. 2. any one of the intestinal lymphatics that take up chyle.

lactic (lak'tik) pertaining to milk.
l. **acid,** a compound formed in the body in anaerobic metabolism of carbohydrate, and also produced by bacterial action on milk.
l. **dehydrogenase,** an enzyme found in high concentrations in a number of tissues. It appears in the blood serum in elevated concentrations when these tissues are severely injured.

lacticemia (lak"tĭ-se'me-ah) lactic acid in the blood.

lactiferous (lak-tif'er-us) conveying milk.

lactifuge (lak'tĭ-fūj) an agent that lessens the secretion of milk.

lactigenous (lak-tij'ĕ-nus) producing milk.

lactigerous (lak-tij'er-us) lactiferous.

lactin (lak'tin) lactose.

lactivorous (lak-tiv'o-rus) subsisting upon milk.

Lactobacillus (lak"to-bah-sil'us) a genus of Schizomycetes, some of which are considered to be etiologically related to dental caries, but are otherwise nonpathogenic.
L. **acidoph'ilus,** a lactobacillus producing the fermented product, acidophilus milk.

lactocele (lak'to-sēl) galactocele.

lactoflavin (lak"to-fla'vin) riboflavin.

lactogenic (lak"to-jen'ik) stimulating the production of milk.
l. **hormone,** one of the gonadotropic hormones of the anterior pituitary; it promotes the growth of breast tissue and is responsible for lactation. Called also prolactin.

lactoglobulin (lak"to-glob'u-lin) a globulin occurring in milk.
immune l's, antibodies occurring in the colostrum of animals.

lactolase (lak'to-lās) an enzyme that produces lactic acid.

lactometer (lak-tom'ĕ-ter) an instrument for measuring the specific gravity of milk.

lactone (lak'tōn) an aromatic liquid from lactic acid.

lactophosphate (lak"to-fos'fāt) a salt of lactic and phosphoric acids.

lactoprecipitin (lak"to-pre-sip'ĭ-tin) a precipitin that precipitates the casein of milk.

lactoprotein (lak"to-pro'te-in) a protein derived from milk.

lactorrhea (lak"to-re'ah) excessive secretion by the mammary gland; galactorrhea.

lactose (lak'tōs) a sugar derived from milk, used in infant formulas.

lactoserum (lak"to-se'rum) the serum of an animal into which milk has been injected.

lactosuria (lak"to-su're-ah) lactose in the urine.

lactotherapy (lak"to-ther'ah-pe) treatment by milk diet.

lactotoxin (lak"to-tok'sin) a toxin found in milk.

lactovegetarian (lak"to-vej"ĕ-ta're-an) a person who subsists on a diet of milk or milk products and vegetables.

lacuna (lah-ku'nah), pl. *lacu'nae* [L.] a small pit or hollow cavity. adj., **lacu'nar.**
absorption l., a pit or groove in developing bone that is undergoing resorption; frequently found to contain osteoclasts.
intervillous l., a blood space of the placenta in which the fetal villi are found.
l. **mag'na,** the largest of the orifices of the glands of Littre.
l. **pharyn'gis,** a depression at the pharyngeal end of the eustachian tube.

lacunule (lah-ku'nūl) a minute lacuna.

lacus (la'kus), pl. *la'cus* [L.] lake.
l. **lacrima'lis,** lacrimal lake.

lae- for words beginning thus, see those beginning *le-*.

Laënnec (la-nek') René Théophile Hyacinthe (1781–1826). French physician. He is known for the invention of the stethoscope in 1819 and his *De l'auscultation médiate,* from which much of our knowledge of chest diseases is derived.
L's **cirrhosis,** atrophic cirrhosis of the liver.

lag (lag) 1. the time elapsing between application of a stimulus and the resulting reaction. 2. the early period after inoculation of bacteria into a culture medium, in which the growth is slow.

lagena (lah-je'nah) the curved, flask-shaped organ of hearing in vertebrates lower than mammals, corresponding to the cochlear duct.

lageniform (lah-jen'ĭ-form) flask-shaped.

lagnosis (lag-no'sis) excessive sexual desire, especially in the male; satyriasis.

lagophthalmos (lag"of-thal'mos) inability to shut the eyes completely.

lake (lāk) 1. a lacuna. 2. to undergo separation of hemoglobin from the erythrocytes.
lacrimal l., the triangular space at the medial angle of the eye, where the tears collect.

lal(o)- (lal'o) word element [Gr.], *speech; babbling.*

laliatry (lal-i'ah-tre) the study and treatment of disorders of speech.

lallation (lah-la'shun) babbling, semi-infantile speech.

lalognosis (lal"og-no'sis) the understanding of speech.

laloneurosis (lal"o-nu-ro'sis) speech disorder of nervous or central origin.

lalopathology (lal"o-pah-thol'o-je) the branch of medicine dealing with disorders of speech.

lalopathy (lah-lop'ah-the) any speech disorder.

lalophobia (lal″o-fo′be-ah) dislike of speaking, often with extreme stuttering.

laloplegia (lal″o-ple′je-ah) paralysis of the organs of speech.

lalorrhea (lal″o-re′ah) an abnormal flow of words.

Lamarck's theory (lah-marks′) the theory that acquired characteristics may be transmitted.

lambda (lam′dah) point of union of lambdoid and sagittal sutures.

lambdacism (lam′dah-sizm) inability to utter the *l* sound.

lambdoid (lam′doid) shaped like the Greek letter lambda, Λ or λ.

lame (lām) incapable of normal locomotion.

lamella (lah-mel′ah), pl. *lamel′lae* [L.] 1. a thin scale or plate. 2. a thin gelatin disk to be placed under the eyelid, containing medication acting on the eye. adj., **lamel′lar.**
　circumferential l., one of the bony plates that underlie the periosteum and endosteum.
　concentric l., haversian lamella.
　endosteal l., one of the bony plates lying beneath the endosteum.
　ground l., interstitial lamella.
　haversian l., one of the concentric bony plates surrounding a haversian canal.
　intermediate l., interstitial l., one of the bony plates that fill in between the haversian systems.
　triangular l., a layer joining the choroid plexuses of the third ventricle.

lamina (lam′ĭ-nah), pl. *lam′inae* [L.] a thin, flat plate or layer; used in anatomic nomenclature to designate such a structure, or a specific portion of a composite structure.
　l. basila′ris, a membrane which with the spiral lamina forms the partition between the scala tympani and scala vestibuli.
　l. cine′rea, the layer of gray matter between the corpus callosum and optic chiasm.
　l. cribro′sa, 1. the fascia covering the opening in the fascia lata for passage of the great saphenous vein. 2. either of the perforated spaces in the brain. 3. the part of sclera that is perforated for passage of the optic nerve.
　epithelial l., the layer of ependymal cells covering the choroid plexus.
　l. fus′ca, the pigmentary layer of the sclera.
　l. pro′pria, 1. the connective tissue layer of mucous membrane. 2. the middle fibrous layer of the tympanic membrane.
　spiral l., a small bony plate projecting from the wall of the cochlea.
　vertebral l., one of the paired dorsal parts of the vertebral arch connected to the pedicles of the vertebra.

laminagraphy (lam″ĭ-nag′rah-fe) laminography.

laminar (lam′ĭ-nar) made up of laminae or layers; pertaining to a lamina.

laminated (lam′ĭ-nāt″ed) made up of laminae or layers.

lamination (lam″ĭ-na′shun) 1. a laminar structure or arrangement. 2. the slicing of the fetal head in embryotomy.

laminectomy (lam″ĭ-nek′to-me) surgical excision

of the posterior arch of a vertebra. The procedure is most often performed to relieve the symptoms of a ruptured intervertebral disk (slipped DISK). When several disks are involved spinal fusion may be done so that the vertebrae in the affected area will remain in a fixed position. Bone grafts, usually taken from the iliac crest, are applied to fuse the affected vertebrae permanently, resulting in limitation of movement of this portion of the spine. Laminectomy is also performed for the removal of an intervertebral or spinal cord tumor.

NURSING CARE. Before surgery the patient will receive treatment for slipped DISK. It should be remembered that when the patient is transported to other departments for various preoperative diagnostic tests, special care must be taken to keep the spine in good alignment.

Postoperatively the patient is placed in a bed with bed boards and a firm mattress. His position is changed by "log-rolling" to prevent motion of the vertebral column. In addition he is observed for signs of hemorrhage or leakage of cerebrospinal fluid on the surgical dressing. Should such signs appear, the surgeon should be notified at once. If necessary the dressings may be reinforced until inspected by the physician, but great care must be exercised in the handling of the operative area lest an infection develop and lead to meningitis.

Pain usually persists for some time after surgery until the local edema and muscle spasms subside. Analgesic medications are given as ordered. Special "bicycle" exercises for the legs may be ordered by the physician to relieve muscle pains of the legs. Early ambulation depends on the desires of the surgeon. If the patient is confined to bed, his position must be changed often to avoid respiratory and pulmonary complications.

laminography (lam″ĭ-nog′rah-fe) a special technique of body-section roentgenography.

laminotomy (lam″ĭ-not′o-me) transection of a vertebral lamina.

lamp (lamp) an apparatus for furnishing heat or light.
　slit l., one embodying a diaphragm containing a slitlike opening, by means of which a narrow flat beam of intense light may be projected into the eye. It gives intense illumination so that microscopic study may be made of the conjunctiva, cornea, iris, lens and vitreous, the special feature being that it illuminates a section through the substance of these structures.
　sun l., ultraviolet lamp.
　ultraviolet l., an electric light bulb that transmits ultraviolet rays; used as a therapeutic device and as a means of obtaining an artificial suntan.

lamprophonia (lam″pro-fo′ne-ah) clearness of voice.

lanatoside (lah-nat′o-sīd) a precurosr of a cardiac glycoside obtained from the leaf of *Digitalis lanata.*
　l. C, a crystalline compound used as a heart stimulant.

Lancefield classification (lans′fēld) the classification of hemolytic streptococci into groups on the basis of serologic action.

lancet (lan′set) a small, pointed, two-edged surgical knife.

lancinating (lan'sĭ-nāt″ing) tearing, darting or sharply cutting; used to describe pain.

Landsteiner's classification (land'sti-nerz) a classification of blood types in which they are designated O, A, B and AB, depending on the presence or absence of agglutinogens A and B in the erythrocytes; called also International classification.

Langerhans' islands (lahng'er-hanz) masses in the pancreas composed of cells smaller than the ordinary cells; they produce the hormone insulin and their degeneration is one of the causes of DIABETES MELLITUS.

lanolin (lan'o-lin) wool fat or wool grease that is refined and incorporated into many commercial preparations. Lanolin is a by-product of the process that accompanies the removal of sheeps' wool from the pelt. In its crude form it is a greasy yellow wax of unpleasant odor. This odor disappears when the lanolin is emulsified and made into salves, creams, ointments and cosmetics. Although lanolin is slightly antiseptic, it has no other medicinal benefits and is valuable principally because of the ease with which it penetrates the skin, and because it does not turn rancid.

Lanoxin (lah-nok'sin) trademark for preparations of digoxin, a cardiotonic.

lanthanum (lan'thah-num) a chemical element, atomic number 57, atomic weight 138.91, symbol La. (See table of ELEMENTS.)

lanugo (lah-nu'go) fine hair, such as that covering the body of the fetus.

laparo- (lap'ah-ro) word element [Gr.], *loin or flank; abdomen.*

laparorrhaphy (lap″ah-ror'ah-fe) suture of the abdominal wall.

laparotomaphilia (lap″ah-rot″o-mah-fil'e-ah) a morbid desire to undergo abdominal surgery for simulated symptoms.

laparotomy (lap″ah-rot'o-me) incision of the abdominal wall.

laparotrachelotomy (lap″ah-ro-tra″kĕ-lot'o-me) low or cervical cesarean section, in which the lower uterine segment is incised.

laqueus (lak'we-us) lemniscus.

lardacein (lar-da'se-in) a protein found in amyloid degeneration.

Largon (lar'gon) trademark for a preparation of propiomazine hydrochloride, a tranquilizer.

larithmics (lah-rith'miks) the study dealing with population in its quantitative aspects.

larva (lar'vah), pl. *lar'vae* [L.] the first or worm-like stage of an insect on issuing from the egg.
  l. mi'grans, a peculiar eruption occurring in a changing pattern on the skin, due to migration beneath its surface of a fly larva or helminth; called also creeping eruption.
  l. mi'grans, visceral, a condition due to prolonged migration of larvae of animal nematodes in human tissue other than skin.

larval (lar'val) 1. pertaining to larvae. 2. larvate.

larvate (lar'vāt) masked; concealed: said of a disease or of a symptom of a disease.

larvicide (lar'vĭ-sīd) an agent destructive to larvae.

larvivorous (lar-viv'o-rus) feeding on or consuming larvae, especially larvae of mosquitoes.

laryng(o)- (lah-ring'go) word element [Gr.], *larynx.*

laryngalgia (lar″in-gal'je-ah) pain in the larynx.

laryngeal (lah-rin'je-al) pertaining to the larynx.

laryngectomee (lar″in-jek'to-me) a person whose larynx has been removed.

laryngectomy (lar″in-jek'to-me) partial or total removal of the larynx by surgery. It is usually performed as treatment for cancer of the larynx. The patient learns afterward to speak without his voice box.

Instruction in the new method of speaking begins as soon as the operative site has healed. At first, patients have difficulty in forming the sounds of speech, but with continued practice, they can learn to speak well.

There are three methods of speaking without use of the larynx. Esophageal speech, the simplest method, is usually the first one the patient learns. He is taught to belch and then to form simple sounds and words while "burping." With careful instruction and persistent practice, he can make sustained belches that cause a column of air to vibrate in his throat and the walls and roof of his pharynx. This air column substitutes for vocal cords as he forms words with his mouth. Esophageal speech is not smooth, and once the patient has mastered it he begins to learn the smoother, more advanced pharyngeal method.

In pharyngeal speech, a person uses only the limited amount of air that enters the nose and mouth when he breathes through the tracheostomy tube. Sound is generated by blocking this air with quick tongue actions, forcing it to vibrate against the roof of the pharynx at the rear of the mouth. The patient's skill in doing this is developed through diligent practice. By controlling the air and expelling it slowly, it is possible to approach the rhythm and phrasing of normal, fluent speech. As he grows in skill and confidence, the pharyngeal speaker sounds like a person with an ordinary, slightly hoarse voice.

The third method is use of an electronic voice box, which connects the opening of the trachea in the neck to the mouth. It can be removed when the patient desires. Experts discourage use of these devices, however, unless the patient cannot or will not learn pharyngeal speech. They are generally awkward to use and very expensive.

NURSING CARE. Before surgery the patient should be given a complete explanation of the surgical procedure and its consequences. Ideally, this is done by the surgeon performing the operation. The nursing personnel can do much to comfort the patient and help him adjust to his condition by showing a willingness to answer questions and discuss plans for his rehabilitation.

It is important for the patient to feel secure and safe in the knowledge that he will not be left alone immediately after surgery when he cannot speak or cry out for help. An explanation of the recovery room, special equipment to be used and type of treatments such as suctioning and administration of oxygen should be given. He will need reassurance that he will never be left without some means of summoning help during the early postoperative period.

After surgery the greatest problem, other than physical needs of the patient, will be one of communication. By close observation of his actions, facial expressions, movements of the hands and so forth, one can usually learn his wishes. It is important that his needs be anticipated whenever possible, to avoid frustration and tension on his part. As the patient recovers he will appreciate having a notebook and pencil to write messages to those caring for him. The patient and his family should be given instructions in the care of the tracheostomy tube after he has been discharged from the hospital. He must be warned against the dangers of aspirating water into the lungs when bathing or showering. Although a dressing is not necessary for covering the tracheal opening in the neck, the patient may wish to cover it with a small square of cotton material or wear a collar or scarf of porous material to hide the wound. These types of coverings are useful in that they act as a filter and remove dust and other irritants from the air being inhaled through the opening.

laryngismus (lar″in-jiz′mus) spasm of the larynx.
   l. strid′ulus, sudden laryngeal spasm with crowing inspiration.

laryngitis (lar″in-ji′tis) inflammation of the mucous membrane of the larynx affecting the voice and breathing. Laryngitis may be acute or chronic, or may occur in other forms.

ACUTE LARYNGITIS. Acute laryngitis may be caused by overuse of the voice, allergies, irritating dust or smoke, hot or corrosive liquids or even violent weeping. It also occurs in viral or bacterial infections, and is frequently associated with other diseases of the respiratory tract.

In adults, a mild case of acute laryngitis begins with a dry, tickling sensation in the larynx, followed quickly by partial or complete loss of the voice. There may be a slight fever, minor discomfort and poor appetite, with recovery after a few days. Other and more uncomfortable symptoms can include a feeling of heat and pain in the throat, difficulty in swallowing and dry cough followed by expectoration; the voice may be either painful to use or absent. Swelling of the larynx and epiglottis may impair breathing. Increasing difficulty in breathing may be a sign of edematous laryngitis, or CROUP.

Treatment for acute laryngitis requires that the patient rest in bed and refrain from talking. The room temperature should be even and warm. The air is kept moist with a humidifier or vaporizer. An ice bag on the throat often is soothing. In severe cases, antibiotics may be necessary.

Children are especially vulnerable to laryngitis because of the smallness of their air passages. Most cases in children subside within a few days, but if inflammation and swelling continue to increase, severe dyspnea occurs.

CHRONIC LARYNGITIS. After repeated attacks of the acute type, chronic laryngitis may develop. This is caused mostly by continual irritation from overuse of the voice, tobacco smoke, dust or chemical vapors, or by a chronic nasal or sinus disorder. Often the moist mucous membrane lining the

larynx becomes granulated. The granulation can proceed to thickening and hardening of the mucous membrane, which changes the voice or makes it hoarse. There is little or no pain, though there may be tickling in the throat and a slight cough.

Chronic laryngitis that has persisted for a number of years may result in chronic hypertrophic laryngitis, a condition in which there is a permanent change in the voice because of hypertrophy of the membrane lining the larynx.

Treatment for chronic laryngitis is the same as for the acute form, with elimination of all sources of irritation and reinfection. Hoarseness that lasts longer than 2 weeks may be a warning of tumor or cancer of the larynx, or of a tumor in the thorax that presses on the recurrent laryngeal nerve, which controls the larynx.

OTHER FORMS OF LARYNGITIS. Paroxysmal laryngitis is a nervous disorder affecting infants that seems to be associated with enlarged adenoids and rickets. It consists of unexplained spasms in which the larynx closes, cutting off the air passage, and then suddenly opens. Sometimes the condition may be fatal. Treatment of this form of laryngitis calls for removal of the adenoids.

Other types include diphtheritic laryngitis, tuberculous laryngitis, traumatic laryngitis and allergic laryngitis. Treatment of diphtheritic laryngitis often involves intubation or tracheostomy in order to admit air. Traumatic laryngitis also often requires tracheostomy. Allergic laryngitis, often caused by smoking or other irritants, is treated in the same way as other allergies.

laryngocele (lah-ring′go-sēl) an anomalous air sac communicating with a cavity of the larynx and producing a tumor-like lesion visible on the outside of the neck.

laryngocentesis (lah-ring″go-sen-te′sis) surgical puncture of the larynx, with aspiration.

laryngofissure (lah-ring″go-fish′er) median laryngotomy.

laryngogram (lah-ring′go-gram) a roentgenogram of the larynx.

laryngography (lar″ing-gog′rah-fe) roentgenography of the larynx.

laryngology (lar″ing-gol′o-je) that branch of medicine which has to do with the throat, pharynx, larynx, nasopharynx and tracheobronchial tree.

laryngopathy (lar″ing-gop′ah-the) any disorder of the larynx.

laryngophantom (lah-ring″go-fan′tom) an artificial model of the larynx.

laryngopharyngeal (lah-ring″go-fah-rin′je-al) pertaining to the larynx and pharynx.

laryngopharyngectomy (lah-ring″go-far″in-jek′-to-me) excision of the larynx and pharynx.

laryngopharyngitis (lah-ring″go-far″in-ji′tis) inflammation of the larynx and pharynx.

laryngopharynx (lah-ring″go-far′ingks) the lower portion of the pharynx.

laryngophony (lar″ing-gof′o-ne) the sound heard in auscultating the larynx.

laryngoplasty (lah-ring′go-plas″te) plastic repair of the larynx.

laryngoplegia (lah-ring″go-ple′je-ah) paralysis of the larynx.

laryngorhinology (lah-ring″go-ri-nol′o-je) the science of the larynx and nose and their diseases.

laryngorrhagia (lah-ring″go-ra′je-ah) hemorrhage from the larynx.

laryngorrhaphy (lar″ing-gor′ah-fe) suture of the larynx.

laryngorrhea (lah-ring″go-re′ah) excessive secretion of mucus from the larynx.

laryngoscope (lah-ring′go-skōp) an endoscope equipped with a light and mirrors for illumination and examination of the larynx.

laryngoscopy (lar″ing-gos′ko-pe) direct visual examination of the larynx with a laryngoscope.

Before direct examination the patient is given a mild sedative to promote relaxation during the procedure which, though not uncomfortable, may be frightening and exhausting for the patient. Immediately before the laryngoscope is passed the throat is anesthetized locally with cocaine spray. The patient lies on his back on the examining table with his head extending over the edge. An attendant stands at his head, holding it in position and supporting its weight.

Following the laryngoscopy, fluids and foods are withheld until the effects of the local anesthetic have worn off and the gag reflex has returned.

Indirect laryngoscopy is examination of the larynx by observation of the reflection of it in a laryngeal mirror.

laryngospasm (lah-ring′go-spazm) spasmodic closure of the larynx.

laryngostenosis (lah-ring″go-stĕ-no′sis) narrowing of the larynx.

laryngostomy (lar″ing-gos′to-me) creation of an artificial opening into the larynx.

laryngotomy (lar″ing-got′o-me) incision of the larynx.
  inferior l., incision of the larynx through the lower part of the fibroelastic membrane of the larynx (cricothyroid membrane).
  median l., incision of the larynx through the thyroid cartilage.
  subhyoid l., incision of the larynx through the fibroelastic membrane attached to the hyoid bone and the thyroid cartilage (thyrohyoid membrane).

laryngotracheitis (lah-ring″go-tra″ke-i′tis) inflammation of the larynx and trachea.

laryngotracheotomy (lah-ring″go-tra″ke-ot′o-me) incision of the larynx and trachea.

laryngoxerosis (lah-ring″go-ze-ro′sis) dryness of the throat.

larynx (lar′ingks) the muscular and cartilaginous structure, lined with mucous membrane, situated at the top of the trachea and below the root of the tongue and the hyoid bone. The larynx contains the vocal cords, and is the source of the sound heard in speech; it is called also the voice box. It is part of the respiratory system, and air passes through the larynx as it travels from the pharynx to the trachea and back again on its way to and from the lungs.

The larynx is composed of cartilages held together by muscles and ligaments. The largest of these cartilages, the thyroid cartilage, forms the Adam's apple, which protrudes in the front of the neck. Two flexible vocal cords reach from the back to the front wall of the larynx and are manipulated by small muscles to produce sound. The epiglottis, a flap or lid at the base of the tongue, closes the larynx as it is lifted up during swallowing and so prevents passage of food or drink into the larynx and trachea.

DISORDERS OF THE LARYNX. Hoarseness is often the result of inflammation of the mucous membrane of the larynx, or LARYNGITIS. Persistent hoarseness or a change of voice without apparent cause may, however, be a warning signal, an indication of tuberculosis, syphilis or a tumor.

In cancer of the larynx the first symptom may be persistent hoarseness or the feeling of a lump in the throat, although this feeling, like other laryngeal symptoms, may be caused by emotional stress. Early diagnosis of laryngeal cancer is essential to effective treatment.

Lasegue's sign (lah-sāgz′) aggravation of pain in the back and leg elicited by passive raising of the heel from the bed with the knee straight.

laser (la′zer) a device that produces an extremely intense, small and nearly nondivergent beam of monochromatic radiation in the visible region, with all the waves in phase; used as a surgical tool, to produce intense heat and energy in a small area.

Lasix (la′siks) trademark for a preparation of furosemide, an oral diuretic.

lassitude (las′ĭ-tūd) weakness; exhaustion.

latency (la′ten-se) a state of seeming inactivity.

latent (la′tent) dormant or concealed; not manifest.

laterad (lat′er-ad) toward the lateral aspect.

lateral (lat′er-al) pertaining to or situated at the side.

lateralis (lat″er-a′lis) [L.] lateral.

laterality (lat″er-al′ĭ-te) a tendency to use preferentially the organs (hand, foot, ear, eye) of the same side in voluntary motor acts.
  crossed l., the preferential use of heterolateral members of the different pairs of organs in voluntary motor acts, e.g., right eye and left hand.
  dominant l., the preferential use of ipsilateral members of the different pairs of organs in voluntary motor acts, e.g., right (dextrality) or left (sinistrality) ear, eye, hand and leg.

lateroflexion (lat″er-o-flek′shun) flexion to one side.

lateroversion (lat″er-o-ver′zhun) abnormal turning to one side.

lathyrism (lath′ĭ-rizm) poisoning due to ingestion of some species of peas of the genus *Lathyrus*.

Latrodectus (lat″ro-dek′tus) a genus of poisonous spiders.

L. mac′tans, a species found in the United States; commonly known as the black widow. Its bite may cause severe symptoms or even death. (For first aid, see INSECT BITES AND STINGS.)

latus (la′tus) [L.] 1. broad, wide. 2. the side or flank.

laughing gas nitrous oxide.

Laurence-Moon-Biedl syndrome (law′rens mōōn be′del) a syndrome composed of obesity, hypogenitalism, retinitis pigmentosa, mental deficiency, skull defects and sometimes syndactyly.

Lauron (law′ron) trademark for a preparation of aurothioglycanide, a gold preparation used in treatment of rheumatoid arthritis.

lavage (lah-vahzh′) irrigation or washing out of an organ or cavity, especially the stomach or intestine.

Gastric lavage, or irrigation of the stomach, is usually done to remove ingested poisons. It also may be employed as an emergency operation if there is danger of vomiting and aspiration during anesthesia, or in cases of persistent vomiting. The solutions used for gastric lavage are physiologic saline, 1 per cent sodium bicarbonate, plain water or a specific antidote for a poison. A nasogastric tube (chilled so that it is more easily swallowed) is passed and then the irrigating fluid is funneled into the tube. It is allowed to flow into the stomach by gravity. The solution is removed by siphonage; when the funnel is lowered, the fluid flows out, bringing with it the contents of the stomach.

Lavema (lah-ve′mah) trademark for preparations of oxyphenisatin, a cathartic.

Lavoisier (lah-vwah-zya′) Antoine Laurent (1743–1794). French chemist, born in Paris and later guillotined by the French Revolutionists. Lavoisier demolished the phlogiston theory (a theory of combustion) and explained the true nature of respiration by his introduction of quantitative relations in chemistry. He was secretary and treasurer of a committee seeking the uniformity of weights and measures in France, which led to the establishment of the metric system.

lawrencium (law-ren′se-um) a chemical element, atomic number 103, atomic weight 257, symbol Lw. (See table of ELEMENTS.)

laxative (lak′sah-tiv) a medicine that loosens the bowel contents and encourages evacuation. A laxative with a mild or gentle effect on the bowels is also known as an aperient; one with a strong effect is referred to as a cathartic or a purgative.

Bland laxatives may be used temporarily in the treatment of CONSTIPATION along with other measures. Mineral oil, or liquid petrolatum, and olive oil act as lubricants. Sometimes mineral oil is used in combination with agar, which is bulk-producing. Cascara sagrada aromatic fluid extract and milk of magnesia are two other mild laxatives. Psyllium hydrophilic mucilloid, which is prepared from a plant seed, helps elimination by encouraging the peristaltic movements.

Saline purges, such as sodium phosphate and magnesium sulfate (Epsom salts), flush the intestinal tract. They do this by preventing the intestines from absorbing water; evacuation takes place as soon as water accumulates.

Castor oil is a strong cathartic that effects complete evacuation of the bowels. Its administration is followed by temporary constipation.

DANGERS OF LAXATIVES. Laxatives should be employed only with the advice of a physician. Constipation may be a symptom of serious organic illness as well as the result of improper diet and habits. Also, laxatives taken regularly tend to deprive the colon of its natural muscle tone. In this way laxatives can be the cause of chronic constipation rather than its cure.

Mineral oil taken regularly tends to dilute certain vitamins derived from the food one eats. It can also seep into the lungs, causing a reaction resembling PNEUMONIA, especially in older people.

Purgative salts can produce DEHYDRATION. Laxatives that produce bulk may cause stonelike balls (bezoars) to develop.

A strong cathartic, such as castor oil, can have fatal results if used when there is nausea, vomiting, abdominal pain or other symptoms of APPENDICITIS. It is also dangerous to use during pregnancy.

Children, in particular, cannot use the same dosage or the strong laxatives taken by adults.

laxator (lak-sa′tor) that which slackens or relaxes.

laxoin (lak′so-in) phenolphthalein, a cathartic.

layer (la′er) a stratum of nearly uniform thickness.
  ameloblastic l., the inner layer of cells of the enamel organ, which forms the enamel of the teeth.
  bacillary l., the rod and cone layer of the retina.
  blastodermic l., germ layer.
  columnar l., 1. layer of rods and cones. 2. mantle layer.
  enamel l., the outermost layer of cells of the enamel organ.
  ganglionic l., a stratum of angular cells in the cerebral cortex.
  germ l., one of the three primary layers of cells formed in the early development of the embryo: ectoderm, entoderm and mesoderm.
  half-value l., that thickness of a filter (copper or aluminum) which will reduce the original intensity of a roentgen ray beam by half.
  malpighian l., the deep part of the epidermis.
  mantle l., the middle layer of the wall of the primitive neural tube, containing primitive nerve cells and later forming the gray matter of the central nervous system.
  nervous l., all of the retina except the pigment layer.
  odontoblastic l., the epithelioid layer of odontoblasts in contact with the dentin of teeth.
  osteogenetic l., the innermost layer of the periosteum.
  palisade l., the basal layer of the rete mucosum, the innermost layer of the epidermis.
  prickle cell l., rete mucosum; the innermost layer of the epidermis.
  l. of rods and cones, a layer of the retina immediately beneath the pigment epithelium, between it and external limiting membrane, containing the rods and cones.
  subendocardial l., the layer of loose fibrous tissue uniting the endocardium and myocardium.
  trophic l., vegetative l., entoderm.

lb. [L.] *li′bra* (pound).

L.D. lethal dose.

L.D.₅₀ median lethal dose.

LDH lactic dehydrogenase.

L-dopa (el-do′pah) an experimental drug that offers promise in the treatment of Parkinson's disease.

L.E. lupus erythematosus.

L.E. cell, a mature neutrophilic polymorphonuclear leukocyte found in lupus erythematosus.

L.E. phenomenon, L.E. test, production of L.E. cells on incubation of normal neutrophils with the serum of affected patients, as a diagnostic test for lupus erythematosus.

lead¹ (led) a chemical element, atomic number 82, atomic weight 207.19, symbol Pb. (See table of ELEMENTS.)

l. acetate, a compound used as an irritant and astringent.

l. monoxide, PbO; used in preparations for local application.

l. poisoning, a form of poisoning caused by the presence of lead or lead salts in the body. Lead poisoning affects the brain, nervous system, blood and digestive system. It can be either chronic or acute.

Chronic lead poisoning (plumbism) was once fairly common among painters, and was called "painter's colic." It became less frequent as paints composed of other chemicals were substituted for lead-based paints and as plastic toys replaced lead ones. The disease is still seen among children with pica (a craving for unnatural articles of food) who may eat lead paint or coatings.

Symptoms include weight loss, anemia, stomach cramp (lead colic), a bluish black line in the gums and constipation. Other symptoms may be mental depression and, in children, irritability and convulsions. In addition to the poisoning, the anemia and weight loss must also be treated, usually by providing an adequate diet. In serious cases, EDTA (calcium disodium edetate) may be prescribed.

Acute lead poisoning, which is rare, can be caused in two ways. Lead may accumulate in the bones, liver, kidneys, brain and muscles and then be released suddenly to produce an acute condition; or large amounts of lead may be inhaled or ingested at one time. Symptoms are a metallic taste in the mouth, vomiting, bloody or black diarrhea and muscle cramps. Diagnosis is made by examination of the blood and urine. Treatment consists of immediate removal of unabsorbed lead in the intestinal tract through the administration of mild saline cathartics and enemas. EDTA is given and in most cases measures must be taken to reduce the increased intracranial pressure that accompanies acute lead poisoning.

lead² (lēd) a specific array (pair) of electrodes used in recording changes in electric potential, created by activity of an organ, such as the heart (electrocardiography) or brain (electroencephalography); applied also to the particular segment of the tracing produced by the potential registered through the specific electrodes; in electrocardiography lead I records the potential differences between the two arms, lead II between the right arm and left leg, lead III between the left arm and left leg and lead V from various sites over the heart.

bipolar l., an array involving two electrodes that experience significant variations in potential.

esophageal l., difference in potential recorded with one electrode inserted in the esophagus.

limb l's, differences in potential recorded with electrodes placed on the arms and left leg.

precordial l's, leads recording electric potential from various sites over the heart, designated V with a subscript numeral indicating the exact site: V_1, fourth intercostal space immediately to the right of the sternum; V_2, fourth intercostal space immediately to the left of the sternum; V_3, midway between V_2 and V_4; V_4, fifth intercostal space in the midclavicular line (the imaginary vertical line on the anterior surface of the body), passing through the center of the nipple; V_5, at the same horizontal level as V_4, in the left anterior axillary line (the imaginary vertical line passing through the middle of the axilla); V_6, left midaxillary line at the same horizontal level as V_4 and V_5.

unipolar l., an array of two electrodes, only one of which experiences considerable potential variation.

lecithin (les′ĭ-thin) a phospholipid consisting of glycerophosphoric acid esters of oleic, stearic or other fatty acid combined with choline, found in many animal tissues, especially nerve tissue, semen and egg yolk.

lecithinase (les′ĭ-thin-ās″) an enzyme that splits up lecithin.

lecitho- (les′ĭ-tho) word element [Gr.], denoting relationship to the yolk of an egg or ovum.

lectin (lek′tin) a term applied to hemagglutinating substances extracted from certain plant seeds.

L.E.D. lupus erythematosus disseminatus.

Ledercillin (led″er-sil′in) trademark for preparations of procaine penicillin G.

leech (lēch) an aquatic segmented worm, *Hirudo medicinalis*, formerly used for drawing blood.

artificial l., Heurteloup's l., a cupping glass or other apparatus for drawing blood by suction.

leeching (lēch′ing) the application of a leech for the withdrawal of blood.

Leeuwenhoek (la′ven-hōok) Antonj van (1632–1723). Dutch microscopist. Born in Delft, Holland, he made many interesting discoveries through his careful observations even though his work was not conducted on a definite scientific plan. He gave the first accurate description of the red blood corpuscles in 1674, and in 1677 he described and illustrated the spermatozoa in animals, although he had been anticipated in this discovery by several months. He investigated the structure of muscle, the crystalline lens and teeth, and was the first to see protozoa and bacteria under the microscope.

leg (leg) the lower extremity, especially the part between the knee and ankle.

Anglesey l., a jointed artificial leg.

baker's l., knock-knee, or genu valgum.

bayonet l., ankylosis of the knee after backward displacement of the tibia and fibula.

bow l., genu varum.

milk l., phlebitis of the femoral vein, especially in women after childbirth; phlegmasia alba dolens.

Legg's disease, Legg-Calvé-Perthes disease (legz), (leg kal-va′per′tēz) osteochrondrosis of the epiphysis of the head of the femur; called also Legg-Calve disease and Legg-Calve-Waldenström disease.

legume (leg′ūm) the pod or fruit of a leguminous plant, such as peas and beans.

legumin (lĕ-gu′min) a globulin characteristically found in the seeds of leguminous plants.

Leiner's disease (li′nerz) erythroderma desquamativum in infants.

leiodermia (li″o-der′me-ah) abnormal smoothness and glossiness of the skin.

leiomyoma (li″o-mi-o′mah) myoma of the nonstriated muscle fibers.

leiomyosarcoma (li″o-mi″o-sar-ko′mah) a sarcoma containing cells of nonstriated muscle.

leiphemia (li-fe′me-ah) thinness of the blood.

Leishman-Donovan bodies (lēsh′man don′o-van) oval bodies found in the spleen in chronic dysentery and certain other diseases.

Leishmania (lēsh-ma′ne-ah) a genus of protozoan organisms, including *L. brasilien′sis*, the cause of American leishmaniasis, *L. donova′ni*, the cause of kala-azar, and *L. trop′ica*, the cause of cutaneous leishmaniasis.

leishmaniasis (lēsh″mah-ni′ah-sis) any disease due to infection with Leishmania.
    American l., infection of the mucous membranes of the nose and throat by *L. brasiliensis*.
    cutaneous l., chronic ulcerative granuloma caused by *L. tropica* and transmitted by the sandfly. It occurs particularly in Asian and African countries and has various names such as Aleppo boil, Delhi sore, Baghdad sore, oriental sore. Treatment consists of parenteral injections of ethylstibamine. Antibiotics are employed to combat secondary infection. Simple lesions may be cleaned, curetted and left to heal.
    visceral l., kala-azar.

lemmoblastic (lem″o-blas′tik) developing into neurolemma tissue.

lemmoblastoma (lem″o-blas-to′mah) spongioblastoma.

lemmocyte (lem′o-sīt) a cell that develops into a neurolemma cell.

lemniscus (lem-nis′kus), pl. *lemnis′ci* [L.] a band or ribbon-like structure, applied especially to collections of nerve fibers in the central nervous system.

lemology (le-mol′o-je) the study of epidemic disease, especially the plague.

length (length) the distance between two extremities or poles.
    basinasal l., the distance from the basion to the center of the suture between the frontal and nasal bones.
    crown-heel l., the distance from the crown of the head to the heel in embryos, fetuses and infants; the equivalent of standing height in older subjects.
    crown-rump l., the distance from the crown of the head to the breech in embryos, fetuses and infants; the equivalent of sitting height in older subjects.

focal l., the distance between a lens and an object from which all rays of light are brought to a focus.

lens (lenz) 1. a glass for converging or scattering rays of light. 2. the crystalline lens, a transparent organ lying behind the pupil and iris and in front of the large vitreous-filled cavity of the eye. The crystalline lens refracts (bends) light rays so that they are focused on the RETINA. In order for the eye to see objects close at hand, light rays from the objects must be bent more sharply to bring them to focus on the retina; light rays from distant objects require much less refraction. It is the function of the lens to "accommodate" or make some adjustment for viewing near objects and objects at a distance. To accomplish this the lens must be highly elastic so that its shape can be changed and made more or less convex. The more convex the lens, the greater the refraction. Small ciliary muscles create tension on the lens, making it less convex; as the tension is relaxed the lens become more spherical in shape and hence more convex.

With increasing age the lenses lose their elasticity; thus their ability to focus light rays in the retina becomes impaired. This condition is called PRESBYOPIA. In farsightedness (HYPEROPIA) the image is focused behind the retina because the refractive power of the lens is too weak or the eyeball axis is too short. Nearsightedness (MYOPIA) occurs when the refractive power of the lens is too strong or the eyeball is too long, so that the image is focused in front of the retina.
    achromatic l., a lens corrected for chromatic aberration.
    apochromatic l., one corrected for chromatic and spheric aberration.
    artificial l., one made of appropriate material, to be inserted in the eyeball after removal of the natural lens.
    biconcave l., one concave on both faces.
    biconvex l., one convex on both faces.
    bifocal l., one made up of two segments, the upper for far vision and the lower for near vision.
    concave l., dispersing lens.
    contact l., a thin, curved shell of glass or plastic that is applied directly to the cornea to correct refractive errors (see also CONTACT LENSES).
    converging l., convex l., one that focuses light.
    convexoconcave l., one that has one convex and one concave face.
    cylindrical l., one which has one surface plane and another concave or convex.
    dispersing l., one that disperses light.
    omnifocal l., a spectacle lens whose power increases regularly in a downward direction, avoiding the discontinuity in field and power inherent in bifocal and trifocal lenses.
    orthoscopic l., one that gives a flat and undistorted field of vision.
    spherical l., one that has a surface that is the segment of a sphere.
    Stokes's l's, an apparatus used in the diagnosis of astigmatism.
    trial l's, lenses used in determining visual acuity.

trifocal l., one made up of three segments, the upper for distant, the middle for intermediate and the lower for near vision.

lentectomy (len-tek′to-me) excision of the lens of the eye.

lenticonus (len″tĭ-ko′nus) a conical protrusion of the substance of the lens of the eye.

lenticular (len-tik′u-lar) 1. pertaining to or shaped like a lens. 2. pertaining to the crystalline lens. 3. pertaining to the lenticular nucleus.

lenticulostriate (len-tik″u-lo-stri′āt) pertaining to the lenticular nucleus and corpus striatum.

lentiform (len′tĭ-form) lens-shaped.

lentiglobus (len″tĭ-glo′bus) exaggerated curvature of the lens of the eye, producing a spherical bulging.

lentigo (len-ti′go), pl. *lentig′ines* [L.] a brownish pigmented spot on the skin due to increased deposition of melanin and an increased number of melanocytes; a freckle.
  l. malig′na, a specialized type that tends to become malignant.

lentitis (len-ti′tis) inflammation of the eye lens.

lentoptosis (len″to-to′sis) hernia of the lens of the eye.

leontiasis (le″on-ti′ah-sis) 1. a bilateral and symmetrical hypertrophy of the bones of the face and cranium, leading to a lion-like facial expression. 2. a form of leprosy with lion-like expression about the face.

leotropic (le″o-trop′ik) running spirally from right to left.

leper (lep′er) a patient with leprosy; the term is officially disapproved of.

lepidic (lĕ-pid′ik) pertaining to, or made up of, scales.

lepidosis (lep″ĭ-do′sis) a scaly eruption.

lepocyte (lep′o-sīt) a nucleated cell having a cell wall.

lepothrix (lep′o-thriks) a condition in which the axillary and sometimes the pubic hairs become covered with scales caused by clumps of bacteria; called also trichomycosis axillaris.

lepra (lep′rah) leprosy; prior to about 1850, psoriasis.

leprid (lep′rid) the cutaneous lesion or lesions of tuberculoid leprosy: hypopigmented or erythematous maculae or plaques, lacking bacilli.

leproma (lep-ro′mah) a superficial granulomatous nodule, rich in bacilli, the characteristic lesion of lepromatous leprosy. adj., **lepro′matous.**

lepromin (lep′ro-min) a repeatedly boiled, autoclaved, gauze-filtered suspension of finely ground lepromatous tissue devised for performing the skin test for tissue resistance to leprosy.

leprosarium (lep′ro-sa′re-um) a hospital or colony for treatment and isolation of patients with leprosy.

leprosy (lep′ro-se) a chronic communicable disease characterized by the production of granulomatous lesions of the skin, upper respiratory and ocular mucous membranes, peripheral nerves and the testes; also called Hansen's disease. Not readily contagious, it often results in severe disability but is rarely fatal. adj., **lep′rous.**

CAUSE. The cause of leprosy is believed to be a species of bacteria, *Mycobacterium leprae* or Hansen's bacillus, which usually attacks the skin and nerves, but not the brain.

FREQUENCY AND TRANSMISSION. Leprosy is essentially a tropical disease, although it has occurred in every country. It is now rare in the United States and in Europe except for the Mediterranean countries. It is still fairly common in Africa, Asia and many of the Pacific islands, as well as in the West Indies and Central and South America. About half of the estimated 3 to 4 million cases in the world are in India and China. Leprosy is most prevalent where economic levels and sanitation standards are low.

Leprosy is not inherited, but the actual means of transmission of the disease have not yet been established. It is known that the source of infection is the discharge from lesions of persons with active cases. It is believed that the bacillus enters the body through the skin or through the mucous membranes of the nose and throat. Leprosy is considered one of the least contagious of infectious diseases; only 3 to 5 per cent of those exposed to it ever contract it.

SYMPTOMS. The incubation period for leprosy is often 5 years or more. Early symptoms consist of the development of red or brown patches on the skin, often with pale white centers appearing later. Along with these, there may be loss of sensation in parts of the body. Nodules appear on the body, often with an accompanying fever. Body hair tends to fall out. There may be neuritis and iritis.

In the lepromatous type, open sores later appear on the face, ear lobes and forehead. Tests show the presence of large numbers of the bacillus in the discharge from these lesions. If the progress of the disease is not checked by treatment, the fingers and toes disintegrate and there may be other disfiguration. Death may occur in extreme cases of this type, but more often it is due to a secondary infection, such as tuberculosis or pneumonia.

In the tuberculoid type, there is loss of sensation on sections of the skin and atrophy of muscles. This often results in the contraction of the hand into a claw.

TREATMENT. Leprosy is most effectively treated with sulfone medications, such as dapsone, developed around 1950. Streptomycin and chlortetracycline hydrochloride (Aureomycin) are also being used.

Treatment continues for several years at least, and sometimes indefinitely. In addition to specific medical therapy, adequate rest, diet and exercise are provided. Physical therapy is employed to retrain affected muscles. Psychiatric help, not only for leprosy patients but for their close contacts and those who only imagine they have been exposed, is invaluable in relieving the anxieties arising from the age-old misconceptions about the disease.

PREVENTION. Measures taken to prevent leprosy include separating infants from leprous parents at birth, and the establishment of clinics and hospitals for diagnosis and treatment. Infected persons are isolated during the contagious period. Many patients return to their homes completely free of symptoms and are able to resume normal living. Cure has been most successful in cases that were diagnosed and treated at an early stage, especially among the young.

Among the public health measures used to prevent leprosy are the laws in most countries requiring that all cases be reported to the local authorities and that all discharged leprous patients be examined at 6-month intervals. Most countries also refuse entry to immigrants known to be infected.

leptazol (lep"tah-zol) pentylenetetrazol, a central nervous system stimulant.

lepto- (lep'to) word element [Gr.], *slender; thin.*

leptocephalus (lep"to-sef'ah-lus) a fetus with a very small head.

leptochromatic (lep"to-kro-mat'ik) having a fine chromatin network.

leptocyte (lep'to-sīt) an erythrocyte characterized by a hemoglobinated border surrounding a clear area containing a center of pigment.

leptocytosis (lep"to-si-to'sis) leptocytes in the blood.

leptodactyly (lep"to-dak'tĭ-le) abnormal slenderness of the digits.

leptodermic (lep"to-der'mik) having a thin skin.

leptomeninges (lep"to-mĕ-nin'jēz) (plural of *leptomeninx*). the two more delicate components of the meninges: the pia mater and arachnoid. adj., **leptomenin'geal.**

leptomeningitis (lep"to-men"in-ji'tis) inflammation of the leptomeninges.

leptopellic (lep"to-pel'ik) having a narrow pelvis.

leptophonia (lep"to-fo'ne-ah) weakness or feebleness of the voice.

leptoscope (lep'to-skōp) an apparatus by which the thickness and composition of an extremely thin layer or membrane can be determined.

Leptospira (lep"to-spi'rah) a genus of spirochetal microorganisms pathogenic for man and other mammals.
  L. icterohaemorrha'giae, the causative agent of leptospiral jaundice, or Weil's disease.

leptospirosis (lep"to-spi-ro'sis) a group of infectious diseases communicated to man by domestic and other animals. The best known is Weil's disease, or leptospiral jaundice; others are mud fever, autumn fever, and swineherd's disease.
  SYMPTOMS. Leptospirosis is usually a short feverish illness which produces a variety of symptoms. It begins with fever, acute headache, chills and sometimes nausea and vomiting. Later, other symptoms may be caused by the effects of the disease upon the kidneys, liver, skin, blood and other organs. These symptoms can include jaundice, skin rashes, hemorrhages of the skin and mucous membranes, inflammation of the eye, hematuria and oliguria.
  Diagnosis is often difficult because the symptoms resemble those of several other diseases. Jaundice is a key symptom that, when present, aids in diagnosis.
  Most cases are mild, consisting only of the early symptoms and having a duration of 1 to 2 weeks. In a few cases, a severe infection may cause damage to the kidneys, liver or heart. Only rarely is the disease fatal.
  CAUSE. The causative organism is Leptospira, a spiral organism that infects the kidneys of cattle, swine, dogs, cats, rats and other animals. The organisms are spread through the animals' urine.
  Usually they are inhaled with the air or taken in food or drink by mouth. The disease is most common among people who handle infected animals or the kidneys and other infected tissues of such animals.
  TREATMENT AND PREVENTION. Treatment is basically symptomatic. Penicillin or other antibiotics may be prescribed.
  Sanitation measures can reduce the spread of the disease in both man and animals. Vaccines for animals are available, but provide only partial immunity to the disease. At the present time there are no vaccines of established value for human beings.

leptothricosis (lep"to-thrĭ-ko'sis) leptotrichosis.

Leptothrix (lep'to-thriks) a genus of microorganisms usually found in fresh water. Some species are found in the human mouth.

leptotrichosis (lep"to-trĭ-ko'sis) infection with Leptothrix.

Leritine (ler'ĭ-tīn) trademark for preparations of anileridine, a narcotic, analgesic and sedative.

lesbianism (lez'be-ah-nizm") female HOMOSEXUALITY, in which a woman chooses another woman as the object of romantic love and sexual interest instead of a man.

lesion (le'zhun) any damage to a tissue. Lesion is a broad term, including wounds, sores, ulcers, tumors, cataracts and any other tissue damage, whether caused by injury or disease. Lesions range from the skin sores associated with eczema to the changes in lung tissue that occur in tuberculosis.

lethal (le'thal) deadly; fatal.

lethargy (leth'ar-je) stupor, or coma, resulting from disease or hypnosis. adj., **lethar'gic.**
  African l., African trypanosomiasis.

Letterer-Siwe disease (let'er-er si'we) a rapidly fatal nonfamilial, nonlipid reticuloendotheliosis of early childhood.

leucine (lu-sēn) a naturally occurring amino acid, one of those essential for human metabolism.

leucinuria (lu"sin-u're-ah) leucine in the urine.

leucismus (lu-siz'mus) whiteness.
  l. pilo'rum, an abnormal streak or spot of white hairs among the hair of the scalp.

leucitis (lu-si'tis) scleritis; inflammation of the sclera.

leuco- (lu'ko) for words beginning thus, see also those beginning *leuko-*.

Leuconostoc (lu"ko-nos'tok) a genus of Schizomycetes found in milk and fruit juices.
  L. citrovo'rum, an organism found in milk and milk products, frequently used in the study of nutritional requirements in bacteria.

leucovorin (lu″ko-vo′rin) a derivative of folic acid; used in megaloblastic anemia.

leuk(o)- (lu″ko) word element [Gr.], *white*.

leukapheresis (lu″kah-fĕ-re′sis) the selective removal of leukocytes from withdrawn blood, which is then retransfused in the patient.

leukasmus (lu-kaz′mus) leukoderma.

leukemia (lu-ke′me-ah) a malignant disease of the tissues in the bone marrow, spleen and lymph nodes. It is characterized by uncontrolled proliferation of leukocytes and their precursors, accompanied by a reduced number of erythrocytes and blood platelets, resulting in anemia and increased susceptibility to infection and hemorrhage. Other typical symptoms include fever, pain in the joints and bones and swelling of the lymph nodes, spleen and liver. adj., **leuke′mic**.

TYPES OF LEUKEMIA. Leukemia is classified clinically on the basis of (1) the duration and character of the disease—acute or chronic; (2) the type of cell involved—myeloid (myelogenous), lymphoid (lymphogenous) or monocytic; and (3) increase or nonincrease in the number of abnormal cells in the blood—leukemic or aleukemic (subleukemic).

In acute leukemia the white cells resemble precursor, or immature, cells. They are larger than normal cells, and they accumulate much more rapidly than in chronic leukemia. They are incapable of performing their normal function of combating infection. In chronic leukemia the white cells are more mature, resembling normal cells and having some limited capacity to oppose invading organisms.

Different types of leukemia dominate in various age groups. Acute lymphoid leukemia occurs in young children, particularly those 3 and 4 years of age. Acute myeloid leukemia affects principally young adults. Chronic lymphoid leukemia is found chiefly in persons 50 to 70 years old, and chronic myeloid leukemia in those 30 to 50 years old. Leukemia ranks high among causes of death in children between 4 and 14 years of age in the United States.

The incidence of the disease is growing, and the increase is only partially explained by increased efficiency of detection.

CAUSE. The precise cause of leukemia is unknown. Much research has been directed toward exploring the possibility of a virus or a genetic defect as the cause. Experiments have produced findings that support viral origin in animals. Evidence of possible viral origin in humans is inconclusive.

That radiation is a factor in myeloid leukemia has been established. When the radiation dose exceeds a certain point, there is a statistical correlation between the size of the dose and the occurrence of leukemia.

It is also known that heredity plays a role in some types of the disease. Leukemia frequency is high among those with Down's syndrome, or mongolism, and the possibility of its development is noticeably greater in a person who has an identical twin with leukemia.

TREATMENT. There is no existing treatment that can permanently control or cure leukemia. Transfusion and replacement of blood cells relieve the symptoms, and various antineoplastic agents temporarily destroy the leukemic cells, prolonging the life of many patients.

Often no treatment is necessary for chronic lymphoid leukemia, except for irradiation to reduce the larger lymph nodes or spleen. The patient may live a normal life.

Treatment of acute leukemia consists of transfusion, antibiotics, steroids and antineoplastic chemicals. Still experimental are the use of massive x-ray treatments and grafting of bone marrow from another person.

NURSING CARE. Most of the nursing problems presented by leukemia result from decrease in the numbers of erythrocytes and platelets, producing a severe anemia and a tendency toward hemorrhage. The patient's energy is conserved by rest in bed and avoidance of activities that produce fatigue. Dyspnea and palpitation occur as the body attempts to compensate for the lack of oxygen supply to the tissue cells. These symptoms may be alarming to the patient and can increase his anxiety. An explanation of the cause of these symptoms may help relieve the anxiety. Rest is also helpful in avoiding symptoms.

Because of constriction of the peripheral blood vessels the patient may experience a continuous feeling of chilliness. Additional warmth should be provided by using warmer clothing or adding an extra lightweight blanket to the bed. Hot water bottles and heating pads are forbidden in most cases because they produce local dilatation of the blood vessels and deprive the vital organs of an adequate blood supply. Decreased sensitivity to heat and cold also present the likelihood of burning the patient without his being aware of it.

The tendency to bleed is common to most leukemia patients and demands careful observation of the patient for signs of hemorrhage. Abnormalities of the urine or stool should be reported. Care must be exercised to avoid trauma that might initiate hemorrhage; for example, if the gums and mouth show a tendency to bleed, brushing of the teeth is discontinued and special mouth care substituted.

Since the patient has a lowered resistance to infection he must be protected from pathogenic microorganisms as much as possible. This may include careful screening of visitors and strict observance of the rules of good personal hygiene.

aleukemic l., leukemia in which the leukocyte count is normal or below normal.

aplastic l., leukemia with diminution of red and white cells and an increase of the proportion of large, atypical leukocytes.

basophilic l., basophilocytic l., leukemia in which many basophilic granulocytes (mast cells) are present in the blood.

embryonal l., stem cell leukemia.

eosinophilic l., leukemia in which eosinophils are the predominating cells.

granulocytic l., myeloid leukemia.

leukopenic l., aleukemic leukemia.

lymphatic l., lymphoblastic l., lymphocytic l., lymphogenous l., lymphoid l., leukemia associated with hyperplasia and overactivity of the lymphoid tissue, in which the leukocytes are lymphocytes or lymphoblasts.

lymphosarcoma cell l., a form of lymphocytoma or lymphoblastoma characterized by the presence of neoplastic lymphocytes in the peripheral blood.

megakaryocytic l., hemorrhagic thrombocythemia.

monocytic l., leukemia in which the predominating leukocytes are monocytes.

myeloblastic l., leukemia in which myeloblasts predominate.

myelocytic l., myelogenous l., myeloid l., leukemia arising from myeloid tissue in which the granular polymorphonuclear leukocytes predominate.

stem cell l., leukemia in which the predominating cell is so immature and primitive that its classification is difficult.

subleukemic l., aleukemic leukemia.

leukemid (lu-ke′mid) a nonspecific skin lesion of leukemia that does not represent cutaneous infiltrations with leukemic cells.

leukemogen (lu-ke′mo-jen) any substance that produces leukemia.

leukemoid (lu-ke′moid) exhibiting blood and sometimes clinical findings resembling those of true leukemia.

leukencephalitis (lūk″en-sef″ah-li′tis) inflammation of the white matter of the brain.

Leukeran (lu′ker-an) trademark for a preparation of chlorambucil, an antineoplastic agent.

leukergy (lu′ker-je) appearance in the blood of peculiar leukocytes characterized by adhesiveness and tendency to gather into a mass; a defense mechanism in infections and other forms of stress.

leukoagglutinin (lu″ko-ah-gloo′tĭ-nin) an agglutinin that acts upon leukocytes.

leukoblast (lu′ko-blast) an immature leukocyte.
  granular l., promyelocyte.

leukoblastosis (lu″ko-blas-to′sis) proliferation of immature leukocytes.

leukocidin (lu″ko-si′din) a substance destructive to leukocytes.

leukocyte (lu′ko-sīt) a colorless blood corpuscle capable of ameboid movement, whose chief function is to protect the body against microorganisms causing disease and which may be one of five types: lymphocytes, monocytes, neutrophils, eosinophils and basophils, the last three often referred to as granulocytes. adj., **leukocyt′ic.**

The leukocytes act by moving through blood vessel walls in order to reach a site of injury. Foreign particles such as bacteria may be engulfed or phagocytosed by the leukocytes, especially the neutrophils and monocytes. It is this process that causes the increase in the number of leukocytes in the blood during infection, and one of the laboratory determinations to diagnose infectious states is based on it. The leukocytes also play some role in the repair of injured tissue, though their function here is not clear.

agranular l's, nongranular l's, lymphoid l's (agranulocytes or lymphocytes), 1. lymphocytes with a round, chromatic nucleus. 2. monocytes with a nucleus indented at the poles.
  granular l's (granulocytes), 3. polymorphonuclear or polynuclear neutrophil leukocytes (heterophil leukocytes) with an irregularly lobed nucleus. 4. eosinophil leukocytes with a two-lobed nucleus. 5. basophil leukocytes with a bent lobed nucleus.
  hyaline l., monocyte.
  leukergic l's, leukocytes that appear in the blood in leukergy.
  mast l., the basophil of the circulating blood.
  transitional l., monocyte.

leukocythemia (lu″ko-si-the′me-ah) leukemia.

leukocytoblast (lu″ko-si′to-blast) a cell that develops into a leukocyte.

leukocytogenesis (lu″ko-si″to-jen′ĕ-sis) the formation of leukocytes.

leukocytolysin (lu″ko-si-tol′ĭ-sin) a lysin that destroys leukocytes.

leukocytolysis (lu″ko-si-tol′ĭ-sis) disintegration of leukocytes.

leukocytoma (lu″ko-si-to′mah) a tumor-like mass of leukocytes.

leukocytopenia (lu″ko-si″to-pe′ne-ah) leukopenia.

leukocytophagy (lu″ko-si-tof′ah-je) ingestion and destruction of leukocytes by cells of the reticuloendothelial system.

leukocytoplania (lu″ko-si″to-pla′ne-ah) wandering of leukocytes; passage of leukocytes through a membrane.

leukocytopoiesis (lu″ko-si″to-poi-e′sis) the formation of leukocytes.

leukocytosis (lu″ko-si-to′sis) increase in the number of leukocytes in the blood.
  mononuclear l., mononucleosis.
  pathologic l., that due to some morbid reaction, e.g., infection or trauma.

leukocytotaxis (lu″ko-si″to-tak′sis) leukotaxis.

leukocytotoxin (lu″ko-si″to-tok′sin) a toxin that destroys leukocytes.

leukocytotropic (lu″ko-si″to-trop′ik) having a selective affinity for leukocytes.

leukocyturia (lu″ko-si-tu′re-ah) leukocytes in the urine.

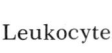
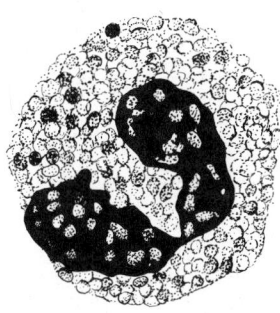
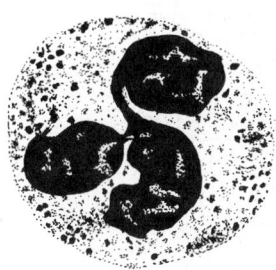

Leukocyte.

leukoderma (lu″ko-der′mah) an acquired condition with localized loss of pigmentation of the skin.
   l. acquisi′tum centrif′ugum, depigmentation of the skin around a pigmented nevus.

leukoedema (lu″ko-ĕ-de′mah) an abnormality of buccal mucosa, consisting of an increase in thickness of the epithelium, with intracellular edema of the malpighian layer.

leukoencephalopathy (lu″ko-en-sef″ah-lop′ah-the) disease of the white matter of the brain.

leukogram (lu′ko-gram) a tabulation of different types of leukocytes in a blood specimen.

leukokeratosis (lu″ko-ker″ah-to′sis) leukoplakia.

leukokinesis (lu″ko-ki-ne′sis) the movement of the leukocytes within the circulatory system.

leukokinetics (lu″ko-ki-net′iks) study of the production, circulation and destruction of leukocytes in the body.

leukokoria (lu″ko-ko′re-ah) appearance of a whitish reflex or mass in the pupillary area behind the lens.

leukolymphosarcoma (lu″ko-lim″fo-sar-ko′mah) lymphosarcoma cell leukemia.

leukolysin (lu-kol′ĭ-sin) leukocytolysin.

leukolysis (lu-kol′ĭ-sis) leukocytolysis.

leukoma (lu-ko′mah) 1. a white corneal opacity; called also walleye. 2. leukosarcoma. adj., **leukom′atous.**
   l. adhae′rens, a white tumor of the cornea enclosing a prolapsed adherent iris.

leukomaine (lu′ko-mān) an alkaloid derived from living animal tissue.

leukomyelitis (lu″ko-mi″ĕ-li′tis) inflammation of white matter of the brain or spinal cord.

leukomyelopathy (lu″ko-mi″ĕ-lop′ah-the) disease of the white matter of the spinal cord.

leukon (lu′kon) the leukocytes and leukocyte-forming tissues of the body.

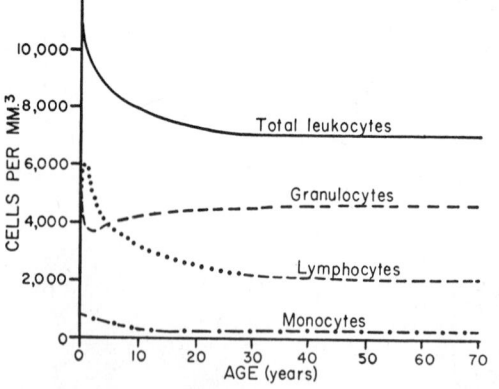

Relative proportions of the different white blood cells at different ages. (From Guyton, A. C.: Textbook of Medical Physiology. 3rd ed. Philadelphia, W. B. Saunders Co., 1966.)

leukonychia (lu″ko-nik′e-ah) abnormal whiteness of the nails, either total or in spots or streaks.

leukopathia (lu″ko-path′e-ah) leukoderma.
   l. un′guium, leukonychia.

leukopedesis (lu″ko-pĕ-de′sis) diapedesis of leukocytes.

leukopenia (lu″ko-pe′ne-ah) deficiency in the number of leukocytes in the blood. adj., **leukope′nic.**
   malignant l., pernicious l., agranulocytosis.

leukophagocytosis (lu″ko-fag″o-si-to′sis) leukocytophagy.

leukoplakia, leukoplasia (lu-ko-pla′ke-ah), (lu″-ko-pla′ze-ah) thickened white patches on the lips, gingivae (gums), tongue or other mucous membranes. They tend to grow into larger patches, or they may take the form of ulcers. Those in the mouth may in time cause pain during the swallowing of food or in speaking. They have a pronounced tendency to become malignant.
   Leukoplakia affects mostly elderly or middle-aged men, often as a result of prolonged irritation of the mouth from such varying factors as badly fitting dentures or immoderate use of tobacco.
   Treatment is aimed at removing any possible cause of physical or chemical irritation. The patient with leukoplakia should give up tobacco and possibly also alcohol and extremely hot food. Dental attention may be necessary if the patient's teeth are uneven or his dentures do not fit properly. A special mouthwash may be prescribed to be used after each meal.
   Surgical removal of the affected area is relatively simple and is frequently the best means of preventing its further development.

leukoplastid (lu″ko-plas′tid) any one of the white granules of plant cells whence the starch-forming elements are formed.

leukopoiesis (lu″ko-poi-e′sis) the production of leukocytes.

leukoprotease (lu″ko-pro′te-ās) an enzyme in the leukocytes that splits up protein.

leukopsin (lu-kop′sin) visual white; the colorless matter into which rhodopsin is changed by exposure to white light.

leukorrhagia (lu″ko-ra′je-ah) profuse leukorrhea.

leukorrhea (lu″ko-re′ah) vaginal discharge, usually white or yellowish in color. Leukorrhea is a symptom of a disorder either in the reproductive organs or elsewhere in the body.
   The glands of the vagina and cervix normally secrete a certain amount of mucus-like fluid that moistens the membranes of the vagina. This discharge is frequently increased at the time of ovulation and before a menstrual period. It is also stimulated by sexual excitement, whether or not coitus takes place.
   Excessive discharge, however, may indicate an abnormal condition. Yellowish or creamy white discharge, especially if it is thick, often contains pus and provides evidence of an infection. Thinner discharge, and the kinds that seem to be clear mucus, usually indicate that the disorder is chronic, but of less significance.
   CAUSES. A frequent cause of leukorrhea is trichomoniasis. The discharge is usually yellowish,

has an unpleasant odor and may be accompanied by itching.

Another cause of leukorrhea is infection of the cervix during childbirth. This infection irritates the mucous glands of the cervix, causing them to secrete an excessive amount of mucus. Venereal diseases, especially gonorrhea, are also a common cause of leukorrhea. When the discharge is profuse, thick and yellowish, and there is a burning sensation during urination, gonorrhea should be suspected.

Other bacteria and fungi may be causes of leukorrhea. Infections of the genital tract that cause leukorrhea may originate from foreign bodies, such as tampons, diaphragms and pessaries, left in the vagina over too long a period.

Leukorrhea sometimes is an early indication of cervical cancer, or of benign conditions, such as polyps or myoma of the uterus. It may also be caused by pelvic congestion associated with heart disease, by malnutrition or by inflammation of the uterine tubes as a result of tuberculosis. In later years, the disorder may be caused by debility.

TREATMENT. Leukorrhea caused by an infection of the reproductive organs is usually treated by douching alone or by douching and medication. The simplest remedy, and usually the first to be prescribed, is a douche of vinegar and water in the proportion of 2 to 4 tablespoonfuls of vinegar to 2 quarts of warm water. If this proves ineffective, a medicated douche may be prescribed, possibly combined with vaginal suppositories. An anti-inflammatory cream or ointment may also be prescribed for irritated external areas.

leukosarcoma (lu″ko-sar-ko′mah) an uncolored or colorless sarcoma.

leukosis (lu-ko′sis) proliferation of leukocyte-forming tissue.

leukotaxine (lu″ko-tak′sin) a crystalline nitrogenous substance that appears when tissue is injured, that can be recovered from inflammatory exudates and that increases capillary permeability and the diapedesis of leukocytes.

leukotaxis (lu″ko-tak′sis) cytotaxis of leukocytes; the tendency of leukocytes to collect in regions of injury and inflammation.

leukothrombin (lu″ko-throm′bin) a fibrin factor formed by leukocytes in the blood.

leukotomy (lu-kot′o-me) incision of the white matter of the frontal lobe of the brain; called also frontal lobotomy.

leukotoxic (lu″ko-tok′sik) destructive to leukocytes.

leukotoxicity (lu″ko-tok-sis′ĭ-te) toxicity for leukocytes.

leukotoxin (lu″ko-tok′sin) a toxin that destroys leukocytes.

leukotrichia (lu″ko-trik′e-ah) whiteness of the hair.

levallorphan (lev″ah-lor′fan) a compound used as an antagonist to narcotics.

levarterenol (lev″ar-tĕ-re′nol) norepinephrine.
l. bitartrate, a compound used as a sympathomimetic and as a pressor agent.

levator (lĕ-va′tor), pl. *levato′res* [L.] that which lifts or elevates, such as a muscle or instrument (elevator) for raising an organ or part.

Levin tube (lĕ-vin′) a nasal gastroduodenal catheter.

levo- (le′vo) word element [L.], *left*.

levocardia (le″vo-kar′de-ah) location of the heart in the left hemithorax, with the apex pointing to the left, associated with transposition of the abdominal viscera and congenital structural anomaly of the heart and usually with absence of the spleen.

Levo-dromoran (le″vo-dro′mo-ran) trademark for preparations of levorphanol tartrate, a narcotic analgesic.

levoduction (le″vo-duk′shun) movement of an eye to the left.

levogram (le′vo-gram) an electrocardiographic tracing showing left axis deviation, indicative of left ventricular hypertrophy.

levogyration (le″vo-ji-ra′shun) rotation to the left.

levonordefrin (le″vo-nor′dĕ-frin) a compound used as a vasoconstrictor.

Levophed (lev′o-fed) trademark for a preparation of levarterenol, a sympathomimetic and pressor agent.

levophobia (le″vo-fo′be-ah) fear of objects on the left side of the body.

levopropoxyphene (le″vo-pro-pok′sĭ-fēn) a compound used for cough.

levorotation (le″vo-ro-ta′shun) a turning to the left.

levorotatory (le″vo-ro′tah-to″re) turning the plane of polarization, or rays of light, to the left.

levorphanol tartrate (lēv-or′fah-nol) a compound used as a narcotic analgesic.

levothyroxine (le″vo-thi-rok′sin) the levorotatory isomer of thyroxine.
sodium l., the sodium salt of levothyroxine, used for replacement therapy in hypothyroidism.

levoversion (le″vo-ver′zhun) a turning toward the left.

levulinic acid (lev″u-lin′ik) an acid from decomposition of pentose sugars of nucleic acid and from the thymus.

levulose (lev′u-lōs) a sugar from fruits, honey and the intestines; called also fructose and fruit sugar.

Leydig cells (li′dig) interstitial cells of the testis, which furnish its internal secretion.

leydigarche (li″dig-ar′ke) establishment or beginning of gonadal function in the male.

L.F.A. left frontoanterior (position of the fetus).

L.F.P. left frontoposterior (position of the fetus).

L.F.T. left frontotransverse (position of the fetus).

LH luteinizing hormone.

Li chemical symbol, *lithium*.

libido (lĭ-be′do, lĭ-bi′do) instinctual energy or drive, often used with special reference to the motive power of the sex life.

Libman-Sacks disease (lib′man saks) nonbacterial verrucous endocarditis.

Librium (lib′re-um) trademark for preparations of chlordiazepoxide, a tranquilizer.

lice (līs) plural of *louse*.

lichen (li′ken) 1. a name applied to many different kinds of papular skin diseases. 2. any species or plant of a group believed to be composed of symbiotic algae and fungi.
  l. al′bus, lichen sclerosus et atrophicus.
  l. amyloido′sus, a condition characterized by localized cutaneous amyloidosis.
  l. chron′icus sim′plex, localized neurodermatitis.
  l. fibromucinoido′sus, lichen myxedematosus.
  l. lepro′sus, a manifestation of lepromatous leprosy, with lichenoid papules appearing in groups.
  l. myxedemato′sus, a skin condition characterized by abnormal deposits of mucin and widespread eruption of soft, pale red or yellowish papules.
  l. nit′idus, a rare skin disease with small, usually flat, sharply margined papules scarcely raised above the level of the skin, pale red or yellowish brown.
  l. pila′ris, lichen spinulosus.
  l. planopila′ris, a variant of lichen planus characterized by formation of acuminate horny papules around the hair follicles, in addition to the typical lesions of ordinary lichen planus.
  l. pla′nus, an inflammatory skin disease with wide flat papules, often in circumscribed patches.
  l. pla′nus et acumina′tus atroph′icans, alopecia cicatrisata with an eruption of follicular spinous papules.
  l. ru′ber monilifor′mis, a variant of lichen simplex chronicus.
  l. ru′ber pla′nus, lichen planus.
  l. sclero′sus et atroph′icus, a skin disorder characterized by alopecia cicatrisata and papules.
  l. scrofulo′sis, a form consisting of reddish papules, peculiar to persons of a tuberculous diathesis.
  l. sim′plex chron′icus, localized neurodermatitis.
  l. spinulo′sus, a condition in which there is a horn or spine in the center of each hair follicle.
  l. stria′tus, a condition characterized by a linear lichenoid eruption, usually in children.
  l. urtica′tus, papular urticaria.

lichenification (li-ken″ĭ-fĭ-ka′shun) thickening and hardening of the skin.

lichenoid (li′kĕ-noid) resembling lichen.

lidocaine (li′do-kān) a compound used as a local anesthetic.

lien (li′en) [L.] spleen. adj., **lie′nal.**
  l. accesso′rius, an accessory spleen.
  l. mo′bilis, an abnormally movable spleen.

lien(o)- (li-e′no) word element [L.], *spleen*.

lienectomy (li″en-ek′to-me) excision of the spleen; splenectomy.

lienitis (li″en-i′tis) splenitis.

lienocele (li-e′no-sēl) hernia of the spleen.

lienography (li″ĕ-nog′rah-fe) roentgenography of the spleen.

lienomalacia (li-e″no-mah-la′she-ah) abnormal softness of the spleen.

lienomedullary (li-e″no-med′u-ler″e) pertaining to the spleen and bone marrow.

lienomyelogenous (li-e″no-mi′ĕ-loj′ĕ-nus) formed in the spleen and bone marrow.

lienomyelomalacia (li-e″no-mi″ĕ-lo-mah-la′she-ah) softening of the spleen and bone marrow.

lienopancreatic (li-e″no-pan″kre-at′ik) pertaining to the spleen and pancreas.

lienopathy (li″ĕ-nop′ah-the) any disease of the spleen.

lienorenal (li″ĕ-no-re′nal) pertaining to the spleen and kidney.

lientery (li′en-ter″e) diarrhea with passage of undigested food. adj., **lienter′ic.**

lienunculus (li″en-ung′ku-lus) a detached mass of splenic tissue; an accessory spleen.

ligament (lig′ah-ment) a tough band of tissue that connects bones at a joint or supports organs. adj., **ligamen′tous.** The injury suffered when a joint is wrenched with sufficient violence to stretch or tear the ligaments is called a SPRAIN.
  accessory l., one that strengthens or supplements another.
  appendiculo-ovarian l., a fold of mesentery extending between the appendix and the broad ligament of the uterus.
  arcuate l's, the arched ligaments that connect the diaphragm with the lowest ribs and the first lumbar vertebra.
  broad l. of liver, the falciform ligament of the liver.
  broad l. of lung, a vertical pleural fold that extends from the hilus down to the base of the lung.
  broad l. of uterus, a broad fold of peritoneum extending from the side of the uterus to the wall of the pelvis; it consists of three parts: supporting the uterus (mesometrium), uterine tube (mesosalpinx) and ovary (mesovarium).
  capsular l., the tough fibrous framework surrounding every joint.
  crural l., inguinal ligament.
  deltoid l., the internal lateral ligament of the ankle joint.
  falciform l. of liver, a sickle-shaped sagittal fold of peritoneum that helps to attach the liver to the diaphragm and separates the right and left lobes of the liver.
  false l., any suspensory ligament that is a peritoneal fold and not of true ligamentous structure.
  Gimbernat's l., a triangular expanse of the aponeurosis of the external oblique muscle, anteriorly jointed to the inguinal ligament, and going to the iliopectineal line; called also lacunar ligament.
  hepatic l's, folds of peritoneum extending from the liver to adjacent structures.

inguinal l., a fibrous band running from the anterior superior spine of the ilium to the spine of the pubis; called also Poupart's ligament.

interarticular l., any ligament situated within the capsule of a joint.

interprocess l., a ligament that connects two processes on the same bone.

lacunar l., Gimbernat's ligament.

nephrocolic l., fasciculi from the fatty capsule of the kidney passing down on the right side to the posterior wall of the ascending colon and on the left side to the posterior wall of the descending colon.

nuchal l., a broad, fibrous, triangular sagittal septum in the back of the neck, separating the right and left sides.

pancreaticosplenic l., a fold of peritoneum extending from the pancreas to the spleen.

Petit's l., uterosacral ligament.

Poupart's l., inguinal ligament.

reinforcing l's, ligaments that serve to reinforce joint capsules.

rhomboid l., the ligament connecting the cartilage of the first rib to the under surface of the clavicle.

round l. of femur, a broad ligament arising from the fatty cushion of the acetabulum and inserted on the head of the femur.

round l. of liver, a fibrous cord from the navel to the anterior border of the liver.

round l. of uterus, a fibromuscular band in the female that is attached to the uterus near the attachment of the uterine tube, passing then along the broad ligament, out through the abdominal ring, and into the labium majus.

suspensory l. of axilla, a layer ascending from the axillary fascia and ensheathing the smaller pectoral muscle.

suspensory l. of lens, ciliary zonule.

sutural l., a band of fibrous tissue between the opposed bones of a suture or immovable joint.

tendinotrochanteric l., a portion of the capsule of the hip joint.

uteropelvic l's, expansions of muscular tissue in the broad ligament of the uterus, radiating from the fascia over the internal obturator muscle to the side of the uterus and the vagina.

uterosacral l., a part of the thickening of the visceral pelvic fascia beside the cervix and vagina.

ventricular l., a false vocal cord.

vesicouterine l., a ligament that extends from the bladder.

vocal l's, the true vocal cords.

ligamentopexy (lig″ah-men′to-pek″se) fixation of the uterus by shortening the ligaments supporting it.

ligamentum (lig″ah-men′tum), pl. *ligamen′ta* [L.] ligament.

ligation (li-ga′shun) application of a ligature.

ligature (lig′ah-tūr) a thread or wire used in SURGERY to tie off blood vessels to prevent bleeding, or to treat abnormalities in other parts of the body by constricting the tissues.

Ligatures are used both inside and outside the body. If a ligature must be left within the body after an operation, the surgeon will most often use one made of animal tissue that will dissolve or become incorporated in the patient's own body tissue. Ligatures used on the outside of the body for stitches or cuts or incisions can be of any durable material, and are removed after they have served their purpose. Special instruments have been developed for the application of ligatures to parts of the body that are difficult for the surgeon's hands to reach or to work in.

light (līt) a form of radiant energy capable of stimulating the special sense organ and giving rise to the sensation of sight.

l. adaptation, adaptation of the eye to vision in the sunlight or in bright illumination (photopia), with reduction in the concentration of the photosensitive pigments of the eye.

axial l., central l., light whose rays are parallel to each other and to the optic axis.

cold l., light from a 750 watt electric bulb that is covered by a wall of circulating water: this lamp may be applied directly to the skin and is used for transillumination of the tissues for cancer diagnosis.

diffused l., light whose rays have been scattered by reflection and refraction.

Finsen l., sunlight passed through a lens containing a solution of copper sulfate in ammonia, which absorbs the yellow, red and infrared rays, leaving the violet and ultraviolet; used in treatment of lupus.

Minin l., a lamp for therapeutic administration of violet and ultraviolet light.

oblique l., light falling obliquely on a surface.

polarized l., light of which the vibrations are made over one plane or in circles or ellipses.

reflected l., light whose rays have bent out of their original course by passing through a transparent medium.

transmitted l., light that passes or has passed through an object.

white l., that produced by a mixture of all wavelengths of electromagnetic energy perceptible as light.

Wood l., light passed through Wood's filter, which eliminates visible light waves and passes ultraviolet waves; used in diagnosis and treatment of skin diseases.

lightening (līt′en-ing) the sensation of decreased abdominal distention caused by descent of the uterus into the pelvic cavity, 2 or 3 weeks before labor begins.

Lignac-Fanconi disease (lēn-yak′ fan-cōn′e) cystinosis.

lignocaine (lig′no-kān) lidocaine, a local anesthetic.

lignoceric acid (lig″no-ser′ik) a saturated fatty acid obtained from kerasin by hydrolysis.

ligula (lig′u-lah) a strip of white matter near the lateral border of the fourth ventricle.

limb (lim) 1. an arm or leg, including all its component parts. 2. a structure or part resembling an arm or leg.

anacrotic l., the ascending portion of a tracing of the pulse wave obtained by the sphygmograph.

catacrotic l., the descending portion of a tracing of the pulse wave obtained by the sphygmograph.

pectoral l., the arm, or a homologous part.

pelvic l., the leg, or a homologous part.

phantom l., an absent part of an arm or leg, subjectively perceived as real and active.

thoracic l., pectoral limb.

limbic (lim′bik) pertaining to a limbus, or margin.

l. system, a system of brain structures common to the brains of all mammals, comprising the cortex and related nuclei; in man its function is thought to be related to emotional response.

limbus (lim′bus), pl. *lim′bi* [L.] an edge or border; used in anatomic nomenclature to designate the edge of the cornea, where it joins the sclera (lim′-bus cor′neae), and other margins in the body.

lime (līm) 1. calcium oxide, a compound occurring in hard white or grayish white masses or granules, or as a white or grayish white powder. 2. the acid fruit of *Citrus aurantifolia.*

l. arsenate, a solution of white arsenic and sodium carbonate in water, used as an insecticide.

chlorinated l., white or grayish granular powder with odor of chlorine; used as a decontaminant and disinfectant.

slaked l., calcium hydroxide.

soda l., a mixture of calcium hydroxide with sodium or potassium hydroxide; used to absorb exhaled carbon dioxide.

sulfurated l., a preparation of lime and sublimed sulfur, used in solution in acute acne vulgaris.

limen (li′men), pl. *lim′ina* [L.] a threshold or boundary.

l. na′si, the upper limit of the vestibule of the nose.

l. of twoness, the distance between two points of contact on the skin necessary for their recognition as giving rise to separate stimuli.

liminal (lim′ĭ-nal) barely perceptible; pertaining to a threshold.

limitans (lim′ĭ-tanz) [L.] limiting.

lindane (lin′dān) a compound used in treatment of scabies and pediculosis, and to rid animals of ectoparasites.

Lindau's disease (lin′dowz) combined hemangioma of the cerebellum and of the retina occurring as a familial disease.

Lindau-von Hippel disease (lin′dow von hip′el) a hereditary condition of unknown origin, with hemangioblastomas of the cerebellum associated with hemangiomas of the skin.

line (lin) a stripe, streak, mark or narrow ridge; often an imaginary line connecting different anatomic landmarks (linea). adj., **lin′ear.**

abdominal l., any line upon the surface of the abdomen, such as one indicating the boundary of a muscle.

absorption l's, dark lines in the spectrum due to absorption of light by the substance through which the light has passed; called also absorption bands.

Beau's l's, transverse lines on the fingernails, seen after wasting disease.

blue l., a characteristic line on the gums showing chronic lead poisoning.

cement l., a line visible in microscopic examination of bone in cross section, marking the boundary of an osteon (haversian system).

cleavage l's, linear clefts in the skin indicative of direction of the fibers.

epiphyseal l., a line of the surface of an adult long bone marking the junction of the epiphysis and diaphysis.

gingival l., 1. a line determined by the level to which the gingiva extends on a tooth. 2. any linear mark visible on the surface of the gingiva.

gum l., gingival line (1).

iliopectineal l., the ridge on the ilium and pubes showing the brim of the true pelvis.

incremental l's, lines supposedly showing the successive layers deposited in a tissue.

intertrochanteric l's (anterior and posterior), traces on the anterior and posterior surfaces of the femur between the trochanters.

lead l., a bluish line at the edge of the gums in lead poisoning.

lip l., a line at the level to which the margin of either lip extends on the teeth.

magnetic l's of force, lines indicating the direction of magnetic force in a magnetic field.

median l., a vertical line dividing the body equally into right and left parts.

milk l., the line of thickened epithelium in the embryo along which the mammary glands are developed.

mylohyoid l., a ridge on the inner surface of the lower jaw.

nuchal l's, three lines (inferior, superior and highest) on the outer surface of the occipital bone.

pectinate l., one marking the junction of the rectal mucosa and the skin lining the anus.

primitive l., primitive streak.

quadrate l., a line on the posterior surface of the femur.

temporal l's, curved lines, inferior and superior, on the external surface of the parietal bone that are continuous with the temporal line of the frontal bone, a ridge that extends upward and backward from the zygomatic process of the frontal bone.

visual l., an imaginary line passing from the midpoint of the visual field to the fovea centralis retinae.

linea (lin′e-ah), pl. *lin′eae* [L.] a narrow ridge or streak on a surface, as of the body or a bone or other organ; a line.

l. al′ba, the tendinous mesial line down the front of the belly.

lin′eae albican′tes, white or colorless lines on the abdomen, breasts or thighs caused by mechanical stretching of the skin, as in pregnancy or obesity, with weakening of the elastic tissue.

l. as′pera, a rough longitudinal line on the back of the femur.

lin′eae atroph′icae, fine reddish lines on the abdomen in Cushing's syndrome.

l. cor′neae seni′lis, a horizontal brown line on the lower part of the cornea in senile degeneration.

l. ni′gra, a name given the tendinous mesial line of the abdomen (linea alba) when it has become pigmented in pregnancy.

lingua (ling′gwah), pl. *lin′guae* [L.] tongue. adj., **lin′gual.**

l. geograph′ica, geographic tongue.

l. ni′gra, black tongue.

linguale (ling-gwa′le) the upper end of the lingual surface of the symphysis of the lower jaw.

lingula (ling′gu-lah), pl. *lin′gulae* [L.] a small, tonguelike structure, such as the projection from the lower portion of the upper lobe of the left lung (lin'gula pulmo'nis sin'istra).

l. of sphenoid, a ridge between the body and greater wing of the sphenoid bone.

linguo- (ling'gwo) word element [L.], *tongue.*

linguopapillitis (ling″gwo-pap″ĭ-li'tis) small painful ulcers around the papillae of the tongue.

liniment (lin'ĭ-ment) an oily, soapy or alcoholic preparation to be rubbed on the skin.

camphor l., a preparation of camphor and cottonseed oil used as a local irritant.

camphor and soap l., mixture of green soap, camphor, rosemary oil, alcohol and purified water, used as a local irritant.

chloroform l., a mixture of chloroform with camphor and soap liniment, used as a local irritant.

medicinal soft soap l., a preparation of medicinal soft soap, lavender oil and alcohol; used as a detergent.

linin (li'nin) the substance of the achromatic nuclear reticulum of the cell.

linitis (lĭ-ni'tis) inflammation of gastric cellular tissue.

plastic l., diffuse hypertrophy of the submucous connective tissue of the stomach, rendering the walls of the stomach rigid, thick and hard, like a leather bag; called also Brinton's disease, hypertrophic gastritis, gastric sclerosis, cirrhosis of the stomach, fibromatosis ventriculi, cirrhotic gastritis and leather bottle stomach.

linkage (lingk'ij) 1. the connection between different atoms in a chemical compound, or the symbol representing it in structural formulae. 2. in genetics, the tendency for a group of genes in a chromosome to remain in continuous association from generation to generation. 3. in psychology, the connection between a stimulus and its response.

linked (lingkt) united; in genetics, referring to characters that are united so as invariably to be inherited together.

linseed (lin'sēd) dried ripe seed of *Linum usitatissimum;* flaxseed. Used as an emollient and in laxatives.

liothyronine (li″o-thi'ro-nēn) the levorotatory isomer of triiodothyronine; used in treatment of hypothyroidism.

sodium l., the sodium salt of triiodothyronine, used in thyroid replacement therapy.

lip (lip) 1. the upper or lower fleshy margin of the mouth. 2. a marginal part.

cleft l., congenital fissure of the upper lip; harelip (see also CLEFT LIP).

double l., redundancy of the submucous tissue and mucous membrane of the lip on either side of the median line.

lip(o)- (lip'o) word element [Gr.], *fat; lipid.*

lipacidemia (lip″as-ĭ-de'me-ah) fatty acid in the blood.

lipaciduria (lip″as-ĭ-du're-ah) fatty acid in the urine.

liparomphalus (lip″ah-rom'fah-lus) fatty tumor of the navel.

liparthritis (li″par-thri'tis) arthritis caused by cessation of ovarian function.

lipase (li'pās, lip'ās) an enzyme that catalyzes the decomposition of fats into glycerin and fatty acids.

lipectomy (lĭ-pek'to-me) excision of fatty tissue or of a lipoma.

lipedema (lip″ĕ-de'mah) an accumulation of excess fat and fluid in subcutaneous tissues.

lipemia (lĭ-pe'me-ah) fat or oil in the blood.

alimentary l., that occurring after ingestion of food.

l. retina'lis, a high level of lipids in the blood, manifested by a milky appearance of the veins and arteries of the retina.

lipfanogen (lip-fan'o-jen) a substance that produces visible fat.

lipid (lip'id) one of a group of naturally occurring substances consisting of the higher fatty acids, their naturally occurring compounds, and substances found naturally in chemical association with them.

lipiduria (lip″ĭ-du're-ah) the presence of lipids in the urine.

lipoarthritis (lip″o-ar-thri'tis) inflammation of the fatty tissue of the joints.

lipoatrophia (lip″o-ah-tro'fe-ah) atrophy of fatty tissues of the body.

lipoblast (lip'o-blast) a connective tissue cell that develops into a fat cell.

lipocaic (lip″o-ka'ik) a substance extracted from the pancreas that prevents deposit of fat in the liver of animals after experimental pancreatectomy.

lipocardiac (lip″o-kar'de-ak) pertaining to fatty degeneration of the heart.

lipocatabolic (lip″o-kat″ah-bol'ik) pertaining to the catabolism of fat.

lipochondrodystrophy (lip″o-kon″dro-dis'tro-fe) Hurler's syndrome.

lipochondroma (lip″o-kon-dro'mah) a chondroma containing fatty elements.

lipochrome (lip'o-krōm) any one of a group of fat-soluble hydrocarbon pigments, such as carotene, lutein, chromophane and the natural yellow coloring material of butter, egg yolk and yellow corn. They are also known as carotenoids.

lipocorticoid (lip″o-kor'tĭ-koid) an adrenocortical hormone effective in causing deposition of fat, especially in the liver.

lipocyte (lip'o-sīt) a fat cell.

lipodieresis (lip″o-di-er'ĕ-sis) the splitting or destruction of fat.

lipodystrophy (lip″o-dis'tro-fe) disturbance of fat metabolism.

intestinal l., a condition marked by deposits of

fats in the intestinal lymphoid tissue, with fatty diarrhea, arthritis and loss of weight.

lipofibroma   (lip″o-fi-bro′mah) a lipoma with fibrous elements.

lipofuscin (lip″o-fus′in) any one of a class of fatty pigments formed by the solution of a pigment in fat. Cf. lipochrome.

lipogenesis (lip″o-jen′ĕ-sis) the formation of fat.

lipogenic (lip″o-jen′ik) producing fat or fatness.

lipoid (lip′oid) 1. fatlike. 2. lipid.

lipoidemia (lip″oi-de′me-ah) lipids in the blood.

lipoidosis (lip″oi-do′sis) any disturbance of lipid metabolism; the presence of lipids in the cells.

lipoiduria (lip″oi-du′re-ah) lipids in the urine.

lipolipoidosis (lip″o-lip″oi-do′sis) both fats and lipids in a tissue.

Lipo-lutin (li″po-lu′tin) trademark for preparations of progesterone, a progestational hormone.

lipolysis (li-pol′ĭ-sis) the splitting up of fat. adj., lipolyt′ic.

lipoma (li-po′mah) a fatty tumor.

lipomatosis (lip″o-mah-to′sis) a condition characterized by abnormal localized, or tumor-like, accumulations of fat in the tissues.

lipomatous (li-po′mah-tus) affected with lipoma.

lipomeria (li″po-me′re-ah) congenital absence of a limb.

lipometabolism (lip″o-mĕ-tab′o-lizm) metabolism of fat.

lipomicron (lip″o-mi′kron) a microscopic fat particle in the blood.

lipomyxoma (lip″o-mik-so′mah) lipoma with myxomatous elements.

lipopenia (lip″o-pe′ne-ah) diminution of the fats in the blood.

lipopeptid (lip″o-pep′tid) a compound of an amino acid and a fatty acid.

lipopexia (lip″o-pek′se-ah) accumulation of fat in the tissues.

lipophage (lip′o-fāj) a cell that absorbs or ingests fat.

lipophagia, lipophagy (lip″o-fa′je-ah), (li-pof′ah-je) 1. destruction of fat. 2. eating of fat. adj., lipopha′gic.
   l. granulomato′sis, intestinal lipodystrophy.

lipophilia (lip″o-fil′e-ah) affinity for fat. adj., lipophil′ic.

lipophrenia (li″po-fre″ne-ah) failure of mental powers.

lipoprotein (lip″o-pro′te-in) a combination of a lipid and a protein, having the general properties (e.g., solubility) of proteins. Practically all of the lipids of the plasma and lipoprotein complexes,

alpha- and beta-lipoproteins being distinguished by electrophoresis.

liposarcoma   (lip″o-sar-ko′mah) sarcoma containing fatty elements.

liposin (li-po′sin) a fat-splitting enzyme in the blood.

liposis (li-po′sis) lipomatosis.

liposoluble (lip″o-sol′u-bl) soluble in fats.

liposome (lip′o-sōm) one of the particles of lipoid matter held emulsified in the tissues in the form of invisible fat.

lipothymia (li″po-thi′me-ah) faintness; syncope.

lipotrophy (li-pot′ro-fe) increase of bodily fat. adj., lipotroph′ic.

lipotropism, lipotropy (li-pot′ro-pizm), (li-pot′ro-pe) affinity for fat or fatty tissue, especially that of certain agents that are capable of decreasing the deposits of fat in the liver. adj., lipotrop′ic.

lipovaccine (lip″o-vak′sēn) a vaccine in a vegetable oil vehicle.

lipoxeny (li-pok′sĕ-ne) desertion of the host by a parasite.

lipoxidemia   (lip″ok-sĭ-de′me-ah) lipacidemia.

Lippes loop (lip′ez) a form of intrauterine contraceptive device.

lip-reading (lip′rēd-ing) perception of speech through the sense of sight, by recognition of the words formed from movement of the lips.

lipsotrichia   (lip″so-trik′e-ah) falling of the hair.

lipuria (li-pu′re-ah) fat or oil in the urine.

Liquaemin (lik′wah-min) trademark for preparations of heparin, an anticoagulant.

Liquamar (lik″wah-mar) trademark for a preparation of phenprocoumon, an anticoagulant.

liquefacient (lik″wĕ-fa′shent) having the quality to convert a solid material into a liquid, producing liquefaction.

liquefaction (lik″wĕ-fak′shun) conversion into a liquid form.

liquescent (li-kwes′ent) tending to become liquid or fluid.

liquid (lik′wid) 1. a substance that flows readily in its natural state. 2. flowing readily; neither solid nor gaseous.
   l. diet, a diet limited to the intake of liquids or foods that can be changed to a liquid state. A liquid diet may be restricted to clear liquids or it may be a full liquid diet (see the table of hospital diets, under DIET).
   CLEAR LIQUID DIET. This is a temporary diet of clear liquids without residue. It is not nutritionally adequate, and is used in some acute illnesses and infections, postoperatively (especially after gastrointestinal surgery) and to reduce fecal matter in the colon. Foods allowed include water, tea, coffee, fat-free broth, carbonated beverages, synthetic fruit juices, ginger ale, plain gelatin and sugar.

THE HUMAN BODY
HIGHLIGHTS of STRUCTURE and FUNCTION

SKELETAL SYSTEM

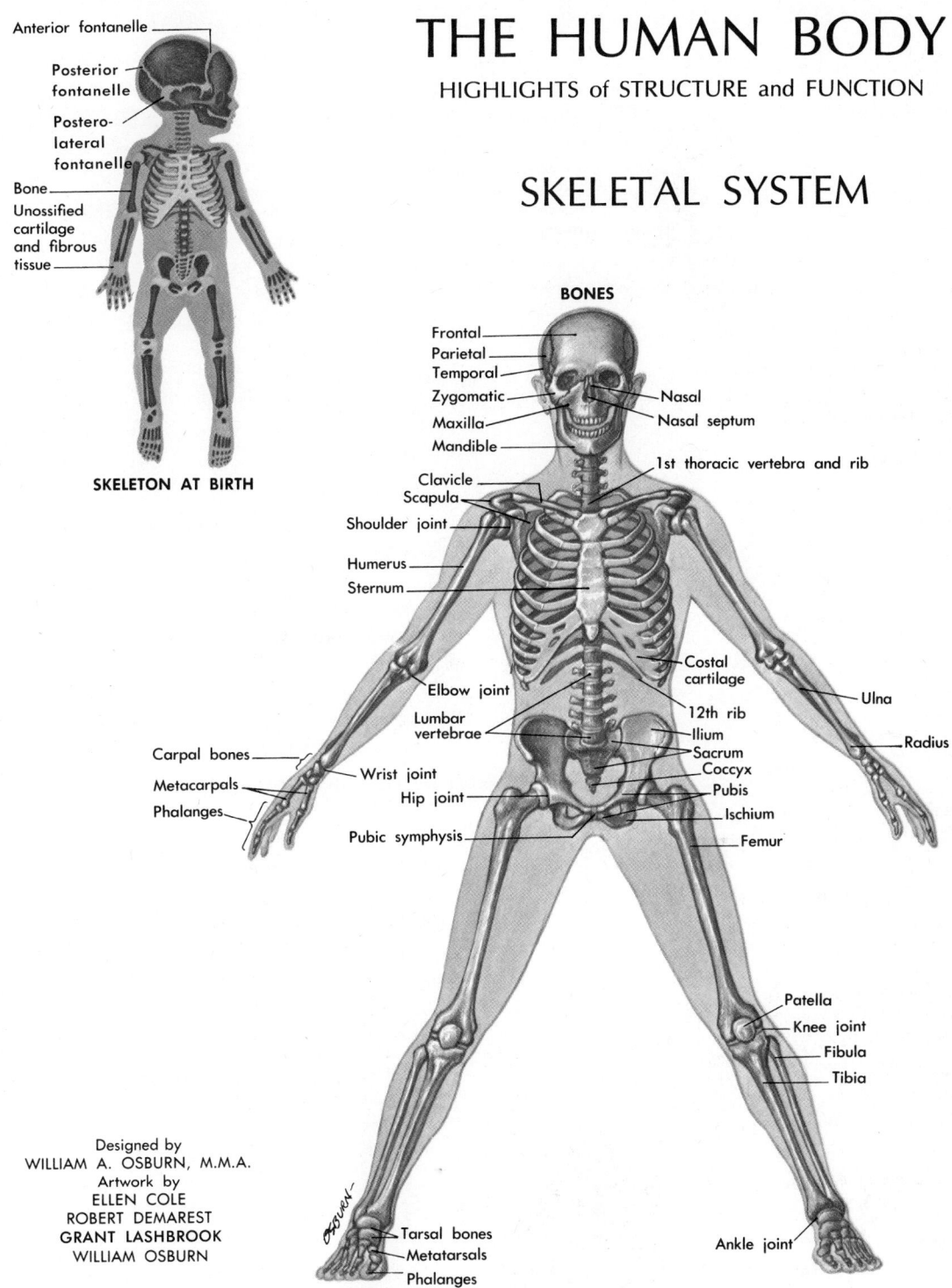

Skeleton at birth (upper left):
- Anterior fontanelle
- Posterior fontanelle
- Postero-lateral fontanelle
- Bone
- Unossified cartilage and fibrous tissue

SKELETON AT BIRTH

BONES

- Frontal
- Parietal
- Temporal
- Zygomatic
- Maxilla
- Mandible
- Nasal
- Nasal septum
- 1st thoracic vertebra and rib
- Clavicle
- Scapula
- Shoulder joint
- Humerus
- Sternum
- Costal cartilage
- 12th rib
- Ilium
- Sacrum
- Coccyx
- Pubis
- Ischium
- Femur
- Ulna
- Radius
- Elbow joint
- Lumbar vertebrae
- Carpal bones
- Metacarpals
- Phalanges
- Wrist joint
- Hip joint
- Pubic symphysis
- Patella
- Knee joint
- Fibula
- Tibia
- Tarsal bones
- Metatarsals
- Phalanges
- Ankle joint

Designed by
WILLIAM A. OSBURN, M.M.A.
Artwork by
ELLEN COLE
ROBERT DEMAREST
GRANT LASHBROOK
WILLIAM OSBURN

W. B. SAUNDERS COMPANY
Philadelphia — London — Toronto

Plate 1

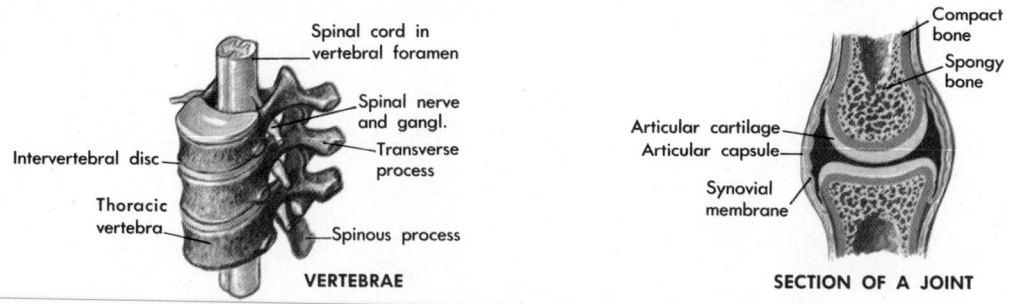

VERTEBRAE

Spinal cord in vertebral foramen
Spinal nerve and gangl.
Transverse process
Spinous process
Intervertebral disc
Thoracic vertebra

SECTION OF A JOINT

Compact bone
Spongy bone
Articular cartilage
Articular capsule
Synovial membrane

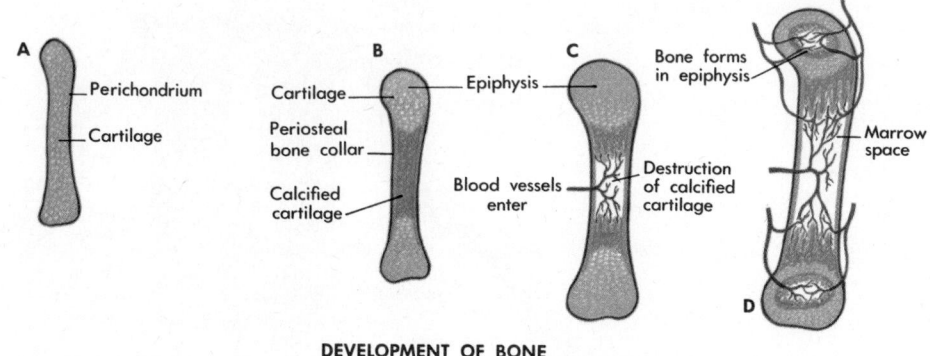

DEVELOPMENT OF BONE

A
Perichondrium
Cartilage

B
Cartilage
Periosteal bone collar
Calcified cartilage

Epiphysis

C
Blood vessels enter
Destruction of calcified cartilage

Bone forms in epiphysis
Marrow space
D

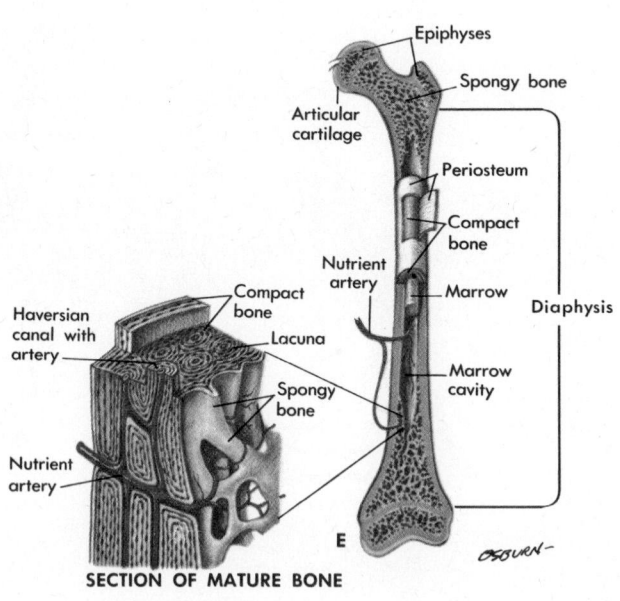

SECTION OF MATURE BONE

Epiphyses
Spongy bone
Articular cartilage
Periosteum
Compact bone
Nutrient artery
Marrow
Diaphysis
Marrow cavity

Haversian canal with artery
Compact bone
Lacuna
Spongy bone
Nutrient artery

E

OSBURN-

Plate 2

SKELETAL MUSCLES

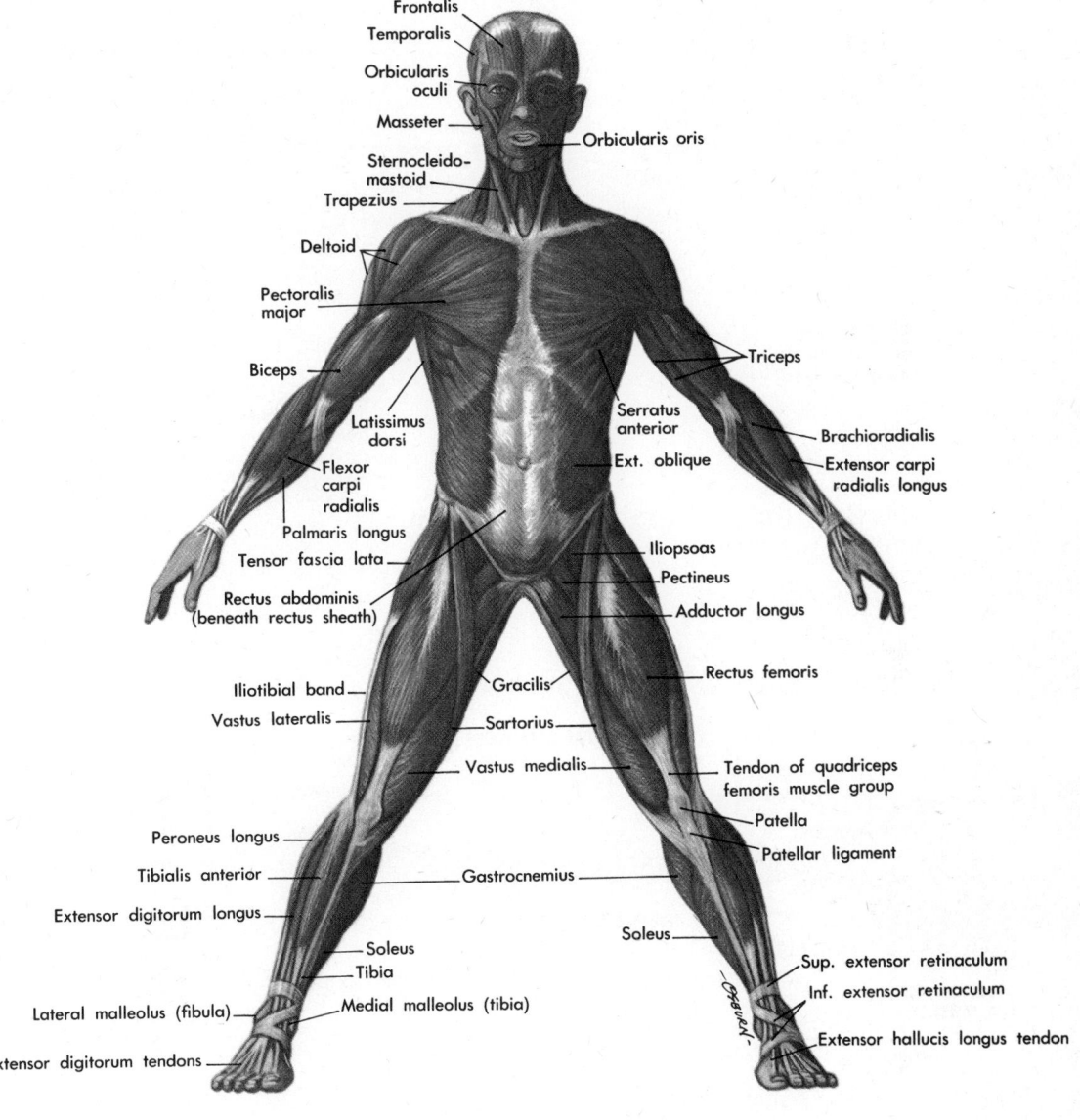

Frontalis
Temporalis
Orbicularis oculi
Masseter
Orbicularis oris
Sternocleido-mastoid
Trapezius
Deltoid
Pectoralis major
Biceps
Triceps
Latissimus dorsi
Serratus anterior
Brachioradialis
Flexor carpi radialis
Ext. oblique
Extensor carpi radialis longus
Palmaris longus
Tensor fascia lata
Iliopsoas
Pectineus
Rectus abdominis (beneath rectus sheath)
Adductor longus
Rectus femoris
Iliotibial band
Gracilis
Vastus lateralis
Sartorius
Vastus medialis
Tendon of quadriceps femoris muscle group
Patella
Peroneus longus
Patellar ligament
Tibialis anterior
Gastrocnemius
Extensor digitorum longus
Soleus
Soleus
Tibia
Sup. extensor retinaculum
Inf. extensor retinaculum
Lateral malleolus (fibula)
Medial malleolus (tibia)
Extensor digitorum tendons
Extensor hallucis longus tendon

Plate 3

HOW A MUSCLE PRODUCES MOVEMENT

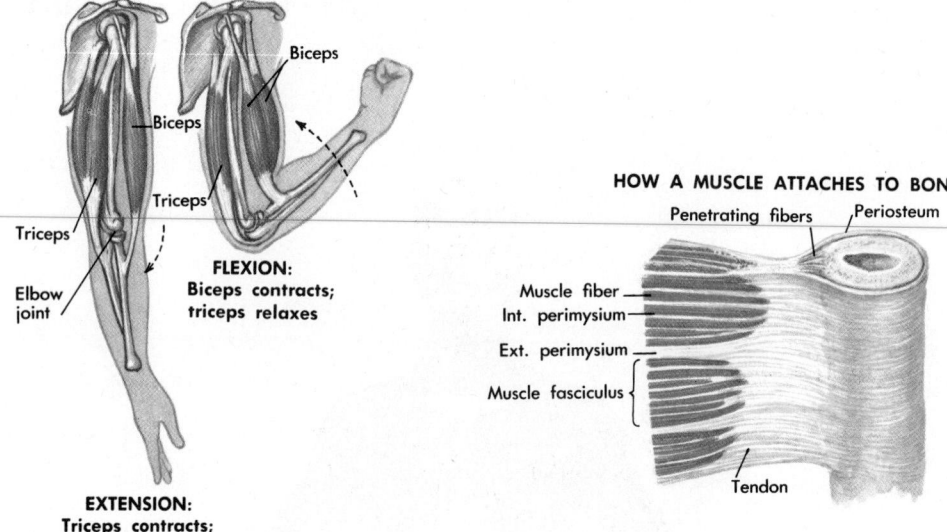

Biceps

Biceps

Biceps

Triceps

Triceps

Elbow joint

**FLEXION:
Biceps contracts;
triceps relaxes**

**EXTENSION:
Triceps contracts;
biceps relaxes**

HOW A MUSCLE ATTACHES TO BONE

Penetrating fibers Periosteum

Muscle fiber
Int. perimysium
Ext. perimysium
Muscle fasciculus

Tendon

The connective tissue which surrounds the muscle fibers and bundles may (1) form a tendon which fuses with the periosteum, or (2) may fuse directly with the periosteum without forming a tendon.

HOW A MUSCLE CONTRACTS

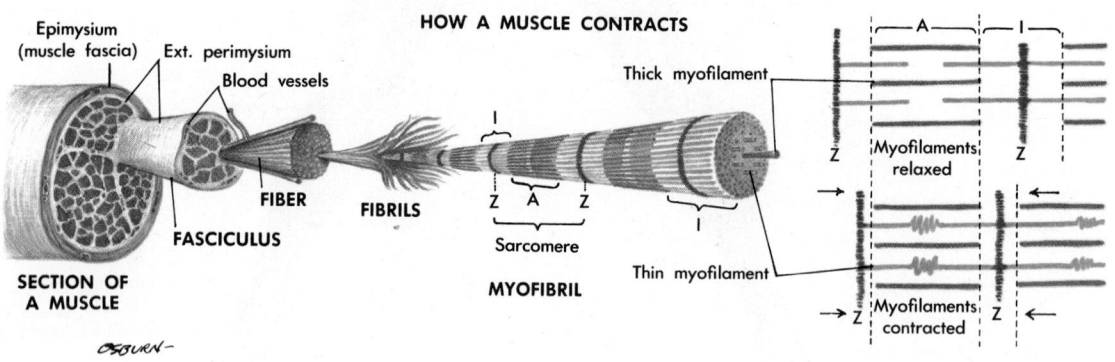

Epimysium (muscle fascia)
Ext. perimysium
Blood vessels

FIBER

FASCICULUS

FIBRILS

**SECTION OF
A MUSCLE**

OSBURN-

I
Z   A   Z

Sarcomere

MYOFIBRIL

Thick myofilament

Thin myofilament

A   I

Z   Z

Myofilaments relaxed

Z   Z

Myofilaments contracted

Plate 4

RESPIRATION AND THE HEART

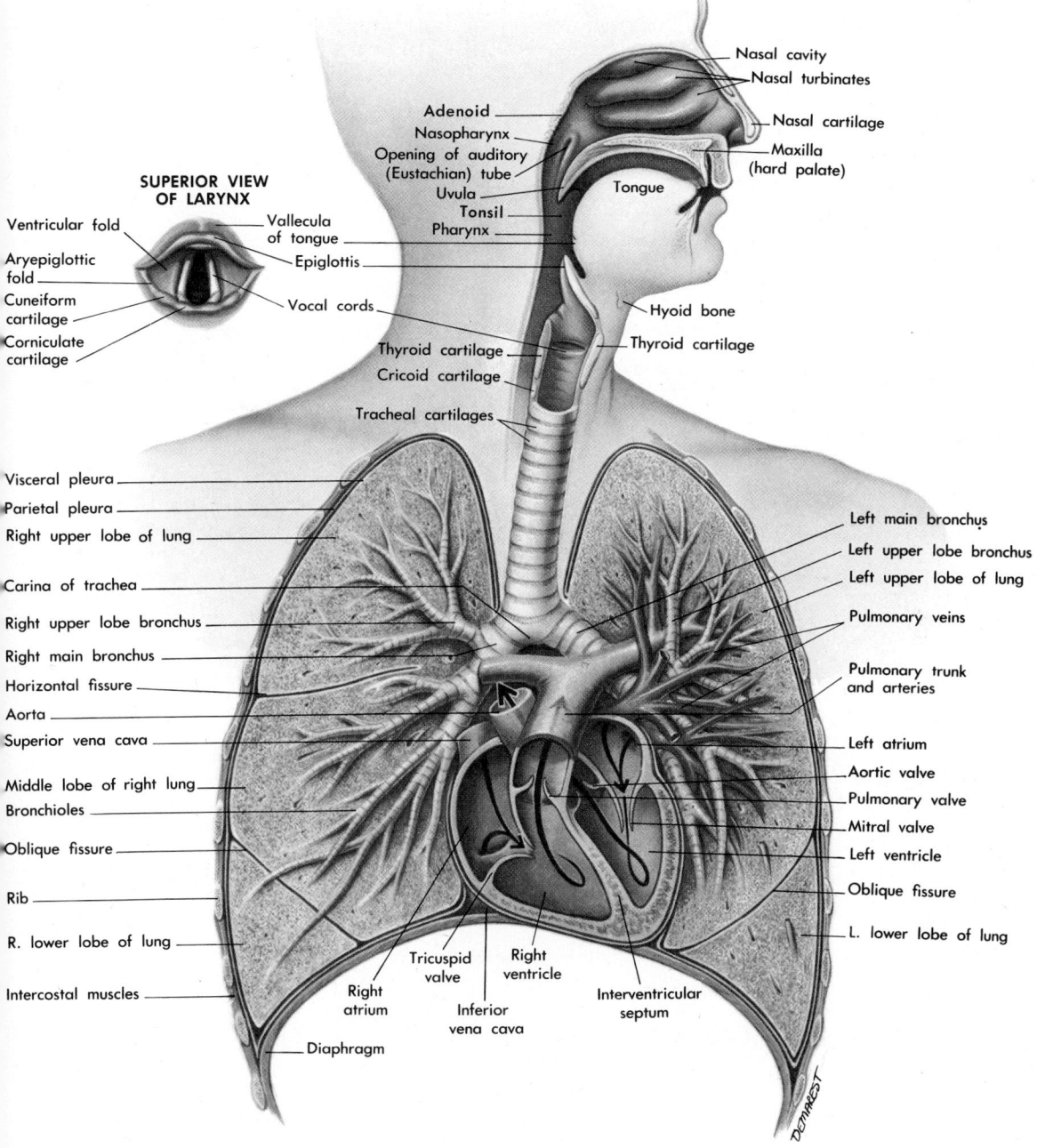

SUPERIOR VIEW OF LARYNX

Ventricular fold
Aryepiglottic fold
Cuneiform cartilage
Corniculate cartilage
Vallecula of tongue
Epiglottis
Vocal cords

Adenoid
Nasopharynx
Opening of auditory (Eustachian) tube
Uvula
Tonsil
Pharynx
Thyroid cartilage
Cricoid cartilage
Tracheal cartilages

Nasal cavity
Nasal turbinates
Nasal cartilage
Maxilla (hard palate)
Tongue
Hyoid bone
Thyroid cartilage

Visceral pleura
Parietal pleura
Right upper lobe of lung
Carina of trachea
Right upper lobe bronchus
Right main bronchus
Horizontal fissure
Aorta
Superior vena cava
Middle lobe of right lung
Bronchioles
Oblique fissure
Rib
R. lower lobe of lung
Intercostal muscles

Left main bronchus
Left upper lobe bronchus
Left upper lobe of lung
Pulmonary veins
Pulmonary trunk and arteries
Left atrium
Aortic valve
Pulmonary valve
Mitral valve
Left ventricle
Oblique fissure
L. lower lobe of lung

Tricuspid valve
Right ventricle
Right atrium
Inferior vena cava
Interventricular septum
Diaphragm

Plate 5

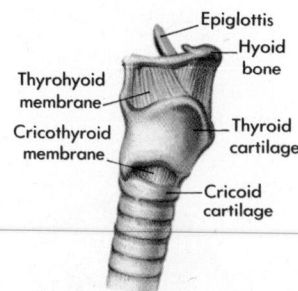

LATERAL VIEW OF THE LARYNX

Epiglottis

Hyoid bone

Thyrohyoid membrane

Cricothyroid membrane

Thyroid cartilage

Cricoid cartilage

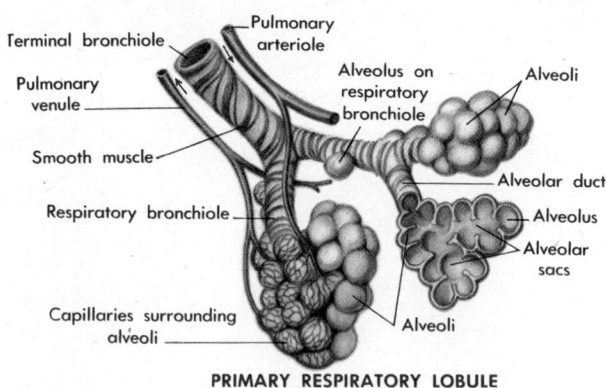

PRIMARY RESPIRATORY LOBULE

Terminal bronchiole

Pulmonary arteriole

Alveolus on respiratory bronchiole

Alveoli

Pulmonary venule

Smooth muscle

Respiratory bronchiole

Alveolar duct

Alveolus

Alveolar sacs

Capillaries surrounding alveoli

Alveoli

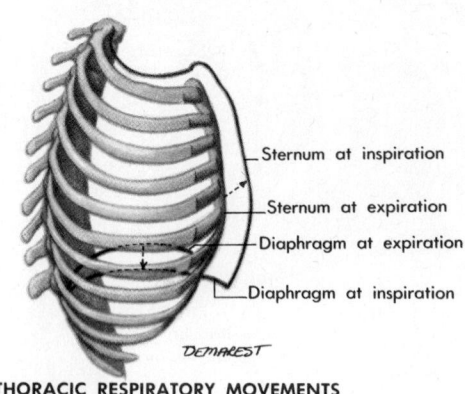

THORACIC RESPIRATORY MOVEMENTS

Sternum at inspiration

Sternum at expiration

Diaphragm at expiration

Diaphragm at inspiration

DEMAREST

Plate 6

BLOOD VASCULAR SYSTEM

VEINS

STRUCTURE

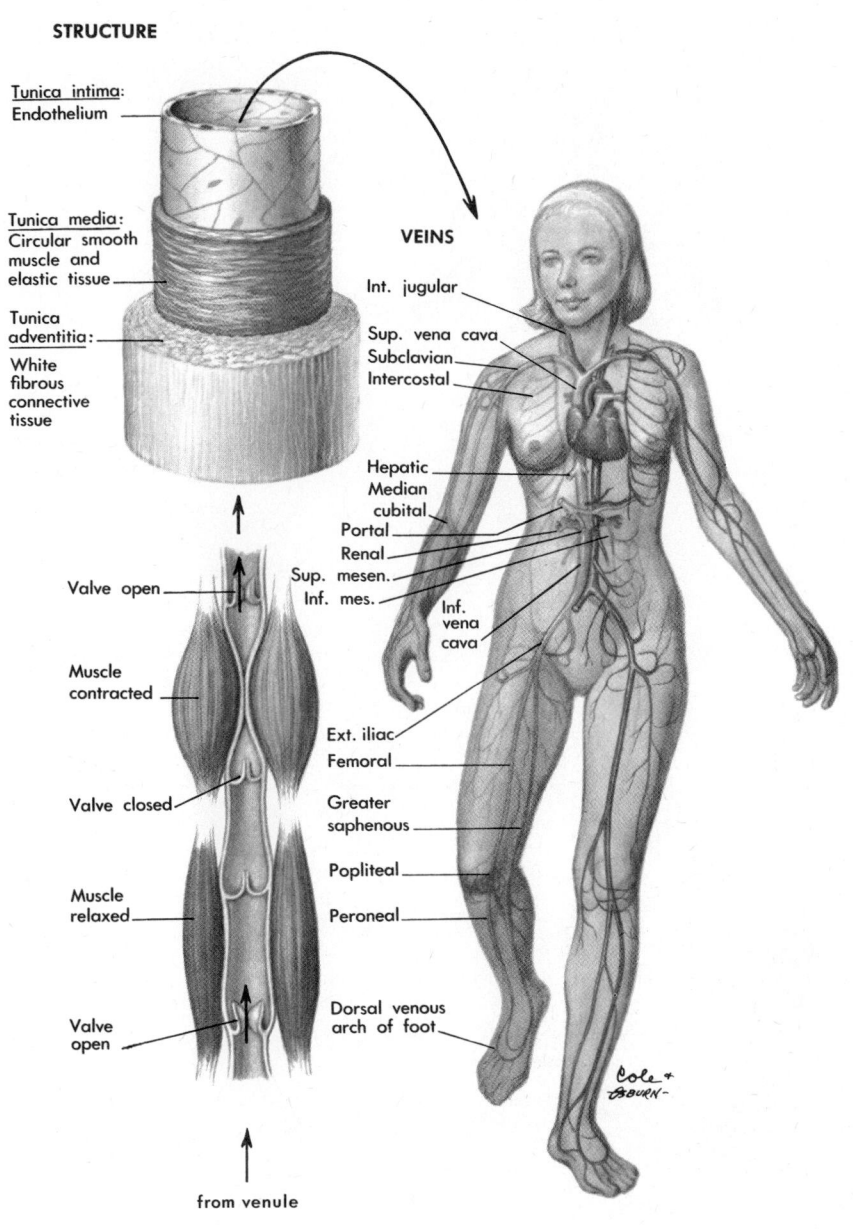

Tunica intima:
Endothelium

Tunica media:
Circular smooth
muscle and
elastic tissue

Tunica
adventitia:

White
fibrous
connective
tissue

VEINS

Int. jugular

Sup. vena cava
Subclavian
Intercostal

Hepatic
Median
  cubital
Portal
Renal
Sup. mesen.
Inf. mes.

Inf.
vena
cava

Valve open

Muscle
contracted

Valve closed

Muscle
relaxed

Valve
open

from venule

Ext. iliac
Femoral

Greater
saphenous

Popliteal

Peroneal

Dorsal venous
arch of foot

Cole &
Osborn

Plate 7

STRUCTURE

ARTERIES

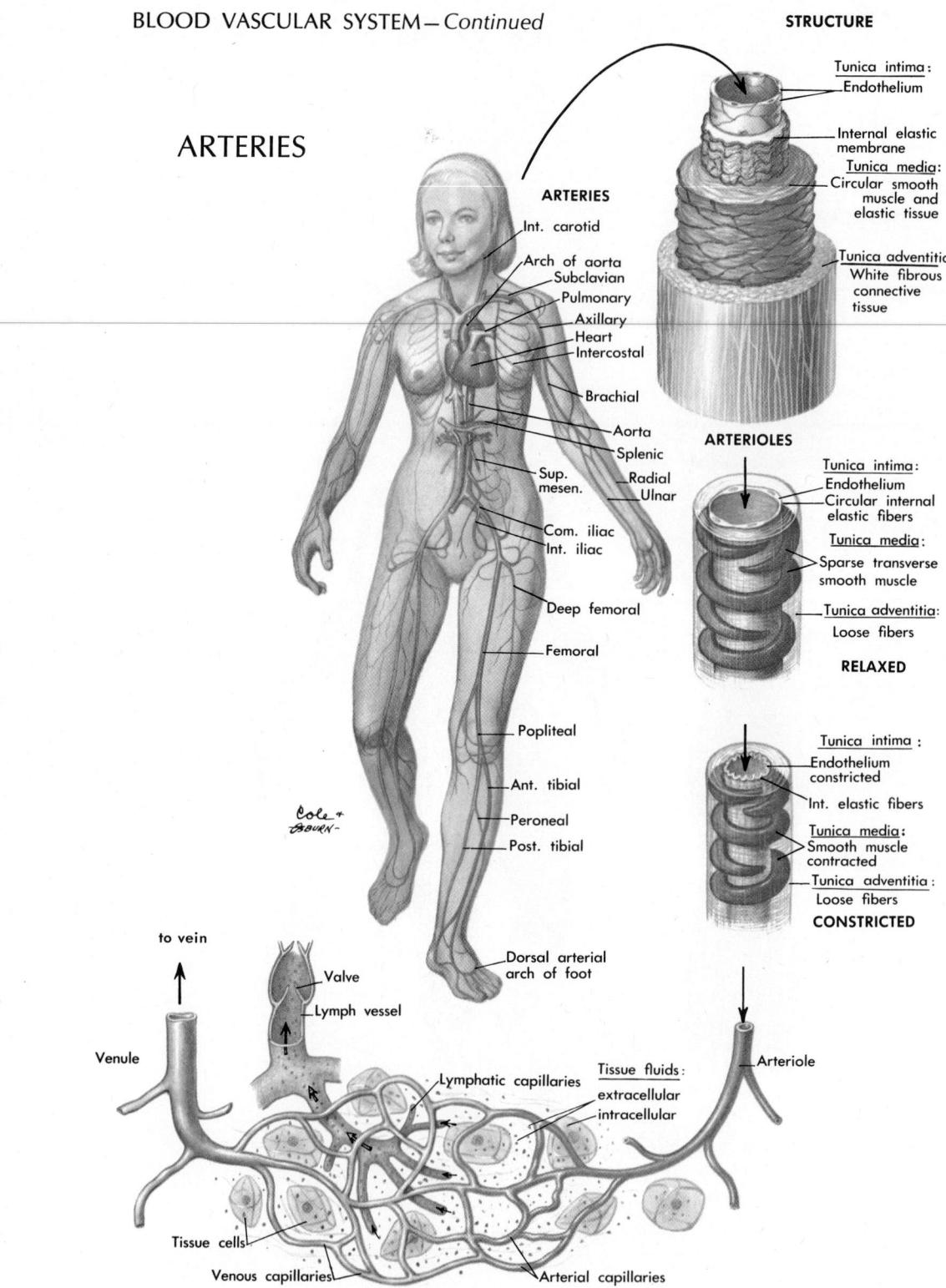

ARTERIES

Int. carotid
Arch of aorta
Subclavian
Pulmonary
Axillary
Heart
Intercostal
Brachial
Aorta
Splenic
Sup. mesen.
Radial
Ulnar
Com. iliac
Int. iliac
Deep femoral
Femoral
Popliteal
Ant. tibial
Peroneal
Post. tibial
Dorsal arterial arch of foot

Tunica intima:
Endothelium
Internal elastic membrane
Tunica media:
Circular smooth muscle and elastic tissue
Tunica adventitia
White fibrous connective tissue

ARTERIOLES

Tunica intima:
Endothelium
Circular internal elastic fibers
Tunica media:
Sparse transverse smooth muscle
Tunica adventitia:
Loose fibers

RELAXED

Tunica intima :
Endothelium constricted
Int. elastic fibers
Tunica media:
Smooth muscle contracted
Tunica adventitia:
Loose fibers

CONSTRICTED

to vein

Valve
Lymph vessel
Venule
Lymphatic capillaries
Tissue fluids:
extracellular
intracellular
Arteriole
Tissue cells
Venous capillaries
Arterial capillaries

A CAPILLARY BED

Plate 8

DIGESTIVE SYSTEM

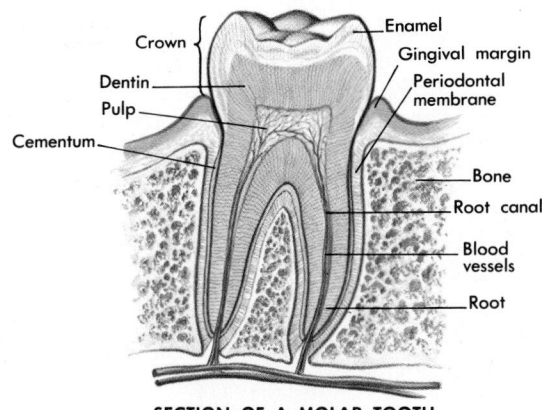

Crown
Enamel
Gingival margin
Dentin
Periodontal membrane
Pulp
Cementum
Bone
Root canal
Blood vessels
Root

SECTION OF A MOLAR TOOTH

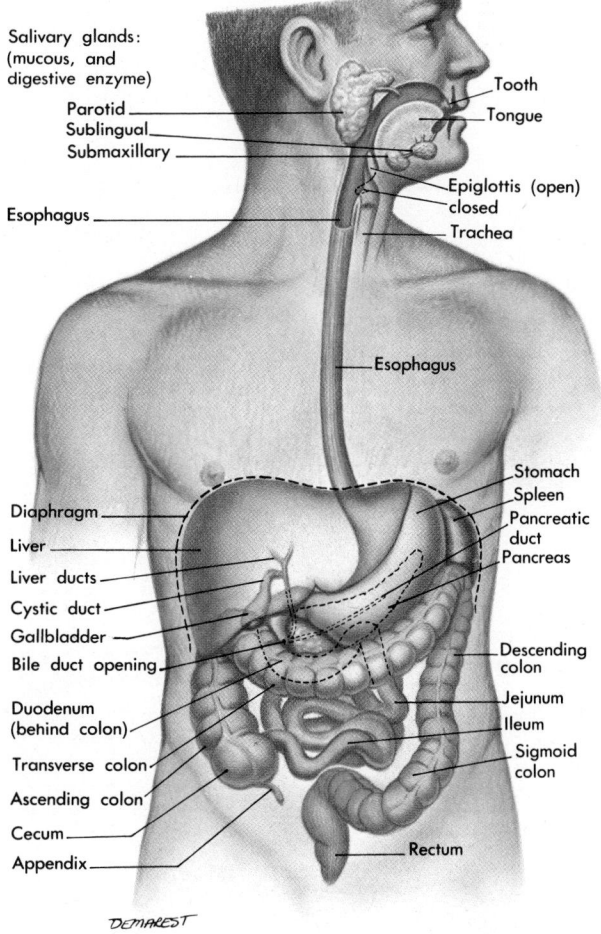

Salivary glands: (mucous, and digestive enzyme)
Parotid
Sublingual
Submaxillary
Esophagus
Tooth
Tongue
Epiglottis (open) closed
Trachea
Esophagus
Stomach
Spleen
Pancreatic duct
Pancreas
Diaphragm
Liver
Liver ducts
Cystic duct
Gallbladder
Bile duct opening
Duodenum (behind colon)
Transverse colon
Ascending colon
Cecum
Appendix
Descending colon
Jejunum
Ileum
Sigmoid colon
Rectum

DEMAREST

Plate 9

DIGESTIVE SYSTEM—*Continued*

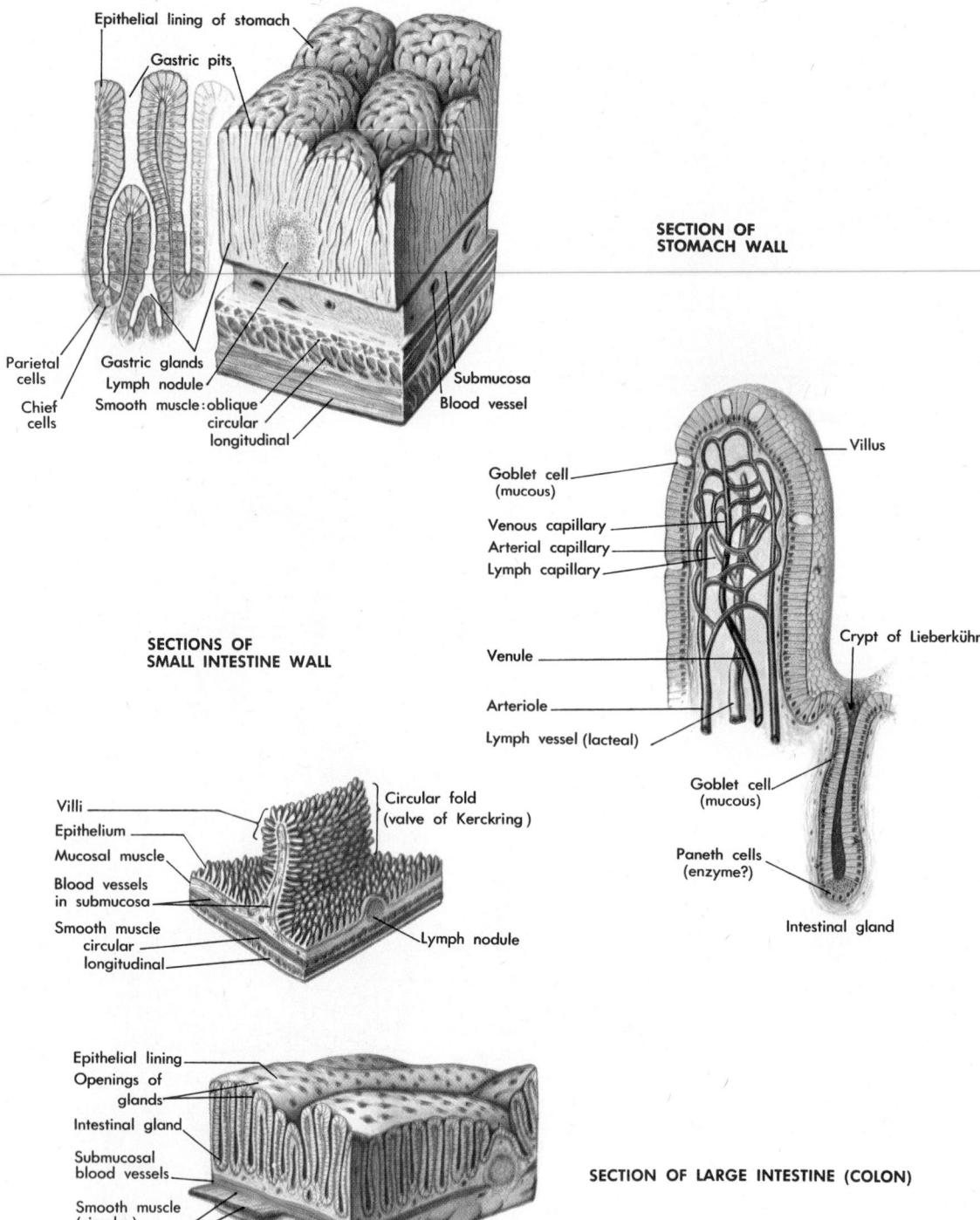

Epithelial lining of stomach

Gastric pits

SECTION OF STOMACH WALL

Parietal cells

Chief cells

Gastric glands
Lymph nodule
Smooth muscle: oblique
circular
longitudinal

Submucosa
Blood vessel

Goblet cell (mucous)

Venous capillary
Arterial capillary
Lymph capillary

Venule

Arteriole

Lymph vessel (lacteal)

Villus

Crypt of Lieberkühn

Goblet cell (mucous)

Paneth cells (enzyme?)

Intestinal gland

SECTIONS OF SMALL INTESTINE WALL

Villi
Epithelium
Mucosal muscle
Blood vessels in submucosa
Smooth muscle circular
longitudinal

Circular fold (valve of Kerckring)

Lymph nodule

Epithelial lining
Openings of glands
Intestinal gland
Submucosal blood vessels
Smooth muscle (circular)
Longitudinal muscle band

DEMAREST

SECTION OF LARGE INTESTINE (COLON)

Plate 10

GENITOURINARY SYSTEM

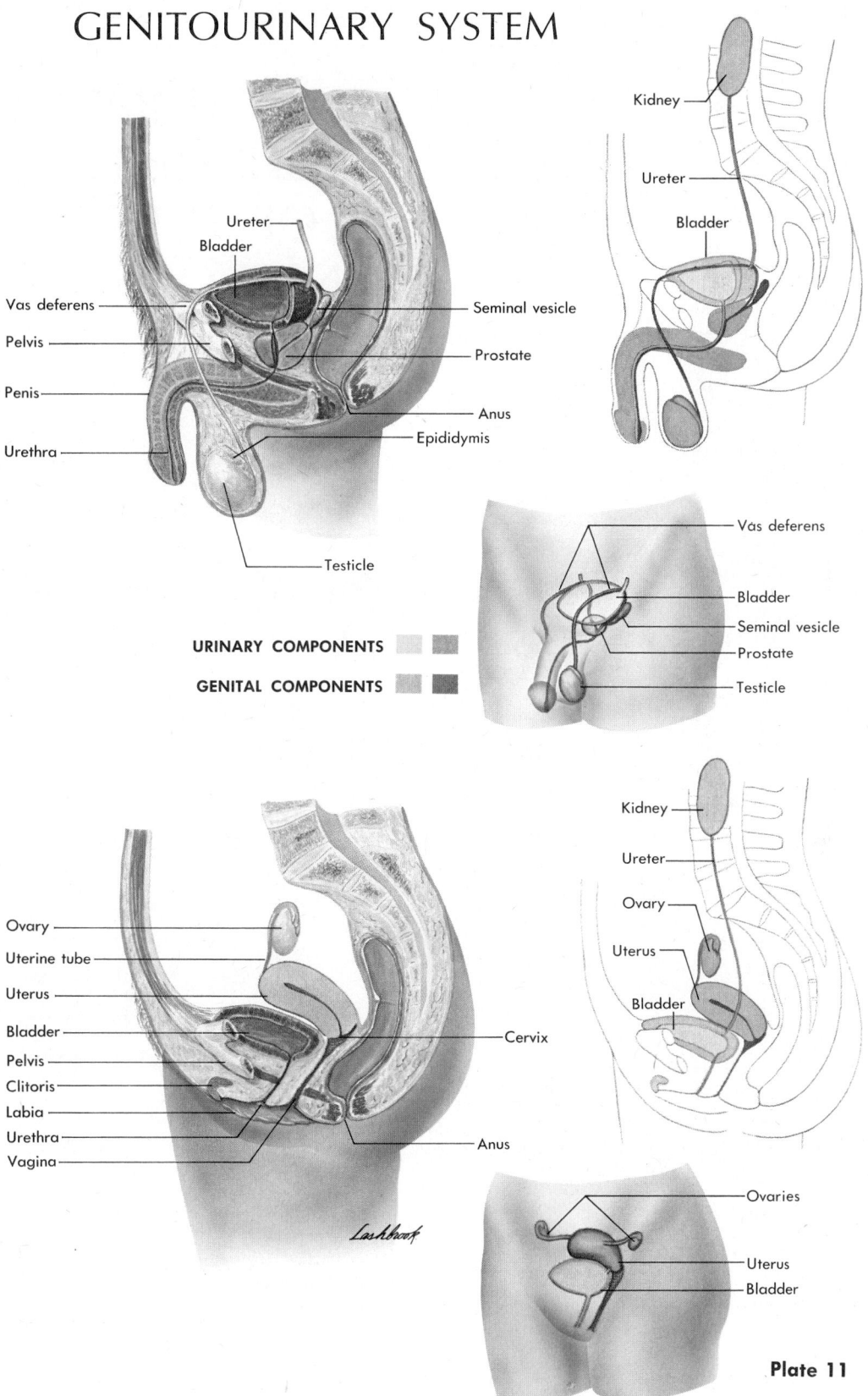

Ureter
Bladder
Vas deferens
Pelvis
Penis
Urethra
Seminal vesicle
Prostate
Anus
Epididymis
Testicle

Kidney
Ureter
Bladder

Vas deferens
Bladder
Seminal vesicle
Prostate
Testicle

URINARY COMPONENTS
GENITAL COMPONENTS

Ovary
Uterine tube
Uterus
Bladder
Pelvis
Clitoris
Labia
Urethra
Vagina
Cervix
Anus

Kidney
Ureter
Ovary
Uterus
Bladder

Ovaries
Uterus
Bladder

Lashbook

Plate 11

STRUCTURAL HIGHLIGHTS OF THE NERVOUS SYSTEM

GENERAL ARCHITECTURE AND PHYSIOLOGY

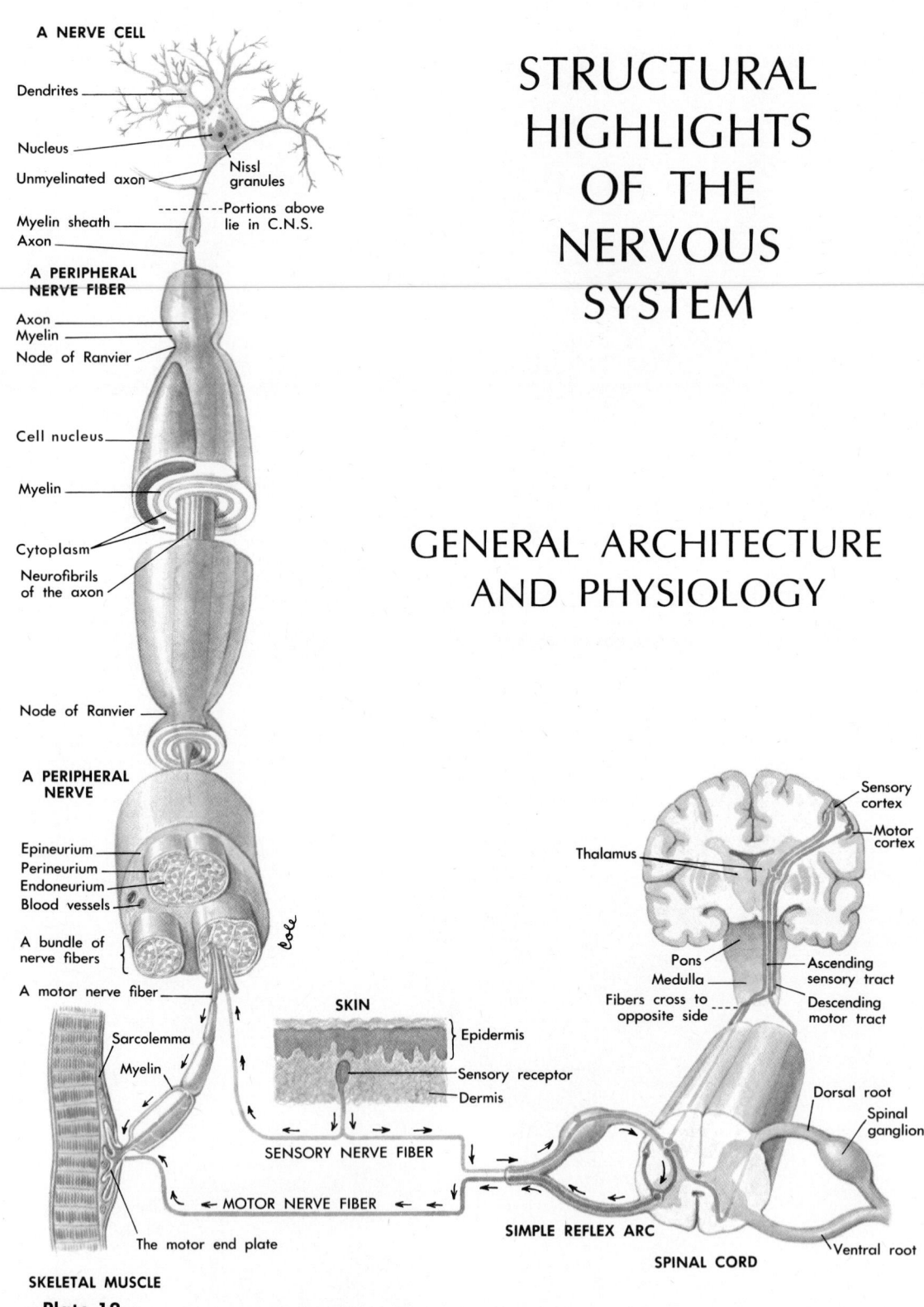

A NERVE CELL

- Dendrites
- Nucleus
- Unmyelinated axon
- Nissl granules
- Myelin sheath
- Portions above lie in C.N.S.
- Axon

A PERIPHERAL NERVE FIBER

- Axon
- Myelin
- Node of Ranvier
- Cell nucleus
- Myelin
- Cytoplasm
- Neurofibrils of the axon
- Node of Ranvier

A PERIPHERAL NERVE

- Epineurium
- Perineurium
- Endoneurium
- Blood vessels
- A bundle of nerve fibers
- A motor nerve fiber
- Sarcolemma
- Myelin
- The motor end plate

SKELETAL MUSCLE

SKIN
- Epidermis
- Sensory receptor
- Dermis

SENSORY NERVE FIBER

← MOTOR NERVE FIBER ← ←

SIMPLE REFLEX ARC

- Thalamus
- Sensory cortex
- Motor cortex
- Pons
- Medulla
- Fibers cross to opposite side
- Ascending sensory tract
- Descending motor tract
- Dorsal root
- Spinal ganglion
- Ventral root

SPINAL CORD

Plate 12

BRAIN AND SPINAL NERVES

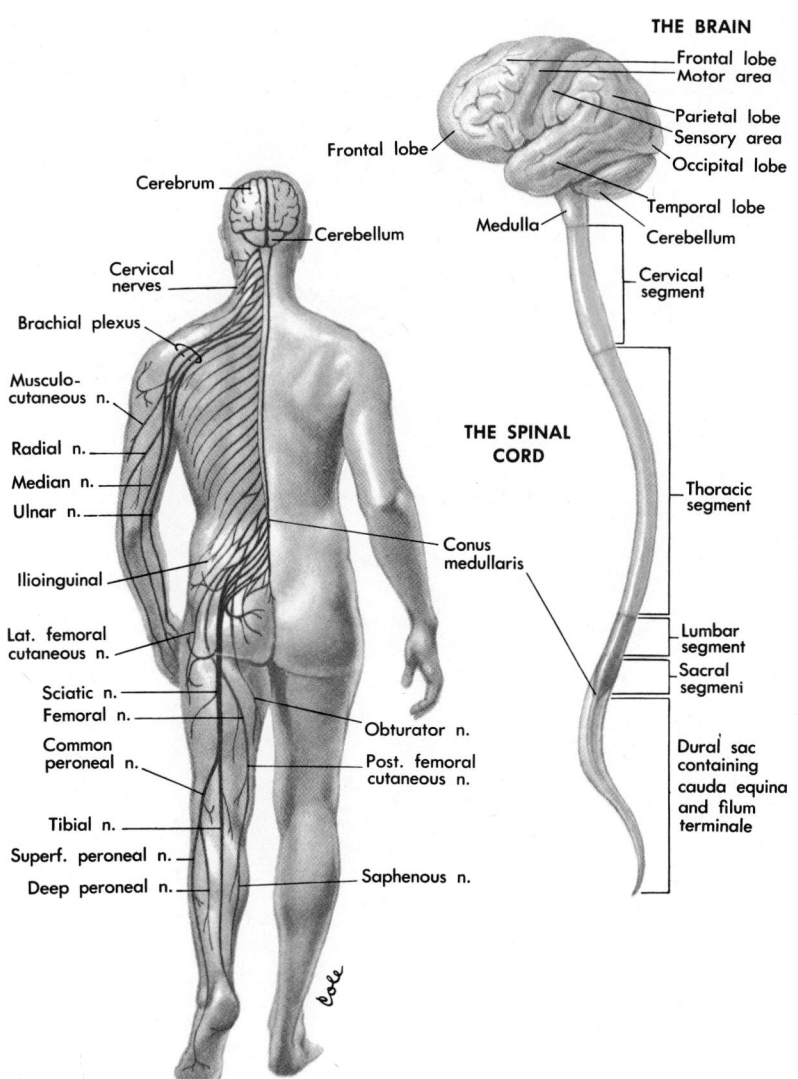

THE BRAIN

Frontal lobe
Motor area
Parietal lobe
Sensory area
Occipital lobe
Temporal lobe
Cerebellum

Frontal lobe

Medulla

Cerebrum

Cerebellum

Cervical nerves

Brachial plexus

Musculo-cutaneous n.

Radial n.

Median n.

Ulnar n.

Ilioinguinal

Lat. femoral cutaneous n.

Sciatic n.
Femoral n.
Common peroneal n.

Tibial n.

Superf. peroneal n.

Deep peroneal n.

THE SPINAL CORD

Cervical segment

Thoracic segment

Conus medullaris

Lumbar segment
Sacral segmeni

Obturator n.

Post. femoral cutaneous n.

Dural sac containing cauda equina and filum terminale

Saphenous n.

THE MAJOR SPINAL NERVES

Plate 13

AUTONOMIC NERVES

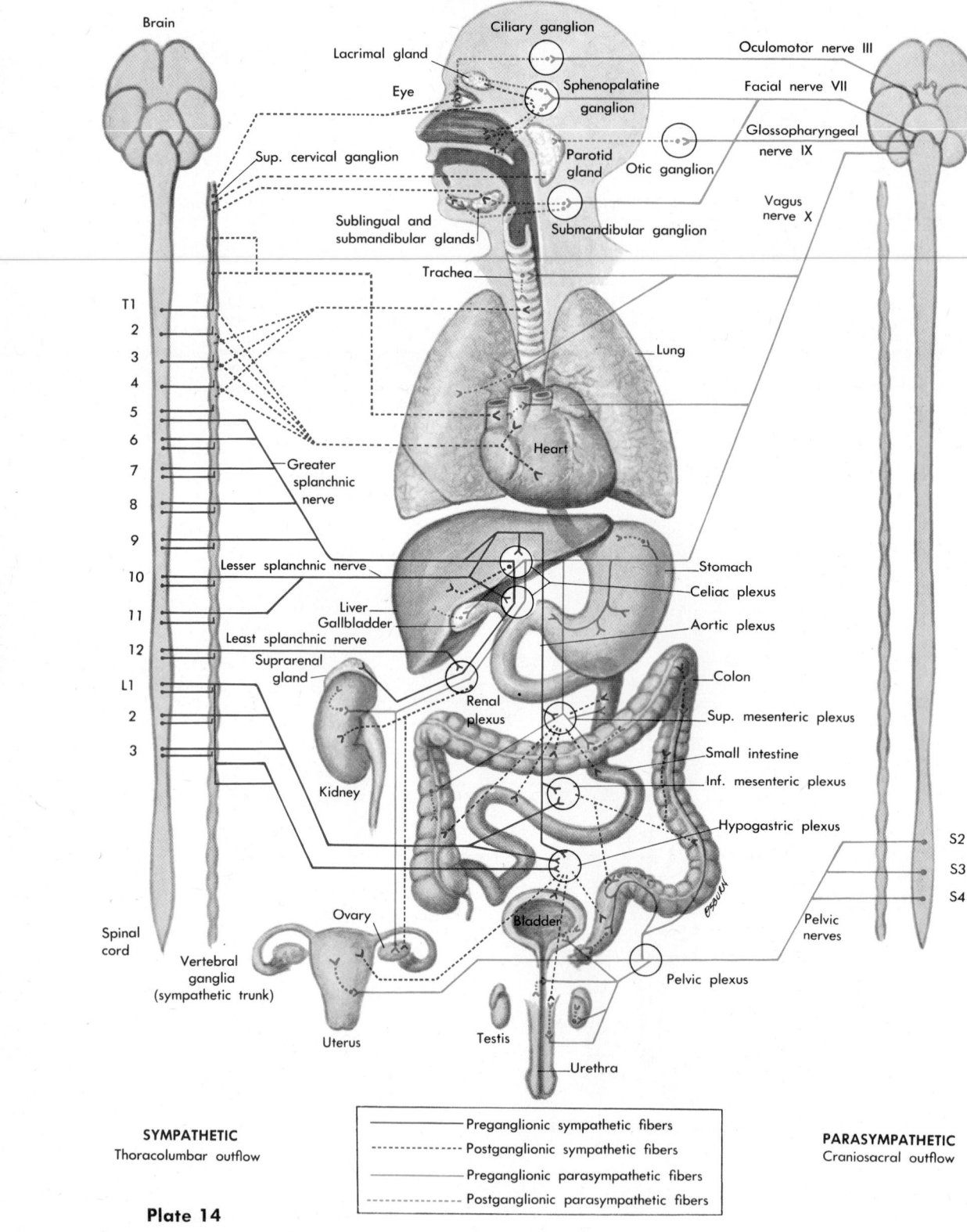

Brain

Ciliary ganglion

Lacrimal gland

Oculomotor nerve III

Eye

Sphenopalatine ganglion

Facial nerve VII

Sup. cervical ganglion

Glossopharyngeal nerve IX

Parotid gland

Otic ganglion

Vagus nerve X

Sublingual and submandibular glands

Submandibular ganglion

Trachea

T1
2
3
4
5
6
7
8
9
10
11
12

L1
2
3

Lung

Heart

Greater splanchnic nerve

Lesser splanchnic nerve

Stomach

Celiac plexus

Liver
Gallbladder

Least splanchnic nerve

Aortic plexus

Suprarenal gland

Renal plexus

Colon

Sup. mesenteric plexus

Kidney

Small intestine

Inf. mesenteric plexus

Hypogastric plexus

S2
S3
S4

Spinal cord

Ovary

Bladder

Pelvic nerves

Vertebral ganglia (sympathetic trunk)

Pelvic plexus

Uterus

Testis

Urethra

————————	Preganglionic sympathetic fibers
- - - - - - - -	Postganglionic sympathetic fibers
————————	Preganglionic parasympathetic fibers
- - - - - - - -	Postganglionic parasympathetic fibers

SYMPATHETIC
Thoracolumbar outflow

PARASYMPATHETIC
Craniosacral outflow

Plate 14

ORGANS OF SPECIAL SENSE

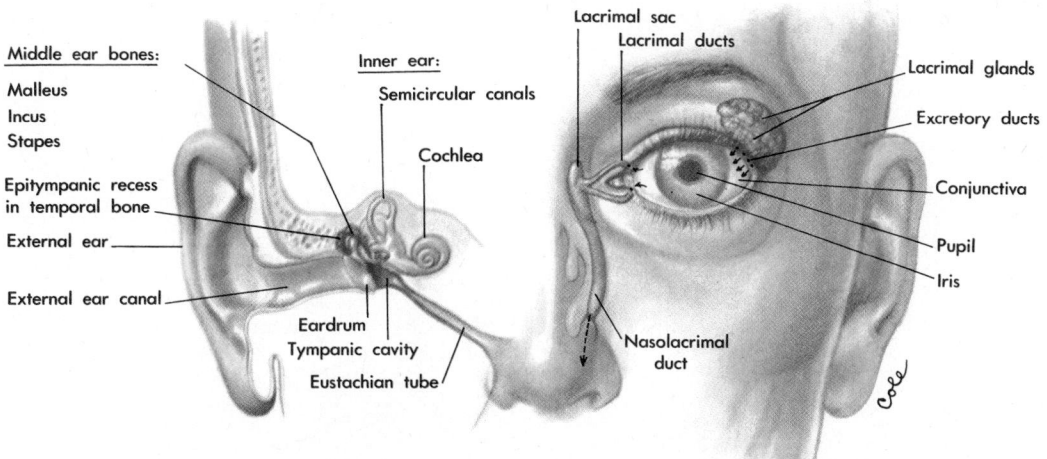

Middle ear bones:

Malleus
Incus
Stapes

Epitympanic recess
in temporal bone

External ear

External ear canal

Semicircular canals

Inner ear:

Cochlea

Eardrum
Tympanic cavity

Eustachian tube

Lacrimal sac
Lacrimal ducts

Lacrimal glands

Excretory ducts

Conjunctiva

Pupil

Iris

Nasolacrimal
duct

THE ORGAN OF HEARING

THE LACRIMAL APPARATUS AND THE EYE

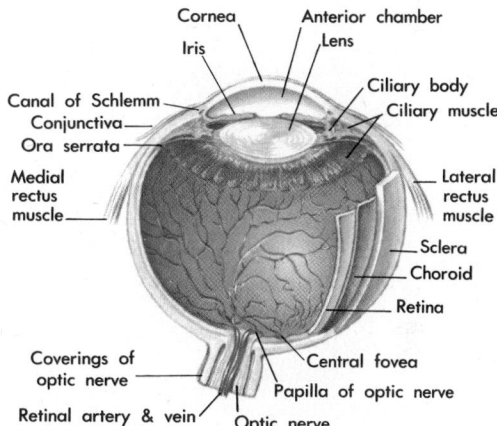

HORIZONTAL SECTION OF THE EYE

Cornea

Iris

Anterior chamber

Lens

Canal of Schlemm
Conjunctiva
Ora serrata

Ciliary body
Ciliary muscle

Medial
rectus
muscle

Lateral
rectus
muscle

Sclera

Choroid

Retina

Coverings of
optic nerve

Central fovea

Papilla of optic nerve

Retinal artery & vein

Optic nerve

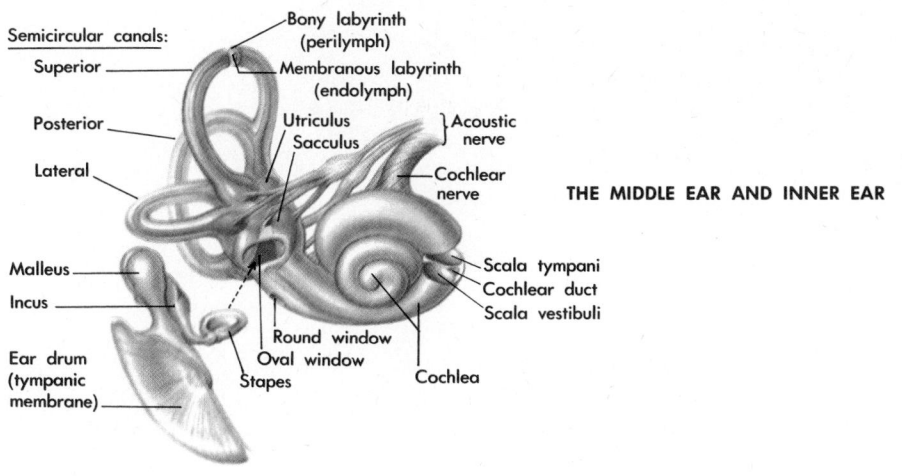

Semicircular canals:

Superior

Posterior

Lateral

Malleus

Incus

Ear drum
(tympanic
membrane)

Bony labyrinth
(perilymph)

Membranous labyrinth
(endolymph)

Utriculus
Sacculus

Acoustic
nerve

Cochlear
nerve

Scala tympani
Cochlear duct
Scala vestibuli

Round window
Oval window
Stapes

Cochlea

THE MIDDLE EAR AND INNER EAR

Plate 15

PARANASAL
SINUSES

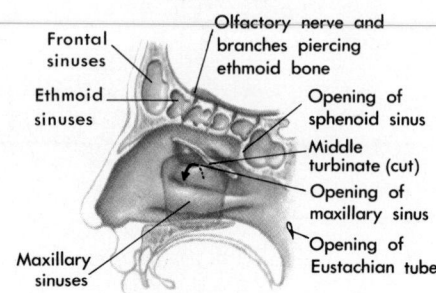

Frontal
sinuses

Olfactory nerve and
branches piercing
ethmoid bone

Ethmoid
sinuses

Opening of
sphenoid sinus

Middle
turbinate (cut)

Opening of
maxillary sinus

Opening of
Eustachian tube

Maxillary
sinuses

SAGITTAL SECTION OF THE NOSE

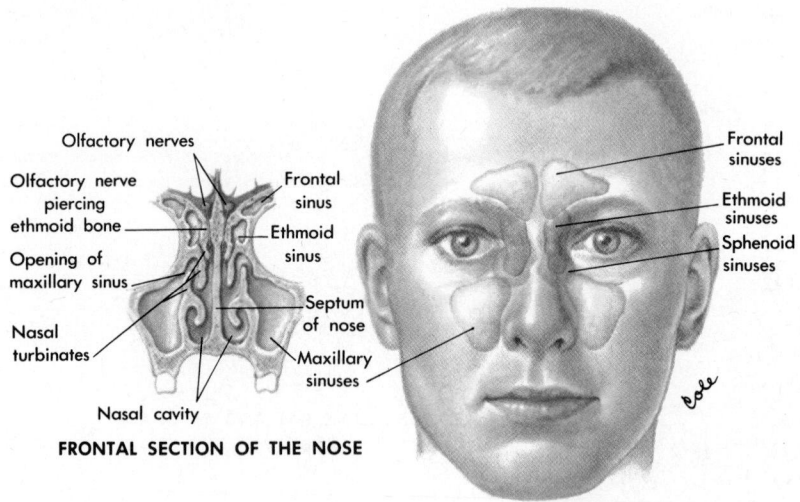

Olfactory nerves

Olfactory nerve
piercing
ethmoid bone

Opening of
maxillary sinus

Nasal
turbinates

Frontal
sinus

Ethmoid
sinus

Septum
of nose

Maxillary
sinuses

Frontal
sinuses

Ethmoid
sinuses

Sphenoid
sinuses

Nasal cavity

FRONTAL SECTION OF THE NOSE

Plate 16

FULL LIQUID DIET. This diet can be nutritionally adequate with careful planning. It is used for acute gastritis, as a transition between clear liquid and soft diet and in conditions in which there is intolerance to solid food. Milk, strained soups and fruit juices are allowed. Foods that liquefy at body temperature, such as ice cream, jello and soft custards, can be included. Cereal gruels and egg nogs are allowed. When a full liquid diet is used as a TUBE FEEDING it must be of a consistency that will allow easy passage through the tube. Most full liquid diets are given in feedings every 2 to 4 hours.

liquor (lik′er, li′kwor) 1. a liquid. 2. a solution of nonvolatile substance in water.

  l. am′nii, amniotic fluid.

  l. cerebrospina′lis, cerebrospinal fluid.

  l. follic′uli, the fluid in the cavity of a developing graafian follicle.

  Morgagni's l., the fluid between the eye lens and its capsule.

  mother l., the liquid remaining after removal of crystals from a solution.

  l. san′guinis, the fluid portion of the blood.

liquorrhea (li″kwo-re′ah) excessive or abnormal flow or discharge of a body fluid, e.g., liquorrhea nasalis.

lissencephalia (lis″en-sĕ-fa′le-ah) absence of gyri on the surface of the brain.

lissive (lis′iv) relieving muscle spasm without interfering with function.

Lister (lis′ter) Baron Joseph (1827–1912). Founder of modern antiseptic surgery. Born at Upton, Essex, England, Lister set out in a scientific manner to apply Pasteur's discoveries to the prevention of the development of microorganisms in wounds. His research was on the early stages of inflammation and blood coagulation, and in 1865 he successfully used carbolic acid in the treatment of an open fracture. Next he turned his attention to the arrest of hemorrhage in aseptic wounds, which led him to adopt a sulfochromic catgut for tying arteries, a material capable of more speedy absorption than silk or flax, which had long been employed. He wrote articles on amputation and anesthetics. Lister was created a baronet in 1883 and raised to the peerage in 1893, but perhaps the greatest memorial to him is the Lister Institute of Preventive Medicine in London.

Listeria (lis-te′re-ah) a genus of bacteria occurring primarily in lower animals. One species, *L. monocytog′enes,* sometimes produces upper respiratory disease or septicemia in man.

listeriosis (lis-tēr″e-o′sis) infection with organisms of the genus Listeria.

listerism (lis′ter-izm) the principles and practice of antiseptic and aseptic surgery.

liter (le′ter) the basic unit of capacity of the metric system, the equivalent of 1.0567 quarts liquid measure.

lith(o)- (lith′o) word element [Gr.], *stone; calculus.*

lithagogue (lith′ah-gog) 1. expelling calculi. 2. an agent that expels calculi.

lithectasy (lĭ-thek′tah-se) removal of calculi through a mechanically dilated urethra.

lithemia (lĭ-the′me-ah) excess of uric (lithic) acid in the blood.

lithiasis (lĭ-thi′ah-sis) the formation of concretions or stones in any hollow structure of the body.

lithic acid (lith′ik) uric acid.

lithium (lith′e-um) a chemical element, atomic number 3, atomic weight 6.939, symbol Li. (See table of ELEMENTS.)

lithoclast (lith′o-klast) an instrument for crushing calculi.

lithocystotomy (lith″o-sis-tot′o-me) incision of the bladder for removal of stone.

lithodialysis (lith″o-di-al′ĭ-sis) the dissolution or crushing of a calculus.

lithogenesis (lith″o-jen′ĕ-sis) formation of calculi, or stones.

litholapaxy (lĭ-thol′ah-pak″se) the crushing of a stone in the bladder and washing out of the fragments.

lithology (lĭ-thol′o-je) the scientific study of calculi.

litholysis (lĭ-thol′ĭ-sis) dissolution of calculi.

lithometra (lith″o-me′trah) ossification of the uterus.

lithonephrotomy (lith″o-nĕ-frot′o-me) excision of a renal calculus.

lithopedion (lith″o-pe′de-on) a stony or petrified fetus.

lithophone (lith′o-fōn) a device for detecting calculi in the bladder.

lithoscope (lith′o-skōp) an instrument for detecting calculi in the bladder by the sound made when the stone is struck.

lithosis (lĭ-tho′sis) disease of the lungs from inhaling fine particles of stone; called also stone grinder's disease.

lithotomy (lĭ-thot′o-me) incision of an organ for removal of calculi.

  l. position, the patient lies on his back, legs flexed on the thighs, thighs flexed on the belly and abducted. Stirrups may be used to support the feet and legs.

lithotresis (lith″o-tre′sis) the drilling or boring of holes in a calculus.

lithotripsy (lith′o-trip″se) the crushing of calculi in the bladder or urethra.

lithotrite (lith′o-trīt) an instrument for crushing calculi.

lithotrity (lĭ-thot′rĭ-te) lithotripsy.

lithous (lith′us) pertaining to a calculus or stone.

lithuresis (lith″u-re′sis) passage of gravel in the urine.

lithuria (lĭ-thu′re-ah) excess of uric acid or urates in the urine.

litmus (lit'mus) a blue stain prepared by enzymatic fermentation of coarsely powdered lichens.

l. **paper,** absorbent paper impregnated with a solution of litmus, dried and cut into strips. It is used to indicate the acidity or alkalinity of solutions. If dipped into alkaline solution it remains blue; acid solution turns it red. It is used to test urine and other body fluids; it has a pH range of 4.5 to 8.3.

livedo (lĭ-ve'do) a discolored patch on the skin.

l. **annula'ris,** l. **racemo'sa,** l. **reticula'ris,** permanent reddish blue mottling of the skin of the extremities.

liver (liv'er) a large gland of red color located in the upper right portion of the abdomen. It has many functions concerned with the process of digestion and with the development of the erythrocytes. It produces bile, helps detoxify harmful substances in the blood and stores food.

STORAGE FUNCTIONS. The liver can store up to 20 per cent of its weight in glycogen and up to 40 per cent of its weight in fats. The basic fuel of the body is a simple form of sugar called glucose. This comes to the liver as one of the products of digestion, and is converted into glycogen for storage. It is reconverted to glucose, when necessary, to keep up a steady level of sugar in the blood. This is normally a slow, continuous process, but in emergencies the liver, responding to epinephrine in the blood, releases large quantities of this fuel into the blood for use by the muscles.

As the chief supplier of glucose in the body, the liver is sometimes called on to convert other substances into sugar. The liver cells can make glucose out of protein and fat. This may also work in reverse: the liver cells can convert excess sugar into fat and send it for storage to other parts of the body.

In addition to these functions, the liver builds many essential proteins and stores up certain necessary vitamins until they are needed by other organs in the body.

PROTECTIVE FUNCTIONS. The liver disposes of worn-out blood cells by breaking them down into their different elements, storing some and sending others to the kidneys for disposal in the urine. It filters and destroys bacteria and also neutralizes poisons.

The liver also helps to maintain the balance of sex hormones in the body. A certain amount of female hormone is normally produced in males, and male hormone in females. When the level of this opposite sex hormone rises above a certain point, the liver takes up the excess and disposes of it.

Finally, the liver polices the proteins that have passed through the digestive system. Some of the amino acids derived from protein metabolism cannot be used by the body; the liver rejects and neutralizes these acids and sends them to the kidneys for disposal.

DISORDERS OF THE LIVER. The liver, with its many complex functions, can be damaged by various disorders and diseases. Often such damage first manifests itself as JAUNDICE. This is a yellowish tinge, best seen in the eyes, that is caused by an excess of bile pigment in the blood. Jaundice is not a disease, it is a symptom of any one of a number of liver disorders or blood dyscrasias.

Besides jaundice, other symptoms of liver disease may be a gradual, unexplained swelling of the abdomen, vomiting of blood and passing of bloody or black tar-like stools.

Infectious, or viral HEPATITIS, is one of the most common diseases of the liver. It is highly contagious and most often affects children and young adults. Its symptoms include jaundice, loss of appetite, fever and abdominal discomfort.

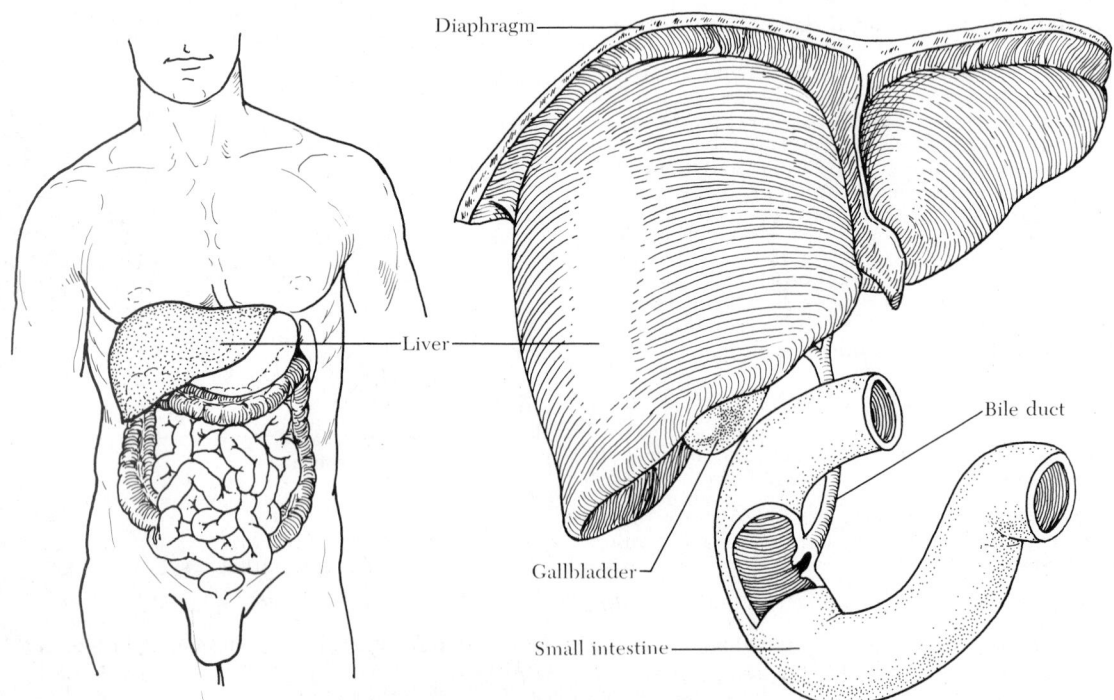

Liver. Bile, manufactured in the liver, is stored in the gallbladder; it passes through the bile duct into the duodenum, the upper end of the small intestine, where it aids in digestion.

The liver may be harmed by excessive use of alcohol and by excessive exposure to poisons such as carbon tetrachloride. Certain disorders of the GALLBLADDER also may damage the liver.

CIRRHOSIS of the liver is a chronic inflammation marked by degeneration of the liver cells and thickening of the surrounding tissue, thought to be caused by severe protein deficiency. The condition often accompanies ALCOHOLISM because of the poor dietary habits of the alcoholic.

Abscess of the liver usually occurs as a complication of peritonitis or abdominal cellulitis, or as an amebic abscess following infection with the *Entamoeba histolytica*.

albuminoid l., amyloid l., one with albuminoid or amyloid degeneration.

biliary cirrhotic l., one in which clogging and distention of the bile ducts is caused by obstruction to the normal flow of bile.

l. extract, a brownish, somewhat hygroscopic powder prepared from mammalian livers; used as a hematopoietic.

fatty l., one affected with fatty degeneration and infiltration.

floating l., wandering liver.

hobnail l., a liver whose surface is marked with nail-like points from atrophic cirrhosis.

iron l., the condition of the liver in hepatic siderosis.

lardaceous l., amyloid liver.

nutmeg l., one presenting a mottled appearance on the cut surface, from passive congestion.

sago l., one affected with amyloid degeneration.

l. spots, a colloquial name for the small brownish patches that appear on the face, neck or back of the hands of many older people. It is a misleading term because these spots have little or nothing to do with the liver. The spots, smooth, flat, irregularly spaced and roundish or oval in shape, are caused by an increase in pigmentation and are entirely harmless. Although liver spots are associated with the process of aging, it is actually not age that is the principal cause but many years of exposure to sun and wind.

l. therapy, treatment of disease, especially pernicious anemia, with extracts of livers of various animals. The extract is injected intramuscularly. Its effect is chiefly due to its vitamin B_{12} content.

wandering l., a displaced and movable liver.

waxy l., albuminoid liver.

livid (liv'id) discolored, as from a contusion or bruise.

lividity (lĭ-vid'ĭ-te) discoloration, as from a bruise or congestion.

livor (li'vor) discoloration.

l. mor'tis, discoloration on dependent parts of the body after death.

lixiviation (lik-siv"e-a'shun) separation of soluble from insoluble material by use of an appropriate solvent, and drawing off the solution.

L.L.L. left lower lobe (of lung).

L.L.Q. left lower quadrant (of abdomen).

L.M. Licentiate in Midwifery.

L.M.A. left mentoanterior (position of the fetus).

L.M.P. left mentoposterior (position of the fetus).

L.M.T. left mentotransverse (position of the fetus).

L.O.A. left occipitoanterior (position of the fetus).

Loa (lo'ah) a genus of parasitic filarial roundworms.

L. lo'a, a threadlike worm commonly found in subcutaneous tissues of man and baboons in Central and South Africa; frequently seen in the eyeball in its migration about the body.

loaiasis (lo"ah-i'ah-sis) infection with worms of the genus Loa.

lobar (lo'ber) pertaining to a lobe.

l. pneumonia, pneumonia affecting one or more lobes of the lungs (see also PNEUMONIA).

lobate (lo'bāt) divided into lobes.

lobe (lōb) a more or less well defined portion of an organ or gland.

azygos l., a small accessory or anomalous lobe at the apex of the right lung.

caudate l., a small lobe of the liver between the inferior vena cava on the right and the left lobe.

ear l., the lower fleshy, noncartilaginous portion of the auricle.

frontal l., the anterior portion of the gray matter of the cerebral hemisphere.

hepatic l., one of the lobes of the liver, designated the right and left and the caudate and quadrate.

occipital l., the most posterior portion of the cerebral hemisphere, forming a small part of its dorsolateral surface.

parietal l., the upper central portion of the gray matter of the cerebral hemisphere, between the frontal and occipital lobes, and above the temporal lobe.

prefrontal l., the anterior part of the frontal lobe.

quadrate l., a small lobe of the liver, between the gallbladder on the right and the left lobe.

Riedel's l., an anomalous tongue-shaped mass of tissue projecting from the right lobe of the liver.

spigelian l., caudate lobe.

temporal l., a long, tongue-shaped process constituting the lower lateral portion of the cerebral hemisphere.

lobectomy (lo-bek'to-me) excision of a lobe, as of the lung, brain or liver.

lobeline (lob'ĕ-lin) an alkaloid, alpha-lobeline, used as a respiratory stimulant: claimed to be a powerful resuscitant in respiratory failure, collapse or shock.

lobitis (lo-bi'tis) inflammation of a lobe, as of the lung.

lobocyte (lo'bo-sīt) a granulocyte with a segmented nucleus.

lobostomy (lo-bos'to-me) incision of a lobe of the lung with drainage.

lobotomy (lo-bot'o-me) cutting of nerve fibers connecting a lobe of the brain with the thalamus. In most cases the affected parts are the prefrontal or frontal lobes, the areas of the brain involved with emotion; thus the operation is referred to as prefrontal, or frontal, lobotomy.

Lobotomy is a form of psychosurgery—a field in which the purpose of an operation is not to remove a growth or repair an injury to the body but to change the patient's mental and emotional state.

Today most physicians regard lobotomy as a last resort and use the operation either for certain violent cases when all else has failed or for people with severe and otherwise untreatable anxiety. Although it can make formerly violent and uncontrollable patients calm and docile, it often seems to lead to emotional emptiness.

Furthermore, in recent years, drugs have been developed that have revolutionized the treatment of severe mental illnesses. Among these are the TRANQUILIZERS, which suppress temporarily the violent symptoms of psychosis.

Lobstein's disease (lōb'stīnz) osteogenesis imperfecta.

lobulated (lob'u-lāt″ed) made up of lobules.

lobule (lob'ūl) a small segment or lobe.
   hepatic l., one of the small vascular units comprising the substance of the liver.
   l. of lung, one of the smaller subdivisions of the lobes of the lungs.
   parietal l., one of two divisions of the parietal lobe of the brain.

lobulus (lob'u-lus), pl. *lob'uli* [L.] lobule.

lobus (lo'bus), pl. *lo'bi* [L.] lobe.

local (lo'kal) restricted to or pertaining to one spot or part.

localization (lo″kah-lĭ-za'shun) 1. the determination of a site or place of any process or lesion. 2. restriction to a circumscribed or limited area.
   cerebral l., determination of areas of the cortex involved in performance of certain functions.
   germinal l., the location on a blastoderm of prospective organs.
   selective l., the tendency of a microorganism to infect a specific variety of tissue.

lochia (lo'ke-ah) the discharge from the birth canal occurring after childbirth. adj., **lo'chial.**
   l. al'ba, that of the final phase after childbirth, containing little blood, but many microorganisms and degenerating cells.
   l. cruen'ta, lochia rubra.
   l. purulen'ta, lochia alba.
   l. ru'bra, that occurring immediately after childbirth, consisting almost entirely of blood.
   l. sanguinolen'ta, l. sero'sa, that of the second phase after childbirth, containing blood and mucus and wound exudation.

lochiocolpos (lo″ke-o-kol'pos) distention of the vagina by retained lochia.

lochiometra (lo″ke-o-me'trah) distention of the uterus by retained lochia.

lochiometritis (lo″ke-o-me-tri'tis) inflammation of the uterus in childbirth.

lochiopyra (lo″ke-o-pi'rah) puerperal fever.

lochiorrhagia, lochiorrhea (lo″ke-o-ra'je-ah), (lo″ke-o-re'ah) abnormally free lochial discharge.

lochioschesis (lo″ke-os'kĕ-sis) retention of the lochia.

loci (lo'si) [L.] plural of *locus.*

Locke's solution (loks) an aqueous solution of sodium chloride, calcium chloride, potassium chloride, sodium bicarbonate and dextrose adjusted to pH 7.4; used in physiologic experiments to keep the excised heart beating.

lockjaw (lok'jaw) tetanus.

locomotor (lo″ko-mo'tor) pertaining to movement.
   l. ataxia, inability to walk properly as a result of damage to the spinal cord by syphilis; called also TABES DORSALIS.

locular (lok'u-lar) containing loculi.

loculus (lok'u-lus), pl. *loc'uli* [L.] 1. a small space or cavity. 2. a local enlargement of the uterus in some mammals, containing an embryo.

locus (lo'kus), pl. *lo'ci* [L.] place; in genetics, the specific site of a gene on a chromosome.

löffleria (lef-le're-ah) the presence of *Corynebacterium diphtheriae* without the ordinary symptoms of diphtheria.

logadectomy (log″ah-dek'to-me) excision of a portion of the conjunctiva.

logaditis (log″ah-di'tis) inflammation of the sclera.

logagnosia (log″ag-no'ze-ah) word defect due to damage to brain centers, as aphasia.

logagraphia (log″ah-graf'e-ah) inability to express ideas in writing.

logamnesia (log″am-ne'ze-ah) sensory aphasia.

logaphasia (log″ah-fa'ze-ah) motor aphasia.

logasthenia (log″as-the'ne-ah) disturbance of the mental processes necessary to the comprehension of speech.

logogram (log'o-gram) the graphic record of the symptoms and signs exhibited by a patient, charted by means of the logoscope.

logoklony (log'o-klon″e) spasmodic repetition of the end syllables of words.

logokophosis (log″o-ko-fo'sis) auditory aphasia.

logoneurosis (log″o-nu-ro'sis) any neurosis with speech disorder.

logopathy (log-op'ah-the) any disorder of speech due to derangement of the central nervous system.

logopedia, logopedics (log″o-pe'de-ah), (log″o-pe'diks) the study and treatment of speech defects.

logoplegia (log″o-ple'je-ah) 1. any paralysis of speech organs. 2. inability to speak, while words are remembered.

logorrhea (log″o-re'ah) excessive or abnormal talkativeness.

logoscope (log'o-skōp) a device in slide rule form designed to facilitate identification of the diseases in which certain signs and symptoms occur.

logoscopy (lo-gos'ko-pe) the use of a logoscope for determining the differential diagnostic possibilities in a case exhibiting certain signs and symptoms.

logospasm (log'o-spazm) the spasmodic utterance of words.

-logy word element [Gr.], *science; treatise; sum of knowledge in a particular subject.*

loin (loin) the part of the back between the thorax and pelvis.

Lomotil (lo′mo-til) trademark for preparations of diphenoxylate hydrochloride, an antidiarrheal.

Long (long), Crawford Williamson (1815–1878). American physician, born at Danielsville, Georgia, who in 1842 administered ether to a patient before removing a neck tumor, the first recorded use of an anesthetic in surgery.

longissimus (lon-jis′ĭ-mus) [L.] longest.

longitudinalis (lon″jĭ-tu″dĭ-na′lis) lengthwise; in official anatomic nomenclature it designates a structure that is parallel to the long axis of the body or an organ.

longus (long′gus) [L.] long.

loop (lŏŏp) a turn or sharp curve in a cordlike structure, especially in the body.
   capillary l′s, minute endothelial tubes that carry blood in the papillae of the skin.
   Henle′s l., the U-shaped loop of the uriniferous tubule of the kidney.
   Lippes l., a form of intrauterine contraceptive device.

L.O.P. left occipitoposterior (position of the fetus).

lophotrichous (lo-fot′rĭ-kus) having a tuft of flagella at one end; said of bacteria.

lordoma (lor-do′mah) lordosis.

lordoscoliosis (lor″do-sko″le-o′sis) lordosis complicated with scoliosis.

lordosis (lor-do′sis) abnormally increased concavity in the curvature of the lumbar spine.

Lorfan (lor′fan) trademark for preparations of levallorphan, an antagonist to narcotics.

L.O.T. left occipitotransverse (position of the fetus).

lotio (lo′she-o) [L.] lotion.
   l. al′ba, white lotion, an astringent.

lotion (lo′shun) a liquid suspension or dispersion for external application to the body, for washing.
   benzyl benzoate l., a preparation of benzyl benzoate, triethanolamine, oleic acid and water; used as a scabicide.
   calamine l., a mixture of calamine, zinc oxide, glycerin, bentonite magma and calcium hydroxide solution; used as an astringent and skin protectant.
   calamine l., phenolated, calamine lotion with liquefied phenol added.
   hydrocortisone l., hydrocortisone in an aqueous vehicle for topical application.
   white l., a preparation of zinc sulfate and sulfurated potash in purified water; astringent and protectant.

Lotusate (lo′tu-sāt) trademark for a preparation of talbutal, a short- to intermediate-acting barbiturate.

loupe (lŏŏp) a convex lens for magnifying or for concentrating light upon an object.

louse (lows), pl. *lice* a general name for various parasitic insects; the true lice, which infest mammals, belong to the suborder Anoplura. They are grayish, wingless insects that vary in length from one-sixth to one-sixteenth of an inch. Those that are parasitic on man are *Pediculus humanus* var. *capitis,* or head louse, which attaches itself to the hairs of the head; *P. humanus* var. *corporis,* the body or clothes louse; and *Phthirus pubis,* or crab louse, which lives in the pubic hair and in the eyelashes and eyebrows.
   Louse infestation is called pediculosis. Lice live on human blood that is obtained by biting the skin. The area bitten itches and may become sore and infected from scratching. Not only are lice an annoyance, but they also transmit some diseases, such as typhus.
   TREATMENT. Head lice hatch eggs in silvery oval-shaped envelopes that attach to the shafts of the hairs. The eggs, called nits, can be removed fairly easily with a mild vinegar solution. The hair is combed with a very fine-toothed comb. The lice are effectively destroyed by applications of 1 per cent benzene hexachloride (lindane) in a cream or shampoo.
   PREVENTION. Cleanliness, frequent bathing and frequent changing of clothing are necessary to avoid contracting lice. When infestation is discovered it is necessary to boil or autoclave all clothing and bed linens used by the infected person. Outer clothing that cannot be boiled or autoclaved should be dry cleaned. Dusting with 10 per cent DDT is usually effective in destroying lice on bedclothing, mattresses and other inanimate objects.

Lowe′s disease (lōz) oculocerebrorenal syndrome.

loxoscelism (lok-sos′sĕ-lizm) a condition resulting from the bite of the brown spider, *Loxosceles reclusa,* which may progress to a gangrenous slough of the affected area; first recognized in South America, but a few cases have been diagnosed in North America.

lozenge (loz′enj) a medicated troche.

L.P.N. Licensed Practical Nurse.

L.R.C.P. Licentiate of the Royal College of Physicians.

L.R.C.S. Licentiate of the Royal College of Surgeons.

L.S.A. left sacroanterior (position of the fetus).

L.Sc.A. left scapuloanterior (position of the fetus).

L.Sc.P. left scapuloposterior (position of the fetus).

LSD a hallucinogenic compound (lysergic acid diethylamide), chemically related to ergot, having consciousness-expanding effects and capable of producing a state of mind in which there is false sense perception (hallucination). The perceptual changes brought about by LSD in normal persons are extremely variable and depend on factors such as age, personality, education, physical make-up and state of health. The danger of the drug lies in the fact that it loosens control over impulsive behavior and may lead to a full-blown psychosis or less serious mental disorder in persons with latent mental illness. LSD is an experimental drug to be used only under the direct supervision of reliable, authorized scientists. Its distribution is regulated by the Food and Drug Administration of the federal government.

LSD was first developed in 1938 and was believed to be potentially useful in the treatment of mental illness. This theory was based on the belief that the drug could produce a schizophrenic syndrome and that psychiatrists and other persons concerned with mental illness could observe the manifestations of a psychosis under controlled conditions. However, competent investigators have shown that the effect of LSD is more closely related to a toxic psychosis such as that produced by fever, stress or drugs of many kinds and is of doubtful use in understanding the mechanism of a true psychosis resulting from severe personality disorder. Authorities are hopeful that LSD may eventually prove useful in the investigation of brain function and the mechanism of mental disease but are not in agreement as to how this will come about.

Abuse of LSD by semiscientific investigators and lay persons has led to much publicity, with the result that a black market now operates to make the drug available to those who wish to "increase their awareness" or attain a state of euphoria. Although LSD is not addictive, the greatest number of persons abusing the drug also have been found to be users of marijuana, amphetamines and barbiturates, and are extremely likely to develop a drug dependence. They apparently use the drug to escape reality rather than for the purpose of helping themselves cope with reality.

L.S.P. left sacroposterior (position of the fetus).

L.S.T. left sacrotransverse (position of the fetus).

LTH luteotropic hormone (lactogenic hormone).

Lu chemical symbol, *lutetium*.

lubb (lub) a syllable used to express the first sound of the heart in auscultation, a dull, prolonged, low sound.

lubb-dupp (lub'dup) syllables used to express the two sounds that mark a complete heart cycle in auscultation.

luciferase (lu-sif'er-ās) an enzyme that catalyzes the bioluminescent reaction in certain animals capable of luminescence.

luciferin (lu-sif'er-in) a heat-stable compound that, when acted on by an enzyme (luciferase), produces bioluminescence.

lucifugal (lu-sif'u-gal) repelled by bright light.

lucipetal (lu-sip'ĕ-tal) attracted by bright light.

Ludwig's angina (lood'vigz) purulent inflammation around the submaxillary gland, beneath the jaw and about the floor of the mouth, usually due to streptococcus infection.

lues (lu'ēz) syphilis. adj., **luet'ic.**

Lugol's solution (loo-golz') strong iodine solution, each 100 ml. containing 4.5 to 5.5 Gm. of iodine and 9.5 to 10.5 Gm. of potassium iodide; sometimes used in the treatment of thyroid disorders.

L.U.L. left upper lobe (of lung).

Lullamin (lul'ah-min) trademark for a preparation of methapyrilene, an antihistamine.

lumb(o)- (lum'bo) word element [L.], *loin.*

lumbago (lum-ba'go) an ache in the lower part (lumbar region) of the back. Lumbago is a popular term for lower back pain. It embraces a number of illnesses. Such pain may be caused by injury, such as back strain, by arthritis, by abuse of the back muscles (from poor posture, a sagging mattress or ill fitting shoes, for example) or by a number of other disorders.

lumbar (lum'bar) pertaining to the loins.

l. **puncture,** insertion of a hollow needle into the subarachnoid space between the third and fourth lumbar vertebrae; called also SPINAL PUNCTURE. A lumbar puncture may be done to obtain a specimen of CEREBROSPINAL FLUID for examination and to measure the pressure within the cerebrospinal cavities. As a therapeutic measure it is sometimes done to relieve intracranial pressure or to remove blood or pus from the subarachnoid space. A lumbar puncture also is necessary for injection of a spinal anesthetic. For certain x-ray examinations of the skull, such as a pneumoencephalogram, air may be injected via a lumbar puncture. For visualization of the spinal canal and course of the spinal cord a radiopaque dye is injected into the subarachnoid space.

l. **vertebrae,** the five vertebrae between the thoracic vertebrae and the sacrum.

lumbarization (lum"bar-ĭ-za'shun) coalescence of the first sacral vertebra with the transverse processes of the fifth lumbar vertebra.

lumbocostal (lum"bo-kos'tal) pertaining to the loin and ribs.

lumbodynia (lum"bo-din'e-ah) lumbago.

lumbosacral (lum"bo-sa'kral) pertaining to the lumbar and sacral region, or to the lumbar vertebrae and sacrum.

l. **plexus,** the lumbar and sacral nerve plexuses, which are continuous in location.

lumbricoid (lum'brĭ-koid) resembling the earthworm; designating the ascaris, or intestinal roundworms.

lumbricosis (lum"brĭ-ko'sis) infection with lumbricoid worms.

lumbricus (lum'brĭ-kus), pl. *lum'brici* [L.] 1. the earthworm. 2. ascaris.

lumbus (lum'bus) [L.] loin.

lumen (lu'men), pl. *lu'mina* [L.] 1. the cavity or channel within a tube or tubular organ, as a blood vessel or the intestine. 2. a unit of light; called also meter candle.

luminal (lu'mĭ-nal) pertaining to a lumen.

luminescence (lu"mĭ-nes'ens) the property of giving off light.

luminophore (lu'mĭ-no-fōr") a chemical group that gives the property of luminescence to organic compounds.

lunate (lu'nāt) moon-shaped or crescentic.

lung (lung) one of the two main organs of respiration, lying on either side of the heart, within the chest cavity. The lungs supply the blood with oxygen inhaled from the outside air, and they dispose of waste carbon dioxide in the exhaled air, as a part of the process known as RESPIRATION.

The lungs are made of elastic tissue filled with interlacing networks of tubes and sacs carrying air, and with blood vessels carrying blood. The bronchi, which bring air to the lungs, branch out within the lungs into many smaller tubes, the bronchioles, which culminate in clusters of tiny air sacs called alveoli, whose total runs into millions. The alveoli are surrounded by a network of capillaries. Through the thin membranes of the capillaries, the air and blood make their exchange of oxygen and carbon dioxide.

The lungs are divided into lobes, the left lung having two lobes and the right lung having three, and further subdivided into bronchopulmonary segments, of which there are about 20. Protecting each lung is the pleura, a two-layered membrane that envelops the lung and contains lubricating fluid between its inner and outer layers. The lungs are inflated and deflated by action of the diaphragm and the intercostal muscles.

DISEASES OF THE LUNGS.   The air brought to the lungs is filtered, moistened and warmed on its way along the respiratory tract but it can nevertheless bring irritants and infectious organisms, and when the body resistance is low for any reason the lungs

may suffer diseases of some seriousness. PNEUMONIA, once a dangerous disease, is now quickly brought under control by antibiotics, but it is still serious and requires prompt medical attention. Viral pneumonia is not effectively treated with antibiotics but is a milder infection than those caused by the pneumococci.

Edema of the lung, or pulmonary edema, usually occurs as a complication of a chronic heart disease of the type that places a strain on the left ventricle. As the left ventricle become weaker it is less able to accommodate and remove blood from the pulmonary vascular bed. This results in congestion and engorgement of the pulmonary vessels with escape of fluid into the alveoli, producing edema of the lung tissue.

PLEURISY is an inflammation of the pleura. Other disorders of the lungs include ASTHMA, BRONCHIECTASIS, ATELECTASIS, EMPHYSEMA, fungal infections and TUBERCULOSIS. SILICOSIS and the other PNEUMOCONIOSES are pulmonary diseases caused by inhalation of dust and are often occupation related.

Lung Abscess.   Lung abscess is an infection of the lung, characterized by a localized accumulation of pus and destruction of tissue. It may be a complication of pneumonia or tuberculosis. A lung abscess may also follow a period of excessive drink-

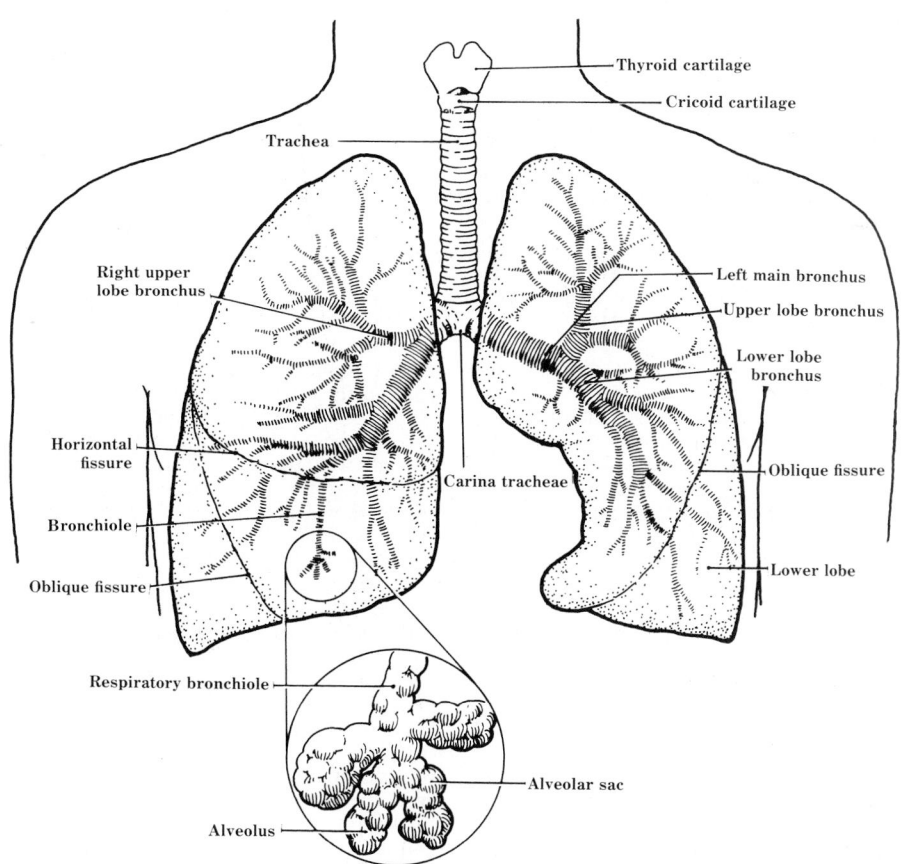

Lungs. (Redrawn from Jacob, S. W., and Francone, C. A.: Structure and Function in Man. 2nd ed. Philadelphia, W. B. Saunders Co., 1970.)

ing by an alcoholic. Infected matter that has been aspirated may lodge in a bronchiole and produce inflammation. Lung cancer may also be responsible for formation of an abscess.

The first symptoms include a dry cough and chest pain. Later these may be followed by fever, chills, productive cough, headache, perspiration, foul-smelling sputum and sometimes dyspnea. If the abscess is a complication of pneumonia, the symptoms tend to be moderated to an exaggeration of the pneumonia symptoms.

When a lung abscess forms, it is in the acute stage and treatment with antibiotics usually is effective. POSTURAL DRAINAGE may be prescribed to assist in drainage of exudate from lungs and bronchioles. In most cases, this treatment produces a cure. If the abscess becomes chronic, surgery may be necessary and usually involves removal of the portion of the lung containing the abscess.

Lung Cancer. Malignant growths of the lung are among the most common types of cancer. Although the exact cause of lung cancer is not known, irritants that are inhaled over a period of time are known to be important predisposing causes. Years ago it was realized that miners of certain ores, men who inhaled the mine dust, developed lung cancer much more often than men in other occupations. Later, other irritants of lung tissue, such as air polluted by fumes from burning fuels or motor exhausts, were singled out as probable causes of the increasing number of cases of the disease in urban and industrial areas. The most obvious irritant, however, and the one most widely encountered, is tobacco smoke, especially cigarette smoke, which is much more frequently and deeply inhaled than the smoke of pipes or cigars.

A study based on autopsies of the lungs of individuals who had died from many varied causes, but whose smoking history was known, showed that unrecognized cancer and precancerous changes in tissue were numerous among smokers and rare among nonsmokers. These findings led the Surgeon General of the United States Public Health Service to appoint a committee to investigate the subject. After an extensive study, the committee issued a report stating that "cigarette smoking is a health hazard of sufficient importance in the United States to warrant appropriate action."

The search for other possible causes of lung cancer has not been neglected. However, no definite findings have been reported thus far.

Since the factors causing lung cancer act slowly and may produce a tumor near the periphery of the lung, early symptoms are vague or may not appear at all, and nearly a third of the cases are in an advanced stage when they are discovered.

The earliest and most common symptom is a cough. Dry at first, this cough later produces sputum which eventually becomes blood-streaked. A wheeze in the chest is frequently a symptom and indicates a partial obstruction in a bronchus. Chest pains, weakness and loss of weight are later symptoms, as is dyspnea.

Diagnosis depends on a careful physical examination, including a chest x-ray. If a suspicious density is seen on the x-ray, samples of sputum will be examined microscopically for the presence of malignant cells. Bronchoscopy is also done, and at the same time a specimen for biopsy can be obtained or the bronchial secretions can be washed out and the cells stained and examined.

When examination indicates lung cancer, prompt treatment is essential. This may involve the surgical removal of the lobe of the lung containing the cancer or of an entire lung if the malignant cells have spread. A significant number of persons affected by lung cancer can be cured by such operations if the surgery is performed in time. In some cases of widespread involvement surgery is not possible; these patients are treated with x-rays or radium or antineoplastic drugs.

For prevention, regular physical examinations are essential. Chest x-rays should be taken at the first suspicion of trouble and, in any case, should be done annually in people 40 years old or older.

The irritants that can trigger lung cancer must be avoided and, when possible, eliminated. Mine workers should take adequate precautions to avoid inhaling harmful dusts. Public health authorities and industry must act more effectively to control air pollution.

The most important step toward protection against lung cancer is the elimination of cigarette smoking.

SURGERY OF THE LUNG. Surgical procedures performed on the lung include removal of the entire lung (pneumonectomy), removal of a lobe of the lung (lobectomy) and removal of only a bronchopulmonary segment (segmental resection). The procedure done depends on the size of the area involved and the type of lesion present.

Pneumonectomy is usually necessary for treatment of cancer, multiple abscesses of the lung or severe bronchiectasis. In this procedure a thoracotomy incision is made and one or two ribs are resected. The large pulmonary vessels (the artery and vein leading to and from the lung) are ligated and cut and the main bronchus serving the lung is closed with sutures. A tube may be inserted to provide for drainage of blood and fluid from the cavity.

Cysts, abscesses or benign tumors that involve only a lobe of the lung are treated by lobectomy. A thoracotomy incision is made and the lung is collapsed before the lobe is removed. The remaining lobes are then reexpanded and catheters are inserted for removal of air and fluid.

Some types of lung surgery are aimed at deliberate collapse of the lung for the purpose of permanently or temporarily reducing the size of the thoracic cavity on one side of the chest. Resection of two or more ribs (thoracoplasty) is done primarily for the treatment of tuberculosis; it also may be done following pneumonectomy, in which case its purpose is to partially fill the space left by removal of the lung.

Artificial pneumothorax involves injection of a measured amount of air into the pleural cavity. Since the pressure within the pleural cavity is normally lower than atmospheric pressure, the introduction of air will collapse the lung. Because the air is gradually absorbed by the tissues over a period of time, injections of air must be repeated at intervals for as long as collapse of the lung is desired. This procedure is done chiefly as a means of treating tuberculous lesions and allows for immobilization of the lung while healing takes place.

Another method used for collapse of the lung is pneumoperitoneum. As the name implies, this procedure involves injection of air into the peritoneal cavity rather than the thoracic cavity. The injected air causes an upward pressure on the diaphragm which in turn pushes against the lung and hinders its expansion.

If there are adhesions between the lung and the lining of the chest wall they may prevent the collapse of the lung. The cutting of these adhesions is called pneumonolysis.

Nursing Care. Before surgery the patient is given an explanation of the procedure to be done and the purpose of the catheters, oxygen therapy and other apparatus to be used postoperatively. Special exercises of the arms, shoulders and chest muscles are often started before surgery and resumed postoperatively. Their purpose is to strengthen the muscles and provide for continued motion of the shoulder and arm and normal functioning of the remaining lung tissue.

Immediately after surgery the patient's pulse, respirations and blood pressure are checked and recorded every 15 minutes until they become stabilized. Oxygen is administered by tent, mask or nasal catheter and the patient is watched closely for signs of respiratory difficulty. Positioning of the patient depends on the specific orders of the surgeon. Generally, the patient is allowed to lie only on his back or the operative side.

After many types of lung surgery the patient returns from the operating room with one or two chest catheters. If there are two catheters the upper one has been inserted for removal of air and the lower one for drainage of serosanguineous fluid from the operative side. The catheters are attached to a closed drainage system. This means that the drainage system must be airtight so that there is no possibility of reflux of air back into the chest cavity. The term pneumothorax is used to denote flow of air from the outside into the pleural cavity. Normally the pleural cavity is under negative pressure and if the cavity is opened air rushes in and fills the thoracic space and causes the lung to collapse. If the pleural cavity is kept airtight, the lung will gradually reexpand as the patient breathes.

There is a variety of equipment used for closed drainage of the pleural cavity; the most frequently used is the underwater drainage system. The catheter leading from the chest is attached to a rubber tube which in turn is connected to a glass tube, the end of which is submerged under water in the drainage bottle. In this way air and fluids can be forced out of the chest cavity as the patient breathes and coughs, but air cannot flow back into the cavity. The drainage in the tube fluctuates slightly each time the patient breathes; if there is no rise and fall of the fluid in the tubing this indicates an obstruction in the drainage system and the physician must be notified immediately. If the obstruction is not relieved, the pressure of accumulating fluid in the chest increases and causes a change in the position of the heart and great vessels. This is known as mediastinal shift and is indicated by dyspnea, a rapid, irregular pulse and symptoms of shock.

Care of the drainage bottles and tubes requires an understanding of the principles of physics involved in a closed drainage system. If the nurse is responsible for emptying the bottles and measuring the amount of drainage, she must clamp off the tubes *before* disconnecting the tubing. The bottles must be kept below the level of the patient's chest as long as they are connected to tubing. If the tubing is accidentally disconnected it must be clamped immediately and the surgeon notified.

Sterile bottles and tubing are always used and must be handled with care to avoid introducing infection into the operative site. (See also THORACIC SURGERY.)

As mentioned before, the orders of the surgeon for positioning of the patient are to be followed. Generally, the patient is permitted to lie on the operative side and back. Lying on the operative side facilitates drainage, and enhances ventilation of the unaffected lung. When turning a patient to the operative side, care must be taken that the catheter is not kinked and the patient's weight is adequately supported with pillows so that the tubes are not obstructed.

Dressings are reinforced but usually they are not changed by the nurse until the drainage tubes have been removed and the incision is closed and healing.

Coughing is encouraged although it may be painful for the patient during the first few postoperative days. Discomfort can be reduced by splinting the chest with the hands or a pillow, or turning the patient onto the operative side during episodes of coughing.

The convalescent period after lung surgery is often long and difficult for the patient. He will need encouragement in continuing his exercises and in other procedures necessary for adequate ventilation and normal function of the remaining lung tissue.

iron l., a type of RESPIRATOR that uses air pressure to expand and contract the lungs of a patient whose respiratory muscles are paralyzed; called also Drinker respirator.

lunula (lu'nu-lah), pl. *lu'nulae* [L.] a small, crescentic or moon-shaped area or structure, e.g., the white area at the base of the nail of a finger or toe, or one of the segments of the valve guarding the opening of the heart into the aorta or the pulmonary trunk.

lupiform (lu'pĭ-form) 1. resembling lupus. 2. resembling a wen.

lupoid (lu'poid) 1. lupiform. 2. a lupiform disease of the skin, ascribed to an acid-fast bacillus.

lupus (lu'pus) tuberculosis of the skin marked by the formation of brownish nodules on the corium; called also lupus vulgaris.

l. erythemato'sus, an inflammatory disease that takes two forms. One, the systemic or disseminated form, causes deterioration of the connective tissues in various parts of the body. This disease may attack the soft internal organs as well as the bones and muscles, and is often fatal. In its other form, the discoid type, it is a fairly mild skin disorder.

Symptoms of the more serious form vary widely, but may include fever, abdominal pains and pains in the muscles and joints. Often the symptoms come and go over a long period of time. Diagnosis of the disease is difficult.

The cause is unknown, but the disease is believed not to be infectious and possibly to be related to the allergies. Lupus erythematosus is one of a group of similar disorders known as the COLLAGEN DISEASES. There is no specific treatment, though corticosteroids may be used to control symptoms.

L.U.Q. left upper quadrant (of abdomen).

luteal (lu'te-al) pertaining to the corpus luteum.

luteectomy (lu″te-ek′to-me) excision of the corpus luteum.

lutein (lu′te-in) a yellow pigment found in the corpus luteum, in fat cells and in the yolk of eggs.
  serum l., yellow coloring matter from serum.

luteinic (lu″te-in′ik) pertaining to the corpus luteum or to lutein.

luteinization (lu″te-in″ĭ-za′shun) the process taking place in the follicle cells of graafian follicles that have matured and discharged their egg: the cells become hypertrophied and assume a yellow color, the follicles becoming corpora lutea.

luteinizing hormone (lu′te-in-īz″ing) a hormone of the anterior pituitary concerned in production of corpora lutea in the ovary and secretion of testosterone by the interstitial cells of the testis; called also interstitial cell-stimulating hormone.

Lutembacher's disease (loo′tem-bak″erz) mitral stenosis associated with atrial septal defect.

luteohormone (lu″te-o-hōr′mōn) progesterone.

luteoma (lu″te-o′mah) a tumor derived from the corpus luteum cells of the ovary.

luteotropic (lu″te-o-trop′ik) stimulating formation of the corpus luteum.
  l. hormone, lactogenic hormone.

luteotropin (lu″te-o-trōp′in) lactogenic hormone.

lutetium (lu-te′she-um) a chemical element, atomic number 71, atomic weight 174.97, symbol Lu. (See table of ELEMENTS.)

Lutocylol (lu″to-si′lol) trademark for preparations of ethisterone, a progestational steroid.

Lutrexin (lu-trek′sin) trademark for a preparation of lututrin, a uterine relaxant.

Lutromone (lu′tro-mōn) trademark for a preparation of progesterone, a progestational hormone.

lututrin (loo′tu-trin) a protein or polypeptide substance from the corpus luteum of sow ovaries; used as a uterine relaxant in treatment of essential dysmenorrhea.

lux (luks) the unit of illumination, being one lumen per square meter.

luxation (luk-sa′shun) dislocation.

luxus (luk′sus) [L.] excess.

Lw chemical symbol, *lawrencium.*

lyase (li′ās) an enzyme that catalyzes the removal of a group of atoms from the substrate.

lycanthropy, lycomania (li-kan′thro-pe), (li″ko-ma′ne-ah) a delusion in which the patient believes himself a wolf.

lying-in (li′ing-in) the puerperal state; childbed.

lymph (limf) the colorless, odorless fluid, slightly alkaline and with a salty taste, circulating within the lymphatic system. It is about 95 per cent water; the remainder consists of plasma proteins and other chemical substances contained in the blood plasma, but in slightly smaller percentage than in plasma. In addition the lymph contains a high concentration of lymphocytes.
  The body contains three main kinds of fluid: blood, tissue fluid and lymph. The blood consists of the blood cells and platelets, the plasma, or fluid portion, and a variety of chemical substances dissolved in the plasma. When the plasma, without its solid particles and some of its dissolved substances, seeps through the capillary walls and circulates among the body tissues, it is known as tissue fluid. When this fluid is drained from the tissues and collected by the lymphatic system, it is called lymph. The LYMPHATIC SYSTEM eventually returns the lymph to the blood, where it again becomes plasma. This movement of fluid through the body is described under CIRCULATORY SYSTEM.
  l. node, one of the accumulations of lymphoid tissue organized as lymphatic organs along the course of lymphatic vessels, consisting of an outer cortical and inner medullary part. Lymph nodes filter and destroy invading bacteria and are the site of production of lymphocytes and certain antibodies. The main lymph nodes are in the neck, axillae and groin. Sometimes called, incorrectly, lymph glands.

lympha (lim′fah) [L.] lymph.

lymphadenectasis (lim-fad″ĕ-nek′tah-sis) dilatation of a lymph node.

lymphadenectomy (lim-fad″ĕ-nek′to-me) excision of a lymph node.

lymphadenia (lim″fah-de′ne-ah) overgrowth of lymphoid tissue.
  l. os′sea, multiple myeloma.

lymphadenitis (lim-fad″ĕ-ni′tis) inflammation of lymph nodes.

lymphadenocyst (lim-fad′ĕ-no-sist″) a degenerated lymph node.

lymphadenogram (lim-fad′ĕ-no-gram″) the film produced by lymphadenography.

lymphadenography (lim″fad-ĕ-nog′rah-fe) roentgenography of lymph nodes after injection of a contrast medium in a lymphatic vessel.

lymphadenoid (lim-fad′ĕ-noid) resembling the tissues of the lymph nodes. Lymphadenoid tissue includes the spleen, bone marrow, tonsils and the lymphoid tissues of the organs and mucous membranes.

lymphadenoleukopoiesis (lim-fad″ĕ-no-lu″ko-poi-e′sis) production of leukocytes by lymphadenoid tissue.

lymphadenoma (lim-fad″ĕ-no′mah) lymphoma.

lymphadenomatosis (lim-fad″ĕ-no″mah-to′sis) lymphomatosis.

lymphadenopathy (lim-fad″ĕ-nop′ah-the) disease of the lymph nodes.
  giant follicular l., a disorder of the lymphatic system, with multiple proliferative follicle-like nodules occurring in the lymph nodes.

lymphadenosis (lim-fad″ĕ-no′sis) proliferation of lymphoid tissue.

lymphadenotomy (lim-fad″ĕ-not′o-me) incision of a lymph node.

lymphagogue (lim′fah-gog) an agent promoting production of lymph.

lymphangiectasis (lim-fan″je-ek′tah-sis) dilatation of a lymphatic vessel.

lymphangiectomy (lim-fan″je-ek′to-me) excision of a lymphatic vessel.

lymphangiitis (lim-fan″je-i′tis) lymphangitis.

lymphangioadenography (lim-fan″je-o-ad″ĕ-nog′rah-fe) lymphography.

lymphangioendothelioma (lim-fan″je-o-en″do-the″le-o′mah) endothelioma arising from lymph channels.

lymphangiofibroma (lim-fan″je-o-fi-bro′mah) fibroma containing lymphangiomatous tissue.

lymphangiogram (lim-fan′je-o-gram″) the film produced by lymphangiography.

lymphangiography (lim-fan″je-og′rah-fe) roentgenography of lymphatic channels after introduction of a contrast medium.

lymphangiology (lim-fan″je-ol′o-je) the scientific study of the lymphatic system.

lymphangioma (lim-fan″je-o′mah) a tumor composed of new-formed lymph spaces and channels. adj., **lymphangio′matous.**
   cavernous l., dilatation of the lymphatic vessels, resulting in cavities filled with lymph.

lymphangiophlebitis (lim-fan″je-o-flĕ-bi′tis) inflammation of lymphatic channels and veins.

lymphangioplasty (lim-fan′je-o-plas″te) surgical restoration of lymphatic channels.

lymphangiosarcoma (lim-fan″je-o-sar-ko′mah) lymphangioma combined with sarcoma.

lymphangiotomy (lim-fan″je-ot′o-me) incision of a lymphatic vessel.

lymphangitis (lim″fan-ji′tis) inflammation of a lymphatic vessel.

lymphatic (lim-fat′ik) 1. pertaining to lymph. 2. a lymphatic vessel, one of the capillaries, collecting vessels and trunks that collect lymph from the tissues and carry it to the blood.
   l. ducts, the two larger vessels into which all lymphatic vessels converge. The right lymphatic duct joins the venous system at the junction of the right internal jugular and subclavian veins and carries lymph from the upper right side of the body. The left lymphatic duct, or thoracic duct, enters the circulatory system at the junction of the left internal jugular and subclavian veins; it returns lymph from the upper left side of the body and from below the diaphragm.
   l. system, all the vessels and structures involved in conveying lymph from the tissues to the blood. It consists of the lymph capillaries, lymphatic vessels, lymphatic ducts and lymph nodes. (See also CIRCULATORY SYSTEM.)
   DISORDERS OF THE LYMPHATIC SYSTEM. Several diseases affect the lymphatic system. LYMPHOGRANULOMA VENEREUM is a viral disease that attacks lymph nodes in the groin and usually is transmitted by sexual contact.
   Lymphadenitis is an inflammation of the lymph nodes, particularly in the neck; swollen tonsils is an example. Generalized lymphadenitis can be a symptom of the secondary stage of syphilis.
   Cancer attacks the lymphatic system, as it does other systems of the body. A tumor of the lymphoid tissue is known as a lymphoma. The general term lymphosarcoma refers to malignant neoplastic disorders of lymphoid tissue.

lymphaticostomy (lim-fat″ĭ-kos′to-me) creation of a permanent opening into the thoracic duct.

lymphatism (lim′fah-tizm) 1. the lymphatic temperament; a slow or sluggish habit. 2. a morbid state due to excessive production or growth of lymphoid tissues, resulting in impaired development and lowered vitality.

lymphatolysin (lim″fah-tol′ĭ-sin) a lysin that acts on lymphoid tissue.

lymphatolysis (lim″fah-tol′ĭ-sis) destruction of lymphoid tissue.

lymphectasia (lim′fek-ta′ze-ah) distention with lymph.

lymphedema (lim″fĕ-de′mah) swelling of subcutaneous tissues due to the presence of excessive lymph fluid.
   congenital l., Milroy's disease, a form of hereditary edema of one or both legs.

lymphemia (lim-fe′me-ah) the presence of an undue number of lymphocytes in the blood; lymphatic leukemia.

lymphenteritis (lim″fen-ter-i′tis) enteritis with serous infiltration.

lymphoadenoma (lim″fo-ad″ĕ-no′mah) a benign tumor of the uterus.

lymphoblast (lim′fo-blast) a lymphocyte in its germinal stage; a developing lymphocyte. Such cells are found in the blood in acute lymphatic leukemia.

lymphoblastic (lim″fo-blas′tik) pertaining to a lymphoblast; producing lymphocytes.

lymphoblastoma (lim″fo-blas-to′mah) malignant lymphoma in which the predominant cell resembles the lymphoblast.

lymphoblastomatosis (lim″fo-blas″to-mah-to′sis) the condition produced by the presence of lymphoblastomas.

lymphoblastosis (lim″fo-blas-to′sis) excess of lymphoblasts in the blood.

lymphocele, lymphocyst (lim′fo-sēl), (lim′fo-sist) a tumor containing lymph.

lymphocystosis (lim″fo-sis-to′sis) formation of cysts containing lymph.

lymphocyte (lim′fo-sīt) a variety of leukocyte that arises in reticular tissue of lymph nodes, generally described as nongranular and including small and large varieties. adj., **lymphocyt′ic.**

lymphocytoblast (lim″fo-si′to-blast) a lymphoblast.

lymphocytoma (lim″fo-si-to′mah) malignant lymphoma in which the predominant cell is the mature type of lymphocyte.

lymphocytopenia (lim″fo-si″to-pe′ne-ah) reduction of the number of lymphocytes in the blood.

lymphocytopoiesis (lim″fo-si″to-poi-e′sis) the formation of lymphocytes.

lymphocytorrhexis (lim″fo-si″to-rek′sis) the rupture or bursting of lymphocytes.

lymphocytosis (lim″fo-si″to′sis) increase in the number of lymphocytes in the blood.

lymphocytotoxin (lim″fo-si″to-tok′sin) a toxin that destroys lymphocytes.

lymphodermia (lim″fo-der′me-ah) any disease of the skin lymphatics.

lymphoduct (lim′fo-dukt) a lymphatic vessel.

lymphogenous (lim-foj′ĕ-nus) producing lymph.

lymphoglandula (lim″fo-glan′du-lah), pl. *lymphoglan′dulae* [L.] a lymph node.

lymphogonia (lim″fo-go′ne-ah) large lymphocytes with a large nucleus, seen in lymphatic leukemia.

lymphogram (lim′fo-gram) a roentgenogram of the lymphatic channels and lymph nodes.

lymphogranuloma (lim″fo-gran″u-lo′mah) Hodgkin's disease.

l. inguina′le, l. vene′reum, a venereal disease caused by a filterable virus. It affects the lymph organs in the genital area, and is the only venereal disease known to be caused by a virus. The virus is usually transmitted by coitus, but may be spread by contaminated articles.

Seven to twelve days or longer after the body is infected, a small, hard sore appears in the genital area. The disease soon spreads from the local sore to the lymph nodes, particularly those in the groin. The lymph nodes may swell to the size of a walnut. As these swellings seldom break open and drain pus, they may remain for months. In women infected with the disease, the vulva may become greatly enlarged. The rectum may become narrowed, so that surgery is necessary for relief.

In the early stages of the disease, there may also be inflammation of the joints, skin rashes and fever. Sometimes the brain and its covering membrane are affected. It is thought that after the initial sore heals, men may no longer transmit the disease. Women, however, may infect sexual partners for years.

Lymphogranuloma venereum may be successfully treated with antibiotics such as tetracycline.

lymphogranulomatosis (lim″fo-gran″u-lo″mah-to′sis) 1. infectious granuloma of the lymphatic system. 2. Hodgkin's disease.

lymphography (lim-fog′rah-fe) roentgenography of the lymphatic channels and lymph nodes, after injection of radiopaque material in a lymphatic vessel.

lymphoid (lim′foid) resembling lymph or lymphoid tissue, or pertaining to the lymphatic system.

l. cell, a mononuclear cell in lymphoid tissue which ultimately is concerned with humoral or cellular immunologic reactivity.

l. tissue, connective tissue with meshes that lodge lymphoid cells.

lymphoidectomy (lim″foi-dek′to-me) excision of lymphoid tissue, such as tonsils and adenoids.

lymphokinesis (lim″fo-ki-ne′sis) movement of endolymph in the semicircular canals.

lympholeukocyte (lim″fo-lu′ko-sīt) a large mononuclear leukocyte.

lymphology (lim-fol′o-je) the study of the lymphatic system.

lymphoma (lim-fo′mah) 1. a primary tumor of lymphoid tissue. 2. any one of various conditions of unknown etiology chiefly affecting lymph nodes, considered to be neoplastic; called also malignant lymphoma.

Burkitt's l., a disease of African children, with rapidly growing osteolytic tumors of the jaw and tumors in the salivary glands, kidneys and other sites; it is fatal if untreated.

clasmocytic l., reticulum cell sarcoma.

giant follicular l., giant follicular lymphadenopathy.

lymphoblastic l., lymphoblastoma.

lymphocytic l., lymphocytoma.

lymphomatosis (lim″fo-mah-to′sis) the formation of multiple lymphomas in the body.

lymphomatous (lim-fo′mah-tus) pertaining to, or of the nature of, lymphoma.

lymphopathia (lim″fo-path′e-ah) lymphopathy.

l. vene′reum, lymphogranuloma venereum.

lymphopathy (lim-fop′ah-the) any disease of the lymphatic system.

lymphopenia (lim″fo-pe′ne-ah) decrease in the number of lymphocytes of the blood.

lymphoplasmia (lim″fo-plaz′me-ah) absence of hemoglobin from the erythrocytes.

lymphopoiesis (lim″fo-poi-e′sis) the development of lymphocytes or of lymphoid tissue. adj., **lymphopoiet′ic.**

lymphoproliferative (lim″fo-pro-lif′er-ah″tiv) pertaining to or characterized by proliferation of lymphoid tissue.

l. syndrome, a general term applied to a group of diseases characterized by proliferation of lymphoid tissue, such as lymphocytic leukemia and malignant lymphoma.

lymphoreticulosis (lim″fo-rĕ-tik″u-lo′sis) proliferation of the reticuloendothelial cells of the lymph nodes.

benign l., cat-scratch disease.

lymphorrhagia, lymphorrhea (lim″fo-ra′je-ah), (lim″fo-re′ah) flow of lymph from cut or ruptured lymphatic vessels.

lymphorrhoid (lim′fo-roid) a localized dilatation of a perianal lymph channel, resembling a hemorrhoid.

lymphosarcoma (lim″fo-sar-ko′mah) a general term applied to malignant neoplastic disorders of lymphoid tissue, but not including Hodgkin's disease.

lymphosarcomatosis (lim″fo-sar-ko″mah-to′sis)

a condition characterized by the presence of multiple lesions of lymphosarcoma.

lymphostasis (lim-fos'tah-sis) stoppage of lymph flow.

lymphotomy (lim-fot'o-me) the anatomy of the lymphatic system.

lymph-vascular (limf-vas'ku-lar) pertaining to lymphatic vessels.

Lynoral (lin'or-al) trademark for a preparation of ethynylestradiol, an estrogenic compound.

lyophil (li'o-fil) a lyophilic substance.

lyophile (li'o-fil) 1. lyophil. 2. lyophilic.

lyophilic (li″o-fil'ik) having an affinity for or stable in solution.

lyophilization (li-of″ĭ-lĭ-za'shun) the creation of a stable preparation of a biologic substance by rapid freezing and dehydration of the frozen product under high vacuum.

lyophobe (li'o-fōb) repelling liquids.

lyophobic (li'o-fo'bik) not having an affinity for or unstable in solution.

lyotropic (li'o-trop'ik) readily soluble.

lypothymia (li″po-thi'me-ah) a depressed state of mind.

lyra (li'rah) a name applied to certain anatomic structures because of their fancied resemblance to a lute or lyre.

lyse (līz) 1. to cause or produce disintegration of a compound, substance or cell. 2. to undergo lysis.

lysemia (li-se'me-ah) disintegration of the blood.

lysergic acid diethylamide (li-ser'jik as'id di-eth'il-am″īd) a hallucinogenic drug better known as LSD.

lysin (li'sin) a substance that causes lysis; an antibody that causes dissolution of cells or other material.

lysine (li'sēn) a naturally occurring amino acid, one of those essential for human metabolism.

lysinogen (li-sin'o-jen) a substance that produces lysins.

lysis (li'sis) 1. destruction or decomposition, as of a cell or other substance, under the influence of a specific agent. 2. solution or separation, as of adhesions binding different anatomic structures. 3. gradual abatement of the symptoms of a disease.

-lysis (li'sis) word element [Gr.], *dissolution*. adj., -lyt'ic.

lysogen (li'so-jen) an antigen causing the formation of lysin.

lysogenesis (li″so-jen'ĕ-sis) 1. the production of lysis or lysins. 2. lysogenicity.

lysogenicity, lysogeny (li″so-jĕ-nis'ĭ-te), (li-soj'ĭ-ne) 1. the ability to produce lysins or cause lysis. 2. the potentiality of a bacterium to produce bacteriophage. 3. symbiosis of a bacterium with a bacteriophage.

lysokinase (li″so-ki'nās) a substance of the fibrinolytic system that activates plasma proactivators.

Lysol (li'sol) a proprietary solution containing phenol derivatives; used as a disinfectant and antiseptic.

lysosome (li'so-sōm) a minute body occurring in a cell and containing various enzymes, mainly hydrolytic.

lysotype (li'so-tīp) 1. the type of a microorganism as determined by its reactions to specific bacteriophages. 2. a taxonomic subdivision of bacteria based on their reactions to specific bacteriophages, or a formula expressing the reactions on which such a subdivision is based.

lysozyme (li'so-zīm) a crystalline, basic protein, which is present in saliva, tears, egg white and many animal fluids and which functions as an antibacterial enzyme.

lyssa (lis'ah) rabies.

lyssoid (lis'oid) resembling rabies.

lyssophobia (lis″o-fo'be-ah) morbid fear of rabies.

lytic (lit'ik) pertaining to lysis or a lysin.

lyze (līz) lyse.

M

M symbol, *molar* (solution); the expressions M/10, M/100, etc., denote the strength of a solution in comparison with the molar, as tenth molar, hundredth molar, etc.

M mega; meter; [L.] *mil'le* (thousand); minim.

m- symbol, *meta-*.

μ symbol, *micron*.

M.A. Master of Arts; meter angle.

ma. milliampere.

maceration (mas″ĕ-ra′shun) the softening of a solid by soaking; wasting away, softening and fraying, as if by action of soaking; in obstetrics, the degenerative changes and eventual disintegration of a fetus retained in the uterus after its death.

macies (ma′she-ēz) [L.] wasting.

macr(o)- (mak′ro) word element [Gr.], *large; long.*

macrencephalia (mak″ren-sĕ-fa′le-ah) hypertrophy of the brain.

macrobiota (mak″ro-bi-o′tah) the macroscopic living organisms of a region.

macroblast (mak′ro-blast) an abnormally large, nucleated erythrocyte; a large young normoblast; a megaloblast.

macrocardius (mak″ro-kar′de-us) a fetus with an extremely large heart.

macrocephalous (mak″ro-sef′ah-lus) having an abnormally large head.

macrocephaly (mak″ro-sef′ah-le) abnormal enlargement of the cranium.

macrocheilia (mak″ro-ki′le-ah) excessive size of the lip.

macrocheiria (mak″ro-ki′re-ah) excessive size of the hands.

macrochemistry (mak″ro-kem′is-tre) chemistry in which the reactions may be seen with the naked eye.

macrocolon (mak″ro-ko′lon) excessive size of the colon.

macrocrania (mak″ro-kra′ne-ah) abnormal increase in size of the skull in relation to the face.

macrocyte (mak′ro-sīt) an erythrocyte of largest type.

macrocythemia, macrocytosis (mak″ro-si-the′-me-ah), (mak″ro-si-to′sis) the presence of abnormally large erythrocytes in the blood.

macrodactylia (mak″ro-dak-til′e-ah) abnormal largeness of the fingers or toes.

macrodystrophia (mak″ro-dis-tro′fe-ah) overgrowth of a part.

　m. lipomato′sa progres′siva, partial gigantism with tumor-like overgrowth of fatty tissue.

macrofauna (mak″ro-faw′nah) the macroscopic animal organisms of a region.

macroflora (mak″ro-flo′rah) the macroscopic vegetable organisms of a region.

macrogamete (mak″ro-gam′ēt) the larger, female gamete of the malarial parasite.

macrogammaglobulin (mak″ro-gam″ah-glob′u-lin) a gamma globulin of extremely high molecular weight.

macrogammaglobulinemia (mak″ro-gam″ah-glob″u-lin-e′me-ah) the presence in the blood of gamma globulins of extremely high molecular weight.

macrogenitosomia (mak″ro-jen″ĭ-to-so′me-ah) excessive bodily development, with unusual enlargement of the reproductive organs.

　m. prae′cox, macrogenitosomia occurring at an early age.

macroglia (mah-krog′le-ah) astroglia.

macroglobulin (mak″ro-glob′u-lin) a protein (globulin) of unusually high molecular weight, in the range of 1,000,000; observed in the blood in a number of diseases.

macroglobulinemia (mak″ro-glob″u-lin-e′me-ah) the presence in the blood serum of macroglobulins.

　Waldenström's m., a form of macroglobulinemia observed chiefly in males past age 50.

macroglossia (mak″ro-glos′e-ah) hypertrophy of the tongue.

macrognathia (mak″ro-nath′e-ah) abnormal overgrowth of the jaw.

macrogyria (mak″ro-ji′re-ah) moderate reduction in the number of sulci of the cerebrum, sometimes with increase in the brain substance, resulting in excessive size of the gyri.

macrolabia (mak″ro-la′be-ah) macrocheilia.

macromastia (mak″ro-mas′te-ah) excessive size of the breasts.

macromelia (mak″ro-me′le-ah) enlargement of one or more extremities.

macromelus (mah-krom′ĕ-lus) a fetus with abnormally large limbs.

macromere (mak′ro-mēr) one of the larger cells formed in unequal cleavage of the fertilized ovum (at the vegetal pole).

macromethod (mak′ro-meth″od) a chemical test in which normal (not minute) quantities are used.

macromolecular (mak″ro-mo-lek′u-lar) composed of large molecules.

macromonocyte (mak″ro-mon′o-sīt) a giant monocyte.

macronormoblast (mak″ro-nor′mo-blast) a very large nucleated erythrocyte; macroblast.

macronormocyte (mak″ro-nor′mo-sīt) a giant erythrocyte.

macronychia (mak″ro-nik′e-ah) abnormally enlarged nails.

macrophage (mak′ro-fāj) a large phagocytic cell.

macrophthalmia (mak″rof-thal′me-ah) abnormal enlargement of the eyeball.

macropodia (mak″ro-po′de-ah) excessive size of the feet.

macropolycyte (mak″ro-pol′e-sīt) a hypersegmented polymorphonuclear leukocyte of greater than normal size.

macroprosopia (mak″ro-pro-so′pe-ah) excessive size of the face.

macropsia (mah-krop′se-ah) a disorder of visual perception in which objects appear larger than their actual size.

macrorrhinia (mak″ro-rin′e-ah) excessive size of the nose.

macroscelia (mak″ro-se′le-ah) excessive size of the legs.

macroscopic (mak″ro-skop′ik) of large size; visible to the unaided eye.

macroscopy (mah-kros′ko-pe) examination with the unaided eye.

macrosigma, macrosigmoid (mak″ro-sig′mah), (mak″ro-sig′moid) excessive size of the sigmoid colon.

macrosomatia, macrosomia (mak″ro-so-ma′she-ah), (mak″ro-so′me-ah) great bodily size.

macrostomia (mak″ro-sto′me-ah) excessive size of the mouth.

macrotia (mah-kro′she-ah) abnormal enlargement of the pinna of the ear.

macula (mak′u-lah), pl. *mac′ulae* [L.] a stain or spot, especially a discolored spot on the skin that is not elevated above the surface; applied also to an opacity of the cornea. adj., **mac′ular.**
  mac′ulae acus′ticae, terminations of the vestibulocochlear nerve in the utricle and saccule.
  m. atroph′ica, a white atrophic patch on the skin.
  m. ceru′lea, a blue patch on the skin seen in pediculosis.
  m. cor′neae, a circumscribed opacity of the cornea.
  m. cribro′sa, a perforated spot or area; an area in the wall of the vestibule of the ear through which branches of the vestibulocochlear nerve pass to the saccule, utricle and semicircular canals.
  m. den′sa, a zone of heavily nucleated cells in the distal renal tubule.

  m. fla′va, a yellow nodule at one end of a vocal cord.
  m. follic′uli, the point on the surface of a vesicular ovarian follicle where rupture occurs.
  m. germinati′va, germinal area; the part of the ovum where the embryo is formed.
  m. lu′tea, m. ret′inae, an irregular yellowish depression on the retina, lateral to and slightly below the optic disk.
  m. sola′ris, a freckle.

maculate (mak′u-lāt) spotted or blotched.

macule (mak′ūl) a macula.

maculopapule (mak″u-lo-pap′ūl) a papule developed on a macula.

madarosis (mad″ah-ro′sis) loss of eyelashes or eyebrows.

Madelung's disease (mah′dĕ-lōōngz) diffuse symmetrical lipomatosis.

Madura foot (mah-du′rah) maduromycosis of the foot.

maduromycosis (mah-du″ro-mi-ko′sis) a chronic fungus disease affecting various body tissues, including the hands, legs and feet; called also mycetoma. The most common form affects the foot (Madura foot) and is characterized by sinus formation, necrosis and swelling.

mafenide (maf′en-īd) a compound used in the topical treatment of superficial infections.

magenta (mah-jen′tah) fuchsin or other salt of rosaniline.

maggot (mag′ot) the soft-bodied larva of an insect, especially one living in decaying flesh.

magma (mag′mah) 1. a suspension of finely divided material in a small amount of water. 2. a thin, pastelike substance composed of organic material.
  bentonite m., a preparation of bentonite and purified water, used as a suspending agent.
  bismuth m., a water suspension of bismuth hydroxide and bismuth subcarbonate, used as an astringent and antacid.
  magnesia m., magnesium hydroxide; used as a laxative and antacid.

Magnacort (mag′nah-kort) trademark for a preparation of hydrocortamate, used in treatment of dermatoses.

magnesia (mag-ne′zhah) magnesium oxide; aperient and antacid.

magnesium (mag-ne′ze-um) a chemical element, atomic number 12, atomic weight 24.312, symbol Mg. (See table of ELEMENTS.)
  m. carbonate, an odorless, stable compound used as an antacid.
  m. citrate, a mild cathartic.
  m. hydroxide, a bulky white powder used as an antacid and cathartic.
  m. oxide, a white powder used as an antacid and cathartic.
  m. phosphate, dibasic, a salt used as a mild saline laxative.
  m. phosphate, tribasic, a white, odorless, tasteless powder used as an antacid.

m. salicylate, a colorless or slightly reddish crystalline powder used as an intestinal antiseptic.

m. stearate, a combination of magnesium with stearic and palmitic acids; used as a dusting powder.

m. sulfate, a crystalline compound used as a cathartic and anticonvulsant.

m. trisilicate, a combination of magnesium oxide and silicon dioxide with varying proportions of water; used as a gastric antacid.

magnet (mag′net) an object having polarity and capable of attracting iron.

magnetism (mag′nĕ-tizm) magnetic attraction or repulsion.

magnetoelectricity (mag-ne″to-e″lek-tris′ĭ-te) electric current induced by a magnet.

magnetotherapy (mag-ne″to-ther′ah-pe) treatment of disease by magnetic currents.

magnetropism (mag-net′ro-pizm) a growth response in a nonmotile organism under the influence of a magnet.

magnification (mag″nĭ-fĭ-ka′shun) apparent increase of the size of an object by means of a lens or a system of lenses.

main (mān) [Fr.] hand.

m. en griffe (ma-non-grif′) clawhand.

Majocchi's disease (mah-yok′ēz) annular telangiectatic purpura.

make (māk) closure and completion of an electric circuit.

makro- for words beginning thus, see those beginning *macro-*.

mal (mal) [Fr.] illness; disease.

grand m., a generalized convulsive seizure attended by loss of consciousness (see also EPILEPSY).

m. de mer, seasickness.

petit m., momentary loss of consciousness without convulsive movements (see also EPILEPSY).

mala (ma′lah) the cheek or cheek bone. adj., **ma′lar.**

malabsorption (mal″ab-sorp′shun) disorder of normal nutritive absorption; disordered anabolism.

malachite green (mal′ah-kīt) a dye used as a stain for bacteria and as an antiseptic for wounds.

malacia (mal-la′she-ah) 1. morbid softening of a part. 2. morbid craving for highly spiced foods.

malacoplakia (mal″ah-ko-pla′ke-ah) a circumscribed area of softening on the membrane lining a hollow organ, as the ureter, urethra or renal pelvis.

m. vesi′cae, a flat yellow growth on the bladder mucosa.

malacosarcosis (mal″ah-ko-sar-ko′sis) softness of muscular tissue.

malacosis (mal″ah-ko′sis) malacia.

malacosteon (mal″ah-kos′te-on) softening of the bones; osteomalacia.

malacotic (mal″ah-kot′ik) soft.

malacotomy (mal″ah-kot′o-me) incision of the abdominal wall.

malady (mal′ah-de) a disease or illness.

malaise (mal-āz′) [Fr.] a feeling of uneasiness or indisposition.

malalignment (mal″ah-līn′ment) displacement of the teeth from their normal relation to the line of the dental arch.

malaria (mah-lār′e-ah) a serious infectious illness characterized by periodic chills and high fever. It responds well to modern drugs but can be chronic. adj., **malar′ial.**

Malaria is found mainly in tropical and subtropical climates. It was once one of the most prevalent diseases in the world; in 1935, malaria cases in the southern United States alone numbered several hundred thousands. It is still common, but mosquito elimination programs and also the antimalarial drugs discovered during and since World War II have caused the number of cases to drop phenomenally.

CAUSE. Malaria is caused by a protozoan parasite, the Plasmodium, which is carried by the Anopheles mosquito. When the mosquito bites an infected person, it sucks in the parasites, which reside in the blood. In the mosquito the plasmodia multiply and travel to the salivary glands from which they are transmitted to the human bloodstream by the mosquito bite. Inside the human host they penetrate the erythrocytes, where they mature, reproduce and at complete maturity burst out of the blood cell. The life cycle varies according to the species of Plasmodium. For *P. vivax* it is 48 hours, *P. malariae* 72 hours and *P. falciparum* 36 to 48 hours.

SYMPTOMS. There are usually no symptoms until several cycles have been completed. Then there is a simultaneous rupturing of cells by the entire brood, causing the characteristic chills followed in a few hours by fever. The temperature may rise to 104 or 105° F. As it subsides, there is profuse perspiring. Other symptoms are headache, nausea, body pains and, after the attack, exhaustion. The symptoms last from 4 to 6 hours and recur at regular intervals, depending upon the parasitic species and its cycle. If the attack occurs every other day, the disease is called tertian malaria; if it occurs at 3 day intervals, it is quartan malaria.

As the disease progresses, the attacks occur less frequently. Bouts of malaria last from 1 to 4 weeks but usually about 2 weeks. Relapses are common, with attacks ceasing and recurring at irregular intervals for several years, especially if untreated. Malaria is not usually fatal; when it is, it is almost always caused by the falciparum species.

TREATMENT. For many years, quinine was the standard treatment for malaria. The intensive research carried on since World War II has provided synthetic medicines such as chloroquine, pentaquine and quinacrine (Atabrine) that are far superior to quinine. They can either relieve the attack promptly or cure the infection.

PREVENTION. There is no effective inoculation against malaria, but antimalarial drugs may be given prophylactically to persons traveling to areas where the disease is widespread. Preventive measures are concentrated on destroying the mosquito. This is done by filling in pools, swamps and places containing stagnant water where mosquitoes breed, and by intensive use of DDT and other insecticides.

malariacidal (mah-lār″e-ah-si′dal) destructive to malarial plasmodia.

malariotherapy (mah-lār″e-o-ther′ah-pe) treatment of paresis by infecting the patient with the parasite of tertian malaria.

Malassezia (mal″ah-se′ze-ah) a genus of fungi. **M. fur′fur,** the causative agent of tinea versicolor.

malassimilation (mal″ah-sim″ĭ-la′shun) defective or faulty assimilation.

malate (ma′lāt) a salt of malic acid.

malaxate (mal′ak-sāt) to knead, as in making pills.

malaxation (mal″ak-sa′shun) an act of kneading.

male (māl) an individual of the sex that produces spermatozoa or begets young.

maleruption (mal″e-rup′shun) eruption of a tooth out of its normal position.

malformation (mal″for-ma′shun) defective formation; deformity.

malic acid (ma′lik) a crystalline acid from juices of many fruits and plants, and an intermediary product of carbohydrate metabolism in the body.

malignancy (mah-lig′nan-se) a tendency to progress in virulence. In popular usage, any condition that, if uncorrected, tends to worsen so as to cause serious illness or death. Cancer is the best known example.

malignant (mah-lig′nant) tending to become progressively worse and to result in death.

malingerer (mah-ling′ger-er) one who is guilty of malingering.

malingering (mah-ling′ger-ing) willful, deliberate and fraudulent feigning or exaggeration of the symptoms of illness or injury to attain a consciously desired end.

malleable (mal′e-ah-bl) susceptible of being beaten out into a thin plate.

malleo-incudal (mal″e-o-ing′ku-dal) pertaining to the malleus and incus.

malleolus (mah-le′o-lus), pl. *malle′oli* [L.] a rounded process, especially either of the two rounded prominences on either side of the ankle joint, at the lower end of the fibula (external, lateral or outer malleolus) or of the tibia (inner, internal or medial malleolus). adj., **malle′olar.**

malleotomy (mal″e-ot′o-me) 1. division of the malleus. 2. operative separation of the malleoli.

malleus (mal′e-us) the largest of the three ossicles of the ear; called also hammer.

malnutrition (mal″nu-trish′un) poor nourishment resulting from improper diet or from some defect in metabolism that prevents the body from using its food properly. Extreme malnutrition may lead to starvation.

CAUSES. Although poverty is still the major cause of malnutrition, the condition is by no means confined to the underdeveloped parts of the world.

Anyone can become undernourished if he seriously neglects his diet. A well balanced diet, the requirements of which vary slightly with a person's age, should include adequate amounts of protein, vitamins, minerals, and carbohydrates. For an explanation of the value of properly balanced diets, see NUTRITION.

Ignorance of the basic principles of nutrition is probably almost as great a cause of undernourishment as poverty. Misplaced faith in vitamin pills as a substitute for food, for example, can, if carried to extremes, cause undernourishment. So can over-reliance on excessively processed foods. Modern methods of processing and refining foods can sometimes cause a loss of valuable nutrients, as happens in the refining of certain grains, such as rice. However, this danger is recognized by both the government and the manufacturers, who try to retain or restore the nutritional value of many foods. ALCOHOLISM, which frequently leads a person to rely on alcohol at the expense of food, is another cause of malnutrition.

People who want to gain or lose weight, or who, like vegetarians, avoid certain foods, may endanger their health by following an unbalanced diet that lacks essential nutrients. Anyone who plans to follow a special diet should talk the matter over with his physician.

Malnutrition can also stem from disease. If the organs of the digestive system that transform food into bone, tissue, blood and energy fail to function properly, the body will not receive adequate nourishment. Such deficiencies can cause diabetes mellitus, certain liver diseases and some anemias. The ENDOCRINE GLANDS and ENZYMES are also vital to the proper use of food by the body, and defects in their functioning may cause forms of malnutrition.

SYMPTOMS. In general, the symptoms of malnutrition are physical weakness, lassitude and an increasing sense of detachment from the world. There are also specific symptoms that vary according to the essential substance lacking in the diet. For example, lack of vitamin A can result in NIGHT BLINDNESS, or poor vision in dim light. In the absence of adequate exposure to sunlight, a lack of vitamin D can cause RICKETS, which results in malformed limbs in infants and children because the bones fail to harden properly. A lack of vitamin C causes SCURVY, with symptoms of bleeding gums and easily bruised skin. Other vitamin deficiency diseases are BERIBERI, PELLAGRA and SPRUE. If there is not enough iron in the diet, ANEMIA develops.

In starvation there are signs of multiple vitamin deficiency. There may be edema, abdominal distention and excessive loss of weight. As starvation progresses, fat cells become small and accumulations of fat are depleted. The liver is reduced in size, the muscles shrivel and the lymphoid tissue, gonads and blood deteriorate.

Because the stomach and the intestinal tract may no longer be capable of digesting food of any bulk, treatment of starvation should begin by feeding the patient easily digested liquids, such as soups, in small quantities. If he is unable to eat or drink, the necessary nutrients can be supplied by intravenous infusion.

malocclusion (mal″ŏ-kloo′zhun) malposition of

the teeth resulting in the faulty meeting of the teeth or jaws. The condition should be corrected because it predisposes to dental caries, may lead to digestive disorders and inadequate nutrition because of difficulty in chewing and can cause serious psychologic effects if there is facial distortion. Corrective treatment is provided by an orthodontist, who may apply appropriate dental braces to improve the position of the teeth.

malonal (mal′o-nal) barbital, a long-acting barbiturate.

malpighian capsule (mal-pig′ĭ-an) a two-layered cellular envelope enclosing the tuft of capillaries constituting the glomerulus of the kidney; called also Bowman's capsule.
   m. corpuscle, the funnel-like structure constituting the beginning of the structural unit of the kidney (nephron) and comprising the malpighian capsule and its partially enclosed glomerulus.
   m. layer, the deep part of the epidermis.

malposition (mal″po-zish′un) abnormal placement.

malpractice (mal-prak′tis) any professional misconduct, unreasonable lack of skill or fidelity in professional duties or illegal or immoral conduct. Malpractice is one form of negligence, which in legal terms can be defined as the omission to do something that a reasonable man, guided by those ordinary considerations which ordinarily regulate human affairs, would do, or the doing of something that a reasonable and prudent man would not do. In medical and nursing practice, malpractice means bad, wrong or injudicious treatment of a patient professionally; it results in injury, unnecessary suffering or death to the patient. The court may hold that malpractice has occurred even though the physician or nurse acted in good faith. Also, malpractice and negligence may occur through omission to act as well as commission of an unwise or negligent act.

malpresentation (mal″prez-en-ta′shun) faulty fetal presentation.

malrotation (mal″ro-ta′shun) abnormal or pathologic rotation, as of the vertebral column.

malt (mawlt) a preparation of grain that contains dextrin, maltose and diastase; it is nutritive and digestant, aiding in the digestion of starchy foods, and is used in the treatment of tuberculosis and other wasting diseases.

Malta fever (mawl′tah) brucellosis.

maltase (mawl′tās) an enzyme that catalyzes the decomposition of maltose to dextrose.

maltodextrin (mawl″to-dek′strin) a dextrin convertible into maltose.

maltose (mawl′tōs) a sugar from malt or digested starch.

malum (ma′lum) [L.] disease.
   m. articulo′rum seni′lis, a painful degenerative state of a joint as a result of aging.
   m. cox′ae seni′lis, osteoarthritis of the hip joint.
   m. per′forans pe′dis, perforating ulcer of the foot.

malunion (mal-ūn′yon) faulty union of the fragments of a fractured bone.

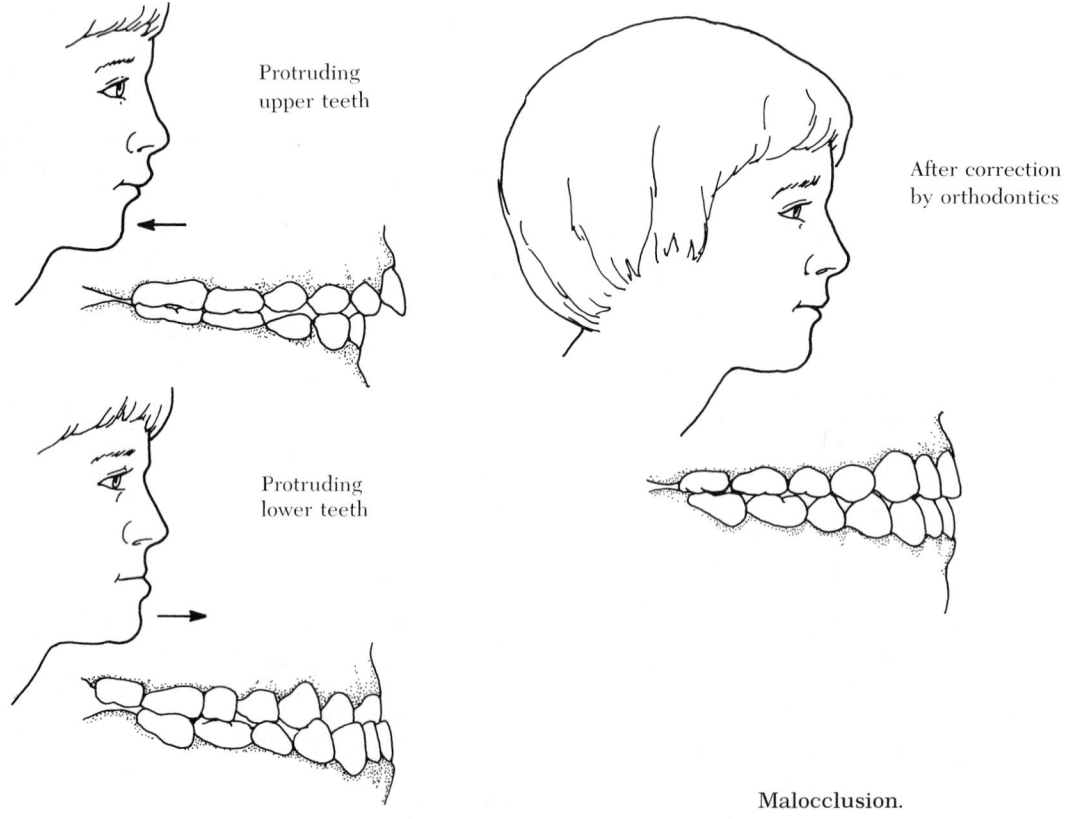

Protruding upper teeth

Protruding lower teeth

After correction by orthodontics

Malocclusion.

mamilla (mah-mil′ah), pl. *mamil′lae* [L.] 1. the nipple of the breast. 2. a nipple-like prominence. adj., **mam′illary.**

mamillated (mam′ĭ-lāt″ed) having nipple-like projections or prominences.

mamillation (mam″ĭ-la′shun) 1. the condition of being mamillated. 2. a nipple-like elevation or projection.

mamilliform (mah-mil′i-form) shaped like a nipple.

mamilliplasty (mah-mil′i-plas″te) theleplasty; plastic reconstruction of the nipples.

mamillitis (mam″i-li′tis) inflammation of the nipple.

mamm(o)- (mam′o) word element [L.], *breast; mammary gland.*

mamma (mam′ah), pl. *mam′mae* [L.] the milk-secreting gland of the female; mammary gland.

mammal (mam′al) an individual of the Mammalia, a division of vertebrates, including all that possess hair and suckle their young. adj., **mammal′ian.**

mammalgia (mah-mal′je-ah) pain in the mammary gland.

mammaplasty (mam′ah-plas″te) mammoplasty.

mammary (mam′ar-e) pertaining to the mamma, or breast.
  m. gland, the collective glandular elements of the BREAST, or mamma, of the female which secrete milk for nourishment of the young. Mammary glands exist in a rudimentary state in the male.

mammectomy (mah-mek′to-me) mastectomy.

mammilla (mah-mil′ah) mamilla.

mammiplasia (mam″ĭ-pla′ze-ah) mammoplasia.

mammiplasty (mam′ĭ-plas″te) mammoplasty.

mammitis (mah-mi′tis) mastitis.

mammography (mah-mog′rah-fe) roentgenography of the breast with or without injection of an opaque substance into its ducts. Simple mammography, without the use of a contrast medium, is sometimes used in the diagnosis of cancer and other disorders of the breast.

mammoplasia (mam″o-pla′ze-ah) development of breast tissue.

mammoplasty (mam′o-plas″te) plastic surgery of the breast.
  augmentation m., plastic surgery to increase the size of the female breast.
  reduction m., plastic surgery to decrease the size of the female breast.

mammose (mam′ōs) having unusually large mammary glands.

mammotomy (mah-mot′o-me) mastotomy.

mammotropic (mam″o-trop′ik) having a stimulating effect on the mammary gland.

mammotropin (mam″o-tro′pin) a hormone of the anterior pituitary that stimulates the mammary gland; called also lactogenic hormone, or prolactin.

Mandelamine (man-del′ah-mēn) trademark for a preparation of methenamine mandelate, a urinary antiseptic.

mandelic acid (man-del′ik) a keto acid used as a urinary antiseptic in nephritis, pyelitis and cystitis. It must be excreted in the urinary tract unchanged in order to have a bacteriostatic effect; therefore, a strongly acid urine should be maintained during its administration. To accomplish this, fluids may be limited and an acidifying agent given (see also ACID-ASH DIET). Citrus fruits and other foods producing an alkaline ash must be restricted. The average dose of mandelic acid or preparations containing this substance depends on the type of preparation used.

mandible (man′dĭ-bl) the horseshoe-shaped bone forming the lower jaw. adj., **mandib′ular.** It consists of a central portion, which forms the chin and supports the lower teeth, and two perpendicular portions, or rami, which point upward from the back of the chin on either side.

mandrin (man′drin) a metal guide for a flexible catheter.

manganese (mang′gah-nēs) a chemical element, atomic number 25, atomic weight 54.938, symbol Mn. (See table of ELEMENTS.)
  m. butyrate, a red powder, used in treatment of some skin diseases.
  m. dioxide, black oxide of manganese; an oxidizing agent.
  m. glycerophosphate, an odorless white powder; hematinic and nerve tonic.

mange (mānj) a skin disease of domestic animals, due to mites.

mania (ma′ne-ah) a disordered mental state of extreme excitement.

maniac (ma′ne-ak) one affected with mania.

manic-depressive (man″ik-de-pres′iv) marked by alternating periods of elation and depression (see also affective PSYCHOSIS).

manipulation (mah-nip″u-la′shun) skillful or dexterous treatment by the hands. In physical therapy, the forceful passive movement of a joint beyond its active limit of motion.

mannitol (man′ĭ-tol) a sugar occurring widely in nature, especially in fungi; used originally in diagnostic tests of kidney function and now therapeutically as a diuretic.
  m. hexanitrate, a crystalline compound used as a vasodilator.

manometer (mah-nom′ĕ-ter) an instrument for ascertaining the pressure of liquids or gases.

Mansonella (man″so-nel′ah) a genus of nematode parasites of the superfamily Filarioidea.
  M. ozzar′di, a species found in man, usually in fatty tissues surrounding organs in the body cavities.

Mansonia (man-so′ne-ah) a genus of mosquitoes comprising some 55 species, distributed primarily in tropical regions, important as vectors of microfilariae and viruses.

mantle (man′tl) an enveloping structure or layer; especially the brain mantle, or pallium.

Mantoux test (man-too′) an intracutaneous test for sensitivity to the tubercle bacillus (*Mycobacterium tuberculosis*), solutions of gradually increasing concentration of purified protein derivative tuberculin being used until a reaction occurs.

manubrium (mah-nu′bre-um), pl. *manu′bria* [L.] 1. the uppermost portion of the sternum (manu′brium ster′ni). 2. the largest process of the malleus, giving attachment to the tendon of the tensor muscle of the tympanum (manu′brium mal′lei).

manus (ma′nus), pl. *ma′nus* [L.] hand.

Mapharsen (mah-far′sen) trademark for a preparation of oxophenarsine hydrochloride, formerly used in the treatment of syphilis.

maple bark disease a granulomatous interstitial pneumonitis due to a rare mold found beneath the bark of maple logs.

maple syrup urine disease a genetic disorder involving deficiency of an enzyme necessary in the metabolism of branched-chain amino acids, and named for the characteristic odor of the urine.

marasmus (mah-raz′mus) progressive wasting, especially in young infants.

marble bones osteopetrosis.

Marchiafava-Micheli syndrome (mar″ke-ah-fah′va me-ka′le) nocturnal paroxysmal hemoglobinuria.

Marezine (mar′ĕ-zēn) trademark for a preparation of cyclizine hydrochloride, an antihistamine.

Marfan's disease (mar-fahnz′) progressive spastic paraplegia in children with congenital syphilis.

M's syndrome, abnormal length of the extremities, especially of the fingers and toes, with subluxation of the lens, congenital anomalies of the heart and other deformities.

margo (mar′go), pl. *mar′gines* [L.] border; margin.

Marie's disease (mah-rēz′) acromegaly.

Marie-Bamberger disease (mah-re′ bahm′berger) hypertrophic osteoarthropathy.

Marie-Strümpell disease (mah-re′ strim′pel) rheumatoid spondylitis.

Marie-Tooth disease (mah-re′ tooth) progressive neuropathic (peroneal) muscular atrophy.

marijuana (mar″ĭ-wahn′ah) the hemp plant, Cannabis, which grows wild in many areas of the world, including the United States and Mexico; an alternative spelling is marihuana. Its cured leaves and flowers, known as "pot," "grass" or "tea," are used in cigarettes for their intoxicating effects. Hashish is a similar preparation.

The marijuana habit is acquired mostly by adolescents or adults who are seeking escape from reality. The user of the drug is exhilarated, loses his inhibitions and may have delusions or hallucinations. His actions may be silly or he may be irritable; his eyelids may droop. If the use of the drug becomes a habit, it often leads to withdrawal from normal activities and unexplained absences from home or job.

Dependence on truly addictive drugs, such as heroin, has a physical basis, and withdrawal of the drug produces severe physical as well as mental disturbances. Addiction to marijuana is psychologic and therefore less difficult to cure; nevertheless, use of marijuana can become a habit. Treatment consists mainly of forbidding the drug (traffic in which is outlawed by federal and state legislation), helping the patient understand himself and his problems and encouraging him to deal with reality in normal ways.

maritonucleus (mar″ĭ-to-nu′kle-us) the nucleus of the ovum after the spermatozoon has entered it.

Marplan (mar′plan) trademark for a preparation of isocarboxazid, an antidepressant.

marrow (mar′o) the soft spongelike material in the cavities of bones. Bone marrow is a network of blood vessels and special connective tissue fibers that hold together a composite of fat and blood-producing cells.

The chief function of marrow is to manufacture erythrocytes, leukocytes and platelets. These blood cells normally do not enter the bloodstream until they are fully developed, so that the marrow contains cells in all stages of growth. If the body's demand for white cells is increased because of infection, the marrow responds immediately by stepping up production. The same is true if more red blood cells are needed, as in hemorrhage or some other types of anemia.

There are two types of marrow, red and yellow. The former produces the blood cells; the latter, which is mainly formed of fatty tissue, normally has no blood-producing function.

During infancy and early childhood all bone marrow is red. But gradually, as one gets older and less blood-cell production is needed, the fat content of the marrow increases to turn some of the marrow from red to yellow. Red marrow continues to be present in adulthood only in the flat bones of the skull, the sternum, ribs, vertebral column, clavicle, humerus and part of the femur. However, under certain conditions, as after hemorrhage, yellow marrow in other bones may again be converted to red and resume its cell-producing functions.

The marrow is occasionally subject to disease, as in aplastic anemia, which may be caused by destruction of the marrow by chemical agents or excessive x-ray exposure. Other diseases that affect the bone marrow are leukemia, pernicious anemia, myeloma and metastatic tumors.

marsupialization (mar-su″pe-ah-lĭ-za′shun) conversion of a closed cavity, such as an abscess or cyst, into an open pouch, by incising it and suturing the edges of its wall to the edges of the wound.

marsupium (mar-su′pe-um), pl. *marsu′pia* [L.] pouch; the scrotum.

masculation (mas″ku-la′shun) the development of male characteristics.

masculine (mas′ku-lin) pertaining to the male sex.

masculinity (mas″ku-lin′ĭ-te) the possession of masculine qualities.

masculinization (mas″ku-lin-ĭ-za′shun) the induction or development of male secondary sex characters in the female.

masculinize (mas'ku-lĭ-nīz) to produce masculine qualities in women.

masculinovoblastoma (mas"ku-lin-o"vo-blas-to'-mah) an ovarian tumor that causes masculinization.

maser (ma'zer) a device that produces an extremely intense, small and nearly nondivergent beam of monochromatic radiation in the microwave region, with all the waves in phase.

mask (mask) 1. to cover or conceal; in audiometry, to obscure or diminish a sound by the presence of another sound of different frequency. 2. an appliance for shading, protecting or medicating the face.
  leutic m., a brownish, blotchy pigmentation over the forehead, temples and cheeks, sometimes occuring in tertiary syphilis.
  m. of pregnancy, brown pigmentation of the forehead, cheeks and nose, sometimes seen in pregnancy.

masochism (mas'o-kizm) 1. the derivation of sexual gratification through the suffering of pain. 2. the passive acceptance of pain.

masochist (mas'o-kist) a person exhibiting or characterized by masochism.

mass (mas) 1. a lump or collection of cohering particles. 2. that characteristic of matter which gives it inertia.
  body cell m., the total weight of the cells of the body, constituting the total mass of oxygen-utilizing, carbohydrate-burning and energy-exchanging cells of the body; regarded as proportional to total exchangeable potassium in the body.
  inner cell m., an internal cluster of cells at one pole of the distended blastocyst which develops into the body of the embryo.
  intermediate cell m., nephrotome.
  lean body m., that part of the body including all its components except neutral storage lipid; in essence, the fat-free mass of the body.
  rest m., the mass of a particle at rest, such as that of a nuclear particle when the atom is neither emitting nor absorbing energy.

massa (mas'ah), pl. *mas'sae* [L.] mass (1).

massage (mah-sahzh') systematic stroking or kneading of the body.
  auditory m., massage of the tympanic membrane.
  cardiac m., intermittent compression of the heart by pressure applied over the sternum (closed cardiac massage) or directly to the heart through an opening in the chest wall (open cardiac massage). (See also CARDIAC MASSAGE.)
  vibratory m., massage by rapidly repeated light percussion with a vibrating hammer or sound.

masseter muscle (mah-se'ter) the muscle that closes the jaws.

masseur (mah-ser') [Fr.] a man who performs massage.

masseuse (mah"sōōs') [Fr.] a woman who performs massage.

massotherapy (mas"o-ther'ah-pe) treatment of disease by massage.

mast cell (mast) a connective tissue cell whose specific physiologic function is unknown. It elaborates granules that contain histamine, heparin and, in the rat and mouse, serotonin.

mastadenitis (mas"tad-ĕ-ni'tis) inflammation of a mammary gland.

mastalgia (mas-tal'je-ah) pain in the breast.

mastatrophy (mas-tat'ro-fe) atrophy of the breast.

mastectomy (mas-tek'to-me) surgical removal of breast tissue. Mastectomy is usually performed to treat malignant breast tumors, although rarely it may be advisable to use the procedure for benign tumors and for other diseases of the breast, such as chronic cystic mastitis. (See also surgery of the BREAST.)
  radical m., amputation of the breast with wide excision of the pectoral muscles and axillary lymph nodes.

Master "2-step" exercise test (mas'ter) a test of coronary circulation, electrocardiographic tracings being recorded while the subject repeatedly ascends and descends two steps, each 9 inches high, as well as immediately and 2 and 6 minutes after cessation of the climbs. The amount of work (number of trips) is standardized for age, weight and sex.

mastication (mas"tĭ-ka'shun) the act of chewing.

masticatory (mas'tĭ-kah-tor"e) 1. pertaining to mastication. 2. a substance to be chewed, but not swallowed.

Mastigophora (mas"tĭ-gof'o-rah) a subphylum of protozoa, including all those that have one or more flagella in their trophozoite form; many are parasitic in both invertebrates and vertebrates, including man.

mastitis (mas"ti'tis) inflammation of the BREAST, occurring in a variety of forms and in varying degrees of severity.
  Chronic cystic mastitis is the most common disorder of the breast resulting from hormonal imbalance. This condition generally occurs in women between the ages of 30 and 50. It is probably related to the activity of the ovaries and is rare after the menopause.
  The disease is characterized by the formation of cysts which give a lumpy appearance to the breast. Symptoms may include pain and tenderness, which are usually aggravated before the menstrual period, at which time the cysts tend to enlarge. There may also be a discharge from the nipple. Periodic change in the size of a lump or its rapid appearance and disappearance is common in cystic mastitis. Since there are times when it may be difficult to distinguish this condition from cancer of the breast, biopsy may be necessary. Treatment may involve removing fluid from the cysts.
  To help relieve the pain associated with cystic mastitis a good supporting brassiere that fits well and is not constricting should be worn day and night. Care should be taken to avoid injury to the breasts.
  Young girls whose breasts are maturing sometimes experience a painful swelling and hardness of the breast, known as puberty mastitis. Occasionally a cloudy liquid may be squeezed from the nipples. The condition, rarely serious, usually

subsides within a few weeks. It is best to wear a brassiere that gives mild support but does not irritate.

Enlargement of one or both breasts, gynecomastia, is sometimes found in adolescent boys and old men. The condition is usually due to excessive estrogenic activity. Secretions may be extruded from the nipple.

A mild inflammation known as stagnation mastitis, or caked breast, may occur during the early lactation period. Glands of the breast can become congested with milk, with formation of painful lumps.

Acute mastitis may occur after childbirth, when it is known as puerperal mastitis. It is an infection resulting usually from the presence of staphylococci and, occasionally, streptococci, which enter through cracks in the skin of the breast, particularly of the nipples. In puerperal mastitis, the breasts are tender, red and warm. They become swollen and painful, and the inflammation responds quickly to sulfonamide medicines or one of the antibiotics, but in some cases an abscess may develop which must be incised and drained.

A milk cyst, galactocele, sometimes develops during lactation. It is probably caused by obstruction of a duct. The cyst can be removed after the baby has been weaned.

There are other types of infectious mastitis not related to lactation. Inflammation of the breast sometimes accompanies mumps, particularly in adults.

Tuberculous mastitis usually occurs in young women and accompanies tuberculosis of the lungs or of the cervical lymph nodes. Treatment is with antibiotics, although surgery is sometimes necessary.

A condition that may occur at the time of the menopause or later in women who have had children is comedomastitis, which is distention of the milk-producing ducts caused by the caking of secretions. Some of the material may be discharged from the nipple. Eventually the condition may develop into plasma cell mastitis. The breast may be tender and painful, with lump formation, nipple retraction, change in the breast contour and possibly a cloudy discharge from the nipple.

Persistent cases of mastitis may require mastectomy.

masto- (mas′to) word element [Gr.], *mammary gland; breast.*

mastocyte (mas′to-sīt) a mast cell.

mastocytoma (mas″to-si-to′mah) a tumor containing mast cells.

mastodynia (mas″to-din′e-ah) mastalgia.

mastography (mas-tog′rah-fe) roentgenography of the breast; mammography.

mastoid (mas′toid) 1. nipple-shaped. 2. the portion of the temporal bone lying behind the meatus of the ear (pars mastoidea), or more specifically the conical projection from it (mastoid process).

m. antrum, an air space in the mastoid portion of the temporal bone communicating with the middle ear and the mastoid cells.

m. cells, hollow spaces of various size and shape in the mastoid process of the temporal bone, communicating with the mastoid antrum and lined with a continuation of its mucous membrane.

mastoidale (mas″toi-da′le) the lowest point of the mastoid process.

mastoidalgia (mas″toi-dal′je-ah) pain in the mastoid region.

mastoidectomy (mas″toi-dek′to-me) surgical removal of mastoid cells. The most frequent indication for mastoidectomy is chronic infection in the mastoid process occurring as a complication of chronic OTITIS MEDIA. The extent of surgery depends on extent of destruction. A radical mastoidectomy involves removal of diseased portions of the mastoid process as well as the incus and malleus of the middle ear and the tympanic membrane. The degree of hearing loss following mastoidectomy depends on the extent of surgery. In some cases tympanoplasty (plastic reconstruction of the middle ear) can preserve much of the hearing. (For nursing care after ear surgery, see EAR.)

mastoideocentesis (mas-toi″de-o-sen-te′sis) paracentesis of the mastoid cells.

mastoiditis (mas″toi-di′tis) inflammation of the mastoid antrum and cells. It is usually the result of an infection of the middle ear, with which the mastoid cells communicate. Mastoiditis most commonly follows sore throat and respiratory infection, but it can also be caused by such diseases as diphtheria, measles and scarlet fever.

The symptoms include earache and a ringing in the ears. The mastoid process may become painful and swollen.

Treatment formerly was limited to mastoidectomy, in which infected cells are removed surgically. Today, however, the development of antibiotics has made it possible to check most cases of mastoiditis at an early stage, so that surgery usually is avoided.

mastoidotomy (mas″toi-dot′o-me) incision of the mastoid process of the temporal bone.

mastology (mas-tol′o-je) study of the mammary gland.

mastoncus (mas-tong′kus) a tumor or swelling of the breast.

masto-occipital (mas″to-ok-sip″ĭ-tal) pertaining to the mastoid process and occipital bone.

mastopathy (mas-top′ah-the) disease of the mammary gland.

mastopexy (mas′to-pek″se) surgical fixation of a pendulous breast.

mastoplasia (mas″to-pla′ze-ah) hyperplasia of breast tissue.

mastoplasty (mas′to-plas″te) mammoplasty.

mastoptosis (mas″to-to′sis) a pendulous condition of the breast.

mastorrhagia (mas″to-ra′je-ah) hemorrhage from the mammary gland.

mastoscirrhus (mas″to-skir′us) hardening of the mammary gland.

mastosis (mas-to′sis) degeneration of breast tissue, with painful nodular swellings.

mastotomy (mas-tot'o-me) incision of a mammary gland.

masturbation (mas"tur-ba'shun) sexual gratification by self-manipulation of the genitalia. Masturbation is too often thought of as shameful and unwholesome. Many harmful effects have mistakenly been attributed to it. We now know that the desire to masturbate is part of the normal process of sexual development. The real harm in masturbation is psychologic because it may evoke deep feelings of guilt, anxiety and fear. A large number of boys and girls have experimented with masturbation during their growing years. Frequent practice by adults, however, may be a sign of some emotional difficulty or maladjustment.

matching (mach'ing) comparison for the purpose of selecting objects having similar or identical characteristics.

m. of blood, comparing the blood of a contemplated donor with that of the recipient to ascertain whether their bloods belong to the same group.

cross m., determination of the compatibility of the blood of a donor and that of a recipient before transfusion by placing erythrocytes of the donor in the recipient's serum and erythrocytes of the recipient in the donor's serum. Absence of agglutination indicates that the two blood samples belong to the same group and are compatible.

materia medica (mah-tēr'e-ah med'ĭ-kah) pharmacology.

maternal (mah-ter'nal) pertaining to the female parent.

matrix (ma'triks), pl. *mat'rices* [L.] a generative, or basic, structure from which a tissue or organ develops, such as the organs from which grow the hair and nail.

nail m., m. un'guis, the end of the nail bed.

matroclinous (mat"ro-kli'nus) resembling the maternal species rather than the paternal; said of a hybrid.

matter (mat'er) physical material having form and weight under ordinary conditions of gravity.

maturation (mat"u-ra'shun) 1. the stage or process of attaining maximal development. In biology, a process of cell division during which the number of chromosomes in the germ cell is reduced to one-half the number characteristic of the species. 2. the formation of pus.

maxilla (mak-sil'ah) pl. *maxil'lae* [L.], *maxil'las* one of two identical bones that form the upper jaw. The maxillae meet in the midline of the face and often are considered as one bone. They have been described as the architectural key of the face because all bones of the face except the mandible touch them. Together the maxillae form the floor of the orbit for each eye, the sides and lower walls of the nasal cavities, and the hard palate. The lower border of the maxilla supports the upper teeth. Each maxilla contains an air space called the maxillary sinus.

maxillectomy (mak"sĭ-lek'to-me) removal of the maxilla.

maxillitis (mak"sĭ-li'tis) inflammation of the maxilla.

maximum (mak'sĭ-mum) 1. the greatest quantity or value possible or achieved under given circumstances. 2. the height of a disease or process.

tubular m. the highest rate in milligrams per minute at which the renal tubules can transfer artificially administered test substances; the maximal tubular excretory capacity. Abbreviated Tm.

Maxitate (mak'sĭ-tāt) trademark for preparations of mannitol hexanitrate, a vasodilator.

maze (māz) a complicated system of intersecting paths used in intelligence tests and in demonstrating learning in experimental animals.

M.B. Bachelor of Medicine.

M.C. [L.] *Ma'gister Chirur'giae* (Master of Surgery); Medical Corps.

Mc megacurie.

mc. millicurie.

μc. microcurie.

McBurney's point (mak-ber'nēz) the point of special tenderness in acute appendicitis; situated about 2 inches from the right anterior superior spine of the ilium, on a line between this spine and the umbilicus. It corresponds with the normal position of the appendix.

M's sign, special tenderness at McBurney's point; indicative of appendicitis.

mcg. microgram.

MCH mean corpuscular hemoglobin, an expression of the average hemoglobin content of a single cell in micromicrograms, obtained by multiplying the hemoglobin in grams by 10 and dividing by the number of erythrocytes (in millions).

MCHC mean corpuscular hemoglobin concentration, an expression of the average hemoglobin concentration in per cent, obtained by multiplying the hemoglobin in grams by 100 and dividing by the hematocrit determination.

mCi millicurie.

μCi microcurie.

McMurray's sign (mak-mur'ēz) occurrence of a cartilage click during manipulation of the knee; indicative of menisceal injury.

MCV 1. mean corpuscular volume, an expression of the average volume of individual cells in cubic microns, obtained by multiplying the hematocrit determination by 10 and dividing by the number of erythrocytes (in millions). 2. mean clinical value, obtained by assigning a numerical value to the response noted in a number of patients receiving a specific treatment, adding these numbers and dividing by the number of patients treated.

M.D. Doctor of Medicine.

Md chemical symbol, *mendelevium.*

M.D.S. Master of Dental Surgery.

meal (mēl) a portion of food or foods taken at some particular and usually stated or fixed time. (See also TEST MEAL.)

mean (mēn) an average; a numerical value intermediate between two extremes.

measles (me'zelz) a highly contagious illness caused by a virus; called also rubeola. Measles is a childhood disease but it can be contracted at any age. Epidemics of measles usually recur every 2 or 3 years and are most common in the winter and spring.

CAUSE. The virus that causes measles is spread by droplet infection. The virus can also be picked up by touching an article, such as a handkerchief, that an infected person has recently used.

The incubation period is usually 11 days, although it may be as few as 9 or as many as 14. The patient can transmit the disease from 3 or 4 days before the rash appears until the rash begins to fade, a total of about 7 or 8 days. One attack of measles usually gives a lifetime immunity to rubeola but not to German measles (RUBELLA), which is somewhat similar to ordinary measles.

SYMPTOMS. Measles symptoms generally appear in two stages. In the first stage the patient feels tired and uncomfortable, and may have a running nose, a cough, a slight fever and pains in the head and back. The eyes may become reddened and sensitive to light. The fever rises a little each day.

The second stage begins at the end of the third or beginning of the fourth day. The patient's temperature is generally between 103 and 104° F. Koplik's spots, small white dots like grains of salt surrounded by inflamed areas, can often be seen on the gums and the inside of the cheeks. A rash appears, starting at the hairline and behind the ears and spreading downward, covering the body in about 36 hours. At first the rash consists of separate pink spots, about a quarter of an inch in diameter, but later some of the spots may run together, giving the patient a blotchy look. The fever usually subsides after the rash has spread. The rash turns brownish and fades after 3 or 4 days.

TREATMENT AND NURSING CARE. The patient should be kept in bed as long as the rash and fever continue, and should get as much rest as possible. Aspirin, nose drops and cough medicine may be prescribed during this stage. Water and fluids can be given for fever. The sickroom should be well ventilated and fairly warm. If the patient's eyes are sensitive to light, strong sunlight should be kept out of the room.

The rash may itch a great deal and prevent the patient from resting. If so, calamine lotion, cornstarch solution or plain cool water will afford some relief. If the itching continues, antihistamine drugs may be necessary.

Measles can greatly lower the body's resistance to other infections such as bronchitis, pneumonia and ear infection. If the patient's temperature remains high for more than 2 days after the rash fades, or if he complains of pain in the ear, throat, chest or abdomen, medical attention should be obtained without delay.

PREVENTION. A vaccine that gives immunity to measles has been developed. Infants are usually given measles vaccine at the age of 9 or 10 months. Until then they are protected by a temporary immunity inherited from the mother. The measles vaccine apparently gives a lifelong immunity to the disease. To be effective, however, it must be given before exposure to the disease.

If an unvaccinated child has already been exposed, he should be given an injection of gamma globulin. If given after exposure to the virus, gamma globulin can often prevent the patient from contracting measles, or at least it makes the course of the disease much milder and lessens the chances of complications.

A child with measles should be isolated from others as long as the disease lasts. Anyone with a cold or cough should be kept away from the patient because another infection can cause serious complications.

The best method is to isolate the child from 3 or 4 days before the rash appears until his temperature is normal and the rash has begun to fade. When the child is well again, the sickroom should be thoroughly cleaned and aired.

meatorrhaphy (me"ah-tor'ah-fe) suture of the cut end of the urethra to the glans penis after incision for enlarging the urinary meatus.

meatoscopy (me"ah-tos'ko-pe) examination of the ureteral orifices by cystoscopy.

meatotomy (me"ah-tot'o-me) incision of the urinary meatus in order to enlarge it.

meatus (me-a'tus), pl. *mea'tus* [L.] an opening or passage. adj., **mea'tal.**
    acoustic m., m. acus'ticus, m. audito'rius, auditory m., a passage in the ear, one leading to the eardrum (external acoustic meatus) and one for passage of nerves and blood vessels (internal acoustic meatus).
    m. na'si, m. of nose, one of the three portions of the nasal cavity on either side of the septum, inferior, middle or superior (mea'tus na'si infe'rior, me'dius, supe'rior).
    m. urina'rius, urinary m., the opening of the urethra on the body surface through which urine is discharged.

Mebaral (meb'ah-ral) trademark for a preparation of mephobarbital, an anticonvulsant with a slight hypnotic action.

mebutamate (meb'u-tam"āt) a compound used to reduce blood pressure and as a mild tranquilizer.

mecamine (mek'ah-min) mecamylamine.

mecamylamine (mek"ah-mil'ah-min) a compound used in blockade of autonomic ganglia and as an antihypertensive.

mechanicoreceptor (mĕ-kan"ĭ-ko-re-sep'tor) a receptor for mechanical stimuli, such as those for sound and touch.

mechanics (mĕ-kan'iks) the science dealing with the motions of material bodies.
    body m., the application of kinesiology to use of the body in daily life activities and to the prevention and correction of problems related to posture.

mechanism (mek'ah-nizm) 1. the combination of mental processes by which a result is obtained. 2. the means unconsciously adopted to gratify a desire.
    defense m., a psychologic reaction or technique for protection against a stressful environmental situation or against anxiety.
    mental m., an unconscious and indirect manner of gratifying a repressed desire.

mechanology (mek"ah-nol'o-je) the science of mechanics or of machines.

mechanoreceptor (mek"ah-no-re-sep'tor) a nerve ending sensitive to mechanical stimuli, e.g., changes in tension or pressure.

mechanotherapy (mek″ah-no-ther′ah-pe) use of mechanical apparatus in treatment of disease or its results, especially in therapeutic exercises.

mechanothermy (mek″ah-no-ther′me) therapeutic heat produced by massage, exercise, etc.

mechlorethamine (me″klōr-eth′ah-mēn) a nitrogen mustard compound used as an antineoplastic agent.

Mecholyl (me′ko-lil) trademark for preparations of methacholine, a parasympathomimetic.

Meckel's diverticulum (mek′elz) a congenital sac or appendage occasionally found in the ileum; a relic of a fetal structure that connects the yolk sac with the intestinal cavity of the embryo.

meclizine (mek′li-zēn) a compound used as an antihistamine and antinauseant.

meconism (mek′o-nizm) opium poisoning; the opium habit.

meconium (me-ko′ne-um) dark green mucilaginous material in the intestine of the full-term fetus; it constitutes the first stools passed by the newborn infant.
   m. ileus, intestinal obstruction in the newborn due to blocking of the bowels with thick meconium.

media (me′de-ah) [L.] 1. plural of *medium.* 2. middle, especially the middle coat of a blood vessel, or tunica media.

medial (me′de-al) pertaining to or situated toward the midline.

medialecithal (me″de-ah-les′i-thal) having a moderate amount of yolk.

medialis (me″de-a′lis) [L.] medial.

median (me′de-an) 1. situated in the median plane or in the midline of a body or structure. 2. the perpendicular line that divides the area of a frequency curve into two equal halves.
   m. nerve, a nerve that originates in the brachial plexus and innervates muscles of the wrist and hand.
   m. plane, an imaginary plane passing longitudinally through the body from front to back and dividing it into right and left halves.

mediastinitis (me″de-as″ti-ni′tis) inflammation of the mediastinum.

mediastinography (me″de-as″ti-nog′rah-fe) roentgenography of the structures of the mediastinum.

mediastinopericarditis (me″de-as″ti-no-per″i-kar-di′tis) inflammation of the mediastinum and pericardium.

mediastinoscopy (me″de-as″ti-nos′ko-pe) endoscopic examination of the mediastinum.

mediastinotomy (me″de-as″ti-not′o-me) incision of the mediastinum.

mediastinum (me″de-ah-sti′num) pl. *mediasti′na* [L.] 1. a median septum or partition. 2. the mass of tissues and organs separating the sternum in front and the vertebral column behind, commonly considered to have three divisions: anterior, middle and superior. adj., **mediasti′nal.**
   m. tes′tis, a partial septum of the testis formed near its posterior border by a continuation of the tunica albuginea.

medicament (me-dik′ah-ment, med′i-kah-ment) a medicinal agent.

medicated (med′i-kāt″ed) imbued with a medicinal substance.

medication (med″i-ka′shun) 1. administration of remedies. 2. a medicinal agent.

medicinal (me-dis′i-nal) having healing qualities.

medicine (med′i-sin) 1. a drug or remedy. 2. the art of healing disease.
   aviation m., that branch of medicine which deals with the physiologic, medical, psychologic and epidemiologic problems involved in flying.
   clinical m., study of medicine at the bedside.
   experimental m., study of the science of healing diseases based on experimentation in animals.
   forensic m., the application of medical knowledge to questions of law; medical jurisprudence. Called also legal medicine.
   internal m., that dealing especially with diagnosis and medical treatment of diseases and disorders of internal structures of the body.
   legal m., forensic medicine.
   patent m., a vernacular term for a nostrum advertised to the public; it is generally of secret composition.
   physical m., the employment of physical means in the diagnosis and treatment of disease. It includes the use of heat, cold, light, water, electricity, manipulation, massage, exercise and mechanical devices.
   preclinical m., the subjects studied in medicine before the student observes actual diseases in patients.
   preventive m., science aimed at preventing disease.
   proprietary m., a remedy whose formula is owned exclusively by the manufacturer and which is marketed usually under a name registered as a trademark.
   psychosomatic m., the study of the interrelations between bodily processes and emotional life.
   socialized m., the practice of medicine under a system in which there is community responsibility for the care of the sick rather than individual responsibility of patient to doctor and doctor to patient.
   space m., that branch of aviation medicine concerned with conditions to be encountered in space.
   state m., a system of medical care in which the government assumes responsibility for the prevention of disease and the care of the sick.
   tropical m., medical science as applied to diseases ordinarily occurring only in hot or tropical countries.
   veterinary m., the diagnosis and treatment of the diseases of animals.

medicolegal (med″i-ko-le′gal) pertaining to medicine and law, or to forensic medicine.

medionecrosis (me″de-o-ne-kro′sis) focal areas of destruction of the elastic tissue and smooth muscle of the tunica media of a blood vessel, especially the aorta or its major branches.

mediopontine (me″de-o-pon′tīn) pertaining to the center of the pons.

mediotarsal (me″de-o-tar′sal) pertaining to the center of the tarsus.

Mediterranean disease thalassemia.
 M. fever, brucellosis.

medium (me′de-um), pl. *me′dia* [L.], *mediums* 1. an agent by which something is accomplished or an impulse is transmitted. 2. a substance providing the proper nutritional environment for the growth of microorganisms; called also culture medium.
 contrast m., a radiopaque substance used in roentgenography to permit visualization of body structures.
 culture m., a substance used to support the growth of microorganisms or other cells.
 dioptric media, refracting media.
 disperse m., dispersion m., the continuous phase of a colloid system; the medium in which a colloid is dispersed, corresponding to the solvent in a true solution.
 refracting media, the transparent tissues and fluid in the eye through which light rays pass and by which they are refracted and brought to a focus on the retina.

medius (me′de-us) [L.] situated in the middle.

Medomin (med′o-min) trademark for a preparation of heptabarbital, a short- to intermediate-acting barbiturate.

Medrol (med′rol) trademark for a preparation of methylprednisolone, an anti-inflammatory steroid.

medroxyprogesterone (med-rok″sĭ-pro-jes′tĕ-rōn) a compound used as a progestational agent.

medulla (mĕ-dul′ah), pl. *medul′lae* [L.] the central or inner portion of an organ. adj., **med′ullary.**
 adrenal m., the inner portion of the ADRENAL GLAND, where epinephrine is produced.
 m. of bone, bone marrow, contained in the medullary canal of bone.
 m. oblonga′ta, that part of the hindbrain lying between the pons above and the spinal cord below; it houses nerve centers for both motor and sensory nerves, where such functions as breathing and the beating of the heart are controlled (see also BRAIN).
 m. os′sium, bone marrow.
 renal m., the inner part of the substance of the kidney, composed chiefly of collecting tubules, and organized into a group of structures called the renal pyramids.
 spinal m., m. spina′lis, spinal cord.

medullated (med′u-lāt″ed) containing or covered by a medullary substance; equipped with myelin sheaths.

medullitis (med″u-li′tis) 1. myelitis. 2. osteomyelitis.

medullization (med″u-lĭ-za′shun) the enlargement of the haversian canals in rarefying osteitis followed by their conversion into marrow channels; also the replacement of bone by marrow cells.

medulloadrenal (mĕ-dul″o-ah-dre′nal) pertaining to the adrenal medulla.

medulloblast (mĕ-dul′o-blast) an undifferentiated cell of the neural tube that may develop into either a neuroblast or spongioblast.

medulloblastoma (mĕ-dul″o-blas-to′mah) a brain tumor composed of medulloblasts.

medulloepithelioma (mĕ-dul″o-ep″ĭ-the″le-o′-mah) a tumor of primitive retinal epithelium and neuroepithelium.

mega- (meg′ah) word element [Gr.], *large;* used in naming units of measurement to designate an amount 10^6 (one million) times the size of the unit to which it is joined, as megacuries (10^6 curies); abbreviation M.

megabacterium (meg″ah-bak-te′re-um) a large bacterium.

megabladder (meg″ah-blad′er) permanent overdistention of the bladder.

megacaryocyte (meg″ah-kar′e-o-sīt″) megakaryocyte.

megacolon (meg″ah-ko′lon) excessive dilatation of the colon.
 acquired m., dilatation of the colon, of unknown etiology, occurring in an adult.
 aganglionic m., a congenital condition characterized by great dilatation of the colon proximal to a narrowed segment in which myenteric plexus ganglion cells are absent.
 congenital m., massive dilatation of the colon proximal to an area that lacks autonomic ganglia.

megacurie (meg″ah-ku′re) a unit of radioactivity, being one million (10^6) curies; abbreviated Mc.

megadyne (meg′ah-dīn) one million dynes.

megaesophagus (meg″ah-e-sof′ah-gus) dilatation and muscular hypertrophy of most of the esophagus, above a constricted, often atrophied, distal segment.

megakaryoblast (meg″ah-kar′e-o-blast) an immature megakaryocyte.

megakaryocyte (meg″ah-kar′e-o-sīt″) the giant cell of bone marrow; it is a large cell with a greatly lobulated nucleus, and is generally supposed to give rise to blood platelets.

megakaryophthisis (meg″ah-kar″e-o-thi′sis) deficiency of megakaryocytes in bone marrow or blood.

megal(o)- (meg′ah-lo) word element [Gr.], *large; abnormal enlargement.*

megalecithal (meg″ah-les′ĭ-thal) containing a large amount of yolk.

megalencephaly (meg″ah-len-sef′ah-le) macrencephalia; hypertrophy of the brain.

megalgia (meg-al′je-ah) a severe pain.

megaloblast (meg′ah-lo-blast″) a primitive erythrocyte of large size. Megaloblasts are found in the blood in pernicious anemia.

megalocardia (meg″ah-lo-kar′de-ah) cardiomegaly; enlargement of the heart.

megalocephaly (meg″ah-lo-sef′ah-le) abnormally increased size of the head.

megalocheiria (meg″ah-lo-ki′re-ah) abnormal largeness of the hands.

megalocornea (meg″ah-lo-kor′ne-ah) a developmental anomaly of the cornea, which is of abnormal size at birth and continues to grow, sometimes reaching a diameter of 14 or 15 mm. in the adult.

megalocyte (meg'ah-lo-sīt") an extremely large erythrocyte.

megalodactylia (meg"ah-lo-dak-til'e-ah) excessive size of the fingers or toes.

megaloenteron (meg"ah-lo-en'ter-on) enlargement of the intestine.

megaloesophagus (meg"ah-lo-e-sof'ah-gus) megaesophagus.

megalogastria (meg"ah-lo-gas'tre-ah) enlargement of the stomach.

megaloglossia (meg"ah-lo-glos'e-ah) macroglossia; hypertrophy of the tongue.

megalohepatia (meg"ah-lo-he-pat'e-ah) enlargement of the liver.

megalomania (meg"ah-lo-ma'ne-ah) a mental state characterized by delusions of exaggerated personal importance, wealth or power.

megalomelia (meg"ah-lo-me'le-ah) abnormal largeness of the limbs.

megalonychosis (meg"ah-lo-nĭ-ko'sis) hypertrophy of the nails and their matrices.

megalopenis (meg"ah-lo-pe'nis) abnormal largeness of the penis.

megalophthalmos (meg"ah-lof-thal'mos) abnormally large size of the eyes.

megalopodia (meg"ah-lo-po'de-ah) abnormal largeness of the feet.

megalopsia (meg"ah-lop'se-ah) macropsia.

megaloscope (meg'ah-lo-skōp") a magnifying speculum.

megalosplenia (meg"ah-lo-sple'ne-ah) enlargement of the spleen.

megalosyndactyly (meg"ah-lo-sin-dak'tĭ-le) a condition in which the digits are large and webbed together.

megaloureter (meg"ah-lo-u-re'ter) enlargement of the ureter.

-megaly (meg'ah-le) word element [Gr.], *enlargement.*

megarectum (meg"ah-rek'tum) enlargement of the rectum.

megavolt (meg'ah-volt) one million volts.

Megimide (meg'ĭ-mīd) trademark for a preparation of bemegride, an analeptic used in barbiturate poisoning.

megohm (meg'ōm) one million ohms.

megophthalmos (meg"of-thal'mos) abnormally large eyes.

megrim (me'grim) migraine.

meibomian cyst (mi-bo'me-an) a small retention cyst of the meibomian gland, a sebaceous follicle of the eyelid; called also CHALAZION.

meiogenic (mi"o-jen'ik) promoting meiosis.

meiosis (mi-o'sis) a special method of cell division occurring in maturation of germ cells, each daughter nucleus receiving half the number of chromosomes typical of the somatic cells of the species.

melalgia (mel-al'je-ah) neuralgic pain in the limbs.

melan(o)- (mel'ah-no) word element [Gr.], *black.*

melancholia (mel"an-ko'le-ah) a mental state characterized by extreme sadness or depression, with inhibition of mental and physical activity. adj., **melanchol'ic.**
  affective m., melancholia corresponding to the depressive phase of manic-depressive psychosis (see also affective PSYCHOSIS).
  involution m., melancholia developing in later life.

melanedema (mel"an-ĕ-de'mah) anthracosis.

mélangeur (ma-lan-zher') [Fr.], an instrument for drawing and diluting specimens of blood for examination.

melaniferous (mel"ah-nif'er-us) containing melanin.

melanin (mel'ah-nin) a dark, sulfur-containing pigment normally found in the hair, skin, ciliary body, choroid of the eye, pigment layer of the retina, and certain nerve cells. It occurs abnormally in certain tumors, known as melanomas, and is sometimes excreted in the urine when such tumors are present (melanuria).

melanism (mel'ah-nizm) excessive deposit of melanin in the skin.

melanoameloblastoma (mel"ah-no-ah-mel"o-blas-to'mah) ameloblastoma with bluish black discoloration due to melanin granules.

melanoblast (mel'ah-no-blast") a cell that develops into a melanophore.

melanoblastoma (mel"ah-no-blas-to'mah) a tumor composed of melanoblasts.

melanocarcinoma (mel"ah-no-kar"sĭ-no'mah) a melanoma attributed to epithelial origin.

melanocyte (mel'ah-no-sīt", mĕ-lan'o-sīt) a cell of the epidermis that synthesizes melanin.
  m.-stimulating hormone, MSH, a substance from the anterior pituitary that influences the formation or deposition of melanin in the body.

malanoderma (mel"ah-no-der'mah) an increased amount of melanin in the skin.

melanodermatitis (mel"ah-no-der"mah-ti'tis) dermatitis with a deposit of melanin in the skin.

melanogen (mĕ-lan'o-jen) a colorless chromogen, convertible into melanin, which may occur in the urine in certain diseases.

melanogenesis (mel"ah-no-jen'ĕ-sis) the production of melanin.

melanoglossia (mel"ah-no-glos'e-ah) blackening

and elongation of the papillae of the tongue; black tongue.

melanoid (mel'ah-noid) resembling melanin.

melanoidin (mel"ah-noi'din) a melanin obtained from the albumins.

melanoleukoderma (mel"ah-no-lu"ko-der'mah) a mottled appearance of the skin.
  m. col'li, a mottled appearance of the skin of the neck and adjacent regions, a rare manifestation of syphilis.

melanoma (mel"ah-no'mah) a tumor characterized by dark pigmentation.
  malignant m., a malignant tumor, usually developing from a nevus and consisting of black masses of cells with a marked tendency to metastasis.

melanomatosis (mel"ah-no-mah-to'sis) the formation of melanomas throughout the body.

melanonychia (mel"ah-no-nik'e-ah) blackness of the nails.

melanopathy (mel"ah-nop'ah-the) any disease characterized by abnormal pigmentation of the skin or tissues.

melanophore (mel'ah-no-fōr") a pigment cell containing melanin.

melanoplakia (mel"ah-no-pla'ke-ah) pigmented patches on the mucous membrane of the mouth.

melanosarcoma (mel"ah-no-sar-ko'mah) a melanoma derived from mesodermal tissues.

melanosis (mel"ah-no'sis) a condition characterized by dark pigmentary deposits.
  m. coli, brown-black discoloration of the mucosa of the colon.

melanotrichia (mel"ah-no-trik'e-ah) abnormally increased pigmentation of the hair.

melanuria (mel"ah-nu're-ah) the discharge of darkly stained urine, usually due to the presence of a melanoma.

melasma (mě-laz'mah) dark pigmentation of the skin.
  m. addiso'nii, Addison's disease.
  m. gravida'rum, discoloration of the skin in pregnancy.

melatonin (mel"ah-to'nin) a compound found in the pineal gland that has a molecular structure similar to that of serotonin; its exact function is uncertain but it appears to have some effect on the ovary.

melena (mě-le'nah) darkening of the feces by blood pigments.

melenemesis (mel"ě-nem'e-sis) vomiting of black matter.

meletin (mel'ě-tin) quercetin, used to reduce capillary fragility.

melioidosis (mel"e-oi-do'sis) a glanders-like disease of rodents, transmissible to man, and caused by *Pseudomonas pseudomallei.*

melitagra (mel"ĭ-tag'rah) eczema with honeycomb crusts.

melitemia (mel"ĭ-te'me-ah) excessive sugar in the blood.

melitoptyalism (mel"ĭ-to-ti'ah-lizm) secretion of saliva containing glucose.

melituria (mel"ĭ-tu're-ah) the presence of any sugar in the urine.

Mellaril (mel'ah-ril) trademark for preparations of thioridazine hydrochloride, a tranquilizer.

melomelus (mě-lom'ě-lus) a fetal monster with supernumerary limbs.

meloplasty (mel'o-plas"te) 1. plastic surgery of a cheek. 2. plastic surgery of the extremities.

melorheostosis (mel"o-re"os-to'sis) a form of osteosclerosis, with linear tracks extending through the long bones.

melotia (mě-lo'she-ah) congenital displacement of the auricle of the ear.

membrana (mem-bra'nah), pl. *membra'nae* [L.] membrane.

membrane (mem'brān) a thin layer of tissue that covers a surface or divides an organ. adj., **mem'branous.**
  abdominal m., peritoneum.
  alveolodental m., periodontium.
  animal m., a thin diaphragm of membrane, as of bladder, used as a dialyzer.
  arachnoid m., arachnoid; one of the layers of the meninges.
  asphyxial m., hyaline membrane (3).
  basement m., the delicate layer underlying the epithelium of mucous membranes and secreting glands.
  basilar m., the lower boundary of the scala media of the ear.
  birth m's, the amnion and placenta.
  cell m., the condensed protoplasm that forms the enveloping capsule of a cell.
  Descemet's m., the posterior lining membrane of the cornea.
  diphtheritic m., the peculiar false membrane characteristic of diphtheria.
  drum m., tympanic membrane.
  false m., a membranous exudate, like that of diphtheria.
  fetal m's, the membranes that protect the embryo and provide for its nutrition, respiration and excretion: the yolk sac (umbilical vesicle), allantois, amnion, chorion, decidua and placenta.
  hyaline m., 1. a membrane between the outer root sheath and inner fibrous layer of a hair follicle. 2. basement membrane. 3. a homogeneous eosinophilic membrane lining alveolar ducts and alveoli, frequently found at necropsy in premature infants (see also HYALINE MEMBRANE DISEASE).
  hyoglossal m., a fibrous lamina connecting the under surface of the tongue with the hyoid bone.
  limiting m., one that constitutes the border of some tissue or structure.
  mucous m., the membrane covered with epithelium lining canals and cavities that communicate with the exterior of the body.
  nuclear m., the outer layer of the nucleoplasm.
  olfactory m., the olfactory portion of the mucous membrane lining the nasal fossa.

oronasal m., a thin epithelial plate separating the nasal pits from the oral cavity of the embryo.

placental m., the semipermeable membrane that separates the fetal from the maternal blood in the placenta.

plasma m., the surrounding membrane of a cell.

Reissner's m., a thin membrane between the cochlear canal and the scala vestibuli.

semipermeable m., one permitting passage through it of some but not all substances.

serous m., the lining membrane of the cavities that have no communication with the exterior of the body.

synovial m., the inner of the two layers of the articular capsule of a synovial joint; composed of loose connective tissue and having a free smooth surface that lines the joint cavity.

tympanic m., the eardrum; the membrane marking the inner termination of the external acoustic meatus, separating it from the middle ear (see also TYMPANIC MEMBRANE).

vernix m., hyaline membrane (3).

virginal m., hymen.

vitelline m., the external envelope of the ovum.

vitreous m., 1. Descemet's membrane. 2. hyaline membrane (1). 3. the transparent inner layer of the choroid of the eye.

membraniform (mem-bran′ĭ-form) resembling a membrane.

membranocartilaginous (mem″brah-no-kar″tĭ-laj′ĭ-nus) pertaining to membrane and cartilage.

membranoid (mem′brah-noid) resembling a membrane.

membrum (mem′brum), pl. *mem′bra* [L.] a limb or member of the body; an entire arm or leg.

m. mulie′bre, clitoris.

m. viri′le, penis.

memory (mem′o-re) the mental faculty that enables one to retain and recall previously experienced sensations, impressions, information and ideas.

The ability of the brain to retain and to use knowledge gained from past experience is essential to the process of learning. Although the exact way in which the brain remembers is not completely understood, it is believed that a portion of the temporal lobe of the brain, lying in part under the temples, acts as a kind of memory center, drawing on memories stored in other parts of the brain.

There are many theories about the way memories are stored. Millions of nerve cells in special patterns are probably involved. One possible explanation for the vast number of memories and the ways the mind has access to them is the chemical one. Brain cells, like other cells in the body, are made up of giant protein molecules. Each living cell contains great numbers of these molecules. The brain alone contains a thousand billion billion (the figure 1 followed by 21 zeros) of them. The impulses that run along the nerves can change these molecules into new combinations, and each cell constantly reproduces these molecules exactly. This, then, could be a chemical way by which memories are stored: the nerves impulses of the experience leave traces in the minutely changed molecules within the cells. These molecules, as they disappear, are steadily reproduced, each according to its pattern. And so the memory trace would, theoretically, remain.

MEMORY THROUGH SENSE IMPRESSIONS. Much of memory is based on the brain's ability to record impressions, images and sensations received by the sense organs. A person remembers only a small portion of the sense impressions he receives; he is more apt to remember impressions that are pleasing to him, but this is only a general rule, and everyone remembers much that is unpleasant as well. But though the brain probably retains only about a tenth of the impressions it receives, even this amount adds up to an enormous store of memories. These memories of touch, taste, smell, sound and sight become raw material that the brain can draw upon in many ways — to recall past experience, to apply it to present situations, to anticipate the nature of future events or to form new thoughts or concepts. As a person continues to have experiences and store up memories, the brain's association of memories becomes increasingly complex.

Sometimes a person may retain certain kinds of sense impressions more efficiently than others. Some persons, for example, have very accurate memories of things they hear, such as conversations or melodies. Others recall visual images more clearly. An extreme example of such aptitude is eidetic memory, in which a person is able to reproduce exact visual images of things he has seen.

OTHER KINDS OF REMEMBERING. The term memory is a general one, and it includes other kinds of remembering besides the collection of simple sense impressions. One of these is the ability to remember events that have just occurred and to add them to one's storehouse of memories. It is thought that this process begins when a new event stimulates a circular chain of electrical impulses in the brain. These impulses then stimulate each other, keeping the event part of one's conscious knowledge. Thinking about the event or mulling it over accentuates the impulses. Eventually the brain turns its attention to something new, but the impulses have left a record and made the event an enduring memory that can be clearly recalled. The ability to form memories of new events seems to be strongest in younger persons. Older persons may recall recent events poorly or with difficulty, while they are still able to remember the past clearly.

Memories of events, actions or facts become stronger if the remembered thing is repeatedly experienced or used. This is why "cramming" may get students through an examination for a day but leave little residue of knowledge. Too much information at once cannot be effectively handled by memory. The repetition of actions contributes to the kind of memory that enables one to perform acts automatically. Many everyday actions and skills are performed in this way.

DISTORTION OF MEMORY. Memories can easily be distorted. Experiments have shown that when a number of people observe an event and are later asked to describe it, no two persons describe it in exactly the same way. When a person has strong emotional feeling about an event, his memory of it is apt to be colored by his emotions. He may remember those aspects of the event that fit in with his own emotions and attitudes, and forget those that do not. Or he may unconsciously add to his recollection details that did not really happen. All of us have probably unconsciously altered the truth in this way at one time or another.

Another distortion of memory that may occur is

the feeling that some situation is familiar and has previously been experienced, when in reality the situation is a completely new one. The person may feel he knows exactly what someone to whom he is talking will say next. It is not known exactly why one suddenly has the feeling called a *déja vu* (literally, "already seen"). Some psychologists suggest that this feeling may be because of some coincidental similarity between the new situation and a past experience.

Loss of Memory. Loss of memory, or AMNESIA, may be a symptom of damage to some area of the brain, or of a decrease in the brain's blood supply. It may also result from psychologic causes; certain experiences may be so distressing to recall that the brain relegates them to the subconscious mind. Only rarely is all memory lost in amnesia. Sometimes an incident or a certain period in the patient's life is forgotten. Or he may recall events in the wrong order but remember each separate event accurately. Amnesia may take different forms, depending on what area of the brain has been injured; in amnesia of hearing, for example, the patient cannot remember his spoken language, while in visual amnesia he has forgotten his written language.

menacme (mĕ-nak′me) the period of a woman's life which is marked by menstrual activity.

menadiol (men″ah-di′ol) a vitamin K analogue.
  m. sodium diphosphate, a compound used to promote the formation of prothrombin.

menadione (men″ah-di′ōn) a compound used as a prothrombinogenic vitamin.

menaphthone (men-af′thōn) menadione.

menarche (mĕ-nar′ke) establishment or beginning of the menstrual function.

mendelevium (men″dĕ-le′ve-um) a chemical element, atomic number 101, atomic weight 256, symbol Md. (See table of ELEMENTS.)

mendelian law (men-de′le-an) in the inheritance of certain traits or characters, offspring are not intermediate in type between the two parents, but the type of one or the other is predominant according to a fixed ratio; called also Mendel's law.
  m. rate, an expression of the numerical relations of the occurrence of distinctly contrasted mendelian characteristics in succeeding generations of hybrid offspring.

Menetrier's disease (men″ĕ-tre-ārz′) excessive proliferation of the gastric mucosa, producing diffuse thickening of the wall of the stomach.

Menformon (men′for-mon) trademark for a preparation of estrone, an estrogenic steroid.

Menière's disease (men″ĕ-ārz′) a disorder of the labyrinth of the inner ear; called also Menière's syndrome and sometimes spelled Meniere and Ménière. It is believed to result from dilatation of the lymphatic channels in the cochlea. In about 90 per cent of cases only one ear is affected. The usual symptoms are tinnitus, heightened sensitivity to loud sounds, progressive loss of hearing, headache and dizziness. In the acute stage there may be severe nausea with vomiting, profuse sweating, disabling dizziness and nystagmus. Some attacks last only minutes, and others continue for hours;

they may occur frequently or only several weeks apart.

The disease usually lasts a few years, with progressive loss of hearing in the affected ear; sometimes the symptoms stop before all hearing is lost. If loss of hearing in the affected ear does become complete, nausea symptoms are likely to disappear.

Menière's disease sometimes develops after an injury to the head or an infection of the middle ear. Many cases, however, have no apparent cause. The disorder is most common among men between the ages of 40 and 60.

A low-salt diet, elimination or restriction of fluids and vasodilating drugs are used in the treatment of this disorder. Sedatives are usually ordered to promote sleep and rest. If the ringing sensation becomes too disturbing to the patient, it may be masked (for example, by music piped in through earphones) to make sleeping easier. In some cases, surgery will give relief.

Care must be taken to avoid injuries due to falls which may occur because of dizziness. Side rails should be used on the bed and during the acute stage the patient should have someone to assist him whenever he is up and about.

mening(o)- (mĕ-ning′go) word element [Gr.], *meninges.*

meningeal (mĕ-nin′je-al) pertaining to the meninges.

meningeorrhaphy (mĕ-nin″je-or′ah-fe) suture of membranes.

meninges (mĕ-nin′jēz), plural of *meninx* [Gr.] the three membranes covering the brain and spinal cord: dura mater, arachnoid and pia mater. adj., **menin′geal.**

meningioma (mĕ-nin″je-o′mah) a tumor of the meninges.
  angioblastic m., angioblastoma.

meningism, meningismus (men′in-jizm), (men″-in-jiz′mus) 1. a condition due to pain in the meningocortical region of the brain, marked by excitation, followed by depression of the cortex, with vomiting, constipation and thermic disorders. 2. a hysterical simulation of meningitis.

meningitis (men″in-ji′tis) inflammation of the meninges, the membranes that cover the brain and spinal cord; called also cerebrospinal meningitis.

There are several varieties of meningitis. The two most important are meningococcal meningitis (the commonest) and tuberculous meningitis. Others include aseptic meningitis and viral meningitis.

CAUSES. Meningococcal meningitis is caused by meningococci. It is generally the epidemic type and is very contagious because the bacteria are present in the throat as well as in the cerebrospinal fluid. It is transmitted by contact and by droplet infection. The incubation period for epidemic meningitis is 2 to 10 days.

In meningococcemia (Waterhouse-Friderichsen syndrome), the bacteria appear in the blood rather than the cerebrospinal fluid. The disease is associated with adrenal hemorrhage and may lead to destruction of the adrenal glands.

Tuberculous meningitis is produced by the same bacteria that cause tuberculosis of the lung. It results in a more chronic inflammation.

Aseptic meningitis occurs principally among

young children during the warm months of the year. It is often referred to as "summer grippe." The infection is caused by enteroviruses (echoviruses) and is usually accompanied by a skin rash.

Viral meningitis in the United States and temperate climates generally is caused chiefly by mumps and poliomyelitis viruses, and less frequently by herpes simplex and other viruses.

SYMPTOMS AND TREATMENT. Whatever the type of infecting agent, the symptoms of meningitis are usually the same. The most characteristic are a violent persistent headache and vomiting, which are caused by increased intracranial pressure.

The patient may be delirious and suffer convulsions. He will hold his neck as rigidly as possible, because any movement of the neck muscles stretches the meninges and increases the pain of the headache.

In tuberculous meningitis, however, the symptoms develop gradually, taking a week or two to appear. Early symptoms are deceptive, particularly in children. They may include sore throat, a dull feeling, fever, general soreness and a rash of red spots on the body.

Diagnosis is confirmed by a LUMBAR PUNCTURE and identification of the causative organism in a sample of cerebrospinal fluid. Treatment is with antibiotics.

NURSING CARE. Isolation of the patient is necessary until the disease has progressed beyond the acute stage (see ISOLATION TECHNIQUE). The environment should be quiet and nonstimulating so as to reduce irritability and promote relaxation. Noise is kept at a minimum and extremely bright lights in the patient's room should be avoided. Disorientation sometimes accompanies meningitis and demands constant attendance so the patient does not injure himself.

Loss of sight or hearing, paralysis and mental retardation are possible complications of meningitis. However, they are usually avoided by prompt treatment with antibiotics which destroy the organisms before permanent damage is done to the nervous system.

meningocele (mĕ-ning'go-sēl) hernial protrusion of meninges through a defect in the skull or vertebral column.

meningocerebritis (mĕ-ning"go-ser"ĕ-bri'tis) inflammation of the brain and meninges.

meningococcemia (mĕ-ning"go-kok-se'me-ah) the presence of meningococci in the blood, producing an acute fulminating disease or an insidious disorder persisting for months or years.

 acute fulminating m., Waterhouse-Friderichsen syndrome.

meningococcidal (mĕ-ning"go-kok-si'dal) destroying meningococci.

meningococcus (mĕ-ning"go-kok'us), pl. *meningococ'ci* [Gr.] a microorganism of the species *Neisseria meningitidis*, the cause of some types of meningitis. adj., **meningococ'cal.**

meningocortical (mĕ-ning"go-kor'tĭ-kal) pertaining to the meninges and cortex of the brain.

meningoencephalitis (mĕ-ning"go-en-sef"ah-li'tis) inflammation of the brain and its membranes.

meningoencephalocele (mĕ-ning"go-en-sef'ah-lo-sēl") hernial protrusion of the meninges and brain substance through a defect in the skull.

meningoencephalomyelitis (mĕ-ning"go-en-sef"ah-lo-mi"ē-li'tis) inflammation of the meninges, brain and spinal cord.

meningoencephalomyelopathy (mĕ-ning"go-en-sef"ah-lo-mi"ē-lop'ah-the) disease involving the meninges, brain and spinal cord.

meningoencephalopathy (mĕ-ning"go-en-sef"-ah-lop'ah-the) noninflammatory disease of the cerebral meninges and brain.

meningomalacia (mĕ-ning"go-mah-la'she-ah) softening of a membrane.

meningomyelitis (mĕ-ning"go-mi"ē-li'tis) inflammation of the spinal cord and its membranes.

meningomyelocele (mĕ-ning-go-mi'e-lo-sēl") hernial protrusion of the meninges and spinal cord through a defect in the vertebral column.

meningomyeloradiculitis (mĕ-ning"go-mi"ē-lo-rah-dik"u-li'tis) inflammation of the meninges, spinal cord and spinal nerve roots.

meningopathy (men"in-gop'ah-the) any disease of the meninges.

meningorhachidian (mĕ-ning"go-rah-kid'e-an) pertaining to the spinal cord and meninges.

meningorrhagia (mĕ-ning"go-ra'je-ah) hemorrhage from cerebral or spinal membranes.

meningorrhea (mĕ-ning"go-re'ah) effusion of blood on the meninges.

meningothelioma (mĕ-ning"go-the"le-o'mah) meningioma.

meninx (me'ningks), pl. *menin'ges* [Gr.] a membrane, especially one of the membranes of the brain or spinal cord—the dura mater, arachnoid and pia mater. adj., **menin'geal.**

meniscectomy (men"ĭ-sek'to-me) excision of a meniscus, as of the knee joint.

meniscitis (men"ĭ-si'tis) inflammation of a semilunar cartilage of the knee joint.

meniscocyte (mĕ-nis'ko-sīt) a crescent- or sickle-shaped erythrocyte.

meniscocytosis (mĕ-nis"ko-si-to'sis) sickle cell anemia.

meniscus (mĕ-nis'kus), pl. *menis'ci* [L.] something of crescent shape, as the concave or convex surface of a column of liquid in a pipet or buret, or a crescent-shaped fibrocartilage (semilunar cartilage) in the knee joint. adj., **menis'ceal.**

meno- (men'o) word element [Gr.], *menstruation.*

menolipsis (men"o-lip'sis) temporary cessation of menstruation.

menometastasis (men"o-mĕ-tas'tah-sis) vicarious menstruation.

menometrorrhagia (men"o-met"ro-ra'je-ah) excessive uterine bleeding at and between menstrual periods.

menopause (men′o-pawz) the span of time during which the menstrual cycle wanes and gradually stops; called also change of life and climacteric. It is the period when ovaries stop functioning and therefore menstruation and childbearing cease. adj., **men′opausal.**

The menopause is a natural physiologic process that results from the normal aging of the ovaries. It occurs when the ovaries can no longer perform the function of ovulation and estrogen production. Because estrogen secretion stops, physiologic changes occur in the woman's body. The uterine tubes shrink in size and become less capable of movement. The uterus, the cavity of the uterus and the cervix also decrease in size. The vagina contracts and its folds become shallower. The clitoris and external sexual organs become smaller. There may be some thinning of the pubic and axillary hair. The breasts usually become less full and firm.

The average age of menopause for American women is between 47 and 49. Almost 75 per cent of women reach it while in their forties, but it may begin as early as 35 and can be delayed until as late as 55. If, for medical reasons, surgery of the reproductive organs becomes necessary, menopause may be brought on before the natural process has begun.

The length of time in which the menopause is completed varies among individual women, but its duration is usually from 6 months to 3 years.

SYMPTOMS AND TREATMENT. Most women pass through the menopause with little discomfort; only about 15 per cent of women experience distress. Occasionally during menopause some existing physical ailments may become exaggerated, and women of nervous temperament may show increased nervousness.

The first and most obvious sign of the menopause is change in the menstrual flow. In the majority of women, bleeding decreases with each period, and the periods are spaced farther apart. In some cases, there may be excessive bleeding during the regular period.

Bleeding may also occur between periods, either as a full flow, or in drops. Vaginal bleeding that occurs after menstruation has definitely stopped is not a normal part of the menopause.

A sensation of heat in the face and upper part of the body, called a "hot flash," is one of the commonest symptoms of menopause. Sometimes hot flashes are followed by sweating or chills. Some women feel just a few of these flashes for a short period of time. Others experience 10 or 20 a day.

Those few women who suffer psychologic reactions at this time may experience fatigue, crying spells, insomnia, inability to concentrate or poor memory. More severe reactions may result in depression. At one time it was thought that the changes in the body's chemistry caused these reactions. Today, many physicians believe that the chemical changes only trigger reactions to other events that may occur at the same time of life. During her forties and fifties, a woman becomes aware of aging. She may be disturbed by the loss of relatives and friends or by her lessened family responsibilities as her children mature. Outside interests and community activities are recommended as a means of helping these women feel wanted and needed.

Hormone injections and mild sedatives or tran-

quilizers may be prescribed to relieve the more distressing symptoms of menopause.

menorrhagia (men″o-ra′je-ah) excessive menstruation. Its causes include uterine tumors, pelvic inflammatory disease and abnormal conditions of pregnancy. Endocrine disturbances may produce functional menorrhagia. Excessive menstruation may cause anemia.

menorrhalgia (men″o-ral′je-ah) pain during menstruation (see also DYSMENORRHEA).

menoschesis, menostasis (mĕ-nos′kĕ-sis, men″o-ske′sis), (mĕ-nos′tah-sis) suppression of menstruation.

menostaxis (men″o-stak′sis) a prolonged menstrual period.

menotoxin (men″o-tok′sin) a toxic substance in the body fluid during menstruation.

menses (men′sēz) menstruation.

menstrual (men′stroo-al) pertaining to menstruation.
  m. cycle, the period of the regularly recurring physiologic changes in the endometrium that culminate in its shedding (menstruation).

Menstrual cycles vary in length; the average is approximately 28 days. The menstrual flow generally lasts about 5 days, although this too varies from person to person. Women menstruate from puberty to menopause, except during pregnancy.

During the first 14 days of the menstrual cycle, a follicle containing an ovum develops in the ovaries. As the menstrual flow ceases, the lining of the uterus is stimulated by estrogen and begins to increase in thickness to prepare for reproduction.

On about the fourteenth day of the cycle, OVULATION takes place and the ovary discharges the ovum. At the time of ovulation, the ruptured follicle is transformed into a yellowish material called the corpus luteum, which in turn secretes progesterone. Progesterone acts on the endometrium, building up tissues with an enriched supply of blood to nourish the future embryo.

If conception does not take place, the estrogen level in the blood falls, the endometrium is no longer stimulated and the uterus again becomes thinner. Blood circulation slows, blood vessels contract and the unused tissue breaks down into the bloody discharge known as menstruation. With its onset, the cycle starts again.

menstruation (men″stroo-a′shun) the periodic discharge from the vagina of blood and tissues from a nonpregnant uterus; the culmination of the MENSTRUAL CYCLE. Menstruation occurs every 28 days or so between puberty and menopause, except during pregnancy, and the flow lasts about 5 days, the times varying from woman to woman.

MENSTRUAL DIFFICULTIES. Some menstrual discomfort is common, but acute discomfort is usually indicative of some disorder. Among the disorders sometimes causing DYSMENORRHEA are myoma of the uterus, endometrial cysts or displacement of the uterus. Menstrual pain may, in some cases, be related to tension or anxiety.

Excessive bleeding, or prolonged periods, called menorrhagia, is sometimes an indication of tumors, polyps, cancer or inflammation.

Menstruation usually starts between the ages of 11 and 14 and continues into the forties. At first the periods may be irregular, but once they are established they usually occur in a fairly definite rhythm, at intervals of 21 to 35 days. In these regular cycles, there may be monthly variations of a few days which are considered to be quite normal. These cycles may be influenced by changes in climate or living conditions, or by emotional factors. Slight irregularities, especially if they occur over a period of time, may be warnings of disturbance of either the thyroid or pituitary glands, or of tumors of the uterus or ovaries.

Occasionally menstruation does not occur at puberty. This condition is known as primary AMEN-ORRHEA. It may be caused by underdevelopment or malformation of the reproductive organs, by glandular disturbances, which generally can be corrected by the administration of hormones.

General ill health, a change in climate or living conditions, emotional shock or, frequently, either the hope or fear of becoming pregnant can sometimes stop menstruation after it has begun. This is called secondary amenorrhea. If this cessation is of short duration, it is not a cause for alarm. If it continues over a long period of time, and there is also the problem of infertility, hormone treatments may be necessary.

anovular m., anovulatory m., periodic uterine bleeding without preceding ovulation.

vicarious m., bleeding from extragenital mucous membrane at the time one would normally expect the menstrual period.

menstruum (men'stroo-um) a solvent medium.

mensuration (men"su-ra'shun) the process of measuring.

mentagra (men-tag'rah) inflammation of the hair follicles; sycosis.

mental (men'tal) 1. pertaining to the mind. 2. pertaining to the chin.

m. hygiene, the science that deals with the development of healthy mental and emotional reactions.

m. mechanism, an unconscious and indirect manner of gratifying a repressed desire.

m. retardation, faulty or inadequate development of the brain which brings with it some degree of inability to learn and to adapt to the needs of everyday life at the usual rate. Occasionally, mental retardation is complete.

Mental retardation is not a disease; it is a general term for a wide range of conditions, resulting from many different causes. Many of these are directly related to various diseases, either in the mother during pregnancy, or in the infant; only some are hereditary. The general health of the mother and the economic situation of the family may also play a role in this condition.

Mental retardation is a relative term. Its meaning depends on what society demands of the individual in learning, skills and social responsibility. Many people who are considered retarded in the complex modern world would get along normally in a simpler society.

DIAGNOSIS. There is no absolute measurement for retardation. At one time the different types were classified only according to the apparent severity of the retardation. Since at that time the most practical standard was intelligence, the degree of retardation was based on the score of the patient on intelligence, or IQ, tests. The average person is considered to have an IQ of between 90 and 110. Those who score below 70 are considered mentally retarded.

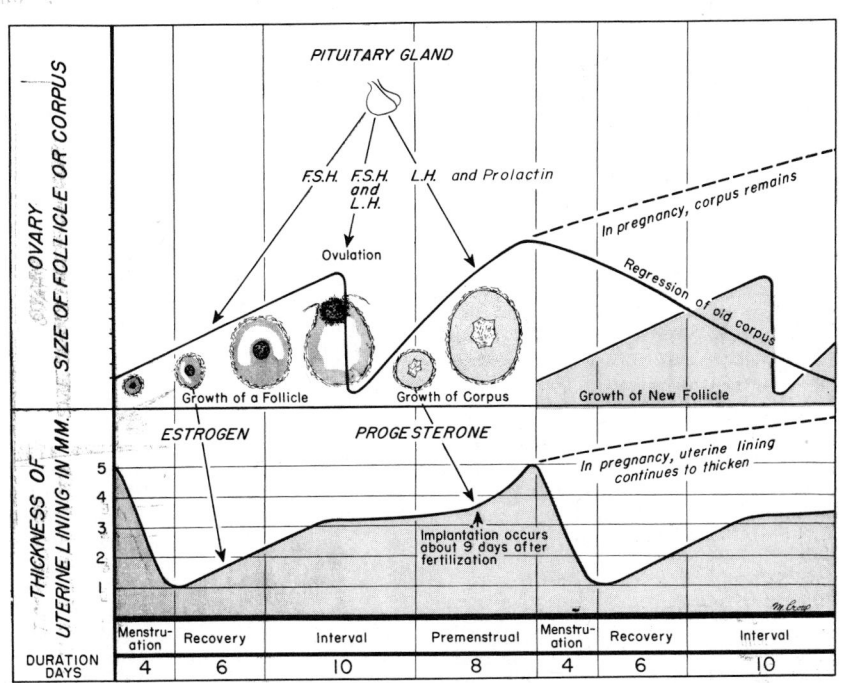

Average 28-day menstrual cycle. The cycle begins when hormones from the pituitary gland stimulate the development of an egg in a follicle inside one of the ovaries. About the fourteenth day, ovulation occurs: The follicle bursts, and the egg is discharged from the ovary. If the egg is not fertilized, the cycle ends in menstruation on the twenty-eighth day. If the egg is fertilized, pregnancy begins. (From Dorland's Illustrated Medical Dictionary. 24th ed. Philadelphia, W. B. Saunders Co., 1965.)

In the past, the different groupings were classified in terms such as feebleminded, idiot, imbecile and moron. Today, most doctors use the following classifications: for IQ's from 50 to 70, mild; 35 to 50, moderate; 20 to 35, severe; under 20, profound. Whatever classifications are used, doctors today recognize that IQ measurements are only one of the factors that have to be considered in determining mental retardation. Others, such as the patient's adaptability to his surroundings and the amount of control he has over his emotions, are also very important.

About 85 per cent of the patients who are considered mentally retarded are in the least severe, or mild, group. Those in this group do not usually have any obvious physical defects and for this reason are not always easy to identify as mentally retarded while they are still infants. Sometimes such a child's mental defects do not show up until he enters school, where he has difficulty in learning and keeping up with others in his age group.

Many of those in the mild category, when they grow up, find employment or a place in society suitable to their abilities, and are no longer identified as mentally retarded. In general, most of those who are mildly retarded are much closer to being normal than abnormal.

Many conditions that can cause severe retardation can be diagnosed during pregnancy, and in some cases proper treatment can lessen or even prevent retardation. Proper care for the mother during pregnancy and for the baby in his first months of life is also important.

CAUSES. There are many causes of mental retardation. Many are known, many are simply suspected. No apparent defect can be found in the vast majority of the mentally retarded. The specific cause of their retardation cannot be pinpointed. There are factors, however, that have been proved by research to contribute to retardation.

A child whose mother did not receive prenatal care is more likely to be retarded. Financial hardship, a broken home, a lack of intellectual stimulation in the family or a deprived environment can play important roles. Unfavorable health factors, such as poor diet or insufficient medical care, can lead to poor physical condition, which may cause a lower level of performance.

Other physical factors may also be involved. A child born prematurely may occasionally not develop entirely normally. Heredity may play a part in some cases when certain combinations of parents' genes may result in faulty metabolism which affects the normal development of the brain.

The conditions that are known to cause mental retardation can occur at any time from conception through early childhood. At the time of conception, there may be genetic irregularities. During pregnancy, certain infections, such as rubella, syphilis or meningitis, and other conditions such as glandular disorder, poor prenatal care, injury or inadequate diet can lead to retardation. At the time of birth, prolonged labor, unusual stress, damage in the course of birth or lack of oxygen can occasionally cause brain damage. During infancy and early childhood, some childhood diseases, glandular imbalances, accidents, such as a blow on the head, and disorders of metabolism may be responsible.

PREVENTION.   Some types of mental retardation can be prevented; others cannot. The causes and diseases that offer some hope of prevention are discussed below.

Metabolism or Hormone Disorders. PHENYLKETONURIA, or PKU, is a congenital defect in the metabolism of the amino acid phenylalanine. If PKU is diagnosed in the first few months of life by means of a urine test and controlled by a special diet, mental retardation can be prevented.

GALACTOSEMIA is a metabolic disorder of milk sugar. This condition can also be detected by a urine test, and mental retardation can be prevented if the infant is given no milk during the first few weeks of life.

A deficiency in a hormone that has a specific effect on the activities of other organs can have various consequences. The best known condition of this kind is HYPOTHYROIDISM, which results in CRETINISM. Hormone imbalances can often be treated by injections of artificial hormones to correct the imbalance.

Erythroblastosis Fetalis (Hemolytic Disease of the Newborn). Occasionally the blood of the mother and that of her unborn child may be incompatible because of a difference in the RH FACTOR. The infant suffering from erythroblastosis fetalis can be treated by exchange or intrauterine fetal TRANSFUSION.

Infections. If the mother contracts RUBELLA during pregnancy, especially during the first 3 months, it may result in defects of the baby's heart and eyes as well as damage to the brain.

SYPHILIS (but not gonorrhea) in the mother can cause mental retardation. This disease can be discovered by blood tests, and if it is treated soon enough, it may not damage the child.

MENINGITIS in childhood can result in severe damage to the brain. Fortunately, modern drugs can usually cure the disease and prevent mental retardation.

TREATMENT.   Some types of mental retardation can be prevented or lessened by proper medical treatment; most, however, cannot. Almost all retarded children can benefit from special education and training which can lead to greater independence.

Parents who believe that their child is not developing at a proper rate or that he shows symptoms of retardation should consult their family physician or local child care clinic at once. It may be very difficult to face the fact that a child may be mentally retarded, but the sooner it is faced the better chance there is of developing a program to help the child make the best adjustment possible. A complete study of the child's condition can be arranged. From this, it will be possible to say how severe the retardation is and what improvement can be expected; a program of education and training for him will be planned. The doctor or agency will also be familiar with the kinds of help that are available in the community. Many public school systems now have special programs for retarded children, and help is available from other agencies, both public and private.

If there does not seem to be any organization in the area that can offer help, there is an office of the National Association for Retarded Children in every state. The national office at 420 Lexington Avenue, New York, N.Y. 10017, can also supply information on the facilities that are available in any local area. The Children's Bureau, U.S. Department of Health, Education and Welfare, Washington, D.C. 20201, can also supply information on schools and other facilities for retarded children.

Today, as a result of increased concern with the problem of mental retardation, every state has clinics that specialize in services to the retarded and their families. Each state department of education offers some programs of special classes for the retarded. Most states also have vocational training programs, such as sheltered workshops where the mentally retarded can be trained to do simple tasks and find employment.

INSTITUTIONS. A very small percentage of children are mentally retarded to such a degree that they cannot learn to care for themselves. In these cases, the child can usually be better cared for in a residential school or other institution.

A decision of this sort should be made by the parents with the help and advice of a professionally qualified person in the community who is familiar with the various alternatives available. Among the factors that must be seriously considered are how disruptive the child is to the home and other children, whether the family can give the child the care and attention he needs, whether an institution could better meet the child's needs and whether the type and location of the institution are suitable.

It is always a difficult decision for parents to send a retarded child to an institution, but with professional guidance all factors can be taken into consideration, and the decision is likely to be one that brings the most benefit to everyone in the family.

menthol (men′thol) an alcohol from various mint oils or produced synthetically, used locally to relieve itching.

mentum (men′tum) [L.] chin.

mepacrine (mep′ah-krin) quinacrine hydrochloride, an antimalarial agent.

mepazine (mep′ah-zēn) a phenothiazine derivative used as a tranquilizer in psychoses and severe neuroses.

mepenzolate (me-pen′zo-lāt) a compound used as an anticholinergic and antispasmodic in hypermotility of the lower bowel.

meperidine hydrochloride (mĕ-per′ĭ-dēn) a fine, white crystalline powder used as a narcotic analgesic.

mephenesin (mĕ-fen′ĕ-sin) a white crystalline powder used as a skeletal muscle relaxant.

mephenoxalone (mef″en-ok′sah-lōn) a compound used in treatment of anxiety and as a calming agent.

mephentermine (mĕ-fen′ter-mēn) a compound used as a sympathomimetic and as a pressor substance.

mephenytoin (mef″en-ĭ′to-in) an anticonvulsant used in the treatment of epilepsy.

mephitic (mĕ-fit′ik) noxious; foul.

mephobarbital (mef″o-bar′bĭ-tal) a white crystalline powder used as an anticonvulsant with a slight hypnotic action.

Mephyton (mef′ĭ-ton) trademark for preparations of vitamin K_1, used as a prothrombinogenic agent.

mepivacaine hydrochloride (mĕ-piv′ah-kān) a compound used as a local anesthetic.

Meprane (me′prān) trademark for preparations of promethestrol, a synthetic estrogen.

meprobamate (mĕ-pro′bah-māt, mep″ro-bam′āt) a bitter white powder used as a tranquilizer.

meprylcaine (mep′ril-kān) a compound used as a local anesthetic.

mepyramine (me-pir′ah-mēn) pyrilamine, an antihistamine.

mEq. milliequivalent.

meralgia (mĕ-ral′je-ah) pain in the thigh.
  m. paresthet′ica, a disease marked by disturbance of sensation in the outer surface of the thigh.

meralluride (mer-al′u-rīd) a mercury compound used as a diuretic.

Meratran (mer′ah-tran) trademark for a preparation of pipradrol hydrochloride, a central nervous system stimulant.

merbromin (mer-bro′min) an antibacterial compound occurring as iridescent green scales or granules.

mercaptan (mer-kap′tan) an alcohol in which oxygen is replaced by sulfur.

mercaptomerin (mer-kap″to-mer′in) an organic mercurial diuretic.
  sodium m., a compound used parenterally as a diuretic.

mercaptopurine (mer-kap″to-pu′rēn) a yellow crystalline compound used as an antineoplastic agent.

Mercuhydrin (mer″ku-hi′drin) trademark for preparations of meralluride, a mercurial diuretic.

mercuramide (mer-kūr′ah-mīd) mersalyl, a mercurial diuretic.

mercurial (mer-ku′re-al) 1. pertaining to mercury. 2. a preparation containing mercury.

mercurialism (mer-ku′re-al-izm″) chronic poisoning from mercury.

mercuric (mer-ku′rik) pertaining to mercury in its higher valence; containing divalent mercury.
  m. chloride, mercury bichloride.
  m. iodide, red, mercury biniodide, used as an antibacterial agent.
  m. oxide, red, an orange-red crystalline powder used as an antiseptic.
  m. oxide, yellow, a yellow to orange-yellow, heavy powder used in ointment form for eye disorders.

Mercurochrome (mer-ku′ro-krōm) trademark for preparations of merbromin, an antibacterial compound.

mercurophylline (mer″ku-ro-fil′in) a white to slightly yellow, odorless powder used as a diuretic.

mercurous (mer′ku-rus) pertaining to mercury in its lower valence; containing monovalent mercury.
  m. chloride, a white, odorless, tasteless powder rarely used in pills or tablets as a cathartic, intestinal antiseptic or to reduce edema, or, in an ointment, as a local antibacterial agent; called also calomel.

mercury (mer'ku-re) a chemical element, atomic number 80, atomic weight 200.59, symbol Hg. (See table of ELEMENTS.) Mercury forms two sets of classes of compounds: mercurous, in which a single atom of mercury combines with a monovalent radical, and mercuric, in which a single atom of mercury combines with a bivalent radical. Mercury and its salts have been employed therapeutically as purgatives; as alternatives in chronic inflammations; and as antisyphilitics, intestinal antiseptics, disinfectants and astringents. They are absorbed by the skin and mucous membranes, causing chronic mercurial poisoning, or hydrargyria. The mercuric salts are more soluble and irritant than the mercurous. See also under mercurous and mercuric.

ammoniated m., a compound used as an antiseptic skin and ophthalmic ointment.

m. bichloride, a poisonous compound occurring as heavy, odorless crystals, crystalline masses or white powder; used in solution as a skin disinfectant.

m. chloride, mild, mercurous chloride.

Mercuzanthin (mer″ku-zan'thin) trademark for a preparation of mercurophylline, a diuretic.

mere (mēr) one of the parts into which a zygote divides.

merergastic (mer″er-gas'tik) pertaining to the simplest type of disorder of psychic function, marked by emotional instability and anxiety.

merethoxylline (mer″ě-thok'sĭ-lēn) a mercury compound used as a diuretic.

meridian (mě-rid′e-an) an imaginary line on the surface of a globe or sphere, connecting the opposite ends of its axis.

meroblastic (mer-o-blas'tik) partially dividing; undergoing cleavage in which only part of the egg participates.

merocele (mer'o-sēl) femoral hernia.

merocoxalgia (mer″o-kok-sal'je-ah) pain in the thigh and hip.

merocrine (mer'o-krin) partly secreting: noting that type of glandular secretion in which the secreting cell remains intact throughout the process of formation and discharge of the secretory products, as in the salivary and pancreatic glands; cf. apocrine and holocrine.

merogenesis (mer″o-jen'ě-sis) cleavage of an ovum.

merogony (mě-rog'o-ne) the development of a portion only of an ovum.

diploid m., development of a fragment of an ovum containing the fused male and female pronuclei.

parthenogenetic m., development of an enucleated portion of an ovum under the influence of an artificial stimulus.

meromicrosomia (mer″o-mi″kro-so'me-ah) unusual smallness of some part of the body.

meroparesthesia (mer″o-par″es-the'ze-ah) alteration of the tactile sense in the extremities.

meropia (mě-ro'pe-ah) partial blindness.

merorachischisis (me″ro-rah-kis'kĭ-sis) fissure of part of the spinal cord.

merosmia (mě-roz'me-ah) inability to perceive certain odors.

merostotic (mer″os-tot'ik) affecting only part of a bone.

merotomy (mě-rot'o-me) a cutting into segments.

merozoite (mer″o-zo'īt) one of the organisms formed by multiple fission (schizogony) of a sporozoite within the body of the host.

Merphene (mer'fēn) trademark for preparations of phenylmercuric nitrate, an antibacterial.

Merphenyl (mer'fen-il) trademark for preparations of phenylmercuric nitrate, an antibacterial.

mersalyl (mer'sah-lil) a white crystalline powder; a mercurial diuretic.

Merthiolate (mer-thi'o-lāt) trademark for preparations of thimerosal, an antibacterial.

mes(o)- (mez'o) word element [Gr.], *middle.*

Mesantoin (mě-san'to-in) trademark for a preparation of mephenytoin, an anticonvulsant.

mesaortitis (mes″a-or-ti'tis) inflammation of the tunica media of the aorta.

mesarteritis (mes″ar-ter-i'tis) inflammation of the tunica media of an artery.

mesatipellic (mes-at″ĭ-pel'ik) having a round pelvis.

mescaline (mes'kah-lēn) a poisonous alkaloid derived from a Mexican cactus, which produces hallucinations of sound and color (see also HALLUCINOGEN).

mescalism (mes'kah-lizm) intoxication due to mescal buttons or mescaline.

mesencephalitis (mes″en-sef″ah-li'tis) inflammation of the mesencephalon, or midbrain.

mesencephalon (mes″en-sef'ah-lon) 1. the midbrain. 2. the middle of the three primary brain vesicles of the embryo.

mesencephalotomy (mes″en-sef″ah-lot'o-me) surgical production of lesions in the midbrain for the relief of intractable pain.

mesenchyma (mě-seng'kĭ-mah) the meshwork of embryonic connective tissue in the mesoderm from which are formed the connective tissues of the body and also the blood vessels and lymph vessels. adj., **mesen'chymal.**

mesenchyme (mes'eng-kīm) mesenchyma.

mesenchymoma (mes″eng-ki-mo'mah) a mixed mesenchymal tumor composed of two or more cellular elements.

mesenterectomy (mes″en-tě-rek'to-me) excision of the mesentery.

mesenteriopexy (mes″en-ter'e-o-pek″se) fixation of a torn mesentery.

mesenteriorrhaphy (mes″en-ter″e-or'ah-fe) suture of the mesentery.

mesenteriplication (mes″en-ter″ĭ-pli-ka'shun)

the operation of taking a tuck in the mesentery to shorten it.

mesenteritis (mes″en-tĕ-ri′tis) inflammation of the mesentery.

mesenterium (mes″en-te′re-um) mesentery.

mesenteron (mes-en′ter-on) the part of the primitive body cavity from which the alimentary canal, lungs, liver and pancreas are derived.

mesentery (mes′en-ter″e) the fold of peritoneum attaching the intestine to the posterior abdominal wall. adj., **mesenter′ic.**

mesiad (me′ze-ad) toward the middle or center.

mesial (me′ze-al) situated in the middle; median; nearer the middle line of the body or nearer the center of the dental arch.

mesially (me′ze-al″e) toward the median line.

mesion (me′ze-on) the plane dividing the body into right and left symmetrical halves.

mesmerism (mez′mer-izm) hypnotism.

mesoappendix (mez″o-ah-pen′diks) the peritoneal fold connecting the appendix to the ileum.

mesobacterium (mez″o-bak-te′re-um), pl. *mesobacte′ria* [L.] a rod-shaped microorganism of medium size.

mesoblast (mez′o-blast) mesoderm.

mesobronchitis (mez″o-brong-ki′tis) inflammation of middle coat of the bronchi.

mesocardia (mez″o-kar′de-ah) location of the heart in the middle line of the thorax.

mesocardium (mez″o-kar′de-um) 1. that part of the embryonic mesentery which connects the embryonic heart with the body wall in front and the foregut behind. 2. myocardium.

mesocecum (mez″o-se′kum) the peritoneal fold that gives attachment to the cecum.

mesocephalon (mez″o-sef′ah-lon) mesencephalon, or midbrain.

mesococcus (mez″o-kok′us), pl. *mesococ′ci* [L.] a spherical microorganism of medium size.

mesocolon (mez″o-ko′lon) the peritoneal process attaching the colon to the posterior abdominal wall.
  pelvic m., sigmoid m., the peritoneum attaching the sigmoid colon to the posterior abdominal wall.
  transverse m., the peritoneum attaching the transverse colon to the posterior abdominal wall.

mesocolopexy, mesocoloplication (mez″o-ko′lo-pek″se), (mez″o-ko″lo-pli-ka′shun) the taking of a tuck in the mesocolon to shorten it.

mesocord (mez′o-kord) an umbilical cord adherent to the placenta.

mesocyst (mez′o-sist) the peritoneal fold attaching the gallbladder to the liver.

mesocytoma (mez″o-si-to′mah) a connective tissue tumor; a sarcoma.

mesoderm (mez′o-derm) an intermediate layer of cells developing between the ectoderm and ento-

derm; from it are formed all types of muscle, connective tissue, bone marrow, blood, lymphoid tissue, and the epithelium of body and joint cavities, blood vessels, etc. adj., **mesoder′mal, mesoder′mic.**
  somatic m., the outer layer of the developing mesoderm.
  splanchnic m., the inner layer of the developing mesoderm.

mesodiastolic (mez″o-di″ah-stol′ik) pertaining to the middle of the diastole.

mesoduodenum (mez″o-du″o-de′num) the mesenteric fold that in early fetal life encloses the duodenum.

meso-epididymis (mez″o-ep″ĭ-did′ĭ-mis) a fold of tunica vaginalis connecting the epididymis and testis.

mesogastrium (mez″o-gas′tre-um) the portion of the primitive mesentery that encloses the stomach and from which the greater omentum develops. adj., **mesogas′tric.**

mesohyloma (mez″o-hi-lo′mah) a tumor developed from the mesothelium.

mesoileum (mez″o-il′e-um) the mesentery of the ileum.

mesojejunum (mez″o-je-ju′num) the mesentery of the jejunum.

mesolecithal (mez″o-les′ĭ-thal) having a moderate amount of yolk.

mesolymphocyte (mez″o-lim′fo-sīt) a medium-sized lymphocyte.

mesomere (mez′o-mēr) 1. a blastomere of size intermediate between a macromere and a micromere. 2. a midzone of the mesoderm between the epimere and hypomere.

mesomerism (mĕ-zom′er-izm) the existence of organic chemical structures differing only in the position of electrons rather than atoms.

mesometritis (mez″o-me-tri′tis) inflammation of the myometrium.

mesometrium (mez″o-me′tre-um) 1. the portion of the broad ligament that supports the uterus. 2. the myometrium.

mesomorphy (mez″o-mor′fe) a type of body build in which tissues derived from the mesoderm predominate. There is relative preponderance of muscle, bone and connective tissue, usually with heavy, hard physique of rectangular outline.

meson (me′zon, mes′on) 1. mesion. 2. any elementary particle having a mass intermediate between the mass of the electron and that of the proton.

mesonephroma (mez″o-nĕ-fro′mah) a tumor arising from the mesonephros.

mesonephron (mez″o-nef′ron) mesonephros.

mesonephros (mez″o-nef′ros), pl. *mesoneph′roi*

[Gr.] the excretory organ of the embryo, arising caudad to the pronephros and using its duct. adj., **mesoneph'ric.**

mesoneuritis (mez″o-nu-ri′tis) 1. inflammation of the substance of a nerve. 2. inflammation of the lymphatics of a nerve.

mesopallium (mez′o-pal′e-um) the portion of the pallium, or gray matter, with stratification and organization that is transitional between archipallium and neopallium.

mesopexy (mez′o-pek″se) repair of the mesentery; mesenteriopexy.

mesophile (mez′o-fīl) a microorganism that grows best at 20 to 55° C.

mesophlebitis (mez″o-flĕ-bi′tis) inflammation of the tunica media of a vein.

Mesopin (mes′o-pin) trademark for a preparation of homatropine methylbromide, a parasympatholytic.

mesopneumon (mez″o-nu′mon) the union of the two layers of the pleura at the hilus of the lung.

mesoporphyrin (mez″o-por′fĭ-rin) a crystalline iron-free porphyrin from heme obtained by a process of reduction.

mesorchium (mez-or′ke-um) the peritoneal fold holding the fetal testis in place.

mesorectum (mez″o-rek′tum) the fold of peritoneum connecting the upper portion of the rectum with the sacrum.

mesoretina (mez″o-ret′ĭ-nah) the middle layer of the retina.

mesoropter (mez″o-rop′ter) the normal position of the eyes with their muscles at rest.

mesorrhaphy (mez-or′ah-fe) suture of the mesentery.

mesosalpinx (mez″o-sal′pinks) the part of the broad ligament of the uterus investing the uterine tube.

mesosigmoid (mez″o-sig′moid) the peritoneal fold by which the sigmoid flexure is attached.

mesosigmoidopexy (mez″o-sig-moi′do-pek″se) fixation of the mesosigmoid in prolapse of the rectum.

mesosternum (mez″o-ster′num) the middle piece or body of the sternum.

mesotendineum, mesotendon (mez″o-ten-din′e-um), (mez″o-ten′don) the connective tissue sheath attaching a tendon to its fibrous sheath.

mesothelial (mez″o-the′le-al) pertaining to the mesothelium.

mesothelioma (mez″o-the″le-o′mah) a tumor made up of cells derived from the mesothelium.

mesothelium (mez″o-the′le-um) the layer of flat cells, derived from the mesoderm, that lines the coelom of the body cavity of the embryo. In the adult it forms the simple squamous-celled layer of the epithelium that covers the surface of all true

serous membranes (peritoneum, pericardium, pleura).

mesothenar (mez-oth′ĕ-nar) the adductor muscle of the thumb.

mesotron (mez′o-tron) meson (2).

mesoturbinate (mez″o-tur′bĭ-nāt) the middle turbinate (nasal concha).

mesovarium (mez″o-va′re-um) the portion of the broad ligament enclosing and holding the ovary in place.

met (met) a unit of measure of metabolic heat, the quantity produced by a resting-sitting subject, or 50 large calories per square meter per hour.

meta- (met′ah) word element [Gr.], (1) *change; transformation; exchange.* (2) *after; next.* (3) the 1,3-position in derivatives of benzene.

metabasis (mĕ-tab′ah-sis) change of disease or place.

metabiosis (met″ah-bi-o′sis) the dependence of one organism upon another for its existence; commensalism.

metabolism (mĕ-tab′o-lizm) the sum total of the physical and chemical processes and reactions taking place among the ions, atoms and molecules of the body. adj., **metabol'ic.** Essentially these processes are concerned with the disposition of the nutrients absorbed into the blood following digestion.

There are two phases of metabolism: the anabolic and the catabolic phase. The anabolic, or constructive, phase is concerned with the conversion of simpler compounds derived from the nutrients into living, organized substances that the body cells can use. In the catabolic, or destructive, phase these organized substances are reconverted into simpler compounds, with the release of energy necessary for the proper functioning of the body cells.

The rate of metabolism can be increased by exercise; by elevated body temperature, as in a high fever, which can more than double the metabolic rate; by hormonal activity, such as that of thyroxine, insulin and epinephrine; and by specific dynamic action that occurs following the ingestion of a meal.

The basal metabolic rate refers to the lowest rate obtained while an individual is at complete physical and mental rest. The BASAL METABOLISM TEST is frequently used in the diagnosis of various diseases, especially in malfunctioning of the thyroid gland.

Congenital defects of metabolic processes, known as inborn errors of metabolism, include AMAUROTIC FAMILIAL IDIOCY, GALACTOSEMIA, GLYCOGENOSIS, PHENYLKETONURIA and many others; all are rare.

metabolite (mĕ-tab′o-līt) any compound produced during metabolism.

metabutethamine (met″ah-bu-teth′ah-min) a compound used as a local anesthetic.

metabutoxycaine (met″ah-bu-tok′sĭ-kān) a compound used as a local anesthetic.

metacarpal (met″ah-kar′pal) pertaining to the metacarpus.

metacarpectomy (met″ah-kar-pek′to-me) excision of a metacarpal bone.

metacarpophalangeal (met″ah-kar″po-fah-lan′-je-al) pertaining to the metacarpus and phalanges.

metacarpus (met″ah-kar′pus) the proximal part of the hand, or the five (metacarpal) bones composing it.

metacentric (met″ah-sen′trik) having the centromere almost at the middle of the replicating chromosome.

metacercaria (met″ah-ser-ka′re-ah), pl. *metacerca′riae* the encysted resting or maturing stage of a trematode parasite in the tissues of an intermediate host.

metachromasia (met″ah-kro-ma′ze-ah) 1. failure to stain true with a given stain. 2. the different coloration of different tissues produced by the same stain. 3. change of color produced by staining. adj., **metachromat′ic.**

metachromatin (met″ah-kro′mah-tin) the basophil part of the chromatin.

metachromatism (met″ah-kro′mah-tizm) metachromasia.

metachromophil (met″ah-kro′mo-fil) not staining normally.

metachromosome (met″ah-kro′mo-sōm) one of two small chromosomes that conjugate only in the last phase of the spermatocyte division.

metachronous (mě-tak′ro-nus) occurring at different times.

metacoele (met′ah-sēl) 1. the fourth ventricle. 2. metacoeloma.

metacoeloma (met″ah-se-lo′mah) that part of the embryonic coelom which develops into the pleuroperitoneal cavity, which is later separated into two cavities by the diaphragm.

metacortandracin (met″ah-kor-tan′drah-sin) prednisone, a steroid used as an anti-inflammatory agent.

metacortandralone (met″ah-kor-tan′drah-lōn) prednisolone, a steroid used as an anti-inflammatory agent.

metacyesis (met″ah-si-e′sis) ectopic pregnancy.

metagaster (met″ah-gas′ter) the permanent intestinal canal of the embryo.

metagenesis (met″ah-jen′ě-sis) alternation of generation.

metagglutinin (met″ah-gloo′tĭ-nin) an agglutinin present in an agglutinative serum that acts on organisms that are closely related to the specific antigen and in a lower dilution; called also partial agglutinin and minor agglutinin.

metagranulocyte (met″ah-gran′u-lo-sīt″) promyelocyte.

metal (met′al) a chemical element or substance marked by luster, malleability, ductility and conductivity of electricity and heat. adj., **metal′lic.**
  alkali m., one of a group of monovalent elements including lithium, potassium, sodium, rubidium and cesium.
  m. fume fever, an occupational disorder occurring in those engaged in welding and other metallic operations and due to the volatilized metals. It includes brass chills, zinc chills, zinc fume fever, brazier's chills and brassfounders' ague.

metalbumin (met″al-bu′min) a substance found in ovarian cysts; pseudomucin.

metalloid (met′ah-loid) 1. a nonmetallic element. 2. any metallic element that has not all the characters of a typical metal. 3. resembling a metal.

metallophobia (met″al-o-fo′be-ah) morbid fear of metallic objects.

metallurgy (met″al-ur′je) the science and art of using metals.

metamer (met′ah-mer) a compound exhibiting, or capable of exhibiting, metamerism.

metamere (met′ah-mēr) one of a series of homologous segments of the body of an animal.

metamerism (mě-tam′er-izm) 1. a type of structural isomerism in which different radicals of the same chemical type are attached to the same polyvalent element and yet give rise to compounds having identical molecular formulae. 2. arrangement into metameres by the serial repetition of a structural pattern.

Metamine (met′ah-mēn) trademark for preparations of trolnitrate, a vasodilator.

metamorphopsia (met″ah-mor-fop′se-ah) defective vision, with distortion of the shape of objects looked at.

metamorphosis (met″ah-mor′fo-sis) change of structure or shape.
  fatty m., any normal or pathologic transformation of fat, including fatty infiltration and fatty degeneration.
  platelet m., a series of progressive, irreversible structural alterations that platelets undergo during coagulation, dependent on the presence of divalent metallic ions.
  retrograde m., conversion into a simpler or more primitive form.
  structural m., viscous m., platelet metamorphosis.

Metamucil (met″ah-mu′sil) trademark for a preparation of psyllium hydrophilic mucilloid, a laxative.

metamyelocyte (met″ah-mi′ě-lo-sīt″) a polymorphonuclear leukocyte in which the nuclear element is a single fragment no longer containing a definite nucleolus.

Metandren (mě-tan′dren) trademark for preparations of methyltestosterone, an androgen.

metanephrine (met″ah-nef′rin) a urinary metabolite of epinephrine.

metanephron (met″ah-nef′ron) metanephros.

metanephros (met″ah-nef′ros), pl. *metaneph′roi* [Gr.] the permanent embryonic kidney, developing later than and caudad to the mesonephros. adj., **metaneph′ric.**

metaneutrophil (met″ah-nu′tro-fil) a cell not staining normally with neutral stains.

metaphase (met'ah-fāz) the second stage of division of the nucleus of a cell in either meiosis or mitosis.

Metaphen (met'ah-fen) trademark for preparations of nitromersol, an antibacterial.

metaphrenia (met"ah-fre'ne-ah) the mental condition in which the interests are withdrawn from the family or group and directed to personal gain or aggrandizement.

metaphysis (mĕ-taf'ĭ-sis), pl. *metaph'yses* [Gr.] the wider part at the end of the shaft of a long bone, adjacent to the epiphyseal disk. adj., **metaphys'eal.**

metaplasia (met"ah-pla'ze-ah) a reversible change in which one adult cell type is replaced by another adult cell type. adj., **metaplas'tic.**

   myeloid m., agnogenic, a condition characterized by foci of extramedullary hematopoiesis and by immature red and white cells in the peripheral blood and mild to moderate anemia.

metaplasm (met'ah-plazm) the inanimate particles of protoplasm; called also deutoplasm.

metaplexus (met"ah-plek'sus) the choroid plexus of the fourth ventricle.

metapneumonic (met"ah-nu-mon'ik) succeeding or following pneumonia.

metapodialia (met"ah-po"de-a'le-ah) the bones of the metacarpus and metatarsus.

metapophysis (met"ah-pof'ĭ-sis) the mammillary process on the superior articular or prearticular processes of certain vertebrae.

metaprotein (met"ah-pro'te-in) a product of the action of an acid or an alkali on a protein.

metaraminol (met"ah-ram'ĭ-nol) an ephedrine compound used as a sympathomimetic and pressor agent.

metargon (met-ar'gon) a name given an isotope of argon, atomic weight 38.

metarubricyte (met"ah-roo"brĭ-sīt) a red cell containing a pyknotic, contracted nucleus, the last stage in erythrocyte development.

metastable (met"ah-sta'bl) capable of undergoing change.

metastasis (mĕ-tas'tah-sis) 1. the transfer of disease from one organ or part to another not directly connected with it. It may be due either to the transfer of pathogenic microorganisms (e.g., tubercle bacilli) or to transfer of cells, as in malignant tumors. 2. pl. *metas'tases* [Gr.] a growth of pathogenic microorganisms or of abnormal cells distant from the site primarily involved by the morbid process. adj., **metastat'ic.**

metastasize (mĕ-tas'tah-sīz) to form new foci of disease in a distant part by metastasis.

metasternum (met"ah-ster'num) the xiphoid process.

metatarsal (met"ah-tar'sal) pertaining to the metatarsus.

metatarsalgia (met"ah-tar-sal'je-ah) pain in the metatarsus.

metatarsectomy (met"ah-tar-sek'to-me) excision of a metatarsal bone.

metatarsophalangeal (met"ah-tar"so-fah-lan'-je-al) pertaining to the metatarsus and the phalanges of the toes.

metatarsus (met"ah-tar'sus) the anterior segment of the foot or, collectively, the five (metatarsal) bones composing it.

   m. pri'mus va'rus, angulation of the first metatarsal bone toward the midline of the body, producing an angle sometimes of 20 degrees or more between its base and that of the second metatarsal bone.

metathalamus (met"ah-thal'ah-mus) the part of the thalamencephalon composed of the medial and lateral geniculate bodies.

metathesis (mĕ-tath'ĕ-sis) 1. artificial transfer of a morbid process. 2. a chemical reaction in which an element or radical in one compound exchanges places with another element or radical in another compound.

Metazoa (met"ah-zo'ah) a phylum of the animal kingdom that includes the multicellular animals, i.e., all animals except the Protozoa.

metazoon (met"ah-zo'on), pl. *metazo'a* [Gr.] an individual organism of the phylum Metazoa.

Metchnikoff theory (mech'nĭ-kof) the theory that bacteria and other harmful elements in the body are attacked and destroyed by cells called phagocytes, and that the contest between such harmful elements and the phagocytes produces inflammation. Named for Elie Metchnikoff (1845–1916), Russian zoologist in Paris and winner, with Ehrlich, of the Nobel prize for medicine and physiology in 1908.

metencephalon (met"en-sef'ah-lon), pl. *metenceph'ala* [Gr.] 1. the part of the central nervous system comprising the pons and cerebellum. 2. the anterior of two brain vesicles formed by specialization of the rhombencephalon in the developing embryo.

meteorism (me'te-o-rizm") tympanites; drumlike distention of the abdomen caused by the presence of gas in the abdomen or intestines.

meteorology (me"te-o-rol'o-je) the science of the atmosphere and its phenomena.

meteorotropic (me"te-or-o-trop'ik) influenced by the weather.

meteorotropism (me"te-o-rot'ro-pizm) the response to influence by meteorologic factors noted in certain biologic events, such as sudden death, attacks of angina, joint pain, insomnia and traffic accidents.

meter (me'ter) the basic unit of linear measure of the metric system, being the equivalent of 39.371 inches; abbreviated M.

-meter (me'ter) word element [Gr.], *instrument for measuring.*

methacholine chloride (meth"ah-ko'lēn) colorless or white crystals; a parasympathomimetic used in cardiovascular disease and as a diagnostic test for pheochromocytoma.

methadone (meth'ah-dōn) a synthetic compound with pharmacologic properties qualitatively similar to those of morphine.

methallenestril (meth″al-ĕ-nes′tril) a nonsteroid estrogenic compound.

methamphetamine (meth″am-fet′ah-mēn) an adrenergic, central nervous system stimulant used in the treatment of narcolepsy, chronic fatigue states, alcoholism and depression. Since it depresses the appetite it is also used in the control of obesity. Its actions are similar to those of amphetamine and so it may produce insomnia, excitement and elevation of blood pressure. Prolonged use can lead to dependence.

methandriol (meth-an′dre-ol) a compound used as an anabolic stimulant.

methandrostenolone (meth-an″dro-sten′o-lōn) a compound used as an anabolic hormone.

methane (meth′ān) a gas from decayed organic matter.

methanol (meth′ah-nol) a mobile, colorless liquid widely used as a solvent; methyl alcohol.

methantheline bromide (mĕ-than′thĕ-lēn) an odorless, bitter, white or nearly white powder used as an anticholinergic and antispasmodic.

methapyrilene (meth″ah-pir′ĭ-lēn) an antihistamine.

metharbital (meth-ar′bĭ-tal) a long-acting barbiturate used as a central nervous system depressant with anticonvulsant action.

methdilazine (meth-di′lah-zēn) a phenothiazine compound used as an antihistamine and antipruritic.

Methedrine (meth′ĕ-drin) trademark for preparations of methamphetamine.

methemoglobin (met-he″mo-glo′bin) a compound formed from hemoglobin by oxidation of the ferrous to the ferric state with essentially ionic bonds. A small amount of methemoglobin is present in the blood normally, but injury or toxic agents convert a larger proportion of hemoglobin into methemoglobin, which is unable to act as a carrier of oxygen.

methemoglobinemia (met-he″mo-glo″bĭ-ne′me-ah) methemoglobin in the blood, usually due to toxic action of drugs or other agents, or to hemolytic processes.

methemoglobinuria (met-he″mo-glo″bĭ-nu′re-ah) methemoglobin in the urine.

methenamine (mĕ-the′nah-min) a white crystalline powder used as a urinary antiseptic.
　m. mandelate, a salt of methenamine and mandelic acid, used in infections of the urinary tract.

Methergine (meth′er-jin) trademark for preparations of methylergonovine, an oxytocic.

methexenyl (meth-ek′sĕ-nil) hexobarbital, an ultra-short-acting barbiturate.

methicillin (meth″ĭ-sil′in) dimethoxyphenyl peni-

cillin, a semisynthetic penicillin that is highly resistant to inactivation by penicillinase.
　sodium m., an antibacterial compound for parenteral administration.

methimazole (meth-im′ah-zōl) a white to pale buff, crystalline powder, used as a thyroid inhibitor.

methiodal sodium (meth-i′o-dal) an odorless, white, crystalline, iodine-containing powder with a slightly saline taste, used as a radiopaque medium for roentgenography of the urinary tract.

methionine (mĕ-thi′o-nin) a sulfur-bearing amino acid essential for optimal growth in infants and for nitrogen equilibrium in adults; used therapeutically as a dietary supplement with lipotropic action.

Methium (meth′e-um) trademark for preparations of hexamethonium, a hypotensive.

methocarbamol (meth″o-kar′bah-mol) a compound used as a skeletal muscle relaxant.

methodology (meth″o-dol′o-je) the science dealing with principles of procedure in research and study.

methohexital (meth″o-hek′sĭ-tal) an ultra-short-acting barbiturate.
　sodium m., a compound used intravenously to produce general anesthesia.

methopromazine (meth″o-pro′mah-zēn) methoxypromazine, a tranquilizer.

methotrexate (meth″o-trek′sāt) a poisonous, orange-brown, crystalline compound used as an antineoplastic agent.

methoxamine (mĕ-thok′sah-mēn) a compound used as a sympathomimetic and vasopressor.

methoxsalen (mĕ-thok′sah-len) a compound used with ultraviolet light in treatment of idiopathic vitiligo.

methoxyflurane (mĕ-thok″se-floo′rān) a compound used as a general anesthetic administered by inhalation.

methoxyphenamine (mĕ-thok″se-fen′ah-mēn) a compound used as a sympathomimetic drug with predominant bronchodilator action.

methoxypromazine (mĕ-thok″se-pro′mah-zēn) a phenothiazine derivative used as a tranquilizer.

methscopolamine (meth″sko-pol′ah-min) a compound used in parasympathetic blockade.

methsuximide (meth-suk′sĭ-mīd) a white to grayish white crystalline powder used as an anticonvulsant to treat petit mal and psychomotor epilepsy.

methyl (meth′il) the monovalent radical, —CH_3.
　m. alcohol, a mobile, colorless liquid used as a solvent and fuel; it is poisonous if taken internally. Called also methanol and wood alcohol.
　m. salicylate, a natural or synthetic wintergreen oil, used as a topical application to inflamed joints.

methylate (meth′ĭ-lāt) a compound of methyl alcohol and a base.

methylation (meth″ĭ-la′shun) treatment with methyl.

methylbenzethonium (meth″il-ben″zĕ-tho′ne-um) an ammonium compound used as a local anti-infective; it is used mainly in prevention of dermatitis in infants. Soap inhibits its action.

methylcellulose (meth″il-sel′u-lōs) a methyl ester of cellulose; used as a bulk laxative and a suspending agent for drugs.

methylcytosine (meth″il-si′to-sin) a pyrimidine occurring in deoxyribonucleic acid.

methyldopa (meth″il-do′pah) an adrenergic-blocking agent, used as an antihypertensive.

methylene blue (meth′ĭ-lēn) a synthetic organic compound, in dark green crystals or lustrous crystalline powder, used as an antidote in cyanide poisoning, as a stain in pathology and bacteriology and as an antiseptic.

methylergonovine (meth″il-er″go-no′vin) a compound used as an oxytocic.

methylhexaneamine (meth″il-hek-sān′ah-min) a compound used as an inhalant to relieve nasal congestion.

methylmelubrin (meth″il-mel′u-brin) dipyrone, an analgesic and antipyretic.

methylparaben (meth″il-par′ah-ben) a compound used as a preservative for drug solutions.

methylparafynol (meth″il-par″ah-fi′nol) a compound used as a hypnotic and sedative.

methylphenidate (meth″il-fen′i-dāt) a compound used as a mild central nervous system stimulant and antidepressant.

methylprednisolone (meth″il-pred-nis′o-lōn) a white, odorless, crystalline powder, a corticosteroid of the glucogenic type, having an anti-inflammatory action similar to that of prednisolone.

methylrosaniline chloride (meth″il-ro-zan′ĭ-lēn) gentian violet, an anthelmintic and anti-infective.

methyltestosterone (meth″il-tes-tos′tĕ-rōn) an orally effective form of testosterone.

methylthionine chloride (meth″il-thi′o-nin) methylene blue.

methylthiouracil (meth″il-thi″o-u′rah-sil) a white, odorless, crystalline powder, used as a thyroid inhibitor.

methyprylon (meth″ĭ-pri′lon) a white, crystalline powder used as a sedative and hypnotic.

Meticortelone (met″ĭ-kor′tĕ-lōn) trademark for preparations of prednisolone, an anti-inflammatory agent.

Meticorten (met″ĭ-kor′ten) trademark for a preparation of prednisone, an anti-inflammatory agent.

metmyoglobin (met-mi″o-glo′bin) a compound formed from myoglobin by oxidation of the ferrous to the ferric state with essentially ionic bonds.

metopagus (mĕ-top′ah-gus) conjoined twins united at forehead.

metopic (mĕ-top′ik) pertaining to the forehead.

metopon (met-o′pon) the anterior metopic lobule of the brain.

metoxenous (mĕ-tok′sĕ-nus) requiring two hosts for the entire life cycle.

metra (me′trah) the uterus.

metralgia (me-tral′je-ah) pain in the uterus.

metrapectic (me″trah-pek′tik) transmitted by the mother, who remains unaffected.

metratonia (me″trah-to′ne-ah) uterine atony.

metratrophia (me″trah-tro′fe-ah) atrophy of the uterus.

Metrazol (met′rah-zol) trademark for preparations of pentylenetetrazol, a central nervous system stimulant.

metrectasia (me″trek-ta′ze-ah) dilatation of the uterus.

metreurynter (me″troo-rin′ter) an inflatable bag for dilating the cervical canal of the uterus.

metreurysis (me-troo′rĭ-sis) dilation of the cervix uteri by means of the metreurynter.

metric (met′rik) pertaining to measures or measurement.
  m. system, a system of weights and measures based on the meter and having all units based on some power of 10. (See also Table of Weights and Measures in the Appendix.)

metritis (me-tri′tis) inflammation of the uterus.

metrocarcinoma (me″tro-kar″sĭ-no′mah) carcinoma of the uterus.

metrocele (me′tro-sēl) hernia of the uterus.

metrocolpocele (me″tro-kol′po-sēl) hernia of the uterus with vaginal prolapse.

metrocyte (me′tro-sīt) 1. a mother cell. 2. a large uninuclear cell containing hemoglobin; supposed to be the mother cell of the red corpuscles of the blood.

metrodynia (me″tro-din′e-ah) pain in the uterus.

metrofibroma (me″tro-fi-bro′mah) myoma (fibroma) of the uterus.

metrology (me-trol′o-je) the science dealing with measurements.

metromalacoma (me″tro-mal″ah-ko′mah) abnormal softening of the uterus.

metronidazole (mĕ″tro-nid′ah-zōl) a compound used as a trichomonacide.

metropathia (me″tro-path′e-ah) disorder of the uterus.
  m. haemorrha′gica, essential uterine hemorrhage.

metropathy (me-trop′ah-the) any uterine disorder.

metroperitoneal (me″tro-per″ĭ-to-ne′al) pertaining to the uterus and peritoneum.

metroperitonitis (me″tro-per″ĭ-to-ni′tis) inflammation of the uterus and peritoneum.

metrophlebitis (me″tro-flĕ-bi′tis) inflammation of the uterine veins.

Metropine (met′ro-pin) trademark for preparations of atropine methylnitrate, an anticholinergic.

metroptosis (me″tro-to′sis) prolapse of the uterus.

metrorrhagia (me″tro-ra′je-ah) uterine bleeding, usually of normal amount, occurring at completely irregular intervals, the period of flow sometimes being prolonged.

metrorrhea (me″tro-re′ah) abnormal uterine discharge.

metrorrhexis (me″tro-rek′sis) rupture of the uterus.

metrosalpingitis (me″tro-sal″pin-ji′tis) inflammation of the uterus and uterine tubes.

metrosalpingography (me″tro-sal″ping-gog′rah-fe) hysterosalpingography; roentgenography of the uterus and uterine tubes.

metroscope (me′tro-skōp) an instrument for examining the uterus.

metrostaxis (me″tro-stak′sis) slow loss of blood from the uterus.

metrostenosis (me″tro-stĕ-no′sis) stenosis of the uterus.

metrotomy (me-trot′o-me) hysterotomy; incision of the uterus.

-metry word element [Gr.], *measurement.*

Metubine (mĕ-tu′bin) trademark for a preparation of dimethyl tubocurarine, a skeletal muscle relaxant.

Metycaine (met′ĭ-kān) trademark for preparations of piperocaine, a local anesthetic.

mev million electron volts.

M.F.D. minimum fatal dose.

Mg chemical symbol, *magnesium.*

mg. milligram.

μg. microgram.

mication (mi-ka′shun) a quick motion, such as winking.

micelle (mi-sel′) a supermolecular colloid particle, most often a packet of chain molecules in parallel arrangement.

micr(o)- (mi′kro) word element [Gr.], *small;* used in naming units of measurement to designate an amount 10^{-6} (one-millionth) the size of the unit to which it is joined, e.g., microcurie.

micrangiopathy (mi-kran″je-op′ah-the) disease of the capillaries.

micrencephaly (mi″kren-sef′ah-le) abnormal smallness and underdevelopment of the brain.

microabscess (mi″kro-ab′ses) an abscess visible only under a microscope.

microaerobic (mi″kro-a″er-o′bik) thriving best or surviving only in the presence of a limited amount of molecular oxygen.

microaerophilic (mi″kro-a″er-o-fil′ik) growing best in the presence of very little free oxygen.

microanalysis (mi″kro-ah-nal′ĭ-sis) the chemical analysis of minute quantities of material.

microanatomy (mi″kro-ah-nat′o-me) histology.

microaneurysm (mi″kro-an′u-rizm) a minute aneurysm occurring on a vessel of small size, as one in the retina of the eye.

microangiopathy (mi″kro-an″je-op′ah-the) a disorder involving the small blood vessels.
   thrombotic m., a condition characterized by fever, hemolytic anemia, thrombocytopenic purpura and neurologic disturbances, with widespread occlusion of small blood vessels.

microbar (mi′kro-bahr) a unit of pressure, being one-millionth (10^{-6}) bar.

microbe (mi′krōb) a microorganism. adj., **micro′bial, micro′bic.**

microbicidal (mi-kro″bĭ-si′dal) destroying microbes.

microbicide (mi-kro′bĭ-sīd) an agent that destroys microbes.

microbioassay (mi″kro-bi″o-as-sa′) determination of the active power of a nutrient or other factor by noting its effect on the growth of a microorganism, as compared with the effect of a standard preparation.

microbiology (mi″kro-bi-ol′o-je) the study of minute living organisms, including bacteria, molds and pathogenic protoza; bacteriology.

microblast (mi′kro-blast) an erythroblast of 5 microns or less in diameter.

microblepharism (mi″kro-blef′ah-rizm) abnormal smallness of eyelids.

microbody (mi′kro-bod″e) a spherical or ovoid organelle surrounded by a single membrane, found in cytoplasm of certain cells.

microbrachius (mi″kro-bra′ke-us) a fetus with abnormally small arms.

microcalorie (mi″kro-kal′o-re) small calorie; the heat required to raise 1 cc. of distilled water from 0 to 1° C.

microcardia (mi″kro-kar′de-ah) abnormal smallness of the heart.

microcentrum (mi″kro-sen′trum) centrosome.

microcephalus (mi″kro-sef′ah-lus) an idiot or fetus with a very small head.

microcephaly (mi″kro-sef′ah-le) small size of the head in relation to the rest of the body.

microcheilia (mi″kro-ki′le-ah) abnormal smallness of the lip.

microcheiria (mi″kro-ki′re-ah) abnormal smallness of the hands.

microchemistry (mi″kro-kem′is-tre) chemistry concerned with exceedingly small quantities of chemical substances.

microcinematography (mi″kro-sin″ĕ-mah-tog′-rah-fe) moving picture photography of microscopic objects.

Micrococcaceae (mi″kro-kok-a′se-e) a family of Schizomycetes containing six genera including Staphylococcus and Micrococcus.

Micrococcus (mi″kro-kok′us) a genus of the family Micrococcaceae found in soil, water etc.

micrococcus (mi″kro-kok′us), pl. *micrococ′ci* [Gr.] a small bacterium occurring predominantly as a single cell rather than in groups or aggregates.

microcolon (mi″kro-ko′lon) abnormal smallness of the colon.

microcoria (mi″kro-ko′re-ah) smallness of the pupil.

microcornea (mi″kro-kor′ne-ah) unusual smallness of the cornea.

microcoulomb (mi″kro-koo′lomb) one-millionth of a coulomb.

microcrania (mi″kro-kra′ne-ah) abnormal smallness of the skull in relation to the face.

microcrith (mi′kro-krith) the weight of one atom of hydrogen.

microcrystalline (mi″kro-kris′tah-lin) made up of minute crystals.

microcurie (mi″kro-ku′re) one-millionth (10^{-6}) curie; abbreviated μCi or μc.

microcurie-hour (mi″kro-ku″re-owr″) a unit of dose equivalent to that obtained by exposure for one hour to radioactive material disintegrating at the rate of 3.7×10^4 atoms per second; abbreviated μc.-hr.

microcyst (mi′kro-sist) a cyst visible only under a microscope.

microcyte (mi′kro-sīt) an erythrocyte 5 microns or less in diameter.

microcythemia, microcytosis (mi″kro-si-the′me-ah), (mi″kro-si-to′sis) a condition in which the erythrocytes are smaller than normal.

microdactylia (mi″kro-dak-til′e-ah) abnormal smallness of the fingers or toes.

microdetermination (mi″kro-de-ter″mĭ-na′shun) chemical examination of minute quantities of substance.

microdissection (mi″kro-dĭ-sek′shun) dissection of tissue or cells under the microscope.

microdontia (mi″kro-don′she-ah) abnormal smallness of the teeth.

microdrepanocytic disease (mi″kro-drep″ah-no-sit′ik) a disorder of the blood hemoglobin in which thalassemia is associated with the sickling trait.

microecology (mi″kro-e-kol′o-je) the branch of the ecology of parasites concerned with the relations of the organisms and the environment provided by the hosts.

microecosystem (mi″kro-e″ko-sis′tem) a miniature ecosystem, occurring naturally or produced in the laboratory for experimental purposes.

microembolus (mi″kro-em′bo-lus), pl. *microem′-boli* [L.] an embolus of microscopic size.

microerythrocyte (mi″kro-ĕ-rith′ro-sīt) microcyte.

microfarad (mi″kro-far′ad) one-millionth (10^{-6}) farad; abbreviated μf.

microfauna (mi″kro-faw′nah) the microscopic animal organisms of a special region.

microfibril (mi″kro-fi′bril) an extremely small fibril.

microfilaria (mi″kro-fĭ-la″re-ah) the prelarval stage of Filarioidea in the blood of man and in the tissues of the vector. This term is sometimes used as a genus name, and is then spelled with a capital M.
    m. bancrof′ti, the microfilaria of *Wuchereria bancrofti.*
    m. streptocer′ca, the larval form of *Onchocerca volvulus,* found in cutaneous lesions of the natives of the Gold Coast.

microflora (mi″kro-flo′rah) the microscopic vegetable organisms of a special region.

microgamete (mi″kro-gam′ēt) the smaller, male gamete of the malarial parasite.

microgastria (mi″kro-gas′tre-ah) congenital smallness of the stomach.

microgenia (mi″kro-je′ne-ah) abnormal smallness of the chin.

microgenitalism (mi″kro-jen′ĭ-tal″izm) smallness of the external genitalia.

microglia (mi-krog′le-ah) non-neural cells forming part of the adventitial structure of the central nervous system. They are migratory and act as phagocytes of waste products of the nervous system.

microglossia (mi″kro-glos′e-ah) abnormal smallness of the tongue.

micrognathia (mi″kro-nath′e-ah) abnormal smallness of the lower jaw.

microgram (mi′kro-gram) one-millionth (10^{-6}) gram, or one-thousandth (10^{-3}) milligram; abbreviated μg. or mcg.

micrograph (mi′kro-graf) a permanent reproduction of the appearance of an object as observed through a microscope.
    electron m., a graphic reproduction of an object as viewed with an electron microscope.

microgyria (mi″kro-ji′re-ah) abnormal smallness of convolutions of the brain.

microgyrus (mi″kro-ji′rus) an abnormally small, malformed convolution of the brain.

microhematocrit (mi″kro-he-mat′o-krit) rapid determination of packed-cell volume of erythrocytes in whole blood, by high-speed centrifugation of a small quantity of blood.

microhepatia (mi″kro-he-pat′e-ah) smallness of the liver.

microhm (mi′krōm) one-millionth (10^{-6}) ohm.

microincineration (mi″kro-in-sin″er-a′shun) the oxidation of a small quantity of material, to eliminate organic matter and leave only the ash, for the purpose of analyzing the elements composing the material.

microlecithal (mi″kro-les′ĭ-thal) having a small amount of yolk.

microlesion (mi′kro-le″zhun) a minute lesion.

microliter (mi′kro-le″ter) one-millionth part of a liter, or one-thousandth of a milliliter; abbreviated μl.

microlith (mi′kro-lith) a minute concretion or calculus.

microlithiasis (mi″kro-lĭ-thi′ah-sis) the formation of minute concretions in an organ.
  m. alveola′ris pulmo′num, pulmonary alveolar m., a condition simulating pulmonary tuberculosis, with deposition of minute calculi in the alveoli of the lungs.

micrology (mi-krol′o-je) the science of microscopy.

micromandible (mi″kro-man′dĭ-bl) extreme smallness of the mandible.

micromastia (mi″kro-mas′te-ah) abnormal smallness of the breast.

micromelia (mi″kro-me′le-ah) abnormal smallness of one or more extremities.

micromelus (mi-krom′ĕ-lus) a fetus with abnormally small limbs.

micromere (mi′kro-mēr) one of the small blastomeres formed by unequal cleavage of a fertilized ovum.

micrometeorology (mi″kro-me″te-o-rol′o-je) that branch of meteorology dealing with the effects on living organisms of the extraorganic aspects of the physical environment within a few inches of the surface of the earth.

micrometer (mi-krom′ĕ-ter) an instrument for making minute measurements.

micromethod (mi′kro-meth″od) a technique dealing with exceedingly small quantities of material.

micrometry (mi-krom′ĕ-tre) measurement of microscopic objects.

micromicro- (mi″kro-mi′kro) word element designating, or 10^{-6} (one-millionth) of 10^{-6} (one-millionth), or 10^{-12} (one-trillionth), part of the unit to which it is joined; now being supplanted by the prefix pico-.

micromicrocurie (mi″kro-mi″kro-ku′re) one-millionth (10^{-6}) microcurie, or 10^{-12} curie; abbreviated $\mu\mu$c.

micromicrogram (mi″kro-mi″kro-gram) one-millionth (10^{-6}) microgram, or 10^{-12} gram; abbreviated $\mu\mu$g. or $\mu\gamma$.

micromicron (mi″kro-mi′kron) one-millionth micron (10^{-9} mm., or 10^{-2} angstroms); abbreviated $\mu\mu$.

micromillimeter (mi″kro-mil′ĭ-me″ter) 1. micron. 2. one-millionth of a millimeter; abbreviated μmm.

micromolecular (mi″kro-mo-lek′u-lar) composed of small molecules.

micromyelia (mi″kro-mi-e′le-ah) abnormal smallness of spinal cord.

micron (mi′kron), pl. *mi′cra, mi′crons* [Gr.] a unit of linear measurement of the metric system, equivalent to 10^{-3} mm., or 10^4 angstroms; abbreviated μ.

micronucleus (mi″kro-nu′kle-us) the smaller of two nuclei of a unicellular organism, associated with reproduction of the cell.

micronutrient (mi″kro-nu′tre-ent) a dietary element essential only in small quantities.

micronychia (mi″kro-nik′e-ah) abnormal smallness of the nails of the fingers or toes.

microorganism (mi″kro-or′gah-nizm) a microscopic animal or plant.

micropathology (mi″kro-pah-thol′o-je) 1. the sum of what is known about minute pathologic change. 2. pathology of diseases caused by microorganisms.

microphage (mi′kro-fāj) a neutrophilic granulocyte.

microphakia (mi″kro-fa′ke-ah) abnormal smallness of the crystalline lens.

microphallus (mi″kro-fal′us) abnormal smallness of the penis.

microphilic (mi″kro-fil′ik) microaerophilic.

microphobia (mi″kro-fo′be-ah) morbid dread of microbes.

microphone (mi′kro-fōn) a device to pick up sound for purposes of amplification or transmission.

microphonia (mi″kro-fo′ne-ah) marked weakness of voice.

microphotograph (mi″kro-fo′to-graf) a photograph of small size.

microphthalmos (mi″krof-thal′mos) abnormal smallness of the eyeball.

microphysics (mi″kro-fiz′iks) the science of the ultimate structure of matter.

microphyte (mi′kro-fīt) a microscopic plant.

micropipet (mi″kro-pi′pet′) a pipet for handling small quantities of liquids (0.1 to 1 ml.).

micropodia (mi″kro-po′de-ah) abnormal smallness of the feet.

micropredator (mi″kro-pred′ah-tor) an organism that derives elements essential for its existence from other species of organisms, larger than itself, without destroying them.

micropsia (mi-krop'se-ah) a disorder of visual perception in which objects appear smaller than their actual size.

micropus (mi-kro'pus) a person with abnormally small feet.

micropyle (mi'kro-pīl) an opening through which a spermatozoon enters the ovum.

microradiography (mi″kro-ra″de-og'rah-fe) radiography under conditions that permit subsequent microscopic examination or enlargement of the radiograph up to several hundred linear magnifications.

microrhinia (mi″kro-rin'e-ah) abnormal smallness of the nose.

microscope (mi'kro-skōp) an instrument used to obtain an enlarged image of small objects and reveal details of structure not otherwise distinguishable.
  binocular m., one with two eyepieces, permitting use of both eyes simultaneously.
  compound m., one consisting of two lens systems whereby the image formed by the system near the object is magnified by the one nearer the eye.
  darkfield m., one so constructed that illumination is from the side of the field so that details appear light against a dark background; used especially in the identification of spirochetal organisms.
  electron m., one in which electrons, instead of light rays, are used to produce an image which may be viewed on a fluorescent screen or photographed. The electron microscope is able to produce much higher magnification than the light microscope.
  light m., one in which the specimen is viewed under ordinary illumination.
  operating m., one designed for use in performance of delicate surgical procedures, e.g., on the middle ear or small vessels of the heart.
  phase m., phase-contrast m., a microscope that alters the phase relationships of the light passing through and that passing around the object, the contrast permitting visualization of the object without the necessity for staining or other special preparation.
  simple m., one that consists of a single lens.
  split lamp m., a corneal microscope with a special attachment that permits examination of the endothelium on the posterior surface of the cornea.
  stereoscopic m., a binocular microscope modified to give a three-dimensional view of the specimen.
  x-ray m., one in which x-rays are used instead of light, the image usually being reproduced on film.

microscopic (mi″kro-skop'ik) of extremely small size; visible only by aid of a microscope.

microscopical (mi″kro-skop'ĭ-kal) pertaining to a microscope or to microscopy.

microscopy (mi-kros'ko-pe) examination with a microscope.
  television m., a special technique in which a magnified image produced by a microscope is projected on a television screen.

microsome (mi'kro-sōm) one of the microscopic particles in the cytoplasm of a cell.

microsomia (mi″kro-so'me-ah) abnormally small size of the body.

microspectroscope (mi″kro-spek'tro-skōp) a spectroscope and microscope combined.

microsphere (mi'kro-sfēr) a rounded mass of microscopic size.

microspherocyte (mi″kro-sfe'ro-sīt) an erythrocyte whose diameter is less than normal, but whose thickness is increased.

microspherocytosis (mi″kro-sfe'ro-si-to'sis) the presence in the blood of an excessive number of microspherocytes.

microsphygmia, microsphyxia (mi″kro-sfig'me-ah), (mi″kro-sfik'se-ah) that condition of the pulse in which it is perceived with difficulty by the finger.

microsplenia (mi″kro-sple'ne-ah) smallness of the spleen.

Microsporum (mi″kro-spo'rum) a genus of fungi that cause various diseases of the skin and hair, including the species *M. audoui'ni, M. ca'nis (lano'sum)* and *M. ful'vum (gyp'seum)*.

microstat (mi'kro-stat) the stage and finder of a microscope.

microstomia (mi″kro-sto'me-ah) abnormally decreased size of the mouth.

microsurgery (mi″kro-ser'jer-e) dissection of minute structures under the microscope, with the use of extremely small instruments.

Microtatobiotes (mi″kro-ta″to-bi-o'tēz) a class of vegetable organisms, dependent on other living organisms for growth and multiplication.

microthrombosis (mi″kro-throm-bo'sis) the presence of many small thrombi in capillaries and other small blood vessels.

microthrombus (mi″kro-throm'bus) a small thrombus in a capillary or other small blood vessel.

microtia (mi-kro'she-ah) abnormal smallness of the pinna of the ear.

microtome (mi'kro-tōm) an instrument for making thin sections for microscopic study.
  freezing m., one for cutting frozen tissues.
  rotary m., one in which wheel action is translated into a back-and-forth movement of the specimen being sectioned.
  sliding m., one in which the specimen being sectioned is made to slide on a track.

microtomy (mi-krot'o-me) the cutting of thin sections.

microtransfusion (mi″kro-trans-fu'zhun) introduction into the circulation of a small quantity of blood of another individual.

microtrauma (mi″kro-traw'mah) a microscopic lesion or injury.

microtubule (mi″kro-tu'būl) a straight, hollow-appearing structure in the cytoplasm of a cell.

microvillus (mi″kro-vil'us) a minute process or protrusion from the free surface of a cell.

microvolt (mi'kro-volt) one-millionth of a volt; abbreviated μv.

microwave (mi'kro-wāv) a wave typical of electromagnetic radiation between far infrared and radiowaves.

microzoon (mi"kro-zo'on), pl. *microzo'a* [Gr.] a microscopic animal organism.

micturate (mik'tu-rāt) urinate.

micturition (mik"tu-rish'un) urination.

midbrain (mid'brān) the short part of the brain stem just above the pons. It contains the nerve pathways between the cerebral hemispheres and the medulla oblongata, and also contains nuclei (relay stations or centers) of the third and fourth cranial nerves. The center for visual reflexes, such as moving the head and eyes, is located in the midbrain. Called also mesencephalon.

middle lobe syndrome atelectasis of the middle lobe of the right lung, with chronic pneumonitis, due to compression of the bronchus by tuberculous hilar lymph nodes.

midfoot (mid'foot) the middle portion of the foot, comprising the region of the navicular, cuboid and cuneiform bones.

midget (mij'et) a normal dwarf; an individual who is undersized but perfectly formed.

midgut (mid'gut) an intermediate region in the embryo between the foregut and hindgut, which is of only brief duration in man.

Midicel (mid'ĭ-sel) trademark for preparations of sulfamethoxypyridazine, a sulfonamide.

midline (mid'līn) the imaginary line that divides the body of an animal into right and left halves.

midwife (mid'wīf) a woman who assists at childbirth.

migraine (mi'grān) a headache, usually severe, often limited to one side of the head, and sometimes accompanied by nausea and vomiting; called also a sick headache.

Although the cause is not completely understood, migraine is thought to be associated with constriction and then dilatation of the cerebral arteries. It is also thought to have a psychologic aspect, since it occurs most often in persons with particular types of personalities and often follows emotional disturbances. Migraine tends to run in families. In women the headaches often occur during the menstrual periods.

The symptoms of migraine vary greatly not only from person to person but also from time to time in the same person. The headaches are usually intense and they frequently occur on one or the other side of the head. They are often accompanied by nausea and vomiting. A typical migraine attack begins with changes in vision, such as a flickering before the eyes, flashes of light or a blacking out of part of the sight.

Aspirin is usually of little help in relieving migraine. Ergotamine tartrate is quite effective but has side effects, and weekly dosages must be limited. Psychotherapy may help to release the tensions that may be an underlying cause.

abdominal m., migraine in which abdominal symptoms are prominent.

Mikedimide (mi-ked'ĭ-mīd) trademark for a preparation of bemegride, an analeptic used in barbiturate poisoning.

mikro- for words beginning thus, see those beginning *micro-*.

Mikulicz's disease (mik'u-lich"ez) chronic lymphocytic infiltration and enlargement of the lacrimal and salivary glands, of unknown origin.

mil (mil) milliliter.

miliaria (mil"e-a're-ah) a cutaneous condition with retention of sweat, which is extravasated at different levels in the skin; called also prickly heat or heat rash. Treatment of miliaria is directed at reducing sweating generally by reducing the external heat load and avoiding irritating agents and tight clothing. Bland powders may be helpful.

miliary (mil'e-er"e) 1. like millet seeds. 2. characterized by the formation of lesions resembling millet seeds.

m. fever, an acute infectious disease characterized by fever, profuse sweating and the formation of a great many papules, succeeded by a crop of pustules; called also sweating sickness.

m. tuberculosis, an acute form of tuberculosis in which minute tubercles are formed in a number of organs of the body, owing to dissemination of the bacilli throughout the body by the bloodstream.

Milibis (mil'ĭ-bis) trademark for preparations of glycobiarsol, a compound used in amebiasis.

milieu (me-lyuh') [Fr.] surroundings; environment.

m. ext'érieur (me-lyuh' ek-sta're-ur") external environment.

m. int'érieur (me-lyuh' an-ta're-ur") internal environment; the blood and lymph in which the cells are bathed.

milium (mil'e-um), pl. *mil'ia* [L.] a small, whitish or yellowish nodule in the skin, usually a retention cyst of a sebaceous gland or hair follicle.

milk (milk) 1. a nutrient fluid produced by the mammary gland of many animals for nourishment of the young. 2. a liquid (emulsion or suspension) resembling the secretion of the mammary gland.

acidophilus m., milk fermented with cultures of *Lactobacillus acidophilus;* used in gastrointestinal disorders to modify the bacterial flora of the intestinal tract.

m.-alkali syndrome, ingestion of milk and absorbable alkali in excess amounts, resulting in kidney damage and elevated blood calcium levels.

casein m., a prepared milk containing very little salts and sugars and a large amount of fat and casein.

certified m., milk whose purity is certified by a committee of physicians or a medical milk commission.

condensed m., milk that has been partly evaporated and sweetened with sugar.

dialyzed m., milk from which the sugar has been removed by dialysis through a parchment membrane.

evaporated m., milk prepared by evaporation of half of its water content.

m. fever, 1. mild puerperal septicemia. 2. a fever

said to attend the establishment of lactation after delivery. 3. an endemic fever said to be caused by the use of unwholesome cow's milk.

fortified m., milk made more nutritious by addition of cream or vitamins.

homogenized m., milk treated so the fats form a permanent emulsion and the cream does not separate.

m. of magnesia, a suspension containing 7 to 8.5 per cent of magnesium hydroxide, used as an antacid and laxative.

modified m., cow's milk made to correspond to composition of human milk.

protein m., milk modified to have a relatively low content of carbohydrate and fat and a relatively high protein content.

Miller-Abbott tube (mil'er ab'ot) a double-channel intestinal tube used for diagnosing and treating obstructive lesions of the small intestine. The tube is inserted via a nostril and gently passed through the stomach and into the small intestine. The Miller-Abbott tube is often used in the treatment of INTESTINAL OBSTRUCTION. Care must be used in irrigating the tube and in attaching it to a suction apparatus because of the possibility of confusing the two lumina. The lumen marked suction is used for irrigations and suction; the other lumen leads to the small rubber bag intended to hold the tube in place. The introduction of too large an amount of fluid into the bag would lead to rupture of the intestine.

milli- (mil'e) word element, *one-thousandth;* used in naming units of measurement to designate an amount 10^{-3} the size of the unit to which it is joined, e.g., milligram (0.001 gm).

milliampere (mil"e-am'pēr) one-thousandth of an ampere.

milliampere-minute (mil"e-am"pēr-min'ut) a unit of electricity equivalent to that delivered by a current of 1 milliampere strength acting for one minute.

millicoulomb (mil"i-koo'lom) one-thousandth (10^{-3}) coulomb; abbreviated mcoul.

millicurie (mil'i-ku're) one-thousandth (10^{-3}) curie; abbreviated mCi or mc.

millicurie-hour (mil'i-ku're-owr") a unit of dose equivalent to that obtained by exposure for one hour to radioactive material disintegrating at the rate of 3.7×10^7 atoms per second; abbreviated mc.-hr.

milliequivalent (mil"e-e-kwiv'ah-lent) the number of grams of a solute contained in 1 milliliter of a normal solution; abbreviated mEq.

milligram (mil'i-gram) one-thousandth of a gram; equivalent of 0.015432 grain avoirdupois or apothecaries' weight; abbreviated mg.

milliliter (mil'i-le"ter) one-thousandth of a liter; equivalent of 16.23 minims; abbreviated ml.

millimeter (mil'i-me"ter) one-thousandth of a meter; equivalent of 0.039 inch; abbreviated mm.

millimicro- (mil"i-mi'kro) word element desig-

nating 10^{-3} (one-thousandth) of 10^{-6} (one-millionth), or 10^{-9} (one-billionth), part of the unit to which it is joined; now being supplanted by the prefix nano-.

millimicrocurie (mil"i-mi"kro-ku're) one-thousandth (10^{-3}) microcurie, or 10^{-9} curie; abbreviated mμc.

millimicrogram (mil"i-mi"kro-gram) one-thousandth (10^{-3}) microgram, or 10^{-9} gram; abbreviated mμg.

millimicron (mil"i-mi'kron) one-thousandth of a micron (10^{-6} mm., or 10 angstroms); abbreviated mμ.

milliosmole (mil"e-oz'mōl) one-thousandth of an osmole.

millirad (mil'i-rad) a unit of absorbed radiation dose, 10^{-3} rad; abbreviated mrad.

milliroentgen (mil"i-rent'gen) a unit of dose equal to one-thousandth (10^{-3}) roentgen; abbreviated mr.

milliunit (mil"e-u'nit) one-thousandth part of a unit (10^{-3}).

millivolt (mil'i-volt) one-thousandth of a volt; abbreviated mv.

Milontin (mi-lon'tin) trademark for preparations of phensuximide, an anticonvulsant.

Milpath (mil'path) trademark for a preparation of meprobamate and tridihexethyl chloride, a tranquilizer.

Milroy's disease (mil'royz) a form of hereditary edema of one or both legs.

Miltown (mil'town) trademark for a preparation of meprobamate, a tranquilizer.

min. minim; minimum; minute.

Minamata disease (min"ah-mah'tah) a severe neurologic disorder due to poisoning by organic mercury and leading to permanent disability or death.

Mincard (min'kard) trademark for a preparation of aminometradine, a diuretic.

mind (mīnd) the faculty by which one is aware of surroundings and by which he is able to experience emotions, remember, reason and make decisions.

mineral (min'er-al) a nonorganic homogeneous substance. There are 19 or more minerals forming the mineral composition of the body; at least 13 are essential to health. These minerals must be supplied in the diet and generally can be supplied by a varied or mixed diet of animal and vegetable products which meet the energy and protein needs. The Food and Nutrition Board of the National Research Council has established recommended daily intakes only for calcium and iron. These two minerals plus iodine are the three elements most frequently missing in the diet. Zinc, iron, copper, magnesium and potassium are the five minerals that are most frequently involved in disturbances of metabolism.

Minerals are electropositive or electronegative. Combinations of electropositive and electronegative elements lead to the formation of salts such as sodium chloride and calcium phosphate.

mineral oil, an oil obtained from petroleum, sometimes used as a laxative. It acts as a lubricant on the intestinal walls. Taken regularly as a laxative, it can be harmful because it prevents absorption of the fat-soluble vitamins. It has also been known to seep into the lungs, causing pneumonia, especially in older people.

mineralization (min″er-al-ĭ-za′shun) the addition of mineral matter to the body.

mineralocorticoid (min″er-al-o-kor′tĭ-koid) any of the hormones of the adrenal cortex having effects on the electrolytes of the extracellular fluid, particularly sodium, potassium and chloride. Aldosterone is the principal mineralocorticoid, and others are desoxycorticosterone and corticosterone, which is also a glucocorticoid. These hormones increase the renal tubular reabsorption of sodium and increase the renal tubular excretion of potassium. Thus, a deficiency of the mineralocorticoids results in excessive loss of sodium (and, consequently, water) in the urine and retention of potassium in the extracellular fluid.

The mineralocorticoids are essential to life because they indirectly affect the fluid and electrolyte balance of the body. Without them there is a decrease in blood volume which soon produces a diminished cardiac output followed by a shocklike state and eventually death.

The body increases the output of mineralocorticoids when the extracellular concentration of sodium falls below normal, or when increased blood pressure is needed to cope with physical stress (see also ALARM REACTION.)

minim (min′im) a unit of volume in the apothecaries system, equivalent to 0.0616 ml.

miocardia (mi″o-kar′de-ah) the contraction of the heart; systole.

Miochol (mi′o-kol) trademark for a preparation of acetylcholine chloride, a miotic.

miopus (mi′o-pus) a fetal monster with two fused heads, one face being rudimentary.

miosis (mi-o′sis) excessive contraction of the pupil.

miotic (mi-ot′ik) 1. pertaining to, characterized by or causing miosis. 2. an agent that causes contraction of the pupil.

miracidium (mi″rah-sid′e-um), pl. *miracid′ia* [Gr.] the free-swimming larva of a trematode parasite which emerges from an egg and penetrates the body of a snail host.

mire (mēr) [Fr.] a figure on the arm of an ophthalmometer the image of which is reflected on the cornea; used to measure corneal astigmatism.

miscarriage (mis-kar′ij) the lay term used to designate loss of the fetus before it is viable (see also ABORTION).

miscible (mis′ĭ-bl) susceptible of being mixed.

misocainia (mis″o-ki′ne-ah) aversion to new ideas.

misogamy (mĭ-sog′ah-me) morbid aversion to marriage.

misogyny (mĭ-soj′ĭ-ne) aversion to women.

misopedia (mis″o-pe′de-ah) morbid dislike of children.

Mitchell's disease (mich′elz) erythromelalgia.

mite (mīt) an arthropod of the order Acarina, characterized by minute size, usually transparent or semitransparent body, and other features distinguishing them from the ticks; they may be free living or parasitic on animals or plants, and may produce various irritations of the skin.
  harvest m., chigger.
  itch m., mange m., *Sarcoptes scabiei.*

mithridatism (mith′rĭ-da″tizm) acquisition of immunity to a poison by ingestion of gradually increasing amounts of it.

miticide (mi′tĭ-sīd) an agent destructive to mites.

mitochondrion (mi″to-kon′dre-on), pl. *mitochon′-dria* [Gr.] a filamentous or granular component (organelle) of cytoplasm, the principal site of oxidative reactions by which the energy in foodstuff is made available for endergonic processes in the cell.

mitogen (mi′to-jen) an agent that induces mitosis.

mitogenesis (mi″to-jen′ĕ-sis) the induction of mitosis in a cell.

mitome (mi′tōm) a thready network of protoplasm.

mitosis (mi-to′sis) the process by which a cell splits into two new cells, each daughter cell having the same number and kind of chromosomes as the parent cell. adj. **mitot′ic.**

The first step in mitosis is duplication of all genes and chromosomes. To accomplish this the cell must double its content of DEOXYRIBONUCLEIC ACID (DNA). Chromosomes are composed of the DNA molecule loosely bound with protein; genes are segments of the DNA molecule. Since the DNA molecule has the ability to duplicate itself (replication), it is possible for the cell to form two identical sets of chromosomes and genes. After they are duplicated they divide between the two separate nuclei that have formed. The final step in mitosis is the splitting of the parent cell into two identical daughter cells, each with a full complement of genes and chromosomes.

Most cells of the body are continually growing and reproducing, so that when the old cells die the new ones take their place; thus, mitosis is a continuous process. It is obvious that this reproduction must take place in an orderly manner, but the exact way in which cell growth and reproduction are regulated is not completely understood. Although certain cells such as the blood-forming cells of the bone marrow and the stratum germinativum of the skin grow and reproduce continually, other cells such as neurons (nerve cells) do not reproduce during a person's lifetime. Neoplastic disorders such as cancer are a result of the abnormal and unrestricted growth and reproduction of certain body cells.

Germ cells reproduce by the process of meiosis.

mitosome (mi′to-sōm) a body formed from the spindle fibers of the preceding mitosis; a spindle remnant.

mitral (mi′tral) shaped like a miter.
  m. stenosis, a narrowing of the left atrioventricular orifice.

m. valve, the valve between the left atrium and the left ventricle of the heart; it is composed of two cusps, anterior and posterior. Called also the bicuspid valve.

mittelschmerz (mit'el-shmerts) [Ger.] pain midway between the menstrual periods.

mixotrophic (mik″so-trof′ik) having nutritional characters of both animals and plants.

mixture (miks′tūr) a combination of different drugs or ingredients, as a fluid with other fluids or solids, or of a solid with a liquid.

ml. milliliter.

M.L.A. Medical Library Association.

M.L.D. minimum lethal dose.

mm. millimeter; muscles.

mμ. millimicron

Mn chemical symbol, *manganese.*

M'Naghten rule (mik-naw′ten) "to establish a defense on the ground of insanity, it must be clearly proved that at the time of committing the act the party accused was laboring under such a defect of reason from disease of the mind as not to know the nature or quality of the act he was doing, or, if he did know it, that he did not know he was doing what was wrong."

mnemonics (ne-mon′iks) cultivation of the memory.

M.O. Medical Officer.

Mo chemical symbol, *molybdenum.*

mobilization (mo″bĭ-lĭ-za′shun) the rendering of a fixed part movable.
   stapes m., surgical correction of immobility of the stapes in treatment of deafness.

modality (mo-dal′ĭ-te) 1. a physical agent used therapeutically. 2. in homeopathy, a condition that modifies a drug action. 3. a specific sensory entity.

mode (mōd) in statistics, the value or item in a variations curve that shows the maximal frequency of occurrence.

Moderil (mod′er-il) trademark for a preparation of rescinnamine, a tranquilizer and antihypertensive.

modiolus (mo-di′o-lus) the central pillar or columella of the cochlea.

Modumate (mod′u-māt) trademark for a preparation of arginine and glutamic acid, a nutrient used for the treatment of ammonia intoxication due to liver failure.

Moebius' disease (me′be-oos) periodic migraine with paralysis of the oculomotor muscles.

M.O.H. Medical Officer of Health.

moiety (moi′ĕ-te) any part or portion.

mol (mol) mole (2).

molality (mo-lal′ĭ-te) the number of moles of a solute per kilogram of pure solvent.

molar (mo′lar) 1. pertaining to a mass. 2. pertaining to a mole. 3. adapted for grinding, as a molar tooth.

molarity (mo-lar′ĭ-te) the number of moles of a solute per liter of solution.

mold (mōld) 1. a true fungus. 2. a matrix or cavity in which something is shaped. 3. to shape, or give form to.

molding (mōld′ing) the shaping of a child's head to the size and shape of the birth canal.

mole (mōl) 1. a fleshy mass formed in the uterus by abortive development of an ovum. 2. that amount of a chemical compound whose mass in grams is equivalent to its formula mass. 3. a fleshy growth or blemish on the skin; a NEVUS.
   hairy m., hairy nevus.
   hydatid m., hydatidiform m., hydatiform m., a mole formed by the proliferation of the chorionic villi, resulting in a mass of cysts that resembles a bunch of grapes.
   pigmented m., nevus pigmentosus.

molecular (mo-lek′u-lar) of, pertaining to or composed of molecules.
   m. biology, study of the biochemical and biophysical aspects of structure and function of genes and other subcellular entities, and of such specific proteins as hemoglobins, enzymes and hormones; it provides knowledge of cellular differentiation and metabolism and of comparative evolution.
   m. weight, the weight of a molecule of a chemical compound as compared with the weight of an atom of hydrogen; it is equal to the sum of the weights of its constituent atoms.

molecule (mol′ĕ-kūl) a very small mass of matter; an aggregation of atoms composing the smallest unit of a compound possessing its characteristic properties.

molimen (mo-li′men) the monthly effort of the menstrual flow.

mollities (mo-lish′e-ēz) abnormal softening.
   m. os′sium, osteomalacia.

molluscum (mŏ-lus′kum) a soft growth. adj., **mollus′cous.**
   m. contagio′sum, a viral infection of the skin and occasionally of the conjunctiva. It is fairly common, usually affects children and is mildly contagious. The source of infection and method of transmission often are unknown.
   The disease is characterized by soft tumor-like lesions which first appear as papules with depressed centers containing a curdlike substance. If untreated the lesions may enlarge to the size of a bean. The lesions may occur over the entire body but affect chiefly the hands, face and genitalia.
   Treatment consists of curettage or light cauterization with an electric cautery.
   m. fibro′sum, m. sim′plex, multiple fibroma of the skin.

mol. wt. molecular weight.

molybdenum (mo-lib′dĕ-num) a chemical element, atomic number 42, atomic weight 95.94, symbol Mo. (See table of ELEMENTS.)

momentum (mo-men′tum) the quantity of motion; the product of mass by velocity.

monad (mo′nad) 1. a single-celled protozoon. 2. a univalent radical or element.

monarthritis (mon″ar-thri′tis) inflammation of a single joint.

monarticular (mon″ar-tik′u-lar) pertaining to one joint.

monathetosis (mon-ath″ĕ-to′sis) athetosis of one part of the body.

monatomic (mon″ah-tom′ik) 1. containing one atom. 2. univalent.

Mondor's disease (mon′dorz) inflammation of a large subcutaneous vein crossing the lateral chest region and breast, the vessel appearing as a tender cord.

monecious (mon-e′shus) requiring only one host for completion of the entire life cycle.

monesthetic (mon″es-thet′ik) affecting a single sense or sensation.

mongolism (mon′go-lizm) a congenital condition involving some degree of mental retardation and various physical malformations. The name is based on characteristic facial traits resembling somewhat those of persons of the Mongolian race. The term mongolism is now considered to be inaccurate and undesirable and is being replaced by the term DOWN'S SYNDROME or trisomy 21. The latter name refers to the presence of three twenty-first chromosomes, found in those with Down's syndrome, instead of the usual pair.

monilethrix (mo-nil′ĕ-thriks) a disease in which the hair becomes brittle and beaded.

Monilia (mo-nil′e-ah) former name of a genus of parasitic fungi, now called Candida.

moniliasis (mo″nĭ-li′ah-sis) candidiasis.

moniliform (mo-nil′i-form) beaded; having the appearance of a string of beads.

monitor (mon′ĭ-tor) 1. to check constantly on a given condition or phenomenon, e.g., blood pressure or heart or respiration rate. 2. an apparatus by which certain conditions or phenomena can be constantly observed and recorded.

mono- (mon′o) word element [Gr.], one.

monoaminomonophosphatide (mon″o-am″ĭ-no-mon″o-fos′fah-tīd) a phosphatide containing one atom of nitrogen and one of phosphorus to the molecule.

monobasic (mon″o-ba′sik) having but one atom of replaceable hydrogen.

monobenzone (mon″o-ben′zōn) a white, crystalline powder used as a melanin-inhibiting agent.

monoblast (mon′o-blast) the cell that is the precursor of the mature monocyte.

monoblastoma (mon″o-blas-to′mah) a tumor containing monoblasts and monocytes.

monoblepsia (mon″o-blep′se-ah) blindness to all colors but one.

monobrachius (mon″o-bra′ke-us) a fetus with but one arm.

monobulia (mon″o-bu′le-ah) concentrated wishing on one thing only.

monocellular (mon″o-sel′u-lar) unicellular.

monocephalus (mon″o-sef′ah-lus) a fetal monster with two bodies and one head.

monochorea (mon″o-ko-re′ah) chorea affecting but one part.

monochorial, monochorionic (mon″o-ko′re-al), (mon″o-ko″re-on′ik) pertaining to or characterized by the presence of a single chorion.

monochromatic (mon″o-kro-mat′ik) pertaining to a single color.

monococcus (mon″o-kok′us) a form of coccus consisting of single cells.

monocontaminated (mon″o-kon-tam′ĭ-nāt″ed) infected by only one species of microorganisms or a single contaminating agent.

monocular (mon-ok′u-lar) pertaining to one eye.

monoculus (mon-ok′u-lus) 1. a bandage for one eye. 2. a cyclops.

monocyclic (mon″o-si′klik) in chemistry, having an atomic structure containing only one ring.

monocyesis (mon″o-si-e′sis) pregnancy with a single fetus.

monocyte (mon′o-sīt) the largest of the leukocytes, 9 to 12 microns in diameter, with a considerably dented nucleus; normally constituting 5 to 10 per cent of the leukocytes of the blood. adj., **monocyt′ic.**

monocytopenia (mon″o-si-to-pe′ne-ah) deficiency of monocytes in the blood.

monocytosis (mon″o-si-to′sis) excess of monocytes in the blood.

monodactylism (mon″o-dak′tĭ-lizm) the presence of only one finger or toe on a hand or foot.

monodiplopia (mon″o-dĭ-plo′pe-ah) double vision in one eye.

Monodral (mon′o-dral) trademark for preparations of penthienate, used in parasympathetic blockade.

monoecious (mon-e′shus) 1. having reproductive organs typical of both sexes in a single individual. 2. requiring only one host for completion of the entire life cycle.

monogenesis (mon″o-jen′ĕ-sis) nonsexual reproduction.

monogenic (mon″o-jen′ik) pertaining to or influenced by a single gene.

monogenous (mon-oj′ĕ-nus) produced asexually.

monogerminal (mon″o-jer′mĭ-nal) developed from one ovum.

monoglyceride (mon″o-glis′er-īd) a compound consisting of one molecule of fatty acid esterified to glycerin.

monoiodotyrosine (mon″o-i-o″do-ti′ro-sēn) a derivative of tyrosine containing one atom of iodine, found in the thyroid gland.

monolocular (mon″o-lok′u-lar) having but one cavity.

monomania (mon″o-ma′ne-ah) a logical system of delusions based on a single false premise.

monomastigote (mon″o-mas′tĭ-gōt) having a single flagellum.

monomelic (mon″o-mel′ik) affecting one limb.

monomer (mon′o-mer) a simple molecule of relatively low molecular weight.
   fibrin m., the material resulting from the action of thrombin on fibrinogen, which then polymerizes to form fibrin.

monomeric (mon″o-mer′ik) pertaining to a single segment.

monometallic (mon″o-mĕ-tal′ik) having one atom of a metal in a molecule.

monomicrobic (mon″o-mi-kro′bik) pertaining to or caused by a single variety of pathogenic microorganisms.

monomorphic (mon″o-mor′fik) existing in only one form.

monomphalus (mon-om′fah-lus) a double fetal monster joined at the navel.

monomyoplegia (mon″o-mi″o-ple′je-ah) paralysis of a single muscle.

monomyositis (mon″o-mi″o-si′tis) inflammation of a single muscle.

mononeural (mon″o-nu′ral) supplied by a single nerve.

mononeuritis (mon″o-nu-ri′tis) inflammation of a single nerve.
   m. mul′tiplex, simultaneous inflammation of several nerves remote from one another.

monont (mon′ont) schizont.

mononuclear (mon″o-nu′kle-ar) having only one nucleus.

mononucleosis (mon″o-nu″kle-o′sis) excess of mononuclear leukocytes in the blood.
   infectious m., an acute infectious disease that causes changes in the leukocytes; called also glandular fever.
   The exact cause of mononucleosis is not yet known, but it is widely considered to be a viral infection. Transmission of the disease is not clearly understood. It occurs more frequently in the spring and affects primarily children and young adults. Although epidemics have been reported, some authorities doubt that the disorder has been the same in all instances.
   SYMPTOMS. Generally, after an incubation period of uncertain duration (1 week to several weeks), headache, sore throat, mental and physical fatigue, severe weakness and symptoms typical of influenza develop. Skin rashes may also occur.
   Diagnosis can be confirmed by the finding of a marked increase in the number of mononuclear leukocytes present in the patient's blood. Another diagnostic test that indicates mononucleosis is the Paul-Bunnell heterophil agglutination test, which demonstrates the presence of certain antibodies

capable of causing clumping of cells in a sample of sheep's blood.
   Occasionally, in about 8 to 10 per cent of all cases of mononucleosis, the liver is involved and jaundice occurs, resulting in a condition that resembles infectious hepatitis. In rare cases, the heart, lungs and central nervous system may also be affected. The spleen may become enlarged; one of the complications, serious but rare, is rupture of the spleen. The lymph nodes and spleen may both remain enlarged for some time after other symptoms have disappeared.
   TREATMENT. Treatment is chiefly symptomatic. Bed rest is especially important in the early stages of the disease, or later if the liver is involved. There is as yet no specific treatment for mononucleosis, and no immunization is available. Headache and sore throat may be relieved by aspirin and gargles.
   Although the more obvious symptoms of mononucleosis may disappear after a period of rest, sufficient rest and curtailed activities must be maintained in order to improve the patient's severely weakened condition and to prevent recurrence of the disease. There is often mental as well as physical fatigue, especially among students, and in these cases some mental depression may accompany convalescence. A rest from schoolwork for a month or two is occasionally advisable in cases of this sort.

mononucleotide (mon″o-nu′kle-o-tīd) a compound of phosphoric acid and a glucoside or pentoside, obtained by the digestion or hydrolytic decomposition of nucleic acid.

monoparesis (mon″o-par′ĕ-sis) paresis of a single part.

monoparesthesia (mon″o-par″es-the′ze-ah) paresthesia of a single part.

monopathy (mo-nop′ah-the) a disease affecting a single part.

monophthalmus (mon″of-thal′mus) a fetus with one eye.

monophyletic (mon″o-fi-let′ik) descended from a single source.

monoplegia (mon″o-ple′je-ah) paralysis of a single part.

monopolar (mon″o-po′lar) having a single pole.

monops (mon′ops) a fetus with a single eye.

monopus (mon′o-pus) a fetus with only one foot.

monorchis (mon-or′kis) a person having only one testis in the scrotum.

monorchism (mon′or-kizm) the condition of having only one descended testis.

monosaccharide (mon″o-sak′ah-rīd) a carbohydrate that cannot be broken down to simpler substances by acid hydrolysis.

monosexual (mon″o-seks′u-al) showing characteristics or traits of one sex only.

monosomy (mon″o-so′me) existence in a cell of only one instead of the normal diploid pair of a particular chromosome. adj., **monoso′mic.**

Monosporium (mon″o-spo′re-um) a genus of fungi.

M. apiosper'mum, a fungus that is one of the causative organisms of maduromycosis.

monostotic (mon″os-tot′ik) affecting a single bone.

monosymptomatic (mon″o-simp″to-mat′ik) having only one symptom.

monosynaptic (mon″o-sĭ-nap′tik) pertaining to or passing through a single synapse.

monoterminal (mon″o-ter′mĭ-nal) using one terminal only in giving electric treatment.

Monotheamin (mon″o-the′ah-min) trademark for preparations of theophylline ethanolamine, a diuretic and bronchodilator.

monothermia (mon″o-ther′me-ah) a condition in which the body temperature remains the same throughout the day.

monotrichous (mon-ot′rĭ-kus) having a single flagellum; applied to a bacterial cell.

monovalent (mon″o-va′lent) 1. having a valence of one. 2. capable of binding one complement only.

monoxenous (mo-nok′sĕ-nus) requiring only one host to complete the life cycle.

monoxide (mon-ok′sīd) an oxide with one oxygen atom in the molecule.

monozygotic (mon″o-zi-got′ik) pertaining to or derived from a single zygote (fertilized ovum); said of TWINS.

mons (mons), pl. *mon'tes* [L.] a prominence.
  m. pu′bis, the rounded fleshy prominence over the symphysis pubis.
  m. ven′eris, a name given the mons pubis in the female.

monster (mon′ster) a fetus that shows developmental anomalies so pronounced that they interfere with the general or local development of the body and cause it to differ from the normal form of the species.

monstriparity (mon″strĭ-par′ĭ-te) the act of giving birth to a monster.

monstrosity (mon-stros′ĭ-te) 1. great congenital deformity. 2. a monster or teratism.

Montgomery straps (mont-gom′er-e) straps made of lengths of adhesive tape, used to secure dressings that must be changed frequently.

monticulus (mon-tik′u-lus) pl. *montic'uli* [L.] a small eminence.
  m. cerebel′li, the projecting part of the superior vermis cerebelli.

mood (mōōd) a prevailing emotional tone or feeling.

Moraxella (mo-rak-sel′ah) a genus of Schizomycetes found as parasites and pathogens in warm-blooded animals.
  M. liquefa′ciens, a form found in conjunctivitis in man.

morbid (mor′bid) 1. pertaining to, characteristic of or characterized by disease or abnormality. 2. pathologic or abnormal.

morbidity (mor-bid′ĭ-te) 1. the condition of being diseased. 2. the proportion of disease to health in a community.

morbific (mor-bif′ik) causing or inducing disease.

morbilli (mor-bil′i) [L.] measles.

morbilliform (mor-bil′ĭ-form) resembling measles.

morbus (mor′bus) [L.] disease.

morcellation (mor″sĕ-la′shun) division of a tumor or organ, followed by piecemeal removal.

mordant (mor′dant) a substance used to fix a stain or dye.

morgue (morg) a place where dead bodies may be temporarily kept, for identification or until claimed for burial.

moria (mo′re-ah) a morbid tendency to joke.

moribund (mor′ĭ-bund) in a dying state.

Mornidine (mor′nĭ-dēn) trademark for preparations of pipamazine, an antiemetic.

morning sickness nausea and vomiting occurring during pregnancy, usually during the early months. Between 50 and 65 per cent of all women experience some degree of morning sickness at some time during pregnancy, and about one-third are affected to the point of vomiting. Morning sickness usually begins during the fifth or sixth week of pregnancy. Some cases may clear up in 1 to 3 weeks; others may persist until the fourteenth or sixteenth week.

In most cases, morning sickness begins with a feeling of nausea on arising. Despite its name, however, morning sickness is not always limited to the morning.

In rare cases—affecting about one woman in 200 —HYPEREMESIS GRAVIDARUM, or pernicious vomiting of pregnancy, may develop. If unchecked, it may result in such symptoms as dehydration and weight loss, and may threaten the life of both mother and the unborn child.

CAUSES. The actual causes of morning sickness are not known. It is believed that hunger is a contributing factor. It is also thought that there may be a metabolic upset that occurs as a result of pregnancy and contributes to this condition. It is likely, however, that morning sickness is often psychologic in origin.

TREATMENT. Morning sickness is little more than a discomfort, and usually requires no treatment. If a woman can be diverted from thinking about it, the condition tends to lessen or to pass away entirely. If possible, a woman should have something light to eat before getting out of bed in the morning. This could be crackers or weak tea, possibly left on the bedside table at night, the tea in a thermos bottle; or better still, she should have breakfast in bed. After eating, she should rest for about 15 minutes before getting up.

Excessive fluid intake should be avoided. At meals, it is best to eat dry foods first. Liquids should be taken last and should be sipped in small quantities. Instead of three large meals, small meals should be eaten at more frequent intervals. It is also advisable to rest after each meal. Dry foods, such as crackers, or soft foods eaten every 2 hours until the nausea is over can also be helpful.

Sights, smells and foods that may be disturbing should be avoided, as should greasy foods, fats and butter. Also to be avoided are those vegetables which are hard to digest, such as cabbage, cauliflower, cucumbers and onions. In certain cases, the physician may prescribe an antinauseant.

moro reflex (mo′ro) flexion of an infant's thighs and knees, fanning and then clenching of fingers, with arms first thrown outward and then brought together as though embracing something; produced by a sudden stimulus, such as striking the table on either side of the child, and seen normally in the newborn. Called also embrace reflex.

moron (mo′ron) a mentally defective person whose mental age is between 8 and 12 years, usually requiring special training and supervision.

morphallaxis (mor″fah-lak′sis) renewal of a lost tissue or part by reorganization of the remaining part of the body of an animal.

morphea (mor-fe′ah) a skin disease marked by pinkish patches bordered by a purplish areola; also called localized scleroderma.

morphine (mor′fēn) an opium alkaloid, a narcotic analgesic and respiratory depressant, usually used as morphine sulfate. The use of morphine carries with it the dangers of addiction (see DRUG ADDICTION) and tolerance, so that increasingly larger doses are needed to achieve the desired effect. Since morphine is a powerful respiratory depressant, the drug should be withheld and the physician notified when the patient's respirations are less than 12 per minute.

morphinism (mor′fĭ-nizm) a morbid state due to morphine.

morphium (mor′fe-um) morphine.

morphodifferentiation (mor″fo-dif″er-en″she-a′-shun) arrangement of formative cells so as to establish the future shape and size of an organ.

morphogenesis (mor″fo-jen′ĕ-sis) the developmental changes of growth and differentiation occurring in the organization of the body and its parts. adj., **morphogenet′ic.**

morphology (mor″fol′o-je) the science of the forms and structure of organized beings. adj., **morpholog′-ic.**

morphometry (mor-fom′ĕ-tre) the measurement of forms.

-morphous (mor′fus) word element [Gr.] indicating the manner of shape or form.

Morquio's disease (mor-ke′oz) familial osteochondrodystrophy.

mors (mors) [L.] death.

morsus (mor′sus) [L.] bite.
  m. diab′oli, the fimbriated end of a uterine tube.

mortal (mor′tal) 1. destined to die. 2. causing or terminating in death.

mortality (mor-tal′ĭ-te) 1. the quality of being mortal. 2. the death rate; the ratio of total number of deaths to the total number of population. The mortality rate of a disease is the ratio of the number of deaths from a given disease to the total number of cases of that disease.

mortar (mor′tar) a vessel with a rounded internal surface, used with a pestle, for reducing a solid to a powder or producing a homogeneous mixture of solids.

Morton's disease (mor′tunz) tenderness or pain in the metatarsophalangeal joint of the third or fourth toe.

morula (mor′u-lah) a solid mass of cells (blastomeres) resembling a mulberry, formed by cleavage of a fertilized ovum.

Morvan's disease (mor′vanz) syringomyelia.

mosaic (mo-za′ik) a pattern made of numerous small pieces fitted together; in genetics, occurrence in an individual of two or more cell populations each having a different chromosome complement.

mosaicism (mo-za′ĭ-sizm) the presence in an individual of cells derived from the same zygote, but differing in chromosomal constitution.

mosquito (mos-ke′to) a blood-sucking winged insect, chiefly of the genus Aedes, Anopheles or Culex. Certain species are responsible for the transmission of disease, including yellow fever and MALARIA.

motile (mo′til) having a spontaneous but not conscious or volitional movement.

motility (mo-til′ĭ-te) the ability to move spontaneously.

motion sickness discomfort felt by some people on a moving boat, train, airplane or automobile, or even on an elevator or a swing. The discomfort is caused by irregular and abnormal motion that disturbs the organs of balance located in the inner ear. There may be mild symptoms of nausea, dizziness or headache, as well as pallor and cold perspiration. In more acute cases, there may be vomiting and sometimes prostration.

Though most people quickly adapt to travel by airplane, ship and automobile, few are wholly immune to motion sickness. Even astronauts become ill if the inner ear organs of balance are continuously stimulated by unusual motion. Fortunately, most cases of motion sickness vanish quickly once the journey is over, leaving no ill effects.

CAUSES. The inner ear possesses three semicircular canals, located at right angles in three different planes. Man is accustomed to movement in the horizontal plane, which stimulates certain semicircular canals; but he is not accustomed to vertical movements, such as the motion of an elevator or a ship pitching at sea. These vertical movements stimulate the semicircular canals in an unusual way, producing the sensation of nausea, or motion sickness.

Anxiety, grief or other emotions can also cause motion sickness. A person unaccustomed to traveling by boat or airplane may be apprehensive or nervous and therefore may develop symptoms of nausea. Some individuals with previous experience of motion sickness become ill on a boat at dock or on an airplane prior to take-off.

Airsickness usually occurs during a bumpy flight caused by stormy weather or turbulent air. However, it may also be triggered by poorly ventilated cabins, hunger, digestive upset, overindulgence in food and drink and unpleasant odors, particularly tobacco smoke.

TREATMENT. Certain antihistamines have proved highly effective in treating symptoms of seasickness. Like nerve depressants, they may be used alone or in combination with mild sedatives. Those who suffer from motion sickness should ask their physician what he recommends before they embark on a trip. Symptoms may also be reduced if the seasick person rests lying down, with his head low, in a comfortable, well aired place.

PREVENTION.   Being rested and in good health prior to a journey helps to prevent motion sickness. A cup of strong coffee taken just before departure may also be helpful. Alcoholic beverages in moderation make some people less nervous and thus help ward off motion sickness; however, in excess they can encourage the condition.

During a voyage by boat, it is advisable for the passenger to remain near the center of the ship, where there will be the least motion. Ample fresh air and exercise and avoidance of stuffy rooms and disagreeable smells are also good precautions. The traveler should keep comfortably warm and avoid overeating and rich foods.

For those traveling by air, a sedative or tranquilizer taken a half hour before departure, and small, easily digested meals taken during the flight help to prevent airsickness. The passenger who experiences motion sickness may benefit from reclining in his seat as far as possible and closing his eyes.

Carsickness is often relieved if the journey is interrupted for short walks in the fresh air and by keeping a window open. Children will frequently find it helpful to glance down, and to refrain from reading. Tobacco smoke can also be an aggravating factor.

motoceptor   (mo′to-sep″tor) any muscle sense receptor.

motoneuron   (mo″to-nu′ron) a motor neuron; an efferent neuron possessing motor function.

motor   (mo′tor) 1. pertaining to motion. 2. a muscle, nerve or center that effects movements.

mottling   (mot′ling) discoloration in irregular areas.

moulage   (moo-lahzh′) [Fr.] a wax model of a structure or lesion.

mould   (mōld) mold.

mounding   (mownd′ing) the rising in a lump of a wasting muscle when struck.

mount   (mownt) to prepare specimens and slides for study.

mountain fever   1. Colorado tick fever. 2. Rocky Mountain spotted fever. 3. brucellosis.

m. sickness, disturbances due to poor adjustment to high altitude. Symptoms include fatigability, shortness of breath, polycythemia, cyanosis and epistaxis.

mouse   (mows) a small rodent, various species of which are used in laboratory experiments.

joint m., a movable fragment of synovial membrane, cartilage or other body within a joint; usually associated with degenerative osteoarthritis and osteochondritis dissecans.

peritoneal m., a free body in the peritoneal cavity, probably a small detached mass of omentum, sometimes visible radiographically.

mouth   (mowth) an opening, especially the oral cavity, forming the beginning of the DIGESTIVE SYSTEM. In it the chewing of food takes place. The mouth is also the site of the organs of taste and the teeth, tongue and lips. Not only is the mouth the entrance to the body for food and sometimes air, but it is a major organ of speech and emotional expression.

STRUCTURE.   Except for the teeth, the interior of the mouth is covered with mucous membrane. This thin lining extends out from the front of the mouth to form the lips. Salivary glands lie above and below the mouth and produce saliva, a liquid that protects the delicate membranes and mixes with food in the first step of digestion of food.

The palate forms the roof of the mouth. The front two-thirds of the palate comprises the hard palate, and the back third, the soft palate. The soft palate is hinged to the hard palate and is flanked on both sides by the tonsils. In the middle of the soft palate is the uvula, a projection pointing down to the tongue. At the root of the tongue, below the uvula, lies the epiglottis.

DISORDERS.   Because of its special functions the mouth is constantly exposed to infection and irritation. These can affect the whole mouth generally or only certain parts, such as the tongue.

Inflammation of the mouth, or STOMATITIS, can indicate the presence of either a mild or severe disease. Local conditions include THRUSH, TRENCH MOUTH, and herpes simplex. Generalized diseases can also give rise to inflammation of the mouth; these include diphtheria, tuberculosis, blood dyscrasias, vitamin deficiencies and syphilis.

CANCER can afflict the sides of the mouth, the lips, the tongue and occasionally the salivary glands. Continued irritation, such as pipe smoking, is thought to be a cause of many mouth cancers. Any persistent sore or swelling should be promptly examined by a physician.

Birth defects affecting the mouth include CLEFT LIP AND CLEFT PALATE. Both have the same cause: failure of adjacent parts of the body to unite properly in fetal life. A cleft lip, or harelip, involves a split in the upper lip. Sometimes the cleft extends into the upper jaw, the floor of the nose and the palate. The resulting deformity of nose and mouth interferes with sucking and speech unless corrected by surgery. A cleft palate, which may cause difficulties in speaking and eating, signifies a cleavage in the uvula and the soft palate. Both conditions are successfully corrected by surgery.

trench m., inflammation of the gingivae and oral mucous membrane (see also TRENCH MOUTH).

mouth-to-mouth resuscitation   a method of ARTIFICIAL RESPIRATION in which the rescuer covers the patient's mouth with his own and breathes out vigorously.

mouthwash   a solution for rinsing the mouth.

movement   (mōōv′ment) an act of moving; motion.

active m., movement produced by the person's own muscles.

ameboid m., movement like that of an ameba, accomplished by protrusion of cytoplasm of the cell.

associated m., movement of parts that act together, as the eyes.

brownian m., molecular m., the peculiar, rapid, oscillatory movement of fine particles suspended in a fluid medium.

passive m., a movement of the body or of the extremities of a patient performed by another person without voluntary motion on the part of the patient.

vermicular m's, the wormlike movements of the intestines in peristalsis.

M.P.D. maximum permissible dose.

M.P.H. Master of Public Health.

mr. milliroentgen.

M.R.L. Medical Record Librarian.

mRNA messenger RNA (ribonucleic acid).

M.S. Master of Science; Master of Surgery.

MSH melanocyte-stimulating hormone.

M.T. Medical Technologist.

μ (mu) micron.

muciferous (mu-sif'er-us) secreting mucus.

muciform (mu'sĭ-form) resembling mucus.

mucigen (mu'sĭ-jen) a substance present in mucous cells, convertible into mucin and mucus.

mucilage (mu'sĭ-lij) an aqueous solution of a gummy substance, used as a vehicle or demulcent. adj., **mucilag'inous.**

mucilloid (mu'sil-oid) a preparation of a mucilaginous substance.

   psyllium hydrophilic m., a powdered preparation of the mucilaginous portion of blond psyllium seeds, used in treatment of constipation.

mucin (mu'sin) a mixture of proteins that is the chief constituent of mucus.

   gastric m., a preparation from the linings of hog's stomach; used in treating peptic ulcer. adj., **mu'-cinous.**

mucinase (mu'sĭ-nās) an enzyme that acts upon mucin.

mucinogen (mu-sin'o-jen) a precursor of mucin.

mucinoid (mu'sĭ-noid) resembling mucin.

mucinosis (mu"si-no'sis) a state with abnormal deposits of mucin in the skin, often associated with hypothyroidism (myxedema).

   follicular m., a disease of unknown cause, characterized by plaques of folliculopapules and usually alopecia.

muciparous (mu-sip'ah-rus) producing mucin.

mucocele (mu'ko-sēl) 1. dilatation of a cavity with accumulated mucous secretion. 2. a mucous polyp.

mucocutaneous (mu"ko-ku-ta'ne-us) pertaining to mucous membrane and skin.

mucoenteritis (mu"ko-en"tě-ri'tis) acute catarrhal enteritis.

mucofibrous (mu"ko-fi'brus) composed of mucous and fibrous tissues.

mucoid (mu'koid) 1. resembling mucus. 2. a conjugated protein of animal origin, differing from mucin in solubility.

mucolytic (mu"ko-lit'ik) destroying or dissolving mucus.

mucomembranous (mu"ko-mem'brah-nus) composed of mucous membrane.

mucoperiosteum (mu"ko-per"e-os'te-um) periosteum having a mucous surface, as in parts of the auditory apparatus.

mucopolysaccharide (mu"ko-pol"e-sak'ah-rīd) a group of polysaccharides that contain hexosamine, that may or may not be combined with protein and that, dispersed in water, form many of the mucins.

mucoprotein (mu"ko-pro'te-in) a compound present in all connective and supporting tissues, containing, as prosthetic groups, mucopolysaccharides; soluble in water and relatively resistant to denaturation.

mucopurulent (mu"ko-pu'roo-lent) marked by an exudate containing both mucus and pus.

mucopus (mu'ko-pus) mucus blended with pus.

Mucor (mu'kor) a genus of saprophytic mold fungi, occasionally pathogenic for man.

mucormycosis (mu"kor-mi-ko'sis) a mycosis due to fungus of the genus Mucor; it is usually a pulmonary infection, but metastatic abscesses may form in various organs.

mucosa (mu-ko'sah), pl. *muco'sae* [L.] mucous membrane. adj., **muco'sal.**

mucosanguineous (mu"ko-sang-gwin'e-us) composed of mucus and blood.

mucoserous (mu"ko-se'rus) composed of mucus and serum.

mucosin (mu-ko'sin) a form of mucin found in tenacious mucus.

mucosocutaneous (mu-ko"so-ku-ta'ne-us) pertaining to a mucous membrane and the skin.

mucous (mu'kus) pertaining to or resembling mucus; also, secreting mucus.

   m. membrane, membrane covered with epithelium lining canals and cavities that communicate with the exterior of the body.

mucoviscidosis (mu"ko-vis"ĭ-do'sis) a condition characterized by accumulation of extremely thick, tenacious mucus in the important mucus-secreting glands, involving especially the exocrine glands of the pancreas; called also CYSTIC FIBROSIS.

mucus (mu'kus) the free slime of the mucous membrane, composed of its secretion, mucin, and various salts and body cells.

müllerian duct (mil-e're-an) either of the two ducts of the embryo that empty into the cloaca, in the female developing into the vagina, uterus and uterine tubes.

multi- (mul'tĭ) word element [L.], *many.*

multiallelic (mul"te-ah-lel'ik) pertaining to or occupied by many different genes affecting the same or different hereditary characters.

multiarticular (mul″te-ar-tik′u-lar) pertaining to many joints.

multibacillary (mul″tĭ-bas′ĭ-la″re) pertaining to or made up of a number of bacilli.

multicellular (mul″tĭ-sel′u-lar) composed of many cells.

multicuspidate (mul″tĭ-kus′pĭ-dāt) having numerous cusps.

multifactorial (mul″tĭ-fak-to′re-al) 1. of or pertaining to, or arising through the action of, many factors. 2. in genetics, arising as the result of the interaction of several genes.

multifocal (mul″tĭ-fo′kal) arising from or pertaining to many foci.

multiform (mul′tĭ-form) occurring in many forms.

multiglandular (mul″tĭ-glan′du-lar) affecting several glands.

multigravida (mul″tĭ-grav′ĭ-dah) a woman pregnant for the third (or more) time.
  grand m., a woman who has had six or more previous pregnancies.

multilobar (mul″tĭ-lo′bar) having numerous lobes.

multilobular (mul″tĭ-lob′u-lar) having many lobules.

multilocular (mul″tĭ-lok′u-lar) having many cells or compartments.

multinodular (mul″tĭ-nod′u-lar) having many nodules.

multinuclear (mul″tĭ-nu′kle-ar) having many nuclei.

multipara (mul-tip′ah-rah) a woman who has had two or more pregnancies resulted in viable offspring. adj., **multip′arous.**
  grand m., a woman who has had seven or more pregnancies that resulted in viable offspring.

multiparity (mul″tĭ-par′ĭ-te) the condition of being a multipara.

multiple (mul′tĭ-pl) manifold; occurring in various parts of the body at once.
  m. myeloma, a primary malignant tumor of bone marrow, marked by circumscribed or diffuse tumorlike hyperplasia of the bone marrow, and usually associated with anemia and with Bence Jones protein in the urine. The patient complains of neuralgic pains; later painful swellings appear on the ribs and skull and spontaneous fractures may occur. Called also Kahler's disease, myelopathic albumosuria, Bence Jones albumosuria, and lymphadenia ossea.
  m. sclerosis, a disease characterized by hardened patches scattered at random throughout the brain and spinal cord, interfering with the nerves in those areas. Multiple sclerosis is one of the most common diseases of the nervous system in the United States, with about 500,000 victims. It generally occurs in young adults.
  Although not a killer, multiple sclerosis can be extremely disabling. Patients may recover almost completely from severely paralyzing attacks, but

medical science has not as yet discovered any way of halting the disease.

Multiple sclerosis is chronic; periods of improvement usually alternate with periods of worsening. The effects of multiple sclerosis vary with the portion of the nervous system affected. Since the location, extent and duration of the injuries vary, it is difficult to describe a typical case of multiple sclerosis.

Often the first sign of the disease is a visual disturbance. The patient may "see double" or lose part of the visual field. Weakness and unusual fatigue are common. There may be a tremor or shaking of the limbs, interfering with fine movements such as writing or sewing. Speech may become slow or monotonous. Balance is sometimes impaired, and walking may be unsteady; or the knees may not bend, causing a stiff gait. There may be loss of bladder and bowel control. Finally, paralysis may occur in any part of the body.

Diagnosis in the early stages may be difficult.
  TREATMENT. Multiple sclerosis seems to grow worse following any illness, and so good general care is necessary to keep up the body's health and resistance to disease. Physical therapy, including massage and exercise, may prevent the affected muscles from being unnecessarily weakened. Because this disease frequently grows worse when there are emotional disturbances, and because patients who are disabled by it may become depressed, psychotherapy may be helpful.

Patients with multiple sclerosis can often lead long, useful lives. The National Multiple Sclerosis Society, 257 Park Avenue South, New York, N.Y. 10010, provides information and assistance concerning all phases of this disease.

multipolar (mul″tĭ-po′lar) having more than two poles or processes.

multisynaptic (mul″tĭ-sĭ-nap′tik) pertaining to or relayed through two or more synapses.

multiterminal (mul″tĭ-ter′mĭ-nal) having several sets of terminals so that several electrodes may be used.

multivalent (mul″tĭ-va′lent) combining with several univalent atoms.

mummying (mum′e-ing) a form of physical restraint in which the entire body is enclosed in a sheet or blanket, leaving only the head exposed.

mumps (mumps) a communicable virus disease that attacks one or both of the parotid glands, the largest of the three pairs of salivary glands; called also epidemic parotitis. Occasionally the submaxillary glands are also affected. Although older people may contract the disease, mumps usually strikes children between the ages of 5 and 15.

Mumps is spread by droplet infection. The disease is contagious in the infected person from 1 to 2 days before symptoms appear until 1 or 2 days after they disappear. The incubation period is usually 18 days, although it may vary from 12 to 26 days. One attack usually gives immunity.
  SYMPTOMS. Often the first noticeable symptom of mumps is a swelling of one of the parotid glands. The swelling is frequently accompanied by pain and tenderness. Occasionally acid foods and beverages

may cause an increase in the pain. In the first stage of mumps, the patient may have a fever of 100 to 104° F. Other common symptoms include loss of appetite, headache and back pain.

The swelling increases for the first 2 or 3 days and then diminishes, disappearing by the sixth or seventh day. The swelling usually appears first on one side and then on the other, with as many as 12 days intervening. Sometimes both sides swell at once; occasionally the second side does not swell at all.

Sometimes the disease occurs virtually without symptoms. This mild form of mumps is responsible for the presence of antibodies and immunity in persons who cannot recall having had the disease and yet seem to be immune to it.

COMPLICATIONS. Mumps may affect other parts of the body as well as the salivary glands. In the male, when the testes are affected, the infection is known as orchitis. It strikes about one-third of those who contract mumps after the age of puberty. Orchitis may occur before the swelling of the parotid glands, but usually does not develop until about 7 to 10 days thereafter.

Involvement of the gonads in females is less common and more difficult to detect. Lower abdominal pain and enlargement of the ovaries are symptoms indicating involvement of the ovaries. The breasts may also be affected.

Mumps may affect the central nervous system. Acute meningoencephalitis is a common complication, causing dizziness, vomiting and headache. It may occur before the parotid glands swell or in the absence of other signs of mumps. No specific treatment is required, and the condition disappears without causing permanent damage.

Pancreatitis is another possible complication.

TREATMENT. Most children with mumps do not feel ill enough to be confined to bed, and it is sufficient if they remain quietly at home, unless there is a rise in temperature or a complication develops. When the swelling of the parotid glands disappears, the child may return to school. If both glands are involved, this time interval is approximately 7 days. A soft diet with plenty of fluids is recommended until fever and swelling vanish.

PREVENTION. Total isolation of the child is not essential. Males over the age of puberty sh uld avoid contact with the patient. The mumps virus cannot survive for any length of time in open air, so it is unnecessary to take special precautions with the patient's clothing, bedding, dishes or utensils.

A vaccine has been developed that gives partial immunity to mumps, but its effectiveness is limited. In children, the disease is so mild that it is considered preferable to allow the child to contract it. The vaccine does not afford protection if it is given during the incubation period following exposure. Moreover, since the immunity provided is partial, repeated doses are required, and they may eventually cause unpleasant reactions.

A mumps gamma globulin serum affords short-term immunity when there is an extraordinary need for protection. Though very expensive, it is useful for male adults who have been exposed to mumps and have reason to be particularly anxious not to contract it. This serum should not be confused with the ordinary commercial gamma globulin used in the treatment of measles.

iodine m., swelling of the salivary and lacrimal glands as a toxic reaction to iodine therapy.

mural (mu'ral) pertaining to a wall of an organ or cavity.

Murel (mu'rel) trademark for preparations of valethamate bromide, an antispasmodic and anticholinergic.

murine (mu'rēn) pertaining to or affecting mice or rats.

murmur (mur'mur) a gentle, blowing auscultatory sound.

aortic m., a sound indicative of disease of the aortic valve.

apex m., one heard over the apex of the heart.

arterial m., one in an artery, sometimes aneurysmal and sometimes hemic.

Austin Flint m., a loud presystolic murmur at the apex usually heard with aortic regurgitation.

blood m., one due to an abnormal, commonly anemic, condition of the blood.

cardiac m., any adventitious sound heard over the region of the heart.

cardiopulmonary m., one produced by the impact of the heart against the lung.

crescendo m., a heart murmur increasing in pitch and force.

diastolic m., one at diastole, due to mitral obstruction or to aortic or pulmonic regurgitation.

direct m., one due to a roughened endocardium and contracted valvular orifice.

Duroziez m., a double murmur heard on compression of the femoral artery with the stethoscope in aortic regurgitation and other conditions.

dynamic m., one caused by irregular pulsation of the heart.

endocardial m., one produced within the heart cavities.

exocardial m., a heart murmur produced outside the heart's cavities.

Flint's m., Austin Flint murmur.

friction m., one due to the rubbing together of two serous surfaces.

functional m., a cardiac murmur occurring in the absence of structural changes in the heart, as with anemia or rapid heart rate.

Graham Steell m., a soft diastolic murmur due to pulmonary insufficiency.

heart m., any adventitious sound heard over the region of the heart.

hemic m., blood murmur.

indirect m., one caused by reversal of the direction of blood current.

inorganic m., one not due to valvular or other lesions.

machinery m., a continuous loud, rough murmur heard in patent ductus arteriosus.

mitral m., one due to disease of the mitral valve.

organic m., one due to structural change in the heart.

prediastolic m., one occurring just before diastole.

presystolic m., one occurring before systole, from mitral or tricuspid obstruction.

pulmonic m., one due to disease of the valves of the pulmonary artery.

regurgitant m., one due to a dilated valvular orifice with consequent regurgitation of blood through the valve.

seagull m., a murmur whose sound resembles the call of a seagull, frequently heard in aortic insufficiency.

systolic m., one occurring at systole, from mitral, aortic, tricuspid or pulmonary obstruction.

tricuspid m., one caused by disease of the tricuspid valve.

vascular m., one heard over a blood vessel.

vesicular m., the murmur of normal breathing.

Murphy's sign (mur'fēz) a sign of gallbladder disease consisting of pain on taking a deep breath when the physician's fingers are on the approximate location of the gallbladder.

Musca (mus'kah) a genus of flies, including the common housefly, *M. domes'tica*.

musca (mus'kah), pl. *mus'cae* [L.] a fly.

mus'cae volitan'tes, specks seen as floating before the eyes.

muscle (mus'l) a bundle of long slender cells, or fibers, that have the power to contract. Muscles are responsible for locomotion and play an important part in performing vital body functions. They also protect the contents of the abdomen against injury and help support the body.

Muscle fibers range in length from a few hundred thousandths of an inch to several inches. They also vary in shape, and in color from white to deep red. Each muscle fiber receives its own nerve impulses, so that fine and varied motions are possible. Each has its small stored supply of glycogen which it uses as fuel for energy. Muscles, especially the heart, also use free fatty acids as fuel. At the signal of an impulse traveling down the nerve, the muscle fiber changes chemical energy into mechanical energy, and the result is muscle contraction.

Some muscles are attached to bones by tendons. Others are attached to other muscles, and to skin—producing the smile, the wink and other facial expressions, for example. All or part of the walls of hollow internal organs, such as the heart, stomach, intestines and blood vessels, are composed of muscles. The last stages of swallowing and of peristalsis are actually series of contractions by the muscles in the walls of the organs involved.

TYPES OF MUSCLE. There are three types of muscle—involuntary, voluntary and cardiac. They are composed respectively of smooth, striated (or striped) and mixed smooth and striated tissue.

Muscles that are not under the control of the conscious part of the brain are called involuntary muscles. They respond to the nerve impulses of the autonomic nervous system. These involuntary muscles are the countless short-fibered, or smooth, muscles of the internal organs. They power the digestive tract, the pupils of the eyes and all other involuntary mechanisms.

The muscles controlled by the conscious part of the brain are called voluntary muscles, and are striated. These are the skeletal muscles that enable the body to move, and there are more than 600 of them in the human body. The fibers of voluntary muscles are grouped together in a sheath of muscle cells. Groups of fibers are bundled together into fascicles and the bundles are surrounded by a tough sheet of connective tissue to form a muscle group like the biceps.

Unlike the involuntary muscles, which can remain in a state of contraction for long periods without tiring and are capable of sustained rhythmic contractions, the voluntary muscles are readily subject to fatigue. They also differ from the involuntary muscles in their need for regular and proper exercise.

The third kind of muscle, cardiac muscle, or the muscle of the heart, is involuntary and consists of striated fibers different from the voluntary muscle fibers. The contraction and relaxation of cardiac muscle continue at a rhythmic pace until death unless the muscle is injured in some way. (See also HEART.)

PHYSIOLOGY OF MUSCLES. No muscle stays completely relaxed, and as long as a person is conscious, it remains slightly contracted. This condition is called tonus, or tone. It keeps the bones in place and enables a posture to be maintained. It allows a person to remain standing, sitting up straight, kneeling or in any other natural position. Muscles also have elasticity. They are capable of being stretched and of performing reflex actions. This is made possible by the motor and sensory nerves which serve the muscles.

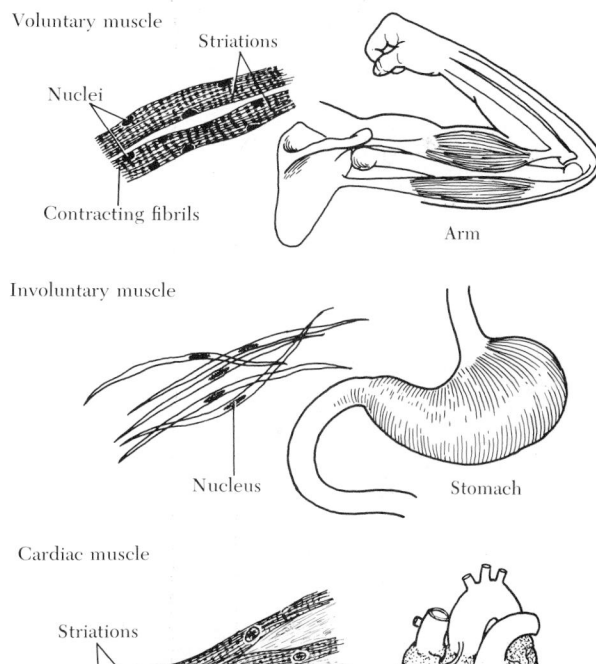

Types of muscle.

Voluntary muscles consist of striated muscle fibers, so called because the contractile fibrils that form them are connected in such a way that they seem to be striped. The nuclei are always on the outer edges.

Involuntary, or smooth, muscle forms the arteries, veins, capillaries, some lymphatic vessels and the organs of the digestive, respiratory and urogenital tracts. Smooth muscle fibers are shaped like spindles and each has a single rod-shaped nucleus.

Cardiac muscle, found only in the heart, is formed by contractile fibrils that differ structurally from those of voluntary muscle.

TABLE OF MUSCLES

COMMON NAME†	NA TERM†	ORIGIN*	INSERTION*	INNERVATION	ACTION
abductor m. of great toe	m. abductor hallucis	medial tubercle of calcaneus, plantar aponeurosis	medial side of base of proximal phalanx of great toe	medial plantar	abducts, flexes great toe
abductor m. of little finger	m. abductor digiti minimi manus	pisiform bone, tendon of ulnar flexor m. of wrist	medial side of base of proximal phalanx of little finger	ulnar	abducts little finger
abductor m. of little toe	m. abductor digiti minimi pedis	lateral tubercle of calcaneus	lateral side of base of proximal phalanx of little toe	lateral plantar	abducts little toe
abductor m. of thumb, long	m. abductor pollicis longus	posterior surfaces of radius and ulna	lateral side of base of first metacarpal bone and trapezium	posterior interosseous	abducts thumb
abductor m. of thumb, short	m. abductor pollicis brevis	tubercles of scaphoid and trapezium, flexor retinaculum of hand	lateral side of base of proximal phalanx of thumb	median	abducts thumb
adductor m., great	m. adductor magnus	*adductor part* – inferior ramus of pubis, ramus of ischium; *extensor part* – ischial tuberosity	*adductor part* – linea aspera of femur; *extensor part* – adductor tubercle of femur	*adductor part* – obturator; *extensor part* – sciatic	*adductor part* – adducts thigh; *extensor part* – extends thigh
adductor m. of great toe	m. adductor hallucis	*oblique head* from long plantar ligament; *transverse head* from plantar ligaments	lateral side of base of proximal phalanx of great toe; sheath of flexor m. of great toe	lateral plantar	flexes and adducts great toe
adductor m., long	m. adductor longus	body of pubis	linea aspera of femur	obturator	adducts, flexes thigh
adductor m., short	m. adductor brevis	body and inferior ramus of pubis	upper part of linea aspera of femur	obturator	adducts, flexes thigh
adductor m. of thumb	m. adductor pollicis	*oblique head* from second metacarpal, capitate and trapezoid; *transverse head* from front of third metacarpal	medial side of base of proximal phalanx of thumb	ulnar	adducts thumb
anconeus m.	m. anconeus	back of lateral epicondyle of humerus	olecranon and posterior surface of ulna	radial	extends forearm
antitragus m.	m. antitragicus	antitragus	caudate process of helix	temporal, posterior auricular branches of facial	
arrector m's of hair	mm. arrectores pilorum	dermis	hair follicles	sympathetic	elevate hairs
articular m. of elbow	m. articularis cubiti	a name applied to a few fibers of the deep surface of the triceps m. of arm that insert into the posterior ligament and synovial membrane of the elbow joint			
articular m. of knee	m. articularis genus	lower part of anterior surface of shaft of femur	suprapatellar bursa	femoral	raises capsule of knee joint
aryepiglottic m.	m. aryepiglotticus	a name applied to inconstant fibers of oblique arytenoid m., from apex of arytenoid cartilage to lateral margin of epiglottis			
arytenoid m., oblique	m. arytenoideus obliquus	muscular process of arytenoid cartilage	apex of opposite arytenoid cartilage	recurrent laryngeal	closes inlet of larynx
arytenoid m., transverse	m. arytenoideus transversus	medial surface of arytenoid cartilage	medial surface of opposite arytenoid cartilage	recurrent laryngeal	approximates arytenoid cartilage
auricular m., anterior	m. auricularis anterior	galea aponeurotica	cartilage of ear	facial	may draw auricle forward
auricular m., posterior	m. auricularis posterior	mastoid process	cartilage of ear	facial	may draw auricle backward
auricular m., superior	m. auricularis superior	galea aponeurotica	cartilage of ear	facial	may raise auricle
biceps m. of arm	m. biceps brachii	*long head* – supraglenoid tubercle of scapula; *short head* – apex of coracoid process	tuberosity of radius and antebrachial fascia	musculocutaneous	flexes and supinates forearm
biceps m. of thigh	m. biceps femoris	*long head* – ischial tuberosity; *short head* – linea aspera of femur	head of fibula, lateral condyle of tibia	sciatic	flexes and rotates leg laterally, extends thigh

Common Name	NA Term	Origin	Insertion	Nerve	Action
brachial m.	m. brachialis	anterior aspect of humerus	coronoid process of ulna	musculocutaneous, radial	flexes forearm
brachioradial m.	m. brachioradialis	lateral supracondylar ridge of humerus	lateral surface of lower end of radius	radial	flexes forearm
bronchoesophageal m.	m. bronchoesophageus	a name applied to muscle fibers arising from wall of left bronchus, reinforcing musculature of esophagus			
buccinator m.	m. buccinator	alveolar processes of maxilla and mandible, pterygomandibular raphe	orbicular m. of mouth and lips	buccal branch of facial	compresses cheek
bulbocavernous m.	m. bulbocavernosus, m. bulbospongiosus	tendinous center of perineum, median raphe of bulb	fascia of penis or clitoris	pudendal	constricts urethra in male, vagina in female
canine m. *See levator m. of angle of mouth*					
ceratocricoid m.	m. ceratocricoideus	a name applied to muscle fibers from cricoid cartilage to inferior horn of thyroid cartilage			
chin m.	m. mentalis	incisive fossa of mandible	skin of chin	facial	wrinkles skin of chin
chondroglossus m.	m. chondroglossus	lesser horn and body of hyoid bone	substance of tongue	hypoglossal	depresses, retracts tongue
ciliary m.	m. ciliaris	*longitudinal division* (Brücke's m's)—junction of cornea and sclera; *circular division* (Müller's m.)—sphincter of ciliary body	outer layers of choroid and ciliary processes	short ciliary	makes lens more convex in visual accommodation
coccygeus m.	m. coccygeus	ischial spine	lower part of lateral border of sacrum, coccyx	third and fourth sacral	supports and raises coccyx
constrictor m. of pharynx, inferior	m. constrictor pharyngis inferior	arch of cricoid, oblique line of thyroid cartilages	median raphe of posterior wall of pharynx	pharyngeal plexus, external branch of superior laryngeal and recurrent laryngeal	constricts pharynx
constrictor m. of pharynx, middle	m. constrictor pharyngis medius	horns of hyoid bone, stylohyoid ligament	median raphe of posterior wall of pharynx	pharyngeal plexus of vagus, glossopharyngeal	constricts pharynx
constrictor m. of pharynx, superior	m. constrictor pharyngis superior	pterygoid hamulus, pterygomandibular raphe, mylohyoid line of mandible, mucous membrane of mouth	median raphe of posterior wall of pharynx	pharyngeal plexus of vagus	constricts pharynx
coracobrachial m.	m. coracobrachialis	coracoid process of scapula	medial border of humerus	musculocutaneous	flexes arm
corrugator m., superciliary	m. corrugator supercilii	medial end of superciliary arch	skin of eyebrow	facial	draws eyebrow downward and medially
cremaster m.	m. cremaster	inferior margin of internal oblique m. of abdomen	pubic tubercle	genital branch of genitofemoral	elevates testis
cricoarytenoid m., lateral	m. cricoarytenoideus lateralis	arch of cricoid cartilage	muscular process of arytenoid cartilage	recurrent laryngeal	approximates vocal folds
cricoarytenoid m., posterior	m. cricoarytenoideus posterior	back of lamina of cricoid cartilage	muscular process of arytenoid cartilage	recurrent laryngeal	separates vocal folds
cricothyroid m.	m. cricothyroideus	arch of cricoid cartilage	lamina and inferior horn of thyroid cartilage	external branch of superior laryngeal	tenses vocal folds
deltoid m.	m. deltoideus	clavicle, acromion, spine of scapula	deltoid tuberosity of humerus	axillary	abducts and flexes or extends arm
depressor m. of angle of mouth	m. depressor anguli oris	external surface of mandible	angle of mouth	facial	pulls down angle of mouth
depressor m. of lower lip	m. depressor labii inferioris	external surface of mandible	orbicular m. of mouth and skin of lower lip	facial	depresses lower lip

*m. = muscle; m's = (pl.) muscles.
†m. = [L.] musculus; mm. = [L.] musculi.

TABLE OF MUSCLES (Continued)

COMMON NAME†	NA TERM†	ORIGIN*	INSERTION*	INNERVATION	ACTION
depressor m. of septum of nose	m. depressor septi nasi	incisive fossa of maxilla	ala and septum of nose	facial	constricts nostril and depresses ala
depressor m., superciliary	m. depressor supercilii	a name applied to a few fibers of orbital part of orbicular m. of eye that are inserted into the eyebrow			
detrusor urinae	detrusor urinae	a collective name applied to muscular coat of urinary bladder			
diaphragm	diaphragma	back of xiphoid process, inner surfaces of lower 6 costal cartilages and lower 4 ribs, medial and lateral arcuate ligaments, bodies of upper lumbar vertebrae	central tendon of diaphragm	phrenic	increases volume of thorax in inspiration
digastric m.	m. digastricus	*anterior belly* – digastric fossa on lower border of mandible near symphysis; *posterior belly* – mastoid notch of temporal bone	by middle tendon to hyoid bone	*anterior belly* – mylohyoid branch of inferior alveolar; *posterior belly* – facial	lowers jaw
dilator m. of pupil	m. dilator pupillae	a name applied to fibers extending radially from free to attached margin of iris			
epicranial m.	m. epicranius	a name applied to muscular covering of scalp, including occipitofrontal and temporoparietal m's and galea aponeurotica			
erector m. of spine	m. erector spinae	a name applied to fibers of more superficial of deep muscles of back, originating from sacrum, spines of lumbar and eleventh and twelfth thoracic vertebrae and iliac crest; it splits into iliocostal, longissimus and spinal m's			
extensor m. of fingers	m. extensor digitorum manus	lateral epicondyle of humerus	extensor expansion of 4 medial fingers	deep branch of radial	extends distal phalanges
extensor m. of great toe, long	m. extensor hallucis long	front of fibula, interosseous membrane	base of distal phalanx of great toe	deep peroneal	extends great toe, dorsiflexes foot
extensor m. of great toe, short	m. extensor hallucis brevis	a name applied to portion of short extensor m. of toes that goes to great toe			
extensor m. of index finger	m. extensor indicis	posterior surface of ulna, interosseous membrane	extensor expansion of index finger	posterior interosseous	extends index finger
extensor m. of little finger	m. extensor digiti minimi manus	lateral epicondyle of humerus	extensor aponeurosis of little finger	deep branch of radial	extends little finger
extensor m. of thumb, long	m. extensor pollicis longus	posterior surface of ulna and interosseous membrane	back of distal phalanx of thumb	posterior interosseous	extends, adducts thumb
extensor m. of thumb, short	m. extensor pollicis brevis	posterior surface of radius	back of proximal phalanx of thumb	posterior interosseous	extends thumb
extensor m. of toes, long	m. extensor digitorum longus pedis	anterior surface of fibula, lateral condyle of tibia, interosseous membrane	extensor expansion of 4 lateral toes	deep peroneal	extends toes
extensor m. of toes, short	m. extensor digitorum brevis pedis	upper surface of calcaneus	extensor tendons of first, second, third, fourth toes	deep peroneal	extends toes
extensor m. of wrist, radial, long	m. extensor carpi radialis longus	lateral supracondylar ridge of humerus	base of second metacarpal bone	radial	extends, abducts hand
extensor m. of wrist, radial, short	m. extensor carpi radialis brevis	lateral epicondyle of humerus, radial collateral ligament	backs of base of second and third metacarpal bones	radial or its deep branch	extends, abducts hand

Common name	Latin name	Origin	Insertion	Nerve	Action
extensor m. of wrist, ulnar	m. extensor carpi ulnaris	*humeral head* – lateral epicondyle of humerus; *ulnar head* – posterior border of ulna	base of fifth metacarpal bone	deep branch of radial	extends, abducts hand
fibular m. *Official alternative for* peroneal m.					
flexor m. of fingers, deep	m. flexor digitorum profundus manus	shaft of ulna, coronoid process, interosseous membrane	bases of distal phalanges of 4 medial fingers	anterior interosseous, ulnar,	flexes distal phalanges
flexor m. of fingers, superficial	m. flexor digitorum sublimis; m. flexor digitorum superficialis manus	*humeroulnar head* – medial epicondyle of humerus, coronoid process of ulna; *radial head* – anterior border of radius	sides of middle phalanges of 4 medial fingers	median	flexes middle phalanges
flexor m. of great toe, long	m. flexor hallucis longus	posterior surface of fibula	base of distal phalanx of great toe	tibial	flexes great toe
flexor m. of great toe, short	m. flexor hallucis brevis	ligaments of sole	both sides of base of proximal phalanx of great toe	medial plantar	flexes great toe
flexor m. of little finger, short	m. flexor digiti minimi brevis manus	hook of hamate bone	medial side of proximal phalanx of little finger	ulnar	flexes little finger
flexor m. of little toe, short	m. flexor digiti minimi brevis pedis	sheath of long peroneal	lateral surface of base of proximal phalanx of little toe	lateral plantar	flexes little toe
flexor m. of thumb, long	m. flexor pollicis longus	anterior surface of radius, medial epicondyle of humerus, coronoid process of ulna	base of distal phalanx of thumb	anterior interosseous	flexes thumb
flexor m. of thumb, short	m. flexor pollicis brevis	tubercle of trapezium, flexor retinaculum	lateral side of base of proximal phalanx of thumb	median	flexes thumb
flexor m. of toes, long	m. flexor digitorum longus pedis	posterior surface of shaft of tibia	distal phalanges of 4 lateral toes	tibial	flexes toes
flexor m. of toes, short	m. flexor digitorum brevis pedis	medial tuberosity of calcaneus	middle phalanges of 4 lateral toes	medial plantar	flexes toes
flexor m. of wrist, radial	m. flexor carpi radialis	medial epicondyle of humerus	bases of second and third metacarpal bones	median	flexes, abducts hand
flexor m. of wrist, ulnar	m. flexor carpi ulnaris	*humeral head* – medial epicondyle of humerus; *ulnar head* – olecranon and posterior border of ulna	pisiform bone, hook of hamate bone, base of fifth metacarpal bone	ulnar	flexes, adducts hand
gastrocnemius m.	m. gastrocnemius	*medial head* – popliteal surface of femur, upper part of medial condyle; *lateral head* – lateral condyle	aponeurosis unites with tendon of soleus to form Achilles tendon	tibial	plantar flexes foot, flexes knee joint
gemellus m., inferior	m. gemellus inferior	tuberosity of ischium	internal obturator tendon	nerve to quadrate m. of thigh	rotates thigh laterally
gemellus m., superior	m. gemellus superior	spine of ischium	internal obturator tendon	nerve to internal obturator	rotates thigh laterally
genioglossus m.	m. genioglossus	superior genial tubercle	hyoid bone, under surface of tongue	hypoglossal	protrudes and depresses tongue
geniohyoid m.	m. geniohyoideus	inferior genial tubercle	body of hyoid bone	a branch of first cervical nerve through hypoglossal	draws hyoid bone forward
glossopalatine m. *See* palatoglossus m.					
gluteus maximus m. (gluteal m., greatest)	m. gluteus maximus	dorsal aspect of ilium, dorsal surface of sacrum and coccyx, sacrotuberous ligament	iliotibial tract band of fascia lata, gluteal tuberosity of femur	inferior gluteal	extends thigh or trunk
gluteus medius m. (gluteal m., middle)	m. gluteus medius	dorsal aspect of ilium between anterior and posterior gluteal lines	greater trochanter of femur	superior gluteal	abducts, rotates thigh medially

Table of Muscles (*Continued*)

Common Name†	NA Term†	Origin*	Insertion*	Innervation	Action
gluteus minimus m. (gluteal m., least)	m. gluteus minimus	dorsal aspect of ilium between anterior and posterior gluteal lines	greater trochanter of femur	superior gluteal	abducts, rotates thigh medially
gracilis m.	m. gracilis	body and inferior ramus of pubis	medial surface of shaft of tibia	obturator	adducts thigh
m. of helix, greater	m. helicis major	spine of helix	anterior border of helix	temporal, posterior auricular branches of facial	tenses skin of acoustic meatus
m. of helix, smaller	m. helicis minor	anterior rim of helix	concha	temporal, posterior auricular branches of facial	
hyoglossus m.	m. hyoglossus	body and greater horn of hyoid bone	side of tongue	hypoglossal	depresses, retracts tongue
iliac m.	m. iliacus	iliac fossa, ala of sacrum	greater psoas tendon, lesser trochanter of femur	femoral	flexes thigh or trunk
iliococcygeus m.	m. iliococcygeus	a name applied to posterior portion of levator ani m., including fibers originating as far forward as obturator canal, and inserting on side of coccyx and in anococcygeal ligaments			
iliocostal m.	m. iliocostalis	a name applied to lateral division of erector m. of spine			
iliocostal m. of loins	m. iliocostalis lumborum	iliac crest	angles of lower ribs	thoracic and lumbar	extends lumbar spine
iliocostal m. of neck	m. iliocostalis cervicis	angles of third, fourth, fifth and sixth ribs	transverse processes of lower cervical vertebrae	cervical	extends cervical spine
iliocostal m. of thorax	m. iliocostalis thoracis	upper borders of angles of 6 lower ribs	angles of upper ribs and transverse process of seventh cervical vertebra	thoracic	keeps thoracic spine erect
iliopsoas m.	m. iliopsoas	a name applied collectively to iliac and greater psoas m's			
incisive m's of upper and lower lip	incisive mm., superior and inferior	incisive fossae of maxilla and mandible	angle of mouth	facial	make vestibule of mouth shallow
m. of incisure of helix	m. incisurae helicis	a name applied to inconstant slips of fibers continuing forward from m. of tragus to bridge notch of cartilaginous part of meatus			
infraspinous m.	m. infraspinatus	infraspinous fossa of scapula	greater tubercle of humerus	suprascapular	rotates arm laterally
intercostal m's	mm. intercostales	a name applied to the layer of muscle fibers separated from the internal intercostal m's by the intercostal nerves and vessels			
intercostal m's, external	mm. intercostales externi	inferior border of rib	superior border of rib below	intercostal	elevate ribs in inspiration
intercostal m's, internal	mm. intercostales interni	inferior border of rib and costal cartilage	superior border of rib and costal cartilage below	intercostal	act on ribs in expiration
interosseous m's of foot, dorsal	mm. interossei dorsales pedis	sides of adjacent metatarsal bones	base of proximal phalanges of second, third and fourth toes	lateral plantar	flex toes
interosseous m's of hand, dorsal	mm. interossei dorsales manus	each by two heads from adjacent sides of metacarpal bones	extensor tendons of second, third and fourth fingers	ulnar	abduct, flex proximal, extend middle and distal phalanges
interosseous m's, palmar	mm. interossei palmares	sides at first, second, fourth and fifth metacarpal bones	extensor tendons of first, second, fourth and fifth fingers	ulnar	adduct, flex proximal, extend middle and distal phalanges
interosseous m's, plantar	mm. interossei plantares	medial side of third, fourth and fifth metatarsal bones	medial side of base of proximal phalanges of third, fourth and fifth toes	lateral plantar	flex toes
interspinal m's	mm. interspinales	a name applied to muscular bands extending on each side between spinous processes of contiguous vertebrae		spinal	extend vertebral column
intertransverse m's	mm. intertransversarii	a name applied to small muscles passing between transverse processes of adjacent vertebrae		spinal	bend vertebral column laterally
ischiocavernous m.	m. ischiocavernosus	ramus of ischium	crus of penis or clitoris	perineal branches of pudendal	maintains erection of penis or clitoris

latissimus dorsi m.	m. latissimus dorsi	spines of lower thoracic vertebrae, thoracolumbar fascia, iliac crest, lower ribs, inferior angle of scapula	floor of intertubercular groove of humerus	thoracodorsal	adducts, extends and rotates humerus medially
levator m. of angle of mouth	m. levator anguli oris	canine fossa of maxilla	orbicular m. of mouth, skin at angle of mouth	facial	raises angle of mouth
levator ani m.	m. levator ani	a name applied collectively to important muscular components of pelvic diaphragm, arising mainly from back of body of pubis and running backward toward coccyx; includes pubococcygeus (levator m. of prostate in male and pubovaginal in female), puborectal and iliococcygeus m's		third and fourth sacral	helps to support pelvic viscera and resist increases in intra-abdominal pressure
levator m. of palatine velum	m. levator veli palatini	apex of pars petrosa of temporal bone and cartilage of auditory tube	aponeurosis of soft palate	pharyngeal plexus	raises and draws back soft palate
levator m. of prostate	m. levator prostatae	a name applied to part of anterior portion of pubococcygeus m., which in male is inserted into prostate and tendinous center of perineum		sacral, pudendal	supports and compresses prostate, helps control micturition
levator m's of ribs	mm. levatores costarum	transverse processes of seventh cervical and first 11 thoracic vertebrae	medial to angle of rib below	intercostal	aid elevation of ribs in respiration
levator m. of scapula	m. levator scapulae	transverse processes of 4 upper cervical vertebrae	vertebral border of scapula	third and fourth cervical	raises scapula
levator m. of thyroid gland	m. levator glandulae thyroideae	isthmus or pyramidal lobule of thyroid gland	body of hyoid bone	external branch of superior laryngeal	
levator m. of upper eyelid	m. levator palpebrae superioris	sphenoid bone above optic foramen	skin and tarsal plate of upper eyelid	oculomotor	raises upper eyelid
levator m. of upper lip	m. levator labii superioris	lower margin of orbit	musculature of upper lip	facial	raises upper lip
levator m. of upper lip and ala of nose	m. levator labii superioris alaeque nasi	frontal process of maxilla	skin and cartilage of ala of nose, upper lip	infraorbital branch of facial	raises upper lip, dilates nostril
long m. of head	m. longus capitis	transverse processes of third to sixth cervical vertebrae	basilar portion of occipital bone	cervical	flexes head
long m. of neck	m. longus colli	*superior oblique portion*—transverse processes of third to fifth cervical vertebrae; *inferior oblique portion*—bodies of first to third thoracic vertebrae; *vertical portion*—bodies of 3 upper thoracic and 3 lower cervical vertebrae	*superior oblique portion*—tubercle of anterior arch of atlas; *inferior oblique portion*—transverse processes of fifth and sixth cervical vertebrae; *vertical portion*—bodies of second to fourth cervical vertebrae	cervical	flexes and supports cervical vertebrae
longissimus m. of head.	m. longissimus capitis	transverse processes of 4 or 5 upper thoracic vertebrae, articular processes of 3 or 4 lower cervical vertebrae	mastoid process of temporal bone	cervical	draws head backward, rotates head
longissimus m. of neck	m. longissimus cervicis	transverse processes of 4 or 5 upper thoracic vertebrae	transverse processes of second or third to sixth cervical vertebrae	lower cervical and upper thoracic	extends cervical vertebrae
longissimus m. of thorax	m. longissimus thoracis	transverse and articular processes of lumbar vertebrae and thoracolumbar fascia	transverse processes of all thoracic vertebrae, 9 or 10 lower ribs	lumbar and thoracic	extends thoracic vertebrae
longitudinal m. of tongue, inferior	m. longitudinalis inferior linguae	undersurface of tongue at base	tip of tongue	hypoglossal	changes shape of tongue in mastication and deglutition
longitudinal m. of tongue, superior	m. longitudinalis superior linguae	submucosa and septum of tongue	margins of tongue	hypoglossal	changes shape of tongue in mastication and deglutition

TABLE OF MUSCLES (Continued)

COMMON NAME†	NA TERM†	ORIGIN*	INSERTION*	INNERVATION	ACTION
lumbrical m's of foot	mm. lumbricales pedis	tendons of long flexor m. of toes	medial side of base of proximal phalanges of 4 lateral toes	medial and lateral plantar	aid in flexing proximal phalanges
lumbrical m's of hand	mm. lumbricales manus	tendons of deep flexor m. of fingers	extensor tendons of 4 lateral fingers	median, ulnar	flex proximal, extend middle and distal phalanges
masseter m.	m. masseter	superficial part–zygomatic process of maxilla, lower border of zygomatic arch; deep part–lower border and medial surface of zygomatic arch	superficial part–angle and ramus of mandible; deep part–upper half of ramus and lateral surface of coronoid process of mandible	masseteric, from mandibular	raises mandible, closes jaws
multifidus m.	m. multifidus	sacrum, sacroiliac ligament, mamillary processes of lumbar, transverse processes of thoracic and articular processes of cervical vertebrae	spines of contiguous vertebrae above	spinal	extends, rotates vertebral column
mylohyoid m.	m. mylohyoideus	mylohyoid line of mandible	body of hyoid bone, median raphe	mylohyoid branch of inferior alveolar	elevates hyoid bone, supports floor of mouth
nasal m.	m. nasalis	maxilla	alar part–ala of nose; transverse part–by aponeurotic expansion with fellow of opposite side	facial	alar part–aids in widening nostril; transverse part–depresses cartilage of nose
oblique m. of abdomen, external	m. obliquus externus abdominus	lower 8 ribs at costal cartilages	crest of ilium, linea alba through rectus sheath	lower thoracic	flexes, rotates vertebral column, compresses abdominal viscera
oblique m. of abdomen, internal	m. obliquus internus abdominis	thoracolumbar fascia, iliac crest, iliac fascia	lower 3 or 4 costal cartilages, linea alba, conjoined tendon to pubis	lower thoracic	flexes, rotates vertebral column, compresses abdominal viscera
oblique m. of auricle	m. obliquus auriculae	cranial surface of concha	cranial surface of auricle above concha	posterior auricular, temporal branches of facial	
oblique m. of eyeball, inferior	m. obliquus inferior bulbi	orbital surface of maxilla	sclera	oculomotor	abducts, elevates and rotates eyeball laterally
oblique m. of eyeball, superior	m. obliquus superior bulbi	lesser wing of sphenoid above optic foramen	sclera	trochlear	abducts, depresses and rotates eyeball
oblique m. of head, inferior	m. obliquus capitis inferior	spinous process of axis	transverse process of atlas	spinal	rotates atlas and head
oblique m. of head, superior	m. obliquus capitis superior	transverse process of atlas	occipital bone	spinal	extends and moves head laterally
obturator m., external	m. obturatorius externus	pubis, ischium, external surface of obturator membrane	trochanteric fossa of femur	obturator	rotates thigh laterally
obturator m., internal	m. obturatorius internus	pelvic surface of hip bone and obturator membrane, margin of obturator foramen	greater trochanter of femur	fifth lumbar, first and second sacral	rotates thigh laterally
occipitofrontal m.	m. occipitofrontalis	frontal belly–galea aponeurotica; occipital belly–highest nuchal line of occipital bone	frontal belly–skin of eyebrow, root of nose; occipital belly–galea aponeurotica	frontal belly–temporal branch of facial; occipital belly–posterior auricular branch of facial	frontal belly–raises eyebrow; occipital belly–draws scalp backward
omohyoid m.	m. omohyoideus	superior border of scapula	body of hyoid bone	ansa cervicalis	depresses hyoid bone
opposing m. of little finger	m. opponens digiti minimi manus	hook of hamate bone	front of fifth metacarpal	ulnar	draws fifth metacarpal forward
opposing m. of thumb	m. opponens pollicis	tubercle of trapezium, flexor retinaculum	lateral side of first metacarpal bone	median	opposes thumb

		Origin	Insertion	Nerve	Action
orbicular m. of eye	m. orbicularis oculi	*orbital part*—medial margin of orbit, including frontal process of maxilla; *palpebral part*—medial palpebral ligament; *lacrimal part*—posterior lacrimal crest	*orbital part*—near origin after encircling orbit; *palpebral part*—orbital tubercle of zygomatic bone; *lacrimal part*—lateral palpebral raphe	facial	closes eyelids, wrinkles forehead, compresses (or dilates?) lacrimal sac
orbicular m. of mouth	m. orbicularis oris	a name applied to complicated sphincter muscle of mouth, comprising 2 parts: *labial part*—consisting of fibers restricted to lips; *marginal part*—consisting of fibers blending with those of adjacent muscles		facial	closes lips
orbital m.	m. orbitalis	bridges inferior orbital fissure		sympathetic fibers	possibly protrudes eye
palatoglossus m.	m. palatoglossus	under surface of soft palate	side of tongue	pharyngeal plexus	elevates tongue, constricts fauces
palatopharyngeus m.	m. palatopharyngeus	soft palate, bony palate	aponeurosis of pharynx, posterior border of thyroid cartilage	pharyngeal plexus	constricts pharynx
palmar m., long	m. palmaris longus	medial epicondyle of humerus	flexor retinaculum, palmar aponeurosis	median	tenses palmar aponeurosis
palmar m., short	m. palmaris brevis	palmar aponeurosis	skin of medial border of hand	ulnar	assists in deepening hollow of palm
papillary m's	mm. papillares	a name applied to conical muscular projections from walls of cardiac ventricles, attached to cusps of atrioventricular valves by chordae tendineae			steady and strengthen atrioventricular valves and prevent eversion of their cusps
pectinate m's	mm. pectinati	a name applied to small muscular ridges projecting from inner walls of auricles of heart, and extending in right atrium from auricle to crista terminalis			
pectineal m.	m. pectineus	pectineal line of pubis	pectineal line of femur	femoral, obturator	flexes, adducts thigh
pectoral m., greater	m. pectoralis major	clavicle, sternum, 6 upper costal cartilages, aponeurosis of external oblique m. of abdomen	greater tubercle of humerus	lateral and medial pectoral	adducts, rotates arm medially
pectoral m., smaller	m. pectoralis minor	second, third, fourth and fifth ribs	coracoid process of scapula	medial pectoral	draws shoulder downward
peroneal m., long	m. peroneus longus	lateral condyle of tibia, lateral surface of fibula	medial cuneiform bone, first metatarsal bone	superficial peroneal	plantar flexes and everts foot
peroneal m., short	m. peroneus brevis	lateral surface of fibula	tuberosity of fifth metatarsal bone	superficial peroneal	everts foot
peroneal m., third	m. peroneus tertius	anterior surface of fibula	fascia or base of fifth metatarsal bone	deep peroneal	aids long extensor m. of toes
piriform m.	m. piriformis	ilium, second to fourth sacral vertebrae	greater trochanter of femur	first and second sacral	rotates thigh laterally
plantar m.	m. plantaris	popliteal surface of femur	Achilles tendon or back of calcaneus	tibial	aids triceps m. of calf
platysma	platysma	a name applied to a platelike muscle originating from the fascia of cervical region and inserting on mandible, and skin around mouth		cervical branch of facial	wrinkles skin of neck, depresses jaw
pleuroesophageal m.	m. pleuroesophageus	a name applied to a bundle of smooth muscle fibers, usually connecting esophagus with left mediastinal pleura			
popliteal m.	m. popliteus	lateral condyle of femur, lateral meniscus	posterior surface of tibia	tibial	rotates leg medially
procerus m.	m. procerus	fascia over nasal bones	skin of forehead	facial	draws eyebrows down
pronator m., quadrate	m. pronator quadratus	anterior surface and border of distal third or fourth of shaft of ulna	anterior surface and border of distal fourth of shaft of radius	anterior interosseous	pronates forearm

TABLE OF MUSCLES (Continued)

COMMON NAME†	NA TERM†	ORIGIN*	INSERTION*	INNERVATION	ACTION
pronator m., round	m. pronator teres	*humeral head*–medial epicondyle of humerus; *ulnar head*–coronoid process of ulna	lateral surface of radius	median	pronates and flexes forearm
psoas m., greater	m. psoas major	lumbar vertebrae	lesser trochanter of femur	second and third lumbar	flexes thigh or trunk
psoas m., smaller	m. psoas minor	last thoracic and first lumbar vertebrae	arcuate line of hip bone	first lumbar	assists greater psoas m.
pterygoid m. lateral (external)	m. pterygoideus lateralis	*upper head*–infratemporal surface of greater wing of sphenoid; infratemporal crest; *lower head*–lateral surface of lateral pterygoid plate	neck of mandible, capsule of temporomandibular joint	mandibular	protrudes mandible, opens jaws, moves mandible from side to side
pterygoid m., medial (internal)	m. pterygoideus medialis	medial surface of lateral pterygoid plate, tuber of maxilla	medial surface of ramus and angle of mandible	mandibular	closes jaws
pubococcygeus m.	m. pubococcygeus	a name applied to anterior portion of levator ani m., originating in front of obturator canal and inserting in anococcygeal ligament and side of coccyx		third and fourth sacral	
puboprostatic m.	m. puboprostaticus	a name applied to smooth muscle fibers contained within medial puboprostatic ligament, which pass from prostate anteriorly to pubis			
puborectal m.	m. puborectalis	a name applied to portion of levator ani m., with a more lateral origin from pubic bone, and continuous posteriorly with corresponding muscle of opposite side		third and fourth sacral	
pubovaginal m.	m. pubovaginalis	a name applied to part of anterior portion of pubococcygeus m., which in female is inserted in walls of urethra and vagina		sacral and pudendal	helps control micturition
pubovesical m.	m. pubovesicalis	a name applied to smooth muscle fibers extending from neck of urinary bladder to pubis			
pyramidal m.	m. pyramidalis	body of pubis	linea alba	last thoracic	tenses abdominal wall
pyramidal m. of auricle	m. pyramidalis auriculae	a name applied to inconstant prolongation of fibers of m. of tragus to spine of helix			
quadrate m. of loins	m. quadratus lumborum	iliac crest, thoracolumbar fascia	twelfth rib, transverse processes of lumbar vertebrae	first and second lumbar, twelfth thoracic	flexes trunk laterally
quadrate m. of lower lip. *See* depressor m. of lower lip					
quadrate m. of sole	m. quadratus plantae	calcaneus, plantar fascia	tendons of long flexor m. of toes	lateral plantar	aids in flexing toes
quadrate m. of thigh	m. quadratus femoris	tuberosity of ischium	intertrochanteric crest and quadrate tubercle of femur	fourth and fifth lumbar, first sacral	rotates thigh laterally
quadrate m. of upper lip. *See* levator m. of upper lip					
quadriceps m. of thigh	m. quadriceps femoris	a name applied collectively to rectus m. of thigh and intermediate, lateral and medial vastus m's, inserting by a common tendon that surrounds patella and ends on tuberosity of tibia		femoral	extends leg
rectococcygeus m.	m. rectococcygeus	a name applied to smooth muscle fibers originating from anterior surface of second and third coccygeal vertebrae and inserting on posterior surface of rectum		autonomic	retracts, elevates rectum
rectourethral m.	m. rectourethralis	a name applied to band of smooth muscle fibers in male, extending from perineal flexure of rectum to membranous part of urethra			
rectouterine m.	m. rectouterinus	a name applied to band of fibers in female, running between cervix uteri and rectum, in rectouterine fold			

English name	Latin name	Origin	Insertion	Nerve supply	Action
rectovesical m.	m. rectovesicalis	a name applied to band of fibers in male, connecting longitudinal musculature of rectum with external muscular coat of bladder			
rectus (straight) m. of abdomen	m. rectus abdominis	xiphoid process, fifth, sixth and seventh costal cartilages	pubic crest and symphysis	lower thoracic	flexes lumbar vertebrae, supports abdomen
rectus (straight) m. of eyeball, inferior	m. rectus inferior bulbi	common tendinous ring	sclera	oculomotor	adducts, depresses and rotates eyeball laterally
rectus (straight) m. of eyeball, lateral	m. rectus lateralis bulbi	common tendinous ring	sclera	abducens	abducts eyeball
rectus (straight) m. of eyeball, medial	m. rectus medialis bulbi	common tendinous ring	sclera	oculomotor	adducts eyeball
rectus (straight) m. of eyeball, superior	m. rectus superior bulbi	common tendinous ring	sclera	oculomotor	adducts, elevates and rotates eyeball medially
rectus (straight) m. of head, anterior	m. rectus capitis anterior	lateral mass of atlas	basilar part of occipital bone	first and second cervical	flexes, supports head
rectus (straight) m. of head, lateral	m. rectus capitis lateralis	transverse process of atlas	jugular process of occipital bone	first and second cervical	flexes, supports head
rectus (straight) m. of head, posterior, greater	m. rectus capitis posterior major	spinous process of axis	occipital bone	suboccipital, greater occipital	extends head
rectus (straight) m. of head, posterior, smaller	m. rectus capitis posterior minor	posterior tubercle of atlas	occipital bone	suboccipital, greater occipital	extends head
rectus (straight) m. of thigh	m. rectus femoris	anterior inferior iliac spine, rim of acetabulum	base of patella, tuberosity of tibia	femoral	extends leg, flexes thigh
rhomboid m., greater	m. rhomboideus major	spinous processes of second, third, fourth and fifth thoracic vertebrae	vertebral margin of scapula	dorsal scapular	retracts and fixes scapula
rhomboid m., smaller	m. rhomboideus minor	spinous processes of seventh cervical and first thoracic vertebrae, lower part of nuchal ligament	vertebral margin of scapula at root of spine	dorsal scapular	retracts and fixes scapula
risorius m.	m. risorius	fascia over masseter	skin at angle of mouth	buccal branch of facial	draws angle of mouth laterally
rotator m's	mm. rotatores	a name applied to a series of small muscles deep in groove between spinous and transverse processes of vertebrae		spinal	extend and rotate vertebral column toward opposite side
sacrococcygeus m., dorsal (posterior)	m. sacrococcygeus dorsalis	a name applied to muscular slip passing from dorsal surface of sacrum to coccyx			
sacrococcygeus m., ventral (anterior)	m. sacrococcygeus ventralis	a name applied to musculotendinous slip passing from lower sacral vertebrae to coccyx			
sacrospinal m. *See* erector m. of spine					
salpingopharyngeus m.	m. salpingopharyngeus	cartilage of auditory tube	posterior part of palatopharyngeus	pharyngeal plexus	raises pharynx
sartorius m.	m. sartorius	anterior superior iliac spine	upper part of medial surface of tibia	femoral	flexes thigh and leg
scalene m., anterior	m. scalenus anterior	transverse processes of third to sixth cervical vertebrae	scalene tubercle of first rib	second to seventh cervical	raises first rib, flexes cervical vertebrae laterally
scalene m., middle	m. scalenus medius	transverse processes of first to seventh cervical vertebrae	upper surface of first rib	second to seventh cervical	raises first rib, flexes cervical vertebrae laterally
scalene m. of pleura. *See* smallest scalene m.					
scalene m., posterior	m. scalenus posterior	transverse processes of fourth to sixth cervical vertebrae	second rib	second to seventh cervical	raises first and second ribs, flexes cervical vertebrae laterally
scalene m., smallest	m. scalenus minimus	a name applied to muscular band occasionally found between anterior and middle scalene m's			

TABLE OF MUSCLES (*Continued*)

Common Name†	NA Term†	Origin*	Insertion*	Innervation	Action
semimembranous m.	m. semimembranosus	tuberosity of ischium	lateral condyle of femur, medial condyle and border of tibia	sciatic	flexes leg, extends thigh
semispinal m. of head	m. semispinalis capitis	transverse processes of upper thoracic and lower cervical vertebrae	occipital bone	suboccipital, greater occipital, branches of cervical	extends head
semispinal m. of neck	m. semispinalis cervicis	transverse processes of upper thoracic vertebrae	spinous processes of second to fifth (or fourth) cervical vertebrae	branches of cervical	extends, rotates vertebral column
semispinal m. of thorax	m. semispinalis thoracis	transverse processes of lower thoracic vertebrae	spinous processes of lower cervical and upper thoracic vertebrae	spinal	extends, rotates vertebral column
semitendinous m.	m. semitendinosus	tuberosity of ischium	upper part of medial surface of tibia	sciatic	flexes and rotates leg medially, extends thigh
serratus m., anterior	m. serratus anterior	8 upper ribs	vertebral border of scapula	long thoracic	draws scapula forward, rotates scapula to raise shoulder in abduction of arm
serratus m., posterior, inferior	m. serratus posterior inferior	spines of lower thoracic and upper lumbar vertebrae	4 lower ribs	ninth to twelfth (or eleventh) thoracic	perhaps lower ribs in expiration
serratus m., posterior, superior	m. serratus posterior superior	nuchal ligament, spinous processes of upper thoracic vertebrae	second, third, fourth and fifth ribs	upper 4 thoracic	perhaps raises ribs in inspiration
soleus m:	m. soleus	fibula, tendinous arch, tibia	calcaneus by Achilles tendon	tibial	plantar flexes foot
sphincter m. of anus, external	m. sphincter ani externus	tip of coccyx, anococcygeal ligament	tendinous center of perineum	inferior rectal, perineal branch of fourth sacral	closes anus
sphincter m. of anus, internal	m. sphincter ani internus	a name applied to a thickening of circular layer of muscular tunic at caudal end of rectum			
sphincter m. of bile duct	m. sphincter ductus choledochi	a name applied to annular sheath of muscle fibers investing bile duct within wall of duodenum			
sphincter m. of hepatopancreatic ampulla	m. sphincter ampullae hepatopancreaticae	a name applied to annular band of muscle fibers investing hepatopancreatic ampulla			
sphincter m. of pupil	m. sphincter pupillae	a name applied to circular fibers of iris		parasympathetic through ciliary	constricts pupil
sphincter m. of pylorus	m. sphincter pylori	a name applied to a thickening of middle layer of stomach musculature around pylorus			
sphincter m. of urethra	m. sphincter urethrae	inferior ramus of pubis	median raphe behind and in front of urethra	perineal	compresses urethra, at least in male
sphincter m. of urinary bladder	m. sphincter vesicae urinariae	a name applied to circular layer of fibers surrounding internal urethral orifice		vesical	closes internal orifice of urethra
spinal m. of head	m. spinalis capitis	spinous processes of upper thoracic and lower cervical vertebrae	occipital bone	spinal	extends head
spinal m. of neck	m. spinalis cervicis	spinous process of seventh cervical vertebra, nuchal ligament	spinous processes of axis	branches of cervical	extends vertebral column
spinal m. of thorax	m. spinalis thoracis	spinous processes of upper lumbar and lower thoracic vertebrae	spinous processes of upper thoracic vertebrae	branches of spinal	extends vertebral column
splenius m. of head	m. splenius capitis	lower half of nuchal ligament, spinous processes of seventh cervical and upper thoracic vertebrae	mastoid part of temporal bone, occipital bone	cervical	extends, rotates head

Common name	Latin name	Origin — Insertion	Nerve	Action
splenius m. of neck	m. splenius cervicis	spinous processes of upper thoracic vertebrae — transverse processes of upper cervical vertebrae	cervical	extends, rotates head and neck
stapedius m.	m. stapedius	interior of pyramidal eminence of tympanic cavity — neck of stapes	facial	dampens movement of stapes
sternal m.	m. sternalis	a name applied to muscular band occasionally found parallel to sternum on sternocostal head of greater pectoral m.		
sternocleidomastoid m.	m. sternocleidomastoideus	mastoid process, superior nuchal line of occipital bone — *sternal head* – manubrium; *clavicular head* – medial third of clavicle	accessory, cervical plexus	flexes vertebral column, rotates head to opposite side
sternocostal m. *See* transverse m. of thorax				
sternohyoid m.	m. sternohyoideus	manubrium sterni and/or clavicle — body of hyoid bone	ansa cervicalis	depresses hyoid bone and larynx
sternothyroid m.	m. sternothyroideus	manubrium sterni — lamina of thyroid cartilage	ansa cervicalis	depresses thyroid cartilage
styloglossus m.	m. styloglossus	styloid process — margin of tongue	hypoglossal	raises and retracts tongue
stylohyoid m.	m. stylohyoideus	styloid process — body of hyoid bone	facial	draws hyoid bone and tongue upward and backward
stylopharyngeus m.	m. stylopharyngeus	styloid process — thyroid cartilage, side of pharynx	glossopharyngeal	raises, dilates pharynx
subclavius m.	m. subclavius	lower surface of clavicle — first rib and its cartilage	nerve to subclavius	depresses lateral end of clavicle
subcostal m's	mm. subcostales	lower border of ribs — upper border of second or third rib below	intercostal	raise ribs in inspiration
subscapular m.	m. subscapularis	subscapular fossa of scapula — lesser tubercle of humerus	subscapular	rotates arm medially
supinator m.	m. supinator	lateral epicondyle of humerus, ligaments of elbow — radius	deep branch of radial	supinates forearm
supraspinous m.	m. supraspinatus	supraspinous fossa of scapula — greater tubercle of humerus	suprascapular	abducts arm
suspensory m.	m. suspensorius	a name applied to flat band of smooth muscle fibers originating from left crus of diaphragm and inserting continuous with muscular coat of duodenum at its junction with jejunum		
tarsal m., inferior	m. tarsalis inferior	inferior rectus m. of eyeball — tarsal plate of lower eyelid	sympathetic	widens palpebral fissure
tarsal m., superior	m. tarsalis superior	levator m. of upper eyelid — tarsal plate of upper eyelid	sympathetic	widens palpebral fissure
temporal m.	m. temporalis	temporal fossa and fascia — coronoid process of mandible	mandibular	closes jaws
temporoparietal m.	m. temporoparietalis	temporal fascia above ear — galea aponeurotica	temporal branches of facial	tightens scalp
tensor m. of fascia lata	m. tensor fasciae latae	iliac crest — iliotibial tract of fascia lata	superior gluteal	flexes, rotates thigh medially
tensor m. of palatine velum	m. tensor veli palatini	scaphoid fossa and spine of sphenoid — aponeurosis of soft palate, wall of auditory tube	mandibular	tenses soft palate, opens auditory tube
tensor m. of tympanum	m. tensor tympani	cartilaginous portion of auditory tube — handle of malleus	mandibular	tenses tympanic membrane
teres major m.	m. teres major	inferior angle of scapula — crest of lesser tubercle of humerus	lower subscapular	adducts arm
teres minor m.	m. teres minor	lateral margin of scapula — greater tubercle of humerus	axillary	rotates arm laterally
thyroarytenoid m.	m. thyroarytenoideus	medial surface of lamina of thyroid cartilage — muscular process of arytenoid cartilage	recurrent laryngeal	shortens vocal folds
thyroepiglottic m.	m. thyroepiglotticus	lamina of thyroid cartilage — epiglottis	recurrent laryngeal	closes inlet to larynx
thyrohyoid m.	m. thyrohyoideus	lamina of thyroid cartilage — greater horn of hyoid bone	ansa cervicalis	raises larynx
tibial m., anterior	m. tibialis anterior	lateral condyle and surface of tibia, interosseous membrane — medial cuneiform, base of first metatarsal	deep peroneal	dorsiflexes and inverts foot
tibial m., posterior	m. tibialis posterior	tibia, fibula, interosseous membrane — bases of second to fourth metatarsal bones and tarsal bones, except talus	tibial	inverts foot
tracheal m.	m. trachealis	a name applied to transverse smooth muscle fibers filling gap at back of each cartilage of trachea	autonomic	lessens caliber of trachea

TABLE OF MUSCLES (Continued)

COMMON NAME†	NA TERM†	ORIGIN*	INSERTION*	INNERVATION	ACTION
m. of tragus	m. tragicus	a name applied to short, flattened vertical band on lateral surface of tragus		temporal, posterior auricular branches of facial	
transverse m. of abdomen	m. transversus abdominis	lower 6 costal cartilages, thoracolumbar fascia, iliac crest	linea alba through rectus sheath, conjoined tendon to pubis	lower thoracic	compresses abdominal viscera
transverse m. of auricle	m. transversus auriculae	cranial surface of auricle	circumference of auricle	posterior auricular branch of facial	retracts helix
transverse m. of chin	m. transversus menti	a name applied to superficial fibers of depressor m. of angle of mouth which turn medially and cross to opposite side			
transverse m. of nape	m. transversus nuchae	a name applied to small muscle often present, passing from occipital protuberance to posterior auricular m.; it may be either superficial or deep to trapezius			
transverse m. of perineum, deep	m. transversus perinei profundus	ramus of ischium	tendinous center of perineum	perineal	fixes tendinous center of perineum
transverse m. of perineum, superficial	m. transversus perinei superficialis	ramus of ischium	tendinous center of perineum	perineal	fixes tendinous center of perineum
transverse m. of thorax	m. transversus thoracis	posterior surface of body of sternum and of xiphoid process	second to sixth costal cartilages	intercostal	perhaps narrows chest
transverse m. of tongue	m. transversus linguae	median septum of tongue	dorsum and margins of tongue	hypoglossal	changes shape of tongue in mastication
transversospinal m.	m. transversospinalis	a name applied collectively to semispinal, multifidus and rotator m's			
trapezius m.	m. trapezius	occipital bone, nuchal ligament, spinous processes of seventh cervical and all thoracic vertebrae	clavicle, acromion, spine of scapula	accessory, cervical plexus	elevates shoulder, rotates scapula to raise shoulder in abduction of arm, draws scapula backward
triangular m. See depressor m. of angle of mouth					
triceps m. of arm (triceps brachii m.)	m. triceps brachii	long head—infraglenoid tubercle of scapula; lateral head—posterior surface of humerus; medial head—posterior surface of humerus below groove for radial nerve	olecranon of ulna	radial	extends forearm
triceps m. of calf (triceps surae m.)	m. triceps surae	a name applied collectively to gastrocnemius and soleus m's			
m. of uvula	m. uvulae	posterior nasal spine of palatine bone and aponeurosis of soft palate	uvula	pharyngeal plexus	raises uvula
vastus (great) m., intermediate	m. vastus intermedius	anterior and lateral surfaces of femur	patella, common tendon of quadriceps m. of thigh	femoral	extends leg
vastus (great) m., lateral	m. vastus lateralis	lateral aspect of femur	patella, common tendon of quadriceps m. of thigh	femoral	extends leg
vastus (great) m., medial	m. vastus medialis	medial aspect of femur	patella, common tendon of quadriceps m. of thigh	femoral	extends leg
vertical m. of tongue	m. verticalis linguae	dorsal fascia of tongue	sides and base of tongue	hypoglossus	changes shape of tongue in mastication and deglutition
vocal m.	m. vocalis	angle between laminae of thyroid cartilage	vocal process of arytenoid cartilage	recurrent laryngeal	causes local variations in tension of vocal fold
zygomatic m., greater	m. zygomaticus major	zygomatic bone	angle of mouth	facial	draws angle of mouth upward and laterally
zygomatic m., smaller	m. zygomaticus minor	zygomatic bone	orbicular m. of mouth, levator m. of upper lip	facial	draws upper lip upward and laterally

Muscles enable the body to perform different types of movement. Those that bend a limb at a joint, raising a thigh or bending an elbow, are called flexors. Those that straighten a limb are called extensors. There are others, the abductors, that make possible movement away from the midline of the body, whereas the abductors permit movement toward the midline. Muscles always act in opposing groups. In bending an elbow or flexing a muscle, for example, the biceps (flexor) contracts and the triceps (extensor) relaxes. The reverse happens in straightening the elbow.

A muscle that has contracted many times, and has exhausted its stores of glycogen and other substances, and accumulated too much lactic acid, becomes unable to contract further and suffers from what is called muscle fatigue. In prolonged exhausting work, fat in the muscles can also be used for energy, and as a consequence the muscles become leaner.

MUSCULAR DISORDERS AND DISEASES. Strenuous physical activity that strains and tears the fibers can cause such muscular disorders including strain, charley horse and muscle cramps.

Muscles may become infected or inflamed by the invasion of organisms, such as the parasite *Trichinella spiralis* which is taken into the body by eating uncooked or poorly cooked pork. It causes the disease called trichinosis. Another type of muscular inflammation is fibrositis.

In poliomyelitis and other diseases of the nervous system, the muscles are disabled because the nerves leading to them have been injured or destroyed. The muscles are not directly harmed, but because they can no longer be stimulated they eventually waste away from disuse. The group of diseases called the progressive muscular atrophies result from wasting.

MYASTHENIA GRAVIS involves primarily the muscles of the face, eyelids, larynx and throat. The cause is an impairment of the conduction of nerve impulses to the muscles.

Some diseases directly disable the muscles. MUSCULAR DYSTROPHY weakens the muscles of the trunk and limbs. The muscles sometimes enlarge or they may weaken and atrophy.

Benign and malignant tumors may (rarely) develop in muscles, producing myomas.

agonistic m., one opposed in action by another muscle, called the antagonist.

antagonistic m., one that counteracts the action of another muscle.

antigravity m's, those that by their tone resist the constant pull of gravity in the maintenance of normal posture.

appendicular m., one of the muscles of a limb.

articular m., one that has one end attached to the capsule of a joint.

cutaneous m., striated muscle that inserts into the skin.

extraocular m's, the extrinsic muscles of the eye.

extrinsic m., one that originates in another part than that of its insertion, as those originating outside the eye, which move the eyeball.

fixation m's, fixator m's, accessory muscles that serve to steady a part.

fusiform m., a spindle-shaped muscle.

hamstring m's, the muscles of the back of the thigh.

intraocular m's, the intrinsic muscles of the eyeball.

intrinsic m., one whose origin and insertion are both in the same part or organ, as those entirely within the eye.

orbicular m., one that encircles a body opening, e.g., the eye or mouth.

organic m., visceral muscle.

Voluntary muscles extend from one bone to another, effect movements by contraction and work on the principle of leverage. For every direct action made by a muscle, an antagonistic muscle effects an opposite movement. To flex the arm, the biceps contracts and the triceps relaxes; to extend the arm, the triceps contracts and the biceps relaxes.

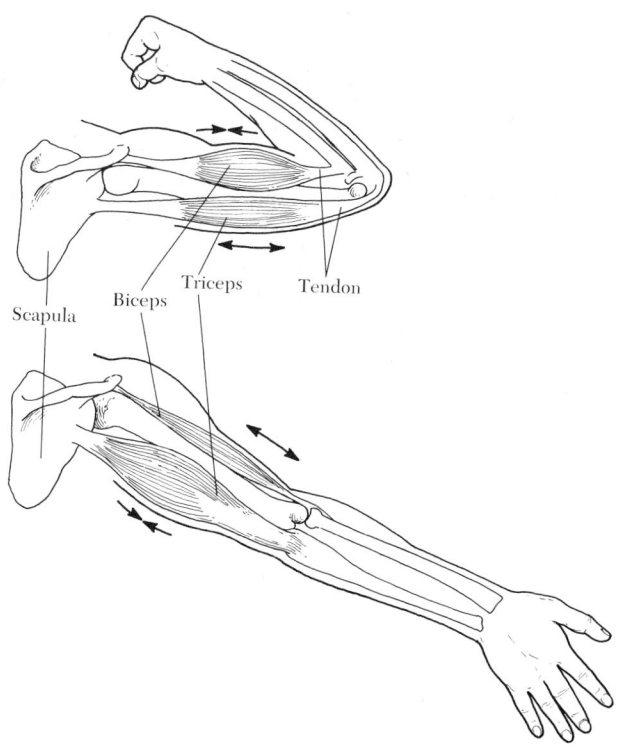

Scapula · Biceps · Triceps · Tendon

postaxial m., one on the dorsal side of an extremity.

preaxial m., one on the ventral side of an extremity.

red m., the darker-colored muscle tissue of some mammals, composed of fibers rich in sarcoplasm, but with only faint cross-striping.

m. relaxant, an agent that specifically aids in reducing muscle tension.

skeletal m's, striated muscles that are attached to bones and typically cross at least one joint.

sphincter m., a ringlike muscle that closes a natural orifice; called also sphincter.

synergic m's, synergistic m's, those that assist one another in action.

thenar m's, the abductor and flexor muscles of the thumb.

vestigial m., one that is rudimentary in man, but well developed in some other mammals.

visceral m., muscle fibers associated chiefly with the hollow viscera.

white m., the paler muscle tissue of some mammals, composed of fibers with little sarcoplasm and prominent cross-striping.

yoked m's, those that normally act simultaneously and equally, as in moving the eyes.

muscular (mus'ku-lar) 1. pertaining to a muscle. 2. having well developed muscles.

m. dystrophy, a group of related muscle diseases that are progressively crippling because muscles are gradually weakened and eventually atrophy. The cause is not known and at present there is no specific cure. The disease can sometimes be arrested temporarily; not all forms of it are totally disabling.

The word dystrophy means faulty or imperfect nutrition. In muscular dystrophy the muscles suffer a vital loss of protein, and muscle fibers are replaced gradually by fat and connective tissue until, in the late stages of the disease, the voluntary muscle system becomes virtually useless. In muscular dystrophy all visible damage occurs in the muscles themselves, and thus the disease is markedly different from MULTIPLE SCLEROSIS, in which the muscles are rendered impotent by damage to the nerves that control them.

Muscular dystrophy, which is believed to affect almost a quarter of a million Americans, is hereditary at least in part, although the way it is inherited is not the same for all types of the disease. The disease (or a propensity for the disease) seems to be carried mainly by women who, while not suffering from it themselves, may pass it on to their offspring, usually their sons. A woman who has conceived a dystrophic child is likely to be a carrier, as may be a woman who has had a dystrophic relative such as an uncle.

CHILDHOOD MUSCULAR DYSTROPHY. Whether or not muscular dystrophy is hereditary, it cannot be detected at birth. In most cases the symptoms begin to be noticeable about the second or third year. The child gradually finds it more difficult to play and get about. Then, as the weakening process of the disease continues, he relies on a wheel chair, and later must spend most of his time in bed. In many cases death comes before the age of 20 from respiratory ailments or heart failure.

This childhood type of disease – unfortunately the most common type – is known as the Duchenne type or progressive muscular dystrophy. It is also sometimes called pseudohypertrophic muscular dystrophy because at the beginning the muscles, especially those in the calves, appear healthy and bulging when actually they are already weakened and their size is due to an excess of fat.

OTHER TYPES. Another type of the disease sometimes begins in childhood but is much more likely to appear during the teens or twenties. When the first symptom is a failure of the musculature of the pelvic girdle, this type is referred to as limb-girdle muscular dystrophy. It usually proceeds more slowly than does the childhood form.

This same type may take the form of facioscapulohumeral muscular dystrophy (referring to the face, shoulder and upper arm muscles), which is likely to manifest itself first in an almost imperceptible weakening of the facial muscles. It is also known as Landouzy-Déjerine muscular dystrophy. Muscle deterioration starts in childhood or early adulthood but it may proceed very gradually over a number of years, sometimes until late in life. Some patients may only be slightly handicapped.

Other, rarer types of muscular dystrophy have been identified, including a distal type that begins in the peripheral muscles of the extremities. Still another type affects only muscles of the eye. Sometimes two or more forms are present in the same patient.

MANAGEMENT OF MUSCULAR DYSTROPHY. There is almost never any pain in muscular dystrophy. The mind is not affected; patients have normal intelligence. As the small muscles often are the last to be damaged, patients may continue to use their fingers. Children with muscular dystrophy are able to enjoy many recreations, even when they must rely on crutches or wheelchairs. The disease is not contagious.

Recent experiments hold out some hope that the progress of the disease can be slowed down, at least temporarily, by the use of certain medications that contribute to a build-up of protein in the patient's body or strengthen his muscle-cell membranes to prevent excessive escape of protein. Physical therapy – exercises, including exercise of the lungs by deep breathing – can sometimes bolster the delaying action against muscular weakness. The aim of such exercise is not to restore muscle power (which cannot be done) but to ensure that the patient makes the best use of the good muscle tissue remaining.

The more active the patient is, the better he will be physically and mentally. Obesity should be avoided.

The Muscular Dystrophy Associations of America, 1790 Broadway, New York, N.Y. 10019, are concerned not only with research but with every aspect of the care and comfort of dystrophic patients and can offer many valuable suggestions.

muscularis (mus"ku-la'ris) [L.] relating to muscle, specifically a muscular layer or coat.

musculature (mus'ku-lah-tūr) the muscular system of the body, or the muscles of a particular region.

musculocutaneous (mus"ku-lo-ku-ta'ne-us) pertaining to muscle and skin.

musculomembranous (mus"ku-lo-mem'brahnus) pertaining to muscle and membrane.

musculophrenic (mus"ku-lo-fren'ik) pertaining to (chest) muscles and the diaphragm.

musculoskeletal (mus″ku-lo-skel′ĕ-tal) pertaining to muscle and skeleton.

musculotendinous (mus″ku-lo-ten′dĭ-nus) pertaining to muscle and tendon.

musculotropic (mus″ku-lo-trop′ik) exerting its principal effect upon muscle.

musculus (mus′ku-lus), pl. *mus′culi* [L.] muscle.

musicotherapy (mu″zĭ-ko-ther′ah-pe) treatment of disease by music.

mustard (mus′tard) an irritant compound derived from dried ripe seed of *Brassica nigra* or *B. juncea*.
nitrogen m's, highly toxic compounds used in treatment of neoplastic disease (see also NITROGEN MUSTARD).
sulfur m., a synthetic compound with vesicant and other toxic properties.

Mustargen (mus′tar-jen) trademark for a preparation of mechlorethamine hydrochloride, an antineoplastic agent.

mutagen (mu′tah-jen) an agent that induces genetic mutation.

mutagenesis (mu″tah-jen′ĕ-sis) the induction of genetic mutation.

mutagenicity (mu″tah-jĕ-nis′ĭ-te) the property of being able to induce genetic mutation.

mutant (mu′tant) in genetics, a variation that breeds true, owing to chromosomal changes.

mutase (mu′tās) 1. an enzyme that produces rearrangement of molecules. 2. a vegetable food preparation rich in proteins.

mutation (mu-ta′shun) change; especially an alteration in a gene that produces a change in later generations of the organism.
induced m., a genetic mutation caused by external factors experimentally or accidentally produced.
somatic m., a genetic mutation occurring in a somatic cell, providing the basis for a mosaic condition.

mute (mūt) 1. unable or unwilling to speak. 2. a person who cannot speak. In most cases, mutes are also deaf (deaf-mute).

mutism (mu′tizm) inability or refusal to speak. In almost all cases, mutes are unable to speak because their deafness has prevented them from hearing the spoken word. Speech is learned by imitating the speech of others. Even the child who is born with normal hearing and then loses it may lose part or all of his power of speech through loss of contact with the speech of others. In certain cases, mutism occurs because the voice organs themselves have been damaged or removed. This is particularly true in the case of cancer of the throat, in which LARYNGECTOMY is performed.
For information about training schools and educational institutions for the deaf-mute, both the National Association of Hearing and Speech Agencies, 919 18th Street, N.W., Washington, D.C. 20006, and the Volta Bureau, 1537 35th Street, N.W., Washington, D.C. 20007, may be consulted. The John Tracy Clinic, 806 West Adams Boulevard, Los Angeles, Calif. 90007, offers a free correspondence course that is designed to give assistance to the parents of deaf children below the age of 6.

akinetic m., a state in which the person makes no spontaneous movement or sound, because of either neurologic or psychologic reasons.
hysterical m., hysterical inability to utter words.

muton (mu′ton) a gene when specified as the smallest hereditary element that can be altered by mutation.

mutualism (mu′tu-al-izm″) the biologic association of two individuals or populations of different species, both of which are benefited by the relationship and sometimes unable to exist without it.

mutualist (mu′tu-al-ist) one of the organisms or species living with another in a mutually beneficial relationship.

M.V. [L.] *Medicus Veterinarius* (veterinary physician).

Mv chemical symbol, *mendelevium*.

mv. millivolt.

M.W.I.A. Medical Women's International Association.

my(o)- (mi′o) word element [Gr.], *muscle*.

myalgia (mi-al′je-ah) muscular pain.
epidemic m., epidemic pleurodynia.

Myanesin (mi-an′ĕ-sin) trademark for mephenesin, a muscle relaxant.

myasthenia (mi″as-the′ne-ah) muscular debility or weakness. adj., myasthen′ic.
angiosclerotic m., excessive muscular fatigue due to vascular changes.
m. gas′trica, weakness and loss of tone in the muscular coats of the stomach; atony of the stomach.
m. gra′vis, a chronic disease characterized by muscular weakness, thought to be caused by a chemical defect at the sites where the nerves and muscles interact (the myoneural junction). There is some evidence that the disease has an immunologic basis.
People with myasthenia gravis find that certain muscles feel weak and tire quickly on exertion. Muscles frequently affected are those of the face, eyelids, larynx and throat. The patient may first detect the onset of myasthenia gravis by the drooping of the eyelids or difficulty in such a relatively simple operation as chewing or even perhaps swallowing water.
There is no true paralysis of the muscles, and usually they do not atrophy. Severe forms of the disease, however, can be seriously disabling or even fatal because the vital muscles of swallowing or breathing may be affected.
Both medical and surgical treatments are helpful to many patients. The drugs neostigmine, physostigmine and pyridostigmine have been used successfully to reverse the disordered chemical reaction at the myoneural junction. Removal of the thymus has also been found effective and in some instances it has even been curative.
NURSING CARE. During acute episodes of myasthenia gravis the patient must be watched closely and his every need anticipated. He may not be able to call for help or do anything to help himself.

Severe muscle weakness throws him completely at the mercy of those assigned to his care. An emergency tracheostomy set is kept at the bedside in case the trachea becomes obstructed with mucus that the patient is unable to remove by coughing. Frequent suctioning is often required, especially before meals.

myatonia (mi″ah-to′ne-ah) defective muscular tone.
m. congen′ita, amyotonia congenita.

myatrophy (mi-at′ro-fe) atrophy of a muscle.

myc(o)- (mi′ko) word element [Gr.], *fungus.*

mycelium (mi-se′le-um) the filamentary part of a fungus.

mycetismus (mi″sĕ-tiz′mus) mushroom poisoning.

mycetogenic (mi-se″to-jen′ik) caused by fungi.

mycetoma (mi″sĕ-to′mah) a chronic disease caused by a variety of fungi, affecting the foot, hands, legs and other parts; called also maduromycosis. The most common form is that of the foot (Madura foot), characterized by sinus formation, necrosis and swelling.

Mycobacterium (mi″ko-bak-te″re-um) a genus of Schizomycetes characterized by acid-fast staining.
M. kansas′ii, the etiologic agent of a tuberculosis-like disease in man.
M. lep′rae, a species considered to be the etiologic agent of leprosy.
M. tuberculo′sis, the causative agent of tuberculosis in man.
M. tuberculo′sis var. bo′vis, the bovine variety of tubercle bacillus, most commonly infecting cattle and acquired by man usually by ingestion of infected milk; uncommon in the United States because of strict testing of cattle.

mycobacterium (mi″ko-bak-te″re-um), pl. *mycobacte′ria* [L.] 1. an individual organism of the genus Mycobacterium. 2. a slender, acid-fast microorganism resembling the bacillus that causes tuberculosis.
anonymous mycobacteria, bacteria resembling the tubercle bacilli, found in pulmonary infections, usually of a chronic nature, in man, for which species names have not been established. Some are affected in color by exposure to light, others are not.

mycodermatitis (mi″ko-der″mah-ti′tis) inflammation of a mucous membrane.

mycogastritis (mi″ko-gas-tri′tis) inflammation of the mucous membrane of the stomach.

mycology (mi-kol′o-je) the study of fungi and fungus diseases.

mycomyringitis (mi″ko-mir″in-ji′tis) fungus inflammation of the eardrum.

Mycoplasma (mi″ko-plaz′mah) a taxonomic name given a genus including the pleuropneumonia-like organisms (PPLO) and separated into 15 species. The organisms are responsible for respiratory illnesses in man.

mycosis (mi-ko′sis) any disease caused by fungi.
m. favo′sa, favus.
m. fungoi′des, a fatal skin disease, with red fungating tumors, cachexia and much pain.
m. interdigita′lis, dermatophytosis.

mycosozin (mi″ko-so′zin) any body protein that destroys fungi.

mycostasis (mi-kos′tah-sis) prevention of growth and multiplication of fungi.

mycostat (mi′ko-stat) an agent that inhibits the growth of fungi.

mycotic (mi-kot′ik) pertaining to a mycosis, or caused by vegetable microorganisms.

mycotoxicosis (mi″ko-tok″sĭ-ko′sis) poisoning due to a fungus.

mydriasis (mĭ-dri′ah-sis) great dilatation of the pupil.

mydriatic (mid″re-at′ik) 1. dilating the pupil. 2. a drug that dilates the pupil.

myectomy (mi-ek′to-me) excision of a muscle.

myectopia (mi″ek-to′pe-ah) displacement of a muscle.

myel(o)- (mi′el-o) word element [Gr.], *spinal cord; bone marrow.*

myelalgia (mi″ĕ-lal′je-ah) pain in the spinal cord.

myelapoplexy (mi″el-ap′o-plek″se) hemorrhage in the spinal cord.

myelatelia (mi″el-ah-te′le-ah) imperfect development of the spinal cord.

myelatrophy (mi″el-at′ro-fe) atrophy of the spinal cord.

myelemia (mi″el-e′me-ah) the presence of myelocytes or neutrophil leukocytes in the blood; myelocytic leukemia.

myelencephalon (mi″el-en-sef′ah-lon) 1. the part of the central nervous system comprising the medulla oblongata and lower part of the fourth ventricle. 2. the posterior of the two brain vesicles formed by specialization of the rhombencephalon in the developing embryo.

myelin (mi′ĕ-lin) 1. the fatlike substance forming a sheath around certain nerve fibers; these nerve fibers are spoken of as myelinated or medullated fibers. 2. a lipoid substance found in the body, especially in certain degenerative diseases. adj., **myelin′ic.**
The myelin sheath is believed to influence the rate at which nerve impulses are conducted; transmission is always more rapid in myelinated fibers than in unmyelinated fibers.
Myelinated nerve fibers occur predominantly in the cranial and spinal nerves and compose the white matter of the brain and spinal cord. In fact, it is the myelin sheath that gives the whitish color to the areas of white matter. Unmyelinated fibers are abundant in the autonomic nervous system. The term gray matter refers to areas in the nervous system in which the nerve fibers are unmyelinated.

myelination, myelinization (mi″ĕ-lĭ-na′shun), (mi″ĕ-lin″ĭ-za′shun) production of myelin around an axon.

myelinoma (mi″ĕ-lĭ-no′mah) a tumor of the myelin.

myelinopathy (mi″ĕ-lĭ-nop′ah-the) degeneration of the white matter of the brain or spinal cord.

myelinosis (mi″ĕ-lĭ-no′sis) fatty degeneration, with formation of myelin.

myelitis (mi″ĕ-li′tis) inflammation of the spinal cord (see also POLIOMYELITIS) or bone marrow (see also OSTEOMYELITIS). adj., **myelit′ic.**
  ascending m., myelitis moving cephalad (upward) along the spinal cord.
  bulbar m., that involving the medulla oblongata.
  central m., myelitis affecting chiefly the gray matter of the spinal cord.
  disseminated m., that which has several distinct foci.
  focal m., myelitis affecting a small area.
  sclerosing m., a form characterized by hardening of the spinal cord and overgrowth of interstitial tissue.
  transverse m., inflammation affecting the entire cross section of the spinal cord at one level.
  traumatic m., myelitis that follows injury to the spinal cord.

myeloarchitecture (mi″ĕ-lo-ar′kĭ-tek″tūr) the organization of the nerve tracts in the spinal cord.

myeloblast (mi′ĕ-lo-blast″) one of the large mononuclear, nongranular cells of bone marrow that develop into myelocytes and also into erythroblasts, according to some hematologists.

myeloblastemia (mi″ĕ-lo-blas-te′me-ah) myeloblasts in the blood.

myeloblastoma (mi″ĕ-lo-blas-to′mah) a focal malignant tumor observed in chronic or acute myelocytic leukemia.

myeloblastosis (mi″ĕ-lo-blas-to′sis) excess of myeloblasts in the blood.

myelocele (mi′ĕ-lo-sēl″) hernial protrusion of the spinal cord through a defect in the vertebral column.

myelocoele (mi′ĕ-lo-sēl″) the central canal of the spinal cord.

myelocyst (mi′ĕ-lo-sist) a cyst developed from rudimentary medullary canals.

myelocystocele (mi″ĕ-lo-sis′to-sēl) hernial protrusion of cystic spinal cord through a defect in the vertebral column.

myelocystomeningocele (mi″ĕ-lo-sis″to-mĕ-ning′go-sēl) protrusion of cystic spinal cord and covering membranes through a defect in the vertebral column.

myelocyte (mi′ĕ-lo-sīt″) one of the typical cells of red bone marrow, giving rise to the granular leukocytes of the blood. They occur in the blood in certain types of LEUKEMIA. adj., **myelocyt′ic.**

myelocytoma (mi″ĕ-lo-si-to′mah) 1. multiple myeloma. 2. chronic myelocytic leukemia.

myelocytosis (mi″ĕ-lo-si-to′sis) increase of myelocytes in the blood.

myelodiastasis (mi″ĕ-lo-di-as′tah-sis) disintegration of the spinal cord.

myelodysplasia (mi″ĕ-lo-dis-pla′ze-ah) defective development of the spinal cord.

myeloencephalic (mi″ĕ-lo-en″se-fal′ik) pertaining to the spinal cord and brain.

myeloencephalitis (mi″ĕ-lo-en-sef″ah-li′tis) inflammation of the spinal cord and brain.

myelofibrosis (mi″ĕ-lo-fi-bro′sis) replacement of bone marrow by fibrous tissue.

myelogenesis (mi″ĕ-lo-jen′ĕ-sis) 1. development of the central nervous system. 2. the deposition of myelin around the axon.

myelogenic, myelogenous (mi″ĕ-lo-jen′ik), (mi″-ĕ-loj′ĕ-nus) produced in the bone marrow.

myelogeny (mi″ĕ-loj′ĕ-ne) development of the myelin sheaths of nerve fibers.

myelogone (mi′ĕ-lo-gōn″) a primitive cell of the myeloid series.

myelogram (mi′ĕ-lo-gram″) a roentgenogram of the spinal cord after the injection of a contrast medium.

myelography (mi″ĕ-log′rah-fe) roentgenography of the spinal cord after injection of a contrast medium into the subarachnoid space.

myeloid (mi′ĕ-loid) 1. pertaining to, derived from or resembling bone marrow. 2. pertaining to the spinal cord. 3. having the appearance of myelocytes, but not derived from bone marrow.
  m. tissue, red bone marrow.

myeloidosis (mi″ĕ-loi-do′sis) formation of myeloid tissue, on red bone marrow.

myeloma (mi″ĕ-lo′mah) 1. a tumor composed of cells of the type normally found in the bone marrow. 2. any medullary tumor. 3. giant cell sarcoma. 4. a slow-growing tumor of a tendinous sheath containing myeloplaxes.
  giant cell m., a tumor of bone marrow containing many giant cells.
  multiple m., plasma cell m., a primary malignant tumor of bone marrow, marked by circumscribed or diffuse tumor-like hyperplasia of the bone marrow, and usually associated with anemia and with Bence Jones protein in the urine. The patient complains of neuralgic pains; later painful swellings appear on the ribs and skull and spontaneous fractures may occur. Called also Kahler's disease, myelopathic albumosuria, Bence Jones albumosuria and lymphadenia ossea.

myelomalacia (mi″ĕ-lo-mah-la′she-ah) morbid softening of spinal cord.

myelomatosis (mi″ĕ-lo-mah-to′sis) 1. the simultaneous presence of many myelomas. 2. any leukemic disease in which myeloblasts are abundant in the blood.

myelomeningitis (mi″ĕ-lo-men″in-ji′tis) inflammation of the spinal cord and meninges.

myelomeningocele (mi″ĕ-lo-mĕ-ning′go-sēl) meningomyelocele.

myelon (mi′ĕ-lon) the spinal cord.

myeloneuritis (mi″ĕ-lo-nu-ri′tis) inflammation of the spinal cord and peripheral nerves.

myeloparalysis (mi″ĕ-lo-pah-ral′ĭ-sis) spinal paralysis.

myelopathy (mi″ĕ-lop′ah-the) any disease of the central nervous system. adj., **myelopath′ic.**

myelophage (mi′ĕ-lo″fāj″) a macrophage that digests myelin.

myelophthisis (mi″ĕ-lo-thi′sis) wasting of the spinal cord.

myeloplast (mi′ĕ-lo-plast″) any leukocyte of the bone marrow.

myeloplax (mi′ĕ-lo-plaks″) a multinuclear giant cell of bone marrow.

myeloplegia (mi″ĕ-lo-ple′je-ah) spinal paralysis.

myelopoiesis (mi″ĕ-lo-poi-e′sis) the formation of marrow or myelocytes.
  extra medullary m., formation of myeloid tissue outside bone marrow.

myeloproliferative (mi″ĕ-lo-pro-lif′er-ah″tiv) pertaining to or characterized by proliferation of myeloid tissue.

myeloradiculitis (mi″ĕ-lo-rah-dik″u-li′tis) inflammation of the spinal cord and spinal nerve roots.

myeloradiculodysplasia (mi″ĕ-lo-rah-dik″u-lo-dis-pla′ze-ah) abnormal development of the spinal cord and spinal nerve roots.

myeloradiculopathy (mi″ĕ-lo-rah-dik″u-lop′ah-the) disease of the spinal cord and spinal nerve roots.

myelorrhagia (mi″ĕ-lo-ra′je-ah) spinal hemorrhage.

myelorrhaphy (mi″ĕ-lor′ah-fe) suture of the spinal cord.

myelosarcoma (mi″ĕ-lo-sar-ko′mah) a sarcomatous growth made up of myeloid tissue or bone marrow cells.

myeloscintogram (mi″ĕ-lo-sin′to-gram) the graphic record of particles counted by a scintillation counter after injection into the subarachnoid space of a solution containing a radioactive isotope.

myelosclerosis (mi″ĕ-lo-sklĕ-ro′sis) 1. sclerosis of the spinal cord. 2. obliteration of the marrow cavity by small spicules of bone. 3. myelofibrosis.

myelosis (mi″ĕ-lo′sis) 1. proliferation of myelocytes. 2. formation of a tumor of the spinal cord.
  erythremic m., a condition characterized by overgrowth of erythroid and reticuloendothelial cells in bone marrow.
  leukemic m., myelosis with a high total white count and with many immature forms.

myelospongium (mi″ĕ-lo-spun′je-um) a network developing into the neuroglia.

myelosuppressive (mi″ĕ-lo-sŭ-pres′iv) 1. inhibitive to the function of bone marrow. 2. an agent that suppresses bone marrow function.

myelotomy (mi″ĕ-lot′o-me) severance of nerve fibers in the spinal cord.

myelotoxin (mi″ĕ-lo-tok′sin) a toxin that destroys marrow cells.

myenteron (mi-en′ter-on) the muscular coat of the intestine. adj., **myenter′ic.**

Myerson's sign (mi′er-sunz) in Parkinson's disease, repeated blinking of the eyes on rapping the forehead.

myesthesia (mi″es-the′ze-ah) muscle sensibility.

myiasis (mi-i′ah-sis) invasion of the body by the larvae of flies, characterized as cutaneous (subdermal tissue), gastrointestinal, nasopharyngeal, ocular or urinary, depending on the region invaded.

myitis (mi-i′tis) inflammation of muscle; myositis.

myko- for words beginning thus, see those beginning *myco-*.

Myleran (mil′er-an) trademark for a preparation of busulfan, an alkylating agent used in the treatment of myelocytic leukemia.

mylohyoid (mi″lo-hi′oid) pertaining to the hyoid bone and molar teeth.

myoalbumin (mi″o-al-bu′min) an albumin in muscle tissue.

myoalbumose (mi″o-al′bu-mōs) a protein from muscle juice.

myoarchitectonic (mi″o-ar″kĭ-tek-ton′ik) pertaining to the structural arrangement of muscle fibers.

myoatrophy (mi″o-at′ro-fe) muscular atrophy.

myoblast (mi′o-blast) an embryonic cell that becomes a cell of muscle fiber.

myoblastoma (mi″o-blas-to′mah) a tumor of muscle made up of cells resembling myoblasts.
  granular cell m., a benign, circumscribed tumor of the mucosa of the lips or other oral structures, made up of large granular cells with small, round nuclei.

myobradia (mi″o-bra′de-ah) slow reaction of muscle to stimulation.

myocardial (mi″o-kar′de-al) pertaining to the muscular tissue of the heart.
  m. infarction, formation of an infarct in the heart muscle, due to interruption of the blood supply to the area (see also CORONARY OCCLUSION).

myocardiograph (mi″o-kar′de-o-graf″) an instrument for making tracings of heart movements.

myocarditis (mi″o-kar-di′tis) inflammation of the muscular walls of the heart. The condition may result from bacterial or viral infections or it may be a toxic inflammation caused by drugs or toxins from infectious agents. Other systemic diseases that may be accompanied by myocarditis are TRICHINOSIS, SERUM SICKNESS, RHEUMATIC FEVER and COLLAGEN DISEASES. In many cases the etiology is unknown.
  SYMPTOMS. The most common symptoms of acute myocarditis are pain in the epigastric region or under the sternum, dyspnea and cardiac arrhythmias. If the condition persists and becomes chronic,

there is pain in the right upper quadrant of the abdomen, owing to hepatic congestion. The latter symptom is a sign of left ventricular failure and often is accompanied by edema and other signs of congestive heart failure.

TREATMENT. Acute myocarditis usually subsides when the primary illness improves. It is considered incidental to the systemic disease and, though it may be a serious manifestation of a systemic illness, acute myocarditis often does not require specific treatment. Steroids and pressor agents such as norephinephrine may be used to reduce the inflammatory process and maintain adequate arterial pressure.

If the heart involvement becomes chronic, treatment then must be aimed at management of the chronic heart failure. (See also congestive HEART FAILURE.)

myocardium (mi″o-kar′de-um) the muscular substance of the heart.

myocardosis (mi″o-kar-do′sis) any myocardial disorder that is not due to an inflammatory condition, but is the result of hypertension, coronary sclerosis and hyperthyroidism.

myocele (mi′o-sēl) hernia of muscle through its sheath.

myocellulitis (mi″o-sel″u-li′tis) myositis with cellulitis.

myoceptor (mi′o-sep″tor) the structure in a muscle fiber that receives the nerve stimulus from the motor end-organ of the nerve.

myocerosis (mi″o-se-ro′sis) amyloid degeneration of muscle.

myochrome (mi′o-krōm) any member of a group of muscle pigments.

Myochrysine (mi″o-kri′sin) trademark for a preparation of gold sodium thiomalate, an antiarthritic.

myoclonus (mi″o-klo′nus) shocklike contractions of part of a muscle, an entire muscle or a group of muscles; usually a manifestation of a convulsive disorder. adj., **myoclon′ic.**
  palatal m., a condition characterized by a rapid rhythmic movement of one side of the palate.

myocyte (mi′o-sīt) a cell of muscular tissue.

myocytoma (mi″o-si-to′mah) a tumor composed of myocytes.

myodemia (mi″o-de′me-ah) fatty degeneration of muscle.

myodiastasis (mi″o-di-as′tah-sis) separation of muscle fibers.

myodynia (mi″o-din′e-ah) myalgia.

myodystonia (mi″o-dis-to′ne-ah) disorder of muscular tone.

myoedema (mi″o-ĕ-de′mah) 1. mounding. 2. edema of a muscle.

myoelectric (mi″o-e-lek′trik) pertaining to the electric properties of muscle.

myoendocarditis (mi″o-en″do-kar-di′tis) combined myocarditis and endocarditis.

myoepithelium (mi″o-ep″ĭ-the′le-um) tissue made up of contractile epithelial cells.

myofascitis (mi″o-fah-si′tis) inflammation of a muscle and its fascia.

myofibril (mi″o-fi′bril) one of the finer contractile elements making up a muscle fiber.

myofibroma (mi″o-fi-bro′mah) myoma combined with fibroma.

myofibrosis (mi″o-fi-bro′sis) replacement of muscle tissue by fibrous tissue.

myofibrositis (mi″o-fi″bro-si′tis) inflammation of the sheath of muscle fiber.

myofilament (mi″o-fil′ah-ment) 1. a myofibril of a smooth muscle cell. 2. one of the ultramicroscopic threadlike structures occurring in bundles in the myofibrils of striated muscle fibers.

myogelosis (mi″o-je-lo′sis) hardening of muscle substance.

myogen (mi′o-jen) an albumin-like protein, constituting 10 per cent of the protein of muscle.

myogenesis (mi″o-jen′ĕ-sis) the formation of muscle fibers and muscles in embryonic development. adj., **myogenet′ic.**

myogenic (mi″o-jen′ik) producing muscle fibers and muscles.

myogenous (mi-oj″ĕ-nus) originating in muscular tissue.

myoglia (mi-og′le-ah) a fibrillar substance formed by muscle cells.

myoglobin (mi″o-glo′bin) a ferrous protoporphyrin globin complex resembling hemoglobin that is present in muscle and that contributes to its color and acts as a storehouse of oxygen.

myoglobulin (mi″o-glob′u-lin) a globulin from muscle serum.

myogram (mi′o-gram) a record produced by myography.

myograph (mi′o-graf) an apparatus for recording the effects of muscular contraction.

myography (mi-og′rah-fe) 1. the use of a myograph. 2. description of muscles.

myohemoglobin (mi″o-he″mo-glo′bin) myoglobin.

myoid (mi′oid) resembling muscle.

myoischemia (mi″o-is-ke′me-ah) local deficiency of blood supply in muscle.

myokinesimeter (mi″o-kin″ĕ-sim′ĕ-ter) an apparatus for measuring muscular contraction from electrical stimulation.

myokinesis (mi″o-ki-ne′sis) 1. muscular movement. 2. operative displacement of muscle fibers. adj., **myokinet′ic.**

myokymia (mi″o-ki′me-ah) persistent quivering of the muscles.

myolemma (mi″o-lem′ah) the sarcolemma.

myolipoma (mi″o-lǐ-po′mah) myoma with fatty elements.

myology (mi-ol′o-je) scientific study or description of the muscles and accessory structures (bursae and synovial sheath).

myolysis (mi-ol′ĭ-sis) degeneration of muscular tissue.

myoma (mi-o′mah) a tumor formed of muscular tissue. adj., **myom′atous.**

m. **of uterus,** a benign tumor of the smooth muscle fibers of the UTERUS; called also fibroid tumor. It is the most common of all tumors found in women. It may occur in any part of the uterus, although it is most frequently in the body of the organ.

Myomas are often multiple, although a single tumor may occur. They are usually small but may grow quite large and occupy most of the uterine wall. After menopause, growth usually ceases. Symptoms vary according to the location and size of the tumors. As they grow they may cause pressure on neighboring organs, painful menstruation, profuse and irregular menstrual bleeding, vaginal discharge or frequent urination, as well as enlargement of the uterus.

In pregnancy, the tumors may interfere with natural enlargement of the uterus with the growing fetus. They may also cause spontaneous abortion and death of the fetus.

Small myomas are usually left undisturbed and are checked at frequent intervals. Larger tumors may be removed surgically. In some instances, hysterectomy is performed.

myomagenesis (mi″o-mah-jen′ě-sis) the development of myomas.

myomalacia (mi″o-mah-la′she-ah) morbid softening of a muscle.

myomatosis (mi″o-mah-to′sis) the formation of myomas throughout the body.

myomectomy (mi″o-mek′to-me) excision of a myoma.

myomelanosis (mi″o-mel″ah-no′sis) melanosis of muscle.

myomere (mi′o-mēr) myotome; the muscle plate or portion of a somite that develops into voluntary muscle.

myometer (mi-om′ě-ter) an apparatus for measuring muscle contraction.

myometritis (mi″o-me-tri′tis) inflammation of the myometrium.

myometrium (mi″o-me′tre-um) the smooth muscle coat of the uterus.

myonecrosis (mi″o-ně-kro′sis) necrosis or death of individual muscle fibers.

myoneural (mi″o-nu′ral) pertaining to both muscle and nerve.

m. **junction,** the point of junction of a nerve fiber with the muscle that it innervates.

myoneuralgia (mi″o-nu-ral′je-ah) neuralgic pain in a muscle.

myoneure (mi′o-nūr) a nerve cell supplying a muscle.

myoneuroma (mi″o-nu-ro′mah) a neuroma containing muscular tissue.

myopachynsis (mi″o-pah-kin′sis) hypertrophy of muscle.

myoparalysis (mi″o-pah-ral′ĭ-sis) paralysis of a muscle.

myopathy (mi-op′ah-the) any disease of a muscle.

myope (mi′ōp) a person affected with myopia.

myopericarditis (mi″o-per″ĭ-kar-di′tis) inflammation of both myocardium and pericardium.

myopia (mi-o′pe-ah) that error of refraction in which rays of light entering the eye parallel to the optic axis are brought to a focus in front of the retina, as a result of the eyeball being too long from front to back, so that vision for near objects is better than for far; called also nearsightedness and shortsightedness (see also VISION). adj., **myop′ic.**

Myopia generally appears before the age of 8, often becoming gradually worse until about the age of 20, when it ceases to change very much. In later years the nearsighted person may find he can read comfortably without his glasses.

In children, the most frequent symptoms of myopia are attempts to brush away blur, frequent rubbing of the eyes and squinting at distant objects.

Myopia can almost always be corrected with eyeglasses. Eye exercises may be useful in helping the eyes adjust to glasses. but they cannot cure myopia.

There is no evidence that reading or watching television can cause or worsen nearsightedness if lighting conditions are satisfactory.

curvature m., myopia due to changes in curvature of the refracting surfaces of the eye.

index m., myopia due to abnormal refractivity of the media of the eye.

malignant m., pernicious m., progressive myopia with disease of the choroid, leading to retinal detachment and blindness.

progressive m., myopia that continues to increase in adult life.

myoplasm (mi′o-plazm) the contractile part of the muscle cell.

myoplasty (mi′o-plas″te) plastic surgery on muscle whereby portions of detached muscles are used, especially in the field of defects or deformities.

myopsychopathy (mi″o-si-kop′ah-the) any neuromuscular affection associated with mental disorder.

myoreceptor (mi″o-re-sep′tor) a receptor situated in skeletal muscle that is stimulated by muscular contraction, providing information to higher centers regarding muscle position.

myorrhaphy (mi-or′ah-fe) suture of a muscle.

myorrhexis (mi″o-rek′sis) rupture of a muscle.

myosalpinx (mi″o-sal′pinks) the muscular tissue of the uterine tube.

myosarcoma (mi″o-sar-ko′mah) myoma blended with sarcoma.

myoschwannoma (mi″o-shwah-no′mah) schwannoma.

myosclerosis (mi″o-sklĕ-ro′sis) hardening of muscle.

myosin (mi′o-sin) one of the two main proteins of muscle. Myosin and actin are the proteins involved in contraction of muscle fibers.

myosinose (mi-os′ĭ-nōs) an albumose produced by digestion of myosin.

myositis (mi″o-si′tis) inflammatory disease of primarily voluntary muscle tissue.
 epidemic m., epidemic pleurodynia.
 m. fibro′sa, a type in which there is a formation of connective tissue in the muscle.
 multiple m., dermatomyositis.
 m. ossif′icans, myositis marked by bony deposits in muscle.
 trichinous m., that which is caused by the presence of *Trichinella spiralis.*

myospasm (mi′o-spazm) spasm of a muscle.

myosteoma (mi-os″te-o′mah) a bony tumor in muscle.

myosynizesis (mi″o-sin″ĭ-ze′sis) adhesion of muscles.

myotactic (mi″o-tak′tik) pertaining to the proprioceptive sense of muscles.

myotasis (mi-ot′ah-sis) stretching of muscle. adj., **myotat′ic.**

myotenositis (mi″o-te″no-si′tis) inflammation of a muscle and tendon.

myotenotomy (mi″o-ten-ot′o-me) surgical division of the tendon of a muscle.

myotome (mi′o-tōm) 1. an instrument for dividing muscles. 2. the muscle plate or portion of a somite that develops into voluntary muscle. 3. a group of muscles innervated from a single spinal nerve.

myotomy (mi-ot′o-me) cutting or dissection of muscular tissue or of a muscle.

myotonia (mi″o-to′ne-ah) increased tone or tension of muscle; tonic spasm of muscle. adj., **myoton′ic.**
 m. atroph′ica, myotonia dystrophica.
 m. congen′ita, a hereditary disease marked by tonic spasm and rigidity of certain muscles when attempts are made to move them. The stiffness tends to disappear as the muscles are used.
 m. dystroph′ica, a rare disease marked by stiffness of the muscles followed in time by atrophy of the muscles of the neck and face, producing hatchet face or tapir mouth. The atrophy extends to the muscles of the trunk and extremities and is associated with cataract. Called also dystrophia myotonica.

myotonometer (mi″o-to-nom′ĕ-ter) an instrument for measuring muscular tonus.

myotonus (mi-ot′o-nus) tonic spasm of a muscle or a group of muscles.

myotrophic (mi′o-tro″fik) 1. increasing weight of muscle. 2. pertaining to myotrophy.

myotrophy (mi-ot′ro-fe) nutrition of muscle.

myotropic (mi″o-trop′ik) having a special affinity for muscle.

myovascular (mi″o-vas′ku-lar) pertaining to muscle and blood vessels.

myria- (mir′e-ah) word element [Gr.] used in naming units of measurement to designate an amount 10^4 times the size of the unit to which it is joined.

Myriapoda (mir″e-ap′o-dah) a class of arthropods, including the millipedes and centipedes.

myring(o)- (mĭ-ring′go) word element [L.], *tympanic membrane.*

myringa (mĭ-ring′gah) the tympanic membrane.

myringectomy (mir″in-jek′to-me) excision of the tympanic membrane; called also myringodectomy.

myringitis (mĭ-rin-ji′tis) inflammation of the tympanic membrane.
 m. bullo′sa, bullous m., a form of viral otitis media in which serous or hemorrhagic blebs appear on the tympanic membrane and adjacent wall of the acoustic meatus.

myringomycosis (mĭ-ring″go-mi-ko′sis) fungus disease of the tympanic membrane.

myringoplasty (mĭ-ring′go-plas″te) surgical reconstruction of the tympanic membrane.

myringorupture (mĭ-ring″go-rup′tūr) rupture of the tympanic membrane.

myringoscope (mĭ-ring′go-skōp) an instrument for inspecting the tympanic membrane.

myringostapediopexy (mĭ-ring″go-stah-pe′de-o-pek″se) fixation of the large lower portion of the tympanic membrane to the head of the stapes.

myringotomy (mir″ing-got′o-me) incision of the tympanic membrane.

myrrh (mer) the oleo-gum-resin from certain trees of Arabia and Africa, used as a protectant.

Mysoline (mi′so-lēn) trademark for preparations of primidone, an anticonvulsant.

mysophilia (mi″so-fil′e-ah) a form of paraphilia in which there is a lustful attitude toward excretions.

mysophobia (mis″o-fo′be-ah) morbid dread of contamination and filth.

Mytelase (mi′tĕ-lās) trademark for a preparation of ambenonium, a cholinesterase inhibitor.

mythomania (mith″o-ma′ne-ah) morbid tendency to lie or exaggerate.

mythophobia (mith″o-fo′be-ah) morbid fear of stating an untruth.

mytilotoxin (mit″ĭ-lo-tok′sin) a poisonous principle from mussels.

myx(o)- (mik′so) word element [Gr.], *mucus; slime.*

myxadenitis (mik″sad-ĕ-ni′tis) inflammation of a mucus-secreting gland.

myxadenoma (mik″sad-ĕ-no′mah) an epithelial tumor with the structure of a mucus-secreting gland.

myxasthenia (mik″sas-the′ne-ah) deficient secretion of mucus.

myxedema (mik″sĕ-de′mah) a condition resulting from advanced hypothyroidism, or deficiency of thyroxine. It is the adult form of the disease known as CRETINISM in children.

Caused by lack of iodine in the diet, by atrophy, surgical removal or a disorder of the thyroid gland, or its destruction by radioactive iodine, or by deficient excretion of thyrotropin by the pituitary gland, myxedema is marked primarily by a growing puffiness and sogginess of the skin.

Because thyroxine plays such an important role in the body's metabolism, lack of this hormone seriously upsets the balance of body processes. Among the symptoms associated with myxedema are excessive fatigue and drowsiness, headaches, weight gain, dryness of the skin, sensitivity to cold and increasing thinness and brittleness of the nails. In women, menstrual bleeding may become irregular. Medical tests reveal slow tendon reflexes, low blood iodine, below-normal metabolism and abnormal uptake of radioactive iodine by the thyroid.

In myxedema the body's defenses against infection are weakened. If the patient has heart disease, this is likely to worsen. Upset of the functions of the adrenal glands may become critical. In time, if myxedema is not brought under control, progressive mental deterioration may result in a psychosis, marked by paranoid delusions.

Myxedema is treated by administration of thyroid extract or similar synthetic preparations. If treatment is begun soon after the symptoms appear, recovery may be complete. Delayed or interrupted treatment may mean permanent deterioration. In most instances, treatment with thyroid or synthetics must be continued throughout the patient's lifetime.

pretibial m., a localized myxedema associated with preceding hyperthyroidism occurring typically on the anterior surface of the legs.

myxoblastoma (mik″so-blas-to′mah) a tumor of mucus connective tissue cells.

myxochondroma (mik″so-kon-dro′mah) myxoma blended with chondroma.

myxocyte (mik′so-sīt) one of the cells of mucous tissue.

myxofibroma (mik″so-fi-bro′mah) myxoma blended with fibroma.

myxoid (mik′soid) resembling mucus.

myxolipoma (mik″so-lĭ-po′mah) myxoma blended with lipoma.

myxoma (mik-so′mah) a tumor composed of mucous tissue. adj., **myxo′matous.**
    odontogenic m., an uncommon tumor of the jaw, possibly produced by myxomatous degeneration of an odontogenic fibroma.

myxomatosis (mik″so-mah-to′sis) 1. the development of multiple myxomas. 2. myxomatous degeneration.

myxomyoma (mik″so-mi-o′mah) a myoma containing myxomatous tissue.

myxoneuroma (mik″so-nu-ro′mah) myxoma blended with neuroma.

myxopapilloma (mik″so-pap″ĭ-lo′mah) combined myxoma with papilloma.

myxopoiesis (mik″so-poi-e′sis) the formation of mucus.

myxorrhea (mik″so-re′ah) a flow of mucus.
    m. intestina′lis, excessive secretion of intestinal mucus.

myxosarcoma (mik″so-sar-ko′mah) a sarcoma containing myxomatous tissue.

myxospore (mik′so-spōr) a spore embedded in a jelly-like mass.

myxovirus (mik″so-vi′rus) a virus of the influenza, parainfluenza, mumps, Newcastle disease or a related group, characteristically causing agglutination of chicken erythrocytes.

Myzomyia (mi″zo-mi′yah) a genus of mosquitoes, several species of which act as carriers of malarial parasites.

Myzorhynchus (mi″zo-ring′kus) a genus of mosquitoes, several species of which act as carriers of malarial parasites.

N

N 1. chemical symbol, *nitrogen.* 2. symbol, *normal* (solution); the expressions 2N (double normal), N/2 or 0.5N (half-normal), N/10 or 0.1N (tenth-normal), etc., denote the strength of a solution in comparison with the normal.

N. nasal.

n. 1. symbol, *index of refraction.* 2. [L.] *ner'vus* (nerve).

NA Nomina Anatomica, the official anatomic terminology approved by the International Congress of Anatomists.

Na chemical symbol, *sodium* (L. *natrium*).

Nabothian cyst (nah-bo'the-an) a cystic dilatation of the uterine cervix caused by inflammatory stenosis of the lumina of the cervical glands.

nacreous (na'kre-us) having a pearl-like luster.

Nacton (nak'ton) trademark for a preparation of poldine methylsulfate, an anticholinergic.

naepaine (ne'pān) a compound used as a local anesthetic.

naevus (ne'vus) nevus.

Nägele's rule (na'gĕ-lēz) a rule for calculating the estimated date of confinement: Subtract 3 months from the first day of the last menstrual period and add 7 days.

nail (nāl) 1. a rod of metal, bone or other material used for fixation of the ends of fractured bones. 2. a hardened or horny cutaneous plate overlying the dorsal surface of the distal end of a finger or toe. The nails are part of the outer layer of the skin. They are composed of hard tissue formed of keratin, the substance that gives skin its toughness.

CARE OF THE NAILS. The main care of the fingernails consists in keeping them trimmed and clean. Trimming may be done with nail scissors or clippers or by filing. With certain types of delicate nail, an emery board is preferable to a metal file. Hand lotion or cream applied to the cuticle helps to keep it soft and avoid hangnails. Wearing rubber gloves for housework and dishwashing helps to protect the nails from breaking.

Toenails seldom give trouble if they are cleaned and trimmed regularly and if shoes fit well. It is advisable to bathe the feet at least once a day and to clean dirt from under the toenails with a nailbrush. The toenails should be trimmed every 2 weeks or so by cutting them straight across rather than rounding them by cutting off their corners. This helps prevent ingrown toenails.

DISORDERS OF THE NAILS. Any change in the basic structure, shape or appearance of the nails — such as softness, brittleness, furrowing or speckling — may be a symptom of a disease affecting the whole body. Marked pallor of the nails may suggest anemia. In certain cases of hemiplegia and poliomyelitis the nails may cease to grow. Curing the disease will cure the condition.

Certain disorders affect the nails themselves. They are readily exposed to outside sources of infection and are particularly vulnerable to injury in the course of daily life. Many of the diseases that afflict the skin may also affect the nail bed and be aggravated by the confining presence of the nail. Congenital defects and metabolic disturbances may affect the nails.

Infections. Most infections involving the nails originate in the folds of tissue around them. Inflammation of this area is called paronychia. It is a fairly common infection by staphylococci, streptococci or other bacteria or fungi, and causes painful swelling around the nail, with red, shiny skin. If untreated, paronychia may spread to the nail bed and cause inflammation there. This condition is known as onychia, and is more serious. The bacteria grow under the nail and can cause severe inflammation and pain. Onychia may also arise when the nail is injured and bacteria or fungi gain entrance to the tissue underneath. If the organisms that penetrate the nail produce pigments, the nail may change color as a result. In extreme cases onychia may also cause the nail to separate from its bed. Among the diseases from which paronychia and onychia may result are tuberculosis, diphtheria and syphilis, and also skin diseases such as psoriasis, fungus diseases and contact dermatitis.

Dermatitis is the most common disorder to involve the nails and often leads to the complete loss of the nail. After treatment the nail will generally grow back, but if the matrix is severely damaged a new nail may be deformed or may fail to grow.

Occasionally toenails become infected with the fungi that cause athlete's foot.

Injuries. A bruise on the nail can be extremely painful and may cause the nail to turn black and blue. Both effects are due to the accumulation of blood underneath. The nail may become detached from its bed or may fall off. Equally painful may be a splinter under the nail. A physician can relieve the pain of these injuries by releasing the accumulated blood with a small incision directly through the nail.

Burns and frostbite can injure the nails and in severe cases may destroy the matrix, so that regrowth is imposible. Too much exposure to radium or x-rays may injure the nail, making it brittle and easily breakable.

Nutritional and Metabolic Disturbances. The general condition of the body is readily reflected in the condition of the nails. Poor circulation may result in weak nails. Digestive disturbances may impair their growth, and vitamin deficiencies may cause them to become inflamed and sometimes to fall out.

Brittle nails may also be caused by metabolic disorders, for example, hypothyroidism.

Hereditary defects. The shape and thickness of nails may be an inherited family trait. A child is sometimes born without nails or with one or more missing. In this case he will remain without them for life; however, hereditary deformities can be treated. For instance, the condition of excessively thick nails can be reduced if it is advisable.

Minor Disorders. Hangnails (shreds of skin at one side of a nail) are unsightly and can best be prevented from forming by gently pushing the cuticle instead of cutting it. A hangnail should be clipped off and treated with antiseptic to avoid the slight danger of infection.

ingrowing n., ingrown n., overlapping of the anterior corners of a nail by the flesh of the digit.

Smith-Petersen n., a nail for fixing the head of the femur in fracture of the femoral neck.

spoon n., a nail with a concave surface.

Nalline (nal'ēn) trademark for a preparation of nalorphine, an antagonist of certain narcotic agents such as morphine.

nalorphine hydrochloride (nal'of-fēn) N-allyl-normorphine; a narcotic antagonist used as an antidote in acute cases of narcotic overdose, but not in drug addiction. Nalorphine is a derivative of morphine and therefore its use is regulated by the Harrison antinarcotic act. It reverses respiratory depression, cardiac arrhythmias and other symptoms of overdosage of morphine, meperidine and methadone, but is ineffective against depression produced by barbiturates and general anesthetics.

The drug may be administered intravenously, intramuscularly or subcutaneously. If the patient receiving the drug experiences serious withdrawal symptoms, he should be given the drug to which he is addicted because nalorphine does not eliminate withdrawal symptoms.

nanism (na'nizm) dwarfishness.

nano- (na'no) word element [Gr.], *dwarf; small size;* used in naming units of measurement to designate an amount 10^{-9} (one-billionth) the size of the unit to which it is joined, e.g., nanocurie.

nanocephalous (na"no-sef'ah-lus) having a very small head.

nanocormia (na"no-kor'me-ah) abnormal smallness of the body or trunk.

nanocurie (na"no-ku're) a unit of radioactivity, being 10^{-9} curie, or the quantity of radioactive material in which the number of nuclear disintegrations is 3.7×10, or 37, per second; abbreviated nc.

nanogram (na'no-gram) one-billionth (10^{-9}) gram.

nanoid (na'noid) dwarfish.

nanomelus (na-nom'ĕ-lus) an individual with undersized limbs.

nanosomia (na"no-so'me-ah) dwarfishness of the body.

nanous (na'nus) dwarfed.

nanus (na'nus) 1. a dwarf. 2. stunted; dwarfish.

nape (nāp) the back of the neck.

naphazoline (naf-az'o-lēn) a sympathomimetic compound used as a vasoconstrictor and nasal decongestant.

naphthalene (naf'thah-lēn) a hydrocarbon from coal tar oil; used as an antiseptic.

naphthol (naf'thol) a crystalline, antiseptic substance from coal tar.

N.A.P.N.E.S. National Association for Practical Nurse Education and Services.

Naqua (nak'wah) trademark for a preparation of trichlormethiazide, a diuretic.

narcissism (nar'sĭ-sizm) sexual attraction toward oneself; self-love. adj., **narcissis'tic.**

narcoanalysis (nar"ko-ah-nal'ĭ-sis) psychoanalysis with use of sedative drugs to help uncover unconscious material.

narcoanesthesia (nar"ko-an"es-the'ze-ah) anesthesia by injection of scopolamine and morphine.

narcohypnia (nar"ko-hip'ne-ah) numbness felt on waking from sleep.

narcohypnosis (nar"ko-hip-no'sis) hypnotic suggestions made while the patient is under the influence of some hypnotic drug.

narcolepsy (nar'ko-lep"se) recurrent attacks of uncontrollable desire for sleep. adj., **narcolep'tic.**

narcomania (nar"ko-ma'ne-ah) a morbid craving for narcotics.

narcose (nar'kōs) 1. somewhat stuporous. 2. drowsy.

narcosine (nar'ko-sēn) noscapine, an antitussive.

narcosis (nar-ko'sis) a stuporous state.

basal n., basis n., narcosis with complete unconsciousness and analgesia.

narcosynthesis (nar"ko-sin'thē-sis) treatment of neuroses by inducing a seminarcosis in which the patient recalls his suppressed memories and resynthesizes his emotions.

narcotic (nar-kot'ic) 1. producing insensibility, stupor or sleep. 2. a drug that produces sleep or stupor.

Medically, the term narcotic includes any drug that has this effect. By legal definition, however, the term refers to habit-forming drugs—for example, opiates such as morphine and heroin and synthetic drugs such as meperidine (Demerol). Narcotics can be legally obtained only with a doctor's prescription. The sale or possession of narcotics for other than medical purposes is strictly prohibited by federal, state and local laws, e.g. the Harrison antinarcotic act.

narcotine (nar'ko-tin) noscapine, an antitussive.

narcotism (nar'ko-tizm) addiction to a narcotic drug.

narcotize (nar'ko-tīz) to put under the influence of a narcotic.

Nardil (nar'dil) trademark for a preparation of phenelzine dihydrogen sulfate, an antidepressant.

naris (na'ris), pl. *na'res* [L.] an opening into the nasal cavity on the exterior of the body (anterior or external naris) or into the nasopharynx (posterior naris).

Narone (nar′ōn) trademark for a preparation of dipyrone, an analgesic and antipyretic.

nasal (na′zal) pertaining to the nose.

  n. septum, a plate of bone and cartilage covered with mucous membrane that divides the cavity of the nose (see also SEPTUM).

nascent (nas′ent, na′sent) being born, or just coming into being; applied especially to a substance or element just escaping from a chemical combination.

nasion (na′ze-on) the middle point of the junction of the frontal and the two nasal bones (frontonasal suture).

nasitis (na-zi′tis) inflammation of the nose.

NAS-NRC National Academy of Sciences – National Research Council.

nasoantritis (na″zo-an-tri′tis) inflammation of the nose and antrum of Highmore (maxillary sinus).

nasociliary (na″zo-sil″e-er″e) affecting the eyes, forehead and root of the nose.

nasofrontal (na″zo-frun′tal) pertaining to the nasal and frontal bones.

nasogastric tube (na″zo-gas′trik) a tube of soft rubber or plastic that is inserted through a nostril and into the stomach. The tube may be inserted for the purpose of instilling liquid foods or other substances, or as a means of withdrawing gastric contents. (See also TUBE FEEDING.)

nasolacrimal (na″zo-lak′rĭ-mal) pertaining to the nose and lacrimal apparatus.

nasopalatine (na″zo-pal′ah-tīn) pertaining to the nose and palate.

nasopharyngitis (na″zo-far″in-ji′tis) inflammation of the nasopharynx.

nasopharynx (na″zo-far′ingks) the part of the pharynx above the soft palate. adj., **nasopharyn′geal.**

nasoseptitis (na″zo-sep-ti′tis) inflammation of the nasal septum.

nasosinusitis (na″zo-si″nŭ-si′tis) inflammation of the paranasal sinuses.

nasus (na′sus) [L.] nose.

natal (na′tal) 1. pertaining to birth. 2. pertaining to the nates (buttocks).

natality (na-tal′ĭ-te) the birth rate.

nates (na′tēz) (L., pl.) the buttocks.

natimortality (na″tĭ-mor-tal′ĭ-te) the proportion of stillbirths to the general birth rate.

National Association for Practical Nurse Education and Service the first national organization concerned solely with practical nurse education and the services rendered by the practical nurse, organized in 1941. Members of N.A.P.N.E.S. include professional and practical nurses, physicians, hospital administrators, other health and welfare workers and interested lay citizens.

The organization maintains an accrediting program for state-approved schools of practical nursing, provides a consulting service for groups interested in starting a practical nurse program, prepares and publishes leaflets, booklets and other educational materials for practical nurses, and sponsors regional workshops and summer school courses on practical nurse education and services.

The official publication of N.A.P.N.E.S. is the *Journal of Practical Nursing.* The headquarters is at 1465 Broadway, New York, N.Y. 10036.

National Federation of Licensed Practical Nurses the only national organization with a membership consisting solely of licensed practical-vocational nurses. The organization was founded in 1949 and has its central office at 250 West 57th Street, New York, N.Y. 10019. Membership is open to licensed practical-vocational nurses who are members of local, state and territorial organizations through which the national organization functions.

N.F.L.P.N. lists its purposes as follows: to establish policy, to speak and act for licensed practical-vocational nurses, to conduct educational workshops and an annual convention, to represent licensed practical-vocational nurses in all affairs of practical nursing and to promote their welfare and nursing skills through its official journal, *Bedside Nurse.*

National League for Nursing a national organization concerned with improving nursing education and nursing service at all levels. In 1952, after 10 years of study of existing nursing organizations, three national organizations and four committees agreed to combine and form the N.L.N. These organizations and committees were: National League of Nursing Education, founded in 1893; National Organization for Public Health Nursing, founded in 1912; Association of Collegiate Schools of Nursing, founded in 1933; Joint Committee on Practical Nurses and Auxiliary Workers in Nursing, founded in 1945; Joint Committee on Careers in Nursing, founded in 1948; National Committee for the Improvement of Nursing Services, founded in 1949; and the National Accrediting Service, founded in 1949.

There are two divisions of the N.L.N., one for individual members and one for agency members. Individual members may be professional and practical nurses, nurses' aides and other professional and lay persons interested in fostering the development and improvement of nursing services or nursing education. An agency membership is available to any organization that provides a nursing service or conducts an educational program in nursing. An allied agency membership, without voting rights, is available as determined by the Board of Directors to interested organizations not engaged in providing nursing service or conducting an educational program in nursing.

The official magazine of the National League for Nursing is *Nursing Outlook.* Offices of the League are located at 10 Columbus Circle, New York, N.Y. 10019.

Natolone (nat′o-lōn) trademark for a preparation of pregnenolone, used as an antiarthritic.

natremia (na-tre′me-ah) the presence of sodium in the blood.

natrium (na′tre-um) [L.] sodium (symbol Na).

natriuresis (na″tre-u-re′sis) the excretion of sodium in the urine.

natriuretic (na″tre-u-ret′ik) 1. pertaining to or promoting natriuresis. 2. an agent that promotes natriuresis.

natruresis (nat″roo-re′sis) natriuresis.

natruretic (nat″roo-ret′ik) natriuretic.

Naturetin (nat″u-re′tin) trademark for preparations of bendroflumethiazide, a diuretic.

naturopath (na′tūr-o-path″) a practitioner of naturopathy.

naturopathy (na″tūr-op′ah-the) a drugless system of healing by the use of physical methods, such as light, air, water, etc.

nausea (naw′ze-ah) the distressing feeling or signal that vomiting may occur. Nausea may be a symptom of a variety of disorders, some minor and some more serious.

Nausea is usually felt when nerve endings in the stomach and other parts of the body are irritated. The irritated nerves send messages to the center in the brain that controls the vomiting reflex. When the nerve irritation becomes intense, vomiting results.

Nausea and vomiting may be set off by nerve signals from many other parts of the body besides the stomach. For example, intense pain in almost any part of the body can produce nausea. The reason is that the nausea-vomiting mechanism is part of the involuntary autonomic nervous system. Nausea can also be precipitated by strong emotions.

nauseant (naw′ze-ant) 1. inducing nausea. 2. an agent causing nausea.

nauseous (naw′shus, naw′ze-us) producing nausea or disgust.

navel (na′vel) the umbilicus, the scar marking the site of entry of the umbilical cord in the fetus.

navicular (nah-vik′u-lar) boat-shaped; applied to certain bones, particularly a bone of the foot.

Nb chemical symbol, *niobium.*

N.B.S. National Bureau of Standards.

nc. nanocurie.

N.C.A. neurocirculatory asthenia.

N.C.I. National Cancer Institute.

N.C.M.H. National Committee for Mental Hygiene.

NCRP National Committee on Radiation Protection and Measurements.

Nd chemical symbol, *neodymium.*

N.D.A. National Dental Association.

Ne chemical symbol, *neon.*

nearsightedness (nēr-sīt′ed-nes) a condition in which vision for near objects is better than for distant ones; called also MYOPIA.

nearthrosis (ne″ar-thro′sis) a false or artificial joint.

nebula (neb′u-lah) 1. slight corneal opacity. 2. cloudiness in urine. 3. a liquid substance prepared for use as a spray.

nebulization (neb″u-lĭ-za′shun) 1. conversion into a spray. 2. treatment by a spray.

nebulizer (neb′u-līz″er) an atomizer; a device for throwing a spray.

Necator (ne-ka′tor) a genus of nematode parasites.

N. america′nus, a species widely distributed in southern United States, Central and South America and the Caribbean area; the New World, or American, HOOKWORM.

necatoriasis (ne-ka″to-ri′ah-sis) infection with organisms of the genus Necator.

neck (nek) a constricted portion, such as the part connecting the head and trunk of the body or the constricted part of an organ, as of the uterus (cervix uteri) or other structure.

anatomic n. of humerus, the constriction of the humerus just below its proximal articular surface.

n. of femur, the heavy column of bone connecting the head of the femur and the shaft.

surgical n. of humerus, the constricted part of the humerus just below the tuberosities.

n. of a tooth, the narrowed part of a tooth between the crown and the root.

uterine n., n. of uterus, cervix uteri.

webbed n., obliteration of the usual angle between the neck and shoulders by an abnormal expanse of tissue.

wry n., torticollis.

necrectomy (nĕ-krek′to-me) excision of necrosed tissue.

necro- (nek′ro) word element [Gr.], *death.*

necrobiosis (nek″ro-bi-o′sis) the physiologic death of cells; a normal mechanism in the constant turnover of many cell populations.

n. lipoi′dica diabetico′rum, a dermatosis characterized by patchy degeneration of the elastic and connective tissue of the skin occurring in diabetes mellitus.

necrocytosis (nek″ro-si-to′sis) death and decay of cells.

necrology (nĕ-krol′o-je, ne-krol′o-je) statistics or records of death.

necromania (nek″ro-ma′ne-ah) morbid interest in death or dead persons.

necroparasite (nek″ro-par′ah-sīt) an organism that lives in dead tissue.

necrophagous (ne-krof′ah-gus) feeding upon dead flesh.

necrophilia (nek″ro-fil′e-ah) morbid attraction to death or to dead bodies; coitus with a dead body.

necrophobia (nek″ro-fo′be-ah) morbid dread of death or of dead bodies.

necropneumonia (nek″ro-nu-mo′ne-ah) gangrene of lung.

necropsy (nek′rop-se) examination of a body after death (see also AUTOPSY).

necrose (ne-krōs′) to undergo necrosis.

necrosin (ne-kro′sin) a toxic substance occurring in inflammatory exudates, producing the signs of inflammation.

necrosis (nĕ-kro′sis, ne-kro′sis) death of a cell or group of cells as the result of disease or injury. adj., **necrot′ic.**

   aseptic n., avascular n., 1. necrosis without infection or inflammation. 2. necrosis occurring as a result of isolation of a part from its blood supply.

   Balser's fatty n., necrosis of the pancreas, spleen and omentum.

   caseous n., necrosis in which the tissue is soft, dry and cheesy, occurring typically in tuberculosis.

   central n., necrosis affecting the central portion of an affected bone, cell or lobule of the liver.

   cheesy n., caseous necrosis.

   coagulation n., coagulative n., death of cells, the protoplasm of the cells becoming fixed and opaque by coagulation of the protein elements, the cellular outline persisting for a long time.

   colliquative n., liquefactive necrosis.

   dry n., that in which the necrotic tissue becomes dry.

   fat n., necrosis of fatty tissue in small white areas.

   liquefactive n., necrosis in which the necrotic material becomes softened and liquefied.

   moist n., necrosis in which the dead tissue is wet and soft.

   superficial n., necrosis affecting the surface of a bone.

   Zenker's n., a particular type of muscular degeneration.

necrospermia (nek″ro-sper′me-ah) a condition in which the spermatozoa are dead.

necrotizing (nek′ro-tīz″ing) causing necrosis.

necrotomy (nĕ-krot′o-me) 1. dissection of a dead body. 2. excision of a sequestrum.

necrotoxin (nek″ro-tok′sin) a factor or substance produced by certain staphylococci that kills tissue cells.

needle (ne′dl) a sharp instrument for sewing or puncturing.

   aneurysm n., one used in ligating blood vessels.

   artery n., aspirating n., a long, hollow needle for removing fluid from a cavity.

   cataract n., one used in removing a cataract.

   discission n., a special form of cataract needle.

   exploring n., a flattened and grooved needle to be thrust into a part where fluid is believed to exist.

   Hagedorn's n's, surgical needles that are flat from side to side and have a straight cutting edge near the point, and a large eye.

   hypodermic n., a hollow, sharp-pointed needle to be attached to a hypodermic syringe for injection of solutions.

   knife n., a cutting-edged needle used in operation.

   ligature n., a slender steel needle having an eye in its curved end, used for passing a ligature underneath an artery.

   Reverdin's n., a surgeon's needle having an eye that can be opened and closed by means of a slide.

   Silverman n., one designed for removal of tissue from an internal organ for study under the microscope.

   stop n., one with a disk that prevents too deep penetration.

negative (neg′ah-tiv) having a value of less than zero; indicating lack or absence, as chromatin-negative or Wassermann-negative; characterized by denial or opposition.

negativism (neg′ah-tī-vizm″) opposition and resistance to suggestion or advice; persistent tendency to contrary behavior.

negatron (neg′ah-tron) a negatively charged electron.

Negri bodies (na′gre) oval or round bodies in the nerve cells of animals dead of rabies.

Neisseria (ni-se′re-ah) a genus of gram-negative, anaerobic organisms.

   N. catarrhal′is, a species found in the respiratory tract.

   N. gonorrhoe′ae, the etiologic agent of gonorrhea.

   N. meningi′tidis, a prominent cause of meningitis and the specific etiologic agent of meningococcal meningitis.

neisserian (ni-se′re-an) pertaining to or caused by organisms of the genus Neisseria, usually *N. gonorrhoea.*

Nema (ne′mah) trademark for a preparation of tetrachloroethylene, an anthelmintic.

nemathelminth (nem″ah-thel′minth) a worm of the phylum Nemathelminthes.

Nemathelminthes (nem″ah-thel-min′thēz) the phylum of helminths, the roundworms, which includes Nematoda.

nemathelminthiasis (nem″ah-thel″min-thi′ah-sis) infection by nematodes or roundworms.

nematoblast (nem′ah-to-blast″) spermatid.

nematocide (nem′ah-to-sīd″) 1. destroying nematodes. 2. an agent that destroys nematodes.

Nematoda (nem″ah-to′dah) a class (or sometimes considered a phylum) of roundworms, some of which are parasitic in man (see also WORM).

nematode (nem′ah-tōd) an individual organism of the class (or phylum) Nematoda.

nematodiasis (nem″ah-to-di′ah-sis) infection by a nematode.

Nembutal (nem′bu-tal) trademark for preparations of pentobarbital, a hypnotic and barbiturate.

neo- (ne′o) word element [Gr.], *new.*

Neo-antergan (ne″o-an′ter-gan) trademark for a preparation of pyrilamine maleate, an antihistamine.

neo-arthrosis (ne″o-ar-thro′sis) nearthrosis.

neoblastic (ne″o-blas′tik) originating in new tissue.

neocerebellum (ne″o-ser″ĕ-bel′um) the more newly developed part of the cerebellum, comprising the lateral lobes.

neocinchophen (ne″o-sin′ko-fen) a white to yellow crystalline powder used as an analgesic and antipyretic.

neocinetic (ne″o-si-net′ik) neokinetic.

neocortex (ne″o-kor′teks) neopallium.

neocyte (ne′o-sīt) an immature form of leukocyte.

neocytosis (ne″o-si-to′sis) the presence of neocytes in the blood.

neodiathermy (ne″o-di″ah-ther′me) short-wave diathermy.

Neo-diloderm (ne″o-di′lo-derm) trademark for a preparation of dichlorisone containing neomycin sulfate, having antipruritic and antibiotic activity.

neodymium (ne″o-dim′e-um) a chemical element, atomic number 60, atomic weight 144.24, symbol Nd. (See table of ELEMENTS.)

neogenesis (ne″o-jen′ĕ-sis) tissue regeneration. adj., **neogenet′ic.**

Neohetramine (ne″o-he′trah-min) trademark for a preparation of thonzylamine hydrochloride, an antihistamine.

Neo-hombreol (ne″o-hom′bre-ol) trademark for preparations of testosterone propionate, an androgen used in replacement therapy.

Neohydrin (ne″o-hi′drin) trademark for a preparation of chlormerodrin, a mercurial diuretic.

Neo-iopax (ne″o-i′o-paks) trademark for a preparation of sodium iodomethamate, used as a contrast medium.

neokinetic (ne″o-ki-net′ik) pertaining to the nervous motor mechanism regulating voluntary muscular control.

neologism (ne-ol′o-jizm) a newly coined word; in psychiatry, a word whose meaning may be known only to the patient using it.

neomembrane (ne″o-mem′brān) a false membrane.

neomycin (ne″o-mi′sin) an antibacterial substance produced by growth of *Streptomyces fradiae;* used as an intestinal antiseptic and in treatment of systemic infections due to gram-negative microorganisms.

neon (ne′on) a chemical element, atomic number 10, atomic weight 20.183, symbol Ne. (See table of ELEMENTS.)

neonatal (ne″o-na′tal) pertaining to the first 4 weeks after birth.

neonate (ne′o-nāt) a newborn infant up to 4 weeks old.

neonatology (ne″o-na-tol′o-je) the art and science of diagnosis and treatment of disorders of the newborn infant.

neopallium (ne″o-pal′e-um) that part of the pallium, or gray matter, showing stratification and organization of the most highly evolved type.

neopathy (ne-op′ah-the) a new disease or a new complication in a disease.

neophilism (ne-of′ĭ-lizm) abnormal love of new things.

neophobia (ne″o-fo′be-ah) morbid dread of new things.

neoplasia (ne″o-pla′ze-ah) a condition characterized by the presence of new growths (tumors).

neoplasm (ne′o-plazm) a mass of new, abnormal tissue; a new growth or TUMOR.

neoplastic (ne″o-plas′tik) 1. pertaining to neoplasia or neoplasm. 2. pertaining to neoplasty.

neoplasty (ne″o-plas″te) replacement of lost parts by plastic methods.

neostigmine (ne″o-stig′min) an acetylcholinesterase inhibitor, used as a cholinergic drug to improve muscle function in myasthenia gravis.
  n. bromide, a white crystalline powder used as a cholinergic and parasympathomimetic.
  n. methylsulfate, a white crystalline powder used as a parasympathomimetic and cholinergic.

neostomy (ne-os′to-me) creation of a new opening into an organ or between two organs.

neostriatum (ne″o-stri-a′tum) the more recently developed part of the corpus striatum.

Neo-synephrine (ne″o-sī-nef′rin) trademark for preparations of phenylephrine, a sympathomimetic.

neothalamus (ne″o-thal′ah-mus) the more lateral, cortical part of the thalamus, of more recent phylogenic origin.

Neothylline (ne″o-thil′in) trademark for preparations of dyphylline, used as a diuretic and as a bronchodilator and peripheral vasodilator.

nephelometer (nef″ĕ-lom′ĕ-ter) an apparatus for measuring minute degrees of turbidity of a solution.

nephralgia (nĕ-fral′je-ah) pain in a kidney.

nephrectasia (nef″rek-ta′ze-ah) dilatation of a renal pelvis.

nephrectomy (nĕ-frek′to-me) surgical removal of a kidney. The procedure is indicated when chronic disease or severe injury produces irreparable damage to the renal cells. Tumors, multiple cysts and congenital anomalies may also necessitate removal of a kidney. A single kidney can carry on the functions formerly done by both kidneys, and thus a patient can survive nephrectomy in good health. (See also surgery of the KIDNEY.)

nephremphraxis (nef″rem-frak′sis) obstruction of the vessels of the kidney.

nephric (nef′rik) pertaining to the kidney.

nephridium (nĕ-frid′e-um), pl. *nephrid′ia* [L.] a rudimentary excretory organ, as found in lower animals, or the embryonic tube from which the kidney develops.

nephrism (nef′rizm) cachexia due to kidney disease.

nephritis (nĕ-fri′tis) inflammation of the kidney; called also Bright's disease. adj., **nephrit′ic.** The most usual form is glomerulonephritis, that is, inflammation of the glomeruli, which are clusters of renal capillaries. Damage to the membranes of the glomeruli results in impairment of the filtering process, so that blood and proteins such as albumin pass out into the urine. Depending on the symptoms it produces, nephritis is classified as acute nephritis, chronic nephritis or NEPHROSIS (called also the nephrotic syndrome).

ACUTE NEPHRITIS. Acute nephritis occurs most frequently in children and young people. The disease seems to strike those who have recently suffered from sore throat, scarlet fever and other infections that are caused by streptococci, and it is believed to originate as an immune response on the part of the kidney.

An attack of acute nephritis may produce no symptoms. More often, however, there are headaches, a rundown feeling, back pain and perhaps slight fever. The urine may look smoky, bloody or wine-colored. Analysis of the urine shows the presence of erythrocytes, albumin and casts. Another symptom is edema. If this occurs, the face or ankles are swollen, more so in the morning than in the evening. The blood pressure usually rises during acute nephritis, and in severe cases hypertension may be accompanied by convulsions.

Treatment consists chiefly of bed rest and a carefully controlled diet. Penicillin is often used if an earlier streptococcal infection is still lingering. Recovery is usually complete. In a small percentage of cases, however, acute nephritis resists complete cure. It may subside for a time and then become active again, or it may develop into chronic nephritis.

CHRONIC NEPHRITIS. Chronic nephritis may follow a case of acute nephritis immediately or it may develop after a long interval during which no symptoms have been present. Many cases of chronic nephritis occur in people who have never had the acute form of the disease.

The symptoms of chronic nephritis are often unpredictable, with great variations in different cases. But in almost every case of the disease there is steady, progressive, permanent damage to the kidneys.

Chronic nephritis generally moves through three stages. In the first stage, the latent stage, there are few outward symptoms, if any. There may be slight malaise, but often the only indication of the disease is the presence of albumin and other abnormal substances in the urine. If a blood count is made during this stage, anemia may be found. There is no special treatment during the latent stage of chronic nephritis. The patient can live a perfectly normal life. He should avoid extremes of fatigue and exposure, and should eat a well balanced diet.

There may be a second stage of chronic nephritis in which edema occurs. Excess body fluids collect in the face, legs or arms. The main treatment in this stage consists of a high-protein, low-sodium diet. Steroid hormones may be helpful.

It is particularly important, at any stage of chronic nephritis, to avoid other infections, which will aggravate the condition.

The final stage of chronic nephritis is UREMIA. At this point damage to the kidneys is so extensive that they begin to fail.

There is no known cure for chronic nephritis, although the progress of the disease can be delayed, so that the patient can live an almost normal life for years. On rare occasions, surgeons have been successful in transplanting a healthy kidney to replace a diseased one. So far, the difficulties in performing this operation are still great. Some patients are being helped by repeated purification of their uremic blood by treatment with an artificial KIDNEY.

diffuse n., nephritis affecting both parenchyma and stroma of the kidney.

fibrous n., nephritis affecting the stroma of the kidney.

glomerular n., nephritis affecting the glomeruli.

interstitial n., nephritis with increase of interstitial tissue and thickening of vessel walls and malpighian corpuscles; sometimes due to alcohol or lead poisoning or gout.

parenchymatous n., nephritis affecting the parenchyma of the kidney.

saturnine n., nephritis due to chronic lead poisoning.

scarlatinal n., an acute nephritis due to scarlet fever.

suppurative n., a form accompanied by abscess of kidney.

tubular n., nephritis especially affecting the tubules.

nephritogenic (nĕ-frit″o-jen′ik) causing nephritis.

nephroblastoma (nef″ro-blas-to′mah) a kidney neoplasm containing embryonic tissue, occurring almost exclusively in children; called also Wilms' tumor.

nephrocalcinosis (nef″ro-kal″sĭ-no′sis) deposition of calcium phosphate in the renal tubules, resulting in renal insufficiency.

nephrocardiac (nef″ro-kar′de-ak) pertaining to the kidney and the heart.

nephrocele (nef′ro-sēl) hernia of a kidney.

nephrocolic (nef″ro-kol′ik) 1. pertaining to the kidney and the colon. 2. renal colic.

nephrocoloptosis (nef″ro-ko″lop-to′sis) downward displacement of the kidney and colon.

nephrogenic (nef″ro-jen′ik) producing kidney tissue.

nephrogenous (nĕ-froj′ĕ-nus) arising in a kidney.

nephrogram (nef′ro-gram) a roentgenogram of the kidney.

nephrography (nĕ-frog′rah-fe) roentgenography of the kidney (see also PYELOGRAPHY).

nephroid (nef′roid) resembling a kidney.

nephrolith (nef′ro-lith) a calculus in a kidney.

nephrolithiasis (nef″ro-lĭ-thi′ah-sis) the presence of renal calculi.

nephrolithotomy (nef″ro-lĭ-thot′o-me) incision of kidney for removal of calculi.

nephrology (nĕ-frol′o-je) scientific study of the kidney.

nephrolysin (nĕ-frol′ĭ-sin) nephrotoxin, a toxin destructive to kidney tissue.

nephrolysis (nĕ-frol′ĭ-sis) 1. freeing of a kidney from adhesions. 2. destruction of kidney substance.

nephroma (nĕ-fro′mah) a tumor of kidney tissue.

nephromegaly (nef″ro-meg′ah-le) enlargement of the kidney.

nephron (nef′ron) the basic functional unit of the KIDNEY, each nephron being capable of forming urine by itself. Each kidney is an aggregation of about a million nephrons. The specific function of the nephron is to remove from the blood plasma certain end products of metabolism, such as urea, uric acid and creatinine, and also any excess sodium, chloride and potassium ions. By allowing for reabsorption of water and some electrolytes back into the blood, the nephron also plays a vital role in the maintenance of normal fluid balance in the body.

The nephron is a complex system of arterioles, capillaries and tubules. Blood is brought to the nephron via the afferent arteriole. As the blood flows through the glomerulus (a network of capillaries), about one-fifth of the plasma is filtered through the glomerular membrane and collects in the malpighian (Bowman's) capsule, which encases the glomerulus. The fluid then passes through the proximal tubule, from there into the loop of Henle, then into the distal tubule and finally into the collecting tubule. As the fluid is making its tortuous journey through these various tubules, most of its water and some of the solutes are reabsorbed into the blood via the peritubular capillaries. The water and solutes remaining in the tubules become urine.

nephropathy (nĕ-frop′ah-the) disease of the kidneys.

nephropexy (nef′ro-pek″se) surgical fixation of a floating or dropped kidney (NEPHROPTOSIS). The care of a patient having this type of surgery is generally the same as that for any type of surgery of the kidney (see also KIDNEY). One important

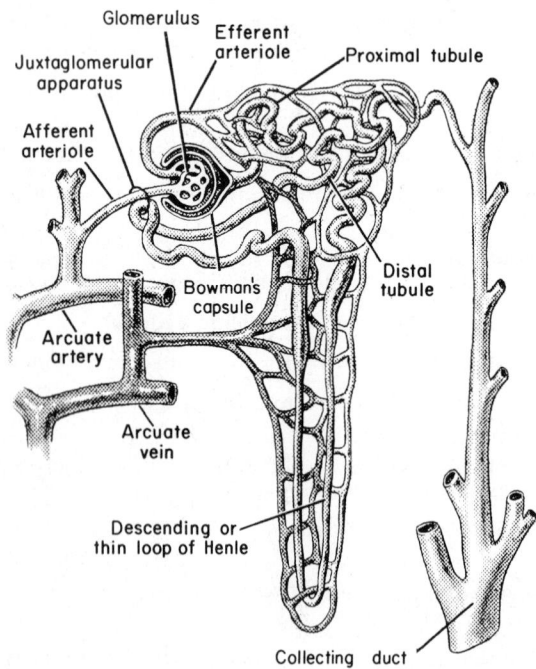

The nephron. (From Guyton, A. C.: Textbook of Medical Physiology. 4th ed. Philadelphia, W. B. Saunders Co., 1971; redrawn from Smith, H. W.: The Kidney. New York, Oxford University Press, 1951.)

point is that after nephropexy the patient is positioned so that his chest is lower than his hips; this position relieves strain on the sutures and helps to maintain the kidney in a normal position.

nephroptosis (nef″rop-to′sis) downward displacement of a kidney; called also floating or dropped kidney. This is found most often in young adult women, especially those who are thin and long waisted. Displacement can occur when the kidney supports are weakened by a sudden strain or blow, or are congenitally defective.

Although the condition may not produce symptoms of a serious nature, it can lead to difficulties if there is kinking of the ureters, producing an obstruction to urinary flow from the kidneys to the bladder. In addition, the patient may have an increased susceptibility to infection.

Correction of nephroptosis is usually by NEPHROPEXY, surgical fixation of the floating kidney.

nephropyelitis (nef″ro-pi″ĕ-li′tis) inflammation of the kidney and its pelvis; pyelonephritis.

nephropyelography (nef″ro-pi″ĕ-log′rah-fe) roentgenography of the kidney (see also PYELOGRAPHY).

nephropyeloplasty (nef″ro-pi′ĕ-lo-plas″te) plastic operation on the renal pelvis.

nephropyosis (nef″ro-pi-o′sis) suppuration of a kidney.

nephrorrhagia (nef″ro-ra′je-ah) hemorrhage from the kidney.

nephrorrhaphy (nef-ror′ah-fe) suture of the kidney.

nephrosclerosis (nef″ro-sklĕ-ro′sis) hardening of the kidney associated with hypertension and disease of the renal arterioles. It is characterized as benign or malignant depending on the severity and rapidity of the hypertension and arteriolar changes.

arteriolar n., nephritis characterized by thickening of the arterioles, degeneration of the renal tubules and thickening of the glomeruli.

nephrosis (nĕ-fro′sis) a disease of the kidneys in which there is malfunction of the kidney tissue without inflammation; called also the nephrotic syndrome.

Nephrosis probably represents one stage of NEPHRITIS. It is marked by excessive accumulation of fluid in the body, apparently due to the inability of the kidneys to regulate the body's water content properly. It is further characterized by a great loss of protein in the urine and decreased serum albumin. The disease may last for many years in children, without fatal result if serious infections and other disorders do not occur. In adults the disease is less common and more likely to become chronic.

The exact cause of nephrosis is not known. The disease may follow acute nephritis, either directly or after an interval as long as a number of years. It may follow or accompany some other disease of the kidneys. It may also occur in a person who has never had any kidney trouble at all. Some cases seem to be brought on by toxins, such as the venom of bees.

The chief symptom of nephrosis is edema, usually settling in the legs at first but then affecting the arms, face and torso. The swelling may be enormous.

Despite his alarming appearance, however, the

nephrosis patient usually recovers completely. Cortisone and related medicines are often very effective in reducing the edema, especially in children. There has also been success with certain immunosuppressive drugs.

amyloid n., chronic nephrosis with amyloid degeneration of the renal epithelium.

lower nephron n., a condition of renal insufficiency leading to uremia. It occurs in severe crush injuries, transfusion reactions, burns, certain kinds of poisoning and other conditions. Damage is mainly to the lower portion of the nephron.

nephrostoma (nĕ-fros′to-mah) one of the funnel-shaped and ciliated orifices of the excretory tubules that open into the coelom in the embryo.

nephrostomy (nĕ-fros′to-me) creation of a permanent opening into the renal pelvis.

nephrotic syndrome (nĕ-frot′ik) a condition marked by massive edema, heavy proteinuria, hypoalbuminemia and unusual susceptibility to intercurrent infections; called also NEPHROSIS.

nephrotome (nef′ro-tōm) a short plate of cells extending ventrolaterally from each somite in the embryo; the source of much of the genitourinary system.

nephrotomography (nef″ro-to-mog′rah-fe) body-section roentgenography for visualization of the kidney.

nephrotomy (nĕ-frot′o-me) incision of a kidney.

nephrotoxicity (nef″ro-tok-sis′ĭ-te) the quality of being toxic or destructive to kidney cells.

nephrotoxin (nef″ro-tok′sin) a toxin destructive to kidney tissue.

nephrotropic (nef″ro-trop′ik) having a special affinity for kidney tissue.

neptunium (nep-tu′ne-um) a chemical element, atomic number 93, atomic weight 237, symbol Np. (See table of ELEMENTS.)

nerve (nerv) a cordlike structure of the body, composed of highly specialized tissue, by which impulses are conveyed from one region of the body to another. For names of specific nerves of the body, see the table.

Depending on their function, nerves are known as sensory, motor or mixed. Sensory nerves, sometimes called afferent nerves, carry information from the outside world to the brain and spinal cord. Sensations of heat, cold and pain are conveyed by the sensory nerves. Motor nerves, or efferent nerves, transmit impulses from the brain and spinal cord to the muscles. Mixed nerves are composed of both motor and sensory fibers, and transmit messages in both directions at once.

Together, the nerves make up the peripheral nervous system, as distinguished from the central nervous system, which consists of the brain and spinal cord. There are 12 pairs of CRANIAL NERVES, which carry messages to and from the brain. Spinal nerves arise from the spinal cord and pass out between the vertebrae; there are 31 pairs, 8 cervical, 12 thoracic, 5 lumbar, 5 sacral and 1 coccygeal. The various nerve fibers and cells that make up the autonomic nervous system serve the glands, heart, blood vessels and involuntary muscles of the internal organs.

accelerator n's, the cardiac sympathetic nerves, which, when stimulated, accelerate the action of the heart.

anabolic n., any nerve, such as the vagus, whose stimulation serves to promote the anabolic processes.

n. block, regional anesthesia secured by making extraneural or paraneural injections in close proximity to the nerve whose conductivity is to be cut off.

calorific n., any nerve whose stimulation causes an increase in body temperature.

depressor n., 1. any afferent nerve whose stimulation depresses a motor center. 2. a nerve that lessens activity of an organ.

excitor n., one that transmits impulses resulting in an increase in functional activity.

excitoreflex n., a visceral nerve that produces reflex action.

frigorific n., any nerve whose stimulation causes a decrease in body temperature.

gangliated n., any nerve of the sympathetic nervous system.

inhibitory n., one that transmits impulses resulting in a decrease in functional activity.

pain n., a sensory nerve whose function is the conduction of stimuli that produce the sensation of pain.

pilomotor n's, those that supply the arrector muscles of hair.

pressor n., an afferent nerve whose irritation stimulates a vasomotor center and increases intravascular tension.

secretory n., an efferent nerve whose stimulation increases vascular activity.

somatic n's, the sensory and motor nerves.

splanchnic n's, those of the blood vessels and viscera.

sudomotor n's, those that control sweating.

sympathetic n's, those of the sympathetic system.

thermic n., thermogenic n., calorific nerve.

trisplanchnic n's, a general name for the system of sympathetic nerves.

trophic n., one concerned with regulation of nutrition.

vasoconstrictor n., one whose stimulation causes contraction of blood vessels.

vasodilator n., one whose stimulation causes dilation of blood vessels.

vasomotor n., one concerned in controlling the caliber of vessels.

vasosensory n., any nerve supplying sensory fibers to the vessels.

nervimotor (ner″vĭ-mo′tor) pertaining to a motor nerve.

nervone (ner′vōn) a cerebroside isolated from nerve tissue.

nervous (ner′vus) 1. pertaining to a nerve or nerves. 2. unduly excitable.

n. breakdown, a popular term for any type of mental illness that interferes with a person's normal activities. The term does not refer to a specific disturbance; a so-called "nervous breakdown" can include any of the mental disorders, including NEUROSIS, PSYCHOSIS or DEPRESSION.

n. system, the chief organ system that correlates the adjustments and reactions of an organism to

TABLE OF NERVES*

COMMON NAME [MODALITY]	NA TERM	ORIGIN	BRANCHES	DISTRIBUTION
abducent n. (6th cranial) [motor]	n. abducens	lower border of pons		lateral rectus muscle of eyeball
accessory n. (11th cranial) [motor]	n. accessorius	medulla oblongata and cervical segments of spinal cord		sternocleidomastoid and trapezius muscles
acoustic n. See vestibulocochlear n.				
alveolar n., inferior [motor, general sensory]	n. alveolaris inferior	mandibular n.	inferior dental and inferior gingival branches; mylohyoid and mental n.'s	teeth and gums of lower jaw, skin of chin and lower lip, mylohyoid muscle and anterior belly of digastric muscle
alveolar nn., superior	nn. alveolares superiores	superior alveolar branches (anterior, middle and posterior) that arise from infraorbital and maxillary nerves, innervating teeth of upper jaw and maxillary sinus, and forming superior dental plexus		
ampullary n., anterior	n. ampullaris anterior	branch of vestibular part of eighth cranial (vestibulocochlear) nerve that innervates ampulla of anterior semicircular duct, ending around hair cells of ampullary crest		
ampullary n., inferior. See ampullary n., posterior				
ampullary n., lateral	n. ampullaris lateralis	branch of vestibular part of eighth cranial (vestibulocochlear) nerve that innervates ampulla of lateral semicircular duct, ending around hair cells of ampullary crest		
ampullary n., posterior	n. ampullaris posterior	branch of vestibular part of eighth cranial (vestibulocochlear) nerve that innervates ampulla of posterior semicircular duct, ending around hair cells of ampullary crest		
ampullary n., superior. See ampullary n., anterior				
anococcygeal nn. [general sensory]	nn. anococcygei	coccygeal plexus		skin region of coccyx
auditory n. See vestibulocochlear n.				
auricular nn., anterior [general sensory]	nn. auriculares anteriores	auriculotemporal n.		skin of anterosuperior part of external ear
auricular n., great [general sensory]	n. auricularis magnus	cervical plexus—C2–C3	anterior and posterior branches	skin of side of head
auricular n., posterior [motor, general sensory]	n. auricularis posterior	facial n.	occipital branch	posterior auricular and occipitofrontal muscles, skin of external acoustic meatus

Common Name [modality]	[L.] Equivalent	Origin	Branches	Distribution
auriculotemporal n. [general sensory, parasympathetic]	n. auriculotemporalis	mandibular n.	anterior auricular n., n. of external acoustic meatus, parotid and superficial temporal branches, branch to tympanic membrane, communicating branch with facial n.	parotid gland, scalp in temporal region, tympanic membrane. *See also* auricular n., anterior, *and* n. of external acoustic meatus
axillary n. [motor, general]	n. axillaris	brachial plexus–C5-C6 through posterior cord	lateral superior brachial cutaneous n., muscular branches	deltoid and teres minor muscles, skin over shoulder
brachial plexus	plexus brachialis	fibers from spinal nerves C5-C8, T1		
buccal n. [general sensory]	n. buccalis	mandibular n.		skin of cheek, mucosa of floor of mouth
cardiac n., cervical inferior [sympathetic (accelerator), visceral afferent]	n. cardiacus cervicalis inferior	cervicothoracic ganglion		heart via cardiac plexus
cardiac n., cervical, middle [sympathetic (accelerator), visceral afferent]	n. cardiacus cervicalis medius	middle cervical ganglion		heart
cardiac n., cervical, superior [sympathetic (accelerator)]	n. cardiacus cervicalis superior	superior cervical ganglion		heart
cardiac n., inferior. *See* cardiac n., cervical, inferior				
cardiac n., middle. *See* cardiac n., cervical, middle				
cardiac n., superior. *See* cardiac n., cervical, superior				
cardiac nn., thoracic [sympathetic (accelerator), visceral afferent]	nn. cardiaci thoracici	ganglia T2-T5 of sympathetic trunk		heart
caroticotympanic nn. [sympathetic]	nn. caroticotympanici	superior cervical sympathetic ganglion	help form tympanic plexus	tympanic region, parotid gland
carotid nn., external [sympathetic]	nn. carotici externi	superior cervical ganglion		cranial blood vessels and glands via external carotid plexus
carotid n., internal [sympathetic]	n. caroticus internus	superior cervical ganglion		cranial blood vessels and glands via internal carotid plexus
cavernous nn. of clitoris [parasympathetic, sympathetic, visceral afferent]	nn. cavernosi clitoridis	uterovaginal plexus		erectile tissue of clitoris

*n. = nerve, [L.] nervus; nn. = (pl.) nerves, [L.] nervi.

TABLE OF NERVES (Continued)

COMMON NAME [MODALITY]	NA TERM	ORIGIN	BRANCHES	DISTRIBUTION
cavernous nn., of penis [sympathetic, parasympathetic, visceral afferent]	nn. cavernosi penis	prostatic plexus		erectile tissue of penis
cervical nn.	nn. cervicales	the 8 pairs of nerves that arise from cervical segments of spinal cord and, except last pair, leave vertebral column above correspondingly numbered vertebra; the ventral branches of upper four, on either side, unite to form cervical plexus; those of lower four contribute most of brachial plexus	superior and inferior branches	
cervical n., transverse [general sensory]	n. transversus colli	cervical plexus—C2-C3		skin and subcutaneous tissue in anterior cervical region
cervical plexus	plexus cervicalis	fibers from spinal nerves C1-C4		
chorda tympani [parasympathetic, special sensory]	chorda tympani	facial n. (intermediate n.)		submandibular and sublingual glands, anterior two thirds of tongue
ciliary nn., long [general sensory]	nn. ciliares longi	nasociliary n., from ophthalmic n.		intraocular structures
ciliary nn., short [parasympathetic, and sympathetic and general sensory from communicating branches with trigeminal n.]	nn. ciliares breves	ciliary ganglion from oculomotor n.		smooth muscle of eye
clunial nn., inferior [general sensory]	nn. clunium inferiores	posterior cutaneous n. of thigh		skin of inferior gluteal region
clunial nn., middle [general sensory]	nn. clunium medii	lateral branch of dorsal branch of sacral n.		skin of middle gluteal region
clunial nn., superior [general sensory]	nn. clunium superiores	lateral branch of dorsal branch of lumbar n.		skin of superior gluteal region
coccygeal n.	n. coccygeus	either of the thirty-first pair of spinal nerves, arising from coccygeal segment of spinal cord		
coccygeal plexus	plexus coccygeus	fibers from spinal nerves S4-S5, Co 1		
cochlear n. See vestibulocochlear n.				
cranial nn.	nn. craniales	the 12 pairs of nerves connected with brain, including olfactory (I), optic (II), oculomotor (III), trochlear (IV), trigeminal (V), abducens (VI), facial (VII), vestibulocochlear (VIII), glossopharyngeal (IX), vagus (X), accessory (XI) and hypoglossal (XII) nerves		

cubital n. *See* ulnar n.

Name	Latin	Origin	Branches	Distribution
cutaneous n. of arm, lateral, inferior [general sensory]	n. cutaneus brachii lateralis inferior	radial n.		skin of back of arm
cutaneous n. of arm, lateral, superior [general sensory]	n. cutaneus brachii lateralis superior	axillary n.		skin of back of arm
cutaneous n. of arm, medial [general sensory]	n. cutaneus brachii medialis	T1 through medial cord		skin on medial and posterior aspects of arm
cutaneous n. of arm, posterior [general sensory]	n. cutaneus brachii posterior	radial n.		skin on dorsal surface of arm
cutaneous n. of calf, lateral [general sensory]	n. cutaneus surae lateralis	common peroneal n.	sural n.	skin of lower dorsal aspect of leg and lateral aspect of foot
cutaneous n. of calf, medial [general sensory]	n. cutaneus surae medialis	tibial n.	sural n.	skin of lower dorsal aspect of leg and lateral aspect of foot
cutaneous n. of foot, dorsal, intermediate [general sensory]	n. cutaneus dorsalis intermedius pedis	superficial peroneal n.	dorsal digital nn. of foot	skin of lateral side of foot and ankle; adjacent sides of third and fourth and of fourth and fifth toes
cutaneous n. of foot, dorsal, lateral [general sensory]	n. cutaneus dorsalis lateralis pedis	sural n.		adjacent sides of fourth and fifth toes, lateral side of fifth toe
cutaneous n. of foot, dorsal, medial [general sensory]	n. cutaneus dorsalis medialis pedis	superficial peroneal n.		skin of medial side of foot and adjacent sides of second and third toes
cutaneous n. of forearm, lateral [general sensory]	n. cutaneus antebrachii lateralis	musculocutaneous n.		skin over radial part of forearm
cutaneous n. of forearm, medial [general sensory]	n. cutaneus antebrachii medialis	brachial plexus – C8–T1 through medial cord	anterior and ulnar branches	skin of front, medial and posteromedial aspects of forearm
cutaneous n. of forearm, posterior [general sensory]	n. cutaneus antebrachii. posterior	radial n.		skin of dorsal aspect of lower half of arm and of forearm
cutaneous n. of thigh, lateral [general sensory]	n. cutaneus femoris lateralis	lumbar plexus – L2–L3		skin of lateral aspect and front of thigh
cutaneous n. of thigh, posterior [general sensory]	n. cutaneus femoris posterior	sacral plexus – S1–S3	inferior clunial nn., perineal branches	skin of inferior gluteal region, back of thigh and leg, external genitalia

digital nn., dorsal, radial. *See* digital nn. of radial n., dorsal

TABLE OF NERVES (Continued)

COMMON NAME [MODALITY]	NA TERM	ORIGIN	BRANCHES	DISTRIBUTION
digital nn., dorsal, ulnar. See digital nn. of ulnar n., dorsal				
digital nn. of foot, dorsal [general sensory]	nn. digitales dorsales pedis	intermediate dorsal cutaneous n.		adjacent sides of third and fourth, and of fourth and fifth toes
digital nn. of lateral plantar n., plantar, common [general sensory]	nn. digitales plantares communes nervi plantaris lateralis	superficial branch of lateral plantar n.	proper plantar digital nn. of lateral plantar n.	(see distribution of nerves listed under branches)
digital nn. of lateral plantar n., plantar, proper [general sensory]	nn. digitales plantares proprii nervi plantaris lateralis	common plantar digital nn. of lateral plantar n.		lateral plantar surface of foot; plantar and adjacent surfaces of fourth and fifth toes
digital nn. of lateral surface of great toe and of medial surface of second toe, dorsal [general sensory, motor]	nn. digitales dorsales hallucis lateralis et digiti secundi medialis	deep peroneal n.		dorsal interosseous muscles, articulations of ankle and foot, skin of adjacent sides of great and second toes
digital nn. of medial plantar n., plantar, common [general sensory]	nn. digitales plantares communes nervi plantaris medialis	medial plantar n.	proper plantar digital nn. of medial plantar n.	(see distribution of nerves listed under branches)
digital nn. of medial plantar n., plantar, proper [general sensory]	nn. digitales plantares proprii nervi plantaris medialis	common plantar digital nn. of medial plantar n.		medial plantar surface of foot; plantar and adjacent surfaces of great and second, and of second and third toes
digital nn. of median n., palmar, common [general sensory]	nn. digitales palmares communes nervi mediani	median n.	proper palmar digital nn. of median n.	(see distribution of nerves listed under branches)
digital nn. of median n., palmar, proper [general sensory]	nn. digitales palmares proprii nervi mediani	common palmar digital nn. of median n.		skin on palmar surface and sides of digits
digital nn. of radial n., dorsal [general sensory]	nn. digitales dorsales nervi radialis	superficial branch of radial n.		ulnar side of thumb, radial side of second finger; adjacent sides of second and third, and of third and fourth fingers
digital nn. of ulnar n., dorsal [general sensory]	nn. digitales dorsales nervi ulnaris	dorsal branch of ulnar n.		skin of ulnar sides of third, fourth and fifth, and of radial sides of fourth and fifth fingers
digital nn. of ulnar n., palmar, common [general sensory]	nn. digitales palmares communes nervi ulnaris	superficial branch of palmar branch of ulnar n.	proper palmar digital nn. of ulnar n.	(see distribution of nerves listed under branches)
digital nn. of ulnar n., palmar, proper [general sensory]	nn. digitales palmares proprii nervi ulnaris	common palmar digital nn. and superficial branch of palmar branch of ulnar n.		skin of adjacent sides of fourth and fifth fingers

		Origin	Branches	Distribution
dorsal n. of clitoris [general sensory, motor]	n. dorsalis clitoridis	perineal nn.		deep transverse muscle of perineum, sphincter muscle of urethra, clitoris
dorsal n. of penis [general sensory, motor]	n. dorsalis penis	perineal nn.		deep transverse muscle of perineum, sphincter muscle of urethra, skin of penis
dorsal scapular n. [motor]	n. dorsalis scapulae	brachial plexus – ventral branch of C5		levator m. of scapula and rhomboid muscle
ethmoidal n., anterior [general sensory]	n. ethmoidalis anterior	nasociliary n., from ophthalmic n.	internal, external, lateral and medial nasal branches	mucosa of nasal septum, lateral wall of nasal cavity, skin of bridge and tip of nose
ethmoidal n., posterior [general sensory]	n. ethmoidalis posterior	nasociliary n., from ophthalmic n.		mucosa of posterior ethmoid cells and of sphenoidal sinus
n. of external acoustic meatus [general sensory]	n. meatus acustici	auriculotemporal n.	branch to tympanic membrane	skin of external acoustic meatus, tympanic membrane
facial n. (7th cranial) [motor, parasympathetic, general sensory, special sensory]	n. facialis	inferior border of pons, between olive and inferior cerebellar peduncle	n. to stapedius; greater petrosal and posterior auricular n.; parotid plexus; digastric, temporal, zygomatic, buccal, lingual, marginal, mandibular and cervical branches, and communicating branch with tympanic plexus	various structures of face, head and neck (see also distribution of individual nerves listed under branches)
femoral n. [general sensory]	n. femoralis	lumbar plexus – L2–L4	saphenous n., muscular and anterior cutaneous branches	anterior thigh muscles, skin on front and medial aspect of thigh and patella (see also distribution of saphenous n.)
fibular n. See entries under peroneal n.	n. fibularis (official alternative for n. peroneus)			
frontal n. [general sensory]	n. frontalis	ophthalmic n.	supraorbital and supratrochlear nn.	(see distribution of nerves listed under branches)
genitofemoral n. [general sensory, motor]	n. genitofemoralis	lumbar plexus – L1–L2	genital and femoral branches	cremaster muscle, skin of scrotum or labium majus and of adjacent area of thigh and femoral triangle
glossopalatine n. See intermediate n.				

TABLE OF NERVES (*Continued*)

COMMON NAME [MODALITY]	NA TERM	ORIGIN	BRANCHES	DISTRIBUTION
glossopharyngeal n. (9th cranial) [parasympathetic, general sensory, special sensory, visceral sensory]	n. glossopharyngeus	medulla oblongata, lateral to olive	tympanic n., pharyngeal, stylopharyngeal, tonsillar and lingual branches, branch to carotid sinus, communicating branch with auricular branch of vagus n.	mucosa of oropharynx, stylopharyngeus muscle, mucosa of palatine tonsil and of adjacent part of soft palate, posterior third of tongue, carotid sinus, carotid body (see also distribution of tympanic n.)
gluteal n., inferior [motor]	n. gluteus inferior	sacral plexus—L5-S2		gluteus maximus muscle
gluteal n., superior [motor]	n. gluteus	sacral plexus—L4-S1		gluteal muscles
hemorrhoidal nn., inferior. *See* rectal nn., inferior				
hypogastric n.	n. hypogastricus (dexter et sinister)	a nerve trunk situated on either side (right and left), interconnecting superior and inferior hypogastric plexuses		
hypoglossal n. (12th cranial) [motor]	n. hypoglossus	lingual branches between pyramid and olive		styloglossus, hyoglossus and genioglossus muscles, intrinsic muscles of tongue
hypoglossal n., lesser. *See* lingual n.				
iliohypogastric n. [general sensory]	n. iliohypogastricus	lumbar plexus—T12	lateral and anterior cutaneous branches	skin over side of buttock and over pubis
ilioinguinal n. [general sensory]	n. ilioinguinalis	lumbar plexus—T12-L1	anterior scrotal branches or anterior labial branches	anterior scrotal or anterior labial region
infraoccipital n. *See* suboccipital n.				
infraorbital n. [general sensory]	n. infraorbitalis	maxillary n.	middle and anterior superior alveolar, inferior palpebral, internal and external nasal and superior labial branches	incisor, cuspid and premolar teeth of upper jaw, skin and conjunctiva of lower eyelid, mobile septum and skin of side of nose, mucous membrane of mouth, skin of upper lip
infratrochlear n. [general sensory]	n. infratrochlearis	nasociliary n., from ophthalmic n.	palpebral branches	root and bridge of nose, conjunctiva and skin of lower eyelid, lacrimal duct
intercostal nn. [general sensory, motor]	nn. intercostales			muscles and skin of back, thorax and upper abdomen
intercostobrachial nn. [general sensory]	nn. intercostobrachiales	second and third intercostal nn.		skin on back and medial aspect of arm
intermediate n. [parasympathetic, special sensory]	n. intermedius	a name given to a small part of facial n., between remainder of facial n. and vestibulocochlear n.	greater petrosal n., chorda tympani	lacrimal, nasal, palatine, submandibular and sublingual glands, and anterior two thirds of tongue

English name	Latin (NA) name	Origin	Branches	Distribution
interosseous n. of forearm, anterior [motor]	n. interosseus antebrachii anterior	median n.		deep muscles on anterior aspect of forearm
interosseous n. of forearm, posterior [motor]	n. interosseus antebrachii posterior	deep branch of radial n.		long abductor muscle of thumb, extensor muscles of thumb and index finger
interosseous n. of leg [general sensory]	interosseus cruris	tibial n.		inferior tibiofibular joint, interosseous membrane
ischiadic n. *See* sciatic n.				
jugular n.	n. jugularis	a name given to sympathetic fibers originating from the superior cervical ganglion and distributed to glossopharyngeal and vagus nn.		
labial nn., anterior [general sensory]	nn. labiales anteriores	ilioinguinal n.		skin of anterior labial region
labial nn., posterior [general sensory]	nn. labiales posteriores	perineal nn.		labium majus
lacrimal n. [general sensory]	n. lacrimalis	ophthalmic n.		lacrimal gland, conjunctiva, lateral commissure of eye, skin of upper eyelid
laryngeal n., inferior [motor]	n. laryngeus inferior	recurrent laryngeal n.		intrinsic muscles of larynx, except cricothyroid muscle
laryngeal n., recurrent [parasympathetic, visceral afferent, motor]	n. laryngeus recurrens	vagus n.	inferior laryngeal, tracheal, esophageal and inferior cardiac branches	tracheal mucosa, esophagus, cardiac plexus (see also distribution of laryngeal n., inferior)
laryngeal n., superior [motor, general sensory, visceral afferent, parasympathetic]	n. laryngeus superior	vagus n.	external and internal branches, branch communicating with inferior laryngeal n.	cricothyroid muscle and inferior constrictor m. of pharynx, mucosa of epiglottis, base of tongue, larynx
lingual n. [general sensory]	n. lingualis	mandibular n.	sublingual n., lingual branches, branch to isthmus of fauces, branch communicating with hypoglossal n. and chorda tympani	anterior two thirds of tongue, adjacent areas of mouth, gums, isthmus of fauces
lumbar nn.	nn. lumbales	the 5 pairs of nerves that arise from lumbar segments of spinal cord, each pair leaving vertebral column below correspondingly numbered vertebrae; ventral branches of these nerves participate in formation of lumbosacral plexus		
lumbar plexus	plexus lumbalis	fibers from spinal nerves L1–L4		
mandibular n. (third division of trigeminal n.) [general sensory, motor]	n. mandibularis	trigeminal ganglion	meningeal branch, masseteric, deep temporal, lateral and medial pterygoid, buccal, auriculotemporal, lingual and inferior alveolar nn.	meningeal branch—accompanies middle meningeal artery to supply dura mater, helps innervate mucosa of mastoid air cells (see also distribution of other nerves listed under branches)

TABLE OF NERVES (*Continued*)

COMMON NAME [MODALITY]	NA TERM	ORIGIN	BRANCHES	DISTRIBUTION
masseteric n. [motor, general sensory]	n. massetericus	mandibular n.		masseter muscle, temporomandibular joint
maxillary n. (second division of trigeminal n.) [general sensory]	n. maxillaris	trigeminal ganglion	middle meningeal branch, zygomatic n., posterior superior alveolar branches, infraorbital n., pterygopalatine n., nasopalatine n. and other branches of pterygopalatine nn. and ganglion	middle meningeal branch – accompanies middle meningeal artery to supply dura mater; posterior superior alveolar branches – maxillary sinus, molar teeth of upper jaw (see also distribution of other nerves listed under branches)
median n. [general sensory]	n. medianus	brachial plexus – C6–T1 through lateral and medial cords	anterior interosseous n. of forearm, common palmar digital nn., and muscular and palmar branches	muscular branches – most of flexor muscles on front of forearm, most of short muscles of thumb; palmar branch – skin of palm (see also distribution of other nerves listed under branches)
mental n. [general sensory]	n. mentalis	inferior alveolar n.	mental and inferior labial branches	skin of chin, lower lip
musculocutaneous n. [general sensory, motor]	n. musculocutaneus	brachial plexus – C5–C7 through lateral cord	lateral cutaneous n. of forearm, muscular branches	biceps and brachialis muscles, skin of radial side of forearm
mylohyoid n. [motor]	n. mylohyoideus	inferior alveolar n.		mylohyoid muscle, anterior belly of digastric muscle
nasociliary n. [general sensory]	n. nasociliaris	ophthalmic n.	long ciliary, posterior ethmoidal, anteriorethmoidal and infratrochlear nn.	(see distribution of nerves listed under branches)
nasopalatine n. [general sensory]	n. nasopalatinus	pterygopalatine ganglion		mucosa of most of nasal septum and anterior part of hard palate
obturator n. [general sensory, motor]	n. obturatorius	lumbar plexus – L3–L4	anterior and posterior branches	gracilis, long and short adductor muscles, sometimes pectineal; skin of medial side of thigh and leg; knee joint, external obturator and great adductor muscles
occipital n., greater [general sensory, motor]	n. occipitalis major	medial branch of dorsal branch of C2		medial portion of scalp of back of head, semispinal muscle of head
occipital n., lesser [general sensory]	n. occipitalis minor	cervical plexus – C2–C3		lateral portion of scalp of back of head

Common name [type]	Latin name	Origin	Branches	Distribution
occipital n., third [general sensory]	n. occipitalis tertius	medial branch of dorsal branch of C3		skin of upper part of back of neck
oculomotor n. (3rd cranial) [motor, proprioceptive, parasympathetic]	n. oculomotorius	midbrain, at medial border of cerebral peduncle	superior and inferior branches	medial and inferior rectus and inferior oblique muscles of eyeball, ciliary muscles, sphincter of pupil; superior rectus muscle, levator muscle of upper eyelid
olfactory nn. (1st cranial) [special sensory]	nn. olfactorii	olfactory bulb		nasal mucosa
ophthalmic n. (first division of trigeminal n.) [general sensory]	n. ophthalmicus	trigeminal ganglion	tentorial branches, frontal, lacrimal, nasociliary nn.	tentorial branches–dura mater of tentorium cerebelli and falx cerebri (see also distribution of other nerves listed under branches)
optic n. (2nd cranial) [special sensory]	n. opticus	optic chiasm		retina
palatine n., anterior. See palatine n., greater				
palatine n., greater [general sensory]	n. palatinus major	pterygopalatine ganglion	posterior inferior lateral nasal n.	gums, mucosa of soft and hard palates, and of inferior concha
palatine nn., lesser [general sensory]	nn. palatini minores	pterygopalatine ganglion		soft palate, uvula, tonsil
perineal nn. [general sensory, motor]	nn. perineales	pudendal n.	posterior scrotal nn., dorsal n. of penis; posterior labial nn., dorsal n. of clitoris	muscles of urogenital diaphragm, skin of external genitalia
peroneal n., common [general sensory, motor]	n. peroneus communis	sciatic n.	lateral cutaneous n. of calf, superficial and deep peroneal nn.	(see distribution of nerves listed under branches)
peroneal n., deep [general sensory, motor]	n. peroneus profundus	common peroneal n.	muscular branches, dorsal digital nn. of lateral surface of great toe and medial surface of second toe	muscular branches–anterior tibial, long extensor of great toe, long extensor of toes, third peroneal
peroneal n., superficial [general sensory, motor]	n. peroneus superficialis	common peroneal n.	muscular branches, medial and intermediate dorsal cutaneous nn. of foot	muscular branches–long and short peroneal muscles (see also distribution of nerves listed under branches)
petrosal n., deep [sympathetic]	n. petrosus profundus	superior cervical sympathetic ganglion		lacrimal, nasal and palatine glands via internal carotid plexus, nerve of pterygoid canal, and branches of pterygopalatine ganglion
petrosal n., greater [parasympathetic, general sensory]	n. petrosus major	intermedate n. via geniculate ganglion		lacrimal, nasal and palatine glands and nasopharynx via pterygopalatine ganglion and its branches

TABLE OF NERVES (Continued)

COMMON NAME [MODALITY]	NA TERM	ORIGIN	BRANCHES	DISTRIBUTION
petrosal n., lesser [parasympathetic]	n. petrosus minor	tympanic plexus of glossopharyngeal n.		otic ganglion and, through communicating branch with auriculotemporal n., parotid gland
phrenic n. [general sensory, motor]	n. phrenicus	cervical plexus—C3–C5	pericardial and phrenicoabdominal branches	diaphragm, pericardium
phrenic nn., accessory	nn. phrenici	contributions of fifth cervical n. to phrenic n. when fifth cervical n. runs separately from rest of phrenic n. throughout a large part of its course		
plantar n., lateral [general sensory]	n. plantaris lateralis	tibial n.	superficial and deep branches	various structures of foot
plantar n., medial [general sensory, motor]	n. plantaris medialis	tibial n.	common plantar digital nn. of medial plantar n.	(see distribution of nerves listed under branches)
pneumogastric n. See vagus n.				
n. to lateral pterygoid [motor]	n. pterygoideus lateralis	mandibular n.		lateral pterygoid muscle
n. to medial pterygoid [motor]	n. pterygoideus	mandibular n.		medial pterygoid muscle
n. of pterygoid canal [parasympathetic, sympathetic, general sensory]	n. canalis pterygoidei	formed by union of deep and greater petrosal nn.		pterygopalatine ganglion and branches
pterygopalatine nn. [general sensory]	nn. pterygopalatini	maxillary n.	nasopalatine and greater and lesser palatine nn., n. of pterygoid canal, orbital, pharyngeal, posterior superior nasal and posterior inferior nasal branches	connect pterygopalatine ganglion with maxillary division of trigeminal n.; branches are usually called "branches of pterygopalatine ganglion"
pudendal n. [general sensory, motor, parasympathetic]	n. pudendus	sacral plexus—S2–S4	inferior rectal and perineal nn., parasympathetic branches to pelvic viscera	organs of pelvis (see also distribution of nerves listed under branches)
radial n. [general sensory, motor]	n. radialis	brachial plexus—C6–C8, and sometimes C5 and T1, through posterior cord	posterior cutaneous and inferior lateral cutaneous nn. of arm, posterior cutaneous n. of forearm, muscular, deep and superficial branches	arm, forearm and hand (see also distribution of nerves listed under branches)
rectal nn., inferior [general sensory, motor]	nn. rectales inferiores	pudendal n.		external sphincter of anus, muscle skin around anus, lining of anal canal

643

recurrent n. *See* laryngeal n., recurrent				
saccular n.	n. saccularis	the branch of vestibular part of eighth cranial (vestibulocochlear) nerve that innervates macula of saccule		
sacral nn.	nn. sacrales	the 5 pairs of nerves that arise from sacral segments of spinal cord; the ventral branches of first 4 pairs participate in formation of sacral plexus		
sacral plexus	plexus sacralis	fibers from spinal nerves L4–L5, S1–S4		
saphenous n. [general sensory]	n. saphenus	femoral n.	infrapatellar and medial crural cutaneous branches	skin of medial aspect of leg and foot
sciatic n. [general sensory]	n. ischiadicus	sacral plexus – L4–S3	common peroneal and tibial nn.	(see distribution of nerves listed under branches)
scrotal nn., anterior [general sensory]	nn. scrotales anteriores	ilioinguinal n.		skin of anterior scrotal region
scrotal nn., posterior [general sensory]	nn. scrotales posteriores	perineal nn.		skin of scrotum
spinal nn. [general sensory]	nn. spinales	the 31 pairs of nerves that arise from spinal cord, including 8 cervical, 12 thoracic, 5 lumbar, 5 sacral and one coccygeal		
splanchnic n., greater [preganglionic sympathetic, visceral afferent]	n. splanchnicus major	thoracic ganglia T5–T10 of sympathetic trunk		celiac ganglion
splanchnic n., lesser [preganglionic sympathetic, visceral afferent]	n. splanchnicus minor	ganglia T9, T10 of sympathetic trunk	renal branch	aorticorenal ganglion
splanchnic n., lowest [sympathetic, visceral afferent]	n. splanchnicus imus	last ganglion of sympathetic trunk, or lesser splanchnic n.		renal plexus
splanchnic nn., lumbar [preganglionic sympathetic, visceral afferent]	nn. splanchnici lumbales	lumbar ganglia of sympathetic trunk		celiac, mesenteric and hypogastric plexuses
splanchnic nn., pelvic [preganglionic, parasympathetic, visceral afferent]	nn. splanchnici pelvini	S2–S4		terminal ganglia in pelvic viscera
splanchnic nn., sacral [preganglionic, sympathetic, visceral afferent]	nn. splanchnici sacrales	sacral part of sympathetic trunk		inferior hypogastric plexus
n. to stapedius [motor]	n. stapedius	facial n.		stapedius muscle
subclavian n. [motor, general sensory]	n. subclavius	brachial plexus – C5–C6 through superior trunk		subclavius muscle, sternoclavicular joint

TABLE OF NERVES (Continued)

COMMON NAME [MODALITY]	NA TERM	ORIGIN	BRANCHES	DISTRIBUTION
subcostal n. [generally sensory, motor]	n. subcostalis	twelfth thoracic n.		abdominal muscles, skin of lower part of abdomen and gluteal region
sublingual n. [general sensory]	n. sublingualis	lingual n.		region of sublingual gland
suboccipital n. [motor]	n. suboccipitalis	C1		rectal and semispinal muscles of head
subscapular n. [motor]	n. subscapularis	brachial plexus—C5 through posterior cord		subscapular and teres major muscles
supraclavicular nn., anterior. See supraclavicular nn., medial				
supracavicular nn., intermediate [general sensory]	mm. supraclaviculares intermedii	cervical plexus—C3–C4		skin over pectoral and deltoid regions
supraclavicular nn., lateral [general sensory]	mm. supraclaviculares laterales	cervical plexus—C3–C4		skin of superior and posterior aspects of shoulder
supraclavicular nn., medial [general sensory]	mm. supraclaviculares mediales	cervical plexus—C3–C4		skin of medial infraclavicular region
supraclavicular nn., middle. See supraclavicular nn., intermediate				
supraclavicular nn., posterior. See supraclavicular nn., lateral				
supraorbital n. [general sensory]	n. supraorbitalis	frontal n., from ophthalmic n.	lateral and medial branches	skin of upper eyelid, forehead, anterior part of scalp (to vertex), mucosa of frontal sinus
suprascapular n. [motor, general sensory]	n. suprascapularis	brachial plexus—C5–C6 through superior trunk		supraspinous and infraspinous muscles, shoulder joint
supratrochlear n. [general sensory]	n. supratrochlearis	frontal n., from ophthalmic n.		medial part of forehead, root of nose, medial commissure of eye, conjunctiva, upper eyelid
sural n. [general sensory]	n. suralis	medial and lateral cutaneous nn. of calf	lateral dorsal cutaneous n. of foot, lateral calcanean branches	skin on back of leg and lateral side of foot and heel
temporal nn., deep [motor]	nn. temporales profundi	mandibular n.		temporal muscles
n. to tensor tympani [motor]	n. tensoris tympani	mandibular n. via otic ganglion		tensor muscle of tympanum

Name	Latin Name	Origin	Branches	Distribution
n. to tensor veli palatini [motor]	n. tensoris veli palatini	mandibular n. via otic ganglion		tensor muscle of palatine velum
thoracic nn.	nn. thoracici	the 12 pairs of spinal nerves that arise from thoracic segments of spinal cord, each pair leaving vertebral column below correspondingly numbered vertebra		body wall of thorax and upper part of abdomen
thoracic n., long [motor]	n. thoracicus longus	brachial plexus – ventral branches of C5–C7		anterior serratus muscle
thoracodorsal n. [motor]	n. thoracodorsalis	brachial plexus–C7–C8 through posterior cord		latissimus dorsi muscle
tibial n. [general sensory, motor]	n. tibialis	sciatic n.	interosseous n. of leg, medial cutaneous n. of calf, sural and medial and lateral plantar nn., and muscular and medial calcanean branches	leg and foot
trigeminal n. (5th cranial)	n. trigeminus	emerges from lateral surface of pons as a motor and a sensory root, the latter expanding into trigeminal ganglion, from which the 3 divisions of nerve arise (see mandibular n., maxillary n. and ophthalmic n.)		
trochlear n. (4th cranial) [motor, proprioceptive]	n. trochlearis	midbrain, below colliculus		superior oblique muscle of eyeball
tympanic n. [general sensory, parasympathetic]	n. tympanicus	glossopharyngeal n.	helps form tympanic plexus	tympanic cavity, tympanic membrane, mastoid air cells, auditory tube
ulnar n. [general sensory, motor]	n. ulnaris	brachial plexus–C7–T1 through medial and lateral cords	muscular, palmar cutaneous, dorsal, palmar, superficial and deep branches	arm and hand
utricular n.	n. utricularis	the branch of vestibular part of eighth cranial (vestibulocochlear) nerve that innervates macula of utricle		
utriculoampullary n.	n. utriculoampullaris	a nerve that arises by peripheral division of vestibular part of eighth cranial (vestibulocochlear) nerve, and supplies utricle and ampullae of semicircular ducts		
vaginal nn. [sympathetic, parasympathetic]	mm. vaginales	uterovaginal plexus from sacral part of sympathetic trunk and parasympathetic branches from pudendal n.		vagina
vagus n. (10th cranial) [parasympathetic, visceral afferent, motor, general sensory]	n. vagus (L. "wandering")	medulla oblongata, lateral to olive	superior and recurrent laryngeal nn., meningeal, auricular, pharyngeal, inferior and superior cardiac, bronchial, anterior and posterior gastric, hepatic, celiac and renal branches	various organs (see also distribution of nerves listed under branches)

TABLE OF NERVES (*Continued*)

COMMON NAME [MODALITY]	NA TERM	ORIGIN	BRANCHES	DISTRIBUTION
vertebral n. [sympathetic]	n. vertebralis	cervicothoracic ganglion		posterior cranial fossa via vertebral plexus
vestibular n. *See* vestibulocochlear n.				
vestibulocochlear n. (8th cranial)	n. vestibulocochlearis	emerges from brain between pons and medulla oblongata, behind facial nerve; it consists of 2 sets of fibers, the vestibular part and the cochlear part, and is connected with the brain by corresponding superior and inferior roots		
vidian n. *See* n. of pterygoid canal				
vidian n., deep. *See* petrosal n., deep				
zygomatic n. [general sensory]	n. zygomaticus	maxillary n.	zygomaticofacial and zygomaticotemporal branches	skin over zygomatic bone and in anterior temporal region

internal and environmental conditions. It is composed of the BRAIN, the spinal cord and the NERVES, which act together to serve as the communicating and coordinating system of the body, carrying information to the brain and relaying instructions from the brain. The system has two main divisions: the central nervous system, composed of the brain and spinal cord; and the peripheral nervous system, which is subdivided into the voluntary and autonomic systems.

THE NERVE CELL. The basic unit of the nervous system is the nerve cell, or NEURON. This highly specialized cell has many fibers extending from it which carry messages in the form of electrical charges and chemical changes. The fibers of some cells are only a fraction of an inch long, but those of others—for example, the sciatic nerve—extend for 2 or 3 feet. These fibers reach into muscles and organs throughout the body, to the ends of the fingers and toes, and cluster by the thousands in areas of the skin no larger than the head of a pin.

The nerve fibers come together from the extremities of the body and gather into cables running to and from the brain. Along the length of the spinal cord are a number of junctions where impulses or messages are sorted or relayed to higher centers.

The fibers of connecting nerve cells do not touch each other. Impulses are relayed from one to another by chemical means across the gap or synapse between them. In most cases an impulse must cross more than one synapse to cause the desired action.

In a REFLEX, the impulse is relayed from one nerve to another by a shortcut that produces a reaction without involving the brain. The knee jerk is an example of the simplest sort of reflex reaction. When the knee is tapped, the impulse travels through the sensory nerve that receives the tap, crosses a single synapse and activates the motor nerve that controls the quadriceps muscle in the thigh, causing the leg to jerk up automatically.

A very different sort of reflex is the conditioned reflex. Conditioning is the process of building links or paths in the nervous system. When an action is done repeatedly the nervous system becomes familiar with the situation and learns to react automatically. A new reflex has been built into the system. Hundreds of daily actions are conditioned reflexes. Walking, running, going up and down stairs and even buttoning a shirt all involve great numbers of complex muscle coordinations that have become automatic.

AUTONOMIC AND VOLUNTARY SYSTEMS. The peripheral nervous system in man evolved over many millennia, developing the ability to perform more and more complicated functions. It is divided into two specialized subsystems. The autonomic nervous system operates without conscious control as the caretaker of the body. The voluntary nervous system, which includes both motor and sensory nerves, controls the muscles and carries information to the brain.

The autonomic system is further specialized into two subsidiary systems: the sympathetic and the parasympathetic. The control centers of these systems lie in the hypothalamus. The sympathetic and parasympathetic nervous systems are continuously operative, functioning to adjust body processes to external and internal demands.

The sympathetic nervous system has in general an excitatory effect, and in response to danger or some other challenge, almost instantly puts body processes into high gear. This is done by the discharge of stimulating secretions at nerve junctions.

These secretions, along with epinephrine discharged into the blood by the adrenal medulla, help start muscle action quickly. Glucose is released from the liver into the blood and thus is made available to all the body's muscles as a source of quick energy. The rates of heart and lung action increase, digestive activity slows down, blood vessels constrict and sweating begins so that the body will be kept cool while under stress. Thus the body is prepared for an extraordinary effort.

The parasympathetic nervous system prevents body processes from accelerating to extremes. Acting more slowly than the sympathetic system, it causes the discharge of secretions that slow the heartbeat and lung action, restore digestive functioning and limit the constriction of the blood vessels. Generally it acts as a damper, so that unless the challenge demands a prolonged effort, body processes will begin returning to normal.

The voluntary nervous system has nerves of two kinds, sensory and motor. The sensory nerves bring messages to the brain from all parts of the body. They are sorted in the spinal cord and sent on to the brain to be analyzed, acted upon, associated with other information and stored as memory.

Messages from the brain, often in response to information received by way of the sensory nerves, are delivered to the muscles by the motor nerves. One motor nerve with its branching fibers may control thousands of muscle fibers.

The different parts of the nervous system are constantly interacting, and are so well coordinated that man can think, feel and act on many different levels and without serious confusion, all at the same time.

DISORDERS OF THE NERVOUS SYSTEM. The various organs of the nervous system may be affected by inflammatory processes, neoplastic disease, degenerative disease and injury. These are referred to as neurologic disorders and may be manifested by paralysis, sensory malfunction and convulsive seizures.

Inflammation of the meninges, the membranes covering the brain and spinal cord, is called MENINGITIS. The brain tissue itself may become inflamed (ENCEPHALITIS), may be deprived of adequate blood supply (cerebral thrombosis, cerebral hemorrhage, CEREBRAL VASCULAR ACCIDENT) or may be damaged by a violent blow to the head (HEAD INJURY, concussion, contusion). Malignant or benign tumors of the BRAIN can produce varying degrees of sensory and motor disorders.

The spinal cord may be affected by viral infections, as POLIOMYELITIS, or bacterial infections. In its late stage SYPHILIS may involve the brain and spinal cord. Accidental injury to the spinal cord can produce paralysis below the site of injury. A ruptured, or slipped, intervertebral DISK causes neurologic symptoms because it presses on the spinal cord.

Degenerative diseases affecting the nervous system include MYASTHENIA GRAVIS, MULTIPLE SCLEROSIS and PARKINSON'S DISEASE.

EPILEPSY, which may or may not be traced to a brain lesion, is another disorder that affects the nervous system.

nervousness (ner'vus-nes) morbid or undue excitability.

nervus (ner'vus), pl. *ner'vi* [L.] nerve.

Nesacaine (nes'ah-kān) trademark for preparations of chloroprocaine, a local anesthetic.

network (net'werk) a structure formed by interlacing fibers.

Neumann's disease (noi'manz) pemphigus vegetans.

neur(o)- (nu'ro) word element [Gr.], *nerve.*

neural (nu'ral) pertaining to nerves.

neuralgia (nu-ral'je-ah) pain in a nerve or along the course of one or more nerves. adj., **neural'gia.** Neuralgia is usually a sharp, spasmlike pain that may recur at intervals. It is caused by inflammation of or injury to a nerve or group of nerves.

Inflammation of a nerve, or NEURITIS, may affect different parts of the body, depending upon the location of the nerve. TIC DOULOUREUX (called also trigeminal neuralgia) is due to involvement of the trigeminal nerve, with neuralgic pain over the jaw, cheek and forehead.

Another form of neuralgia is SCIATICA, or pain occurring along the sciatic nerve. This pain is felt in the back and down the back of the thigh to the ankle. It may result from inflammation of or injury to the sciatic nerve, and is often associated with conditions such as arthritis of the spine, slipped intervertebral disk, diabetes mellitus and gout.

    degenerative n., neuralgia occurring in advanced age, and marked by signs of degeneration in the central nervous system.

    epileptiform n., tic douloureux (trigeminal neuralgia).

    n. facia'lis ve'ra, geniculate neuralgia.

    Fothergill's n., tic douloureux (trigeminal neuralgia).

    geniculate n., Hunt's n., neuralgia involving the geniculate ganglion, producing pain in the middle ear and external acoustic meatus.

    idiopathic n., neuralgia not accompanied by any structural change.

    intercostal n., neuralgia of the intercostal nerves, causing pain in the side.

    mammary n., neuralgic pain in the breast.

    Morton's n., pain in the metatarsus of the foot.

    nasociliary n., pain in the eyes, forehead and root of the nose.

    otic n., geniculate neuralgia.

neurapophysis (nu″rah-pof'ĭ-sis) a structure forming either side of the neural arch, or the dorsal wall of the spinal canal.

neurapraxia (nu″rah-prak'se-ah) a nerve lesion producing paralysis in the absence of peripheral degeneration.

neurarthropathy (nūr″ar-throp'ah-the) combined disease of joints and nerves.

neurasthenia, neurataxia (nu″ras-the'ne-ah), (nu″rah-tak'se-ah) a group of symptoms including fatigue, loss of appetite, lack of energy and aches and pains, resulting from a functional disorder of the nervous system, due usually to prolonged and excessive expenditure of energy; popularly called nervous prostration.

neuratrophia (nu″rah-tro'fe-ah) impaired nutrition of the nervous system.

neuratrophic (nu″rah-trof'ik) characterized by atrophy of the nerves.

neuraxis (nu-rak'sis) 1. the cerebrospinal axis, or central nervous system. 2. axon.

neuraxitis (nu'rak-si'tis) encephalitis.

neuraxon (nu-rak'son) axon.

neure (nūr) a neuron.

neurectasia, neurectasis (nu″rek-ta'ze-ah), (nu-rek'tah-sis) the surgical stretching of a nerve.

neurectomy (nu-rek'to-me) excision of a nerve.

neurectopia (nu″rek-to'pe-ah) displacement or abnormal situation of a nerve.

neurergic (nu-rer'jik) pertaining to nerve action.

neurexeresis (nūr″ek-ser-e'sis) the operation of tearing out a nerve.

neurilemma (nu″rĭ-lem'ah) the sheath of a nerve fiber; neurolemma.

neurilemoma (nu″rĭ-lĕ-mo'mah) a tumor of a peripheral nerve sheath; neurolemmoma.

neurinoma (nu″rĭ-no'mah) a nodular enlargement or tumor on a peripheral nerve.

neurinomatosis (nu″rĭ-no'mah-to'sis) a condition characterized by the presence of multiple neurinomas.

neurite (nu'rīt) axon.

neuritis (nu-ri'tis) inflammation of a nerve. adj., **neurit'ic.** There are many forms with different effects. Some increase or decrease the sensitivity of the body part served by the nerve; others produce paralysis; some cause pain and inflammation. The cases in which pain is the chief symptom are generally called neuralgia.

Neuritis and neuralgia attack the peripheral nerves, the nerves that link the brain and spinal cord with the muscles, skin, organs and all other parts of the body. These nerves usually carry both sensory and motor fibers; hence both pain and some paralysis may result. Treatment varies with the specific form of neuritis involved.

GENERALIZED NEURITIS. Certain toxic substances such as lead, arsenic and mercury may produce a generalized poisoning of the peripheral nerves, with tenderness, pain and paralysis of the limbs. Other causes of generalized neuritis include alcoholism, vitamin-deficiency diseases such as beriberi and diabetes mellitus, thallium poisoning, some types of allergy and some viral and bacterial infections, such as diphtheria, syphilis and mumps.

Some attacks of generalized neuritis begin with fever and other symptoms of an acute illness. However, neuritis caused by lead or alcohol poisoning comes on very slowly over the course of weeks or months.

Usually an attack of generalized neuritis will subside by itself when the toxic substance is eliminated. Rest and a nutritious diet containing extra vitamins, especially of the B group, are helpful. Physical therapy may relieve the pain and paralysis. Generalized neuritis may be prevented through knowledge of the dangers of poor nutrition, industrial hazards, chronic alcoholism and infections.

SPECIAL TYPES OF NEURITIS. Frequently, instead of a generalized irritation of the nerves, only one nerve is affected. BELL'S PALSY, or facial paralysis, results when the facial nerve is affected. It usually lasts only a few days or weeks. Sometimes, however, the cause is a tumor pressing on the nerve, or injury to the nerve by a blow, cut or bullet. In that event, recovery depends on the success in treating the tumor or injury.

Sciatica. The sciatic nerve, which runs from the spinal cord down each leg, is the widest nerve in the body and one of the longest. It is exposed to many different kinds of injury in the back, in the pelvis and along its course in the leg.

Inflammation of or injury to the sciatic nerve, with resultant SCIATICA, causes pain that travels down from the back or thigh into the feet and toes. Certain muscles of the leg may be partly or completely paralyzed, so that it is difficult to move the thigh or leg. A back injury, irritation from arthritis of the spine or pressure on the nerve that occurs during certain types of work may be the cause. Certain diseases such as diabetes mellitus or gout may be the inciting factor. The most common cause is probably a herniated or slipped intervertebral disk.

Some cases of sciatica are idiopathic—that is, without known cause. However, because of the long, painful and disabling course of severe sciatica, it is worth considerable time and money to have every possible cause investigated and the underlying trouble corrected if possible. Sedatives and physical therapy may also be required to relieve the pain or disability.

Neuritis of the Spinal Nerves. Injury or disease may affect any of the many nerves traveling out from the spine. For example, inflammation of the nerves between the ribs causes pain in the chest that may resemble pleurisy or even coronary occlusion (heart attack). This is called intercostal neuritis or intercostal neuralgia. Similarly, the nerves traveling down the neck to the arm may be subject to various injuries or diseases. For example, too vigorous pulling on the nerves in the neck, as might occur in difficult obstetrical deliveries, causes the condition known as brachial paralysis.

Saturday Night Palsy. This is a pressure neuritis that afflicts alcoholics. It usually commences after a sound night's sleep or after anesthesia in thin persons. The superficial nerves that are pressed against bones at the elbow and knee and the humerus are most commonly affected.

Neuritis of the Cranial Nerves. Bell's palsy results from inflammation of the seventh cranial, or facial nerve. Another nerve, the fifth cranial, or trigeminal, nerve, also ends in the face and jaws, and may be the source of a neuralgia that causes spasms of pain on one side of the face. This is called TIC DOULOUREUX or trigeminal neuralgia. It may be set off by a draft of cold air, by chewing or by other factors. Medicines and, if necessary, surgery can relieve this painful malady.

The nerves leading to the retina of the eye may be involved in various ailments. This condition, optic neuritis, is potentially dangerous to vision and requires immediate treatment. Any of the other cranial nerves may be affected by infections, tumors and toxins. The antibiotic streptomycin occasionally causes damage to the eighth cranial nerve, which helps control the sense of balance in the inner ear. Any disturbance of vision, hearing, balance, swallowing, taste or speech may be a

sign of trouble in the cranial nerves, and should be brought to a physician's attention at once.

HERPES ZOSTER, or shingles, is also a nerve ailment, with symptoms of pain and small blisters following the path of the affected nerve.

ascending n., that which progresses toward the central nervous system.

axial n., inflammation of the central part of a nerve.

degenerative n., neuritis marked by degeneration of the parenchyma.

descending n., that which progresses toward the periphery.

endemic n., beriberi.

facial n., Bell's palsy.

interstitial n., inflammation of the connective tissue of a nerve trunk.

multiple n., neuritis affecting several nerves at once; polyneuritis.

parenchymatous n., neuritis affecting primarily the medullary substance and axons.

peripheral n., neuritis of the terminal nerves.

postocular n., retrobulbar n., inflammation of that part of the optic nerve posterior to the eyeball.

toxic n., neuritis due to some poison.

traumatic n., neuritis due to injury.

neuroanastomosis (nu″ro-ah-nas″to-mo′sis) surgical anastomosis of one nerve to another.

neuroanatomy (nu″ro-ah-nat′o-me) anatomy of the nervous system.

neuroarthropathy (nu″ro-ar-throp′ah-the) joint disease associated with disease of the central nervous system.

neurobiology (nu″ro-bi-ol′o-je) biology of the nervous system.

neurobiotaxis (nu″ro-bi″o-tak′sis) the alleged tendency of bodies and dendrites of nerve cells to grow toward the source of their stimulation.

neuroblast (nu′ro-blast) any embryonic cell that develops into a nerve cell or neuron; an immature nerve cell.

neuroblastoma (nu″ro-blas″to′mah) a malignant tumor made up of neuroblasts.

n. sympath′icum, a tumor of sympathetic nerve cell origin.

neurocanal (nu″ro-kah-nal′) the central canal of the spinal cord.

neurocardiac (nu″ro-kar′de-ak) pertaining to the nervous system and the heart.

neurocentrum (nu″ro-sen′trum) one of the embryonic vertebral elements from which the spinous processes of the vertebrae develop.

neuroceptor (nu′ro-sep″tor) one of the terminal elements of a dendrite that receives the stimulus from the neuromittor of the adjoining neuron.

neurochemistry (nu″ro-kem′is-tre) scientific study of the chemical processes taking place in the nervous system.

neurochondrite (nu″ro-kon′drīt) an embryonic cartilaginous element that develops into the neural arch of the vertebra.

neurochorioretinitis (nu″ro-ko″re-o-ret″ĭ-ni′tis) inflammation of optic nerve, choroid and retina.

neurochoroiditis (nu″ro-ko″roi-di′tis) inflammation of the optic nerve and choroid.

n. **asthenia,** a symptom-complex characterized by easy fatigability, breathlessness and pain in the region of the heart; it is a form of NEUROSIS.

neurocirculatory (nu″ro-ser″ku-lah-to″re) pertaining to the nervous and circulatory systems.

neurocladism (nu-rok′lah-dizm) the formation of new branches by the process of a neuron; especially the force by which, in regeneration of divided nerves, the newly formed axons become attracted by the peripheral stump, so as to form a bridge between the two ends.

neuroclonic (nu″ro-klon′ik) marked by nervous spasm.

neurocranium (nu″ro-kra′ne-um) the part of the cranium enclosing the brain.

neurocutaneous (nu″ro-ku-ta′ne-us) pertaining to nerves and skin.

neurocyte (nu′ro-sīt) a nerve cell of any kind.

neurocytology (nu″ro-si-tol′o-je) scientific study of the cellular components of the nervous system.

neurocytoma (nu″ro-si-to′mah) 1. a brain tumor consisting of undifferentiated cells of nervous origin (neural epithelium). 2. neuroblastoma.

neurodendrite, neurodendron (nu″ro-den′drīt), (nu″ro-den′dron) dendrite.

neurodermatitis (nu″ro-der″mah-ti′tis) a type of skin disorder characterized by a thickened, well circumscribed, scaly plaque that is pigmented and lichenified. There is persistent itching at the site of the lesion. Called also lichen simplex chronicus.

The condition is particularly common in persons of Oriental extraction who live in the United States, and is more common in women over 40 years of age. The lesions may arise from normal skin or they may occur as a complication of other forms of DERMATI-TIS.

Treatment consists of administration of corticosteroids applied locally as a cream or given by injection. The area should be protected by light dressings and the patient encouraged to avoid mental stress, emotional upsets and irritation of the affected area.

The condition tends to become chronic with unexplained remissions and reappearance of lesions in a different part of the body.

neurodermatosis (nu″ro-der″mah-to′sis) a skin disease of nervous origin.

neurodiagnosis (nu″ro-di″ag-no′sis) diagnosis of neurologic diseases.

neurodynamic (nu″ro-di-nam′ik) pertaining to nervous energy.

neurodynia (nu″ro-din′e-ah) pain in a nerve.

neuroelectricity (nu″ro-e″lek-tris′ĭ-te) electric current generated in the nervous system.

neuroencephalomyelopathy (nu″ro-en-sef″ah-lo-mi″ē-lop′ah-the) disease involving the nerves, brain and spinal cord.

neuroendocrine (nu″ro-en′do-krin) pertaining to the nervous and endocrine systems in anatomic or functional relationship.

neuroepithelioma (nu″ro-ep″ĭ-the″le-o′mah) neurocytoma.

neuroepithelium (nu″ro-ep″ĭ-the′le-um) epithelium containing specialized sensory cells that receive external stimuli.

neurofibril, neurofibrilla (nu″ro-fi′bril), (nu″ro-fi-bril′ah) one of the delicate threads traversing the cytoplasm of nerve cells in every direction.

neurofibroma (nu″ro-fi-bro′mah) a connective tissue tumor of the nerve fiber fascicle.

neurofibromatosis (nu″ro-fi″bro-mah-to′sis) a familial condition characterized by developmental changes in the nervous system, muscles, bones and skin, and marked by the formation of neurofibromas over the entire body associated with patches of tan pigmentation; called also von Recklinghausen's disease.

neurofibrositis (nu″ro-fi″bro-si′tis) inflammation of muscle fibers involving sensory nerve filaments.

neurogenesis (nu″ro-jen′ē-sis) formation of the nervous system in embryonic development.

neurogenic (nu″ro-jen′ik) forming nervous tissue, or generating nervous energy.

neurogenous (nu-roj′ē-nus) arising from the nervous system.

neuroglia (nu-rog′le-ah) the supporting structure of the brain and spinal cord, composed of specialized cells and their processes; called also glia.

neurogliocyte (nu-rog′le-o-sīt) one of the cells composing the neuroglia.

neuroglioma (nu″ro-gli-o′mah) 1. a tumor of glia cells. 2. glioma in which there are nerve cells.

n. **gangliona′re,** glioma in which ganglion cells are embedded.

neurogliosis (nu-rog″le-o′sis) a condition marked by numerous neurogliomas.

neurogram (nu′ro-gram) the imprint left on the brain by past mental experiences.

neurohistology (nu″ro-his-tol′o-je) histology of the nervous system.

neurohormone (nu′ro-hor″mōn) a hormone stimulating the neural mechanism.

neurohumor (nu″ro-hu′mor) a chemical substance secreted by a neuron.

neurohypophysis (nu″ro-hi-pof′ĭ-sis) the main part of the posterior lobe of the hypophysis cerebri (see also PITUITARY GLAND).

neuroid (nu′roid) resembling a nerve.

neurokeratin (nu″ro-ker′ah-tin) a scleroprotein present in neuroglia fibrils (supporting elements) of nervous tissue.

neurolemma (nu″ro-lem′ah) a thin membranous

sheath spirally enwrapping myelin layers of myelinated nerves or axons of unmyelinated nerves; called also sheath of Schwann.

neurolemmitis   (nu″ro-lĕ-mi′tis) inflammation of the neurolemma.

neurolemmoma   (nu″ro-lĕ-mo′mah) a tumor of a peripheral nerve sheath.

neuroleptic   (nu″ro-lep′tik) 1. producing symptoms resembling those of disorders of the nervous system. 2. an agent that produces symptoms resembling those of nervous system disorders.

neurolipomatosis   (nu″ro-lī-po″mah-to′sis) a condition characterized by the formation of multiple fat deposits, with involvement of the nervous system because of pressure on the nerves.

neurologist   (nu-rol′o-jist) a specialist in neurology.

neurology   (nu-rol′o-je) scientific study of the nervous system, its functions and its disorders. adj., **neurolog′ic.**

neurolysis   (nu-rol′ĭ-sis) 1. liberation of a nerve from adhesions. 2. relief of tension upon a nerve obtained by stretching. 3. exhaustion of nervous energy. 4. destruction of nerve tissue. adj., **neurolyt′ic.**

neuroma   (nu-ro′mah) a tumor largely made up of nerve cells and fibers. adj., **neurom′atous.**
   amputation n., one formed at the end of a nerve severed in amputation of a limb.
   amyelinic n., one containing only nonmedullated nerve fibers.
   n. cu′tis, neuroma in the skin.
   cystic n., a false neuroma, or a neuroma that has become cystic.
   false n., one that does not contain genuine nerve fibers.
   ganglionated n., ganglionic n., one composed of true nerve cells.
   myelinic n., one containing medullated nerve fibers.
   plexiform n., one marked by multiple nodular enlargements along the course of the cutaneous nerves.
   n. telangiecto′des, one containing an excess of blood vessels.

neuromalacia   (nu″ro-mah-la′she-ah) softening of the nerves.

neuromatosis   (nu″ro-mah-to′sis) a disease condition characterized by the presence of many neuromas.

neuromechanism   (nu″ro-mek′ah-nizm) the structure and arrangement of the nervous system in regard to the regulation of the function of an organ.

neuromere   (nu′ro-mēr) one of the segments of the rhombencephalon in the developing embryo.

neuromittor   (nu″ro-mit′or) one of the terminal elements at the peripheral end of a neuron that transfers a stimulus to the neuroceptor of the adjoining neuron.

neuromuscular, neuromyal   (nu″ro-mus′ku-lar), (nu″ro-mi′al) pertaining to the nerves and muscles.

neuromyelitis   (nu″ro-mi″ĕ-li′tis) inflammation of the nerves and spinal cord.

neuromyositis   (nu″ro-mi″o-si′tis) neuritis complicated by myositis.

neuron   (nu′ron) a nerve cell with its processes, collaterals and terminations, regarded as a structural unit of the nervous system. Neurons are highly specialized cells having two characteristic properties: irritability, which means they are capable of being stimulated; and conductivity, which means they are able to conduct impulses. They are composed of a cell body (neurosome) and one or more processes (nerve fibers) extending from the body.

The processes or nerve fibers are actually extensions of the cytoplasm surrounding the nucleus of the neuron. A nerve cell may have only one such slender fiber extending from its body, in which case it is classified as unipolar. A neuron having two processes is bipolar, and one with three or more processes is multipolar. Most neurons are multipolar, this type of neuron being widely distributed throughout the central nervous system and autonomic ganglia. The multipolar neurons have a single process called an axon and several branched extensions called dendrites. The dendrites receive stimuli from other nerves or from a receptor organ, such as the skin or ear, and transmit them through the neuron to the axon. The axon conducts the impulses to the dendrite of another neuron or to an effector organ that is thereby stimulated to action.

Many processes are covered with a layer of lipid material called MYELIN. Peripheral nerve fibers have a thin outer covering called neurolemma.

TYPES OF NEURONS. Neurons that receive stimuli from the outside environment and transmit them toward the brain are called afferent or sensory neurons. Neurons that carry impulses in the opposite direction, away from the brain and other nerve centers to muscles, are called efferent or motor neurons. Another type of nerve cell, the association or internuncial neuron, or interneuron, is found in the brain and spinal cord; these neurons conduct impulses from afferent to efferent neurons.

SYNAPSES. The point at which an impulse is transmitted from one neuron to another is called a synapse. The transmission is chemical in nature; that is, there is no direct contact between the axon of one neuron and the dendrites of another. The cholinergic nerves (parasympathetic nervous system) liberate at their axon endings a substance called acetylcholine, which acts as a stimulant to the dendrites of adjacent neurons. In a similar manner, the adrenergic nerves (sympathetic nervous system) liberate sympathin, a substance that closely resembles epinephrine and probably is identical to norepinephrine.

The synapse may involve one neuron in chemical contact with many adjacent neurons, or it may involve the axon terminals of one neuron and the dendrites of a succeeding neuron in a nerve pathway. There are many different patterns of synapses.

RECEPTOR END-ORGANS. The dendrites of the sensory neurons are designed to receive stimuli from various parts of the body. These dendrites are called receptor end-organs and are of three general types: exteroceptors, interoceptors and proprioceptors. Their names give a clue to their specific function. The exteroceptors are located near the external surface of the body and receive impulses from the skin. They transmit information about the senses of touch, heat, cold and other factors in the external environment. The interoceptors are located in the internal organs and receive information from the viscera, e.g., pressure, tension and pain. The proprioceptors are found in muscles, tendons and joints and transmit "muscle sense," by which one is aware of the position of his body in space.

NEURONS AND EFFECTORS. The axons of motor neurons form synapses with skeletal muscle fibers to produce motion. These junctions are called motor end-plates or myoneural junctions. The axon of a motor neuron divides just before it enters the muscle fibers and forms synapses near the nuclei of muscle fibers. These motor neurons are called somatic efferent neurons. Visceral efferent neurons form synapses with smooth muscle, cardiac muscle and glands.

connector n., one whose dendrites and axon both synapse with other neurons.

lower motor n's, the peripheral neurons whose cell bodies lie in the ventral gray column of the spinal cord and whose terminations are in the skeletal muscles. Cf. upper motor neurons.

peripheral motor n., the neuron in a peripheral reflex arc that receives the impulse from an interneuron (internuncial neuron) and transmits it to a voluntary muscle.

postganglionic n's, neurons whose cell bodies are situated in the autonomic ganglia and whose purpose is to relay impulses beyond the ganglia.

preganglionic n's, neurons whose cell bodies lie in the central nervous system and whose efferent fibers terminate in the autonomic ganglia.

upper motor n's, the neurons in the cerebral cortex that conduct impulses from the motor cortex to the motor nuclei of the cerebral nerves or to the ventral gray columns of the spinal cord. Cf. lower motor neurons.

neuronitis (nu″ro-ni′tis) inflammation of a neuron.

neuronophage (nu-ron′o-fāj) a phagocyte that destroys nerve cells.

neuronophagia (nu″ron-o-fa′je-ah) phagocytic destruction of nerve cells.

neuronyxis (nu″ro-nik′sis) surgical puncture of a nerve.

neuro-ophthalmology (nu″ro-of″thal-mol′o-je) that branch of ophthalmology dealing with portions of the nervous system related to the eye.

neuropapillitis (nu″ro-pap″ĭ-li′tis) optic neuritis.

neuroparalysis (nu″ro-pah-ral′ĭ-sis) paralysis due to disease of a nerve or nerves.

neuropathogenicity (nu″ro-path″o-jĕ-nis′ĭ-te) the quality of producing or the ability to produce pathologic changes in nerve tissue.

neuropathology (nu″ro-pah-thol′o-je) the study of diseases of the nervous system.

neuropathy (nu-rop′ah-the) any disease of the nervous system, especially a degenerative (noninflammatory) disease of a nerve or nerves. adj., neuropath′ic.

diabetic n., a disease of the peripheral nerves primarily occurring as a consequence of diabetes mellitus. Sensory nerves are most often involved.

ischemic n., nerve degeneration due to circulatory obstruction.

progressive hypertrophic interstitial n., a familial disease characterized by chronic interstitial neuritis, hypertrophy of the peripheral nerves and posterior nerve roots and sclerosis of the posterior columns.

neurophage (nu′ro-fāj) neuronophage.

neuropharmacology (nu″ro-far″mah-kol′o-je) scientific study of the effects of drugs on the nervous system.

neurophthisis (nu-rof′thĭ-sis) wasting of nerve tissue.

neurophysiology (nu″ro-fiz″e-ol′o-je) physiology of the nervous system.

neuropil (nu′ro-pil) a dense feltwork of interwoven cytoplasmic processes of nerve cells (dendrites and axons) and of glia cells in the central nervous system and some parts of the peripheral nervous system.

neuroplasm (nu′ro-plazm) the protoplasm of a nerve cell. adj., neuroplas′mic.

neuroplasty (nu′ro-plas″te) plastic surgery of a nerve.

neuropodium (nu″ro-po′de-um) a bulbous termination of an axon in a synapse.

neuropore (nu′ro-pōr) an opening in the anterior or posterior end of the neural tube of the developing embryo that closes eventually.

neuropotential (nu″ro-po-ten′shal) nerve energy; nerve potential.

neuropsychiatrist (nu″ro-si-ki′ah-trist) a specialist in neuropsychiatry.

neuropsychiatry (nu″ro-si-ki′ah-tre) a branch of medicine combining neurology and psychiatry.

neuropsychopathy (nu″ro-si-kop′ah-the) a combined nervous and mental disease.

neuropsychosis (nu″ro-si-ko′sis) nervous disease complicated with mental disorder; a psychosis.

neuroradiology (nu″ro-ra″de-ol′o-je) the branch of radiography concerned especially with visualization of the contents of the skull and vertebral column.

neurorecurrence (nu″ro-re-ker′ens) neurorelapse.

neuroregulation (nu″ro-reg″u-la′shun) regulation and control of nervous activity.

neurorelapse (nu″ro-re-laps′) acute nervous symptoms following insufficient treatment of syphilis with arsenicals.

neuroretinitis (nu″ro-ret″ĭ-ni′tis) inflammation of the optic nerve and retina.

neuroretinopathy (nu″ro-ret″ĭ-nop′ah-the) pathologic involvement of the optic disk and retina.

neuroroentgenography (nu″ro-rent″gen-og′rah-fe) neuroradiology.

neurorrhaphy (nu-ror′ah-fe) suture of a divided nerve.

neurosarcocleisis (nu″ro-sar″ko-kli′sis) an operation for neuralgia, done by relieving pressure on the affected nerve by partial resection of the bony canal through which it passes and transplanting the nerve among soft tissues.

neurosarcoma (nu″ro-sar-ko′mah) a sarcoma derived from cells of the nervous system.

neurosclerosis (nu″ro-sklĕ-ro′sis) hardening of nerve tissue.

neurosecretion (nu″ro-se-kre′shun) secretory activities of nerve cells.

neurosensory (nu″ro-sen′so-re) pertaining to a sensory nerve.

neurosis (nu-ro′sis) an emotional disorder that can interfere with a person's ability to lead a normal, useful life, or can impair his physical health; sometimes called psychoneurosis.

A neurosis is generally a milder form of mental illness than a PSYCHOSIS. Those persons with neurotic symptoms are usually in contact with reality; they are able to function in society even though they may feel uncomfortable or their efficiency may be impaired. By contrast, psychotic persons tend to withdraw from the real world into one of their own, or to act in strange, even bizarre, ways, and are often not aware of their illness.

CAUSES. Current theories agree that neuroses arise from mental conflicts rooted in a person's childhood. The budding personality handles these ever present conflicts by means of mental and defense mechanisms, including IDENTIFICATION, RATIONALIZATION, REPRESSION, PROJECTION and others.

How each child uses these defense mechanisms in the process of maturing determines whether he will be healthy or neurotic. Symptoms such as obsessions, compulsions, phobias and other behavior represent unsuccessful attempts to master these conflicts. These symptoms can be so mild as to be barely noticeable. They can sometimes even be useful: A compulsion for neatness makes a good craftsman. It is a rare person who does not at some time show some trace of neurotic symptoms or behavior. At the other extreme, neurotic patterns can be severe enough to warrant intensive treatment.

TYPES OF NEUROSES. Psychiatrists today prefer to call neuroses "reactions" because these conditions result from, or are reactions to, psychologic factors. At the time the word "neurosis" came into use, it was thought that disorders of the nervous system were responsible for neurotic symptoms, and the term is still very widely used to describe these conditions.

Types of neurosis include the neurotic character and the various specific neuroses. Specific neuroses may take a number of different forms, which are not necessarily clearly defined as separate. A person may have several different neurotic symptoms but usually one tends to dominate.

Neurotic Character. Practically everyone has unconscious conflicts to some extent. Most people take them in their stride. Some people, however, develop a neurotic character, and suffer from a general maladjustment to society. In most cases the neurotic cannot sustain satisfactory relationships in the world around him, though some of them are charming, attractive people. A neurotic character is more difficult to treat than a specific neurotic symptom. The patient with a specific neurosis usually senses that there is something wrong with him, but the patient with a neurotic character structure may not, since he has convinced himself his ways of behavior are reasonable.

Anxiety Neurosis. In this condition, the patient has periods of anxiety which can vary from mild uneasiness ("free-floating anxiety") to blind panic. The anxiety can produce a variety of physical symptoms such as sweating, dizziness and shortness of breath.

Everyone occasionally experiences anxiety as a normal response to a dangerous or unusual situation. In anxiety neurosis the person feels the same emotion without any apparent reason. He cannot identify the source of the threat that produces his anxiety. The symptoms are the result of unconscious fears, which often are triggered by an apparently harmless stimulus that the patient unconsciously links with a deeply buried anxiety-producing experience.

Phobic Neurosis (Phobias). Phobic neurosis is an exaggerated fear. The feared objects, ideas or situations are often symbolic of the unconscious conflict. They divert attention from the conflict, and thus help to keep it unconscious. The neurotic may make elaborate changes in his life to avoid the object of his fear, often with severe effects on his family and friends.

Before the roots of neurosis in psychologic conflicts were discovered, it was believed that the different phobias were separate conditions. Names were assigned to an almost endless list of fears. Some of these, such as claustrophobia, fear of enclosed spaces, have become fairly common words. Today, however, the treatment of phobic neurosis is concerned more with discovering and resolving the unconscious conflict that causes the fear than with the specific object that is feared.

Obsessive-Compulsive Neurosis. There are actually two different symptoms in this neurosis, although they are closely related and are often found in the same person. The obsessive symptom is an overwhelming intrusion of certain thoughts or desires into the mind. The patient does not know why these thoughts or desires keep intruding, but it is very difficult for him to eliminate them from his mind. The compulsive symptom is an uncontrollable urge to act in certain patterns. He does not know why he follows these patterns, but he is very uncomfortable if he does not.

The mild forms of these symptoms are familiar to most people. For example, most children play the game of avoiding the cracks on a sidewalk. As adults, they may find themselves doing this occasionally, perhaps when they are thinking over a problem. The neurotic who follows this pattern, however, will feel real anxiety if he steps on a crack in the sidewalk.

In phobias and obsessive-compulsive neurosis, the patient deflects, or displaces, the unresolved conflict onto an external object or action as a substitute. By doing this, the person tries to control the conflict magically and to eliminate his anxiety. The obsession or ritual probably represents a smokescreen which the mind throws up to keep the inner conflict from becoming conscious.

Depressive Neurosis. This is an excessively deep and long-lasting depression. It may be set off by an external event, such as the death of a loved one, or there may be no apparent cause.

Depression as such is not abnormal. The well-adjusted person, however, works out and absorbs his grief. He is soon able to resume his activities and reestablish social relationships. The neurotic is not able to escape his depression for any length of time.

The depressive neurotic suffers from a general slowing down of mental and physical activity. He may have symptoms such as insomnia, loss of appetite and lack of interest in outside activities. The condition can vary from very mild to extremely severe; in severe cases, the person may even attempt suicide.

Neurotic depression is closely associated with a lack of confidence and self-esteem and with an inability to express strong feelings. Repressed anger is thought to be a powerful contribution to depression. The person feels inadequate to cope with the situations that arise in everyday life and feels that he is insecure.

Dissociative Neurosis. In this condition, parts of the personality and memory become cut off from each other. At times, anxiety causes the person to forget who he is or what he is doing. When he regains his self-awareness, he does not recall what has taken place. An example of this is amnesia; a less severe form is sleepwalking.

A dissociative neurosis is very likely an attempt by the mind to shield itself from anxiety caused by an unresolved conflict. When the patient encounters a situation that may be symbolic of his inner conflict, he goes into a form of trance to avoid experiencing the conflict.

In a few extreme cases, dissociative neurosis may take the form of multiple personality. The change from one personality to another, with no conscious awareness of the other, takes place in situations of extreme emotional stress.

Conversion Neurosis. Conversion neurosis, or conversion reaction, is a severe form of hysteria, in which the person unconsciously converts his anxiety into a physical symptom. This symptom may be blindness, deafness, inability to speak or paralysis of one or several limbs. The symptom is real, but there is no physical explanation for it. The symptom may disappear with as little apparent cause as it appeared.

The symptom in a conversion neurosis serves to spare the patient from dealing with an anxiety-producing situation that is too difficult to face. The best-known examples of this are shell shock and combat fatigue, in which the soldier becomes paralyzed and cannot participate in battle. The part of the body affected by conversion neurosis often has an important symbolic relationship to the patient's unconscious conflict. It may also be a part of the body which the patient considers weak.

Because the symptom is so obvious, a conversion neurosis is easily detected and diagnosed. It is a comparatively rare condition today.

PREVENTION. The formation of neurotic symptoms can be prevented to some extent. There is no doubt that a warm, secure home life, parental affection and the proper balance between understanding and discipline promote a healthy soil for the sound development of the child. The overall solidity of the parents' relationship to their child is of enormous importance. However, other elements also play a role: Each child is born with different possibilities of reaction to the world around him. School and community influences are also meaningful. All these are also responsible to some degree for the mental health of everyone.

PSYCHOSOMATIC DISORDERS. Illnesses that result from the interaction of mind and body are known as psychosomatic disorders. They are an exaggerated physical reaction to emotional stress. Psychosomatic disorders usually affect only organs under the control of the autonomic nervous system, such as the digestive tract, the endocrine glands, the heart, the genitourinary, circulatory and respiratory systems and the skin. Among illnesses known to be partly or completely psychosomatic illnesses are MIGRAINE, mucous COLITIS and ULCERATIVE COLITIS, peptic ULCER, SKIN allergies and perhaps ASTHMA. Treatment must be directed at both the physical symptoms and the underlying psychologic cause.

TREATMENT. All neuroses are in part or entirely the result of unconscious conflicts and can be treated, even though the neurotic is entirely unaware of the conflicts. The form of treatment, PSYCHOTHERAPY, tries through many different methods to make the patient conscious of his unresolved conflict. Once he is aware of it, the therapist can help him resolve it.

neuroskeletal   (nu″ro-skel′ĕ-tal) pertaining to nervous tissue and skeletal muscular tissue.

neuroskeleton   (nu″ro-skel′ĕ-ton) endoskeleton.

neurosome (nu′ro-sōm) 1. the body of a nerve cell. 2. a small particle in the ground substance of the protoplasm of neurons.

neurospasm (nu′ro-spazm) nervous twitching of a muscle.

neurospongioma   (nu″ro-spun″je-o′mah) neuroglioma.

neurospongium (nu″ro-spun′je-um) 1. the fibrillar component of neurons. 2. a meshwork of nerve fibrils.

neurosurgery   (nu″ro-ser′jer-e) surgery of the nervous system.

neurosuture (nu′ro-su″tūr) neurorrhaphy.

neurosyphilis   (nu″ro-sif′ĭ-lis) syphilis of the nervous system.
    paretic n., dementia and paralysis caused by neurosyphilis.
    tabetic n., tabes dorsalis.

neurotension (nu″ro-ten′shun) nerve stretching.

neurothecitis   (nu″ro-the-si′tis) inflammation of a nerve sheath.

neurotherapy (nu″ro-ther′ah-pe) 1. the treatment of nervous disorders. 2. psychotherapy.

neurothlipsis   (nu″ro-thlip′sis) pressure on a nerve.

neurotic   (nu-rot′ik) 1. pertaining to or affected with a neurosis. 2. pertaining to the nerves. 3. a nervous person in whom emotions predominate over reason.

neuroticism (nu-rot′ĭ-sizm) perverted or excessive nervous action.

neurotization (nu-rot″ĭ-za′shun) 1. regeneration of a nerve after its division. 2. the operation of implanting a nerve into a paralyzed muscle.

neurotmesis (nu″rot-me′sis) damage to a nerve, producing complete division of all the essential structures.

neurotomy (nu-rot′o-me) dissection or cutting of nerves.

neurotony (nu-rot′o-ne) stretching of a nerve.

neurotoxicity (nu″ro-tok-sis′ĭ-te) the quality of exerting a destructive or poisonous effect upon nerve tissue. adj., **neurotox′ic.**

neurotoxin (nu″ro-tok′sin) a substance that is poisonous or destructive to nerve tissue.

neurotrauma (nu″ro-traw′mah) wounding of a nerve.

neurotripsy (nu′ro-trip″se) crushing or bruising of a nerve.

neurotrophy (nu-rot′ro-fe) nutrition of nerve tissue.

neurotropism (nu-rot′ro-pizm) 1. the quality of having a special affinity for nervous tissue. 2. the alleged tendency of regenerating nerve fibers to grow toward specific portions of the periphery. adj., **neurotrop′ic.**

neurovaccine (nu″ro-vak′sēn) vaccine virus prepared by growing the virus in the brain of a rabbit.

neurovascular (nu″ro-vas′ku-lar) both nervous and vascular.

neurovirulence (nu″ro-vir′u-lens) the competence of an infectious agent to produce pathologic effects on the nervous system.

neurula (nu′roo-lah) the stage of development in the embryo marked by appearance of elements of the nervous system.

neurulation (nu″roo-la′shun) formation in the early embryo of the neural plate, followed by its closure with development of the neural tube.

neutral (nu′tral) neither basic nor acid.

neutralize (nu′tral-īz) to counteract and thereby destroy acid or alkaline qualities.

Neutrapen (nu′trah-pen) trademark for a lyophilized preparation of penicillinase, an enzyme sometimes used to treat allergic reactions to penicillin.

neutrino (nu-tre′no) a hypothetical elementary particle with an extremely small mass and no electric charge.

neutrocyte (nu′tro-sīt) a neutrophil leukocyte.

neutrocytopenia (nu″tro-si″to-pe′ne-ah) neutropenia.

neutrocytophilia, neutrocytosis (nu″tro-si″to-fil′e-ah), (nu″tro-si-to′sis) neutrophilia.

neutroflavine (nu″tro-fla′vin) acriflavine, an antiseptic dye.

neutron (nu′tron) an electrically neutral or uncharged particle of matter existing along with protons in the atoms of all elements except the mass 1 isotope of hydrogen.

neutropenia (nu″tro-pe′ne-ah) diminished number of neutrophils in the blood.

   chronic n. of childhood, a condition in which granulocytopenia, recurrent infections, lymphadenopathy and hepatosplenomegaly may be present for a considerable time, with subsequent spontaneous remission.

   chronic hypoplastic n., a syndrome resembling primary splenic neutropenia, but with hypocellular bone marrow.

   cyclic n., diminution or disappearance of neutrophils of circulating blood occurring at regular intervals.

   hypersplenic n., deficiency of neutrophils in the blood as the result of their increased destruction by the spleen.

   idiopathic n., malignant n., agranulocytosis.

   periodic n., cyclic neutropenia.

   peripheral n., decrease of neutrophils in the circulating blood.

   primary splenic n., a syndrome marked by splenomegaly, destruction of granular leukocytes of the blood, and overactive bone marrow.

neutrophil (nu′tro-fil) a medium-sized mature leukocyte, with a three- to five-lobed nucleus, and cytoplasm containing small granules which stain a pale lavender, normally constituting 60 to 70 per cent of the leukocytes of the blood.

   filamented n., a neutrophilic leukocyte that has two or more lobes connected by a filament of chromatin.

   nonfilamented n., a neutrophilic leukocyte whose lobes are connected by thick strands of chromatin.

   rod n., stab n., a neutrophilic leukocyte whose nucleus is not divided into segments.

neutrophilia (nu″tro-fil′e-ah) increase in the neutrophilic leukocytes of the blood.

neutrophilic (nu″tro-fil′ik) stainable by neutral dyes.

nevoid (ne′void) resembling a nevus.

nevoxanthoendothelioma (ne″vo-zan″tho-en″do-the″le-o′mah) a condition in which groups of yellow-brown papules or nodules occur on the extensor surfaces of the extremities of infants.

nevus (ne′vus), pl. *ne′vi* [L.] a small, flat, elevated or pedunculated lesion of the skin, pigmented or nonpigmented, and with or without hair growth, characterized by a specific type of cell; called also mole.

Most moles are either brown, black or flesh-colored; they may appear on any part of the skin. They vary in size and thickness, and occur in groups or singly. Usually they are not disfiguring.

A nevus is usually not troublesome unless it is unsightly or unless it becomes inflamed or cancerous. Fortunately, nevi seldom become cancerous; when they do, the cause is often constant irritation. Any change in size, color or texture of a mole, or any excessive itching or any bleeding, should be reported to a physician. Moles can be removed by surgery or by one of several other methods, such as the application of solid carbon dioxide, injections and radium treatment.

n. arachnoi′deus, n. araneo′sus, n. ara′neus, one composed of dilated blood vessels radiating from a point in branches resembling the legs of a spider.

blue n., a papular to nodular solitary growth composed of masses of dermal melanoblasts in the corium, developing in childhood, and occurring on the face, forearms or hands.

capillary n., one that involves the skin capillaries.

n. caverno′sus, cavernous angioma, or erectile tumor.

n. flam′meus, a diffuse, poorly defined area varying from pink to dark bluish red, involving otherwise normal skin; port-wine stain.

hairy n., a more or less pigmented nevus with hairs growing from its surface.

junction n., nests of cells at the junction of the epidermis and dermis. It is slightly raised, flat, nonhairy and pigmented.

n. lipomato′sus, one that contains a mass of fat.

n. pigmento′sus, a congenital dark-colored spot on the skin.

sebaceous n., a benign sebaceous tumor with highly differentiated cells, found after middle age and sometimes simulating early basal cell carcinoma.

spider n., nevus arachnoideus.

n. spi′lus, a smooth, flat nevus.

n. spongio′sus al′bus, a white spongy nevus.

n. u′nius latera′lis, an epithelial nevus occurring as a transverse band around one side of the trunk.

n. vascular′is, n. vasculo′sus, a reddish swelling or patch on the skin due to hypertrophy of the skin capillaries: the term includes nevus flammeus, the elevated strawberry marks, nevus araneus and cavernous angioma (erectile tumor).

n. veno′sus, venous n., a complex form of capillary hemangioma occurring most often on the face and having the deep purple color of port wine.

New Drugs an annual publication of the Council on Drugs of the American Medical Association, listing and describing drugs introduced recently.

newborn (nu′born) 1. recently born. 2. a human infant during the first 4 weeks after birth.

Newcastle disease a viral disease of birds, including domestic fowl, characterized by respiratory and gastrointestinal and encephalitic symptoms; also transmissible to man.

newton (nu′ton) a unit of force; the force that, when acting continuously upon a mass of 1 kilogram, will impart to it an acceleration of 1 meter per second per second.

N.F. National Formulary, a publication of the American Pharmaceutical Association, revised at 5-year intervals, establishing official standards for therapeutically useful drugs.

N.F.L.P.N. National Federation of Licensed Practical Nurses.

ng. nanogram.

N.H.L.I. National Heart and Lung Institute.

N.H.M.R.C. National Health and Medical Research Council.

Ni chemical symbol, *nickel.*

niacin (ni′ah-sin) the antipellagra vitamin, a vitamin of the B complex. It is a constituent of several different foods, especially liver, yeast, bran, peanuts, lean meats, fish and poultry. A well balanced diet usually supplies more than the daily requirement. Niacinamide, a related compound, is usually used as the vitamin supplement, because niacin produces peripheral vasodilation with flushing of the skin. These effects are useful in some conditions, however, and niacin is used to improve peripheral circulation in MENIÈRE′S DISEASE, MIGRAINE and peripheral vascular disease. It is also used to depress the blood cholesterol level.

niacinamide (ni″ah-sin-am′īd) a white, crystalline powder, the amide of niacin; used in prophylaxis and treatment of pellagra.

NIAID National Institute of Allergy and Infectious Diseases.

nialamide (ni-al′ah-mīd) a compound with antidepressant action, used in psychoses.

NIAMD National Institute of Arthritis and Metabolic Diseases.

Niamid (ni′ah-mid) trademark for a preparation of nialamide, an antidepressant.

niche (nich) a small recess, depression or indentation, especially a recess in the wall of a hollow organ that tends to retain contrast media, as revealed by roentgenography.

NICHHD National Institute of Child Health and Human Development.

nickel (nik′el) a chemical element, atomic number 28, atomic weight 58.71, symbol Ni. (See table of ELEMENTS.)

Nicolas-Favre disease (ne-ko-lah′ fav′r) lymphogranuloma venereum.

Niconyl (ni′ko-nil) trademark for a preparation of isoniazid, used in the treatment of tuberculosis.

nicotinamide (nik″o-tin′ah-mīd) niacinamide.

nicotine (nik′o-tēn, nik′o-tin) an alkaloid that in its pure state is a colorless, pungent, oily and highly poisonous liquid, having an acrid burning taste. It is a constituent of tobacco. In water solution, it is sometimes used as an insecticide and plant spray.

Although nicotine is highly toxic, the amount inhaled while smoking tobacco is too small to cause death. The nicotine in tobacco can, however, cause indigestion and increase in blood pressure, and dull the appetite. It also acts as a vasoconstrictor. Medical authorities link SMOKING with heart disease, lung cancer and other diseases.

nicotinic acid (nik″o-tin′ik) niacin, the antipellagra factor of the vitamin B complex.

nicotinism (nik′o-tin-izm″) poisoning by tobacco or by nicotine.

nicoumalone (ni-koo′mah-lōn) acenocoumarol, an anticoagulant.

nictitation (nik″tĭ-ta′shun) the act of winking.

nidation (ni-da′shun) implantation of the fertilized ovum (zygote) in the endometrium of the uterus in pregnancy.

NIDR National Institute of Dental Research.

nidus (ni'dus), pl. *ni'di* [L.] a nest; point of origin or focus of a morbid process.

Niemann-Pick disease (ne'man pik) a fatal heredofamilial disease with massive enlargement of the liver and spleen, brownish yellow discoloration of the skin and nervous system dysfunction. Foamy reticular cells containing phospholipids infiltrate the liver, spleen, lungs, lymph nodes and bone marrow. It is rare and occurs chiefly in Jewish children.

nifuroxime (ni"fūr-ok'sim) a white to yellow crystalline powder used as a local antibacterial and antiprotozoan agent.

night blindness inability or a reduced ability to see in dim light. In night blindness, the eyes not only see more poorly in dim light, but are slower to adjust from brightness to dimness.

Depending on its brightness, light is perceived by either of two sets of visual cells located in the retina of the eye. One set, the cones, perceive bright light primarily; the other set, the rods, perceive dim light primarily. Dim light produces a change in a pigment called rhodopsin in the rods. This change causes nerve impulses to travel to the brain, where they register as visual impressions. Night blindness occurs when the rods lack rhodopsin.

One cause of night blindness is a deficiency of vitamin A – the primary source of rhodopsin. The defect in vision usually can be cured by proper diet plus therapeutic doses of the deficient vitamin.

In the elderly, there is sometimes a diminution of rhodopsin, with resulting night blindness. Other losses in vision may follow. Diminished blood supply to the eyes is thought to be a cause of this form of the condition. Treatment generally is only of limited effectiveness.

Night blindness sometimes accompanies glaucoma.

Nightingale (nīt'in-gāl") Florence (1820–1910). Founder of modern nursing. Born in Florence, Italy, of wealthy English parents, Miss Nightingale in 1854 led a group of nurses to the Crimea to care for English troops, and proceeded to reorganize military nursing and sanitation in England and later in India. She contributed to the field of dietetics, and her skill as a statistician in gathering data won her election to the Royal Statistical Society and honorary membership in the American Statistical Association.

Nightingale Pledge an oath frequently taken by nurses at capping ceremonies or upon graduation from a school of nursing. It was written in 1893 by a committee of which Mrs. Lystra E. Gretter was chairman and was first administered to the 1893 graduating class of the Farrand Training School, Harper Hospital, Detroit, Michigan. It is as follows:

I solemnly pledge myself before God and in the presence of this assembly:

To pass my life in purity and to practice my profession faithfully.

I will abstain from whatever is deleterious and mischievous, and will not take or knowingly administer any harmful drug.

I will do all in my power to elevate the standard of my profession, and will hold in confidence all personal matters committed to my keeping and all family affairs coming to my knowledge in the practice of my profession.

With loyalty will I endeavor to aid the physician in his work, and devote myself to the welfare of those committed to my care.

nightmare (nīt'mār) a frightening dream, especially one that is so terrifying or disturbing that it causes the sleeper to wake up.

nightshade (nīt'shād) a plant of the genus Solanum.

   deadly n., belladonna leaf.

NIGMS National Institute of General Medical Sciences.

nigra (ni'grah) [L. black] substantia nigra. adj., ni'gral.

nigrities (ni-grish'e-ēz) blackness.

   n. lin'guae, black tongue.

N.I.H. National Institutes of Health.

nihilism (ni'ĕ-lizm) 1. a doctrine of meaninglessness or nothingness. 2. a delusion of nonexistence of the self or part of the self.

nikethamide (nĭ-keth'ah-mīd) clear colorless to yellowish crystals; a central nervous system stimulant used in circulatory and respiratory failure.

Nikolsky's sign (nĭ-kol'skēz) a condition in which the outer layer of the skin is easily rubbed off by slight injury.

Nilevar (ni'le-var) trademark for preparations of norethandrolone, a synthetic androgen.

NIMH National Institute of Mental Health.

NINDB National Institute of Neurological Diseases and Blindness.

ninhydrin (nin-hi'drin) a chemical compound used as a test for amino acids.

niobium (ni-o'be-um) a chemical element, atomic number 1, atomic weight 92.906, symbol Nb. (See table of ELEMENTS.)

Nionate (ni'o-nāt) trademark for a preparation of ferrous gluconate, a hematinic.

niperyt (ni'per-it) pentaerythritol tetranitrate, a vasodilator used in the treatment of angina pectoris.

niphablepsia (nif"ah-blep'se-ah) snow blindness.

nipple (nip'l) a round or cone-shaped projection at the tip of each breast, or a similarly shaped structure. The nipples are located slightly to the side rather than in the middle of the breasts. Usually, the size of the nipple is in proportion to the size of the breast, but large nipples may be found on small breasts and vice versa. In men, the nipple is smaller than in women.

Surrounding the nipple is a pigmented area called the areola. The color of the areola varies with the complexion. In childless women, it is usually reddish. During pregnancy it increases in size and darkens in color, becoming almost black in brunettes. The color fades after the milk-producing period ends.

The tip of the female nipple contains tiny depressions that are openings of the lactiferous ducts. During pregnancy special care should be given the nipples. Any secretion that accumulates should be gently washed off. If the nipples are tender, the physician will advise the use of cold cream, cocoa butter, lanolin or another emollient to increase their pliability.

If nipples are inverted, a woman may make them protrude by gently pressing with the fingers while applying cream or oil. It may be necessary to use a breast pump to evert the nipples.

Paget's disease of the breast, a rare type of breast cancer, causes ulceration and itching of the nipple. It should be treated immediately.

Nisentil (ni'sen-til) trademark for a preparation of alphaprodine, a synthetic narcotic and analgesic.

Nissl bodies (nis'l) large granular protein bodies that stain with basic dyes, forming the substance of the reticulum of the cytoplasm of a nerve cell. Ribonucleoprotein is one of the main constituents.

Nisulfazole (ni-sul'fah-zōl) trademark for a preparation of para-nitrosulfathiazole, a sulfonamide.

nit (nit) the egg of a louse.

nitavirus (ni″tah-vi'rus) a minute infectious agent probably consisting of deoxyribonucleic acid and generally associated with an eosinophilic body occupying most of the central area of the affected cell.

niter (ni'ter) potassium nitrate.

niton (ni'ton) radon.

Nitranitol (ni'trah-ni″tol) trademark for preparations of mannitol hexanitrate, a vasodilator.

nitrate (ni'trāt) a salt of nitric acid.

nitre (ni'ter) potassium nitrate.

nitremia (ni-tre'me-ah) excess of nitrogen in the blood.

Nitretamin (ni-tre'tah-min) trademark for preparations of trolnitrate, a vasodilator.

nitric (ni'trik) pertaining to or containing nitrogen in one of its higher valences.

n. acid, a highly caustic, fuming acid sometimes used in the immediate treatment of animal bites to prevent rabies, and as a cauterizing agent in the eradication of various kinds of warts. It can be fatal if swallowed, and large amounts of nitric acid applied to the skin can cause necrosis. The antidote for nitric acid poisoning is an alkali or sodium bicarbonate applied liberally.

nitrification (ni″tri-fi-ka'shun) the bacterial oxidation of ammonia and organic nitrogen to nitrites and nitrates.

nitrile (ni'trīl) a compound containing the monovalent −CN radical.

nitrite (ni'trīt) a salt of nitrous acid. Nitrites are used as antispasmodics and arterial vasodilators.

Nitrobacter (ni″tro-bak'ter) a genus of Schizomycetes containing microorganisms that oxidize nitrites to nitrates.

Nitrobacteraceae (ni″tro-bak″te-ra'se-e) a family of Schizomycetes known informally as the nitrifying bacteria.

nitrobacteria (ni″tro-bak-te're-ah) bacteria capable of oxidizing ammonia into nitrogen acids.

nitrocellulose (ni″tro-sel'u-lōs) pyroxylin, a base that is dissolved in alcohol or ether to form collodion.

Nitrocystis (ni″tro-sis'tis) a genus of Schizomycetes that oxidize nitrites to nitrates.

nitrofurantoin (ni″tro-fu-ran'to-in) an antibacterial agent used in treatment of urinary tract infections.

nitrofurazone (ni″tro-fu'rah-zōn) an odorless, lemon-yellow, crystalline powder used as a local antibacterial agent.

nitrogen (ni'tro-jen) a chemical element, atomic number 7, atomic weight 14.007, symbol N. (See table of ELEMENTS.) It is a gas constituting about four-fifths of common air; chemically it is almost inert.

amide n., amino n., that portion of the nitrogen in protein that exists in the form of acid amides.

n. balance, the state of the body in regard to ingestion and excretion of nitrogen. In negative nitrogen balance the amount of nitrogen excreted is greater than the quantity ingested; in positive nitrogen balance the amount excreted is smaller than the amount ingested.

n. cycle, the steps by which nitrogen is extracted from the nitrates of soil and water, incorporated as amino acids and proteins in the body of living organisms and ultimately reconverted to nitrates.

n. monoxide nitrous oxide, an anesthetic.

n. mustards, a group of toxic, blistering alkylating agents, including nitrogen mustard itself (mechlorethamine hydrochloride) and related compounds; used to destroy diseased tissue in certain forms of cancer. Nitrogen mustards do not cure these conditions, but ease their effects by destroying mitotic cells — those newly formed by division — thereby affecting malignant tissue in its early stage of development, and leaving normal tissue unaffected. They are especially useful in the treatment of leukemia, in which they reduce the leukocyte count, and in cases in which the malignant disease is widespread throughout the body and therefore cannot be effectively treated locally by surgery or radiotherapy. In cases of lung cancer, mechlorethamine hydrochloride is usually injected directly into the lungs via the pulmonary circulation. Side effects, which tend to limit the usefulness of these drugs, include nausea, vomiting and a decrease in bone marrow production.

nonprotein n., NPN, the nitrogenous constituents of the blood exclusive of the protein bodies, consisting of the nitrogen of urea, uric acid, creatine, creatinine, amino acids, polypeptides and an undetermined part known as rest nitrogen.

Measurement of nonprotein nitrogen is used as a test of renal function. Normally nonprotein nitrogen substances are excreted by the kidneys as end products of protein metabolism; their accumulation in the blood may indicate kidney disease, urinary retention, decrease in urinary output or circulatory disease that impairs the supply of blood to the kidneys. The normal range for nonprotein nitrogen is 15 to 35 mg. per 100 ml. of blood. No special preparation is necessary for this test.

nitrogenous (ni-troj'ĕ-nus) containing nitrogen.

nitroglycerin (ni″tro-glis'er-in) a chemical well known as an explosive but also possessing medical uses; called also glyceryl trinitrate.

Nitroglycerin is a vasodilator and is used medically to relieve certain types of pain, especially in cases of ANGINA PECTORIS. Generally the nitroglycerin tablet is placed under the tongue when the attack occurs; it quickly dissolves and gives relief within 1 or 2 minutes. It may cause transient palpitation, flushing, faintness and perhaps headache.

Since nitroglycerin reduces blood pressure, it can be dangerous if used when a patient is already in a state of shock.

Nitroglyn (ni′tro-glin) trademark for a preparation of glyceryl trinitrate (nitroglycerin), a vasodilator.

Nitrol (ni′trol) trademark for preparations of glyceryl trinitrate (nitroglycerin), a vasodilator.

nitromannite (ni″tro-man′ĭt) mannitol hexanitrate, a vasodilator.

nitromersol (ni″tro-mer′sol) brownish yellow to yellow granules or powder used as a local antibacterial.

nitrosification (ni-tro″sĭ-fĭ-ka′shun) the oxidation of ammonia into nitrites.

nitrosobacterium (ni-tro″so-bak-te′re-um), pl. *nitrosobacte′ria* [L.] a microorganism that oxidizes nitrites to nitrates.

Nitrosococcus (ni″tro-so-kok′us) a genus of Schizomycetes that oxidize ammonia to nitrite.

Nitrosocystis (ni″tro-so-sis′tis) a genus of Schizomycetes that oxidize ammonia to nitrite.

Nitrosogloea (ni″tro-so-gle′ah) a genus of Schizomycetes that oxidize ammonia to nitrite.

Nitrosomonas (ni″tro-so-mo′nas) a genus of Schizomycetes that oxidize ammonia to nitrite.

Nitrosospira (ni″tro-so-spi′rah) a genus of Schizomycetes that oxidize ammonia to nitrite.

nitrous (ni′trus) pertaining to or containing nitrogen in one of its lower valences.
   n. acid, an unstable compound with which free amino groups react to form hydroxyl groups and liberate gaseous nitrogen.
   n. oxide, a colorless gas used by inhalation as a general anesthetic; called also laughing gas. (See also ANESTHETIC.)

Nitrovas (ni′tro-vas) trademark for a preparation of glyceryl trinitrate (nitroglycerin), a vasodilator.

N.L.N. National League for Nursing.

N.M.A. National Medical Association.

N.M.R.I. Naval Medical Research Institute, part of the National Naval Medical Center.

nn. [L. pl.] *ner′vi* (nerves).

N.N.D. New and Nonofficial Drugs, a former publication of the American Medical Association, listing and describing drugs evaluated by the Council on Pharmacy and Chemistry.

No chemical symbol, *nobelium.*

nobelium (no-be′le-um) a chemical element, atomic number 102, atomic weight 253, symbol No. (See table of ELEMENTS.)

Nocardia (no-kar′de-ah) a genus of microorganisms of the family Actinomycetaceae; pathogenic species are *N. asteroi′des, N. farci′nica, N. madu′rae* and *N. tenu′is.*

noci- (no′se) word element [L.], *harm; injury.*

nociassociation (no″se-ah-so″se-a′shun) unconscious discharge of nervous energy under the stimulus of injury.

nociceptor (no″se-sep′tor) receiving injury; said of a receptive neuron for painful sensations. adj., **nocicep′tive.**

nociperception (no″se-per-sep′shun) the perception of traumatic stimuli.

noctalbuminuria (nok″tal-bu″mĭ-nu′re-ah) excess of albumin in the urine secreted at night.

Noctec (nok′tek) trademark for preparations of chloral hydrate, a hypnotic and sedative.

noctiphobia (nok″tĭ-fo′be-ah) morbid dread of night.

nocturia (nok-tu′re-ah) excessive urination at night.

node (nōd) a swelling, knot or protuberance. adj., **no′dal.**
   n. of Aschoff and Tawara, atrioventricular node.
   atrioventricular n., A-V n., a collection of cardiac muscle fibers at the base of the interatrial septum that transmits the cardiac impulse initiated by the sinoatrial node (see also ATRIOVENTRICULAR NODE).
   Bouchard's n's, nodules on the second joints of the fingers, considered symptomatic of dilatation of the stomach.
   Delphian n., a lymph node encased in the fascia in the midline just above the thyroid isthmus, so called because it is exposed first at operation and, if diseased, is indicative of the condition to be found in the thyroid gland.
   Flack's n., sinoatrial node.
   gouty n., one due to gouty inflammation.
   Haygarth's n's, joint swellings in rheumatoid arthritis.
   Heberden's n's, nodular protrusions on the phalanges at the distal interphalangeal joints of the fingers in osteoarthritis.
   Keith's n., Keith-Flack n., sinoatrial node.
   Legendre's n's, Bouchard's nodes.
   lymph n., one of the accumulations of lymphoid tissue organized as lymphatic organs along the course of lymphatic vessels, consisting of an outer cortical and inner medullary part. Lymph nodes filter and destroy invading bacteria and are the site of production of lymphocytes and certain antibodies. The main lymph nodes are in the neck, axillae and groin. Sometimes called, incorrectly, lymph glands.
   Meynet's n's, nodules in the capsules of joints and in tendons in rheumatic conditions, especially in children.
   Osler's n's, small, raised, swollen, tender areas, bluish or sometimes pink or red, occurring commonly in the pads of the fingers or toes, in the thenar or hypothenar eminences or the soles of the

feet; they are practically pathognomonic of sub-acute bacterial endocarditis.

Parrot's n., a syphilitic node on the outer table of the skull.

n's of Ranvier, the periodic interruptions in the myelin sheath of myelinated nerve fibers.

Rotter's n's, lymph nodes occasionally found between the greater and smaller pectoral muscles which often contain metastases from breast cancer.

Schmorl's n., an irregular or hemispherical bone defect in the upper or lower margin of the body of a vertebra into which the nucleus pulposus of the intervertebral disk herniates.

sentinel n., signal n., a firm node just above the left clavicle, behind inserting fibers of the sterno-cleidomastoid muscles, frequently evidencing metastases from a visceral carcinoma.

singer's n., a small, white nodule on the vocal cord; the condition occurs in persons who use their voices excessively.

sinoatrial n., S-A n., a collection of atypical muscle fibers in the wall of the right atrium where the rhythm of cardiac contraction is usually established; therefore also referred to as the pacemaker of the heart.

syphilitic n., a swelling on a bone due to syphilitic periostitis.

n. of Tawara, atrioventricular node.

teacher's n., singer's node.

Troisier's n., Virchow's n., sentinel node.

vital n., the respiratory center.

nodose (no'dōs) having nodes or projections.

nodosity (no-dos'ĭ-te) 1. a node. 2. the quality of being nodose.

nodular (nod'u-lar) marked with, or resembling, nodules.

nodule (nod'ūl) a small boss or node that is solid and can be detected by touch.

Albini's n's, gray nodules sometimes seen on the free edges of the mitral and tricuspid valves of infants; they are remains of fetal structures.

apple jelly n's, cutaneous nodules of apple-jelly color in lupus vulgaris.

Aschoff's n's, Aschoff's bodies.

Gamna n's, brown or yellow pigmented nodules seen in the spleen in certain cases of enlargement.

Jeanselme's n's, juxta-articular n's, nodules on the limbs near the joints due to treponemal infection.

Koster's n., a tubercle composed of one giant cell enclosed by a double layer of cells.

Leishman's n's, the pinkish nodules seen in the nonulcerative keloid-like type of cutaneous leishmaniasis.

lymphatic n's, a term applied to lymph nodes, as well as to one of the small collections of lymphoid tissue situated deep to epithelial surfaces, and also to temporary small accumulations of lymphocytes in the cortex of a lymph node.

rheumatic n's, small, mostly subcutaneous nodules made up of a mass of Aschoff bodies and seen in rheumatic fever.

typhus n's, minute skin nodules formed by perivascular infiltration of mononuclear cells in typhus.

nodulus (nod'u-lus), pl. nod'uli [L.] nodule.

nodus (no'dus), pl. no'di [L.] node.

Noguchi's reaction (no-goo'chēz) a modification of the Wassermann test for syphilis.

Noguchia (no-goo'che-ah) a genus of Schizomycetes found in the conjunctiva of man and animals having a follicular disease.

Noludar (nol'u-dar) trademark for preparations of methyprylon, a sedative and hypnotic.

noma (no'mah) a rare acute gangrenous disease starting in the oral mucous membrane, penetrating underlying tissue and perforating the skin.

n. puden'di, n. vul'vae, destructive ulceration of the external genitalia in the female.

nomen (no'men), pl. no'mina [L.] name.

No'mina Anatom'ica, the official body of anatomic nomenclature; abbreviated NA.

nomenclature (no'men-kla″tūr) terminology; a classified system of technical terms.

anatomic n., a scheme presenting the names of all the structures of the body.

binomial n., the system of designating plants and animals by two latinized words designating the genus and species.

taxonomic n., a scheme presenting the names of categories, or taxa, into which living organisms are grouped.

nomogram (nom'o-gram) the graphic representation produced in nomography; a chart or diagram on which a number of variables are plotted, forming a computation chart for the solution of complex numerical formulae.

nomography (no-mog'rah-fe) a graphic method of representing the relation between any number of variables.

nonan (no'nan) recurring on the ninth day (every eight days).

nonapeptide (non″ah-pep'tīd) a peptide containing nine amino acids.

non compos mentis (non kom'pos men'tis) [L.] not of sound mind.

nonconductor (non″kon-duk'tor) a substance that does not readily transmit electricity, light or heat.

nondisjunction (non″dis-jungk'shun) failure of a pair of chromosomes to separate during meiosis, so that both members of the pair are carried to the same daughter nucleus, and the other daughter cell lacks that chromosome.

nonelectrolyte (non″e-lek'tro-līt) a compound which, dissolved in water, does not separate into charged particles and is incapable of conducting an electric current.

nonphotochromogen (non″fo-to-kro'mo-jen) a microorganism that is not conspicuously affected in color by exposure to light; specifically, a member of the anonymous mycobacteria.

nonprotein nitrogen (non-pro'te-in) NPN; the nitrogenous constituents of the blood exclusive of the protein bodies; measurement of NPN is used as a test of renal function. (See also under NITROGEN.)

nonsecretor (non″se-kre'tor) a person with A or B

type blood whose body secretions do not contain the particular (A or B) substance.

nontaster (non-tās'ter) a person unable to taste a particular substance, such as phenylthiocarbamide, which is used in certain genetic studies.

nonunion (non-ūn'yun) failure of the ends of a fractured bone to unite.

nonviable (non-vi'ah-bl) not capable of living.

noopsyche (no'o-si"ke) the intellectual processes of the mind.

noothymopsychic (no"o-thi"mo-si'kik) pertaining to intellectual and affective processes of the mind.

noradrenaline (nor"ah-dren'ah-lin) norepinephrine.

noramidopyrine (nor-am"ĭ-do-pi'rēn) dipyrone, an analgesic and antipyretic.

nordefrin (nor'dĕ-frin) a compound used as a sympathomimetic agent.

norepinephrine (nor"ep-ĭ-nef'rin) a hormone secreted by the adrenal medulla in response to splanchnic stimulation. It also is formed at the endings of certain nerve fibers of the sympathetic nervous system and takes part in the transmission of impulses from one nerve ending to another. It is prepared synthetically and used as a sympathomimetic and pressor agent, under the name levarterenol.

norethandrolone (nor"eth-an'dro-lōn) a synthetic androgen equal to testosterone in anabolic activity, but having less androgenic activity.

norethindrone (nor-eth'in-drōn) a compound used as a progestational agent.

Norisodrine (nor-i'so-drin) trademark for preparations of isoproterenol, a sympathomimetic, cardiac stimulant and antispasmodic.

Norlutin (nor-lu'tin) trademark for a preparation of norethindrone, a progestational agent.

norm (norm) a fixed or ideal standard.

norm(o)- (nor'mo) word element [L.], *normal; usual; conforming to the rule.*

normal (nor'mal) agreeing with the regular and established type. When said of a solution, it denotes one containing in each liter 1 Gm. equivalent weight of the active substance; designated N/1 or 1 N.

normetanephrine (nor"met-ah-nef'rin) a urinary metabolite of norepinephrine.

normoblast (nor'mo-blast) a late stage in the development of an erythrocyte characterized by a pyknotic nucleus and abundant hemoglobin in the cytoplasm.

   intermediate n., polychromatophilic erythroblast.

normoblastosis (nor"mo-blas-to'sis) excessive production of normoblasts in the bone marrow.

normocalcemia (nor"mo-kal-se'me-ah) a normal level of calcium in the blood.

normocapnia (nor"mo-kap'ne-ah) a normal level of carbon dioxide in the blood.

normochromasia (nor"mo-kro-ma'ze-ah) a normal staining reaction in a cell or tissue.

normochromia (nor"mo-kro'me-ah) normal color of erythrocytes.

normochromocyte (nor"mo-kro'mo-sīt) an erythrocyte having the normal amount of hemoglobin.

normocyte (nor'mo-sīt) an erythrocyte that is normal in size, shape and color.

Normocytin (nor"mo-si'tin) trademark for preparations of concentrated crystalline vitamin B_{12}.

normocytosis (nor"mo-si-to'sis) a normal state of the erythrocytes.

normoglycemia (nor"mo-gli-se'me-ah) normal sugar content of the blood.

normokalemia (nor"mo-kah-le'me-ah) a normal level of potassium in the blood.

normotension (nor"mo-ten'shun) normal tone, tension or pressure.

normotensive (nor"mo-ten'siv) 1. characterized by normal tension or blood pressure. 2. a person with normal blood pressure.

normothermia (nor"mo-ther'me-ah) a normal state of temperature.

normotonia (nor"mo-to'ne-ah) normal tone or tension.

normotopic (nor"mo-top'ik) normally located.

normotrophic (nor"mo-trof'ik) of normal development; not exhibiting either hypertrophy or hypotrophy.

normovolemia (nor"mo-vo-le'me-ah) normal blood volume.

Norodin (nor'o-din) trademark for a preparation of methamphetamine hydrochloride, a central nervous system stimulant.

Norpramin (nor'prah-min) trademark for a preparation of desipramine hydrochloride, an antidepressant.

norsulfazole (nor-sul'fah-zōl) sulfathiazole, a sulfonamide.

nos(o)- (nos'o) word element [Gr.], *disease.*

noscapine (nos'kah-pēn) an alkaloid present in opium; used as a nonaddictive antitussive.

nose (nōz) the specialized structure of the face that serves both as the organ of smell and as a means of bringing air into the lungs. Air breathed in through the nose is warmed and filtered; that breathed through the mouth is not.

   The nostrils, which form the external entrance of the nose, lead into the two nasal cavities, which are separated from each other by a partition (the nasal septum) formed of cartilage and bone. Three bony ridges project from the outer wall of each nasal cavity and partially divide the cavity into three air passages. At the back of the nose these passages lead into the pharynx. The passages also are connected by openings with the paranasal sinuses. One of the functions of the nose is to drain fluids discharged from the sinuses. The nasal cavities also have a connection with the ears by the eustachian tubes, and with the region of the eyes by the naso-lacrimal ducts.

The interior of the nose is lined with *mucous membrane*. Most of this membrane is covered with minute hairlike projections called cilia. Moving in waves these cilia sweep out from the nasal passages the nasal mucus, which may contain pollen, dust and bacteria from the air. The mucous membrane also acts to warm and moisten the inhaled air.

High in the interior of each nasal cavity is a small area of mucous membrane that is not covered with cilia. In this pea-sized area are located the endings of the nerves of smell, the olfactory receptors. These receptors sort out odors. Unlike the taste buds of the tongue, which distinguish between only four different tastes (salt, sweet, sour and bitter), the olfactory receptors can detect innumerable different odors. This ability to smell contributes greatly to what we usually think of as taste, because much of what we consider flavor is really odor. (See also SMELL.)

DISORDERS OF THE NOSE. The mucous membrane of the nose is subject to inflammation; any such inflammation is called RHINITIS, a term derived from the Greek word *rhinos,* meaning nose. Rhinitis is often caused by an infection, as in the COMMON COLD, or by an allergy, particularly HAY FEVER. In both cases the symptoms are similar, including runny eyes, sneezing, a nasal discharge and temporary stopping-up of the nasal passages. In such an infection, the nasal mucus is white or yellow in color.

Nasal polyps may obstruct the nasal passages and limit breathing through the nose. Enlarged adenoids also may interfere with nasal breathing.

Nosebleed may be caused by injury to the nose, or it may be a symptom of various diseases. (See also EPISTAXIS.)

Frequently the nasal septum may grow irregularly or be deflected to one side by an injury. This condition is known as deviated SEPTUM.

nosebleed   (nōz'blēd) bleeding from the nose (called also EPISTAXIS).

FIRST AID FOR NOSEBLEED

1. Have the patient sit up with his head tilted back.
2. Grasp the nose firmly between the thumb and forefinger.
3. If bleeding continues, gently insert small wads of cotton or gauze into the nose, and then press the nostrils firmly together again.
4. If a clot fails to form, apply cold compresses to the nose, lips and back of the neck.
5. If bleeding still persists, consult a physician.

nosocomial   (nos"o-ko'me-al) pertaining to a hospital or infirmary.

nosogeny   (no-soj'ĕ-ne) the development of a disease; pathogenesis.

nosography   (no-sog'rah-fe) a description of diseases.

nosology   (no-sol'o-je) the science of the classification of diseases.

nosomania   (nos"o-ma'ne-ah) the insane belief that one is diseased.

nosomycosis   (nos"o-mi-ko'sis) a disease caused by a parasitic fungus.

nosonomy   (no-son'o-me) the classification of diseases.

nosoparasite   (nos"o-par'ah-sīt) an organism found in a disease that it is able to modify, but not to produce.

nosophilia   (nos"o-fil'e-ah) morbid desire to be sick.

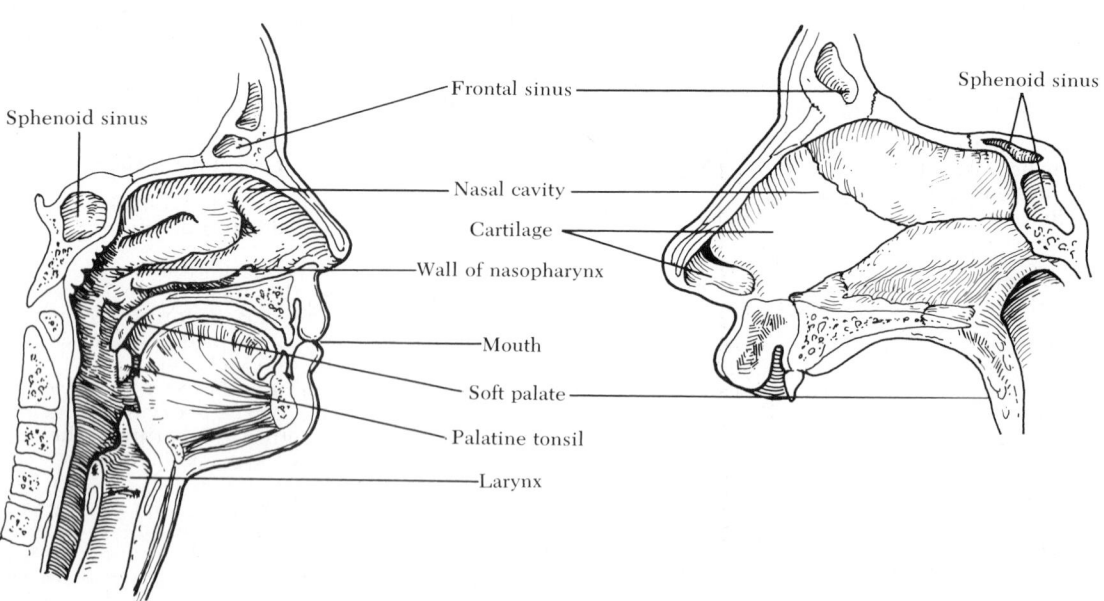

Nose and related structures.

nosophobia (nos″o-fo′be-ah) morbid dread of sickness.

nosopoietic (nos″o-poi-et′ik) causing disease.

Nosopsyllus (nos″o-sil′us) a genus of fleas. N. fascia′tus, the rat flea, a carrier of murine typhus and plague.

nosotaxy (nos′o-tak″se) the classification of disease.

nosotherapy (nos″o-ther′ah-pe) the treatment of one disease by means of another.

nostril (nos′tril) either aperture of the nose.

nostrum (nos′trum) a quack, patent or secret remedy.

Nostyn (nos′tin) trademark for a preparation of ectylurea, a central nervous system depressant.

notal (no′tal) pertaining to the back; dorsal.

notalgia (no-tal′je-ah) pain in the back.

notch (noch) an indentation, especially one on the edge of a bone or other organ.
    aortic n., dicrotic n., the depression on the sphygmogram due to closure of the aortic valves.
    parotid n., the notch between the ramus of the mandible and the mastoid process of the temporal bones.
    preoccipital n., one on the lower edge of the external surface of a cerebral hemisphere, between the occipital and temporal lobes.
    sacrosciatic n., the large notch on the posterior border of the hip bone, where the posterior borders of the ilium and ischium become continuous.
    trigeminal n., one in the superior border of the pars petrosa of the temporal bone, near the apex, for transmission of the trigeminal nerve.

notencephalocele (no″ten-sef′ah-lo-sēl″) hernial protrusion of brain at the back of the head.

notencephalus (no″ten-sef′ah-lus) a fetus affected with notencephalocele.

notifiable (no″tĭ-fi′ah-bl) necessary to be reported to the board of health.

notochord (no′to-kord) a cylindrical cord of cells on the dorsal side of an embryo, marking its longitudinal axis.

noumenal (noo′mĕ-nal) pertaining to pure thought, independent of sensory perception.

Novaldin (no-val′din) trademark for preparations of dipyrone, an analgesia and antipyretic.

novobiocin (no″vo-bi′o-sin) an antibiotic derived from Streptomyces. It should be kept in reserve to be used only when necessary, that is, when resistance to other agents has developed. It is effective against infections caused by penicillin-resistant microorganisms. However, organisms have been able to develop resistance to novobiocin rapidly. Leukopenia has been observed in some patients receiving the drug. Jaundice not uncommonly occurs in infants after novobiocin administration.

Novocaine (no′vo-kān) trademark for preparations of procaine hydrochloride, a local anesthetic.

Novrad (nov′rad) trademark for preparations of levopropoxyphene, used for cough.

noxa (nok′sah) an injurious agent, act or influence.

noxious (nok′shus) hurtful; injurious.

Np chemical symbol, *neptunium*.

NPN nonprotein nitrogen.

N.S.A. Neurosurgical Society of America.

N.S.C.C. National Society for Crippled Children.

N.S.N.A. National Student Nurse Association.

N.S.P.B. National Society for the Prevention of Blindness.

nucha (nu′kah) the nape of the neck.

nuclear (nu′kle-ar) pertaining to a nucleus.

nuclease (nu′kle-ās) an enzyme that decomposes nucleic acids.

nucleated (nu′kle-āt″ed) having a nucleus or nuclei.

nucleic acids (nu-kle′ik) substances found in the cells of all living tissue. They are extremely complex and of high molecular weight, containing phosphoric acid, sugars, and purine and pyrimidine bases. Two pentose sugars are involved as constituents of the nucleic acids: ribose and deoxyribose. Thus are derived the names of the nucleic acids RIBONUCLEIC ACID (RNA) and DEOXYRIBONUCLEIC ACID (DNA).
    The nucleic acids and their derivatives are of great importance in metabolism, and though all of their functions are not yet completely understood, they appear to be concerned with controlling the general pattern of metabolism and acting as catalysts in many chemical reactions within the cell. The synthesis of proteins necessary for growth and development is affected by the nucleic acids, as are the intermediate steps in the metabolism of other foodstuffs.
    The nucleic acids are also of great biologic significance. For example, DNA and RNA are the chemical repositories of genetic information and therefore affect the transmission of individual characteristics and functions from cell to cell and also from individual persons to their offspring.

nuclein (nu′kle-in) a decomposition product of nucleoprotein consisting of nucleic acids and bases.

nucleofugal (nu″kle-of′u-gal) moving away from a nucleus.

nucleohistone (nu″kle-o-his′tōn) a complex nucleoprotein made up of deoxyribonucleic acid and a histone, found in the nucleus of various cells.

nucleolonema (nu″kle-o″lo-ne′mah) a threadlike element appearing as a tangled skein within the nucleolus of a cell.

nucleolus (nu-kle′o-lus), pl. *nucle′oli* [L.] a rounded, basophilic body, rich in ribonucleic acid, within the nucleus of a cell.

nucleolymph (nu′kle-o-limf″) karyolymph; the fluid part of a cell nucleus, in which the other elements are dispersed.

nucleomitophobia (nu″kle-o-mi″to-fo′be-ah) morbid fear of an atomic explosion.

nucleon (nu′kle-on) a particle of an atomic nucleus; a proton or neutron, the total number of which constitutes the mass number of the isotope.

nucleonics (nu″kle-on′iks) the study of nucleons or of atomic nuclei, especially their practical applications.

nucleopetal (nu″kle-op′ĕ-tal) moving toward a nucleus.

nucleophilic (nu″kle-o-fil′ik) having an affinity for nuclei.

nucleoplasm (nu′kle-o-plazm″) karyoplasm; the protoplasm of the nucleus of a cell.

nucleoprotein (nu″kle-o-pro′te-in) one of a class of conjugated proteins, consisting of nucleic acids and simple proteins.

nucleosidase (nu″kle-o-si′dās) an intracellular enzyme that is capable of causing the decomposition of nucleosides.

nucleoside (nu′kle-o-sīd″) one of a class of compounds produced by hydrolysis of nucleotides, consisting of a sugar (a pentose or a hexose) and a purine or pyrimidine base.

nucleotide (nu′kle-o-tīd″) one of a group of compounds obtained by hydrolysis of nucleic acids, consisting of purine or pyrimidine bases linked to sugars, which in turn are esterified with phosphoric acid.

diphosphopyridine n., a coenzyme widely distributed in nature and involved in many enzymatic reactions.

triphosphopyridine n., a coenzyme similar to diphosphopyridine nucleotide, but involved in a smaller number of reactions.

nucleotoxin (nu″kle-o-tok′sin) a toxin from cell nuclei, or one that affects cell nuclei.

nucleus (nu′kle-us), pl. *nu′clei* [L.] 1. a spheroid body within a cell. The nucleus contains large quantities of DEOXYRIBONUCLEIC ACID (DNA), a nucleic acid that controls the synthesis of protein enzymes of the cytoplasm and also cellular reproduction. Because of its DNA content the nucleus is considered to be the control center of the cell. 2. a mass of gray matter in the central nervous system, especially such a mass marking the central termination of a cranial nerve. 3. in chemistry, the dense core of an atom. It has two major components: protons and neutrons. Traveling in orbit around the nucleus is a cloud of negatively charged particles called ELECTRONS. The number of protons in the atomic nucleus gives a substance its identity as a particular ELEMENT. adj., **nu′clear.**

n. ambig′uus, the nucleus of the glossopharyngeal, vagus and accessory nerves in the medulla oblongata.

basal nuclei, basal ganglia.

caudate n., n. cauda′tus, a long, horseshoe-shaped mass of gray matter that forms part of the corpus striatum and is closely related to the lateral ventricle of the brain.

cochlear nuclei, dorsal and ventral, the nuclei of termination of the sensory fibers of the eighth cranial (vestibulocochlear) nerve; located at the junction of the medulla oblongata and the pons.

conjugation n., fertilization nucleus.

dentate n., n. denta′tus, a crumpled mass of gray matter in each cerebellar hemisphere.

diploid n., a cell nucleus containing the number of chromosomes typical of the somatic cells of the particular species.

n. fasti′gii, a flat mass of gray matter in the cerebellum, over the roof of the fourth ventricle.

fertilization n., one produced by fusion of the male and female pronuclei in the fertilized ovum.

free n., a cell nucleus from which the other elements of the cell have disappeared.

germ n., germinal n., pronucleus.

gonad n., the reproductive nucleus of a cell.

gray n., gray matter of the spinal cord.

haploid n., a cell nucleus containing half of the number of chromosomes typical of the somatic cells of a particular species.

intraventricular n., caudate nucleus.

large cell n., nucleus ambiguus.

laryngeal n., the nucleus of origin of nerve fibers to the larynx.

lenticular n., lentiform n., the part of the corpus striatum comprising the putamen and globus pallidus.

motor n., any collection of cells in the central nervous system giving origin to a motor nerve.

nerve n., a collection of cells in the nervous system directly related to a peripheral nerve.

n. oliva′ris, olivary n., a folded band of gray matter enclosing a white core and producing the elevation on the medulla oblongata known as the olive.

n. of origin, any collection of nerve cells giving origin to the fibers, or a part of the fibers, of a peripheral nerve.

paraventricular n. of hypothalamus, a group of nerve cell bodies in the anterior part of the hypothalamus, a source of the posterior pituitary hormones.

polymorphic n., a cell nucleus that assumes an irregular form or splits up into lobes.

n. pulpo′sus, the pulpy mass in the center of an intervertebral disk.

red n., nucleus ruber.

reproductive n., micronucleus.

ring nuclei, ringed nuclei, ringlike nuclei in the polymorphonuclear leukocytes in the stools of patients with bacillary dysentery.

n. ru′ber, an oval mass of gray matter in the anterior part of the tegmentum and extending into the posterior part of the hypothalamus; it receives fibers from the cerebellum.

sacral n., a mass of gray matter in the spinal cord opposite the site of origin of the second and third sacral nerves.

segmentation n., the fertilization nucleus after cleavage has begun.

sensory n., the nucleus of termination of the afferent (sensory) fibers of a peripheral nerve.

sperm n., the male pronucleus.

striate n., corpus striatum.

supraoptic n. of hypothalamus, a group of closely packed nerve cell bodies overlying the beginning of the optic tract, a source of the posterior pituitary hormones.

tegmental n., 1. nucleus fastigii. 2. nucleus ruber.

vesicular n., a cell nucleus with a visible nuclear membrane and chromatin material usually lightly diffused throughout the karyolymph.

vestibular n., the four cellular masses in the floor

of the fourth ventricle, in which the branches of the eighth cranial (vestibulocochlear) nerve terminate.

yolk n., the area of the cytoplasm of an ovum in which the synthetic activities leading to the accumulation of food supplies in the oocyte are initiated.

zygote n., fertilization nucleus.

nuclide (nu′klīd) any atomic configuration capable of existing for a measurable lifetime, usually more than 10^{-9} seconds.

nudomania (nu″do-ma′ne-ah) a morbid desire to be nude.

nudophobia (nu″do-fo′be-ah) a morbid dread of being nude.

nullipara (nu-lip′ah-rah) a woman who has not produced a viable offspring; para 0. adj., **nullip′- arous.**

nulliparity (nul″ĭ-par′ĭ-te) the state of being a nullipara.

number (num′ber) a symbol, as a figure or word, expressive of a certain value or a specified quantity.

atomic n., a number expressive of the number of protons in an atomic nucleus, or the positive charge of the nucleus expressed in terms of the electronic charge.

Avogadro's n., the number of particles of the type specified by the chemical formula of a certain substance in 1 gram-molecule of the substance.

mass n., the number expressive of the mass of a nucleus, being the total number of nucleons — protons and neutrons — in the nucleus of an atom or nuclide.

numbness (num′nes) a paresthesia of touch insensibility in a part.

nummular (num′u-lar) 1. coin shaped. 2. arranged like a stack of coins.

Numorphan (nu-mor′fan) trademark for preparations of oxymorphone hydrochloride, a narcotic analgesic.

Nupercaine (nu′per-kān) trademark for preparations of dibucaine, a local and spinal anesthetic.

nurse (ners) 1. a person who makes a profession of caring for the sick, disabled or enfeebled, or of aiding in the maintenance of a state of health (see also NURSING PRACTICE). 2. to care for a sick or disabled person or to aid in the maintenance of health. 3. to nourish at the breast (see also BREAST FEEDING).

community health n., one whose work combines elements of both nursing and public health practice and takes place primarily outside the therapeutic institution (see also PUBLIC HEALTH NURSING).

licensed practical n., one who is licensed to perform for compensation selected acts in the care of the ill, injured or infirm under the direction of a registered professional nurse or a licensed physician or a licensed dentist, and not requiring the substantial specialized skill, judgment and knowledge required in professional nursing.

public health n., a professional title being replaced in the United States by community health nurse (see also PUBLIC HEALTH NURSING).

registered n., a graduate nurse registered and licensed to practice by a State Board of Nurse Examiners or other state authority.

nursery (ner′sĕ-re) the department in a hospital where newborn infants are cared for.

nursing (ners′ing) the profession of performing the functions of a NURSE.

n. history, a written record providing data for assessing the nursing care needs of a patient.

n. practice, the performance for compensation of any act in the observation, care and counsel of the ill, injured or infirm, or in the maintenance of health or prevention of illness of others, or in the supervision and teaching of other personnel, or in the administration of medications and treatments as prescribed by a licensed physician or dentist, requiring substantial specialized judgment and skill and based on knowledge and application of the principles of biologic, physical and social sciences.

n. process, the series of operations constituting nursing care, usually conceptualized in three phases: assessment, intervention and evaluation. Additional components often designated are observation, inference and validation.

nutation (nu-ta′shun) nodding.

nutrient (nu′tre-ent) 1. nourishing; aiding nutrition. 2. a nourishing substance, or food.

nutriment (nu′trĭ-ment) nourishment; nutritious material.

nutriology (nu″tre-ol′o-je) the study of foods and their use in diet and therapy.

nutrition (nu-trish′un) the nourishment of the body by food. adj., **nutrit′ional, nu′tritive.** It includes all the processes by which the body uses food for energy, maintenance and growth. Nutrition is particularly concerned with those properties of food that build sound bodies and promote health. In this sense, good nutrition means a balanced diet containing adequate amounts of the essential nutritional elements that the body must have to function normally.

THE BALANCED DIET. To form the foundation for a good diet the Institute of Home Economics, United States Department of Agriculture, recommends the Basic Four Food Groups.

The essential ingredients of a balanced diet are proteins, vitamins, minerals, fats and carbohydrates. The body can manufacture sugars from fats, and fats from sugars and proteins, depending on the need. But it cannot manufacture proteins from sugars and fats.

The most important constituents of proteins are the AMINO ACIDS. These complex organic compounds of nitrogen play a vital role in nutrition. The best sources of complete proteins — that is, proteins containing all the essential amino acids — are meat, fish, eggs and dairy products. The amount of protein that a person actually needs, however, is much smaller than many people suppose.

Vitamins are special substances that are present, in varying amounts, in all food. Their absence from the diet can cause such diseases as beriberi (lack of vitamin B_1, or thiamine), pellagra (lack of the B vitamin niacin) and scurvy (lack of vitamin C, or ascorbic acid). (See also VITAMINS.)

The principal minerals needed by the body are calcium and phosphorus (to build bones and teeth) and iron (to assure a sufficient supply of erythrocytes). All three are plentiful in eggs, dairy products, lean meat and enriched flour. Some sources of calcium are American cheese, Swiss cheese, molasses, turnip tops and dandelion greens; of phosphorus, cereals, meat and fish; of iron, kidney beans, navy beans, liver and other meats, beet greens, spinach and whole-wheat bread.

The trace of iodine needed to prevent goiter is easily provided by iodized table salt. The minute amounts of magnesium, manganese and copper that are necessary are found in any balanced diet.

For quick energy, the body should have sugars (carbohydrates) and starches (which the body converts into sugars). Fats and proteins can also provide energy and can be stored for future use, whereas sugars and starches cannot. Since the body can manufacture most of its own fat, fats are of secondary importance in a balanced diet.

AGE AND NUTRITION.   Because the body's needs change as it grows and develops, good nutrition for a child or teenager is not the same as good nutrition for a mature or older person. Growing bodies need plentiful supplies of calcium, phosphorus and other minerals to build strong bones and teeth, and abundant protein for firm muscles, energy and stamina.

For children especially, breakfast is the key meal of the day. Expending as much energy as they do, children need a hearty morning meal, rich in vitamin C, calcium, iron and thiamine, in order to offset the physical and mental fatigue that they usually feel before lunch time.

SPACING AND SERVING OF MEALS.   Nutritionists generally consider breakfast the most important meal of the day because it ends the body's overnight fast and supplies the "fuel" for a person to get under way at top efficiency. If possible, meals should be spaced at regular intervals. They should never be rushed. This is especially true of the main daily meal.

nutritious   (nu-trish'us) affording nourishment.

nutriture   (nu'trĭ-tūr) the status of the body in relation to nutrition.

Nutting   (nut'ing) M. Adelaide (1858–1948). A pioneer in establishing the foundations on which

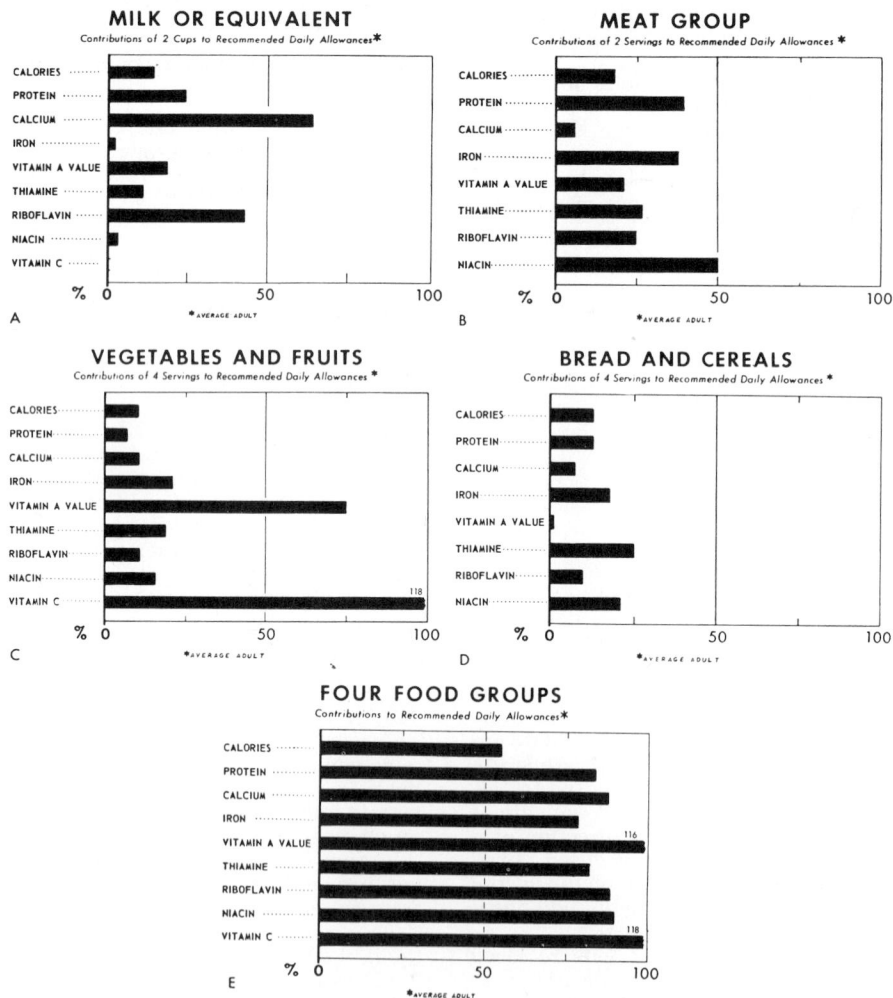

Nutrients provided by four food groups, taken singly (A, B, C, D) and together (E). The equivalent of milk is cheese or ice cream; the equivalent of meat is fish, poultry, eggs, dry beans and peas, or nuts. The vegetables are dark green and deep yellow; the fruits are citrus; the cereals and bread are whole grain, enriched, restored. (From Essentials of an Adequate Diet. Washington, D.C., U.S. Department of Agriculture, 1957.)

nursing as a modern profession rests. She was in the first graduating class at Johns Hopkins Hospital School of Nursing and eventually became Superintendent of Nurses and Principal of the School of Nursing. At Johns Hopkins Miss Nutting instituted many reforms and advances in nursing education. She eliminated the 12-hour-duty day, abolished the monthly stipend for students and instituted a 3-year course. Her purposes in instigating these changes were to release the student from financial obligation to the hospital so that exploitation of the student as a source of cheap labor could be abolished, and to provide the student with more time for study and learning.

nux (nuks) [L.] nut.
   n. vom'ica, the dried ripe seed of *Strychnos nux-vomica;* used as a tincture, extract or fluidextract for its bitter tonic properties.

nyctalgia (nik-tal'je-ah) pain that occurs only in sleep.

nyctalope (nik'tal-lōp) a person affected with nyctalopia.

nyctalopia (nik"tah-lo'pe-ah) night blindness.

nycterine (nik'ter-in) occurring at night.

nyctohemeral (nik"to-hem'er-al) pertaining to both day and night.

nyctophilia (nik"to-fil'e-ah) a preference for darkness or for night.

nyctophobia (nik"to-fo'be-ah) morbid dread of darkness.

nyctophonia (nik"to-fo'ne-ah) loss of voice during the day.

nyctotyphlosis (nik"to-tif-lo'sis) night blindness.

Nydrazid (ni'drah-zid) trademark for preparations of isoniazid, used in treatment of tuberculosis.

nylidrin (nil'ĭ-drin) a compound used as a peripheral vasodilator.

nympha (nim'fah), pl. *nym'phae* [L.] labium minus.

nymphectomy (nim-fek'to-me) excision of the nymphae.

nymphitis (nim-fi'tis) inflammation of a nympha.

nymphomania (nim"fo-ma'ne-ah) excessive sexual desire in a woman, which may lead to promiscuous sexual behavior. This form of sexual deviation is usually the result of a psychologic inability to achieve sexual satisfaction. Since the condition originates in emotional rather than physical disturbance, it is the underlying emotional problem that should be treated.

nymphoncus (nim-fong'kus) swelling or enlargement of the nymphae.

nymphotomy (nim-fot'o-me) surgical incision of the nymphae or clitoris.

nystagmiform (nis-tag'mĭ-form) resembling nystagmus.

nystagmograph (nis-tag'mo-graf) an instrument for recording the movements of the eyeball in nystagmus.

nystagmoid (nis-tag'moid) resembling nystagmus.

nystagmus (nis-tag'mus) involuntary rhythmic oscillation of the eyball, either horizontal, vertical or rotatory. adj., **nystag'mic.**
   aural n., a form due to labyrinthine disturbance.
   Cheyne's n., a peculiar rhythmical eye movement resembling Cheyne-Stokes respiration in rhythm.
   disjunctive n., nystagmus in which the eyes move away from each other.
   labyrinthine n., vestibular nystagmus.
   lateral n., horizontal movement of the eyes.
   optokinetic n., nystagmus induced by looking at a moving object.
   rotatory n., rotation of the eyes about the visual axis.
   vertical n., up-and-down movement of the eyes.
   vestibular n., nystagmus due to vestibular disease.

nystatin (nis'tah-tin) an antibiotic substance produced by growth of *Streptomyces noursei;* used in treatment of infections due to *Candida albicans.*

nystaxis (nis-tak'sis) nystagmus.

nyxis (nik'sis) puncture or pricking.

O

O chemical symbol, *oxygen*.

O. [L.] *oc'ulus* (eye); [L.] *octa'rius* (pint).

o- symbol, *ortho-*.

O₂ 1. chemical symbol, molecular (diatomic) oxygen. 2. symbol, both eyes.

O₃ chemical symbol, *ozone* (triatomic oxygen).

O.B. obstetrics.

ob- (ob) word element [L.], *against; in front of; toward.*

obdormition (ob″dor-mish'un) local numbness from nerve pressure.

obesity (o-bēs'ĭ-te) excessive accumulation of fat in the body; increase in weight beyond that considered desirable with regard to age, height and bone structure. adj., **obese'**.

EFFECTS OF OBESITY. Being overweight can affect physical and mental health. Too many extra pounds are a strain on the body, and can eventually shorten the span of life. Obesity is also unattractive, and this may create psychologic problems.

The overweight person is inviting a number of unnecessary complications. Some of these are an overworked heart; shortness of breath; a tendency to arteriosclerosis and high blood pressure or to diabetes mellitus; chronic back and joint pains from increased strain on joints and ligaments; a greater tendency to contract infectious diseases; and a reduced ability to exercise or enjoy sports. Carefully compiled statistics show that mortality from circulatory conditions is about 45 per cent higher in seriously overweight men than in those whose weight is reasonably close to normal, and death from such conditions is apt to occur sooner. Because of this increased risk, life insurance companies are reluctant to grant insurance to people greatly overweight.

Psychologically, too, the obese person is at a disadvantage. The show of good cheer sometimes associated with obese people usually masks unconscious — or even conscious — unhappiness and disappointment. Obesity can cause personality problems; in turn, emotional difficulties such as those caused by persistent loneliness, tension or boredom sometimes find an outlet in compulsive overeating.

CAUSES OF OBESITY. Many overweight people delude themselves into believing that their extra pounds are caused by glandular disturbances. This is very rarely the case, although some types of obesity do result from improper functioning of glands that secrete the hormones that control metabolism, appetite and the body's utilization of fat. Such cases can usually be controlled or cured by hormones given under a physician's direction.

Most often, however, obesity is caused simply by eating or drinking too much. Unable to "burn" all the "fuel" it takes in and does not eliminate as waste, the body stores the surplus as fat. And fat, it has been discovered, is not simply inactive stored material; fat works busily making more fat. The common observation that "the more you eat, the more you need to eat" is true enough, superficially, since the heart and other muscles of an obese person have to work harder than those of a person of normal weight, and consequently require more "fuel." Thus overindulgence leads to further overindulgence in a vicious circle.

CONTROL OF OBESITY. The most important factor in losing weight is the determination to do so, and the will to remain reduced when weight has been lost. In general, it is unwise to try to lose a great deal of weight in a short time. The right procedure depends largely on how much overweight one is. If it is only a few pounds, and the program has been worked out with the physician, a person can usually succeed on his own. He should inform his doctor at once of any unusual symptom, such as diarrhea. On the other hand, one who is seriously overweight should keep in close touch with the doctor throughout the recommended reducing course.

Height and weight charts such as those compiled by the Metropolitan Life Insurance Company (see Appendix) list the weights considered desirable for men and women of various heights and builds. The minimal and maximal figures, in pounds, are for persons wearing their regular indoor clothing, including shoes.

MENU FOR ONE DAY: 995 CALORIES

Food	Number of Calories
Breakfast	
Orange juice (½ cup)	85
Soft-boiled egg	75
Toast, 1 slice	75
Butter (1 teaspoonful)	30
Coffee	0
with cream (1 tablespoonful)	30
	295
Luncheon	
Consommé (1 cup)	25
Lamb chop	130
Broccoli (1 large stalk)	40
Carrots (½ cup)	25
Pineapple slice	50
Coffee or tea	0
with cream	30
	300
Dinner	
Crabmeat (3 ounces)	90
Green peas (½ cup)	55
Cole slaw	15
with vinegar	0
Apple	75
Cookie	75
Skimmed milk (1 cup)	90
	400

Calorie Diets. For most overweight people, a balanced low-calorie diet provides the most straightforward way to lose weight. Diets of this kind vary according to the food preferences and special requirements of the individual; for example, some people need more than the average amount of bulk to keep the intestinal tract clear.

A menu for one day, totaling 995 calories, taken from a typical reducing diet is given in the table. Vitamin supplements may be required with some low-calorie diets. See also CALORIE.

Diet and Exercise. While exercise can be very beneficial to health, it is not in itself an effective way to lose weight. It has been estimated, for example, that the average overweight person would have to walk 36 miles to lose a single pound. On the other hand, exercise can be a valuable adjunct to dieting, as it keeps the dieter fit and helps him lose weight in the right places. Many physicians recommend a course of exercises along with a diet, varying the program according to the patient's age and physical condition.

OTHER REDUCING METHODS. A variety of pills, powders and other preparations sold commercially do curb the appetite, making it easier for overweight people to refrain from overeating. Such preparations should never be taken except on the prescription or advice of a physician; some contain thyroid extract, which can be harmful to the heart and other parts of the body. Furthermore, even preparations that are harmless to most people can harm a few.

obex (o'beks) the thickening of the ependyma at the caudal angle of the roof of the fourth ventricle of the brain.

objective (ob-jek'tiv) 1. perceptible by the external senses. 2. a result for whose achievement an effort has been made. 3. the lens or system of lenses of a microscope nearest the object that is being examined.
　　achromatic o., one in which the chromatic aberration is corrected for two colors.
　　apochromatic o., one in which chromatic aberration is corrected for three colors.
　　semiapochromatic o., one in which the chromatic aberration for three colors is almost entirely overcome.

obligate (ob'lĭ-gāt) imposed by necessity; incapable of adaptation to different conditions.

oblique (o-blēk') slanting; inclined.

obliquity (ŏ-blik'wĭ-te) the state of being oblique or slanting.

obliteration (ŏ-blit"ĕ-ra'shun) complete removal, whether by disease and degeneration or by a surgical operation.

oblongata (ob"long-gah'tah) medulla oblongata (see also BRAIN).

obsession (ob-sesh'un) preoccupation with an idea that morbidly dominates the mind constantly.

obsessive-compulsive (ob-ses'iv-kom-pul'siv) marked by a compulsion to repeatedly perform certain acts or carry out certain rituals. Obsessive-compulsive reaction is a type of NEUROSIS in which there is the intrusion of insistent, repetitious and unwanted ideas or impulses to perform certain acts. The patient may feel compelled to wash his hands repeatedly, to utter certain words or phrases over and over again or to carry out ritualistically other acts that interfere with his normal daily activities.

obstetrician (ob"stĕ-trish'an) one who practices obstetrics.

obstetrics (ob-stet'riks) the branch of medicine dealing with pregnancy, labor and the puerperium. adj., **obstet'ric, obstet'rical.**

obstipation (ob"stĭ-pa'shun) intractable constipation.

obstruction (ob-struk'shun) the act of blocking or clogging; state of being clogged.
　　intestinal o., any hindrance to the passage of feces (see also INTESTINAL OBSTRUCTION).

obstruent (ob'stroo-ent) 1. causing obstruction. 2. any agent or agency that causes obstruction.

obtund (ob-tund') to dull or blunt, especially sensitivity to pain.

obtundent (ob-tun'dent) a soothing or partially anesthetic agent.

obturator (ob"tu-ra'tor) a disk or plate that closes an opening.
　　o. foramen, the large opening between the pubic bone and the ischium.
　　o. muscle, the muscle that rotates the thigh laterally.
　　o. sign, pain on outward pressure on the obturator foramen as a sign of inflammation in the sheath of the obturator nerve probably caused by appendicitis.

obtusion (ob-tu'zhun) a deadening or blunting of sensitivity.

occipital (ok-sip'ĭ-tal) pertaining to the back part of the head.
　　o. bone, the unpaired bone constituting the back and part of the base of the skull.
　　o. lobe, the posterior portion of the cerebral hemisphere.

occipitalization (ok-sip"ĭ-tal-ĭ-za'shun) fusion of the first cervical vertebra with the skull (occiput).

occiput (ok'sĭ-put) the back part of the head.

occlude (o-klood') to fit close together; to close tight.

occlusion (ŏ-kloo'zhun) 1. the act of closure or state of being closed. 2. the contact of the teeth of both jaws when closed or during the movements of the mandible in mastication. adj., **occlu'sal.**
　　abnormal o., malocclusion.
　　anatomic o., occlusion in which all the teeth are present and occlude properly.
　　capsular o., surgical closure of the renal capsule for the relief of floating kidney (nephroptosis).
　　central o., centric o., occlusion of the teeth with the jaws closed in normal position.
　　coronary o., obstruction to the flow of blood through an artery of the heart (see also CORONARY OCCLUSION).
　　eccentric o., occlusion of the teeth when the lower jaw has moved from the position of rest.

occult   (ŏ-kult′) obscure or hidden from view.

o. blood test, examination, microscopically or by a chemical test, of a specimen of feces, urine, gastric juice, etc., to determine the presence of blood not otherwise detectable. Feces are tested when intestinal bleeding is suspected but there is no visible evidence of blood in the stools.

occupational diseases   (ok″u-pa′shun-al) abnormal conditions of the body caused or aggravated by the occupation of the individual. The disorders vary with the type of work involved.

Dusts are a common cause of occupational diseases. Fine particles of silica can lead to SILICOSIS among miners, glassworkers and persons involved in the manufacture of cement and similar materials. Another cause of occupational disease is poisonous gases and vapors, which can result in respiratory disorders and may also involve the blood and other body systems. Certain kinds of chemicals can affect the skin, causing some forms of DERMATITIS. Working conditions, such as high temperatures or humidity, excessive noise, changes in air pressure or continuous exposure to sun and wind, can cause varied disorders such as HEAT EXHAUSTION, impaired hearing or vision, BENDS, or skin conditions.

Control and prevention of occupational diseases is very much a major concern of the individual worker, management, the community health service and the state and federal governments. It involves education of the worker on how to protect himself against occupational hazards; management's cooperation in supplying proper equipment and conditions; inspection and testing services performed by the government; the existence of adequate medical and first-aid services at the location of the work; adequate hospitalization facilities, insurance and compensation; and research into methods to provide safety and good health.

occupational therapy   the teaching of useful skills or hobbies to sick or handicapped persons in order to promote their rehabilitation and recovery or to facilitate their ability to make a living.

Occupational therapy aims to meet the universal human need to be occupied, to exercise body and mind, to be useful and creative and as far as possible to care for oneself. This constructive focus may be vital for patients who have become disabled by such disorders as rheumatoid arthritis, paralyzing strokes or heart disease, or by the loss of limbs, sight or hearing.

The recovery of the ill or injured generally occurs faster if their outlook is positive, and if they are active mentally and physically. Persons who are busy with interesting activities are less likely to brood about their illness, and the activity itself helps to restore the ability to function. Secondarily, such activities may form a foundation for later vocational rehabilitation.

Most large hospitals have departments of occupational therapy staffed by professionals trained in this field. The therapist collaborates with the physician and also with the psychologist, if one is involved. After carefully investigating the interests and abilities of the person, the therapist sets up a suitable activity program. Physical activities encourage the use of affected muscles and ligaments. Recreation is gauged to meet special aptitudes whenever possible. The activities should give the patient the satisfaction of success without over-taxing him. The ideal is the maximal use of the person's capacities in a program that will meet his mental and emotional needs.

When a patient leaves the hospital, therapy can be continued at home. In some communities, institutions specializing in occupational therapy have been set up to teach the handicapped on a broader or more intensive basis than is possible in hospital or home.

ochrodermatosis   (o″kro-der″mah-to′sis) a condition marked by yellowness of the skin.

ochrodermia   (o″kro-der′me-ah) yellowness of the skin.

ochrometer   (o-krom′ĕ-ter) an instrument for measuring capillary blood pressure.

ochronosis   (o″kro-no′sis) a peculiar discoloration of body tissues caused by deposit of alcapton bodies as the result of a metabolic disorder.

exogenous o., ochronosis allegedly due to exposure to a noxious substance.

ocular o., brown or gray discoloration of the sclera, sometimes involving also the conjunctivae and eyelids.

octa-   (ok′tah) word element [Gr. L.], *eight.*

octan   (ok′tan) occurring on the eighth day (every seven days).

octaploidy   (ok′tah-ploi″de) the state of having eight sets of chromosomes (8n).

Octin   (ok′tin) trademark for preparations of isometheptene, a sympathomimetic and antispasmodic.

octipara   (ok-tip′ah-rah) a woman who has had eight pregnancies that resulted in viable offspring; para VIII.

ocul(o)-   (ok′u-lo) word element [L.], *eye.*

ocular   (ok′u-lar) 1. pertaining to the eye. 2. eyepiece (of a microscope).

oculist   (ok′u-list) a general term referring to a professional person who treats the eyes; commonly used to designate an ophthalmologist.

oculocerebrorenal syndrome   (ok″u-lo-sĕ-re″bro-re′nal) vitamin D-resistant rickets associated with glaucoma, mental retardation and faulty reabsorption of certain elements in the renal tubules; called also Lowe's disease.

oculocutaneous   (ok″u-lo-ku-ta′ne-us) pertaining to or affecting both the eyes and the skin.

oculofacial   (ok″u-lo-fa′shal) pertaining to the eyes and face.

oculogyration   (ok″u-lo-ji-ra′shun) the movement of the eyeball.

oculomotor   (ok″u-lo-mo′tor) pertaining to eye movements.

o. nerve, the third cranial nerve; it is mixed, that is, it contains both sensory and motor fibers. Various branches of the oculomotor nerve provide for muscle sense and movement in most of the muscles of the eye, for constriction of the pupil and for accommodation of the eye.

oculomotorius   (ok″u-lo-mo-to′re-us) the oculomotor nerve.

oculonasal (ok″u-lo-na′zal) pertaining to the eye and the nose.

oculopupillary (ok″u-lo-pu′pĭ-ler″e) pertaining to the pupil of the eye.

oculus (ok′u-lus), pl. *oc′uli* [L.] eye.

O.D. 1. Doctor of Optometry. 2. [L.] *oc′ulus dex′ter* (right eye).

odont(o)- (o-don′to) word element [Gr.], *tooth.*

odontalgia (o″don-tal′je-ah) toothache.

odontectomy (o″don-tek′to-me) excision of a tooth.

odontexesis (o″don-tek′sĕ-sis) cleaning, scraping and polishing of the teeth.

odontiasis (o″don-ti′ah-sis) eruption of the teeth, or any disorder caused thereby.

odontic (o-don′tik) pertaining to the teeth.

odontinoid (o-don′tĭ-noid) a tumor composed of tooth substance.

odontitis (o″don-ti′tis) inflammation of a tooth.

odontoblast (o-don′to-blast) one of the connective tissue cells forming the outer surface of the dental pulp adjacent to the dentin.

odontoblastoma (o-don″to-blas-to′mah) a tumor made up of odontoblasts.

odontoclasis (o″don-tok′lah-sis) breaking of a tooth.

odontoclast (o-don′to-klast) a multinucleated giant cell associated with absorption of roots of deciduous teeth.

odontodynia (o-don″to-din′e-ah) odontalgia.

odontogen (o-don′to-jen) the substance that develops into the dentin of the teeth.

odontogenesis (o-don″to-jen′ĕ-sis) the origin and development of the teeth. adj., **odontogenet′ic.**
   o. imperfec′ta, imperfect formation of dentin.

odontogenic (o-don″to-jen′ik) originating from a tooth or tooth-forming tissue.

odontogeny (o″don-toj′ĕ-ne) odontogenesis.

odontoid (o-don′toid) like a tooth.

odontolith (o-don′to-lith) a concretion on a tooth; dental calculus.

odontology (o″don-tol′o-je) scientific study of the teeth.

odontoma (o″don-to′mah) a tumor derived from tissues involved in tooth formation.
   ameloblastic o., an odontogenic tumor characterized by simultaneous occurrence of ameloblastoma and a composite odontoma.
   composite o., one consisting of both enamel and dentin in an abnormal pattern.
   coronary o., one attacking the crown of a tooth.
   radicular o., one attacking the root of a tooth.

odontopathy (o″don-top′ah-the) any disease of the teeth.

odontoperiosteum (o-don″to-per″e-os′te-um) periodontium.

odontorrhagia (o-don″to-ra′je-ah) hemorrhage following extraction of a tooth.

odontoscope (o-don′to-skōp) a dental mirror for examining the teeth.

odontosis (o″don-to′sis) formation or eruption of the teeth.

odontotomy (o″don-tot′o-me) incision of a tooth.

odontotrypy (o″don-tot′rĭ-pe) the boring or drilling of a tooth.

odynacusis (o-din″ah-ku′sis) painful hearing.

-odynia (o-din′e-ah) word element [Gr.], *pain.*

odynometer (o″din-om′ĕ-ter) an instrument for measuring pain.

odynophagia (o-din″o-fa′je-ah) painful swallowing of food.

oe- for words beginning thus, see also those beginning *e-*.

Oedipus complex (ed′ĭ-pus) a term used originally in PSYCHOANALYSIS to signify the complicated conflicts and emotions felt by a child when, during a stage of his normal development as a member of the family circle, he becomes aware of a particularly, strong, sexually tinged attachment to his mother; the term also applies to a similar attachment felt by a girl to her father (called also Electra complex). At the same time, the child tends to view the other parent as a rival and yearns to take that parent's place. This pattern, which was described by Sigmund Freud, is named from the legend of the mythical Greek hero, King Oedipus of Thebes, who unknowingly killed his father and married his mother.
   According to psychoanalysts, a child enters the oedipal phase at about the third year and usually has solved his largely unconscious conflicts in a satisfactory way by the age of 5 or 6. He does this by turning his feelings of possessiveness toward one parent and competitiveness toward the other into a wish to be like them and to be liked by both of them. Eventually, a child who has worked out his conflicts well can focus his affection on members of the opposite sex outside the family circle and can establish satisfactory marital relationships as an adult.
   Freud's theory is generally accepted by psychiatrists, although many have developed supplementary theories for the behavior pattern he described.

Oesophagostomum (e-sof″ah-gos′to-mum) a genus of nematode worms found in the intestines of various animals.

Oestrus (es′trus) a genus of flies whose larvae parasitize the nasal cavities and sinuses of ruminants.
   O. o′vis, a widespread species that deposits its larvae on the nostrils of sheep and goats, and which may cause ocular myiasis in man.

Of. official.

official (ŏ-fish′al) authorized by pharmacopeias and recognized formularies.

officinal (o-fis'ĭ-nal) regularly kept for sale in druggists' shops.

Oguchi's disease (o-goo'chēz) a form of hereditary night blindness common in Japan.

OH symbol, *hydroxyl ion.*

ohm (ōm) a unit of electric resistance, being that of a column of mercury 1 sq. mm. in cross section and 106.25 cm. long.

Ohm's law (ōmz) the strength of an electric current varies directly as the electromotive force and inversely as the resistance.

oidiomycosis (o-id″e-o-mi-ko'sis) candidiasis.

oil (oil) a generally combustible substance that is not miscible with water, but is soluble in ether. Such substances, depending on their origin, are classified as animal, mineral or vegetable oils. Depending on their behavior on heating, they are classified as volatile or fixed.
    essential o., ethereal o., volatile oil.
    fixed o., an oil that does not evaporate on warming and occurs as a solid, semisolid or liquid.
    volatile o., an oil that evaporates readily; such oils occur in aromatic plants, to which they give odor and other characteristics.

ointment (oint'ment) a semisolid preparation for external application to the body. Official ointments consist of medicinal substances incorporated in suitable vehicles (bases).
    white o., a mixture of white wax and white petrolatum; used as a vehicle for medications to be applied to the skin.
    yellow o., a mixture of yellow wax and petrolatum; used as a vehicle for medications.

O.L. [L.] *oc'ulus lae'vus* (left eye).

-ol word termination indicating an alcohol or a phenol.

oleaginous (o″le-aj'ĭ-nus) oily; greasy.

oleandomycin (o″le-an″do-mi'sin) an antibiotic substance produced by growth of *Streptomyces antibioticus;* used chiefly in treatment of infections by gram-positive organisms.

oleate (o'le-āt) 1. a salt of oleic acid. 2. a solution of a substance in oleic acid.

olecranarthritis (o-lek″ran-ar-thri'tis) inflammation of the elbow joint.

olecranarthrocace (o-lek″ran-ar-throk'ah-se) tuberculosis of the elbow joint.

olecranarthropathy (o-lek″ran-ar-throp'ah-the) disease of the elbow joint.

olecranoid (o-lek'rah-noid) resembling the olecranon.

olecranon (o-lek'rah-non) the bony projection of the ulna at the elbow. adj., **olec'ranal.**

oleic acid (o-le'ik) a long-chain unsaturated fatty acid found in animal and vegetable fats.

oleoresin (o″le-o-rez'in) an extract containing the resinous and oily constituents of a drug, obtained by evaporating ethereal acetone, or alcoholic percolates.

oleotherapy (o″le-o-ther'ah-pe) treatment by injections of oil.

oleothorax (o″le-o-tho'raks) intrapleural injection of oil.

oleovitamin (o″le-o-vi'tah-min) a preparation of fat-soluble vitamins in fish liver or edible vegetable oil.

oleum (o'le-um), pl. *o'lea* [L.] oil.

olfact (ol'fakt) a unit of odor, the minimal perceptible odor, being the minimal concentration of a substance in solution that can be perceived by a large number of normal individuals, expressed in terms of grams per liter.

olfactie (ol-fak'te) a unit of odor.

olfaction (ol-fak'shun) 1. the act of smelling. 2. the sense of smell.

olfactology (ol″fak-tol'o-je) the science of the sense of smell.

olfactometer (ol″fak-tom'ĕ-ter) an instrument for testing the sense of smell.

olfactory (ol-fak'to-re) pertaining to the sense of smell.
    o. bulb, the bulblike extremity of the olfactory nerve on the under surface of each anterior lobe of the cerebrum.
    o. nerve, the first cranial nerve: it is purely sensory and is concerned with the sense of smell. The nerve cell bodies are situated in the olfactory area of the mucous membrane of the nose. The nerve fibers lead upward through openings in the ethmoid bone and connect with the cells of the olfactory bulb. From there the fibers pass inward to the cerebrum.

olig(o)- (ol'ĭ-go) word element [Gr.], *few; little; scanty.*

oligemia (ol″ĭ-ge'me-ah) deficiency in volume of the blood. adj., **olige'mic.**

oligidria (ol″ig-id're-ah) deficiency in sweat secretion.

oligocholia (ol″ĭ-go-ko'le-ah) deficiency of bile.

oligochromemia (ol″ĭ-go-kro-me'me-ah) deficiency of hemoglobin in blood.

oligochylia (ol″ĭ-go-ki'le-ah) deficiency of chyle.

oligochymia (ol″i-go-ki'me-ah) deficiency of chyme.

oligocythemia (ol″i-go-si-the'me-ah) scarcity of erythrocytes in the blood.

oligodactylia (ol″ĭ-go-dak-til'e-ah) congenital absence of a digit of a hand or foot.

oligodendrocyte (ol″ĭ-go-den'dro-sīt) a cell of oligodendroglia.

oligodendroglia (ol″ĭ-go-den-drog'le-ah) nonnervous tissue of ectodermal origin forming part of the outer structure of the central nervous system.

oligodendroglioma (ol″ĭ-go-den″dro-gli-o′mah) a tumor composed of oligodendroglia.

oligodipsia (ol″ĭ-go-dip′se-ah) abnormally diminished thirst.

oligodontia (ol″ĭ-go-don′she-ah) congenital absence of some of the teeth.

oligodynamic (ol″ĭ-go-di-nam′ik) active in a small quantity.

oligogalactia (ol″ĭ-go-gah-lak′she-ah) deficient secretion of milk.

oligogenic (ol″ĭ-go-jen′ik) produced by a few genes at most; used in reference to certain hereditary characters.

oligohemia (ol″ĭ-go-he′me-ah) oligemia.

oligohydramnios (ol″ĭ-go-hi-dram′ne-os) deficiency of the amniotic fluid in pregnancy.

oligohydruria (ol″ĭ-go-hi-droo′re-ah) abnormally high concentration of urine.

oligomania (ol″ĭ-go-ma′ne-ah) disordered mental activity on a few subjects; impairment of a few of the mental faculties.

oligomenorrhea (ol″ĭ-go-men″o-re′ah) infrequent or scanty menstrual flow.

oligo-ovulation (ol″ĭ-go-o″vu-la′shun) maturation and discharge of fewer than the normal number of ova from the ovaries.

oligophosphaturia (ol″ĭ-go-fos″fah-tu′re-ah) deficiency of phosphates in the urine.

oligophrenia (ol″ĭ-go-fre′ne-ah) mental deficiency.
  phenylpyruvic o., o. phenylpyru′vica, mental deficiency due to a genetically determined inability to convert phenylalanine to tyrosine, with accumulation of phenylalanine in body fluids and excretion of abnormally large amounts of its metabolites in the urine (PHENYLKETONURIA).

oligoplasmia (ol″ĭ-go-plaz′me-ah) deficiency of blood plasma.

oligopnea (ol″ĭ-gop′ne-ah) retarded breathing.

oligoposia (ol″ĭ-go-po′ze-ah) abnormally diminished intake of fluids.

oligoptyalism (ol″ĭ-go-ti′ah-lizm) diminished secretion of saliva.

oligoria (ol″ĭ-go′re-ah) abnormal indifference toward persons or objects.

oligospermia (ol″ĭ-go-sper′me-ah) deficiency of spermatozoa in the semen.

oligotrichia (ol″ĭ-go-trik′e-ah) congenital thinness of growth of the hair.

oligotrophia, oligotrophy (ol″ĭ-go-tro′fe-ah), (ol″ĭ-got′ro-fe) a state of poor (insufficient) nutrition.

oliguria (ol″ĭ-gu′re-ah) diminution of urinary secretion to between 100 and 400 ml. in 24 hours. adj., **oligu′ric.**

olivary (ol′ĭ-ver″e) shaped like an olive.

olive (ol′iv) a rounded elevation lateral to the upper part of each pyramid of the medulla oblongata.

Ollier's disease (ol″e-āz′) dyschondroplasia.

-oma (o′mah) word element [Gr.], *tumor.*

omagra (o-mag′rah) gout in the shoulder.

omalgia (o-mal′je-ah) pain in the shoulder.

omarthritis (o″mar-thri′tis) inflammation of the shoulder joint.

omentectomy (o″men-tek′to-me) excision of omentum.

omentitis (o″men-ti′tis) inflammation of the omentum.

omentofixation, omentopexy (o-men″to-fik-sa′-shun), (o-men′to-pek″se) fixation of the omentum, to establish collateral circulation in portal obstruction or in coronary occlusion.

omentorrhaphy (o″men-tor′ah-fe) suture of the omentum.

omentum (o-men′tum), pl. *omen′ta* [L.] a fold of peritoneum extending from stomach to adjacent abdominal organs. adj., **omen′tal.**
  gastrocolic o., greater omentum.
  gastrohepatic o., lesser omentum.
  greater o., a peritoneal fold attached to the anterior surface of the transverse colon.
  lesser o., a peritoneal fold joining the lesser curvature of the stomach and the first part of the duodenum to the porta hepatis.
  o. ma′jus, greater omentum.
  o. mi′nus, lesser omentum.

omitis (o-mi′tis) inflammation of the shoulder.

omocephalus (o″mo-sef′ah-lus) a fetal monster with no arms and an incomplete head.

omodynia (o″mo-din′e-ah) pain in the shoulder.

omoplata (o″mo-plat′ah) the scapula.

omphalectomy (om″fah-lek′to-me) excision of the umbilicus.

omphalic (om-fal′ik) pertaining to the umbilicus.

omphalitis (om″fah-li′tis) inflammation of the umbilicus.

omphalocele (om′fal-o-sēl″) protrusion, at birth, of part of the intestine through a defect in the abdominal wall at the umbilicus.

omphaloncus (om″fah-long′kus) tumor of the umbilicus.

omphalophlebitis (om″fah-lo-flĕ-bi′tis) inflammation of the umbilical veins.

omphaloproptosis (om″fah-lo-prop-to′sis) prolapse of the umbilical cord.

omphalorrhagia (om″fah-lo-ra′je-ah) hemorrhage from the umbilicus.

omphalorrhea (om″fah-lo-re′ah) effusion of lymph at the umbilicus.

omphalorrhexis (om"fah-lo-rek'sis) rupture of the umbilicus.

omphalosite (om'fal-o-sīt") a fetal monster with no heart, which cannot live after the umbilical cord is cut.

omphalotaxis (om"fah-lo-tak'sis) replacement of prolapsed umbilical cord.

omphalotomy (om"fah-lot'o-me) the cutting of the umbilical cord.

omphalotripsy (om-fal'o-trip"se) separation of the umbilical cord by crushing.

onanism (o'nah-nizm) incomplete sexual relations with withdrawal just before emission; sometimes used as a synonym for masturbation.

Onchocerca (ong"ko-ser'kah) a genus of filarial worms, parasitic on humans and animals.
 O. vol'vulus, a species causing human infection, dwelling in tumors in subcutaneous connective tissue and often affecting the eyes.

onchocerciasis (ong"ko-ser-ki'ah-sis) infection by worms of the genus Onchocerca.

oncogenesis (ong"ko-jen"ĕ-sis) the production of tumors. adj., **oncogenet'ic.**

oncogenic (ong"ko-jen'ik) causing tumor formation.

oncogenous (ong-koj'ĕ-nus) arising in or originating from a tumor.

oncology (ong-kol'o-je) sum of knowledge regarding tumors.

oncolysis (ong-kol'ĭ-sis) destruction or dissolution of a neoplasm. adj., **oncolyt'ic.**

oncoma (ong-ko'mah) a tumor; a swelling.

oncometer (ong-kom'ĕ-ter) an instrument for measuring variations in size of the viscera.

oncosis (ong-ko'sis) the formation of multiple tumors.

oncosphere (ong"ko-sfēr) the larva of a tapeworm in the spherical stage.

oncotherapy (ong"ko-ther'ah-pe) the treatment of tumors.

oncothlipsis (ong"ko-thlip'sis) pressure caused by a tumor.

oncotic (ong-kot'ik) pertaining to swelling.

oncotomy (ong-kot'o-me) the incision of an abscess or tumor.

oncotropic (ong"ko-trop'ik) having special affinity for tumor cells.

oneiric (o-ni'rik) pertaining to dreams.

oneirism (o-ni'rizm) a waking dream state.

oneiroanalysis (o-ni"ro-ah-nal'ĭ-sis) exploration of conscious and unconscious personality by interpretation of drug-induced dreams.

oneirogenic (o"ni-ro-jen'ik) producing a dream-like state.

oneirology (o"ni-rol'o-je) the science of dreams.

oneiroscopy (o"ni-ros'ko-pe) analysis of dreams for diagnosis of a patient's mental state.

oniomania (o"ne-o-ma'ne-ah) insane desire to make purchases.

onomatology (on"o-mah-tol'o-je) the science of names and nomenclature.

onomatomania (on"o-mat"o-ma'ne-ah) mental derangement with regard to words or names.

onomatophobia (on"o-mat"o-fo'be-ah) morbid aversion to a certain word or name.

ontogeny (on"toj'ĕ-ne) the complete developmental history of an individual organism.

onychalgia (on"ĭ-kal'je-ah) pain in the nails.

onychatrophia (o-nik"ah-tro'fe-ah) atrophy of the nails.

onychectomy (on"ĭ-kek'to-me) excision of a fingernail or toenail.

onychia (o-nik'e-ah) inflammation of the nail bed, resulting in loss of the nail.
 o. latera'lis, paronychia.
 o. malig'na, onychia with fetid ulceration.
 o. parasit'ica, onychomycosis.

onychitis (on"ĭ-ki'tis) inflammation of the matrix of a nail.

onychogenic (on"ĭ-ko-jen'ik) producing nail substance.

onychograph (o-nik'o-graf) an instrument for recording variations of blood pressure in the capillaries of the fingertips.

onychogryposis (on"ĭ-ko-grĭ-po'sis) abnormal elongation and twisting of the nails, giving a claw-like appearance.

onychoid (on'ĭ-koid) resembling a fingernail.

onycholysis (on"ĭ-kol'ĭ-sis) loosening or separation of a nail from its bed.

onychomadesis (on"ĭ-ko-mah-de'sis) complete loss of the nail.

onychomalacia (on"ĭ-ko-mah-la'she-ah) softening of the fingernail.

onychomycosis (on"ĭ-ko-mi-ko'sis) fungus infection of the nails.

onychopathy (on"ĭ-kop'ah-the) disease of the nails.

onychophagy (on"ĭ-kof'ah-je) biting of the nails.

onychorrhexis (on"ĭ-ko-rek'sis) spontaneous splitting and brittleness of the nails.

onychoschizia (on"ĭ-ko-skiz'e-ah) loosening of the nail from its bed.

onychosis (on"ĭ-ko'sis) disease or malformation of the nails.

onychotillomania (on"ĭ-ko-til"o-ma'ne-ah) neurotic picking or tearing at the nails.

onychotomy (on"ĭ-kot'o-me) incision into a fingernail or toenail.

onychotrophy (on″ĭ-kot′ro-fe) nutrition of the nails.

onyx (on′iks) 1. a variety of hypopyon. 2. a fingernail or toenail.

onyxitis (on″ik-si′tis) onychitis.

ooblast (o′o-blast) a cell from which an ovum is developed.

oocyst (o′o-sist) the membrane surrounding a zygote after union of the gametes.

oocyte (o′o-sīt) a growing or full-grown oogonial cell that has not yet completed its maturation process.
  primary o., the original large cell into which an oogonium develops.
  secondary o., the large cell produced by unequal meiotic division of a primary oocyte.

oogenesis (o″o-jen′ĕ-sis) the development of mature ova from oogonia.

oogonium (o″o-go′ne-um), pl. *oogo′nia* [Gr.] the primordial cell from which the ovarian egg arises, at any stage of its growth, to become a primary oocyte.

oophor(o)- (o-of′o-ro) word element [Gr.], *ovary.*

oophoralgia (o″of-o-ral′je-ah) pain in an ovary.

oophorectomy (o″of-o-rek′to-me) excision of an ovary. Bilateral oophorectomy refers to the removal of both ovaries. The procedure is done for tumors, severe infection or other disorders of the ovary. Removal of the ovaries from a girl who has not yet reached puberty prevents the development of secondary sex characters. However, if the ovaries are removed from an adult woman, there is no significant loss of femininity. Reproduction is not possible after removal of the ovaries, and the female sex hormones estrogen and progesterone are no longer produced.

oophoritis (o″of-o-ri′tis) inflammation of an ovary.
  mumps o., involvement of the ovaries in epidemic parotitis (mumps).

oophorocystectomy (o-of″o-ro-sis-tek′to-me) excision of an ovarian cyst.

oophorocystosis (o-of″o-ro-sis-to′sis) formation of an ovarian cyst.

oophorohysterectomy (o-of″o-ro-his″ter-ek′to-me) excision of the ovaries and uterus.

oophoroma (o-of″o-ro′mah) a malignant tumor of the ovary.

oophoron (o-of′o-ron) an ovary.

oophoroplasty (o-of′o-ro-plas″te) plastic repair of an ovary.

oophororrhaphy (o″of-o-ror′ah-fe) suture of an ovary.

oosperm (o′o-sperm) a fertilized ovum.

ootid (o′o-tid) a ripe ovum; one of four cells derived from the two consecutive divisions of the primary oocyte.

opacity (o-pas′ĭ-te) 1. the condition of being opaque. 2. an opaque area.

opalescent (o″pal-es′ent) showing various colors like an opal.

opaque (o-pāk′) impervious to light rays, or by extension to roentgen rays or other electromagnetic vibrations; neither translucent nor transparent.

operation (op″er-a′shun) any action performed with instruments or by the hands of a surgeon.
  cosmetic o., one for correction of an unsightly defect.
  exploratory o., opening of the body for determination of the cause of otherwise unexplainable symptoms.
  radical o., one by which all diseased or involved tissue is removed, effecting complete cure without effort to preserve body structures.

operative (op′er-a″tiv) 1. pertaining to an operation. 2. acting to produce an effect.

operculum (o-per′ku-lum), pl. *oper′cula* [L.] a lid or covering, especially folds from the frontal, parietal and temporal lobes of the cerebrum overlying the insula. adj., **oper′cular.**
  dental o., the hood of gingival tissue overlying the crown of an erupting tooth.
  trophoblastic o., the plug of trophoblast that helps close the gap in the endometrium made by the implanting blastocyst.

operon (op′er-on) a system of adjacent genes on a chromosome, one of which, the operator gene, interacts with repressor in the cell and controls activity of the remaining structural genes of the system.

ophiasis (o-fi′ah-sis) baldness in winding streaks across the head.

ophidiophobia (o-fid″e-o-fo′be-ah) morbid dread of snakes.

ophidism (o′fĭ-dizm) poisoning by snake venom.

Ophthaine (of′thān) trademark for a preparation of proparacaine hydrochloride, a local anesthetic.

ophthalm(o)- (of-thal′mo) word element [Gr.], *eye.*

ophthalmectomy (of″thal-mek′to-me) excision of an eye.

ophthalmia (of-thal′me-ah) severe inflammation or infection of the eye or conjunctiva.
  Egyptian o., trachoma.
  gonorrheal o., acute and severe purulent conjunctivitis due to gonorrheal infection.
  o. neonato′rum, purulent opthalmia of the newborn, usually caused by the gonococcus. It is prevented by instilling silver nitrate or other chemical in the eyes of the newborn.
  phlyctenular o., a form with vesicles on the epithelium of the cornea or conjunctiva.
  sympathetic o., inflammation of a sound eye accompanying involvement of the other.

ophthalmic (of-thal′mik) pertaining to the eye.

ophthalmitis (of″thal-mi′tis) inflammation of the eye.

ophthalmoblennorrhea (of-thal″mo-blen″o-re′-ah) gonorrheal ophthalmia.

ophthalmocele (of-thal′mo-sēl) exophthalmos.

ophthalmodynamometry (of-thal″mo-di″nah-mom′ĕ-tre) determination of the blood pressure in the retinal artery.

ophthalmodynia (of-thal″mo-din′e-ah) neuralgic pain of the eye.

ophthalmo-eikonometer (of-thal″mo-i″ko-nom′-ĕ-ter) an instrument used to determine both the refraction of the eye and the relative size and shape of the ocular images.

ophthalmofunduscope (of-thal′mo-fun′dŭ-skōp) an instrument for examining the fundus of the eye.

ophthalmography (of″thal-mog′rah-fe) description of the eye and its diseases.

ophthalmogyric (of-thal″mo-ji′rik) causing movements of the eye.

ophthalmolith (of-thal′mo-lith) a lacrimal calculus.

ophthalmologist (of″thal-mol′o-jist) a physician who specializes in diagnosing and prescribing treatment for defects, injuries and diseases of the EYE, and is skilled at delicate eye surgery, such as that required to remove cataracts; called also oculist or eye specialist.

ophthalmology (of″thal-mol′o-je) the study of the eye and its diseases.

ophthalmomalacia (of-thal″mo-mah-la′she-ah) abnormal softness of the eyeball.

ophthalmometer (of″thal-mom′ĕ-ter) an instrument for measuring the refractive power of the eye.

ophthalmometry (of″thal-mom′ĕ-tre) determination of the refractive power of the eye.

ophthalmomycosis (of-thal″mo-mi-ko′sis) any disease of the eye caused by a fungus.

ophthalmomyotomy (of-thal″mo-mi-ot′o-me) division of the muscles of the eyes.

ophthalmoneuritis (of-thal″mo-nu-ri′tis) inflammation of the optic nerve.

ophthalmopathy (of″thal-mop′ah-the) any disease of the eye.

ophthalmophthisis (of″thal-mof′thĭ-sis) abnormal softness of the eye.

ophthalmoplasty (of-thal′mo-plas″te) plastic surgery of the eye.

ophthalmoplegia (of-thal″mo-ple′je-ah) paralysis of the eye muscles.
  o. exter′na, paralysis of the extraocular muscles.
  o. inter′na, paralysis of the intraocular muscles.
  nuclear o., that due to a lesion of nuclei of motor nerves of eye.
    partial o., that affecting some of the eye muscles.
    progressive o., gradual paralysis of all the eye muscles.
  total o., paralysis of all the eye muscles, both intraocular and extraocular.

ophthalmoptosis (of-thal″mop-to′sis) exophthalmos.

ophthalmoreaction (of-thal″mo-re-ak′shun) local reaction of the conjunctiva after instillation into the eye of toxins or organisms causing typhoid fever and tuberculosis.

ophthalmorrhagia (of-thal″mo-ra′je-ah) hemorrhage from the eye.

ophthalmorrhea (of-thal″mo-re′ah) oozing of blood from the eye.

ophthalmorrhexis (of-thal″mo-rek′sis) rupture of an eyeball.

ophthalmoscope (of-thal′mo-skōp) an instrument for examining the interior of the eye. It sends a bright, narrow beam of light through the lens of the eye, and contains a lens through which the physician can examine interior parts of the eye. It is helpful in detecting possible disorders of the eyes, as well as disorders of other organs that are reflected in the condition of the eyes.

ophthalmoscopy (of″thal-mos′ko-pe) examination of the eye by means of the ophthalmoscope.

ophthalmotomy (of″thal-mot′o-me) incision of the eye.

ophthalmotrope (of-thal′mo-trōp) a mechanical eye that moves like a real eye.

ophthalmoxerosis (of-thal″mo-ze-ro′sis) xerophthalmia; abnormal dryness of the surface of the conjunctiva, due to vitamin A deficiency.

opian (o′pe-an) noscapine, an antitussive.

opianine (o-pi′ah-nin) noscapine, an antitussive.

opiate (o′pe-āt) 1. a remedy containing opium. 2. any drug that induces sleep.

opiomania (o″pe-o-ma′ne-ah) intense craving for opium.

opisthorchiasis (o″pis-thor-ki′ah-sis) infection by flukes of the genus Opisthorchis.

Opisthorchis (o″pis-thor′kis) a genus of flukes parasitic in the liver and biliary tract of various birds and mammals, including man.
  O. sinen′sis, a species widely distributed in China, Japan, Korea, Vietnam and parts of India; called also *Clonorchis sinensis.*

opisthotonos (o″pis-thot′o-nos) tetanic spasm that flexes the head and feet backward.

opium (o′pe-um) a narcotic drug obtained from the juice of the opium poppy (*Papaver somniferum*). It is the source from which morphine and heroin are derived. Opium induces sleep and relieves pain, but is poisonous in large doses. Since it is addictive, its sale or possession for other than medical uses is strictly prohibited by federal, state and local laws. (See also DRUG ADDICTION.)

opiumism (o′pe-ŭ-mizm″) habitual misuse of opium, and its consequences.

opocephalus (o″po-sef′ah-lus) a fetal monster with ears fused, one orbit, no mouth and no nose.

opodidymus (o″po-did′ĭ-mus) a fetal monster with two fused heads and sense organs partly fused.

Oppenheim's disease (op′en-hīmz) amyotonia congenita.

Oppenheim-Urbach disease (op′en-hīm ur′-bahkh) necrobiosis lipoidica diabeticorum.

oppilative (op′ĭ-la″tiv) 1. closing the pores. 2. constipating.

opsinogen (op-sin′o-jen) a substance that forms opsonins.

opsiuria (op″se-u′re-ah) excretion of urine more rapidly during fasting than after a meal.

opsogen (op′so-jen) opsinogen.

opsomania (op″so-ma′ne-ah) an abnormal craving for some special food.

opsonification (op-son″ĭ-fĭ-ka′shun) the rendering of bacteria and other cells subject to phagocytosis.

opsonin (op-so′nin) an antibody that renders bacteria and other cells susceptible to phagocytosis. adj., **opson′ic.**

immune o., an antibody that sensitizes a particulate antigen to phagocytosis, after combination with the homologous antigen in vivo or in vitro.

opsonocytophagic (op″so-no-si″to-fa′jik) pertaining to the phagocytic activity of blood in the presence of serum opsonins and homologous leukocytes.

opsonoid (op′so-noid) an opsonin in which the active element has been destroyed.

opsonology (op″so-nol′o-je) the study of opsonins and opsonic action.

opsonometry (op″so-nom′ĕ-tre) measurement of the amount of opsonin present.

opsonophilia (op″so-no-fil′e-ah) affinity for opsonins. adj., **opsonophil′ic.**

opsonotherapy (op″so-no-ther′ah-pe) treatment by use of bacterial vaccines to increase the opsonic action of the blood.

optesthesia (op″tes-the′ze-ah) visual sensibility.

optic (op′tik) pertaining to the eye.

o. nerve, the second cranial nerve; it is purely sensory and is concerned with carrying impulses for the sense of sight. The rods and cones of the RETINA are connected with the optic nerve which leaves the eye slightly to the nasal side of the center of the retina. The point at which the optic nerve leaves the eye is called the blind spot because there are no rods and cones in this area. The optic nerve passes through the optic foramen of the skull and into the cranial cavity. It then passes backward and undergoes a division; those nerve fibers leading from the nasal side of the retina cross to the opposite side while those from the temporal side continue to the thalamus uncrossed. After synapsing in the thalamus the neurons convey visual impulses to the occipital lobe of the brain.

Degenerative and inflammatory lesions of the optic nerve occur as a result of infections, toxic damage to the nerve, metabolic or nutritional disorders or trauma. Syphilis is the most frequent cause of infectious disorders of the optic nerve. Methanol (methyl alcohol) is highly toxic to the optic nerve and can cause total blindness. Diabetes mellitus and anemia are examples of metabolic and nutritional disorders that can lead to damage to the optic nerve and produce serious loss of vision.

Treatment of optic neuritis is aimed at control of the primary cause of the disorder. Cortisone and similar steroids are often used to relieve symp-

toms; however, nothing can be done to regain sight lost through damage to the nerve.

optical (op′tĭ-kal) pertaining to vision.

optician (op-tish′an) a person who measures and grinds eyeglasses to prescription. Although this is a very exact and intricate science, the optician does not need a state license to practice. He is not qualified to examine eyes or to prescribe the correct eyeglasses.

opticist (op′tĭ-sist) a specialist in the science of optics.

opticociliary (op″tĭ-ko-sil′e-er″e) pertaining to the optic and ciliary nerves.

opticokinetic (op″tĭ-ko-ki-net′ik) pertaining to movement of the eyes.

opticopupillary (op″tĭ-ko-pu′pĭ-ler″e) pertaining to the optic nerve and pupil.

optics (op′tiks) the science of light and vision.

optogram (op′to-gram) the visual image formed on the retina by bleaching of the rhodopsin.

optometer (op-tom′ĕ-ter) a device for measuring the power and range of vision.

optometrist (op-tom′ĕ-trist) a professional person trained to examine the eyes and prescribe eyeglasses to correct irregularities in the vision. The optometrist uses various devices such as eye charts to determine the strength of the vision and to discover any irregularities such as ASTIGMATISM. He then prescribes the necessary correction. The optometrist is not a physician and is not qualified to diagnose or treat diseases or injuries of the eye, or perform surgery.

optometry (op-tom′ĕ-tre) measurement of the powers of vision and the adaptation of lenses for the aid thereof, utilizing any means other than drugs.

optostriate (op″to-stri′āt) pertaining to the optic thalamus and corpus striatum.

O.R. operating room.

ora (o′rah) 1. plural of os [L.], mouth. 2. pl. o′rae [L.] an edge or margin.

o. serra′ta ret′inae, the zigzag margin of the retina of the eye.

orad (o′rad) toward the mouth.

oral (o′ral) pertaining to the mouth.

Oranixon (or″ah-nik′son) trademark for a prepration of mephenesin, a skeletal muscle relaxant.

orbicular (or-bik′u-lar) circular; rounded.

orbit (or′bit) 1. the bony cavity containing the eyeball and its associated muscles, vessels and nerves; the ethmoid, frontal, lacrimal, nasal, palatine, sphenoid and zygomatic bones and the maxilla contribute to its formation. 2. the path of an electron around the nucleus of an atom. adj., **or′bital.**

orbitonometer (or″bĭ-to-nom′ĕ-ter) an instrument for measuring backward displacement of the eyeball produced by a given pressure on its anterior aspect.

orbitotomy (or″bĭ-tot′o-me) incision into the orbit.

orchi(o)- (or′ke-o) word element [Gr.], *testis.*

orchialgia (or″ke-al′je-ah) pain in a testis.

orchichorea (ok″ke-ko-re′ah) twitching or jerking of a testis.

orchidectomy (or″kĭ-dek′to-me) orchiectomy.

orchidic (or-kid′ik) pertaining to a testis.

orchidoptosis (or″kĭ-dop-to′sis) falling or relaxation of the testis.

orchidorrhaphy (or″kĭ-dor′ah-fe) orchiopexy.

orchidotherapy (or″kĭ-do-ther′ah-pe) treatment with testicular extract.

orchidotomy (or″kĭ-dot′o-me) incision and drainage of a testis.

orchiectomy (or″ke-ek′to-me) excision of a testis. This procedure is sometimes necessary when a testis is seriously diseased or injured. It may be performed, also, in order to control cancer of the prostate.

If both testes are removed the ability to reproduce is ended. There is also a diminution in the production of the hormone testosterone. Orchiectomy does not interfere with the ability to have coitus but removal of the testes usually reduces sexual desire.

Removal of both testes before puberty prevents the development of secondary sex characters because of the deficiency of testosterone. If the procedure is performed after puberty, when the masculine characteristics are already developed, the changes that occur are much less extreme.

orchiepididymitis (or″ke-ep″ĭ-did″ĭ-mi′tis) inflammation of a testis and epididymis.

orchiocele (or′ke-o-sēl″) hernial protrusion of a testis.

orchiodynia (or″ke-o-din′e-ah) pain in a testis.

orchiomyeloma (or″ke-o-mi″ĕ-lo′mah) myeloma of a testis.

orchioncus (or″ke-ong′kus) tumor of a testis.

orchioneuralgia (or″ke-o-nu-ral′je-ah) pain in a testis.

orchiopathy (or″ke-op′ah-the) any disorder of the testes.

orchiopexy (or′ke-o-pek″se) surgical fixation of an undescended testis in the scrotum. An incision is made over the inguinal canal and the testis is brought down into the scrotum. In most cases the surgeon applies traction by placing a suture in the lower scrotum and attaching the suture to the inner thigh by a piece of adhesive tape. This traction is continued for about 1 week.

NURSING CARE. Preoperative care of the child is routine. During the postoperative period care must be taken to avoid disturbing the tension mechanism. Contamination of the suture line should be avoided, and if the child is not toilet trained, this usually requires leaving an indwelling catheter in place until the incision has healed.

orchioplasty (or′ke-o-plas″te) plastic surgery of a testis.

orchioscheocele (or″ke-os′ke-o-sēl) scrotal tumor with scrotal hernia.

orchioscirrhus (or″ke-o-skir′us) hardening of a testis.

orchitis (or-ki′tis) inflammation of a testis. Orchitis is not a common disorder, but it can occur in a variety of infectious diseases, including syphilis, tuberculosis, glanders, leprosy and certain of the parasitic diseases. It usually accompanies EPIDIDYMITIS. Acute orchitis may also occur in such diseases as typhoid fever, pneumonia or mumps in adult males.

The symptoms of acute orchitis are swelling of one or both testes with pain and sensitivity to touch. In chronic orchitis there is no pain but the testes swell slowly and become hard.

order (or′der) a taxonomic category subordinate to a class and superior to a family (or suborder).

orderly (or′der-le) a male hospital attendant who does general work, attending especially to needs of male patients.

ordinate (or′dĭ-nāt) one of the lines in a graph along which is plotted one of the factors considered in the study, as temperature in a time-temperature study. The other line is called the abscissa.

Oretic (o-ret′ik) trademark for a preparation of hydrochlorothiazide, a diuretic and antihypertensive.

Oreton (or′e-ton) trademark for preparations of testosterone, a male sex hormone.

orexigenic (o-rek″sĭ-jen′ik) increasing the appetite.

orf (orf) a contagious pustular dermatitis of sheep, communicable to man.

organ (or′gan) a structural unit of a plant or animal body that serves a specific function or functions.

 acoustic o., organ of Corti.

 cell o., a structural part of a cell having some definite function in its life or reproduction, as a nucleus or a centrosome.

 cement o., the embryonic tissue that develops into the cementum of the tooth.

 o. of Corti, the terminal acoustic apparatus within the scala media of the inner ear, including the rods of Corti and the auditory cells, with their supporting elements.

 enamel o., a process of epithelium forming a cap over a dental papilla and developing into the enamel.

 o. of Giraldès, the paradidymis.

 Golgi tendon o., one of the mechanoreceptors arranged in series with muscle in the tendons of mammalian muscles, being the receptor for stimuli responsible for the lengthening reaction.

 gustatory o., the organ concerned with the perception of taste; the taste buds.

 Meyer's o., an area of papillae on either side of the posterior part of the tongue.

 olfactory o's, the specialized structures concerned with the perception of odors.

 reproductive o's, those concerned with reproduction (see also REPRODUCTIVE ORGANS).

 segmental o., the pronephros, mesonephros and metanephros together.

sense o's, sensory o's, specialized structures containing receptors that are remarkably sensitive to the appropriate stimulus.

target o., the organ affected by a particular hormone.

terminal o., the organ at either end of a reflex arc.

vestigial o., one that was functional in some earlier animal but which, through a change in environment or mode of life in the species, has become unnecessary to survival.

o's of Zuckerkandl, two rounded masses of chromaffin cells about the root of the inferior mesenteric artery, formed before birth and persisting to puberty. Tumors of these structures produce symptoms similar to those of PHEOCHROMOCYTOMA.

organelle (or″gah-nel′) a minute structure serving a specific function in the life processes of a cell, e.g., a specific particle of organized living substance contained in the cytoplasm (mitochondria, lysosomes, ribosomes and centrioles), or a flagellum of a protozoon.

organic (or-gan′ik) 1. pertaining to or having organs. 2. pertaining to substances derived from living organisms.

o. acid, an acid containing the carboxyl group, COOH.

o. chemistry, the scientific study of compounds containing carbon.

organicist (or-gan′ĭ-sist) one who believes that the symptoms of disease are due to organic changes.

organism (or′gah-nizm) an individual animal or plant.

organization (or″gah-nĭ-za′shun) 1. the process of organizing or being organized, especially the conversion of a plastic mass, such as a blood clot or inflammatory exudate, into fibrous tissue. 2. an organism or organized body.

organizer (or′gah-nīz″er) a special region of the embryo that is capable of determining the differentiation of other regions.

organogenesis, organogeny (or″gah-no-jen′ĕ-sis), (or″gah-noj′ĕ-ne) the segregation of tissues into different organs in embryonic development.

organography (or″gah-nog′rah-fe) 1. description of organs. 2. roentgenographic visualization of body organs.

organoleptic (or″gah-no-lep′tik) making an impression on or affecting an organ or the entire organism.

organotherapy (or″gah-no-ther′ah-pe) therapeutic administration of animal organs or their extracts.

organotropism (or-gah-not′ro-pizm) the special affinity of chemical compounds or pathogenic agents for particular tissues or organs of the body. adj., **organotrop′ic.**

organum (or′gah-num), pl. *or′gana* [L.] a somewhat independent part of the body that performs a special function.

orgasm (or′gazm) the climax of sexual excitement.

orientation (o″re-en-ta′shun) the recognition of one's position in relation to time and space.

orientomycin (o-re-en″to-mi′sin) cycloserine, an antibiotic.

orifice (or′ĭ-fis) 1. the entrance or outlet of any body cavity. 2. any foramen, meatus or opening.

origin (or′ĭ-jin) a beginning, as of a nerve or blood vessel, or the end of a skeletal muscle that remains relatively fixed when the muscle contracts.

Orinase (or′ĭ-nās) trademark for a preparation of tolbutamide, an oral hypoglycemic agent.

ornithine (or′nĭ-thēn) a naturally occurring amino acid isolated from the urine and excrement of fowls.

Ornithodoros (or″nĭ-thod′o-ros) a genus of arthropods (family Argasidae), including *O. mouba′ta,* a vector of the organism causing relapsing fever, and many other species that transmit pathogenic microorganisms.

ornithosis (or″nĭ-tho′sis) a viral infection of birds that is occasionally transmitted to man, to produce an acute viral pneumonitis; that transmitted by parrots is commonly called PSITTACOSIS.

orolingual (o″ro-ling′gwal) pertaining to the mouth and tongue.

oronasal (o″ro-na′zal) pertaining to the mouth and nose.

oropharynx (o″ro-far′ingks) the part of the pharynx behind the mouth and tongue.

Oroya fever (o-ro′yah) the acute febrile anemic stage of Carrión's disease.

orphenadrine (or-fen′ah-drēn) a compound used as an antihistaminic, antitremor and antispasmodic agent for relaxation of skeletal muscle spasm and tremor.

orrhology (or-rol′o-je) scientific study of serums.

orrhomeningitis (or″o-men″in-ji′tis) inflammation of a serous membrane.

orrhorrhea (or″o-re′ah) a watery or serous discharge.

orrhotherapy (or″o-ther″ah-pe) serotherapy.

orth(o)- (or′tho) word element [Gr.], *straight; normal; correct.*

orthesis (or-the′sis) orthosis.

orthetics (or-thet′iks) orthotics.

ortho- (or′tho) in chemistry, a prefix indicating an isomer; also a cyclic derivative that has two substituents in adjacent positions. Abbreviated *o-.*

orthobiosis (or″tho-bi-o′sis) proper and hygienic living.

orthocephalic (or″tho-sĕ-fal′ik) having a head with a vertical index of 70.1 to 75.

orthochorea (or″tho-ko-re′ah) choreic movements in the erect posture.

orthochromatic (or″tho-kro-mat′ik) staining normally.

orthocrasia (or″tho-kra′ze-ah) normal reaction of the body to drugs, proteins, etc.

orthodiagraphy (or″tho-di′ag′rah-fe) the recording of outlines of organs as seen by the fluoroscope.

orthodontia, orthodontics (or-tho-don′she-ah), (or″tho-don′tiks) that branch of dentistry concerned with irregularities of teeth and malocclusion, and associated facial problems.

   corrective o., that concerned with correction of existing malocclusion and its sequelae.

   interceptive o., that concerned with elimination of conditions that might lead to malocclusion.

   preventive o., that concerned with preservation of the integrity of normal occlusion.

orthodontist (or″tho-don′tist) a dentist who specializes in orthodontics.

orthodromic (or″tho-drom′ik) traveling or conducting impulses forward or in the normal direction.

orthogenics (or″tho-jen′iks) eugenics.

orthoglycemic (or″tho-gli-se′mik) having the normal amount of sugar in the blood.

orthograde (or′tho-grād) carrying the body upright in walking.

orthometer (or-thom′ĕ-ter) an instrument for determining the relative protrusion of the eyeballs.

orthopedic (or″tho-pe′dik) pertaining to the correction of deformities or to orthopedics.

orthopedics (or″tho-pe′diks) the art and science of prevention, diagnosis and treatment of diseases and abnormalities of the musculoskeletal system.

orthopedist (or-tho-pe′dist) a specialist in orthopedics.

orthopercussion (or″tho-per-kush′un) percussion with the distal phalanx of the finger held perpendicularly to the body wall.

orthophoria (or″tho-fo′re-ah) normal equilibrium of the eye muscles, or muscular balance.

orthopnea (or″thop-ne′ah) ability to breathe only in the upright position.

orthopneic position (or″thop-ne′ik) the patient's head and arms rest on an overbed table that is padded with pillows and placed across his lap.

orthopsychiatry (or″tho-si-ki′ah-tre) that branch of psychiatry that deals with mental and emotional development, embracing child psychiatry and mental hygiene.

orthoptic (or-thop′tik) pertaining to correction of deviation of the visual axes.

orthoptics (or-thop′tiks) treatment of strabismus by exercise of the ocular muscles.

orthoptoscope (or-thop′to-skōp) an instrument for exercising the ocular muscles in treating strabismus.

orthoroentgenography (or″tho-rent″gen-og′-rah-fe) orthodiagraphy.

orthoscope (or′tho-skōp) an apparatus that neutralizes the corneal refraction by means of a layer of water; used in ocular examinations.

orthoscopic (or″tho-skop′ik) affording a correct and undistorted view.

orthoscopy (or-thos′ko-pe) examination by means of an orthoscope.

orthosis (or-tho′sis), pl. *ortho′ses* [Gr.] a brace or other orthopedic device that is applied to an existing segment of the body for the purpose of protecting the segment or assisting in restoration or improvement of its function.

orthostatic (or″tho-stat′ik) pertaining to the upright position.

orthostatism (or′tho-stat″izm) an erect standing position of the body.

orthotic (or-thot′ik) serving to protect or to restore or improve function; pertaining to the use or application of an orthosis.

orthotics (or-thot′iks) the field of knowledge relating to orthoses and their use.

orthotist (or′tho-tist) a person skilled in orthotics and practicing its application in individual cases.

orthotonos (or-thot′o-nos) tetanic spasm that fixes the head, body and limbs in a rigid straight line.

Orthoxine (or-thok′sēn) trademark for preparations of methoxyphenamine, a sympathomimetic drug.

orthuria (or-thoo′re-ah) normal frequency of urination.

O.S. [L.] *oc′ulus sinis′ter* (left eye).

Os chemical symbol, *osmium.*

os[1] (os), pl. *o′ra* [L.] an opening or mouth.

os[2] (os), pl. *os′sa* [L.] a bone (see table of BONES).
   o. cox′ae, hip bone.

osazone (o′sah-zōn) any one of a series of compounds obtained by heating sugars with phenylhydrazine and acetic acid.

osche(o)- (os′ke-o) word element [Gr.], *scrotum.*

oscheitis (os″ke-i′tis) inflammation of the scrotum.

oscheocele (os′ke-o-sēl″) a swelling or tumor of the scrotum.

oscheoma (os″ke-o′mah) tumor of the scrotum.

oscheoplasty (os′ke-o-plas″te) plastic repair of the scrotum.

oscillation (os″ĭ-la′shun) a backward and forward motion, like a pendulum; also vibration, fluctuation or variation.

oscillogram (ŏ-sil′o-gram) a graphic record made by an oscillograph.

oscillograph (ŏ-sil′o-graf) an instrument for recording electric oscillations; such an instrument, working on the plan of a string galvanometer, is used in recording the action of the heart.

oscillometer (os″ĭ-lom′ĕ-ter) an instrument for

measuring oscillations of any kind, such as changes in the volume of the arteries accompanying the heartbeat.

oscillometry (os″ĭ-lom′ĕ-tre) the measurement of oscillations, as by the string galvanometer.

oscillopsia (os″ĭ-lop′se-ah) a visual sensation that stationary objects are swaying back and forth.

oscilloscope (ŏ-sil′o-skōp) an instrument for displaying the shape or wave form of transient or recurrent electrical signals. It is used in the electronic monitoring of heart action and other body functions.

oscitation (os″ĭ-ta′shun) the act of yawning.

osculum (os′ku-lum) an aperture or little opening.

Osgood-Schlatter disease (oz′good shlat′er) osteochondrosis of the tuberosity of the tibia.

-osis (-o′sis) word element [Gr.], *disease, morbid state; abnormal increase.*

Osler's disease (ōs′lerz) 1. polycythemia vera. 2. hereditary hemorrhagic telangiectasia.

Osler-Vaquez disease (ōs′ler vah-ka′) polycythemia vera.

osmatic (oz-mat′ik) pertaining to the sense of smell.

osmesthesia (oz″mes-the′ze-ah) the sense by which odors are perceived and distinguished.

osmics (oz′miks) the science dealing with the sense of smell.

osmidrosis (oz″mĭ-dro′sis) the secretion of foul-smelling sweat; bromhidrosis.

osmium (oz′me-um) a chemical element, atomic number 76, atomic weight 190.2, symbol Os. (See table of ELEMENTS.)

osmolality (oz″mo-lal′ĭ-te) the concentration of the solute in a solution per unit of solvent.

osmolarity (oz″mo-lar′ĭ-te) the concentration of the solute in a solution per unit of total volume of solution.

osmole (oz′mōl) the standard unit of osmotic pressure, being the amount produced by one mole of solute in a liter of water.

osmometer (oz-mom′ĕ-ter) 1. a device for testing the sense of smell. 2. an instrument for measuring osmotic pressure.

osmophilic (oz″mo-fil′ik) readily subject to osmosis.

osmophore (oz′mo-fōr) the group of atoms in a molecule of a compound that is responsible for its odor.

osmoreceptor (oz″mo-re-sep′tor) 1. a specialized sensory nerve ending sensitive to stimulation giving rise to the sensation of odors. 2. a specialized sensory nerve ending that is stimulated by changes in osmotic pressure of the surrounding medium.

osmoregulation (oz″mo-reg″u-la′shun) adjustment of internal osmotic pressure of a simple organism in relation to that of the surrounding medium.

osmoregulator (oz″mo-reg′u-la′tor) an instrument for regulating the penetrating power of roentgen rays.

osmoregulatory (oz″mo-reg′u-lah-to″re) pertaining to or accomplishing adaptation to the osmotic pressure of the surrounding medium.

osmose (oz′mōs) to pass through a membrane by osmosis.

osmosis (oz-mo′sis) the diffusion of water through a semipermeable membrane, the principal flow

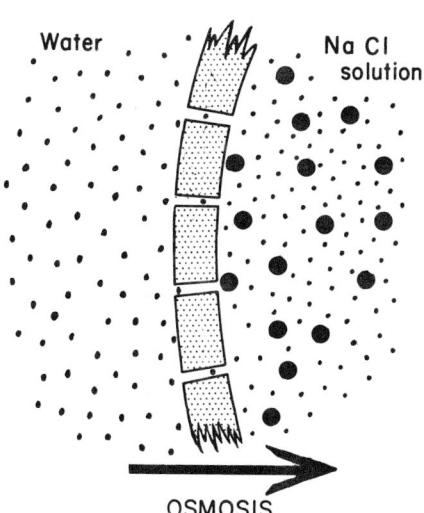

Osmosis at a cell membrane when a sodium chloride solution is placed on one side of the membrane and water on the other side. (From Guyton, A. C.: Textbook of Medical Physiology. 4th ed. Philadelphia, W. B. Saunders Co., 1971.)

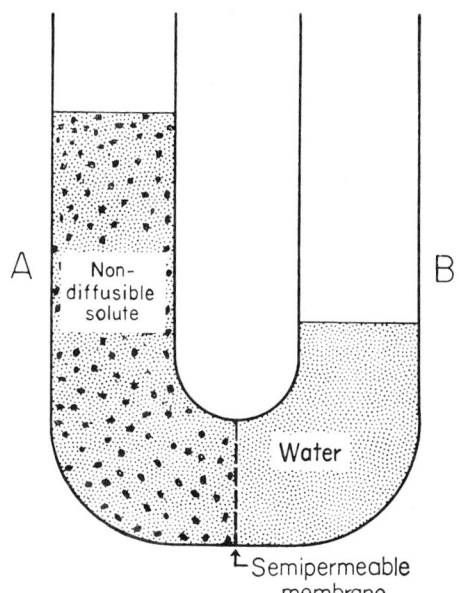

Demonstration of osmotic pressure on the two sides of a semipermeable membrane. (From Guyton, A. C.: Textbook of Medical Physiology. 4th ed. Philadelphia, W. B. Saunders Co., 1971.)

being from the less dense solution (that with a greater percentage of water) to the more dense solution. adj., **osmot'ic.**

The semipermeable membrane referred to in the definition is permeable to water and to some but not all of the dissolved solutes. The process of osmosis and the factors that influence it are important clinically in the maintenance of adequate body fluids and in the proper balance between volumes of extracellular and intracellular fluids.

The term osmotic pressure refers to the amount of pressure necessary to stop the flow of water across the membrane. The hydrostatic pressure of the water exerts an opposite effect; that is, it exerts pressure in favor of the flow of water across the membrane. The osmotic pressure of the particles in a solute depends on the relative concentrations of the solutions on either side of the membrane, and on the area of the membrane. The osmotic pressure exerted by the nondiffusible particles in a solution is determined by the numbers of particles in a unit of fluid and not by the mass of the particles.

osmosity (oz-mos'ĭ-te) a measure of the osmotic pressure of a solution, expressed numerically by the molarity.

osphresiology (os-fre″ze-ol'o-je) the science of odors and sense of smell.

osphresiometer (os-fre″ze-om'ĕ-ter) an instrument for measuring acuteness of the sense of smell.

osphresis (os-fre'sis) the sense of smell. adj., **osphret'ic.**

ossein (os'e-in) the animal matter of bone.

osseofibrous (os″e-o-fi'brus) made up of fibrous tissue and bone.

osseous (os'e-us) composed of bone.

ossicle (os'ĭ-kl) a small bone, especially one of those in the middle ear. adj., **ossic'ular.**
    auditory o's, the small bones of the middle ear: incus, malleus and stapes.

ossiculectomy (os″ĭ-ku-lek'to-me) excision of one or more of the ossicles of the middle ear.

ossiculum (ŏ-sik'u-lum), pl. *ossic'ula* [L.] ossicle.

ossiferous (ŏ-sif'er-us) producing bone.

ossific (ŏ-sif'ik) forming bone.

ossification (os″ĭ-fĭ-ka'shun) formation of or conversion into BONE.
    cartilaginous o., endochondral o., ossification that occurs in and replaces cartilage.
    intramembranous o., development of bone in and replacing connective tissue.
    perichondral o., periosteal o., that which occurs in a layered manner beneath the perichondrium, or, later, the periosteum.

ostalgia (os-tal'je-ah) pain in the bones.

oste(o)- (os'te-o) word element [Gr.], *bone.*

osteanagenesis (os″te-an″ah-jen'ĕ-sis) regeneration or reproduction of bone.

ostearthritis (os″te-ar-thri'tis) inflammation of bones and joints (see also OSTEOARTHRITIS).

ostearthrotomy (os″te-ar-throt'o-me) excision of an articular end of a bone.

ostectomy (os-tek'to-me) excision of a bone.

osteectopia (os″te-ek-to'pe-ah) displacement of a bone.

ostein (os'te-in) ossein.

osteitis (os″te-i'tis) a general term for inflammation of bone tissue. It is used to describe a number of conditions; for instance, advanced cases of syphilis can lead to syphilitic osteitis.
    o. defor'mans, a chronic bone disease of unknown origin that causes certain bones to become abnormally soft and large, and eventually deformed. The bones most commonly affected are the long bones of the legs, the lower spine, the pelvis and the skull. Called also Paget's disease.

The disease is not common and usually does not occur in persons under the age of 30. Often symptoms are so mild they are unnoticed. When symptoms do occur, the earliest one is usually pain in the affected bone. The disease disturbs the growth of new bone tissue, with the result that bones often thicken, become soft and coarsen in texture. In an advanced case, the weakened bone may be fractured by even a light blow. If the bones of the leg are affected, they become bowed under the body's weight. The person is stooped forward from spinal deformity. If the skull is affected, it may enlarge, causing headache. Nerves may be pinched by protruding bone, causing neuralgia or even deafness or blindness.

In most cases of Paget's disease of the bone, no treatment is necessary. When there are complications, these can be treated, but almost all patients with this form of osteitis can expect to live out their normal life span.
    o. fibro'sa cys'tica, bone inflammation with fibrous changes in the marrow spaces and replacement of bone by fibrous tissue. When the disease is generalized, all the bones are affected (von Recklinghausen's disease). The cause frequently is overfunctioning of the parathyroid glands, or an active tumor (adenoma) of these glands, in which case treatment includes surgical removal of the tumor. Orthopedic surgery may be necessary to correct severe bone deformities.
    o. fragil'itans, osteogenesis imperfecta.
    gummatous o., a chronic form with syphilitic gummas.
    rarefying o., a bone disease in which the inorganic matter is diminished and the hard bone becomes cancellated.
    vascular o., rarefying osteitis in which the spaces formed become occupied by blood vessels.

ostempyesis (ost″em-pi-e'sis) suppuration within a bone.

osteoarthritis (os″te-o-ar-thri'tis) hypertrophic degeneration of joints that is part of the normal aging process; called also degenerative joint disease.

Osteoarthritis, as part of aging, is most likely to strike the joints that receive the most use or stress over the years. These include the knees, the joints of the big toes and those of the lower part of the spine. Another common form of osteoarthritis affects the distal joints of the fingers; this form usually occurs in women.

Symptoms vary from mild to severe, depending on the amount of degeneration that has taken place.

Osteoarthritis is caused by disintegration of the cartilage that covers the ends of the bones. As the cartilage wears away, the roughened surface of the bone is exposed, and pain and stiffness result. In severe cases the center of the bone wears away and a bony ridge is left around the edges. This ridge may restrict movement of the joint. Osteoarthritis is less crippling than rheumatoid arthritis, in which two bone surfaces may fuse, completely immobilizing the joint.

Treatment is aimed at preventing crippling deformities, relieving pain and maintaining motion of the joint (see also treatment of ARTHRITIS).

osteoarthropathy (os"te-o-ar-throp'ah-the) any disease of the joints and bones.

hypertrophic o., osteoarthritis associated with clubbing of fingers and toes and periostosis of shafts of cylindrical bones of the extremities, often secondary to chronic conditions of the lungs and heart; called also pulmonary or secondary hypertrophic osteoarthropathy.

osteoarthrotomy (os"te-o-ar-throt'o-me) ostearthrotomy.

osteoblast (os'te-o-blast") an immature bone-producing cell.

osteoblastoma (os"te-o-blas-to'mah) a tumor whose cells tend to differentiate into bone cells.

osteocampsia (os"te-o-kamp'se-ah) curvature of a bone.

osteocarcinoma (os"te-o-kar'sĭ-no'mah) 1. osteoma combined with carcinoma. 2. carcinoma of a bone.

osteochondritis (os"te-o-kon-dri'tis) inflammation of bone and cartilage.

o. defor'mans juveni'lis, degeneration of the epiphysis of a bone due to interference with its blood supply.

o. defor'mans juveni'lis dor'si, osteochondrosis of vertebrae.

o. dis'secans, osteochondritis resulting in the splitting of pieces of cartilage into the joint, particularly the knee joint or shoulder joint. The fragment of cartilage is called a joint mouse.

osteochondrodystrophy (os"te-o-kon"dro-dis'-tro-fe) a disorder of bone and cartilage formation.

familial o., a disorder of bone and cartilage appearing between the ages of 1 and 4 years, causing shortness of stature, and thought to be transmitted by a recessive gene.

osteochondrofibroma (os"te-o-kon"dro-fi-bro'-mah) a tumor containing osseous, cartilaginous and fibrous elements.

osteochondrolysis (os"te-o-kon-drol'ĭ-sis) osteochondritis dissecans.

osteochondroma (os"te-o-kon-dro'mah) a benign bone tumor consisting of projecting adult bone capped by cartilage.

osteochondromatosis (os"te-o-kon"dro-mah-to'-sis) the occurrence of multiple osteochondromas.

synovial o., a condition in which cartilage bodies are formed in the synovial membrane of the joints, tendon sheaths or bursae, and later undergo secondary calcification and ossification.

osteochondropathy (os"te-o-kon-drop'ah-the)

any morbid condition involving both bone and cartilage, or marked by abnormal endochondral ossification.

osteochondrophyte (os"te-o-kon'dro-fīt) a tumor of cartilage and bone.

osteochondrosarcoma (os"te-o-kon"dro-sar-ko'-mah) an osteosarcoma containing considerable cartilage.

osteochondrosis (os"te-o-kon-dro'sis) a disorder of a bony epiphysis due to interference with the blood supply in children; known by various names, depending on the bone involved.

osteoclasis (os"te-ok'lah-sis) surgical fracture of a bone.

osteoclast (os'te-o-klast") 1. a surgical instrument used for fracturing bone. 2. a large, multinuclear cell frequently associated with resorption of bone.

osteoclastoma (os"te-o-klas-to'mah) a bone tumor composed of giant cells.

osteocope (os'te-o-kōp") severe pain in a bone, a symptom of syphilitic bone disease.

osteocranium (os"te-o-kra'ne-um) the fetal skull during the period of ossification, from early in the third month of gestation.

osteocystoma (os"te-o-sis-to'mah) a cystic tumor in bone.

osteocyte (os'te-o-sīt") one of the cells lodged in flat, oval cavities in bone, communicating with each other by cytoplasmic processes.

osteodentin (os"te-o-den'tin) dentin that resembles bone.

osteodermia (os"te-o-der'me-ah) a condition characterized by bony deposits in the skin.

osteodynia (os"te-o-din'e-ah) pain in a bone.

osteodystrophy (os"te-o-dis'tro-fe) abnormal development of bone.

renal o., a condition due to chronic renal disease, and marked by hyperactivity of the parathyroid glands, resulting in deossification of previously normally mineralized bone.

osteo-epiphysis (os"te-o-e-pif'ĭ-sis) a bony epiphysis.

osteofibroma (os"te-o-fi-bro'mah) a tumor of osseous and fibrous tissues.

osteogen (os'te-o-jen") the substance composing the inner layer of the periosteum, from which bone is formed.

osteogenesis (os"te-o-jen'ĕ-sis) the development of the bones.

o. imperfec'ta, a congenital condition with skeletal deformity due to imperfect formation and mineralization of bone. The bones are abnormally brittle and fracture easily.

osteogenic (os"te-o-jen'ik) 1. forming bone. 2. arising from bone.

osteogeny (os"te-oj'ĕ-ne) osteogenesis.

osteography (os″te-og′rah-fe) description of the bones.

osteohalisteresis (os″te-o-hah-lis″ter-e′sis) deficiency in mineral elements of bone.

osteoid (os′te-oid) 1. resembling bone. 2. the organic matrix of bone; young bone that has not undergone calcification.

osteology (os″te-ol′o-je) scientific study of the bones.

osteolysis (os″te-ol′ĭ-sis) dissolution of bone; applied especially to the removal or loss of calcium from the bone.

osteoma (os″te-o′mah) a tumor, benign or malignant, composed of bone.

BENIGN OSTEOMA. Benign tumors of bone are slow growing and often cause no symptoms. They frequently are first noticed as a swelling in the area; if they involve the joints symptoms result from decreased mobility. As the tumor develops, the patient experiences pain and tenderness, and pathologic fractures are not uncommon with large tumors. Treatment includes surgical removal of the tumor and repair of the affected bone. Some benign tumors require no treatment.

MALIGNANT OSTEOMA. Malignant bone tumors that arise from the bone (sarcoma) are rare, only about 15 occurring per million persons. They are found most often in children and young adults.

Cancer that spreads to bone tissue from other parts of the body usually is carcinoma rather than sarcoma.

Cancer of the bone can spread to other organs of the body through the blood and lymph channels. It tends to metastasize to the lungs, and from the lungs to the brain or the organs of the abdomen.

Symptoms. Symptoms of bone cancer are pain, swelling and disability in the area of the diseased bones. The pain at first is mild, stops and starts again and then becomes increasingly severe. Swelling may appear soon after the first signs of pain, but often it cannot be seen until later. The disability may affect a nearby joint, such as the knee, shoulder or hip. There may also be a hard, painful lump over which the skin moves freely. The skin temperature in the area may be slightly elevated.

Diagnosis and Treatment. Diagnosis of bone tumor is made after examination of x-ray film and a microscopic study of the suspected tissue. Malignant tumors can be treated by radiotherapy and surgery during the early stage of development. The prognosis for these tumors is grave, however. Hormone therapy and medication can also be helpful in certain types of the disease.

   o. du′rum, o. ebur′neum, one containing hard bony tissue.

   o. medulla′re, one containing marrow spaces.

   osteoid o., a benign bone tumor consisting of osteoid tissue surrounded by sclerotic, reactive bone.

   o. spongio′sum, one containing cancellated bone.

osteomalacia (os″te-o-mah-la′she-ah) softening of the bones, resulting from a disturbance of calcium and phosphorus metabolism caused by a vitamin D deficiency in adults. A similar condition in children is called RICKETS. The deficiency may be due to lack of exposure to ultraviolet rays, inadequate intake of vitamin D in the diet or failure to absorb or utilize vitamin D.

The disease is characterized by decalcification of the bones, particularly those of the spine, pelvis and lower extremities. X-ray examination reveals transverse, fracture-like lines in the affected bones and areas of demineralization in the matrix of the bone. As the bones soften they become bent, flattened or otherwise deformed.

Treatment consists of administration of large daily doses of vitamin D and dietary measures to insure adequate calcium and phosphorus intake.

osteomatoid (os″te-o′mah-toid) resembling an osteoma.

osteomere (os′te-o-mēr″) one of a series of similar bony structures, such as the vertebrae.

osteometry (os″te-om′ĕ-tre) measurement of the bones.

osteomyelitis (os″te-o-mi″ĕ-li′tis) inflammation of bone caused by a pyogenic microorganism. It may result in bone destruction, in stiffening of joints if the infection spreads to the joints and, in extreme cases occurring before the end of the growth period, in the shortening of a leg if the growth center is destroyed.

Acute osteomyelitis is caused by bacteria that enter the body through a wound, spread from an infection near the bone or come from a skin or throat infection. The infection usually affects the long bones of the arms and legs and causes acute pain and fever. It most often occurs in children and adolescents, particularly boys.

The onset may be quite sudden, with chills, high fever and severe pain. Signs and symptoms include a marked increase in leukocytes, tenderness, swelling and redness of the skin over the bone involved and bacteremia. About 10 to 14 days after the onset of symptoms, x-rays show signs of the bone infection.

Usually, antibiotic treatment will clear the infection. If not, the infection destroys areas of the bone involved and an abscess forms. Acute osteomyelitis may become chronic, especially if the patient has a low resistance to infection.

Tuberculous osteomyelitis is caused by tubercle bacilli that enter the bloodstream and settle in a bone. The disease progresses slowly and is chronic. Any bone may be infected but those most commonly involved are the vertebrae. Spinal tuberculosis, or POTT'S DISEASE, causes bone destruction and often spinal deformities. Other bones that may be affected are the long bones of the hands or feet.

TREATMENT. Treatment of acute osteomyelitis consists of administration of antibiotics and sometimes surgical drainage of the abscess. Fragments of dead bone (sequestra) that remain and prevent healing must be removed surgically. If the blood supply to the bone is not obstructed, the bone can grow back. Treatment of chronic osteomyelitis is similar to that for the acute type.

Tuberculous osteomyelitis is treated like other forms of TUBERCULOSIS and sometimes by surgical drainage and immobilization of the bones involved.

NURSING CARE. Absolute rest of the affected part is essential to proper healing and prevention of deformity. Because of pain and local tenderness one must be very gentle in handling the patient. Proper positioning with pillows and sandbags helps relieve the discomfort and also keeps the affected limb in good alignment. When a cast has been applied to insure immobilization, the nursing care is the same as for any patient in a cast (see CAST). Drainage from the infected bone must be considered grossly contaminated and requires special precautions so that the infection is not spread to others.

Since most patients with osteomyelitis are children, some form of occupational therapy or diversionary activities must be devised to insure adequate rest for the affected bone. The parents must also be cautioned against letting the child indulge in strenuous exercise during the convalescent period at home. At all times during both the acute stage and the convalescent period the patient must be protected from other infections, which may result in a recurrence of symptoms. A well balanced diet, adequate periods of rest and other measures to promote the general well-being of the patient are important in overcoming the infection and preventing complications.

osteomyelodysplasia (os″te-o-mi″ĕ-lo-dis-pla′ze-ah) a condition characterized by thinning of the osseous tissue of bones, increase in size of the marrow cavities and associated leukopenia and fever.

osteomyelography (os″te-o-mi″ĕ-log′rah-fe) roentgenographic examination of bone marrow.

osteon (os′te-on) the basic unit of structure of compact bone, comprising a haversian canal and its concentrically arranged lamellae.

osteoncus (os″te-ong′kus) tumor of a bone.

osteonecrosis (os″te-o-nĕ-kro′sis) necrosis of a bone.

osteopath (os′te-o-path″) one who treats diseases by manipulation of the bones; a practitioner of OSTEOPATHY.

osteopathia (os″te-o-path′e-ah) osteopathy(1).
　o. **conden′sans dissemina′ta,** osteopoikilosis.
　o. **stria′ta,** an asymptomatic condition characterized radiographically by multiple condensations of cancellous bone tissue, giving a striated appearance.

osteopathology (os″te-o-pah-thol′o-je) any disease of bone.

osteopathy (os″te-op′ah-the) 1. any disease of a bone. 2. a system of therapy utilizing generally accepted physical, medicinal and surgical methods of diagnosis and therapy, and emphasizing the importance of normal body mechanics and manipulative methods of detecting and correcting faulty structure. adj., **osteopath′ic.**

Osteopathy is founded on the theory that the body will produce the remedies necessary to protect itself so long as the bones are aligned properly and do not press on nerves.

During the past few decades, many changes have been made in the practice of osteopathy, bringing it closely into line with conventional medical practices. While still holding to the tenet that the body is a unit that possesses the inherent ability to overcome most curable diseases, osteopaths recognize that physical, chemical and nutritional factors influence the state of health and that medicines and surgery are necessary in the treatment of disease. Disorders that can be recognized are treated as

distinct diseases, and manipulation may or may not be used as an adjunct to other treatment.
　hunger o., disturbances of the skeletal system observed in famine areas, characterized by a reduction in the amount of normally calcified bone.

osteopecilia (os″te-o-pe-sil′e-ah) osteopoikilosis.

osteopedion (os″te-o-pe′de-on) a dead fetus that has become stony or petrified.

osteoperiosteal (os″te-o-per″e-os′te-al) pertaining to bone and periosteum.

osteoperiostitis (os″te-o-per″e-os-ti′tis) inflammation of a bone and its periosteum.

osteopetrosis (os″te-o-pĕ-tro′sis) a condition in which there are bandlike areas of condensed bone at the epiphyseal lines of long bones and condensation of the edges of smaller bones; called also Albers-Schönberg disease and marble bones.

osteophage (os′te-o-fāj) osteoclast.

osteophlebitis (os″te-o-flĕ-bi′tis) inflammation of the veins of a bone.

osteophyma (os″te-o-fi′mah) a tumor or outgrowth of a bone.

osteophyte (os′te-o-fīt″) a bony excrescence or outgrowth.

osteoplasty (os′te-o-plas″te) plastic surgery of the bones.

osteopoikilosis (os″te-o-poi″kī-lo′sis) a mottled condition of bones, apparent radiographically and due to the presence of multiple sclerotic foci.

osteoporosis (os″te-o-po-ro′sis) a metabolic bone disease in which there is a failure of osteoblasts to lay down bone matrix. adj., **osteoporot′ic.** The condition leads to thinning of the skeleton and decreased precipitation of lime salts. There also may be inadequate calcium absorption into the bone and excessive bone resorption.

The principal causes are lack of physical activity, lack of estrogens or androgens and possibly a chronic low intake of calcium. There is almost always some degree of osteoporosis in senility. The condition may accompany endocrine disorders, bone marrow disorders and nutritional disturbances.

Symptoms include pathologic fractures and collapse of the vertebrae without compression of the spinal cord. The latter is often discovered "accidentally" on x-ray examination made for some other reason.

Treatment varies with the cause but hormone therapy is helpful in most cases. Measures are taken to improve the nutritional status, and a diet high in protein and calcium is recommended. Patients should be kept active and those confined to bed must be given passive and active exercises. Prognosis usually is good when treatment is carried out diligently.
　adipose o., that in which the enlarged spaces are filled with fat.
　o. **circumscrip′ta,** demineralization occurring in localized areas of bone, especially in the skull.
　o. **of disuse,** that occurring when the normal laying down of bone is slowed because of lack of the normal stimulus of functional stress on the bone.

osteopsathyrosis (os″te-op-sath″ĭ-ro′sis) osteogenesis imperfecta.

osteoradionecrosis (os″te-o-ra″de-o-nĕ-kro′sis) necrosis of bone as a result of excessive exposure to radiation.

osteorrhagia (os″te-o-ra′je-ah) hemorrhage from bone.

osteorrhaphy (os″te-or′ah-fe) fixation of fragments of bone with sutures or wires.

osteosarcoma (os″te-o-sar-ko′mah) a malignant tumor arising from undifferentiated fibrous tissue of bone. adj., **osteosarco′matous.**

osteosclerosis (os″te-o-sklĕ-ro′sis) abnormal hardness of bone; osteopetrosis. adj., **osteosclerot′ic.**
    o. **congen′ita,** achondroplasia.
    o. **frag′ilis,** osteopetrosis; so called because of frequency of pathologic fracture of affected bones.
    o. **frag′ilis generalisa′ta,** osteopoikilosis.
    o. **myelofibrosis,** a condition of excessive erythroblastic activity of the bone marrow characterized by fibrotic changes in the blood vessels of the marrow and calcification of the bones.

osteoseptum (os″te-o-sep′tum) the bony part of the nasal septum.

osteosis (os″te-o′sis) the formation of bony tissue.

osteospongioma (os″te-o-spun″je-o′mah) a spongy tumor of bone.

osteostixis (os″te-o-stik′sis) surgical puncture of a bone.

osteosuture (os″te-o-su′tūr) osteorrhaphy.

osteosynovitis (os″te-o-sin″o-vi′tis) synovitis with osteitis of neighboring bones.

osteosynthesis (os″te-o-sin′thĕ-sis) surgical fastening of the ends of a fractured bone.

osteotabes (os″te-o-ta′bēz) a disease, chiefly of infants, in which bone marrow cells are destroyed and the marrow disappears.

osteothrombophlebitis (os″te-o-throm″bo-flĕ-bi′tis) inflammation through intact bone by a progressive thrombophlebitis of small venules.

osteothrombosis (os″te-o-throm-bo′sis) thrombosis of the veins of a bone.

osteotome (os′te-o-tōm″) a knife or chisel for cutting bone.

osteotomy (os″te-ot′o-me) the surgical cutting of a bone.
    cuneiform o., removal of a wedge of bone.
    linear o., the sawing or simple cutting of a bone.

osteotrite (os′te-o-trīt″) an instrument for scraping away diseased bone.

ostitis (os-ti′tis) osteitis.

ostium (os′te-um), pl. *os′tia* [L.] a door, or opening; used in anatomic nomenclature as a general term to designate an opening into a tubular organ, or between two distinct body cavities. Called also orifice and opening. adj., **os′tial.**

o. **abdomina′le,** the fimbriated end of the uterine tube.
    o. **inter′num,** the uterine end of the uterine tube.
    o. **pharyn′geum,** the nasopharyngeal end of the eustachian tube.
    o. **pri′mum,** an opening in the lower portion of the membrane dividing the embryonic heart into right and left sides.
    o. **secun′dum,** an opening in the upper portion of the membrane dividing the embryonic heart into right and left sides, appearing later than the ostium primum.
    o. **tympan′icum,** the tympanic end of the eustachian tube.
    o. **u′teri,** the opening of the cervix of the uterus into the vagina.
    o. **vagi′nae,** the external orifice of the vagina.

O.T. occupational therapy; old tuberculin.

otalgia (o-tal′je-ah) pain in the ear.

OTC over the counter; applied to drugs not required by law to be sold on prescription only.

otectomy (o-tek′to-me) excision of tissues of internal and middle ear.

othelcosis (ōt″hel-ko′sis) suppuration of the ear.

othemorrhea (ōt″hem-o-re′ah) flow of blood from the ear.

otiatrics (o″te-at′riks) the science and treatment of ear diseases.

otic (o′tik) pertaining to the ear.

oticodinia (o″tĭ-ko-din′e-ah) vertigo from ear disease.

otitis (o-ti′tis) inflammation of the ear. adj., **otit′ic.**
    aviation o., inflammation of the middle ear due to changes in air pressure; called also aero-otitis media.
    o. **exter′na,** inflammation of external ear.
    furuncular o., the formation of furuncles in the external acoustic meatus.
    o. **inter′na,** inflammation of the inner ear.
    o. **labyrin′thica,** inflammation of the labyrinth.
    o. **mastoi′dea,** inflammation of the mastoid antra.
    o. **me′dia,** inflammation of the middle ear. It occurs most commonly in infants and young children and frequently follows or accompanies an upper respiratory infection. The condition may be acute or chronic.
    ACUTE OTITIS MEDIA. The principal symptoms are earache, loss of hearing, fever and a feeling of fullness and pressure in the ear. As the infection progresses pressure builds up behind the tympanic membrane (eardrum) and may cause perforation or rupture of it. This is followed by drainage of exudate into the external acoustic meatus.
    Treatment consists of bed rest, analgesics to relieve the pain and systemic antibiotics. Surgical incision into the eardrum (myringotomy) may be necessary to relieve pressure and promote drainage. If acute otitis media is treated promptly it resolves with rare exception. If it is not treated successfully it will develop into chronic otitis media and the infection may spread to the mastoid cells, causing mastoiditis.
    CHRONIC OTITIS MEDIA. This condition is almost always associated with perforation of the ear-

drum. It may complicate an upper respiratory disease or be associated with mastoiditis. Drainage from the ear, ringing in the ear and loss of hearing are frequent symptoms.

Treatment is aimed at relief of the primary source of infection, which may be chronic sinusitis, enlarged tonsils and adenoids, nasal polyps or nasal allergy. Antibiotic drugs and antiseptic or antibiotic ear drops are used to treat the infection. If suppuration continues and the mastoid process becomes involved, MASTOIDECTOMY is done.

o. sclerot'ica, otitis marked by hardening of the ear structures.

otoantritis (o″to-an-tri'tis) inflammation of the attic of the tympanum and the mastoid antrum.

Otobius (o-to'be-us) a genus of arthropods (family Argasidae) parasitic in the ears of various animals and known also to bite man.

otoblennorrhea (o″to-blen″o-re'ah) mucous discharge from the ear.

otocephalus (o″to-sef'ah-lus) a fetal monster lacking the lower jaw and having ears united below the face.

otocleisis (o″to-kli'sis) closure of the auditory passages.

otoconia (o″to-ko'ne-ah) a dustlike substance made up of calcium carbonate, found in the membranous labyrinth of the inner ear.

otocyst (o'to-sist) 1. the auditory vesicle of the embryo. 2. the organ of hearing in invertebrates.

Otodectes (o″to-dek'tēz) a genus of mites that may be parasitic on man.

otodynia (o″to-din'e-ah) pain in the ear; earache.

otoencephalitis (o″to-en-sef″ah-li'tis) inflammation of brain extending from the middle ear.

otoganglion (o″to-gang'gle-on) the otic ganglion.

otography (o-tog'rah-fe) description of the ear.

otolaryngology (o″to-lar″ing-gol'o-je) otology and laryngology regarded as a single specialty.

otolith (o'to-lith) otoconia.

otologist (o-tol'o-jist) a specialist in otology.

otology (o-tol'o-je) the branch of medicine dealing with the ear and its diseases.

otomassage (o″to-mah-sahzh') massage of the middle ear and ossicles.

Oto-microscope (o″to-mi'kro-skop) trademark for an operating microscope devised to improve visualization of the surgical field in operations on the ear.

Otomyces (o″to-mi'sēz) a genus of fungi infecting the ear.

otomycosis (o″to-mi-ko'sis) a fungal infection of the outer ear. The infection thrives in warm, moist climates and is encouraged by poor local hygiene and swimming. Symptoms include itching, which may be intense, pain and a stinging sensation in the external acoustic meatus.

The condition is treated with antibiotics to prevent secondary infection and the administration of ear drops containing neomycin or polymyxin B sulfate. The area should be cleaned locally with dilute aluminum acetate solution combined with acetic acid before ear drops are applied.

otopathy (o-top'ah-the) any disease of the ear.

otoplasty (o'to-plas″te) plastic repair of the ear.

otopolypus (o″to-pol'ĭ-pus) a polyp in the ear.

otopyorrhea (o″to-pi″o-re'ah) purulent discharge from the ear.

otorhinolaryngology (o″to-ri″no-lar″ing-gol'o-je) the branch of medicine dealing with the ear, nose and throat.

otorhinology (o″to-ri-nol'o-je) the branch of medicine dealing with the ear and nose.

otorrhagia (o″to-ra'je-ah) hemorrhage from the ear.

otorrhea (o″to-re'ah) a discharge from the ear.

otosalpinx (o″to-sal'pinks) the auditory tube, or eustachian tube.

otosclerosis (o″to-sklĕ-ro'sis) the formation of spongy bone in the inner ear, often causing the auditory ossicles to become fixed and less able to pass on vibrations when sound enters the ear. adj., **otosclerot'ic.** The ossicle chiefly involved in the condition is the stirrup or stapes, which becomes fixed to the oval window.

The cause of otosclerosis is still unknown. It may be hereditary, or perhaps related to vitamin deficiency or otitis media. An early symptom is ringing in the ears, but the most noticeable symptom is progressive loss of hearing.

This disease usually begins in the teens or early twenties. It strikes women about twice as often as men, and may be worsened by pregnancy. Approximately 10 million people in the United States are affected to a greater or lesser degree by otosclerosis.

Although no cure is known, recently developed surgical techniques can often restore hearing by freeing the stirrup or replacing it with other tissue. In this operation, STAPEDECTOMY, the stirrup is removed and replaced with grafted body tissue attached to a stainless steel wire or plastic tube.

In some cases of otosclerosis the hearing loss may be relieved by the use of a hearing aid.

otoscope (o'to-skōp) an instrument for inspecting or auscultating the ear.

otoscopy (o-tos'ko-pe) examination of the external acoustic meatus with an otoscope.

otosteal (o-tos'te-al) pertaining to the small bones of the ear.

ototomy (o-tot'o-me) dissection of the ear.

ototoxic (o″to-tok'sik) having a deleterious effect upon the eighth cranial (vestibulocochlear) nerve or on the organs of hearing and balance.

ototoxicity (o″to-tok-sis'ĭ-te) the property of exerting deleterious effects upon the ear or the sense of hearing.

Otrivin (o'trĭ-vin) trademark for preparations of xylometazoline hydrochloride, a nasal decongestant.

O.U. 1. [L.] *oc'uli u'nitas* (both eyes together). 2. [L.] *oc'uli uter'que* (each eye).

ouabain (wah-ba'in) a glycoside obtained from a plant, used for its stimulating effect upon the heart. Its effect is similar to that of digitalis.

ounce (owns) a measure of weight in both the avoirdupois and the apothecaries' system; abbreviation oz. The ounce avoirdupois is one-sixteenth of a pound, or 437.5 grains (28.3495 Gm.). The apothecaries' ounce is one-twelfth of a pound, or 480 grains (31.103 Gm); symbol ℥. (See also Table of Weights and Measures in the Appendix.)
    fluid o., a unit of liquid measure of the apothecaries' system, being 8 fluid drams, or the equivalent of 29.57 ml.

outlay (owt'la) a graft applied to the surface of an organ or structure.

outlimb (owt'lim) the distal part or segment of an extremity.

outpatient (owt-pa'shent) a patient who comes to the hospital, clinic or dispensary for diagnosis and/or treatment but does not occupy a bed.

outpocketing (owt-pok'et-ing) 1. evagination. 2. enclosure of the distal end of a pedicle flap within an opening made in the body tissues.

output (owt'poot) the yield or total of anything produced; substance eliminated from the body, usually expressed as quantity per unit of time.
    cardiac o., the quantity of blood ejected from the heart per unit of time, being the product of stroke volume times the number of beats in the interval.
    energy o., the energy a body is able to manifest in work or activity.
    stroke o., the amount of blood ejected by each ventricle at each beat of the heart.
    urinary o., the amount of urine secreted by the kidneys.

ova (o'vah) plural of *ovum.*

ovalbumin (ov"al-bu'min) albumin from the whites of eggs.

ovalocyte (o'vah-lo-sīt") elliptocyte, an oval erythrocyte.

ovari(o)- (o-va're-o) word element [L.], *ovary.* See also words beginning *oophor(o)-*.

ovarialgia (o-va"re-al'je-ah) pain in an ovary.

ovarian (o-va're-an) pertaining to an ovary.

ovariectomy (o-va"re-ek'to-me) excision of an ovary (see also OOPHORECTOMY).

ovariocele (o-va're-o-sēl") hernia of an ovary.

ovariocentesis (o-va"re-o-sen-te'sis) surgical puncture of an ovary.

ovariocyesis (o-va"re-o-si-e'sis) ovarian pregnancy.

ovariorrhexis (o-va"re-o-rek'sis) rupture of an ovary.

ovariosalpingectomy (o-va"re-o-sal"pin-jek'to-me) excision of an ovary and uterine tube.

ovariostomy (o-va"re-os'to-me) incision of an ovary, with drainage.

ovariotomy (o-va"re-ot'o-me) surgical removal of an ovary, or removal of an ovarian tumor.

ovariotubal (o-va"re-o-tu'bal) pertaining to an ovary and uterine tube.

ovaritis (o"vah-ri'tis) inflammation of an ovary.

ovarium (o-va're-um), pl. *ova'ria* [L.] ovary.

ovary (o'var-e) the sex gland in the female in which the ova are formed. Almond-shaped and about the size of large walnuts, the two ovaries are located in the lower abdomen on either side of the uterus.
    FUNCTIONS OF THE OVARIES. The ovaries have two basic functions: ovulation and the production of hormones, chiefly estrogen and progesterone, which influence a woman's feminine physical characteristics and affect the reproductive process. (See also OVULATION and REPRODUCTION.)
    DISORDERS OF THE OVARIES. One of the commonest disorders of the ovary is a cyst. Not all so-called ovarian cysts are true cysts; many are tumors. Ovarian cysts occur frequently and in a variety of sizes and types.
    The commonest ovarian cysts are simple follicle retention cysts, small and frequently numerous cysts containing a clear fluid. Ordinarily follicle cysts disappear without treatment within 2 months. They do not change into malignant growths.
    Another type of ovarian cyst, the mucinous cystadenoma, is in reality a tumor. These tumors may reach enormous size, creating pressure within the abdominopelvic cavity. Although these tumors are benign, they may become malignant.
    DERMOID CYSTS of the ovary are usually benign although they may be subject to malignant change. They grow slowly and when opened after removal are found to be filled with a thick, yellow sebaceous fluid. Hair, teeth, bone and other kinds of tissues are often found partially developed in the cyst.
    Oophoritis (inflammation of an ovary) may be caused by infection reaching the ovary by way of the uterine tube. Tuberculous and streptococcal infections of the ovary are common, and the ovary may also become infected in GONORRHEA. Fever and pain, sometimes accompanied by swelling, are the usual symptoms. Sulfonamides and antibiotics usually can eliminate the infection, but if it fails to respond to treatment, surgery may become necessary. Surgical removal of an ovary is called OOPHORECTOMY, or ovariectomy.
    Tumors of the ovary are generally classified as malignant or benign. They may arise from misplaced endometrial tissue or from the ovarian tissues. Malignant cells from other organs may travel to the ovary and set up a secondary malignant tumor in the ovary; an example is Krukenberg's tumor, which usually originates in the stomach.
    Symptoms of an ovarian tumor usually do not present themselves until the tumor is fairly well advanced. Tumors in the early stage are usually found during a routine examination. Treatment of these tumors in all stages involves surgical removal or the use of radiotherapy or a combination of the two.

overbite (o'ver-bīt) extension of incisal ridges of the upper anterior teeth below the incisal ridges of the anterior teeth in the lower jaw when the jaws are closed normally.

overcompensation (o″ver-kom″pen-sa′shun) exaggerated correction of a real or imagined physical or psychologic defect.

overhydration (o″ver-hi-dra′shun) a state of excess fluids in the body.

overjet (o′ver-jet) extension of the incisal or buccal cusp ridges of the upper teeth labially or buccally to the ridges of the teeth in the lower jaw when the jaws are closed normally.

overlay (o′ver-la) a later component superimposed on a preexisting state or condition.
   psychogenic o., an emotionally determined increment to a preexisting symptom or disability of organic or physically traumatic origin.

overventilation (o″ver-ven″tī-la′shun) hyperventilation.

ovi (o′vi) [L.] genitive of *ovum.*
   o. albu′min, the white of an egg.
   o. vitel′lus, the yolk of an egg.

oviduct (o′vĭ-dukt) a tube for the passage of ova; a UTERINE TUBE. adj., **ovidu′cal.**

oviferous (o-vif′er-us) producing or conveying ova.

ovigenesis (o″vĭ-jen′ĕ-sis) oogenesis. adj., **ovigenet′ic.**

ovine (o′vīn) pertaining to or derived from sheep.

oviparous (o-vip′ah-rus) producing eggs in which the embryo develops outside of the maternal body.

ovisac (o′vĭ-sak) a graafian follicle.

Ovocylin (o″vo-sil′in) trademark for a preparation of estradiol, an estrogenic compound.

ovoflavin (o″vo-fla′vin) riboflavin derived from eggs.

ovoglobulin (o″vo-glob′u-lin) the globulin of white of egg.

ovolytic (o″vo-lit′ik) splitting up egg albumin.

ovomucoid (o″vo-mu′koid) a mucoid principle from egg albumin.

ovotestis (o″vo-tes′tis) a gonad containing both testicular and ovarian tissue.

ovoviviparous (o″vo-vi-vip′ah-rus) bearing living young that hatch from eggs inside the body of the maternal organism, the embryo being nourished by food stored in the egg.

ovulation (o″vu-la′shun) the process in which an ovum is discharged from an ovary. Normally, in an adult woman, ovulation occurs at intervals of about 28 days and alternates between the two ovaries. As a rule, only one ovum is produced, but occasionally ovulation produces two or more ova; if such ova subsequently become fertilized, the result may be multiple births, such as twins or triplets.
   Ovulation takes place approximately at the midpoint of the menstrual cycle, 14 days after the onset of menstruation. During the preceding weeks, a GRAAFIAN FOLLICLE, or cell cluster in the ovary containing the ovum, grows from the size of a pinhead to that of a pea. At the moment of ovulation, the follicle bursts open and the ovum is discharged.
   The discharged ovum enters the uterine tube adjoining the ovary and moves toward the uterus; if it encounters a spermatozoon while it is still alive (about 48 hours), the two merge. Fertilization usually takes place in the uterine tube. The fertilized ovum then makes its way to the uterus where it becomes embedded in the prepared wall as the first stage of growth of the new infant (see also

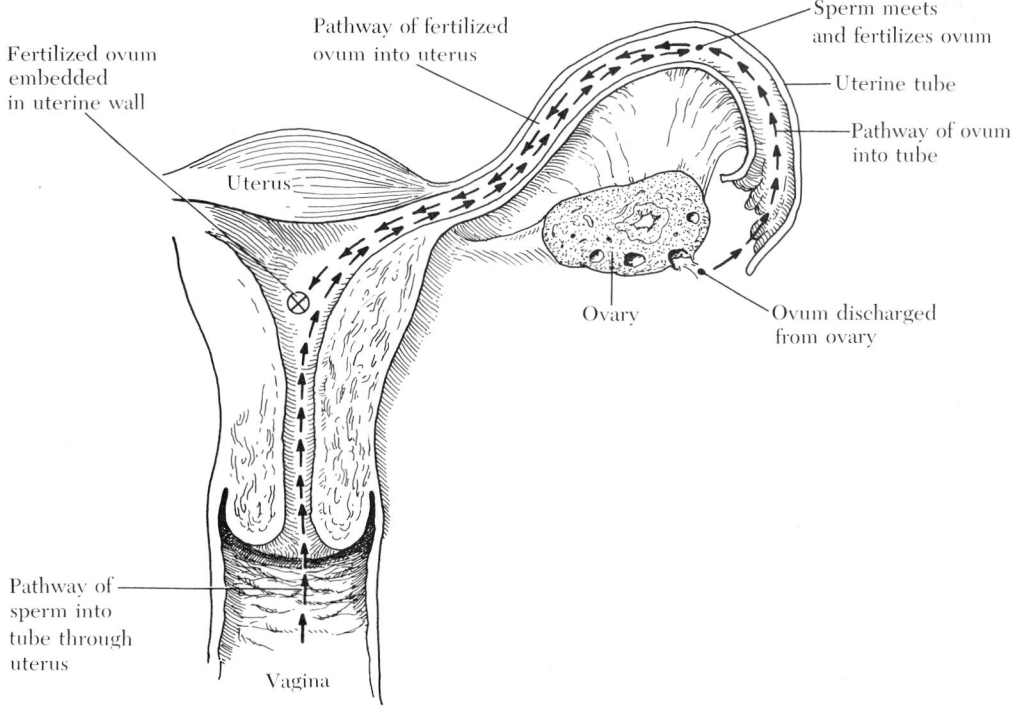

Ovulation.

REPRODUCTION). If fertilization does not take place the ovum loses its vitality and the blood and tissue lining the uterus are shed in the menstrual flow.

ovule (o'vūl) the ovum in the ovary, or any small egglike structure.
　primitive o., primordial o., a rudimentary ovum in the ovary.

ovulum (ov'u-lum), pl. *ov'ula* [L.] an ovule.

ovum (o'vum), pl. *o'va* [L.] egg; the female reproductive element that may develop into a new organism; sometimes applied to any stage of the fertilized germ cell during cleavage and even until hatching or birth of the new individual. The human ovum consists of protoplasm that contains some yolk, enclosed by a cell wall consisting of two layers, an outer one (zona pellucida, zona radiata) and an inner, thin one (vitelline membrane). There is a large nucleus (germinal vesicle), within which is a nucleolus (germinal spot). adj., **o'vular.**
　alecithal o., one with no or very little food yolk.
　blighted o., a fertilized ovum in which development has become arrested.
　centrolecithal o., one with the yolk concentrated at the center of the egg, surrounded by a thin layer of cytoplasm.
　holoblastic o., one that undergoes total cleavage.
　isolecithal o., one with a small amount of yolk evenly distributed throughout the cytoplasm.
　meroblastic o., one that undergoes partial cleavage.
　permanent o., the mature ovum ready for fertilization.
　primitive o., primordial o., any egg cell that may eventually become an oocyte within the graafian follicle.
　telolecithal o., one with a comparatively large amount of yolk massed at one pole.

Owren's disease (ow'renz) parahemophilia.

oxacillin (ok″sah-sil'in) a semisynthetic penicillin that is relatively stable in an acid medium and resistant to inactivation by penicillinase, and therefore effective against staphylococci.

Oxaine (ok'sān) trademark for a preparation of oxethazine, a gastric mucosal anesthetic, antacid and demulcent.

oxalate (ok'sah-lāt) a salt of oxalic acid.
　potassium o., colorless, odorless crystals used extensively as a reagent.
　sodium o., a white, odorless, crystalline powder, formerly used as an anticoagulant in collection of blood for laboratory examination.

oxalemia (ok″sah-le'me-ah) excess of oxalates in the blood.

oxalic acid (ok-sal'ik) a poisonous, crystalline, dibasic acid found in various fruits and vegetables, and formed in the metabolism of ascorbic acid in the body; used as a disinfectant for the skin (especially by surgeons "scrubbing" for surgery) and in removing such stains as iron rust and ink. It is highly toxic and if ingested should be neutralized by the administration of lime water (calcium hydroxide solution) or other convenient source of calcium, which reacts with the acid to form insoluble calcium oxalate.

oxalism (ok'sah-lizm) poisoning by oxalic acid or by an oxalate.

oxalosis (ok″sah-lo'sis) a metabolic disorder with deposits of oxalate crystals in the kidneys and other body tissues.

oxaluria (ok″sah-lu're-ah) oxalic acid or oxalates in the urine.

oxanamide (ok-san'ah-mīd) a compound used as a tranquilizer.

oxethazaine (ok-seth'ah-zān) a compound used as a gastric mucosal anesthetic, antacid and demulcent.

oxidant (ok'sĭ-dant) the electron acceptor in an oxidation-reduction (redox) reaction.

oxidase (ok'sĭ-dās) an enzyme that catalyzes oxidation.
　cytochrome o., an oxidation-catalyzing enzyme that receives electrons transferred by a cytochrome.

oxidation (ok″sĭ-da'shun) the act of oxidizing or state of being oxidized. adj., **oxida'tive.** Chemically it consists in the increase of positive charges on an atom or the loss of negative charges. Univalent oxidation indicates loss of one electron; divalent oxidation, the loss of two electrons. The opposite reaction to oxidation is reduction.

oxide (ok'sīd) a compound of oxygen with an element or radical.

oxidize (ok'sĭ-dīz) to cause to combine with oxygen.

oxidoreductase (ok″sĭ-do-re-duk'tās) an enzyme that catalyzes the reversible transfer of electrons from one substance to another.

oxidosis (ok″sĭ-do'sis) acidosis.

oximeter (ok-sim'ĕ-ter) a photoelectric device for determining the oxygen saturation of the blood.

oxophenarsine (ok″so-fen-ar'sin) a compound formerly used in the treatment of syphilis, largely replaced by penicillin.

Oxsoralen (ok-sor'ah-len) trademark for preparations of methoxsalen, a pigment stimulant.

oxtriphylline (oks-trif'ĭ-lēn) a compound used as a mild diuretic, myocardial stimulant and smooth muscle relaxant.

oxybenzene (ok″sĭ-ben'zēn) phenol.

oxyblepsia (ok″sĭ-blep'se-ah) unusual acuity of vision.

oxybutyric acid (ok″sĭ-bu-tir'ik) an acid found in the urine and blood in diabetes mellitus.

oxycephaly (ok-sĭ-sef'ah-le) a high, pointed condition of the skull, with a vertical index of 77 or more. adj., **oxycephal'ic.**

oxychloride (ok″sĭ-klo'rīd) an element or radical combined with oxygen and chlorine.

oxychromatic (ok″sĭ-kro-mat'ik) staining with acid dyes.

oxychromatin (ok″sĭ-kro'mah-tin) that part of chromatin that stains with acid dyes.

oxycinesia (ok″sĭ-si-ne'ze-ah) pain on motion.

oxyesthesia (ok″se-es-the′ze-ah) abnormal acuteness of the senses.

oxygen (ok′sĭ-jen) a chemical element, atomic number 8, atomic weight 15.999, symbol O. (See table of ELEMENTS.) It is a colorless and odorless gas that makes up about 20 per cent of the atmosphere. In combination with hydrogen, it forms water; by weight, 90 per cent of water is oxygen. It is the most abundant of all the elements of nature. Large quantities of it are distributed throughout the solid matter of the earth, because the gas combines readily with many other elements. With carbon and hydrogen, oxygen forms the chemical basis of much organic material.

Oxygen is essential in sustaining all kinds of life. Among the higher animals, it is obtained from the air and drawn into the lungs by the process of RESPIRATION.

OXYGEN BALANCE AND "OXYGEN DEBT." The need of every cell for oxygen requires a balance in supply and demand. But this balance need not be exact at all times. In fact, in strenous exercise the oxygen needs of muscle cells are greater than the amount the body can absorb even by the most intense breathing. Thus, during athletic competition, the participants make use of the capacity of muscles to function even though their needs for oxygen are not fully met. When the competition is over, however, the athletes will continue to breathe heavily until the muscles have been supplied with sufficient oxygen. This temporary deficiency is called oxygen debt.

EFFECTS AND TREATMENT OF OXYGEN LACK. Total deprivation of the supply of oxygen to the body causes death within minutes. Severe curtailment of oxygen, as during ascent to high altitudes or in certain illnesses, may bring on a variety of symptoms of HYPOXIA, or oxygen lack. A number of poisons, among them cyanide and carbon monoxide, and also large overdoses of sedatives disrupt the oxygen distribution system of the body. Such disruption occurs also in various illnesses, such as anemia and diseases of lungs, heart, kidneys and liver. Oxygen lack due to any condition may give rise to cyanosis, a state marked by bluishness of body extremities, lips and earlobes. Other symptoms of hypoxia are physical discomfort, dyspnea and emotional upset.

To revive or treat a person suffering from hypoxia, it is usual to administer oxygen artificially. A victim of heart disease or pneumonia may be placed in an oxygen tent containing a mixture of carbon dioxide with a large proportion of oxygen. Victims of carbon monoxide poisoning are also treated with this kind of mixture. Oxygen can also be administered by means of the oxygen mask, which is placed over mouth and nose, and by nasal catheter.

NURSING CARE DURING OXYGEN THERAPY. Certain properties of oxygen require special precautions during the administration of this gas. Since oxygen supports combustion all sources of sparks or fire must be eliminated from the environment. This requires prohibition of smoking in the area, use of cotton blankets instead of wool blankets which might produce static electricity, frequent checking of all electrical equipment in the patient's room so that electric sparks are avoided and use of a hand bell instead of the electric call bell. Oxygen is heavier than air and will readily seep through holes in an oxygen tent or under the edges of a tent that is not securely tucked under the mattress.

When oxygen is administered by mask the mask should fit snugly and follow the contour of the face. The mask should be removed periodically so that the face can be washed and powdered to prevent irritation of the skin.

Nasal catheters have a tendency to produce irritation of the nasal mucosa and therefore require frequent changing, using alternate nostrils. The patient may be more comfortable if some type of nonoily lubricant is applied to the nasal mucosa. Oil-based lubricants cannot be used because they may be aspirated into the lungs and produce pneumonia.

A form of oxygen therapy in which the oxygen is administered under a pressure higher than atmospheric pressure is called HYPERBARIC OXYGENATION. The oxygen is administered in a hyperbaric chamber. As the atmospheric pressure within the chamber is increased, a proportionately greater amount of oxygen is dissolved in the blood. Nursing personnel working inside the hyperbaric chamber must enter a decompression chamber when leaving the hyperbaric chamber so that they will not suffer from decompression sickness (see also BENDS).

oxygenase (ok′sĭ-jen-ās″) an enzyme that transfers oxygen from the air.

oxygenation (ok″sĭ-jĕ-na′shun) saturation with oxygen.

   hyperbaric o., exposure to oxygen under conditions of greatly increased pressure (see also HYPERBARIC OXYGENATION).

oxygenator (ok′sĭ-jĕ-na″tor) an apparatus by which oxygen is introduced into the blood during circulation outside the body, as during open-heart surgery. (See also HEART-LUNG MACHINE.)

   bubble o., a device in which pure oxygen is introduced into an extracorporeal reservoir of blood, either directly or through a filter.

   film o., a device, encased in a container of oxygen, that makes possible reduction of a thin film of blood to facilitate the exchange of gases.

   rotating disk o., a type of film oxygenator in which a series of parallel disks rotate through an extracorporeal pool of venous blood in a container of oxygen; gaseous exchange occurs between the thin film of blood on the exposed surface of the disks and the oxygen in the container.

   screen o., a type of film oxygenator in which the venous blood is passed over a series of screens in a container of oxygen, gaseous exchange taking place in the thin film of blood produced on the screens.

oxygeusia (ok″sĭ-gu′ze-ah) extreme acuteness of the sense of taste.

oxyhemoglobin (ok″sĭ-he″mo-glo′bin) hemoglobin combined with oxygen.

oxyhemoglobinometer (ok″sĭ-he″mo-glo″bĭ-nom′ĕ-ter) an instrument for measuring the oxygen content of the blood.

oxyhemograph (ok″sĭ-he′mo-graf) an apparatus for determining the oxygen content of the blood.

oxyhydrocephalus (ok″sĭ-hi″dro-sef′ah-lus) hydrocephalus with the top of the head pointed.

oxyhyperglycemia (ok″sĭ-hi″per-gli-se′me-ah) a

condition in which there is slight glycosuria and an oral glucose tolerance curve that rises to about 180 to 200 mg. per 100 ml., but returns to fasting values $2\frac{1}{2}$ hours after ingestion of the glucose.

oxyiodide (ok″se-i′o-dīd) an element or radical combined with oxygen and iodine.

oxylalia (ok″sĭ-la′le-ah) rapidity of speech.

Oxylone (ok′sĭ-lōn) trademark for a preparation of fluorometholone, an anti-inflammatory agent.

oxymetholone (ok″sĭ-meth′o-lōn) a steroid compound used to treat patients with wasting effects after a long illness.

oxymorphone (ok″sĭ-mor′fōn) a compound used as a narcotic analgesic.

oxymyoglobin (ok″sĭ-mi″o-glo′bin) myoglobin combined with oxygen.

oxyopia (ok″se-o′pe-ah) abnormal acuteness of sight.

oxyosis (ok″se-o′sis) acidosis.

oxyosmia (ok″se-oz′me-ah) extreme acuteness of the sense of smell.

oxypathia (ok″sĭ-path′e-ah) 1. acuteness of sensation. 2. oxypathy.

oxypathy (ok-sip′ah-the) inability of the body to eliminate unoxidizable acids.

oxyphenbutazone (ok″sĭ-fen-bu′tah-zōn) a compound used as an anti-inflammatory agent and in treatment of joint diseases.

oxyphencyclimine (ok″sĭ-fen-si′klĭ-mēn) a compound used in parasympathetic blockade.

oxyphenisatin (ok″sĭ-fĕ-ni′sah-tin) a compound used as an enema for cleansing the colon.

oxyphenonium (ok″sĭ-fĕ-no′ne-um) a compound used as an anticholinergic.

oxyphil (ok′sĭ-fil) a structure or element readily stainable with an acid dye. adj., **oxyphil′ic, oxyph′-ilous.**

oxyphonia (ok″sĭ-fo′ne-ah) an abnormally sharp quality of the voice.

oxypurine (ok″sĭ-pu′rēn) a purine containing oxygen.

oxyrhine (ok′sĭ-rīn) having a sharp-pointed nose.

oxytetracycline (ok″sĭ-tet-rah-si′klēn) an antibiotic substance isolated from the elaboration products of *Streptomyces rimosus,* effective against a wide range of microorganisms.

oxytocic (ok″sĭ-to′sik) 1. hastening the process of childbirth. 2. an agent that accelerates childbirth.

oxytocin (ok″sĭ-to′sin) a hormone produced by the posterior lobe of the pituitary gland (neurohypophysis) or prepared synthetically. It acts as a powerful stimulant to the pregnant uterus, especially toward the end of gestation. The hormone also causes milk to be expressed from the alveoli into the lactiferous ducts during suckling.

Injection of oxytocin may be used to induce labor or strengthen the uterine contractions during labor. It is administered with care so as to avoid trauma to the mother or infant by hyperactivity of the uterine muscles during labor. Oxytocin also may be administered intravenously by slow drip and it is sometimes applied to the mucous membranes of the nasal cavity and absorbed into the bloodstream.

oxyuriasis (ok″se-u-ri′ah-sis) infection with Oxyuris.

oxyuricide (ok″se-u′rĭ-sīd) a drug destructive to Oxyuris.

oxyurid (ok″se-u′rid) a seatworm or threadworm; an individual organism of the genus Oxyuris.

oxyurifuge (ok″se-u′rĭ-fūj) an agent that promotes expulsion of worms of the genus Oxyuris.

Oxyuris (ok″se-u′ris) a genus of nematode intestinal parasites.

O. **vermicula′ris,** *Enterobius vermicularis.*

oz. ounce.

ozena (o-ze′nah) an offensive-smelling discharge from the nose.

ozone (o′zōn) an allotropic and more active form of oxygen, O_3; antiseptic and disinfectant.

ozonometer (o″zo-nom′ĕ-ter) an apparatus for measuring the ozone in the atmosphere.

ozostomia (o″zo-sto′me-ah) foulness of the breath.

P

P chemical symbol, *phosphorus*.

P. position; presbyopia; [L.] *prox'imum* (near); pulse; [L.] *punc'tum* (point); pupil.

p- symbol, *para-*.

P₁ parental generation.

P₂ pulmonic second sound (see HEART SOUNDS).

Pa chemical symbol, *protactinium*.

PAB, PABA para-aminobenzoic acid, an antirickettsial agent.

pabulum (pab'u-lum) food or aliment.

Pacatal (pak'ah-tal) trademark for a preparation of mepazine, a sedative used in psychoses and neuroses.

pacemaker (pās'māk-er) a center or a substance that controls the rhythm of a body process; the term usually refers to the cardiac pacemaker.

The so-called "normal pacemaker" of the HEART is the sinotrial node, a small mass of specialized muscle tissue in the heart near the junction with the superior vena cava. It sets a rhythm of contraction and relaxation that is followed by the other portions of the heart. Thus the heartbeat is established.

The normal rhythm, 60 to 100 contractions per minute, is increased by physical or emotional stress, and decreases during rest. The pace varies from person to person and is affected by abnormal conditions such as heart injuries and generalized infections. If the normal pacemaker fails to function, its regulating task may be taken over by another small mass of special muscular tissue, the atrioventricular node.

In some cases of heart disorder, the heart becomes unable to regulate its own pace. This disorder may be remedied by the use of an electronic device to regulate the heartbeat. The artificial pacemaker is a built-in battery for persons whose failing hearts will respond to the stimulus of the 5-milliampere jolt needed to maintain a proper beat. The impulse from the battery is delivered to the heart via a soft plastic cable sewn into the heart. The batteries usually last 2 or 3 years; when they run down they are replaced by a new pacemaker.

In women, the uterus contains two pacemakers that control uterine contractions. These regulating centers are located near the openings of the uterine tubes. When the child is ready to be born, the pacemakers set off a series of rhythmic contractions in the uterus that gradually force the baby out into the birth canal.

pachy- (pak'e) word element [Gr.], *thickened; thickening.*

pachyblepharon (pak"ĭ-blef'ah-ron) thickening of the eyelids.

pachycephalia (pak"ĭ-se-fa'le-ah) abnormal thickness of the bones of the skull.

pachychromatic (pak"ĭ-kro-mat'ik) having thick chromatin threads.

pachydactylia (pak"ĭ-dak-til'e-ah) enlargement of the fingers and toes.

pachyderma (pak"ĭ-der'mah) abnormal thickening of the skin. adj., **pachyder'matous.**
    p. laryn'gis, warty thickenings on the vocal cords.
    p. ves'icae, thickening of the mucous membrane of the bladder.

pachydermatocele (pak"ĭ-der-mat'o-sēl) hypertrophy of the skin and subcutaneous tissues, with a tendency of the skin to hang in folds; called also cutis laxa and dermatolysis.

pachydermatosis (pak"ĭ-der"mah-to'sis) chronic pachyderma.

pachydermia (pak"ĭ-der'me-ah) pachyderma.

pachydermoperiostosis (pak"ĭ-der"mo-per"e-os-to'sis) thickening of the skin associated with periostosis.

pachyglossia (pak"ĭ-glos'e-ah) abnormal thickness of the tongue.

pachygyria (pak"ĭ-ji're-ah) a condition in which the cerebral convolutions are broad and flat.

pachyhematous (pak"ĭ-hem'ah-tus) having thickened blood.

pachyleptomeningitis (pak"ĭ-lep"to-men"in-ji'tis) inflammation of dura mater and pia mater.

pachylosis (pak"ĭ-lo'sis) a thickened, dry, scaly state of the skin, particularly of the legs.

pachymeningitis (pak"ĭ-men"in-ji'tis) inflammation of the dura mater.

pachymeningopathy (pak"ĭ-men"in-gop'ah-the) noninflammatory disease of the dura mater.

pachymeninx (pak"ĭ-me'ninks) the dura mater.

pachymeter (pah-kim'ĕ-ter) an instrument for measuring the thickness of objects.

pachynsis (pah-kin'sis) thickening.

pachyonychia (pak"e-o-nik'e-ah) abnormal thickening of the nails.
    p. congen'ita, a rare congenital disorder characterized by the presence, at birth, of massively thickened, clawlike nails.

pachyostosis (pak"e-os-to'sis) hypertrophy of the bones.

pachyotia (pak"e-o'she-ah) marked thickness of the ears.

pachypelviperitonitis (pak″ĭ-pel″vĭ-per″ĭ-to-ni′-tis) pelvic peritonitis with thickening of the peritoneum.

pachyperiostitis (pak″ĭ-per″e-os-ti′tis) periostitis of long bones resulting in abnormal thickness of the bones.

pachyperitonitis (pak″ĭ-per″ĭ-to-ni′tis) inflammation and thickening of the peritoneum.

pachypleuritis (pak″ĭ-ploo-ri′tis) inflammation and thickening of the pleura.

pachysalpingitis (pak″ĭ-sal″pin-ji′tis) chronic interstitial inflammation of the muscular coat of the oviduct producing thickening; called also mural salpingitis and parenchymatous salpingitis.

pachysalpingo-oothecitis, pachysalpingo-ovaritis (pak″ĭ-sal-ping″go-o″o-the-si′tis), (pak″ĭ-sal-ping″go-o″var-i′tis) inflammation of the ovary and oviduct, with thickening.

pachysomia (pak″ĭ-so′me-ah) thickening of parts of the body.

pachyvaginalitis (pak″ĭ-vaj″ĭ-nal-i′tis) inflammation and thickening of the tunica vaginalis of the testis.

pachyvaginitis (pak″ĭ-vaj″ĭ-ni′tis) chronic vaginitis with thickening of the vaginal walls.

pack (pak) 1. treatment by wrapping a patient in blankets, wet or dry and either hot or cold; referred to as wet, dry, hot or cold pack, respectively. Also the blankets in which a patient is wrapped. 2. a dressing is inserted firmly into a wound or body cavity, as the nose, uterus or vagina, principally for stopping hemorrhage.

packer (pak′er) an instrument for introducing a dressing into the vagina or other body cavity.

packing (pak′ing) 1. the filling of a wound or cavity with gauze, sponge or other material. 2. the substance used for filling a cavity. 3. treatment with the pack.

pad (pad) a cushion-like mass of soft material.
  abdominal p., a pad for the absorption of discharges from abdominal wounds.
  dinner p., a pad placed over the stomach before a plaster jacket is applied; the pad is then removed to leave space under the jacket to take care of expansion of the stomach after eating.
  fat p., 1. a large pad of fat lying behind and below the patella. 2. sucking pad.
  kidney p., a pad held in place by a belt for support of movable kidney.
  Malgaigne's p's, adipose pads in the knee joint immediately above the articular surface of the femur and on either side of the upper end of the patella.
  Mikulicz's p., a pad made of folded gauze, for packing off viscera in surgical procedures.
  sucking p., suctorial p., a lobulated mass of fat that occupies the space between the masseter muscle and the external surface of the buccinator muscle. It is well developed in infants.
  surgical p., a rubber sheet for the carrying off of fluids in surgical operation.

pae- for words beginning thus, see those beginning *pe-*.

Paget's disease (paj′ets) either of two entirely different diseases named after Sir James Paget (1814–1899), the British surgeon who first described them. One is a rare type of cancer of the nipple of the breast; the other is a bone disease that is called also OSTEITIS DEFORMANS.

Pagitane (paj′ĭ-tān) trademark for a preparation of cycrimine, used to produce parasympathetic blockade and in treating Parkinson's disease.

-pagus (pa′gus) word element [Gr.], *twin fetal monster.*

PAH, PAHA para-aminohippuric acid, used in testing renal function.

pain (pān) a feeling of distress, suffering or agony, caused by stimulation of specialized nerve endings. Its purpose is chiefly protective; it acts as a warning that early tissue damage is taking place somewhere in the body.

The receptors for the stimulus of pain are specific groups of myelinated and unmyelinated nerve fibers abundantly distributed near the surface of the body, and to a lesser degree in the internal organs. Some of the internal organs such as the lungs and uterus have comparatively few receptors, and therefore are relatively insensitive to painful stimuli. The distribution of pain receptors in the mucosa of the intestinal tract apparently is similar to that in the skin, and the mucosa is quite sensitive to irritation or other painful stimuli.

Superficial pain is felt when a stimulus reaches the cutaneous receptors near the surface of the body. It is felt as a sudden, sharp pain at the site of the stimulation. Deep pain arises from stimulation of receptors in the internal structures such as the muscles and viscera, and tends to be duller, of longer duration and less localized.

When the receptors are stimulated, the impulses are transmitted along nerve fibers that feed into the spinal ganglia. They then travel upward along nerve fibers to the thalamus. Here the pain impulses are integrated and the individual becomes aware of the painful stimulus. The impulses are finally transmitted to the sensory portion of the cerebral cortex where the pain is analyzed and its location and intensity are determined.

REACTIONS TO PAIN. There are two types of reaction to pain; physical and psychologic. The physical reaction is usually an automatic response to superficial pain resulting from stimulation of the sympathetic nervous system and producing an outpouring of epinephrine. There is a shift of blood from the skin, brain and intestinal tract toward the muscles; the blood pressure increases and the pulse rate rises. This reaction soon subsides if the pain persists and remains intense. The individual then becomes weak, shows signs of shock and may become nauseated and vomit. He most often seeks rest and quiet and becomes withdrawn.

The psychologic aspects of pain are more complex and difficult to determine. An individual's reaction to pain depends on many factors, such as his previous experience with pain, his training in regard to proper and acceptable responses to pain and discomfort, his state of health and the presence or absence of fatigue. Anxiety and tension generally increase sensitivity to pain. A person's attention to, or degree of distraction from, the presence of painful stimuli can also affect his reaction to the pain.

NURSING CARE. Pain is a subjective symptom; that is, the nurse or physician must rely on the patient to determine and describe the intensity, location and characteristics of the pain he is feeling. By observation of the patient's general posture, facial expressions and outward symptoms of physical reaction to pain it is sometimes possible to determine whether or not discomfort or distress is present. By being aware of the psychologic aspects of pain such as anxiety and tension, one can do much to relieve or lessen to some degree the distress suffered by a patient. Denying or expressing doubt that the pain actually exists, or implying that a patient is not acting in an acceptable manner when something is causing him suffering, only serves to increase his discomfort. His anxiety and tension can be greatly reduced if one shows appreciation of the fact that pain is present and indicates a willingness to try to help him gain relief. Simple measures such as smoothing the bed linen, rearranging the pillows or changing the patient's position can show such a willingness. It also may help the patient if he is allowed to talk about his feelings toward the pain or the cause of it.

When analgesic drugs have been ordered "as needed" the patient should know that they are available to him and that they will be given promptly if he requests them. If he is forced to wait until the nurse decides when he needs them, he may become resentful, angry and tense, and the effect of the medication when it is finally given will be diminished. Of course, one must guard against addiction or habituation in patients with chronic disorders necessitating frequent administration of narcotics and analgesics. However, this is essentially the responsibility of the physician prescribing the drugs; the nurse's responsibility lies in reporting to him indications that the patient is becoming overly dependent on the drug.

Since pain is a symptom and therefore of value in diagnosis, it is important to keep accurate records of the observations of the patient having pain. These observations should include the following: the nature of the pain, that is, whether it is described by the patient as being sharp, dull, burning, aching, etc.; the location of the pain, if the patient is able to determine this; the time of onset and the duration, and whether or not certain nursing measures and drugs are successful in obtaining relief; and the relation to other circumstances, such as the position of the patient, occurrence before or after eating and stimuli in the environment such as heat or cold that may trigger the onset of pain.

abdominal p., pain occurring in the area between the chest and pelvis; it is usually a signal that something is wrong with one of the organs within the abdominal cavity.

One of the most frequent causes of abdominal pain is stomach or intestinal distress caused by some indiscretion such as overeating, eating too much rich food or eating when one is tired or emotionally upset. Pain from such a cause is usually transient and will clear up as soon as the digestive disorder resolves. Whenever abdominal pain is severe or persistent, or whenever it is accompanied by fever, vomiting, rectal bleeding or diarrhea, there are urgent reasons for seeking medical attention.

There are certain questions a doctor will usually ask about abdominal pain in order to find its cause:

1. Is the pain a new one or has it occurred before, and if so, how often?

2. Is there any specific area of the abdomen where the pain began, and has it remained there or moved elsewhere?

3. Does the pain ease or disappear after eating?

4. Is it accompanied by nausea or diarrhea?

5. Is it a dull pain, a sharp pain or a crampy pain?

6. Is the pain eased by walking about or by lying down?

bearing-down p., a variety of pain in childbirth.

boring p., a sensation as of being pierced with a gimlet.

false p's, pains in the latter part of pregnancy that simulate those of labor; Braxton Hicks contractions.

fulgurant p., intense shooting pain.

gas p., pain caused by distention of the stomach or intestines by accumulations of air or gas.

growing p., a rheumatic-type pain peculiar to youth.

hunger p., pain coming on at the time for feeling hunger for a meal; a symptom of gastric disorder.

labor p's, the rhythmic pains of increasing severity and frequency due to contraction of the uterus at childbirth.

lancinating p., sharp darting pain.

lightning p's, the cutting pains of locomotor ataxia (tabes dorsalis).

osteocopic p., pain in the bones, peculiar to syphilis.

parenchymatous p., pain at the peripheral end of a nerve.

phantom p., pain felt as if it were in the patient's limb, after AMPUTATION of the limb.

referred p., pain in a part other than that in which the cause that produced it is situated.

root p., pain caused by disease of the sensory nerve roots and occurring in the cutaneous areas supplied by the affected roots.

terebrant p., terebrating p., boring pain.

painter's colic lead colic.

palat(o)- (pal′ah-to) word element [L.], *palate.*

palate (pal′at) the roof of the mouth. adj., **pal′atal.** The front portion braced by the upper jaw bones (maxillae) is known as the hard palate and forms the partition between the mouth and the nose. The fleshy part arching downward from the hard palate to the throat is called the soft palate and separates the mouth and the upper throat cavity, or pharynx. When one swallows, the rear of the soft palate swings up against the back of the pharynx and blocks the passage of food and air to the nose. A fleshy lobe called the uvula hangs from the middle of the soft palate.

artificial p., a prosthesis to close a cleft palate.

bony p., the rigid framework of the hard palate, formed by parts of the maxilla and the palatine bone.

cleft p., congenital fissure of median line of palate (see also CLEFT LIP).

palatine (pal′ah-tīn) pertaining to the palate.

palatitis (pal″ah-ti′tis) inflammation of the palate.

palatognathus (pal″ah-tog′nah-thus) congenital fissure of the hard and soft palates.

palatoplasty (pal'ah-to-plas"te) plastic repair of the palate.

palatoplegia (pal"ah-to-ple'je-ah) paralysis of the palate.

palatorrhaphy (pal"ah-tor'ah-fe) suture of the palate.

palatoschisis (pal"ah-tos'ki-sis) fissure of the palate.

palatum (pal-ah'tum) [L.] palate.

pale(o)- (pa'le-o) word element [Gr.], *old.*

paleencephalon (pa"le-en-sef'ah-lon) the phylogenetically old part of the brain; all of the brain except the cerebral cortex and its dependences.

paleocerebellum (pal"e-o-ser"ĕ-bel'um) the phylogenetically older parts of the cerebellum.

paleocortex (pa"le-o-kor'teks) the phylogenetically older portion of the cerebral cortex; the olfactory cortex.

paleogenesis (pa"le-o-jen'ĕ-sis) palingenesis (2).

paleogenetic (pa"le-o-jĕ-net'ik) originated in the past.

paleokinetic (pa"le-o-ki-net'ik) a term applied to the nervous motor mechanism concerned in automatic associated movements.

paleontology (pa"le-on-tol'o-je) the study of life in the early eras of the earth's history.

paleopathology (pa"le-o-pah-thol'o-je) study of disease in bodies that have been preserved from ancient times.

paleostriatum (pa"le-o-stri-a'tum) the more early formed portion of the corpus striatum, represented by the globus pallidus.

paleothalamus (pa"le-o-thal'ah-mus) the medial (noncortical) portion of the thalamus.

pali(n)- (pal'in) word element [Gr.], *again; pathologic repetition.*

palikinesia (pal"ĭ-ki-ne'ze-ah) pathologic repetition of movements.

palilalia (pal"ĭ-la'le-ah) a disorder of enunciation in which a phrase or word is repeated with increasing rapidity.

palinal (pal'ĭ-nal) directed or moved backward.

palindromia (pal"in-dro'me-ah) a recurrence or relapse.

palinesthesia (pal"in-es-the'ze-ah) the return of sensation after anesthesia or coma.

palingenesis (pal"in-jen'ĕ-sis) 1. regeneration or restoration. 2. reappearance of ancestral characters; atavism.

palingraphia (pal"in-graf'e-ah) repetition of words or letters in writing.

palinphrasia (pal"in-fra'ze-ah) repetition of words or phrases in speaking.

palladium (pah-la'de-um) a chemical element, atomic number 46, atomic weight 106.4, symbol Pd. (See table of ELEMENTS.)

pallanesthesia (pal"an-es-the'ze-ah) insensibility of bone to vibrations of a tuning fork.

pallesthesia (pal"es-the'ze-ah) sensibility of bone to vibrations of a tuning fork.

palliative (pal'e-a"tiv) relieving symptoms without curing the disease.

pallidectomy (pal"ĭ-dek'to-me) surgical excision of the globus pallidus or extirpation of it by other means (chemopallidectomy).

pallidofugal (pal"ĭ-dof'u-gal) conducting impulses away from the globus pallidus.

pallidotomy (pal"ĭ-dot'o-me) creation of lesions in the globus pallidus; used in treatment of certain involuntary movement disorders.

pallidum (pal'ĭ-dum) the globus pallidus of the brain. adj., **pal'lidal.**

pallium (pal'e-um) the gray matter covering the cerebral hemispheres, characterized by a distinctive layering of the cellular elements; the cerebral cortex.

pallor (pal'or) absence of skin coloration.

palm (pahm) the hollow or flexor surface of the hand. adj., **pal'mar.**

palma (pahl'mah), pl. *pal'mae* [L.] palm.
  pal'mae plica'tae, the branching folds of the mucosa of the vagina.

palmaris (pahl-ma'ris) palmar.

palmitic acid (pal-mit'ik) a fatty acid found in most of the common fats and oils.

palmus (pahl'mus) 1. palpitation. 2. clonic spasm of leg muscles, producing a jumping motion.

palpate (pal'pāt) to perform palpation; to feel with the fingers or hand.

palpation (pal-pa'shun) feeling with the fingers or hand, to determine by use of the tactile senses the physical characteristics of tissues or organs.

palpebra (pal'pĕ-brah), pl. *pal'pebrae* [L.] eyelid. adj., **pal'pebral.**

palpebritis (pal"pĕ-bri'tis) inflammation of the eyelid.

palpitation (pal"pĭ-ta'shun) a heartbeat that is unusually rapid, strong or irregular enough to make a person aware of it—usually over 120 per minute, as opposed to the normal 60 to 100 per minute. In most cases, palpitation is the result of excitement or nervousness, of strong exertion or of taking certain medications. There are also palpitations that result from various types of heart disorders such as paroxysmal tachycardia and flutter, abnormal rhythms in which the heart executes runs of rapid beats. Another is atrial fibrillation, in which the beats are rapid but irregular, seeming to occur at random.
  These palpitations may be caused by organic heart disease, but they also can result from other factors. Similarly, emotional pressures rather than organic changes may cause the so-called "nervous heart," or functional heart disease.

palsy (pawl'ze) paralysis.

Bell's p., neuropathy of the facial nerve; facial paralysis (see also BELL'S PALSY).

birth p., obstetric paralysis.

cerebral p., a persisting qualitative motor disorder appearing before age 3, due to nonprogressive damage of the brain (see also CEREBRAL PALSY).

Erb's p., paralysis of the muscles of the arm and chest wall in the newborn, due to injury of the nerve roots of the brachial plexus occurring in delivery.

shaking p., paralysis agitans, or PARKINSON'S DISEASE.

paludism (pal'u-dizm) malaria.

Paludrine (pal'u-drin) trademark for a preparation of proguanil hydrochloride, an antimalarial drug.

pamaquine naphthoate (pam'ah-kwin naf'tho-āt) an odorless yellow powder used as an antimalarial.

Pamine (pam'ēn) trademark for preparations of methscopolamine, used in parasympathetic blockade.

Pamisyl (pam'ĭ-sil) trademark for preparations of aminosalicylic acid, used in treatment of tuberculosis.

pampiniform (pam-pin'ĭ-form) shaped like a tendril.

pampinocele (pam-pin'o-sēl) varicocele.

pan- (pan) word element [Gr.], *all.*

panacea (pan"ah-se'ah) a remedy for all diseases.

panagglutinin (pan"ah-gloo'tĭ-nin) an agglutinin that agglutinates the corpuscles of all groups.

panangiitis (pan"an-je-i'tis) inflammation involving all the coats of a vessel.

necrotizing p., diffuse, extensive inflammation involving both arteries and veins, with cutaneous and visceral manifestations.

panarteritis (pan"ar-ter-i'tis) periarteritis nodosa.

panarthritis (pan"ar-thri'tis) inflammation of all the joints.

panatrophy (pan-at'ro-fe) atrophy of several parts.

pancarditis (pan"kar-di'tis) general inflammation of the heart, involving pericardium, myocardium and endocardium.

panchromia (pan-kro'me-ah) the condition of staining with various dyes.

Pancoast's syndrome (pan'kōsts) roentgenographic shadow at the apex of the lung, neuritic pain in the arm, atrophy of the muscles of the arm and hand and Horner's syndrome; observed in tumor near the apex of the lung.

pancolectomy (pan"ko-lek'to-me) excision of the entire colon, with creation of an outlet from the ileum on the body surface.

pancrealgia (pan"kre-al'je-ah) pain in the pancreas.

pancreas (pan'kre-as) a large gland located be-

low and behind the stomach and the liver. It is composed of both endocrine and exocrine tissue. The islands of Langerhans, being endocrine in nature, secrete two hormones: insulin, which plays a major role in carbohydrate metabolism, and glucagon, which has an effect opposite to that of insulin. The exocrine cells of the pancreas secrete pancreatic juice, which contains enzymes essential to the digestive processes. A system of ducts within the organ collects these secretions and empties them into the duodenum.

DISORDERS OF THE PANCREAS. Failure of the islands of Langerhans to produce sufficient amounts of insulin results in DIABETES MELLITUS. Disturbances in the exocrine functions of the pancreas produce serious digestive disorders. The pancreas can also be the seat of cancerous growth, and occasionally the pancreatic ducts are blocked by stones; either condition may require surgery. Various factors, not yet fully understood, may result in acute pancreatitis, a condition in which the fluids digest the tissue of the organ itself. This self-digesting may also be set off if the flow in the ducts is reversed and bile enters the pancreas, activating the enzymes in its secretions. Sudden severe abdominal pain, vomiting and fever can accompany pancreatitis. Treatment may involve surgery, though bed rest and antibiotics are frequently prescribed. Chronic pancreatitis, a less serious disorder, sometimes occurs after gallbladder diseases.

CYSTIC FIBROSIS, a serious congenital disease, is characterized by a deficiency in the secretion of pancreatic juice, and an increase in its viscosity.

annular p., a developmental anomaly in which the pancreas forms a ring entirely surrounding the duodenum.

pancreatalgia (pan"kre-ah-tal'je-ah) pain in the pancreas.

pancreatectomy (pan"kre-ah-tek'to-me) excision of the pancreas.

pancreatemphraxis (pan"kre-ah-tem-frak'sis) congestion of the pancreas from stoppage of the pancreatic duct.

pancreathelcosis (pan"kre-ath"el-ko'sis) ulceration of the pancreas.

pancreatic (pan"kre-at'ik) pertaining to the pancreas.

p. duct, the main excretory duct of the pancreas, which usually unites with the common bile duct before entering the duodenum at the major duodenal papilla.

pancreatico- (pan"kre-at'ĭ-ko) word element [Gr.], *pancreatic duct.*

pancreaticoduodenostomy (pan"kre-at"ĭ-ko-du-o-de-nos'to-me) anastomosis of the pancreatic duct to a different site on the duodenum.

pancreaticogastrostomy (pan"kre-at"ĭ-ko-gas-tros'to-me) anastomosis of the pancreatic duct to the stomach.

pancreaticojejunostomy (pan"kre-at"ĭ-ko-je-joo-nos'to-me) anastomosis of the pancreatic duct to the jejunum.

pancreatin (pan'kre-ah-tin) a substance from the pancreas of the hog or ox containing enzymes, principally pancreatic amylase, trypsin and pancreatic lipase.

pancreatism (pan'kre-ah-tizm″) activity of the pancreas.

pancreatitis (pan″kre-ah-ti'tis) inflammation of the PANCREAS.
acute hemorrhagic p., a form due to hemorrhage into the gland.
chronic p., fibrosis of the pancreas.

pancreato- (pan'kre-ah-to) word element [Gr.], *pancreas.*

pancreatoduodenectomy (pan″kre-ah-to-du″o-de-nek'to-me) resection of the head of the pancreas, part of the common bile duct, the pyloric portion of the stomach, and the duodenum.

pancreatoenterostomy (pan″kre-ah-to-en″ter-os'to-me) anastomosis of the pancreas to the intestinal tract.

pancreatogenous (pan″kre-ah-toj'ĕ-nus) arising in the pancreas.

pancreatography (pan″kre-ah-tog'rah-fe) roentgenography of the pancreas, performed during surgery by injecting contrast medium into the pancreatic duct.

pancreatolithectomy (pan-kre″ah-to-li-thek'to-me) excision of a calculus from the pancreas.

pancreatolithiasis (pan-kre″ah-to-li-thi'ah-sis) the presence of calculi in the ductal system or parenchyma of the pancreas.

pancreatolithotomy (pan-kre″ah-to-li-thot'o-me) incision of the pancreas for the removal of calculi.

pancreatolysis (pan″kre-ah-tol'ĭ-sis) destruction of pancreatic tissue.

pancreatoncus (pan″kre-ah-tong'kus) tumor of the pancreas.

pancreatotomy (pan″kre-ah-tot'o-me) incision of the pancreas.

pancreatotropic (pan-kre″ah-to-trop'ik) having a special influence on the pancreas.

pancreolithotomy (pan″kre-o-li-thot'o-me) pancreatolithotomy.

pancreolysis (pan″kre-ol'ĭ-sis) pancreatolysis.

pancreotherapy (pan″kre-o-ther'ah-pe) the therapeutic use of pancreas tissue.

pancreozymin (pan″kre-o-zi″min) a hormone of the duodenal mucosa that stimulates the external secretory activity of the pancreas.

pancytopenia (pan″si-to-pe'ne-ah) abnormal depression of all the cellular elements of the blood.

pandemic (pan-dem'ik) a widespread epidemic.

panendoscope (pan-en'do-skōp) a cystoscope that gives a wide view of the bladder.

panesthesia (pan″es-the'ze-ah) the sum of the sensations experienced.

pangenesis (pan-jen'ĕ-sis) the doctrine that in reproduction each cell of the parent body is represented by a particle, which during development gives rise to parts similar to those of their origin.

panhematopenia (pan″hem-ah-to-pe'ne-ah) abnormal decrease of all the cellular elements of the blood.
primary splenic p., a form of hypersplenism with indiscriminate elimination of all circulating elements of the blood.

panhidrosis (pan″hi-dro'sis) perspiration of the whole surface of the body.

panhypopituitarism (pan-hi″po-pĭ-tu'ĭ-tar-izm″) anterior pituitary insufficiency; Simmonds's disease.

panhysterectomy (pan″his-tĕ-rek'to-me) complete excision of the uterus and cervix.

panhystero-oophorectomy (pan″his-ter-o-o″of-o-rek'to-me) excision of the entire uterus and ovaries.

panhysterosalpingectomy (pan″his-ter-o-sal″pin-jek'to-me) excision of the entire uterus and oviducts.

panhysterosalpingo-oophorectomy (pan″his-ter-o-sal-ping″go-o″of-o-rek'to-me) excision of the uterus, cervic, oviducts and ovaries.

panic (pan'ik) an episode of acute anxiety, with abandonment of reason.

panimmunity (pan″ĭ-mu'nĭ-te) immunity to several infections.

Panmycin (pan-mi'sin) trademark for preparations of tetracycline; an antibiotic.

panmyeloid (pan-mi'ĕ-loid) pertaining to all elements of the bone marrow.

panmyelophthisis (pan-mi″ĕ-lof'thĭ-sis) general aplasia of the bone marrow.

panmyelosis (pan-mi″ĕ-lo'sis) proliferation of all the elements of the bone marrow.

panneuritis (pan″nu-ri'tis) general or multiple neuritis.
p. epidem'ica, beriberi.

panniculitis (pah-nik″u-li'tis) inflammation of the panniculus adiposus.
nodular nonsuppurative p., a disease marked by painful nodules in the subcutaneous fatty tissue; called also Weber-Christian disease.

panniculus (pah-nik'u-lus), pl. *pannic'uli* [L.] a layer of tissue.
p. adipo'sus, subcutaneous tissue containing large amounts of fat.
p. carno'sus, a muscular layer in superficial fascia.

pannus (pan'us) a membrane-like structure, as produced by (1) superficial vascularization of the cornea with infiltration of granulation tissue, or (2) exudate overlying synovial cells on the inside of a joint capsule, usually occurring in rheumatoid arthritis or related articular rheumatism.

panophobia (pan"o-fo'be-ah) fear of everything; vague and persistent dread of an unknown evil.

panophthalmitis (pan"of-thal-mi'tis) inflammation of all the eye structures.

panosteitis (pan"os-te-i'tis) inflammation of every part of a bone.

panotitis (pan"o-ti'tis) inflammation of all the parts or structures of the ear.

Panparnit (pan-par'nit) trademark for a preparation of caramiphen hydrochloride, used in parasympathetic blockade, as an antispasmodic and in treatment of Parkinson's disease.

panphobia (pan-fo'be-ah) panophobia.

panproctocolectomy (pan-prok"to-ko-lek'to-me) excision of the entire rectum and colon, with creation of an outlet from the ileum on the body surface.

pansinusitis (pan"si-nŭ-si'tis) inflammation of all the accessory sinuses of the nose.

Panstrongylus (pan-stron'ji-lus) a genus of arthropods (order Hemiptera), species of which are vectors of trypanosomes.

pantalgia (pan-tal'je-ah) pain over the whole body.

pantomography (pan-to-mog'rah-fe) a method of body-section roentgenography used for visualization of curved surfaces at any depth. adj., **pantomograph'ic.**

pantophobia (pan"to-fo'be-ah) panophobia.

pantothenate (pan-to'then-āt) a salt of pantothenic acid.

pantothenic acid (pan"to-then'ik) a vitamin of the B complex present in all living tissues, almost entirely in the form of a coenzyme A (CoA). This coenzyme has many metabolic roles in the cell and a lack of pantothenic acid can lead to depressed metabolism of both carbohydrates and fats. The daily requirement for this vitamin is not known and no definite deficiency syndrome has been recognized in man, perhaps because of its wide occurrence in almost all foods. However, some symptoms attributed to deficiency of other B-complex vitamins may be due to a lack of pantothenic acid.

pantotropic, pantropic (pan"to-trop'ik), (pan-trop'ik) having affinity for tissues derived from all three of the germ layers (ectoderm, entoderm and mesoderm).

panturbinate (pan-tur'bĭ-nāt) the entire structure of a nasal concha, including bone and soft tissue.

panzootic (pan"zo-ot'ik) occurring pandemically among animals.

papain (pah-pa'in, pah-pi'in) a digestant from papaw fruit.

Papanicolaou smear test (pap"ah-nik"o-la'oo) a simple, painless test used most commonly to detect cancer of the uterus and cervix; often called Pap test or smear. The test is based on the discovery by Dr. George N. Papanicolaou (1883–1962) that malignant uterine tumors slough off cancerous cells into surrounding vaginal fluid.

The Papanicolaou technique is used also in diagnosis of lung, stomach and bladder cancers. The test can be performed on any body excretion (urine, feces), secretion (sputum, prostatic fluid, vaginal fluid) or tissue scraping (as from the uterus or the stomach). The sample is removed from the area being examined, placed on a glass slide, stained and then studied under a microscope for evidence of abnormal, or cancerous, cells.

In 5 minutes, the Pap test can reveal uterine or cervical cancer at a stage in which it produces no visible symptoms, has done no damage and usually can be completely cured. The American Cancer Society recommends that all women over 30 have a routine Papanicolaou test once a year.

papaverine (pah-pav'er-in) an alkaloid obtained from opium and prepared synthetically.

p. hydrochloride, a white, crystalline compound used as a smooth muscle relaxant.

papilla (pah-pil'ah), pl. *papil'lae* [L.] a small, nipple-shaped projection or elevation. adj., **pap'-illary.**

circumvallate p., vallate papilla.

papillae of corium, small conical masses projecting from the corium up into grooves in the overlying epidermis.

dental p., dentinal p., the small mass of condensed mesenchyma capped by each of the enamel organs.

duodenal p., either of the small elevations (major and minor) on the mucosa of the duodenum, the major at the entrance of the conjoined pancreatic and common bile ducts, the minor at the entrance of the accessory pancreatic duct.

filiform p., one of the threadlike elevations covering most of the tongue surface.

foliate p., one of the parallel mucosal folds on the tongue margin at the junction of its body and root.

fungiform p., one of the knoblike projections of the tongue scattered among the filiform papillae.

gingival p., the triangular pad of the gingiva filling the space between the proximal surfaces of two adjacent teeth.

hair p., a mass within the corium beneath each hair bulb.

incisive p., an elevation at the anterior end of the raphe of the palate.

lacrimal p., an elevation on the margin of either eyelid, near the medial angle of the eye.

lingual papillae, elevations on the surface of the tongue; they contain the taste buds.

mammary p., the nipple of the mammary gland.

nervous papillae, papillae of the skin enclosing special nerve terminations.

optic p., optic disk.

palatine p., incisive papilla.

p. pi'li, hair papilla.

renal p., the blunted apex of a renal pyramid.

tactile p., a papilla on the corium enclosing a tactile corpuscle.

urethral p., a slight elevation in the vestibule of the vagina at the external orifice of the urethra.

vallate p., one of the 8 to 12 large papillae arranged in a V near the base of the tongue.

vascular papillae, the papillae of the corium that contain loops of blood vessels.

p. of Vater, Vater's p., major duodenal papilla.

papillectomy (pap"ĭ-lek'to-me) excision of a papilla.

papilledema (pap″il-ĕ-de′mah) edema and hyperemia of the optic disk (choked disk), usually associated with increased intracranial pressure.

papillitis (pap″ĭ-li′tis) inflammation of a papilla, especially of the optic disk.

papilloadenocystoma (pap″ĭ-lo-ad″ĕ-no-sis-to′-mah) a tumor containing elements of papilloma, adenoma and cystoma.

papillocarcinoma (pap″ĭ-lo-kar″sĭ-no′mah) 1. a carcinoma in which there are papillary excrescences. 2. a malignant papilloma.

papilloma (pap″ĭ-lo′mah) a benign tumor derived from epithelium. Papillomas may arise from skin, mucous membranes or glandular ducts. adj., **papillo′matous.**

papillomatosis (pap″ĭ-lo″mah-to′sis) development of multiple papillomas.

papilloretinitis (pap″ĭ-lo-ret″ĭ-ni′tis) inflammation of the optic nerve and disk.

papillosphincterotomy (pap″ĭ-lo-sfingk″ter-ot′o-me) partial incision of the sphincter of the major duodenal papilla.

papulation (pap″u-la′shun) the formation of papules.

papule (pap′ūl) a circumscribed, solid, elevated lesion of the skin, up to 5 mm. in diameter. adj., **pap′ular.**

papyraceous (pap″ĭ-ra′shus) like paper.

par (par) [L.] pair.

para- (par′ah) [L.] a woman who has produced living young. Used with numerals to designate the number of pregnancies that have resulted in the birth of viable offspring, as para 0 (none—nullipara), para I (one—unipara), para II (two—bipara), para III (three—tripara), para IV (four—quadripara). The number is not indicative of the number of offspring produced in the event of a multiple birth.

para- (par′ah) word element [Gr.], *beside; beyond; accessory to; apart from; against.* In chemistry, a prefix indicating the substitution in a derivative of the benzene ring of two atoms linked to opposite carbon atoms in the ring; abbreviated *p-.*

para-agglutinin (par″ah-ah-gloo′tĭ-nin) partial agglutinin.

para-aminobenzoic acid (par″ah-am″ĭ-no-ben-zo′ik) PABA; a derivative of benzoic acid, classified as a vitamin of the B complex group but not yet proved essential in the diet of human beings. It depresses the activity of certain rickettsial infections and therefore is used in their treatment. PABA antagonizes the action of sulfonamides and should not be used in combination with them. Derivatives of para-aminobenzoic acid include local anesthetics such as procaine (Novocaine).

para-aminohippuric acid (par″ah-am″ĭ-no-hĭ-pu′rik) PAH or PAHA; a compound used to measure the effective renal plasma flow and to determine the functional capacity of the renal tubular excretory mechanism.

para-aminosalicylic acid (par″ah-am″ĭ-no-sal″ĭ-sil′ik) PAS; a derivative of benzoic acid used in treatment of tuberculosis. It enhances the potency of streptomycin and delays development of bacilli resistant to streptomycin. Gastrointestinal irritation accompanied by anorexia, nausea and vomiting may be reduced by administering the drug together with food at mealtime.

para-anesthesia (par″ah-an″es-the′ze-ah) anesthesia of the lower part of the body.

para-appendicitis (par″ah-ah-pen″dĭ-si′tis) appendicitis involving nearby structures.

parabion, parabiont (par″ah-bi′on), (par″ah-bi′-ont) one of two organisms living in a condition of parabiosis.

parabiosis (par″ah-bi-o′sis) the cooperative association of two distinct organisms, or the anatomic and physiologic union of two animals as created surgically for experimental purposes or as occurs naturally in Siamese twins. adj., **parabiot′ic.**
dialytic p., the separate circulation of the blood of two animals through a dialyzer to eliminate harmful factors from the blood of one and add to it essential factors from the blood of the other.

parablepsia (par″ah-blep′se-ah) false or perverted vision.

parabulia (par″ah-bu′le-ah) perversion of will.

paracarbinoxamine (par″ah-kar″bin-ok′sah-min) carbinoxamine, an antihistamine.

paracasein (par″ah-ka′se-in) the compound into which casein is converted in the stomach by rennin or pepsin, before undergoing complete digestion.

paracenesthesia (par″ah-sen″es-the′ze-ah) any disturbance of the general sense of well-being.

paracentesis (par″ah-sen-te′sis) surgical puncture and drainage of a cavity.
abdominal p., insertion of a trocar through a small incision and into the abdominal cavity, to remove fluids or inject a therapeutic agent. The procedure is most often done to remove excess fluid in the peritoneal cavity of a patient with cirrhosis of the liver.
Before the procedure the patient is instructed to empty his bladder, to reduce the danger of accidental puncture of the bladder. The skin below the umbilicus and overlying the rectus muscle is cleansed with an antiseptic. A local anesthetic is used to anesthetize the skin and underlying tissues at the site of insertion of the trocar. During the procedure the patient may be placed in a sitting position with his feet resting on a foot stool or on the floor. His back and arms should be well supported. The container for collecting the drainage is placed at the patient's feet. As the fluid is being withdrawn the patient is observed for symptoms of fainting or shock.
The amount and character of the fluid obtained is recorded and a specimen is saved if the physician requests laboratory examination of the fluid. After the trocar is removed a sterile dressing is applied to the site.
thoracic p., surgical puncture and drainage of the thoracic cavity (see also THORACENTESIS).

paracephalus (par″ah-sef′ah-lus) a fetus with a defective head and imperfect sense organs.

paracetaldehyde (par-as″et-al′dĕ-hīd) paraldehyde, a hypnotic and sedative.

paracetamol (par-as″et-am′ol) acetaminophen, an analgesic and antipyretic.

parachloramine (par″ah-klor′ah-mēn) meclizine, an antihistamine and antinauseant.

parachlorophenol (par″ah-klo″ro-fe′nol) a crystalline compound used as a topical antibacterial agent.

paracholia (par″ah-ko′le-ah) disordered bile secretion.

parachordal (par″ah-kor′dal) beside the notochord.

parachroma (par″ah-kro′mah) skin discoloration.

parachromatopsia (par″ah-kro″mah-top′se-ah) color blindness.

parachromophoric (par″ah-kro″mo-for′ik) secreting coloring matter, but retaining it in the organism.

paracinesia (par″ah-si-ne′se-ah) parakinesia.

paracoccidioidomycosis (par″ah-kok-sid″e-oi″-do-mi-ko′sis) a skin infection due to *Blastomyces* (*Paracoccidioides*) *brasiliensis*.

Paracolobactrum (par″ah-ko″lo-bak′trum) a genus of Schizomycetes found in the intestinal tract of animals, including man.

Paracort (par′ah-kort) trademark for a preparation of prednisone, an anti-inflammatory agent.

Paracortol (par″ah-kor′tol) trademark for a preparation of prednisolone, an anti-inflammatory agent.

paracusis (par″ah-ku′sis) derangement of the hearing.

paracyesis (par″ah-si-e′sis) ectopic pregnancy.

paradental (par″ah-den′tal) 1. having some connection with or relation to the science or practice of dentistry. 2. periodontal.

paradidymis (par″ah-did′ĭ-mis) a small, vestigial structure found occasionally in the adult in the lower part of the spermatic cord.

Paradione (par″ah-di′ōn) trademark for preparations of paramethadione, an anticonvulsant.

paradipsia (par″ah-dip′se-ah) a perverted appetite for fluids.

paraffin (par′ah-fin) a purified mixture of solid hydrocarbons obtained from petroleum.
　liquid p., liquid petrolatum (mineral oil).

paraffinoma (par″ah-fĭ-no′mah) a swelling forming around a deposit of paraffin in the tissues.

Paraflex (par′ah-fleks) trademark for a preparation of chlorzoxazone, a skeletal muscle relaxant.

paragammacism (par″ah-gam′ah-sizm) faulty enunciation of *g, k* and *ch* sounds.

paraganglioma (par″ah-gang″gle-o′mah) a tumor of the tissue composing the paraganglia.
　medullary p., pheochromocytoma.
　nonchromaffin p., carotid body tumor.

paraganglion (par″ah-gang′gle-on), pl. *paragan′-glia* [Gr.] a collection of chromaffin cells derived from neural ectoderm, occurring outside the adrenal medulla. Most secrete epinephrine or norepinephrine.

parageusia (par″ah-gu′ze-ah) perversion of the sense of taste.

paraglobulin (par″ah-glob′u-lin) a globulin from blood serum, blood cells, lymph and various tissues.

paraglossa (par″ah-glos′ah) swelling of the tongue.

paragonimiasis (par″ah-gon″ĭ-mi′ah-sis) infection with flukes of the genus Paragonimus.

Paragonimus (par″ah-gon′ĭ-mus) a genus of trematode parasites.
　P. westerman′i, the lung fluke, a species occurring primarily in Asia, but also in Africa and South and Central America; found in the lungs of man and crab-eating mammals.

paragrammatism (par″ah-gram′ah-tizm) a disorder of speech, with confusion in the use and order of words and grammatical forms.

paragraphia (par″ah-graf′e-ah) impairment of ability to express thoughts in writing.

parahemophilia (par″ah-he″mo-fil′e-ah) a condition resembling hemophilia, but due to lack of a different blood clotting factor.

parahormone (par″ah-hōr′mōn) a substance, not a true hormone, that has a hormone-like action in controlling the functioning of some distant organ.

parainfluenza virus (par″ah-in″floo-en′zah) one of a group of viruses isolated from patients with upper respiratory tract disease of varying severity.

parakeratosis (par″ah-ker″ah-to′sis) 1. any disorder of the stratum corneum of the skin. 2. retention of the nuclei in the cells of the keratin or stratum corneum, normally seen in true mucous membrane.

parakinesia (par″ah-ki-ne′se-ah) perversion of motor powers.

paralalia (par″ah-la′le-ah) a disorder of speech, especially the production of a vocal sound different from the one desired, or the substitution in speech of one letter for another.

paralambdacism (par″ah-lam′dah-sizm) faulty enunciation of the *l* sound.

paralbumin (par″al-bu′min) an albumin showing characteristics differing from those of the normal compound.

paralbuminemia (par″al-bu″mĭ-ne′me-ah) the presence in the blood of abnormal albumins (paraalbumins).

paraldehyde (pah-ral′dĕ-hīd) a colorless, transparent liquid with an unpleasant odor and taste; hypnotic and sedative.

paralepsy (par′ah-lep″se) psycholepsy; a condition characterized by sudden changes of mood.

paralexia (par″ah-lek′se-ah) impairment of the ability to comprehend written language.

paralgesia (par″al-je′ze-ah) an abnormal and painful sensation.

parallagma (par″ah-lag′mah) displacement of a bone or of the fragments of a broken bone.

parallax (par′ah-laks) an apparent displacement of an object due to change in the observer's position.

parallergy (par-al′er-je) a predisposition to allergy produced by previous sensitization.

paralogia (par″ah-lo′je-ah) derangement of the reasoning faculty, marked by illogical or delusional speech.

paralysis (pah-ral′ĭ-sis) loss or impairment of the ability to move parts of the body. Paralysis is a symptom of a wide variety of physical and emotional disorders rather than a disease in itself.

TYPES OF PARALYSIS. Paralysis results from damage to parts of the nervous system. The kind of paralysis resulting, and the degree, depend on whether the damage is to the central nervous system or the peripheral nervous system.

If the central nervous system is damaged, paralysis frequently affects the movement of a limb as a whole, not the individual muscles. The more common forms of central paralysis are hemiplegia, in which the whole of one side of the body, including the face, arm and leg, is affected, and paraplegia, in which both legs and possibly the trunk are affected. In central paralysis the tone of the muscles is increased (spasticity).

If the peripheral nervous system is damaged, individual muscles or groups of muscles in a particular part of the body, rather than a whole limb, are more likely to be affected. The muscles are flaccid, and there is often impairment of sensation.

CAUSES OF CENTRAL PARALYSIS. A CEREBROVAS-CULAR ACCIDENT, or stroke, is one of the commonest causes of central paralysis. Although there is usually some permanent disability, much can be done to rehabilitate the patient.

Paralysis produced by damage to the spinal cord can be the result of direct injuries, tumors and infectious diseases.

Paralysis in children may be a result of failure of the brain to develop properly in intrauterine life or of injuries to the brain, as in the case of cerebral palsy. Congenital syphilis may also leave a child partially paralyzed.

There is no organic basis for the paralysis resulting from hysteria. This type of paralysis is a result of emotional disturbance or mental illness.

CAUSES OF PERIPHERAL PARALYSIS. Until the recent development of immunizing vaccines, the most frequent cause of peripheral paralysis in children was poliomyelitis. NEURITIS, inflammation of a nerve, can produce paralysis. Causes can be physical, as with cold or injury; chemical, as in lead poisoning; or disease states, such as diabetes mellitus or infection. Paralysis caused by neuritis frequently disappears when the disorder causing it is corrected.

abducens p., lesion of the abducens nerve causing paralysis of the external rectus muscle of the eye.

p. of accommodation, paralysis of the ciliary muscles of the eye so as to prevent accommodation.

p. ag′itans, a progressive disease of late life, with masklike facies, tremor, slowing of voluntary movements, festinating gait, peculiar posture and muscle weakness (see also PARKINSON'S DISEASE).

ascending p., spinal paralysis that progresses upward.

birth p., that due to injury received at birth.

brachial p., paralysis of an arm from damage to the brachial plexus.

brachiofacial p., paralysis of the face and arm.

bulbar p., paralysis and atrophy of the muscles of the lips, tongue, mouth, pharynx and larynx due to changes in motor centers of the medulla oblongata.

cerebral p., paralysis caused by some intracranial lesion (see also CEREBRAL PALSY).

cerebrospinal p., hereditary, a hereditary condition that develops usually in early middle life, with gradually developing paralyses in the upper or lower extremities, in the two extremities on one side, or in all four extremities.

creeping p., locomotor ataxia (tabes dorsalis).

crossed p., paralysis affecting one side of the face and the other side of the body.

decubitus p., paralysis due to pressure on a nerve from lying for a long time in one position.

diver's p., decompression sickness (bends).

Duchenne's p., progressive bulbar paralysis.

emotional p., inaction due to opposing psychic drives of equal strength.

facial p., Bell's palsy.

familial periodic p., a rare disease marked by recurring attacks of rapidly progressive flaccid paralysis, often associated with a marked fall of serum potassium. It occurs in young people, usually in several members of a family.

infantile p., poliomyelitis.

ischemic p., local paralysis due to stoppage of circulation.

Landry's p., acute ascending myelitis.

mixed p., combined motor and sensory paralysis.

motor p., paralysis of the voluntary muscles.

obstetric p., paralysis of the newborn resulting from injuries received at birth.

pseudobulbar p., paralysis simulating bulbar paralysis, but due to a lesion in the cerebrum. It is marked especially by spasmodic laughing and crying.

pseudohypertrophic p., paralysis with enlargement and fatty degeneration of the affected muscles.

sensory p., loss of sensation resulting from a morbid process.

spastic p., paralysis with rigidity of the muscles and heightened deep muscle reflexes.

spinal p., paraplegia.

spinal p., spastic, congenital lateral sclerosis of the spinal cord, producing atrophy and rigidity of the muscles of the extremities.

Volkmann's p., ischemic paralysis.

paralytic (par″ah-lit′ik) 1. pertaining to paralysis. 2. a person affected with paralysis.

paralytogenic (par″ah-lit″o-jen′ik) causing paralysis.

paralyzant (par′ah-līz″ant) 1. causing paralysis. 2. a drug that causes paralysis.

paramania (par″ah-ma′ne-ah) a condition in which the patient exhibits joy by complaining.

Paramecium (par″ah-me′she-um) a genus of ciliate protozoans.

paramedical (par″ah-med′ĭ-kal) having some connection with or relation to the science or practice of medicine; adjunctive to the practice of medicine in the maintenance or restoration of health and normal functioning. The paramedical services include physical, occupational and speech therapy, and the activity of social workers.

paramenia (par″ah-me′ne-ah) disordered or difficult menstruation.

parameter (pah-ram′ĕ-ter) an arbitrary constant whose values characterize the mathematical expressions into which it enters.

paramethadione (par″ah-meth″ah-di′ōn) a compound used as an anticonvulsant in petit mal epilepsy.

paramethasone (par″ah-meth′ah-sōn) a compound used as a corticosteroid with anti-inflammatory action.

parametric (par″ah-met′rik) around the uterus.

parametrismus (par″ah-me-triz′mus) painful spasm of muscle in the broad ligament of the uterus.

parametritis (par″ah-me-tri′tis) inflammation of the parametrium.

parametrium (par″ah-me′tre-um) loose connective tissue and smooth muscle within the broad ligaments and near the uterus.

paramimia (par″ah-mim′e-ah) faulty use of gestures and movements.

paramnesia (par″am-ne′ze-ah) 1. perversion of memory in which the person believes he remembers events or circumstances that never happened; called also retrospective falsification. 2. a state in which words are remembered, but are used without a comprehension of their meaning.

paramorphia (par″ah-mor′fe-ah) abnormality of form.

paramyoclonus (par″ah-mi-ok′lo-nus) a condition characterized by myoclonic contractions of various muscles.

   p. mul′tiplex, a condition characterized by sudden shocklike contractions.

paramyotonia (par″ah-mi″o-to′ne-ah) a disease marked by tonic spasms due to impairment of muscular tonicity.

   p. congen′ita, myotonia congenita.

paranasal sinuses (par″ah-na′zal) mucosa-lined air cavities in bones of the skull, communicating with the nasal cavity (see also SINUS).

paranephric (par″ah-nef′rik) 1. near the kidney. 2. pertaining to the adrenal gland.

paranephros (par″ah-nef′ros), pl. *paranephʹroi* [Gr.] an adrenal gland.

paranesthesia (par″an-es-the′ze-ah) para-anesthesia.

paraneural (par″ah-nu′ral) alongside a nerve.

para-nitrosulfathiazole (par″ah-ni″tro-sul″fah-thi′ah-zōl) a sulfonamide compound used as an antibacterial.

paranoia (par″ah-noi′ah) a mental disorder characterized by delusions of persecution, illusions of grandeur or a combination of both. It is a chronic disease that develops over months and years and for which there is usually no cure.

In the acute stage of the disease, the paranoiac regards himself as being very important and distinguished, or he believes he is being plotted against by others, and in his imagination he builds up an elaborate system of "evidence" to support this belief. This imaginary system is kept separate from the paranoiac's everyday attitudes and activities; hence his outward behavior may appear normal. The extent of his illness remains mostly hidden, though it may erupt occasionally into crimes of violence.

Symptoms of paranoia sometimes appear in lesser degrees in schizophrenia. In slight to moderate form paranoid personality traits are found in many neurotic persons who are excessively suspicious of other people's motives and are quick to take offense at imagined wrongs. (See also PSYCHOSIS.)

paranoiac (par″ah-noi′ak) a person affected with paranoia.

paranoic (par″ah-no′ik) pertaining to or characterized by paranoia.

paranoid (par′ah-noid) 1. resembling paranoia. 2. a person afflicted with paranoia.

paranomia (par″ah-no′me-ah) aphasia in which the names of objects seen (visual paranomia) or touched (myotactic paranomia) are not recollected.

paranosis (par″ah-no′sis) the primary advantage that is to be gained by illness.

paranucleus (par″ah-nu′kle-us) a body sometimes seen in cell protoplasm near the nucleus.

paraparesis (par″ah-pah-re′sis) a partial paralysis of the lower extremities.

parapertussis (par″ah-per-tus′is) a disease caused by *Bordetella parapertussis* that resembles pertussis (whooping cough) but is much milder.

paraphasia (par″ah-fa′ze-ah) a defect in the ability to comprehend, elaborate or express speech concepts, characterized by the misuse of words.

paraphemia (par″ah-fe′me-ah) aphasia marked by the employment of the wrong words.

paraphia (par-a′fe-ah) a disorder of the sense of touch.

paraphilia (par″ah-fil′e-ah) expression of the sexual instinct in practices that are socially unacceptable or biologically undesirable (see also SEXUAL DEVIATION).

paraphiliac (par″ah-fil′e-ak) a person who exhibits paraphilia.

paraphimosis (par″ah-fi-mo′sis) retraction and constriction of the foreskin behind the glans penis.

paraphobia (par″ah-fo′be-ah) a mild phobia.

paraphrasia (par″ah-fra′ze-ah) disorderly arrangement of spoken words.

paraphrenia (par″ah-fre′ne-ah) a term formerly applied to any of a group of psychoses now called paranoid states.

paraplasm (par′ah-plazm) 1. any abnormal growth. 2. hyaloplasm (1).

paraplastic (par″ah-plas′tik) 1. having perverted formative power. 2. misshapen.

paraplectic (par″ah-plek′tik) paraplegic.

paraplegia (par″ah-ple′je-ah) paralysis of the legs and, in some cases, the lower part of the body. adj., **paraple′gic.** Paraplegia is a form of central nervous system paralysis, in which the paralysis affects all the muscles of the parts involved.

In the majority of cases, paraplegia results from disease or injury of the spinal cord that causes interference with nerve paths connecting the brain and the muscles. Conditions that may result in such interference include physical injuries, hemorrhage, tuberculosis, tumor and syphilis.

In paraplegia, the loss of ability to use the legs may be accompanied by a loss of sensation in them and, in some cases, by loss of control over the bowels and bladder. Fortunately, much has been learned about the techniques of restoring paraplegics to normal activity, and today many are able to resume useful and productive lives.

NURSING CARE. Because rehabilitation is the ultimate goal for a paraplegic patient, the nursing care during the early stages of the disorder must be particularly concerned with preventing complications that may stand in the way of successful rehabilitation. These complications include DECU-BITUS ULCERS, respiratory disorders, orthopedic deformities, urinary infections or calculi and gastrointestinal disorders.

The psychologic and emotional aspects of paraplegia also must be considered. Many times the paraplegic patient is suddenly thrust into the role of dependence because of accidental injury to the spinal cord. This means that he must make a tremendous adjustment to his condition in a short time. His mental attitude and emotional response to paralysis will greatly affect the success of attempts at rehabilitation.

During the early stages of his illness the patient may not be able to assist in his daily personal care, but as his condition improves and the physician allows more physical activity he must be encouraged to do as much as possible for himself. As he learns to become less dependent on others, his attitude toward his future will improve.

Care of the Skin. The type of bed used and the positioning of the patient with paraplegia will depend on the cause and extent of the paralysis and the preference of the physician. Patients with spinal cord injuries may be placed in traction or the spinal cord may be hyperextended by placing the patient's head at the foot of the bed and adjusting the bed. In some cases the physician may request a special orthopedic frame such as the STRYKER FRAME or other special bed. These devices facilitate nursing care but the patient still must be turned frequently (as allowed by the physician) and receive special skin care to avoid the development of decubitus ulcers (pressure sores).

Since the patient has no feeling below the point of damage to the spinal cord, he will not be aware of discomfort or other signs of pressure. Injections should not be given in the area of paralysis because of limited absorption of the drug and decreased circulation to the part.

Respiratory Disorders. Hypostatic pneumonia and other respiratory problems are guarded against by deep breathing exercises. Coughing and frequent changing of position may be contraindicated and the physician must be consulted before these measures are taken. The patient should be protected from respiratory infections, such as the common cold, which can have serious complications in a paraplegic who is confined to bed.

Orthopedic Deformities. Until the patient is allowed out of bed and can engage in some form of physical activity his joints should be put through their full range of motion at least once a day. Proper positioning of the feet and legs will help prevent contractures, footdrop and ankylosis. The physical therapist usually supervises exercises but the nursing staff must assist in carrying out the physician's orders.

Urinary Complications. Urinary infections and the formation of calculi, particularly in the bladder, frequently develop in the patient with paralysis of the lumbar area. Since he has no control over urination, an indwelling catheter may be inserted. This measure keeps the patient dry but it also predisposes him to infection since the catheter serves as a ready means of entrance for pathogenic organisms. Aseptic technique must be used in handling the catheter, drainage tubing and collecting apparatus.

The formation of bladder stones results from incomplete emptying of the bladder with a pooling of urine and inadequate elimination of wastes. Frequent bladder irrigations and the forcing of fluids to at least 3000 ml. daily will help eliminate this problem. Since an alkaline urine supports the growth of bacteria and the formation of stones, the juices of citrus fruits are not allowed. An ACID-ASH DIET will lower the pH of urine.

Various methods have been devised for collecting urine when the patient is incontinent. The effectiveness of rubber urinals, penile clamps or other collecting devices will depend on the individual patient. As the patient becomes more independent he must learn by trial and error the method best suited for him.

Gastrointestinal Complications. A flaccid bowel produces abdominal distention and predisposes the patient to fecal impaction. If the bowel paralysis is temporary, the distention may be relieved by a rectal tube and injections of neostigmine or other drugs to stimulate peristalsis. If the lumbar region is permanently paralyzed, the patient will have fecal incontinence as well as frequent accumulations of flatus and fecal material in the lower intestine. Rehabilitation of the patient then requires working out some method of bowel control so that regularity of defecation can be accomplished. This will involve some dietary restrictions to control the amount of residue in the colon and to avoid diarrhea and excessive flatus. Rectal suppositories or small enemas may be used regularly to stimulate evacuation at a time convenient for the patient.

paraplexus (par″ah-plek′sus) the choroid plexus of the lateral ventricle of the brain.

parapoplexy (par-ap′o-plek″se) slight apoplexy.

parapraxia (par″ah-prak′se-ah) inability to perform purposive movements properly.

paraprotein (par″ah-pro′te-in) an abnormal type of serum globulin.

paraproteinemia (par″ah-pro″te-ĭ-ne′me-ah) the presence in the blood of an abnormal serum globulin, such as a cryoglobulin or a macroglobulin.

parapsis (par-ap′sis) perversion of the sense of touch.

parapsoriasis (par″ah-so-ri′ah-sis) a chronic red, scaly, skin eruption resembling psoriasis.

parapsychology (par″ah-si-kol′o-je) the study of psychic phenomena, i.e., relations between persons and events which apparently occur without the intervention of the five human senses.

parapsychosis (par″ah-si-ko′sis) perversion of the function of thought.

parareflexia (par″ah-re-flek′se-ah) any disorder of the reflexes.

pararhotacism (par″ah-ro′tah-sizm) faulty enunciation of *r* sound.

pararrhythmia (par″ah-rith′me-ah) cardiac arrhythmia with two separate rhythms at one time.

pararthria (par-ar′thre-ah) imperfect utterance of words.

Parasal (par′ah-sal) trademark for preparations of para-aminosalicylic acid, used in treatment of tuberculosis.

parasigmatism (par″ah-sig′mah-tizm) faulty enunciation of *s* and *z* sounds.

parasite (par′ah-sīt) an organism that lives in or on another organism, from which it gains its nourishment. adj., **parasit′ic.** Among the many parasites in nature, a few feed upon human hosts, causing diseases ranging from the mildly annoying to the severe and even fatal. Parasites include multicelled and single-celled animals, funguses and bacteria. Viruses are sometimes considered to be parasites.
   erratic p., one that invades an organ of the host in which it is not usually found.
   facultative p., one that is not entirely dependent on a host for its survival, but can adapt itself to a parasitic way of life.
   incidental p., an organism that accidentally acquires an unnatural host and survives.
   obligatory p., one that is entirely dependent upon a host for its survival.
   pathogenic p., one that causes disease in the host.
   periodic p., sporadic p., one that intermittently visits a host to obtain some benefit.
   temporary p., one that lives free of its host during part of its life cycle.

parasiticide (par″ah-sit′ĭ-sīd) a substance destructive to parasites.

parasitism (par′ah-si″tizm) the biologic association of two individuals or populations of different species, one of which nourishes itself at the expense of the other, which it often affects adversely, but does not rapidly destroy.

parasitogenic (par″ah-si″to-jen′ik) due to parasites.

parasitology (par″ah-si-tol′o-je) the scientific study of parasites.
   medical p., that particularly concerned with the study of disease-causing parasites.

parasitophobia (par″ah-si″to-fo′be-ah) morbid dread of parasites.

parasitotropic (par″ah-si″to-trop′ik) having affinity for parasites.

paraspadias (par″ah-spa′de-as) a developmental anomaly in which the urethra opens on one side of the penis.

paraspasm (par′ah-spazm) spasm of the corresponding muscles on both sides of the body.

parasteatosis (par″ah-ste″ah-to′sis) disorder of sebaceous secretions.

parasternal (par″ah-ster′nal) beside the sternum.

parasympathetic nervous system (par″ah-sim″-pah-thet′ik) part of the autonomic NERVOUS SYSTEM, the preganglionic fibers of which leave the central nervous system with cranial nerves III, VII, IX and X and the first three sacral nerves; postganglionic fibers are distributed to the heart, smooth muscles and glands of the head and neck, and the thoracic, abdominal and pelvic viscera.

parasympatholytic (par″ah-sim″pah-tho-lit′ik) producing effects resembling those of interruption of the parasympathetic nerve supply of a part; having a destructive effect on the parasympathetic nerve fibers or blocking the transmission of impulses by them.

parasympathomimetic (par″ah-sim″pah-tho-mi-met′ik) producing effects resembling those of stimulation of the parasympathetic nerve supply of a part.

parasystole (par″ah-sis′to-le) an abnormally prolonged interval between systole and diastole.

paratenon (par″ah-ten′on) the fatty areolar tissue filling the interstices of the fascial compartment in which a tendon is situated.

paratherapeutic (par″ah-ther″ah-pu′tik) caused by treatment of some other disease.

parathion (par″ah-thi′on) an insecticide compound, which may cause fatal poisoning in man.

Parathormone (par″ah-thōr′mōn) trademark for a preparation of parathyroid extract.

parathymia (par″ah-thi′me-ah) perverted, contrary or inappropriate emotions.

parathyroid (par″ah-thi′roid) 1. situated beside the thyroid gland. 2. pertaining to the parathyroid glands.
   p. glands, two pairs of small glands located near or attached to the thyroid gland, two on each side of it. They are sometimes embedded in the thyroid tissue. They are part of the endocrine system. Their secretion, parathyroid hormone, controls the metabolism of CALCIUM and PHOSPHORUS in the body.
   The parathyroid glands are subject to two major disorders: HYPERPARATHYROIDISM and HYPOPARATHYROIDISM.

SOME ANIMAL PARASITES HARMFUL TO MAN

PARASITE (Approximate Length) Areas of Occurrence	CONDITION CAUSED	USUAL SOURCE OF INFECTION	PREVENTION
INTERNAL PARASITES			
AMEBA (1/25,000 in.—microscopic) Tropics; occasionally U.S.	Amebic dysentery	Contaminated food and drink	Avoiding unsanitary food and drink
MALARIA PARASITE (1/3,000 in.—microscopic) Tropics; southern U.S.	Malaria	Mosquito bites	Mosquito control; protection against bites
BLOOD FLUKE (1/4–1/2 in.) Tropics; rare in U.S.	Schistosomiasis (disease of liver, intestine, bladder)	Water (organism can penetrate skin)	Avoiding contaminated water
TAPEWORM (6–60 ft.) Most countries; beef tapeworm common in U.S.	Tapeworm (in intestine)	Raw or poorly cooked beef, pork or fish	Cooking meat and fish
HOOKWORM (1/4–1/2 in.) Warm regions; common in southern U.S.	Hookworm disease (ancylostomiasis)	Contaminated soil	Wearing shoes; avoiding direct contact with infected soil
ASCARIS ROUNDWORM (6–12 in.) Parts of southern U.S.; wherever sanitation is poor	Intestinal disorder (ascariasis)	Raw vegetables and fruits	Cooking fruits and vegetables
PINWORM (1/12–1/2 in.) Throughout world	Pinworm infection (enterobiasis)	Contaminated food; contact with infected person	Personal cleanliness
TRICHINA WORM (1/16–1/6 in.) Throughout world; common in U.S.	Trichinosis	Poorly cooked pork	Thorough cooking of pork products
FILARIA WORM (1 1/2–4 in.) Tropics	Filariasis	Mosquito bites	Avoiding mosquito bites
SKIN PARASITES			
ITCH MITE (1/100 in.) Most countries, including U.S.	Scabies	Contact with infected person	Cleanliness of body and clothing; avoiding contact with infected person
LICE (1/25–1/8 in.) Most countries, including U.S.	Itching of skin (pediculosis); also may carry disease germ	Contact with human carrier, clothing, bedding	Cleanliness of body and clothing; avoiding contact with infected person
TICKS (1/10–1/2 in.) Most countries, including U.S.	Skin infestation; also may carry rabbit fever, other diseases	Tick-infested areas	Avoiding tick-infested areas or wearing heavy tight-fitting clothing
FLEAS (1/12–1/8 in.) Most countries, including U.S.	Skin irritation; also may carry disease germs	Animal and human carriers	Cleanliness; avoiding close contact with carriers

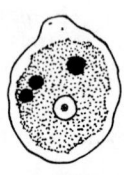

AMEBA

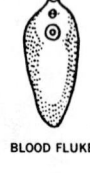

BLOOD FLUKE

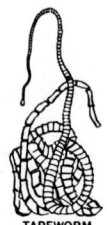

TAPEWORM

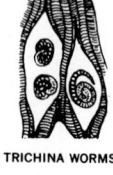

TRICHINA WORMS

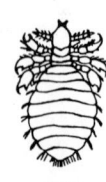

LOUSE

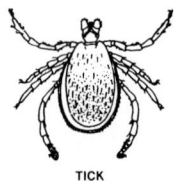

TICK

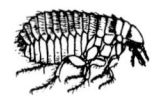

FLEA

parathyroidectomy (par″ah-thi″roi-dek′to-me) excision of a parathyroid gland.

parathyroidoma (par″ah-thi″roi-do′mah) a tumor arising from or composed of tissue resembling the parathyroid gland.

parathyroprivia (par-ah-thi″ro-pri′ve-ah) the condition due to absence of functioning parathyroid glands.

paratrachoma (par″ah-trah-ko′mah) conjunctivitis resembling trachoma.

paratrichosis (par″ah-trĭ-ko′sis) 1. growth of hair in abnormal situations. 2. abnormality of the hair itself.

paratrophy (par-at′ro-fe) 1. bacterial nutrition in which the growth energy is obtained from the host. 2. dystrophy.

paratyphoid (par″ah-ti′foid) an acute generalized infection that can be caused by several different species of Salmonella, although the strains of *S. paratyphi* are the most common causative microorganisms. The disease is usually milder and has a shorter incubation period and more abrupt onset than typhoid fever. Clinically and pathologically, the two diseases cannot be distinguished. (See also TYPHOID FEVER.)

paravaccinia (par″ah-vak-sin′e-ah) an eruption of tubercles sometimes following vaccination.

paravertebral (par″ah-ver′tĕ-bral) near the vertebrae.

paravitaminosis (par″ah-vi″tah-mĭ-no′sis) vitamin deficiency without the usual symptoms.

Paré (par-a′) Ambroise (1510–1590). French surgeon. As an army surgeon treating gunshot wounds, Paré discontinued the application of boiling oils as was customary at that time. He invented many new surgical instruments and reintroduced the use of ligatures to tie off the blood vessels for amputation. He described carbon monoxide poisoning, and has been cited as probably the first to think of flies as transmitters of infectious disease. In obstetrics he did podalic versions and induced labor for uterine hemorrhage. He introduced reimplantation of the teeth in dentistry, and wrote a small book on medical jurisprudence.

Paredrine (par′ah-drēn) trademark for preparations of hydroxyamphetamine, a sympathomimetic nasal decongestant, pressor and mydriatic.

paregoric (par″ĕ-gor′ik) a mixture of powdered opium, anise oil, benzoic acid, camphor and glycerin, in diluted alcohol, used in the treatment of abdominal cramps and diarrhea.

parenchyma (pah-reng′kĭ-mah) the essential or functional elements of an organ, as distinguished from its stroma or framework. adj., **paren′chymal, parenchym′atous.**

Parenogen (par-en′o-gen) trademark for a preparation of fibrinogen, a substance essential for blood clotting.

parenteral (pah-ren′ter-al) not through the alimentary canal, e.g., by subcutaneous, intramuscular, intrasternal or intravenous injection.

parepididymis (par″ep-ĭ-did′ĭ-mis) paradidymis.

parergasia (par″er-ga′ze-ah) a psychic disorder marked by incongruities and mannerisms.

paresis (pah-re′sis, par′ĕ-sis) incomplete paralysis. adj., **paret′ic.**
    general p., syphilitic p., a chronic disease of the brain characterized by degeneration of the cortical neurons and by progressive loss of mental and physical power, and resulting from antecedent syphilitic infection; called also paralytic dementia.

paresthesia (par″es-the′ze-ah) an abnormal or perverted sensation such as burning or tingling due to a disorder of the sensory nervous system.

pareunia (pah-ru′ne-ah) coitus.

paridrosis (par″ĭ-dro′sis) any disorder of the perspiration.

paries (pa′re-ez), pl. *pari′etes* [L.] a wall, as of an organ or cavity.

parietal (pah-ri′ĕ-tal) of or pertaining to the walls of an organ or cavity.
    p. bone, one of two quadrilateral bones forming the sides and roof of the cranium.
    p. lobe, the upper central lobe of the cerebral cortex. It is the receptive area for fine sensory stimuli, and the highest integration and coordination of sensory information is carried on in this area. Damage to the parietal lobe can produce defects in vision and aphasia.

parietography (pah-ri″ĕ-tog′rah-fe) roentgenographic visualization of the walls of an organ.

parity (par′ĭ-te) the condition of a woman with respect to her having borne viable offspring.

Parkinson's disease (par′kin-sunz) a progressive disease of the brain occurring in later life, characterized by stiffness of muscles and tremors; called also parkinsonism, paralysis agitans and shaking palsy.
    SYMPTOMS. Parkinson's disease usually appears gradually and progresses slowly. At first the victim may be troubled by mild tremors of the hands and nodding of the head. He may notice that his movements are somewhat slower and more difficult than usual. Then loss of mobility in the face produces the characteristic masklike facies. As the disease advances, the tremors increase and may involve the whole body, although generally they are not apparent with intentional movements. The muscles become stiffer, making movement increasingly difficult. The gait becomes shuffling and festinating. The back tends to become bent forward in a stooped position. Parkinson's disease does not affect the mental capacity.
    CAUSE. The disease is caused by damage to several small areas of the brain, the substantia nigra, the globus pallidus and the thalamus. In some cases the damage may be the result of a viral infection or of carbon monoxide poisoning. In later life, the cause may be cerebral arteriosclerosis. When the cause is known, the condition is usually called parkinsonism. However, in a large number of patients the cause is not apparent; in these patients the condition is called Parkinson's disease.
    TREATMENT. Physical therapy is an important part of the treatment. Regular active exercise and light massage are helpful. Special muscle exercises

to lessen stiffness and discomfort may be prescribed.

Several medicines are helpful in controlling the symptoms. They include atropine sulfate and related drugs; trihexyphenidyl (Artane); and antihistamines, such as diphenhydramine (Benadryl). Experimental use of the new drug L-dopa indicates that it offers great promise.

In certain cases brain surgery may be helpful in relieving the condition. A surgical technique in which a needle-like device is cooled to a very low temperature and inserted into the brain, destroying a tiny portion of the globus pallidus or thalamus, has had excellent results in some cases. Destruction of such a tiny area by chemical means has also been employed.

parkinsonian (par″kin-sun′e-an) pertaining to or resembling Parkinson's disease.

parkinsonism (par′kin-sun-izm″) a condition marked by rigidity and tremor characteristic of Parkinson's disease. The term parkinsonism is usually restricted to cases in which the condition is known to be secondary to some other disorder.

Parnate (par′nāt) trademark for a preparation of tranylcypromine, an antidepressant.

paroccipital (par″ok-sip′ĭ-tal) beside the occipital bone.

paromomycin (par′o-mo-mi″sin) a stable antibiotic derived from a strain of Streptomyces and effective against Entamoeba, Salmonella, Shigella, Proteus, Aerobacter and *Escherichia coli.*

paromphalocele (par″om-fal′o-sēl) hernia near the navel.

paronychia (par″o-nik′e-ah) infection involving the folds of tissue surrounding the fingernail. The causative organisms may be bacteria or fungi, which usually gain entrance through a hangnail or break in the skin due to improper manicuring. Acute infections are treated with hot compresses and the application of an antibiotic or fungicidal ointment. A pocket of purulent material may require incision with a scalpel to promote drainage and healing. Chronic infections are more difficult to cure and may require the application of a corticosteroid ointment. If the infection is widespread and difficult to treat topically, removal of the nail may be necessary. (See also NAIL.)

paroophoron (par″o-of′o-ron) a small, vestigial structure found between the layers of the mesosalpinx.

parophthalmia (par″of-thal′me-ah) inflammation of the connective tissue around the eye.

paropsis (par-op′sis) a disorder of vision.

parorchidium (par″or-kid′e-um) displacement of a testis.

parorexia (par″o-rek′se-ah) nervous perversion of the appetite, with craving for special articles of food.

parosmia (par-oz′me-ah) perversion of the sense of smell.

parostosis (par″os-to′sis) ossification of tissues outside of the periosteum.

parotid (pah-rot′id) near the ear.

p. glands, the largest of the three main pairs of salivary glands, located on either side of the face, just below and in front of the ears. From each gland a duct, the parotid duct (sometimes called Stensen's duct), runs forward across the cheek and opens on the inside surface of the cheek opposite the second molar of the upper jaw.

The parotid glands are made up of groups of cells clustered around a globular cavity, resembling a bunch of grapes. Small ducts draining each cavity join the ducts of neighboring cavities to form larger ducts, which in turn join the parotid duct.

From the system of ducts flows the thin, watery secretion of the parotid glands called saliva, which plays an important role in the process of digestion. As food is chewed the saliva with which it is mixed and moistened makes it possible for the food to be reduced to a substance that can be swallowed.

Controlled by the autonomic nervous system, the secretion of the salivary glands begins whenever the sensory nerves of the mouth, or in some cases nerves located elsewhere in the body, are stimulated.

Salivation may be an involuntary reflex, as when food or even inedible material placed in the mouth starts the flow of the secretion from the glands, or it may be a conditioned reflex, as when the flow is started by the sight, smell or thought of food.

DISORDERS OF THE PAROTID GLANDS. The most common disease affecting the parotid glands is MUMPS, or epidemic parotitis.

Swelling and tenderness may also result from infections caused by other viruses or bacteria in the glands. Less often, these symptoms indicate a blockage of a duct by either infection or a calculus, in which case the swelling is likely to fluctuate, especially at mealtimes. Though stubborn or recurring cases sometimes require surgery, stones often can be removed by massage. For infections, antibiotics and warm compresses are the usual treatment.

Occasionally additional glandular masses grow in or near a parotid gland. The majority of such growths are mixed tumors, so called because they contain cartilage or other material as well as the usual glandular material. Usually they are benign; occasionally they may be malignant and require surgery.

parotidectomy (pah-rot″i-dek′to-me) excision of a parotid gland.

parotiditis, parotitis (pah-rot″i-di′tis), (par″o-ti′-tis) inflammation of the parotid gland.

contagious p., epidemic p., mumps; an acute, communicable viral disease involving chiefly the parotid gland, but frequently affecting other oral glands or the pancreas or gonads (see also MUMPS).

parovarian (par″o-va′re-an) beside the ovary.

parovarium (par″o-va′re-um) epoophoron; a vestigial structure associated with the ovary.

paroxysm (par′ok-sizm) an episode or occurrence of abrupt onset and termination. adj., **paroxys′mal.**

parrot fever a viral infection transmitted to man by birds; called also PSITTACOSIS.

Parry's disease (par′ēz) exophthalmic goiter.

pars (pars), pl. *par′tes* [L.] a division or part.

p. mastoi′dea, the mastoid portion of the temporal bone, being the irregular, posterior part.

p. petro'sa, the petrous portion of the temporal bone, containing the inner ear and wedged in at the base of the skull between the sphenoid and occipital bones.

p. squamo'sa, the flat, scalelike, anterior and superior portion of the temporal bone.

p. tympan'ica, the tympanic portion of the temporal bone, the curved plate lying below the squama and in front of the mastoid process.

Parsidol (par'sĭ-dol) trademark for a preparation of ethopropazine, used to produce parasympathetic blockade and in treatment of Parkinson's disease.

parthenogenesis, parthogenesis (par″thĕ-no-jen'ĕ-sis), (par″tho-jen'ĕ-sis) development of an ovum not initiated by combination with a male gamete; it may occur as a natural phenomenon or be induced by chemical or mechanical stimulation (artificial parthenogenesis). adj., **parthenogenet'ic, parthogenet'ic.**

partial thromboplastin time a one-stage clotting test to detect deficiencies of the components of the intrinsic thromboplastin system, performed by measuring the clotting time of recalcified plasma after addition of crude cephalin brain extract; abbreviated PTT.

particle (par'tĭ-kl) an extremely small mass or portion of substance or matter. (See also ALPHA PARTICLES and BETA PARTICLES.)

particulate (par-tik'u-lāt) composed of separate particles.

parturient (par-tu're-ent) giving birth or pertaining to birth; by extension, a woman at childbirth.

parturifacient (par-tu″rĭ-fa'shent) a medicine that facilitates childbirth.

parturiometer (par-tu″rĭ-om'ĕ-ter) a device used in measuring the expulsive power of the uterus.

parturition (par″tu-rish'un) expulsion or delivery of the fetus from the body of the maternal organism.

parulis (pah-roo'lis) abscess of the gingiva.

parumbilical (par″um-bil'ĭ-kal) near the navel.

parvicellular (par″vĭ-sel'u-lar) composed of small cells.

PAS, PASA para-aminosalicylic acid, used in treatment of tuberculosis.

Pasteur (pas-ter') Louis (1822–1895). French chemist and bacteriologist, founder of microbiology and developer of the method of vaccination by attenuated virus. He was born at Dôle, Jura.

By optical investigation of racemic acid, he discovered a new class of isomeric substances which led to work by others on stereochemistry and for which he received the ribbon of the Legion of Honor. Pasteur came to the rescue of the wine industry by his interest in fermentation, and showed that spoiling of wine caused by microorganisms could be prevented by partial heat sterilization (pasteurization), a process now applied to all perishable foods. Experimental foundation was given to his ideas of fermentation and the long-accepted theory of spontaneous generation was disposed of once and for all. Later he came to the rescue of the silkworm industry and found methods for detecting and preventing pébrine and flâcherie, the two diseases that were destroying it. He turned his attention then to anthrax, chicken cholera and hydrophobia (rabies), and developed preventive inoculations against them. The Pasteur Institute was opened shortly thereafter and institutions were founded all over the world for inoculation against rabies.

Pasteurella (pas″tĕ-rel'ah) a genus of Schizomycetes.

P. pes'tis, the etiologic agent of plague.

P. tularen'sis, the etiologic agent of tularemia.

pasteurellosis (pas″ter-ĕ-lo'sis) infection with organisms of the genus Pasteurella.

pasteurization (pas″tūr-ĭ-za'shun) exposure of milk or other substances to a temperature of 60° C. for 30 minutes, killing pathogenic bacteria and delaying other bacterial development.

patch (pach) a small area differing from the rest of a surface.

Peyer's p's, whitish patches of lymphatic follicles in mucous and submucous layers of the small intestine.

p. test, a test for hypersensitivity in which filter paper or gauze saturated with the substance in question is applied to the skin, usually on the forearm. A positive reaction is reddening or swelling at the site. (See also SKIN TEST.)

patella (pah-tel'ah), pl. *patel'lae* [L.] a triangular bone at the knee; the kneecap.

patellapexy (pah-tel'ah-pek″se) surgical fixation of the patella to the lower end of the femur.

patellar (pah-tel'ar) of or pertaining to the patella.

p. ligament, the continuation of the central portion of the tendon of the quadriceps muscle of the thigh; called also patellar tendon.

p. reflex, involuntary contraction of the quadriceps muscle and jerky extension of the leg when the patellar ligament is tapped with a mallet. It is often used as a test of nervous system function. Called also KNEE JERK and quadriceps reflex.

patellectomy (pat″ĕ-lek'to-me) excision of the patella.

patelliform (pah-tel'ĭ-form) shaped like the patella.

patellofemoral (pah-tel″o-fem'o-ral) pertaining to the patella and femur.

patency (pa'ten-se) the condition of being wide open.

patent (pa'tent) 1. open, unobstructed or not closed. 2. apparent, evident.

p. ductus arteriosus, a congenital heart defect, persistence of the opening between the aorta and pulmonary artery. The ductus arteriosus is open during prenatal life, allowing most of the blood of the fetus to bypass the lungs, but normally this channel closes shortly before birth. When the ductus arteriosus remains open, it places special burdens on the left ventricle and causes a diminished blood flow in the aorta.

The symptoms of patent ductus arteriosus are usually so slight they are not noticed until the child is older and more active. He then begins to experience dyspnea on exertion. If the ductus is large there may be retardation of growth.

Treatment is surgical, preferably when the child is from 4 to 10 years of age. The open ductus arteriosus is ligated. Prognosis for this condition, when not accompanied by other congenital heart defects, is excellent.

p. medicine (pat'ent), vernacular term for a nostrum advertised to the public. It is generally of secret composition.

path(o)- (path'o) word element [Gr.] *disease; morbid condition.*

pathergasia (path"er-ga'ze-ah) mental malfunction, implying functional or structural damage.

pathergy (path'er-je) 1. a condition in which the application of a stimulus leaves the body abnormally susceptible to subsequent stimuli. 2. a condition of being allergic to several antigens.

pathic (path'ik) pertaining to disease.

Pathilon (path'ĭ-lon) trademark for preparations of tridihexethyl, used in parasympathetic blockade.

patho-anatomy (path"o-ah-nat'o-me) pathologic anatomy.

pathobiology (path"o-bi-ol'o-je) pathology.

pathogen (path'o-jen) any disease-producing agent or microorganism. adj., **pathogen'ic.**

pathogenesis (path"o-jen'ĕ-sis) the development of disease or of a morbid or pathologic state. adj., **pathogenet'ic.**

pathogenicity (path"o-jĕ-nis'ĭ-te) the quality of producing or the ability to produce pathologic changes or disease.

pathogeny (pah-thoj'ĕ-ne) pathogenesis.

pathoglycemia (path"o-gli-se'me-ah) sugar in the blood as a result of some disease.

pathognomonic (path"og-no-mon'ik) specifically distinctive or characteristic of a disease or pathologic condition.

pathologic (path'o-loj'ik) 1. pertaining to or caused by disease. 2. pertaining to pathology.

pathologist (pah-thol'o-jist) a specialist in pathology.

pathology (pah-thol'o-je) the scientific study of the alterations produced by disease.
   behavior p., psychopathology.
   clinical p., pathology applied to the solution of clinical problems; especially the use of laboratory methods in clinical diagnosis.
   comparative p., that which considers human disease processes in comparison with those of the lower animals.
   experimental p., the study of artificially induced pathologic processes.
   oral p., that which treats of conditions causing or resulting from morbid anatomic or functional changes in the structures of the mouth.
   surgical p., the study of the pathology of diseases accessible to operative intervention.

patholysis (pah-thol'ĭ-sis) dissolution of tissues by disease.

pathomimesis (path"o-mi-me'sis) malingering.

pathomorphism (path"o-mor'fizm) abnormal morphology.

pathonomia, pathonomy (path"o-no'me-ah), (pah-thon'o-me) the science of the laws of disease.

pathophobia (path"o-fo'be-ah) morbid fear of disease.

pathophoresis (path"o-fo-re'sis) the transmission of disease.

pathophysiology (path"o-fiz"e-ol'o-je) the physiology of disordered function.

pathopleiosis (path"o-pli-o'sis) the tendency to magnify the gravity of one's disease.

pathopsychology (path"o-si-kol'o-je) the psychology of mental disease.

pathosis (pah-tho'sis) a diseased condition.

pathway (path'wa) a course usually followed. In neurology, the nerve structures through which a sensory impression is conducted to the cerebral cortex (afferent pathway), or through which an impulse passes from the brain to the skeletal musculature (efferent pathway).
   biosynthetic p., the sequence of enzymatic steps in the synthesis of a specific end product in a living organism.

-pathy (path'e) word element [Gr.], *morbid condition* or *disease;* generally used to designate a noninflammatory condition.

patient (pa'shent) a person who is undergoing treatment for disease.

patroclinous (pat"ro-kli'nus) inheriting or inherited from the father.

patulous (pat'u-lus) spread widely apart; open.

Paul-Bunnell test (pawl bun-el') a method of testing for the presence of heterophil antibodies in the blood: the blood of patients with infectious mononucleosis contains antibodies for the erythrocytes of sheep.

Paveril (pav'er-il) trademark for preparations of dioxyline, a vasodilator.

pavor (pa'vor) an extreme fear reaction; terror.
   p. diur'nus, an extreme fear reaction in a child during a daytime nap.
   p. noctur'nus, an extreme fear reaction in a child during sleep or at night.

P.B. *Pharmacopoeia Britannica* (British pharmacopoeia).

Pb chemical symbol, lead (L. *plumbum*).

PBI protein-bound iodine (see PROTEIN-BOUND IODINE TEST).

p.c. [L.] *post ci'bum* (after meals).

PCG phonocardiogram.

pCO$_2$ carbon dioxide tension (see RESPIRATION).

P.C.V. packed-cell volume, the volume of the blood corpuscles in a centrifuged sample of blood, especially the volume of packed red cells in cubic centimeters per 100 cc. of blood.

Pd chemical symbol, *palladium*.

peanut oil (pe′nut) a refined fixed oil from seed kernels of cultivated varieties of *Arachis hypogaea;* used as a solvent for drugs administered by injection.

pearl (perl) 1. a small medicated granule. 2. a glass globule with a single dose of volatile medicine.
epithelial p., a form of granule found in epithelioma.
Laennec's p's, round masses of sputum in bronchial asthma.

pecazine (pe′kah-zēn) mepazine, a tranquilizer.

peccant (pek′ant) unhealthy; causing ill health.

pectase (pek′tās) an enzyme that catalyzes the demethylation of pectin, thus producing pectic acid.

pectin (pek′ten), pl. *pec′tines* [L.] a narrow zone in the anal canal distal to the line separating the rectal mucosa and the skin of the canal. adj., **pectin′eal.**
p. os′sis pu′bis, the sharp anterior border of the pubic bone (os pubis).

pectenitis (pek″tĕ-ni′tis) inflammation of the pecten of the anus.

pectenosis (pek″tĕ-no′sis) stenosis of the anal canal due to an inelastic ring of tissue.

pectin (pek′tin) a purified carbohydrate product from the dilute acid extract of the inner portion of the rind of citrus fruits or from apple pulp; used as a plasma substitute or an emulsifying or gelling agent.

pectinate, pectiniform (pek′tĭ-nāt), (pek-tin′ĭ-form) shaped like a comb.

pectoral (pek′tor-al) 1. pertaining to the chest or breast. 2. effective in diseases of the chest.
p. muscles, four muscles of the chest (see table of MUSCLES).

pectoralgia (pek″to-ral′je-ah) pain in the chest.

pectoralis (pek″to-ra′lis) pertaining to the chest or breast.

pectoriloquy (pek″to-ril′o-kwe) transmission of the sound of spoken words through the chest wall, indicating the presence of a cavity or solidification of pulmonary structures.

pectorophony (pek″to-rof′o-ne) exaggeration of vocal resonance heard on auscultation.

pectus (pek′tus) the breast, chest or thorax.
p. carina′tum, a malformation of the chest wall in which the sternum is abnormally prominent; called also pigeon chest or chicken breast.
Moderate cases cause no difficulties and require no treatment. In severe cases, the deformity of the chest may interfere with lung and heart action, causing dyspnea on exercise and increased susceptibility to respiratory infections. Serious malformations can usually be corrected by surgery.
p. excava′tum, a congenital malformation of the chest wall characterized by a pronounced funnel-shaped depression with its apex over the lower end of the sternum; called also funnel chest.

The condition is caused by a shortening of the central portion of the diaphragm, which pulls the sternum backward during inhalation, and by the growth of ribs. Except in mild cases, it decreases the ability of the child to engage in sustained exercise. It delays recovery from coughs and colds, reduces the ability to eat a full meal, so that most patients are underweight, and often produces a functional heart murmur. Noisy breathing may occur during sleep. A child may also develop an emotional problem because of embarrassment over the deformity.

The deformity can be satisfactorily corrected by surgery.

ped(o)- (pe′do) word element, (1) [Gr.] *child;* (2) [L.] *foot.*

pedal (ped′al) pertaining to the foot or feet.

pederasty (ped″er-as′te) sexual intercourse per anum; usually applied to that between human males, especially between an adult and a youth.

pediatric (pe″de-at′rik) pertaining to diseases of children.

pediatrician (pe″de-ah-trish′an) a specialist in pediatrics.

pediatrics (pe″de-at′riks) the department of medicine dealing especially with problems and diseases of young children.

pedicellation (ped″ĭ-sĕ-la′shun) the development of a pedicle.

pedicle (ped′ĭ-kl) a footlike or stemlike part, such as a narrow strip by which a graft of tissue remains attached to the donor site.
vertebral p., one of the paired parts of the vertebral arch that connect a lamina to the vertebral body.

pediculation (pĕ-dik″u-la′shun) 1. the process of forming a pedicle. 2. infestation with lice.

pediculicide (pĕ-dik′u-lĭ-sīd) an agent that destroys lice.

pediculophobia (pĕ-dik″u-lo-fo′be-ah) morbid dread of lice.

pediculosis (pĕ-dik″u-lo′sis) infestation with lice. (See also LOUSE.)

Pediculus (pĕ-dik′u-lus) a genus of lice.
P. huma′nus, a species that feeds on human blood and is an important vector of relapsing fever, typhus and trench fever; included in the species are *P. humanus* var. *capitis,* occurring in the head, and *P. humanus* var. *corporis,* occurring elsewhere on the body.
P. inguina′lis, P. pu′bis, *Phthirus pubis.*

pediophobia (pe″de-o-fo′be-ah) morbid dread of children or dolls.

pedodontia, pedodontics (pe″do-don′she-ah), (pe″do-don′tiks) the department of dentistry dealing with the teeth and mouth conditions of children.

pedodontist (pe″do-don′tist) a dentist who specializes in pedodontics.

pedograph (ped′o-graf) an imprint of the weight-bearing surface of the foot.

pedomorphism (pe″do-mor′fizm) retention in adult organisms of bodily characters that in early evolutionary history were only infantile.

pedophilia (pe″do-fil′e-ah) abnormal fondness for children.

pedophobia (pe″do-fo′be-ah) fear or dread of children.

peduncle (pe-dung′kl) a stemlike part; applied to collections of nerve fibers coursing between different regions in the central nervous system. adj., **pedun′cular.**
  cerebellar p's, three sets of paired bundles (superior, middle and inferior) connecting the cerebellum to the midbrain, pons and medulla oblongata, respectively.
  cerebral p's, two massive bundles, one on each side, constituting the ventral portion of the midbrain.
  pineal p., a slender band going forward on either side from the pineal gland.

pedunculated (pe-dung′ku-lāt″ed) having a peduncle.

pedunculotomy (pe-dung″ku-lot′o-me) incision of a peduncle of the brain.

pedunculus (pe-dung′ku-lus) peduncle.

Peganone (peg′ah-nōn) trademark for a preparation of ethotoin, an anticonvulsant.

Pel-Ebstein disease (pel eb′stīn) Hodgkin's disease.

peladophobia (pel″ah-do-fo′be-ah) morbid fear of baldness.

pelage (pel′ij) the hairy covering of the body.

peliosis (pe″le-o′sis) purpura.

pella (pel′ah) cutis; the skin.

pellagra (pĕ-la′grah, pĕ-lag′rah) a disease caused by a diet seriously deficient in niacin, or nicotinic acid. Most persons with pellagra also suffer from deficiencies of vitamin B$_2$ (riboflavin) and other essential vitamins and minerals. adj., **pellag′rous.**
  Pellagra occurs in many areas of the world. Until recent years, it was the major form of acute vitamin deficiency in the southeastern United States. It is now sharply on the decline in the United States, largely as a result of the efforts of the Public Health Service. The disease also occurs in persons suffering from alcoholism and drug addiction.
  SYMPTOMS. Chief symptoms of pellagra are various skin, digestive, and mental disturbances. The mouth becomes inflamed and the tongue red and sore; cracks and sores appear in the skin around the mouth. The skin on the back of the hands may become red, thick and scaly, as may that of the neck and chest—areas exposed to sunlight and the chafing of clothes.
  Vomiting and loss of appetite occur. Diarrhea often appears early and becomes worse as the dis-

ease progresses, thus hampering treatment by preventing effective absorption of essential vitamins.
  Mental symptoms are variable. In some cases, there may be only insomnia and minor depression. In other cases, the sufferer may become stuporous, or on the contrary become violent and irrational. Headache, irritability and general anxiety may also be present.
  TREATMENT. Treatment of pellagra consists of an improved diet, often combined with large doses of niacinamide. In acute cases, niacinamide must be administered by injection and must be accompanied by large doses of other vitamins.
  The patient's diet should include meat (particularly liver), whole-grain cereals and peanuts, all of which are especially good sources of niacin. In severe cases of pellagra, bed rest is required. Skin lesions are treated with antibiotics.

pellagrin (pĕ-la′grin, pĕ-lag′rin) a person affected with pellagra.

pellagroid (pĕ-lag′roid) resembling pellagra.

Pellegrini's disease (pel″a-gre′nēz) calcification of the medial collateral ligament of the knee due to trauma; called also Pellegrini-Stieda disease.

pellet (pel′et) a small pill or granule.

pellicle (pel′ĭ-kl) a thin scum forming on the surface of liquids.

pellicula (pĕ-lik′u-lah) epidermis.

pellucid (pĕ-lu′sid) translucent.

pelvic (pel′vik) pertaining to the pelvis.
  p. bone, hip bone, comprising the ilium, ischium and pubis.
  p. diameters, imaginary lines connecting opposite points of the pelvis; the most important are: *anteroposterior* (of inlet), that joining the sacrovertebral angle and the symphysis pubis; *anteroposterior* (of outlet), that joining the tip of the coccyx and the subpubic ligament; *conjugate,* the anteroposterior diameter of the inlet; *diagonal conjugate,* that joining the sacrovertebral angle and the subpubic ligament; *external conjugate,* that joining the depression above the spine of the first sacral vertebra and the middle of the upper border of the symphysis pubis; *internal conjugate,* that joining the sacral promontory and the upper edge of the symphysis pubis; *true conjugate,* that joining the sacrovertebral angle and the most prominent portion of the posterior aspect of the symphysis pubis; *transverse* (of inlet), that joining the two most widely separated points of the pelvic inlet; *transverse* (of outlet), that joining the ischial tuberosities.
  p. inlet, the superior opening of the pelvis.
  p. outlet, the inferior opening of the pelvis.

pelvicephalometry (pel″vĭ-sef″ah-lom″ĕ-tre) roentgenographic measurement of the fetal head in relation to the maternal pelvis.

pelvimeter (pel-vim′ĕ-ter) an instrument for measuring the pelvis.

pelvimetry (pel-vim′ĕ-tre) measurement of the capacity and diameter of the pelvis, either internally or externally or both, with the hands or with a pelvimeter.

pelvioileoneocystostomy (pel″ve-o-il″e-o-ne″o-sis-tos'to-me) anastomosis of the renal pelvis to an isolated segment of the ileum, which is then anastomosed to the urinary bladder.

pelviotomy (pel"ve-ot'o-me) 1. incision or transection of a pelvic (hip) bone. 2. pyelotomy; incision of the renal pelvis.

pelviperitonitis (pel"vĭ-per"ĭ-to-ni'tis) inflammation of the pelvic peritoneum.

pelviroentgenography (pel"vĭ-rent"gĕ-nog'rah-fe) roentgenography of the organs of the pelvis.

pelvis (pel'vis) 1. the expanded, proximal portion of the ureter, usually contained in the substance of the kidney, in which the calices of the kidney open. 2. the basin formed by the hip bones and lower portion of the vertebral column, constituting the lowest part of the trunk.

The bony pelvis is formed by the sacrum, the coccyx and the ilium, pubis and ischium, bones that form the hip and pubic arch. These bones are separate in the child, but become fused by adulthood.

The pelvis is subjected to more stress than any other body structure. The upper part of the pelvic girdle, which is somewhat flared, supports the weight of internal organs in the upper part of the body.

Pelvic structures in men and women differ both in shape and in relative size. The male pelvis is heart shaped and narrow and proportionately heavier and stronger than the female, so that it is better suited for lifting and running. The female pelvis is constructed to accommodate the fetus during pregnancy and to facilitate its downward passage through the pelvic cavity in childbirth. The most obvious difference between the male and female pelvis is in the shape. A woman's hips are wider and her pelvic cavity is round and relatively large. Even among women, moreover, there are differences in the shape of the pelvis, and these differences must be taken into account in childbirth. During pregnancy the capacity of the pelvis and the PELVIC DIAMETERS are measured, so that possible complications during labor can be avoided.

android p., one with a wedge-shaped inlet and narrow anterior segment typically found in the male.

anthropoid p., one whose anteroposterior diameter equals or exceeds the transverse diameter.

assimilation p., one in which the sacrum articulates with the vertebral column higher (high assimilation pelvis) or lower (low assimilation pelvis) than normal, the number of lumbar vertebrae being correspondingly decreased or increased.

brachypellic p., a short oval type of pelvis, in which the transverse diameter exceeds the anteroposterior diameter by 1 to 3 cm.

contracted p., one showing a decrease of 1.5 to 2 cm. in an important diameter.

dolichopellic p., a long, oval pelvis with the anteroposterior diameter greater than the transverse diameter.

false p., part of the pelvic cavity above a plane determined by a line on the inner surface of the ilium extending from the sacroiliac joint to the eminence at the junction of the ilium and the superior ramus of the pubis.

flat p., one in which the anteroposterior dimension is abnormally reduced.

frozen p., a condition in which the fornices of the uterus are filled with a hardened exudate.

gynecoid p., one with a rounded, oval shape, typical of the normal female.

infantile p., a generally contracted pelvis with an oval shape, a high sacrum and inclination of the walls.

inverted p., split pelvis.

juvenile p., infantile pelvis.

kyphotic p., one marked by increase of the conjugate diameter at the brim with decrease of the transverse diameter at the outlet.

p. ma'jor, false pelvis.

malacosteon p., one deformed as a result of rickets.

mesatipellic p., a round type of pelvis, in which the transverse diameter is equal to the anteroposterior diameter or exceeds it by no more than 1 cm.

p. mi'nor, true pelvis.

Nägele's p., one contracted in an oblique diameter, with complete ankylosis of the sacroiliac joint on one side, rotation of the sacrum toward the same side and deviation of the symphysis pubis to the opposite side.

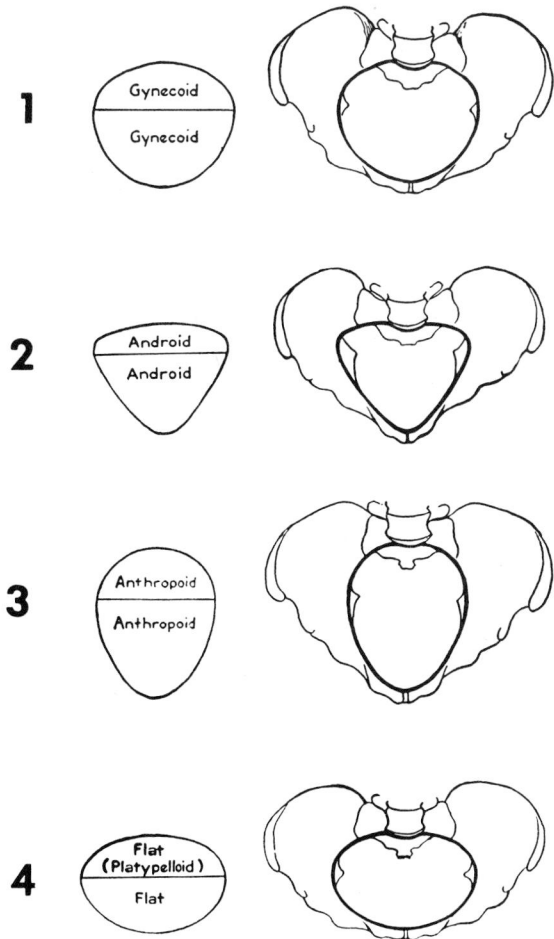

1 Gynecoid / Gynecoid

2 Android / Android

3 Anthropoid / Anthropoid

4 Flat (Platypelloid) / Flat

Pure types of pelvic inlets according to Caldwell, Moloy and D'Esopo. (From Davis, M. E., and Rubin, R.: De Lee's Obstetrics for Nurses. 18th ed. Philadelphia, W. B. Saunders Co., 1966.)

platypellic p., a broad pelvis, in which the transverse diameter exceeds the anteroposterior diameter by 3 cm. or more.

platypelloid p., one shortened in the anteroposterior aspect, with a flattened transverse, oval shape.

rachitic p., one affected with rickets.

Robert's p., one with a rudimentary sacrum and great reduction of the transverse diameter.

scoliotic p., one tilted as a result of scoliosis.

split p., one with a congenital separation at the symphysis pubis.

spondylolisthetic p., one deformed by sliding of the lower lumbar vertebrae over the sacrum and into the pelvis.

true p., the part of the pelvic cavity below a plane determined by a line on the inner surface of the ilium, extending from the sacroiliac joint to the eminence at the junction of the ilium and the superior ramus of the pubis.

pelvospondylitis (pel″vo-spon″dĭ-li′tis) inflammation of the pelvic portion of the spine.

p. ossif′icans, rheumatoid spondylitis.

pemphigoid (pem′fĭ-goid) 1. resembling pemphigus. 2. a group of skin disorders similar to but clearly distinguishable from pemphigus.

bullous p., a chronic, usually nonfatal, bullous skin disorder seen in middle-aged or elderly persons.

pemphigus (pem′fĭ-gus) a skin disease characterized by large "water blisters." The disease owes its name to the Greek word for blister: *pemphix*. A rare disease, it is also a serious one that requires prompt treatment. It can occur in acute or chronic form. The term pemphigus generally refers to pemphigus vulgaris, the chronic form.

Clusters of blisters usually appear first near the nose and mouth—sometimes inside them—and then gradually spread over the skin of the rest of the body. When the blisters burst, they leave round patches of raw and tender skin. The skin itches, burns and gives off an offensive odor. The patient loses appetite and weight. If the disease is allowed to progress, it may cause extreme weakness, prostration and shock, accompanied by chills, sweating, fever and often pneumonia.

The cause of pemphigus is unknown. It seems to occur only in adults.

The patient must be hospitalized from the beginning and given antibiotics and sometimes blood transfusions. He suffers intense discomfort and may need to suck anesthetic tablets to allay pain around the mouth while eating.

Progress has been made in the treatment of this disease through the persistent use of cortisone, administered orally, and of the pituitary extract ACTH, administered intramuscularly. Fatalities, once fairly common, now can usually be averted. The disease is difficult to control, however, and therapy sometimes must be maintained for years to prevent continuing attacks.

benign chronic familial p., a genetically transmitted condition that resembles pemphigus but heals spontaneously.

Brazilian p., a condition resembling pemphigus foliaceus endemic in Brazil.

bullous p., a chronic, generalized bullous eruption occurring in elderly adults predominantly, and usually not fatal.

p. erythemato′sus, pemphigus in which the lesions resemble lupus erythematosus and are limited to the face and chest.

p. folia′ceus, pemphigus characterized by widespread flaky, slightly exudative lesions, resembling exfoliative dermatitis.

hemorrhagic p., a condition characterized by the presence of bullae filled with hemorrhagic fluid.

South American p., Brazilian pemphigus.

p. veg′etans, a variant of bullous pemphigus in which wartlike hypertrophic vegetative masses replace many of the bullous lesions.

p. vulga′ris, chronic pemphigus.

wildfire p., Brazilian pemphigus.

pendulous (pen′du-lus) hanging loosely.

penetrance (pen′ĕ-trans) the frequency with which a heritable trait is manifested by individuals carrying the principal gene or genes conditioning it.

penetrometer (pen″ĕ-trom′ĕ-ter) 1. an instrument for measuring the penetrating power of x-rays. 2. a device for registering the resistance of semisolid material to penetration.

-penia (pe′ne-ah) word element [Gr.], *scarcity*.

penicillamine (pen″ĭ-sil-am′in) an amino acid obtained from penicillin by treatment with hot mineral acids; used in the treatment of diseases characterized by excess copper deposition in the body, as Wilson's disease.

penicillin (pen″ĭ-sil′in) an antibiotic substance extracted from cultures of certain molds of the genus Penicillium that have been grown on special media.

Penicillin was discovered by Sir Alexander Fleming in 1929 at St. Mary's Hospital in London. During World War II it came into general use and was hailed as a "wonder drug" because of its ability to control certain types of infections. Since the discovery of penicillin many other antibiotics have been developed, some of them more effective than penicillin against certain types of organisms. Penicillin is known as a narrow-spectrum antibiotic, which means that it is effective against relatively few organisms. (See also ANTIBIOTIC.)

Many different preparations of penicillin are available today; the choice of preparation depends on the specific needs in a particular case. Penicillin is prepared in a number of salts, but aluminum, calcium, potassium and sodium are the most common. It exists in several types: F, G, K, O, V and X. Type G is most commonly used. Type V is a synthetic penicillin. Procaine penicillin G is a preparation modified to prolong its effectiveness. Dimethoxyphenyl penicillin (methicillin) and oxacillin are semisynthetic penicillins that are highly resistant to inactivation by penicillinase. Phenoxymethyl penicillin (phenethicillin) is a preparation for oral administration.

Penicillin is administered intramuscularly, orally in liquid or tablet form and topically in ointments. Oral administration requires larger doses of the drug because absorption is incomplete.

Allergic reaction to penicillin occurs in some persons. The reaction may be slight—a stinging or burning sensation at the site of injection—or it can be more serious—severe dermatitis or even anaphylactic shock, which may be fatal.

penicillinase (pen″ĭ-sil′ĭ-nās) an enzyme produced by bacteria that inactivates penicillin; it is sometimes used to treat allergic reactions to penicillin.

Penicillium (pen″ĭ-sil′e-um) a genus of fungi.

penis (pe′nis) the external male organ of urination and coitus.

The body of the penis consists of three cylindrical-shaped masses of erectile tissue which run the length of the penis. Two of the masses lie alongside each other and end behind the head of the penis. The third mass lies underneath them. This latter mass contains the urethra. The penis terminates in an oval or cone-shaped body, the glans penis, which contains the exterior opening of the urethra.

The glans penis is covered by a loose skin, the foreskin or prepuce, which enables it to expand freely during erection. The skin ends just behind the glans penis and folds forward to cover it. The inner surface of the foreskin contains glands that secrete a lubricating fluid called smegma which makes it easy for the penis to expand and retract past the foreskin.

DISORDERS OF THE PENIS. Disorders of the penis are rare. One of the most common complaints is phimosis, due to tight foreskin, which may make erection painful. This condition can be easily remedied by circumcision.

Among the most common diseases of the penis are those caused by venereal infections, such as syphilis and gonorrhea. Cancer of the penis is rare and virtually never occurs in a person who has been circumcised.

penitis (pe-ni′tis) inflammation of the penis.

penniform (pen′ĭ-form) shaped like a feather.

Penrose drain (pen′rōz) a cigarette drain consisting of a piece of rubber tubing through which gauze has been pulled.

penta (pen′tah) word element [Gr.], *five.*

pentachlorin (pen″tah-klo′rin) chlorophenothane, a DDT compound used as an insecticide.

pentad (pen′tad) an element or radical with a valence of five.

pentaerythritol tetranitrate (pen″tah-e-rith′rĭ-tol tĕ″trah-ni′trāt) a vasodilator, used in treatment of angina pectoris.

pentamethylenetetrazol (pen″tah-meth″ĭ-lēn-tĕ′trah-zol) pentylenetetrazol, a central nervous system stimulant.

pentamidine isethionate (pen-tam′ĭ-dēn i″sĕ-thi′o-nāt) a compound used as an antiprotozoan and local anesthetic.

pentapeptide (pen″tah-pep′tīd) a polypeptide containing five amino acids.

pentaploidy (pen″tah-ploi″de) the state of having five sets of chromosomes (5n).

pentapyrrolidinium (pen″tah-pĭ-ro″lĭ-din′e-um) pentolinium tartrate, a ganglionic blocking agent.

pentaquine (pen′tah-kwin) an antimalarial compound.

pentavalent (pen″tah-va′lent, pen-tav′ah-lent) having a valence of five.

penthienate (pen-thi′ĕ-nāt) a compound used in parasympathetic blockade.

Penthrane (pen′thrān) trademark for a preparation of methoxyflurane, an anesthetic.

Pentids (pen′tidz) trademark for preparations of potassium penicillin G.

pentobarbital, pentobarbitone (pen″to-bar′bĭ-tal), (pen″to-bar′bĭ-tōn) a short- to intermediate-acting barbiturate.

   p. sodium, a hypnotic compound used orally, rectally or intravenously.

pentolinium tartrate (pen″to-lin′e-um tar′trāt) a ganglionic blocking agent used primarily as an antihypertensive. Dosage is adjusted according to observations of blood pressure as well as toxic effects. These side effects include cardiovascular collapse and must be treated immediately with epinephrine or levarterenol.

pentolysis (pen-tol′ĭ-sis) the disintegration or splitting up of pentose.

pentose (pen′tōs) any sugar or hydrocarbon of formula $C_5H_{10}O_5$.

pentoside (pen′to-sīd) a compound (glycoside) of pentose with another substance.

pentosuria (pen″to-su′re-ah) pentose in the urine.

Pentothal sodium (pen′to-thal) trademark for a preparation of thiopental sodium, a hypnotic given by intravenous injection or rectally. The intravenous route is used when it is desirable to produce ANESTHESIA quickly for short duration. Psychiatrists use the drug as a sedative or sometimes in narcoanalysis.

pentylenetetrazol (pen″tĭ-lēn-te′trah-zol) a compound used as a central nervous system stimulant.

Pen-vee (pen′ve) trademark for preparations of penicillin V.

peonin (pe′o-nin) a dye used as an indicator for alkalis and acids.

peppermint (pep′er-mint) the dried leaves and flowering tops of *Mentha piperita,* used as a flavoring vehicle for drugs.

pepsin (pep′sin) a proteolytic enzyme that is the principal digestive component of gastric juice. It acts as a catalyst in the chemical breakdown of protein. Pepsin also has a milk-clotting action similar to that of rennin and thereby facilitates the digestion of milk protein. A preparation from the fresh stomach of the hog is used therapeutically.

pepsinogen (pep-sin′o-jen) the inactive precursor of pepsin, secreted by the chief cells of the stomach and converted to pepsin under the influence of hydrogen ions.

peptic (pep′tik) pertaining to pepsin or to digestion.

   p. ulcer, a sore on the inner wall of the digestive tract in or near the stomach. There are two kinds of peptic ulcers: *Gastric* ulcers occur in the stomach; duodenal ulcers occur in the duodenum, the part of the small intestine nearest the stomach.

It is estimated that 3 out of every 1000 people have peptic ulcers. Ulcers develop at any age, though rarely in children under ten. They occur in people of all races and occupations; in men more than in women; and most frequently in tense, hard-driving or anxious persons. (See also ULCER.)

peptid (pep'tid) peptide.

peptidase (pep'tĭ-dās) an enzyme that catalyzes the hydrolysis of peptide linkages in polypeptides.

peptide (pep'tīd, pep'tid) a compound of low molecular weight that yields two or more amino acids on hydrolysis; known as di-, tri-, tetra-, etc., peptides, depending on the number of amino acids.

peptidolytic (pep"tĭ-do-lit'ik) splitting up peptides.

peptogenic (pep"to-jen'ik) producing pepsin or peptones.

peptoid (pep'toid) a product of proteolytic digestion that does not give the biuret reaction.

peptolysis (pep-tol'ĭ-sis) the splitting up of peptone. adj., **peptolyt'ic.**

peptone (pep'tōn) an intermediate product formed in the digestion of protein.

Peptostreptococcus (pep"to-strep"to-kok'us) a genus of Schizomycetes occurring as parasitic inhabitants of the intestinal tract.

peptotoxin (pep"to-tok'sin) any toxin developed from a peptone; also a toxin that develops from putrefying proteins.

peracidity (per"ah-sid'ĭ-te) excessive acidity.

peracute (per"ah-kūt') very acute or sharp.

Perandren (per-an'dren) trademark for a preparation of testosterone, a male sex hormone.

per anum (per a'num) [L.] through the anus.

Perazil (per'ah-zil) trademark for preparations of chlorcyclizine, an antihistamine.

percentile (per-sen'tĭl, per-sen'til) one of the values establishing the division of a series of variables into hundredths, or the range of items included in such a segment.

percept (per'sept) the impression registered in the brain as the result of stimulation of a sense organ.

perception (per-sep'shun) recognition and proper interpretation of stimuli received in the brain, especially from the organs of special sense.
    depth p., the ability to recognize depth or the relative distances to different objects in space.
    extrasensory p., awareness gained otherwise than through the usual physical senses.

perceptive (per-sep'tiv) related to or important in the function of perception.

perceptivity (per"sep-tiv'ĭ-te) ability to receive sense impressions.

percolate (per'ko-lāt) 1. to submit to percolation. 2. any solution obtained by percolation. 3. to trickle slowly through a substance.

percolation (per"ko-la'shun) the extraction of soluble parts of a drug by passing a solvent liquid through it.

Percorten (per-kor'ten) trademark for preparations of desoxycorticosterone, a corticosteroid.

percuss (per-kus') to perform percussion.

percussion (per-kush'un) in medical diagnosis, tapping a part of the body with the fingers in order to determine the size, position and density of the organs underneath. Percussion is most commonly used on the chest and back for examination of the heart and lungs. For example, since the heart is not resonant and the adjacent lungs are, when the physician's fingers strike the chest over the heart the sound waves will change in pitch. This serves as a guide to the precise location and size of the heart.
    auscultatory p., percussion combined with auscultation.
    immediate p., that in which the blow is struck directly against the body surface.
    instrumental p., that in which the blow is delivered by an instrument rather than the examiner's hand or fingers.
    mediate p., that in which the blow is struck against another object or material placed on the surface of the body.
    palpatory p., a combination of palpation and percussion, affording tactile rather than auditory impressions.

percussor (per-kus'or) an instrument for performing percussion.

percutaneous (per"ku-ta'ne-us) performed through the skin.

perencephaly (per"en-sef'ah-le) porencephalia.

perflation (per-fla'shun) the blowing of air into a space to force secretions out.

perforans (per'fo-rans) [L.] penetrating; a term applied to various muscles and nerves.

perforating (per'fo-rāt"ing) piercing or passing through a part.

perforation (per"fo-ra'shun) a hole or break in the containing walls or membranes of an organ or structure of the body. Perforation occurs when erosion, infection or other factors create a weak spot in the organ and internal pressure causes a rupture. It also may result from a deep penetrating wound caused by trauma.
    A perforated ulcer is a complication of duodenal and gastric ulcers. It requires immediate surgical correction to prevent hemorrhage, shock and peritonitis.
    Perforation of the eardrum occurs when an infectious process of the middle ear creates an increase in pressure behind the tympanic membrane. Although perforation may occur spontaneously in OTITIS MEDIA, and is advantageous because it allows for adequate drainage of exudate and relieves pain, it is not desirable because the ragged edges of the perforation may not heal as they should for the eardrum to remain intact. Surgical incision of the eardrum (myringotomy) is preferred to spontaneous perforation.
    The eardrum also may be perforated when a sharp object is inserted into the external acoustic meatus or when extreme pressure from the outside, such

as occurs when swimming or diving in deep water, causes the tympanic membrane to rupture.

Gallbladder perforation sometimes occurs as a complication of CHOLECYSTITIS and GALLSTONES. When the gallbladder is infected, necrosis may progress to the point of destroying the wall of the gallbladder, so that the bile spills out into the abdominal cavity. Gallstones may cause complete obstruction of the cystic duct so that the flow of bile is dammed up and the gallbladder becomes inflamed and eventually ruptures. Treatment of gallbladder perforation usually involves cholecystectomy.

Intestinal perforation is a complication of typhoid fever, ULCERATIVE COLITIS, INTESTINAL OBSTRUCTION and other disorders in which there is inflammation of the intestinal wall or obstruction of the intestinal lumen. The condition is treated surgically with resection of the affected portion of intestine.

perfrication (per″fri̇-ka'shun) rubbing with an ointment or topical medicine.

perfusion (per-fu'zhun) the act of pouring through or into; especially the passage of a fluid through the vessels of a specific organ or body part.

peri- (per'e) word element [Gr.], *around; near.* See also words beginning *para-*.

Periactin (per″e-ak'tin) trademark for preparations of cyproheptadine hydrochloride, an antihistamine and antiserotonin.

periadenitis (per″e-ad″ĕ-ni'tis) inflammation of tissues around a gland.

perianal (per″e-a'nal) around the anus.

periangiitis (per″e-an″je-i'tis) inflammation of the tissue around a blood or lymph vessel.

periangiocholitis (per″e-an″je-o-ko-li'tis) inflammation of tissues around the bile ducts.

periaortitis (per″e-a″or-ti'tis) inflammation of tissues around the aorta.

periapical (per″e-a'pi̇-kal) surrounding the root apex of a tooth.

periappendicitis (per″e-ah-pen″di̇-si'tis) inflammation of the appendix and surrounding tissues.

periarterial (per″e-ar-te're-al) around an artery.

periarteritis (per″e-ar″ter-i'tis) inflammation of the outer coat of an artery.
   p. gummo'sa, accumulation of gummas in the blood vessels in syphilis.
   p. nodo'sa, an inflammatory disease of the coats of small and medium-sized arteries with inflammatory changes around the vessels and marked by symptoms of systemic infection (see also COLLAGEN DISEASES).

periarthritis (per″e-ar-thri'tis) inflammation around a joint.

periarticular (per″e-ar-tik'u-lar) situated around a joint.

periaxial (per″e-ak'se-al) around an axis.

periaxillary (per″e-ak'si̇-ler″e) around the axilla.

peribronchiolitis (per″i̇-brong″ke-o-li'tis) inflammation around the bronchioles.

peribronchitis (per″i̇-brong-ki'tis) inflammation of an entire lobe of the lung with bronchitis in that portion of the lung and thickening of the peribronchial tissue.

pericardiac (per″i̇-kar'de-ak) pertaining to the pericardium; around the heart.

pericardial (per″i̇-kar'de-al) pertaining to the pericardium.

pericardicentesis (per″i̇-kar″di̇-sen-te'sis) puncture of the pericardial cavity with aspiration of fluid.

pericardiectomy (per″i̇-kar″de-ek'to-me) excision of the pericardium.

pericardiocentesis (per″i̇-kar″de-o-sen-te'sis) pericardicentesis.

pericardiolysis (per″i̇-kar″de-ol'i̇-sis) the freeing of adhesions between the visceral and parietal pericardium.

pericardiomediastinitis (per″i̇-kar″de-o-me″de-as″ti̇-ni'tis) inflammation of the pericardium and mediastinum.

pericardiophrenic (per″i̇-kar″de-o-fren'ik) pertaining to the pericardium and diaphragm.

pericardiopleural (per″i̇-kar″de-o-ploo'ral) pertaining to the pericardium and pleura.

pericardiorrhaphy (per″i̇-kar″de-or'ah-fe) suture of the pericardium.

pericardiostomy (per″i̇-kar″de-os'to-me) creation of an opening into the pericardial cavity through the chest wall for drainage of effusions.

pericardiosymphysis (per″i̇-kar″de-o-sim'fi̇-sis) adhesion between visceral and parietal pericardium.

pericardiotomy (per″i̇-kar″de-ot'o-me) incision of pericardium.

pericarditis (per″i̇-kar-di'tis) inflammation of the pericardium, the fibroserous sac that encloses the heart.
   TYPES OF PERICARDITIS. There are many forms of pericarditis. Acute pericarditis is usually secondary to some other bacterial infection, for example, osteomyelitis, lung abscess or pneumonia. It may also occur without bacterial infection, resulting from a tumor, rheumatic heart disease, uremia or coronary thrombosis, or it may be the aftermath of a chest wound in which the pericardium is pierced. Acute pericarditis may be dry, or fibrinous, in which a fibrinous exudate forms on the serous membrane, or it may occur with effusion, that is, with accumulation of fluid in the pericardial cavity.
   Occasionally the pericardium is affected directly by what appears to be a virus; this condition is called acute nonspecific pericarditis. Another form, chronic pericarditis, is usually adhesive— that is, the heart is anchored to surrounding tissues by adhesions. It sometimes follows acute pericarditis, but often the cause is unknown. In the constrictive form of chronic pericarditis, which may be tuberculous in origin, calcium and fibrous deposits may form around the heart and interfere

with its movements. This form may be extremely serious and difficult to cure.

SYMPTOMS AND TREATMENT. The symptoms of acute pericarditis vary with the cause but usually include chest pain and dyspnea, an increase in the pulse rate and a rise in temperature. In dry pericarditis distinct sounds of friction caused by deposits of fibrin may be heard through a stethoscope. In the effusive form, the excess accumulation of pericardial fluid can be detected by x-rays or electrocardiography. The excess fluid is sometimes drained by pericardicentesis.

Treatment of acute pericarditis is directed mainly at curing its original cause. Antibiotics have proved successful in treating bacterial pericarditis. Many patients with nonspecific pericarditis with effusion are helped dramatically by cortisone medications.

In the constrictive form of chronic pericarditis there may be dyspnea and pain in the heart region, plus symptoms elsewhere in the body, such as edema, enlargement of the liver or distention of the neck veins. The best means of treatment is surgery to remove the constrictions and permit free heart action.

pericardium (per″ĭ-kar′de-um) the fibroserous sac enclosing the heart, composed of external (fibrous) and internal (serous) layers.

   adherent p., one abnormally connected with the heart by dense fibrous tissue.

   fibrous p., the external layer of the pericardium, consisting of dense fibrous tissue.

   parietal p., the parietal layer of the serous pericardium, which is in contact with the fibrous pericardium.

   serous p., the inner, serous portion of pericardium, consisting of two layers, visceral and parietal, enclosing a potential space, the pericardial cavity.

   visceral p., the inner layer of the serous pericardium, which is in contact with the heart.

pericardosis (per″ĭ-kar-do′sis) disease of the pericardium.

pericecal (per″ĭ-se′kal) around the cecum.

pericecitis (per″ĭ-se-si′tis) inflammation around the cecum.

pericementitis (per″ĭ-se″men-ti′tis) periodontitis.

pericementum (per″ĭ-se-men′tum) the tissue between the root of a tooth and the dental alveolus.

pericholangitis (per″ĭ-ko″lan-ji′tis) inflammation of tissues surrounding the bile ducts.

pericholecystic (per″ĭ-ko″le-sis′tik) around the gallbladder.

pericholecystitis (per″ĭ-ko″le-sis″ti′tis) inflammation of tissues around the gallbladder.

perichondritis (per″ĭ-kon-dri′tis) inflammation of the perichondrium.

perichondrium (per″ĭ-kon′dre-um) the membrane covering the surface of a cartilage.

perichondroma (per″ĭ-kon-dro′mah) a tumor of the perichondrium.

perichordal (per″ĭ-kor′dal) surrounding the notochord.

perichoroidal (per″ĭ-ko-roi′dal) surrounding the choroid of the eye.

Periclor (per′ĭ-klōr) trademark for a preparation of petrichloral, a hypnotic and sedative.

pericolic (per″ĭ-kol′ik) around the colon.

pericolitis, pericolonitis (per″ĭ-ko-li′tis), (per″ĭ-ko″lon-i′tis) inflammation around the colon.

pericolpitis (per″ĭ-kol-pi′tis) inflammation of tissues around the vagina.

periconchal (per″ĭ-kong′kal) around the concha.

pericorneal (per″ĭ-kor′ne-al) around the cornea.

pericoronal (per″ĭ-kŏ-ro′nal) around the crown of a tooth.

pericranitis (per″ĭ-kra-ni′tis) inflammation of the pericranium.

pericranium (per″ĭ-kra′ne-um) the periosteum of the skull.

pericystitis (per″ĭ-sis-ti′tis) inflammation of tissues about the bladder.

pericyte (per′ĭ-sīt) a peculiar elongated cell found wrapped around capillaries.

pericytial (per″ĭ-si′shal) around a cell.

periderm (per′ĭ-derm) a layer of epidermis in the fetus that generally disappears before birth.

peridesmitis (per″ĭ-dez-mi′tis) inflammation of the peridesmium.

peridesmium (per″ĭ-dez′me-um) the membrane sheathing a ligament.

perididymis (per″ĭ-did′ĭ-mis) the tunica vaginalis testis, the membrane covering the front and sides of the testis and epididymis.

perididymitis (per″ĭ-did″ĭ-mi′tis) inflammation of the tunica vaginalis testis.

peridiverticulitis (per″ĭ-di″ver-tik″u-li′tis) inflammation around an intestinal diverticulum.

periductal (per″ĭ-duk′tal) around a duct.

periduodenitis (per″ĭ-du″o-dĕ-ni′tis) inflammation around the duodenum.

periencephalitis (per″e-en-sef″ah-li′tis) inflammation of the surface of the brain.

periencephalomeningitis (per″e-en-sef″ah-lo-men″in-ji′tis) inflammation of the cerebral cortex and meninges.

perienteritis (per″e-en″tĕ-ri′tis) inflammation of the peritoneal coat of the intestines.

periepithelioma (per″e-ep″ĭ-the″le-o′mah) a tumor that sometimes affects the adrenal gland and may lead to a large metastatic growth of the liver.

periesophagitis (per″e-e-sof″ah-ji′tis) inflammation of the tissues around the esophagus.

perifascicular (per″ĭ-fah-sik′u-lar) surrounding a fascicle of nerve or muscle fibers.

perifistular (per″ĭ-fis′tu-lar) around a fistula.

perifolliculitis (per″ĭ-fŏ-lik″u-li′tis) inflammation around the hair follicles.

perigangliitis (per″ĭ-gang″gle-i′tis) inflammation around a ganglion.

perigastric (per″ĭ-gas′trik) around the stomach.

perigastritis (per″ĭ-gas-tri′tis) inflammation of the peritoneal coat of the stomach.

periglossitis (per″ĭ-glŏ-si′tis) inflammation of the tissues around the tongue.

perihepatitis (per″ĭ-hep″ah-ti′tis) inflammation of the tissues around the liver.

perijejunitis (per″ĭ-je″joo-ni′tis) inflammation around the jejunum.

perilabyrinthitis (per″ĭ-lab″ĭ-rin-thi′tis) inflammation of the tissues around the labyrinth.

perilaryngitis (per″ĭ-lar″in-ji′tis) inflammation of the tissues around the larynx.

perilymph (per′ĭ-limf) fluid contained in the space separating the membranous and osseous labyrinths of the ear.

perilymphadenitis (per″ĭ-lim″fad-ĕ-ni′tis) inflammation of tissues around a lymph node.

perilymphangitis (per″ĭ-lim″fan-ji′tis) inflammation around a lymphatic vessel.

perimeningitis (per″ĭ-men″in-ji′tis) pachymeningitis; inflammation of the dura mater.

perimeter (pĕ-rim′ĕ-ter) 1. the boundary of a two-dimensional figure. 2. an apparatus for determining the extent of the peripheral visual field.

perimetrium (per″ĭ-me′tre-um) the serous membrane enveloping the uterus.

perimetry (pĕ-rim′ĕ-tre) measurement of the visual field.

perimyelitis (per″ĭ-mi″ĕ-li′tis) 1. spinal meningitis. 2. inflammation of the endosteum.

perimyelography (per″ĭ-mi″ĕ-log′rah-fe) roentgenography of the spine after injection of a contrast medium into the subarachnoid space.

perimyositis (per″ĭ-mi″o-si′tis) inflammation of connective tissue around a muscle.

perimysiitis (per″ĭ-mis″e-i′tis) inflammation of the perimysium.

perimysium (per″ĭ-mis′e-um) connective tissue binding together the fascicles of skeletal muscle.

perinatal (per″ĭ-na′tal) relating to the period shortly before and after birth; from the twenty-ninth week of gestation to 1 to 4 weeks after birth.

perineal (per″ĭ-ne′al) pertaining to the perineum.

perineocele (per″ĭ-ne′o-sēl) a hernia between the rectum and the prostate or between the rectum and the vagina.

perineoplasty (per″ĭ-ne′o-plas″te) plastic repair of the perineum.

perineorrhaphy (per″ĭ-ne-or′ah-fe) suture of the perineum.

perineotomy (per″ĭ-ne-ot′o-me) incision of the perineum.

perineovaginal (per″ĭ-ne″o-vaj′ĭ-nal) pertaining to the perineum and vagina.

perinephric (per″ĭ-nef′rik) around the kidney.

perinephritis (per″ĭ-nĕ-fri′tis) inflammation of the peritoneal envelope of the kidney.

perinephrium (per″ĭ-nef′re-um) the peritoneal envelope and other tissues around the kidney.

perineum (per″ĭ-ne′um) the pelvic floor; in the female, the region between the vaginal orifice and the anus, and in the male, the region between the scrotum and the anus. During childbirth the perineum may be torn, resulting in possible damage to the urinary meatus and anal sphincter. To avoid a perineal tear, the obstetrician often cuts the perineum just before delivery and sutures the incision after delivery of the infant and the placenta. This procedure is called an episiotomy. Surgical repair of a torn or lacerated perineum is called perineorrhaphy.

perineuritis (per″ĭ-nu-ri′tis) inflammation of the perineurium.

perineurium (per″ĭ-nu′re-um) the connective tissue sheath surrounding each bundle of nerve fibers (fascicle) in a peripheral nerve.

periocular (per″e-ok′u-lar) around the eye.

periodic (pe″re-od′ik) repeated or recurring at intervals; applied to disease, designating a condition occurring at intervals, separated by periods of freedom from symptoms.
  p. disease, a condition characterized by regularly recurring intermittent episodes of fever, edema, arthralgia or gastric pain and vomiting, continuing for years in otherwise healthy persons.

periodicity (pe″re-o-dis′ĭ-te) the recurrence of certain phenomena at approximately regular intervals.

periodontal (per″e-o-don′tal) around a tooth.
  p. disease, a disease process affecting the tissues about a tooth.

periodontics (per″e-o-don′tiks) the branch of dentistry dealing with periodontal tissue and its diseases.

periodontist (per″e-o-don′tist) a dentist who specializes in periodontics.

periodontitis (per″e-o-don-ti′tis) inflammation of the tissues around a tooth. The condition is caused by residual food, bacteria and calcium deposits (tartar) that collect in the spaces between the gum and lower part of the tooth crown. If it continues unchecked the infection will spread to the bone in which the teeth are rooted. The bone then resorbs and the teeth are slowly detached from their supporting tissues.
  Periodontitis is treated with local cleansing and scraping of the area, establishment of drainage for exudate and oxygenating mouthwashes. Antibiotic drugs are indicated if the symptoms are severe. Extraction of the affected teeth may be necessary if the lesion is advanced.

periodontium (per″e-o-don′she-um) the tissues investing and supporting the teeth.

periodontoclasia (per″e-o-don″to-kla′ze-ah) a degenerative or destructive disease of the periodontium.

periodontology (per″e-o-don-tol′o-je) the science and study of the periodontium and its diseases.

periodontosis (per″e-o-don-to′sis) noninflammatory diseases of the periodontium, characterized by destruction of the periodontium and by bone resorption.

periomphalic (per″e-om-fal′ik) situated around the umbilicus.

perionychium (per″e-o-nik′e-um) the epidermis bordering a nail.

perionyxis (per″e-o-nik′sis) inflammation of the skin around a nail.

perioophoritis (per″e-o″of-o-ri′tis) inflammation of the tissues around the ovary.

perioophorosalpingitis (per″e-o-of″o-ro-sal″pin-ji′tis) inflammation of the tissues around ovary and oviduct.

perioptometry (per″e-op-tom′ĕ-tre) measurement of acuity of peripheral vision or of the limits of the visual field.

perioral (per″e-o′ral) situated or occurring around the mouth.

periorbita (per″e-or′bĭ-tah) the periosteal covering of the bones forming the orbit, or eye socket.

periorbital (per″e-or′bĭ-tal) around the eye socket.

periorbitis (per″e-or-bi′tis) inflammation of the periorbita.

periorchitis (per″e-or-ki′tis) inflammation of the tunica vaginalis testis, the membrane covering the front and sides of the testis and epididymis.

periosteitis (per″e-os″te-i′tis) periostitis.

periosteo-edema (per″e-os″te-o-ĕ-de′mah) edema of the periosteum.

periosteomyelitis (per″e-os″te-o-mi″ĕ-li′tis) inflammation of the entire bone, including periosteum and marrow.

periosteophyte (per″e-os′te-o-fīt″) a bony growth on the periosteum.

periosteorrhaphy (per″e-os″te-or′ah-fe) suture of the periosteum.

periosteotomy (per″e-os″te-ot′o-me) incision of the periosteum.

periosteum (per″e-os′te-um) a specialized connective tissue covering all bones of the body, and possessing bone-forming potentialities. Periosteum also serves as a point of attachment for certain muscles. The connective tissues of the muscle fuse with the fibrous layers of periosteum. adj., **perios′teal.**

periostitis (per″e-os-ti′tis) inflammation of the periosteum.

dental p., periodontitis.
  diffuse p., widespread periostitis of the long bones.

periostoma (per″e-os-to′mah) a bony growth around bone.

periostosis (per″e-os-to′sis) abnormal deposition of periosteal bone.

periotic (per″e-o′tik) situated around the ear.

peripachymeningitis (per″ĭ-pak″ĭ-men″in-ji′tis) inflammation of the substance between the dura mater and the bony covering of the central nervous system.

peripancreatitis (per″ĭ-pan″kre-ah-ti′tis) inflammation of tissues around the pancreas.

peripericarditis (per″ĭ-per″ĭ-kar-di′tis) inflammation of tissues around the pericardium.

periphacitis (per″ĭ-fah-si′tis) inflammation of the capsule of the eye lens.

peripherad (pĕ-rif′er-ad) toward the periphery.

peripheral (pĕ-rif′er-al) pertaining to or situated at or near the periphery.
  p. nervous system, the portion of the NERVOUS SYSTEM consisting of the nerves and ganglia outside the brain and spinal cord.

peripheroceptor (pĕ-rif″er-o-sep′tor) any one of the receptors at the peripheral ends of the sensory neuron which receives the stimulus.

periphery (pĕ-rif′er-e) an outward part or surface.

periphlebitis (per″ĭ-flĕ-bi′tis) inflammation of the external coat of a vein.

periphoria (per″ĭ-fo′re-ah) deviation of an eye around the anteroposterior axis only when fusion is prevented.

periphrenitis (per″ĭ-frĕ-ni′tis) inflammation of the diaphragm and adjoining structures.

periplast (per′ĭ-plast) the protoplasm of a cell outside the nucleus; cytoplasm.

peripleural (per″ĭ-ploo′ral) surrounding the pleura.

peripleuritis (per″ĭ-ploo-ri′tis) inflammation of tissues around the pleura.

periportal (per″ĭ-por′tal) situated around the portal vein.

periproctitis (per″ĭ-prok-ti′tis) inflammation of tissues around the rectum and anus.

periprostatic (per″ĭ-pros-tat′ik) around the prostate.

periprostatitis (per″ĭ-pros″tah-ti′tis) inflammation of substance around the prostate.

peripylephlebitis (per″ĭ-pi″le-flĕ-bi′tis) inflammation of tissues around the portal vein.

peripylic (per″ĭ-pi′lik) around the portal vein.

peripyloric (per″ĭ-pi-lo′rik) around the pylorus.

perirectal (per″ĭ-rek′tal) around the rectum.

perirectitis (per″ĭ-rek-ti′tis) periproctitis.

perirenal (per″ĭ-re′nal) around the kidney.

perirhinal (per″ĭ-ri′nal) around the nose.

perisalpingitis (per″ĭ-sal″pin-ji′tis) inflammation of tissues around the uterine tube.

perisigmoiditis (per″ĭ-sig″moi-di′tis) inflammation of the peritoneum of the sigmoid flexure.

perisinusitis (per″ĭ-si″nŭ-si′tis) inflammation of the substance about a sinus.

perispermatitis (per″ĭ-sper″mah-ti′tis) inflammation of tissues about the spermatic cord.

perisplanchnic (per″ĭ-splangk′nik) around a viscus or the viscera.

perisplanchnitis (per″ĭ-splangk-ni′tis) inflammation of tissues around the viscera.

perisplenic (per″ĭ-splen′ik) around the spleen.

perisplenitis (per″ĭ-sple-ni′tis) inflammation of the peritoneal surface of the spleen.

perispondylitis (per″ĭ-spon″dĭ-li′tis) inflammation of tissues around a vertebra.

peristalsis (per″ĭ-stal′sis) a wavelike progression of alternate contraction and relaxation of the muscle fibers of the esophagus and intestines, by which contents are propelled along the alimentary tract. adj., **peristal′tic.**

When food is swallowed, it passes into the esophagus. Muscular contractions in the wall of the esophagus work the food downward, pushing it into the stomach. Here peristaltic contractions not only move the food in small amounts into the intestine but also aid in the disintegration of the food and help mix it with gastric juice. Peristalsis forces the food through the intestine for further digestion until the food waste finally reaches the rectum, from which it is periodically discharged from the body. The waves of peristalsis are irregular; they are stronger at some times than others. They are also weaker in some people, notably the elderly.

Although the normal peristaltic wave is downward, it is sometimes reversed. Reverse peristaltic action may be triggered by mild digestive upsets or more serious disorders, such as an obstruction in the stomach or intestines.

peristole (pĕ-ris′to-le) the capacity of the walls of the digestive tract to surround or grasp its contents after the ingestion of food.

perisynovial (per″ĭ-sĭ-no′ve-al) around a synovial structure.

peritectomy (per″ĭ-tek′to-me) excision of a ring of conjunctiva around the cornea in treatment of pannus.

peritendineum (per″ĭ-ten-din′e-um) connective tissue investing larger tendons and extending between fibers composing them.

peritendinitis, peritenonitis (per″ĭ-ten″dĭ-ni′tis), (per″ĭ-ten″o-ni′tis) inflammation of the sheath of a tendon.

perithelioma (per″ĭ-the″le-o′mah) a tumor of the perithelium.

perithelium (per″ĭ-the′le-um) the fibrous layer around the capillaries.

perithyroiditis (per″ĭ-thi″roi-di′tis) inflammation of the capsule of the thyroid.

peritomy (pĕ-rit′o-me) 1. surgical incision of the conjunctiva and subconjunctival tissue about the whole circumference of the cornea. 2. circumcision.

peritoneal (per″ĭ-to-ne′al) pertaining to the peritoneum.

p. cavity, the space between the parietal and visceral layers of the peritoneum.

p. dialysis, the employment of the peritoneum surrounding the abdominal cavity as a dialyzing membrane for the purpose of removing waste products or toxins accumulated as a result of renal failure. Certain crystalloids such as urea; creatinine; electrolytes; and some drugs, such as the salicylates, bromides and barbiturates, can be removed. Peritoneal dialysis is used as an alternative to the artificial KIDNEY.

Fluid equal in osmolarity and chemical content with normal blood and tissue fluid is introduced into the peritoneal cavity via a catheter. The dialyzing fluid is left in the peritoneal cavity for 20 minutes to 1 hour. This period is referred to as the equalization period or dialysis phase and is followed by drainage of the fluid from the peritoneum. Then a new exchange is begun. The exchange is continued for a variable period of time, depending on the diagnosis and the patient's symptoms. Dialysis is usually discontinued after the patient's blood chemistry reaches a normal level.

INDICATIONS. Renal failure, whether acute or chronic, is the most frequent indication for peritoneal dialysis. Since certain drugs can be removed by dialysis, some types of acute drug poisoning are treated by this method.

Peritoneal dialysis cannot be employed when there is severe abdominal trauma, adhesions or severe coagulation defects. Such complications as peritonitis, bleeding, intestinal perforation and excessive loss of plasma protein may occur. Peritoneal dialysis is more expensive and time-consuming and less efficient than the artificial kidney.

NURSING CARE. To avoid complications strict adherence to aseptic technique is essential. If there is any break in the tubing connections during the procedure the peritoneal cavity must be considered contaminated. If the tubing becomes blocked the physician should be notified immediately.

Intake and output of fluids must be recorded accurately to avoid DEHYDRATION or overhydration. Daily weight measurement on a stretcher scale facilitates calculation of fluid loss or gain.

The peritoneal drainage fluid is observed for cloudiness and the presence of blood or other abnormal constituents. The vital signs are recorded at frequent intervals so that early signs of shock or the development of an infection can be discovered.

As in any type of treatment that employs mechanical devices, it is most important to avoid preoccupation with the machinery at the expense of the patient. One must always consider the patient as a person, recognizing his emotional problems, and providing him with warmth, understanding and kindness.

peritonealgia (per″ĭ-to″ne-al′je-ah) pain in the peritoneum.

peritoneocentesis (per"ĭ-to"ne-o-sen-te'sis) paracentesis of the abdominal (peritoneal) cavity.

peritoneoclysis (per"ĭ-to"ne-ok'lĭ-sis) injection of fluid into the peritoneal cavity.

peritoneopathy (per"ĭ-to"ne-op'ah-the) any disease of the peritoneum.

peritoneoscope (per"ĭ-to'ne-o-skōp") an endoscope for use in peritoneoscopy.

peritoneoscopy (per"ĭ-to"ne-os'ko-pe) visual examination of the organs of the abdominal (peritoneal) cavity with a peritoneoscope.

peritoneotomy (per"ĭ-to"ne-ot'o-me) incision into the peritoneum.

peritoneum (per"ĭ-to-ne'um) the serous membrane lining the walls of the abdominal and pelvic cavities (parietal peritoneum) and investing contained viscera (visceral peritoneum), the two layers enclosing a potential space, the peritoneal cavity.

peritonitis (per"i-to-ni'tis) inflammation of the peritoneum.

ACUTE PERITONITIS. Acute peritonitis may be produced by inflammation of abdominal organs; by irritating substances from a perforated gallbladder or gastric ulcer; by rupture of a cyst; or by irritation from blood, as in cases of internal bleeding.

Symptoms and Diagnosis. Immediate and intense pain is felt at the site of infection, followed usually by fever, vomiting and extreme weakness. The abdomen becomes rigid and sensitive to the touch. The patient may suffer mental confusion, fever, prostration or shock. Although antibiotics have greatly reduced the mortality rate of acute peritonitis, the infection should be treated and controlled immediately; it can be fatal if neglected.

Diagnosis is based on manual examination, x-ray films and blood tests.

Treatment. The basic treatment for acute peritonitis is a combination of surgery, antibiotics and other measures. The peritoneal cavity often must be opened and the toxic material removed. The original source of infection, such as an inflamed appendix, may have to be removed, or an abscess caused by the peritonitis may have to be drained. Antibiotics such as penicillin, streptomycin or tetracycline are used to fight the infection itself.

The patient usually takes nothing by mouth. Fluids are given intravenously. Narcotics and sedatives are often used to relieve pain and ensure rest. Treatment may also include blood transfusions and suction through a nasogastric tube to relieve abdominal pressure and to prevent accumulation of gas in the intestines.

CHRONIC PERITONITIS. The chronic form of this disease is comparatively rare, and is often associated with tuberculosis. Less frequently it may result from longstanding irritation caused by the presence in the abdomen of a foreign body such as gunshot.

In general, symptoms of chronic peritonitis are milder than those of acute peritonitis. Symptoms of tuberculous peritonitis are abdominal pain, low-grade fever, constipation and general ill health, including loss of weight and appetite. Treatment depends on the underlying cause and the severity of the condition.

adhesive p., peritonitis characterized by adhesions between peritoneal structures.

bile p., that due to the presence of bile in the peritoneum.

silent p., acute peritonitis causing death without symptoms.

peritonsillar (per"ĭ-ton'sĭ-lar) around a tonsil.

peritonsillitis (per"ĭ-ton"sĭ-li'tis) inflammation of peritonsillar tissues.

Peritrate (per'ĭ-trāt) trademark for a preparation of pentaerythritol tetranitrate, a vasodilator used in treatment of angina pectoris.

peritrichous (pĕ-rit'rĭ-kus) having flagella distributed over the whole surface.

perityphlitis (per"ĭ-tif-li'tis) inflammation of tissues around the cecum.

periureteral (per"ĭ-u-re'ter-al) around the ureter.

periureteritis (per"ĭ-u-re"tĕ-ri'tis) inflammation of tissues around the ureter.

periurethral (per"ĭ-u-re'thral) around the urethra.

periuterine (per"ĭ-u'ter-in) around the uterus.

perivaginal (per"ĭ-vaj'ĭ-nal) around the vagina.

perivaginitis (per"ĭ-vaj"ĭ-ni'tis) inflammation of tissues around the vagina.

perivascular (per"ĭ-vas'ku-lar) situated around a vessel.

perivasculitis (per"ĭ-vas"ku-li'tis) inflammation of a perivascular sheath.

perivesical (per"ĭ-ves'ĭ-kal) around the bladder.

perivesiculitis (per"ĭ-vĕ-sik"u-li'tis) inflammation of tissues around the seminal vesicles.

perlèche (per-lesh') a form of oral candidiasis at the labial commissures in children.

permeability (per"me-ah-bil'ĭ-te) the rate at which a substance moves through a permeable layer under a given force.

permeable (per'me-ah-bl) not impassable; allowing the passage of fluids.

permease (per'me-ās) a stereospecific membrane transport system.

permeation (per"me-a'shun) the act of spreading through or penetrating a substance, tissue or organ, as by a disease process, such as cancer.

pernicious (per-nish'us) fatal.

p. anemia, a form of anemia caused by lack of the intrinsic factor, which normally is produced by the stomach mucosa. The deficiency results in inadequate and abnormal formation of erythrocytes, and failure to absorb vitamin B_{12}. Some persons with pernicious anemia show only mild symptoms and are not particularly aware of the illness; in others the condition becomes very serious and, if it remains untreated, it can be fatal.

SYMPTOMS. A pale, colorless complexion is typical of all anemias, including pernicious anemia. Jaundice also occurs in pernicious anemia, with soreness and reddening of the tongue, difficulty in swallowing and digestive disturbances including diarrhea. Other symptoms may include fatigability, heart palpitation and dyspnea. Changes in the nerves and spinal cord may produce numbness and tingling in the fingers and toes, and the gait may become unsteady. The involvement of the nerves can be completely cured if it has existed for less than 6 months, but may be incurable if it is of longer standing. In advanced cases, mental disturbances may also occur. Laboratory tests reveal abnormalities in the erythrocytes in the blood and in the bone marrow. Gastric analysis shows an absence of hydrochloric acid and perhaps even an absence of gastric juice.

TREATMENT. Pernicious anemia is successfully treated by regular injections of vitamin B_{12}, given several times a week at first and monthly after the condition has been brought under control. This treatment must be lifelong to prevent relapse. The injections do not cure the disease but arrest it by providing the body directly with the necessary vitamin that it fails to absorb from the digestive tract. Special diets, liver extract and other medications taken by mouth usually are not required since the basic defect is not dietary deficiency but improper use of food ingested.

Pernicious anemia is believed to be inherited. The disease occurs usually after the age of 35, and it is more common in persons of Scandinavian, Irish and English descent. Although no cure is known, most patients who continue with treatments can look forward to a normal life span with good health and normal activities.

See also ANEMIA for nursing care.

pernio (per′ne-o) chilblain.

perniosis (per′ne-o′sis) chilblain affecting several areas of the body.

pero- (pe′ro) word element [Gr.], *deformity.*

perobrachius (pe″ro-bra′ke-us) a fetus with deformed feet and arms.

perocephalus (pe″ro-sef′ah-lus) a fetus with a deformed head.

perochirus (pe″ro-ki′rus) a fetus with deformed hands.

peromelia (pe″ro-me′le-ah) congenital deformity of the limbs.

peromelus (pe″rom′ĕ-lus) a fetus with deformed limbs.

peroneal (per″o-ne′al) pertaining to the fibula.
   p. nerve, common, a nerve originating in the sciatic nerve and innervating the calf and foot.

Per. op. emet. [L.] *perac′ta operatio′ne emet′ici* (when the action of the emetic is over).

peropus (pe′ro-pus) a fetus with malformed legs and feet.

peroral (per-o′ral) performed or administered through the mouth.

per os (per os) [L.] by mouth.

peroxidase (pĕ-rok′si-dās) an enzyme that catalyzes the decomposition of peroxides, by catalyzing the transfer of oxygen from peroxide to another substance.

peroxide (pĕ-rok′sīd) an oxide with more than the normal proportion of oxygen.

hydrogen p., H_2O_2, an antiseptic with a mildly antibacterial action. A 3 per cent solution foams on touching skin or mucous membrane and appears to have a mechanical cleansing action.

perphenazine (per-fen′ah-zēn) a phenothiazine compound used as a tranquilizer and antiemetic.

per primam intentionem (per pri′mam in-ten″-she-o′nem) [L.] by first intention (see HEALING).

per rectum (per rek′tum) through the rectum.

persalt (per′sawlt) any salt that contains a greater amount of the acid radical than a protosalt.

Persantin (per-san′tin) trademark for preparations of dipyridamole, a drug used to increase coronary blood flow.

per secundam intentionem (per se-kun′dam in-ten″she-o′nem) [L.] by second intention (see HEALING).

perseveration (per-sev″er-a′shun) persistence of one reply or one idea in response to various questions; continuance of activity after cessation of the causative stimulus.

persona (per-so′nah) in psychology, a term for the personality "mask" or facade presented by a person to the outside world, as opposed to the anima, the unconscious, or inner being, of a person.

personality (per″sŏ-nal′ĭ-te) the sum of the behavior, attitudes and character traits of an individual. Many factors that determine personality are inherited; they are shaped and modified by the individual's environment. Students of human behavior have long debated whether inherited traits or life experiences play the greater role in molding personality. They all agree, however, on the influence of the early years on personality development.

EARLY LIFE AND PERSONALITY. The infant comes into the world completely dependent on others for his basic needs. His feeling of security in a relationship with his mother, or an adequate substitute, is the cornerstone of his mental health in later years.

As a child develops, he needs to learn and to meet the day-to-day problems of life, and to master them. In resolving these challenges, he chooses his solutions from many possibilities. He must substitute other ways of behavior for his many natural antisocial impulses. Psychologists have studied how these choices are made and use technical terms to describe them, such as repression and sublimation. The behavior patterns chosen result in certain character traits which will influence a child's way of meeting the world — whether he will lead or follow, be conscientious or reckless, imitate his parents or prefer to be as different from them as possible, or take a realistic, flexible path between these extremes. The sum total of these traits represents the personality.

THE WELL ADJUSTED PERSONALITY. A well adjusted individual is one who adjusts himself to his surroundings, the world he lives in, and the people in it. If he cannot, he makes realistic efforts to change the situation. He also uses his abilities constructively and successfully.

The well adjusted person is realistic. He faces facts whether they are pleasant or unpleasant and deals with them instead of merely worrying about them or denying them.

The mature person is independent. He forms reasoned opinions and then acts on them. He seeks a reasonable amount of information and advice before making a decision. Once the decision is made, he is willing to face the consequences of it. He does not attempt to force others to make decisions for him.

An ability to love others is typical of the well adjusted individual. On the other hand, the mature person is also able to enjoy receiving love and affection. He can accept a reasonable dependence on others.

The well adjusted individual has the ability to make long-range choices and to forego immediate pleasures for the sake of these long-range goals. He is also able to reevaluate these goals and change them if necessary.

The mature person can get angry, but his anger is directed at rational targets. When the occasion demands, he can be stirred to fierce anger, but he never loses sight of the reason for his anger or of what he hopes to accomplish with it. He is not a chronic worrier. He usually likes his work and does it well, but it is not his entire life.

Finally, the mature person has the capacity for continued emotional growth. He continues to deepen his understanding of others throughout his life.

Naturally, few people meet all these qualifications of the ideally developed personality, just as few people are in perfect physical health.

DISORDERS OF PERSONALITY. In addition to specific types of mental illness, such as NEUROSIS and PSYCHOSIS, there are a number of what are known as personality or character disorders. In general these are difficult both to diagnose and to treat.

Terms that are often used to describe persons with disturbed personalities are neurotic or neurotic character. Such persons are able to function in their daily life, but are emotionally and psychologically "crippled" by inadequate or unstable personalities, and their chances of forming good relationships and fulfilling their potentialities are poor. Among the patterns often encountered in such persons are either passive or aggressive reactions to life, in which the person is excessively dependent on other people or hostile to them. Sometimes his behavior represents a combination of both attitudes. Other personality types have traits that show some similarity to the symptoms of the three major types of psychosis—schizophrenia, paranoia and affective psychosis—although these people are not psychotic. They are referred to as schizoid, paranoid or cyclothymic personalities.

A special form of personality disorder is the PSYCHOPATHIC PERSONALITY, or sociopathic personality. A person with this disorder shows abnormal behavior patterns, although they differ from the patterns observed in neurosis and psychosis. He may have a greatly exaggerated sense of self-importance, and his emotions are often very shallow. Some of the problems of the psychopathic personality can include sexual deviation, alcoholism and drug addiction. Certain kinds of criminals belong in this group.

Although personality disorders are more difficult to treat than other forms of mental illness, a great deal can be done in many cases. Since these disorders are the result of unresolved emotional conflicts, often dating back to childhood, the treatment attempts to uncover the roots of these conflicts and to help the patient resolve them. The various techniques for doing this are included under the term PSYCHOTHERAPY.

alternating p., double p., dual p., a state of disordered consciousness in which the subject leads two lives, alternately, with amnesia for the other.

multiple p., a state of disordered consciousness in which the subject leads three or more lives, alternatively, with amnesia for those not lived at the moment.

perspiration (per″spĭ-ra′shun) 1. the excretion of moisture through the pores of the skin. 2. the salty fluid, consisting largely of water, excreted by the sweat glands in the skin; called also sweat.

The body has approximately 2 million sweat glands. The secretory portion is located in the corium and is connected to the epidermis by a long straight duct. The largest of these glands are in the armpits and groin, but the greatest number per square inch is found on the soles of the feet and the palms of the hands.

In midsummer temperatures—or during strenuous exertion or unusual emotional stress—the body's perspiration output may exceed several quarts per day. On a cool day without exertion or emotional stress, the body loses well over a pint of perspiration. This kind of sweating is known medically as "insensible" perspiration because it is virtually unnoticeable; as the sweat reaches the surface of the skin, it evaporates immediately. When sweating becomes noticeable, it is known as "sensible" perspiration.

FUNCTIONS. The chief role of the sweat glands and perspiration is to maintain the body temperature at a constant level. Thus the skin is cooled as perspiration evaporates. The blood in the capillaries of the skin likewise is cooled before it courses back into the body.

The sweat glands have a minor excretory function. Perspiration contains water, sodium chloride and small amounts of urea, lactic acid and potassium ions. It also contains antibacterial substances that defend the body against infection.

ABNORMAL PERSPIRATION. Malfunctioning of the sweat glands is somewhat unusual and seldom is cause for alarm unless accompanied by another disease. For example, profuse sweating (diaphoresis) may accompany such diseases as tuberculosis, rickets and malaria. Night sweats may be a sign of serious disease. Excessive perspiration may also be generated temporarily by shock or by motion sickness or hormonal changes during menopause.

The commonest serious problem from excessive sweating is probably the temporary loss of salt, resulting in a sodium deficiency.

Excessive sweating, or hyperhidrosis, that is not accompanied by disease is sometimes hereditary and is difficult to treat. Diminished or total absence of sweating, or anhidrosis, may occur in the elderly and in those with pronounced thyroid deficiency or severe skin disease. In treating anhidrosis the primary step is to try to cure the condition causing it.

In CYSTIC FIBROSIS the sweat contains an abnormally high content of sodium chloride, and excessive sweating in these patients must be guarded against. In the rare malady called chromhidrosis, the perspiration turns black, blue, green, red, yellow or a combination of colors. The cause is unknown, although certain bacteria may be responsible.

persulfate (per-sul′fāt) a sulfate that contains more sulfuric acid than the ordinary sulfate.

per tertiam intentionem (per ter′she-am in-ten″-she-o′nem) [L.] by third intention (see HEALING).

Perthes' disease (per′tēz) osteochondrosis of the epiphysis of the head of the femur.

Pertophrane (per′to-frān) trademark for a preparation of desipramine hydrochloride, an antidepressant.

per tubam (per tu′bam) [L.] through a tube.

pertussis (per-tus′is) an infectious disease due to *Bordetella pertussis*, and characterized by coryza, bronchitis and a typical explosive cough ending in crowing inspiration (see also WHOOPING COUGH).

pertussoid (per-tus′oid) 1. resembling whooping cough. 2. an influenzal cough resembling that of whooping cough.

per vaginam (per vah-ji′nam) [L.] through the vagina.

perversion (per-ver′zhun) deviation from the normal course.
   sexual p., sexual deviation.

pervert (per′vert) a person who deviates from a normal course, especially a sexual deviate.

pes (pes), pl. *pe′des* [L.] foot; the terminal organ of the leg, or lower limb; any footlike part.
   p. abduc′tus, a deformity in which the anterior part of the foot is displaced and lies laterally to the vertical axis of the leg.
   p. adduc′tus, a deformity in which the anterior part of the foot is displaced and lies medially to the vertical axis of the leg.
   p. ca′vus, a foot with an abnormally high longitudinal arch, either congenital or caused by contractures or disturbed muscle balance.
   p. corvi′nus, a set of wrinkles radiating from the lateral canthus of the eye; crow's foot.
   p. pla′nus, flatfoot; one with an abnormally low longitudinal arch.
   p. supina′tus, a deformity in which the inner border of the anterior part of the foot is higher than the outer border.
   p. val′gus, flatfoot.
   p. va′rus, a permanent toeing-in position of the foot; pigeon toe.

pessary (pes′ah-re) 1. an instrument placed in the vagina to support the uterus or rectum. 2. a medicated vaginal suppository.

pesticide (pes′tĭ-sīd) a poison used to destroy pests of any sort.

pestiferous (pes-tif′er-us) causing a pestilence.

pestilence (pes′tĭ-lens) 1. a virulent epidemic contagious disease. 2. an epidemic of a virulent contagious disease. adj., **pestilen′tial.**

pestle (pes′el) an instrument with a rounded end, used in a mortar to reduce a solid to a powder or produce a homogeneous mixture of solids.

-petal word element [L.], *directed* or *moving toward.*

petechia (pe-te′ke-ah), pl. *pete′chiae* [L.] a small, pinpoint, nonraised, perfectly round, purplish red spot caused by intradermal or submucous hemorrhage, which later turns blue or yellow. adj., **pete′chial.**

pethidine hydrochloride (peth′ĭ-dēn) meperidine hydrochloride, a narcotic analgesic drug.

petit mal (pĕ-te′ mahl) a relatively mild epileptic attack occurring in children, contrasting with grand mal, a major attack. In petit mal, the affected person loses consciousness only momentarily. Often the only outward signs of the attack are twitching of the eyes and mouth and a brief lapse of attention. The facial expression is blank and empty. (See also EPILEPSY).

petrichloral (pet″rĭ-klo′ral) a derivative of chloral used as a hypnotic and sedative.

pétrissage (pa-trĭ-sahzh′) [Fr.] a kneading action in massage.

petrolatum (pet″ro-la′tum) a purified mixture of hydrocarbons obtained from petroleum; used as a base for ointments and as a soothing application to the skin. It occurs in semisolid and liquid form. The liquid form (called also mineral oil) is used as a lubricant laxative.

petroleum (pĕ-tro′le-um) a thick natural oil obtained from wells and springs especially dug in the earth. It consists of a mixture of various hydrocarbons. It has been used as an expectorant, diaphoretic, and vermifuge and in skin diseases.
   p. jelly, petrolatum.

petrolization (pet″rol-ĭ-za′shun) spreading of petroleum on bodies of water to destroy mosquito larvae.

petromastoid (pet″ro-mas′toid) pertaining to the pars petrosa and the pars mastoidea of the temporal bone.

petrosal (pĕ-tro′sal) pertaining to the pars petrosa, or petrous portion of the temporal bone.

petrosalpingostaphylinus (pet″ro-sal-ping″go-staf″ĭ-li′nus) the levator muscle of the palatine velum.

petrosectomy (pet″ro-sek′to-me) excision of the cells of the apex of the pars petrosa of the temporal bone.

petrositis (pet″ro-si′tis) inflammation of the pars petrosa of the temporal bone.

petrous (pet′rus) resembling rock or stone.
   p. bone, the pars petrosa, or petrous portion of the temporal bone.

pexis (pek′sis) 1. the fixation of matter by a tissue. 2. surgical fixation, usually by suturing. adj., **pex′ic.**

-pexy (pek′se) word element [Gr.], *surgical fixation.* adj., **-pec′tic.**

Peyer's patches (pi′erz) whitish patches of lymphatic follicles in mucous and submucous layers of the small intestine.

peyote (pa-o′te) a drug obtained from the Mexican cactus, Anhalonium; sometimes used to produce an intoxication marked by feelings of ecstasy (see also HALLUCINOGEN).

Peyronie's disease (pa-ron-ēz′) induration of the corpora cavernosa of the penis, with proliferation of connective tissue and possible presence of cartilage or bone.

Pfeiffer's disease (pfi′ferz) infectious mononucleosis.

pg. picogram.

PGA pteroylglutamic (folic) acid.

pH symbol, *hydrogen ion concentration*. It expresses the degree to which a solution is acidic or alkaline. The pH range extends from 0 ("pure" acid) to 14 ("pure" base). pH 7.0 indicates neutrality; a pH of less than 7 indicates acidity, and a pH of more than 7 indicates alkalinity.

phac(o)- (fak′o) word element [Gr.], *lens*. See also words beginning *phako-*.

phacitis (fah-si′tis) inflammation of the eye lens.

phacoanaphylaxis (fak″o-an″ah-fi-lak′sis) anaphylaxis to protein of the eye lens.

phacocele (fak′o-sēl) hernia of the eye lens.

phacocystectomy (fak″o-sis-tek′to-me) excision of part of the lens capsule for cataract.

phacocystitis (fak″o-sis-ti′tis) inflammation of the capsule of the eye lens.

phacoerysis (fak″o-er′ĭ-sis) removal of the eye lens in cataract by suction.

phacoglaucoma (fak″o-glaw-ko′mah) lens changes produced by glaucoma.

phacohymenitis (fak″o-hi″men-i′tis) inflammation of the capsule of the eye lens.

phacoid (fak′oid) shaped like a lens.

phacoiditis (fak″oi-di′tis) inflammation of the eye lens.

phacoidoscope (fah-koi′do-skōp) phacoscope.

phacolysis (fah-kol′ĭ-sis) dissolution of the crystalline lens by operation or by medical means. adj., **phacolyt′ic.**

phacomalacia (fak″o-mah-la′she-ah) soft cataract, that is, without a hard nucleus.

phacometachoresis (fak″o-met″ah-ko-re′sis) displacement of the eye lens.

phacosclerosis (fak″o-sklĕ-ro′sis) hardening of the eye lens; cataract with a hard nucleus.

phacoscope (fak′o-skōp) an instrument for viewing accommodative changes of the eye lens.

phacotoxic (fak″o-tok′sik) exerting a deleterious effect upon the crystalline lens.

phag(o)- (fag′o) word element [Gr.], *eating; ingestion.*

phage (fāj) bacteriophage.

phagedena (faj″ĕ-de′nah) rapidly spreading and sloughing ulceration.

phagocyte (fag′o-sīt) any cell, such as a polymorphonuclear leukocyte, that destroys microorganisms or harmful cells. adj., **phagocyt′ic.**

phagocytin (fag-″o-si′tin) a bactericidal substance from neutrophilic leukocytes.

phagocytoblast (fag″o-si′to-blast) a cell giving rise to phagocytes.

phagocytolysis (fag″o-si-tol′ĭ-sis) destruction of phagocytes. adj., **phagocytolyt′ic.**

phagocytose (fag″o-si′tōs) to envelop and destroy bacteria and other foreign material.

phagocytosis (fag″o-si-to′sis) the uptake or envelopment of solid particles by living cells.

phagodynamometer (fag″o-di″nah-mom′ĕ-ter) an apparatus for measuring the force exerted in chewing food.

phagokaryosis (fag″o-kar″e-o′sis) phagocytosis allegedly effected by the cell nucleus.

phagomania (fag″o-ma′ne-ah) an insatiable craving for food or an obsessive preoccupation with the subject of eating.

phagotherapy (fag″o-ther′ah-pe) treatment by feeding.

phakoma (fah-ko′mah) a lenslike mass or tumor.

phakomatosis (fak″o-mah-to′sis) a heredofamilial tumorous state, with formation of lenslike masses, spots, tumefactions and cysts. There are three syndromes: tuberous sclerosis, Lindau-von Hippel disease and neurofibromatosis.

phalangeal (fah-lan′je-al) pertaining to a phalanx.

phalangectomy (fal″an-jek′to-me) excision of a phalanx.

phalangitis (fal″an-ji′tis) inflammation of one or more phalanges.

phalangosis (fal″an-go′sis) a condition in which the eyelashes grow in rows.

phalanx (fa′langks), pl. *phalan′ges* [Gr.] any bone of a finger or toe. adj., **phalan′geal.**

phallectomy (fal-ek′to-me) amputation of the penis.

phallic (fal′ik) pertaining to the penis.

phallitis (fal-i′tis) inflammation of the penis.

phallocampsis (fal″o-kamp′sis) curvature of the penis during erection.

phallodynia (fal″o-din′e-ah) pain in the penis.

phallotomy (fal-ot′o-me) incision of the penis.

phallus (fal′us) the penis.

phaneromania (fan″er-o-ma′ne-ah) abnormal attention to some external growth, as picking at a wart, etc.

phanerosis (fan″er-o′sis) the process of becoming visible.

phanic (fan′ik) visible; apparent.

Phanodorn (fan′o-dorn) trademark for a preparation of cyclobarbital, a short- to intermediate-acting barbiturate.

phantasm (fan′tazm) an impression or image not evoked by actual stimuli.

phantasy (fan′tah-se) 1. the faculty of receiving and reproducing unreal notions or sensations. 2. an image or daydream. 3. a mental mechanism by which a harsh reality is converted into an imaginary experience that satisfies the patient's subjective demands. Also spelled fantasy.

phantom (fan′tom) 1. a shadowy image or impression. 2. a model of the body or of a specific part, used for demonstration or other purposes; in nuclear medicine, a device that simulates conditions encountered in vivo, to permit accurate determination of radiation received from a radioactive source.
   anatomic p., one used in nuclear medicine that corresponds as closely as possible to the configuration of the organ it represents.
   basic p., one used in nuclear medicine, constructed in a geometric configuration, with little resemblance to the organ it represents.
   intermediate p., one used in nuclear medicine that has a strong geometric flavor, but bears some resemblance to the organ it represents.
   p. pain, pain felt as if it were in a limb, after AMPUTATION of the limb.

pharmacal (far′mah-kal) pertaining to pharmacy.

pharmaceutical (far″mah-su′tĭ-kal) 1. pertaining to pharmacy or drugs. 2. a medicinal drug.

pharmaceutics (far″mah-su′tiks) the apothecary's art.

pharmacist (far′mah-sist) a person licensed to compound or dispense drugs.

pharmacodiagnosis (far″mah-ko-di″ag-no′sis) use of drugs in diagnosis.

pharmacodynamics (far″mah-ko-di-nam′iks) the study of the action of drugs.

pharmacogenetics (far″mah-ko-jĕ-net′iks) study of the effects of genetic factors on the individual organism's response to drugs.

pharmacognosy (far″mah-kog′no-se) the study of crude medicines.

pharmacology (far″mah-kol′o-je) the science that deals with the study of drugs in all its aspects.

pharmacomania (far″mah-ko-ma′ne-ah) abnormal fondness for taking or administering medicines.

pharmacopeia (far″mah-ko-pe′ah) an authoritative treatise on drugs and their preparations.

pharmacophobia (far″mah-ko-fo′be-ah) morbid dread of medicines.

pharmacophore (far′mah-ko-for″) the group of atoms in the molecule of a drug that causes the therapeutic effect.

pharmacopoeia (far″mah-ko-pe′ah) pharmacopeia.

pharmacopsychosis (far″mah-ko-si-ko′sis) a mental disease due to alcohol, drugs or poisons.

pharmacoroentgenography (far″mah-ko-rent″-gĕ-nog′rah-fe) roentgenographic examination of a body or organ under influence of a drug that best facilitates such examination.

pharmacotherapy (far″mah-ko-ther′ah-pe) treatment of disease with medicines.

pharmacy (far′mah-se) 1. the art of preparing and compounding medicines. 2. a shop for the compounding and dispensing of drugs and medical supplies.

pharyng(o)- (fah-ring′go) word element [Gr.], *pharynx.*

pharyngalgia (far″ing-gal′je-ah) pain in the pharynx.

pharyngeal (fah-rin′je-al) pertaining to the pharynx.

pharyngectomy (far″in-jek′to-me) excision of part of pharynx.

pharyngemphraxis (far″in-jem-frak′sis) obstruction of the pharynx.

pharyngismus (far″in-jiz′mus) muscular spasm of pharynx.

pharyngitis (far″in-ji′tis) inflammation of the pharynx.
   Acute pharyngitis usually appears suddenly and runs its course in a few days or a week. Symptoms, more severe in children, are dry, sore throat, fatigue and mild fever. Often, swallowing is painful, the head aches and there is a harsh cough and a persistent desire to clear the throat. The throat frequently becomes swollen and covered with a thick mucous material. Sometimes there is pain in the ears, or hoarseness. In most cases, treatment is similar to that for a cold: rest, liquids, aspirin and, when prescribed, antibiotics.
   Chronic pharyngitis is the result of continuous reinfection or chronic irritation of exposed parts of the throat. It is similar to acute pharyngitis, but less severe. The simple catarrhal form can be caused by smoking, dust, smog or constant breathing through the mouth.
   Symptomatic treatment includes hot saline gargles, liquid diet and an increase in fluid intake. Sulfonamides or antibiotics may be prescribed when a bacterial infection is present.
   The symptoms of pharyngitis can occur during the early stages of such diseases as scarlet fever, measles and whooping cough.

pharyngocele (fah-ring′go-sēl) a hernial pouch or cystic deformity of the pharynx.

pharyngoconjunctival fever (fah-ring″go-kon″-jung-ti′val) a febrile disease of viral origin occurring in epidemic form and characterized by fever, pharyngitis, rhinitis, conjunctivitis and enlarged cervical lymph nodes.

pharyngoconjunctivitis (fah-ring″go-kon-jungk″tĭ-vi′tis) inflammation involving the pharynx and conjunctiva, the result of a virus infection.

pharyngodynia (fah-ring″go-din′e-ah) pain in the pharynx.

pharyngoesophageal (fah-ring″go-e-sof″ah-je′-al) pertaining to the pharynx and esophagus.

pharyngoglossal (fah-ring″go-glos′al) pertaining to the pharynx and tongue.

pharyngolaryngitis (fah-ring″go-lar″in-ji′tis) inflammation of the pharynx and larynx.

pharyngology (far″ing-gol′o-je) scientific study of the pharynx.

pharyngomycosis (fah-ring″go-mi-ko′sis) fungus disease of the pharynx.

pharyngoparalysis (fah-ring″go-pah-ral′ĭ-sis) paralysis of the pharyngeal muscles.

pharyngopathy (far″ing-gop′ah-the) disease of the pharynx.

pharyngoperistole (fah-ring″go-pĕ-ris′to-le) narrowing of the pharynx.

pharyngoplasty (fah-ring′go-plas″te) plastic repair of the pharynx.

pharyngoplegia (fah-ring″go-ple′je-ah) paralysis of the pharyngeal muscles.

pharyngorhinitis (fah-ring″go-ri-ni′tis) inflammation of the nasopharynx.

pharyngorrhea (far″ing-go-re′ah) mucous discharge from the pharynx.

pharyngoscope (fah-ring′go-skōp) an instrument for inspecting the pharynx.

pharyngoscopy (far″ing-gos′ko-pe) examination of the pharynx.

pharyngospasm (fah-ring′go-spazm) spasm of the pharyngeal muscles.

pharyngostenosis (fah-ring″go-stĕ-no′sis) narrowing of the pharynx.

pharyngotomy (far″ing-got′o-me) incision of the pharynx.

pharynx (far′ingks) the musculomembranous cavity, about 5 inches long, behind the nasal cavities, mouth and larynx, communicating with them and with the esophagus.

The pharynx includes many individual structures and may be divided into three areas: the nasopharynx (top), oropharynx (center, behind the mouth) and laryngopharynx (bottom). The nasopharynx, connected with the nasal cavities, provides a passage for air during breathing; it also contains the openings of the eustachian tubes through which air enters the middle ear. The oropharynx and laryngopharynx provide passageways for both air and food. The pharynx also functions as a resonating organ in speech.

The pharynx is separated from the mouth by the soft palate and its fleshy V-shaped extension or flap, the uvula, which hangs from the top of the back of the mouth, above the root of the tongue. In swallowing, the uvula lifts up, closing off the nasopharynx as food passes from the mouth through the lower parts of the pharynx to the esophagus. On each side of the entrance to the pharynx from the mouth, and behind the nasal passage, are the TONSILS and ADENOIDS, masses of lymphoid tissue.

The most common disorders of the pharynx are PHARYNGITIS and the inflammation and discomfort resulting from TONSILLITIS.

phase (fāz) 1. one of the aspects or stages through which a varying entity may pass. 2. In physical chemistry, a component that is homogeneous of itself, bounded by an interface, and mechanically separable from other phases of the system.

continuous p., in a heterogeneous system, the component in which the disperse phase is distributed, corresponding to the solvent in a true solution.

disperse p., the discontinuous portion of a heterogeneous system, corresponding to the solute in a true solution.

phatnorrhagia (fat″no-ra′je-ah) hemorrhage from a tooth socket.

Phe-mer-nite (fe′mer-nīt) trademark for preparations of phenylmercuric nitrate, local antibacterial.

Phemerol (fe′mer-ol) trademark for preparations of benzethonium, an antiinfective.

phemitone (fem′ĭ-tōn) mephobarbital, an anticonvulsant.

phenacaine (fen′ah-kān) a compound used as a local anesthetic.

phenacemide (fĕ-nas′e-mīd) phenacetylurea, used as an anticonvulsant in psychomotor and grand mal epilepsy.

phenacetin (fĕ-nas′ĕ-tin) acetophenetidin, an antipyretic and analgesic.

phenadone (fen′ah-dōn) methadone, a synthetic compound with properties similar to those of morphine.

phenaglycodol (fen″ah-gli′ko-dol) a compound used as a tranquilizer.

phenanthrene (fe-nan′thrēn) a colorless, crystalline hydrocarbon.

phenate (fe′nāt) a salt formed by union of a base with phenic acid (phenol).

phenazocine (fĕ-naz′o-sēn) a compound used as an analgesic.

phenelzine (fen′el-zēn) a compound used as an antidepressant.

Phenergan (fen′er-gan) trademark for preparations of promethazine hydrochloride, an antihistamine.

phenethicillin (fĕ-neth″ĭ-sil′in) phenoxymethyl penicillin.

phenformin (fen-for′min) a synthetic hypoglycemic drug sometimes used in the treatment of diabetes mellitus. Its action is not yet completely understood; it is not related to other hypoglycemic agents such as tolbutamide or chlorpropamide in activity and chemical structure.

phenindamine (fĕ-nin′dah-min) a compound used as an antihistamine.

phenindione (fen-in′di-ōn) a compound used as an anticoagulant.

pheniramine (fĕ-nir′ah-min) a compound used as an antihistamine.

phenmetrazine (fen-met′rah-zēn) a compound used to reduce the appetite.

phenobarbital (fe″no-bar′bĭ-tal) a long-acting barbituric-acid compound used as a hypnotic anticonvulsant and sedative.

phenocopy (fe′no-kop″e) 1. an individual whose phenotype mimics that of another genotype, but whose character is determined by environment and is not hereditary. 2. the simulated trait in a phenocopy individual.

phenol (fe′nol) 1. an extremely poisonous antiseptic, germicide and disinfectant. 2. a type of organic compound containing one or more hydroxyl groups attached to an aromatic or carbon ring.
  p. coefficient, a measure of the bactericidal activity of a chemical compound in relation to phenol. The activity of the compound is expressed as the ratio of dilution in which it kills in 10 minutes but not in 5 minutes under the specified conditions. It can be determined in the absence of organic matter, or in the presence of a standard amount of added organic matter.
  liquefied p., phenol maintained in liquid state by the presence of 10 per cent of water; used in diluted form in preparations for use on the skin.
  p. red, phenolsulfonphthalein.
  p. salicylate, phenyl salicylate.

phenolphthalein (fe″nol-thal′ēn) a compound used as a cathartic.

phenolsulfonphthalein (fe″nol-sul″fōn-thal′ēn) PSP, a dye used in testing kidney function, particularly renal blood flow and tubular function. The PSP test is less accurate than some other renal function tests because damage to the kidney cells must be rather extensive before positive results are obtained. The dye is given intravenously or intramuscularly; in both instances the patient may have a light breakfast and one glass of water, but no coffee or tea. In the intravenous test, the patient first drinks a glass of water and a urine specimen is collected 15 minutes later. At this time he drinks another glass of water, and then urine specimens are collected 1 hour and 2 hours after the dye has been administered. The intramuscular test is similar except that the last two urine specimens are collected 1 hour and 10 minutes, and 2 hours and 10 minutes, after injection of the dye.

phenomenon (fĕ-nom′ĕ-non), pl. *phenom′ena* [Gr.] an unusual or distinctive event whose occurrence is considered indicative of a certain quality or condition.

phenopropazine (fe″no-pro′pah-zēn) ethopropazine, used to produce parasympathetic blockade and to reduce tremors in Parkinson's disease.

phenothiazine (fe″no-thi′ah-zēn) a compound used as a veterinary drug. Its derivatives are widely used as tranquilizers.

phenotype (fe′no-tīp) the outward, visible expression of the hereditary constitution of an organism. adj., **phenotyp′ic.**

Phenoxene (fĕ-nok′sēn) trademark for a preparation of chlorphenoxamine; an antihistamine.

phenoxybenzamine (fĕ-nok″se-ben′zah-mēn) a compound used in adrenergic blockade to reduce blood pressure and as a vasodilator.

phenprocoumon (fen-pro′koo-mon) an anticoagulant of the coumarin type.

phensuximide (fen-suk′sĭ-mīd) a whitish crystalline powder used as an anticonvulsant in petit mal epilepsy.

phentermine (fen′ter-mēn) a sympathomimetic amine, used as an anorexigenic agent.

phentolamine (fen-tol′ah-mēn) a compound used as an antihypertensive and adrenolytic agent for the diagnosis of pheochromocytoma.

Phenurone (fen′u-rōn) trademark for a preparation of phenacemide, an anticonvulsant.

phenyl (fen′il, fe′nil) the monovalent radical, C_6H_5. adj., **phenyl′ic.**
  p. salicylate, a compound used as an enteric coating for tablets.
  p. tertiary butylamine, phentermine, an anorexigenic agent.

phenylalanine (fen″il-al′ah-nīn) a naturally occurring amino acid essential for optimal growth in infants and for nitrogen equilibrium in human adults.

phenylbutazone (fen″il-bu′tah-zōn) a compound used as an analgesic and antipyretic.

phenylephrine (fen″il-ef′rin) a compound with sympathomimetic action used mainly as a nasal decongestant, mydriatic, a local vasoconstrictor or a pressor agent in hypotensive states.

phenylhydrazine (fen″il-hi′drah-zēn) a compound used in the treatment of polycythemia vera because it causes hemolysis of erythrocytes. It is used also as a reagent for detection of sugar in the urine.

phenylketonuria (fen″il-ke″to-nu′re-ah) PKU, a congenital disease due to a defect in the metabolism of the amino acid phenylalanine. The condition is hereditary and results from lack of an enzyme, phenylalanine hydroxylase, necessary for the conversion of the amino acid phenylalanine into tyrosine. Thus there is accumulation of phenylalanine in the blood with eventual excretion of phenylpyruvic acid in the urine. If untreated, the condition results in mental retardation and other abnormalities.
  Persons with phenylketonuria are usually blue-eyed and blond, with defective pigmentation, the skin being excessively sensitive to light and tending to eczema. Other manifestations besides mental retardation are tremors, poor muscular coordination, excessive perspiration and perhaps convulsions.
  The disorder can be detected at or shortly after birth by a simple test of the infant's urine (now required by law in several states). A special diet, begun in the first few weeks of life and continued, permits the infant to grow and develop normally. Thus, although the disease is not curable, its effects can be counteracted. Even if a person has had this disease for years, proper diet can improve his physical condition. The diet is designed to restrict the intake of phenylalanine. Since few nutrients con-

Exchange Lists for Low Phenylalanine Diet

Food	Amount	Food	Amount
List I – Lofenalac		Prunes	
30 Mg. Phenylalanine – 2 Equivalents†		Cooked	2 large
Lofenalac‡ (dry)	4 tbsp.	Juice	⅓ c.
Lofenalac (reconstituted)	1 c.	Strained	3 tbsp.
		Raisins	2 tbsp.
List II – Vegetables		Strawberries	3 large
15 Mg. Phenylalanine – 1 Equivalent		Tangerine	⅔ small
Beans, green		Watermelon	⅔ c.
Strained and chopped	1½ tbsp.		
Regular	3 tbsp.	*List IV – Breads*	
Beets		*30 Mg. Phenylalanine – 2 Equivalents*	
Strained	2 tbsp.	Barley cereal, Gerber's, dry	2⅓ tbsp.
Regular	3 tbsp.	Biscuits[a]	1 small
Cabbage, raw, shredded	4 tbsp.	Cereal food, Gerber's, dry	2 tbsp.
Carrots		Cookies, arrowroot	1½
Strained and chopped	3 tbsp.	Corn	2 tbsp.
Raw	¼ large	Cornflakes	⅓ c.
Canned	4 tbsp.	Crackers	
Celery, raw	1½ small	Barnum animal	6
	stalks	Saltines	3
Cucumber, raw	⅓ medium	Cream of Wheat, cooked	2 tbsp.
Lettuce, head	2 leaves	Farina, cooked	2½ tbsp.
Spinach, creamed – strained		Mixed cereal, pablum, dry	1⅔ tbsp.
and chopped	1½ tbsp.	Oatmeal	
Squash		Gerber's strained	1⅔ tbsp.
Winter		Pablum, dry	1⅔ tbsp.
Strained	3 tbsp.	Potatoes, Irish	2½ tbsp.
Chopped	6 tbsp.	Rice Flakes, Quaker	⅓ c.
Cooked	2 tbsp.	Rice Krispies, Kellogg's	⅓ c.
Summer, cooked	4 tbsp.	Rice, Puffed, Quaker	½ c.
Tomato		Sugar Crisps	¼ c.
Raw	¼ small	Sweet potatoes or yams	
Canned	2 tbsp.	Cooked	3 tbsp.
Juice	2½ tbsp.	Strained	4 tbsp.
		Wafers, sugar, Nabisco	6
List III – Fruits		Wheat, Puffed, Quaker	⅓ c.
15 Mg. Phenylalanine – 1 Equivalent			
Apple	2 medium-	*List V – Fats*	
	large	*5 Mg. Phenylalanine – ⅓ Equivalent*	
Apricots, dried	4 large	Butter	1 tsp.
	halves	Cream, heavy	1 tsp.
Banana	½ med.	Margarine	1 tbsp.
Cantaloupe	½ c. diced	Mayonnaise	1½ tbsp.
Dates, dried	2	Olives, ripe	1 large
Fruit cocktail, canned	2½ tbsp.		
Grapefruit		*List VI – Desserts*	
Sections	⅓ c.	*30 Mg. Phenylalanine – 2 Equivalents*	
Juice	⅓ c.	Cookies	
Orange	1 medium	Rice flour	2
Sections	⅔ c.	Corn starch	2
Juice	3 tbsp.	Ice cream[a]	
Grape juice	⅓ c.	Chocolate	⅓ c.
Lemon juice	3 tbsp.	Pineapple	⅓ c.
Nectarine	1 medium	Strawberry	⅓ c.
Peaches		Vanilla	⅓ c.
Raw	1 medium	Puddings[a]	⅓ c.
Canned in syrup	1½ halves	Sauce, Hershey syrup	2 tbsp.
Strained	5 tbsp.		
Chopped	7 tbsp.	*List VII – Free Foods; Little or No*	
Pears		*Phenylalanine; May Be Used as Desired*	
Raw	1⅓ medium	Candy	
Canned in syrup	3 halves	Butterscotch	—
Strained and chopped	10 tbsp.	Cream mints	—
Pears and pineapple, strained		Fondant	—
and chopped	7 tbsp.	Gum drops	—
Pineapple		Hard	—
Raw	⅓ c.	Jelly beans	—
Canned in syrup	1½ small	Lollipops	—
	slices	Cornstarch	—
Juice	½ c.	Guava butter	—
Plums, canned in syrup	1½ medium	Honey	—
Plums with tapioca		Jams, jellies, and marmalades	—
Strained	5 tbsp.	Molasses	—
Chopped	7 tbsp.	Oil	—

EXCHANGE LISTS FOR LOW PHENYLALANINE DIET (*Continued*)

FOOD	AMOUNT	FOOD	AMOUNT
Sauces		*List VIII—Foods to Avoid; High Phenylalanine*	
Lemon[a]	—	*Content; May Be Used Only Occasionally*	
White[a]	—	*in Very Small Portions*	
Syrups		Breads, most	—
Corn	—	Cheeses of all kinds	—
Maple	—	Eggs	—
Sugar		Legumes, dried	—
Brown	—	Meat, poultry, fish	—
White	—	Milk#	—
Tapioca	—	Nuts	—
		Nut butters	—

From Krause, M. V.: Food, Nutrition and Diet Therapy. 4th ed. Philadelphia, W. B. Saunders Co., 1966; adapted from Phenylketonuria. Children's Bureau Pub. No. 388, U. S. Department of Health, Education, and Welfare, Social Security Adm., Washington, D.C., 1961, and Miller, G. T., et al.: Phenylalanine content of fruit. J. Amer. Diet. Ass., 46:43, 1965.

†One equivalent may be defined as providing 15 mg. phenylalanine.

‡Mead Johnson & Company.

[a]Special recipe must be used.

#Milk is high in phenylalanine (1 oz. contains 50 mg.), but it may be ordered in infants to keep phenylalanine blood levels up to normal.

tain proteins lacking phenylalanine, synthetic preparations of protein supplements are used.

The defect is a recessive trait that is transmitted through apparently healthy parents, who if tested will show signs of the disease.

phenylmercuric (fen″il-mer-ku′rik) denoting a compound containing the radical C_6H_5Hg-, some of which have bacteriostatic and bactericidal properties.

p. nitrate, a compound of phenol, mercury and nitric acid; used as a local antibacterial.

phenylpropanolamine hydrochloride (fen″il-pro″pah-nol′ah-min) a compound with actions similar to those of ephedrine; used by spray or instillation as a bronchodilator and local vasoconstrictor.

phenylpropylmethylamine (fen″il-pro″pil-meth″il-am′ēn) a compound used as a nasal decongestant.

phenylpyruvic acid (fen″il-pi-roo′vik) an intermediate product of the metabolism of phenylalanine in the body.

phenylthiocarbamide (fen″il-thi″o-kar-bam′īd) a compound used in genetics research, the ability to taste it being determined by a single dominant gene. The compound is intensely bitter to approximately 70 per cent of the population, and nearly tasteless to the rest.

phenyltoloxamine (fen″il-to-lok′sah-mēn) a compound used as an antihistamine.

phenylurea (fen″il-u-re′ah) a hypnotic compound prepared from urea and aniline.

phenyramidol (fen″ĭ-ram′ĭ-dol) a benzyl alcohol compound suggested as an analgesic.

phenytoin (fen′ĭ-to-in) diphenylhydantoin, an anticonvulsant.

pheochrome (fe′o-krōm) staining dark with chromium salts; chromaffin.

pheochromoblast (fe″o-kro′mo-blast) an embryonic structure that develops into pheochromocytes.

pheochromocyte (fe″o-kro′mo-sīt) a chromaffin cell; a cell of the adrenal or sympathetic tissue that stains darkly with chromium salts.

pheochromocytoma (fe″o-kro″mo-si″to′mah) a small chromaffin cell tumor, usually located in the adrenal medulla but occasionally occurring in chromaffin tissue of the sympathetic paraganglia. It is relatively rare and has a tendency to occur in families. The tumor is potentially fatal, but the condition can be cured if diagnosed early, before there has been irreparable damage to the cardiovascular system.

SYMPTOMS. Because the tumor is composed of cells similar to the secreting cells of the adrenal medulla, it is capable of secreting epinephrine and norepinephrine. The symptoms of the tumor are therefore directly related to excessive amounts of these two hormones in the tissues and blood.

The cardinal symptom is hypertension. In some cases the blood pressure is consistently high with slight fluctuations, and in others the hypertension is intermittent with periods of normal blood pressure. Other symptoms include severe headache, sweating, visual blurring, apprehension, tachycardia, and postural hypotension.

DIAGNOSIS. Pheochromocytoma must be differentiated from several other disorders such as essential hypertension and thyrotoxicosis, which it closely resembles. Diagnosis is based on the patient's symptoms and the findings of specific chemical and pharmacologic tests. The test considered most reliable is direct assay of epinephrine and norephinephrine in the plasma and urine following an attack. Another test involving measurement of vanillylmandelic acid (VMA) and of metanephrine and normetanephrine in urine is considered satisfactory. The level of these substances in the urine in patients with pheochromocytoma is almost twice the upper limits of normal.

Two types of pharmacologic tests are used; one provokes an increase in blood pressure, the other causes a fall in blood pressure. The provocative test uses histamine or methacholine to stimulate action of the tumor and thereby provoke an attack. This test must be given with extreme caution and only when the patient is between attacks and his blood pressure is near normal (less than 170/110 mm. of mercury). An antihypertensive drug such as phentolamine hydrochloride (Regitine) must be on hand when the test is done. If the blood pressure increases too rapidly, phentolamine is given intravenously.

For the patient with sustained hypertension the test of choice involves the administration of an adrenolytic agent such as phentolamine which will produce hypotension. If, after administration of the drug, the blood pressure decreases to near normal within 3 to 4 minutes and remains depressed for several minutes more, the diagnosis of pheochromocytoma is confirmed. During this test a hypertensive drug must be on hand in the event the blood pressure falls too rapidly and there is danger of shock.

For at least 24 hours prior to either of these pharmacologic tests the patient must not receive any sedatives or antihypertensive drugs. Immediately before the test reliable blood pressure readings are taken and a basic average established. The patient should remain in bed during the test, resting quietly and with a needle already inserted in a vein so that at the time the drug is administered he will not be unduly disturbed.

TREATMENT. Surgical removal of the tumor, or tumors if there are more than one, is necessary for complete remission of symptoms. There are two possible complications of surgery: a sudden rise in blood pressure and development of tachycardia due to discharge of pressor agents as the tumor is being manipulated, and severe hypotension and shock following removal of the tumor. These hazards have been substantially reduced in recent years by the preoperative administration of sedatives and antihypertensive drugs, and the use of blood or plasma to maintain adequate blood volume.

If surgery has involved resection of a portion of the adrenal cortex, it may be necessary for the patient to receive adrenocortical hormones by injection.

NURSING CARE. Once the diagnosis of pheochromocytoma has been established, the patient is prepared for surgery. The preoperative period may extend for several weeks while attempts are made to stabilize the blood pressure and hormonal imbalances. The patient should be kept in a quiet atmosphere and usually is given sedatives, such as phenobarbital, to promote rest. His blood pressure is taken at frequent intervals and recorded. These readings are used later as a basis for comparison during the postoperative period. They also alert the physician to extremes in blood pressure that are characteristic in this disorder.

When assisting with either of the pharmacologic tests used in diagnosing pheochromocytoma, the nurse must know the action of the specific drug being used and assist in the measurement and recording of the patient's blood pressure. She also observes the patient for signs of shock when an antihypertensive drug is being used. Equipment for administration of drugs necessary for combating severe reactions to the test drugs must be at hand.

Postoperatively the patient must again be watched for the development of severe hypertension, which can lead to cerebral vascular accident, and for extreme hypotension with circulatory collapse and profound shock.

If the adrenal cortex has been resected during surgery, hormonal imbalances are likely to occur. These include HYPOGLYCEMIA, addisonian crisis and extreme diuresis and electrolyte and fluid imbalance. The hypoglycemia is most likely to occur in patients who have had symptoms of diabetes mellitus prior to surgery, and is treated with infusions of glucose solution. Adrenocortical hormones may be administered by slow intravenous drip, the rate of flow being adjusted according to blood pressure readings and other reactions of the patient. The nurse's responsibility lies in close observation of the patient so that disturbances in electrolyte and fluid balance, extremes in blood pressure and disorders of metabolism can be recognized early and treated promptly.

Ph.G. Graduate in Pharmacy.

-phil(e) (fil) word element [Gr.], *entity (person or thing) having affinity for or morbid fondness for something.* adj., **-phil'ic.**

-philia (fil'e-ah) word element [Gr.], *affinity for; morbid fondness of.* adj., **phil'ic.**

philtrum (fil'trum) the vertical groove in the median portion of the upper lip.

phimosis (fi-mo'sis) tightness of the foreskin, which cannot be drawn back from the glans penis.

pHisoHex (fi'so-heks) trademark for an emulsion containing hexachlorophene; used as a skin cleanser.

phleb(o)- (fleb'o) word element [Gr.], *vein.*

phlebangioma (fleb"an-je-o'mah) a venous aneurysm.

phlebarteriectasia (fleb"-ar-te"re-ek-ta'ze-ah) dilatation of veins and arteries.

phlebectasia (fleb"ek-ta'ze-ah) dilatation of a vein or veins.

phlebectomy (flĕ-bek'to-me) excision of a vein.

phlebemphraxis (fleb"em-frak'sis) stoppage of a vein by a plug or clot.

phlebismus (flĕ-biz'mus) obstruction and turgescence of veins.

phlebitis (flĕ-bi'tis) inflammation of a vein. It is relatively common, especially in the veins of the lower limbs.

Phlebitis is not serious when the inflammation is located in a superficial vein since these veins are numerous enough to permit the flow of blood to be rechanneled, so that the inflamed vein is bypassed. When a deep vein is involved, however, phlebitis is potentially more dangerous. It can also have serious consequences if it occurs in certain areas such as the veins of the cranium, where it may lead to cerebral abscesses.

CAUSES. The causes of phlebitis are uncertain. The disease sometimes occurs for no apparent reason; at other times, it seems to follow a variety of other disorders—for example, circulatory difficulties, blood disorders and obesity. Phlebitis may be a complication of pneumonia, typhoid fever or other general infections. It may also be a result of injury to a vein, either after an accident or occasionally as an aftermath of surgery.

Once in about a hundred births phlebitis develops in a newly delivered mother; in such cases it usually appears about 10 days after delivery. This form of phlebitis is commonly called "milk leg," because it is associated with the onset of milk production by the mother.

Phlebitis may also develop when circulation is sluggish after long periods of staying in bed without proper exercising of the limbs and frequent changing of position.

SYMPTOMS AND TREATMENT. When phlebitis occurs in a superficial vein, there is usually pain and tenderness. This may be so slight at first that the tenderness is felt only when pressure is applied to the painful area. As the inflammation increases, the pain becomes more acute, especially during walking or other exercise.

The inflamed area swells and becomes red and warm. A tender cordlike mass may form under the skin; it may grow smaller as the condition subsides, but occasionally lasts for some time.

When the inflammation occurs in a deep vein and affects the vein's inner lining, there may be formation of a thrombus on the vein wall. This condition is known as thrombophlebitis. When clots in the veins interfere with the normal flow of blood, fluid accumulates and causes edema.

If phlebitis is superficial, the patient usually does not have to be confined to bed. Frequently, a supportive elastic dressing is used until the vein is healed.

When deeper veins are affected, however, or if the inflammation is severe, bed rest is required to prevent the clot from being dislodged. Antibiotics are sometimes prescribed to combat infection. Anticoagulants are used and the extremity is elevated to prevent further clots or propagation of the existing clot. In some extreme cases, or when an embolism is likely to occur, surgery may be necessary as a preventive measure.

In persons prone to thrombophlebitis, anticoagulation is used as a preventive measure, particularly when long periods of bed rest are required, such as after surgery.

phleboclysis (flē-bok'lĭ-sis) introduction of a solution into a vein.

phlebogram (fleb'o-gram) 1. a sphygmographic tracing of a venous pulse. 2. a film obtained at phlebography.

phlebography (flē-bog'rah-fe) roentgenography of the veins after introduction of a contrast medium.

phlebolith (fleb'o-lith) a venous calculus or concretion.

phlebomanometer (fleb"o-mah-nom'ĕ-ter) an instrument for the direct measurement of venous blood pressure.

phlebophlebostomy (fleb"o-flē-bost'to-me) anastomosis of two veins, as of the portal vein and inferior vena cava.

phleboplasty (fleb'o-plas"te) plastic repair of a vein.

phleborrhaphy (flē-bor'ah-fe) suture of a vein.

phleborrhexis (fleb"o-rek'sis) rupture of a vein.

phlebosclerosis (fleb"o-sklĕ-ro'sis) abnormal thickening and hardening of the walls of veins.

phlebostasis (flĕ-bos'tah-sis) 1. retardation of blood flow in veins. 2. temporary removal of a portion of blood from the general circulation by compressing the veins of an extremity.

phlebothrombosis (fleb"o-throm-bo'sis) the development of venous thrombi in the absence of antecedent inflammation of the vessel wall, as opposed to thrombophlebitis, in which there are inflammatory changes in the vessel wall.

phlebotome (fleb'o-tōm) a lancet for venesection.

Phlebotomus (fle-bot'o-mus) a genus of flies, called sandflies, the females of which are blood sucking; various species are vectors of various disease-producing organisms.
  p. fever, a febrile disease of short duration, resembling dengue in many of its symptoms, occurring in Mediterranean countries, caused by a virus that is transmitted by a species of sandfly; called also sandfly fever.
  P. papatas'ii, the sandfly, an insect of India and the Mediterranean countries, believed to convey the causative organism of phlebotomus fever.

phlebotomy (flĕ-bot'o-me) incision of a vein for the purpose of withdrawing blood.

phlegm (flem) mucus.

phlegmasia (fleg-ma'ze-ah) inflammation with fever.
  p. al'ba do'lens, phlebitis of the femoral vein, with resultant painful swelling of the leg.
  p. al'ba do'lens puerpera'rum, phlebitis of the femoral vein in puerperal women.
  p. ceru'lea do'lens, an acute fulminating form of deep venous thrombosis, with pronounced edema and severe cyanosis of the extremity.

phlegmatic (fleg-mat'ik) of dull and sluggish temperament.

phlegmon (fleg'mon) inflammation of the connective tissue, leading to ulceration or abscess; cellulitis. adj., **phleg'monous.**
  bronze p., cellulitis with bronze-colored spots.
  diffuse p., diffuse cellulitis with septic symptoms.
  gas p., cellulitis in which gas is formed; gas gangrene.
  ligneous p., woody p., inflammation causing induration of the involved tissues.

phlog(o)- (flo'go) word element [Gr.], *inflammation.*

phlogistic (flo-jis'tik) inflammatory.

phlogogenic (flo"go-jen'ik) producing inflammation.

phlorhizin (flo-ri'zin) a bitter glycoside that causes glycosuria by blocking the renal tubular reabsorption of glucose.

P.H.L.S. Public Health Laboratory Service (British).

phlyctena (flik-te'nah) a vesicle containing a thin ichor or lymph, especially a blister caused by a burn.

phlyctenoid (flik′tĕ-noid) resembling a phlyctena.

phlyctenosis (flik″tĕ-no′sis) any pustular disease or lesion.

phlyctenule (flik′ten-ūl) a minute vesicle; an ulcerated nodule of the cornea or conjunctiva. adj., **phlyctenʹular.**

phlyctenulosis (flik-ten″u-lo′sis) a condition marked by formation of phlyctenules.

-phobe (fōb) word element [Gr.], *entity* (person or thing) *having antipathy toward or morbid fear of something.*

phobia (fo′be-ah) any persistent abnormal fear that appears to result from repressed inner conflicts of which the affected person is not aware. Used as a word ending designating abnormal or morbid fear of or aversion to the subject indicated by the stem to which it is affixed. adj. **phoʹbic.**
   A person with a phobia reacts uncontrollably and unreasonably to the situation of which he is afraid. A wide variety of exaggerated fears can exist in neurotic persons (see also NEUROSIS).
   Some typical phobias are: acrophobia–fear of heights; agoraphobia–fear of open or public places; astraphobia–fear of lightning; cenotophobia–morbid fear of new things or new ideas; claustrophobia–morbid fear of closed places; hemophobia –fear of blood; xenophobia–morbid dread of strangers.

phobophobia (fo″bo-fo′be-ah) morbid fear of one's own fears.

phocomelus (fo-kom′ĕ-lus) a fetus with hands and feet, but no legs or arms

phonal (fo′nal) pertaining to the voice.

phonarteriogram (fōn″ar-te′re-o-gram″) a tracing or graphic record of arterial sounds obtained in phonarteriography.

phonarteriography (fōn″ar-te″re-og′rah-fe) the recording of arterial sounds by phonocardiography.

phonasthenia (fo″nas-the′ne-ah) weakness of the voice from fatigue.

phonation (fo-na′shun) the utterance of vocal sounds.

phone (fōn) a speech sound.

phoneme (fo′nēm) 1. an auditory hallucination. 2. the smallest distinct unit of sound in a language.

phonendoscope (fo-nen′do-skōp) a stethoscope that intensifies auscultatory sounds.

phonetics (fo-net′iks) the science of vocal sounds.

phonic (fon′ik, fo′nik) pertaining to the voice.

phonism (fo′nizm) a sensation of hearing produced by the effect of something seen, felt, tasted, smelled or thought of.

phonocardiogram (fo″no-kar′de-o-gram″) the record produced by phonocardiography.

phonocardiography (fo″no-kar″de-og′rah-fe) the graphic registration of the sounds produced by action of the heart. adj., **phonocardiographʹic.**

phonocatheter (fo″no-kath′ĕ-ter) a catheter with a device in its tip for picking up and transmitting sound.

phonocatheterization (fo″no-kath″ĕ-ter-ĭ-za′-shun) use of a phonocatheter for detection of sounds produced in the circulatory system.
   intracardiac p., detection of sounds by means of a phonocatheter passed into the heart as an aid in the diagnosis of cardiac defects.

phonogram (fo′no-gram) a graphic record of a sound.

phonology (fo-nol′o-je) phonetics.

phonomassage (fo″no-mah-sahzh′) alternating pressure and suction in the external ear in order to exercise and stimulate the tympanic membrane and ossicles.

phonometer (fo-nom′ĕ-ter) a device for measuring the intensity of vocal sounds.

phonomyography (fo″no-mi-og′rah-fe) the recording of sounds produced by muscle contraction.

phonopathy (fo-nop′ah-the) disease of the organs of speech.

phonophobia (fo″no-fo′be-ah) morbid dread of sounds or of speaking aloud.

phonophore (fo′no-fōr) 1. a form of stethoscope. 2. an ossicle of the middle ear.

phonophotography (fo″no-fo-tog′rah-fe) photographic recording of sound waves.

phonopneumomassage (fo″no-nu″mo-mah-sahzh′) air massage of the middle ear.

phonopsia (fo-nop′se-ah) a visual sensation caused by the hearing of sounds.

phonoreception (fo″no-re-sep′shun) the reception of stimuli perceived as sound.

phonoreceptor (fo″no-re-sep′tor) a receptor for sound stimuli.

phonorenogram (fo″no-re′no-gram) a record of the sounds produced by pulsation of the renal artery obtained by a phonocatheter passed through a ureter into the renal pelvis.

phonostethograph (fo″no-steth′o-graf) an instrument by which chest sounds are amplified, filtered and recorded.

-phore (fōr) word element [Gr.], *a carrier.*

phoresis (fo-re′sis) introduction of chemical ions into the tissues by passage of an electric current.

phoria (fo′re-ah) tendency of the visual axis of one eye to deviate when the other eye is covered.

phorology (fo-rol′o-je) study of disease carriers and the transmission of disease.

phorometer (fo-rom′ĕ-ter) an instrument for measuring heterophoria, and more generally the relative strength of the ocular muscles.

phose (fōz) a visual sensation, as of light or color.

phosgene (fos′jēn) a toxic gas, carbonyl chloride, $COCl_2$, used in warfare.

phosphagen (fos′fah-jen) a compound, such as

phosphocreatine and phosphoarginine, that is present in tissue and that yields high-energy phosphate.

Phosphaljel (fos'fal-jel) trademark for a preparation of aluminum phosphate gel, an antacid.

phosphatase (fos'fah-tās) an enzyme that hydrolyzes monophosphoric esters, with liberation of inorganic phosphate, found in practically all tissues, body fluids and cells, including erythrocytes and leukocytes.

   acid p., a phosphatase that is active in an acid environment; found in erythrocytes, prostatic tissue, spleen, kidney and other tissues.

   alkaline p., a phosphatase that is active in an alkaline environment; found in bone, liver, kidney, leukocytes, adrenal cortex and other tissues.

phosphate (fos'fāt) a salt of phosphoric acid. adj., **phosphat'ic.**

   Phosphates are widely distributed in the body, the largest amounts being in the bones and teeth. They are continually excreted in the urine and feces, and must be replaced in the diet. Inorganic phosphates function as buffer salts to maintain the ACID-BASE BALANCE in blood, saliva, urine and other body fluids. The principal phosphates in this buffer system are monosodium and disodium phosphate. Organic phosphates, in particular adenosine triphosphate (ATP), take part in a series of reversible reactions involving phosphoric acid, lactic acid, glycogen and other substances, which furnish the energy expended in muscle contraction. This is thought to occur through the hydrolysis of the so-called high-energy phosphate bond present in ATP, phosphocreatine and certain other body compounds.

   acid p., a salt of phosphoric acid in which only one or two of the hydrogen atoms have been replaced.

   calcium p., a compound containing calcium and the phosphate radical; used as an antacid and laxative.

   creatine p., phosphocreatine.

   ferric p., a yellowish white powder insoluble in water or acetic acid.

   ferric p., soluble, ferric phosphate rendered soluble by the presence of sodium citrate; used as a hematinic.

   magnesium p., a salt of phosphoric acid used as a laxative or antacid.

   normal p., a phosphate in which all the hydrogen atoms of the acid have been replaced.

phosphatemia (fos"fah-te'me-ah) phosphates in the blood.

phosphatide (fos'fah-tīd) a fatty acid ester of a phosphorylated polyvalent alcohol.

   prothromboplastic p's, substances that are believed to function as parts of both thromboplastin and antithromboplastin.

phosphaturia (fos"fah-tu're-ah) excess of phosphates in the urine.

phosphene (fos'fēn) an objective visual sensation that occurs with the eyes closed, and in the absence of retinal stimulation by visible light.

phosphide (fos'fīd) a binary compound of phosphorus.

phosphite (fos'fīt) a salt of phosphorous acid.

phosphoarginine (fos"fo-ar'ji̇-nin) an arginine-

phosphoric acid compound found in invertebrate muscles; similar to phosphocreatine in mammals.

phosphocreatine (fos"fo-kre'ah-tin) a creatine-phosphoric acid compound occurring in muscle, being the most important storage form of high-energy phosphate, the energy source in muscle contraction.

phospholipid, phospholipin (fos"fo-lip'id), (fos"-fo-lip'in) a compound of an alcohol, fatty acids and phosphoric acid. Lecithin, cephalin and sphingomyelin are examples.

phosphonecrosis (fos"fo-nĕ-kro'sis) necrosis of the jaw bone occurring in persons who work with phosphorus; called also phossy jaw.

phosphopenia (fos"fo-pe'ne-ah) deficiency of phosphorus in the body.

phosphoprotein (fos"fo-pro'te-in) a protein containing phosphoric acid conjugated with an amino acid.

phosphorated (fos'fo-rāt"ed) charged or combined with phosphorus.

phosphorescence (fos"fo-res'ens) the emission of light without appreciable heat; the property of continuing luminous in the dark after exposure to light or other radiation.

phosphorhidrosis (fos"for-hi̇-dro'sis) secretion of phosphorescent or luminous sweat.

phosphoric acid (fos-for'ik) a crystalline compound or clear, syrupy liquid whose salts are called phosphates.

phosphorism (fos'fo-rizm) poisoning by phosphorus.

phosphorolysis (fos"fo-rol'ĭ-sis) the reversible combination and separation of sugar and phosphoric acid in carbohydrate metabolism.

phosphorous acid (fos'for-us) a white, hygroscopic, crystalline compound whose salts are called phosphites.

phosphoruria (fos"for-u're-ah) phosphorus in the urine.

phosphorus (for'for-us) a chemical element, atomic number 15, atomic weight 30.974, symbol P. (See table of ELEMENTS.) Phosphorus, in combination with calcium, oxygen and hydrogen, forms the substance of bones. It also plays an important role in cell metabolism. It is obtained by the body from milk products, cereals, meat and fish, and its use by the body is controlled by vitamin D and calcium.

   Phosphorus is very inflammable and exceedingly poisonous. Inhalation of its vapor by workers in chemical industries may cause necrosis of the mandible. Free phosphorus causes fatty degeneration of the liver and other viscera.

   ordinary p., a waxy solid, exceedingly poisonous.

   ^{32}P, radioactive p., the RADIOISOTOPE with an atomic weight of 32; used in treating leukemia and allied disorders.

phosphorylase (fos-for'ĭ-lās) an enzyme that

catalyzes the conversion of glycogen into glucose-1-phosphate.

phosphorylation (fos"for-ĭ-la'shun) the process of introducing the trivalent PO (phosphoryl) group into an organic molecule.

phosphotransferase (fos"fo-trans'fer-ās) an enzyme that catalyzes the transfer of a phosphate group.

phosphuresis (fos"fu-re'sis) the urinary excretion of phosphorus (phosphates). adj., **phosphuret'ic.**

phot(o)- (fo'to) word element [Gr.], *light.*

photalgia (fo-tal'je-ah) pain, as in the eye, caused by light.

phote (fōt) a unit of illumination, being 1 lumen per square centimeter.

photechy (fo'tek-e) the power shown by certain substances of becoming radioactive after having been exposed to radiation.

photic (fo'tik) pertaining to light.

photism (fo'tizm) a visual sensation produced by the effect of something heard, felt, tasted, smelled or thought of.

photoallergy (fo"to-al'er-je) allergic sensitivity to light. adj., **photoaller'gic.**

photobiology (fo"to-bi-ol'o-je) the branch of biology dealing with the effect of light on organisms.

photobiotic (fo"to-bi-ot'ik) living only in the light.

photocatalysis (fo"to-kah-tal'ĭ-sis) promotion or stimulation of a reaction by light. adj., **photocatalyt'ic.**

photochemistry (fo"to-kem'is-tre) the branch of chemistry that deals with the chemical properties or effects of light rays.

photochromogen (fo"to-kro'mo-jen) a microorganism whose pigmentation develops as a result of exposure to light. adj., **photochromogen'ic.**

photocoagulation (fo"to-ko-ag"u-la'shun) condensation of protein material by controlled use of light rays, as in treatment of pathologic conditions of the eye, such as retinal detachment.

photodermatitis (fo"to-der"mah-ti'tis) an abnormal state of the skin in which light is an important causative factor.

photodynamics (fo"to-di-nam'iks) the science of the activating effects of light.

photodynia (fo"to-din'e-ah) photalgia.

photoelectric (fo"to-e-lek'trik) pertaining to the electric effects of light or other radiation.

photofluorography (fo"to-floo"or-og'rah-fe) the photographic recording of fluoroscopic images on small films, a procedure used in mass roentgenography of the chest.

photogene (fo'to-jēn) after-image; a retinal impression remaining after cessation of the stimulus causing it.

photogenic (fo"to-jen'ik) produced by light, or producing light.

photokinetic (fo"to-ki-net'ik) moving in response to the stimulus of light.

photolysis (fo-tol'ĭ-sis) decomposition by light.

photolyte (fo'to-līt) a substance decomposed by light.

photomania (fo"to-ma'ne-ah) mania developed under the influence of light.

photometer (fo-tom'ĕ-ter) a device for measuring the intensity of light.

photometry (fo-tom'ĕ-tre) measurement of the intensity of light.

photomicrograph (fo"to-mi'kro-graf) a photograph of an object as seen through an ordinary light microscope.

photon (fo'ton) a particle (quantum) of electromagnetic radiation.

photonosus (fo-ton'o-sus) any disease due to excessive light.

photo-ophthalmia (fo"to-of-thal'me-ah) ophthalmia caused by intense light, such as electric light, rays of welding arc or reflection from snow.

photoperceptive (fo"to-per-sep'tiv) able to perceive light.

photoperiodicity (fo"to-pe"re-o-dis'ĭ-te) regularly recurrent changes in the relation of light and darkness noted in the annual passage of the earth about the sun; applied also to the rhythm of certain biologic phenomena as determined by those changes.

photophilic (fo"to-fil'ik) fond of or thriving in light.

photophobia (fo"to-fo'be-ah) abnormal intolerance of light.

photophthalmia (fo"tof-thal'me-ah) photo-ophthalmia.

photopia (fo-to'pe-ah) the adjustment of the eye for light.

photopsia, photopsy (fo-top'se-ah), (fo'top-se) an appearance as of sparks or flashes, in retinal disease.

photoptarmosis (fo"to-tar-mo'sis) sneezing caused by the influence of light.

photoptometer (fo"top-tom'ĕ-ter) a device for measuring visual acuity.

photoreception (fo"to-re-sep'shun) the process of detecting radiant energy, usually of wavelengths between 3900 and 7700 angstroms, being the range of visible light.

photoreceptive (fo"to-re-sep'tiv) able to perceive light.

photoreceptor (fo"to-re-sep'tor) a nerve endorgan or receptor that responds to stimulation of light rays.

photoscan (fo'to-skan) a two-dimensional representation (map) of the gamma rays emitted by a radioisotope, revealing its varying concentration in a body tissue, differing from a scintiscan only in that the printout mechanism is a light source exposing a photographic film.

photosensitive (fo″to-sen′sĭ-tiv) sensitive to light.

photostable (fo′to-sta″bl) unchanged by the influence of light.

photosynthesis (fo′to-sin′thē-sis) a chemical combination caused by the action of light; specifically the formation of carbohydrates from carbon dioxide and water in the chlorophyll tissue of plants under the influence of light. adj., **photosynthet′ic.**

phototaxis (fo′to-tak′sis) movement of a freely motile organism in response to the stimulation of light. adj., **phototac′tic.**

phototherapy (fo″to-ther′ah-pe) treatment of disease by light rays.

phototoxic (fo″to-tok′sik) having a toxic effect triggered by exposure to light.

phototrophic (fo″to-trof′ik) utilizing light in metabolism, as in certain plants and bacteria.

phototropism (fo-tot′ro-pizm) 1. the tendency of an organism to turn or move toward (positive phototropism) or away from (negative phototropism) light. 2. change of color produced in a substance by the action of light.

photuria (fo-tu′re-ah) phosphorescence of the urine.

phren (fren) 1. the mind or heart. 2. the diaphragm.

phrenalgia (frĕ-nal′je-ah) 1. pain in the diaphragm. 2. melancholia.

phrenasthenia (fren″as-the′ne-ah) feebleness of mind.

phrenemphraxis (fren″em-frak′sis) crushing of the phrenic nerve, a form of collapse therapy used in tuberculosis.

phrenetic (frĕ-net′ik) affected with mania.

phrenic (fren′ik) pertaining to the diaphragm or to the mind.
    p. nerve, a major branch of the cervical plexus. It extends through the thorax to provide innervation of the diaphragm. Nerve impulses from the inspiratory center in the brain travel down the phrenic nerve, causing contraction of the diaphragm, and inspiration occurs.

phrenicectomy (fren″ĭ-sek′to-me) resection of the phrenic nerve.

phrenicoexeresis (fren″ĭ-ko-ek-ser′ĕ-sis) avulsion of the phrenic nerve.

phrenicotomy (fren″ĭ-kot′o-me) surgical division of the phrenic nerve, causing a one-sided paralysis of the diaphragm with immobilization and compression of a diseased lung.

phrenicotripsy (fren″ĭ-ko-trip′se) surgical crushing of the phrenic nerve.

phrenitis (frĕ-ni′tis) delirium or frenzy.

phrenocardia (fren″o-kar′de-ah) a psychic con-

dition marked by pain in the cardiac region, dyspnea and palpitations.

phrenocolic (fren″o-kol′ik) pertaining to the diaphragm and colon.

phrenodynia (fren″o-din′e-ah) pain in the diaphragm.

phrenology (frĕ-nol′o-je) study of the faculties and qualities of mind from the shape of the skull.

phrenopathy (frĕ-nop′ah-the) any mental disease.

phrenoplegia (fren″o-ple′je-ah) a sudden attack of mental disorder. 2. paralysis of the diaphragm.

phrenosin (fren′o-sin) a cerebroside containing cerebronic acid attached to the sphingosine; obtained from the brain.

phrenotropic (fren″o-trop′ik) exerting its principal effect upon the mind.

phrynoderma (frin″o-der′mah) a dry dermatosis, probably due to deficiency of vitamin A.

phthalylsulfacetamide (thal″il-sul″fah-set′ah-mĭd) a compound used as an intestinal anti-infective.

phthalylsulfathiazole (thal″il-sul″fah-thi′ah-zōl) a compound used as an intestinal antibacterial.

phthalylsulfonazole (thal″il-sul-fon′ah-zōl) phthalylsulfacetamide.

phthiriasis (thĭ-ri′ah-sis) infestation with lice of the species *Phthirus pubis.*

Phthirus (thir′us) a genus of lice.
    P. pu′bis, a species of louse that infests the pubic hair and sometimes the eyebrows and eyelashes.

phthisic (tiz′ik) 1. affected with phthisis. 2. a popular name for asthma.

phthisiology (tiz″e-ol′o-je) the scientific study of tuberculosis.

phthisiophobia (tiz″e-o-fo′be-ah) morbid fear of tuberculosis.

phthisis (thi′sis) 1. a wasting of the body. 2. tuberculosis.
    p. bul′bi, shrinkage of the eyeball.
    grinder's p., a combination of tuberculosis and silicosis of the lungs occurring in grinders in the cutlery trade.
    miner's p., anthracosis.
    pulmonary p., tuberculosis.
    p. ventric′uli, atrophy of the mucous membrane of the stomach and alimentary canal.

phylaxin (fi-lak′sin) any substance that protects against disease and its consequences.

phylaxis (fi-lak′sis) the bodily defense against infection. adj., **phylac′tic.**

phylloquinone (fil′o-kwin′ōn) phytonadione, a vitamin K preparation.

phylogeny (fi-loj′ē-ne) the complete developmental history of a race or group of organisms. adj., **phylogenet′ic, phylogen′ic.**

phylum (fi′lum), pl. *phy′la* [L., Gr.] a primary

division of the plant or animal kingdom, including organisms that are assumed to have a common ancestry.

phyma (fi′mah), pl. *phy′mata* [Gr.] any skin tumor.

phymatiasis   (fi″mah-ti′ah-sis)   tuberculosis.

phymatosis (fi″mah-to′sis) a disease characterized by the presence of skin tumors.

physiatrics (fiz″e-ah′triks) that branch of medicine using physical agents, such as light, heat, water and electricity, and mechanical apparatus, in the diagnosis, prevention and treatment of bodily disorders (see also PHYSICAL THERAPY).

physiatrist   (fiz″e-ah′trist)   a physician who specializes in physiatrics.

physic (fiz′ik) 1. the art of medicine and of therapeutics. 2. a medicine, especially a cathartic.

physical (fiz′ĭ-kal) pertaining to nature or to the body.
  p. examination, examination of the bodily state of a patient by ordinary physical means, as inspection, palpation, percussion and auscultation.
  p. therapist, a person skilled in the techniques of physical therapy and qualified to administer treatments prescribed by a physician.
  There are approximately 40 schools of physical therapy in the United States that are approved by the American Medical Association. They are usually affiliated with medical schools, hospitals or universities having training hospitals. Although requirements vary, in most cases an applicant must have had 2 years of college, with courses in anatomy, biology and the physical sciences, or be a graduate of an accredited school of nursing.
  p. therapy, the treatment of bodily ailments by various physical or nonmedicinal means. This usually includes the use of heat, water, exercise, massage and electric current.
  Physical therapy attempts to relieve pain and to improve or restore muscular function. Its ultimate goal is to train the disabled individual in the safest and most effective means of performing essential activities.
  Exercise is the most widely used means of treatment in physical therapy. Methods may vary widely because exercises are designed to fit the patient's individual needs and abilities. Exercise makes it possible to increase the mobility of a joint, to strengthen a muscle and to train a voluntary muscle to contract and relax in coordination with other muscles. Exercise may be either active or passive.
  In some instances, exercises are carried out under water (hydrotherapy). This is particularly true in cases of poliomyelitis. Special pools are often used to train muscles because the buoyancy of the water requires less effort from weakened muscles and allows a greater range of movement.
  HEAT is a very important agent in many types of physical therapy. It stimulates circulation and relieves pain in the area being treated. Heat may be applied by means of infrared rays, high-frequency electric currents (diathermy), hot moist compresses, immersion in hot water or through the use of melted paraffin. Heat is of particular value in the treatment of arthritis.
  Massage is frequently used as an adjunct of exer-

cise. It helps improve circulation and relieves local pain or muscle spasms. Electrotherapy, or the use of electrical currents of low intensity, is sometimes employed to make muscles contract spontaneously. This is important in training weakened muscles.

physician   (fĭ-zish′un)   an authorized practitioner of medicine.
  attending p., one who attends a hospital at stated times to visit the patients and give directions as to their treatment.
  resident p., a graduate and licensed physician learning a specialty through in-hospital training.

physicochemical (fiz″ĭ-ko-kem′ĭ-kal) pertaining to both physics and chemistry.

physics (fiz′iks) the study of the laws and phenomena of nature, especially of forces and general properties of matter.

physinosis (fiz″ĭ-no′sis) a disease due to physical agents.

physio- (fiz′e-o) word element [Gr.], *nature; physiology.*

physiochemical (fiz″e-o-kem′ĭ-kal) pertaining to both physiology and chemistry.

physiognomy (fiz″e-og′no-me) 1. the determination of mental or moral character and qualities by the face. 2. the face.

physiologic (fiz″e-o-loj′ik) 1. normal; not pathologic. 2. pertaining to physiology.

physiology   (fiz″e-ol′o-je)   the science dealing with the function of various parts and organs of living organisms.
  cell p., scientific study of phenomena involved in cell growth and maintenance, self-regulation and division of cells, interactions between nucleus and cytoplasm, and general behavior of protoplasm.
  comparative p., that concerned with many different types of organisms.
  general p., that concerned with establishment of the general principles of functional mechanisms underlying life processes of all organisms.
  morbid p., pathologic p., the study of disordered functions or of function in diseased tissues.
  special p., that concerned with a specific group of animals, e.g., mammals or insects.

physiometry (fiz″e-om′ĕ-tre) measurement of physiologic functions by physiologic or serologic methods.

physiotherapist (fiz″e-o-ther′ah-pist) physical therapist.

physiotherapy (fiz″e-o-ther′ah-pe) physical therapy.

physique (fĭ-zēk′) the body organization, development and structure.

physis (fi′sis) the segment of tubular bone concerned mainly with growth.

physohematometra (fi″so-hem″ah-to-me′trah) gas and blood in the uterine cavity.

physohydrometra (fi″so-hi″dro-me′trah) gas and serum in the uterine cavity.

physometra (fi″so-me′trah) gas in the uterine cavity.

physopyosalpinx (fi″so-pi″o-sal′pinks) gas and pus in the oviduct.

physostigmine (fi″so-stig′min) an alkaloid usually obtained from dried ripe seed of *Physostigma venenosum.*

p. salicylate, a cholinesterase inhibitor, used topically in the conjunctival sac to produce miosis; it has been used in the treatment of myasthenia gravis.

phyt(o)- (fi′to) word element [Gr.], *plant; an organism of the vegetable kingdom.*

phytalbumin (fi″tal-bu′min) albumin of vegetable origin.

phytobezoar (fi″to-be′zōr) a bezoar composed of vegetable fibers.

phytochemistry (fi″to-kem′is-tre) study of chemical processes occurring in plants, the nature of plant chemicals and various applications of such chemicals to science and industry.

phytogenous (fi-toj′ĕ-nus) derived from plants.

phytoglobulin (fi″to-glob′u-lin) a plant globulin.

phytohemagglutinin (fi″to-hem″ah-gloo′tĭ-nin) a hemagglutinin of plant origin.

phytohormone (fi″to-hōr′mōn) a plant hormone.

phytoid (fi′toid) resembling a plant.

phytomelin (fi″to-mel′in) rutin, a bioflavonoid obtained from buckwheat and other sources; used to reduce capillary fragility.

phytomenadione (fi″to-men″ah-di′ōn) phytonadione, a vitamin K preparation.

phytomitogen (fi″to-mi′to-jen) a substance of plant origin that induces mitosis in human cells.

phytonadione (fi″to-nah-di′ōn) a vitamin K preparation used as a prothrombinogenic agent.

phytoparasite (fi″to-par″ah-sīt) a parasitic vegetable organism.

phytopathology (fi″to-pah-thol′o-je) 1. the pathology of plants. 2. pathology of diseases caused by schizomycetes.

phytophotodermatitis (fi″to-fo″to-der″mah-ti′tis) a morbid condition of the skin due to contact with certain plants and subsequent exposure to light.

phytoplankton (fi″to-plangk′ton) minute plant organisms, mostly algae, found floating free in practically all natural waters.

phytoplasm (fi′to-plazm) protoplasm of plants.

phytosis (fi-to′sis) any disease caused by a phytoparasite.

phytosterol (fi″to-ste′rol) one of a group of compounds that are closely related to cholesterol, found in plants.

phytotoxin (fi″to-tok′sin) an exotoxin produced by certain species of higher plants.

pia (pi′ah) [L.] soft; tender.

p. ma′ter, the innermost of the three membranes covering the brain and spinal cord.

pia-arachnitis (pi″ah-ar″ak-ni′tis) leptomeningitis; inflammation of the leptomeninges, or pia mater and arachnoid.

pia-arachnoid (pi″ah-ah-rak′noid) the pia mater and arachnoid considered together as one organ.

pial (pi′al) pertaining to the pia mater.

piarachnitis (pi″ar-ak-ni′tis) pia-arachnitis.

piarachnoid (pi″ar-ak′noid) pia-arachnoid.

piarrhemia (pi″ah-re′me-ah) lipemia; the presence of fat or oil in the blood.

pica (pi′kah) craving for unnatural articles of food; an abnormal appetite, such as is seen in hysteria and in pregnancy.

pico- (pi′ko) word element [It.], *small;* used to designate an amount 10^{-12} (one-trillionth) the size of the unit to which it is joined, e.g., picocurie.

picocurie (pi″ko-ku′re) a unit of radioactivity, 10^{-12} curie or 10^{-6} microcurie.

picogram (pi′ko-gram) a unit of mass, 10^{-12} gram or 10^{-6} microgram.

picornavirus (pi-kor″nah-vi′rus) one of a group of extremely small, ether-resistant ribonucleic acid viruses, subdivided into the enteroviruses (poliovirus, Coxsackie virus, echovirus) and the rhinoviruses.

picounit (pi″ko-u′nit) one-trillionth part of a unit (10^{-12}).

picrate (pik′rāt) a salt of picric acid.

picric acid (pik′rik) a pale yellow crystalline substance used as an antiseptic, astringent and stimulant of epithelial growth; called also trinitrophenol.

picrotoxin (pik″ro-tok′sin) an active principle from the seed of *Anamirta cocculus,* used as a central nervous system stimulant and as an antidote in barbiturate poisoning.

piedra (pe-a′drah) a hair disease in which nodules form on the shafts; caused by certain species of the fungus Piedraia.

piesesthesia (pi-e″zes-the′ze-ah) the sense by which pressure stimuli are felt.

piesimeter (pi″e-sim′ĕ-ter) instrument for testing the sensitiveness of the skin to pressure.

piezocardiogram (pi-e″zo-kar′de-o-gram″) a graphic tracing of the changes in pressure caused by pulsation of the heart against the esophageal wall, recorded through the esophagus.

pigeon chest prominence of the sternum and rib cartilage; called also PECTUS CARINATUM and pigeon breast.

pigeon toe a foot condition in which the toes turn inward; called also pes varus. Severe cases are considered a form of CLUBFOOT.

pigment (pig′ment) a coloring matter or dye-stuff. adj., **pig′mentary.**

bile p., any one of the coloring matters of the bile; they are bilirubin, biliverdin, bilifuscin, biliprasin, choleprasin, bilihumin and bilicyanin.

blood p., any one of the pigments derived from hemoglobin; they are heme, hematoidin, hemosiderin, hematoporphyrin, methemoglobin and hemofuscin.

respiratory p., a substance in the blood or body fluid of animals that carries oxygen to the various tissues of the body for use in the oxidative processes of the cells, such as the hemoglobin of human blood.

pigmentation (pig″men-ta′shun) the deposition of coloring matter; the coloration or discoloration of a part by a pigment.

hematogenous p., pigmentation derivatives, such as hematoidin or hemosiderin.

malarial p., pigmentation due to accumulation, especially in the spleen and liver, of dark brown pigment liberated from erythrocytes destroyed by malarial parasites.

pigmented (pig′ment-ed) containing pigment.

pigmentolysin (pig″men-tol′ĭ-sin) a lysin that destroys pigment.

pigmentolysis (pig″men-tol′ĭ-sis) destruction of pigment.

piitis (pi-i′tis) inflammation of the pia mater.

pilary (pil′ar-e) pertaining to the hair.

pile (pīl) 1. hemorrhoid. 2. in nucleonics, a chain-reacting fission device for producing slow neutrons and radioisotopes.

sentinel p., an edematous tag of skin, usually in the midline and posteriorly, marking the outer limit of a fissure in the wall of the anus.

pileous (pil′e-us) hairy.

pileus (pil′e-us) 1. one of the cerebellar hemispheres. 2. a membrane that sometimes covers an infant's head at birth.

pill (pil) a small globular or oval medicated mass to be swallowed.

enteric-coated p., one enclosed in a substance that dissolves only when it has reached the intestines.

pillar (pil′ar) a supporting structure.

p's of the fauces, folds of mucous membrane at the sides of the oropharynx.

pilleus (pil′e-us) pileus.

pillion (pil′yon) a temporary artificial leg.

pilocarpine (pi″lo-kar′pin) an alkaloid from leaves of *Pilocarpus jaborandi* and *P. microphyllus;* used as a cholinergic and miotic.

p. hydrochloride, p. nitrate, salts of pilocarpine used to produce constriction of the pupil.

pilocystic (pi″lo-sis′tik) cystic and containing hair.

piloerection (pi″lo-e-rek′shun) erection of the hair.

pilojection (pi″lo-jek′shun) introduction of one or more hairs into an aneurysmal sac, to promote formation of a blood clot.

pilology (pi-lol′o-je) the study of the hair.

pilomotor (pi″lo-mo′tor) causing movements of the hairs.

pilonidal (pi″lo-ni′dal) having a nidus of hairs.

p. cyst, a congenital lesion in the midline of the sacral region, overlying the junction of the sacrum and coccyx. The cyst is believed to result from an infolding of skin in which hair continues to grow. These cysts cause no symptoms unless they become infected, which is quite likely because of their location. Pain and swelling, with the formation of an abscess, are the symptoms of an infected pilonidal cyst. Treatment consists of surgical removal.

pilose (pi′lōs) hairy; covered with hair.

pilosebaceous (pi″lo-se-ba′shus) pertaining to hair and sebaceous glands.

pilous (pi′lus) pilose.

pilus (pi′lus), pl. *pi′li* [L.] hair.

p. annula′tus, (pl. *pi′li annula′ti*), ringed hair.

p. cunicula′tus, (pl. *pi′li cunicula′ti*), burrowing hair.

p. incarna′tus (pl. *pi′li incarna′ti*), ingrown hair.

pi′li multigem′ini, the growth of several hairs from the same follicle.

pimelosis (pim″ĕ-lo′sis) 1. conversion into fat. 2. obesity.

piminodine (pi-min′o-dēn) a compound used as a narcotic analgesic.

pimple (pim′pl) a papule or pustule.

pin (pin) a slender, elongated piece of metal used for securing fixation of parts.

Steinmann p., a pin driven through the distal part of a fractured bone as a means of applying traction, or used to immobilize the fragments of a fractured bone.

pincement (pans-maw′) [Fr.] pinching of the flesh in massage.

pineal (pin′e-al) 1. like a pine cone. 2. pertaining to the pineal gland.

p. gland, a small gland in the central part of the brain, believed by many researchers to be an endocrine gland. In certain amphibians and reptiles the gland is thought to function as a light receptor. Its role in human physiology is largely unknown. It secretes melatonin. Clinically, if calcified, the pineal gland is an important radiologic landmark. Called also pineal body.

pinealectomy (pin″e-ah-lek′to-me) excision of the pineal gland.

pinealoma (pin″e-ah-lo′mah) a tumor of the pineal gland.

pinealopathy (pin″e-ah-lop′ah-the) disease of the pineal gland.

Pinel (pe-nel′) Philippe (1745–1826). French physician, born at Saint-André, Tarn. In his *Traité médico-philosophique sur l'aliénation mentale* he advocated more humane treatment of the insane. As head physician first of the Bicêtre and then of Salpêtrière, he abandoned the use of restraining chains and was able to put into practice a number of other reforms.

pinguecula, pinguicula (ping-gwek′u-lah), (ping-gwik′u-lah), pl. *pinguec′ulae, pinguic′ulae* [L.] a small, yellowish spot on the cornea, seen usually in the elderly.

piniform (pin'ĭ-form) shaped like a pine cone.

pink disease acrodynia.

pinkeye (pink'ī) a contagious inflammation of the conjunctiva caused by bacteria; called also acute contagious conjunctivitis.

pinna (pin'ah) the projecting part of the ear lying outside the head; auricle.

pinocyte (pin'o-sīt) a cell that absorbs and digests tissue fluids.

pinocytosis (pin″o-si-to'sis) the uptake of fluid material by a living cell, particularly by means of invagination of the cell membrane and vacuole formation.

pinosome (pin'o-sōm) a small, fluid-filled vacuole occurring in the cytoplasm of a cell after the breakdown of the canal-like intrusions formed during pinocytosis.

pint (pīnt) a unit of liquid measure in the apothecaries' system, 16 fluid ounces or equivalent to 473.17 milliliters.

pinta (pin'tah) a treponemal infection characterized by bizarre pigmentary changes, occurring in Cuba and hot lowlands of the American continent, and effectively treated by penicillin.
   p. fever, a disease observed in northern Mexico, identical with Rocky Mountain spotted fever.

pinworm (pin'werm) a name applied to various nematode parasites, especially to individuals of the species *Enterobius vermicularis,* but also to those parasitic in other animals than man (see also WORMS).

pionemia (pi″o-ne'me-ah) fat in the blood.

pipamazine (pi-pam'ah-zēn) a phenothiazine compound used as an antiemetic.

Pipanol (pip'ah-nol) trademark for a preparation of trihexyphenidyl, used as an anticholinergic and in treatment of Parkinson's disease.

pipenzolate (pi-pen'zo-lāt) a compound used in parasympathetic blockade.

piperazine (pi-per'ah-zēn) a compound, various salts of which are used as anthelmintics.

piperidolate (pi″per-id'o-lāt) a compound used in parasympathetic blockade.

piperocaine (pi'per-o-kān″) a compound used as a local anesthetic.

pipet (pi-pet') 1. a heavy-walled glass tube of small bore, with a slightly beveled end, used to draw up by suction small quantities of liquid. 2. to draw into and discharge from a pipet.
   diluting p., one incorporating a bulbous expansion in which the liquid under study can be diluted with the appropriate solution.
   measuring p., one with a graduated scale, permitting accurate measurement of a quantity of liquid.

pipethanate (pi-peth'ah-nāt) a compound used as a mild tranquilizer and peripheral anticholinergic.

pipette (pi-pet') pipet.

Pipizan (pi'pĭ-zan) trademark for a preparation of piperazine, an anthelmintic.

pipradrol (pi'prah-drol) a compound used as a central nervous system stimulant.

Piptal (pip'tal) trademark for preparations of pipenzolate methylbromide, an anticholinergic.

piroplasmosis (pi″ro-plaz-mo'sis) babesiosis.

Pirquet's reaction (per-kāz') a local inflammatory reaction of the skin following inoculation with tuberculin, more marked in tuberculous subjects than in normal ones; called also scarification test.

pisiform (pi'sĭ-form) resembling a pea in size and shape.

pit (pit) a depressed area or hollow.
   anal p., proctodeum.
   auditory p., a cuplike depression in an auditory placode, a stage in development of the auditory vesicle.
   ear p., a slight depression in front of the helix, and above the tragus, sometimes leading to a congenital preauricular cyst or fistula.
   nasal p., olfactory p., a depression appearing in the olfactory placodes in the early stages of development of the nose.

pitch (pich) 1. a black viscous substance derived from tar. 2. the quality of sound dependent on the frequency of vibration of the waves producing it.

pithecoid (pith'ĕ-koid) apelike.

pithing (pith'ing) destruction of the brain and spinal cord by thrusting a blunt needle into the vertebral canal and cranium; done on animals to destroy sensibility preparatory to experimenting on their living tissue.

Pitocin (pĭ-to'sin) trademark for a solution of oxytocin for injection; used to stimulate uterine contraction.

Pitressin (pĭ-tres'in) trademark for a solution of vasopressin for injection. It has the pressor actions of posterior pituitary extract.

pitting (pit'ing) the formation of depressions or hollows.

pituita (pĭ-tu'ĭ-tah) glutinous mucus or phlegm.

pituitarigenic (pĭ-tu″ĭ-tar″ĭ-jen'ik) produced by secretions of the pituitary gland.

pituitarism (pĭ-tu'ĭ-tar-izm″) disorder of pituitary function.

pituitary gland (pĭ-tu'ĭ-tār″e) the master gland of the endocrine system, so called because it controls hormone production of other endocrine glands; called also hypophysis cerebri.
   This pea-sized gland lies in a small recess (the sella turcica) at the base of the brain and is connected to the HYPOTHALAMUS by the hypophyseal (pituitary) stalk. The hypothalamus controls many of the secretory functions of the pituitary gland by secreting hormonal substances which in turn stimulate production of pituitary hormones. Information concerned with the well-being of an individual and gathered by the nervous system is transmitted to the hypothalamus which then regu-

lates secretion of pituitary hormones. The activities of the nervous system and the endocrine system are thereby correlated.

The pituitary gland is divided physiologically into two portions, each portion producing a number of different hormones. The adenohypophysis, called also the anterior lobe, produces at least seven hormones, six of which have their primary action on other endocrine glands. The neurohypophysis, called also the posterior lobe, is not as well understood, but is known to secrete two important hormones. All the endocrine glands interact with one another to some extent, but only the pituitary has the special function of stimulating other members of the system to produce their particular hormones.

HORMONES OF THE ADENOHYPOPHYSIS (ANTERIOR LOBE). *Growth Control.* The hormones from the adenohypophysis exert their influence indirectly, except for growth hormone (somatotropin), which acts directly on the tissues of the body. This hormone insures proper growth and development of the skeleton.

Overproduction of growth hormone, which is usually due to a tumor of the pituitary gland, leads to GIGANTISM, a disorder that produces overly tall but well proportioned persons who are usually of normal strength and mental ability. If the overproduction of growth hormone occurs after a person has reached adulthood, he will grow no taller, but certain parts of his bony structure will grow abnormally, especially the cheek bones, jaw bone, hands and feet. This condition is called ACROMEGALY. Treatment for it, and for gigantism, is by IRRADIATION or surgical removal (hypophysectomy) of the pituitary gland.

At the other end of the scale is DWARFISM. Although dwarfism may be the result of other disorders, underproduction of growth hormone of the pituitary gland is one of the more common causes.

Weight Control. Failure of the pituitary to produce sufficient hormones can lead to a rare condition of malnourishment and premature senility known as SIMMONDS' DISEASE. A slightly different kind of pituitary deficiency can cause a rare condition called Fröhlich's syndrome in children; the symptoms are obesity, mental laziness and underdevelopment of the reproductive organs. If the condition occurs after puberty, fat may accumulate around certain portions of the body, particularly the hips.

Treatment of pituitary underproduction is by the administration of pituitary extract.

Control of Other Glands. In addition to growth hormone, six other hormones have been isolated from the adenohypophysis.

Thyrotropin (called also thyroid-stimulating hormone, or TSH) controls secretion of the hormone thyroxine from the thyroid gland. ACTH (adrenocorticotropic hormone) controls secretion of cortisol (hydrocortisone) from the cortex of the ADRENAL GLAND. By way of a feedback device, the secretion of cortisol from the adrenal cortices regulates the release of ACTH from the adenohypophysis. Thus a high level of cortisol in the blood inhibits the secretion of ACTH.

Follicle-stimulating hormone (FSH) affects the reproductive organs of both the female and the male. It stimulates the growth of the ovarian follicle and secretion of estrogen in the female and maintains the formation of spermatozoa in the male. FSH is called a gonadotropic hormone because it controls the GONADS. Another gonadotropic hormone is luteinizing hormone (LH). In the female, LH acts with FSH to bring about maturation of the ovarian follicle; it also initiates rupture of the mature follicle so that the ovum is released, acts upon the cells of the capsule surrounding the follicle to cause formation of the corpus luteum and stimulates these cells to produce progesterone. In the male, LH is called interstitial cell-stimulating hormone (ICSH) and it stimulates the development

HYPOPHYSEAL HORMONES

NAME AND SOURCE	SYNONYMS	FUNCTION
Adenohypophysis (anterior lobe)		
TSH	Thyroid-stimulating hormone; thyrotropin	Stimulates thyroid growth and secretion.
ACTH	Adrenocorticotropic hormone; corticotropin	Stimulates adrenocortical growth and secretion
STH	Growth hormone; somatotropin	Accelerates body growth
FSH	Follicle-stimulating hormone	Stimulates growth of ovarian follicle and estrogen secretion in the female and spermatogenesis in the male
LH	Luteinizing hormone (in the female); interstitial cell-stimulating hormone, ICSH (in the male)	Stimulates ovulation and luteinization of ovarian follicles in the female and production of testosterone in the male
LTH	Luteotropic hormone, luteotropin, prolactin, mammotropin, lactogenic hormone	Maintains the corpus luteum and stimulates secretion of milk
MSH	Melanocyte-stimulating hormone	Stimulates melanocytes causing pigmentation
Neurohypophysis (posterior lobe)		
Antidiuretic Hormone (ADH)	Vasopressin	Promotes water retention by way of the renal tubules and stimulates smooth muscle of blood vessels and digestive tract
Oxytocin		Stimulates contraction of smooth muscle in the uterus

From Jacob, S. W., and Francone, C. A.: Structure and Function in Man. 2nd ed. Philadelphia, W. B. Saunders Co., 1970.

and functioning of the Leydig or interstitial cells of the testes and thereby controls testicular production of testosterone.

Lactogenic or luteotropic hormone (LTH) is also known by such names as luteotropin, prolactin and mammotropin. It has two known functions in the female. It stimulates the corpus luteum to produce progesterone and stimulates the production of milk in the mammary glands. (The ejection of milk from the mammary glands is controlled by oxytocin, a secretion of the neurohypophysis.)

Melanocyte-stimulating hormone (MSH) is believed to influence the formation or deposition of melanin in the body.

HORMONES OF THE NEUROHYPOPHYSIS (POSTERIOR LOBE). The neurohypophysis produces two hormones. Vasopressin, or antidiuretic hormone (ADH), decreases the rate of urine formation by stimulating reabsorption of water by the renal tubules, and therefore is important in the maintenance of fluid balance; it also increases blood pressure (pressor effect), stimulates contraction of the intestinal musculature and increases peristalsis, and exerts some influence on the uterus. Underproduction of this hormone results in excessive urination and a rare disorder called diabetes insipidus (not to be confused with diabetes mellitus).

The other hormone produced by the neurohypophysis is oxytocin. It is necessary for contraction of the uterus during labor and delivery; the exact mechanism responsible for its release at the time it is needed is not known. Oxytocin also is secreted during suckling and causes ejection of milk from the mammary glands.

Both vosapressin and oxytocin are available for therapeutic use. Vasopressin is used as a test substance in diagnosing and treating diabetes insipidus. Oxytocin is given to induce labor, and also to cause contraction of the uterus after delivery of the placenta. A powdered preparation of posterior pituitary is occasionally used as a nasal snuff to treat diabetes insipidus, and posterior pituitary injection is available for subcutaneous injection.

Pituitrin (pǐ-tu'ǐ-trin) trademark for a preparation of posterior pituitary injection.

pityriasis (pit″ǐ-ri'ah-sis) a skin condition with formation of branny scales.

p. al'ba, a chronic condition with patchy scaling and hypopigmentation of the skin of the face.

p. ro'sea, a self-limited papulosquamous eruption of the back primarily. The lesions are pinkish oval patches and may be accompanied by mild to moderate pruritus.

p. ru'bra, a rare condition marked by scarlatiniform patches beginning on the forearms and spreading to the entire body, with scaling of the skin and shedding of hair.

p. ru'bra pila'ris, a rare chronic dermatitis with the formation of scaly patches.

p. versic'olor, tinea versicolor.

pityroid (pit'ǐ-roid) like bran; branny.

Pityrosporon (pit″ǐ-ros'po-ron) a genus of fungi, some species of which may be pathogenic for man.

PKU phenylketonuria.

placebo (plah-se'bo) an inactive substance resembling a medication that may be given experimentally or for its psychologic effects.

placenta (plah-sen'tah) a spongy structure that grows on the wall of the uterus during pregnancy, and through which the unborn child is nourished; called also afterbirth. adj., **placen'tal.**

In anatomic nomenclature the placenta consists of a uterine and a fetal portion. The chorion, the superficial or fetal portion, is surfaced by a smooth, shining membrane continuous with the sheath of the umbilical cord (amnion). The deep, or uterine, portion is divided by deep sulci into lobes of irregular outline and extent (the cotyledons). Over the maternal surface of the placenta is stretched a delicate, transparent membrane of fetal origin. Around the periphery of the placenta is a large vein (the marginal sinus), which returns a part of the maternal blood from the organ.

The major function of the placenta is to allow diffusion of nutrients from the mother's blood into the fetus's blood and diffusion of waste products from the fetus back to the mother. This two-way exchange takes place across the placental membrane, which is semipermeable; that is, it acts as a selective filter, allowing some materials to pass through and holding back others.

In the early months of pregnancy the placenta acts as a nutrient storehouse and helps to process some of the food substances that nourish the fetus. Later, as the fetus grows and develops, these metabolic functions of the placenta are gradually taken on by the fetal liver.

The placenta secretes both estrogens and progesterone. After birth of the infant the placenta is cast off from the uterus and expelled via the birth canal.

abruptio placentae (ah-brup'she-o plah-cen'te), premature separation of a normally situated placenta. Mild abruptio placentae usually occurs during labor when the cervix uteri is partially dilated. Symptoms include change in the character of the patient's labor, external bleeding and fetal distress.

Serious abruptio placentae occurs must often before the onset of labor. Symptoms include sudden, severe pain in the region of the uterus, some external bleeding and indications of fetal distress. Treatment is symptomatic unless there is an indication of severe hemorrhage or fetal death, in which case a cesarean section is indicated.

p. accre'ta, one abnormally adherent to the uterine wall, with partial or complete absence of the decidua basalis.

battledore p., one with the umbilical cord inserted at the edge.

p. circumvalla'ta, one encircled with a raised white nodular ring, the attached membranes being doubled back over the edge of the placenta.

p. fenestra'ta, one that has spots where placental tissue is lacking.

p. incre'ta, one abnormally adherent and penetrating the uterine wall.

p. membrana'cea, one spread over an unusually large area of the uterine wall.

p. nappifor'mis, placenta circumvallata.

p. percre'ta, one abnormally adherent with invasion of the uterine wall to the serosal layer.

p. prae'via, one located in the lower uterine segment, near the cervix uteri, instead of in the proper position higher on the uterine wall. Any expansion of the cervix may cause tearing of placental tissue and bleeding. This condition is life threatening to both mother and fetus, and may require delivery by cesarean section.

p. reflex'a, one in which the margin is thickened, appearing to turn back on itself.

p. spu'ria, an accessory portion without blood vessels connecting it with the placenta.

p. succenturia'ta, an accessory portion with blood vessels connecting it with the placenta.

placentation (plas″en-ta'shun) the manner of formation and attachment of the placenta.

placentitis (plas″en-ti'tis) inflammation of the placenta.

placentography (plas″en-tog'rah-fe) radiography of the pregnant uterus to determine the position of the placenta.

placentoid (plah-sen'toid) resembling the placenta.

placentology (plas″en-tol'o-je) scientific study of the development, structure and functioning of the placenta.

placentolysin (plas″en-tol'ĭ-sin) an antibody capable of destroying placental cells.

placentoma (plas″en-to'mah) a neoplasm derived from retained placenta.

Placidyl (plas'ĭ-dil) trademark for a preparation of ethchlorvynol, a hypnotic and sedative.

placode (plak'ōd) a platelike structure, especially a thickening of the ectoderm marking the site of future development in the early embryo of an organ of special sense, e.g., the *auditory placode* (ear), *lens placode* (eye) and *olfactory placode* (nose).

pladarosis (plad″ah-ro'sis) a soft tumor on the eyelid.

plagiocephaly (pla″je-o-sef'ah-le) bizarre distortion of the shape of the skull resulting from irregular closure of the cranial sutures.

plague (plāg) an acute febrile, infectious, highly fatal disease caused by the bacillus *Pasteurella pestis*. It is primarily a disease of rats, and is usually spread to human beings by fleas. The more common form of plague is the bubonic. There is also a pneumonic type, which can be spread directly from man to man by droplet infection.

Plague is a devastating disease. Three outbreaks of plague in history have wiped out whole populations. The first of these spread over Europe in the sixth century A.D. in a tremendous cycle of pestilence that lasted for more than 50 years. The second, called the Black Death, was perhaps the most deadly outbreak the world has known. It swept over Europe in the 14th century, and more than one-quarter of the European population—25 million people—perished. The Great Plague of London in 1665 was a relatively minor outbreak. A third great epidemic raged in the Orient at the turn of the 20th century. The greatest toll was in India, where there were more than 12 million deaths from 1896 to 1933.

Some cases have spread to the United States. Extensive epidemics have been prevented in this country by strict quarantines and by sanitation measures that have been enforced since the disease was traced to rat and wild rodent fleas.

BUBONIC PLAGUE. Bubonic plague is characterized by acutely inflamed and painful swellings of the lymph nodes, or buboes, usually in the groin.

The disease strikes suddenly with chills and fever. Children may have convulsions. There is vomiting and thirst, generalized pain, headache and mental dullness. Delirium may also be present.

After the third day, black spots, which give the disease the name "black death," may appear. Tender, enlarged lymph nodes are usually seen between the second and fifth days. Some cases of bubonic plague are mild. The more virulent cases last 5 or 6 days, and are usually fatal. If the patient survives past the tenth or twelfth day, there is a good chance of recovery.

The mortality rate for untreated cases runs between 25 and 50 per cent, but has reached as high as 90 per cent. Until recently, little could be done for the disease. Today, however, streptomycin, when used early enough, has cut the mortality rate to 5 per cent. Sulfadiazine is less effective.

PNEUMONIC PLAGUE. Pneumonic plague usually occurs during outbreaks of bubonic plague and may be a direct complication of it. There is extensive involvement of the lungs and the sputum contains many organisms. Until recently, pneumonic plague was always fatal. Now, with streptomycin, the chances of recovery are good if treatment is begun within 24 hours.

PREVENTION. The most important measure in controlling plague is the extermination of rats. This is especially necessary around shipping areas, in warehouses and on docks. Rat control for ships arriving from plague areas is vital.

Where there is an outbreak of plague, strict quarantine measures are called for, as well as the use of insecticides to protect inhabitants of the stricken area against fleas. Immunization with plague vaccine is desirable. Persons who have been in contact with active cases of plague are given preventive medicines.

murine p., infection in domestic rodents due to *Pasteurella pestis*.

septicemic p., that occurring with *Pasteurella pestis* in the bloodstream, with death before the appearance of buboes or of pulmonary manifestations.

sylvatic p., plague in wild rodents, such as the ground squirrel, which serve as a reservoir from which man may be infected.

plane (plān) 1. a flat surface. 2. a specified level, as the plane of anesthesia.

coronal p., frontal plane.

datum p., a given horizontal plane from which craniometric measurements are made.

frontal p., any plane passing longitudinally through the body from side to side, at right angles to the median plane and dividing the body into front and back parts.

horizontal p., one passing through the body at right angles to the median and frontal planes, and dividing the body into upper and lower parts.

median p., one passing longitudinally through the body from front to back and dividing it into right and left halves.

sagittal p., a vertical plane through the body parallel to the median plane and dividing the body into left and right portions.

transverse p., one passing horizontally through the body, at right angles to the sagittal and frontal planes, and dividing the body into upper and lower portions.

planigraphy (plah-nig′rah-fe) a method of body-section roentgenography that shows in detail structures lying in a predetermined plane of the body while blurring structures in other planes, produced by movement of the film and x-ray tube in certain specified directions. adj., **planigraph′ic.**

plankton (plangk′ton) the minute, free-floating organisms living in practically all natural waters.

planned parenthood birth control.

planoconcave (pla″no-kon′kāv) flat on one side and concave on the other.

planoconvex (pla″no-kon′veks) flat on one side and convex on the other.

planocyte (plan′o-sīt) a wandering cell.

planography (plah-nog′rah-fe) planigraphy.

planta (plan′tah) the sole of the foot.

plantalgia (plan-tal′je-ah) pain in the sole of the foot.

plantar (plan′tar) pertaining to the sole of the foot.
   p. wart, a common WART located on the sole of the foot. Plantar warts are caused by a virus which may be picked up by going barefoot. Unlike other warts, this type is usually sensitive to pressure; it may feel tender when touched and may be painful during walking.

plantaris (plan-ta′ris) [L.] plantar.

plantation (plan-ta′shun) insertion or application of material into or on the human body, including implantation, replantation and transplantation.

plantigrade (plan′tī-grād) walking or running flat on the lower surface of the foot; characteristic of man and of such quadrupeds as the bear.

planula (plan′u-lah) the embryo in the stage when it consists of two primary layers.

planum (pla′num), pl. *pla′na* [L.] plane.

plaque (plak) a patch or flat area.
   atheromatous p., a deposit of predominantly fatty material in the lining of blood vessels occurring in atherosclerosis.
   bacterial p., a collection of bacteria growing in a deposit of material on the surface of a tooth.
   blood p., a blood platelet.
   dental p., a deposit of material on the surface of a tooth.

Plaquenil (pla′kwĕ-nil) trademark for a preparation of hydroxychloroquine, an antimalarial.

plasm (plazm) 1. plasma. 2. formative substance (cytoplasm, hyaloplasm, etc.)
   germ p., the reproductive and hereditary substance that is passed on from the germ cell in which an individual originates in direct continuity to the germ cells of succeeding generations.

plasma (plaz′mah) 1. the fluid portion of the blood in which corpuscles are suspended. Plasma is to be distinguished from serum, which is plasma from which the fibrinogen has been separated in the process of clotting. 2. cytoplasm or protoplasm. adj., **plasmat′ic.**

   Of the total volume of blood, 55 per cent is made up of plasma. It is a clear, straw-colored liquid, 2 per cent water, in which are contained plasma proteins, inorganic salts, foods, gases, waste materials from the cells and various hormones, secretions and enzymes. These substances are transported to or from the tissues of the body by the plasma.

   Plasma obtained from blood donors is given to those suffering from loss of blood or from shock to help maintain adequate blood pressure. Since plasma can be dried and stored in bottles, it can be transported almost anywhere, ready for immediate use after addition of the appropriate fluid. Plasma can be given to anyone, regardless of blood type. (See also BLOOD, SERUM and TRANSFUSION.)
   antihemophilic human p., normal human plasma that has been processed promptly to preserve the antihemophilic properties, being frozen within 6 hours and dispensed in frozen or dried state.
   normal human p., sterile plasma obtained by pooling approximately equal amounts of the liquid portion of citrated whole blood from eight or more adult humans, used as a blood volume replenisher.
   p. volume expander, a solution transfused instead of blood to increase the volume of fluid circulating in the blood vessels.

plasmacytoma (plaz″mah-si-to′mah) a primary tumor of bone marrow, composed of mature, well differentiated or more anaplastic plasmocytes; a type of myeloma.

plasmagene (plaz′mah-jēn) a self-reproducing copy of a nuclear gene persisting in the cytoplasm of a cell.

plasmapheresis (plaz″mah-fĕ-re′sis) removal of blood, separation of the plasma by centrifugation and reinjection of the cells into the body; used as a means of obtaining plasma and in the treatment of certain pathologic conditions.

plasmasome (plaz′mah-sōm) a leukocyte granule.

plasmic (plaz′mik) plasmatic; pertaining to or of the nature of plasma.

plasmin (plaz′min) the active principle of the fibrinolytic or clot-lysing system, a proteolytic enzyme with a high specificity for fibrin and the particular ability to dissolve formed fibrin clots.

plasminogen (plaz-min′o-jen) the inactive precursor of plasmin, occurring in the beta globulin fraction of the plasma; profibrinolysin.

Plasmochin naphthoate (plaz′mo-kin naf′tho-āt) trademark for a preparation of pamaquine naphthoate, an antimalarial.

plasmocyte (plaz′mo-sīt) a mononuclear cell of bone marrow, responsible, in part, for the manufacture of antibodies.

Plasmodium (plaz-mo′de-um) a multispecies genus of sporozoa parasitic in the erythrocytes of various animals; four species, *P. falcip′arum, P. mala′riae, P. ova′le* and *P. vi′vax,* cause the four specific types of malaria in man.

plasmogen (plaz′mo-jen) bioplasm; the essential part of protoplasm.

plasmology (plaz-mol′o-je) the science of the most minute particles of living matter.

plasmolysis (plaz-mol′ĭ-sis) contraction of cell protoplasm due to loss of water by osmosis.

plasmorrhexis (plaz″mo-rek′sis) a morphologic change in erythrocytes, consisting in the escape from the cells of round, shining granules and splitting off of particles; called also erythrocytorrhexis.

plasmoschisis (plaz-mos′kĭ-sis) the splitting up of cell protoplasm.

plasmosome (plaz′mo-sōm) the true nucleolus of a cell.

plasmotropism (plaz-mot′ro-pizm) solution or destruction of erythrocytes in the liver, spleen or marrow, as contrasted with their destruction in the circulation.

plasmozyme (plaz′mo-zīm) prothrombin.

plaster (plas′ter) 1. a mixture of materials that hardens; used for immobilizing or making impressions of body parts. 2. an adhesive substance spread on fabric or other suitable backing material, for application to the skin, often containing some medication, such as an anodyne or rubefacient.

  adhesive p., fabric spread with pressure-sensitive adhesive mixture, for application to the skin.

  p. of paris, calcium sulfate dihydrate, reduced to a fine powder; the addition of water produces a porous mass used in making casts and bandages to support or immobilize body parts, and in dentistry for taking dental impressions.

  salicylic acid p., a mixture of 10 to 40 per cent salicylic acid in a suitable base; used as a keratolytic.

plastic (plas′tik) 1. tending to build up tissues. 2. capable of being molded. 3. a substance produced by chemical condensation or by polymerization.

  p. surgery, surgery performed to improve the appearance or function of exposed parts of the body that are defective, deformed or damaged. This kind of surgery has been practiced for thousands of years. Artificial noses and ears have been found on Egyptian mummies. Medical records show that the ancient Hindus reconstructed noses by using skin flaps lifted from the cheek or forehead—a technique that was often practiced, since it was a custom to mutilate the noses of persons who broke the laws.

  SKIN GRAFTING. The most common procedure of plastic surgery is skin GRAFTING. This is the replacement of severely damaged skin in one area with healthy skin obtained from another area of the patient's body or from the body of a skin donor. Some grafting is done to prevent the formation of disfiguring scars, such as those that may form on the face from bad burns. If burns or other injuries are extensive, grafting can prevent extensive scarring with tissue that is unsightly and cannot perform all the necessary functions of normal skin. Skin contractures can thus be avoided.

  A skin graft can sometimes be made by the simple procedure of cutting a piece of healthy skin from one part of the body, such as the back or the thigh, and stitching it to the injured area. Small arteries from the tissues surrounding the injured area then grow into the graft, nourish it with blood and promote normal growth. If the area to be covered is large, a number of separate patches may be stitched to it, forming islands of skin that will enlarge with healing until the entire area is covered. This is called "postage stamp" or pinch grafting.

  In some cases, in order to ensure a good blood supply to the patch, or for other reasons, the surgeon may employ a modern version of the technique used by the ancient Hindus—the pedicle graft. He cuts a flap of skin only partly free from the healthy area in the patient's body, then attaches the loose end to the damaged area. Still fed by its natural blood supply, the flap remains healthy while its cut edge grows into and begins to cover the area of damaged skin. Meanwhile, the area from which the flap was cut and folded away is healing and growing new skin. Soon the surgeon can cut the flap free, and both the graft and the area from which the flap was taken can heal completely.

  When the damaged area and the flap are awkwardly located, this technique can involve inconvenience to the patient. His arm, for example, may have to be strapped against his head to provide a skin flap for his face. This sometimes can be avoided by a delayed graft, a plate of skin moved from the healthy area to the damaged one by stages, without at any stage being entirely cut loose from the blood supply.

  REPAIRING MOUTH AND OTHER DEFECTS. Among common defects that can be corrected by plastic surgery are CLEFT LIP AND CLEFT PALATE. Others are webbed fingers and toes, protruding or missing ears, receding chins and injured noses. In addition, the shape of various types of noses can be altered for the sake of appearance.

  FACIAL RECONSTRUCTION. In facial reconstruction, missing bone and muscle, and sometimes skin, are replaced by substitutes. Sometimes the reconstruction is made with bone or cartilage taken from another part of the body, or sometimes it is made by artificial means.

  Use of Prostheses. Often the substitute for missing tissue is a *prosthesis*, a replacement not made from living tissue. A prosthesis may be inserted beneath the skin (to build out a receding chin, for instance) or attached to the skin surface (for example, to replace an ear).

  Prostheses attached to, not inserted beneath, the skin frequently are employed to fill out depressed or missing facial areas, the after effects of accidents, cancer or war injuries. In building such a replacement, the surgeon first makes an impression of the face and a plaster cast of the impression. The substitute part is molded in wax or clay in the plaster cast, and from this model the actual replacement part is made. Such parts, molded and painted to match the texture and color of the skin, have been used to replace many structures, including missing ears and noses.

  Use of Cartilage, Skin and Bone. Noses and ears also have been reconstructed with rib cartilage and skin grafts. Eyebrows have been made by the use of skin grafts from the scalp, and chest deformities repaired by the use of bone chips from other parts of the body.

  Sometimes a nose is remodeled to correct a hump or hook, or a saddle nose (a depression on the ridge), or a twisted nose. Incisions are made inside to avoid causing outside scars, and the surgeon either removes excess cartilage or bone, or inserts it, according to the improvement wanted. Cartilage and bone may be obtained from other parts of the body, usually the ribs or hip. After the operation, the skin over the nose adapts to the new structure.

Dermabrasion. Skin blemishes such as acne scars and pits can be "sandpapered" or planed. This technique, called dermabrasion, seeks to correct superficial blemishes and to remove superficial accumulations of pigment. However, as dermabrasion can occasionally cause increased scarring or introduce variation in skin color and texture, such treatment is infrequently performed today.

FACE LIFTING. To the layman, the term "plastic surgery" often conveys an operation performed to make an aging face look younger. The technical term for this is rhytidoplasty, or plastic surgery for the removal of wrinkles. If such an operation is performed by a reputable surgeon it can be moderately successful, but only temporarily. Reoperation is often necessary. The operation is usually done by opening skin flaps in the region around the ears and undermining the skin of the cheeks and jaws. The eyelids and the area of the eyebrows may be operated on in association with the primary operation.

plasticity (plas-tis'ĭ-te) the quality of being plastic, or capable of being molded.

plastid (plas'tid) any cell or constructive unit.

-plasty (plas'te) word element [Gr.], *formation or plastic repair of.*

plate (plāt) a flat structure or layer, chiefly of bone.

approximation p., a disk of bone, or the like, used in intestinal surgery.

axial p., the primitive streak of the embryo.

deck p., roof plate.

dental p., a plate of acrylic resin, metal or other material that is fitted to the shape of the mouth, and serves for the support of artificial teeth.

dorsal p., roof plate.

epiphyseal p., the thin plate of cartilage between the epiphysis and the shaft of a bone; it is the site of growth in length and is obliterated by epiphyseal closure.

floor p., the unpaired ventral longitudinal zone of the neural tube.

foot p., the flat portion of the stapes.

growth p., the area between the epiphysis and diaphysis of long bones within which growth in length occurs.

medullary p., neural plate.

muscle p., myotome (2).

neural p., a thickened band of ectoderm in the midbody region of the developing embryo, which develops into the nervous system.

roof p., the unpaired dorsal longitudinal zone of the neural tube.

sole p., a mass of protoplasm in which a motor nerve ending is embedded.

tarsal p., the substance that gives firmness to the eyelid.

ventral p., floor plate.

platelet (plāt'let) a small disk or platelike structure, especially the smallest of the formed elements in blood. Blood platelets (called also thrombocytes) are disk-shaped, non-nucleated blood elements with a very fragile membrane; they tend to adhere to uneven or damaged surfaces. They average about 250,000 per cubic millimeter of blood and are principally concerned with coagulation of blood and the contraction of a blood clot. They are formed in red bone marrow and the rate of their formation

seems to be governed by the amount of oxygen in the blood and the presence of nucleic acid derivatives from injured tissue.

direct p. count, estimation of the number of platelets per cubic millimeter of blood directly from whole blood.

p. factors, factors important in hemostasis which are contained in or attached to the platelets.

indirect p. count, the count of the total number of platelets per cubic millimeter of blood by counting the platelets on a stained blood film.

platinectomy (plat"ĭ-nek'to-me) excision of the footplate in surgical mobilization of the stapes, in treatment of hearing loss.

platinum (plat'ĭ-num) a chemical element, atomic number 78, atomic weight 195.09, symbol Pt. (See table of ELEMENTS.)

platy- (plat'e) word element [Gr.], *broad; flat.*

platybasia (plat"ĭ-ba'ze-ah) malformation of the base of the skull, with upward displacement of the upper cervical vertebrae and bony impingement on the brain stem. It is accompanied by neurologic signs referable to the medulla oblongata, cervical spinal cord and cranial nerves.

platycelous (plat"ĭ-se'lus) having one surface flat and the other concave, referring to vertebrae.

platycephalous (plat"ĭ-sef'ah-lus) having a wide, flat head.

platycoria (plat"ĭ-ko're-ah) a dilated condition of the pupil of the eye.

platycrania (plat"ĭ-kra'ne-ah) artificial flattening of the skull.

Platyhelminthes (plat"ĭ-hel-min'thēz) a phylum of dorsoventrally flattened, bilaterally symmetrical animals, commonly known as flatworms.

platyhieric (plat"ĭ-hi-er'ik) having a wide sacrum.

platypellic, platypelloid (plat"ĭ-pel'ik), (plat"ĭ-pel'oid) having a broad pelvis.

platypodia (plat"ĭ-po'de-ah) flatness of the sole of the foot.

platyrrhine (plat'ĭ-rīn) having a broad nose.

platysma (plah-tiz'mah) a subcutaneous neck muscle extending from the neck to the clavicle; it acts to wrinkle the skin of the neck and to depress the jaw.

Plaut-Vincent disease (plowt vin'sent) trench mouth (Vincent's angina).

pledget (plej'et) a small compress or tuft.

pleiotropy (pli-ot'ro-pe) 1. the quality of having affinity for tissues derived from the different germ layers. 2. ability of a gene to manifest itself in many ways. adj., pleiotrop'ic.

pleochromatic (ple"o-kro-mat'ik) showing various colors under varying circumstances.

pleochromocytoma (ple"o-kro"mo-si-to'mah) a tumor composed of tissues of varying colors.

pleocytosis (ple"o-si-to'sis) the presence of a

greater than normal number of cells, as of more than the normal number of lymphocytes in cerebrospinal fluid.

pleomastia (ple″o-mas′te-ah) the presence of supernumerary mammary glands or nipples.

pleomorphic (ple″o-mor′fik) occurring in various distinct forms.

pleomorphism (ple″o-mor′fizm) the quality of being pleomorphic.

pleonasm (ple′o-nazm) an excess of parts.

pleonemia (ple″o-ne′me-ah) increased volume of blood in a part. adj., **pleone′mic.**

pleonexia (ple″o-nek′se-ah) 1. morbid greediness. 2. a condition in which circulating hemoglobin holds more firmly than normal to its oxygen and consequently gives off to the tissues less oxygen than normal.

pleoptics (ple-op′tiks) a technique of eye exercises designed to develop fuller vision of an amblyopic eye and assure proper binocular cooperation.

plessesthesia (ples″es-the′ze-ah) palpatory percussion.

plessimeter (plĕ-sim′ĕ-ter) pleximeter.

plessor (ples′or) plexor.

plethora (pleth′o-rah) a condition marked by vascular turgescence, excess of blood and fullness of pulse. It is attended by a feeling of tension in the head, a florid complexion and a liability to nosebleed. adj., **plethor′ic.**

plethysmograph (plĕ-thiz′mo-graf) an instrument for determining and registering variations in the size of an organ, part or limb and in the amount of blood present or passing through it for recording variations in the size of parts and in the blood supply.

plethysmography (pleth″iz-mog′rah-fe) the recording of the changes in the size of a part as modified by the circulation of blood in it.

pleur(o)- (ploo′ro) word element [Gr.], *pleura; rib; side.*

pleura (ploo′rah), pl. *pleu′rae* [Gr.] the serous membrane investing the lungs (pulmonary pleura) and lining the walls of the thoracic cavity (parietal pleura), the two layers enclosing a potential space, the pleural cavity. adj., **pleu′ral.**

pleuracotomy (ploo″rah-kot′o-me) incision into the pleural cavity.

pleuralgia (ploo-ral′je-ah) pain in the pleura or in the side.

pleurapophysis (ploo″rah-pof′ĭ-sis) a rib or its homologue.

pleurectomy (ploo-rek′to-me) excision of a portion of the pleura.

pleurisy, pleuritis (ploo′rĭ-se), (ploo-ri′tis) inflammation of the pleura; it may be caused by infection, injury or tumor. It may be a complication of lung diseases, particularly of pneumonia, or sometimes of tuberculosis, lung abscess or influenza. The symptoms are cough, fever, chills, sharp, sticking pain that is worse on inspiration, and rapid shallow breathing. adj., **pleurit′ic.**

TYPES OF PLEURISY. The membranous pleura that encases each lung is composed of two close-fitting layers; between them is a lubricating fluid. If the fluid content remains unchanged by the disease, the pleurisy is said to be dry. If the fluid increases abnormally, it is a wet pleurisy, or pleurisy with effusion.

In dry pleurisy the two layers of membrane may become congested and swollen and rub against each other with a grating effect as the lungs inflate and deflate with breathing. This can be painful. Although only the outer layer causes pain (the inner layer has no pain nerves), the pain may be severe enough to necessitate the use of a strong analgesic.

Wet pleurisy is less likely to cause pain, because there usually is no chafing. But the fluid may interfere with breathing by compressing the lung. In some cases the lung is permanently displaced, failing to return to full capacity because of thickening of the pleura.

If the excess fluid of wet pleurisy becomes infected, with formation of pus, the condition is known as purulent pleurisy or EMPYEMA.

Inflammation of the part of the pleura that covers the diaphragm is called diaphragmatic pleurisy.

TREATMENT. The most effective measures against pleurisy are antibiotics, heat applications and bed rest. When there is intense pain on breathing, the physician may strap the chest to limit its movement.

pleurocele (ploo′ro-sēl) hernia of lung tissue or of pleura.

pleurocentesis (ploo″ro-sen-te′sis) surgical puncture and drainage of the pleural cavity.

pleurocentrum (ploo″ro-sen′trum) the lateral element of the vertebral column.

pleurocholecystitis (ploo″ro-ko″le-sis-ti′tis) inflammation of the pleura and gallbladder.

pleuroclysis (ploo-rok′lĭ-sis) injection of fluids into the pleural cavity.

pleurodesis (ploo-rod′ĕ-sis) production of adhesions between the parietal and the visceral pleura.

pleurodynia (ploo″ro-din′e-ah) pain of the intercostal muscles or of the pleural nerves.
  epidemic p., epidemic diaphragmatic p., an epidemic viral disease marked by a sudden attack of pain in the chest, fever and a tendency to recrudescence on the third day; called also devil's grip and Bornholm disease.

pleurogenic (ploo″ro-jen′ik) originating in the pleura.

pleurography (ploo-rog′rah-fe) roentgenographic examination of the pleural cavity.

pleurohepatitis (ploo″ro-hep″ah-ti′tis) hepatitis with inflammation of the pleura near the liver.

pleurolith (ploo′ro-lith) a concretion in the pleura.

pleurolysis (ploo-rol′ĭ-sis) surgical separation of the pleura from its attachments.

pleuroparietopexy (ploo″ro-pah-ri′ĕ-to-pek″se)

the operation of fixing the visceral pleura to the parietal pleura, thus binding the lung to the chest wall.

pleuropericarditis   (ploo″ro-per″ĭ-kar-di′tis) inflammation involving the pleura and the pericardium.

pleuropexy (ploo″ro-pek′se) surgical induction of fusion between the visceral and parietal pleura.

pleuropneumonia   (ploo″ro-nu-mo′ne-ah) pneumonia accompanied by pleurisy.

pleuropneumonia-like organisms (ploo″ro-nu-mo′nyah-lĭk) PPLO, a group of filterable microorganisms without cell walls; in man they generally produce a clinically mild pneumonitis or bronchitis. They are transmissible from man to man. Treatment is with tetracycline. Called also Mycoplasma.

pleuropneumonolysis   (ploo″ro-nu″mo-nol′ĭ-sis) collapse of a tuberculous lung by removal of ribs from one side.

pleurorrhea   (ploo″ro-re′ah) a pleural effusion.

pleuroscopy   (ploo-ros′ko-pe) direct examination of the pleural cavity by incision of the chest wall.

pleurothotonos (ploo″ro-thot′o-nus) tetanic bending of the body to one side.

pleurotomy   (ploo-rot′o-me) incision of the pleura.

pleurovisceral   (ploo″ro-vis′er-al) pertaining to the pleura and viscera.

plexiform   (plek′sĭ-form) resembling a plexus or network.

pleximeter   (plek-sim′ĕ-ter) 1. a plate to be struck in mediate percussion. 2. a glass plate used to show the condition of the skin under pressure.

plexitis   (plek-si′tis) inflammation of a nerve plexus.

plexor   (plek′sor) a hammer used in diagnostic percussion.

plexus   (plek′sus), pl. *plex′us* [L.] *plex′uses* a network or tangle, chiefly of veins or nerves.

brachial p., a nerve plexus originating from the ventral branches of the last four cervical and the first thoracic spinal nerves. It gives off many of the principal nerves of the shoulder, chest and arms.

cardiac p., the plexus around the base of the heart, beneath and behind the arch of the aorta, formed by cardiac branches from the vagus nerves and the sympathetic trunks and ganglia, and made up of sympathetic, parasympathetic and visceral afferent fibers that innervate the heart.

celiac p., solar plexus.

cervical p., a network of nerve fibers formed by the first four cervical spinal nerves and supplying the structures in the region of the neck. One important branch is the phrenic nerve, which supplies the diaphragm.

choroid p., the ependyma lining the ventricles of the brain with the vascular fringes of the pia mater invaginating them; it is concerned with formation of the cerebrospinal fluid.

cystic p., a nerve plexus near the gallbladder.

lumbar p., a plexus originating from the ventral branches of the twelfth thoracic and the first four lumbar spinal nerves.

myenteric p., a nerve plexus situated in the muscular layers of the intestines.

nerve p., a distinct network formed by fibers from several adjacent spinal nerves.

pampiniform p., 1. in the male, a plexus of veins from the testis and the epididymis, constituting part of the spermatic cord. 2. in the female, a plexus of ovarian veins in the broad ligament of the uterus.

sacral p., a plexus arising from the ventral branches of the last two lumbar and first four sacral spinal nerves.

solar p., a network of ganglia and nerves supplying the abdominal viscera (see also SOLAR PLEXUS).

plica   (pli′kah), pl. *pli′cae* [L.] a plait or fold.

pli′cal circula′res, pli′cae conniven′tes, the permanent transverse folds of the small intestine.

pli′cae gas′tricae, the series of folds in the mucous membrane of the stomach.

p. muco′sa, a fold of mucous membrane.

pli′cae palma′tae, folds of the anterior and posterior walls of the canal of the cervix uteri.

p. polon′ica, a matting of the hair with crusts and vermin.

plicate   (pli′kāt) plaited or folded.

plication   (pli-ka′shun) the process of taking a fold or plait, for shortening or decreasing the size of an organ or structure.

plicotomy   (pli-kot′o-me) surgical division of the posterior fold of the tympanic membrane.

plombage   (plom-bahzh′) [Fr.] the filling of a space or cavity in the body with inert material.

plug   (plug) an obstructing mass.

epithelial p., a mass of ectodermal cells that temporarily closes the external naris of the fetus.

mucous p., a plug formed by secretions of mucous glands, especially one formed by those of the cervix uteri and closing the cervical canal during pregnancy.

plumbic   (plum′bik) pertaining to lead.

plumbism   (plum′bizm) a chronic form of poisoning caused by absorption of lead or lead salts (see also LEAD POISONING).

plumbum   (plum′bum) [L.] lead (symbol Pb).

Plummer-Vinson syndrome   (plum′er vin′son) difficulty in swallowing, with atrophy of buccal, glossophryngeal and esophageal mucosa, deficiency of iron in plasma and often anemia.

pluri-   (ploor′e) word element [L.], *many.*

pluriglandular   (ploor″ĭ-glan′du-lar) pertaining to, derived from or affecting several glands.

plurigravida   (ploor″ĭ-grav′ĭ-dah) multigravida; a woman pregnant for the third (or more) time.

plurilocular   (ploor″ĭ-lok′u-lar) multilocular; having many cells or compartments.

plurimenorrhea   (ploor″ĭ-men″o-re′ah) increased frequency of menstrual periods.

pluripara   (ploo-rip′ah-rah) multipara; a woman

who has had two or more pregnancies that resulted in viable offspring.

pluriparity (ploor″ĭ-par′ĭ-te) multiparity; the condition of being a pluripara (multipara).

pluripotentiality (ploor″ĭ-po-ten″she-al′ĭ-te) ability to develop or act in any one of several different ways.

plutonium (ploo-to′ne-um) a chemical element, atomic number 94, atomic weight 242, symbol Pu. (See table of ELEMENTS.)

Pm chemical symbol, *promethium.*

-pnea (ne′ah) word element [Gr.], *respiration; breathing.* adj., **-pne′ic.**

pneodynamics (ne″o-di-nam′iks) the dynamics of respiration.

pneograph (ne′o-graf) a device for registering respiratory movements.

pneometer (ne-om′ĕ-ter) pneumometer.

pneoscope (ne′o-skōp) a device for determining movements of the chest wall in respiration.

pneum(o)- (nu′mo) word element [Gr.], *air or gas; lung.*

pneumarthrogram (nu-mar′thro-gram) a roentgenogram of a joint after it has been injected with air.

pneumarthrography (nu″mar-throg′rah-fe) roentgenography of a joint after it has been injected with air.

pneumarthrosis (nu″mar-thro′sis) gas or air in a joint.

pneumat(o)- (nu′mah-to) word element [Gr.] *air or gas; lung.*

pneumatic (nu-mat′ik) pertaining to air or respiration.

pneumatization (nu″mah-tĭ-za′shun) the formation of air cavities in tissue, especially such formation in the temporal bone.

pneumatocele (nu-mat′o-sēl) 1. hernia of lung tissue. 2. a tumor or sac containing gas.

pneumatodyspnea (nu″mah-to-disp′ne-ah) difficulty in breathing due to emphysema.

pneumatogram (nu-mat′o-gram) a tracing made by a pneumatograph.

pneumatograph (nu-mat′o-graf) a device for registering movements of the chest wall in respiration.

pneumatology (nu″mah-tol′o-je) the science of gases and air and of their therapeutic use.

pneumatometer (nu″mah-tom′ĕ-ter) pneumometer.

pneumatometry (nu″mah-tom′ĕ-tre) measurement of the air inspired and expired.

pneumatorrhachis (nu″mah-tor′ah-kis) the presence of gas in the vertebral canal.

pneumatosis (nu″mah-to′sis) air or gas in an abnormal location in the body.
  p. cystoi′des intestina′lis, p. cystoi′des intestino′rum, a condition characterized by the presence of thin-walled, gas-containing cysts in the wall of the intestines.

pneumatotherapy (nu″mah-to-ther′ah-pe) treatment by rarefied or condensed air.
  cerebral p., injection of pure oxygen into the subarachnoid space, in treatment of psychoses.

pneumaturia (nu″mah-tu′re-ah) gas or air in the urine.

pneumectomy (nu-mek′to-me) pneumonectomy.

pneumoamnios (nu″mo-am′ne-os) gas in the amniotic fluid.

pneumoangiography (nu″mo-an″je-og′rah-fe) roentgenography of the blood vessels of the lungs.

pneumoarthrography (nu″mo-ar-throg′rah-fe) roentgenography of a joint after injection of air or gas into the articular capsule.

pneumocephalus (nu″mo-sef′ah-lus) air in the cerebral ventricles.

pneumococcemia (nu″mo-kok-se′me-ah) pneumococci in the blood.

pneumococcidal (nu″mo-kok-si′dal) destroying pneumococci.

pneumococcosis (nu″mo-kok-o′sis) infection with pneumococci.

pneumococcosuria (nu″mo-kok″o-su′re-ah) pneumococci in the urine.

pneumococcus (nu″mo-kok′us), pl. *pneumococ′ci* the organism, *Diplococcus pneumoniae,* which causes lobar pneumonia; it is a small, slightly elongated, encapsulated coccus, one end of which is pointed or lance-shaped, and commonly occurs in pairs; 80 serologic strains or types have been differentiated. adj., **pneumococ′cal.**

pneumoconiosis (nu″mo-ko″ne-o′sis) any of a group of lung diseases resulting from inhalation of particles of industrial substances, such as the dust of iron ore or coal, and retention of them in the lungs. The diseases vary in severity but all are occupational diseases, acquired by workers in the course of their jobs.
  Symptoms of the pneumoconioses include shortness of breath, chronic cough and expectoration of mucus containing the offending particles.
  SILICOSIS is probably the best known and most severe of these diseases. Asbestosis, caused by inhalation of asbestos fibers, is probably second only to silicosis in severity. Prevention and early diagnosis are important, for no effective treatment is available. Anthracosilicosis is caused by the inhalation of coal dust and silica and is similar in its development and its effects to silicosis. Beryllium lung disease or berylliosis is found in workers exposed to beryllium in the manufacture of fluorescent lamps, and in members of their families who are contaminated by the chemicals in the worker's clothing. Other types of pneumoconiosis

include aluminum pneumoconiosis, cadmium worker's disease and siderosis.

pneumocystography (nu″mo-sis-tog′rah-fe) roentgenography of the urinary bladder after injection of air or gas.

pneumocystotomography (nu″mo-sis″to-to-mog′rah-fe) body-section roentgenography after inflation of the bladder with air.

pneumoderma (nu″mo-der′mah) subcutaneous emphysema; air or gas beneath the skin.

pneumoencephalogram (nu″mo-en-sef′ah-lo-gram″) the film produced by pneumoencephalography.

pneumoencephalography (nu″mo-en-sef″ah-log′rah-fe) radiography of the intracranial contents after injection of air or gas into the subarachnoid space, usually by spinal puncture, permitting visualization of the ventricles.

pneumoencephalomyelogram (nu″mo-en-sef′-ah-lo-mi′el-o-gram″) the roentgenogram obtained by pneumoencephalomyelography.

pneumoencephalomyelography (nu″mo-en-sef″ah-lo-mi′ĕ-log′rah-fe) the making of x-ray films of the brain and spinal cord after injection of air or gas into the subarachnoid space.

pneumography (nu-mog′rah-fe) 1. description of the lungs. 2. roentgenography of a part after injection of oxygen. 3. graphic recording of respiratory movements.

pneumohemopericardium (nu″mo-he″mo-per″ĭ-kar′de-um) air and blood in the pericardium.

pneumohemothorax (nu″mo-he″mo-tho′raks) gas or air and blood in the pleural cavity.

pneumohydrometra (nu″mo-hi″dro-me′trah) gas and fluid in the uterus.

pneumohydropericardium (nu″mo-hi″dro-per″ĭ-kar′de-um) air or gas with fluid in the pericardium.

pneumohydrothorax (nu″mo-hi″dro-tho′raks) air or gas with fluid in the thoracic cavity.

pneumohypoderma (nu″mo-hi″po-der′mah) air or gas in the subcutaneous tissues.

pneumolith (nu′mo-lith) a pulmonary concretion.

pneumolithiasis (nu″mo-lĭ-thi′ah-sis) the presence of concretions in the lungs.

pneumology (nu-mol′o-je) the study of diseases of the air passages.

pneumomediastinogram (nu″mo-me″de-as-ti′no-gram) the film produced by pneumomediastinography.

pneumomediastinography (nu″mo-me″de-as″-tĭ-nog′rah-fe) roentgenography of the mediastinum after injection of air or gas.

pneumomediastinum (nu″mo-me″de-ah-sti′num) the presence of air or gas in tissues of the mediastinum, occurring pathologically or introduced intentionally.

pneumometer (nu-mom′ĕ-ter) spirometer; an

instrument for measuring the volume of air inspired and expired.

pneumomyelography (nu″mo-mi″ĕ-log′rah-fe) roentgenography of the vertebral canal after injection of air or gas.

pneumonectasis (nu″mo-nek′tah-sis) emphysema of the lungs.

pneumonectomy (nu″mo-nek′to-me) resection of lung tissue: of an entire lung (total pneumonectomy) or less (partial pneumonectomy), or of a single lobe (lobectomy). (See also surgery of the LUNG.)

pneumonemia (nu″mo-ne′me-ah) pulmonary congestion.

pneumonia (nu-mo′ne-ah) acute inflammation or infection of the lung. Pneumonia once was a common cause of death and killed one out of four victims. It is still a serious disease, especially in infants and the elderly, who are most vulnerable. The general mortality rate has been drastically reduced, however, because of new medicines and modern methods of treatment.

TYPES, SYMPTOMS AND TREATMENT. Infectious pneumonia may be caused by either bacteria or viruses. It may be primary or secondary (a complication of another disease) and may involve one or both lungs. It is most frequently caused by the pneumococcus. The microorganisms that give rise to pneumonia are always present in the upper respiratory tract. They cause no harm unless resistance is severely lowered by some other factor, such as a severe cold, disease, alcoholism or general poor health. Age is also a factor. When resistance is lowered or the conditions are favorable, the pneumococci invade the lungs.

Lobar Pneumonia. Pneumonia that affects a segment or an entire lobe of the lung is called lobar pneumonia. When both lungs are affected, the disease is called bilateral, or double, pneumonia. Whole sections of the lung tissue become solidified by inflammatory material, so that air cannot enter the alveoli. A chest x-ray is usually made to confirm the diagnosis and determine the extent of the disease.

Lobar pneumonia strikes suddenly. The symptoms are a cough, sharp chest pains (due to accompanying PLEURISY), blood-streaked or brownish sputum and a high fever that generally starts with a chill. Pulse and respiration increase to almost twice their normal rates.

Antibiotics and sulfonamides have greatly reduced the seriousness of lobar pneumonia. These drugs are usually administered for at least a week after the disease subsides to prevent the return of the infection.

Bronchial Pneumonia (Bronchopneumonia). Bronchopneumonia is a less dramatic form of pneumonia that is more prevalent than lobar pneumonia. The area affected is usually smaller than in the lobar type. The inflammation is localized in or around the bronchi, and causes the lung to be spotted with clusters of infected tissue. The symptoms appear gradually and are usually milder than in lobar pneumonia. The temperature rises more slowly and does not go as high, and there is no crisis as in lobar pneumonia.

Bronchopneumonia is rarely fatal except in patients with heart disease or other complications. It is often more difficult to treat, however; relapses are common and can be serious. Diagnosis is also more difficult because the causes are varied.

If the disease is bacterial, antibiotics such as penicillin are usually employed effectively. If it is viral, however, antibiotics are not effective and the disease may have to run its course. Viral pneumonia may be caused by the influenza virus or by the virus causing psittacosis.

Staphylococcic pneumonia is a very serious form of the disease and is occasionally fatal.

Primary Atypical Pneumonia. This type of pneumonia occurs chiefly in young adults who are otherwise healthy. It is often found in military camps and is due to various viruses or to pleuro-pneumonia-like organisms (Mycoplasma).

In the past this type of pneumonia often went undetected. The symptoms are similar to those of a cold. There may be headache, fever, a dry cough, generalized aches and a feeling of extreme fatigue. X-ray examination of the lungs will reveal evidence of infection.

Antibiotics such as tetracycline are used in treatment, and general measures are the same as for lobar pneumonia. The fever usually disappears in 10 days if there are no complications.

Other Types. Other kinds of pneumonia are caused by inhalation of poisonous gases (chemical pneumonia), accidental inhalation of food or liquids while unconscious (aspiration pneumonia), a blow or injury to the chest that interferes with normal respiration (traumatic pneumonia) or inhalation of oily substances (oil or lipoid pneumonia). Hypostatic pneumonia, which is due to lying on the back, frequently occurs in elderly bedridden patients. Interstitial pneumonia is a chronic form in which there is an increase of the interstitial tissue and a decrease of the proper lung tissue, with induration.

NURSING CARE. Bed rest is of primary importance in assisting the body to combat the infection and in preventing unnecessary strain on the lungs and respiratory system. The fever presents problems of dehydration. Fluids are given frequently by mouth, or intravenously if necessary. An accurate record must be kept of the patient's intake and output. Bowel elimination must be checked regularly since the peristaltic action of the intestines may be affected in severe pneumonia. Delirium is not uncommon because of the high fever and requires careful observation of the patient and measures to prevent self-injury (see also DELIRIUM).

Mouth care is given regularly to combat dryness and cracking of the lips, which occur as a result of fever and dehydration.

To relieve the chest pain caused by pleurisy in pneumonia, it may help to have the patient lie on the affected side so that the side is splinted during coughing episodes. It is also helpful to place the hands on the patient's chest and apply pressure as a means of splinting the chest as the patient coughs.

The temperature, pulse and respiration are checked and recorded at least every 4 hours. When the temperature falls the patient usually perspires profusely, requiring frequent changing of his gown and the bed linens. He must be protected from drafts and kept warm during this time.

pneumonic (nu-mon'ik) pertaining to the lung or to pneumonia.

p. plague, a form of PLAGUE with extensive involvement of the lungs.

pneumonitis (nu"mo-ni'tis) inflammation of lung tissue.

pneumonocentesis (nu-mo"no-sen-te'sis) surgical puncture of a lung for drainage of a cyst or abscess.

pneumonocirrhosis (nu-mo"no-sĭ-ro'sis) cirrhosis of the lung.

pneumonoconiosis (nu-mo"no-ko"ne-o'sis) pneumoconiosis.

pneumonograph (nu-mon'o-graf) a roentgenogram of the lungs.

pneumonography (nu"mo-nog'rah-fe) roentgenography of the lungs.

pneumonolysis (nu"mo-nol'ĭ-sis) division of tissues attaching the lung to the wall of the chest cavity, to permit collapse of the lung.

extraperiosteal p., that in which the separation is between the inner surface of the ribs and the periosteum, which, with the intercostal muscle bundles, remains attached to the parietal pleura.

extrapleural p., pneumonolysis in which the separation is between the parietal pleura and the chest wall.

intrapleural p., that in which the separation is between the visceral and the parietal pleura.

pneumonometer (nu"mo-nom'ĕ-ter) pneumometer.

pneumonomycosis (nu-mo"no-mi-ko'sis) fungus disease of the lungs.

pneumonopathy (nu"mo-nop'ah-the) any lung disease.

pneumonopexy (nu-mo'no-pek"se) fixation of the lung to the thoracic wall.

pneumonophthisis (nu"mon-of-thi'sis) pulmonary tuberculosis.

pneumonorrhaphy (nu"mon-or'ah-fe) suture of the lung.

pneumonosis (nu"mo-no'sis) any lung disease.

pneumonotomy (nu"mo-not'o-me) incision of the lung.

pneumopericardium (nu"mo-per"ĭ-kar'de-um) the presence of air or gas in the pericardial cavity.

pneumoperitoneum (nu"mo-per"ĭ-to-ne'um) the presence of air or gas in the peritoneal cavity, occurring pathologically or introduced intentionally.

pneumoperitonitis (nu"mo-per"ĭ-to-ni'tis) peritonitis with formation of gas.

pneumophone (nu'mo-fōn) an instrument for measuring pressure in the middle ear.

pneumopleuritis (nu"mo-ploo-ri'tis) inflammation of the lungs and pleura.

pneumopyelography (nu"mo-pi"ĕ-log'rah-fe) roentgenography after infection of oxygen or air into the renal pelvis.

pneumopyopericardium (nu″mo-pi″o-per″ĭ-kar′-de-um) air or gas and pus in the pericardium.

pneumopyothorax (nu″mo-pi″o-tho′raks) air or gas and pus in the pleural cavity.

pneumoradiography (nu″mo-ra″de-og′rah-fe) radiography of a part after injection of oxygen or other gas as contrast material.

pneumoresection (nu″mo-re-sek′shun) removal of a portion of the lung.

pneumoretroperitoneum (nu″mo-ret″ro-per″ĭ-to-ne′um) the presence of air or gas in the retroperitoneal space.

pneumorrhagia (nu″mo-ra′je-ah) hemorrhage from the lungs.

pneumosilicosis (nu″mo-sil″ĭ-ko′sis) the deposit of silica particles in the lungs (see also SILICOSIS).

pneumotherapy (nu″mo-ther′ah-pe) 1. treatment of disease of the lungs. 2. pneumatotherapy.

pneumothorax (nu″mo-tho′raks) accumulation of air or gas in the pleural cavity, resulting in collapse of the lung on the affected side. The condition may occur spontaneously, as in the course of a pulmonary disease, or it may follow trauma to, and perforation of, the chest wall. Artificial pneumothorax is a surgical procedure sometimes used in the treatment of tuberculosis or following pneumonectomy; it involves the injection of measured amounts of air into the pleural cavity to collapse the lung and immobilize it while healing takes place (see also surgery of the LUNG).

SPONTANEOUS PNEUMOTHORAX. This condition sometimes occurs when there is an opening on the surface of the lung allowing leakage of air from the bronchi into the pleural cavity. Most often it occurs when an emphysematous bulla or other weakened area on the lung ruptures. Normally the pleural cavity is an airtight compartment with a negative pressure. When air enters the pleural cavity the lung collapses, producing shortness of breath, and the heart and mediastinum shift toward the unaffected side.

Other symptoms of spontaneous pneumothorax are a sudden sharp chest pain, fall in blood pressure, weak and rapid pulse and cessation of normal respiratory movements on the affected side of the chest.

Spontaneous pneumothorax may require no specific treatment beyond bed rest and the administration of oxygen to relieve dyspnea. The patient usually is more comfortable if he is allowed to sit up. In some cases THORACENTESIS and aspiration of air from the pleural cavity may be necessary. This allows for reexpansion of the lung. If air continues to leak from the defect in the lung surface a continuous closed-drainage apparatus is set up. As soon as the lung lesion heals and the lung is reexpanded, the patient is allowed to resume his usual activities.

Tension pneumothorax is a particularly dangerous form of pneumothorax that occurs when air escapes into the pleural cavity from a bronchus but cannot regain entry into the bronchus. As a result, continuously increasing air pressure in the pleural cavity causes progressive collapse of the lung tissue. Emergency treatment—aspiration of air from the pleural cavity—is necessary in this disorder.

pneumotomography (nu″mo-to-mog′rah-fe) body-section roentgenography after injection of air or other gas into the region or organ being visualized.

pneumotomy (nu-mot′o-me) pneumonotomy.

pneumotoxin (nu″mo-tok′sin) a toxin produced by the bacteria of pneumonia.

pneumotropic (nu″mo-trop′ik) 1. having a special affinity for lung tissue. 2. having a selective affinity for pneumococci.

pneumotropism (nu-mot′ro-pizm) predilection of an agent or organism for lung tissue.

pneumoventriculography (nu″mo-ven-trik″u-log′rah-fe) pneumoencephalography.

P.O. [L.] *per os* (by mouth).

Po chemical symbol, *polonium*.

pO₂ oxygen pressure (tension).

pock (pok) a pustule, especially of smallpox.

podagra (po-dag′rah) gouty pain in the great toe.

podalgia (po-dal′je-ah) pain in the feet.

podalic (po-dal′ik) accomplished by means of the feet, as podalic version.

podarthritis (pod″ar-thri′tis) inflammation of the joints of the feet.

podencephalus (pod″en-sef′ah-lus) a fetal monster without a cranium, the brain hanging by a pedicle.

podiatrist (po-di′ah-trist) a specialist in treating the feet for minor ailments, such as corns, bunions, calluses and fungal infections; called also chiropodist. Podiatrists are not graduate physicians, and their treatments should be confined to minor foot conditions. Such treatments may include minor surgical procedures and prescription of corrective shoes or special exercises.

podiatry (po-di′ah-tre) the scientific study and care of the feet.

podium (po′de-um) a footlike part, such as an extension of the protoplasm of a cell.

podobromidrosis (pod″o-brom″ĭ-dro′sis) fetid perspiration of the feet.

pododynamometer (pod″o-di″nah-mom′ĕ-ter) a device for determining the strength of the leg muscles.

pododynia (pod″o-din′e-ah) pain in the feet.

podology (po-dol′o-je) study of the foot.

podophyllin (pod″o-fil′in) the yellow purgative resin of plants of the genus Podophyllum.

podophyllum (pod″o-fil′um) the dried rhizome and roots of *Podophyllum peltatum;* used as a caustic agent for certain skin tumors.

pogoniasis (po″go-ni′ah-sis) excessive or abnormal growth of the beard.

pogonion (po-go′ne-on) the anterior midpoint of the chin.

-poiesis (-poi-e′sis) word element [Gr.], *formation.* adj., **-poiet′ic.**

poikilionia (poi″kil-e-o′ne-ah) variation in the ionic content of the blood.

poikilo- (poi′kĭ-lo) word element [Gr.], *varied; irregular.*

poikiloblast (poi′kĭ-lo-blast″) an abnormally shaped erythroblast.

poikilocyte (poi′kĭ-lo-sīt″) an erythrocyte showing abnormal variations in shape.

poikilocytosis (poi″kĭ-lo-si-to′sis) the presence of poikilocytes in the blood.

poikiloderma (poi″kĭ-lo-der′mah) a condition characterized by pigmentary and atrophic changes in the skin, giving it a mottled appearance.

poikiloplastocyte (poi″kĭ-lo-plas′to-sīt) an irregularly shaped blood platelet.

poikiloploidy (poi′kĭ-lo-ploi″de) the state of having different numbers of chromosomes in different cells.

poikilosmosis (poi″kil-oz-mo′sis) adjustment by a cell, tissue, organ or organism of the tonicity of its fluid milieu to the tonicity of the surrounding medium. adj., **poikilosmot′ic.**

poikilotherm (poi′kĭ-lo-therm″) an organism whose temperature varies with that of the external environment; a "cold-blooded" organism.

poikilothermy (poi″kĭ-lo-ther′me) the state of having body temperature that varies with that of the environment. adj., **poikilother′mal, poikilother′mic.**

point (point) 1. a small area or spot; the sharp end of an object. 2. to approach the surface, like the pus of an abscess, at a definite spot.
    auricular p., the center of the opening of the external acoustic meatus.
    boiling p., the temperature at which a liquid will boil: at sea level, 100° C., or 212° F.
    boiling p., normal, the temperature at which a liquid boils at one atmosphere pressure.
    cardinal p's, the points on the different refracting media of the eye that determine the direction of the entering or emerging light rays.
    craniometric p's, the established points of reference for measurement of the skull.
    dew p., the temperature at which moisture in the atmosphere is deposited as dew.
    disparate p's, points on the two retinas on which incident light rays do not produce the same impression.
    far p., the remotest point at which an object is clearly seen when the eye is at rest.
    fixation p., the point for which accommodation of the eye is momentarily adjusted and where vision is clearest.
    freezing p., the temperature at which a liquid begins to freeze; for water, 0° C., or 32° F.
    isoelectric p., the pH of a solution at which a dipolar ion does not migrate in an electric field.

    isoionic p., the pH of a solution at which the number of cations equals the number of anions.
    lacrimal p., a small aperture situated on a slight elevation at the medial end of the eyelid margin, through which tears from the lacrimal lake enter the lacrimal canaliculi.
    McBurney's p., a point of special tenderness in appendicitis, on a line connecting the umbilicus and anterior superior spine of the right ilium, about 2 inches from the latter.
    melting p., the temperature at which a solid becomes liquefied by heat.
    near p., the nearest point of clear vision, the absolute near point being that for either eye alone, and the relative near point that for the two eyes together.
    nodal p's, two points on the axis of an optical system situated so that a ray falling on one will produce a parallel ray emerging through the other.

pointillage (pwahn-te-yahzh′) [Fr.] massage with the points of the fingers.

poison (poi′zun) a substance that, on ingestion, inhalation, absorption, application, injection or development within the body, in relatively small amounts, produces injury to the body by its chemical action.
    Corrosives are poisons that destroy tissues directly. They include the mineral acids, such as nitric acid, sulfuric acid and hydrochloric acid; the caustic alkalis, such as ammonia, sodium hydroxide (lye), sodium carbonate and sodium hypochlorite; and carbolic acid (phenol).
    Irritants are poisons that inflame the mucous membranes by direct action. These include arsenic, copper sulfate, salts of lead, zinc and phosphorus, and many others.
    Nerve toxins act on the nerves or affect some of the basic cell processes. This large group includes the narcotics, such as opium, heroin and cocaine, and the barbiturates, anesthetics and alcohols.
    Blood toxins act on the blood and deprive it of oxygen. They include carbon monoxide, carbon dioxide, hydrocyanic acid and the gases used in chemical warfare. Some blood toxins destroy the blood cells or the platelets.
    See also POISONING and names of individual poisons.
    p. ivy, oak and sumac, common plants of the genus Rhus (or Toxicodendron) that cause allergic skin reactions. The poison contained in their leaves, roots and berries is an oily substance called urushiol. It has no effect on some people; in others, momentary or even indirect contact may cause painful rashes and blisters.
    POISON IVY. Poison ivy (*Rhus toxicodendron*) grows in the form of climbing vines, shrubs that trail on the ground and shrubbery that grows upright without any support. The vine clings to stone and brick houses and climbs trees and poles. It flourishes abundantly along fences, paths and roadways, and is often partly hidden by other foliage.
    Recognition. The poison ivy plant is attractive and is often picked as a decoration by unsuspecting flower gatherers. Although poison ivy comes in many forms and displays seasonal changes, it has one constant characteristic: The leaves always grow in clusters of three, one at the end of the stalk, the other two opposite one another.
    Transmission. The plant is particularly potent in the spring and early summer when it is full of oily resinous sap. This forms an invisible film upon

POISONS, SIGNS AND SYMPTOMS AND EMERGENCY TREATMENT

POISON	SOURCES	SIGNS AND SYMPTOMS	EMERGENCY TREATMENT
Acetanilid	Headache remedies	Gastrointestinal disturbances; anemia; methemoglobinemia; antipyresis; collapse	Gastric lavage; cathartics; enema; oxygen; artificial respiration; transfusions.
Acids (e.g., hydrochloric and nitric acids)	Cleaning solutions	Pain in throat, esophagus and stomach; dysphagia; diarrhea; shock; collapse. If topical, skin is first white, then turns yellow or brown.	Give milk of magnesia, aluminum hydroxide, mild soap solution, milk or water with egg whites. Apply sodium bicarbonate solution to skin.
Ammonia	Household ammonia	Burning sensation in mouth and stomach; nausea; vomiting; abdominal pain; respiratory failure.	Give weak acids, olive oil, fluids.
Aniline dyes	Crayons, shoe polish	Apathy; dyspnea; cyanosis due to methemoglobinemia.	1% methylene blue solution I.V. (2mg./kg.); lavage with water; oxygen; blood.
Amphetamines	Stimulants, anti-obesity preparations	Irrational behavior; cerebral stimulation; shock; cardiac arrhythmias; tremors; convulsions; coma.	Pentobarbital (100 mg.) or Amytal (250 mg.) I.M.
Antihistamines	Cold compounds, anti-allergic drugs	Vomiting; convulsions; hyperpyrexia; generalized depression; hallucinations; unconsciousness.	Gastric lavage; symptomatic treatment (paraldehyde or ether during convulsions; caffeine or coramine during depressed state). Histamine 0.1 mg./kg.
Arsenic	Insecticides, weed killer, rodenticides	Odor of garlic on breath and in stools; faintness; nausea; difficulty in swallowing; thirst; vomiting; gastric pain; oliguria; albuminuria; cold, clammy skin; "rice water stools"; collapse.	Universal antidote followed by lavage with sodium bicarbonate solution or emetic; intravenous fluids; sedation; dimercaprol (BAL). Conserve body heat.
Barbiturates	Sedatives	Somnolence; stupor; coma; respiratory and circulatory collapse.	Bemegride; fluids; oxygen; peritoneal dialysis.
Bromides	Bromo Seltzer, sedatives	Acute poisoning; stupor; ataxia; muscular weakness; collapse. Chronic poisoning: bromide acne; foul breath; gastrointestinal disturbances; depression; apathy; ataxia; muscular weakness; anemia.	Large doses of normal saline solution; diuretics (ammonium chloride or mercuhydrin).
Caffeine	Coffee, No-Doz	Gastrointestinal distress; diuresis; photophobia; premature systoles; tremors; convulsions; hallucinations.	Gastric lavage; central depressants (pentobarbital); fluids.
Camphor	Camphorated oil, moth balls	Odor on breath; headache; excitement; delirium; convulsions.	Gastric lavage with water; sedation with barbiturates, but no opiates.
Carbon monoxide	Coal gas, illuminating gas, exhaust from motor vehicles	Skin is cherry red; headache; dizziness; impaired hearing and vision; drowsiness; confusion; loss of consciousness; slow respiration; rapid pulse.	Move victim to fresh air; artificial respiration; mixture of 90% oxygen and 10% carbon dioxide; bed rest for 48 hours. Conserve body heat.
Carbon tetrachloride	Spot removers, some fire extinguishers, solvents	Nausea; vomiting; headache; inebriation; convulsions; coma; dark colored urine; jaundice; diarrhea; disturbance of hearing and vision.	If poison has been swallowed, lavage with 1:10,000 potassium permanganate solution. If inhaled give oxygen–carbon dioxide mixture. High protein and carbohydrate diet; fluids.
Chlorophenothane (DDT)	Insecticides	Headache, nausea; vomiting; diarrhea; paresthesias of lips and tongue; numbness of extremities; malaise; sore throat; tremor; convulsions; respiratory failure.	Lavage with water; saline cathartic; force fluids (tea or coffee); give calcium gluconate. Avoid fats, fat solvents and opiates. Wash skin with soap and water.
Cyanide	Rodenticides, metal polish	Odor of bitter almond oil on breath; headache; rapid breathing; dyspnea; heart palpitation; tightness in chest; cyanosis; convulsions. Death may occur within a few minutes.	Immediately after ingestion, lavage with 1:10,000 potassium permanganate solution. Inhale several amyl nitrite perles followed by 10% sodium nitrite I.V. May follow with 50% sodium thiosulfate I.V. (Principle of therapy is to form methemoglobin in blood, which combines with cyanide.) Oxygen and blood transfusion.

POISONS, SIGNS AND SYMPTOMS AND EMERGENCY TREATMENT (*Continued*)

POISON	SOURCES	SIGNS AND SYMPTOMS	EMERGENCY TREATMENT
Ethyl alcohol	Liquors	Central depression; disturbance in gait; incoherence; excitement; stupor; coma; respiratory depression.	Excitement treated with paraldehyde, chloral hydrate or tranquilizers. Drowsiness treated with caffeine sodium benzoate, dextroamphetamine or methylphenidate. Intravenous infusions with dextrose; vitamins; artificial respiration if necessary.
Fluoride	Insecticides	Excessive salivation; abdominal pain; hematemesis; diarrhea; muscle weakness; difficulty swallowing; facial paralysis; respiratory failure; circulatory collapse.	Calcium chloride or milk orally. Lavage with 1% calcium chloride or milk.
Hydrocarbons	Kerosene, gasoline, cleaning fluids	Burning sensation in mouth, esophagus and stomach; vomiting; dizziness; tremor; muscular cramps; confusion; fever; cold, clammy skin; weak pulse; thirst; coma; respiratory failure.	Avoid lavage. Oxygen; fluids; antibiotics; saline cathartics.
Iodine	Tincture of iodine	Brown stain on lips, tongue, and in mouth; odor of iodine in vomitus; thirst, fainting; giddiness; vomiting; abdominal pain; diarrhea; shock.	Water with starch, flour or mashed potatoes. Lavage with starch or 5% sodium thiosulfate solution, milk or egg whites.
Lead	Paint	Gastrointestinal irritation; pain; vomiting; diarrhea; headache; insomnia; visual disturbances; irritability; delirium; convulsions. In chronic poisoning, "lead-lines" on gums.	Gastric lavage; papaverine or calcium gluconate for relief of colic; surgery to correct encephalopathy in children. Edathamil calcium-disodium I.V. Barbiturates to control central excitation.
Lye	Drain and toilet bowl cleanser	Burning pain in mouth, throat and stomach; mucous membranes ulcerated; bloody vomitus; constricted throat; difficult respirations; cold, clammy skin; rapid pulse; violent purging; anxiety.	Emetics and lavage not recommended; give large amounts of weak acids, such as lemon or vinegar followed by demulcents such as egg whites, gruel, olive oil, salad oil. Analgesics; parenteral fluids.
Mercury	Antiseptics, fireworks, insect spray	Abdominal pain, vomiting; bloody diarrhea; constriction of throat and esophagus; ashen gray color of mucous membranes; circulatory collapse; kidney damage; oliguria; anuria.	Universal antidote. Lavage with copious milk, egg white or 5% sodium formaldehyde sulfoxylate, followed by sodium bicarbonate solution. Dimercaprol; fluids. Conserve body heat.
Morphine	Opium derivative	Slow, shallow respiration; pinpoint pupils; weak pulse; muscle twitching; spasm; cyanosis; coma; respiratory paralysis.	Keep respiratory passages clear; administer oxygen; nalorphine.
Nicotine	Insecticides, tobacco	Nausea; vomiting; confusion; salivation; abdominal cramps; convulsions; diarrhea; sweating; headache; weakness; perspiration; dilation of pupils; faintness; respiratory paralysis.	Universal antidote; lavage with 0.5% tannic acid or 1:5000 potassium permanganate solution; artificial respiration. Wash contaminated skin with cold water; stimulants if needed.
Paris Green (Copper arsenite + copper acetate)	Pesticides	Vomiting of green material followed by gastric and abdominal pain; diarrhea with dark and sometimes bloody stools; metallic taste in mouth; neuromuscular weakness; thirst; oliguria→anuria; cold, clammy skin; coma; convulsions; death.	Potassium ferrocyanide 10 gr. in water (to form an insoluble salt of copper) followed by lavage with sodium bicarbonate solution; demulcents (milk, egg white in water, gelatin, etc.).
Phenols	Phenol liquefied, cresol, Lysol, creosote	Corrosion of mucous membranes; pain; vomiting; bloody diarrhea; headache; dizziness; cold, clammy skin; oliguria; hematuria; unconsciousness; slow respiration; respiratory failure; dark urine.	Lavage with olive oil, egg white and milk; parenteral fluids; oxygen and carbon dioxide; analgesics. Remove from skin with 50% solution of alcohol or olive oil.

POISONS, SIGNS AND SYMPTOMS AND EMERGENCY TREATMENT (*Continued*)

POISON	SOURCES	SIGNS AND SYMPTOMS	EMERGENCY TREATMENT
Phosphorus	Rodenticides, roach poison, fireworks, matches	Nausea; vomiting; abdominal pain; diarrhea; shock; garlic odor on breath; liver and kidney damage.	Lavage with 2% copper sulfide then 1:10,000 potassium permanganate; give fluids.
Salicylates	Aspirin, oil of wintergreen	Hyperpnea; listlessness; vomiting; dizziness; mental confusion; acidosis; hemorrhagic manifestations.	Lavage with milk or 1:10,000 potassium permanganate solution. Instill saline cathartic in stomach after lavage; oral or parenteral fluid. Watch electrolyte and acid-base balance.
Sodium hypophosphite or hypochlorite	Bleaching agents, washing powders	Vomiting; corrosive burns of lips, mouth and tongue.	Gastric lavage; give fluids.
Strychnine	Cathartics, insecticides, rodenticides	Central nervous system stimulation; hyperreflexia, stiffness of face or neck; convulsions; opisthotonos; death due to asphyxia.	Lavage with 1:10,000 potassium permanganate (unless convulsing). Universal antidote; barbiturates to control convulsions; keep patient in quiet room away from stimulation; oxygen.
Quaternary ammonium compounds	Zephiran, etc.	Burning pain in mouth and throat; nausea; vomiting; apprehension; restlessness; muscle weakness; collapse; coma; convulsions.	Lavage or induce vomiting. Give mild soap solution as antidote; cathartic.

From Asperheim, M. K.: The Pharmacologic Basis of Patient Care. Philadelphia, W. B. Saunders Co., 1968.

the human skin on contact. Direct contact is not always necessary. Some cases of poison ivy dermatitis are caused by the handling of clothing or garden implements that have been contaminated by the sap, sometimes months earlier; dogs and cats may carry it on their fur. Many people are so sensitive that smoke from a brush fire containing poison ivy brings on a rash.

Symptoms. After exposure, the symptoms of poison ivy dermatitis may develop in a matter of hours, though sometimes they do not appear for several days. There is reddening on the hands, neck, face, legs or whatever parts of the body have been exposed, with considerable itching. Small blisters form which later become larger and eventually exude a watery fluid. The skin then becomes crusty and dry. After a few weeks all symptoms spontaneously disappear.

Treatment. An attack of poison ivy dermatitis can sometimes be avoided if the skin is scrubbed immediately after contact with ordinary yellow laundry soap, which has a high alkaline content. The skin should be lathered several times and rinsed each time in running water. This may remove all or at least part of the poison ivy film before it is able to penetrate the skin.

If, despite precautions, dermatitis does develop, various treatments may relieve the itching. One is to apply a compress soaked in Burow's solution (obtainable at any drugstore), diluted in the proportion of one part solution to 15 parts cool water. Another standard remedy is calamine lotion.

If the inflammation becomes unusually severe or is accompanied by fever, a physician should be consulted. He may prescribe one of the cortisone preparations, which may be taken orally, injected or applied locally as a cream.

Immunization. In general, programs of desensitizing and immunization must be started well in advance of potential contact with poison ivy, and must be repeated at regular intervals, often weekly for 4 or 5 weeks. There is some doubt as to their effectiveness.

POISON OAK. Poison oak (*Rhus diversiloba*), sometimes known as oakleaf ivy, is not related to the oak tree but does bear a close kinship to poison ivy. The eastern and western varieties resemble each other quite closely.

Poison oak is usually a low-growing shrub and seldom a climbing vine. It has three leaves, like poison ivy, but they are lobed and bear a slight resemblance to small oak leaves. The berries are white and small, resembling those of poison ivy.

Poison oak causes the same symptoms as poison ivy, except that they are usually milder. There is redness of the skin, but blisters are less frequent.

Prevention, treatment and immunization are the same as for poison ivy dermatitis.

POISON SUMAC. Although poison sumac (*Rhus venenata*) goes by other names, such as swamp sumac, poison elder, poison ash, poison dogwood and thunderwood, there is only one variety of it. Sometimes, however, poison sumac is confused with the several harmless kinds of sumac.

Poison sumac is a coarse woody shrub or small tree, and it has white berries, which distinguish it from the several harmless varieties of sumac, which have red berries.

Symptoms and treatment are similar to those of poison ivy dermatitis.

poisoning (poi'zun-ing) the morbid condition produced by a poison. (See also CARBON MONOXIDE POISONING, FOOD POISONING and LEAD POISONING.)

SYMPTOMS. The symptoms of poisoning vary greatly according to the poison taken and the time that has elapsed. Some poisons cause no immediate symptoms. In general, poisoning should be suspected in the following instances: (1) a revealing odor such as alcohol on the breath; (2) discoloration of the mouth or lips; (3) evidence of eating leaves or wild berries; (4) severe pain or a burning sensation in the mouth and throat; (5) nausea or vomiting; (6) convulsions; (7) confusion or disturbance of sight; (8) unconsciousness or deep sleep; (9) sudden illness, when an open bottle or container of medicine or poisonous chemicals is found nearby.

FIRST AID. In all cases of poisoning, speed in treatment is essential. First aid should be started immediately and, if possible, another person should call the physician or the nearest poison center.

Swallowed Poisons. General first aid treatment consists of diluting the poison by giving one or more large glasses of fluids (water or milk) and emptying the stomach by inducing vomiting. When vomiting begins, the victim should be placed face down with head lower than hips to prevent vomitus from entering the lungs. When the vomiting is ended, the person should be helped to sit up and given one or two glasses of milk. If milk is not available, tea or water may be substituted.

The poison container and any remaining poison should be saved to help in identification and in estimation of dosage. If there is no evidence of the poison, the vomitus should be saved for examination.

If the poison has a label, administer the antidote as directed. If the poison is unknown, activated charcoal is recommended as first choice for antidote; however, it is not effective against caustic alkalis, cyanide, mineral acids and alcohol.

Do not induce vomiting in the following cases:

1. If the victim has swallowed a corrosive poison, such as a strong acid or alkali, in which case there is severe pain, a burning sensation in the mouth and throat and vomiting.

2. If the victim has swallowed a petroleum product, such as gasoline, kerosene or cigarette lighter fluid.

3. If the victim has swallowed iodine or strychnine.

4. If the victim has convulsions, is in a coma or is unconscious.

For strong acids, give lots of milk. If milk is not easily available, water, or a solution of a tablespoon of milk of magnesia in a cup of water, may be used. For alkali, milk is also the preferred antidote, but water or any fruit juice may be substituted. One to two cups is sufficient for a child under 5; in older persons, up to four cups should be given.

In strychnine poisoning, fluids should be given and vomiting induced only if the poison has just been taken. Once it has entered the system, even the slightest movement may bring on convulsions. Immediate medical attention is necessary.

In overdose of sleeping pills or morphine, the patient should be kept lying down and warm until medical help arrives.

Inhaled Poisons. General first-aid treatment for poisoning by such gases as carbon monoxide, hydrocyanic acid and methane consists of dragging or carrying the victim to fresh air and administering artificial respiration, if breathing is irregular or has stopped. The rescuer should be careful not to risk being overcome himself. In telephoning the hospital, police or fire department for help, one should specify the nature of the accident so that the proper emergency equipment may be brought. The victim should be wrapped in blankets to maintain body temperature, and be kept quiet. If he has convulsions, he should be kept in a semidark room and care should be taken to avoid jarring him.

External Poisons. If the skin has been contaminated by a chemical, the poison should be washed off immediately with water from a faucet, shower or hose, and any contaminated clothing should be removed at the same time.

If the poison is in the eye, the eyelids should be held open while a gentle, continuous stream of water is poured into the eye.

PREVENTION OF POISONING. *In poisoning, prevention is far better than any treatment.* To prevent poisoning, the American Medical Association recommends the following precautions:

1. Keep all medicines, household chemicals and other poisonous substances locked up. There is no place "out of reach of children."

2. Never transfer poisonous substances to unlabeled containers, or food containers such as milk or soda bottles, or cereal boxes.

3. Never reuse containers of chemical products.

4. Never store poisonous substances on the same shelves used for storing food. Confusion might be fatal.

5. Never leave discarded medicines within the reach of children or pets. Pour contents down the drain or toilet or incinerator. Rinse the container.

6. Always read the label before using any chemical product.

7. Do not give or take medicines in the dark.

8. Never tell children the medicine you are giving them is candy.

9. When preparing the baby's formula, taste the ingredients. Never store boric acid, salt or talcum near the formula ingredients.

There are more than 500 Poison Control Centers throughout the United States. In case of poisoning, information concerning antidotes can be obtained by telephone from the nearest center.

blood p., septicemia.

Polaramine (po-lar′ah-mēn) trademark for preparations of dexchlorpheniramine maleate, an antihistamine.

polarimeter (po″lah-rim′ĕ-ter) a device for measuring the rotation of polarized light.

polarimetry (po″lah-rim′ĕ-tre) measurement of the rotation of polarized light.

polariscope (po-lar′ĭ-skōp) an instrument for the study of polarization.

polarity (po-lar′ĭ-te) the condition of having poles or of exhibiting opposite effects at the two extremities.

polarization (po″lar-ĭ-za′shun) the production of that condition in light in which its vibrations are parallel to each other in one plane, or in circles and ellipses.

poldine (pol′dēn) a compound used in parasympathetic blockade and to reduce acid formation in the stomach.

pole (pōl) 1. either extremity of any axis, as of the fetal ellipse or eye lens. 2. either one of two points that have opposite physical qualities (electric or other). adj., **po′lar.**

animal p., that pole at which the cytoplasm is concentrated in an ovum.

anterior p., the front or facial end of the anteroposterior axis of the eye.

antigerminal p., vegetal pole.

cephalic p., the end of the fetal ellipse at which the head of the fetus is situated.

frontal p., the most prominent part of the anterior end of each hemisphere of the brain.

germinal p., animal pole.

negative p., the terminal of an electric cell that has the lower potential, and toward which the current flows; cathode.

nutritive p., vegetal pole.

occipital p., the posterior end of the occipital lobe of the brain.

pelvic p., the end of the fetal ellipse at which the breech of the fetus is situated.

positive p., the terminal of an electic cell that has the higher potential, and from which the current flows; anode.

posterior p., the retinal end of the anteroposterior axis of the eye, usually between the macula lutea and the optic disk.

temporal p., the prominent anterior end of the temporal lobe of the brain.

vegetal p., vegetative p., vitelline p., that pole at the end of an ovum at which the yolk is massed.

poli(o)- (po′le-o) word element [Gr.], *gray matter.*

poliencephalitis (po″le-en-sef″ah-li′tis) polioencephalitis.

poliencephalomyelitis (po″le-en-sef″ah-lo-mi″ĕ-li′tis) polioencephalomyelitis.

polioclastic (po″le-o-klas′tik) destroying gray matter of the nervous system.

polioencephalitis (po″le-o-en-sef″ah-li′tis) inflammatory disease of the gray matter of the brain.

inferior p., bulbar paralysis.

polioencephalomeningomyelitis (po″le-o-en-sef″ah-lo-mĕ-ning″go-mi″ĕ-li′tis) inflammation of the gray matter of the brain and spinal cord and of the meninges.

polioencephalomyelitis (po″le-o-en-sef″ah-lo-mi″ĕ-li′tis) inflammation of the gray matter of the brain and spinal cord.

polioencephalopathy (po″le-o-en-sef″ah-lop′ah-the) disease of the gray matter of the brain.

poliomyelencephalitis (po″le-o-mi″el-en-sef″ah-li′tis) polioencephalomyelitis.

poliomyelitis (po″le-o-mi″ĕ-li′tis) a contagious viral disease that attacks the central nervous system, injuring or destroying the nerve cells that control the muscles and sometimes causing paralysis; called also polio and infantile paralysis. Paralysis most often affects the legs but can involve any muscles, including those that control breathing and swallowing. Since the development and use of vaccines against poliomyelitis, the disease has become far less common. However, the number of cases among very young infants who have not been immunized is on the rise.

Poliomyelitis is a very serious disease, but it is not often fatal. Paralysis develops in about half of all patients with polio, and of these about half recover completely. Only a small percentage of patients have serious symptoms; many cases are so mild that they are undiagnosed and never reported.

There are three known types of poliovirus, each causing a different type of the disease. Most paralytic cases are caused by type 1. Poliovirus is found in the throat of a patient for the first few days of the disease, and in his intestines for a longer period, sometimes as long as 17 weeks. The disease spreads by means of droplets of moisture from an infected person's throat or by waste products from his intestines. The contagious period is 7 or more days from the time of onset of the disease.

The poliovirus is short-lived, and cannot survive long in the air. The incubation period of polio is from 1 to 2 weeks, and occasionally as long as 3 weeks. Members of the family or other contacts may be carriers, but only for a short period of time.

SYMPTOMS. The early symptoms of polio include fever, headache, vomiting, sore throat, pain and stiffness in the back and neck and drowsiness. In the nonparalytic type, the fever usually lasts about 7 days, and the stiffness fades away in 3 to 5 days. In paralytic polio, some weakness or paralysis of the arms or legs begins 1 to 7 days after the first symptoms. The first sign of bulbar polio, which affects the muscles of swallowing and breathing, is difficulty in swallowing, speaking and breathing. This usually occurs in the first 3 days of the disease.

TREATMENT. There is at present no cure for polio; once the disease begins, it must be allowed to run its course. However, proper symptomatic treatment can often prevent crippling aftereffects. Applications of warm packs often reduce pain and promote relaxation. The patient is kept warm and quiet during the acute stage of the disease. Good bed posture is essential to prevention of deformities.

PREVENTION. The first safe, effective vaccine against polio was developed under the direction of Dr. Jonas E. Salk, and is usually referred to by his name. The Salk vaccine, which came into use in 1955, uses killed poliovirus to stimulate the production and release of antibodies into the bloodstream. The Salk method requires three injections 6 weeks apart, followed by a fourth booster about 6 months later. For infants, the vaccine is often combined with vaccines against diphtheria, tetanus and whooping cough. The first injection of the series is given at about the age of 6 weeks. Many physicians recommend that additional boosters of Salk vaccine be given, but the vaccine has not been in use long enough to determine how necessary this may be.

The second vaccine developed against polio was the oral type, which contains weakened but live strains of the poliovirus and is swallowed. Several scientists were responsible for the development of the oral vaccine; the most widely used type is that developed by Dr. Albert B. Sabin. The Sabin vaccine, which is usually swallowed on a sugar cube, is given in three doses, one of each type of virus, 6 weeks apart. It is recommended that infants be given a fourth booster dose of all three types, about 6 months after the third dose.

There are still many people who have not been immunized against polio. Also, it is rare for any vaccine to be 100 per cent effective. For these reasons, general good hygiene and health precautions are still important in the fight against polio.

REHABILITATION. A person who has been paralyzed by an acute case of polio can often be restored to activity through proper treatment. New techniques of physical therapy have been remarkably successful in educating patients to use individual muscles again. In some cases, reconstructive surgery on the affected limb is valuable. Orthopedic devices, such as braces, supports and special shoes, may also be helpful.

The National Foundation (formerly the National Foundation for Infantile Paralysis) can give advice on all aspects of treatment and rehabilitation for polio victims. The Foundation also gives financial aid to polio patients who are unable to afford proper treatment. The headquarters of the National Foundation are at 800 Second Avenue, New York, N.Y. 10017; there are local offices in many communities across the country.

NURSING CARE. During the early stages of poliomyelitis the patient is isolated, individually or in a group. ISOLATION TECHNIQUE is continued until the acute stage has passed and the patient is no longer a source of infection.

Complete bed rest is ordered during the acute stage of the illness. The patient should lie on a firm mattress and be properly positioned so that his body is in good alignment at all times. When his position is changed he must be turned gently, with his joints supported, and care must be taken not to grasp the muscles, which are extremely tender and painful and have a tendency toward spasms when stimulated. The paralysis of the affected limbs is a result of involvement of the motor nerves; the sensory nerves are not involved and thus the patient has no loss of sensory perception and can experience pain.

Warm, moist packs are applied to the affected limbs to reduce muscle spasm and relieve pain. Later, as the acute symptoms subside, the physician may order physical therapy measures such as massage and passive exercises to avoid contractures and maintain muscle tone.

If the poliomyelitis is of the bulbar type, affecting the muscles of respiration, a RESPIRATOR will be used to maintain adequate ventilation of the lungs. A TRACHEOSTOMY is sometimes necessary to facilitate breathing and maintain a patent airway. Swallowing difficulties may require TUBE FEEDING or intravenous infusion to provide adequate nutrition. The patient with bulbar poliomyelitis must have someone in constant attendance during the acute stage of his illness.

Fears and anxieties about the outcome of his illness are quite common in a patient with poliomyelitis. Most persons, even children, are usually aware of the crippling effects of this disease. The nursing staff must help the patient and his family in their adjustment to the changes poliomyelitis may bring about in their lives.

poliomyelopathy (po"le-o-mi"ĕ-lop'ah-the) disease of the gray matter of the spinal cord.

polioplasm (po'le-o-plazm") protoplasm.

poliosis (po"le-o'sis) premature grayness of the hair.

poliovirus (po"le-o-vi'rus) the causative agent of poliomyelitis, separable, on the basis of specificity of neutralizing antibody, into three serotypes designated types 1, 2 and 3.

pollen (pol'en) the male fertilizing element of flowering plants.

pollenogenic (pol"ĕ-no-jen'ik) caused by the pollen of plants.

pollenosis (pol"ĕ-no'sis) pollinosis.

pollex (pol'eks) [L.] thumb.
p. pe'dis, great toe; hallux.

pollinosis (pol"ĭ-no'sis) an allergic reaction to pollen; hay fever.

pollution (pŏ-lu'shun) defiling or making impure, especially contamination by noxious substances.

polonium (po-lo'ne-um) a chemical element, atomic number 84, atomic weight 210, symbol Po. (See table of ELEMENTS.)

poloxalkol (pol-ok'sal-kol) a compound used as a fecal softener.

polus (po'lus), pl. po'li [L.] pole.

poly (pol'e) a polymorphonuclear leukocyte.

poly- (pol'e) word element [Gr.], many.

polyadenia (pol"e-ah-de'ne-ah) pseudoleukemia.

polyadenomatosis (pol"e-ad"ĕ-no"mah-to'sis) multiple adenomas in a part.

polyadenosis (pol"e-ad"ĕ-no'sis) disorder of several glands, particularly endocrine glands.

polyadenous (pol"e-ad'ĕ-nus) having or affecting many glands.

polyagglutinability (pol"e-ah-gloo"tĭ-nah-bil'ĭ-te) susceptibility to agglutination by a number of agents.

polyamine-methylene resin (pol"e-am'in-meth'-ĭ-lēn) an anion-exchange resin used as a gastric antacid.

polyandry (pol"e-an'dre) 1. concurrent marriage of a woman to more than one man. 2. union of two or more male pronuclei with a female pronucleus, resulting in polyploidy of the zygote.

polyangiitis (pol"e-an"je-i'tis) inflammation involving multiple blood or lymph vessels.

polyarteritis (pol"e-ar"ter-i'tis) inflammation of several arteries.
p. nodo'sa, periarteritis nodosa.

polyarthric (pol"e-ar'thrik) polyarticular.

polyarthritis (pol"e-ar-thri'tis) inflammation of several joints.
p. rheumat'ica, rheumatic fever.

polyarticular (pol"e-ar-tik'u-lar) affecting many joints.

polyatomic (pol"e-ah-tom'ik) made up of several atoms.

polybasic (pol"e-ba'sik) having several replaceable hydrogen atoms.

polyceptor (pol"e-sep'tor) an amboceptor capable of binding several different complements.

polychemotherapy (pol"e-ke"mo-ther'ah-pe) simultaneous administration of several chemotherapeutic agents.

polycholia (pol"e-ko'le-ah) excessive secretion of bile.

polychondritis (pol″e-kon-dri′tis) inflammation of many cartilages of the body.

chronic atrophic p., p. chron′ica atro′phicans, relapsing p., an acquired disease of unknown origin, chiefly involving various cartilages and showing both chronicity and a tendency to recurrence.

polychondropathy (pol″e-kon-drop′ah-the) relapsing polychondritis.

polychrest (pol′e-krest) 1. useful in many conditions. 2. a remedy that is useful in many diseases.

polychromatic (pol″e-kro-mat′ik) many-colored.

polychromatophil (pol″e-kro-mat′o-fil) a cell or other element stainable with many kinds of stain.

polychromatophilia (pol″e-kro-mat″o-fil′e-ah) 1. the property of being stainable with various stains or tints; affinity for all sorts of stains. 2. a condition in which the erythrocytes, on staining, show various shades of blue combined with tinges of pink.

polyclinic (pol″e-klin′ik) a hospital or infirmary treating patients with many kinds of diseases.

polyclonia (pol″e-klo′ne-ah) a disease marked by many clonic spasms.

Polycycline (pol″e-si′klēn) trademark for preparations of tetracycline hydrochloride, an antibiotic.

polycyesis (pol″e-si-e′sis) multiple pregnancy.

polycystic (pol″e-sis′tik) containing many cysts or cavities.

polycyte (pol′e-sīt) a hypersegmented polymorphonuclear leukocyte of normal size.

polycythemia (pol″e-si-the′me-ah) abnormal increase in the erythrocyte count or in hemoglobin concentration.

There are two distinct forms of the disease. In primary polycythemia (called also polycythemia vera), the cause for the red cell increase is not understood. There is hyperplasia of the cell-forming tissues of the bone marrow, with resultant elevation of the erythrocyte count and hemoglobin level, and an increase in the number of leukocytes and platelets. The condition has been compared to leukemia and regarded as a malignant neoplastic disease.

Secondary polycythemia is a physiologic condition resulting from a decreased oxygen supply to the tissues. The body attempts to compensate for the oxygen deficiency by manufacturing more hemoglobin and red blood cells. Living at high altitudes can produce polycythemia, as can severe chronic lung and heart disorders, especially congenital heart defects.

SYMPTOMS. The symptoms of both primary and secondary polycythemia are much the same. The increased erythrocyte production results in thickening of the blood and an increased tendency toward clotting. The viscosity of the blood limits its ability to flow properly, diminishing the supply of blood to the brain and to other vital tissues. This may cause mental sluggishness, irritability, headache, dizziness, fainting, disturbances of sensation in the hands and feet and a feeling of fullness in the head. There may be episodes of acute pain as spontaneous clots occur in the blood vessels.

The spleen becomes enlarged. The smaller veins become more prominent, so that the skin has a bluish hue. The secondary form is often accompanied by enlargement of the tips of the fingers (clubbing).

In another form, polycythemia hypertonica, called also Gaisböck's disease, there is no spleen enlargement, but hypertrophy of the heart and increased blood pressure.

TREATMENT. Treatment is aimed at reducing the red cell count and decreasing the blood volume. It includes both the modern techniques of radiation therapy and the ancient practice of bloodletting. In mild cases periodic bloodletting may be the only treatment necessary. More recent methods use radioactive phosphorus or nitrogen mustard and other alkylating agents.

In secondary polycythemia, successful treatment of the causative illness will relieve the polycythemia.

polycytosis (pol″e-si-to′sis) excess of cells in the blood.

polydactylia (pol″e-dak-til′e-ah) the presence of supernumerary fingers or toes.

polydentia (pol″e-den′she-ah) polydontia; presence of supernumerary teeth.

polydipsia (pol″e-dip′se-ah) excessive thirst.

polydysspondylism (po,″e-dis-spon′dĭ-lizm) malformation of several vertebrae and the sella turcica, with dwarfed stature and low intelligence.

polyembryony (pol″e-em-bri′o-ne) the production of two or more embryos from a single ovum.

polyemia (pol″e-e′me-ah) excessive blood in the body.

p. hyperalbumino′sa, excess of albumin in the blood plasma.

p. polycythem′ica, an increase in the number of red corpuscles in the blood.

p. sero′sa, increase in the amount of blood serum.

polyesthesia (pol″e-es-the′ze-ah) a sensation as if several points were touched on application of a stimulus to a single point.

polyesthetic (pol″e-es-thet′ik) affecting several senses.

polyethylene (pol″e-eth′ĭ-lēn) a synthetic plastic material formed by polymerization of ethylene, used in reparative surgery.

p. glycol, a polymer of ethylene oxide and water, available in liquid form (polyethylene glycol 300 or 400) or as waxy solids (polyethylene glycol 1540 or 4000), used in various pharmaceutical preparations as a water-soluble ointment base.

polygalactia (pol″e-gah-lak′she-ah) excessive secretion of milk.

polygenic (pol″e-jen′ik) pertaining to or influenced by several different genes.

polyglandular (pol″e-glan′du-lar) affecting many glands.

polygnathus (po-lig′nah-thus) a double monster united by the jaws.

polygram (pol′e-gram) a tracing made by a polygraph.

polygraph (pol'e-graf) an apparatus for simultaneously recording several mechanical or electrical impulses, such as blood pressure, pulse and respiration, and variations in electrical resistance of the skin; used frequently as a lie detector.

polygyny (po-lij'ĭ-ne) 1. concurrent marriage of a man to more than one woman. 2. union of two or more female pronuclei with one male pronucleus, resulting in polyploidy of the zygote.

polygyria (pol″e-ji're-ah) a condition in which there is more than the normal number of convolutions in the brain.

polyhedral (pol″e-he'dral) having many sides or surfaces.

polyhidrosis (pol″e-hĭ-dro'sis) excessive secretion of sweat.

polyhydramnios (pol″e-hi-dram'ne-os) excess of amniotic fluid in pregnancy, usually defined as greater than 2000 ml.

polyhydruria (pol″e-hi-droo're-ah) abnormal dilution of the urine.

polyinfection (pol″e-in-fek'shun) infection with more than one organism.

polykaryocyte (pol″e-kar'e-o-sīt″) a giant cell containing several nuclei.

Polykol (pol'e-kol) trademark for preparations of poloxalkol, a fecal softener.

polyleptic (pol″e-lep'tik) having many remissions and excerbations.

polymastia (pol″e-mas'te-ah) the presence of more than two breasts.

polymelus (po-lim'ĕ-lus) a fetus with supernumerary limbs.

polymenia, polymenorrhea (pol″e-me'ne-ah), (pol″e-men″o-re'ah) abnormally frequent menstruation.

polymer (pol'ĭ-mer) a compound, usually of high molecular weight, formed by combination of simpler molecules.
    addition p., one formed by repeated combination of the smaller molecules (monomers) without formation of any other product.
    condensation p., one formed by repeated combination of the smaller molecules, with simultaneous elimination of water or other simple compound, e.g., nylon.

polymeria (pol″ĭ-me're-ah) the presence of supernumerary parts of the body.

polymeric (pol″ĭ-mer'ik) characterized by polymerism.

polymerism (po-lim'ĕ-rizm, pol'ĭ-mĕ-rizm″) the phenomenon or process that results in the formation of a polymer.

polymerization (po-lim″er-ĭ-za'shun, pol″ĭ-mer″-ĭ-za'shun) the formation of a compound, usually of high molecular weight, by the combination of several identical molecules (monomers).

polymicrobial (pol″e-mi-kro'be-al) pertaining to or caused by several varieties of pathogenic microorganisms.

polymorph (pol'e-morf) a polymorphonuclear leukocyte.

polymorphism (pol″e-mor'fizm) the quality of existing in several different forms. adj., **polymor'-phic, polymor'phous.**

polymorphocellular (pol″e-mor″fo-sel'u-lar) having cells of many forms.

polymorphonuclear (pol″e-mor″fo-nu'kle-ar) having a nucleus so deeply lobed or so divided as to appear to be multiple.
    p. leukocyte, a type of granular leukocyte with an irregularly lobed nucleus.

polymyalgia (pol″e-mi-al'je-ah) pain involving many muscles.

polymyoclonus (pol″e-mi-ok'lo-nus) 1. a fine or minute muscular tremor. 2. polyclonia.

polymyopathy (pol″e-mi-op'ah-the) disease affecting several muscles simultaneously.

polymyositis (pol″e-mi″o-si'tis) inflammation of many muscles.

polymyxin (pol″e-mik'sin) an antibiotic substance derived from culture of various strains of *Bacillus polymyxa,* several closely related compounds being designated by letters.
    p. B sulfate, a bacteriostatic and bactericidal, effective mainly against gram-negative organisms. It is especially effective against *Pseudomonas aeruginosa,* which may cause septicemia, meningitis, urinary tract infections and middle ear infections. Toxicity is low but there may be some damage to kidney and nerve cells.
    Polymyxin is administered parenterally or orally. Oral preparations are not used for systemic infections because the drug is poorly absorbed from the intestinal tract. It may be administered topically in the ear; before application the external acoustic meatus should be cleaned and dried thoroughly.

polynesic (pol″ĭ-ne'sik) affecting many separate locations.

polyneural (pol″e-nu'ral) pertaining to many nerves.

polyneuralgia (pol″e-nu-ral'je-ah) neuralgia of several nerves.

polyneuritis (pol″e-nu-ri'tis) inflammation involving many peripheral nerves.
    acute febrile p., acute infectious p., a disease beginning with fever followed by paralysis of the face, trunk and proximal segments of the limbs.
    diabetic p., polyneuritis seen in diabetes mellitus variously affecting sensory or motor nerves.

polyneuromyositis (pol″e-nu″ro-mi-o-si'tis) inflammation involving several muscles, with loss of reflexes, sensory loss and paresthesias.

polyneuropathy (pol″e-nu-rop'ah-the) a disease involving several nerves.
    erythredema p., a condition occurring in infants, marked by swollen bluish red hands and feet and disordered digestion, followed by multiple arthritis and muscular weakness; called also acrodynia.

polyneuroradiculitis (pol″e-nu″ro-rah-dik″u-li′-tis) inflammation of spinal ganglia, nerve roots and peripheral nerves.

polynuclear (pol″e-nu′kle-ar) 1. polynucleate. 2. polymorphonuclear.

polynucleate (pol″e-nu′kle-āt) having many nuclei.

polyodontia (pol″e-o-don′she-ah) presence of supernumerary teeth.

polyonychia (pol″e-o-nik′e-ah) presence of supernumerary nails.

polyopia (pol″e-o′pe-ah) visual perception of several images of a single object.

polyorchidism (pol″e-or′kĭ-dizm) the presence of more than two testes.

polyorchis (pol″e-or′kis) a person exhibiting polyorchidism.

polyorchism (pol″e-or′kizm) polyorchidism.

polyorrhymenitis (pol″e-or″hi-mĕ-ni′tis) malignant inflammation of serous membranes.

polyostotic (pol″e-os-tot′ik) affecting several bones.

polyotia (pol″e-o′she-ah) the presence of more than two ears.

polyovulatory (pol″e-ov′u-lah-tor″e) normally discharging several ova in one ovarian cycle.

polyp (pol′ip) a growth extending outward from a mucous membrane. Polyps may be attached to a membrane by a thin stalk, in which case they are known as pedunculated polyps, or may have a broad base (sessile polyps). They are usually an overgrowth of normal tissue, but sometimes polyps are true tumors – that is, masses of new tissue separate from the supporting membrane. Usually benign, they may lead to complications or eventually become malignant.

Polyps may occur wherever there is mucous membrane: in the nose, ears, mouth, lungs, heart, stomach, intestines, urinary bladder, uterus and cervix.

Polyps are most commonly found in the uterus, where they may cause excessive menstrual flow and sometimes sterility. They are often removed by surgery.

Cervical polyps are more dangerous than uterine polyps since they are more likely to become malignant.

Nasal polyps grow in the nasal cavity or in the sinuses. They are produced by local irritation, sometimes as a result of an allergy. They are not dangerous, but if they grow large enough to extend into the nose, they sometimes cause stuffiness and headaches. It is necessary to treat the allergy or any other source of irritation responsible for the growth of polyps. If the polyps continue to be troublesome, surgery may be necessary.

Polyps occasionally occur on the gingiva between the teeth. Here again, the only problem is discomfort; they may easily be removed. Much the same is true of the raspberry-shaped polyp occasionally found in the ear.

Polyps in the stomach are rarer but more serious. A polyp can cause pain if the stalk is sufficiently long for the polyp to be drawn into the duodenum. Usually, however, no pain is felt. When stomach polyps are discovered, they should be removed by surgery. Although usually benign, they may become malignant in time.

Polyps also form in the intestines. Usually they appear there in middle age, but some infants are born with polyps in the large intestine. Multiple intestinal polyps may be a hereditary disorder. In most cases they cause no symptoms unless they become large enough to obstruct the intestine or become ulcerated so that they bleed. When they do, symptoms may include cramping pains in the lower abdomen, diarrhea and the passage of blood and mucus.

Whether or not they cause symptoms, intestinal polyps should be removed by surgery, since any one of them may become malignant. Although all causes of intestinal cancer have not yet been discovered, it is believed that polyps are often a contributing factor.

In males, polyps sometimes occur in the urethra, usually as the result of some disorder of the prostate. They are not likely to develop into cancer, but they may cause a discharge from the urethra and make urination difficult or frequent. They do not affect sexual potency or vigor. Although these polyps can be removed by surgery, they are more often removed by fulguration.

In women, a urethral polyp, or caruncle, is a small growth on the mucous membrane of the urethra. It may cause pain on urination, vaginal discharge or bleeding. Caruncles are easily removed by fulguration.

polyparesis (pol″e-pah-re′sis) general paresis.

polypathia (pol″e-path′e-ah) the presence of several diseases at one time.

polypectomy (pol″e-pek′to-me) surgical excision of a polyp.

polypeptidase (pol″e-pep′tĭ-dās) an enzyme that catalyzes the hydrolysis of polypeptides.

polypeptide (pol″e-pep′tīd) a compound containing two or more amino acids linked by a peptide bond; called dipeptide, tripeptide, etc., depending on the number of amino acids present.

polyperiostitis (pol″e-per″e-os-ti′tis) inflammation of the periosteum of several bones.
  p. hyperesthet′ica, a chronic disease of the periosteum with extreme tenderness of the skin and soft parts.

polyphagia (pol″e-fa′je-ah) excessive ingestion of food.

polyphalangia (pol″e-fah-lan′je-ah) excess of phalanges in a finger or toe.

polypharmacy (pol″e-far′mah-se) the simultaneous administration of several therapeutic agents in combination or separately.

polyphasic (pol″e-fa′zik) having or existing in many phases; containing colloids of several types.

polyphobia (pol″e-fo′be-ah) abnormal fear of many things.

polyphrasia (pol″e-fra′ze-ah) excessive talkativeness.

polyplastic (pol″e-plas′tik) 1. containing many structural or constituent elements. 2. undergoing many changes of form.

polyplegia (pol″e-ple′je-ah) paralysis of several muscles.

polyploid (pol′e-ploid) 1. characterized by polyploidy. 2. an individual or cell characterized by polyploidy.

polyploidy (pol′e-ploi″de) the state of having more than two sets of homologous chromosomes.

polypnea (pol″ip-ne′ah) rapid or panting respiration.

polypodia (pol″e-po′de-ah) the presence of supernumerary feet.

polypoid (pol′y-poid) resembling a polyp.

polyposia (pol″ĭ-po′ze-ah) ingestion of abnormally increased amounts of fluids for long periods of time.

polyposis (pol″ĭ-po′sis) the formation of numerous polyps.
    familial p., the appearance in childhood of innumerable adenomatous polyps in the lower bowel, tending to occur in several members of the same family.

polypus (pol′ĭ-pus), pl. *pol′ypi* [L.] polyp.

polyradiculitis (pol″e-rah-dik″u-li′tis) inflammation of the nerve roots.

polyradiculoneuritis (pol″e-rah-dik″u-lo-nu-ri′-tis) acute infectious polyneuritis that involves the peripheral nerves, the spinal nerve roots and the spinal cord.

polyribosome (pol″e-ri′bo-sōm) a cluster of ribosomes in the cytoplasm of a cell, the site of protein synthesis.

polysaccharide (pol″e-sak′ah-rīd) a carbohydrate which, on acid hydrolysis, yields 10 or more monosaccharides.
    immune p's, polysaccharides that can function as specific antigens, such as bacterial capsular substances.

polysarcous (pol″e-sar′kus) corpulent; too fleshy.

polyscelia (pol″e-se′le-ah) the presence of more than two legs.

polyserositis (pol″e-se″ro-si′tis) general inflammation of serous membranes.

polysinusectomy (pol″e-si″nŭ-sek′to-me) excision of diseased mucous membrane of several paranasal sinuses.

polysinusitis (pol″e-si″nŭ-si′tis) inflammation of several sinuses.

polysome (pol′e-sōm) polyribosome.

polysomia (pol″e-so′me-ah) a developmental anomaly with doubling or tripling of the body.

polysomus (pol″e-so′mus) a fetal monster exhibiting polysomia.

polysomy (pol″e-so′me) an excess of a particular chromosome.

polysorbate 80 (pol″e-sor′bāt) an oleate ester of sorbitol and its anhydride condensed with polymers of ethylene oxide; used as a surfactant.

polyspermia (pol″e-sper′me-ah) 1. excessive secretion of semen. 2. polyspermy.

polyspermy (pol″e-sper′me) fertilization of an ovum by more than one spermatozoon; occurring normally in certain species (physiologic polyspermy) and sometimes abnormally in others (pathologic polyspermy).

polystichia (pol″e-stik′e-ah) two or more rows of eyelashes on an eyelid.

polytene (pol′e-tēn) composed of or containing many strands of chromatin (chromonemata).

polyteny (pol″e-te′ne) reduplication of chromonemata in the chromosome without separation into distinct daughter chromosomes.

polythelia (pol″e-the′le-ah) the presence of supernumerary nipples.

polytocous (po-lit′ŏ-kus) giving birth to several offspring at one time.

polytrichia (pol″e-trik′e-ah) hypertrichosis; excessive hairiness.

polytrophia (pol″e-tro′fe-ah) excessive nutrition.

polytropic (pol″e-trop′ik) affecting many kinds of bacteria or several kinds of tissue.

polyunguia (pol″e-ung′gwe-ah) the presence of supernumerary nails on the fingers or toes; polyonychia.

polyuria (pol″e-u′re-ah) excessive excretion of urine.

polyvalent (pol″e-va′lent) having more than one valence.
    p. vaccine, one prepared from more than one strain or species of microorganisms.

polyvinylpyrrolidone (pol″e-vi″nil-pi-rol′ĭ-dōn) PVP, a polymer of formaldehyde, sometimes used as a plasma volume expander.

Pompe's disease (pomps) generalized glycogenosis.

pompholyx (pom′fo-liks) a skin disease with small, deep-seated vesicles on the palms and soles and between the digits.

pomphus (pom′fus) a wheal.

pomum (po′mum), pl. *po′ma* [L.] apple.
    p. ada′mi, the prominence on the throat caused by thyroid cartilage; Adam's apple.

ponophobia (po″no-fo′be-ah) abnormal fear of pain or fatigue.

ponos (po′nos) infantile kala-azar.

pons (ponz) 1. that part of the hindbrain lying above the medulla oblongata and below the midbrain or mesencephalon; with the cerebellum and middle part of the fourth ventricle, constituting the metencephalon. 2. a slip of tissue connecting two parts of an organ.

p. tari′ni, the floor of the posterior perforated substance, an area on the ventral surface of the brain.

p. varo′lii, pons (1).

ponticulus (pon-tik′u-lus), pl. *pontic′uli* [L.] propons. adj., **pontic′ular.**

pontine (pon′tīn) pertaining to the pons.

Pontocaine (pon′to-kān) trademark for preparations of tetracaine, a topical anesthetic.

pontocerebellar (pon″to-ser″ĕ-bel′ar) pertaining to the pons and cerebellum.

popliteal (pop″lī-te′al) pertaining to the area behind the knee.

poradenitis (pōr″ad-ĕ-ni′tis) suppurative inflammation of lymph nodes with formation of draining fistulas.

p. nos′tras, lymphogranuloma venereum.

porcine (pōr′sīn) pertaining to, characteristic of or derived from swine.

porcupine disease ichthyosis.

pore (pōr) a small opening or empty space.

porencephalia (po″ren-sĕ-fa′le-ah) the development or presence of abnormal cavities in the brain tissue.

porencephalitis (po″ren-sef″ah-li′tis) porencephalia with inflammation of the brain.

porencephalous (po″ren-sef′ah-lus) characterized by porencephalia.

porencephaly (po″ren-sef′ah-le) porencephalia.

porocele (po′ro-sēl) scrotal hernia with thickening of the coverings.

porokeratosis (po″ro-ker″ah-to′sis) hypertrophy of the stratum corneum of the skin, followed by its atrophy.

porosis (po-ro′sis) 1. formation of the callus at the ends of fractured bones. 2. cavity formation.

porosity (po-ros′ĭ-te) the condition of being porous.

porotomy (po-rot′o-me) meatotomy.

porous (po′rus) penetrated by pores and open spaces.

porphin (por′fīn) the fundamental ring structure of four linked pyrrole nuclei around which porphyrins and chlorophyll are built.

porphobilinogen (por″fo-bi-lin′o-jen) an intermediary product in the biosynthesis of heme.

porphobilinogenuria (por″fo-bi-lin″o-jen-u′re-ah) excretion of porphobilinogen in the urine.

porphyria (por-fēr′e-ah) a genetic disorder characterized by a disturbance in porphyrin metabolism with resultant increase in the formation and excretion of porphyrins (uroporphyrin and coproporphyrin) or their precursors; called also hematoporphyria. Porphyrins, in combination with iron, form hemes, which in turn combine with specific proteins to form hemoproteins. Hemoglobin is a hemoprotein, as are many other substances that are essential to normal functioning of the cells and tissues of the body.

Two general types of porphyria are known: erythropoietic porphyrias, which are concerned with the formation of erythrocytes in the bone marrow; and hepatic porphyrias, which are responsible for liver dysfunction.

The manifestations of porphyria include gastrointestinal, neurologic and psychologic symptoms, cutaneous photosensitivity, pigmentation of the face (and later of the bones) and anemia with enlargement of the spleen. Large amounts of porphyrins are excreted in the urine and feces.

Treatment of this condition has been primarily symptomatic and varies in its effectiveness. Photosensitivity may be controlled by avoiding exposure to light. Removal of the spleen is useful in some cases of the erythropoietic type of porphyria. Drug therapy includes the use of phenothiazines, chlorpromazine and promazine in particular. These drugs allay pain and nervousness and apparently allow a period of remission from symptoms. Corticotropin has been successful in some cases.

Patients with porphyria must not be given barbiturates, sulfonamides, alcohol or chloroquine as these chemicals may precipitate or intensify attacks. It is recommended that patients with this disease carry with them at all times some means of identifying themselves as having porphyria so that in an emergency they will not be given a drug that may precipitate an attack, and possibly cause death.

porphyrin (por′fĭ-rin) one of a group of complex cyclic compounds that are important components of hemoglobin, myoglobin, cytochrome and catalase.

porphyrinogen (por″fĭ-rin′o-jen) a colorless, fully hydrogenated compound giving rise to the corresponding porphyrin by oxidation.

porphyrinopathy (por″fĭ-rĭ-nop′ah-the) a disorder of porphyrin metabolism.

porphyrinuria (por″fĭ-rĭ-nu′re-ah) excretion of an abnormal type or quantity of porphyrin in the urine.

porrigo (por′ĭ-go) ringworm or other disease of the scalp.

p. decal′vans, alopecia areata.

p. favo′sa, favus.

p. larva′lis, eczema with impetigo of the scalp.

porta (por′tah), pl. *por′tae* [L.] an entrance or gateway, especially the site where blood vessels and other supplying or draining structures enter an organ.

p. hep′atis, the transverse fissure of the liver, where the portal vein and hepatic artery enter and the hepatic ducts leave.

portacaval (por″tah-ka′val) pertaining to or connecting the portal vein and inferior vena cava.

portal (por′tal) 1. an avenue of entrance. 2. pertaining to an entrance, especially the porta hepatis.

p. circulation, a general term denoting the circulation of blood through larger vessels from the capillaries of one organ to those of another; applied especially to the passage of blood from the gastrointestinal tract and spleen through the portal vein to the liver. (See also CIRCULATORY SYSTEM.)

p. of entry, the pathway by which bacteria or other pathogenic agents gain entry to the body.

p. vein, a short, thick trunk formed by the union of the superior mesenteric and splenic veins behind the neck of the pancreas; it ascends to the right end of the porta hepatis, where it divides into successively smaller branches, following branches of the hepatic artery, until it forms a capillary system of sinusoids that permeates the entire substance of the liver.

portio (por'she-o), pl. *portio'nes* [L.] a part or division; used in names of parts of various structures of the body.

p. du'ra, the facial nerve.

p. interme'dia, a fascicle that joins the facial and vestibulocochlear nerves; called also intermediate nerve.

p. mol'lis, vestibulocochlear nerve.

p. vagina'lis, the portion of the uterus that projects into the vagina.

portogram (por'to-gram) the film obtained by portography.

portography (por-tog'rah-fe) roentgenography of the portal vein after injection of opaque material.

portal p., portography after injection of opaque material into the superior mesenteric vein or one of its branches, the abdomen being opened.

splenic p., portography after percutaneous injection of opaque material into the substance of the spleen.

port-wine stain a diffuse, poorly defined area varying from pink to dark bluish red, involving otherwise normal skin; nevus flammeus.

porus (po'rus), pl. *po'ri* [L.] an opening; used in names of various openings in the body.

p. acus'ticus exter'nus, the outer end of the external acoustic meatus.

p. acus'ticus inter'nus, the opening of the internal acoustic meatus in the cranial cavity.

p. op'ticus, the opening in the sclera for passage of the optic nerve.

-posia (po'ze-ah) word element [Gr.], *drinking; intake of fluids.*

position (po-zish'un) 1. the placement of body members, as a particular position assumed by the patient to achieve comfort in certain conditions, or the particular arrangement of body parts to facilitate the performance of certain diagnostic or therapeutic procedures. 2. in obstetrics, the relation of the body of the fetus to the maternal pelvis at the beginning of parturition (see table).

anatomic p., that of the human body, standing erect, with palms facing forward, used as the position of reference in designating the site or direction of structures of the body.

decubitus p., that of the body lying on a horizontal surface, designated according to the aspect of the body touching the surface as dorsal decubitus (on the back), left or right lateral decubitus (on the left or right side) and ventral decubitus position (on the anterior surface).

dorsal recumbent p., the patient lies on his back with his legs slightly separated, thighs slightly flexed on the body and legs on the thighs with the soles of the feet resting on the bed.

Fowler's p., the head of the patient's bed is raised 18 to 20 inches above the level.

genupectoral p., knee-chest p., the patient rests on his knees and chest. The head is turned to one side, and the arms are extended on the bed, the elbows flexed and resting so that they partially bear the weight of the patient. The abdomen remains unsupported, though a small pillow may be placed under the chest.

lithotomy p., the patient lies on his back with the legs well separated, the thighs acutely flexed on the abdomen and the legs on the thighs. Stirrups may be used to support the feet and legs.

orthopneic p., the patient's head and arms rest on an overbed table padded with pillows and placed across his lap. The table is elevated to a comfortable height, and the back is supported with pillows. Used when the patient has difficulty breathing in any position other than sitting up.

recumbent p., the patient lies on his back with

VARIOUS FETAL POSITIONS IN UTERO

IN CEPHALIC PRESENTATION
Vertex — occiput the point of direction
  Left occipitoanterior (L.O.A.)
  Left occipitotransverse (L.O.T.)
  Right occipitoposterior (R.O.P.)
  Right occipitotransverse (R.O.T.)
  Right occipitoanterior (R.O.A.)
  Left occipitoposterior (L.O.P.)
Face — chin the point of direction
  Right mentoposterior (R.M.P.)
  Left mentoanterior (L.M.A.)
  Right mentotransverse (R.M.T.)
  Right mentoanterior (R.M.A.)
  Left mentotransverse (L.M.T.)
  Left mentoposterior (L.M.P.)
Brow — the point of direction
  Right frontoposterior (R.F.P.)
  Left frontoanterior (L.F.A.)
  Right frontotransverse (R.F.T.)
  Right frontoanterior (R.F.A.)
  Left frontotransverse (L.F.T.)
  Left frontoposterior (L.F.P.)

IN BREECH PRESENTATION
Complete breech — sacrum, the point of direction
  (feet crossed and thighs flexed on abdomen)
  Left sacroanterior (L.S.A.)
  Left sacrotransverse (L.S.T.)
  Right sacroposterior (R.S.P.)
  Right sacroanterior (R.S.A.)
  Right sacrotransverse (R.S.T.)
  Left sacroposterior (L.S.P.)
Incomplete breech — sacrum the point of direction.
  Same designations as above, adding the qualifications footling, knee, etc.

IN TRANSVERSE PRESENTATION
Shoulder — scapula the point of direction

Left scapuloanterior (L. Sc. A.) Right scapuloanterior (R. Sc. A.)	Back anterior positions
Right scapuloposterior (R. Sc. P.) Left scapuloposterior (L. Sc. P.)	Back posterior positions

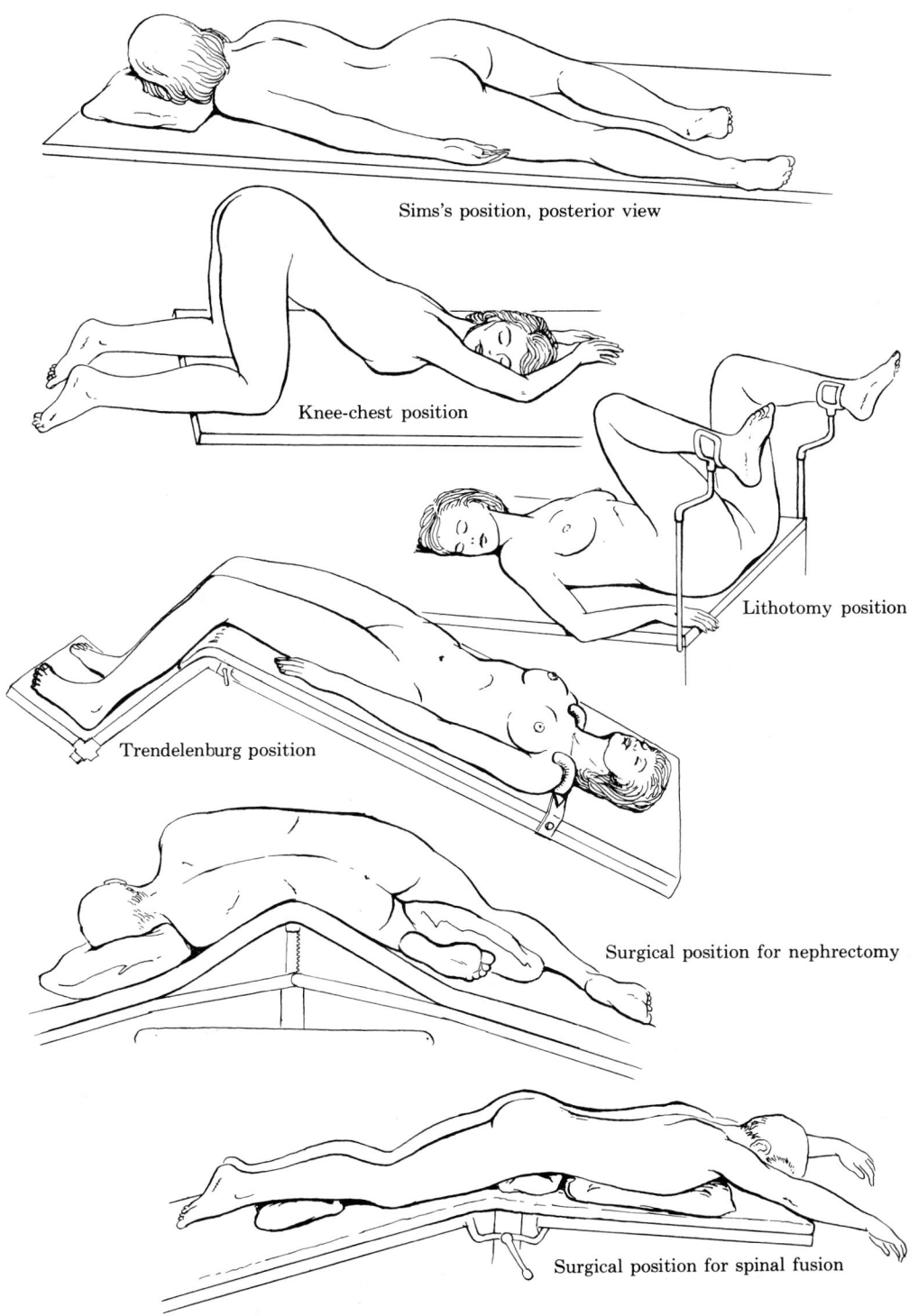

Sims's position, posterior view

Knee-chest position

Lithotomy position

Trendelenburg position

Surgical position for nephrectomy

Surgical position for spinal fusion

Positions. (From Dorland's Illustrated Medical Dictionary. 24th ed. Philadelphia, W. B. Saunders Co., 1965.)

legs extended or slightly flexed to relax the abdominal muscles.

Sims's p., the patient lies on his left side with the left thigh slightly flexed, and the right thigh acutely flexed on the abdomen. The left arm is drawn behind the body with the body inclined forward. The right arm may be positioned according to the patient's comfort. Called also left lateral position.

Trendelenburg's p., the patient lies on his back, on a plane inclined 45 degrees with the head lower than the rest of the body. The legs and knees flexed over the adjustable lower section of the table or bed, which is lowered. The patient is well supported to prevent slipping.

positive (poz'ĭ-tiv) having a value greater than zero; indicating existence or presence, as chromatin-positive or Wassermann-positive; characterized by affirmation or cooperation.

positron (poz'ĭ-tron) a positively charged electron.

posology (po-sol'o-je) the science of dosage or a system of dosage.

post (pōst) [L.] preposition, *after*.

post- (pōst) word element [L.] *after; behind* (in time or space).

postalbumin (pōst"al-bu'min) a serum protein that has an electrophoretic mobility between albumin and alpha-globulin at pH 8.6.

postcardiotomy (pōst-kar"de-ot'o-me) occurring after or as a consequence of open-heart surgery.

postcava (pōst-ka'vah) the inferior vena cava. adj., **postca'val.**

postcibal (pōst-si'bal) after eating.

postclavicular (pōst"klah-vik'u-lar) behind the clavicle.

postclimacteric (pōst"kli-mak'ter-ik) after the climacteric.

postcommissure (pōst-kom'ĭ-shūr) the posterior commissure of the brain.

postcommissurotomy syndrome (pōst-kom"ĭ-shūr-ot'o-me) fever, chest pain, pneumonitis and cardiomegaly, occurring frequently in patients who have undergone mitral commissurotomy and attributed by some to reactivation of rheumatic fever.

postdiastolic (pōst-di"as-tol'ik) after diastole.

postdicrotic (pōst"di-krot'ik) after the dicrotic elevation of the sphygmogram.

postencephalitis (pōst"en-sef"ah-li'tis) a condition sometimes remaining after recovery from epidemic encephalitis.

postepileptic (pōst"ep-ĭ-lep'tik) following an epileptic attack.

posterior (pos-tēr'e-or) directed toward or situated at the back; opposite of anterior.
 p. chamber, that part of the aqueous humor-containing space of the eyeball between the iris and the lens.

postero- (pos'ter-o) word element [L.], *the back; posterior to.*

posteroanterior (pos"ter-o-an-tēr'e-or) directed from the back toward the front.

posteroexternal (pos"ter-o-ek-ster'nal) situated on the outside of a posterior aspect.

posterolateral (pos"ter-o-lat'er-al) situated on the side and toward the posterior aspect.

posteromedian (pos"ter-o-me'de-an) situated on the middle of a posterior aspect.

posterosuperior (pos"ter-o-su-pēr'e-or) situated behind and above.

postesophageal (pōst"e-sof"ah-ge'al) behind the esophagus.

postethmoid (pōst-eth'moid) behind the ethmoid bone.

postganglionic (pōst"gang-gle-on'ik) distal to a ganglion.

postglomerular (pōst"glo-mer'u-lar) distal to a glomerulus of the kidney.

posthepatitic (post"hep-ah-tit'ik) occurring after or as a consequence of hepatitis.

posthioplasty (pos'the-o-plas"te) plastic repair of the prepuce.

posthitis (pos-thi'tis) inflammation of the prepuce.

postictal (pōst-ik'tal) following a seizure or stroke.

postligation (pōst"li-ga'shun) occurring after or as a consequence of ligation of a blood vessel

postmaturity (pōst"mah-tu'rĭ-te) overdevelopment; the condition of a postmature infant.

postmedian (pōst-me'de-an) behind a median line or plane.

postmeiotic (pōst"mi-ot'ik) occurring after or pertaining to the time following meiosis.

postminimus (pōst-min'ĭ-mus) an appendage attached to the proximal phalanx of the fifth finger or toe.

postmitotic (pōst"mi-tot'ik) occurring after or pertaining to the time following mitosis.

post mortem (pōst mor'tem) after death.

postmortem (pōst-mor'tem) performed or occurring after death.

postnatal (pōst-na'tal) occurring after birth.

postoblongata (pōst"ob-long-gah'tah) the part of the medulla oblongata below the pons.

postoperative (pōst-op'er-ah-tiv, pōst-op'er-a"tiv) after a surgical operation.
 p. care, care of the patient following a surgical procedure. Immediately after surgery the patient usually is transferred to a recovery room. This is a special unit within the operating room suite, designed to facilitate management of the patient recovering from anesthesia, and staffed with personnel experienced in this type of nursing care.
 Immediately after surgery, the patient requires constant attendance. A patent airway must be maintained so that respiration is adequate and of normal character. An endotracheal tube and RESPIRATOR may be used to assist the patient with respiratory

difficulties. The skin is observed for color, turgor and dryness. A flaccid, parchment-like skin indicates dehydration; cold clammy skin may be symptomatic of shock, and cyanosis and local discoloration are indicative of oxygen deficiency as a result of an obstructed airway or impaired circulation. The pulse, respirations and blood pressure are checked every 15 minutes or oftener; notes are made as to their quality, rate and rhythm.

The position of the patient may be governed by the type of surgery done, but ideally the patient should be placed on his side with a pillow to his back for support. The uppermost leg is slightly flexed to relieve tension on the abdominal muscles and may be supported with a small pillow. The side position allows for drainage of mucus or other material in the mouth and lessens the danger of aspiration of vomitus. During vomiting the head is kept turned to the side and suctioning is used as necessary to clear the air passages. The patient's position should be changed at least every 2 hours unless there is a contraindication, and pressure areas are gently massaged. When repositioning the patient, all movements should be gentle and slow, as sudden overstimulation can cause a drop in blood pressure.

While the patient is awakening from anesthesia the hospital personnel must use caution in their conversations and statements made about the patients in the unit. With his senses dulled and his reasoning hampered by drugs and anesthesia, the patient may misinterpret the sounds and statements he hears. Noise must be kept at a minimum, voices should be kept low and whispering (which is rude at any time) is especially disturbing to the patient recovering from anesthesia.

In many cases a catheter, nasogastric tube or drainage tube is inserted during surgery. The purposes of these should be understood by the nurse and it is usually her responsibility to connect them to the proper drainage and suction apparatus. Dressings around drainage tubes should be observed for excess drainage or bleeding and reinforced as necessary.

Other physical aspects of postoperative care are outlined in the table. See also specific operative procedures (e.g., COLOSTOMY) and specific organs (e.g., surgery of the KIDNEY or LUNG). For complications that may arise during the postoperative period, see also SHOCK, HEMORRHAGE, THROMBOSIS, EMBOLISM and CARDIAC ARREST.

postoral (pōst-o'ral) in the back part of the mouth.

postparalytic (pōst"par-ah-lit'ik) following an attack of paralysis.

POSTOPERATIVE CARE

I. Control of pain	Nursing measures to provide maximum comfort and reassurance of the patient Analgesic drugs
II. Maintenance of drainage	Urinary catheters Gastric suction Thoracic drainage Bile drainage Drainage from surgical wounds
III. Maintenance of fluid and electrolyte balance	Intravenous fluids and minerals Oral intake Observation and recording of output
IV. Relief of abdominal distention, nausea and vomiting	Rectal tube Gastric suction Ice collar Antiemetic drugs
V. Prevention of complications: A. Shock B. Hemorrhage	Close observation for signs of shock and hemorrhage
C. Blood clots in vascular system	Frequent turning Early ambulation
D. Hypostatic pneumonia	Encourage coughing and deep breathing and turn frequently
E. Decubitus ulcers	Frequent turning Skin care
F. Contractures	Proper positioning Exercise
G. Wound infection	Adherence to the basic principles of cleanliness and asepsis

From Keane, C. B.: Essentials of Nursing. 2nd ed. Philadelphia, W. B. Saunders Co., 1969.

post partum (pōst par'tum) after parturition.

postpartum (pōst-par'tum) occurring after childbirth or after delivery.

postpontile (pōst-pon'tīl) behind the pons.

postprandial (pōst-pran'de-al) after a meal.

postpubescent (pōst″pu-bes'ent) after puberty.

postsynaptic (pōst″sĭ-nap'tik) situated distal to a synapse, or occurring after the synapse is crossed.

postulate (pos'tu-lāt) anything assumed or taken for granted.

    Koch's 's, a statement of the kind of experimental evidence required to establish the causative relation of a given microorganism to a given disease. The conditions are: 1, the microorganism is present in every case of the disease; 2, it is to be cultivated in pure culture; 3, inoculation of such culture must produce the disease in susceptible animals; 4, it must be obtained from such animals, and again grown in a pure culture.

postural (pos'tu-ral) pertaining to posture or position.

    p. drainage, a form of physical therapy used to remove secretions from the lungs. The patient assumes a position in which the upper trunk is lower than the rest of the body; the force of gravity, in conjunction with the action of the cilia of the bronchial airways, moves secretions upward toward the trachea, so that the patient can cough them up more easily.

    Postural drainage is usually done three times a day: in the morning before breakfast, in the mid-afternoon and before retiring at night. At these times the stomach is likely to be empty, and nausea, gagging and vomiting are less likely to occur. The treatment usually lasts no more than 20 to 30 minutes, depending on the patient's tolerance. Mouth care is given after each treatment to remove the foul taste frequently accompanying removal of the stagnant mucus from the lower bronchial tree.

    "Clapping" and "vibrating" are often done in conjunction with postural drainage. These techniques require specific instructions from a physical therapist. In general they involve placing a cupped hand over the chest wall and gently tapping and vibrating the chest to assist in dislodging the plugs

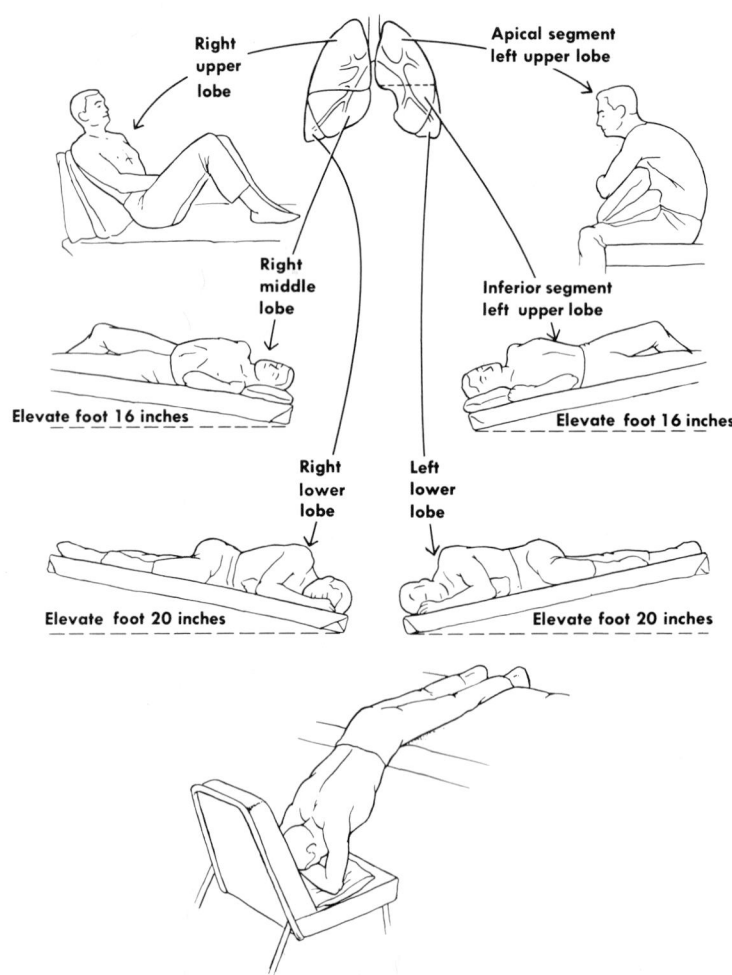

Postural drainage. Position for drainage of various portions of the lung. At bottom, a less specific position that is frequently used. (From Shafer, K. N., et al.: Medical-Surgical Nursing. 4th ed. St. Louis, C. V. Mosby Co., 1967.)

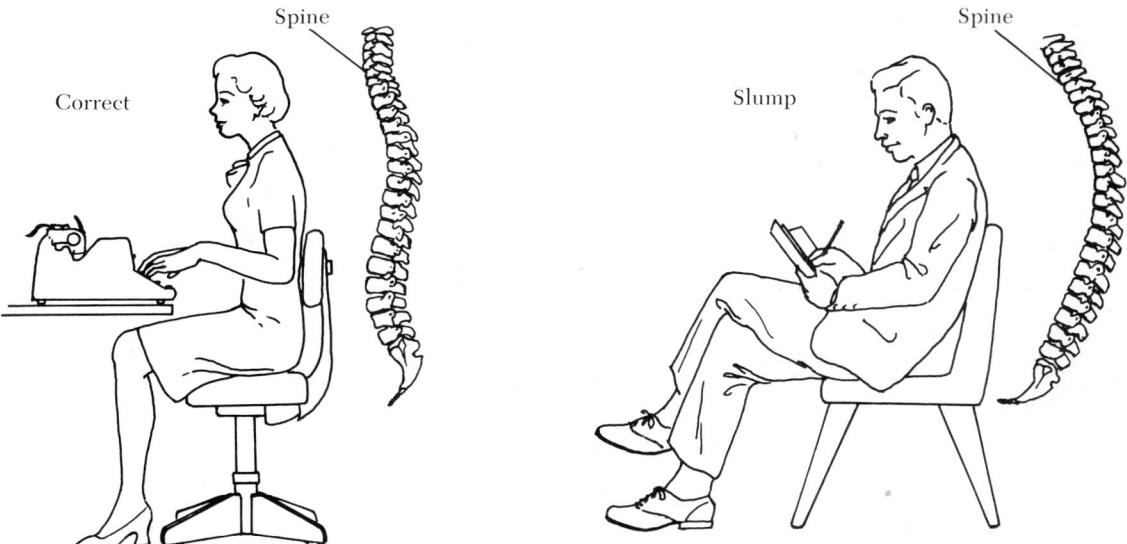

Left, good sitting posture: the spine and feet are in normal positions and the weight of the body is equally distributed. Right, slouching puts too much weight on the end of the spine, compresses internal organs, strains muscles and interferes with the circulation in the legs.

Correct standing posture, center, is easy and natural. The chest is slightly raised and the buttocks are tucked in. Left, too-rigid posture. Keeping the spine unnaturally straight can cause strain on the knees and back muscles. Right, slumping can lead to backache and round shoulders.

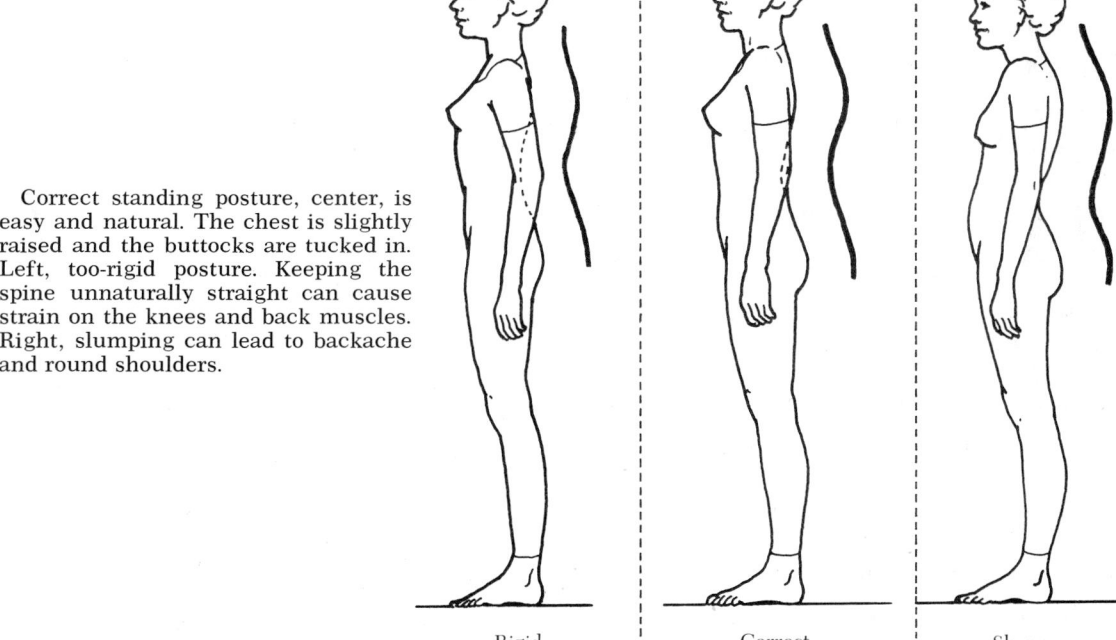

of mucus, allowing air to penetrate behind the secretions and thus helping in their removal.

Postural drainage is most helpful to patients with chronic bronchitis and bronchiectasis, and to certain postoperative patients.

posture (pos'tūr) an attitude of the body. Good posture cannot be defined by any rigid formula. It is usually considered to be the natural and comfortable bearing of the body in normal, healthy persons. This generally means that in a standing position the body is naturally, but not rigidly, straight, and that in a sitting position the back is comfortably straight.

Good standing and sitting posture helps promote normal functioning of the body's organs and increases the efficiency of the muscles, thereby minimizing fatigue. Good posture is also important to good appearance. Clothes fit better, movements become more graceful and an impression of poise is achieved.

Maintenance of good posture for a patient confined to bed or wheelchair is essential to the patient's general well-being and also is important in the prevention of deformities of the muscles and bones. The patient should be observed for evidence of "slumping," in which the normal curves of the spine are exaggerated. The rib cage should be supported so that the ribs are elevated and there is no constriction of the chest wall. Pillows are arranged under the shoulders and head so that the chin is not forced downward on the chest. Excessive extension of the ankles should be avoided by adequate support against the soles of the feet. The legs should be supported so that the weight of one does not fall on the other. The arms are supported so that they do not lie across the chest or pull the shoulders into a "rounded" position. Frequent changing of position and adequate exercise of the limbs are also essential to the maintenance of good posture and the prevention of deformities.

postuterine (pōst-u'ter-in) behind the uterus.

postvaccinal (pōst-vak'sĭ-nal) occurring after vaccinia or after inoculation of vaccinia virus.

postvermis (pōst-ver'mis) the lower surface of the vermis of the cerebellum.

postvital (pōst-vi'tal) following cessation of life.

postzygotic (pōst"zi-got'ik) occurring after or pertaining to the time following the union of the gametes (formation of the zygote).

potable (po'tah-bl) fit to drink.

potamophobia (po"tah-mo-fo'be-ah) a dread of large bodies of water.

potash (pot'ash) impure potassium carbonate.
  caustic p., potassium hydroxide.

potassa (po-tas'ah) potassium hydroxide.

potassemia (pot"ah-se'me-ah) excess of potassium in the blood.

potassic (po-tas'ik) containing potassium.

potassium (po-tas'e-um) a chemical element, atomic number 19, atomic weight 39.102, symbol K. (See table of ELEMENTS.) In combination with other minerals in the body, potassium forms alkaline salts that are important in body processes and play an essential role in maintenance of the acid-base and water balance in the body. All body cells, especially muscle tissue, require a high content of potassium. A proper balance between sodium, calcium and potassium in the blood plasma is necessary for proper cardiac function.

Since most foods contain a good supply of potassium, potassium deficiency (hypokalemia) is unlikely to be caused by an unbalanced diet. Possible causes include Cushing's syndrome (due to an adrenal gland disorder) and Fanconi's syndrome (the result of a congenital kidney defect). The cause could also be an excessive dose of cortisone or prolonged vomiting or diarrhea. Signs of potassium deficiency can include weakness and lethargy, rapid pulse, nausea, diarrhea and tingling sensations.

If the body absorbs enough potassium but the element is not distributed properly, various disorders may develop. Thus an abnormally low content of potassium in the blood may result in an intermittent temporary paralysis of the muscles, known as familial periodic paralysis.

Potassium deficiency can be treated by means of medication containing potassium salts. If the difficulty lies in the body's use of potassium, treatment is concerned with the primary cause of the deficiency.

p. acetate, a compound used as a systemic and urinary alkalizer.

p. bicarbonate, a compound used as a gastric antacid and to replenish electrolytes in the body.

p. bitartrate, a white crystalline salt used as a diuretic, cathartic and refrigerant.

p. bromide, a compound used as a sedative and antiepileptic.

p. carbonate, a salt used chiefly in pharmaceutical and chemical manufacturing procedures.

p. chlorate, a highly toxic compound used as an oxidizing germicide and for hemorrhoids and proctitis.

p. chloride, a compound used orally or intravenously as an electrolyte replenisher.

p. citrate, a white, granular powder used as a diuretic, expectorant, sudorific and systemic alkalizer.

p. gluconate, a compound used in the prophylaxis and treatment of hypokalemia.

p. hydroxide, a white, crystalline compound with alkaline and caustic properties.

p. iodide, a colorless, transparent compound used as an expectorant and in the prophylaxis of goiter.

p. nitrate, a salt used as a diuretic and as a topical mucous membrane antiseptic; called also niter and saltpeter.

p. permanganate, a dark purple, crystalline salt used as an oxidant and local anti-infectant.

p. sodium tartrate, a compound used as a saline cathartic and also in combination with sodium bicarbonate and tartaric acid (Seidlitz powders, a cathartic).

p. tartrate, a compound used as a diuretic, diaphoretic and cathartic.

potency (po'ten-se) power; especially (1) the ability of the male to perform coitus; (2) the power of a medicinal agent to produce the desired effects; (3) the ability of an embryonic part to develop and complete its destiny. adj., **po'tent.**

prospective p., the total developmental possibilities of an embryonic part.

potential (po-ten′shal) 1. existing and ready for action, but not active. 2. electric tension or pressure.

action p., the temporary change in electrical energy between stimulated and resting portions of a cell.

membrane p., the electric potential that exists on the two sides of a membrane or across the wall of a cell.

resting p., the potential present within the resting cell.

potentiation (po-ten″she-a′shun) enhancement of one agent by another so that the combined effect is greater than the sum of the effects of each one alone.

potion (po′shun) a large dose of liquid medicine.

Pott's disease (pots) tuberculous spondylitis, usually beginning as a tuberculous osteomyelitis of the vertebrae and progressing to damage of the intervertebral disks. If erosion continues unchecked, there is complete destruction of the affected vertebrae.

Symptoms include stiffness of the back, pain on motion, prominence of the spinous process of certain vertebrae and occasionally abscess formation, paralysis and abdominal pain. Diagnosis is confirmed by demonstration of *Mycobacterium tuberculosis* (the tubercle bacillus) in the affected bone.

Treatment includes administration of antibacterial drugs such as isoniazid and streptomycin. Para-aminosalicylic acid (PAS) may be used instead of streptomycin if streptomycin is contraindicated. Surgical fixation of the affected vertebrae (spinal fusion) may be required for correction of orthopedic deformities such as KYPHOSIS (hunchback) which may occur as a result of Pott's disease.

P's fracture, fracture of the lower part of the fibula with serious injury of the lower tibial articulation.

pouch (powch) a pocket-like space, cavity or sac, e.g., one formed by bending back of the peritoneum on the surfaces of adjoining organs.

abdominovesical p., the pouchlike reflection of the peritoneum from the abdominal wall to the anterior surface of the bladder.

Rathke's p., a diverticulum from the embryonic buccal cavity from which the anterior lobe of the pituitary gland is developed.

poudrage (poo-drahzh′) [Fr.] application of a powder (e.g., talc or asbestos) to a surface, as done to promote fusion of serous membranes (e.g., two layers of pericardium or pleura).

poultice (pōl′tis) a soft, moist mass to be placed hot upon the skin, for the purpose of supplying heat and moisture.

pound (pownd) a unit of weight in the avoirdupois (453.6 Gm., or 16 ounces) or apothecaries' (373.2 Gm., or 12 ounces) system.

povidone-iodine (po′vĭ-dōn-i′o-dīn) a complex produced by reacting iodine with the polymer polyvinylpyrrolidone; used as a mild anti-infective agent.

powder (pow′der) an aggregation of particles obtained by grinding or triturating a solid.

Dover's p., powder of ipecac and opium, a diaphoretic.

dusting p., an absorbent, antiseptic, astringent or soothing powder for external use.

effervescent p., compound, (1) a mixture of sodium bicarbonate and potassium tartrate and (2) tartaric acid, each to be dissolved in water and the solutions mixed as the effervescence subsides; an aperient.

Seidlitz p's, a mixture of sodium bicarbonate, potassium sodium tartrate and tartaric acid; used as a cathartic.

senna p., compound, a powder prepared from fennel oil, sucrose, powdered senna, powdered glycyrrhiza and washed sulfur; a laxative.

p. of tragacanth, compound, a mixture of powdered tragacanth, acacia, starch and sucrose; a demulcent.

pox (poks) an eruptive disease.

poxvirus (poks-vi′rus) one of a group of morphologically similar and immunologically related agents, including the viruses of vaccinia and variola (smallpox).

P.P.D. purified protein derivative (tuberculin).

PPLO pleuropneumonia-like organisms.

p.p.m. parts per million.

Pr chemical symbol, *praseodymium*.

prae- for words beginning thus, see those beginning *pre-*.

pragmatagnosia (prag″mat-ag-no′ze-ah) loss of ability to recognize objects.

pragmatamnesia (prag″mat-am-ne′ze-ah) loss of power of remembering the appearance of objects.

pramoxine (pram-ok′sēn) a compound used as a local anesthetic.

prandial (pran′de-al) pertaining to a meal.

Pranone (pra′nōn) trademark for a preparation of ethisterone, a progestational steroid.

Prantal (pran′tal) trademark for preparations of diphemanil methylsulfate, an anticholinergic used in the treatment of peptic ulcer.

praseodymium (pra″ze-o-dim′e-um) a chemical element, atomic number 59, atomic weight 140.907, symbol Pr. (See table of ELEMENTS.)

Prausnitz-Küstner reaction (prows′nits kist′ner) the production of local hypersensitiveness by the intradermal injection of the serum of an allergic person.

praxiology (prak″se-ol′o-je) the science of conduct.

praxis (prak′sis) the doing or performance of action.

pre- (pre) word element [L.], *before* (in time or space).

preagonal (pre-ag′o-nal) immediately before the death agony.

prealbumin (pre″al-bu′min) one of a group of serum proteins that have an electrophoretic mobility slightly faster than albumin at pH 8.6.

preanesthetic (pre″an-es-thet′ik) before anesthesia.

preauricular (pre″aw-rik′u-lar) situated in front of the ear.

precancerous (pre-kan′ser-us) pertaining to an early stage in the development of a CANCER.

precava (pre-ka′vah) the superior vena cava. adj., **preca′val.**

preceptor (pre′sep-tor) a practicing physician whom a student accompanies, observes and assists, as one facet of his education in medicine.

prechordal (pre-kor′dal) in front of the notochord.

precipitant (pre-sip′ĭ-tant) a substance that causes precipitation.

precipitate (pre-sip′ĭ-tāt) 1. to cause settling in solid particles of a substance in solution. 2. a deposit of solid particles settled out of a solution. 3. occurring with undue rapidity, as precipitate labor.

precipitation (pre-sip″ĭ-ta′shun) the act or process of precipitating.

precipitin (pre-sip′ĭ-tin) an antibody produced by immunization and able to precipitate from solution the antigen producing it.

　p. reaction, a reaction involving the specific serologic precipitation of an antigen in solution with its specific antiserum in the presence of electrolytes. The reaction is used in the typing of pneumococcus strains, in testing whether blood is human or animal and for diagnostic purposes.

precipitinogen (pre-sip″ĭ-tin′o-jen) a soluble antigen that stimulates the formation of a precipitin.

precipitinoid (pre-sip′ĭ-tin-oid″) a precipitin whose activity has been destroyed by heat, so that although it still retains its affinity for the antigen, it no longer precipitates.

precipitophore (pre-sip′ĭ-to-fōr″) the group in a precipitin that is the active cause of precipitation.

preclinical (pre-klin′ĭ-kal) 1. before the appearance or development of disease. 2. preceding the study of diseases in living patients.

precocity (pre-kos′ĭ-te) unusually early development of mental or physical traits. adj., **preco′cious.**

precognition (pre″kog-nish′un) the extrasensory perception of a future event.

precommissure (pre-kom′ĭ-shūr) the anterior commissure of the brain.

preconscious (pre-kon′shus) not present in consciousness, but readily recalled into it.

preconvulsive (pre″kon-vul′siv) preceding convulsions.

precordia, precordium (pre-kor′de-ah), (pre-kor′-de-um) the region over the heart and stomach; the epigastrium and lower part of the thorax. adj., **precor′dial.**

precuneus (pre-ku′ne-us), pl. *precu′nei* [L.] a small convolution on the medial surface of the parietal lobe of the cerebrum.

precursor (pre-ker′sor) an agent or disease that normally precedes or may develop into another, as a premalignant lesion or an intermediate compound in a metabolic or synthetic process.

predation (prĕ-da′shun) the biologic association of two individuals or populations of different species, one of which feeds upon the other.

predator (pred′ah-tor) an individual or species that feeds upon and destroys organisms of another species, on which it is dependent for survival.

prediabetes (pre-di″ah-be′tēz) a state of latent impairment of carbohydrate metabolism in which the criteria for diabetes mellitus are not all satisfied.

prediastole (pre″di-as′to-le) the interval immediately preceding diastole.

prediastolic (pre″di-ah-stol′ik) 1. pertaining to the beginning of diastole. 2. occurring just before the diastole.

predicrotic (pre″di-krot′ik) occurring before the dicrotic wave of the sphygmogram.

predigestion (pre″di-jes′chun) partial artificial digestion of food before its ingestion into the body.

predisposition (pre-dis″po-zish′un) a special tendency toward some disease.

prednisolone (pred-nis′o-lōn) a compound used as a glucocorticoid.

prednisone (pred′nĭ-sōn) a compound used as a glucocorticoid.

preeclampsia (pre″e-klamp′se-ah) a toxemia of late pregnancy, characterized by hypertension, albuminuria and edema, but without convulsions (see also ECLAMPSIA).

prefrontal (pre-frun′tal) 1. situated in the anterior part of the frontal region or lobe. 2. the central part of the ethmoid bone.

preganglionic (pre″gang-gle-on′ik) proximal to a ganglion.

pregenital (pre-jen′ĭ-tal) pertaining to the early infantile stage of sexual life before the genitalia have become the dominant zone.

preglomerular (pre″glo-mer′u-lar) proximal to a glomerulus of the kidney.

pregnancy (preg′nan-se) the condition of having a developing embryo or fetus in the body, after union of an ovum and spermatozoon. Human pregnancy lasts about 9 months, although it may vary considerably from that average.

　CONCEPTION. Once a month an ovum matures in one of the ovaries and travels down the nearby uterine tube to the uterus. This process is called ovulation. If coitus takes place within a day or two of ovulation, one of the spermatozoa may unite with the ovum and fertilize it. The fertilized ovum then implants itself in the wall of the uterus, which is richly supplied with blood, and begins to grow. (See also OVULATION, REPRODUCTION and UTERINE TUBE.)

SIGNS OF PREGNANCY. Usually the first indication of pregnancy is a missed menstrual period. Unless the period is more than 10 days late, however, this is not a definite indication, since many factors, including a strong fear of pregnancy, can delay menstruation. Nausea, or "morning sickness," usually begins in the fifth or sixth week of pregnancy. About 4 weeks after conception, changes in the breasts become noticeable: there may be a tingling sensation in the breasts, the nipples enlarge and the areolae (the darkened areas around the nipples) may become darker. Frequent urination, another early sign, is the result of expansion of the uterus, which presses on the bladder.

Other signs of pregnancy include softening of the cervix and filling of the cervical canal with a plug of mucus. Early in labor this plug is expelled and there is slight bleeding; expulsion of the mucous plug is known as "show" and indicates the beginning of cervical dilatation. Chadwick's sign of pregnancy refers to a bluish color of the vagina which is a result of increased blood supply to the area.

When the abdominal wall becomes stretched there may be a breaking down of elastic tissues resulting in depressed areas in the skin which are smooth and reddened. These markings are called striae gravidarum. In subsequent pregnancies the old striae appear as whitish streaks and frequently do not disappear completely.

There are several fairly accurate laboratory tests for pregnancy. The so-called "rabbit" and "frog" tests are based on the fact that a pregnant woman's urine contains a hormone that causes certain changes in the test animal (see also PREGNANCY TESTS).

GROWTH OF THE FETUS. The average pregnancy lasts about 280 days, or 40 weeks, from the date of conception to childbirth. Since the exact date of conception usually is not known, the physician determines an approximate date of birth by taking the date of the beginning of the last menstrual period, adding 7 days, counting back 3 months and advancing the date arrived at to the following year. This is approximate, since pregnancy may be shorter than the average or can last as long as 300 days.

The stages of growth of the fetus are fairly well defined. At the end of the first month, the fetus has grown beyond microscopic size. After 2 months, it is a little over an inch long, its face is formed and its limbs are partly formed. By the end of the third month, the fetus is 3 inches long and weighs about an ounce. The limbs, fingers, toes and ears are fully formed, and the sex can be distinguished.

After 4 months, the fetus is about 8 inches long and weighs nearly half a pound. The mother can feel its movements, and usually the physician can hear its heartbeat. The eyebrows and eyelashes are formed, and the skin is pink and covered with fine hair. By the end of the fifth month, the fetus is 12 inches long and weighs 1 lb. It now has hair on its head. At the end of the sixth month, the fetus is 14 inches long and weighs nearly 2 lb. Its skin is very wrinkled.

After 7 months, the fetus is 16 inches long and weighs about 3 lb., with more fat under its skin. In the male, the testes have descended into the scrotum. By the end of the eighth month, the fetus is 18 inches long, weighs about 5 lb., and has a good chance of survival if it is born at that time. At the end of 9 months, the average length of the fetus is 20 inches, and the average weight is 7 lb.

CARE OF THE UNBORN CHILD. There is little the expectant mother must or can do specifically for the baby. Her thoughts, activities and emotional experiences have no effect on the child. The fetus is well protected within the amnion and the mother need not worry if she happens to bump her abdomen, nor need she try to avoid certain sleeping positions for fear of crushing the child.

There are a few diseases, however, that can seriously harm the unborn child. Rubella (German measles) may be responsible for many types of birth defects, particularly if the mother contracts it in the first 3 months of pregnancy. A pregnant woman who has been exposed to the disease should inform her physician immediately. Her blood can be tested for antibodies to the rubella virus, and if she has none, the physician may administer an injection of immune serum globulin to help raise the body's resistance to the disease.

Venereal diseases can have tragic effects on the baby, even though the symptoms in the mother are minor at the time of pregnancy. Syphilis is particularly dangerous, since it is one of the few diseases that can be transmitted to the fetus in the uterus. The child is either stillborn or born infected, and rarely escapes mental or physical defects. Successful treatment of the mother before the fifth month of pregnancy will prevent infection of the infant. Gonorrhea may infect the infant's eyes during its passage through the birth canal, causing blindness. At birth, penicillin or silver nitrate drops are instilled in the eyes of all infants to prevent this infection.

A rare danger is ERYTHROBLASTOSIS FETALIS, a serious blood dyscrasia in the newborn infant caused by Rh incompatibility; in most cases the mother is Rh negative and the infant is Rh positive. (See also RH FACTOR.) The first child of an Rh-negative mother is not at risk, but subsequent Rh-positive fetuses are. An infant with erythroblastosis fetalis is given an exchange transfusion immediately after birth, so that his Rh-positive blood is replaced with Rh-negative blood. In certain cases, if the life of the fetus is thought to be in danger, it is given an intrauterine TRANSFUSION.

ABORTION (often called miscarriage by laymen) is termination of pregnancy before the fetus is viable, that is, before the 20th week of pregnancy, according to official terminology. A baby born dead after the 20th week of pregnancy is said to be stillborn. An infant born alive between the 20th and 35th weeks of pregnancy is considered premature, although the official criterion of prematurity is the weight of the infant (less than 2500 Gm.).

PRENATAL CARE. The care of the mother during her entire pregnancy is important to her well-being and that of her unborn infant. It will help provide ease and safety during pregnancy and childbirth. The physician learns about the patient's physical condition and medical history, and can detect possible complications before they become serious.

On the first prenatal visit the physician takes the patient's medical history in considerable detail, including any diseases or operations she has had, the course of previous pregnancies, if any, and whether there is a family history of multiple births or of diabetes mellitus or other chronic diseases. The first visit also includes a thorough physical examination and measurement of the pelvis. Blood samples are taken for a serologic test for syphilis and for laboratory tests such as an erythrocyte count, hemoglobin determination and blood typing. Urine is tested for albumin and sugar and examined microscopically. On subsequent visits the patient brings a urine specimen, collected upon arising that morning, to be tested for albumin. At each prenatal visit her blood pressure is taken and recorded and she is weighed. The physician supervises the patient's diet, advises her on the amount and kind of activity she may engage in and answers her questions about other aspects of her daily life.

Diet and Weight. In the first few weeks of pregnancy there may be slight loss of weight, especially if there is morning sickness. Then weight increase begins and it usually becomes a problem to keep weight down. Being overweight puts an extra strain on the pregnant woman, and it is much easier to avoid adding pounds during pregnancy than it is to get rid of them afterward. Women of normal weight should gain about 20 pounds during pregnancy. Others may be put on special diets to lose or gain weight.

The pregnant woman should consume about 2000 calories a day, mainly in meats and other proteins, green vegetables and fruits. Starches, fats and sugars are usually restricted. Supplemental iron and vitamins may be prescribed, and the physician may advise the patient to drink at least a quart of milk a day to provide an adequate supply of calcium.

The pregnant woman should consume at least eight glasses of fluid (water or other liquids) a day; this helps reduce the danger of infection in the urinary tract.

Many women, when pregnant, experience acute cravings for certain foods, such as lobster, pickles or candy. Aside from the risk of gaining weight, eating such foods will do no harm, nor will not eating them.

Discomforts and Complications. MORNING SICKNESS usually appears in the early months of pregnancy and rarely lasts beyond the third month. Often it requires no treatment, or can be relieved by such simple measures as eating dry crackers and tea before rising. Indigestion and heartburn are best prevented by avoiding foods that are difficult to digest, such as cucumbers, cabbage, cauliflower, spinach and onions, and rich foods. Milk of magnesia may provide relief. Constipation usually can be corrected by diet or a mild laxative like milk of magnesia. Stronger laxatives should not be used unless prescribed by the physician.

A visit to a dentist early in pregnancy is a good idea to forestall any possibility of infection arising from tooth decay. Pregnancy does not encourage tooth decay.

No unnecessary medication should be taken during pregnancy. If x-rays are necessary for any reason, the physician in charge of the procedure must be aware of the pregnancy.

HEMORRHOIDS sometimes occur in pregnancy because of pressure from the enlarged uterus on the veins in the rectum. The physician should be consulted for treatment.

VARICOSE VEINS also result from pressure of the uterus, which restricts the flow of blood from the legs and feet. Lying flat with the feet raised on a pillow several times a day will help relieve swelling and pain in the legs. In more difficult cases the physician may prescribe an eleastic bandage or support stockings.

Backache during pregnancy is caused by the heavy abdomen pulling on muscles that are not normally used, and can be relieved by rest, a maternity corset and sensible shoes.

Swelling of the feet and ankles usually is relieved by rest and by remaining off the feet for a day or two. If the swelling does not disappear, the physician should be informed since it may be an indication of a more serious complication.

Shortness of breath is common in the later stages of pregnancy. If at any time it becomes so extreme that the woman cannot climb a short flight of stairs without discomfort, the physician should be consulted. If mild shortness of breath interferes with sleep, lying in a half-sitting position, supported by several pillows, may help. The physician may prescribe a sedative if shortness of breath causes insomnia.

SERIOUS COMPLICATIONS. *Cystitis and Pyelitis.* The symptoms of CYSTITIS (inflammation of the urinary bladder) are a frequent desire to urinate and pain and burning sensations during urination. The disease responds quickly to antibiotics, and to drinking large quantities of fluids. It should be treated immediately, as it may lead to PYELITIS, inflammation of the kidney pelvis, which, if not treated, can become very serious. Pyelitis responds to treatment with sulfonamides and antibiotics. The symptoms are frequency and urgency of urination, pain on urination (dysuria), chills and fever and back pain in the region of the kidneys.

Hyperemesis Gravidarum. Excessive and pernicious vomiting of pregnancy, called HYPEREMESIS GRAVIDARUM, is more serious and much less common than simple morning sickness. Hyperemesis gravidarum is characterized by persistent vomiting, inability to take any food by mouth, exhaustion, loss of weight, dehydration and sometimes jaundice and nerve involvement. It is rarely fatal, but is serious and requires prompt treatment, in the hospital, consisting of sedation to ensure rest and correction of dehydration and nutritional deficiencies by intravenous administration of fluids and nutrients. Since psychologic factors are thought to contribute to the cause of hyperemesis gravidarum, psychotherapy is sometimes included in treatment.

Ectopic Pregnancy. An ectopic pregnancy takes place when the fertilized egg implants itself outside the uterus instead of in the wall of the uterus. Usually ectopic pregnancy is tubal; that is, the site of implantation is one of the uterine tubes. The tube is small, and the growing fetus ruptures it. The resulting symptoms are vaginal bleeding and severe pain on one side of the abdomen. Prompt surgery is necessary for removal of the fetus and the tube, to stop the bleeding. Removal of one uterine tube does not prevent further pregnancies.

Any vaginal bleeding during pregnancy must be reported immediately to the physician; it may indicate ectopic pregnancy, abortion or premature labor, and delay in reporting it may endanger the life of the mother or baby.

Toxemia; Preeclampsia; Eclampsia. Toxemia of pregnancy is a term used to describe a syndrome of excessive fluid retention (edema), hypertension, albuminuria and, in severe cases, convulsions and coma. The condition is rare, and little is known about its cause. It occurs during the last 3 months of pregnancy, as a rule, and is more common in women who are pregnant for the first time.

The early and milder form, preeclampsia, often is detected during a routine prenatal visit from blood pressure readings and urinalysis. The symptoms are puffiness about the face and hands, persistent vomiting, severe, persistent headache, disturbances in vision (blurring, dimness and spots before the eyes) and very rapid gain in weight; if they occur, the physician should be notified immediately. Treatment varies in individual cases, but usually includes restriction of salt intake, diuretics and rest.

If preeclampsia goes undiagnosed or is not satisfactorily controlled, convulsions and coma may result, and the condition is then called ECLAMPSIA. Patients with eclampsia are critically ill and must be hospitalized. Treatment is aimed at controlling the convulsions, lowering the blood pressure, minimizing the edema and terminating the pregnancy at the time most favorable for mother and child.

Placenta Praevia and Abruptio Placentae. These complications are rare, and little is known about their causes. Both occur in the last 3 months of pregnancy and are accompanied by vaginal bleeding.

In placenta praevia, the PLACENTA, through which the fetus is nourished, is attached near the cervix uteri instead of in the normal position higher on the uterine wall. If some of the placental tissue is torn by expansion of the cervix, pain, bleeding and premature labor will result.

Abruptio placentae is premature separation of the normally implanted placenta. It results in sudden, severe pain in the region of the uterus, vaginal bleeding and indications of fetal distress.

Both conditions require immediate medical treatment because they threaten the life of the fetus. Transfusions may be given to the mother to replace blood lost, and in some cases cesarean section must be resorted to.

abdominal p., development of the fetus in the abdominal cavity.

cervical p., development of the fetus in the cervix uteri.

ectopic p., extrauterine p., development of the fetus outside the cavity of the uterus.

false p., development of all the signs of pregnancy without the presence of an embryo.

hydatid p., pregnancy with formation of a hydatid mole.

interstitial p., development of the fetus in that part of the uterine tube within the wall of the uterus.

molar p., conversion of the ovum into a mole.

multiple p., the presence of more than one fetus in the uterus at the same time.

mural p., interstitial pregnancy.

ovarian p., pregnancy occurring in an ovary.

oviducal p., tubal pregnancy.

phantom p., false pregnancy.

p. tests, laboratory procedures for early determination of pregnancy. Within 2 weeks after the first missed menstrual period, CHORIONIC GONADOTROPIN (CG), a hormone secreted by the placenta, is present in the blood and urine of a pregnant woman. It can be detected by biologic tests, in which urine (or serum) is injected into laboratory animals, and by immunologic tests.

In the Aschheim-Zondek (AZ) test, immature female mice are used, and changes in their ovaries are observed within 100 hours if CG is present in the urine injected.

The Friedman test makes use of a female rabbit, and ovarian changes are observed within 48 hours after injection of urine from a pregnant woman.

Male frogs are used in the Galli Mainini test; sperm are found in their urine 1 to 4 hours after injection of urine containing CG.

In the immunologic tests, urine is mixed with antihuman chorionic gonadotropin serum; if the urine does *not* contain CG (absence of pregnancy), an antigen-antibody reaction (agglutination) will occur. These tests take only a few minutes or a few hours.

Another method sometimes used is administration to the woman of an estrogenic hormone, by injection or orally. If a menstrual period does not follow within a certain length of time (depending on the hormone used), the likelihood of pregnancy is about 95 per cent.

No test is 100 per cent reliable. Very occasionally certain reproductive disorders can result in the presence of CG in the urine and blood when there is no pregnancy. In some cases, especially in the early weeks of pregnancy, not enough CG is produced to cause a positive test reaction. The accuracy of the tests increases with the length of the pregnancy. For most women, however, the tests are 95 to 99 per cent accurate and, considered with the presence or lack of other symptoms, make it possible to say with certainty that a tested patient is or is not pregnant.

tubal p., development of the embryo within a uterine tube.

tuboabdominal p., development of the products of conception partly in the fimbriated end of the uterine tube and partly in the abdominal cavity.

pregnant (preg′nant) having a developing ovum within the body.

pregnene (preg′nēn) a compound that forms the chemical nucleus of progesterone.

pregneninolone (preg″nēn-in′o-lōn) ethisterone, a progestational steroid.

pregnenolone (preg-nēn′o-lōn) a compound used as an antiarthritic.

pregravidic (pre″grah-vid′ik) preceding pregnancy.

prehallux (pre-hal′uks) a supernumerary bone of the foot growing from the inner border of the navicular bone.

prehemiplegic (pre″hem-ĭ-ple′jik) preceding hemiplegia.

prehensile (pre-hen′sil) adapted for grasping or seizing.

prehension (pre-hen′shun) the act of grasping.

prehypophysis (pre″hi-pof′ĭ-sis) the anterior lobe of the hypophysis cerebri, or pituitary gland.

preictal (pre-ik′tal) occurring before a stroke, seizure or attack.

preimmunization (pre″im-u-nĭ-za′shun) artificial immunization produced in very young infants.

preinvasive   (pre″in-va′siv) not yet invading tissue outside the site of origin.

Preludin (pre-lu′din) trademark for preparations of phenmetrazine hydrochloride, used to reduce the appetite.

premalignant   (pre″mah-lig′nant) preceding malignancy.

premature   (pre″mah-tūr′) born or interrupted before the state of maturity; occurring before the proper time.

p. infant, an infant weighing between 1000 and 2500 Gm. (between 2¹⁄₅ and 5¹⁄₂ lb.) at birth; also, any infant born before the 35th week of pregnancy, although weight is considered more important as a criterion than length of gestation. An infant weighing less than 2¹⁄₅ lb. at birth is called immature.

A premature infant whose weight approaches 5¹⁄₂ lb. has nearly the average chances of survival, but a very premature infant begins life with serious handicaps. His breathing is difficult, he cannot nurse and he cannot maintain his body temperature without artificial aid. His limbs are underdeveloped and his neck seems abnormally long, with the head appearing to be attached loosely to the body. The skin is wrinkled and the flesh flabby. Development of the kidneys, liver and other organs is inadequate for proper functioning, and the baby's resistance to infection is low.

Most premature infants are placed in an incubator immediately after birth. An incubator provides the baby with the proper warmth, humidity and atmosphere, corresponding somewhat to conditions within the uterus. It also provides protection against infection, and handling of the baby can be kept to a minimum. If the child is unable to nurse and swallow, he is fed by nasogastric tube. He is kept in the incubator until he reaches the level of development of a full-term infant.

NURSING CARE.   The nursing staff in the nursery must wear special gowns and caps and carefully wash their hands after each contact with an infant and before handling the infant or equipment used in his care.

The temperature within the incubator is regulated so that the infant's temperature is maintained between 96 and 98° F. Humidity is kept at 50 to 60 per cent; if the infant has respiratory difficulty it is raised as high as 85 to 100 per cent. When the infant is cyanotic, oxygen is added but the oxygen content should not exceed 40 per cent because excessive amounts of oxygen produce retrolental fibroplasia, which results in blindness in the infant. Some incubators are designed so that they rock rhythmically, to facilitate respiration and circulation.

The premature infant should be handled as little as possible, and then with extreme gentleness to avoid stimulating him. When the infant is fed by bottle he must be watched for cyanosis, fatigue, vomiting or other difficulties in sucking, swallowing and retaining the formula.

prematurity   (pre″mah-tūr′ĭ-te) underdevelopment; the condition of a premature infant.

premaxillary   (pre-mak′sĭ-ler″e) in front of the maxilla.

p. bone, incisive bone; a separate bone in the upper jaw of the fetus which later fuses with the maxilla on either side.

premedication   (pre″med-ĭ-ka′shun) administration of drugs to produce basal narcosis before giving a general anesthetic.

premeiotic   (pre″mi-ot′ik) occurring before or pertaining to time preceding meiosis.

premenarchal   (pre″mĕ-nar′kal) occurring before establishment of menstruation.

premenstrual (pre-men′stroo-al) preceding menstruation.

p. tension, a complex of symptoms sometimes occurring in the 10 days before menstruation, including emotional instability and irritability, pain in the breasts, headache, nausea, anorexia, constipation, pelvic discomfort, edema and abdominal distention.

The causes of these symptoms are not fully understood but are believed to be associated with a disturbed salt balance, resulting in the accumulation of water in the tissues just before menstruation. Psychogenic factors may contribute. Emotional and physical symptoms usually disappear with the onset of menstruation. If symptoms are habitually troublesome, restriction of fluid and salt intake and a diuretic may be prescribed. Tranquilizers and reassurance that the condition is not serious are also helpful.

premenstruum   (pre-men′stroo-um) the period before menstruation.

premitotic   (pre″mi-tot′ik) occurring before or pertaining to the time preceding mitosis.

premolar (pre-mo′lar) in front of the molar teeth.

premorbid   (pre-mor′bid) occurring before the development of disease.

premortal (pre-mor′tal) occurring before death.

premunition   (pre″mu-nish′un) infection immunity; resistance to hyperinfection by the same organism, sometimes stimulated by and existing during the presence of the specific infecting organism in the host.

premyeloblast (pre-mi′ĕ-lo-blast″) an early precursor of a myelocyte.

premyelocyte (pre-mi′ĕ-lo-sīt″) promyelocyte.

prenarcosis   (pre″nar-ko′sis) narcosis induced preliminary to general or local anesthesia.

prenatal (pre-na′tal) preceding birth.

p. care, care of the pregnant woman before delivery of the infant (see also PREGNANCY).

preneoplastic   (pre″ne-o-plas′tik) before the formation of a tumor.

preoperative   (pre-op′er-ah-tiv, pre-op′er-a″tiv) preceding an operation.

p. care, the psychologic and physiologic preparation of a patient before operation. The preoperative period may be extremely short, as with an emergency operation, or it may encompass several weeks during which diagnostic tests, specific medications and treatments and measures to improve the patient's general well-being are employed in preparation for surgery.

PSYCHOLOGIC ASPECTS.   Although each patient reacts in his own unique way to the news that he is going to have surgery, all patients experience some degree of anxiety and fear—fear of the unknown, worry over disability or death and apprehension about the insecurity of his and his family's future.

Much of this anxiety can be relieved if the various aspects of his preoperative and postoperative care and the type of surgery planned are explained to the patient. The surgeon usually explains the surgical procedure and assists the patient in planning rehabilitation. The anesthesiologist usually reviews the type of anesthesia to be used and the general effects it will have on the patient. The nursing staff explains the hospital routine, specific nursing procedures necessary, the purpose of diagnostic tests required and the types of equipment that will be used during the preoperative and postoperative periods. The nurse can demonstrate her interest in the patient and his family by answering questions (or referring them to the surgeon), and giving them a general idea of how long the patient will be away from his room during surgery and recovery from anesthesia. It is reassuring for them to know, for example, that oxygen administration, blood transfusions and the use of a nasogastric tube or catheter do not necessarily indicate a critical situation. The use of various pieces of equipment that seem "routine" to the hospital staff may be extremely upsetting to the patient and his family if they do not understand why the equipment is necessary.

Spiritual reinforcement during this period may be very important to some patients, and though the nurse must be careful not to give the impression of prying into the patient's private affairs, she must also show a willingness to assist him and his family in obtaining a spiritual advisor if they indicate a desire for her to do so. She must always respect the individual patient's beliefs and convictions even though she may not share them, and she must support him in his search for spiritual reassurance and guidance.

PHYSIOLOGIC ASPECTS. Except in emergency situations every effort is made to have the patient in a state of optimal health before surgery is performed. Specific diets, protein and vitamin supplements and other measures to improve the nutritional status may be employed. Intravenous infusions and transfusions of whole blood or plasma may be necessary to improve the fluid and electrolyte status and blood volume. Infections should be brought under control before surgery if they cannot be eliminated completely. Accurate records of the patient's vital signs, blood pressure and urinary output will assist the surgeon in diagnosing and correcting conditions that may adversely affect the patient's physiologic response to an operative procedure.

More specific measures, such as CATHETERIZATION and administration of OXYGEN, will depend on the organ or system involved.

PHYSICAL PREPARATION. The skin and hair are harborers of infection and require special attention before surgery. The particular area to be shaved and cleansed will depend on the wishes of the surgeon and the accepted hospital procedure. Generally, it is desirable to shave and cleanse with an antiseptic an area larger than the proposed incision. An exception may be the head or face, especially the eyebrows, which are never shaved. If large amounts of hair must be removed from the head, the hair should be saved so that it can be used for a hairpiece later if the patient so desires.

In some types of orthopedic surgery preparation of the skin may start as much as 24 hours before the operation. The operative site is wrapped in sterile towels or dressings; in some cases the dressings are removed at regular intervals and an antiseptic is applied. This type of skin preparation must be done according to specific directions from the surgeon.

Restriction of food and fluids varies. Usually the patient is allowed a light evening meal and then given nothing by mouth after midnight the night before surgery.

PREOPERATIVE MEDICATIONS. Generally there are three types of drugs used prior to surgery: sedatives, such as one of the barbiturates, to promote relaxation and rest and to stabilize the blood pressure and pulse; drying agents, such as atropine and scopolamine, which decrease secretion of mucus in the mouth and throat; and narcotics, such as morphine and meperidine hydrochloride (Demerol), which promote relaxation and enhance the effects of the anesthetic.

Preoperative medications must be given at the exact time ordered because their strength, action and duration are planned according to the type of anesthesia used.

IMMEDIATE PREOPERATIVE CARE. Most institutions use a check list or clearance record for surgical procedures. This eliminates the danger of overlooking some aspect of the immediate preoperative preparation. Such an omission might delay surgery or result in legal problems. The operative permit must be signed by the patient or his guardian or legal representative. This permit is necessary to protect the surgeon against claims of unauthorized surgery, and to protect the patient against surgery he would not willingly endorse.

The preoperative check list includes such items as laboratory tests and their findings, history and physical examination records, disposal of valuables, removal of dentures and their disposition, vital signs and blood pressure of the patient immediately before he goes to the operating room and other specific information such as consultation for sterilization.

Unless a urinary catheter has been inserted, the patient is offered the bedpan just before he is taken to the operating room. Hairpins, bobbie pins and combs are removed from the hair and the head is covered with a cap or scarf. As the patient leaves the unit he is reassured that everything is in order and that everyone concerned with his care is interested in him and the outcome of his operation.

preoral (pre-o'ral) in front of the mouth.

prepallium (pre-pal'e-um) the cerebral cortex in front of the fissure of Rolando.

preparalytic (pre″par-ah-lit′ik) preceding paralysis.

prepatellar (pre″pah-tel′ar) in front of the patella.

preprandial (pre-pran′de-al) before meals.

prepuce (pre′pūs) a cutaneous fold over the glans penis or glans clitoridis. adj., **prepu′tial.**

preputiotomy (pre-pu″she-ot′o-me) incision of the prepuce of the penis to relieve phimosis.

preputium (pre-pu′she-um) prepuce.

prepyloric (pre″pi-lor′ik) anterior to the pylorus; that area of the stomach proximal to the pylorus.

presacral (pre′sa-kral) anterior to the sacrum.

presby- (pres′be) word element [Gr.], *old age.*

presbyatry (pres″be-ah′tre) treatment of the diseases of old age.

presbycardia (pres″bĭ-kar′de-ah) impairment of cardiac function with advancing years, with senescent changes in the body and no evidence of other cause of heart disease.

presbycusis (pres″bĭ-ku′sis) impairment of hearing due to old age.

presbyesophagus (pres″be-e-sof′ah-gus) a condition characterized by alteration in motor function of the esophagus as a result of degenerative changes occurring with advancing age.

presbyophrenia (pres″be-o-fre′ne-ah) disorientation and confabulation occurring in old age.

presbyopia (pres″be-o′pe-ah) impaired vision as a result of the aging process of the body; the impairment usually consists of hyperopia, or farsightedness. Presbyopia is caused by a loss of elasticity in the crystalline lens of the eye. The lens focuses images on the retina with the aid of muscles that stretch it to make it less convex or relax it to make it more spherical and thus more convex. As it ages, the lens may lose its ability to become convex enough to accommodate to nearby objects. This condition usually begins around the age of 40. Presbyopia can most often be comfortably corrected through the use of eyeglasses.

prescription (pre-skrip′shun) a written directive, as for the compounding or dispensing and administration of drugs, or for other service to a particular patient.

Federal law divides medicines into two main classes: prescription medicines and over-the-counter medicines. Dangerous, powerful or habit-forming medicines to be used under a physician's supervision can be sold only by prescription. The prescription must be written by a physician; otherwise the pharmacist is forbidden to prepare and fill it.

There are four parts to a drug prescription. The first is the symbol ℞ from the Latin *recipe,* meaning "take." This is the superscription. The second part is the inscription, specifying the ingredients and their quantities. The third part is the subscription, which tells the pharmacist how to compound the medicine. The signature is the last part, and it is usually preceded by an S to represent the Latin *signa,* meaning "mark." The signature is where the physician indicates what instructions are to be put on the outside of the package to tell the patient when and how to take the medicine and in what quantities.

The pharmacist keeps a file of all the prescriptions he fills.

presenile (pre-se′nīl) pertaining to a condition resembling senility, but occurring in early or middle life.

presentation (prez″en-ta′shun) the particular part of the body of the fetus appearing at the ostium uteri or, during labor, bounded by the girdle of resistance.

breech p., presentation of the buttocks of the fetus in labor.

breech p., complete, presentation of the buttocks of the fetus in labor, with the feet alongside the buttocks.

breech p., frank, presentation of the buttocks of the fetus in labor, with the legs extended against the trunk and the feet lying against the face.

breech p., incomplete, presentation of the fetus with one or both feet or knees prolapsed into the maternal vagina.

cephalic p., presentation of any part of the fetal head in labor, whether the vertex, face or brow.

compound p., prolapse of an extremity of the fetus alongside the head in cephalic presentation or of

PRESCRIPTION ABBREVIATIONS

a̅a̅	of each
a.c. (ante cibum)	before meals
aq. (aqua)	water
aq. dest.	distilled water
b.i.d. (bis in die)	twice a day
caps	capsules
hora	an hour
h.s. (hora somni)	at bedtime
liq.	a liquor
M. (misce)	mix
mist. (mistura)	a mixture
m. dict. (modo dictu)	as directed
mollis	soft
non. rep. (non repetatur)	do not repeat (do not refill)
omn. hor. (omni hora)	every hour
omn. man. (omni mane)	every morning
omn. noct. (omni nocte)	every night
p.c. (post cibum)	after meals
p.r.n. (pro re nata)	as needed
pulv. (pulvis)	a powder
q.s. (quantum sufficit)	a sufficient quantity
q.i.d. (quater in die)	four times a day
q.	every
℞	take (thou) a recipe
Sig. (signa)	directions
statim	immediately
t.i.d. (ter in die)	three times a day
ut dict.	as directed

From the SK&F Pocket Book of Medical Tables. 15th ed. Philadelphia, Smith, Kline & French Laboratories, 1966.

one or both arms alongside a presenting breech at the beginning of labor.

footling p., presentation of the fetus with one foot (single footling) or two feet (double footling) prolapsed into the maternal vagina.

placental p., placenta praevia.

transverse p., presentation of any portion of the side of the fetal body at the ostium uteri in labor.

preservative (pre-zer′vah-tiv) a substance added to a product to destroy or inhibit multiplication of microorganisms.

presomite (pre-so′mīt) referring to embryos before the appearance of somites.

presphenoid (pre-sfe′noid) the anterior portion of the body of the sphenoid bone.

presphygmic (pre-sfig′mik) preceding the pulse wave.

prespinal (pre-spi′nal) in front of the spine.

pressor (pres′or) increasing blood pressure and vasomotor activity.

pressoreceptive (pres″o-re-sep′tiv) sensitive to stimuli due to vasomotor activity.

pressoreceptor (pres″o-re-sep′tor) a receptor or nerve ending sensitive to stimuli of vasomotor activity.

pressosensitive (pres″o-sen′sĭ-tiv) pressoreceptive.

pressure (presh′ur) stress or strain, by compression, expansion, pull, thrust or shear.

arterial p., the blood pressure in the arteries.
atmospheric p., the pressure exerted by the atmosphere, about 15 lb. to the square inch at sea level.

blood p., the tension in the walls of blood vessels derived from the heart action, the elasticity of the walls of the arteries, the resistance of the arterioles, and the volume and viscosity of the blood (see also BLOOD PRESSURE).

capillary p., the blood pressure in the capillaries.
cerebrospinal p., the pressure of the cerebrospinal fluid, normally 100 to 200 mm. of water.

diastolic p., arterial pressure during diastole.
hydrostatic p., the pressure exerted by a liquid at rest, with respect to adjacent bodies.

intracranial p., the pressure in the space between the skull and the brain.

intraocular p., the pressure exerted against the outer coats by the contents of the eyeball.

negative p., pressure less than that of the atmosphere.

oncotic p., the osmotic pressure of a colloid system.

osmotic p., the pressure required to stop diffusion between solutions of different concentration or between a solute and the fluid in which it is dissolved (see also OSMOSIS).

partial p., pressure exerted by each of the constituents of a mixture of gases.

p. points, various locations at which digital pressure may be applied for the control of hemorrhage.

positive p., pressure greater than that of the atmosphere.

pulse p., the difference between the systolic and diastolic pressures.

p. sore, decubitus ulcer.

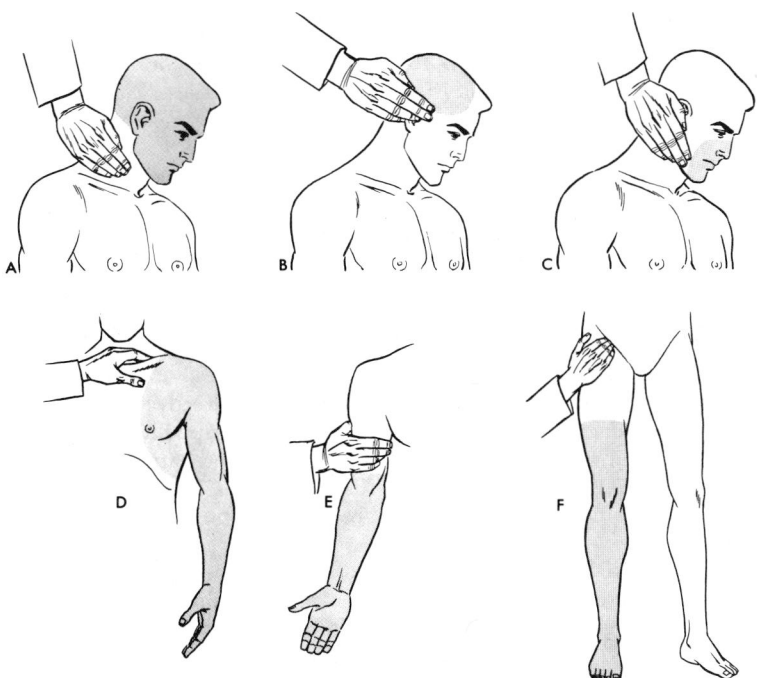

Digital pressure points. The shaded areas are those within which hemorrhage may be controlled by pressure on the specific artery. *A,* Carotid artery; *B,* temporal artery; *C,* external maxillary artery; *D,* subclavian artery; *E,* brachial artery; *F,* femoral artery. (From Crawford, S. S.: The emergency duties of the industrial nurse. Nursing Clin. N. Amer., 2:271, 1967.)

systolic p., arterial pressure during systole.

venous p., the blood pressure in the veins.

presternum (pre-ster′num) the manubrium; the upper part of the sternum.

presuppurative (pre-sup′u-ra″tiv) preceding suppuration.

presynaptic (pre″sĭ-nap′tik) situated proximal to a synapse, or occurring before the synapse is crossed.

presystole (pre-sis′to-le) the interval just before systole.

presystolic (pre″sis-tol′ik) preceding systole.

pretarsal (pre-tar′sal) in front of the tarsus.

pretibial (pre-tib′e-al) in front of the tibia.

p. fever, a disease marked by rash on the front of the tibial region, by pain in the lumbar region and by fever and coryza.

prevalence (prev′ah-lens) the number of cases of a specific disease in existence in a given population at a certain time.

preventive (pre-ven′tiv) serving to avert the occurrence of.

p. medicine, science aimed at preventing disease.

prevertebral (pre-ver′tĕ-bral) in front of a vertebra.

prevesical (pre-ves′ĭ-kal) anterior to the bladder.

previable (pre-vi′ah-bl) not yet viable; said of a fetus incapable of extrauterine existence.

previtamin (pre-vi′tah-min) a precursor of a vitamin.

prezygotic (pre″zi-got′ik) occurring before or pertaining to the time preceding union of the gametes (formation of the zygote).

prezymogen (pre-zi′mo-jen) a substance in the cell that is converted into zymogen.

priapism (pri′ah-pizm) persistent abnormal erection of the penis, usually without sexual desire. It is seen in diseases and injuries of the spinal cord, and may be caused by vesical calculus and certain injuries to the penis.

prickle cell (prik′l) a dividing keratinocyte in the stratum germinativum of the epidermis, with delicate radiating processes connecting with other similar cells.

prickly heat miliaria.

primaquine (pri′mah-kwin) a compound used as an antimalarial agent.

primate (pri′māt) an individual belonging to the highest order of mammals, Primates (pri-ma′tēz), which contains man and the apes, monkeys, etc.

primer (prīm′er) a substance that prepares for or facilitates the action of another.

primidone (pri′mĭ-dōn) a compound used as an anticonvulsant.

primigravida (pri″mĭ-grav′ĭ-dah) a woman pregnant for the first time; gravida I.

primipara (pri-mip′ah-rah) unipara; a woman who has had one pregnancy that resulted in viable offspring, para I. adj., **primip′arous.**

primiparity (pri″mĭ-par′ĭ-te) the state of being a primipara.

primordial (pri-mor′de-al) original or primitive; of the simplest and most undeveloped character.

primordium (pri-mor′de-um) the first beginnings of an organ or part in the developing embryo.

Prinadol (prin′ah-dol) trademark for a preparation of phenazocine, an analgesic.

principle (prin′sĭ-pl) 1. a chemical component. 2. a substance on which certain of the properties of a drug depend. 3. a law of conduct.

active p., any constituent of a drug that helps to confer upon it a medicinal property.

antianemia p., the constituent in liver and certain other tissues that produces the hematopoietic effect in pernicious anemia.

pleasure p., the automatic instinct or tendency to avoid pain and secure pleasure.

proximate p., any one of the definite compounds into which a substance may be directly or readily resolved.

reality p., the mental activity that develops to control the pleasure principle under the pressure of necessity or the demands of reality.

Priodax (pri′o-daks) trademark for a preparation of iodoalphionic acid, used as a contrast medium in cholecystography.

Priscoline (pris′ko-lēn) trademark for preparations of tolazoline, a vasodilator and sympatholytic.

Privine (pri′vēn) trademark for preparations of naphazoline, a nasal decongestant.

p.r.n. [L.] *pro re na′ta* (according as circumstances may require).

pro- (pro) word element [L., Gr.], *before; in front of; favoring.*

proaccelerin (pro″ak-sel′er-in) clotting factor V.

proactivator (pro-ak′tĭ-va″tor) a precursor of an activator; a factor that reacts with an enzyme to form an activator.

proamnion (pro-am′ne-on) that part of the embryonal area at the front and sides of the head that remains without mesoderm for some time.

proarrhythmic (pro″ah-rith′mik) 1. tending to produce cardiac arrhythmia. 2. an agent that tends to produce cardiac arrhythmia.

proband (pro′band) propositus.

probang (pro′bang) a flexible rod with a ball, tuft or sponge at the end; used in diseases of the esophagus or larynx.

Pro-banthine (pro-ban-thīn′) trademark for preparations of propantheline bromide, an anticholinergic.

probarbital (pro-bar′bĭ-tal) an intermediate-acting barbiturate compound used as a sedative and hypnotic.

probe (prōb) a long, slender instrument for exploring wounds or body cavities or passages.

probenecid (pro-ben′ĕ-sid) a white, crystalline compound, used in the treatment of GOUT to promote excretion of uric acid, and in some forms of arthritis.

procainamide hydrochloride (pro-kān′ah-mīd) a compound used in the treatment of cardiac arrhythmia.

procaine (pro′kān) a compound used to produce local anesthesia.
   p. hydrochloride, a white crystalline powder used for infiltration and spinal anesthesia, and nerve block.

procephalic (pro″sĕ-fal′ik) pertaining to the anterior part of the head.

procercoid (pro-ser′koid) a larval stage of fish tapeworms.

process (pros′es) 1. a prominence or projection, as from a bone. 2. a series of operations or events leading to achievement of a specific result.
   acromial p., acromion.
   alveolar p., the thick curved ridge that projects downward and forms the free lower border of the maxilla and bears the teeth.
   basilar p., a forward projection of the occipital bone, articulating with the sphenoid bone.
   capitular p., the articular process on a vertebra for the head of a rib.
   caudate p., the portion connecting the right lobe and caudate lobe of the liver.
   ciliary p's, fringelike processes encircling the margin of the eye lens.
   coracoid p., a projection from the anterior and upper edge of the scapula.
   coronoid p., 1. a projection on the ulna that articulates in the coronoid fossa of the humerus. 2. a process of the mandible.
   ensiform p., xiphoid process.
   epiphyseal p., epiphysis.
   ethmoid p., a projection from the upper border of the inferior nasal concha.
   frontonasal p., an expansive facial process in the embryo that develops into the forehead and bridge of the nose.
   malar p., an eminence by which the superior maxilla articulates with the zygoma; zygomatic process.
   mamillary p., a tubercle on each superior articular process of a lumbar vertebra.
   mastoid p., a conical projection at the base of mastoid portion of temporal bone.
   odontoid p., a toothlike projection of the axis that articulates with the atlas.
   pterygoid p., one of the wing-shaped processes of the sphenoid bone.
   spinous p. of vertebrae, a part of the vertebrae projecting backward from the arch, giving attachment to muscles of the back.
   styloid p., a long, pointed projection, particularly a long spine projecting downward from the inferior surface of the temporal bone.
   xiphoid p., the pointed process of cartilage, supported by a core of bone, connected with the lower end of the sternum.
   zygomatic p., a projection from the frontal or

temporal bone, or from the maxilla, by which they articulate with the zygoma.

processus (pro-ses′us), pl. *proces′sus* [L.] process; used in official names of various anatomic structures.

procheilon (pro-ki′lon) the central prominence of the mucocutaneous margin of the upper lip.

prochlorpemazine, prochlorperazine (pro″klōr-pem′ah-zēn), (pro″klōr-per′ah-zēn) a phenothiazine derivative used as a tranquilizer and antiemetic.

procidentia (pro″sī-den′she-ah) a falling down, or state of prolapse, especially prolapse of the uterus.

procoagulant (pro″co-ag′u-lant) tending to favor the occurrence of coagulation.

proconceptive (pro″kon-sep′tiv) aiding or promoting conception.

proconvertin (pro″kon-ver′tin) prothrombinogen; clotting factor VII.

procreation (pro″kre-a′shun) the act of begetting or generating.

proct(o)- (prok′to) word element [Gr.], *rectum.*

proctagra, proctalgia (prok-tag′rah), (prok-tal′-je-ah) pain in the rectum.

proctatresia (prok″tah-tre′ze-ah) imperforation of the anus.

proctectasia (prok″tek-ta′ze-ah) dilatation of the rectum or anus.

proctectomy (prok-tek′to-me) excision of the rectum.

procteurynter (prok″tu-rin′ter) an instrument for dilating the anus.

proctitis (prok-ti′tis) inflammation of the rectum.

proctocele (prok′to-sēl) hernial protrusion of part of the rectum into the vagina; rectocele.

proctoclysis (prok-tok′lĭ-sis) slow injection of liquid into the rectum.

proctocolectomy (prok″to-ko-lek′to-me) excision of the rectum and colon.

proctocolonoscopy (prok″to-ko″lon-os′ko-pe) inspection of interior of the rectum and lower colon.

proctocolpoplasty (prok″to-kol′po-plas″te) repair of a rectovaginal fistula.

proctocystotomy (prōk″to-sis-tot′o-me) removal of a bladder calculus through the rectum.

proctodeum (prok″to-de′um) the ectodermal depression of the caudal end of the embryo, which becomes the anal canal.

proctodynia (prok″to-din′e-ah) pain in the rectum.

proctogenic (prok″to-jen′ik) derived from the anus or rectum.

proctology (prok-tol′o-je) the branch of medicine treating of the rectum and its diseases.

proctoparalysis (prok″to-pah-ral′ĭ-sis) paralysis of the anal sphincter.

proctoperineoplasty (prok″to-per″ĭ-ne′o-plas″te) plastic repair of the rectum and perineum.

proctoperineorrhaphy (prok″to-per″ĭ-ne-or′ah-fe) suture of the rectum and perineum.

proctopexy (prok′to-pek″se) surgical fixation of the rectum.

proctophobia (prok″to-fo′be-ah) mental apprehension in patients with rectal disease.

proctoplasty (prok′to-plas″te) plastic repair of the rectum and anus.

proctoplegia (prok″to-ple′je-ah) proctoparalysis.

proctoptosis (prok″top-to′sis) prolapse of the rectum.

proctorrhaphy (prok-tor′ah-fe) suture of the rectum.

proctorrhea (prok″to-re′ah) a mucous discharge from the anus.

proctoscope (prok′to-skōp) an endoscope specially designed for passage through the anus to permit inspection of the lower part of the intestine.

proctoscopy (prok-tos′ko-pe) rectal examination with a proctoscope. The examination is usually done prior to rectal surgery, and it may be a part of the physical examination of a patient with hemorrhoids, rectal bleeding or other symptoms of a rectal disorder.
NURSING CARE. Before the examination, the lower bowel must be cleansed so that visualization of the rectal mucosa will be possible. Cleansing is done by enema or insertion of a rectal suppository or both. Cathartics are not given as they tend to cause collection of liquid stool in the area being examined. The patient is instructed to eat a light meal the evening before proctoscopy is scheduled, and breakfast is omitted or limited to liquids.
For the examination the patient is placed in knee-chest position and draped so that the rectal orifice is exposed. If the patient cannot maintain this position, the physician may allow him to lie on his side in Sims's position. The proctoscope is lubricated before insertion. Although the procedure may be uncomfortable and tiring for the patient there should be no pain associated with proctoscopy.
After the examination is completed the patient should be allowed to rest before returning to his home or hospital room.

proctosigmoid (prok″to-sig′moid) the rectum and sigmoid colon.

proctosigmoidectomy (prok″to-sig″moi-dek′to-me) excision of the rectum and sigmoid.

proctosigmoiditis (prok″to-sig″moi-di′tis) inflammation of the rectum and sigmoid.

proctosigmoidoscopy (prok″to-sig″moi-dos′ko-pe) direct visual examination of the rectum and sigmoid.

proctospasm (prok′to-spazm) spasm of the rectum.

proctostat (prok′to-stat) a radium-containing tube for insertion into the rectum.

proctostenosis (prok″to-stĕ-no′sis) stricture of the rectum.

proctostomy (prok-tos′to-me) surgical creation of a new opening of the rectum on the body surface.

proctotomy (prok-tot′o-me) incision of the rectum, usually for anal or rectal stricture.

proctovalvotomy (prok″to-val-vot′o-me) incision of the rectal valves.

procumbent (pro-kum′bent) prone; lying on the face.

procursive (pro-ker′siv) tending to run forward.

procyclidine (pro-si′klĭ-dēn) tricyclamol, an anticholinergic.

prodrome (pro′drōm) a premonitory symptom, indicating the onset of disease.

proencephalus (pro″en-sef′ah-lus) a fetus with a protrusion of the brain through a frontal fissure.

proenzyme (pro-en′zīm) zymogen; an inactive precursor of an enzyme.

proerythroblast (pro″ĕ-rith′ro-blast) an early precursor of an erythrocyte.

profenamine (pro-fen′ah-mēn) ethopropazine, used in parasympathetic blockade and in Parkinson's disease.

profibrillatory (pro-fib′rĭ-lah-to″re) tending to produce cardiac fibrillation.

profibrinolysin (pro-fi″brĭ-nol′ĭ-sin) plasminogen, the precursor of fibrinolysin.

proflavin (pro-fla′vin) a reddish brown, crystalline powder used in the treatment of infected wounds.

profundus (pro-fun′dus) [L.] deep.

progenitor (pro-jen′ĭ-tor) a parent or ancestor.

progeny (proj′ĕ-ne) offspring, or descendants.

progeria (pro-je′re-ah) premature development of the characteristics usually associated with old age.

progestational (pro″jes-ta′shun-al) preceding gestation; referring to changes in the endometrium preparatory to implantation of the developing ovum should fertilization occur.
p. **agent**, a synthetic compound having the physiologic effects of PROGESTERONE. Such compounds are used therapeutically to treat functional uterine bleeding, dysmenorrhea, threatened abortion and some cases of infertility. Called also progestogen.
p. **hormones**, substances, including PROGESTERONE, that are concerned mainly with preparing the endometrium for nidation of the fertilized ovum if conception has occurred.

progesteroid (pro-jes′tĕ-roid) a progesterone-like compound, or one having progestational effects.

progesterone (pro-jes′tĕ-rōn) a steroid with progestational activity, isolated from human ovaries, adrenal cortex and placenta.

Progesterone plays a major part in the menstrual cycle. During the maturation of the ovum, estrogen, the principal female sex hormone, is produced at a high rate. At ovulation estrogen production is sharply reduced, and the ovary then creates within itself a special endocrine structure called the corpus luteum whose sole function is to produce progesterone. Unless fertilization takes place, the corpus luteum disappears when it has performed its function.

The progesterone produced by the corpus luteum is promptly carried by the blood to the uterus, as was the estrogen that preceded it. Both hormones now work to prepare the uterus for possible conception.

In pregnancy, progesterone acts in a way that protects the embryo and fosters growth of the placenta. By decreasing the frequency of uterine contractions it helps to prevent expulsion of the implanted ovum. It also promotes secretory changes in the mucosa of the uterine tubes, thereby helping to provide nutrition for the fertilized ovum as it travels through the tube on its way to the uterus.

Another function of progesterone is promotion of the development of the mammary glands in preparation for lactation. Lactogenic hormone, from the anterior lobe of the PITUITARY GLAND, stimulates production of the milk, and progesterone prepares the glands for secretion.

Progesterone also has an indirect effect on the fluid and electrolyte balance of the body by blocking the effect of aldosterone.

Diminished secretion of progesterone can lead to menstrual difficulties in nonpregnant women and spontaneous abortion in pregnant women.

Commercial preparations of progesterone are used in the treatment of threatened abortion and for relief of various menstrual disorders such as dysmenorrhea, menorrhagia and metrorrhagia.

progestin (pro-jes'tin) a trade name for preparations of progesterone.

progestogen (pro-jes'to-jen) a substance that induces progestational changes.

proglossis (pro-glos'is) the tip of the tongue.

proglottid, proglottis (pro-glot'id), (pro-glot'is) one of the segments making up the body of a tapeworm.

prognathism (prog'nah-thizm) abnormal protrusion of the lower jaw. adj., **prognath'ic.**

prognathous (prog'nah-thus, prog-na'thus) having projecting jaws.

prognosis (prog-no'sis) the probable outcome of an attack of a disease. adj., **prognos'tic.**

progranulocyte (pro-gran'u-lo-sīt") promyelocyte.

proguanil (pro-gwan'il) a compound used as an antimalarial.

Progynon (pro-jin'on) trademark for preparations of estradiol, an estrogen.

proiomenorrhea (pro"e-o-men"o-re'ah) early or premature menstruation.

proiosystole (pro"e-o-sis'to-le) a contraction of the heart occurring before its normal time; a premature heartbeat.

proiotia (pro"e-o'she-ah) sexual or genital precocity.

projection (pro-jek'shun) 1. a throwing forward, especially the reference of impressions made on the sense organs to their proper source. 2. the act of extending or jutting out, or a part that juts out. 3. a mental mechanism whereby emotionally unacceptable traits are denied by a person as his own and attributed (projected) to another. It is often called the "blaming" mechanism because in using it one seeks to place the blame for his inadequacies upon someone else. In its extreme form projection can lead to hostility and physical attack upon others when the person mistakenly perceives these persons as responsible for his mental anguish.

prokaryocyte (pro-kar'e-o-sīt") an immature erythrocyte intermediate between a karyoblast and a karyocyte.

prokaryosis (pro"kar-e-o'sis) the state of not having a true nucleus, the nuclear material being scattered in the protoplasm of the cell.

prolabium (pro-la'be-um) the prominent central part of the upper lip.

prolactin (pro-lak'tin) a hormone secreted by the anterior pituitary that promotes the growth of breast tissue and stimulates milk production in the mammary gland; called also lactogenic hormone, luteotropic hormone and LTH.

prolamine (pro-lam'in) one of a class of simple proteins insoluble in water and absolute alcohol, but soluble in 70 to 80 per cent ethyl alcohol; obtained principally from cereal seeds.

prolan (pro'lan) gonadotropic hormone.

prolapse (pro'laps) the falling down, or downward displacement, of a part or viscus.

  p. of cord, protrusion of the umbilical cord ahead of the presenting part of the fetus in labor.

  frank p., prolapse of the uterus in which the vagina is inverted and hangs from the vulva.

  p. of the iris, protrusion of the iris through a wound in the cornea.

  rectal p., p. of rectum, protrusion of the rectal mucous membrane through the anus.

  p. of uterus, protrusion of the uterus through the vaginal orifice.

prolapsus (pro-lap'sus) [L.] prolapse.

prolepsis (pro-lep'sis) recurrence of a paroxysm before the expected time. adj., **prolep'tic.**

proliferation (pro-lif"ĕ-ra'shun) the reproduction or multiplication of similar forms, especially of cells and morbid cysts.

proligerous (pro-lij'er-us) producing offspring.

proline (pro'lēn) a naturally occurring amino acid.

Proluton (pro-lu'ton) trademark for preparations of progesterone.

promazine (pro'mah-zēn) a phenothiazine derivative used as a tranquilizer.

promethazine (pro-meth'ah-zēn) a phenothiazine derivative used as an antihistamine.

promethestrol (pro-meth′es-trol) a compound used as an estrogenic substance.

promethium (pro-me′the-um) a chemical element, atomic number 61, atomic weight 147, symbol Pm. (See table of ELEMENTS.)

Promin (pro′min) trademark for a preparation of glucosulfone sodium, used in treatment of leprosy.

promine (pro′mēn) a substance widely distributed in animal cells that is characterized by its ability to promote cell division and growth.

prominence (prom′ĭ-nens) a conspicuously elevated area.

promonocyte (pro-mon′o-sīt) a cell of the monocytic series intermediate between the monoblast and monocyte, with coarse chromatin structure and one or two nucleoli.

promontory (prom′on-tor″e) a projecting process or eminence.
   p. of the sacrum, the upper, projecting part of the sacrum.

promoxolane (pro-mok′so-lān) a compound used as a tranquilizer.

promyelocyte (pro-mi′ĕ-lo-sīt″) a cell intermediate between myeloblast and myelocyte, containing a few undifferentiated cytoplasmic granules.

pronate (pro′nāt) to place in or assume a prone position.

pronation (pro-na′shun) the act of assuming the prone position; placing or lying face downward. Applied to the hand, turning the palm backward (posteriorly) or downward, performed by medial rotation of the forearm. Applied to the foot, a combination of eversion and abduction movements taking place in the tarsal and metatarsal joints and resulting in lowering of the medial margin of the foot, hence of the longitudinal arch.

prone (prōn) lying face downward, or on the ventral surface.

pronephros (pro-nef′ros), pl. *proneph′roi* [Gr.] the earliest and simplest excretory organ in the embryo; although it serves no purpose in many vertebrates, its development precedes that of a mesonephros.

Pronestyl (pro-nes′til) trademark for preparations of procainamide hydrochloride, used in treatment of cardiac arrhythmia.

pronormoblast (pro-nor′mo-blast) a name given early forms of the erythrocytic series; proerythroblast.

pronucleus (pro-nu′kle-us) the nucleus of an ovum or spermatozoon before their fusion in the fertilized ovum.
   female p., the nucleus of an ovum before it unites with that of the spermatozoon that has penetrated its cytoplasm.
   male p., the nucleus of the spermatozoon after it has penetrated the cytoplasm of an ovum.

prootic (pro-ot′ik) in front of the ear.

Propadrine (pro′pah-drēn) trademark for a preparation of synthetic alkaloid, resembling ephedrine in composition and action.

propagation (prop″ah-ga′shun) reproduction.

propalinal (pro-pal′ĭ-nal) having a backward and forward motion or direction.

propane (pro′pān) a volatile hydrocarbon from petroleum.

propantheline bromide (pro-pan′thĕ-lēn) a compound used as an anticholinergic.

proparacaine (pro-par′ah-kān) a compound used as a local anesthetic.

propedeutics (pro″pĕ-du′tiks) the introduction to an art or science.

propepsin (pro-pep′sin) pepsinogen; the inactive precursor of pepsin.

properdin (pro-pār′din) a euglobulin isolated from normal serum that is capable of destroying bacteria and viruses.

prophase (pro′fāz) the first stage of division of the nucleus of a cell in either meiosis or mitosis.

prophenpyridamine (pro″fen-pi-rid′ah-mēn) pheniramine, an antihistaminic.

prophylactic (pro″fĭ-lak′tik) tending to ward off disease.

prophylactodontics (pro″fĭ-lak″to-don′tiks) the branch of dentistry concerned with prevention of dental and oral diseases.

prophylaxis (pro″fĭ-lak′sis) prevention of disease.

propiodal (pro-pi′o-dal) an iodide compound used as a source of iodine.

propiomazine (pro″pe-o-ma′zēn) a phenothiazine derivative used to potentiate the sedative action of barbiturates and as an adjunct to ether anesthesia.

propionic acid (pro″pe-on′ik) a compound produced by oxidation of normal propyl alcohol or by action of certain bacteria on hexoses, pentoses, lactic acid and glycerin.

proplexus (pro-plek′sus) the choroid plexus of the lateral ventricle of the brain.

propons (pro′pons) delicate plates of white matter passing across the anterior end of the pyramid of the cerebellum and just below the pons.

propositus (pro-poz′ĭ-tus), pl. *propos′iti* [L.] a person whose hereditary disorder stimulates genetic study in his family; called also proband.

propoxycaine (pro-pok′se-kān) a compound used as a local anesthetic.

propoxyphene (pro-pok′se-fēn) dextropropoxyphene, an analgesic.

proprietary medicine (pro-pri′ĕ-ter″e) any chemical, drug or similar preparation used in the treatment of diseases, if such article is protected against free competition as to name, product, composition or process of manufacture by secrecy, patent, trademark or copyright, or by other means.

proprioceptive (pro"pre-o-sep'tiv) receiving stimuli within the body.

proprioceptor (pro"pre-o-sep'tor) one of the specialized nerve endings in muscles, tendons and joints that are sensitive to changes in tension of muscle or tendon, and thereby provide information concerning body movements and position.

proptometer (pro-tom'ĕ-ter) an instrument for measuring exophthalmos.

proptosis (prop-to'sis) downward or forward displacement of an organ or part.

propulsion (pro-pul'shun) 1. a tendency to fall forward in walking. 2. festination.

propylene glycol (pro'pĭ-lēn gli'kol) a colorless, viscous liquid, used as a substitute for glycerin.

propylhexedrine (pro"pil-hek'sĕ-drēn) a compound used as an inhalant to decongest nasal mucosa.

propyliodone (pro"pil-i'o-dōn) a compound used as a radiopaque medium in bronchography.

propylparaben (pro"pil-par'ah-ben) a compound used as an antifungal preservative.

propylthiouracil (pro"pil-thi"o-u'rah-sil) a compound used as a thyroid inhibitor.

pro re nata (pro ra nah'tah) [L.] according as circumstances may require; abbreviated p.r.n.

prorennin (pro-ren'in) a precursor of rennin; renninogen.

prorubricyte (pro-roo'brĭ-sīt) proerythroblast.

prosecretin (pro"se-kre'tin) the supposed precursor of secretin.

prosector (pro-sek'tor) one who dissects anatomic subjects for demonstration.

prosencephalon (pros"en-sef'ah-lon) 1. the forebrain, comprising the cerebral hemispheres, diencephalon, hypothalamus and thalamencephalon. 2. the most anterior of the three primary divisions of the neural tube of the embryo, which later divides into the telencephalon and the diencephalon.

prosodemic (pros"o-dem'ik) passing from one person to another instead of reaching a large number at once, through such means as water supply: said of a disease progressing in that way.

prosogaster (pros"o-gas'ter) foregut.

prosopagnosia (pros"o-pag-no'se-ah) inability to recognize the faces of other people or one's own features in a mirror.

prosopalgia (pros"o-pal'je-ah) neuralgia of the trigeminal nerve (TIC DOULOUREUX).

prosopantritis (pros"o-pan-tri'tis) inflammation of the frontal sinuses.

prosopectasia (pros"o-pek-ta'ze-ah) oversize of the face.

prosoplasia (pros"o-pla'ze-ah) development into a higher state of organization.

prosopodiplegia (pros"o-po-di-ple'je-ah) paralysis of the face and one lower extremity.

prosoponeuralgia (pros"o-po-nu-ral'je-ah) facial neuralgia.

prosopoplegia (pros"o-po-ple'je-ah) facial paralysis.

prosoposchisis (pros"o-pos'kĭ-sis) congenital fissure of the face.

prosopospasm (pros'o-po-spazm") spasm of the face.

prosoposternodymia (pros"o-po-ster"no-dim'e-ah) a double monster joined face to face and sternum to sternum.

prosopothoracopagus (pros"o-po-tho"rah-kop'-ah-gus) twin fetuses joined in the thorax, face and neck.

prosopotocia (pros"o-po-to'she-ah) face presentation in labor.

prostaglandin (pros"tah-glan'din) a substance, first found in semen of man and sheep, that causes strong contraction of smooth muscle and dilation of certain vascular beds.

prostatalgia (pros"tah-tal'je-ah) pain in the prostate.

prostate (pros'tāt) an accessory reproductive organ in the male, located next to and under the bladder and completely surrounding the urethra. It is about the size of a walnut and consists of a median and two lateral lobes. adj., **prostat'ic.**

The prostate secretes a thin, slightly alkaline fluid that flows through ducts into the urethra. This fluid is secreted continuously, and the excess passes from the body in the urine. The rate of secretion increases greatly during sexual stimulation and the fluid contributes to the bulk of the semen.

DISORDERS OF THE PROSTATE. Enlargement of the prostate (benign prostatic hypertrophy) is a common complaint in men over 50 years of age. Because of its position around the urethra, enlargement of the prostate quickly interferes with the

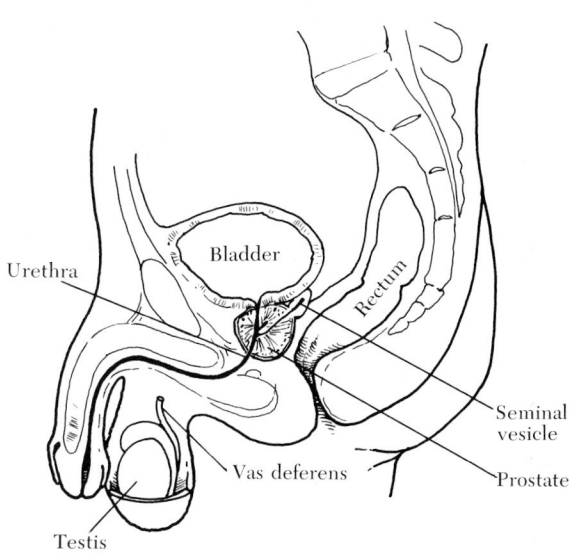

Prostate.

normal passage of urine from the bladder. Urination becomes increasingly difficult, and the bladder never feels completely emptied. If left untreated, continued enlargement of the prostate eventually obstructs the bladder completely, and emergency measures become necessary to empty the bladder. If the prostate is markedly enlarged, chronic constipation may result. The usual remedy is PROSTATECTOMY.

In men over 60 years of age, cancer of the prostate may occur. The symptoms are similar to those of prostatic enlargement. If the malignancy is discovered in time, the gland can be removed before the cancer has a chance to spread. Symptoms of cancer of the prostate usually respond to estrogens or to orchiectomy.

Inflammation of the prostate (prostatitis) usually responds to antibiotics; if it does not, a prostatic abscess may form, which can be incised and drained surgically.

prostatectomy (pros″tah-tek′to-me) excision of the prostate. There are several alternate methods of performing this surgical procedure. In suprapubic prostatectomy the gland is removed through an abdominal incision. The bladder is also incised and the gland is removed from above. This procedure is preferred when the prostate is greatly enlarged. In perineal prostatectomy an incision is made into the perineum and the gland is removed from below. Disadvantages of this method include frequent contamination of the wound and the likelihood of incontinence and rectal injury as complications. The most popular and least traumatic method of removal of an enlarged prostate is transurethral resection. A surgical incision is not involved since the surgeon approaches the prostate via the urethra, using a cystoscope and removing small pieces of obstructing gland tissue with an electric wire.

NURSING CARE. Preoperatively the patient must be watched for signs of urinary retention and bladder distention. An indwelling catheter is often inserted to prevent this difficulty; if so, its purpose should be explained to the patient. Care must be used in the administration of sedatives and hypnotics since many of these patients are elderly and are likely to suffer from mental confusion and other adverse effects from drugs of this type. It may be necessary to use side rails on the bed, especially at night, to prevent accidents and injury to the patient.

Immediately after surgery the patient is observed for signs of hemorrhage, a primary danger of prostatectomy. Though the urinary drainage can be expected to be bright red for the first 24 hours after surgery, excessive bleeding must be reported immediately. An increasingly darker color may indicate an increase in blood content in the drainage.

In addition, special attention is given the catheter leading from the bladder to insure adequate drainage at all times. Severe pain in the bladder region may indicate obstruction of the catheter by blood clots or bits of tissue. Irrigations, when done to remove the obstruction, demand strict aseptic technique to avoid the introduction of infectious microorganisms into the urinary tract and the surgical wound. Severe abdominal pain and rigidity may indicate perforation of the bladder.

The surgical wound of a suprapubic prostatectomy demands frequent attention since the bladder has been incised and there is almost constant drainage of urine onto the surgical dressings. Frequent changing of these dressings is necessary to prevent irritation of the surrounding skin and the development of unpleasant odors. Infection is a particular hazard in both suprapubic and perineal prostatectomy patients.

prostaticovesiculectomy (pros-tat″ĭ-ko-vě-sik″u-lek′to-me) excision of the prostate and seminal vesicles.

prostatism (pros′tah-tizm) the condition resulting from obstruction to urination due to prostatic hypertrophy.

prostatitis (pros″tah-ti′tis) inflammation of the prostate.

prostatocystitis (pros″tah-to-sis-ti′tis) inflammation of the prostate and the bladder.

prostatocystotomy (pros″tah-to-sis″tot′o-me) incision of the bladder and prostate.

prostatodynia (pros″tah-to-din′e-ah) pain in the prostate.

prostatolith (pros-tat′o-lith) a calculus in the prostate.

prostatolithotomy (pros″tah-to-lĭ-thot′o-me) incision of the prostate for removal of a calculus.

prostatomegaly (pros″tah-to-meg′ah-le) hypertrophy of the prostate.

prostatomyomectomy (pros″tah-to-mi″o-mek′to-me) excision of a prostatic myoma.

prostatorrhea (pros″tah-to-re′ah) catarrhal discharge from the prostate.

prostatotomy (pros″tah-tot′o-me) surgical incision of the prostate.

prostatovesiculectomy (pros″tah-to-vě-sik″u-lek′to-me) excision of the prostate and seminal vesicles.

prostatovesiculitis (pros″tah-to-vě-sik″u-li′tis) inflammation of the prostate and seminal vesicles.

prosthesis (pros′thĕ-sis, pros-the′sis), pl. *prosthe′ses* [Gr.] 1. the replacement of an absent part by an

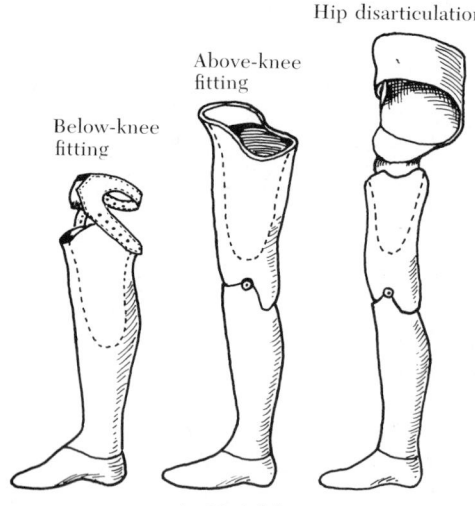

Artificial legs.

artificial substitute. 2. an artificial substitute for a missing part, such as an eye, leg or denture; the term is also applied to any device by which performance of a natural function is aided or augmented, such as a hearing aid or eyeglasses. adj., **prosthet'ic.**

ARTIFICIAL LIMB. Recent advances in the field of surgical amputation and the art of designing artificial limbs have made it possible for a person who has lost a limb to be equipped with a prosthesis that functions so efficiently, and so closely resembles the original in appearance, that he is able to resume normal activities with his handicap passing virtually unnoticed.

Fitting an Artificial limb. There are two stages in the fitting of an artificial limb. First, the surgeon prepares a stump that will be suitable for the particular type of limb required. The form of the stump will depend on a number of factors, chiefly the occupation of the person and his enthusiasm and ability to adapt to the limb and use it to the best advantage. The surgeon aims to make the stump long enough to retain some muscular strength and (in the case of legs) short enough to be able to bear weight. It is usually found that the limb is easier to control if the amputation is made in the middle of one of the long bones rather than at a joint. In the second stage, the limb-maker fits and shapes the limb.

Materials Used in the Limb. A variety of materials can be used for the manufacture of artificial limbs. Wood, especially willow, is the most popular. It is comparatively light and resilient, and is easily shaped. If necessary, for example in the artificial limb for a growing child, it can be added to. Aluminum or an aluminum alloy is used when lightness is particularly desirable – in a limb for an aged person, for example. Plastic limbs are also being developed. Leather and various metals are used for reinforcement and control.

Powering the Limb. Most artificial limbs are powered by the muscles, either those remaining in the stump or other available muscles. The muscles of the stump often can be considerably strengthened by physical therapy. Muscle power can be reinforced by means of springs, straps, gears, locks, levers or, in some cases, hydraulic mechanisms.

The Artificial Leg. The most commonly fitted artificial limb is the knee-jointed leg, used by persons whose legs have been amputated above the knee. This prosthesis is powered by the hip and remaining thigh muscles, which kick the leg forward. The key points in such a limb are the socket, where it fits onto the stump, the knee and the ankle. The possibility of walking with a normal gait depends primarily on the successful alignment of the socket joint; the knee usually consists of a joint centered slightly behind that of the natural leg, as this has been found to afford greater stability; sometimes the ankle joint is omitted and the flexibility of the ankle achieved by the use of a rubber foot.

The Artificial Arm. The choice of a particular artificial arm depends largely on the person's occupation. There is a wide variety of types, ranging from the purely functional, which will enable a person to perform heavy work, to the purely cosmetic, which aims only at looking as natural as possible. Those persons whose work requires them to do heavy lifting are often fitted with a "pegarm," a short arm without an elbow joint, which is easily controlled and has great leverage.

The Artificial Hand. There are a great many different types of artificial hands. Many artificial arms are so constructed that they can be fitted with a selection of different hands, depending on the type of work to be done. It is generally agreed by experts that the various types of hooks offer the greatest functional efficiency. These reproduce the most powerful function of natural hands – the pressure between thumb and forefinger. But there are hands that combine a certain amount of utility with cosmetic value, often by means of a cosmetic glove covering a mechanical hand; and there are also hands designed simply for appearance, though these usually offer some support as well.

Most hooks and hands are mechanically connected to the opposite shoulder and operated by a

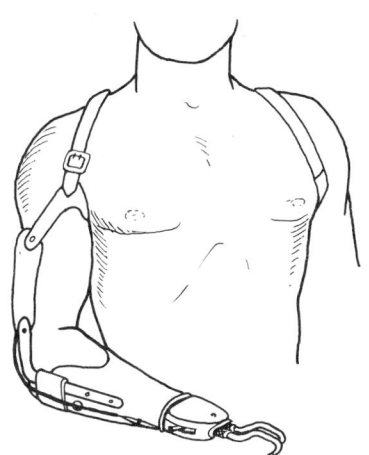

Below-elbow amputee fitting

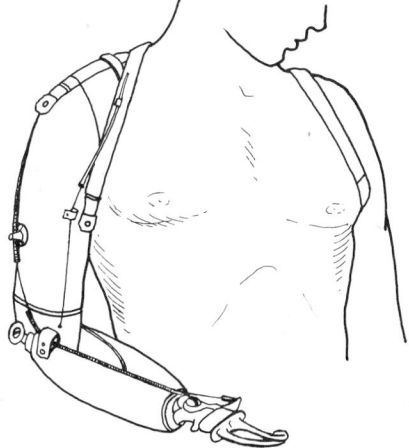

Above-elbow amputee fitting

Artificial arms. Most are mechanically controlled and are connected by straps to the opposite shoulder.

shrugging motion. However, a procedure known as kineplasty employs the person's own arm and chest muscles to work the device. In this method, selected muscles are tunneled under by surgery and lined by skin. Pegs adapted to the tunnels can then be made to move an artificial hand mechanism Kineplasty is employed when skill rather than strength is desired.

PROTECTING THE STUMP. In a person with an artificial limb, there is always a danger that the stump will become irritated or infected. He will probably wear a sock to cover the stump, and this should be washed daily; the stump itself should also be washed regularly and carefully, particularly between skin folds. And when the artificial limb is not being used the stump should, if possible, be exposed to the fresh air.

cleft palate p., an appliance used to restore the integrity of the roof of the mouth in patients with cleft palate.

dental p., artificial substitutes for missing teeth or parts of teeth.

internal p., a substitute for a diseased or non-functioning internal structure of the body, as the head of the femur or a valve of the heart.

maxillofacial p., a replacement for parts of the upper jaw or the face missing because of disease or injury.

prosthetics (pros-thet′iks) the art and science of replacing, by artificial means, body parts that may be missing or defective as a result of surgical intervention, trauma, disease or developmental anomaly.

prosthodontics (pros″tho-don′tiks) the branch of dental art and science concerned with construction of artificial appliances to replace missing teeth, and sometimes other parts of the oral cavity and face.

Prostigmin (pro-stig′min) trademark for prepa-

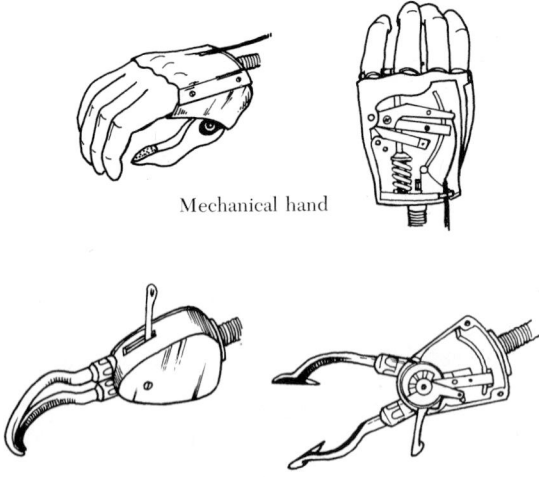

Mechanical hand

Hook

Artificial hands. The hook is the more efficient, but the mechanical hand, sometimes covered by a glove, provides both cosmetic value and utility.

rations of neostigmine, a parasympathomimetic and cholinergic.

prostration (pros-tra′shun) extreme exhaustion or lack of energy or power.

heat p., a condition caused by exposure to excessive heat; see also HEAT EXHAUSTION.

nervous p., neurasthenia.

protactinium (pro″tak-tin′e-um) a chemical element, atomic number 91, atomic weight 231, symbol Pa. (See table of ELEMENTS.)

Protalba (pro-tal′bah) trademark for preparations of protoveratrine A, an antihypertensive agent.

protamine (pro′tah-min) one of a class of simple proteins, soluble in water, not coagulated by heat, and precipitated from aqueous solution by addition of alcohol; found combined with nucleic acids in ripe fish sperm. Protamine sulfate is used to neutralize heparin, the anticoagulant.

protandry (pro-tan′dre) hermaphroditism in which the male gonad matures before the female gonad.

protanopia (pro″tah-no′pe-ah) blindness to red and green.

protean (pro′te-an) changing form or assuming many shapes.

protease (pro′te-ās) a proteolytic enzyme.

protectant, protective (pro-tek′tant), (pro-tek′tiv) a preparation that affords protection against a noxious agent or influence.

protein (pro′te-in) a compound containing carbon, hydrogen, oxygen, nitrogen and usually sulfur and phosphorus, the characteristic element being nitrogen. Protein compounds are of high molecular weight and consist largely of chains of AMINO ACIDS.

Protein substances in the body are essential to its structure and function. For example, such structures as cell walls, various membranes, connective tissue and muscles are mainly protein. None of the cells of the body can survive without an adequate supply of protein; in fact, proteins constitute about 20 per cent of the cell mass. The hormones, which are so important in the regulation of metabolism, are proteins, as are many of the enzymes that act as catalysts in the chemical reactions of metabolism.

The proteins in blood plasma are divided into three major types: ALBUMIN, GLOBULINS and FIBRINOGEN. Albumin plays an important role in the maintenance of normal distribution of water in the various compartments of the body by exerting osmotic pressure at the capillary membrane. This pressure prevents fluid of the plasma from leaking out of the capillaries and into the space between the tissue cells. (See also body FLUIDS.) Albumin is also a transport substance. The globulins are vital to the process of immunity (nearly all ANTIBODIES are gamma globulin molecules) and also act as transporters of various substances from one part of the body to another. Fibrinogen is essential to the blood clotting mechanism.

Food proteins are of great nutritional importance since they are necessary for the building and repair of all kinds of body tissues, especially of muscles and organs such as the heart, liver and kidneys. Major sources of protein are animal products such as meat, eggs, fish and milk.

The digestion of protein foods begins in the stomach, is continued in the duodenum and is completed in the small intestine. The end products of protein digestion, amino acids, pass into the blood, some to be used as structural proteins for the building of body tissues, others to be used as enzymes and the rest to be carried to various parts of the body as a reserve. If a ready supply of carbohydrates is not available, some proteins may be converted into needed energy.

SYMPTOMS OF PROTEIN DEFICIENCY. Severe protein deficiency undermines general health, and is usually manifest in weakness, poor resistance and swelling of body tissues (nutritional edema) due to accumulation of fluid in the tissue spaces. Protein starvation can result from lack of protein in the diet —in persons who, from lack of available supplies of protein foods or through ignorance, satisfy their hunger with large amounts of carbohydrates and little else. Kwashiorkor is a disorder of infants and young children whose diet is deficient in protein. The illness develops soon after weaning when the child no longer receives a protein supply from his mother's milk.

Sometimes deficiency develops when digestive disorders or infections interfere with proper digestion. A congenital defect in metabolism such as PHENYLKETONURIA may lead to inability to make proper use of the protein that is available in the diet.

The first step in treatment of protein deficiency is correction of the deficiency in the diet. If the protein deficiency is secondary to another disorder, treatment is aimed at relief of the primary cause of the deficiency.

Bence Jones p., a low-molecular-weight, heat-sensitive urinary protein found in patients with multiple myeloma.

compound p., a protein that on hydrolysis yields a simple protein and a nonprotein matter.

conjugated p's, those that contain the protein molecule united to some other molecule or molecules.

C-reactive p., a protein found in the serum of persons in whom inflammation or necrosis is present. It forms a precipitate with the C-polysaccharide of the pneumococcus, and a nonspecific test (C-reactive protein test) based on this fact is sometimes used in diagnosing or determining the progress of inflammatory diseases and widespread malignancies.

defensive p., any protein formed within the body and serving as a protection against disease.

derived p's, derivatives of the protein molecule formed by hydrolytic changes.

immune p's, proteins formed by the combination of albuminous matters of the body with the enzymes of pathogenic bacteria.

native p., an unchanged, naturally occurring animal or vegetable protein.

plasma p's, proteins found in the blood plasma.

protective p., defensive protein.

serum p., any protein found in the serum of the blood.

simple p's, those that yield only α-amino acids or their derivatives on hydrolysis.

protein-bound iodine test PBI; a laboratory test done to determine thyroid function by measuring the amount of iodine precipitated with plasma proteins. The hormone thyroxine contains iodine which is bound to blood proteins (protein-bound).

Thus measurement of the amount of protein-bound iodine in the blood aids in determining the thyroid's production of thyroxine. The normal range is from 4 to 8 mcg. per 100 ml. of blood. In hypothyroidism the amount is less than normal and in hyperthyroidism it is elevated.

Preparation for the test is minimal; neither restriction of food and fluids nor limitation of physical activity is required. It is important, however, that for several weeks prior to the test the patient does not receive iodine in any artificial form, as in dyes used for x-ray studies or in cough syrups, gargles or other patent medicines. Estrogens must also be withheld because they cause an abnormally high reading.

proteinase (pro′te-ĭ-nās″) an enzyme that splits protein.

proteinemia (pro″te-ĭ-ne′me-ah) excess of protein in the blood.

proteinivorus (pro″te-ĭ-niv′o-rus) feeding on protein.

proteinogram (pro″te-in′o-gram) a graphic representation of proteins present in a solution, such as blood serum.

proteinosis (pro″te-ĭ-no′sis) the accumulation of protein in the tissues.

lipid p., a disturbance of lipid metabolism marked by yellowish deposits of a lipid-protein mixture on the inner surface of the lips, under the tongue and on the fauces.

pulmonary alveolar p., a pulmonary disease of unknown etiology characterized by the deposit of protein material in the alveoli and causing respiratory insufficiency. It is usually fatal.

tissue p., amyloidosis.

proteinuria (pro″te-ĭ-nu′re-ah) protein in the urine.

proteoclastic (pro″te-o-klas′tik) splitting up proteins.

proteolipid, proteolipin (pro″te-o-lip′id), (pro″te-o-lip′in) a combination of a protein and a lipid, having the solubility characteristics of a lipid.

proteolysin (pro″te-ol′ĭ-sin) a specific substance causing proteolysis.

proteolysis (pro″te-ol′ĭ-sis) the breaking down of proteins into simpler compounds. adj., **proteolyt′ic.**

proteometabolism (pro″te-o-mĕ-tab′o-lizm) the metabolism of protein.

proteopeptic (pro″te-o-pep′tik) digesting protein.

proteopexy (pro′te-o-pek″se) the fixation of protein within the organism.

proteose (pro′te-ōs) any albumose or other substance intermediate between a protein and a peptone.

proteosuria (pro″te-o-su′re-ah) the presence of proteose in the urine.

proteuria (pro″te-u′re-ah) proteinuria.

Proteus (pro'te-us) a genus of Schizomycetes usually found in fecal and other putrefying material. Certain species are primarily saprophytes; others may be pathogenic when there is reduced host resistance.

P. vulga'ris, the type species of Proteus, occurring, often as a secondary invader, in a variety of localized suppurative pathologic processes, and being a common cause of cystitis.

prothipendyl (pro-thi'pen-dil) a compound used as a tranquilizer.

prothrombin (pro-throm'bin) a glycoprotein present in the plasma that is converted into thrombin by extrinsic thromboplastin during the second stage of blood clotting; called also clotting factor II.

prothrombinase (pro-throm'bin-ās) thromboplastin.

prothrombinogen (pro'throm-bin'o-jen) a heat- and storage-stable material, present in serum but not in plasma, participating only in the formation of extrinsic thromboplastin; called also clotting factor VII and serum prothrombin conversion accelerator (SPCA).

prothrombinogenic (pro-throm"bī-no-jen'ik) promoting the production of prothrombin.

prothrombinokinase (pro-throm"bī-no-ki'nās) prothrombinogen.

prothrombinopenia (pro-throm"bī-no-pe'ne-ah) deficiency of prothrombin in the blood.

protistology (pro"tis-tol'o-je) microbiology.

proto- (pro'to) word element [Gr.], *first.*

protobiology (pro"to-bi-ol'o-je) scientific study of the simplest forms of living organisms, primarily viruses.

protoblast (pro'to-blast) a cell with no cell wall; an embryonic cell.

protochrome (pro'to-krōm) a substance derived from proteins giving reactions identical with urochrome.

protocol (pro'to-kol) a written statement of the history and treatment of any particular patient, especially one made for a medicolegal purpose.

protocooperation (pro"to-ko-op"er-a'shun) symbiosis in which populations (or individuals) gain from the association but are able to survive without it.

protodiastolic (pro"to-di"ah-stol'ik) immediately following the second heart sound.

protoduodenum (pro"to-du"o-de'num) the first portion of the duodenum, developed from the embryonic foregut.

protogaster (pro"to-gas'ter) foregut.

protogyny (pro-toj'ĭ-ne) hermaphroditism in which the female gonad matures before the male gonad.

protokylol (pro"to-ki'lol) a compound used as a sympathomimetic agent and as a bronchodilator.

proton (pro'ton) an elementary particle of mass number 1, with a positive charge equal to the negative charge of the electron; a constituent particle of every nucleus, the number of protons in the nucleus of each ATOM of a chemical element being indicated by its atomic number.

protonephros (pro"to-nef'ros), pl *protoneph'roi* [Gr.] pronephros.

protoneuron (pro"to-nu'ron) the first neuron in a peripheral reflex arc.

Protophyta (pro-tof'ĭ-tah) the lowest division of the vegetable kingdom, made up of unicellular organisms and including the algae, bacteria and viruses.

protophyte (pro'to-fīt) a unicellular plant or vegetable organ; an individual belonging to the Protophyta.

protophytology (pro"to-fi-tol'o-je) scientific study of the simplest forms of plants.

protoplasm (pro'to-plazm) the viscid translucent colloid material, the essential constituent of the living cell. It is composed mainly of proteins, lipids, carbohydrates and inorganic salts. adj., **protoplas'mic.**

protoplast (pro'to-plast) a bacterial or plant cell deprived of its rigid wall and dependent for its integrity on an isotonic or hypertonic medium.

protoporphyria (pro"to-por-fēr'e-ah) porphyria in which protoporphyrin is the compound present.

erythropoietic p., a form in which excessive amounts of free protoporphyrin are found in erythrocytes, plasma and bone marrow, with sensitivity of skin to sunlight and sometimes liver damage.

protoporphyrin (pro"to-por'fī-rin) a porphyrin whose iron complex united with protein occurs in hemoglobin, myoglobin and certain respiratory pigments.

protoporphyrinuria (pro"to-por"fī-rī-nu're-ah) protoporphyrin in the urine.

protosalt (pro'to-sawlt) that one of a series of salts of the same base which contains the smallest amount of the combining substance.

protospasm (pro'to-spazm) a spasm that begins in a limited area and extends to other parts.

prototoxin (pro'to-tok'sin) the most virulent of a series of toxins.

protoveratrine (pro"to-ver'ah-trēn) an antihypertensive alkaloid isolated from *Veratrum album.* There are two forms, A and B; B is less potent.

protovertebra (pro"to-ver'tĕ-brah) somite.

protoxide (pro-tok'sīd) that one of a series of oxides of the same element which contains the least amount of oxygen.

Protozoa (pro"to-zo'ah) a phylum of the animal kingdom, comprising the lowest forms and made up of microscopic, unicellular organisms. Pathogenic protozoa include the Plasmodium of human malaria, *Trypanosoma gambiense* of African trypanosomiasis (African sleeping sickness), *Entamoeba histolytica* of amebic dysentery and

Balantidium coli and *Isospora belli*, both of which cause diarrhea in man. adj., **protozo'an.**

protozoacide (pro"to-zo'ah-sīd) destructive to protozoa.

protozoiasis (pro"to-zo-i'ah-sis) infection with protozoa.

protozoology (pro"to-zo-ol'o-je) scientific study of the simplest forms of animals (protozoa).

protozoon (pro"to-zo'on), pl. *protozo'a* [Gr.] a unicellular animal organism; an individual belonging to the Protozoa.

protozoophage (pro"to-zo'o-fāj) a phagocyte that consumes protozoa.

protraction (pro-trak'shun) a forward extension in space or time.

protractor (pro-trak'tor) an instrument for extracting foreign bodies from wounds.

protrusion (pro-troo'zhun) extension beyond the usual limits, or above a plane surface.

protuberance (pro-tu'ber-ans) a projecting part, or prominence.

protuberantia (pro-tu"ber-an'she-ah), pl. *protuberan'tiae* [L.] protuberance.

proud flesh soft, edematous, unhealthy-looking granulation tissue.

Provell (pro-vel') trademark for a preparation of protoveratrines A and B.

Provera (pro-ver'ah) trademark for preparations of medroxyprogesterone acetate, a progestational agent.

provertebra (pro-ver'tĕ-brah) somite.

Provest (pro'vest) trademark for a combination of medroxyprogesterone and ethynylestradiol; an oral contraceptive.

provitamin (pro-vi'tah-min) the precursor of a vitamin.

provocative (pro-vok'ah-tiv) stimulating the appearance of a sign, reflex, reaction or therapeutic effect.

proximad (prok'sī-mad) in a proximal direction.

proximal (prok'sī-mal) nearest to a point of reference, as to a center or median line or to the point of attachment or origin.

proximalis (prok"sī-ma'lis) [L.] proximal.

proximate (prok'sī-mit) immediate; nearest.

proximoataxia (prok"sī-mo-ah-tak'se-ah) ataxia of the proximal part of an extremity.

prozymogen (pro-zi'mo-jen) prezymogen.

pruriginous (proo-rij'ĭ-nus) of the nature of prurigo.

prurigo (proo-ri'go) a chronic skin disease marked by small, pale papules and intense itching.
 p. estiva'lis, a form occurring during warm weather.
 p. fe'rox, prurigo of a severe type with large papules and lymphadenopathy.

 p. mi'tis, prurigo of a mild type.
 p. nodula'ris, a form marked by intense itching and formation of discrete, firm, erythematous nodules.
 p. sim'plex, a mild form with crops of papules tending to recur in cycles.
 summer p., prurigo estivalis.

pruritogenic (proo"rĭ-to-jen'ik) causing pruritus, or itching.

pruritus (proo-ri'tus) itching. adj., **prurit'ic.** It is common in many types of skin disorders, especially allergic inflammation and parasitic infestations. Systemic diseases that may cause pruritus include DIABETES MELLITUS (pruritus vulvae) and liver disorders with jaundice. Hemorrhoids are often accompanied by rectal pruritus. Emotional distress plays an important role in the development and control of this disturbing symptom. Unless pruritus is relieved the patient may become exhausted from lack of sleep.
 Cleanliness, soothing ointments or lotions, sodium bicarbonate baths and sometimes tranquilizing drugs are used in the relief of pruritus. Since it is a symptom of some other disorder, complete cure of pruritus depends on cure of the primary illness.
 p. a'ni, itching in the anal region.
 essential p., that occurring without known cause.
 p. seni'lis, itching in the aged, due to degeneration of the skin.
 symptomatic p., that which occurs secondarily to another condition.
 p. vul'vae, itching of the external genitalia in the female.

prussiate (proo'she-āt) cyanide.

p.s. per second.

psammoma (sah-mo'mah) a tumor (especially of brain or ovary) containing granular material, called psammoma bodies.

psammosarcoma (sam"o-sar-ko'mah) a sarcoma containing granular material.

pseud(o)- (su'do) word element [Gr.], *false.*

pseudacousma (su"dah-kōōz'mah) an auditory defect with sounds seemingly altered in quality or pitch.

pseudarthritis (su"dar-thri'tis) a hysterical joint affection.

pseudarthrosis (su"dar-thro'sis) a pathologic entity characterized by deossification of a weight-bearing long bone, followed by bending and pathologic fracture, with inability to form normal callus leading to existence of the "false joint" that gives the condition its name.

pseudencephalus (su"den-sef'ah-lus) a fetus with a tumor in place of the brain.

pseudesthesia (su"des-the'ze-ah) a sensation occurring in the absence of the appropriate stimuli; an imaginary sensation.

pseudoacromegaly (su"do-ak"ro-meg'ah-le) acropachyderma.

pseudoagraphia (su″do-a-graf′e-ah) a condition in which the patient can copy writing, but cannot write except in a meaningless and illegible manner.

pseudoallele (su″do-ah-lēl′) one of two or more genes that are seemingly allelic, but which can be shown to have distinctive loci on the chromosome. adj., **pseudoallel′ic.**

pseudoanemia (su″do-ah-ne′me-ah) a condition marked by paleness without true anemia.

pseudoaneurysm (su″do-an′u-rizm) an appearance resembling an aneurysm, but due to enlargement and tortuosity of a vessel.

pseudoangina (su″do-an′ji-nah) a syndrome resembling angina, but without organic heart disease.

pseudoangioma (su″do-an″je-o′mah) a venous thrombus that has become canalized.

pseudoapoplexy (su″do-ap′o-plek″se) a condition like apoplexy, but without cerebral hemorrhage.

pseudoataxia (su″do-ah-tak′se-ah) general incoordination resembling ataxia.

pseudoatheroma (su″do-ath″er-o′mah) a sebaceous cyst.

pseudoblepsis (su″do-blep′sis) perversion of vision, objects appearing different from what they really are.

pseudobulbar (su″do-bul′bar) apparently, but not really, due to a bulbar lesion.

pseudocartilaginous (su″do-kar″tĭ-laj′ĭ-nus) resembling cartilage.

pseudocast (su′do-kast) an accidental formation of urinary sediment resembling a true cast.

pseudocele (su′do-sēl) pseudocoele.

pseudocholesteatoma (su″do-ko″lĕ-ste″ah-to′-mah) a horny mass of epithelial cells in the middle ear, resembling cholesteatoma.

pseudochorea (su″do-ko-re′ah) a state of general incoordination resembling chorea.

pseudochromesthesia (su″do-kro″mes-the′ze-ah) a sensation of color experienced on hearing sounds.

pseudochromhidrosis (su″do-krōm″hĭ-dro′sis) discoloration of sweat by surface contaminants, such as pigment-producing bacteria or chemical substances on the skin.

pseudocide (su′do-sīd) the deliberate taking of measures to harm one's self without wishing to die.

pseudocirrhosis (su″do-sĭ-ro′sis) apparent cirrhosis of the liver, due to severe hepatic congestion as in severe heart failure or pericarditis.

pseudocoarctation (su″do-ko″ark-ta′shun) a condition resembling coarctation, without narrowing of the lumen.

pseudocoele (su′do-sēl) the fifth ventricle of the brain.

pseudocoloboma (su″do-kol″o-bo′mah) a scar on the iris resembling a coloboma.

pseudocopulation (su″do-kop″u-la′shun) the fertilization of animal ova by the spermatozoa of the male without sexual union.

pseudocrisis (su″do-kri′sis) a false crisis.

pseudocroup (su′do-krōōp) laryngismus stridulus; sudden laryngeal spasm with crowing inspiration.

pseudocyesis (su″do-si-e′sis) false pregnancy; development of all the signs of pregnancy without the presence of an embryo.

pseudocyst (su′do-sist) a dilated space resembling a cyst.
   pancreatic p., an accumulation of pancreatic juice in the retroperitoneal space as a result of necrosis and rupture of a pancreatic duct.

pseudodementia (su″do-de-men′she-ah) a state of general apathy resembling dementia, but with no actual defect of intelligence.

pseudodiphtheria (su″do-dif-the′re-ah) a condition resembling diphtheria, but not due to *Corynebacterium diphtheriae.*

pseudodipsia (su″do-dip′se-ah) false thirst; thirst that is not associated with a bodily need for water and is not satisfied by the intake of water.

pseudoedema (su″do-ĕ-de′mah) a puffy state resembling edema.

pseudoemphysema (su″do-em″fĭ-se′mah) a condition resembling emphysema, but due to temporary obstruction of the bronchi.

pseudoephedrine (su″do-ĕ-fed′rin) one of the isomers of ephedrine; used as a nasal decongestant.

pseudoerysipelas (su″do-er″ĭ-sip′ĕ-las) an inflammatory subcutaneous disease resembling erysipelas.

pseudofracture (su″do-frak′tūr) the roentgenographic appearance of a thickened periosteum and new bone formation over what looks like an incomplete fracture.

pseudoganglion (su″do-gang′gle-on) an enlargement on a nerve resembling a ganglion.

pseudogeusesthesia (su″do-gūs″es-the′ze-ah) a false sensation of taste associated with a sensation of another modality.

pseudogeusia (su″do-gu′ze-ah) a sensation of taste occurring in the absence of a stimulus or inappropriate to the exciting stimulus.

pseudoglaucoma (su″do-glaw-ko′mah) ophthalmoscopic characteristics and visual field defects typical of glaucoma but not due to elevated intraocular pressure.

pseudoglottis (su″do-glot′is) the space between the false vocal cords.

pseudogout (su′do-gowt) a condition resembling gout, but with calcium salt rather than urate crystals in the synovia.

pseudohaustration (su″do-hos-tra′shun) a false appearance of normal sacculation of the wall of the colon.

pseudohemophilia (su″do-he″mo-fil′e-ah) angiohemophilia; Von Willebrand's disease.

pseudohemoptysis (su″do-he-mop′tĭ-sis) spitting of blood that comes from some source other than the lungs.

pseudohermaphrodite (su″do-her-maf′ro-dīt) an individual exhibiting pseudohermaphroditism.
   female p., one whose gonads are ovaries.
   male p., one whose gonads are testes.

pseudohermaphroditism (su″do-her-maf′ro-ditizm″) a state in which the gonads are of one sex, but the morphologic criteria of sex are ambiguous or contradictory, owing to an endocrine disorder. Pseudohermaphroditism is not to be confused with hermaphroditism, in which the individual possesses both ovarian and testicular tissue.

pseudohernia (su″do-her′ne-ah) an inflamed sac or gland simulating strangulated hernia.

pseudohydrocephalus (su″do-hi″dro-sef′ah-lus) abnormally large appearance of a normal-sized head, due to smallness of the face and body.

pseudohypertrichosis (su″do-hi″per-trĭ-ko′sis) persistence after birth of the fine hair present during fetal life, due to inability of the skin to throw it off.

pseudohypoparathyroidism (su″do-hi″po-par″-ah-thi′roi-dizm) a condition clinically resembling hypoparathyroidism, but caused by failure of response to parathyroid hormone, rather than deficiency of it.

pseudoisochromatic (su″do-i″so-kro-mat′ik) seemingly of the same color throughout: applied to solutions or cards for testing color blindness, containing two pigments or colors which will be distinguished by the normal eye, but not by the color blind.

pseudojaundice (su″do-jawn′dis) yellowness of the skin due to other than liver disease.

pseudoleukemia (su″do-lu-ke′me-ah) a condition clinically resembling leukemia, but without its characteristic blood findings.

pseudologia (su″do-lo′je-ah) the writing of anonymous letters to people of prominence, to one's self, etc.
   p. fantas′tica, a tendency to tell extravagant and fantastic falsehoods centered about one's self.

pseudomania (su″do-ma′ne-ah) 1. false or pretended mental disorder. 2. pathologic lying.

pseudomelanosis (su″do-mel″ah-no′sis) pigmentation of tissues after death.

pseudomelia (su″do-me′le-ah) phantom limb.
   p. paresthet′ica, the perception of morbid or perverted sensations as occurring in an absent or paralyzed limb.

pseudomembrane (su″do-mem′brān) a layer of gray-white exudate, resembling a true membrane, formed on the mucosa in certain diseases. adj., **pseudomem′branous.**

Pseudomonas (su″do-mo′nas) a genus of Schizomycetes, found in soil and fresh or salt water.
   P. aerugino′sa, the only species of Pseudomonas

that is pathogenic for man; it causes a great variety of suppurative and other infections.
   P. pseudomal′lei, the causative agent of melioidosis, a disease of rodents occasionally transmitted to man.

pseudomucin (su″do-mu′sin) a variety of mucin from ovarian cysts.

pseudomyxoma (su″do-mik-so′mah) a colloid growth on the peritoneum, often secondary to an ovarian cyst.
   p. peritone′i, the presence in the peritoneal cavity of mucoid material from a ruptured ovarian cyst or appendiceal mucocele.

pseudo-obstruction (su″do-ob-struk′shun) a condition simulating obstruction.
   intestinal p., a condition characterized by constipation, colicky pain and vomiting, but without evidence of organic obstruction at laparotomy.

pseudopapilledema (su″do-pap″il-ĕ-de′mah) anomalous elevation of the optic disk.

pseudoparalysis (su″do-pah-ral′ĭ-sis) loss of muscular power without real paralysis, caused by voluntary inhibition of motor impulses because of pain in coordination, etc.

pseudoparaphrasia (su″do-par″ah-fra′ze-ah) complete general incoherence in which the patient calls everything by a wrong name.

pseudoparaplegia (su″do-par″ah-ple′je-ah) paralysis of the lower limbs, but with normal reflexes.

pseudoparesis (su″do-pah-re′sis) a hysterical condition simulating paresis.

pseudopelade (su″do-pe′lād) alopecia with formation of small white scars.

pseudophakia (su″do-fa′ke-ah) failure of development of the crystalline lens, its place being occupied by tissue of abnormal type.

pseudoplegia (su″do-ple′je-ah) hysterical paralysis.

pseudopodium (su″od-po′de-um) a temporary protrusion of the protoplasm of an ameba, for purposes of locomotion or to engulf food.

pseudopolyp (su″do-pol′ip) a hypertrophied tab of mucous membrane resembling a polyp, but caused by ulceration surrounding intact mucosa.

pseudopolyposis (su″do-pol″ĭ-po′sis) numerous pseudopolyps in the colon and rectum, due to longstanding inflammation.

pseudopregnancy (su″do-preg′nan-se) false pregnancy; development of all the signs of pregnancy without the presence of an embryo.

pseudo-pseudohypoparathyroidism (su″do-su″-do-hi″po-par″ah-thi′roi-dizm) a condition resembling pseudohypoparathyroidism, but with normal levels of calcium and phosphorus in the blood serum.

pseudopterygium (su″do-tĕ-rij′e-um) a fold of conjunctiva attached to any part of the cornea, following ulceration of the cornea.

pseudoptosis (su″do-to′sis) decrease in the size of the palpebral aperture.

pseudoreaction (su″do-re-ak′shun) a false or deceptive reaction; in intradermal skin tests, a reaction not due to the specific protein being tested but due to impurities or to other proteins in the medium in which the toxin is suspended or dissolved.

pseudorickets (su″do-rik′ets) renal osteodystrophy.

pseudoscarlatina (su″do-skar″lah-te′nah) a septic condition with fever and eruption resembling scarlet fever.

pseudosclerosis (su″do-sklĕ-ro′sis) a condition with the symptoms but without the lesions of multiple sclerosis; a form of hepaticolenticular degeneration.

pseudoscrotum (su″do-skro′tum) a solid partition with a median raphe, resembling the scrotum in the male, obliterating the opening into the vagina in female pseudohermaphroditism.

pseudosmia (su-doz′me-ah) a sensation of odor without the appropriate stimulus.

pseudosyphilis (su″do-sif′ĭ-lis) a condition resembling syphilis, but not caused by *Treponema pallidum.*

pseudotabes (su″do-ta′bēz) tabes dorsalis not due to syphilis and without Argyll Robertson pupils.

pseudotetanus (su″do-tet′ah-nus) persistent muscular contractions not associated with *Clostridium tetani.*

pseudotuberculosis (su″do-tu-ber″ku-lo′sis) a condition like tuberculosis, but not caused by *Mycobacterium tuberculosis.*

pseudotumor (su″do-tu′mor) phantom tumor.
  p. cer′ebri, a benign, nontumorous condition producing signs of increased intracranial pressure.

pseudotyphoid (su″do-ti′foid) a disease showing the symptoms of typhoid fever, but without the characteristic lesions of that disease and without typhoid bacilli.

pseudoxanthoma elasticum (su″do-zan-tho′mah e-las′tĭ-kum) a rare skin disease characterized by yellowish papules and plaques occurring along the sides of the neck, the axilla and lower abdomen. It is produced by degeneration of the elastic fibers of the skin and may be hereditary.

p.s.i. pounds per square inch.

psilocin (si′lo-sin) a hallucinogenic substance closely related to psilocybin.

psilocybin (si″lo-si′bin) a hallucinogenic crystalline compound isolated from a species of mushrooms (see also HALLUCINOGEN).

psilosis (si-lo′sis) 1. sprue. 2. falling out of the hair.

psittacosis (sit″ah-ko′sis) a viral infection transmitted by birds of the psittacine family, e.g., parrots and parakeets. A similar infection can be transmitted by chickens, ducks, pigeons and other fowl; this type is usually called ornithosis. These conditions are highly contagious but are seldom transmitted from one person to another.

The virus is inhaled into the body and attacks the respiratory tract. The first symptoms appear after an incubation period of 6 to 15 days and include fever, sore throat, headache, loss of appetite, chills and profuse sweating. Later there may be coughing, difficulty in breathing and abdominal distress. Prostration may occur. Infiltrates may appear in the chest x-ray. Special laboratory tests are necessary for accurate diagnosis.

Psittacosis usually runs its course in 2 or 3 weeks. Complications may be avoided by the administration of such antibiotics as tetracycline and penicillin. Fatalities are uncommon.

psoas (so′as) one of two muscles of the loins.

psodymus (sod′ĭ-mus) a fetal monster with two heads and two trunks, but united below.

psoitis (so-i′tis) inflammation of a psoas muscle or its sheath.

psora (so′rah) 1. scabies. 2. psoriasis.

psorelcosis (sor″el-ko′sis) ulceration due to scabies.

psoriasis (so-ri′ah-sis) a chronic, recurrent skin disease marked by bright red patches covered with silvery scales. The lesions appear most often on the knees, elbows and scalp, and sometimes in the form of dot-shaped marks on the fingernails. The chest, abdomen, backs of arms and legs, palms of hands and soles of feet are other locations frequently affected. adj., **psoriat′ic.**

The cause of psoriasis is not known, although the fact that it seems to occur in families with a previous history of the disease suggests a hereditary factor. It may also occur with rheumatoid arthritis, although the connection is not clear.

Some cases of psoriasis are acute; most cases are chronic and recurrent. Early attacks may respond well to treatment, only to reappear.

TREATMENT. There is at present no cure available. Acute attacks are usually treated with a soothing lotion or ointment, or by warm baths. In some cases sunlight or special ultraviolet-ray therapy is prescribed. Chronic cases frequently respond to cortisone-containing ointments. A warm climate and freedom from anxiety often seem to help psoriasis patients.

Psorophora (so-rof′o-rah) a genus of large, annoying mosquitoes, the larvae of which prey on the larvae of other kinds of mosquitoes.

psorous (so′rus) affected with itch.

PSP phenolsulfonphthalein, a dye used in testing kidney function.

psych(o)- (si′ko) word element [Gr.], *mind.*

psychalgia (si-kal′je-ah) pain due to psychic causes, e.g., anxiety or depression.

psychalia (si-ka′le-ah) a morbid state in which voices seem to be heard and images to be seen.

psychanalysis (si″kah-nal′ĭ-sis) psychoanalysis.

psychanopsia (si″kah-nop′se-ah) psychic blindness.

psychasthenia (si″kas-the′ne-ah) a functional neurosis marked by anxiety, pathologic fears and obsessions.

psychataxia (si″kah-tak′se-ah) a disordered mental state with confusion, agitation and inability to fix the attention.

psyche (si′ke) the human faculty for thought, judgment and emotion; the mental life, including both conscious and unconscious processes.

psycheclampsia (si″ke-klamp′se-ah) acute mania.

psychedelic (si″kĕ-del′ik) pertaining to or characterized by freedom from anxiety, and by relaxation, enjoyable perceptual changes and highly creative thought patterns. By extension, applied to a type of drug that produces these effects. Psychedelic drugs such as LSD and mescaline cause hallucinations and altered mental function. They are highly controversial and potentially dangerous and should be used for experimental purposes only, and under the direct supervision of a competent authorized investigator. (See also HALLUCINOGEN.)

psychiatrist (si-ki′ah-trist) a specialist in psychiatry.

psychiatry (si-ki′ah-tre) the branch of medicine that deals with the diagnosis, treatment and prevention of disorders of the mind. adj., **psychiat′ric.**

descriptive p., that based on observation and study of external factors that can be seen, heard or felt.

dynamic p., the study of emotional processes, their origins and the mental mechanisms underlying them.

psychic (si′kik) pertaining to the mind or psyche.

psychoallergy (si″ko-al′er-je) a condition of sensitization to certain words, ideas, people and other symbols of emotional patterns.

psychoanaleptic (si″ko-an″ah-lep′tik) stimulating the mind.

psychoanalysis (si″ko-ah-nal′ĭ-sis) a technique for diagnosing and treating mental illness originally developed by Dr. Sigmund Freud. adj., **psychoanalyt′ic.** Psychoanalysis is a well known form of PSYCHOTHERAPY, a term that covers all psychologic techniques used in the treatment of mental illness.

Psychoanalysis is based on Freud's theories of the way the mind develops and functions. Briefly, these theories state that during early childhood the child has a number of instinctual impulses and desires that are in conflict with what is expected of him by his family and the society in which he lives. In the process of resolving these conflicts he represses the feelings he must curb, or blocks them out of his conscious mind. Some of these repressed desires continue to exist in his unconscious mind, however. When they continue to exist as conflicts, they may erupt into NEUROSIS.

A neurotic adult will tend to respond to people in terms of his childhood feelings toward members of his family, even though these responses are not appropriate to the situation. Without realizing it, he is going through adult life still fighting the battles of childhood. His unresolved conflicts prevent him from seeing others as they are and reacting to them in an appropriate way.

Psychoanalysis attempts, in Freud's words, "to make the unconscious conscious." Its goal is to help the patient become aware of and resolve his childhood conflicts, so that he can react to his life situation as it is and not in terms of these conflicts. The psychoanalyst does not instruct or advise the patient; he helps him to instruct himself.

TECHNIQUES. One of the techniques that Freud developed to aid this process is free association. When a person is trying to focus on an emotional disturbance, he often has stray thoughts that seem to be meaningless but offer clues to the real nature of this difficulty. These thoughts can be organized by the analyst and interpreted to indicate the unconscious process involved. In psychoanalysis, the patient is asked to say whatever comes to his mind, however trivial or "unspeakable" it may seem. In order to make free association easier, the patient lies in a relaxed position on a couch facing away from the analyst.

Another important technique of psychoanalysis is interpretation of dreams. A person's dreams are an expression of his unconscious wishes and drives, which are disguised, appear as symbols and give valuable indications of unconscious fears and conflicts. With the help of the analyst, the patient free-associates about his dreams, and tries to understand their real content and to learn what is behind the disguise.

Hypnosis is sometimes used to elicit experiences that have been repressed.

During the course of analysis, the patient tends to react to the analyst in terms of his childhood conflicts. This is called transference. Since the analyst is a neutral figure, when the patient reacts to his analyst in unreasonable ways, accusing him, for example, of being cruel, the analyst can point out to the patient that this is how he must have felt about his father. Again, the patient might be able to find excuses for his fear of his neighbors in various ways, but be unable to find an excuse for his similar fear of the analyst. He may then realize that others of his fears are also groundless and based on unconscious conflicts.

Psychoanalysis is ordinarily a very prolonged, intensive form of treatment. It usually involves several sessions a week for a year or more.

psychobiology (si″ko-bi-ol′o-je) study of the interrelations of body and mind in the formation and functioning of personality.

psychocoma (si″ko-ko′mah) melancholic stupor.

psychocutaneous (si″ko-ku-ta′ne-us) pertaining to the relations between mental or emotional factors and skin disorders.

psychodelic (si″ko-del′ik) psychedelic.

psychodiagnosis (si″ko-di″ag-no′sis) the use of psychologic testing in the diagnosis of disease.

psychodrama (si″ko-drah′mah) the psychiatric technique of having a patient act out conflicting situations of his daily life.

psychodynamics (si″ko-di-nam′iks) the science of human behavior and motivation.

psychodysleptic (si″ko-dis-lep′tik) inducing a delusional state of mind.

psychogalvanometer (si″ko-gal″vah-nom′ĕ-ter) a galvanometer for recording the electrical agitation produced by emotional stresses.

psychogenesis (si″ko-jen′ĕ-sis) mental development; origin within the mind.

psychogenic (si″ko-jen′ik) originating in the mind; having an emotional or psychologic origin (in relation to a symptom), rather than an organic basis.

psychogeriatrics (si″ko-jer″e-at′riks) psychologic and psychiatric treatment of the aged.

psychogram (si′ko-gram) 1. psychograph. 2. a visual sensation associated with a mental idea, as of a certain number that appears visualized when it is thought of.

psychograph (si′ko-graf) 1. a chart for recording graphically the personality traits of an individual. 2. a written description of the mental functioning of an individual.

psychokinesis (si″ko-ki-ne′sis) the influence of mind on matter without the intermediation of physical force.

psycholepsy (si″ko-lep′se) a condition characterized by sudden changes of mood.

psycholeptic (si″ko-lep′tik) exerting a relaxing effect on the mind.

psychology (si-kol′o-je) the scientific study of mental processes and behavior. adj., **psycholog′ic.**
  abnormal p., the study of derangements or deviations of mental functions.
  analytic p., psychology by introspective methods, as opposed to experimental psychology.
  clinical p., the use of psychologic knowledge and techniques in the treatment of persons with emotional difficulties.
  criminal p., the study of the mentality, the motivation and the social behavior of criminals.
  depth p., the psychology of the unconscious; psychoanalysis.
  dynamic p., a school of psychology that stresses the element of energy in mental processes.
  experimental p., the study of the mind and mental operations by the use of experimental methods.
  genetic p., that branch of psychology that deals with the development of mind in the individual and with its evolution in the race.
  gestalt p., gestaltism; the theory that the objects of mind, as immediately presented to direct experience, come as complete unanalyzable wholes or forms that cannot be split into parts.
  physiologic p., that branch of psychology that applies the facts taught in neurology to show the relation between the mental and the neural.
  social p., that branch of psychology that treats of the social aspects of mental life.

psychometrician (si″ko-mĕ-trish′an) a person skilled in psychometry.

psychometrics (si″ko-met′riks) the testing and measuring of mental and psychologic ability, efficiency, potentials and functioning.

psychometry (si-kom′ĕ-tre) measurement of work done and of time consumed in mental operations.

psychomotor (si″ko-mo′tor) pertaining to motor effects of cerebral or psychic activity.

psychoneurosis (si″ko-nu-ro′sis) mental disorder that is of psychogenic origin but presents the essential symptoms of functional nervous disease, as hysteria, neurasthenia, psychasthenia (see also NEUROSIS). adj., **psychoneurot′ic.**

psychonomy (si-kon′o-me) the science of the laws of mental activity.

psychopath (si′ko-path) a person who has a psychopathic personality.
  sexual p., one whose sexual behavior is manifestly antisocial and criminal.

psychopathic personality (si″ko-path′ik) a type of personality disorder, characterized by a conspicuous disregard for the rights or needs of others; called also sociopathic personality. The behavior patterns of the psychopath are not typical of either NEUROSIS or PSYCHOSIS, and differ somewhat from those of other types of personality disorders.
  There is no sharp dividing line between the normal and the psychopathic personality. The psychopath shows a lack of emotional maturity, an unwillingness to take responsibility and emotional instability. Unlike the neurotic person, he expresses his conflict in antisocial acts so that society suffers, rather than the psychopath himself.
  CHARACTERISTICS. The chief characteristic of a psychopath is an apparent lack of conscience. He expresses his conflicts in various ways, including compulsive lying, stealing and certain other types of antisocial or criminal activity. He may suffer from alcoholism or drug addiction; sexual deviation may also be an expression of psychopathic personality.
  Like other types of mental illness, a psychopathic personality probably has many roots in the emotions and experiences of early childhood, but their form of expression is different. A psychopathic personality affects the entire structure of the character, so that the person feels that everyone else is out of step. If the patient is a criminal, he may honestly believe that anyone who is not a criminal is merely stupid. Those with psychopathic personalities often seem to be unable to learn from experience.
  TREATMENT. Unfortunately, it is extremely difficult to treat a patient with a psychopathic personality. The techniques of PSYCHOTHERAPY depend on the cooperation of the patient, and this in turn depends on his willingness to admit that something is wrong with him. This is an admission that those with psychopathic personalities are rarely willing or able to make. They seldom accept psychiatric help, and since they are legally sane, they cannot be compelled to undergo treatment.

psychopathology (si″ko-pah-thol′o-je) the study of abnormal behavior, its manifestations, development and causation.

psychopathy (si-kop′ah-the) any disease of the mind.

psychopharmacology (si″ko-far″mah-kol′o-je) the study of the action of drugs on the psychologic functions.

psychophylaxis (si″ko-fi-lak′sis) mental hygiene.

psychophysical (si″ko-fiz′ĭ-kal) pertaining to the mind and its relation to physical manifestations.

psychophysics (si″ko-fiz′iks) scientific study of the quantitative relations between characteristics or patterns of physical stimuli and the sensations induced by them.

psychophysiology (si″ko-fiz″e-ol′o-je) scientific study of the interaction and interrelations of psychic and physiologic factors.

psychoplegic (si″ko-ple′jik) an agent lessening cerebral excitability.

psychoprophylaxis (si″ko-pro″fĭ-lak′sis) psychophysical training aimed at suppression of all painful sensation associated with normal childbirth.

psychorrhea (si″ko-re′ah) an incoherent stream of thought.

psychosensory (si″ko-sen′so-re) perceiving and interpreting sensory stimuli.

psychosexual (si″ko-seks′u-al) pertaining to the psychic or emotional portion of the sex instinct.

psychosis (si-ko′sis), pl. *psycho′ses* [Gr.] a major emotional disorder with derangement of the personality and loss of contact with reality, often with delusions, hallucinations or illusions. adj., **psychot′ic.**

A psychotic person may live in his own private world, completely out of touch with reality. He cannot cope with the demands of the real world, and he withdraws from it. In general, this loss of contact with reality is one of the more obvious differences between psychosis and NEUROSIS.

About half the hospital beds in the United States today are occupied by patients with mental illness, almost all of them sufferers from psychosis. Psychosis disables as many Americans per year as heart disease and cancer combined.

TYPES OF PSYCHOSIS. Psychoses are usually classified as functional psychoses, those for which no physical cause has been discovered, and organic psychoses, which are the result of organic damage to the brain.

The main types of functional psychosis are schizophrenia, paranoia, affective psychosis and involutional reaction.

Schizophrenia. This is the most widespread form of psychosis. About half of all patients hospitalized for mental illness are schizophrenics. This condition was formerly called dementia praecox, or "early insanity," because it usually appears between the ages of 15 and 30.

The schizophrenic is apt to be shy, dreamy, bored and lacking in physical and mental energy. When he becomes unable to find a solution for a painful situation, he retreats into a world he imagines as he would like it to be. The schizophrenic becomes unable to distinguish fact from imagination and uninterested in doing so. As a result, his actions may seem very strange unless they are understood as the product of a dream world. For example, one symptom of schizophrenia is the use of neologisms, or made-up words that are meaningless to the listener. Hallucinations and delusions may occur, as may CATALEPSY.

Certain types of schizophrenia respond more readily to treatment than do others. In all types, early treatment is extremely important, as the prospects for recovery seem to be closely connected with the duration of the condition.

Paranoia. This psychosis, which is much less common than schizophrenia, is characterized by delusions of persecution or grandiose delusions. A person suffering from it becomes more and more deluded, seeing hidden meanings to support his conviction that others are plotting against him, or to substantiate his belief that he is a person of great importance. He often uses an intricate form of logic to try to explain his delusions.

There are many degrees of paranoid reaction. Paranoid attitudes also appear in one type of schizophrenia.

In paranoia, unlike other psychoses, the entire personality is not affected; the patient does not lose contact with reality, but tends rather to misinterpret reality in terms of his delusion.

Affective Psychosis. This psychosis is characterized by greatly exaggerated emotional reactions. It is called a manic-depressive reaction because of the conspicuous mood swings that are characteristic of the condition. Although there are two possible phases, manic and depressive, the disorder takes many forms, sometimes entirely manic, or entirely depressive, with many variations. In an extremely mild form the affective reaction is not a true psychosis.

During the manic phase, the patient's energy and optimism seem boundless, mental activity and talking are accelerated, physical activity becomes greatly increased; lack of judgment, combined with over-enthusiasm, may make the patient dangerous to himself and to others. During the depressive phase, the patient's mental activity is greatly retarded, he may sit or lie inert, scarcely able to move or speak (see also CATALEPSY). The danger of suicide may be present. In some cases the patient appears greatly agitated even though he is extremely depressed.

Affective psychosis tends to recur. Many patients seem to recover spontaneously and then exhibit symptoms again after a period of more or less normal behavior.

Involutional Reaction. This is a psychotic reaction that occurs in late middle age. It was formerly thought to be related to the menopause in women and its emotional counterpart, the climacteric, in men. Characteristics of this type of psychosis include agitation, depression, feelings of guilt, paranoia, preoccupation with minor symptoms of physical disorders, severe insomnia and suicidal tendencies. The course of the illness tends to be prolonged.

CAUSES. There is still much to be learned about the causes of functional psychoses. The roots of these conditions may be in the patient's early emotional experiences, or in his physical make-up, or in his environment. The high incidence of psychosis in certain families with a history of mental illness suggests that heredity may also play some role. However, it should be remembered that children whose parents are mentally disturbed and untreated may absorb psychotic ways of responding emotionally and viewing reality, in the same way that young children learn healthy ways of dealing with the real world from their environment.

The causes of organic psychoses are much better understood. Among the physical causes that can lead to psychosis are infectious diseases which involve the brain, certain deficiency diseases, lead poisoning, tumors, interference with the brain's blood supply and wounds and blows that injure the brain. In a very few cases, epilepsy may lead to some mental deterioration. These organic psychoses are more resistant to treatment than are those with a functional basis.

TREATMENT.   In most cases, patients with psychosis must be treated in a mental hospital. The major form of treatment is PSYCHOTHERAPY, in which the patient is helped to understand and deal with his condition. However, this method will not work when the patient is out of contact with reality, and completely absorbed in his own fantasies and hallucinations.

In such cases, chemotherapy, the use of drugs to control the patient's emotions and behavior, may be very helpful. Important among these drugs are chlorpromazine hydrochloride (Thorazine) and certain other phenothiazine derivatives. They act to calm the patient and often to help him become more rational.

The treatment of psychosis has been revolutionized by the development of two other types of drugs, the tranquilizers and the antidepressants or "psychic elevators." These medicines do not cure the conditions; they merely control the symptoms. In many cases, they make it possible to treat the patients while they continue to live at home.

Another type of treatment that is sometimes used is SHOCK THERAPY. The patient is rendered unconscious briefly by electric shock or drugs. This treatment often helps bring patients with melancholia or schizophrenia back to reality, thus making it possible to use the techniques of psychotherapy.

In a very few cases that are not helped by any other form of treatment, psychosurgery may be used. In this treatment, the connection between different parts of the brain is surgically severed. The result is a lessening of emotional reactions and tensions. Many doctors object to psychosurgery because of the negative aspects of its results, and the operation is used as a last resort.

alcoholic p., mental disorder caused by excessive use of alcohol.

depressive p., one characterized by mental depression, melancholy, despondency, inadequacy and feelings of guilt.

drug p., a toxic psychosis due to the ingestion of drugs.

exhaustion p., a psychosis due to some exhausting or depressing occurrence, as an operation.

gestational p., a psychosis developing during pregnancy.

Korsakoff's p., a syndrome marked by amnesia, confabulation and peripheral neuritis, usually associated with alcoholism and vitamin deficiencies (see also KORSAKOFF'S SYNDROME).

periodic p., a condition in which intermittent periods of depression or hypomania recur regularly in a seemingly mentally healthy or nearly healthy person.

polyneuritic p., Korsakoff's psychosis.

senile p., mental deterioration of old age, with tendency to confabulation, loss of memory of recent events, irritability and assaultiveness.

situational p., a transitory psychosis caused by an unbearable situation over which the patient has no control.

toxic p., psychosis due to the ingestion of toxic agents or to the presence of toxins within the body.

psychosolytic (si″ko-so-lit′ik) relieving or abolishing psychotic symptoms.

psychosomatic (si″ko-so-mat′ik) pertaining to the interrelations of mind and body.

p. illness, an illness that can be traced to an emotional cause. The term psychosomatic comes from the Greek words *psyche*, meaning mind, and *soma*, body. A psychosomatic illness, although its origin is partly or completely emotional, has obvious physical symptoms, usually affecting organs under control of the autonomic nervous system.

TYPES.   There are a number of physical conditions in which emotional factors are known to play an important part. Physicians suspect that certain others, such as ASTHMA, may similarly be affected by emotional causes, but the evidence is not yet clear-cut.

Possibly the most widely known psychosomatic illness, and the first to be proved to be of emotional origin, is gastric or duodenal ULCER. Other conditions of the digestive system can also be traced wholly or in part to emotional causes. Among these are regional enteritis and ULCERATIVE COLITIS.

MIGRAINE is frequently a psychosomatic illness. Certain medicines may prevent attacks of this illness, but some form of psychotherapy may be necessary as well if the underlying causes are emotional.

Other conditions that appear to be in some cases psychosomatic include hypertension, hyperthyroidism, arthritis and certain skin disorders.

TREATMENT.   Both the physical symptoms and the psychologic causes of psychosomatic illness must be treated. Emotional disturbances are treated by different types of PSYCHOTHERAPY. Some patients may respond well to PSYCHOANALYSIS, but in many cases of psychosomatic illness this intensive and extended form of treatment is not required.

psychosomimetic (si-ko″so-mi-met′ik) psychotomimetic.

psychosurgery (si″ko-ser′jer-e) the performance of operations on the brain as a means of treating emotional or mental disorder.

psychotherapy (si″ko-ther′ah-pe) any of a number of related techniques for treating mental illness by psychologic methods. These techniques are similar in that they all rely mainly on establishing communication between the therapist and the patient as a means of understanding and modifying the patient's behavior. On occasion, drugs may be used, but only in order to make this communication easier.

FORMS OF PSYCHOTHERAPY.   Perhaps the best known form of psychotherapy is PSYCHOANALYSIS, the technique developed by Dr. Sigmund Freud. Psychoanalysis attempts, through free association and dream interpretation, to reveal and resolve the unconscious conflicts that are at the root of mental illness.

Closely related to psychoanalysis is analytically oriented therapy, or "brief therapy." This uses some of the techniques of psychoanalysis, but tends to concentrate on the patient's present-life difficulties rather than on the unconscious roots of these difficulties.

One recently developed technique that has become popular is group therapy. Six to ten patients meet regularly to discuss their problems under the guidance of a group therapist. Group therapy is based on the principle of transference—that is, a patient tends to react to others in terms of his childhood attitudes toward family members. During group therapy, he may react to one member of the group as a hated rival brother, and to another as a dominating mother. In the give-and-take of discussion, he will begin to recognize the distortions in these reactions, and to see similar distortions in his day-to-day relationships with other people. Group therapy is generally combined with individual therapy and can help reduce the cost to each patient. It is also widely used in mental hospitals, where it has helped relieve the great shortage of trained therapists.

Adjunctive therapy, such as occupational therapy and music therapy, is helpful in relieving tensions and emotional problems that are associated with a feeling of uselessness. Psychodrama, in which patients act out phantasies or real-life situations, may provide a means of communication for patients who are not capable of expressing their problem by speech.

Play therapy is a form of psychotherapy adapted to children. It is very difficult to induce an emotionally disturbed or even a normal child to talk about his problems. Play therapy provides an alternative. The child reveals himself when he plays with toys provided by the therapist and acts out his phantasies. The therapist helps him "get things out of his system," accepting him warmly as he is, and guiding him toward a solution to his problems. Since these are closely related to the way he is treated at home, play therapy is usually combined with some form of therapy for the parents. Recently experiments have been made with family group therapy, in which the entire family meets regularly with the therapist. This new technique sometimes appears to have remarkable results.

psychotogenic (si-kot″o-jen′ik) producing a psychosis.

psychotomimetic (si-kot″o-mi-met′ik) characterized by or producing symptoms similar to those of a psychosis.

psychotonic (si″ko-ton′ik) elevating or stimulating the mind.

psychotropic (si″ko-trop′ik) exerting an effect upon the mind.

psychr(o)- (si′kro) word element [Gr.], *cold.*

psychroalgia (si″kro-al′je-ah) a painful sensation of cold.

psychrometer (si-krom′ĕ-ter) an instrument for measuring the moisture of the atmosphere.

psychrophile (si′kro-fīl) a microorganism that grows best at 15 to 20° C. adj., **psychrophil′ic.**

psychrophobia (si″kro-fo′be-ah) morbid dread of cold.

psychrotherapy (si″kro-ther′ah-pe) treatment of disease by applying cold.

psyllium (sil′e-um) the plant *Plantago psyllium,* the seed of which is used as a laxative.

Pt chemical symbol, *platinum.*

pt. pint.

PTA plasma thromboplastin antecedent, clotting factor XI.

ptarmic (tar′mik) causing sneezing.

ptarmus (tar′mus) spasmodic sneezing.

PTC plasma thromboplastin component, clotting factor IX.

pteroylglutamic acid (ter″o-il-gloo-tam′ik) folic acid.

pterygium (tĕ-rij′e-um) a winglike structure, especially a patch of thickened conjunctiva originating in the palpebral fissure and extending over part of the cornea, or an abnormal extension and adherence of the cuticle over the proximal portion of the nail plate.
  p. col′li, a band of tissue from the mastoid region to the region of the sternum.

pterygoid (ter′ĭ-goid) shaped like a wing.
  p. process, either of the two processes of the sphenoid bone descending from the points of junction of the great wings and body of the bone, and each consisting of a lateral and medial plate.

pterygomandibular (ter″ĭ-go-man-dib′u-lar) pertaining to the pterygoid process and the mandible.

pterygomaxillary (ter″ĭ-go-mak′sĭ-ler″e) pertaining to a pterygoid process and the maxilla.

pterygopalatine (ter″ĭ-go-pal′ah-tīn) pertaining to a pterygoid process and the palatine bone.

ptilosis (ti-lo′sis) falling out of the eyelashes.

ptomaine (to′mān, to-mān′) a basic substance derived from putrefying tissues.
  p. poisoning, a term commonly misapplied to FOOD POISONING. Contrary to popular belief, ptomaines are not injurious to the human digestive system, which is quite capable of reducing them to harmless substances. Decomposed foods are often responsible for food poisoning, however, because they may harbor certain forms of poison-producing bacteria.

ptosis (to′sis) abnormal downward displacement of an organ or body structure, especially paralytic drooping of the upper eyelid. adj., **ptot′ic.**

-ptosis (to′sis) word element [Gr.], *downward displacement.* adj., **-ptot′ic.**

PTT partial thromboplastin time.

ptyalagogue (ti-al′ah-gog) sialagogue.

ptyalectasis (ti″ah-lek′tah-sis) 1. a state of dilatation of a salivary gland duct. 2. surgical dilation of a salivary gland duct.

ptyalin (ti′ah-lin) an enzyme found in saliva that converts starch into maltose and dextrose.

ptyalism (ti′ah-lizm) excessive secretion of saliva.

ptyalocele (ti-al′o-sēl) a cystic tumor containing saliva.

ptyalogenic (ti″ah-lo-jen′ik) formed from saliva.

ptyaloreaction (ti″ah-lo-re-ak′shun) a reaction occurring in or performed on the saliva.

ptyalorrhea (ti″ah-lo-re′ah) ptyalism.

Pu chemical symbol, *plutonium.*

pubarche (pu-bar′ke) the first appearance of pubic hair.

puberty (pu′ber-te) the stage of growth at which the reproductive organs become capable of functioning. Puberty in a girl is marked by broadening of the hips, development of the breasts, the appearance of pubic hair and the onset of menstruation. At puberty a boy's shoulders broaden, his voice deepens and pubic and facial hair appears. Girls usually reach puberty between the ages of 11 and 13, and boys between 13 and 15; the timing varies widely among individuals, however.

pubes (pu′bēz) 1. the hair on the external genitalia, or the region covered with it. 2. plural of *pubis*.

pubescence (pu-bes′ens) 1. puberty. 2. lanugo.

pubescent (pu-bes′ent) 1. arriving at the age of puberty. 2. covered with down or lanugo.

pubic (pu′bik) pertaining to the pubes, or pubic bones.

pubiotomy (pu″be-ot′o-me) transection of the symphysis pubis.

pubis (pu′bis), pl. *pu′bes* [L.] the anterior portion of the hip bone, a distinct bone in early life; called also pubic bone.

public health (pub′lik) the field of medicine that is concerned with safeguarding and improving the physical, mental and social well-being of the community as a whole.

The United States Public Health Service (U.S.P.H.S.) is a tax-supported federal health agency that is a unit of the Department of Health, Education and Welfare. State and county public health agencies function under the supervision of and with financial support from the national Public Health Service.

Programs carried out by the U.S.P.H.S. include research programs, quarantine regulations, medical and psychiatric examinations of immigrants, Civil Defense programs and financial and technical aid to local health departments to support training programs for personnel and improve the health of citizens of the community.

p.h. nursing, the branch of nursing concerned with providing nursing care and health guidance to individuals and families in the home and school, at work and at medical and health centers. The public health nurse is employed by a local agency or the United States Public Health Service. She works to implement such programs as school and preschool health programs, immunization and treatment of communicable diseases, maternal and child health clinics and home visits for the purpose of providing health education and nursing care. She frequently participates in educational programs for nurses, allied professional workers and civic organizations, and is involved in studying and planning and putting into action local and national health programs.

pubofemoral (pu″bo-fem′o-ral) pertaining to the pubis and femur.

puboprostatic (pu″bo-pros-tat′ik) pertaining to the pubis and prostate.

pubovesical (pu″bo-ves′ĭ-kal) pertaining to the pubis and bladder.

pudendum (pu-den′dum), pl. *puden′da* [L.] the external structures of the reproductive system in the female, including the mons pubis and the labia majora and minora. adj., **puden′dal, pu′dic.**

puericulture (pu′er-ĭ-kul″tūr) the art of rearing children.

puerile (pu′er-il) pertaining to a child or to childhood.

puerilism (pu′er-il-izm″) reversion of the mind to the state of childhood.

puerpera (pu-er′per-ah) a woman who has just given birth to a child.

puerperal (pu-er′per-al) pertaining to a puerpera or to the puerperium.

p. fever, an infectious disease of childbirth; called also puerperal sepsis and childbed fever.

Until the mid-19th century, this dreaded, then mysterious illness sometimes swept through a hospital maternity ward, killing most of the new mothers. Today strict aseptic hospital techniques have made the disease uncommon in most parts of the world, except in unusual circumstances such as illegally induced abortion.

Puerperal fever results from an infection originating in the birth canal and affecting the endometrium. This infection can spread throughout the body, causing septicemia. The preliminary symptoms are fever, chills, excessive bleeding, foul lochia and abdominal and pelvic pain. In acute stages, the pain spreads to the legs and chest; complications may be serious or even fatal.

Treatment consists mainly of administration of antibiotics, and in most instances they promptly clear up the infection. If the disease has progressed to an acute stage before treatment begins, blood transfusions may be necessary.

puerperalism (pu-er′per-al-izm″) a disease condition incident to childbirth.

puerperium (pu″er-pe′re-um) the period or state of confinement after childbirth, usually 4 to 6 weeks.

Pulex (pu′leks) a genus of fleas, several species of which transmit the microorganism causing plague.

P. ir′ritans, a widely distributed species, known as the human flea, which infests domestic animals as well as man.

pulicicide (pu-lis′ĭ-sīd) an agent destructive to fleas.

pulicosis (pu″lĭ-ko′sis) irritation of the skin caused by flea bites.

pullulation (pul″u-la′shun) development by sprouting, or budding.

pulmo-aortic (pul″mo-a-or′tik) pertaining to the lungs and aorta.

pulmometer (pul-mom′ĕ-ter) an apparatus for measuring lung capacity; spirometer.

pulmometry (pul-mom′ĕ-tre) measurement of lung capacity.

pulmonary (pul′mo-ner″e) pertaining to the lungs, or to the pulmonary artery.

p. artery, the large artery originating from the superior surface of the right ventricle and passing diagonally upward to the left across the route of the aorta. The pulmonary trunk divides between the fifth and sixth thoracic vertebrae, forming the right pulmonary artery, which enters the right lung, and the left pulmonary artery, which enters the left lung.

p. circulation, the circulation of blood to and from the lungs. Unoxygenated blood from the right ventricle flows through the right and left pulmonary arteries to the right and left lung. After entering the lungs, the branches subdivide, finally emerging as capillaries which surround the alveoli and release the carbon dioxide in exchange for a fresh supply of oxygen. The capillaries unite gradually and assume the characteristics of veins. These veins join to form the pulmonary veins, which return the oxygenated blood to the left atrium.

p. valve, the pocket-like structure that guards the orifice between the right ventricle and the pulmonary artery.

p. vein, the large vein (right and left branches) that carries oxygenated blood from the lungs to the left atrium of the heart.

pulmonectomy (pul″mo-nek′to-me) pneumonectomy.

pulmonic (pul-mon′ik) 1. pertaining to the lungs; pulmonary. 2. pertaining to the pulmonary artery.

pulmonitis (pul″mo-ni′tis) inflammation of the lung; pneumonitis; pneumonia.

pulmonohepatic (pul-mo″no-hĕ-pat′ik) pertaining to or communicating with the lung and liver.

pulmonology (pul″mo-nol′o-je) the science concerned with the anatomy, physiology and pathology of the lungs.

pulmonoperitoneal (pul-mo″no-per″ĭ-to-ne′al) pertaining to or communicating with the lung and peritoneum.

pulmotor (pul′mo-tor) an apparatus for forcing oxygen into the lungs, and, when they are distended, for sucking out air.

pulp (pulp) soft, juicy animal or vegetable tissue. adj., **pul′pal.**

dental p., the richly vascularized and innervated connective tissue inside a tooth.

digital p., a cushion of soft tissue on the palmar or plantar surface of the distal phalanx of a finger or toe.

tooth p., dental pulp.

white p., sheaths of lymphatic tissue surrounding the arteries of the spleen.

pulpa (pul′pah) pl. *pul′pae* [L.] pulp.

pulpalgia (pul-pal′je-ah) pain in the dental pulp.

pulpectomy (pul-pek′to-me) removal of dental pulp.

pulpefaction (pul″pĕ-fak′shun) conversion into pulp.

pulpy (pul′pe) soft; of the consistency of pulp.

pulsatile (pul′sah-tīl) characterized by a rhythmic pulsation.

pulsation (pul-sa′shun) a throb, or rhythmic beat, as of the heart.

pulse (puls) the beat of the heart as felt through the walls of the arteries. What is usually meant by pulse is the pulsation felt in the radial artery at the wrist. Other sites of pulsation include the side of the neck (carotid artery), the elbow (brachial artery), the temple (temporal artery), the anterior side of the hip bone (femoral artery), the back of the knee (popliteal artery) and the instep (dorsalis pedis artery).

What is felt is not the blood pulsing through the arteries (as is commonly supposed) but a shock wave that travels along the fibers of the arteries as the heart contracts. This shock wave is generated by the pounding of the blood as it is ejected from the heart under pressure. It is analogous to the hammering sound heard in steampipes as the steam is admitted into the pipes under pressure. A pulse in the veins is too weak to be felt, although sometimes it is measured by sphygmograph; the tracing obtained is called a phlebogram.

The pulse is usually felt just inside the wrist below the thumb by placing two or three fingers lightly upon the radial artery. The thumb is never used to take a pulse because its own pulse is likely to be confused with the one being taken. Pressure should be light; if the artery is pressed too hard, the pulse will disappear entirely. The number of beats felt in exactly 1 minute is the pulse rate.

In taking a pulse, the rate, rhythm and force of the pulse are noted. The average rate in an adult is between 60 and 80 beats per minute. The rhythm is checked for possible irregularities, which may be an indication of heart disease; the force of the pulse is an indication of the general condition of the heart and the circulatory system.

An instrument for registering the movements, form and force of the arterial pulse is called a sphygmograph. The sphygmographic tracing (or pulse tracing) consists of a curve having a sudden rise (primary elevation) followed by a sudden fall, after which there is a gradual descent marked by a number of secondary elevations.

abdominal p., that in the abdominal aorta.

abrupt p., one that strikes the finger rapidly.

anacrotic p., one that makes a break in the ascending limb of the sphygmogram.

ardent p., one that appears to strike the finger at a single point.

bigeminal p., one in which two beats occur in rapid succession, the groups of two being separated by a longer interval.

catacrotic p., one that makes a break in the descending limb of the sphygmogram.

cordy p., a tense, firm pulse.

Corrigan's p., a jerky pulse with full expansion and sudden collapse.

dicrotic p., one in which the tracing shows two marked expansions in one beat of the artery; seen in increased arterial tension.

full p., one with copious volume of blood.

hard p., one characterized by high tension.

hyperdicrotic p., one showing a dicrotic notch below the base line of the sphygmogram; a sign of extreme exhaustion.

jerky p., one in which the artery is suddenly and markedly distended.

paradoxical p., one that is weaker during inspiration, as in some cases of adherent pericardium.

pistol-shot p., one in which the arteries are subject to quick distention and collapse.

plateau p., a pulse that is slowly rising and sustained.

p. pressure, the difference between the systolic and diastolic pressures.

quick p., one that strikes the finger smartly and leaves it quickly.

Quincke's p., reddening of the nail bed with each systole; seen in aortic insufficiency.

radial p., that felt over the radial artery.

Riegel's p., one that is smaller during expiration.

thready p., one that is very fine and scarcely perceptible.

tricrotic p., one showing three sphygmographic waves to the pulse beat.

undulating p., one giving the sensation of successive waves.

unequal p., one in which some beats are strong and others weak.

vagus p., a slow pulse caused by influence of the vagus nerve on the heart.

water-hammer p., Corrigan's pulse.

wiry p., a small, tense pulse.

pulseless disease (puls'les) absence of the pulse and of perceptible blood pressure in the arms, with changes in the fundus of the eye and hypertension in the lower extremities.

pulsimeter (pul-sim'ĕ-ter) an apparatus for measuring the force of the pulse.

pulsus (pul'sus) [L.] pulse.

p. alter'nans, a pulse in which there is regular alteration of weak and strong beats.

p. bigem'inus, bigeminal pulse.

p. ce'ler, a swift, abrupt pulse.

p. dif'ferens, inequality of the pulse observable at corresponding sites on either side of the body.

p. paradox'us, paradoxical pulse.

p. par'vus et tar'dus, a small hard pulse that rises and falls slowly.

p. ra'rus, a slow pulse due to prolongation of the heartbeat.

p. tar'dus, an abnormally slow pulse.

pultaceous (pul-ta'shus) like a poultice; pulpy.

pulverulent (pul-ver'u-lent) powdery; dusty.

pulvinar (pul-vi'nar) the posterior inner part of the optic thalamus.

pump (pump) an apparatus for drawing or forcing liquid or gas.

air p., one for exhausting or forcing in air.

blood p., a machine used to propel blood through the tubing of extracorporeal circulation devices.

breast p., a pump for taking milk from the breast.

dental p., a device for removing saliva during dental operations.

p.-oxygenator, heart-lung machine.

stomach p., a pump for removing the contents from the stomach.

punctate (pungk'tāt) spotted; marked with points or punctures.

punctiform (pungk'tĭ-form) like a point.

punctum (pungk'tum), pl. *punc'ta* [L.] point.

p. cae'cum, blind spot.

punc'ta doloro'sa, painful spots along a nerve.

p. lacrima'le (pl. *punc'ta lacrima'lia*), an opening of a lacrimal duct on the edge of the eyelid.

p. lu'teum, macula lutea.

p. ossificatio'nis, center of ossification.

p. prox'imum, near point.

p. remo'tum, far point.

punc'ta vasculo'sa, minute red spots that mark the cut surface of white matter of the brain.

puncture (pungk'tūr) 1. the piercing of an organ or other body structure with a hollow needle for the withdrawal of fluid or the removal of tissue for microscopic study. 2. a wound made by a pointed instrument.

cisternal p., puncture of the cisterna cerebellomedullaris just below the occipital bone to obtain a specimen of cerebrospinal fluid (see also CISTERNAL PUNCTURE).

lumbar p., puncture of the subarachnoid space in the region of the lumbar vertebrae in order to obtain cerebrospinal fluid (see also LUMBAR PUNCTURE).

spinal p., puncture of the spinal canal (see also SPINAL PUNCTURE).

sternal p., removal of bone marrow from the manubrium of the sternum through a spinal puncture needle (see also STERNAL PUNCTURE).

P.U.O. pyrexia of unknown origin.

pupil (pu'pil) the opening in the center of the iris. adj., **pu'pillary.**

Adie's p., abnormality in the size of the pupil, and delay in reaction to light and accommodation. (See also ADIE'S SYNDROME.)

Argyll Robertson p., one that is miotic and responds to accommodation effort, but not to light.

fixed p., a pupil that does not react to light, accommodation or on convergence.

Hutchinson's p., a condition of the pupils in which one is dilated and the other not.

pupilla (pu-pil'ah) [L.] pupil.

pupillatonia (pu″pil-ah-to'ne-ah) failure of the pupil to react to light.

pupillometry (pu″pĭ-lom'ĕ-tre) measurement of the diameter or width of the pupil of the eye.

pupilloplegia (pu″pĭ-lo-ple'je-ah) pupillatonia.

pupilloscopy (pu″pĭ-los'ko-pe) skiametry; a method for evaluating refractive errors of the eye.

pupillostatometer (pu″pĭ-lo-stah-tom'ĕ-ter) an instrument for measuring the distance between the pupils.

pupillotonia (pu″pĭ-lo-to'ne-ah) abnormal tonic reaction of the pupil, as in ADIE'S SYNDROME.

purgation (per-ga'shun) catharsis; purging effected by a cathartic medicine.

purgative (per'gah-tiv) 1. effecting purgation; cathartic. 2. a medicine that causes purgation.

purge (perj) 1. a purgative medicine or dose. 2. to cause free evacuation of feces.

purine (pu'rēn) a colorless, crystalline compound not found in nature but synthesized by chemists, or one of a group of compounds of which it is the base, such as uric acid, adenine, xanthine and theobromine.

p.-free diet, a diet sometimes used in the treatment of GOUT, omitting meat, fowl and fish, but using eggs, cheese and vegetables. The following foods are especially high in purines: kidney, liver, sweetbreads, sardines, anchovies and meat extracts.

Purinethol (pu'rēn-thol) trademark for a preparation of mercaptopurine, an antineoplastic agent.

Purkinje's cells (pur-kin'jēz) large, branched cells of the middle layer of the brain.

p's fibers, beaded muscular fibers forming a network in the subendocardial tissue of the ventricles of the heart. They are thought to be concerned in the conduction of stimuli from the atria to the ventricles.

Purodigin (pu″ro-dij'in) trademark for a preparation of crystalline digitoxin, a heart stimulant.

purpura (per'pu-rah) a hemorrhagic disease characterized by extravasation of blood into the tissues, under the skin and through the mucous membranes, and producing spontaneous ecchymoses (bruises) and petechiae (small red patches) on the skin. The disorder is accompanied by a marked decrease in circulating platelets and hence is sometimes called thrombocytopenic purpura. adj., **purpu'ric.**

There are two general types of purpura: primary or idiopathic purpura, in which the cause is unknown, and secondary or symptomatic purpura, which may be associated with exposure to drugs or other chemical agents, systemic diseases such as anemia and leukemia, diseases affecting the bone marrow or spleen and infectious diseases such as rubella (German measles).

SYMPTOMS. The outward manifestations and laboratory findings of primary and secondary purpura are similar. There is evidence of bleeding under the skin, with easy bruising and the development of petechiae. In the acute form there may be bleeding from any of the body orifices, such as hematuria, nosebleed, vaginal bleeding and bleeding gums. The PLATELET count is below 100,000 per cubic millimeter of blood and may go as low as 10,000 per cubic millimeter (normal count is about 250,000 per cubic millimeter). The bleeding time is prolonged and clot retraction is poor. Coagulation time is normal.

TREATMENT. Differential diagnosis is necessary to determine the type of purpura present and to eliminate the cause if it can be determined. General measures include protection of the patient from trauma, elective surgery and tooth extractions, any one of which may lead to severe or even fatal hemorrhage. Corticosteroids may be administered when the purpura is moderately severe and of short duration. Splenectomy is indicated when other, more conservative measures fail and is successful in a majority of cases. In some instances, especially in children, there may be spontaneous and permanent recovery from idiopathic purpura.

allergic p., anaphylactic p., a form of nonthrombocytopenic purpura of unknown origin, associated with increased capillary permeability and one or more allergic symptoms.

annular telangiectatic p., a rare form in which punctate erythematous lesions coalesce to form an annular or serpiginous pattern.

p. ful'minans, a severe nonthrombocytopenic purpura observed mainly in children, usually following an infectious disease, and often associated with extensive extravascular thromboses and gangrene.

p. hemorrha'gica, idiopathic thrombocytopenic purpura.

Henoch's p., nonthrombocytopenic purpura with acute visceral symptoms such as vomiting, diarrhea, hematuria and renal colic.

nonthrombocytopenic p., purpura without any decrease in the platelet count of the blood. In such cases the cause of purpura is either abnormal capillary fragility or a clotting factor deficiency.

Schönlein-Henoch p., idiopathic purpura in which there may be concomitant articular symptoms (Schönlein's disease) and intestinal symptoms.

p. seni'lis, purpuric eruption on the legs of elderly or debilitated persons.

thrombocytopenic p., purpura associated with a decrease in the number of platelets in the blood.

thrombotic thrombocytopenic p., thrombocytopenic purpura associated with thrombosis in terminal arterioles and capillaries, prominent signs being neurologic disturbance, anemia and azotemia.

purpureaglycoside (per-pu″re-ah-gli'ko-sīd) a cardiac glycoside from the leaves of *Digitalis purpurea.*

p. C, deslanoside.

purpurin (per'pu-rin) 1. a red coloring matter of the urine; called also uroerythrin. 2. a dye used as a nuclear stain.

purulence (pu'roo-lens) the formation or presence of pus.

purulent (pu'roo-lent) containing or consisting of pus.

puruloid (pu'roo-loid) resembling pus.

pus (pus) a thick fluid composed of viable and necrotic polymorphonuclear leukocytes, with necrotic tissue debris partially liquefied by enzymes liberated from the dead leukocytes, and other tissue breakdown products, characteristically produced in infections due to certain bacteria.

pustula (pus'tu-lah), pl. *pus'tulae* [L.] pustule.

pustulant (pus'tu-lant) causing pustulation.

pustulation (pus″tu-la'shun) the formation of pustules.

pustule (pus'tūl) a circumscribed, pus-containing lesion of the skin. adj., **pus'tular.**

malignant p., anthrax.

pustulosis (pus″tu-lo'sis) a condition marked by an eruption of pustules.

putamen (pu-ta'men) the outer part of the lenticular nucleus.

putrefaction (pu″trĕ-fak'shun) decomposition of animal or vegetable matter effected largely by action of microorganisms. adj., **putrefac'tive.**

putrefy (pu'trĕ-fi) to decompose, with the production of foul-smelling compounds; applied especially to the decomposition of proteins and organic matter.

putrescent (pu-tres'ent) undergoing putrefaction.

PVP polyvinylpyrrolidone, a plasma volume expander.

pyarthrosis (pi"ar-thro'sis) suppurative inflammation of a joint; suppurative arthritis.

pyel(o)- (pi'ĕ-lo) word element [Gr.], *renal pelvis*.

pyelectasis (pi"ĕ-lek'tah-sis) dilatation of the renal pelvis.

pyelephlebitis (pi"ĕ-lĕ-flĕ-bi'tis) pylephlebitis.

pyelitis (pi"ĕ-li'tis) inflammation of the renal pelvis, the outer basin-like portion of the kidney at the attachment of the ureter.

Pyelitis is a fairly common disease, and usually can be diagnosed and cured without great difficulty. Prompt and effective treatment is necessary to prevent the spread of infection and the development of pyelonephritis, a severely disabling disease in the chronic form, in which damage to the kidney cells may lead to high blood pressure and uremia.

CAUSE. Pyelitis is usually caused by a microorganism such as *Escherichia coli* or (less often) streptococcus or staphylococcus, which may invade the kidneys by way of the blood. Pyelitis may also arise from an infection of the bladder (CYSTITIS).

The disease is most common among young children, affecting females far more often than males because the urethra is considerably shorter in the female than in the male. This favors ascending infections from the outside to enter the bladder. Female children not properly trained in their toilet habits will, after bowel movements, rub the toilet tissue from the anus forward toward the vagina rather than vice versa. In this way the bacteria so commonly found in fecal matter find their way into the urinary bladder and from there to the pelvis of the kidney.

Any urinary obstruction can sharply increase the chances of the development of pyelitis, since obstruction interferes with the normal ability of the kidney to rid the body of harmful bacteria.

SYMPTOMS. Probably the most common symptoms of pyelitis are frequency and urgency of urination and dysuria. Other possible symptoms include fever, chills, headache and pain in one or both sides of the lower back. Pyelitis may also be present without any outward symptoms, but urinalysis will reveal many pus cells and occasionally erythrocytes.

TREATMENT. Pyelitis and pyelonephritis can usually be treated quite successfully with sulfonamides. Certain antibiotics are also helpful, and so are the urinary antiseptics. If the disease is treated promptly, the patient can look forward to early and complete recovery.

pyelocaliectasis (pi"ĕ-lo-kal"e-ek'tah-sis) dilatation of the kidney pelvis and calices.

pyelocystitis (pi"ĕ-lo-sis-ti'tis) inflammation of the renal pelvis and bladder.

pyelogram (pi'ĕ-lo-gram") the film produced by pyelography.

pyelography (pi"ĕ-log'rah-fe) roentgenography of the kidney and ureter after injection of a contrast medium, introduced by the intravenous or retrograde method. Preparation of the patient for pyelography includes clearing the intestinal tract of as much fecal material and gas as possible so that there can be adequate visualization of the urinary tract structures. Usually this is accomplished by administration of castor oil and enemas. The evening before the examination the patient is given a light meal and then all foods and fluids are restricted after 9:00 P.M.

In the intravenous method the contrast medium is injected intravenously at designated intervals and x-ray films are taken to observe the rate of excretion, the concentration of the contrast medium in the pelves and calices of the kidney and the outline of the ureters and urinary bladder. The possibility of an allergic reaction to the contrast medium must always be considered. Drugs such as epinephrine and hydrocortisone should be on hand for use in the event of a serious allergic reaction. The patient may experience a mild transitory sensation of warmth, flushing of the face or a salty taste in the mouth, but these should last only a few moments. Symptoms of ANAPHYLACTIC SHOCK demand immediate treatment.

Retrograde pyelography involves introduction of the contrast medium by way of ureteral catheters. This procedure may be done when special studies of certain parts of the urinary tract are indicated, or when adequate concentration of the contrast medium cannot be achieved by the intravenous method.

pyelolithotomy (pi"ĕ-lo-lĭ-thot'o-me) incision of the renal pelvis for removal of calculi.

pyelometer (pi"ĕ-lom'ĕ-ter) pelvimeter.

pyelometry (pi"ĕ-lom'ĕ-tre) 1. measurement of the changes in pressure in the renal pelvis. 2. pelvimetry.

pyelonephritis (pi"ĕ-lo-nĕ-fri'tis) inflammation of the kidney and renal pelvis (see also PYELITIS and NEPHRITIS).

pyelonephrosis (pi"ĕ-lo-nĕ-fro'sis) any disease of the kidney and its pelvis.

pyelopathy (pi"ĕ-lop'ah-the) any disease of the renal pelvis.

pyelophlebitis (pi"ĕ-lo-flĕ-bi'tis) inflammation of the veins of the renal pelvis.

pyeloplasty (pi'ĕ-lo-plas"te) plastic repair of the renal pelvis.

pyelostomy (pi"ĕ-los'to-me) the operation of forming an opening in the renal pelvis for the purpose of temporarily diverting the urine from the ureter.

pyelotomy (pi"ĕ-lot'o-me) incision of the renal pelvis.

pyemesis (pi-em'ĕ-sis) the vomiting of pus.

pyemia (pi-e'me-ah) the presence of pyogenic microorganisms in the bloodstream and the formation of secondary abscesses wherever these microorganisms lodge; called also metastatic infection. adj., **pye'mic.**

arterial p., a form due to the dissemination of emboli from a cardiac thrombosis.

cryptogenic p., that in which the source of infection is in a deep body tissue.

Pyemotes (pi"ĕ-mo'tēz) a genus of mites.

P. ventrico'sus, a species parasitic on various insect pests which occasionally causes a dermatitis in man (grain itch).

pyencephalus (pi″en-sef′ah-lus) abscess of the brain.

pygal (pi′gal) pertaining to the buttocks.

pygalgia (pi-gal′je-ah) pain in the buttocks.

pygoamorphus (pi″go-ah-mor′fus) a fetal monster with a teratoma in the sacral region.

pygodidymus (pi″go-did′ĭ-mus) a fetal monster with double hips and pelvis.

pygomelus (pi-gom′ĕ-lus) a fetal monster with extra limbs on the buttocks.

pygopagus (pi-gop′ah-gus) a twin fetal monster joined at the buttocks.

pykn(o)- (pik′no) word element [Gr.], *thick; compact; frequent.*

pyknemia (pik-ne′me-ah) thickening of the blood.

pyknic (pik′nik) having a short, thick, stocky build.

pyknolepsy (pik′no-lep″se) a form of idiopathic epilepsy in which momentary lapses of consciousness may occur as frequently as hundreds of times daily.

pyknometer (pik-nom′ĕ-ter) 1. an instrument for measuring the thickness of parts. 2. an instrument for determining the specific gravity of the urine.

pyknomorphous (pik″no-mor′fus) having the stained portions of the cell body compactly arranged.

pyknophrasia (pik″no-fra′ze-ah) thickness of speech.

pyknosis (pik-no′sis) thickening and shrinkage of the nucleus after death of a cell. adj., pyknot′ic.

pyle- (pi′le) word element [Gr.], *portal vein.*

pylemphraxis (pi″lem-frak′sis) obstruction of the portal vein.

pylephlebectasis (pi″le-flĕ-bek′tah-sis) dilatation of the portal vein.

pylephlebitis (pi″le-flĕ-bi′tis) inflammation of the portal vein.

pylethrombophlebitis (pi″le-throm″bo-flĕ-bi′tis) thrombosis and inflammation of the portal vein.

pylethrombosis (pi″le-throm-bo′sis) thrombosis of the portal vein.

pyloralgia (pi″lo-ral′je-ah) pain and spasm of the pylorus.

pylorectomy (pi″lo-rek′to-me) excision of the pylorus.

pyloric (pi-lor′ik) pertaining to the pylorus.
 p. stenosis, increase in the size of the pyloric muscle; the lumen of the pylorus is obstructed and emptying of the stomach is impeded. The condition is congenital and there is a familial tendency toward it.
 The initial symptom is vomiting, mild at first but becoming increasingly more forceful. It can occur both during and after feedings. Diagnosis may be confirmed by x-ray examination using a barium meal.

Treatment is usually surgical, involving longitudinal splitting of the muscle (pyloromyotomy).

pylorodiosis (pi-lor″o-di-o′sis) dilatation of a pyloric stricture by the fingers or an instrument.

pyloroduodenitis (pi-lor″o-du″o-dĕ-ni′tis) inflammation of the pyloric and duodenal mucosa.

pyloromyotomy (pi-lor″o-mi-ot′o-me) incision of the longitudinal and circular muscles of the pylorus.

pyloroplasty (pi-lor′o-plas″te) plastic surgery of the pylorus, especially for pyloric stricture, to provide a larger communication between the stomach and duodenum.

pyloroscopy (pi″lor-os′ko-pe) inspection of the pylorus.

pylorospasm (pi-lor′o-spazm) spasm of the pylorus or of the pyloric portion of the stomach.
 congenital p., spasm of the pylorus in infants from birth.
 reflex p., pylorospasm due to extragastric conditions.

pylorostenosis (pi-lor″o-stĕ-no′sis) pyloric stenosis.

pylorostomy (pi″lor-os′to-me) formation of an opening into the pylorus through the abdominal wall.

pylorotomy (pi″lor-ot′o-me) 1. gastrotomy. 2. pyloromyotomy.

pylorus (pi-lor′us) the junction of the stomach and the duodenum. A ring of muscles, the pyloric sphincter, serves as a "gate," closing the opening from the stomach to the intestine. It opens periodically, allowing the contents of the stomach to move into the duodenum. The pylorus contains many glands that help produce hydrochloric acid.
 Occasionally, in infants, the pyloric muscle is greatly enlarged and thickened, so that emptying of the stomach is prevented. This condition, hypertrophic pyloric obstruction or PYLORIC STENOSIS, can be corrected by surgery.

pyo- (pi′o) word element [Gr.], *pus.*

pyocalix (pi″o-ka′liks) pus in the calix of the kidney pelvis.

pyocele (pi′o-sēl) a collection of pus about the testis.

pyocelia (pi″o-se′le-ah) pus in the abdominal cavity.

pyocephalus (pi″o-sef′ah-lus) the presence of purulent fluid in the cerebral ventricles.

pyochezia (pi″o-ke′ze-ah) the presence of pus in the feces.

pyococcus (pi″o-kok′us) a micrococcus that causes suppuration.

pyocolpos (pi″o-kol′pos) pus in the vagina.

pyocyanase (pi″o-si′ah-nās) an antibacterial substance from cultures of *Pseudomonas aeruginosa.*

pyocyanin (pi″o-si′ah-nin) an antibiotic from *Pseudomonas aeruginosa.*

pyocyst (pi′o-sist) a cyst containing pus.

pyoderma (pi″o-der′mah) a purulent skin disease.
   p. gangreno′sum, a cutaneous ulcer originating in an operative or traumatic wound, with undermining of the border. It is frequently associated with ulcerative colitis.

pyodermatitis (pi″o-der″mah-ti′tis) a purulent inflammation of the skin.

pyodermatosis (pi″o-der″mah-to′sis) any skin disease of pyogenic origin.

pyodermia (pi″o-der′me-ah) pyoderma.

pyofecia (pi″o-fe′se-ah) pus in the feces.

pyogenesis (pi″o-jen′ĕ-sis) the formation of pus.

pyogenic (pi″o-jen′ik) producing suppuration.

pyohemia (pi″o-he′me-ah) pyemia.

pyohemothorax (pi″o-he″mo-tho′raks) pus and blood in the pleural cavity.

pyoid (pi′oid) resembling or like pus.

pyolabyrinthitis (pi″o-lab″ĭ-rin-thi′tis) inflammation of the labyrinth of the ear, with suppuration.

pyometra (pi″o-me′trah) an accumulation of pus within the uterus.

pyometritis (pi″o-me-tri′tis) purulent inflammation of the uterus.

pyonephritis (pi″o-nĕ-fri′tis) purulent inflammation of the kidney.

pyonephrolithiasis (pi″o-nef″ro-lĭ-thi′ah-sis) pus and calculi in the kidney.

pyonephrosis (pi″o-nĕ-fro′sis) suppurative destruction of the renal parenchyma, with total or almost complete loss of kidney function.

pyonychia (pi″o-nik′e-ah) pyogenic infection of the fold surrounding a nail.

pyo-ovarium (pi″o-o-va′re-um) an abscess of the ovary.

pyopericarditis (pi″o-per″ĭ-kar-di′tis) purulent pericarditis.

pyopericardium (pi″o-per″ĭ-kar′de-um) pus in the pericardium.

pyoperitoneum (pi″o-per″ĭ-to-ne′um) pus in the peritoneal cavity.

pyoperitonitis (pi″o-per″ĭ-to-ni′tis) purulent inflammation of the peritoneum.

pyophthalmitis (pi″of-thal-mi′tis) purulent inflammation of the eye.

pyophysometra (pi″o-fi″so-me′trah) pus and gas in the uterus.

pyoplania (pi″o-pla′ne-ah) wandering of pus from one place to another.

pyopneumocholecystitis (pi″o-nu″mo-ko″le-sis-ti′tis) inflammation of the gallbladder, with the presence of pus and gas.

pyopneumohepatitis (pi″o-nu″mo-hep″ah-ti′tis) abscess of the liver with pus and gas in the abscess cavity.

pyopneumopericardium (pi″o-nu″mo-per″ĭ-kar′de-um) pus and gas in the pericardium.

pyopneumoperitonitis (pi″o-nu″mo-per″ĭ-to-ni′tis) peritonitis with the presence of pus and gas.

pyopneumothorax (pi″o-nu″mo-tho′raks) the presence of both purulent exudates and air or gas within the pleural cavity.

pyoptysis (pi-op′tĭ-sis) expectoration of purulent matter.

pyopyelectasis (pi″o-pi″ĕ-lek′tah-sis) dilatation of the renal pelvis with pus.

pyorrhea (pi″o-re′ah) a copious discharge of pus.
   p. alveola′ris, a purulent inflammation of the dental periosteum, with progressive necrosis of the alveoli and looseness of the teeth (see also PERIODONTITIS).

pyosalpingitis (pi″o-sal″pin-ji′tis) inflammation of the uterine tube with formation of pus.

pyosalpingo-oophoritis (pi″o-sal-ping″go-o″of-o-ri′tis) purulent inflammation of the uterine tube and ovary.

pyosalpinx (pi″o-sal′pinks) an accumulation of pus in a uterine tube.

pyosis (pi-o′sis) suppuration.

pyospermia (pi″o-sper′me-ah) pus in the semen.

pyostatic (pi″o-stat′ik) arresting suppuration.

pyostomatitis (pi″o-sto″mah-ti′tis) inflammation of the mucous membrane of the mouth, with suppuration.

pyothorax (pi″o-tho′raks) an accumulation of pus in the thorax; empyema.

pyoureter (pi″o-u-re′ter) pus in the ureter.

pyovesiculosis (pi″o-vĕ-sik″u-lo′sis) pus in the seminal vesicles.

pyoxanthose (pi″o-zan′thōs) a yellow pigment from pus.

pyramid (pir′ah-mid) a pointed or cone-shaped structure or part.
   p. of the cerebellum, the central portion of the inferior vermis cerebelli.
   p. of light, a triangular reflection seen upon the tympanic membrane.
   malpighian p., renal pyramid.
   p's of the medulla, two anterior and two posterior columns within the medulla oblongata.
   renal p., one of the wedge-shaped masses constituting the medulla of the kidney, the base toward the cortex and culminating at the summit in the renal papilla.
   p. of tympanum, the elevation in the middle ear that contains the stapedius muscle.

pyramidal (pi-ram′ĭ-dal) shaped like a pyramid.

p. tracts, collections of motor nerve fibers arising in the brain and passing down through the spinal cord to motor cells in the anterior horns.

pyramis (pir'ah-mis), pl. *pyram'ides* [Gr.] pyramid.

pyrathiazine (pi″rah-thi'ah-zēn) a phenothiazine compound used as an antihistamine.

pyrazinamide (pi″rah-zin'ah-mīd) a compound used as a tuberculostatic agent.

pyrectic (pi-rek'tik) pertaining to fever; feverish.

pyretic (pi-ret'ik) pertaining to fever.

pyretogenesis (pi-re″to-jen'ĕ-sis) the origination of fever.

pyretogenous (pi″rĕ-toj'ĕ-nus) producing fever.

pyretolysis (pi″rĕ-tol'ĭ-sis) reduction of fever.

pyretotherapy (pi-re″to-ther'ah-pe) treatment by artificially increasing the patient's body temperature.

pyrexia (pi-rek'se-ah) fever; elevated body temperature. adj., **pyrex'ial.**

Pyribenzamine (pir″ĭ-ben'zah-mēn) trademark for preparations of tripelennamine, an antihistamine.

pyridine (pir'ĭ-dēn, pir'ĭ-din) a coal tar compound used chiefly as a solvent; it is the parent of many naturally occurring organic compounds.

pyridostigmine (pir″ĭ-do-stig'mēn) a compound used as a cholinesterase inhibitor in the treatment of myasthenia gravis.

pyridoxine, pyridoxol (pir″ĭ-dok'sēn), (pir″ĭ-dok'-sol) a component of the vitamin B complex (vitamin B₆), sometimes used in the treatment of nausea and vomiting of pregnancy and in radiation sickness.

pyrilamine (pi-ril'ah-mēn) a compound used as an antihistamine.

pyrimethamine (pi″rĭ-meth'ah-mēn) a compound used as an antimalarial.

pyrimidine (pi-rim'ĭ-dēn) an organic compound that is the fundamental form of several bases (the pyrimidine bases) present in nucleic acids.

pyrogen (pi'ro-jen) an agent that causes fever. adj., **pyrogen'ic.**
   bacterial p., a fever-producing agent of bacterial origin.

pyroglobulin (pi″ro-glob'u-lin) a blood globulin that precipitates from serum on heating.

pyroglobulinemia (pi″ro-glob″u-lin-e'me-ah) the presence in the blood of an abnormal globulin constituent that is precipitated by heat.

pyroligneous (pi″ro-lig'ne-us) obtained by destructive distillation of wood.

pyrolysis (pi-rol'ĭ-sis) the decomposition of a substance at high temperatures in the absence of oxygen.

pyromania (pi″ro-ma'ne-ah) a morbid compulsion to start fires.

pyrometer (pi-rom'ĕ-ter) a device for measuring high degrees of heat.

Pyronil (pi'ro-nil) trademark for a preparation of pyrrobutamine, an antihistamine.

pyronine (pi'ro-nin) a red aniline histologic stain.

pyrophobia (pi″ro-fo'be-ah) morbid dread of fire.

pyrosis (pi-ro'sis) heartburn; a burning sensation in the esophagus and stomach, with sour eructation.

pyrotic (pi-rot'ik) caustic.

pyrotoxin (pi″ro-tok'sin) a toxin developed during fever.

pyroxylin (pi-rok'sĭ-lin) a product of the action of a mixture of nitric and sulfuric acids on cotton, consisting chiefly of cellulose tetranitrate. It is dissolved in alcohol or ether to form collodion.

pyrrobutamine (pir″o-bu'tah-min) a compound used as an antihistamine.

pyrrole (pir'ōl) a compound, found in coal tar and tars, obtained by distillation of waste animal matter.

pyruvate (pi'roo-vāt) a salt or ester of pyruvic acid.

pyruvic acid (pi-roo'vik) a compound formed in the body in aerobic metabolism of carbohydrate.

pyrvinium (pir-vin'e-um) a compound used as an anthelmintic.

pyuria (pi-u're-ah) excretion of urine containing pus.

PZI protamine zinc insulin.

Q

Q. quadrant.

q.d. [L.] *qua'que di'e* (every day).

Q fever a febrile rickettsial infection caused by *Coxiella burnetii.* The causative microorganisms are found on the hides of sheep and cattle, and it is thought that human beings contract the disease by breathing in the dried microorganisms carried in dust particles in the air. In Australia, where the disease was first described, it is transmitted by ticks. Symptoms include sudden high fever, chills, headache, muscle pains and coughing. The disease usually is quickly brought under control by antibiotics. The Q stands for query.

q.h. [L.] *qua'que ho'ra* (every hour).

q.i.d. [L.] *qua'ter in di'e* (four times a day).

q.q.h. [L.] *qua'que quar'ta ho'ra* (every 4 hours).

QRS complex a group of waves depicted on an electrocardiogram; called also the QRS wave. It actually consists of three distinct waves created by the passage of the cardiac electrical impulse through the ventricles and occurring at the beginning of each contraction of the ventricles. In a normal ELECTROCARDIOGRAM the R wave is the most prominent of the three; the Q and S waves may be extremely weak and sometimes are absent.

One abnormality of the QRS complex is increased voltage resulting from enlargement of heart muscle, which produces increased quantities of electric current. This enlargement is caused by an excessive work load for some part of the heart and usually is due to a defect in the heart valves or great vessels near the heart.

A low-voltage QRS complex may result from local intraventricular block, toxic conditions of the heart and fluid in the pericardium. Pleural effusion and emphysema also can cause a decrease in the voltage of the QRS complex.

q.s. [L.] *quan'tum sa'tis* (a sufficient amount).

qt. quart.

quack (kwak) one who misrepresents his ability and experience in diagnosis and treatment of disease or the effects to be achieved by his treatment.

quackery (kwak'er-e) misrepresentation of one's ability to diagnose and treat disease.

quadr(i)- (kwod're) word element [L.], *four.*

quadrangular (kwod-rang'gu-lar) having four angles.

quadrant (kwod'rant) 1. one-fourth of the circumference of a circle. 2. one of four corresponding parts, or quarters, as of the surface of the abdomen or of the field of vision.

quadrantanopia (kwod"ran-tah-no'pe-ah) loss of vision in one fourth of the visual field.

quadrate (kwod'rāt) square or squared.

quadriceps (kwod'rĭ-seps) having four heads. **q. muscle,** a name applied collectively to four muscles, the rectus of the thigh and the intermediate lateral and medial great muscles, inserting by a common tendon that surrounds the patella and ends on the tuberosity of the tibia, and acting to extend the leg upon the thigh.

quadrigemina (kwod"rĭ-jem'ĭ-nah) the corpora quadrigemina.

quadrigeminal (kowd"rĭ-jem'ĭ-nal) fourfold; in four parts.

quadrilateral (kwod"rĭ-lat'er-al) having four sides.

quadrilocular (kwod"rĭ-lok'u-lar) having four cavities.

quadripara (kwod-rip'ah-rah) a woman who has had four pregnancies that resulted in viable offspring; para IV.

quadripartite (kwod"rĭ-par'tīt) divided into four.

quadriplegia (kwod"rĭ-ple'je-ah) paralysis of all four limbs; tetraplegia.

quadrisect (kwod'rĭ-sekt) to cut into four parts.

quadritubercular (kwod"rĭ-tu-ber'ku-lar) having four tubercles or cusps.

quadrivalent (kwod"rĭ-va'lent, kwod-riv'ah-lent) having a valence of four.

quadruplet (kwah-drup'let, kwah-droo'plet, kwod'roo-plet) one of four offspring produced at one birth.

qualimeter (kwah-lim'ĕ-ter) an instrument for measuring the penetrating power of roentgen rays.

quantimeter (kwon-tim'ĕ-ter) an instrument for measuring the quantity of roentgen rays generated by a Coolidge tube.

quantivalence (kwon-tiv'ah-lens) valence (1).

quantum (kwon'tum), pl. *quan'ta* [L.] an elemental unit of energy; the amount emitted or absorbed at each step when energy is emitted or absorbed by atoms or molecules.

quarantine (kwor'an-tēn) 1. a place or period of detention of ships coming from infected or suspected ports. 2. restrictions placed on entering or leaving premises where a case of communicable disease exists.

quart (kwort) one-fourth of a gallon (946 cc.).

quartan (kwor'tan) 1. recurring in 4-day cycles (every third day). 2. a variety of intermittent fever of which the paroxysms recur on every third day (see MALARIA).

double q., a quartan fever of which the recurrences are alternately severe and relatively mild.

triple q., a fever in which the paroxysms occur every day because of infection with three different groups of quartan parasites.

quartile (kwor′tīl, kwor′til) one of the values establishing the division of a series of variables into fourths, or the range of items included in such a segment.

quartipara (kwor-tip′ah-rah) quadripara; a woman who has had four pregnancies that resulted in viable offspring; para IV.

quater in die (kwah′ter in de′a) [L.] four times a day.

quaternary (kwah′ter-ner″e, kwah-ter′ner-e) 1. fourth in a series. 2. made up of four elements or radicals.

Queckenstedt′s test (kwek′en-stets″) when the veins in the neck are compressed on one or both sides there is a rapid rise in the pressure of the cerebrospinal fluid of healthy persons, and this rise quickly disappears when pressure is taken off the neck. But when there is a block in the spinal canal the pressure of the cerebrospinal fluid is affected little or not at all by the maneuver.

Quelicin (kwel′ĭ-sin) trademark for a preparation of succinylcholine, a muscle relaxant.

quercetin (kwer′sĕ-tin) a form of rutin and other glycosides, used to reduce abnormal capillary fragility.

Quervain′s disease (kār′vanz) inflammation of the long abductor and short extensor tendons of the thumb, with swelling and tenderness.

Quiactin (kwi-ak′tin) trademark for a preparation of oxanamide, a tranquilizer.

Quick hippuric acid excretion test (kwik) measurement of hippuric acid in the urine after ingestion of a standard dose of benzoic acid; formerly used as a test of liver function.

Q. one-stage prothrombin time test, a method of determining the integrity of the prothrombin complex in the blood; used in controlling anticoagulant therapy.

Q. tourniquet test, estimation of capillary fragility by counting the number of petechiae appearing in a limited area on the flexor surface of the forearm after obstruction to the circulation by a blood pressure cuff applied to the upper arm.

quickening (kwik′en-ing) the first perceptible movement of the fetus in the uterus, appearing usually in the sixteenth to eighteenth week of pregnancy.

quinacrine (kwin′ah-krin) a compound used as an antimalarial and anthelmintic.

quinalbarbitone (kwin″al-bar′bĭ-tōn) secobarbital, a short- to intermediate-acting barbiturate.

Quincke′s disease (kwink′ez) angioneurotic edema.

quinic acid (kwin′ik) a crystalline compound from cinchona.

quinidine (kwin′ĭ-din) an isomer of quinine, used in treatment of cardiac arrhythmias.

quinine (kwi′nīn) a white, bitter alkaloid usually obtained from cinchona; an analgesic, antipyretic, bitter tonic and effective antimalarial.

q. and urea hydrochloride, a double salt of quinine and urea hydrochlorides; used in treatment of malaria and as a sclerosing agent for internal hemorrhoids.

q. and urethan injection, a sterile solution containing quinine hydrochloride and urethan; a sclerosing agent for varicose veins.

q. salicylate, a salt used as an antipyretic and antirheumatic.

q. sulfate, a white crystalline salt, more largely used as a remedy than any other of the cinchona alkaloid salts.

quininism (kwin′ĭ-nizm) cinchonism; poisoning from cinchona bark or its alkaloids.

quinone (kwi-nōn′, kwin′ōn) a principle obtained by oxidizing quinic acid.

quinquevalent (kwing″kwĕ-va′lent, kwing-kwev′ah-lent) pentavalent; having a valence of five.

quinsy (kwin′ze) acute suppurative inflammation of the tonsil and the surrounding tissue.

quint- (kwint) word element [L.] *five.*

quintan (kwin′tan) recurring every 5 days (every fourth day).

q. fever, trench fever.

quintipara (kwin-tip′ah-rah) a woman who has had five pregnancies that resulted in viable offspring; para V.

quintuplet (kwin′too-plet) one of five offspring produced at one birth.

Quotane (kwo′tān) trademark for preparations of dimethisoquin hydrochloride, a local anesthetic.

quotid. [L.] *quotid′ie* (every day).

quotidian (kwo-tid′e-an) 1. recurring every day. 2. a form of intermittent malarial fever with daily recurrent paroxysms.

double q., a fever having two daily paroxysms.

quotient (kwo′shent) a number obtained by division.

achievement q., the achievement age divided by the mental age, indicating the progress in learning.

caloric q., the heat evolved (in calories) divided by the oxygen consumed (in milligrams) in a metabolic process.

intelligence q., I.Q., a numerical expression of intellectual capacity obtained by multiplying the mental age of the subject, ascertained by testing, by 100 and dividing by his chronologic age.

respiratory q., an expression of the ratio of the carbon dioxide produced to the oxygen consumed by an organism.

R

R 1. symbol, *roentgen*. 2. a symbol used in general chemical formulae to represent an organic radical.

R. Réaumur; rectal; [L.] *remo'tum* (far); respiration; right.

℞ symbol [L.], *rec'ipe* (take).

Ra chemical symbol, *radium*.

rabbit fever tularemia.

rabiate, rabid (ra'be-āt), (rab'id) affected with rabies.

rabies (ra'bēz, ra'be-ēz) an acute infectious viral disease communicated to man by the bite of an infected animal and affecting the brain and the nervous system; called also hydrophobia.

Rabies is transmitted by warm-blooded animals, especially dogs and foxes. The virus is often present in the saliva of affected animals and is transmitted chiefly through bite wounds and occasionally through open wounds or sores.

After the virus enters the body it travels along the nerve trunk to the brain; the farther the bite is from the head, the longer it takes to reach the brain. The incubation period varies from 2 weeks to as long as 6 months. The bitten person must start treatment with antirabies vaccine and serum before the virus reaches the brain. The disease must be prevented because it is always fatal in man.

PREVENTION. All warm-blooded family pets—including dogs, cats and monkeys—should be vaccinated against rabies periodically.

It is also essential to learn to recognize a rabid animal. In the early "anxiety" stages, a rabid animal may have a change of temperament. Many, including wild animals, may become unusually friendly. The rabid animal may next enter a "furious" stage in which it wanders about biting everything that moves, and even some things that do not move, such as sticks and stones. It then develops paralysis of the throat, which makes swallowing difficult. The name hydrophobia, "fear of water," was given to the disease because it was observed that stricken animals avoid water. Actually, they do not do so because of fear, but because they cannot swallow. Saliva often drips from the animal's mouth and may may be whipped into a foam.

Some animals pass directly from the anxiety stage to paralysis without becoming violent. This is called the "dumb" form of rabies. The animal may appear to have something caught in his throat. Usually, a dog with something in his throat tries to remove it himself, but a rabid dog will not. Eventually all of the rabid animal's muscles become paralyzed and it dies.

TREATMENT. When a person is bitten by an animal the wound should be washed thoroughly with soap and water, and then treated like any other wound. It is extremely important to go to a physician immediately. If at all possible, steps should be taken to find out if the biting animal has rabies.

The animal should be confined for observation. When the biting animal must be killed in order to capture it, care must be taken to see that the head is not damaged, so that the brain can be examined to establish a diagnosis. There are times when the biting animal cannot be caught for observation. If so, the bitten person must be given antirabies treatment immediately.

Preventive treatment of suspected rabies is based on immunization by a series of vaccine injections. When bites are in areas close to the head or in areas with many nerve endings, such as the hands, the virus may reach the brain very quickly. In such cases treatment should start immediately, even though the suspected animal is still being observed. Along with the vaccine, such patients are often given immune serum to establish passive immunity.

In man, rabies causes pain, fever, mental derangement, vomiting, profuse secretion of sticky saliva, convulsions and difficulty in breathing and swallowing. Treatment is palliative and consists of sedation to keep the patient in a coma. Death occurs in 2 to 5 days.

race (rās) a class or breed of animals; a group of individuals having certain characteristics in common, owing to a common inheritance.

racemic (ra-se'mik) made up of two enantiomorphic isomers and therefore optically inactive.

racemization (ras"ĕ-mĭ-za'shun) the transformation of one-half of the molecules of an optically active compound into molecules that possess exactly the opposite (mirror-image) configuration, with complete loss of rotatory power because of the statistical balance between equal numbers of dextrorotatory and levorotatory molecules.

racemose (ras'ĕ-mōs) shaped like a bunch of grapes.

racephedrine (ra-sef'ĕ-drin) the racemic mixture of ephedrine; used as a sympathomimetic.

-rachia (ra'ke-ah) word element [Gr.], *state of the spinal fluid;* also sometimes spelled *-rrhachia.*

rachialgia (ra"ke-al'je-ah) pain in the vertebral column.

rachianesthesia (ra"ke-an"es-the'ze-ah) loss of sensation produced by injection of an anesthetic into the spinal canal.

rachicentesis (ra"kĭ-sen-te'sis) puncture into the spinal canal (see also SPINAL PUNCTURE).

rachidial, rachidian (rah-kid'e-al), (rah-kid'e-an) pertaining to the spine.

rachigraph (ra'kĭ-graf) an instrument for recording the outlines of the spine and back.

rachilysis (rah-kil'ĭ-sis) correction of lateral

curvature of the spine by combined traction and pressure.

rachiocampsis (ra″ke-o-kamp′sis) spinal curvature.

rachiometer (ra″ke-om′ĕ-ter) an apparatus for measuring spinal curvature.

rachiomyelitis (ra″ke-o-mi″ĕ-li′tis) inflammation of the spinal cord.

rachioplegia (ra″ke-o-ple′je-ah) spinal paralysis.

rachiotomy (ra″ke-ot′o-me) incision of the vertebral column.

rachipagus (ra-kip′ah-gus) a double fetal monster joined at the vertebral column.

rachis (ra′kis) the vertebral column.

rachischisis (rah-kis′kĭ-sis) congenital fissure of the vertebral column.
  r. poste′rior, spina bifida.

rachitic (rah-kit′ik) pertaining to rickets.

rachitis (rah-ki′tis) rickets.

rachitogenic (rah-kit″o-jen′ik) causing rickets.

rachitomy (rah-kit′o-me) the surgical or anatomic opening of the spinal canal.

rad (rad) acronym for *radiation absorbed dose;* a unit of measurement of the absorbed dose of ionizing radiation. It corresponds to an energy transfer of 100 ergs per gram of any absorbing material (including tissue).

rad. [L.] *ra′dix* (root).

radectomy (rah-dek′to-me) excision of a portion of the root of a tooth.

radiability (ra″de-ah-bil′ĭ-te) the state of being susceptible to penetration by radiant energy (as x-rays or gamma rays).

radiad (ra′de-ad) toward the radial side or aspect.

radial (ra′de-al) 1. pertaining to the radius. 2. radiating; spreading outward from a common center.
  r. artery, an artery in the forearm, wrist and hand; the one usually used for taking the PULSE.

radialis (ra″de-a′lis) [L.] radial.

radiant (ra′de-ant) 1. diverging from a center. 2. emitting rays of light.

radiatio (ra″de-a′she-o), pl. *radiatio′nes* [L.] a radiating structure. In anatomy, a collection of nerve fibers connecting different portions of the brain.

radiation (ra″de-a′shun) 1. divergence from a common center. 2. a structure made up of diverging elements, especially a tract of the central nervous system made up of diverging fibers. 3. electromagnetic waves, such as those of visible light, infrared rays, ultraviolet rays, x-rays and gamma rays, or streams of atomic particles such as alpha and beta particles.
  Sources of radiation include natural or "background" radiation, such as cosmic rays from outer space, and the naturally occurring radioactive sub-

stances found in the earth. Man-made radiations result from artificially produced nuclear reactions in stable elements which are then changed to radioactive substances. (See also RADIOACTIVITY.)

KINDS OF RADIATION. Radiations are particulate and nonparticulate; that is, they may be made up of particles such as neutrons and protons which are fragments of the nuclei of disintegrating atoms, or they may consist of electromagnetic waves, which have no mass. Particulate radiations may consist of ALPHA PARTICLES or BETA PARTICLES. Most radioactive isotopes (RADIOISOTOPES) emit particulate radiations and at the same time also release electromagnetic rays (GAMMA RAYS).

Both particulate and nonparticulate radiations are capable of penetrating and being absorbed into matter. Alpha particles are the least penetrating; beta particles slightly more penetrating; and the gamma rays, like x-rays, are capable of completely penetrating the body. This ability to penetrate matter and change the basic structure of cells of the body is used beneficially in the treatment of tumors and other medical conditions.

X-rays, called also roentgen rays, are a form of radiation consisting of energy waves of very short wavelength, which gives them their special penetrating power. They are produced by bombarding a tungsten target with highspeed electrons in a Coolidge tube. They are not visible to the human eye, but, like ordinary light, they may be captured as a visible image on film, or on the specially coated screen of a FLUOROSCOPE. The degree of penetration of x-rays depends partly on the density of the matter at which they are aimed and partly on the voltage used. Equipment used for x-ray diagnosis is usually lower in voltage than that used for x-ray therapy.

The application of radiation, whether by x-ray or radioactive substances, for treatment of various illnesses is called RADIOTHERAPY or therapeutic radiation.

RADIATION HAZARDS. Harmful effects of uncontrolled radiation include serious disturbances of bone marrow and other blood-forming organs, burns and sterility. There may be permanent damage to the germ plasm or GENES, which results in genetic mutations. The mutations can be transmitted to future generations. Radiation also may produce harmful effects on the embryo or fetus, bringing about fetal death or malformations. Studies of groups of persons exposed to long-term radiation have shown that radiation acts as a carcinogen; that is, it can produce cancer, especially leukemia. Radiation also apparently shortens the life span of those exposed to it over a period of time, and predisposes persons to the development of cataracts.

Exposure to large doses of radiation over a short period of time produces a group of symptoms known as the acute radiation syndrome. These symptoms include general malaise, nausea and vomiting, followed by a period of remission of symptoms. Later, the patient develops more severe symptoms such as fever, hemorrhage, fluid loss, anemia and central nervous system involvement. The symptoms then gradually subside or become more severe, and may lead to death.

RADIATION PROTECTION. In order to avoid the radiation hazards mentioned above, one must be aware of three basic principles of time, distance and shielding involved in protection from radiation.

Obviously, the longer one stays near a source of radiation the greater will be his exposure. The same is true of proximity to the source; the closer one gets to a source of radiation the greater the exposure.

Shielding is of special importance when, as in the case of physicians and hospital personnel involved in radiotherapy, time and distance cannot be completely utilized as safety factors. In such instances lead, which is an extremely dense material, is utilized as a protective device. The walls of diagnostic x-ray rooms are lined with lead, and lead containers are used for radium, cobalt-60 and other radioactive materials used in radiotherapy. X-ray therapists, radiologists and other personnel concerned with use of x-rays can obtain additional protection by wearing lead aprons and gloves.

Monitoring devices such as the film badge or pocket monitor are worn by persons working near sources of radiation. These devices contain special photographic film that is sensitive to radiation and thus serve as a guide to the amount of radiation to which a person has been exposed. For monitoring large areas in which radiation hazards may pose a problem, survey meters such as the Geiger counter may be used. The survey meter also is useful in finding sources of radiation such as a radium implant, which might be lost.

Sensible use of these protective and monitoring devices can greatly reduce unnecessary exposure to radiation and allow for full realization of the many benefits of radiation.

corpuscular r., particles emitted in nuclear disintegration, including alpha and beta particles, protons, neutrons, positrons and deuterons.

electromagnetic r., energy, unassociated with matter, that is transmitted through space by means of waves (electromagnetic waves) traveling in all instances at 3×10^{10} cm., or 186,284 miles per second, but ranging in length from 10^{11} cm. (electrical waves) to 10^{-12} cm. (cosmic rays) and including radio waves, infrared, visible light and ultraviolet, x-rays and gamma rays.

infrared r., the portion of the spectrum of electromagnetic radiation of wavelengths ranging between 7700 and 120,000 angstroms (see also INFRARED RAYS).

interstitial r., energy emitted by radium or radon inserted directly into the tissue.

ionizing r., corpuscular or electromagnetic radiation that is capable of producing ions, directly or indirectly, in its passage through matter.

pyramidal r., fibers extending from the pyramidal tract to the cortex.

r. sickness, a condition sometimes occurring in patients who have received therapeutic doses of radiation. Its severity varies with the individual and his physical condition, the body areas exposed and the amount, kind and intensity of the exposure. The disease may be so slight that the exposed person scarcely notices it, or it may cause severe symptoms. With modern techniques and increased knowledge about radiation, there is a lower incidence of severe radiation sickness than formerly. The systemic reactions to radiation include a general feeling of malaise, loss of appetite or nausea and vomiting and headache. These symptoms tend to subside when the therapy is discontinued, leaving no permanent effect on the patient.

r. striothalam'ica, a fiber system joining the thalamus and the hypothalamic region.

tegmental r., fibers radiating laterally from the nucleus ruber.

thalamic r., fibers streaming out through the lateral surface of the thalamus, through the internal capsule to the cerebral cortex.

ultraviolet r., the portion of the spectrum of electromagnetic radiation of wavelengths ranging between 1800 and 3900 angstroms (see also ULTRAVIOLET RAYS).

radical (rad'ĭ-kal) 1. directed to the cause; going to the root or source of a morbid process. 2. a group of atoms that enters into and goes out of chemical combination without change, and that forms one of the fundamental constituents of a molecule.

acid r., the electronegative element that combines with hydrogen to form an acid.

alcohol r., all of the alcohol molecule except the hydroxyl group ($-OH$).

radicle (rad'ĭ-kl) one of the smallest branches of a vessel or nerve.

radicotomy (rad"ĭ-kot'o-me) rhizotomy; division or transection of a nerve root.

radiculalgia (rah-dik"u-lal'je-ah) neuralgia of the nerve roots.

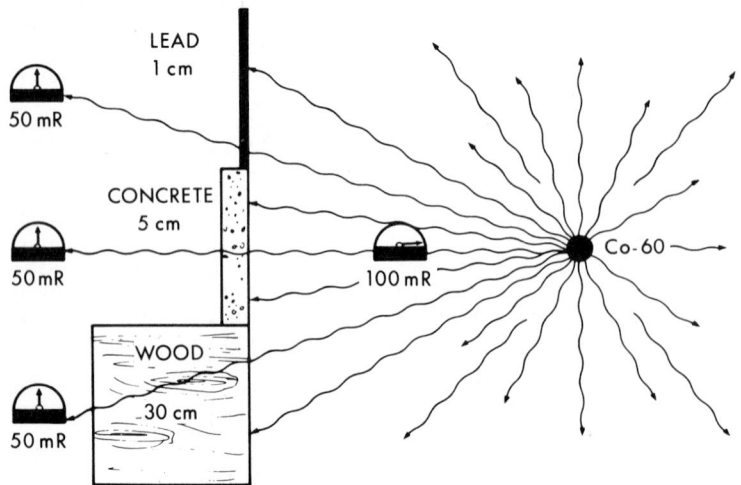

Comparison of efficacy of various materials for radiation shielding. (From Boeker, E. H.: The nurse in radiation protection. Nursing Clin. N. Amer., 2:23, 1967.)

radicular (rah-dik'u-lar) pertaining to a root or radicle.

radiculitis (rah-dik"u-li'tis) inflammation of a spinal nerve root, especially of the portion of the root that lies between the spinal cord and the spinal canal.

radiculoganglionitis (rah-dik"u-lo-gang"gle-o-ni'tis) inflammation of the posterior spinal nerve roots and their ganglia.

radiculomedullary (rah-dik"u-lo-med'u-ler"e) affecting the nerve roots and spinal cord.

radiculomeningomyelitis (rah-dik"u-lo-mĕ-ning"go-mi"ĕ-li'tis) inflammation of the nerve roots, meninges and spinal cord.

radiculomyelopathy (rah-dik"u-lo-mi"ĕ-lop'ah-the) disease of the nerve roots and spinal cord.

radiculoneuritis (rah-dik"u-lo-nu-ri'tis) Guillain-Barré syndrome.

radiculoneuropathy (rah-dik"u-lo-nu-rop'ah-the) disease of the nerve roots and spinal nerves.

radiculopathy (rah-dik"u-lop'ah-the) disease of the nerve roots.

radiectomy (ra"de-ek'to-me) excision of the root of a tooth.

radio- (ra'de-o) word element [L.], *radiation; radium; radius;* affixed to the name of a chemical element to designate a radioactive isotope of that element, as radiocarbon, radioiodine, etc.

radioactinium (ra"de-o-ak-tin'e-um) a substance formed by the disintegration of actinium.

radioactive (ra"de-o-ak'tiv) characterized by radioactivity.

radioactivity (ra"de-o-ak-tiv'ĭ-te) the emission of particulate or electromagnetic radiations consequent to the disintegration of the nuclei of unstable or radioactive elements. These emissions or radiations include ALPHA PARTICLES, BETA PARTICLES and GAMMA RAYS.

The property of radioactivity occurs naturally in a number of elements. In general, the chemical elements of atomic number above 83 are radioactive. Stable elements that are not naturally radioactive can be made so by bombarding isotopes of the element with high-velocity particles. When an element is unstable, whether naturally or artificially, the ratio of protons to neutrons in its atoms is uneven. Each atom attempts to achieve stability by giving off particles from its nucleus and thus it begins to disintegrate, releasing both nuclear particles and electromagnetic radiations. Since these radiations interact with matter, including the cells of the body, they can be used in medical therapy. (See also RADIATION and RADIOTHERAPY.)

The amount of radioactivity of a given substance can be measured by determining the rate at which a given number of atoms disintegrate in a given period of time. The basic unit of measurement used for radioactivity is the curie (Ci). One-thousandth of a curie is a millicurie; one-millionth of a curie is a microcurie; and one-trillionth of a curie is a picocurie. These units of measure are used to calculate the dosage of radioactivity needed for various therapeutic procedures in much the same way that units

of measure such as the gram or milligram are used to measure dosage of medications.

radioautogram (ra"de-o-aw'to-gram) autoradiogram.

radioautography (ra"de-o-aw-tog'rah-fe) autoradiography.

radiobicipital (ra"de-o-bi-sip'ĭ-tal) pertaining to the radius and biceps muscle of the arm.

radiobiologist (ra"de-o-bĭ-ol'o-jist) an expert in radiobiology.

radiobiology (ra"de-o-bi-ol'o-je) the branch of science concerned with effects of light and of ultraviolet and ionizing radiations on living tissue or organisms.

radiocalcium (ra"de-o-kal'se-um) a radioactive isotope of calcium, ^{45}Ca, with a half-life of 180 days; used as a tracer in the study of calcium metabolism.

radiocarbon (ra"de-o-kar'bon) a radioactive isotope of carbon; the isotope of mass 14 (^{14}C) is used in many diagnostic procedures and physiologic investigations; with a half-life of 5568 years, it has provided a means of determining the age of many ancient substances and articles.

radiocarcinogenesis (ra"de-o-kar"sĭ-no-jen'ĕ-sis) cancer formation due to exposure to radiation.

radiocardiogram (ra"de-o-kar'de-o-gram") the graphic record produced by radiocardiography.

radiocardiography (ra"de-o-kar"de-og'rah-fe) graphic recording of variation with time of the concentration, in a selected chamber of the heart, of a radioactive isotope, usually injected intravenously.

radiocarpal (ra"de-o-kar'pal) pertaining to the radius and carpus.

radiochemistry (ra"de-o-kem'is-tre) chemistry dealing with radioactive compounds and their properties and uses.

radiocinematograph (ra"de-o-sin"ĕ-mat'o-graf) an apparatus combining the moving picture camera and the roentgen ray machine, making possible moving pictures of the internal organs.

radiocurable (ra"de-o-kūr'ah-bl) curable by radiation.

radiode (ra'de-ōd) an apparatus for therapeutic application of radioactive substances.

radiodermatitis (ra"de-o-der"mah-ti'tis) cutaneous reaction to exposure to excessive quantities of ionizing or corpuscular radiation.

radiodiagnosis (ra"de-o-di"ag-no'sis) diagnosis by means of x-rays or gamma rays.

radioecology (ra"de-o-e-kol'o-je) the science dealing with the effects of radiation on species of plants and animals in natural communities or ecosystems.

radioelectrocardiogram (ra"de-o-e-lek"tro-kar'-de-o-gram") the tracing obtained by radioelectrocardiography.

radioelectrocardiograph (ra"de-o-e-lek"tro-kar'-

de-o-graf") the apparatus used in radioelectrocardiography.

radioelectrocardiography (ra"de-o-e-lek"tro-kar"de-og'rah-fe) the recording of alterations in the electric potential of the heart, with impulses beamed by radio waves from the subject to the recording device by means of a small transmitter attached to the patient.

radioelement (ra"de-o-el'ĕ-ment) a radioactive element.

radioencephalogram (ra"de-o-en-sef'ah-lo-gram") a curve showing the passage of an injected tracer through the cerebral blood vessels as revealed by an external scintillation counter.

radioencephalography (ra"de-o-en-sef"ah-log'-rah-fe) the recording of changes in the electric potential of the brain without direct attachment between the recording apparatus and the subject, the impulses being beamed by radio waves from the subject to the receiver.

radiogram (ra'de-o-gram") a picture of internal structures of the body produced by the action of x-rays or gamma rays on a specially sensitized film.

radiograph (ra'de-o-graf") the film produced by radiography.

radiography (ra"de-og'rah-fe) the taking of pictures (radiograms) of internal structures of the body by exposure of specially sensitized film to x-rays or gamma rays.

radiohumeral (ra"de-o-hu'mer-al) pertaining to the radius and humerus.

radioimmunity (ra"de-o-ĭ-mu'nĭ-te) a condition of decreased sensitivity to radiation sometimes produced by repeated irradiation.

radioiodine (ra"de-o-i'o-dīn) a radioactive isotope of iodine; ^{131}I is frequently used in thyroid investigation and in treatment of exophthalmic goiter.

radioisotope (ra"de-o-i'so-tōp) a radioactive form of an element. A radioisotope consists of unstable atoms that emit rays of energy or streams of atomic particles. Radioisotopes occur naturally, as in the cases of radium and uranium, or may be created artificially.

Scientists create artificial radioisotopes by bombarding stable atoms of an element with subatomic particles in a nuclear reactor or in an atom smasher, or cyclotron. When the nucleus of a stable atom is charged by bombarding particles, the atom usually becomes unstable, or radioactive, and is said to be "labeled" or "tagged."

Radioisotopes are used in medicine for both diagnosis and treatment. In general, the therapeutic use of radioisotopes is reserved for older persons, aged 40 and over, because of the possible danger of radiation-induced chromosomal change. (See also RADIOTHERAPY.)

The most widely used radioisotopes in medicine are forms of iodine, phosphorus, gold, iron and cobalt.

RADIOACTIVE IODINE. When taken into the body, iodine salts concentrate in the thyroid gland. The amount of ^{131}I (radioactive iodine) absorbed by the gland, as measured by a Geiger counter or similar instrument, can reveal whether the gland is functioning normally or is underactive or overactive. In exophthalmic GOITER and HYPERTHYROIDISM, radiation from ^{131}I is used to destroy excessive thyroid tissue. Similarly, ^{131}I is used to destroy malignant cells in some kinds of cancer of the thyroid.

RADIOACTIVE PHOSPHORUS. Radioactive phosphorus (^{32}P) gravitates to actively growing tissues, particularly those involved in manufacturing blood cells; its radiation is therefore used to destroy erythrocytes in polycythemia vera. Phosphorus-32 is also useful in the treatment of chronic leukemia and some other forms of cancer.

RADIOACTIVE GOLD. A radioisotope of gold (^{198}Au) is used to relieve some types of cancer that are not subject to surgery, such as inoperable cancer of the prostate. A further use is the treatment of certain malignant conditions in body cavities of the chest and abdominal regions. Gold-198 may also be used to reduce or destroy a tumor of the pituitary gland.

RADIOACTIVE IRON. Since iron forms part of hemoglobin, radioactive iron (^{59}Fe) is useful in studying the dynamics of hemoglobin formation and breakdown, as in anemia.

RADIOACTIVE COBALT. Radioactive cobalt (^{60}Co) is used in radiotherapy for localized cancer. It can be produced relatively cheaply and in compact equipment, and provides radiation of high intensity. Cobalt-60 is also used in measuring vitamin B_{12} absorption in pernicious anemia.

radiologist (ra"de-ol'o-jist) a specialist in radiology.

radiology (ra"de-ol'o-je) the branch of medical science dealing with use of x-rays, radioactive substances and other forms of radiant energy in diagnosis and treatment of disease. adj., **radiolo'gic.**

radiolucent (ra"de-o-lu'sent) permitting the passage of radiant energy, such as x-rays, yet offering some resistance to it, the representative areas appearing dark on the exposed film.

radiometer (ra"do-om'ĕ-ter) an instrument for measuring the penetrating power of radiant energy.

radiomimetic (ra"de-o-mi-met'ik) producing effects similar to those of ionizing radiations.

radion (ra'de-on) a particle given off by radioactive matter.

radionecrosis (ra"de-o-nĕ-kro'sis) necrosis from exposure to radiant energy.

radioneuritis (ra"de-o-nu-ri'tis) neuritis from exposure to radiant energy.

radionuclide (ra"de-o-nu'klīd) a radioactive nuclide; one that disintegrates with the emission of corpuscular or electromagnetic radiations.

radiopacity (ra"de-o-pas'ĭ-te) the quality or property of obstructing the passage of radiant energy, such as x-rays (roentgenopacity) or gamma rays. adj., **radiopaque'.**

radioparent (ra"de-o-par'ent) permitting the passage of radiant energy.

radiopathology (ra"de-o-pah-thol'o-je) the pathology of radiation effects on tissues.

radiopelvimetry (ra″de-o-pel-vim′ĕ-tre) measurement of the pelvis by radiography.

radiophosphorus (ra″de-o-fos′fo-rus) a radioactive isotope of phosphorus; ^{32}P is used in treatment of polycythemia vera and chronic leukemia and in erythrocyte studies.

radioreceptor (ra″de-o-re-sep′tor) a receptor for the stimuli that are excited by radiant energy, such as light and heat.

radioresistance (ra″de-o-re″zis′tans) resisting the effects of radiation, especially in reference to the treatment of malignancy.

radioscopy (ra″de-os′ko-pe) fluoroscopy.

radiosensibility (ra″de-o-sen″sĭ-bil′ĭ-te) sensibility to irradiation.

radiosensitive (ra″de-o-sen′sĭ-tiv) sensitive to irradiation.

radiosodium (ra″de-o-so′de-um) a radioactive isotope of sodium; ^{24}Na has been used in the study of blood flow, water balance and peripheral vascular diseases.

radiosurgery (ra″de-o-ser′jer-e) surgical treatment by the use of radium.

radiotelemetry (ra″de-o-tĕ-lem′ĕ-tre) measurement based on data transmitted by radio waves from the subject to the recording apparatus.

radiotherapy (ra″de-o-ther′ah-pe) the use of x-rays, radiation from radioactive substances and other similar forms of radiant energy in the treatment of cancer and other diseases.

X-RAYS, or roentgen rays, are energy waves of very short wavelength that have many properties, including the power to injure or destroy tissue, such as the growths produced by cancer. Therapeutic radiation ordinarily does not destroy cancer cells directly; only the very highest dose will kill the cells outright. Radiation somehow alters the cell so that it cannot reproduce. The irradiated cell eventually ages and dies, leaving no new cells behind. Radium, the first radioactive substance to be used in medical treatment, spontaneously gives off rays that affect the growth of tissue. Other substances not normally radioactive, such as cobalt, can be made radioactive (see RADIOISOTOPE), and are widely used in medicine.

The purpose of radiotherapy is to deliver a definite amount of radiation to a specific location. The prescribed dosage should be sufficient to treat the lesion, but not great enough to damage permanently the normal tissue surrounding the lesion. Radiotherapy is often used in conjunction with surgical treatment or with drugs, or with a combination of the two, especially in the treatment of cancer.

Certain sources of radioactivity lend themselves to specific locations or types of malignant disease or other medical disorders. Radium, for example, can be utilized as an implant directly into a malignant tumor located in the mouth or uterine cavity. Cobalt-60 and cesium-137 emit high-energy gamma rays and are often housed in shielded units that are located a distance from the patient. The unit, called a teletherapy unit, is designed so that a beam of gamma radiation can be aimed at a designated part of the patient's body. This type of radiotherapy is particularly useful in the treatment of deep-seated malignancies that are not readily accessible for implantation. Liquid radioisotopes, such as colloid suspensions of radioactive gold or phosphorus, can be instilled into the pleural or peritoneal cavity for local irradiation. Other radioisotopes in liquid form, such as radioactive iodine, are administered on the basis of the affinity of a body organ for a particular element.

X-rays are employed for a variety of disorders. High-voltage x-rays can be used for deep-seated malignancies; low-voltage x-rays are useful in the treatment of skin lesions that require only surface penetration over a relatively large area.

NURSING CARE. Hospital personnel concerned with the care of patients receiving radiotherapy must be aware of the hazards of radiation and the protective policies and procedures established to reduce these hazards. Most institutions and clinics provide a safety program under the leadership of a radiation physicist or radiation safety officer. Since radiation cannot be seen or felt, it is extremely important to observe all rules outlined in the program.

Sources of radiation that may be of particular concern to nursing personnel include: radioactive substances such as radium and cobalt-60 that are used as implants and serve as internal sources of radiation; external sources of radiation such as x-ray machines and cobalt-60 therapy units; and liquid radioisotopes such as iodine-131 and suspensions of radioactive gold or phosphorus.

Generally speaking, the degree of exposure to radiation depends on three factors: (1) the distance between the source of radiation and the individual, (2) the amount of time an individual is exposed to radiation and (3) the type of shielding provided. (See also RADIATION.)

When a nurse must remain with a patient while he receives diagnostic or therapeutic x-rays, she should wear a lead apron and lead gloves. She must be aware of, and observe carefully, the policies and procedures established for personnel in and around x-ray rooms and the rooms that house teletherapy units. After the treatment is finished the patient will not serve as a source of radiation.

Internal implants can present certain hazards to those involved in bedside care of patients receiving this type of radiotherapy. The nursing staff should be instructed in the amount of time it is safe to remain close to the patient.

Another factor to be considered is accidental removal or dislodgment of a radioactive implant. Most patients are confined to bed and refused bathroom privileges, but it is still possible for a radium needle or radon seeds, for example, to be accidentally removed from the body. Should an implant become dislodged the physician or radiation safety officer must be notified immediately. Under no circumstances should a radioactive substance be handled with the bare hands. A lead container and long-handled forceps should be kept at the patient's bedside in the event an implant should become dislodged. It can then be picked up immediately and placed in the container. Dressings, bed linen, bedpans and emesis basins should be checked with a radiation detection instrument after each use or before disposal.

Liquid radioactive substances require additional precautions since these substances can enter the body of a worker through the skin, or by ingestion or inhalation. Not all types of radioactive materials require the same precautions. For example, radioactive iodine is excreted in the urine for several days after it has been administered to the patient. In addition it appears in the patient's sweat, tears and saliva; thus all articles such as bed linens and toothbrush used by the patient must be considered a possible radiation hazard. Radiophosphorus acts in the same way. Colloidal gold usually is instilled into a body cavity and is not absorbed as are iodine and phosphorus. However, the radioactive gold emits gamma rays that penetrate beyond the patient's body and present a radiation hazard.

Care of the skin is of particular importance when a patient is receiving radiation from x-ray or teletherapy unit. Before the series of treatments is begun, the skin is washed with soap and water to remove all traces of ointments or lotions from the skin. Powders, ointments and other applications containing metals such as zinc absorb x-rays and increase damage to the skin.

Once the treatments are begun, the areas marked as "ports" or areas of entry for radiation are not washed or rubbed with alcohol or lotion. These ports of entry are extremely sensitive and subject to breakdown as would be a minor burn. It is important to avoid any friction or pressure on the area. No medications, lotions or powders may be applied to the area without written orders from the physician.

Local reactions to radiation from internal sources include irritation of mucous membranes lining the mouth, pharynx, vagina or bladder. The affected area becomes inflamed and tender. If the irritation continues, a grayish white membrane may form over the area. Bleeding also may occur as the underlying tissues become irritated.

In most cases the oral and pharyngeal mucosa heals rapidly once the radiation is discontinued. During radiotherapy frequent mouth washes, good oral hygiene and soothing gargles may help eliminate the distressing symptoms.

If the vaginal mucosa is irritated, the physician may order douches to cleanse the area and promote healing. Because the area is greatly irritated, douching must be done with extreme gentleness. The occurrence of bleeding is usually a contraindication to douching and should be reported to the physician.

Irritation of the bladder mucosa may result in difficulty in voiding and painful urination. This should be reported so that urinary antiseptics may be ordered to relieve the symptoms and reduce the danger of infection.

Diarrhea, constipation or blood in the stool indicates irritation of the bowel mucosa in patients receiving radiotherapy for conditions of the lower abdomen or pelvis. An oil retention enema or analgesic suppository may be ordered to relieve the irritation.

Since nausea frequently occurs in patients receiving radiotherapy a high-calorie liquid diet given in small frequent feedings is usually best. Patients unable to swallow because of involvement of the mouth or throat are fed by nasogastric tube.

The distressing side effects of radiotherapy are often aggravated by the patient's mental attitude toward this type of treatment. It is often helpful to have the patient and his family discuss their feelings and express their anxieties about radiation. They should be given a simple explanation of the purpose of the treatment and helped to understand that the discomforts associated with radiotherapy are not indicative of a lack of success or an unusual reaction to radiotherapy. This type of treatment may be more acceptable to the patient if it is pointed out to him that surgery and other types of therapy are also accompanied by discomforts and inconveniences and that these side effects are only temporary.

radiothermy (ra″de-o-ther′me) short-wave diathermy.

radiotoxemia (ra″de-o-tok-se′me-ah) toxemia produced by a radioactive substance, or resulting from radiotherapy.

radiotransparent (ra″de-o-trans-pār′ent) offering no obstruction to transmission of radiant energy, such as x-rays.

radiotropic (ra″de-o-trop′ik) influenced by radiation.

radio-ulnar (ra″de-o-ul′nar) pertaining to the radius and ulna.

radium (ra′de-um) a chemical element, atomic number 88, atomic weight, 226, symbol Ra. (See table of ELEMENTS.) Radium is highly radioactive and is found in uranium minerals. Radium salts emit, besides heat and light, three distinct kinds of radiation (alpha, beta and gamma rays) and also a radioactive gas called radon.

Radium is used in the treatment of malignant diseases, particularly those that are readily accessible, for example, tumors of the cervix uteri, mouth or tongue. In the form of needles or pellets, it can be inserted in the tumorous tissue (interstitial implantation) and left in place until its rays penetrate and alter the structure of the malignant cells. It also can be used in the form of plaques applied to the diseased tissue. Large amounts of radium are used as a source of GAMMA RAYS, which are capable of deep penetration of matter. Radium rays have been used in the treatment of lupus, eczema, psoriasis, xanthoma, mycosis fungoides and other skin diseases; for the removal of papillomas, granulomas and nevi; for palliative treatment in carcinoma and sarcoma; and in myelogenous and lymphatic leukemia. (See also RADIOTHERAPY.)

radius (ra′de-us), pl. *ra′dii* [L.] 1. a line radiating from a center, or a circular limit defined by a fixed distance from an established point or center. 2. in anatomy, the bone on the outer or thumb side of the forearm.

radix (ra′diks), pl. *rad′ices* [L.] root.

radon (ra′don) a chemical element, atomic number 86, atomic weight 222, symbol Rn. (See table of ELEMENTS.) Radon is a colorless, gaseous, radioactive element produced by the disintegration of radium.

rage (rāj) a violently aggressive emotional state.
   sham r., an outburst of motor activity resembling the outward manifestations of fear and anger, occurring in decorticated animals and in certain pathologic conditions in man.

rale (rahl) an abnormal respiratory sound heard

in auscultation and indicating some pathologic condition.

amphoric r., a musical, tinkling sound.

clicking r., a small, sticky sound, heard in early pulmonary tuberculosis.

crackling r., subcrepitant rale.

crepitant r., a fine, dry crackling sound resembling the sound produced by rubbing hairs between the fingers; heard in the early stages of pneumonia.

dry r., a whistling, musical or squeaky sound, heard in asthma and bronchitis.

moist r., a sound produced by fluid in the bronchial tubes.

sibilant r., a high-pitched hissing sound produced by viscid secretions in the bronchioles or by bronchiolar spasm.

subcrepitant r., a fine, moist rale associated with fluid in the bronchioles.

Ramibacterium (ra″me-bak-te′re-um) a genus of Schizomycetes found in the intestinal tract and occasionally associated with purulent infections.

ramification (ram″ĭ-fĭ-ka′shun) 1. distribution in branches. 2. a branch or set of branches.

ramify (ram′ĭ-fi) to branch; to diverge in different directions.

ramisectomy (ram″ĭ-sek′to-me) rhizotomy; division or transection of a nerve root.

ramitis (rah-mi′tis) inflammation of a nerve root.

ramose (ra′mōs) branching; having many branches.

ramus (ra′mus), pl. *ra′mi* [L.] a branch, as of a nerve, vein or artery.

r. commu′nicans (pl. *ra′mi communican′tes*), a branch of a spinal nerve given off mesially to the autonomic ganglion.

dorsal r., a branch given off by a spinal nerve, just beyond the union of its dorsal and ventral roots, usually supplying the skin, muscle and bone of the dorsal part of the neck and trunk.

ventral r., the continuation of a spinal nerve after the branching off of the dorsal ramus and the ramus communicans, dividing ultimately into the lateral and ventral divisions, supplying the limbs and ventral and lateral parts of the trunk.

rancid (ran′sid) having a musty, rank taste or smell; applied to fats that have undergone decomposition, with the liberation of fatty acids.

range (rānj) the difference between the upper and lower limits of a variable or of a series of values.

r. of accommodation, the alteration in the refractive state of the eye produced by accommodation. It is the difference in diopters between the refraction by the eye adjusted for its far point and that when adjusted for its near point. Called also amplitude of accommodation.

r. of audibility, the range between the extremes of vibration beyond which the human ear perceives no sound: lower limit, 16 to 20 cycles per second; upper limit, 18,000 to 20,000 cycles per second.

r. of motion, the range, measured in degrees of a circle, through which a joint can be extended and flexed.

ranine (ra′nīn) pertaining to a ranula, or to the lower surface of the tongue.

ranula (ran′u-lah) a cystic tumor beneath the

tongue due to obstruction and dilatation of the sublingual or submaxillary gland or of a mucous gland.

pancreatic r., a retention cyst of the pancreatic duct.

raphe (ra′fe) a seam; used in anatomic nomenclature as a general term to designate the line of union of the halves of various symmetrical parts.

abdominal r., linea alba.

rapport (rah-por′) an understanding between two persons, especially between patient and physician.

rarefaction (rar″ĕ-fak′shun) the condition of being or becoming less dense.

rash (rash) an outbreak of lesions on the skin; a skin eruption or exanthem.

heat r., miliaria.

raspberry mark congenital hemangioma.

ratbite fever either of two distinct diseases that may be transmitted to man by the bite of an infected rat and less commonly by the bite of an infected squirrel, weasel, dog, cat or pig. The more common of the two fevers in the United States is Haverhill fever, so named because the first epidemic to be studied occurred in Haverhill, Mass. The other form, sodoku, rarely occurs in the United States but is observed frequently in Japan and other Eastern countries. Although when both diseases were originally identified they followed the bite of a rat or similar animal, there are also other modes of transmission.

Haverhill fever is caused by *Streptobacillus moniliformis*. If the disease follows a rat bite, a fluid-filled sore appears at the site of the bite within 10 days. High fever alternates with periods of normal temperature at intervals of 24 to 48 hours, and there is swelling of regional lymph nodes. The joints—usually the large joints—become reddened, swollen and painful. There may be back pain, and a spotty, measles-like skin rash.

Sodoku, or spirillar ratbite fever, is caused by *Spirillum minus*. The original bite heals promptly but within 5 to 28 days the site becomes swollen and takes on a dusky, purplish hue. In sodoku, there is usually no joint inflammation and the rash is patchy rather than spotty. Otherwise the symptoms are similar to those characteristic of Haverhill fever.

Treatment for both forms of ratbite fever is with penicillin, streptomycin or other antibiotics.

rate (rāt) the speed or frequency with which an event or circumstance occurs per unit of time, population or other standard of comparison.

attack r., the rate at which new cases of a specific disease occur.

basal metabolic r., an expression of the rate of which oxygen is utilized in a fasting subject at complete rest as a percentage of a value established as normal for such a subject (see also BASAL METABOLISM TEST).

birth r., the number of births during one year for the total population (crude birth rate), for the female population (refined birth rate) or for the female population of childbearing age (true birth rate).

case r., morbidity rate.

case fatality r., the number of deaths due to a specific disease as compared to the total number of cases of the disease.

death r., the number of deaths per stated number of persons (1000 or 10,000 or 100,000) in a certain region in a certain year.

dose r., the amount of any therapeutic agent administered per unit of time.

erythrocyte sedimentation r., an expression of the extent of settling of erythrocytes in a vertical column of blood per unit of time (see also SEDIMENTATION RATE).

fatality r., the number of deaths caused by a specific circumstance or disease, expressed as the absolute or relative number among individuals encountering the circumstance or having the disease.

growth r., an expression of the increase in size of an organic object per unit of time.

heart r., the number of contractions of the cardiac ventricles per unit of time.

metabolic r., an expression of the amount of oxygen consumed by the body cells.

morbidity r., the number of cases of a given disease occurring in a specified period per unit of population.

mortality r., death rate; the mortality rate of a disease is the ratio of the number of deaths from a given disease to the total number of cases of that disease.

pulse r., the number of pulsations noted in a peripheral artery per unit of time; normally between 60 and 80 per minute in an adult.

respiration r., the number of movements of the chest wall per unit of time, indicative of inspiration and expiration; normally 16 to 20 per minute in an adult.

sedimentation r., an expression of the extent of settling of erythrocytes in a vertical column of blood per unit of time (see also SEDIMENTATION RATE).

ratio (ra'she-o) a numerical expression of the quantitative relations between different factors or elements.

A-G r., albumin-globulin r., the ratio of albumin to globulin in blood serum, plasma, cerebrospinal fluid or urine.

arm r., a figure expressing the relation of the length of the longer arm of a mitotic chromosome to that of the shorter arm.

cardiothoracic r., the ratio of the transverse diameter of the heart to the internal diameter of the chest at its widest point just above the dome of the diaphragm.

sex r., the number of females in a population per number of males, usually stated as the number of females per 1000 males.

rational (rash'un-al) accordant with reason.

rationalization (rash"un-al-ĭ-za'shun) a defense mechanism in which a person finds logical reasons (justification) for his behavior while ignoring the real reasons. It is a form of self-deception and is unconsciously employed to make tolerable certain feelings, behavior and motives that would otherwise be intolerable. Everyone employs rationalization at some time or other and in most instances it is a relatively harmless behavior pattern; the danger lies in deceiving oneself habitually so that eventually harmful or destructive behavior can be justified in one's mind.

Rau-sed (row'sed) trademark for a preparation of reserpine, an antihypertensive.

Rauwiloid (row'wi-loid) trademark for preparations of alseroxylon, an antihypertensive.

Rauwolfia (raw-wol'fe-ah) a genus of climbing shrubs indigenous to Asia, including over 100 species and providing numerous alkaloids of medical interest.

rauwolfia (raw-wol'fe-ah) an alkaloid derived from shrubs of the genus Rauwolfia.
r. serpentina, the dried root of *Rauwolfia serpentina,* used chiefly as an antihypertensive.

ray (ra) a line of light, heat or other form of radiant energy, emanating from an object or substance.

actinic r., a light ray that produces chemical changes.

alpha r's, high-speed helium nuclei ejected from radioactive substances (see also ALPHA PARTICLES).

Becquerel's r's, emanations given off by radium, uranium and other radioactive substances.

beta r's, electrons ejected from radioactive materials with moderate velocity and power (see also BETA PARTICLES).

border r's, grenz rays.

caloric r., radiant energy that is converted into heat when applied to the body.

cathode r., a ray resembling x-rays, but carrying negative electricity and capable of being deflected by the magnet.

cosmic r's, penetrating radiations that apparently move through interplanetary space in every direction.

delta r's, secondary beta rays produced in a gas by the passage of alpha particles.

digital r., a digit of the hand or foot and corresponding metacarpal or metatarsal bone, regarded as a continuous unit.

gamma r's, electromagnetic radiation of short wavelengths emitted during nuclear reaction, of high energy and velocity and having no electric charge or mass (see also GAMMA RAYS).

grenz r's, very soft electromagnetic radiation of wavelengths of 1 to 5 angstroms.

hertzian r's, electromagnetic waves with a greater wavelength than a light wave, used in wireless transmission of signals, speech, etc.

infrared r's, rays beyond the red end of the visible spectrum, of 7700 to 120,000 angstroms wavelength (see also INFRARED RAYS).

medullary r., a cortical extension of a bundle of tubules from a renal pyramid.

Millikan r's, cosmic rays.

roentgen r's, x-rays.

transition r's, grenz rays.

ultraviolet r's, radiant energy beyond the violet end of the visible spectrum, of 3900 to 1800 angstroms wavelength (see also ULTRAVIOLET RAYS).

x-r's, electromagnetic radiation of wavelengths ranging between 0.05 and 5 angstroms (including grenz rays). (See also X-RAYS.)

x-r's, diagnostic, x-rays of wavelengths of 0.12 to 0.30 angstrom.

x-r's, therapeutic, x-rays of wavelength of 0.05 to 0.12 angstrom.

Raynaud's disease (ra-nōz') a primary or idiopathic vasospastic disorder characterized by bilateral and symmetrical pallor and cyanosis of the fingers, with or without local gangrene. In some cases both the hands and feet may be affected, and rarely the disease may involve the nose, chin or cheeks. The cause of Raynaud's disease is unknown. Attacks are precipitated by cold or emotional upset and relieved by warmth. The condition occurs almost exclusively in young women, especially those who are experiencing tension and emotional pressure.

Attacks often end spontaneously or upon application of warmth. As the disease progresses, however, small gangrenous ulcers may develop on the fingertips and, eventually, permanent disability of the hands can result from contractures, severe pain and changes in the skin. The latter condition (sclerodactylia) is characterized by a tightening of the skin so that it appears stretched over the fingers, a decrease of mobility and a smoothness and abnormal shine to the skin.

Mild cases of Raynaud's disease can be controlled by avoidance of cold and injury to the fingers, high-calorie diet, relief of mental stress and, if necessary, elimination of the habit of smoking. More severe cases may require sympathectomy to prevent conduction of sympathetic nerve impulses which stimulate constriction of the local blood vessels. Vasodilating drugs are sometimes useful in preventing attacks if they are taken before exposure to cold, but they are not successful in all cases and act primarily to provide only a temporary relief of symptoms.

R's phenomenon, episodic, symmetrical constriction of small arteries of the extremities, resulting in cyanosis or pallor of the part, followed by hyperemia, producing a red color.

Rb chemical symbol, *rubidium.*

RBC red blood cells; red blood (cell) count (see BLOOD COUNT).

R.B.E. relative biological effectiveness; effectiveness of other types of radiation compared with that of one roentgen of gamma rays or x-rays.

R.D.S. respiratory distress syndrome.

Re chemical symbol, *rhenium.*

react (re-akt′) 1. to respond to a stimulus. 2. to enter into chemical action with.

reaction (re-ak′shun) 1. opposite action or counteraction; the response of a part to stimulation. 2. the phenomena caused by the action of chemical agents; a chemical process in which one substance is transformed into another substance or substances. 3. in psychology, the mental or emotional state that develops in any particular situation.

adjustment r., one elicited by a change in situation or environment, sometimes evidenced as a transient personality disorder.

alarm r., the response of the adrenal cortex in stress, resulting in production of certain adrenocortical hormones (see also ALARM REACTION.)

allergic r., a reaction, local or general, of the body to contact with a substance to which the subject has an idiosyncrasy (see also ALLERGY).

antigen-antibody r., the combination of antigen with homologous antibody with the formation of a complex (see also ANTIGEN).

anxiety r., a neurotic reaction characterized by abnormal apprehension or uneasiness.

biuret r., a chemical test used to demonstrate the presence of protein.

chain r., one that is self-propagating; a chemical process in which each time a free radical is destroyed a new one is formed.

conversion r., a loss or alteration of a sensory or motor function as an expression of anxiety (see also CONVERSION REACTION).

cross r., one between an antigen and an antibody of closely related but not identical species.

defense r., a mental reaction that shuts out from consciousness ideas not acceptable to the ego.

r. of degeneration, loss of response to a faradic stimulation in a muscle, and to galvanic and faradic stimulation in a nerve.

delayed-blanch r., pallor instead of erythema appearing 5 to 10 minutes after intradermal injection of acetylcholine or methacholine and persisting for 15 to 30 minutes; associated with atopic disease.

depressive r., a response to an environmental loss or stress characterized by morbid sadness or melancholy.

dissociative r., a neurotic reaction in which amnesia, fugue, somnambulism or splitting of the personality occurs.

dyssocial r., disregard by a person of the normal codes of social behavior.

false negative r., an erroneously negative reaction to a test.

false positive r., an erroneously positive reaction to a test, especially a positive response to a test for syphilis due to some disease other than syphilis.

r.-formation, a mental mechanism by which one assumes an attitude that is the reverse of, and a substitute for, a repressed antisocial impulse.

immune r., the response of an organism to elements recognized as nonself, with production of plasmocytes, lymphocytes and antibodies, leading to ultimate rejection of the foreign material.

involutional psychotic r., a reaction occurring in late middle life, with severe depression and sometimes with paranoid thinking (see also PSYCHOSIS).

lengthening r., reflex elongation of extensor muscles that permits flexion of a limb.

leukemoid r., a blood picture resembling leukemia with immature leukocytes in the blood but due to another disorder.

near-point r., constriction of the pupil when the gaze is fixed on a near point.

transfusion r., a group of symptoms due to agglutination of the recipient's blood cells when blood for transfusion is incorrectly matched, or when the recipient has a hypersensitivity to some element of the donor blood (see also TRANSFUSION).

reactivity (re″ak-tiv′ĭ-te) the process or property of reacting.

Reactrol (re-ak′trol) trademark for a preparation of clemizole hydrochloride, an antihistaminic.

reagent (re-a′jent) a substance used to produce a chemical reaction.

reagin (re′ah-jin) an antibody or substance behaving like an antibody in complement-fixation tests and similar reactions.

atopic r., the antibody responsible for hypersensitivity reactions to specific substances with manifestations such as asthma and eczema.

Réaumur thermometer (ra″o-mer′) a thermometer on which the freezing point of water is 0 and the boiling point is 80 degrees.

recapitulation (re″kah-pit″u-la′shun) repetition in the development and growth of an individual of the evolutionary stages through which the species evolved.

receiver (re-se′ver) a vessel for collecting a gas or distillate.

receptaculum (re″sep-tak′u-lum), pl. *receptac'ula* [L.] a vessel or receptable.
   r. chy′li, an expansion at the lower end of the thoracic duct that receives several lymph-collecting vessels.

receptor (re-sep′tor) a sensory nerve terminal that responds to stimulation by transmitting impulses to the central nervous system.

recess (re-ses′) a small, empty space or cavity.

recessive (re-ses′iv) tending to recede; in genetics, incapable of expression unless carried by both members of a set of homologous chromosomes.

recessus (re-ses′us), pl. *reces'sus* [L.] a recess.

recidivation (re-sid″ĭ-va′shun) 1. the relapse or recurrence of a disease. 2. the repetition of an offense or crime.

recidivism (re-sid′ĭ-vizm) a tendency to relapse, especially the tendency to return to a life of crime.

recidivist (re-sid′ĭ-vist) a person who tends to relapse, especially one who tends to return to criminal habits after treatment or punishment.

recipe (res′ĭ-pe) 1. [L.] take: used at the head of a prescription and written as ℞. 2. a formula for the preparation of a combination of ingredients.

recipient (re-sip′e-ent) the person who receives blood or other body tissue by transfusion or grafting.
   universal r., a person thought to be able to receive blood of any "type" without precipitation or agglutination of the cells.

Recklinghausen's disease (rek′ling-how″zenz) 1. neurofibromatosis. 2. osteitis fibrosa cystica.

recombination (re″kom-bĭ-na′shun) the reunion, in the same or different arrangement, of formerly united elements; in genetics, the formation of new combinations of genes in fertilization.

recompression (re″kom-presh′un) return to normal environmental pressure after exposure to greatly diminished pressure.

recon (re′kon) a hereditary unit indivisible by genetic recombination.

recrement (rek′rĕ-ment) saliva, or other secretion, that is reabsorbed into the blood.

recrudescence (re″kroo-des′ens) recurrence of symptoms after temporary abatement; a recrudescence occurs after some days or weeks, a relapse after weeks or months. adj., **recrudes′cent**.

recruitment (re-kroot′ment) 1. the gradual increase to a maximum in a reflex when a stimulus of unaltered intensity is prolonged. 2. in audiology, an abnormal increase in loudness caused by a very slight increase in sound intensity, as in Menière's disease.

rect(o)- (rek′to) word element [L.], *rectum*. See also words beginning *proct(o)-*.

rectal (rek′tal) pertaining to the rectum.

rectalgia (rek-tal′je-ah) proctalgia; pain in the rectum.

rectectomy (rek-tek′to-me) excision of the rectum.

rectification (rek″tĭ-fĭ-ka′shun) the process of purifying or correcting.

rectified (rek′tĭ-fīd) brought to an established standard of purity.

rectitis (rek-ti′tis) proctitis; inflammation of the rectum.

rectocele (rek′to-sēl) hernial protrusion of part of the rectum into the vagina.

rectocolitis (rek″to-co-li′tis) inflammation of the rectum and colon.

rectolabial (rek″to-la′be-al) pertaining to or communicating with the rectum and a labium majus, as a rectolabial fistula.

rectopexy (rek′to-pek″se) proctopexy.

rectoplasty (rek′to-plas″te) proctoplasty.

rectoscope (rek′to-skōp) proctoscope.

rectosigmoid (rek″to-sig′moid) the lower portion of the sigmoid colon and the upper portion of the rectum.

rectosigmoidectomy (rek″to-sig″moi-dek′to-me) excision of the rectosigmoid colon.

rectostomy (rek-tos′to-me) the operation of forming a permanent opening into the rectum for the relief of stricture of the rectum.

rectourethral (rek″to-u-re′thral) pertaining to the rectum and urethra.

rectouterine (rek″to-u′ter-in) pertaining to the rectum and uterus.

rectovaginal (rek″to-vaj′ĭ-nal) pertaining to the rectum and vagina.

rectovesical (rek″to-ves′ĭ-kal) pertaining to the rectum and bladder.

rectovestibular (rek″to-ves-tib′u-lar) pertaining to or communicating with the rectum and the vestibule of the vagina.

rectovulvar (rek″to-vul′var) pertaining to or communicating with the rectum and vulva.

rectum (rek′tum) the distal portion of the large intestine, beginning anterior to the third sacral vertebra as a continuation of the sigmoid and ending at the anal canal. The feces, the solid waste products of digestion, are formed in the large intestine and are gradually pushed down into the rectum by the muscular action of the intestine. Distention of the rectum by the accumulating feces sets up nerve impulses that indicate to the brain the need to empty the bowels.

The rectum is between 6 and 8 inches long, with the anal canal making up the last inch. The anus is kept closed—except during the evacuation process—by muscular rings, the anal sphincters.

In a rectal examination, the physician palpates the rectum by inserting a gloved and lubricated finger into the rectum. The examination helps in determining whether there are masses in the rectum or pelvic region, and in determining the size and texture of the prostate in men. More extensive examination of the interior surface of the rectum may be done by PROCTOSCOPY.

rectus (rek′tus) [L.] straight.

recumbent (re-kum′bent) lying down.

recurrence (re-ker′ens) the return of symptoms after a temporary absence.

recurrent (re-ker′ent) returning after a remission; reappearing.

red (red) 1. one of the primary colors produced by the longest waves of the visible spectrum. 2. a dye of the color of blood.
   r. blood cell, erythrocyte.
   Congo r., a dark red or brownish powder; used as a diagnostic aid in amyloidosis.
   phenol r., phenolsulfonphthalein.
   scarlet r., a dye that stimulates wound healing.

redia (re′de-ah), pl. *re′diae* [L.] the second or third larval stage of certain trematode parasites, which develops in the body of a snail host.

redintegration (red″in-tĕ-gra′shun) 1. restitution of a part. 2. a psychic process in which part of a complex stimulus provokes the complete reaction that was previously made to the complex stimulus as a whole.

Redisol (red′ĭ-sol) trademark for a preparation of crystalline vitamin B_{12}.

redox (red′oks) oxidation-reduction.

reduce (re-dūs′) 1. to replace in normal position, as to reduce a fracture. 2. to decrease in size. 3. to deprive of oxygen.

reductant (re-duk′tant) the electron donor in an oxidation-reduction (redox) reaction.

reductase (re-duk′tās) an enzyme that has a reducing action on chemicals.

reduction (re-duk′shun) 1. restoration of the normal relation of parts, as in fracture, dislocation or hernia. 2. in chemistry, the subtraction of oxygen from, or the addition of hydrogen to, a substance; the loss of positive charges or the gain of negative charges; the opposite of oxidation.
   r. of chromosomes, the passing of the members of a chromosome pair to the daughter cells during meiosis, each daughter cell receiving half the diploid number.
   closed r., restoration of the proper position of the fragments of a fractured bone by external manipulation, and application of a cast to maintain immobilization.
   open r., restoration of the proper position of the fragments of a fractured bone under direct visualization at operation, with some form of internal or external fixation.

reduplication (re-du″plī-ka′shun) 1. a doubling back. 2. a developmental anomaly resulting in the doubling of an organ or part, with a connection between them at some point and the excess part usually a mirror image of the other.

Reed (rēd) Walter (1851–1902). American bacteriologist, born in Gloucester County, Virginia. As a military physician, Reed was appointed during the Spanish-American War chief of a committee to investigate typhoid fever epidemic in the army camps. In 1899, when yellow fever was particularly severe in Cuba, he again was appointed chairman of a committee to study its method of transmission, and he proved by thorough experimentation that yellow fever was carried only by a certain species of mosquito, *Aedes aegypti*.

refection (re-fek′shun) recovery; repair.

refine (re-fīn′) to purify or free from foreign matter.

reflection (re-flek′shun) a turning or bending back, as the folds produced when a membrane passes over the surface of an organ and then passes back to the body wall that it lines.

reflector (re-flek′tor) a device for reflecting light or sound waves.

reflex (re′fleks) 1. directed backward; produced by deflection of a nerve impulse that does not penetrate the level of consciousness. 2. a reflection. 3. an automatic response to a given stimulus, depending only on the anatomic relations of the neurons involved.

A reflex is built into the nervous system and does not need the intervention of conscious thought to take effect.

The knee jerk is an example of the simplest type of reflex. When the knee is tapped, the nerve that receives this stimulus sends an impulse to the spinal cord, where it is relayed to a motor nerve. This causes the quadriceps muscle at the front of the thigh to contract and jerk the leg up. This reflex, or simple reflex arc, involves only two nerves and one synapse. The leg begins to jerk up while the brain is just becoming aware of the tap.

Other simple reflexes, the stretch reflexes, help the body maintain its balance. Every time a muscle is stretched, it reacts with a reflex impulse to contract. As a person reaches or leans, the skeletal muscles tense and tighten, tending to hold him and keep him from falling. Even in standing still, the stretch reflexes in the skeletal muscles make many tiny adjustments to keep the body erect.

The "hot-stove" reflex is more complex, calling into play many different muscles. Before the hand is pulled away, an impulse must go from the sensory nerve endings in the skin to a center in the spinal cord, from there to a motor center, and then out along the motor nerves to shoulder, arm and hand muscles. Trunk and leg muscles respond to support the body in its sudden change of position, and the head and eyes turn to look at the cause of the injury. All this happens while the person is becoming aware of the burning sensation. A reflex that protects the body from injury, as this one does, is called a nociceptive reflex. Sneezing, coughing and gagging are similar reflexes in response to foreign bodies in the nose and throat, and the wink reflex helps protect the eyes from injury.

A conditioned reflex is one acquired as the result of experience. When an action is done repeatedly the nervous system becomes familiar with the situation and learns to react automatically, and a new reflex is built into the system. Walking, running and typewriting are examples of activities that require large numbers of complex muscle coordinations that have become automatic.

abdominal r's, contractions about the navel on sharp downward friction of the abdominal wall. It indicates that the spinal cord from the eighth to the twelfth dorsal nerve is intact.

accommodation r., the coordinated changes that occur when the eye adapts itself for near vision; they are constriction of the pupil, convergence of the eyes and increased convexity of the lens.

Achilles r., plantar extension of the foot elicited by a tap on the Achilles tendon, preferably while the patient kneels on a bed or chair, the feet hanging free over the edge; called also ankle jerk and triceps surae reflex.

anal r., momentary contraction of sphincter muscles when the skin around the anus is touched.

ankle r., Achilles reflex.

auditory r., any reflex caused by stimulation of the auditory nerve; especially momentary closure of both eyes produced by a sudden sound.

Babinski r., dorsiflexion of the big toe and fanning of the other toes when the sole of the foot is scraped (see also BABINSKI REFLEX).

biceps r., tensing of the tendon of the biceps muscle felt on percussion over the tendon with the arm and forearm relaxed.

carotid sinus r., slowing of the heartbeat on pressure on the carotid artery at the level of the cricoid cartilage.

chain r., a series of reflexes, each serving as a stimulus to the next.

ciliary r., the movement of the pupil in accommodation.

ciliospinal r., dilation of the ipsilateral pupil on scratching or pinching the skin at the side of the neck.

clasp-knife r., lengthening reaction; reflex elongation of extensor muscles which permits flexion of a limb.

conditioned r., one acquired as the result of experience.

conjunctival r., closure of the eyelid when the conjunctiva is touched.

convergency r., convergence of the visual axes with fixation on a near point.

corneal r., blinking of the ipsilateral eyelids (direct corneal reflex) or of the eyelids of the opposite eye (consensual corneal reflex) when the cornea is touched lightly.

cremasteric r., contraction of the ipsilateral cremaster muscle, drawing the testis upward, when the upper inner aspect of the thigh is stroked longitudinally.

deep r., one elicited by stimulation of a deep body structure, as a tendon or the periosteum of a bone.

digital r., Hoffmann's sign.

embrace r., Moro reflex.

gag r., elevation of the soft palate and retching elicited by touching the back of the tongue or the wall of the pharynx.

gastrocolic r., stimulation of emptying of the colon resulting from filling of the stomach.

gastroileac r., relaxation of the ileocecal valve in response to the stimulus of food in the stomach.

grasp r., flexion or clenching of the fingers or toes on stimulation of the palm of the hand or sole of the foot.

jaw-jerk r., closure of the mouth on tapping the passively opened chin; seen occasionally in health and frequently in upper motor neuron disease.

knee r., knee jerk.

light r., 1. constriction of the pupil when a light is shown into the same (direct light reflex) or the opposite eye (indirect or consensual light reflex). 2. a luminous image reflected when light strikes the normal tympanic membrane.

Magnus-DeKleijn r., tonic neck reflex.

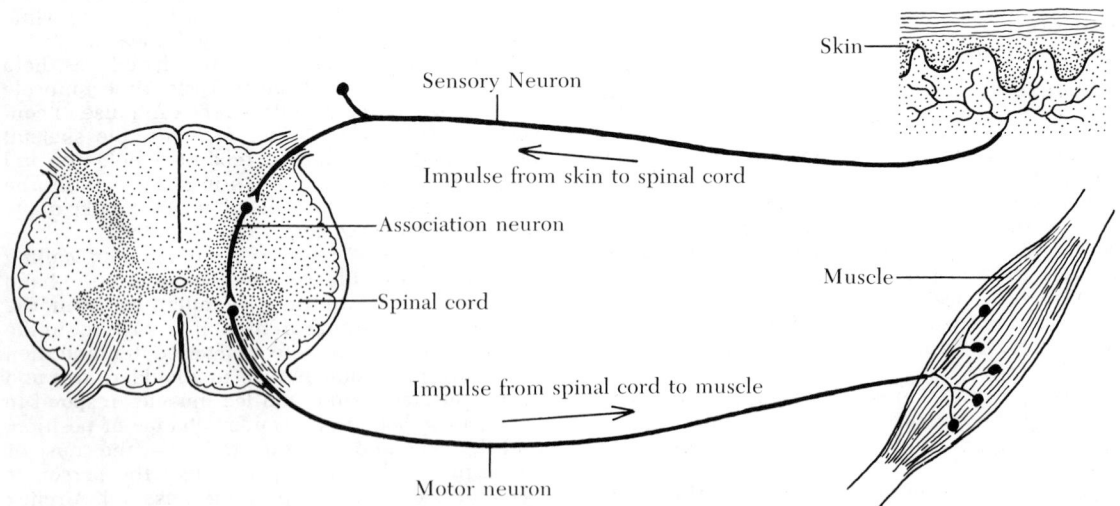

Nerve pathway of a simple reflex. When the sensory nerve ending is stimulated, a nerve impulse travels along a sensory (afferent) neuron to the spinal cord. Here an association neuron transfers the impulse to a motor (efferent) neuron. The motor neuron carries the impulse to a muscle, which contracts and moves a body part.

Mayer's r., adduction of the thumb on downward pressure of the index finger.

Moro r., flexion of an infant's thighs and knees, fanning and then clenching of fingers, with arm first thrown outward and then brought together as though embracing something; produced by a sudden stimulus and seen normally in the newborn.

myotatic r., stretch reflex.

nociceptive r's, reflexes initiated by painful stimuli.

patellar r., knee jerk.

perianal r., anal reflex.

pharyngeal r., gag reflex.

pilomotor r., contraction of the arrector muscles of the hair (producing cutis anserina, or goose flesh) on stroking of the nape of the neck or the axillary region.

plantar r., plantar flexion of the foot when the ankle is grasped firmly and the lateral border of the sole is stroked or scratched from the heel toward the toes.

proprioceptive r., a reflex that is initiated by stimuli arising from some function of the reflex mechanism itself.

pupillary r., a change in size of the pupil in response to various stimuli (change in illumination or point of fixation, or emotional stimulation).

quadriceps r., contraction of the quadriceps muscle and extension of the leg elicited by tapping the patellar ligament when the leg hangs loosely flexed at a right angle (see also KNEE JERK).

red r., the usually bright red appearance of the pupil when viewed through the ophthalmoscope at a distance of a foot or less.

righting r., the ability to assume an optimal position when there has been a departure from it.

spinal r., any reflex action mediated through a center of a spinal cord.

startle r., Moro reflex.

stretch r., reflex contraction of a muscle in response to passive longitudinal stretching.

sucking r., sucking movements of the lips of an infant elicited by touching the lips or the skin near the mouth.

superficial r., one elicited by stimulation of superficial nerve endings, as in the skin.

swallowing r., stimulation of the palate causes swallowing; called also palatal reflex.

tendon r., contraction of a muscle caused by percussion of its tendon.

tonic neck r., extension of the arm and sometimes of the leg on the side to which the head is forcibly turned, with flexion of the contralateral limbs.

triceps r., contraction of the belly of the triceps muscle and slight extension of the arm when the tendon of the muscle is tapped directly, with the arm flexed and fully supported and relaxed.

triceps surae r., Achilles reflex.

reflexogenic (re-flek″so-jen′ik) producing reflex action.

reflexograph (re-flek′so-graf) an instrument for graphically recording a reflex.

reflux (re′fluks) a return flow.

hepatojugular r., swelling of the jugular vein induced by pressure over the liver seen in heart failure.

refract (re-frakt′) to ascertain errors of ocular refraction.

refraction (re-frak′shun) 1. the deviation of light in traversing obliquely a medium of differing density. 2. determination of the refractive errors of the eye and their correction by glasses.

double r., refraction in which incident rays are divided into two refracted rays.

dynamic r., refraction of the eye when at rest.

ocular r., the refraction of light produced by the media of the normal eye and resulting in the focusing of images upon the retina.

static r., refraction of the eye when its accommodation is paralyzed.

refractionist (re-frak′shun-ist) one skilled in determining errors of refraction of the eye.

refractive (re-frak′tiv) pertaining to or subserving a process of refraction; having the power to refract.

refractometer (re″frak-tom′ĕ-ter) an apparatus for measuring the refractive power of the eye.

refractory (re-frak′to-re) not readily yielding to treatment.

r. period, a short period succeeding the time at which a nerve or muscle enters into a condition of functional activity during which the nerve or muscle does not respond to a second stimulation.

refrangible (re-fran′jĭ-bl) susceptible of being refracted.

refresh (re-fresh′) to freshen or make raw again; to denude of an epithelial covering.

refrigerant (re-frij′er-ant) 1. relieving fever and thirst. 2. a cooling remedy.

refrigeration (re-frij″ĕ-ra′shun) therapeutic application of low temperature (see also HYPOTHERMIA).

refusion (re-fu′zhun) the temporary removal and subsequent return of blood to the circulation (see also HEART-LUNG MACHINE).

regeneration (re-jen″ĕ-ra′shun) the natural replacement of a lost or injured organ or part.

regimen (rej′ĭ-men) a strictly regulated scheme of diet, exercise or other activity designed to achieve certain ends.

regio (re′je-o), pl. regio′nes [L.] a plane area with more or less definite boundaries; used in anatomic nomenclature as a general term to designate certain areas on the surface of the body within certain defined boundaries.

region (re′jun) a plane with more or less definite boundaries; called also regio.

abdominal r., the various anatomic regions of the abdomen, including the hypochondriac, epigastric, lateral, umbilical, inguinal and pubic regions.

lumbar r., the region of the back lying lateral to the lumbar vertebrae.

pubic r., the middle portion of the most inferior region of the abdomen, located below the umbilical region and between the inguinal regions.

regional (re′jun-al) pertaining to a certain region or regions.

r. anesthesia, insensibility caused by interrupting

the sensory nerve conductivity of any region of the body (see also ANESTHETIC).

r. enteritis, inflammation of the terminal portion of the ileum; called also regional ileitis and Crohn's disease.

registry (rej'is-tre) 1. an office where a nurse may have her name listed as being available for duty. 2. a central agency for collection of pathologic material and related data, so organized that the data can be properly processed and made available for study.

Regitine (rej'ĭ-tēn) trademark for a preparation of phentolamine, an adrenolytic used to test for the presence of pheochromocytoma.

regression (re-gresh'un) 1. return to an earlier or primitive state. 2. subsidence of symptoms or of a disease process. 3. in biology, the tendency in successive generations toward mediocrity. 4. a mental mechanism utilized to resolve conflict or frustration by returning to a behavior that was successful in earlier years. Everyone uses this mechanism at some time, usually when under stress, resorting to tears, tantrums or other childish behavior to obtain certain goals or relieve frustrations. Some degree of regression frequently accompanies physical illness and can be expected in patients who are hospitalized for a physical disorder. Patients who are mentally ill may exhibit regression to an extreme degree, reverting all the way back to infantile behavior (atavistic regression).

regurgitant (re-ger'jĭ-tant) flowing back.

regurgitation (re-ger'jĭ-ta'shun) abnormal backward progression of fluids or other vessel contents, as the return of undigested food from the stomach to the oral cavity, or of blood through valves of the heart.

aortic r., reverse passage of blood from the aorta into the left ventricle in insufficiency of the valve guarding its entrance.

mitral r., backflow of blood from the left ventricle to the left atrium through an imperfectly functioning mitral valve.

pulmonic r., backflow of blood through the pulmonary valve.

tricuspid r., backflow of blood through the tricuspid valve from the right ventricle to the right atrium and venae cavae.

rehabilitation (re"hah-bil"ĭ-ta'shun) the process of restoring a person's ability to live and work as normally as possible after a disabling injury or illness. It aims to help the patient achieve maximum possible physical and psychologic fitness and regain the ability to care for himself. It offers assistance with the learning or relearning of skills needed in everyday activities, with occupational training and guidance and with psychologic readjustment.

Rehabilitation is an integral part of convalescence. Proper food, medication and hygiene and suitable exercise provide the physical basis for recovery. The patient is encouraged to be active physically and mentally to the extent recommended by the physician. PHYSICAL THERAPY, OCCUPATIONAL THERAPY and vocational training are used extensively in the rehabilitation of severely handicapped individuals.

rehabilitee (re"hah-bil'ĭ-te) the subject of rehabilitation.

rehalation (re"hah-la'shun) rebreathing.

rehydration (re"hi-dra'shun) the restoration of water or fluid content to a body or to a substance that has become dehydrated.

reimplantation (re"im-plan-ta'shun) replacement of a structure in a site from which it was dislodged.

reinfection (re"in-fek'shun) a second infection by the same agent.

reinforcement (re"in-fors'ment) the increasing of force or strength.

r. of reflex, strengthening of a reflex response by the patient's performance of some unrelated action during elicitation of the reflex.

reinnervation (re"in-er-va'shun) the operation of grafting a live nerve to restore the function of a paralyzed muscle.

Reiter's disease (ri'terz) a disease of males marked by initial diarrhea followed by urethritis, conjunctivitis and migratory polyarthritis and frequently accompanied by keratotic lesions of the skin.

rejection (re-jek'shun) the immune reaction of the recipient to foreign tissue cells (antigens) after homograft TRANSPLANTATION, with the production of antibodies and ultimate destruction of the transplanted organ.

relapse (re-laps') the return of a disease weeks or months after its apparent cessation.

relapsing fever (re-laps'ing) any one of a group of similar infectious diseases transmitted to man by the bites of lice and ticks, and marked by alternating periods of normal temperature and periods of fever relapse. The diseases in the group are caused by several different species of spirochetes belonging to the genus Borrelia.

SYMPTOMS AND DIAGNOSIS. Generally, relapsing fever starts with a sudden high fever of 104 to 105° F., accompanied by chills, headache, muscle aches, nausea and vomiting. There may also be jaundice and a rash. The attack lasts 2 or 3 days, after which the symptoms disappear by crisis, with profuse sweating accompanying the rapid drop in temperature. In elderly people this may be accompanied by collapse, in which the heart and respiratory system function poorly. After 3 or 4 days there is a relapse and the symptoms return in their former severity. The cycle continues through four or more attacks before the disease has run its course. Relapsing fevers are rarely fatal, but they can be serious.

TREATMENT AND PREVENTION. Treatment is with antibiotics. Sponge baths and aspirin help to control the fever and comfort the patient.

Although tick-borne relapsing fever still occurs in the western United States as well as in other parts of the world, the louse-borne fever is now largely confined to underdeveloped parts of Asia, Africa, and Latin America. Improved public sanitation and louse and tick control account for the decline in the incidence of the disease.

relaxant (re-lak'sant) 1. causing relaxation. 2. an agent that causes relaxation.

muscle r., an agent that specifically aids in reducing muscle tension.

relaxation (re″lak-sa′shun) a lessening of tension.

relaxin (re-lak′sin) a factor that produces relaxation of the symphysis pubis and dilation of the cervix uteri in certain animal species. A pharmaceutical preparation, extracted from the ovaries of pregnant sows, has been used in treatment of dysmenorrhea and premature labor, and to facilitate labor at term.

Releasin (re-le′sin) trademark for a preparation of relaxin.

REM rapid eye movement, a phase of SLEEP associated with dreaming and characterized by rapid movements of the eyes.

rem (rem) the amount of any ionizing radiation that has the same biologic effectiveness as 1 rad of x-rays.

remedy (rem′ĕ-de) anything that cures, palliates or prevents disease. adj., **reme′dial.**
    specific r., one that is invariably effective in treatment of a certain condition.

remission (re-mish′un) improvement or abatement of the symptoms of a disease.

remittence (re-mit′ens) temporary abatement, without actual cessation, of symptoms.

remittent (re-mit′ent) having periods of abatement and of exacerbation.

ren (ren), p. *re′nes* [L.] kidney.
    r. mo′bilis, wandering kidney; nephroptosis.

renal (re′nal) pertaining to the kidney.

Rendu-Weber-Osler disease (ron-du′ web′r ōs′-ler) hereditary hemorrhagic telangiectasia.

reniform (ren′ĭ-form) kidney-shaped.

renin (re′nin) an enzyme elicited by ischemia of the kidneys or by diminished pulse pressure, which converts hypertensinogen into angiotensin.

renipelvic (ren″ĭ-pel′vik) pertaining to the renal pelvis.

reniportal (ren″ĭ-por′tal) pertaining to the portal system of the kidney.

renipuncture (ren″ĭ-pungk′tūr) surgical incision of the capsule of the kidney; done for relief of albuminuric pain.

rennet (ren′et) a preparation of calf's stomach that contains rennin and is used for curdling the milk in cheese-making.

rennin (ren′in) a powerful milk-clotting enzyme of gastric juice of infants; in the adult its function is assumed by pepsin and chymotrypsin. Rennin catalyzes the conversion of casein from a soluble to an insoluble form (paracasein or curd).

renninogen (rĕ-nin′o-jen) the proenzyme in the gastric glands that is converted into rennin.

renogastric (re″no-gas′trik) pertaining to the kidney and stomach.

renography (re-nog′rah-fe) roentgenographic study of the kidney.

renointestinal (re″no-in-tes′tĭ-nal) pertaining to the kidney and intestine.

renopathy (re-nop′ah-the) any disease of the kidneys.

renoprival (re″no-pri′val) pertaining to or caused by lack of kidney function.

renotropic (re″no-trop′ik) having a special affinity for kidney tissue.

reovirus (re″o-vi′rus) (respiratory and enteric origin) one of a subgroup of the echoviruses.

rep (rep) roentgen-equivalent-physical, a unit of radiation equivalent to the absorption of 93 ergs per gram of tissue.

repair (re-pār) the physical or mechanical restoration of damaged tissues, especially the replacement of dead or damaged cells in a body tissue or organ by healthy new cells.
    plastic r., restoration of anatomic structure by means of tissue transferred from other sites or derived from other individuals, or by other substance.

repellent (re-pel′ent) 1. capable of dispersing a swelling. 2. capable of driving away, as insects or mosquitoes. 3. a substance that repels insects or mosquitoes.

repercussion (re″per-kush′un) 1. the driving in of an eruption or the scattering of a swelling. 2. ballottement.

replantation (re″plan-ta′shun) restoration of an organ or other body structure to its original site.

replication (rĕ″plī-ka′shun) 1. a turning back of a part so as to form a duplication. 2. repetition of an experiment to ensure accuracy.

repolarization (re″po-lar-ĭ-za′shun) the reestablishment of polarity, or the restoration of the exhibition of opposite effects at the two extremities.

repositor (re-poz′ĭ-tor) an instrument for replacing displaced parts.

repression (re-presh′un) a defense mechanism whereby a person unconsciously banishes unacceptable ideas, feelings or impulses from consciousness. A person using repression to obtain relief from mental conflict is unaware that he is "forgetting" unpleasant situations as a way of avoiding them. If employed to extreme, repression may lead to increased tension and irresponsible behavior that the person himself cannot understand or explain. Psychoanalysis frequently is employed to explore the causes and relieve tension resulting from repressed feelings of guilt, hostility or rejection.
    enzyme r., interference, usually by the end product of a pathway, with synthesis of the enzymes of that pathway.

repressor (re-pres′or) a compound that represses the formation of a specific enzyme.

reproduction (re″pro-duk′shun) the process by which a living entity or organism produces a new individual of the same kind. The gonads, or sex glands—the ovaries in the female and the testes in the male—produce the germ cells that unite and grow into a new individual. Reproduction begins

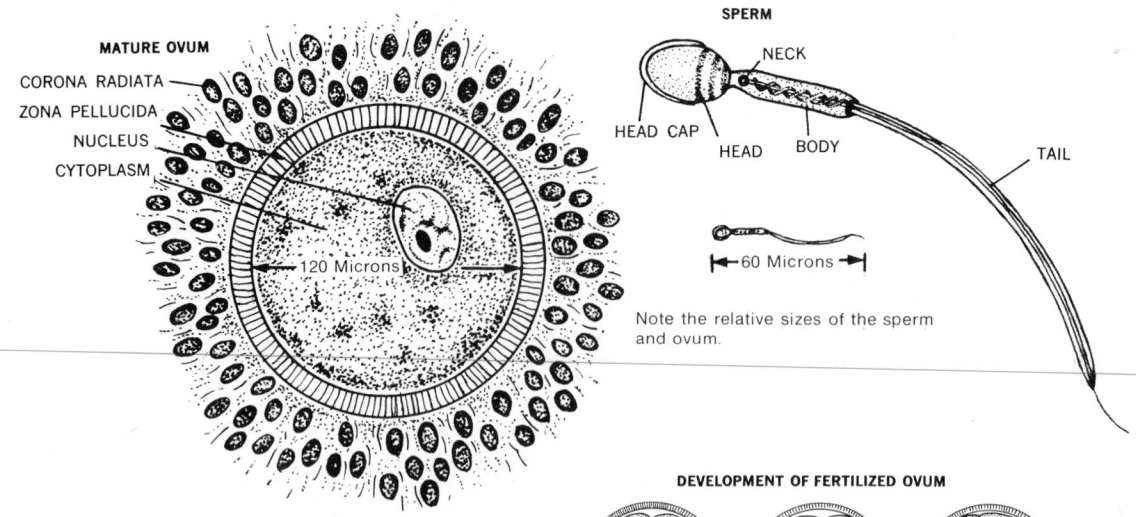

MATURE OVUM

CORONA RADIATA
ZONA PELLUCIDA
NUCLEUS
CYTOPLASM

120 Microns

SPERM

NECK
HEAD CAP
HEAD
BODY
TAIL

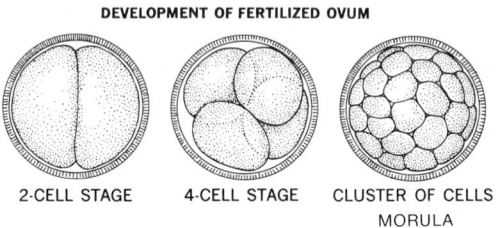

60 Microns

Note the relative sizes of the sperm and ovum.

Only one of millions of sperm cells that the male introduces into the female actually fertilizes an ovum, shown here in diagrammatic cross section. The sperm propel themselves with their tails. The fertilized ovum rapidly divides and redivides; the resulting cell mass is called the morula.

DEVELOPMENT OF FERTILIZED OVUM

2-CELL STAGE   4-CELL STAGE   CLUSTER OF CELLS
MORULA

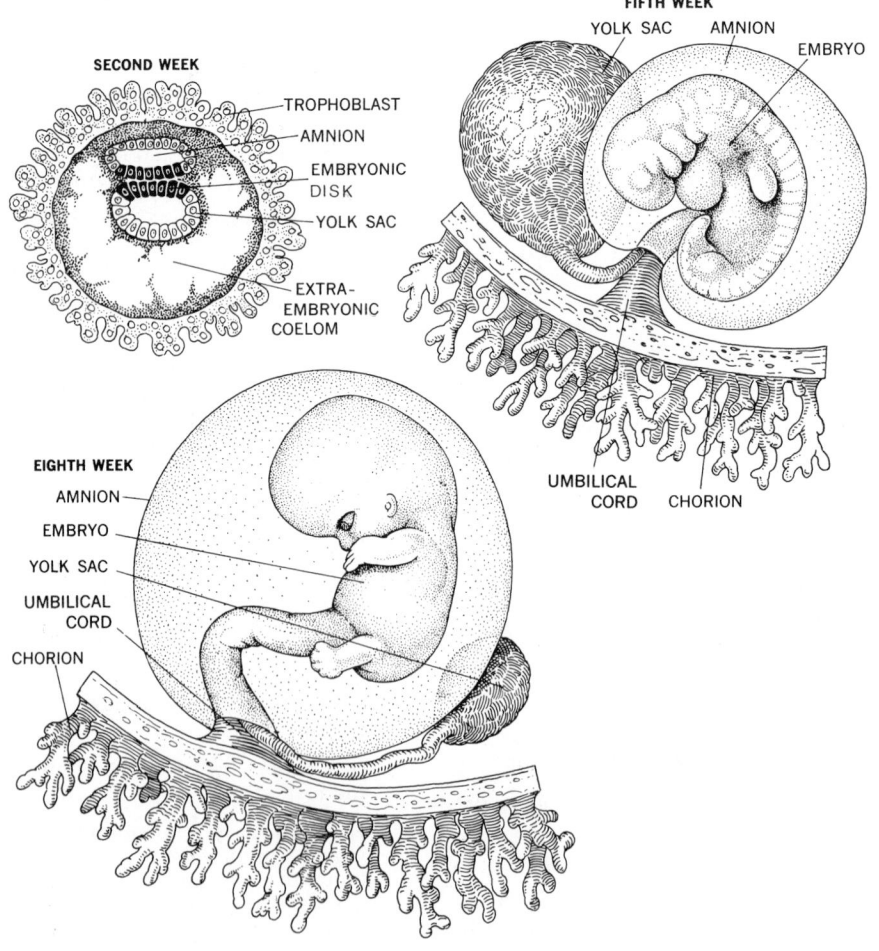

SECOND WEEK

TROPHOBLAST
AMNION
EMBRYONIC DISK
YOLK SAC
EXTRA-EMBRYONIC COELOM

FIFTH WEEK

YOLK SAC
AMNION
EMBRYO
UMBILICAL CORD
CHORION

EIGHTH WEEK

AMNION
EMBRYO
YOLK SAC
UMBILICAL CORD
CHORION

when the germ cells unite, a process called fertilization.

PRODUCTION OF GERM CELLS. The germ cells are the male spermatozoon and the female ovum, or egg. The mature ovum is a comparatively large round cell that is just visible to the naked eye. Spermatozoa can be seen only under a microscope, where each appears as a small, flattened head with a long whiplike tail used for locomotion.

Maturation of an ovum is a remarkable process controlled by hormones secreted by the female's endocrine glands. The MENSTRUAL CYCLE is ordinarily 28 days long, measured from the beginning of one menstrual period to the beginning of the next. During the first 2 weeks of the usual cycle, one of the ova becomes mature enough to be released from the ovary. At the time of OVULATION the mature ovum is released and at this point can be fertilized.

The ovum is discharged into the abdominal cavity. Somehow, by mechanisms that are not clear, it moves into a uterine tube. Then it begins the descent toward the uterus. If the ovum remains unfertilized, menstrual bleeding occurs about 2 weeks later.

There is no sexual cycle in the male comparable to the cyclical activity of ovulation in the female. Mature sperm are constantly being made in the testes of the adult male and stored there in the duct system.

FERTILIZATION, OR CONCEPTION. During coitus, semen is ejaculated from the penis into the back of the vagina near the cervix uteri. About a teaspoonful of semen is discharged with each ejaculation, containing several hundred millions of spermatozoa. Of this enormous number of sperm, only one is needed to fertilize the egg. Yet the obstacles to be overcome are considerable. Many of the sperm are deformed and cannot move. Others are killed by the acid secretions of the vagina (the semen itself is alkaline). The sperm must then swim against the current of secretions flowing out of the uterus.

The sperm swim on the average between an eighth of an inch to a full inch in a minute. When one or more vigorous sperm are able to reach the ovum, which is normally in the outer half of the uterine tube, fertilization occurs. The head end of the sperm plunges through the thick wall of the egg, leaving its tail outside. The genetic materials, the chromosomes, are injected into the egg, where they unite with the chromosomes inherited from the mother (see HEREDITY). The sex of the child is determined at this instant; it depends on the sex chromosome carried by the sperm.

If by chance two eggs have been released and are fertilized by two sperm, fraternal TWINS are formed. Identical twins are produced by a single fertilized egg that divides into two eggs early in its development.

Ovulation and Fertilization. Fertilization can occur only on the average of 4 days of every menstrual cycle. The mature ovum lives only 1 or 2 days after ovulation, and the sperm have only about the same amount of time before they perish in the female reproductive tract. To fertilize the ovum, coitus must take place within the period that begins 1 or 2 days before ovulation and lasts until 1 or 2 days after ovulation. There is much variation, however, in the time when ovulation occurs. Most women ovulate between the twelfth and the sixteenth days after the beginning of the last period,

but others ovulate as early as 8 or as late as 20 days after the first day of the period.

PREGNANCY. The egg begins to change immediately after fertilization. The membrane surrounding the egg becomes impenetrable to other sperm. Soon the egg is dividing into a cluster of two, then four, then more cells, as it makes its way down the uterine tube toward the uterus. At first it looks like a bunch of grapes. By the time the egg reaches the uterus, in 3 to 5 days, the cells are formed in the shape of a minute ball, hollow on the inside with an internal bump at one side where the embryo will form. This aggregation of cells, called a blastocyst, quickly buries itself in the lining of the uterus (implantation). On rare occasions, implantation takes place not in the uterine lining, but elsewhere in an ectopic, or abnormal, site. This produces an ECTOPIC PREGNANCY.

As soon as the blastocyst is implanted, its wall begins to change into a structure that eventually develops into the placenta. Through the placenta the fetus secures nourishment from the mother and rids itself of waste products. Essentially the placenta is a filtering mechanism by which the mother's blood is brought close to the fetal blood without the actual mixing of blood cells.

During the early stages of pregnancy, the future child grows at an extremely rapid rate. The mother's body must undergo profound changes to support this organism. The muscles of the uterus grow, vaginal secretions change, the blood volume expands, the work of the heart increases, the mother gains weight, the breasts prepare for nursing and other adjustments are made throughout the mother's body. (See also PREGNANCY and LABOR.)

asexual r., reproduction without the fusion of germ cells.

cytogenic r., production of a new individual from a single germ cell or zygote.

sexual r., reproduction by the fusion of a female germ cell with a male germ cell or by the development of an unfertilized egg.

somatic r., production of a new individual from a multicellular fragment by fission or budding.

reproductive (re″pro-duk′tiv) serving purposes of reproduction.

r. organs, female, the ovaries, which produce the ova, or eggs; the uterine tubes; the uterus; the vagina, or birth canal; and the vulva, comprising the external genitalia. The breasts are a secondary sex character, enclosing the mammary glands.

The reproductive system is linked to the body's system of endocrine glands by the ovaries. Besides producing the ova, the ovaries secrete the female sex hormones ESTROGEN and PROGESTERONE, which influence the body's development and general functioning as well as the sexual function.

The two ovaries, each about the size of a small plum, lie one on each side of the pear-shaped uterus at its wide upper part. When a female is born, her undeveloped ovaries already contain the specialized cells that can eventually become ova. At puberty these ova begin to ripen, one a month; usually the ovaries alternate in producing them. As the undeveloped egg cell, called a follicle, begins to ripen, it makes its way to the ovary's surface, breaks through its own outer covering, and is released. Release of an egg cell, called OVULATION, occurs about once in 28 days.

After its separation from the ovary the ovum is drawn into the nearby uterine tube through its fringed, flared opening, and is moved along by rhythmic contractions of the tube's walls and by the cilia of its mucous membrane lining. In the course of its passage the ovum ripens fully, and if fertilization occurs it usually takes place while the ovum is moving through the uterine tube.

The other end of the tube opens directly into the uterus. This muscular organ is capable of stretching to contain a fertilized ovum as it grows through the 9 months of pregnancy. Its mucous membrane lining is also specially adapted to hold the unborn infant securely and to nourish it. When the ovum arrives, the hormones estrogen and progesterone produced in the ovary have previously stimulated the uterus to prepare its lining with extra blood vessels. If the egg has not been fertilized, it loses its vitality, the hormone supply ceases and the extra blood and tissues are discharged from the body through the vagina, in the menstrual flow. If fertilization, or conception, has taken place, the growth of a new life has begun; menstruation does not occur, and in fact ceases entirely during the 9 months (approximately 280 days) of pregnancy.

The lower end of the uterus forms an opening called the cervix, or neck, which protrudes into the birth canal or vagina. Enclosed by muscles and lined with mucous membrane, the vagina measures on the average about 3 inches in length. In coitus it receives the male copulatory organ, the penis, and the discharge of sperm during ejaculation. Like the uterus, the vagina undergoes changes during pregnancy that enable it to stretch to many times its usual size, allowing the infant to pass through it in childbirth.

The exterior opening of the vagina and the surrounding organs make up the vulva. The vulva consists of the labia majora (the major lips), the labia minora (the minor lips), the vestibule and the clitoris. Somewhat anterior to the vulva lies a tri-

angular fatty pad covered with pubic hair, the mons veneris. Between the clitoris and the entry to the vagina is the opening of the urethra, from which urine is excreted. The anus lies to the rear of the vaginal opening. In a virgin, a membrane called the hymen usually closes off a part of the opening to the vagina.

The labia majora envelop the labia minora, and these join together at the clitoris, a rudimentary, diminutive, penis-like organ that has a purely erotic function. Like the penis, the clitoris has a foreskin and many nerve endings. The area that surrounds the entry to the vagina and lies within the labia minora is the vestibule. At each side of the vaginal opening and elsewhere in the vestibule, glands secrete lubricating fluids to facilitate coitus.

A woman's breasts serve to provide milk for the newborn infant. At puberty the breasts increase in size; during pregnancy they become much larger and start to secrete milk shortly after childbirth.

DISORDERS OF THE FEMALE REPRODUCTIVE ORGANS. Bacterial and other infections, tumors and birth injuries can affect the female reproductive organs. Growths, or tumors, can develop in all parts of the female reproductive tract. These are most often benign, and may not require treatment, but they should be examined periodically in case they grow large and affect the organs, or become malignant.

In the OVARY, cysts or tumors can develop without symptoms. When diagnosed, an ovarian tumor is usually removed surgically; cysts, however, often remain without excessive harm or pain. The neighboring uterine tubes may also be the site of growths, though such tumors usually result from the involvement of some other organ. The UTERUS, particularly the cervix, is one of the most frequent locations of tumors. In the uterus they are usually myomas, which may attain considerable size. These are, however, quite readily diagnosed and, when found early enough, are treated successfully by surgery.

In the reproductive system, the BREASTS are the most common site of growths of all kinds, both

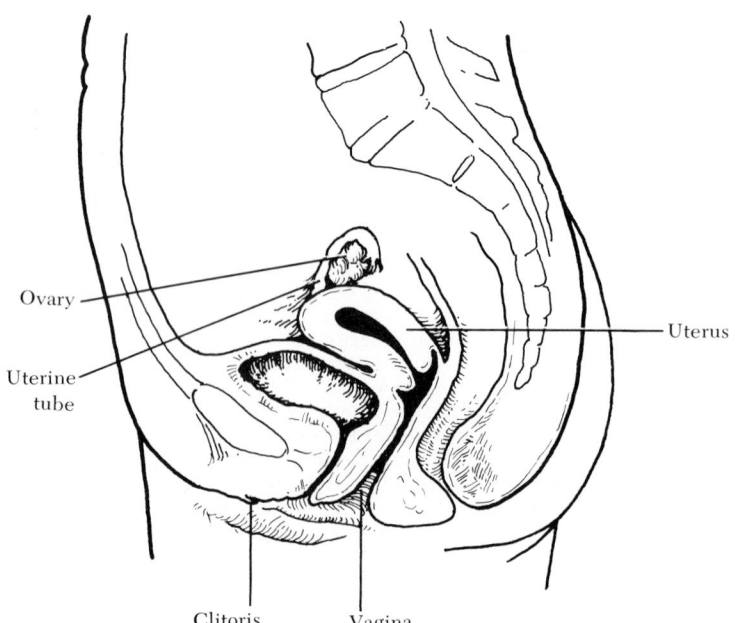

Ovary

Uterine tube

Uterus

Clitoris   Vagina

Female reproductive organs.

cysts and tumors, the latter both benign and malignant. A variety of sores and abscesses may afflict the breasts, especially in their milk-producing periods. Any lump or other irregularity within or on a breast should receive prompt medical attention.

The most prevalent bacterial diseases of a woman's reproductive organs are the venereal infections. Of these the most serious are SYPHILIS and GONORRHEA. Venereal diseases are almost always contracted through coitus.

A number of bacterial protozoa and fungus infections can occur within the vagina or in the area of the vulva. These cause discharges and irritation and can usually be readily treated following a correct diagnosis.

Difficult childbirth can produce deformations of the reproductive organs, particularly of the uterus.

r. organs, male, the external genitalia, accessory glands that secrete special fluids and the ducts through which these organs and glands are connected to each other and through which the spermatozoa are ejaculated during coitus.

EXTERNAL GENITALIA. The penis, testes and scrotum (the sac that contains the testes) are together known as the external genitalia. The penis is the organ through which semen is transferred into the female during coitus. Semen is a carrier for the spermatozoa, which are produced in the testes. The testes also produce the male hormone testosterone, which gives a sexually mature male his distinctively masculine characteristics and his sexual energy and drive.

The testes are suspended from the spermatic cord, which also connects the testes with the other parts of the reproductive system. This cord consists of blood vessels, nerves and ducts, all enclosed in connective tissue.

ACCESSORY GLANDS. The accessory reproductive glands include the prostate, two seminal vesicles and two bulbourethral glands, known also as Cowper's glands.

The PROSTATE is located below and against the urinary bladder. It completely surrounds the urethra. It produces a thin, clear, slightly alkaline fluid that neutralizes the normal acidity of the

urethra caused by the continual passage of urine. This fluid enables the spermatozoa to pass through the urethra unharmed.

The seminal vesicles are two glands located just above and to the rear of the prostate. These glands consist of many small sacs, or pockets, in which is produced and stored the thick, milky fluid that is ejaculated during the male orgasm. The fluid serves as the carrier for the sperm and is the major constituent of the semen.

The two bulbourethral glands, which are about the size of peas, secrete a clear, sticky fluid that lubricates the urethra, thus making it easier for the semen to pass through it during ejaculation.

DUCTS. The spermatozoa are led from the testes to the urethra through a system of ducts. First, there are two convoluted tubes, one lying on top of each testis and connected directly to it. Each tube is called an epididymis. Mature spermatozoa produced in the testes are stored in each epididymis.

Each epididymis is connected to a vas deferens, a part of the spermatic cord that conducts the spermatozoa to the duct lying close to the bladder.

The vasa deferentia join with ducts leading from the seminal vesicles just before the urethra. The combined duct is called the ejaculatory duct. This duct passes through the prostate and joins with the urethra. The urethra then conducts the semen through the penis.

DISCHARGE OF SEMEN. The tissues that form the mass of the penis are called erectile tissue. This tissue is spongy in nature and filled with innumerable hollow spaces. There is also a network of veins and arteries within the penis. Sexual excitement causes the muscles surrounding the veins to contract, thereby restricting the flow of blood from the penis. At the same time, the muscles surrounding the arteries relax, permitting the free flow of blood into the penis at the full pressure of the circulatory system. The result is that the spongy tissue fills with blood and the penis swells in size and becomes stiff and erect.

Sexual excitement also stimulates the accessory glands to secrete larger amounts of their fluids. When the sexual tension becomes acute enough, as a result of coitus, masturbation or purely mental stimulation (as in "wet dreams"), there is a series of reflex contractions of the reproductive organs. The muscles surrounding the seminal ducts, the prostate and the seminal vesicles contract convulsively; this causes the semen to be ejaculated forcibly from the penis. There is first an ejaculation of the fluid from the prostate, followed immediately by the semen. About 2 or 3 cc. of semen is ejaculated. This volume of semen is believed to contain between 200 and 500 million sperm, only one of which is necessary to fertilize the ovum.

DISORDERS OF THE MALE REPRODUCTIVE ORGANS. For disorders that affect particular organs, see PENIS, PROSTATE and CRYPTORCHIDISM. Since the male reproductive organs are connected so closely with each other, an infection in one is likely to spread throughout the entire reproductive system. This is particularly true of venereal diseases, such as SYPHILIS and GONORRHEA, which are contracted almost always through coitus.

R.E.S. reticuloendothelial system.

rescinnamine   (re-sin'ah-min) an alkaloid from

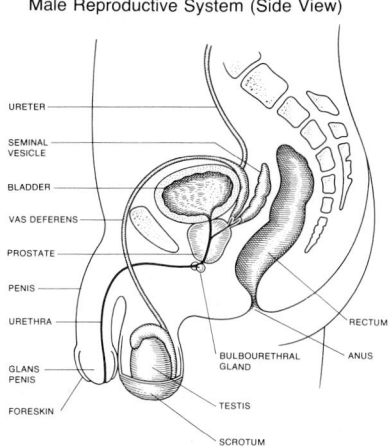

Male Reproductive System (Side View)

URETER

SEMINAL VESICLE

BLADDER

VAS DEFERENS

PROSTATE

PENIS

URETHRA

RECTUM

GLANS PENIS

BULBOURETHRAL GLAND

ANUS

FORESKIN

TESTIS

SCROTUM

Male reproductive organs. (From Burt, J. J., and Brower, L. A.: Education for Sexuality. Philadelphia, W. B. Saunders Co., 1970.)

various species of Rauwolfia; used as an anti-hypertensive and tranquilizer.

resection (re-sek'shun) surgical removal of a considerable portion of an organ or body part.

    gastric r., partial gastrectomy.

    submucous r., excision of a portion of a deflected nasal septum after first laying back a flap of mucous membrane.

    transurethral r., removal of the prostate by means of an instrument passed through the urethra.

    wedge r., removal of a triangular mass of tissue, as from the ovary.

    window r., submucous resection.

resectoscope (re-sek'to-skōp) an instrument for transurethral prostatic resection.

resectoscopy (re″sek-tos'ko-pe) transurethral resection of the prostate.

reserpine (res'er-pēn) an active alkaloid from *Rauwolfia serpentina,* used as an antihypertensive, tranquilizer and sedative.

reserve (re-zerv') 1. to hold back for future use. 2. a supply, beyond that ordinarily used, that may be utilized in emergency.

    alkali r., alkaline r., the amount of buffer compounds in the blood that are capable of neutralizing acids, such as sodium bicarbonate and proteins. Since the bicarbonates are the most important of these buffers, the term blood bicarbonate is often preferred to alkali reserve.

    cardiac r., the potential ability of the heart to perform work beyond that necessary under basal conditions.

reservoir (rez'er-vwar) a storage space.

    biologic r., the animals capable of harboring, without injury to themselves, pathogenic microorganisms that may at any time be transmitted to man and produce disease.

    r. of infection, a source of pathogenic organisms in permanent hosts or healthy carriers, from which they spread to cause disease.

residual (re-zid'u-al) remaining or left behind.

    r. urine, urine remaining in the bladder after voiding; seen with bladder outlet obstruction and disorders affecting nerves controlling bladder function.

residue (rez'ĭ-doo) a remainder; that which remains after the removal of other substances.

residuum (re-zid'u-um), pl. *resid'ua* [L.] a residue or remainder.

resin (rez'in) 1. a naturally occurring solid, brittle, amorphous substance, as an exudate from plants and trees, soluble in alcohol and volatile oils and insoluble in water. 2. a precipitate obtained by mixing an alcohol solution with water. adj., **res'inous.**

    acrylic r's, products of the polymerization of acrylic or methacrylic acid or their derivatives, used in fabrication of medical prostheses and dental restorations and appliances.

    heat-curing r., one that requires the use of heat to effect its polymerization.

    ion-exchange r., a high-molecular-weight, insoluble polymer of simple organic compounds capable of exchanging its attached ions for other ions in the surrounding medium; classified as *cation-* or

anion-exchange resin, depending on the charge of the ion exchanged. Cation-exchange resins are used to restrict absorption of sodium in edematous states. Anion-exchange resins are used as antacids in treatment of ulcers.

    podophyllum r., an amorphous powder obtained by percolation of podophyllum with alcohol; used in treatment of condyloma acuminatum.

    quick-cure r., self-curing r., any resin that can be polymerized by addition of an activator and a catalyst without the use of external heat.

    synthetic r., an amorphous, organic solid or semisolid substance produced by polymerization of simple compounds.

Resinat (rez'ĭ-nat) trademark for preparations of polyamine-methylene resin, an anion-exchange resin used as a gastric antacid.

resistance (re-zis'tans) 1. opposition of a conductor to passage of electricity or other energy or substance. 2. the ability of an organism to withstand a noxious influence. 3. in studies of respiration, an expression of the opposition to flow of air produced by the tissues of the air passages, in terms of pressure per amount of air per unit of time. 4. in psychoanalysis, opposition to the coming into consciousness of repressed material.

    peripheral r., resistance to the passage of blood through the small blood vessels, especially the capillaries.

resolution (rez″o-lu'shun) 1. subsidence of a pathologic state, as the subsidence of an inflammation, or the softening and disappearance of a swelling. 2. perception as separate of two adjacent points; in microscopy, the smallest distance at which two adjacent objects can be distinguished as separate.

resolvent (re-zol'vent) promoting resolution.

resolving power (re-zol'ving) the ability of the eye or of a lens to make small objects that are close together separately visible, thus revealing the structure of an object.

resonance (rez'o-nans) 1. a rich quality of sound produced by the transmission of its vibrations to a cavity. Decrease of resonance is called dullness; its absence, flatness.

    amphoric r., resembling the sound produced by blowing over the mouth of an empty bottle.

    skodaic r., resonance of a tympanic quality over the upper part of the thorax when the lower portion of a lung is entirely compressed by pleuritic effusion.

    tympanic r., drumlike reverberation of a cavity filled with air.

    tympanitic r., the peculiar sound elicited by percussing a tympanitic abdomen.

    vesicular r., normal pulmonary resonance.

    vocal r., the sound of ordinary speech as heard through the chest wall.

resonant (rez'o-nant) giving an intense, rich sound on percussion.

resonator (rez'o-na″tor) 1. an instrument used to intensify sounds. 2. an electric circuit in which oscillations of a certain frequency are set up by oscillations of the same frequency in another circuit.

resorcin (rĕ-zor'sin) resorcinol.

resorcinism (rĕ-zor′sĭ-nizm) chronic poisoning by resorcinol.

resorcinol (rĕ-zor′sĭ-nol) a compound used as a local anti-infective.

 r. monoacetate, a viscous, pale yellow or amber liquid; used as a local irritant and antibacterial and antifungal agent.

resorcinolphthalein (rĕ-zor″sĭ-nol-thal′ēn) fluorescein, a dye used in certain diagnostic procedures, as for example the detection of corneal abrasions.

resorption (re-sorp′shun) removal by absorption of something already secreted or formed in the body, as reabsorption in the kidney of certain elements from the urine, or destruction of bone or of cementum or dentin of teeth.

respirable (rĕ-spīr′ah-bl) suitable for respiration.

respiration (res″pĭ-ra′shun) the exchange of oxygen and carbon dioxide in the body (1) in the lungs, (2) between the cell and its environment, and (3) in the metabolism of the cell.

THE RESPIRATORY SEQUENCE. The sequence of the respiration process begins as air enters the corridors of the nose or mouth, where it is warmed and moistened. The air then passes through the pharynx, larynx and trachea and into the bronchi.

The bronchi branch in the lungs into smaller and smaller bronchioles, ending in clusters of tiny air sacs. There are 750 million of these alveoli, as they are called, in the lungs. The blood flows through the lungs in the pulmonary circulation. Through the thin membrane of the network of capillaries around the alveoli, the air and the blood exchange oxygen and carbon dioxide. The carbon dioxide molecules migrate from the erythrocytes in the capillaries through the porous membrane into the air in the alveoli, while the oxygen molecules cross from the air into the red blood cells.

The erythrocytes proceed through the circulatory system, carrying the oxygen in loose combination with HEMOGLOBIN and giving it up to the body cells that need it. In cellular respiration the blood cells release oxygen and pick up carbon dioxide. The lungs dispose of the carbon dioxide, left there by the red blood cells, in the process of breathing. With each breath, about one-sixth of the air in the lungs is exchanged for new air.

BREATHING. The lungs inflate and deflate some 16 to 20 times a minute. Their elastic tissue allows them to expand and contract like a bellows worked by the diaphragm and the intercostal muscles. The diaphragm contracts, flattening itself downward, and thus enlarges the thoracic cavity. At the same time the ribs are pulled up and outward by the action of the narrow but powerful intercostal muscles that expand and contract the rib cage. As the chest expands, the air rushes in.

Exhalation occurs when the respiratory muscles relax and the chest returns automatically to its minimum size, expelling the air.

Automatic Breathing Controls. The automatic control of breathing stems from poorly defined areas known as the respiratory centers, located in the medulla oblongata and pons. From there, impulses are sent down the spinal cord to the nerves that control the diaphragm, and to the intercostal muscles. Chemical and reflex signals control these nerve centers.

The chemical controls of breathing are mainly dependent on the level of carbon dioxide in the blood. The response is so sensitive that if the carbon dioxide in the blood increases two-tenths of 1 per cent, the respiratory rate increases automatically to double the amount of air taken in, until the excess of carbon dioxide is eliminated. It is not lack of oxygen but excess of carbon dioxide that causes this instant and powerful reaction.

The pCO_2, or carbon dioxide tension, of arterial blood normally is 38 to 40 mm. of mercury. When the pCO_2 increases, the respiratory centers are stimulated and breathing becomes more rapid; conversely, decrease of the pCO_2 slows the rate of respiration. The pCO_2 acts both directly on the respiratory centers of the brain and on the carotid and aortic bodies, chemoreceptors that are responsive to changes in blood pCO_2, pO_2 and pH.

PROTECTIVE RESPIRATORY MECHANISMS. The lungs are constantly exposed to the surrounding atmosphere. Twenty times a minute, more or less, they take in a gaseous mixture, along with whatever foreign particles happen to be floating in it and at whatever temperature it may be. To compensate, the lungs have some remarkable protective devices.

On its way through the nasal passage, the cold air from outside is preheated by a large supply of blood, which gives off warmth through the thin mucuous membrane that lines the respiratory tract. This same mucous lining is always moist, and dry air picks up moisture as it passes.

Dust, soot and bacteria are filtered out by a barrier of cilia, tiny threadlike growths that line the passageways of the respiratory tract. The cilia catch not only foreign particles but also mucus produced by the respiratory passages themselves. Since the movement of the cilia is always toward the outside, they push the interfering matter upward, away from the delicate lung tissues, so that it can be expectorated or swallowed. Particles that are too large for the cilia to dispose of usually stimulate a sneeze or a cough, which forcibly expels them.

Sneezing and coughing are reflex acts in response to stimulation of nerve endings in the respiratory passages. The stimulus for a cough comes from the air passages in the throat; for a sneeze, from those in the nose.

 abdominal r., the inspiration and expiration of air by the lungs accomplished mainly by the abdominal muscles and diaphragm.

 aerobic r., oxidative transformation of substances utilizing oxygen.

 anaerobic r., chemical reactions in which free oxygen takes no part.

 artificial r., that maintained artificially (see also ARTIFICIAL RESPIRATION).

 Cheyne-Stokes r., rhythmic waxing and waning of the depth of respiration due to disease affecting the respiratory centers.

 diaphragmatic r., that performed mainly by the diaphragm.

 external r., the exchange of carbon dioxide and oxygen by diffusion between the external environment and the bloodstream.

 internal r., the exchange of oxygen and carbon dioxide between the bloodstream and the cells of the body.

respirator (res′pĭ-ra″tor) a mechanical device used to substitute for or assist with the respirations of a patient with pulmonary insufficiency. Respirators work either on the principle of intermittent positive pressure breathing (IPPB)—they inflate the lungs at regular intervals by providing positive pressure—or on the principle of delivering a specified volume of air. Once the lungs are inflated, expiration is passive. However, when necessary, the respirator also can use negative pressure and actually suck the air out of the lungs.

There is a wide variety of respirators available; the three most popular models are the Bird respirator and the Bennett respirator (pressure type) and the Emerson respirator (volume type). These models can be adjusted so that the patient's respirations can trigger the apparatus, or they can be set at controlled breathing, in which case the machine provides a certain number of respirations per minute independently of the patient. The older types of respirators, such as the Drinker respirator (iron lung) and other chamber respirators provide only controlled, automatic breathing and are used only when paralysis prohibits respiration.

NORMAL PHYSIOLOGY OF RESPIRATION AND INDICATIONS FOR USE OF THE RESPIRATOR. Under normal circumstances the rhythmic movements of the diaphragm and of the intercostal muscles produce breathing. The lungs themselves have no muscles. During inhalation the diaphragm contracts and flattens. At the same time, the intercostal and chest muscles draw the ribs upward and outward. These movements enlarge the thoracic cavity. Just as when a bellows is expanded, this enlargement reduces the air pressure inside the thoracic cavity. Outside, the normal air pressure of approximately 15 lb. per square inch pushes air into the cavity. Use of the respirator is indicated when pathologic conditions reduce or completely eliminate the patient's ability to ventilate the lungs adequately.

Conditions in which a respirator may be used include structural defects or injuries to the chest or lungs, paralysis of the muscles of respiration and structural diseases of the lungs, such as emphysema, chronic bronchitis, asthma and cancer of the lung.

Nonautomatic, patient-controlled ventilation is most often used in various types of therapy when aerosol medications are administered. The respirator, by forcing air into the lungs, helps deliver medication to the deep, poorly ventilated areas of the lungs, thus relieving congestion, reducing bronchospasm and liquefying mucus. The deep breathing brought about by use of the respirator assists the patient in coughing up secretions without extreme fatigue, and also helps stretch the respiratory muscles and alveolar walls so that their elastic tone is improved.

An automatic cycling rate can be set according to the patient's respiration when irregular or shallow respirations do not provide adequate ventilation of the lungs. The rate is set slightly below the patient's usual respiratory rate so that respiration will continue when and if he ceases to breathe properly. The respirator assists his breathing by providing positive pressure, thus reducing the work load of the respiratory muscles.

Controlled ventilation is used when the patient is totally unable to breathe for himself. The machine is set on an automatic cycle. If a tracheostomy tube or endotracheal tube has been inserted to maintain a patent airway, the respirator is attached to the tube; otherwise, a mask is used.

NURSING CARE. Although the specific nursing care of the patient during use of a respirator depends on the type of apparatus used and its purpose, there are some general rules that apply in all cases.

The effectiveness of the apparatus in delivering air depends on an airtight connection between the machine and the patient's air passages. Leakage of air and other gases must therefore be controlled as much as possible. When a mouthpiece is used the patient is instructed in its use and told that he should bite down gently on the mouthpiece, seal the edges with his lips and refrain from breathing through his nose during the treatment. If a mask is used, it should fit the contours of the face. Before the mask is applied the skin is cleansed of facial oils so that slippage of the mask is reduced to a minimum. Tracheostomy and endotracheal tubes are outfitted with a cuff that is attached to the tube and acts as a seal around the edges of the tube. Finally, all connections for the tubing must be checked for leaks.

The respirator is continually checked to see that it is functioning properly. By listening to the rhythmic cycle and observing the unit, one can determine whether the apparatus is working correctly. This requires a thorough understanding of the particular machine and the purposes for which it is being used. No one should attempt to care for a patient using a respirator without prior instruction in the use of that particular apparatus.

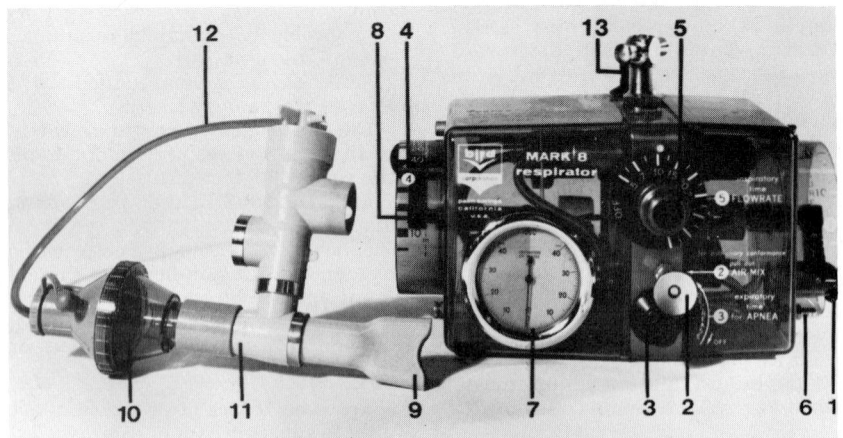

Bird respirator. (From McCallum, H. P.: The nurse and the respirator. Nursing Clin. N. Amer., *1*:597, 1966.)

While the patient is using the machine, he is observed for signs of respiratory difficulty, changes in color and change in pulse volume. A reduction of pulse volume may indicate circulatory difficulties arising from failure of the right heart to fill properly because of prolonged expansion of the lungs. When this occurs the situation may be controlled by lengthening the expiration phase.

When a patient is being maintained on the respirator for a long period of time he is obviously critically ill and requires continual observation and care. HYPERVENTILATION may occur as a result of too rapid removal of carbon dioxide via the respiratory system (see also respiratory ALKALOSIS). Another possibility is gastric distention, which can develop when the patient is in a coma or unconscious and air escapes into the stomach. Gastric suction may be necessary to remove the air from the stomach.

TRACHEOSTOMY care is of vital importance when the patient is being maintained on a respirator with controlled ventilation and positive pressure is being delivered via a tracheostomy tube. Suction is applied as necessary and some method for moisturizing the air is provided. In fact, whether the patient has a tracheostomy or not, the air passages must be kept moist whenever a respirator is used for a prolonged period.

If aerosol medications are administered by use of a respirator, it is important to know the type of medication being used, its desired effects and the signs and symptoms of overdosage or toxic side effects. When such symptoms appear the rate of nebulization requires adjustment.

The psychologic implications of the use of a respirator are manifold. If he is conscious or semiconscious, the patient is aware that the machine is concerned with maintaining his very "breath of life" and he is understandably apprehensive about its use and effects on his breathing. When a respirator is used for a brief period as a means of therapy, the patient can be told that he can control the cycle by the slightest effort on his part. Once he understands the way the machine works and his questions are answered to his satisfaction his fears can be allayed. The patient who is partially or totally dependent on a respirator will need more reassurance. He should be assured that someone will be

Bennett respirator. (Courtesy of Puritan-Bennett Corp.)

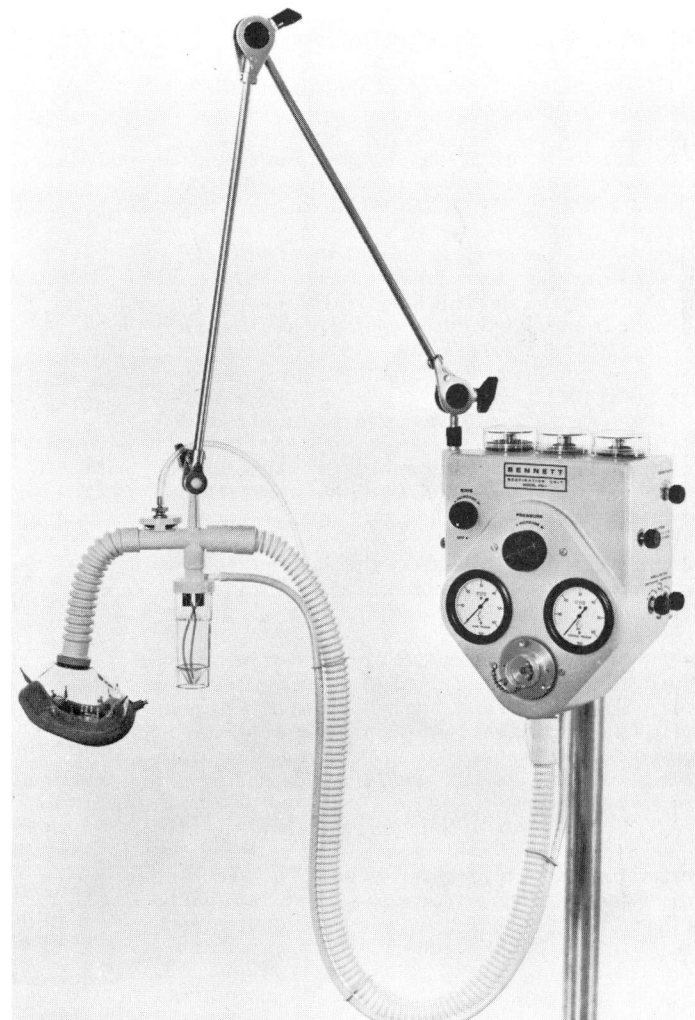

near at all times in case the apparatus needs adjusting. Much of his panic and fear can be relieved if the nursing staff exercises patience and maintains a calm attitude when helping him adjust to the respirator.

Another problem that may develop from continued use of the respirator is overdependence on the machine once the patient has adjusted to it. He learns that breathing is maintained without any effort on his part and he becomes loath to discontinue the respirator and expose himself to the harrowing experience of struggling for breath. Much of this anxiety is unwarranted and the patient must be helped to understand that some effort on his part is necessary while he is being "weaned" from the apparatus. This requires much patience and understanding on the part of the nurse and she must emphasize that the process will be gradual, that the respirator will be kept available at the bedside and ready for use if needed, and that it can be put to use immediately whenever there is an indication for its need.

respiratory   (re-spi'rah-to″re, res'per-ah-to″re) pertaining to respiration.

r. distress syndrome, a condition of the newborn characterized by acute difficulty in breathing, occurring most frequently in premature infants, infants of diabetic mothers or infants delivered by cesarean section.

r. quotient, an expression of the ratio of the carbon dioxide produced to the oxygen consumed by an organism.

r. syncytial virus, a virus isolated from children with bronchopneumonia and bronchitis, characteristically causing syncytium formation in tissue culture.

r. system, the group of specialized organs whose specific function is to provide for the transfer of oxygen from the air to the blood and of waste carbon dioxide from the blood to the air. The organs of the system include the NOSE, the PHARYNX, the LARYNX, the TRACHEA, the bronchi and the LUNGS. (See also RESPIRATION.)

RESPIRATORY DISORDERS.   Of the numerous disorders that affect the respiratory system, the most frequent is the COMMON COLD, a virus infection of the upper respiratory tract. Common upper respiratory disorders also include HAY FEVER and other allergic reactions.

Other diseases that affect the respiratory tract include INFLUENZA, WHOOPING COUGH and DIPHTHERIA. Some more generalized diseases, such as MEASLES, are also accompanied by respiratory symptoms. A respiratory inflammation or infection, such as a cold, may spread to other parts of the respiratory system and may be a cause of a number of related symptoms and disorders. For example, one condition that may stem from a cold or from other causes is SINUSITIS, inflammation of the paranasal sinuses.

In children in particular, enlarged ADENOIDS may block the rear of the nasal passages and make breathing through the nose difficult. The tonsils at the sides of the throat are also very susceptible to infection and enlargement (see also TONSILLITIS). When inflammation affects the larynx, or voice box, the condition is known as LARYNGITIS, and if it attacks the bronchial tubes, it is called BRONCHITIS. Another disorder that affects the bronchial tubes is

ASTHMA, which causes contraction and mucous plugging of the tubes and hinders breathing. Asthma is frequently an allergic reaction.

Some of the most serious respiratory disorders arise as complications in a number of types of heart disease. Pulmonary embolism also causes serious respiratory distress.

Inflammation of the lungs is known as PNEUMONIA. PLEURISY occurs when the coverings of the lungs, the pleurae, become inflamed. A serious infectious disease that may attack the lungs is TUBERCULOSIS. A LUNG ABSCESS, an inflammation in which there is localized accumulation of pus and destruction of tissue, may sometimes be a complication of tuberculosis or pneumonia.

A very serious disease that has become increasingly prevalent in the 20th century is LUNG CANCER. Other parts of the respiratory system may also be affected by cancer. For information on other respiratory disorders, see the separate articles on the various respiratory organs.

respirometer (res″pĭ-rom'ĕ-ter) an instrument for determining the nature of the respiration.

response (re-spons') any action or change of condition evoked by a stimulus.

reticulocyte r., increase in the formation of reticulocytes in response to a bone marrow stimulus.

rest (rest) 1. repose after exertion. 2. a fragment of embryonal tissue retained within the adult.

restenosis (re″stĕ-no'sis) recurrent stenosis, especially of a cardiac valve after surgical correction of the primary condition.

false r., stenosis recurring after failure to divide either commissure of a cardiac valve beyond the area of incision of the papillary muscles.

restibrachium (res″tĭ-bra'ke-um) the inferior peduncle of the cerebellum.

restiform (res'tĭ-form) shaped like a rope.

restim (res'tim) a biologically derived nonpyrogenic, nontoxic lipid material that has a stimulating effect on the reticuloendothelial system.

restoration (res″to-ra'shun) 1. induction of a return to a previous state, as a return to health or replacement of a part to normal position. 2. partial or complete reconstruction of a body part, or the device used in its place.

restorative (rĕ-stōr'ah-tiv) 1. promoting a return of health. 2. a remedy that aids in restoring health.

restraint (re-strānt') forcible control.

chemical r., control of the behavior of a disturbed psychotic patient by means of sedatives.

mechanical r., control of the behavior of a disturbed psychotic patient by mechanical means.

resuscitation (rĕ-sus″ĭ-ta'shun) restoration to life or consciousness of one apparently dead, or whose respirations have ceased (see also ARTIFICIAL RESPIRATION).

resuscitator (rĕ-sus'ĭ-ta″tor) an apparatus for initiating respiration in persons whose breathing has stopped.

retardate (rĕ-tar'dāt) a mentally retarded person.

retardation (re″tar-da'shun) hindrance or delay in

any process, as in mental or physical development (see also MENTAL RETARDATION).

retardin (rĕ-tar′din) a hormone from the pancreas that regulates fat metabolism and neutralizes the toxic action of thyroxine.

retching (rech′ing) a strong involuntary effort to vomit.

rete (re′te), pl. *re′tia* [L.] a network; usually applied to an anastomosing network of small arteries or veins or of other channels.
   r. malpig′hii, the innermost stratum of epidermis.
   r. mirab′ile, a network of small anastomosing blood vessels, chiefly from a single trunk, that subsequently reunite into a single vessel.
   r. muco′sum, rete malpighii.
   r. tes′tis, the network of channels formed in the mediastinum of the testis by the vasa recta.

retention (rĕ-ten′shun) the process of holding back or keeping in a position, as persistence in the body of material normally excreted.
   r. of urine, accumulation of urine within the bladder because of inability to urinate.

reticular, reticulated (rĕ-tik′u-lar), (rĕ-tik′u-lat″ed) resembling a network.

reticulation (rĕ-tik″u-la′shun) the formation of a network.

reticulemia (rĕ-tik″u-le′me-ah) the presence in the blood of increased numbers of immature erythrocytes.

reticulin (rĕ-tik′u-lin) a scleroprotein present in connective tissue closely related to collagen in composition.

reticulocyte (rĕ-tik′u-lo-sīt″) a young non-nucleated cell of the erythrocytic series, grossly indistinguishable from an erythrocyte, but, on special staining, showing granules or a diffuse network of fibrils.

reticulocytogenic (rĕ-tik″u-lo-si″to-jen′ik) causing the formation of reticulocytes.

reticulocytopenia (rĕ-tik″u-lo-si″to-pe′ne-ah) deficiency of reticulocytes in the blood.

reticulocytosis (rĕ-tik″u-lo-si-to′sis) excess of reticulocytes in the blood.

reticuloendothelial (rĕ-tik″u-lo-en″do-the′le-al) pertaining to tissues having both reticular and endothelial attributes.
   r. system, a network of cells and tissues found throughout the body, especially in the blood, general connective tissue, spleen, liver, lungs, bone marrow and lymph nodes. Some of the reticuloendothelial cells found in the blood and in the general connective tissue are unusually large in size. These cells are concerned in blood cell formation and destruction, storage of fatty materials and metabolism of iron and pigment, and play a role in inflammation and immunity. Some of the cells are motile—that is, capable of spontaneous motion—and phagocytic—they can ingest and destroy unwanted foreign material.
   The reticuloendothelial cells of the SPLEEN possess the ability to dispose of disintegrated erythrocytes. They do not, however, destroy hemoglobin, which is liberated in the process.
   The reticuloendothelial cells located in the blood

cavities of the LIVER are called Kupffer cells. These cells, together with the cells of the general connective tissue and bone marrow, are capable of transforming into bile pigment the hemoglobin released by disintegrated erythrocytes.
   DISORDERS OF THE RETICULOENDOTHELIAL SYSTEM. The reticuloendothelial system can be the site of a variety of diseases, all of which are rare. They are generally treated by x-ray therapy and steroids, among other methods. The prospects for recovery cannot always be predicted.
   The disorders include Gaucher's disease, Letterer-Siwe disease, eosinophilic granuloma and HAND-SCHÜLLER-CHRISTIAN DISEASE. A rare illness called Niemann-Pick disease strikes mainly children of Jewish origin.

reticuloendothelioma (rĕ-tik″u-lo-en″do-the″le-o′mah) a tumor of the reticuloendothelial system.

reticuloendotheliosis (rĕ-tik″u-lo-en″do-the″le-o′sis) hyperplasia of reticuloendothelium.

reticuloendothelium (rĕ-tik″u-lo-en″do-the′le-um) the tissue of the reticuloendothelial system.

reticuloma (rĕ-tik″u-lo′mah) a tumor composed of cells of reticuloendothelial origin (monocytes).

reticulopenia (rĕ-tik″u-lo-pe′ne-ah) reticulocytopenia.

reticulopodium (rĕ-tik″u-lo-po′de-um) a threadlike, branching pseudopodium.

reticulosarcoma (rĕ-tik″u-lo-sar-ko′mah) a sarcoma composed of reticulum cells.

reticulosis (rĕ-tik″u-lo′sis) an abnormal increase in cells of the reticuloendothelial system.

reticulum (rĕ-tik′u-lum), pl. *retic′ula* [L.] a small network.
   endoplasmic r., a system of membrane-bounded cavities in the cytoplasm of a cell, occurring in two types, granular, or rough-surfaced, and agranular, or smooth-surfaced; it is involved in cellular protein production and the secretion of cellular products.
   sarcoplasmic r., a network of smooth-surfaced tubules surrounding the myofibrils of striated muscle fibers.

retiform (rĕ′tī-form, ret′ī-form) reticular.

retina (ret′ĭ-nah) the innermost of the three tunics of the eyeball, surrounding the vitreous body and continuous posteriorly with the optic nerve. adj., **retinal.** The retina is composed of light-sensitive neurons arranged in three layers; the first layer is made up of rods and cones and the other two transmit impulses from the rods and cones to the OPTIC NERVE. The rods are sensitive in dim light, and the cones are sensitive in bright light and are responsible for color vision. (See also EYE.)
   Retinopathies are pathologic conditions of the retina; they occur in conjunction with certain systemic disorders, such as hypertension, nephritis, toxemia of pregnancy and diabetes mellitus.
   DETACHMENT OF THE RETINA is complete or partial separation of the retina from the choroid, the middle coat of the eyeball. It occurs most often in

persons with MYOPIA (nearsightedness), but it also can result from trauma to the head.

retinaculum (ret″ĭ-nak′u-lum), pl. *retinac′ula* [L.] a structure or device for holding a thing in place, as an anatomic structure or a surgical instrument.
flexor r. of hand, a fibrous band forming the carpal canal through which pass the tendons of the flexor muscles of the hand and fingers.
r. morgag′ni, a ridge formed by the coming together of segments of the ileocecal valve.
r. ten′dinum, a tendinous restraining structure, such as an annular ligament.
Weitbrecht's r., retinacular fibers attached to the neck of the femur.

retine (ret′ēn) a substance widely distributed in animal cells, capable of inhibiting cell division and growth.

retinene (ret′ĭ-nēn) an ocular pigment derived from vitamin A and formed by the bleaching action of light on rhodopsin.

retinitis (ret″ĭ-ni′tis) inflammation of the retina.
r. circina′ta, retinitis with white spots surrounding the macula lutea.
r. haemorrha′gica, retinitis with profuse retinal hemorrhages.
r. pigmento′sa, progressive retinal sclerosis with pigmentation and atrophy. There are star-shaped deposits of pigment in the retina and the retinal vessels become obliterated. Visual impairment is progressive.
r. prolif′erans, a condition that may result from intraocular hemorrhage, with the formation of fibrous bands extending into the vitreous from the retina; retinal detachment may result.
suppurative r., retinitis due to pyemic infection.

retinoblastoma (ret″ĭ-no-blas-to′mah) glioma of the retina.

retinochoroiditis (ret″ĭ-no-ko″roi-di′tis) inflammation of the retina and choroid.

retinoid (ret′ĭ-noid) resembling the retina.

retinomalacia (ret″ĭ-no-mah-la′she-ah) softening of the retina.

retinopapillitis (ret″ĭ-no-pap″ĭ-li′tis) inflammation of retina and optic disk (papilla).

retinopathy (ret″ĭ-nop′ah-the) any noninflammatory disease of the retina.
diabetic r., retinal manifestations of diabetes mellitus, including microaneurysms and punctate exudates.
exudative r., deposits of white or yellowish exudates in the fundus of the eye, with deposition of cholesterol and blood debris.
hypertensive r., exudates, hemorrhages and vascular sclerosis in the retina due to hypertension.

retinoschisis (ret″ĭ-nos′kĭ-sis) 1. a congenital cleft of the retina. 2. cleavage of retinal layers with the formation of holes, due to degenerative changes occurring with age.

retinoscope (ret′ĭ-no-skōp″) skiascope; an instrument used in skiametry.

retinoscopy (ret″ĭ-nos′ko-pe) skiametry; observation of the pupil and retina under a beam of light projected into the eye, as a means of determining refractive errors of the eye.

retinosis (ret″ĭ-no′sis) any degenerative noninflammatory condition of the retina.

retinotoxic (ret″ĭ-no-tok′sik) having a deleterious effect upon the retina.

retisolution (ret″ĭ-so-lu′shun) dissolution of the Golgi apparatus.

retort (rĕ-tort′) a globular, long-necked vessel used in distillation.

retothelioma (re″to-the″le-o′mah) a tumor composed of reticuloendothelium.

retothelium (re″to-the′le-um) reticuloendothelium.

retractile (rĕ-trak′til) susceptible of being drawn back.

retraction (rĕ-trak′shun) the act of drawing back, or condition of being drawn back.

retractor (rĕ-trak′tor) instrument for holding open the edges of a wound.

retribution (rĕ-trī-bu′shun) the unconscious granting or inflicting of one's desserts as requital for good or evil.

retro- (ret′ro, re′tro) word element [L.], *behind; posterior to.*

retroaction (ret″ro-ak′shun) action in a reversed direction.

retroauricular (ret″ro-aw-rik′u-lar) behind the auricle.

retrobulbar (ret″ro-bul′bar) behind the eyeball or medulla oblongata.

retrocecal (ret″ro-se′kal) behind the cecum.

retrocedent (ret″ro-se′dent) going back; coming back or returning.

retrocervical (ret″ro-ser′vĭ-kal) behind the cervix uteri.

retrocession (ret″ro-sesh′un) a going back, or return; specifically, a dropping backward of the entire uterus.

retrocolic (ret″ro-kol′ik) behind the colon.

retrocollic (ret″ro-kol′ik) pertaining to the back of the neck.

retrocollis (ret″ro-kol′is) spasmodic torticollis in which the head is drawn back.

retrocursive (ret″ro-ker′siv) marked by stepping backward.

retrodeviation (ret″ro-de″ve-a′shun) a bending backward.

retrodisplacement (ret″ro-dis-plās′ment) backward displacement.

retroesophageal (ret″ro-e-sof″ah-je′al) behind the esophagus.

retroflexion (ret″ro-flek′shun) the bending of an

organ so that its top is thrust backward: specifically, the bending backward of the body of the uterus upon the cervix.

retrognathia (ret″ro-nath′e-ah) position of the jaws behind the frontal plane of the forehead.

retrognathic (ret″ro-nath′ik) having a receding lower jaw.

retrograde (ret′ro-grād) going backward; retracing a former course.
   r. pyelography, radiography of the kidney after introduction of contrast medium through the ureter.

retrography (rĕ-trog′rah-fe) mirror writing.

retrogression (ret″ro-gresh′un) 1. degeneration. 2. catabolism.

retroinfection (ret″ro-in-fek′shun) infection of a mother by the fetus in utero.

retroinsular (ret″ro-in′su-lar) behind the island of Reil of the cerebral cortex.

retrolabyrinthine (ret″ro-lab″ĭ-rin′thin) behind the labyrinth of the ear.

retrolental (ret″ro-len′tal) behind the lens of the eye.
   r. fibroplasia, a condition peculiar to premature infants and characterized by the presence of opaque tissue behind the lens, leading to detachment of the retina and arrest of growth of the eye. It is the chief cause of blindness in the newborn. The cause of the condition is oxygen poisoning; a high concentration of oxygen causes spasm of the retinal vessels, which eventually leads to exudation of blood and serum through the vessel walls. To prevent this occurrence it is recommended that concentration of oxygen in the incubator not exceed 40 per cent, and that addition of oxygen be discontinued as soon as possible.

retrolingual (ret″ro-ling′gwal) behind the tongue.

retromammary (ret″ro-mam′ar-e) behind the mammary gland.

retromandibular (ret″ro-man-dib′u-lar) behind the lower jaw.

retromastoid (ret″ro-mas′toid) behind the mastoid process.

retromorphosis (ret″ro-mor-fo′sis) reversion to an earlier or more primitive form; catabolism.

retronasal (ret″ro-na′zal) pertaining to the back part of the nose.

retro-ocular (ret″ro-ok′u-lar) behind the eye.

retroparotid (ret″ro-pah-rot′id) behind the parotid gland.

retropatellar (ret″ro-pah-tel′ar) behind the patella.

retroperitoneal (ret″ro-per′ĭ-to-ne′al) behind the peritoneum.

retroperitoneum (ret″ro-per″ĭ-to-ne′um) the retroperitoneal space; the space between the peritoneum and the posterior abdominal wall.

retroperitonitis (ret″ro-per″ĭ-to-ni′tis) inflammation in the retroperitoneal space.

retropharyngeal (ret″ro-fah-rin′je-al) behind the pharynx.

retropharyngitis (ret″ro-far″in-ji′tis) inflammation of posterior part of the pharynx.

retroplasia (ret″ro-pla′ze-ah) change of a cell to an earlier type.

retroposed (ret″ro-pōsd′) displaced backward.

retroposition (ret″ro-po-zish′un) background displacement.

retropulsion (ret″ro-pul′shun) 1. a driving back, as of the fetal head in labor. 2. tendency to walk backward, as in some cases of tabes dorsalis.

retrotarsal (ret″ro-tar′sal) behind tarsus of the eye.

retrouterine (ret″ro-u′ter-in) behind the uterus.

retroversion (ret″ro-ver′zhun) the tipping backward of an entire organ, as of the uterus.

Reuss's color charts (rois′ez) charts with colored letters printed on colored backgrounds; used for testing color vision.

reversal (rĕ-ver′sal) a turning or change in the opposite direction.
   sex r., a change in characteristics from those typical of one sex to those typical of the other.

reversion (rĕ-ver′zhun) 1. a returning to a previous condition. 2. in genetics, inheritance from some remote ancestor of a character that has not been manifest for several generations.

revulsant (rĕ-vul′sant) 1. causing revulsion. 2. an agent causing revulsion.

revulsion (rĕ-vul′shun) the drawing of blood from one part to another part.

revulsive (rĕ-vul′siv) 1. causing revulsion. 2. an agent causing revulsion.

Rezipas (rez′ĭ-pas) trademark for a preparation of para-aminosalicylic acid, used in treatment of tuberculosis.

Rf. chemical symbol, *rutherfordium.*

R.F.A. right frontoanterior (position of the fetus).

R.F.P. right frontoposterior (position of the fetus).

R.F.T. right frontotransverse (position of the fetus).

Rf chemical symbol, *rutherfordium.*

Rh factor one of many types of substances called agglutinogens that may be present in the erythrocytes (red blood cells). There are at least eight different variations of these agglutinogens, and each of the agglutinogens is called an Rh factor (named for the rhesus monkey used in early experiments). If any one of these factors is present in an individual's red blood cells, he is said to be Rh positive; if the factor is absent he is said to be Rh negative. Approximately 85 per cent of all Caucasoids are Rh positive, and 15 per cent are Rh negative. Other races, such as Indians of North America, Negroes, Japanese and Chinese, are 99 to 100 per cent Rh positive.

The presence or absence of an Rh factor is especially important in blood transfusions and in pregnancy because mixing of two types of blood may result in the agglutination (clumping together) of red blood cells, with plugging of the capillaries and destruction of the red blood cells. This agglutination is an immune reaction and depends on the formation of antibodies against the specific agglutinogen (Rh factor) present in the erythrocytes. It should be pointed out that this immune reaction does not occur immediately, but depends on the gradual formation of antibodies; the response also is more severe in some persons than in others. Thus there may be no difficulty in the first transfusion of Rh-incompatible blood, but on repeated exposure to the Rh factor, the Rh-negative individual becomes "sensitized" to the agglutinogens in Rh-positive blood and builds up a greater quantity of antibodies.

In pregnancy difficulty may arise when the mother is Rh negative and the fetus is Rh positive. The Rh antigens (agglutinogens) in the fetal tissues diffuse through the placental membrane and enter the mother's blood. Her body reacts by forming anti-Rh agglutinins, which diffuse back through the placental membrane into the fetal circulation and cause clumping of the fetal erythrocytes. This condition is called ERYTHROBLASTOSIS FETALIS, or hemolytic disease of the newborn. When the erythrocytes are destroyed, hemoglobin leaks into the plasma, producing jaundice and anemia. In utero, the hemoglobin is metabolized by the mother mainly; however, post partum, the neonate cannot detoxify the excess hemoglobin pigments (bilirubin) and they may destroy nerve tissue and produce brain damage—a condition called kernicterus. The antibodies also may damage many other cells of the body.

The fetal-maternal reaction is similar to an Rh-produced transfusion reaction in that the agglutination varies in severity and usually occurs gradually. An Rh-negative mother having her first Rh-positive child usually does not build up sufficient antibodies (agglutinins) to cause harm to the fetus, but in subsequent pregnancies with Rh-positive infants she may. The incidence of erythroblastosis fetalis in infants of Rh-negative mothers depends on the number of Rh-positive children she has. If the father of the children is Rh positive and heterozygous (about 55 per cent are) about one-fourth of the offspring will be Rh negative, and will not stimulate the production of antibodies in the mother.

Scientific advances have helped reduce the risk to the Rh-positive infants of Rh-negative mothers. (See also AMNIOCENTESIS and exchange and intrauterine TRANSFUSION.) Recently it has become possible to immunize Rh-negative mothers after their first pregnancy against future Rh-incompatibility reactions. Immediately after parturition, anti-Rh antibody is injected into the mother; it combines with Rh-positive erythrocytes or substances from the fetus that have entered the maternal circulation, and renders them inert—that is, no longer capable of eliciting maternal antibody formation. Immunization must be repeated after each birth.

rhabd(o)- (rab′do) word element [Gr.], *rod; rod-shaped.*

Rhabditis (rab-di′tis) a genus of parasitic nematode worms.

rhabdium (rab′de-um) a voluntary muscle fiber.

rhabdocyte (rab′do-sīt) metamyelocyte.

rhabdoid (rab′doid) resembling a rod; rod-shaped.

rhabdomyoblastoma (rab″do-mi″o-blas-to′mah) a tumor whose cells tend to differentiate into striated muscle cells.

rhabdomyolysis (rab″do-mi-ol′ĭ-sis) disintegration of striated muscle fibers with excretion of myoglobin in the urine.

rhabdomyoma (rab″do-mi-o′mah) a tumor derived from striated muscle.

Rhabdonema (rab″do-ne′mah) Rhabditis.

rhabdophobia (rab″do-fo′be-ah) morbid dread of a stick or of a beating.

rhabdosarcoma (rab″do-sar-ko′mah) a sarcoma containing striated muscle fibers.

rhachi- for words beginning thus, see those beginning *rachi-*.

rhacoma (rah-ko′mah) 1. excoriation. 2. a pendulous scrotum.

rhagades (rag′ah-dēz) painful fissures in the skin.

-rhage see *-rrhage.*

rhaphe (ra′fe) raphe.

-rhaphy see *-rrhaphy.*

rhenium (re′ne-um) a chemical element, atomic number 75, atomic weight 186.2, symbol Re. (See table of ELEMENTS.)

rheo- (re′o) word element [Gr.], *flow; relation to electricity.*

rheobase (re′o-bās) the minimum potential of electric current necessary to produce stimulation.

rheocardiogram (re″o-kar′de-o-gram″) the graphic record obtained by rheocardiography.

rheocardiography (re″o-kar″de-og′rah-fe) a recording of the variation occurring during the cardiac cycle in the total resistance to the flow of an alternating current sent through the body.

rheochord (re′o-kord) rheostat.

rheology (re-ol′o-je) the science of the deformation and flow of matter, such as the flow of blood through the heart and blood vessels.

rheometer (re-om′ĕ-ter) 1. galvanometer. 2. an instrument for measuring rapidity of the blood current.

rheonome (re′o-nōm) an apparatus for determining the effect of irritation on a nerve.

rheophore (re′o-fōr) electrode.

rheoscope (re′o-skōp) a device indicating the presence of an electric current.

rheostat (re′o-stat) an apparatus for regulating resistance in an electric circuit.

rheostosis (re″os-to′sis) a condition of hyperostosis marked by the presence of streaks in the bones.

rheotaxis (re"o-tak'sis) orientation of a longitudinal body in a stream of liquid, with its long axis parallel with the direction of flow, designated negative (moving in the same direction) or positive (moving in the opposite direction).

rheotome (re'o-tōm) a device for breaking an electric circuit.

rheotrope (re'o-trōp) an instrument for reversing an electric current.

rhestocythemia (res"to-si-the'me-ah) the occurrence of broken-down erythrocytes in the blood.

rheum (rōōm) a watery discharge from the nose, eyes or sores.

rheumarthritis (roo"mar-thri'tis) rheumatism of the joints.

rheumatalgia (roo"mah-tal'je-ah) rheumatic pain.

rheumatic (roo-mat'ik) pertaining to or affected with rheumatism.

r. fever, a disease associated with the presence of hemolytic streptococci in the body. It is called rheumatic fever because two of the commonest symptoms are fever and pain in the joints similar to that of rheumatism. Rheumatic fever is relatively common and occurs particularly among children between 5 and 15 years of age. Young adults in the early twenties are also susceptible, although less so.

CAUSES. Rheumatic fever is believed to be a complication of an infection caused by the streptococcus that causes such common childhood illnesses as scarlet fever, tonsillitis, "strep throat" and ear infections. Rheumatic fever is only one of several complications that can result from a streptococcal infection.

The connection between rheumatic fever and a previous streptococcal infection has been proved only indirectly. That is, in almost all cases of rheumatic fever there is evidence of a previous streptococcal infection; and when these infections have been treated promptly, the occurrence of rheumatic fever has declined sharply. There is evidence that the symptoms of rheumatic fever may result from an antigen-antibody reaction to one or more of the products of the hemolytic streptoccus, but the exact way in which this occurs is not known.

Rheumatic fever tends to run in families, and there may be a hereditary predisposition to the disease. Economic and environmental conditions such as damp, cold climate and poor health habits may be contributing factors.

SYMPTOMS. The initial symptoms usually appear 1 to 4 weeks after the streptococcal infection has occurred. The actual onset of the disease may be either gradual or sudden. The symptoms vary widely and may be of any degree of severity.

The commonest initial complaints are a slight fever, a feeling of tiredness, a vague feeling of pain in the limbs and nosebleeds. If the disease takes an acute form, the fever may reach 104° F. by the second day and continue for several weeks, although the usual course of the fever is about 2 weeks. On the other hand, the fever may be quite mild.

Joint pain develops at any stage of the disease and lasts from a few hours to several weeks. The joints swell and are tender to the touch. The pain and swelling often subside in one group of joints and arise in another. As the pain subsides, the joints return to normal.

Other symptoms may include spasmodic twitching movements known as Sydenham's chorea, often called St. Vitus's dance; it is most common in girls between the ages of 6 and 11. A rash caused by the fever may appear upon the body. Nodules may be seen or felt under the skin at the elbow, knee and wrist joints, and along the spine. Among the most serious signs is the development of a heart murmur and cardiac decompensation.

HEART DAMAGE. The seriousness of rheumatic fever lies primarily in the permanent damage it can do to the heart. The disease tends to recur; and these recurrent attacks may further weaken the heart.

The usual cardiac complication of rheumatic fever is endocarditis — inflammation of the inner lining of the heart, including the membrane over the valves. As a valve heals, its edges may become so scarred and stiff that they fail to close properly. As a result, blood leaks through the valve when it is closed, producing the sound characteristic of a heart murmur. The valves may become thickened with scar tissue, so that the amount of blood that can flow through the heart is restricted. If there is severe stenosis of the mitral valve and the patient develops symptoms of congestive heart failure, surgery to enlarge the valve (COMMISSUROTOMY) may be indicated.

TREATMENT. The main purpose of treatment is to reduce the fever and pain; no means have yet been discovered for fighting the disease directly. Until the introduction of antibiotics and hormone extracts, the chief medications were aspirin and other salicylates. Antibiotics are now prescribed if there is evidence of a ongoing streptococcal infection or the chance of exposure to streptococcal infection. ACTH or cortisone may be prescribed to reduce the pain and swelling in the joints, but their effect on the ultimate course of the disease is controversial. If pain is severe, analgesic drugs may be given.

Bed rest is an important part of the treatment, particularly if the disease has caused heart damage. Depending upon the severity of the disease, the patient may be kept in bed for months, and prolonged convalescence may be needed.

NURSING CARE. In the acute phase of rheumatic fever rest is most important to reduce the work load of the heart. The patient should be made as comfortable as possible and disturbed only when necessary. Nursing care should be planned so that long periods of complete rest are possible. Proper positioning with adequate support of the limbs and maintenance of good body alignment is essential to rest and the prevention of complications.

The temperature, pulse and respirations are checked and recorded at least every 4 hours during the day. The volume and rhythm as well as the rate of the pulse should be noted. The blood pressure is taken once a day. Fluid intake may be restricted if there is edema, and sodium intake may also be limited; in either case the reason for the restriction should be explained to the patient. A record is kept of the intake and output.

Frequent back care and good oral hygiene are needed to promote comfort and relaxation. When turning the patient, one should be gentle and slow, avoiding unnecessary handling of the joints, which may be tender and swollen.

During the convalescence period the patient is allowed a gradual return to physical activities. The amount of activity depends on the physician's orders and is based on the patient's pulse rate, erythrocyte sedimentation rate and C-reaction protein test. Measures must be taken to avoid respiratory infections, which will retard the progress of the patient. Small, frequent feedings that provide a well balanced diet are usually preferred to three meals a day, which may be only partially eaten by a patient who is not engaging in a normal amount of physical activity.

As the need for rest is decreased some provision must be made for diversional activities that will help eliminate boredom and keep the child content. The psychologic effects of a prolonged period of enforced dependence on others must also be considered. The parents and the child will need encouragement and help in the transition from total dependence to relative independence.

PREVENTION. Preventive care is extremely important, especially when rheumatic fever has once occurred, since it tends to return unless precautionary steps are taken. The patient is given penicillin, orally every day or by intramuscular injection once a month, for many years in order to prevent streptococcal infection. A good nutritious diet and sufficient sleep are important. Administration of antibiotics to all patients with a history of rheumatic fever undergoing even minor surgery, including tooth extraction, is important in preventing bacterial endocarditis.

It is believed that prompt and effective treatment of "strep throat" among the general population will prevent many cases of rheumatic fever.

r. heart disease, the most important and constant manifestation of rheumatic fever, consisting of inflammatory changes with valvular deformations and other residua.

rheumatid (roo'mah-tid) a skin lesion or eruption occurring in rheumatism.

rheumatism (roo'mah-tizm) a disease marked by pain in joints or muscles; a term applied by laymen to such disorders as ARTHRITIS, OSTEOARTHRITIS, BURSITIS and SCIATICA.

acute articular r., rheumatic fever.

rheumatoid (roo'mah-toid) resembling rheumatism.

r. arthritis, a form of arthritis, the cause of which is unknown, although infection, hypersensitivity, hormone imbalance and psychologic stress have been suggested as possible causes. The disease is most common in persons 20 to 40 years old (it is relatively uncommon in children), and more than two-thirds of the patients are women.

SYMPTOMS. Rheumatoid arthritis is marked by stiff, sore joints, usually in the fingers, wrists, knees, ankles or toes. Swelling, redness and tenderness occur in the soft tissue surrounding the affected joints. In acute stages, the patient may feel severe pain, fatigue and general weakness caused by rheumatoid changes in the muscles, and there may be fever. The affected joints become painful, swollen and stiff, and the pain tends to migrate to other joints. Later, nodules may develop under the skin at sites of bony prominences.

The course of rheumatoid arthritis is unpredictable. Symptoms may stop abruptly for reasons as little understood as the causes of the disease; they usually recur just as unexpectedly. In general, joint and muscle symptoms are particularly troublesome after the patient has been inactive physically, and lessen when he resumes normal activity. Chronic rheumatoid arthritis may result in permanent deformity and immobility of joints.

TREATMENT. Proper care and early treatment are essential to recovery and to the prevention of permanent damage to the joints. Though no specific cure has been found for rheumatoid arthritis, most patients respond well to treatment involving salicylates, cortisone and gold salts and carefully regulated programs of alternating rest and therapeutic exercise (see ARTHRITIS). The disease is progressive and likely to recur, sometimes with increasing intensity. In about 15 per cent of the cases, some degree of permanent stiffness eventually develops.

RHEUMATOID ARTHRITIS IN CHILDREN. About 5 per cent of all patients with rheumatoid arthritis are children, with the onset of the illness occurring between the ages of 2 and 4 years. The disease is self-limited, usually lasting about 3 years. It begins quite abruptly with a spiking fever to as high as 106° F., pain and swelling of joints and a rash. During the clinical course there often are periods of remission followed by sudden exacerbations of symptoms. Treatment is the same as for adults.

Because of the nature of the disease and the age of the patient, a long-term plan of home care is necessary. The parents, local physician and community agencies concerned with chronic illness should participate in the planning and care of the child so that a coordinated and disciplined program can be carried out.

r. factor, a protein of high molecular weight in the serum of most patients with rheumatoid arthritis, detectable by serologic tests.

rheumatology (roo"mah-tol'o-je) the study of rheumatic conditions.

rheumatosis (roo"mah-to'sis) any disorder of rheumatic origin.

rheumic (roo'mik) pertaining to a rheum or flux.

rhexis (rek'sis) the rupture of a blood vessel or of an organ.

rhigosis (rĭ-go'sis) the perception of cold.

rhin(o)- (ri'no) word element [Gr.], *nose; noselike structure.*

rhinal (ri'nal) pertaining to the nose.

rhinalgia (ri-nal'je-ah) pain in the nose.

rhinencephalon (ri"nen-sef'ah-lon) the portion of the brain concerned with the sense of smell.

rhinesthesia (ri"nes-the'ze-ah) the sense of smell.

rhineurynter (ri"nu-rin'ter) a dilatable bag for distending a nostril.

rhinion (rin'e-on) the lower end of the suture between the nasal bones.

rhinitis (ri-ni'tis) inflammation of the mucous membrane of the nose. It may be mild and chronic, or acute and of short duration.

Viruses, bacteria and allergens are responsible

for the varied manifestations of rhinitis. Often a viral rhinitis is complicated by a bacterial infection caused by streptococci, staphylococci and pneumococci or other bacteria. Hay fever, an acute type of allergic rhinitis, is also subject to bacterial complications. Many factors assist the invasion of the mucous membranes by bacteria, including allergens, excessive dryness, exposure to dampness and cold, excessive inhalation of dust and injury to the nasal cilia due to viral infection.

In general, rhinitis is not serious but some forms may be contagious. The mucous membrane of the nose becomes swollen and there is a nasal discharge. Some types are accompanied by fever, muscle aches and general discomfort with sneezing and running eyes. Breathing through the nose may become difficult or impossible. Often rhinitis is accompanied by inflammation of the throat and sinuses. If bacterial infection develops, the nasal discharge is thick and contains pus.

In acute rhinitis, the medical term for the COMMON COLD, the best treatment consists of rest, preferably in bed, a well balanced diet, and sufficient fluids. Aspirin will relieve headache and fever.

Chronic rhinitis may result in a permanent thickening of the nasal mucosa. Treatment is aimed at eliminating the primary cause of rhinitis and administration of decongestants to relieve nasal congestion.

rhinoantritis (ri″no-an-tri′tis) inflammation of the mucous membrane of the nose and maxillary sinus (antrum of Highmore).

rhinocheiloplasty (ri″no-ki′lo-plas″te) plastic surgery of the nose and lip.

rhinocleisis (ri″no-kli′sis) obstruction of the nasal passage.

rhinodacryolith (ri″no-dak′re-o-lith″) a lacrimal concretion in the nasal duct.

rhinodynia (ri″no-din′e-ah) pain in the nose.

rhinogenous (ri-noj′ĕ-nus) arising in the nose.

rhinolalia (ri″-no-la′le-ah) a nasal quality of speech from a defect or disease of the nasal passages.
　　r. aper′ta, that due to too great opening of the nasal passages.
　　r. clau′sa, that due to undue closure of the nasal passages.

rhinolaryngitis (ri″no-lar″in-ji′tis) inflammation of the mucous membrane of the nose and larynx.

rhinolith (ri′no-lith) a nasal calculus.

rhinolithiasis (ri″no-lĭ-thi′ah-sis) the formation of nasal calculi.

rhinometer (ri-nom′ĕ-ter) an apparatus for measuring the nose or its cavities.

rhinomycosis (ri″no-mi-ko′sis) fungus infection of the nasal mucosa.

rhinonecrosis (ri″no-nĕ-kro′sis) necrosis of the nasal bones.

rhinopathy (ri-nop′ah-the) any disease of the nose.

rhinopharyngitis (ri″no-far″in-ji′tis) inflammation of the nasopharynx.

rhinopharyngocele (ri″no-fah-ring′go-sēl) a tumor of the nasopharynx.

rhinophonia (ri″no-fo′ne-ah) a nasal twang or quality of voice.

rhinophore (ri′no-fōr) a nasal cannula to facilitate breathing.

rhinophyma (ri″no-fi′mah) nodular congestion and enlargement of the nose.

rhinoplasty (ri′no-plas″te) plastic reconstruction of the nose.

rhinopolypus (ri″no-pol′ĭ-pus) a nasal polyp.

rhinorrhagia (ri″no-ra′je-ah) nosebleed; epistaxis.

rhinorrhea (ri″no-re′ah) copious mucous discharge from the nose.
　　cerebrospinal r., discharge of cerebrospinal fluid through the nose, usually due to skull fracture.

rhinosalpingitis (ri″no-sal″pin-ji′tis) inflammation of the mucosa of the nose and eustachian tube.

rhinoscleroma (ri″no-sklĕ-ro′mah) a granulomatous disease involving the nose and nasopharynx. The growth forms hard patches or nodules, which tend to increase in size and are painful on pressure. The disease occurs in Egypt, eastern Europe and Central and South America.

rhinoscope (ri′no-skōp) a speculum for nasal examination.

rhinoscopy (ri-nos′ko-pe) examination of the nose with a speculum, through either the anterior nares or the nasopharynx.

rhinostegnosis (ri″no-steg-no′sis) obstruction of the nasal passages.

rhinotomy (ri-not′o-me) incision into the nose.

rhinovirus (ri″no-vi′rus) one of a group of viral agents found associated with the common cold.

rhizo- (ri′zo) word element [Gr.], *root.*

rhizoblast (ri′zo-blast) a delicate fibril connecting the basal granule and nucleus of a protozoan.

rhizode (ri′zōd) a rootlike structure, such as a projection from a colony of microorganisms into the medium on which it is grown.

rhizome (ri′zōm) the subterraneous root stock of a plant.

rhizomelic (ri″zo-mel′ik) pertaining to the hips and shoulders (the roots of the limbs).

rhizomeningomyelitis (ri″zo-mĕ-ning″go-mi″ĕ-li′tis) radiculomeningomyelitis; inflammation of the nerve roots, meninges and spinal cord.

rhizoneure (ri′zo-nūr) a nerve cell forming a nerve root.

Rhizopoda (ri-zop′o-dah) a division of protozoa that includes the amebae.

rhizopodium (ri″zo-po′de-um), pl. *rhizopo′dia* [Gr.] a filamentous pseudopodium, characterized by branching and anastomosis of the branches.

rhizotomy (ri-zot′o-me) division or transection of a nerve root, either within the spinal canal or outside it.

rhod(o)- (ro′do) word element [Gr.], *red.*

rhodium (ro′de-um) a chemical element, atomic number 45, atomic weight 102.905, symbol Rh. (See table of ELEMENTS.)

rhodocyte (ro′do-sīt) erythrocyte.

rhodogenesis (ro″do-jen′ĕ-sis) restoration of the purple tint to rhodopsin after its bleaching by the light.

rhodophylaxis (ro″do-fi-lak′sis) the supposed property of the retinal epithelium of protecting and increasing the power of rhodopsin to regain its color after bleaching.

rhodoporphyrin (ro″do-por′fĭ-rin) a porphyrin derived from chlorophyll.

rhodopsin (ro-dop′sin) the visual purple: a photosensitive purple-red chromoprotein in the retinal rods. Lack of rhodopsin results in NIGHT BLINDNESS. Vitamin A is the primary source of rhodopsin.

rhombencephalon (romb″en-sef′ah-lon) 1. the hindbrain, including the medulla oblongata, pons and cerebellum. 2. the most caudal of the three primary vesicles formed in embryonic development of the brain, which later divides into the metencephalon and the myelencephalon.

rhombocoele (rom′bo-sēl) the terminal expansion of the canal of the spinal cord.

rhomboid (rom′boid) shaped like a rhomb or kite.

rhonchus (rong′kus) a coarse dry rale in the bronchial tubes. adj., **rhon′chal, rhon′chial.**

rhotacism (ro′tah-sizm) faulty enunciation or overuse of *r* sounds.

rhubarb (roo′barb) the dried rhizome and root of *Rheum officinale*; used in fluidextract or aromatic tincture as a cathartic.

Rhus (rus) a genus of trees and shrubs, many of them poisonous. Contact with certain species produces a severe dermatitis. The most important poisonous species are *R. diversilo′ba*, or poison oak, *R. toxicoden′dron*, or poison ivy, and *R. venena′ta*, or poison sumac. Most species of Rhus are sometimes classified in the genus Toxicodendron. (See also POISON IVY, OAK AND SUMAC.)

rhypophagy (ri-pof′ah-je) the eating of filth.

rhypophobia (ri″po-fo′be-ah) morbid fear of filth.

rhythm (rithm) regularity of occurrence, as of variation of energy, electrical discharge, muscular contraction or other phenomenon. adj., **rhyth′mic, rhyth′mical.**
    alpha r., in electroencephalography, the dominant 8 to 12 per second rhythm seen in the normal resting adult.
    biologic r., the established regularity with which certain phenomena recur in living organisms.
    circadian r., the regular recurrence in cycles of approximately 24 hours from one stated point to another, e.g., certain biologic activities that occur at that interval regardless of constant darkness or other conditions of illumination.
    coupled r., an abnormal relation between pulse and heartbeat, every other beat of the heart producing no pulse at the wrist.
    delta r., the rhythm of 6 per second seen in the electroencephalogram with sleep.
    gallop r., a cardiac cycle with an accentuated extra sound, creating an auscultatory effect like the sound of a galloping horse.
    nodal r., heart rhythm initiated by the atrioventricular node of the heart.
    sinus r., the normal heart rhythm originating in the sinoatrial node.
    ventricular r., the ventricular contractions occurring in complete heart block.

rhythmicity (rith-mis′ĭ-te) a state of rhythmic contraction.

rhytidoplasty (rit′ĭ-do-plas″te) plastic surgery for the elimination of wrinkles from the skin.

rhytidosis (rit″ĭ-do′sis) a wrinkling, as of the cornea.

rib (rib) any one of the paired bones, 12 on either side, extending from the thoracic vertebrae toward the median line on the ventral aspect of the trunk.
    abdominal r′s, asternal r′s, false ribs.
    cervical r., a supernumerary rib arising from a cervical vertebra.
    false r′s, the five lower ribs on either side, not attached directly to the sternum.
    floating r′s, the two lower false ribs on either side, attached only to the vertebrae.
    slipping r., one whose attaching cartilage is repeatedly dislocated.
    true r′s, the seven upper ribs on either side, attached to both vertebrae and sternum.
    vertebral r′s, floating ribs.
    vertebrocostal r′s, the three upper false ribs on either side, attached to vertebrae and costal cartilages.
    vertebrosternal r′s, true ribs.

riboflavin (ri″bo-fla′vin) vitamin B$_2$, a yellow crystalline powder, apparently concerned in the metabolism of all living cells; called also lactoflavin.
    Symptoms of riboflavin deficiency (ariboflavinosis) include general weakness, weight loss, lesions at the corners of the mouth, on the lips and around the nose, reddening and soreness of the tip and edges of the tongue, corneal and other eye changes and seborrheic dermatitis.
    Foods with the highest content of riboflavin are liver, kidney, heart, brewer's yeast, milk, greens and enriched cereals. Riboflavin deficiency is most common among people of the southeastern United States and other regions, such as Asia and the West Indies, where the diet is likely to contain relatively large quantities of corn, potatoes and rice, which lack riboflavin. A well balanced diet will prevent riboflavin deficiency; it will also correct the disorder, with the help of supplementary doses of riboflavin and other vitamins.

ribonuclease (ri″bo-nu′kle-ās) an enzyme that catalyzes the depolymerization of ribonucleic acid.

ribonucleic acid (ri″bo-nu-kle′ik) RNA, a nucleic acid found in all living cells which on hydrolysis yields adenine, guanine, cytosine, uracil, ribose and phosphoric acid; it takes part in protein synthesis in the cell. Messenger RNA is an RNA fraction of intermediate molecular weight that transfers information from deoxyribonucleic acid (DNA) in the nucleus to the protein-forming system of the cell. Ribosomal RNA is nonspecific RNA present in ribosomes with almost equal proportions of protein. Soluble RNA, or transfer RNA, is an RNA fraction of low molecular weight that combines with one amino acid species, transferring it from activating enzyme to ribosome to facilitate synthesis of a specific polypeptide.

ribonucleoprotein   (ri″bo-nu″kle-o-pro′te-in) a nucleoprotein that yields a ribonucleic acid on hydrolysis.

ribose (ri′bōs) an aldopentose found in and characteristic of ribonucleic acid.
   r. nucleic acid, ribonucleic acid.

ribosome   (ri′bo-sōm) a submicroscopic ribonucleic acid-containing particle in the cytoplasm of a cell, sometimes closely associated with endoplasmic reticulum, and the site of cellular protein synthesis.

Richards (rich′ardz) Melinda Ann (1841–1930). "America's first trained nurse," the first graduate of the Training School of the New England Hospital in Boston, in 1873. She devoted her life to active nursing and to the training of other nurses.

ricinism (ri′si-nizm) intoxication due to inhalation or ingestion of a poisonous principle (ricin) of castor bean, producing superficial inflammation of the respiratory mucosa with hemorrhages into the lung, or edema of the gastrointestinal tract with hemorrhages.

Ricinus communis (ris′i-nus kom-u′nis) the plant whose seeds afford castor oil.

rickets (rik′ets) a condition of infancy and childhood caused by deficiency of vitamin D, which leads to altered calcium and phosphorus metabolism and consequent disturbance of ossification of bone. Because of the widespread use of vitamin D-fortified milk, together with the additional vitamins that most infants are given, the disease is now uncommon in the United States.
   Since the action of sunlight on the skin produces vitamin D in the human body, rickets often occurs in parts of the world where the winter is especially long, and where smoke and fog constantly intercept the sun. Negroes and other dark-skinned people are somewhat more susceptible to the disease if they live in areas with little sunlight, since the pigment in the skin blocks absorption of the sun's rays.
   When a vitamin D deficiency occurs in adults, it produces a condition known as OSTEOMALACIA, softening of the bone.
   SYMPTOMS.   A major symptom of rickets is softening (decalcification) of the bones. In children, this can produce various degrees of deformity, including nodules on the ribs and flexibility and bending of bones. Bowleg and knock-knee and an improperly developed or misshapen skull of a squared or boxed appearance are typical. The ability of the bones to support the body is seriously impaired.
   PREVENTION.   A proper diet that includes vitamin D-fortified milk is usually sufficient to prevent rickets. Ordinary milk contains adequate amounts of calcium but is a poor source of vitamin D. Small amounts of the vitamin are present in eggs, and in such fish as cod, herring, tuna, sardines and salmon.

Sunlight and other sources of ultraviolet light are beneficial.
   TREATMENT.   Treatment of an active case of rickets involves the administration of vitamin D concentrate. The response to treatment usually is rapid.
   There is a type of vitamin D-resistant rickets in which excessive loss of calcium and phosphorus does not respond to the usual doses of vitamin D. This condition is often familial. Treatment involves massive doses of vitamin D and calcium supplements in the diet.
   fetal r., achondroplasia.

Rickettsia (ri-ket′se-ah) a genus of small, rod-shaped to round microorganisms found in the cytoplasm of tissue cells of lice, fleas, ticks and mites, and transmitted to man by their bites.
   The diseases caused by rickettsiae can be classified in five groups: the spotted fever group (Rocky Mountain spotted fever, boutonneuse fever and rickettsialpox); the typhus group (epidemic typhus and endemic typhus); a tsutsugamushi group (scrub typhus); Q fever; and trench fever.
   Rickettsial diseases are not common in communities with high sanitary standards, since prevention depends on controlling the rodent and insect populations. Major epidemics have occurred, especially in times of war when standards of sanitation drop.

rickettsial (ri-ket′se-al) pertaining to or caused by rickettsiae.

Rickettsiales (ri-ket″se-a′lez) an order of Microtatobiotes, parasitic in both vertebrates and invertebrates.

rickettsialpox (ri-ket′se-al-poks″) a febrile disease with vesiculopapular eruption, caused by rickettsiae and transmitted by mites carried by house mice; called also Kew Gardens fever.

rickettsicidal   (ri-ket″si-si′dal) destructive to rickettsiae.

ridge (rij) a linear projection or elevation, as on a bone, or a linear thickening of other tissue, as in the embryo.
   dental r., any linear elevation on the crown of a tooth.
   germ r., an epithelial ridge on the embryonic mesonephros, giving rise to the sexual elements.
   mammary r., an ectodermal thickening in early embryos, along which the mammary glands subsequently develop.

Rift Valley fever a febrile disease of viral origin; its symptoms resemble those of dengue, and it is rarely fatal.

rigidity (ri-jid′i-te) inflexibility or stiffness.
   clasp-knife r., increased tension in the extensors of a joint when it is passively flexed, giving way suddenly on exertion of further pressure; seen especially in upper motor neuron disease.
   cogwheel r., tension in a muscle that gives way in little jerks when the muscle is passively stretched; seen in paralysis agitans.

rigor (rig′or, ri′gor) a chill; rigidity.
   r. mor′tis, rigidity of skeletal muscles, developing 6 to 10 hours after death and persisting for 3 or 4 days.

rima (ri'mah), pl. *ri'mae* [L.] a linear opening between two more or less parallel borders.

r. **glot'tidis,** the opening between the vocal cords.

r. **o'ris,** the opening of the mouth.

r. **palpebra'rum,** the slit between the eyelids.

r. **puden'di,** the space between the labia majora; called also pudendal fissure.

Rimifon (rim'ĭ-fon) trademark for a preparation of isoniazid, used in treatment of tuberculosis.

rimula (rim'u-lah), pl. *rim'ulae* [L.] a minute fissure.

ring (ring) a circular or continuous structure, as one surrounding an opening in an organ or in the body wall, or, in chemistry, a collection of atoms united in a continuous or closed chain.

abdominal r., external, an opening in the aponeurosis of the external oblique muscle for the spermatic cord or round ligament.

abdominal r., internal, an aperture in the transverse fascia for the spermatic cord or round ligament.

benzene r., the hexagon representing the arrangement of carbon atoms in a molecule of benzene, different compounds being derived by replacement of the hydrogen atoms by different elements or compounds.

constriction r., a thickened area of myometrium during labor, over a point of depression in the fetal body or at a point just below it.

retraction r., pathologic, a complication of prolonged labor marked by failure of relaxation of the circular fibers at the internal opening of the cervix, obstructing delivery of the infant.

retraction r., physiologic, the demarcation between the upper, contracting portion of the uterus in labor and the lower, dilating part.

umbilical r., the orifice in the abdominal wall of the fetus for transmission of the umbilical vein and arteries.

vascular r., a congenital anomaly of the aortic arch and its tributaries, the vessels forming a ring about the trachea and esophagus and causing varying degrees of compression.

Ringer's solution (ring'erz) a sterile solution of sodium chloride, potassium choride and calcium chloride in purified water, a physiologic salt solution for topical use.

ringworm (ring'werm) the popular name for a fungus infection of the skin, even though it is not caused by a worm and is not always ring-shaped in appearance.

Ringworm is caused by a group of related fungi of different types. These parasites feed on the body's waste products of dead skin and perspiration. They attack the skin in various areas, especially in body folds, such as the armpit and crotch. One type found between the toes is called ATHLETE'S FOOT; another affects the soles and toenails.

Some forms of ringworm, usually found in children and frequently traced to exposure to infected pets, attack the scalp and exposed areas of the body, particularly the arms and legs. These infections appear as reddish patches, often scaly or blistered, and may cause destruction of the hair shaft. They sometimes become ring-shaped as the infection spreads out while its center heals or seems to heal. There is itching and soreness.

The fungi are highly contagious and are spread by humans, animals and even objects, such as combs or towels handled by infected persons. Scratching is almost certain to pass the infection from one part of the body to another.

Ringworm is treated with antifungal drugs. Prevention is largely a matter of cleanliness. All parts of the body should be washed with soap and water, especially hairy areas and body folds where perspiration is likely to collect. Thorough drying is as important as bathing, for the fungi thrive in warm dampness.

Rinne test (rin'nĕ) a test of hearing made with tuning forks, comparing the duration of perception by bone conduction and by air conduction. In the normal ear, the fork is heard twice as long by air conduction as by bone conduction.

RISA (ri'sah) trademark for a preparation of radioiodinated serum albumin, used for measuring blood volume and cardiac output.

ristocetin (ris"to-se'tin) an antibiotic substance derived from culture of *Nocardia lurida*; used in treatment of infections by gram-positive cocci.

risus (ri'sus) [L.] laughter.

r. **sardon'icus,** a grinning expression produced by spasm of the facial muscles.

Ritalin (rit'ah-lin) trademark for preparations of methylphenidate, a mild central nervous system stimulant and antidepressant.

Ritter's disease (rit'erz) exfoliative dermatitis of infants.

riziform (riz'ĭ-form) resembling grains of rice.

R.L.L. right lower lobe (of lung).

R.L.Q. right lower quadrant (of abdomen).

R.M.A. right mentoanterior (position of the fetus).

R.M.P. right mentoposterior (position of the fetus).

R.M.T. right mentotransverse (position of the fetus).

R.N. Registered Nurse.

Rn chemical symbol, *radon.*

RNA ribonucleic acid.

R.O.A. right occipitoanterior (position of the fetus).

Robalate (ro'bah-lāt) trademark for preparations of dihydroxyaluminum aminoacetate, an antacid.

Robaxin (ro-bak'sin) trademark for preparations of methocarbamol, a skeletal muscle relaxant.

Robb (rob) Isabel Hampton (1860–1910). An early leader in nursing education, the first "principal" of Johns Hopkins School of Nursing in Baltimore and a founder of the forerunner of the American Nurses' Association.

Roccal (ro'kal) trademark for a preparation of benzalkonium chloride, a disinfectant and germicide.

Rocky Mountain spotted fever an infectious disease marked by fever, headache, muscle pain, rash and mental symptoms; called also tick fever.

Rocky Mountain spotted fever belongs to a group

of insect-borne fevers caused by microscopic parasites known as rickettsiae, which attack the cells lining small blood vessels. The strain responsible for Rocky Mountain spotted fever is transmitted from rodent to man by the wood tick. In the eastern and southern states, it is transmitted by the dog tick, and is sometimes called Eastern spotted fever.

SYMPTOMS. After the bite of the infected tick, there is an incubation period of 3 to 10 days before the major symptoms set in. Within a day or two after the bite, the victim may feel somewhat ill and lose his appetite. The actual onset is marked by chills or chilly sensations, fever, headache, pain behind the eyes, joint and muscle pain and photophobia. Other symptoms are nausea, vomiting, sore throat and abdominal pain. Some patients become highly irritable and delirious, or so lethargic that they may lapse into a stupor or coma. Usually 3 to 5 days after the onset a rash appears on the wrists and ankles, then spreads to the trunk and limbs and occasionally to the face.

The appearance and progress of small red spots that eventually become larger sores distinguish Rocky Mountain spotted fever from the several diseases it resembles in its other symptoms (measles, typhoid fever, typhus).

TREATMENT AND PREVENTION. Like other rickettsial diseases, Rocky Mountain spotted fever responds readily to treatment with tetracyclines and chloramphenicol. If untreated, it can be extremely serious and often fatal. Preventive measures are directed mainly against the disease-carrying ticks and rodents.

rod (rod) a straight, slim mass of substance; specifically, one of the retinal rods, highly specialized cylindrical neuroepithelial cells containing rhodopsin, which, with the retinal cones, form the light-sensitive elements of the retina.

Corti's r's, stiff, pillar-like structures forming two rows in the organ of Corti.

Heidenhain's r's, rodlike epithelial striations in the tubules of the kidney.

rodenticide (ro-den′tĭ-sīd) an agent destructive to rodents.

rodonalgia (ro″do-nal′je-ah) erythromelalgia.

Roentgen (rent′gen) Wilhelm Conrad (1845–1923). German physicist, born at Lennep (Rhineland). For his accidental discovery of x-rays in 1895, while experimenting with a cathode-ray tube, he received the first Nobel prize for physics in 1901.

roentgen (rent′gen) a special unit (2.58×10^{-4} coulomb per kilogram of air) used in expressing the amount of exposure to x-rays or gamma rays; symbol R.

r. ray, x-ray.

roentgenism (rent′gen-izm) 1. the therapeutic application of x-rays. 2. disease due to excessive exposure to x-rays.

roentgenkymogram (rent″gen-ki′mo-gram) the film obtained by roentgenkymography.

roentgenkymograph (rent″gen-ki′mo-graf) the apparatus used in roentgenkymography.

roentgenkymography (rent″gen-ki-mog′rah-fe) a technique of graphically recording the movements of an organ by means of x-rays.

roentgenogram (rent′gen-o-gram″) a film produced by roentgenography.

roentgenography (rent″gĕ-nog′rah-fe) the taking of pictures (roentgenograms) of internal structures of the body by passage of x-rays through the body to act on specially sensitized film.

body-section r., x-ray visualization of structures lying in a particular plane of the body by various techniques which cause blurring of the images of structures in other planes.

miniature r., the taking of radiograms on small films, to screen for certain diseases.

mucosal relief r., a technique for revealing any abnormality of the intestinal mucosa, involving injection and evacuation of a barium enema, followed by inflation of the intestine with air under light pressure. The light coating of barium on the inflated intestine in the roentgenogram reveals clearly even small abnormalities.

serial r., the making of several exposures of a particular area at arbitrary intervals.

spot film r., the recording on film of any desired area at any time during fluoroscopic examination.

roentgenologist (rent″gĕ-nol′o-jist) a specialist in roentgenology.

roentgenology (rent″gĕ-nol′o-je) the scientific study of the diagnostic and therapeutic use of x-rays.

roentgenolucent (rent″gen-o-lu′sent) permitting the passage of x-rays.

roentgenometry (rent″gĕ-nom′ĕ-tre) measurement of the penetrating or therapeutic power of x-rays.

roentgenopaque (rent″gen-o-pāk′) not permitting the passage of x-rays.

roentgenoscope (rent′gen-o-skōp′) a fluoroscope; an apparatus for examining the body by means of the fluorescent screen excited by x-rays.

roentgenoscopy (rent″gĕ-nos′ko-pe) fluoroscopy.

roentgenotherapy (rent″gen-o-ther′ah-pe) treatment by x-rays.

Roger's disease (ro-zhāz′) an abnormal congenital communication between the ventricles of the heart.

Rokitansky's disease (ro″kĭ-tan′skēz) acute yellow atrophy of the liver.

Rolicton (ro-lik′ton) trademark for a preparation of amisometradine, a diuretic.

rolitetracycline (ro″le-tet″rah-si′klēn) an antibiotic compound used for intravenous or intramuscular injection.

rombergism (rom′berg-izm) the tendency of a patient to sway when he stands still with feet close together and eyes closed; associated with loss of position sense.

Romilar (ro′mil-ar) trademark for preparations of dextromethorphan hydrobromide, an antitussant.

rongeur (ron-zher′) [Fr.] a forceps designed for use in cutting bone.

room (rōōm) a place in a building enclosed and set apart for occupancy.

delivery r., a hospital room to which an obstetric patient is taken for delivery.

intensive therapy r., intensive care unit, a hospital unit in which are concentrated special equipment and skilled personnel for seriously ill patients requiring immediate and continuous care and observation.

labor r., predelivery room.

operating r., a room in a hospital used for surgical operations.

postdelivery r., a recovery room for the care of obstetric patients immediately after delivery.

predelivery r., a hospital room where an obstetric patient remains during the first stage of labor, i.e., from the time contractions begin until she is ready for delivery.

recovery r., a hospital unit adjoining operating or delivery rooms, with special equipment and personnel for the care of postoperative or obstetric patients until they may safely be returned to general duty nursing care in their own room or ward.

root (root) 1. the descending and subterranean part of a plant. 2. that portion of an organ, such as a tooth, hair or nail, that is buried in the tissues, or by which it arises from another structure.

nerve r., anterior, the structure composed of efferent (motor) fibers emerging from the anterior aspect of the spinal cord and, with the fibers of the posterior root, forming the spinal NERVE; called also motor root and ventral root.

nerve r., posterior, the structure composed of afferent (sensory) fibers emerging from a spinal NERVE and entering the dorsolateral aspect of the spinal cord; called also dorsal root and sensory root.

R.O.P. right occipitoposterior (position of the fetus).

Rorschach test (ror'shahk) one for disclosing personality traits and conflicts by the patient's interpretation of 10 cards bearing symmetrical ink blots in various colors and shading.

rosacea (ro-za'she-ah) a chronic disease affecting the skin of the nose, forehead and cheeks, marked by flushing, followed by red coloration due to capillary dilatation, with the appearance of papules and acne-like pustules; called also acne rosacea and brandy face.

rosaniline (ro-zan'ĭ-lin) a substance from coal tar, the basis of various dyes and stains.

rosary (ro'zah-re) a structure resembling a string of beads.

rachitic r., a series of palpable or visible prominences at the points where the ribs join their cartilages: seen in certain cases of rickets.

roseola (ro-ze'o-lah) a rose-colored rash; specifically, epidemic roseola, or rubeola.

r. choler'ica, an eruption sometimes seen in cholera.

epidemic r., rubeola.

r. infantum, a fairly common acute viral disease that usually occurs in children less than 24 months old; called also exanthem subitum, it attacks suddenly but disappears in a few days, leaving no permanent marks.

Diagnosis is difficult because the sole symptom at first, beyond irritability and drowsiness, is fever. There may be convulsions, and generally the fever is very high; 104° F. is not unusual. Despite the high fever, the disease is quite mild. Treatment consists only of such standard measures as aspirin and tepid sponge baths to allay the fever..

As the fever subsides, in 3 or 4 days, and the disease is apparently at an end, a pink-reddish rash breaks out, usually on the body. This is completely unlike the course of other childhood diseases, such as measles, scarlet fever and chickenpox, in which the rash is present during the most intense phase of the illness.

The rash of roseola infantum does not persist for more than a few days, and, in fact, may disappear in a few hours. Very often it is so transitory that it is entirely missed. Once the disease is over, the child is believed to be immune for life against further attacks.

syphilitic r., an eruption of rose-colored spots in early secondary syphilis.

r. typho'sa, the eruption of typhoid fever or typhus.

r. vacci'nia, a rash sometimes occurring after vaccination.

rosette (ro-zet') any structure or formation resembling a rose, such as (1) the clusters of polymorphonuclear leukocytes around a globule of lysed nuclear material, as observed in the test for disseminated lupus erythematosus, or (2) a figure formed by the chromosomes in an early stage of mitosis (spireme).

rosin (roz'in) the solid resin obtained from species of Pinus, a genus of trees; used in preparation of ointments and plasters.

rostellum (ros-tel'um) the hook-bearing part of the head of worms.

rostral (ros'tral) 1. resembling a rostrum. 2. directed toward the front end of the body.

rostrum (ros'trum), pl. *ros'tra* [L.], a beak-shaped process.

R.O.T. right occipitotransverse (position of the fetus).

rot (rot) decay.

rotation (ro-ta'shun) the process of turning around an axis. In obstetrics, the turning of the fetal head or presenting part 90 degrees so as to accommodate to the pelvic outlet. It should occur naturally, but if it does not it must be accomplished manually or instrumentally by the obstetrician.

rotenone (ro'tĕ-nōn) a poisonous compound from derris root and other roots; used as an insecticide and as a scabicide.

rotula (rot'u-lah) 1. the patella. 2. a lozenge or troche.

rotular (rot'u-lar) pertaining to the patella.

roughage (ruf'ij) coarse, largely indigestible material, such as bran, cereals, fruit and vegetable fibers, that acts as an irritant to stimulate intestinal evacuation.

rouleau (roo-lo'), pl. *rouleaux'* [Fr.], a role of erythrocytes resembling a pile of coins.

roundworm (round'werm) one of various types of parasitic nematode worms, somewhat resembling the common earthworm, which sometimes invade the human intestinal tract and multiply there. Very common among them is the pinworm, or seatworm, which infects 10 per cent of the population of North America. Others include the ascarids, the hookworm and the trichina, which causes TRICHINOSIS. These worms can all impair health to varying degrees, but proper treatment will generally eliminate them. (See also WORMS.)

R.P.F. renal plasma flow.

rpm revolutions per minute.

R.Q. respiratory quotient.

-rrhachia (ra′ke-ah) word element [Gr.], *state of the spinal fluid*; spelled also *-rachia*.

-rrhachis (ra′kis) word element [Gr.], *spinal cord*.

-rrhage, -rrhagia (rāj), (ra′je-ah) word element [Gr.], *excessive flow*. adj., **-rrhag′ic.**

-rrhaphy (rah′fe) word element [Gr.], *stitching; suture*. adj., **-rrhaph′ic.**

-rrhea (re′ah) word element [Gr.], *profuse flow*; adj., **-rrhe′ic.**

-rrhexis (rek′sis) word element [Gr.], *rupture; bursting*. adj., **-rrhec′tic.**

rRNA ribosomal RNA (ribonucleic acid).

R.S.A. right sacroanterior (position of the fetus).

R.Sc.A. right scapuloanterior (position of the fetus).

R.Sc.P. right scapuloposterior (position of the fetus).

R.S.N.A. Radiological Society of North America.

R.S.P. right sacroposterior (position of the fetus).

R.S.T. right sacrotransverse (position of the fetus).

Ru chemical symbol, *ruthenium*.

rubber-dam (rub′er-dam) a sheet of thin latex rubber used by dentists to isolate a tooth from the fluids of the mouth during dental treatment, and in some surgical procedures to isolate certain tissues or structures.

rubedo (roo-be′do) redness of the skin.

rubefacient (roo″bĕ-fa′shent) 1. reddening the skin. 2. an agent that reddens the skin.

rubella (roo-bel′ah) a mild systemic disease caused by a virus and characterized by fever and a transient rash; called also German measles and 3-day measles.

Rubella can be dangerous to a pregnant woman because the virus can damage the developing embryo. The danger is greatest during the first trimester, although recent research has shown that the virus can be harmful at any stage of pregnancy. The location and extent of congenital anomaly that can result are determined in large measure by the developmental stage of the embryo at the time the virus attacks. Congenital heart defects, cataract, mental retardation and deafness are some of the more common defects resulting from maternal rubella.

Rubella is not as contagious as chickenpox or measles, but there are frequent epidemics among school children, usually during the spring and early summer. The virus is spread by direct contact and

by droplet infection. The patient can transmit the disease from the first appearance of symptoms until the rash disappears, usually a total of 3 or 4 days. The incubation period of rubella is usually 16 to 18 days.

Rubella begins with a slight cold, some fever and a sore throat. The lymph nodes just behind the ears and at the back of the neck may swell, causing some soreness or pain when the head is moved. The rash appears first on the face and scalp, and spreads to the body and arms the same day. Rubella rash is similar to that of MEASLES, although the spots usually do not run together. The rubella rash fades after 2 or 3 days, although in a few cases the disease may last as long as a week.

TREATMENT AND PREVENTION. Except for complications that may result if the disease is contracted during pregnancy, other complications are quite rare. The patient may be kept in bed for the duration of the illness, but no special treatment, medicine or diet is necessary unless the patient has a high fever. One attack of German measles usually gives lifetime immunity to the disease, although a second attack does occasionally occur.

A vaccine against rubella is available. It is given in a single subcutaneous injection to children more than a year old. It is never given to a pregnant woman, or to any woman who might become pregnant in the succeeding 2 months.

rubeola (roo-be′o-lah, ru″be-o′lah) 1. measles. 2. rubella.

rubeosis (roo″be-o′sis) redness.
  r. i′ridis, a condition characterized by a new formation of vessels and connective tissue on the surface of the iris frequently seen in diabetics.

rubescent (roo-bes′ent) growing red.

rubidium (roo-bid′e-um) a chemical element, atomic number 37, atomic weight 85.47, symbol Rb. (See table of ELEMENTS.)

Rubin test (roo′bin) a test for patency of the uterine tubes, made by transuterine inflation with carbon dioxide gas.

rubor (roo′bor) [L.] redness, one of the cardinal signs of inflammation.

Rubramin (roo′brah-min) trademark for preparations of vitamin B_{12} activity concentrate.

rubriblast (roo′brĭ-blast) a cell of the erythrocytic series having a fine chromatin structure in the nucleus, and usually discernible nucleoli.

rubric (roo′brik) red; specifically, pertaining to the nucleus ruber.

rubricyte (roo′brĭ-sīt) a young cell of the erythrocytic series having a definite chromatin structure in the nucleus, but no discernible nucleoli.

rubrospinal (roo″bro-spi′nal) pertaining to the nucleus ruber and the spinal cord.

rubrum (roo′brum) [L.] red.
  r. scarlati′num, scarlet red.

rudiment (roo′dĭ-ment) 1. an organ or part having little or no function but which has functioned at an earlier stage of the same individual or in his ancestors. 2. primordium.

rudimentary (roo″dĭ-men′ter-e) incompletely developed.

ruga (roo′gah), pl. *ru′gae* [L.] a ridge or fold.

rugose (roo′gōs) marked by ridges; wrinkled.

rugosity (roo-gos′ĭ-te) 1. the condition of being rugose. 2. a ridge or ruga.

R.U.L. right upper lobe (of lung).

rumbatron (rum′bah-tron) a high efficiency radio oscillator in which atoms are shattered and which employs electrons as the bombarding particles.

ruminant (roo′mĭ-nant) an animal that has a stomach with four complete cavities, and that characteristically regurgitates undigested food from the rumen, the first stomach, and masticates it when at rest.

rumination (roo″mĭ-na′shun) 1. in man, the regurgitation of food after almost every meal, part of it being vomited and the rest swallowed; a condition seen in infants. 2. persistent meditation on a certain subject.

rump (rump) the buttock or gluteal region.

runt disease (runt) a syndrome produced by immunologically competent cells in a foreign host that is unable to reject them, resulting in gross retardation of host development and in death.

rupia (roo′pe-ah) an eruption in tertiary syphilis, with formation of bullae.

rupture (rup′tūr) 1. to break apart or disrupt. 2. the bursting or breaking of a part. 3. hernia.

R.U.Q. right upper quadrant (of abdomen).

Rush (rush) Benjamin (1745–1813). American physician, born in Philadelphia, and educated at Princeton and the University of Edinburgh. He helped found the Philadelphia Dispensary in 1786, and was physician to Pennsylvania Hospital, where he introduced clinical instruction. Rush protested against improper treatment to the insane until the legislature made provision for construction of a ward for them at Pennsylvania Hospital. He served as a surgeon in the Continental army, and founded with James Pemberton the first anti-slave society in America. As a member of the Continental Congress, Rush was a signer of the Declaration of Independence, and in 1787 he was a member of the Pennsylvania convention that adopted the Federal Constitution. He was appointed Treasurer of the United States Mint in Philadelphia in 1799.

rush (rush) a rapid movement.
  peristaltic r's, vigorous peristaltic movements, propelling intestinal contents 20 to 50 cm. before dying out.

ruthenium (roo-the′ne-um) a chemical element, atomic number 44, atomic weight 101.07, symbol Ru. (See table of ELEMENTS.)

rutherford (ruth′er-ford) a unit of radioactive disintegration, representing one million disintegrations per second.

rutherfordium (ruth″er-for′de-um) a chemical element, atomic number 104, atomic weight 261, symbol Rf. (See table of ELEMENTS.)

rutin, rutoside (roo′to-sīd) a bioflavonoid obtained from buckwheat and other sources; used to reduce capillary fragility.

R.V. residual volume.

rye (ri) the cereal plant *Secale cereale*, and its nutritious seed.
  ergotized r., spurred r., rye affected with the fungus *Claviceps purpurea*, from which ergot is derived.

S

S chemical symbol, *sulfur*.

S. [L.] *se'mis* (half); sight; [L.] *sig'na* (mark); [L.] *sin'ister* (left).

S.A.B. Society of American Bacteriologists.

Sabin (sa'bin) Albert Bruce (1906–   ). American virologist, born in Bialystok, Russia; he came to the United States in 1921, and is known for his discovery of an oral vaccine against poliomyelitis.

S. vaccine, an oral vaccine against POLIOMYELITIS consisting of three types of live, attenuated polioviruses. It is given in a capsule, in candy, on a lump of sugar, in milk or by medicine dropper, and is especially convenient for administration to children and large groups of people.

A unique advantage of the Sabin vaccine is its potential effectiveness in checking the transmission of paralytic viruses from one person to another. Polioviruses reside first in the intestinal tract, from which they spread to other areas, eventually reaching the nervous system and causing paralysis. In a person who has been vaccinated by injection (with Salk vaccine), the viruses are destroyed by antibodies before they reach the nervous system but after they have moved out of the intestine; viruses in the intestine are not destroyed and, still infectious, pass out of the body.

Sabin vaccine, taken orally, stimulates the production of antibodies in the digestive system as well as in other systems of the body; viruses in the intestine are destroyed, not passed on. Thus persons who have received the Sabin vaccine become neither infected nor carriers, whereas those who have received the Salk vaccine can be carriers of the viruses even though they are not themselves infected.

sabulous (sab'u-lus) gritty or sandy.

saburra (sah-bur'ah) sordes; foulness of the mouth or stomach.

saburral (sah-bur'al) 1. pertaining to saburra. 2. gritty; gravelly.

sac (sak) a pouch; a baglike organ or structure.
air s., an alveolus of the lung.
alveolar s., the spaces into which the alveolar ducts open distally, and with which the alveoli communicate.
amniotic s., the sac enclosing the fetus suspended in the amniotic fluid.
conjunctival s., the potential space, lined by conjunctiva, between the eyelids and the eyeball.
endolymphatic s., the blind, flattened cerebral end of the endolymphatic duct.
heart s., the pericardium.
hernial s., the peritoneal pouch that encloses protruding intestine.
lacrimal s., a membranous reservoir into which the lacrimal duct drains and which is continuous with the nasolacrimal duct.
vitelline s., yolk s., a membranous structure formed in early embryonic development, connected with the midgut.

saccate (sak'āt) 1. shaped like a sac. 2. contained in a sac.

saccharase (sak'ah-rās) invertin.

saccharate (sak'ah-rāt) a salt of saccharic acid.

saccharated (sak'ah-rāt″ed) sugary; charged with sugar.

saccharic acid (sah-kar'ik) a dibasic acid formed by the action of nitric acid on dextrose or carbohydrates containing dextrose.

saccharide (sak'ah-rīd) one of a series of carbohydrates, including the sugars; they are divided into monosaccharides, disaccharides, trisaccharides and polysaccharides according to the number of saccharide groups composing them.

sacchariferous (sak″ah-rif'er-us) containing sugar.

saccharin (sak'ah-rin) a white, crystalline compound several hundred times sweeter than sucrose; used as a noncaloric sweetening agent.
calcium s., an artificial sweetening agent.

saccharogalactorrhea (sak″ah-ro-gah-lak″to-re'ah) secretion of milk containing an excess of sugar.

saccharolytic (sak″ah-ro-lit'ik) capable of splitting up sugar.

saccharometabolic (sak″ah-ro-met″ah-bol'ik) pertaining to the metabolism of sugar.

saccharometabolism (sak″ah-ro-mĕ-tab'o-lizm) the metabolism of sugar.

saccharometer (sak″ah-rom'ĕ-ter) an apparatus for measuring the proportion of sugar in a solution.

Saccharomyces (sak″ah-ro-mi'sēz) a genus of protophytes, the yeast fungi. They are oval, unicellular organisms characterized by budding. Only two species are pathogenic for man: *S. al'bicans* (*Candida albicans*) and *S. neofor'mans* (*Cryptococcus neoformans*).

saccharomycosis (sak″ah-ro-mi-ko'sis) 1. any disease due to yeast fungi. 2. a skin disease marked by the presence of nodules containing Saccharomyces.

saccharorrhea (sak″ah-ro-re'ah) glycosuria.

saccharose (sak'ah-rōs) ordinary cane sugar, or sucrose.

saccharosuria (sak"ah-ro-su're-ah) saccharose in the urine.

saccharum (sak'ah-rum) [L.] sugar, especially sucrose.
 s. lac'tis, lactose.

sacciform (sak'sĭ-form) shaped like a bag or sac.

saccular (sak'u-lar) pertaining to or resembling a sac.

sacculated (sak'u-lāt"ed) containing saccules.

saccule (sak'ūl) a little bag or sac; a small, pouch-like cavity, especially the smaller of the two divisions of the membranous labyrinth of the inner ear.

sacculus (sak'u-lus), pl. *sac'culi* [L.] a saccule.
 s. laryn'gis, a diverticulum extending upward from the front of the ventricle of the larynx.

saccus (sak'us), pl. *sac'ci* [L.] a sac.

sacr(o)- (sa'kro) word element [L.], *sacrum.*

sacrad (sa'krad) toward the sacrum.

sacral (sa'kral) pertaining to the sacrum.

sacralgia (sa-kral'je-ah) pain in the sacrum.

sacralization (sa"kral-ĭ-za'shun) fusion of the fifth lumbar vertebra with the sacrum.

sacrectomy (sa-krek'to-me) excision or resection of the sacrum.

sacrococcygeal (sa"kro-kok-sij'e-al) pertaining to the sacrum and coccyx.

sacrocoxalgia (sa"kro-kok-sal'je-ah) a painful condition of the sacrum and coccyx.

sacrocoxitis (sa"kro-kok-si'tis) inflammation of the sacroiliac joint.

sacrodynia (sa"kro-din'e-ah) pain in the sacral region.

sacroiliac (sa"kro-il'e-ak) pertaining to the sacrum and the ilium, and the joint formed by these two bones, or to the lower part of the back where these bones meet on both sides of the back. The ilium is the upper part of the hip bone. The sacrum, near the end of the spine, forms a wedge-shaped joint within the open portion of the ilium.
 The tight joint allows little motion and is subject to great stress, as the body's weight pushes downward and the legs and pelvis push upward against the joint. The sacroiliac joint must also bear the leverage demands made by the trunk of the body as it turns, twists, pulls and pushes. When these motions, especially during weight lifting, place an excess of stress on the ligaments that bind the joint and on the connecting muscles, strain may result.
 s. disease, chronic tuberculosis of the sacroiliac joint.

sacroiliitis (sa"kro-il"e-i'tis) inflammation of the sacroiliac joint.

sacrolumbar (sa"kro-lum'bar) pertaining to the sacrum and loins.

sacrosciatic (sa"kro-si-at'ik) pertaining to the sacrum and ischium.

sacrospinal (sa"kro-spi'nal) pertaining to the sacrum and vertebral column.

sacrouterine (sa"kro-u'ter-in) pertaining to the sacrum and uterus.

sacrovertebral (sa"kro-ver'tĕ-bral) pertaining to the sacrum and vertebrae.

sacrum (sa'krum) the triangular-shaped bone at the base of the spine formed usually by five fused vertebrae that are wedged dorsally between the two hip bones.

sadism (sad'izm) a form of sexual perversion in which sexual satisfaction is gained by inflicting pain on others. adj., **sadis'tic.** It can manifest itself in many ways other than during the sexual act. Sadism is a mental disturbance and should be treated by psychotherapy.

sadist (sad'ist) a person exhibiting or characterized by sadism.

sadomasochism (sad"o-mas'o-kizm) a state characterized by both sadistic and masochistic tendencies. adj., **sadomasochis'tic.**

sadomasochist (sad"o-mas'o-kist) a person exhibiting sadomasochism.

sagittal (saj'ĭ-tal) 1. shaped like an arrow. 2. situated in the direction of the sagittal suture; said of an anteroposterior plane or section coinciding with (median sagittal plane) or parallel to the long axis of the body.

sagittalis (saj"ĭ-ta'lis) [L.] sagittal.

sago (sa'go) starch from the pith of various palm trees.

Saint Anthony's fire 1. ergotism. 2. an infection of the skin and subcutaneous tissues; called also ERYSIPELAS.

Saint Vitus's dance Sydenham's chorea.

sal (sal) [L.] salt.
 s. ammo'niac, ammonium chloride.
 s. so'da, sodium carbonate.
 s. volat'ile, ammonium carbonate.

salicylamide (sal"ĭ-sil-am'īd) a white, crystalline powder used as an analgesic.

salicylanilide (sal"ĭ-sil-an'ĭ-līd) a white or slightly pink crystalline compound used as an antifungal agent.

salicylate (sal'ĭ-sil"āt, sah-lis'ĭ-lāt) a salt of salicylic acid.

salicylated (sal'ĭ-sil-āt"ed) impregnated or charged with salicylic acid.

salicylazosulfapyridine (sal"ĭ-sil"ah-zo-sul"fah-pir'ĭ-din) a sulfonamide-related salicylic acid compound used in treatment of chronic ulcerative colitis.

salicylic acid (sal"ĭ-sil'ik) a hydroxyl derivative of benzoic acid. In its pure form it is used as a keratolytic agent to induce peeling of skin or skin lesions. It is prepared in ointments, creams and collodions containing from 3 to 20 per cent salicylic acid, depending on the effect desired.

The sodium salt of salicylic acid, sodium salicylate, is used mainly as an antirheumatic and antipyretic. Acetylsalicylic acid (ASPIRIN) is a widely used analgesic, antipyretic and antirheumatic.

Since salicylic acid is an irritant to skin and mucous membranes, preparations taken internally may produce gastrointestinal upsets with prolonged use or overdosage.

salicylide (sal'ĭ-sil″īd) an anhydride of salicylic acid.

salicylism (sal'ĭ-sil″izm) toxic symptoms caused by salicylic acid.

salicyltherapy (sal″ĭ-sil-ther'ah-pe) treatment with salicylic acid and the salicylates.

salifiable (sal″ĭ-fi'ah-bl) capable of combining with an acid to form a salt.

salimeter (sah-lim'ĕ-ter) an instrument for determining the strength of saline solutions.

saline (sa'līn) salty; of the nature of a salt.

s. solution, a solution of salt (sodium chloride) in purified water. Physiologic saline solution is a 0.9 per cent solution of sodium chloride and water and is of the same osmotic pressure as blood serum. It is sometimes given intravenously to replace lost sodium and chloride. Excessive quantities may cause edema, elevated blood sodium levels and loss of potassium from the tissue fluid.

saliva (sah-li'vah) the enzyme-containing secretion of the salivary glands.

salivant (sal'ĭ-vant) causing an excessive flow of saliva.

salivary (sal'ĭ-ver-e) pertaining to the saliva.

s. gland, one of the glands in the mouth that secrete saliva. The major ones are the three pairs of glands known as the parotid, submaxillary and sublingual glands. There are other smaller salivary glands within the cheeks and tongue.

The largest of the salivary glands are the parotids, located below and in front of each ear. Saliva secreted by these is discharged into the mouth through openings in the cheeks on each side opposite the upper teeth. The submaxillary glands, located inside the lower jaw, discharge saliva upward through openings into the floor of the mouth. The sublingual glands, beneath the tongue, also discharge saliva into the floor of the mouth.

The saliva is needed to moisten the mouth, to lubricate food for easier swallowing and to provide the enzymes necessary to begin food breakdown in the preliminary stage of digestion. The salivary glands produce about 3 pints of saliva daily.

The salivary glands are controlled by the nervous system. Normally they respond by producing saliva within 2 or 3 seconds after being stimulated by the sight, smell or taste of food. This quick response is a reflex action.

In mumps (parotitis), the parotids become inflamed and swollen. Occasionally, salivary glands produce too much saliva; this condition is called ptyalism, and is the result of local irritation from dental appliances or of disturbances of digestion or of the nervous system or other causes. Certain diseases, drugs such as morphine or atropine and nutritional deficiency of vitamin B can result in decreased secretion of saliva.

s. gland inclusion disease, cytomegalic inclusion disease.

salivation (sal″ĭ-va'shun) 1. the secretion of saliva. 2. ptyalism.

Salk (sawlk) Jonas Edward (1914–   ). American physician, born in New York City. He developed a vaccine for the prevention of poliomyelitis, and is director of the Salk Institute for Biological Studies.

S. vaccine, a preparation of killed polioviruses of three types given in a series of intramuscular injections to immunize against POLIOMYELITIS.

Salla's cells (sal'ahz) star-shaped cells of connective tissue in the fibers that form the sensory nerve endings situated in the pericardium.

salmiac (sal'me-ak) ammonium chloride.

Salmonella (sal″mo-nel'ah) a genus of Schizomycetes including the typhoid-paratyphoid bacilli and bacteria usually pathogenic for lower animals which are often transmitted to man.

S. enterit'idis, a common cause of gastroenteritis in man.

S. paraty'phi, the etiologic agent of paratyphoid.

S. ty'phi, the causative organism of typhoid fever, occurring only in man.

salmonellosis (sal″mo-nel-o'sis) infection with Salmonella, especially (1) paratyphoid and (2) a form of food poisoning due to certain species of the genus Salmonella.

salping(o)- (sal-ping'go) word element [Gr.], *tube* (*eustachian tube* or *uterine tube*).

salpingectomy (sal″pin-jek'to-me) excision of a uterine tube.

salpingemphraxis (sal″pin-jem-frak'sis) 1. obstruction of a uterine tube. 2. obstruction of a eustachian tube.

salpingian (sal-pin'je-an) pertaining to the eustachian or the uterine tube.

salpingion (sal-pin'je-on) a point at the apex of the petrous bone on the lower surface.

salpingitis (sal″pin-ji'tis) 1. inflammation of a uterine tube. 2. inflammation of the eustachian tube.

salpingocele (sal-ping'go-sēl) hernial protrusion of a uterine tube.

salpingocyesis (sal-ping″go-si-e'sis) development of the embryo within a uterine tube; tubal pregnancy.

salpingography (sal″ping-gog'rah-fe) roentgenologic visualization of the uterine tubes after intrauterine injection of a radiopaque medium.

salpingolithiasis (sal-ping″go-lĭ-thi'ah-sis) the presence of calcareous deposits in the wall of the uterine tubes.

salpingolysis (sal″ping-gol'ĭ-sis) surgical separation of adhesions involving the uterine tubes.

salpingo-oophorectomy (sal-ping″go-o″of-o-rek'to-me) excision of a uterine tube and ovary.

salpingo-oophoritis (sal-ping″go-o″of-o-ri'tis) inflammation of a uterine tube and ovary.

salpingo-oophorocele (sal-ping″go-o-of′o-ro-sēl″) hernia of a uterine tube and ovary.

salpingo-ovariotripsy (sal-ping″go-o-va′re-o-trip″se) ablation of uterine tube, ovary and adnexa.

salpingopexy (sal-ping′go-pek″se) fixation of a uterine tube.

salpingoplasty (sal-ping′go-plas″te) plastic repair of a uterine tube.

salpingoscope (sal-ping′go-skōp) an instrument for examination of nasopharynx and eustachian tube.

salpingostomy (sal′ping-gos′to-me) restoration of the patency of a uterine tube.

salpingotomy (sal″ping-got′o-me) surgical incision of a uterine tube.

salpinx (sal′pinks) 1. a uterine tube. 2 a eustachian tube.

salt (sawlt) 1. sodium chloride. 2. any compound of a base or radical and an acid. 3. (plural, *salts*) a saline purgative.
  acid s., a salt in which some of the replaceable hydrogen atoms remain in the molecule, giving it the properties of an acid.
  baker's s., ammonium carbonate.
  basic s., a salt with hydroxyl groups in the molecule, giving it the properties of a base.
  bile s's, compounds formed in the liver that aid in digestion and absorption of fats and absorption of fat-soluble vitamins.
  buffer s., a salt in the blood that is able to absorb slight excesses of acid or alkali with little or no change in the hydrogen ion concentration.
  double s., a salt in which the hydrogen atoms of the acid have been replaced by two metals.
  Epsom s., magnesium sulfate.
  Glauber's s., sodium sulfate.
  haloid s., a binary compound of a halogen—i.e., of chlorine, iodine, bromine, fluorine.
  neutral s., normal s., a salt in which all the hydrogen of the acid has been replaced; it is neither acid nor basic.
  Rochelle s., potassium sodium tartrate.
  smelling s., aromatic ammonium carbonate.

saltation (sal-ta′shun) 1. leaping or dancing as in chorea. 2. in genetics, an abrupt variation in species; a mutation.

salubrious (sah-lu′bre-us) conducive to health; wholesome.

saluresis (sal″u-re′sis) excretion of sodium and chloride in the urine.

saluretic (sal″u-ret′ik) an agent that promotes saluresis.

salutary (sal′u-tār″e) healthful.

salve (sav) ointment.

Salyrgan (sal′er-gan) trademark for a preparation of mersalyl, a mercurial diuretic.

S.A.M.A. Student American Medical Association.

samarium (sah-ma′re-um) a chemical element, atomic number 62, atomic weight 150.35, symbol Sm. (See table of ELEMENTS.)

sanative (san′ah-tiv) curative; healing.

sanatorium (san″ah-to′re-um) an institution for treatment of sick persons, especially a private hospital for convalescents or patients who are not extremely ill; often applied to an institution for the treatment of tuberculosis.

sanatory (san′ah-tor″e) conducive to health.

sand (sand) a substance composed of fine gritty particles.
  brain s., acervulus cerebri; sandy matter about the pineal gland and other parts of the brain.

Sander's disease (san′derz) epidemic keratoconjunctivitis.

sandfly (sand′fli) various two-winged flies, especially those of the genus Phlebotomus, which are important vectors in the transmission of leishmaniasis and phlebotomus fever, which is known also as sandfly fever.

Sandril (san′dril) trademark for preparations of reserpine, an antihypertensive and tranquilizer.

sane (sān) sound in mind.

sangui- (sang′gwe) word element [L.], *blood.*

sanguicolous (sang-gwik′o-lus) living in the blood.

sanguifacient (sang″gwĭ-fa′shent) forming blood.

sanguimotor (sang″gwĭ-mo′tor) pertaining to circulation of the blood.

sanguinaria (sang″gwĭ-na′re-ah) the dried rhizome of *Sanguinaria canadensis;* a local irritant and sternutatory.

sanguine (sang′gwin) 1. abounding in blood. 2. ardent, hopeful.

sanguineous (sang-gwin′e-us) bloody; abounding in blood.

sanguinolent (sang-gwin′o-lent) of a bloody tinge.

sanguirenal (sang″gwĭ-re′nal) pertaining to the blood and kidneys.

sanguis (sang′gwis) [L.] blood.

sanguivorous (sang-gwiv′o-rus) blood-eating; said of female mosquitoes that prefer blood to other nutrients.

sanies (sa′ne-ēz) a fetid ichorous discharge containing serum, pus and blood. adj., **sa′nious.**

saniopurulent (sa″ne-o-pu′roo-lent) purulent, with serum and blood.

sanioserous (sa″ne-o-se′rus) serous, with pus and blood.

sanitarium (san″ĭ-ta′re-um) an institution for the promotion of health. The word was originally coined to designate the institution established by the Seventh Day Adventists at Battle Creek, Michigan, to distinguish it from institutions providing care for mental or tuberculous patients.

sanitary (san'ĭ-tār″e) promoting or pertaining to health.

sanitation (san″ĭ-ta′shun) the establishment of conditions favorable to health.

sanitization (san″ĭ-tĭ-za′shun) the process of making or the quality of being made sanitary.

sanitize (san'ĭ-tīz) to clean and sterilize.

sanity (san″ĭ-te) soundness, especially soundness of mind.

San Joaquin Valley fever coccidioidomycosis.

santonin (san'to-nin) a lactone from the unexpanded flower heads of *Artemisia cina;* used as an anthelmintic.

sap (sap) the natural fluid substance of animal or vegetable tissue.
   cell s., hyaloplasm.
   nuclear s., karyolymph.

saphena (sah-fe′nah) either of two large superficial veins of the leg.

saphenous (sah-fe′nus) pertaining to or associated with a saphena; applied to certain arteries, nerves, veins, etc.
   great s. vein, the longest vein in the body, extending from the dorsum of the foot to just below the inguinal ligament, where it opens into the femoral vein.
   small s. vein, a vein in the back of the ankle passing up the back of the leg to the knee joint.

sapid (sap′id) having taste or flavor.

sapo (sa′po) [L.] soap; a compound of fatty acids with an alkali.

saponaceous (sa″po-na′shus) soapy; of soaplike feel or quality.

saponification (sah-pon″ĭ-fĭ-ka′shun) conversion of an oil or fat into a soap by combination with an alkali. In chemistry, the term now denotes the hydrolysis of an ester by an alkali, resulting in the production of a free alcohol and an alkali salt of the ester acid.

saponin (sap′o-nin) a group of glycosides, widely distributed in the plant world and characterized by (1) their property of forming durable foam when their watery solutions are shaken, (2) their ability to dissolve erythrocytes even in high dilutions and (3) their having the compound sapogenin as their aglycones.

sapophore (sap′o-fōr) the group of atoms in the molecule of a compound that gives the substance its characteristic taste.

sapphism (saf′izm) homosexual behavior in the female; lesbianism.

sapr(o)- (sap′ro) word element [Gr.], *rotten; putrid; decay; decayed material.*

sapremia (sah-pre′me-ah) intoxication due to the presence in the blood of products of saprophytic and nonpathogenic bacteria; called also septic intoxication.

saprogen (sap′ro-jen) an agent that causes putrefaction.

saprogenic (sap″ro-jen′ik) causing putrefaction.

saprogenous (sah-proj′ĕ-nus) arising or resulting from putrefaction.

saprophilous (sah-prof′ĭ-lus) living on dead matter; applied mainly to microorganisms.

saprophyte (sap′ro-fīt) a plant organism, such as yeasts, molds and most bacteria, that absorbs required nutrients directly through the cell membrane, from decomposing animal or plant bodies or from masses of plant and animal by-products. adj., **saprophyt′ic.**

saprozoic (sap″ro-zo′ik) living on decayed organic matter; said of animals, especially protozoa.

sarc(o)- (sar′ko) word element [Gr.], *flesh.*

sarcitis (sar-si′tis) inflammation of muscle tissue.

sarcoadenoma (sar″ko-ad″ĕ-no′mah) adenosarcoma.

sarcoblast (sar′ko-blast) a primitive cell that develops into a muscle cell.

sarcocarcinoma (sar″ko-kar″sĭ-no′mah) carcinosarcoma.

sarcocele (sar′ko-sēl) a fleshy swelling or tumor of the testis.

Sarcocystis (sar″ko-sis′tis) a genus name applied to parasitic organisms of uncertain taxonomic status found in muscle tissue of various animals. *S. lindeman′ni* is a species that rarely infects man.

Sarcodina (sar″ko-di′nah) a subphylum of Protozoa, including all the amebas, characterized by an extremely flexible plasma membrane covering the body surface, permitting body cytoplasm to flow in all directions, with constant alteration in the outline of the body.

sarcogenic (sar″ko-jen′ik) forming flesh.

sarcoid (sar′koid) 1. resembling flesh; fleshy. 2. a sarcoma-like tumor; a general term applied to a group of skin lesions generally credited with being of tuberculous nature.
   Boeck's s., a type of multiple benign sarcoid characterized by its superficial nature and showing a predilection for the face, arms and shoulders.

sarcoidosis (sar″koi-do′sis) a disorder that may affect any part of the body but most frequently involving the lymph nodes, liver, spleen, lungs, skin, eyes and small bones of the hands and feet, characterized by the presence in all affected organs or tissues of epithelioid cell tubercles, which become converted, in the older lesions, into a rather hyaline featureless fibrous tissue.
   s. cor′dis, involvement of the heart in sarcoidosis, with lesions ranging from a few asymptomatic granulomas to widespread infiltration of the myocardium by large masses of sarcoid tissue.
   muscular s., sarcoidosis involving the skeletal muscles, with sarcoid tubercles, interstitial inflammation with fibrosis, and disruption and atrophy of the muscle fibers.

sarcolemma (sar″ko-lem′ah) the delicate elastic sheath covering every striated muscle fiber.

sarcoleukemia (sar″ko-lu-ke′me-ah) lymphosarcoma cell leukemia.

sarcology (sar-kol′o-je) scientific study of the soft tissues of the body.

sarcolysis (sar-kol′ĭ-sis) disintegration of the soft tissues.

sarcolyte (sar′ko-līt) a cell concerned in disintegration of soft tissues.

sarcoma (sar-ko′mah) a tumor, often highly malignant, composed of cells derived from connective tissue such as bone and cartilage, muscle, blood vessel or lymphoid tissue. These tumors usually develop rapidly and metastasize through the lymph channels. adj., **sarco′matous.**
   The different types of sarcomas are named for the specific tissue they affect: fibrosarcoma—in fibrous connective tissue; lymphosarcoma—in lymphoid tissues; osteosarcoma—in bone; chondrosarcoma—in cartilage; rhabdosarcoma—in muscle; liposarcoma—in fat cells.
   giant cell s., one that contains giant cells, or myeloplaxes.
   Kaposi's s., multiple soft bluish nodules of the skin with hemorrhages, similar to infectious granulomas, which may become neoplastic.
   reticulum cell s., a form of malignant lymphoma in which the dominant cell type is derived from the reticuloendothelium.

sarcomagenesis (sar-ko″mah-jen′ĕ-sis) the production of sarcoma.

sarcomatoid (sar-ko′mah-toid) resembling a sarcoma.

sarcomatosis (sar-ko″mah-to′sis) a condition characterized by development of many sarcomas.

sarcomatous (sar-ko′mah-tus) of the nature of a sarcoma.

sarcomere (sar′ko-mēr) the unit of length of a myofibril.

sarcomphalocele (sar″kom-fal′o-sēl) a fleshy tumor of the umbilicus.

sarcoplasm (sar′ko-plazm) the cytoplasm of a striated muscle fiber, filling the spaces between myofibrils, and presumably responsible for the inception and coordination of muscle fiber contraction.

sarcoplast (sar′ko-plast) an interstitial cell of a muscle, itself capable of being transformed into a muscle.

sarcopoietic (sar″ko-poi-et′ik) forming muscle.

Sarcoptes (sar-kop′tēz) a widely distributed genus of mites, including the species *S. scabie′i,* the itch mite, the cause of scabies in man; different varieties of the organism cause mange in different animals.

sarcosis (sar-ko′sis) 1. the presence of multiple fleshy tumors. 2. abnormal increase of flesh.

sarcosome (sar′ko-sōm) the darker contractile part of a muscle fibril.

sarcostosis (sar″kos-to′sis) ossification of fleshy tissue.

sarcostyle (sar′ko-stīl) a fibril of an elementary muscle fiber.

sarcous (sar′kus) pertaining to flesh or muscle tissue.

sardonic (sar-don′ik) noting a kind of spasmodic or satanic grin or involuntary smile, the risus sardonicus.

sat. saturated.

satellite (sat′ĕ-līt) 1. in genetics, a knob of chromatin connected by a stalk to the short arm of certain chromosomes. 2. a minor, or attendant, lesion situated near a large one.

satellitosis (sat″ĕ-li-to′sis) a gathering of phagocytic neuroglial cells around the ganglion cells of the brain cortex in general paresis.

saturated (sat′u-rāt″ed) 1. having all affinities of its elements satisfied (saturated compound). 2. holding all of a solute that can be held in a solution by the solvent (saturated solution).

saturation (sat″u-ra′shun) 1. the state of a solvent that holds in solution all of a substance it can possibly contain. 2. in radiotherapy, the delivery of an erythema dose within a short time and then maintaining this effect for some time by administering additional smaller doses.

saturnine (sat′ur-nīn) pertaining to lead.

saturnism (sat′urn-izm) lead poisoning; plumbism.

satyriasis, satyromania (sat″ĭ-ri′ah-sis), (sat″ĭ-ro-ma′ne-ah) insatiable sexual desire in the male.

saucerization (saw″ser-ĭ-za′shun) the formation of a shallow depression, as by excavation or injury.

sauriderma (saw″rĭ-der′mah) a variety of ichthyosis.

sauriosis (saw″re-o′sis) keratosis follicularis.

Sb chemical symbol, *antimony* (L. *stibium*).

Sc chemical symbol, *scandium.*

s.c. subcutaneously.

scab (skab) 1. the crust of a superficial sore. 2. to become covered with a crust or scab.

scabicide (ska′bi-sid) an agent used in treating scabies.

scabies (ska′bēz, ska′be-ēz) a contagious skin disease caused by the itch mite, *Sarcoptes scabiei.* Scabies, sometimes called "the itch," is most likely to erupt in folds of the skin, as in the groin, beneath the breasts or between the toes or fingers.
   The adult itch mite has a rounded body about one-fiftieth of an inch long. Scabies is caused by the female, which burrows beneath the skin and digs a short tunnel parallel to the surface, in which it lays its eggs. The eggs hatch in a few days, after which the baby mites find their way to the skin surface, where they live their brief lives until they too are ready to burrow and lay their eggs.

SYMPTOMS. During the initial tunnel-digging and egg-laying the human host may be oblivious to what is happening. There is little itching. The very slight skin discoloration may be mistaken for any one of numerous other skin disorders.

In about a week, the itching becomes intense because of hypersensitivity to the mite. The itch is much worse at night. The tunnels in the skin can now be discerned as slightly elevated grayish white lines. The mite itself can often be seen — with the aid of a magnifying glass — as an infinitesimal white speck at the end of the tunnel. Blisters and pustules also may develop on the skin near the tunnel.

TRANSMISSION. Scabies is easily transmitted from person to person by direct skin contact or to a limited extent by contact with clothing of infected persons. Epidemics are fairly common in such places as camps, barracks and institutions. It is unusual for one member of a family not to communicate it to the others.

The period of communicability lasts until the itch mites and eggs are totally destroyed, a period of 1 to 2 weeks, depending on the effectiveness of the treatment used.

TREATMENT AND PREVENTION. The usual therapy begins with a hot bath and thorough scrubbing to open and expose the burrows. This is followed by the application of some type of DDT preparation.

The patient's underwear and bedclothing must be changed and laundered daily until all the itch mite eggs are hatched out and the mites eliminated.

Good personal hygiene and wearing fresh and clean clothing are the two most effective ways to prevent scabies.

Norwegian s., a variety characterized by immense numbers of mites and marked scaling of the skin.

scabieticide (ska″be-et′ĭ-sīd) scabicide.

scabiophobia (ska″be-o-fo′be-ah) morbid dread of scabies.

scabrities (ska-brish′e-ēz) a scabby or rough state of the skin.

scala (ska′lah), pl. *sca′lae* [L.] a ladder-like structure, applied especially to various passages of the cochlea.

s. me′dia, a space in the ear between Reissner's membrane and the basilar membrane.

s. tym′pani, the part of the cochlea below the spiral lamina.

s. vestib′uli, the part of the cochlea above the spiral lamina.

scald (skawld) a burn caused by a hot liquid or a hot, moist vapor.

scale (skāl) 1. a thin flake or compacted platelike body, as of epithelial cells. 2. a scheme or device by which some property may be measured (as hardness, weight, linear dimension). 3. to remove incrustations or other material from a surface, as from the enamel of teeth.

absolute s., a temperature scale with zero at the absolute zero of temperature.

Baumé s., a graduated scale for indicating the density of a liquid.

Celsius s., a temperature scale with zero at the freezing point of water and the normal boiling point of water at 100 degrees.

centigrade s., one with 100 gradations or steps between two fixed points, as the Celsius scale.

Fahrenheit s., a temperature scale with the freezing point of water at 32 and the normal boiling point of water at 212 degrees.

French s., one used for denoting the size of catheters, sounds and other tubular instruments, each unit being approximately 0.33 mm. in diameter.

Réaumur s., a temperature scale on which zero represents the freezing point and 80 degrees the boiling point of water.

scalene muscles (ska′lēn) four muscles (anterior, middle, posterior, smallest) of the upper thorax that raise the first and second ribs and thus aid in respiration.

scalenectomy (ska″le-nek′to-me) resection of a scalene muscle.

scalenotomy (ska″le-not′o-me) division of the scalene muscles for the purpose of restricting respiratory activity of the upper part of the thorax; used in treatment of pulmonary tuberculosis.

scall (skawl) a crusty disease, as of the scalp.

scalp (skalp) that area of the head (exclusive of the face) which is usually covered by a growth of hair.

scalpel (skal′pel) a straight knife with convex edge.

scalpriform (skal′prĭ-form) shaped like a chisel.

scaly (skāl′e) characterized by scales.

scan (skan) scintiscan.

scandium (skan′de-um) a chemical element, atomic number 21, atomic weight 44.956, symbol Sc. (See table of ELEMENTS.)

scanning (skan′ing) 1. close visual examination of a small area or of different isolated areas. 2. a manner of utterance characterized by somewhat regularly recurring pauses.

radioisotope s., production of a two-dimensional record of the emissions of a radioactive isotope concentrated in a specific organ or tissue of the body, as brain, kidney or thyroid gland.

scanography (skan-og′rah-fe) a method of making radiographs by the use of a narrow slit beneath the tube in such a manner that only a line or sheet of x-rays is employed and the x-ray tube moves over the object so that all the rays of the central beam pass through the part being radiographed at the same angle.

scapha (ska′fah), pl. *sca′phae* [L.] the curved depression separating the helix and antihelix.

scaphocephalia, scaphocephaly (skaf″o-sĕ-fa′le-ah), (skaf″o-sef′ah-le) abnormal length and narrowness of the skull as a result of premature closure of the sagittal suture; usually accompanied by mental retardation. adj., **scaphocephal′ic.**

scaphoid (skaf′oid) shaped like a boat; applied to one of the carpal bones.

scaphoiditis (skaf″oi-di′tis) inflammation of the scaphoid bone.

scapula (skap′u-lah), pl. *scap′ulae* [L.] the flat triangular bone in the back of the shoulder; the shoulder blade.

winged s., one having a prominent vertebral border usually owing to weakness of one of the muscles holding the scapula in place.

scapulalgia (skap″u-lal′je-ah) pain in the scapula.

scapular (skap′u-lar) pertaining to the scapula.

scapulectomy (skap″u-lek′to-me) excision of the scapula.

scapuloclavicular (skap″u-lo-klah-vik′u-lar) pertaining to the scapula and clavicle.

scapulohumeral (skap″u-lo-hu′mer-al) pertaining to the scapula and humerus.

scapulopexy (skap′u-lo-pek″se) surgical fixation of the scapula.

scapulothoracic (skap″u-lo-tho-ras′ik) pertaining to the scapula and thorax.

scar (skar) cicatrix; a mark remaining after the healing of a wound, such as one caused by injury, illness, smallpox vaccination or surgery.

Beneath the skin is a fibrous connective tissue known as subcutaneous tissue and composed of cells called fibroblasts, which after injury are stimulated to grow into granulation tissue, which knits the wound together. Dense masses of granulation tissue form scar tissue. (See also HEALING and KELOID.)

scarification (skar″ĭ-fĭ-ka′shun) production in the skin of many small superficial scratches or punctures, as for introduction of vaccine.

scarificator (skar′ĭ-fĭ-ka″tor) an instrument for scarifying.

scarifier (skar′ĭ-fi″er) an instrument with many sharp points, used in scarification.

scarlatina (skar″lah-te′nah) scarlet fever. adj., **scarlat′inal.**

s. angino′sa, scarlet fever with severe throat symptoms.

s. haemorrha′gica, a form in which there is extravasation of blood into the skin and mucous membranes.

s. malig′na, a variety with severe symptoms and great prostration.

scarlatinella (skar-lat″ĭ-nel′ah) mild scarlet fever without fever.

scarlatiniform (skar″lah-tin′ĭ-form) resembling scarlet fever.

scarlet fever (skar′let) an acute contagious childhood disease caused by a hemolytic streptococcus; called also scarlatina. Scarlet fever follows a streptococcal infection of the throat, skin, middle ear or some other part of the body. The disease is most common in late winter and spring.

Scarlet fever is usually spread by droplet infection. Objects the infected person has used, such as clothers, dishes or toys, may carry the streptococcus but this mode of transmission is rare. Occasionally a widespread outbreak may be caused by milk or food that has been infected by a person carrying the streptococcus.

Scarlet fever was formerly a very common and serious disease. In recent years, the number and severity of cases have greatly decreased. Complications are much less common, largely as a result of the development and use of antibiotics.

SYMPTOMS. The incubation period is usually 2 to 5 days, although it may be as few as 1 or as many as 7 days. Symptoms vary a great deal. In some patients there is only sore throat and swelling of the lymph nodes of the neck. The tonsils may be covered by a patchy purulent discharge. The bright red rash from which the disease takes its name appears on the second day; it may be mild or widely spread, depending on the strain of the causative streptococcus. There may be nausea and vomiting. The skin usually feels hot and dry, and there also may be headache and chills. In mild cases the temperature may rise to about 101° F. and in severe cases to 103 or even 105° F.

If there are no complications, the temperature will slowly return to normal. The rash fades in about a week, and the skin peels; this peeling is usually most pronounced on the palms and soles. In all, the active stage of the disease lasts about 7 days.

TREATMENT. Because of the contagious nature of the disease, the patient should be isolated. Antibiotics, usually penicillin, are administered. This treatment is continued for about 10 days to avoid relapse. Aspirin may be used to relieve headache, fever and sore throat.

COMPLICATIONS. Among the possible complications of scarlet fever are swelling of the lymph nodes of the neck, infection of the ears and sinuses, kidney disease, pneumonia and rheumatic fever. Any of these complications may be serious. However, since the development of antibiotics, they have become increasingly rare. Prompt and adequate treatment greatly reduces the danger of complications.

PREVENTION. If a child who has not had scarlet fever is exposed to it, prompt treatment with antibiotics may prevent the disease altogether. The short incubation period of scarlet fever makes immediate treatment necessary.

A person who has been exposed to scarlet fever and has not developed symptoms by the end of 7 days can assume that he was not infected. If symptoms do develop, he should be treated immediately. Cases of scarlet fever must be reported to local health authorities.

A vaccine that gives some immunity to scarlet fever has been developed but it confers immunity for only about 6 months. Since scarlet fever has become a much less serious disease, this vaccine is not often necessary.

Contact with a patient with scarlet fever or with any objects he uses should be avoided. The patient's clothes and bedding should be washed separately immediately after use, or soaked in a disinfectant for 2 hours if they are to be washed with those of other members of the family. Any toys, books or other objects that the patient uses should be thoroughly aired or washed with soap and hot water.

The active stage of scarlet fever is over as soon as the fever is gone. The patient's skin may peel during the convalescent period but he can no longer pass the disease on to others. If the case was mild, the patient can usually return to his normal activities in 7 to 10 days.

If there is any persistent discharge from a body opening, such as a running ear, contagion may still be possible, although if the patient has been treated properly with antibiotics, the streptococci will usually have been destroyed.

After the patient has recovered, his room should be thoroughly cleaned and aired. Dust-catching surfaces, such as floors, tables and window sills, should be washed with soap and hot water. If the patient has been using a private bathroom, it should be washed and disinfected as well. (See also ISOLATION TECHNIQUE.)

SCAT sheep cell agglutination test, a test for infectious mononucleosis.

scatacratia (skat″ah-kra′she-ah) incontinence of feces.

scatology (skah-tol′o-je) study and analysis of the feces.

scatophagy (skah-tof′ah-je) the eating of dung.

scatoscopy (skah-tos′ko-pe) examination of the feces.

scatter (skat′er) the diffusion or deviation of x-rays produced by a medium through which the rays pass.
  back s., backward diffusion of x-rays.

scattergram (skat′er-gram) a graph in which the values found in a statistical study are represented by disconnected, individual symbols.

Sc.D. Doctor of Science.

schema (ske′mah) a plan, outline or arrangement.

schematogram (ske-mat′o-gram) a tracing in reduced form of the outline of the body.

Schenck's disease (shenks) sporotrichosis.

Scheuermann's disease (shoi′er-manz) osteochondrosis of the vertebrae.

Schick text (shik) intracutaneous injection of diluted diphtheria toxin equal to one-fiftieth of the minimum lethal dose. Lack of immunity to diphtheria is indicated by redness and edema at the injection site on the fifth to seventh day.

Schilder's disease (shil′derz) progressive subcortical encephalopathy.

Schilling test (shil′ing) a test for gastrointestinal absorption of vitamin B_{12}; a measured amount of radioactive vitamin B_{12} is given orally, followed by a parenteral flushing dose of the nonradioactive vitamin, and the percentage of radioactivity is determined in the urine excreted over a 24-hour period. A low urinary excretion that becomes normal after the test is repeated with intrinsic factor is diagnostic of primary pernicious anemia.

Schimmelbusch's disease (shim′el-boosh″ez) a form of mastitis marked by the production of many small cysts.

schindylesis (shin″dī-le′sis) an articulation in which a thin plate of one bone is received into a cleft in another, as in the articulation of the perpendicular plate of the ethmoid bone with the vomer.

Schirmer's test (sher′merz) a test for keratocon-junctivitis sicca; a piece of filter paper is inserted into the conjunctival sac over the lower eyelid with the end of the paper hanging down on the outside. If the projecting paper remains dry after 15 minutes, deficient tear formation is indicated.

schist(o)- (skis′to) word element [Gr.], *cleft; split.*

schistasis (skis′tah-sis) a splitting; specifically, any congenital split condition of the body.

schistocelia (skis″to-se′le-ah) congenital fissure of the abdomen.

schistocephalus (skis″to-sef′ah-lus) a fetal monster with a cleft head.

schistocormus (skis″to-kor′mus) a fetal monster with a cleft trunk.

schistocyte (skis′to-sīt) a fragment of an erythrocyte, commonly observed in the blood in hemolytic anemia.

schistocytosis (skis″to-si-to′sis) excess of schistocytes in the blood.

schistoglossia (skis″to-glos′e-ah) cleft tongue.

schistomelus (skis-tom′ĕ-lus) a fetal monster with a cleft limb.

schistoprosopus (skis″to-pros′o-pus) a fetal monster with fissure of the face.

Schistosoma (skis″to-so′mah) a genus of trematodes, including several species parasitic in the blood of man and domestic animals. The organisms are called schistosomes or blood flukes. Larvae (cercariae) enter the body of the host by way of the digestive tract, or through the skin from contact with contaminated water, and migrate in the blood to small blood vessels of organs of the intestinal or urinary tract; they attach themselves to the blood vessel walls and mature and reproduce. The intermediate host is snails of various species.
  S. haemato′bium, a species endemic in north, central and west Africa and the Near East; the organisms are found in the venules of the urinary bladder wall, and eggs may be isolated from the urine.
  S. japon′icum, a species geographically confined to the Far East, and found chiefly in the venules of the intestine.
  S. manso′ni, a species widely distributed in Africa and parts of South America; the organisms are found in the host's mesenteric veins, and eggs may be found in the feces.

schistosome dermatitis (skis′to-sōm) dermatitis caused by penetration of the skin by larvae (cercariae) of organisms of the genus Schistosoma.

schistosomiasis (skis″to-so-mi′ah-sis) infection with flukes of the genus Schistosoma; called also bilharziasis. The disease is rare in North America, but is a significant health problem in many parts of the world, including the Near East, Africa, the Far East, South America and the West Indies, and Puerto Rico. The various species cause different forms of the disease; *S. mansoni* and *S. japonicum* produce intestinal symptoms, and *S. haematobium* produces hematuria and other urinary symptoms.
  Treatment includes correction of anemia and

other nutritional disorders caused by the parasites, and destruction of adult worms by administration of antimony and stibophen. Improvement in sanitation and snail control are the chief preventive measures.

schistosomicide (skis″to-so′mĭ-sīd) an agent that destroys schistosomes.

schistosomus (skis″to-so′mus) a fetal monster with a cleft abdomen.

schistothorax (skis″to-tho′raks) a developmental anomaly with fissure of the chest or sternum.

schiz(o)- (skiz′o) word element [Gr.], *divided; division.* See also words beginning *schist(o)-*.

schizaxon (skiz-ak′son) an axon that divides into two nearly equal branches.

schizogenesis (skiz″o-jen′ĕ-sis) reproduction by fission.

schizogony (skĭ-zog′o-ne) the asexual reproduction of a sporozoan parasite (sporozoite) by multiple fission within the body of the host, giving rise to merozoites, as in malaria.

schizogyria (skiz″o-ji′re-ah) a condition in which the cerebral convolutions have wedge-shaped cracks.

schizoid (skiz′oid) 1. resembling schizophrenia: a term applied to a shut-in, unsocial, introspective personality. 2. a person of schizoid personality.

schizomycete (skiz″o-mi-sēt′) an organism of the class Schizomycetes.

Schizomycetes (skiz″o-mi-se′tēz) a class of vegetable organisms (division Protophyta), including organisms that usually contain no photosynthetic pigments and usually reproduce by fission.

schizomycosis (skiz″o-mi-ko′sis) any disease due to Schizomycetes.

schizont (skiz′ont) the stage in the development of the malarial parasite following the trophozoite whose nucleus divides into many smaller nuclei.

schizonychia (skiz″o-nik′e-ah) splitting of the nails.

schizophasia (skiz″o-fa′ze-ah) incomprehensible, disordered speech.

schizophrenia (skiz″o-fre′ne-ah) a chronic mental disorder characterized by inability to distinguish between fantasy and reality, and often accompanied by hallucinations and delusions. adj., **schizophren′ic.**
  Schizophrenia, formerly called dementia praecox, is the most common form of PSYCHOSIS, it usually develops between the ages of 15 and 30. It can vary from a mild disorder, at times undetected, to one so severe as to require prolonged hospitalization. The chances of recovery are best if the condition is treated early.
  catatonic s., a psychotic reaction characterized by uncooperative or impulsive behavior and motor disturbances, especially excitement, stupor or CATALEPSY.

hebephrenic s., a psychotic state characterized by inappropriate affect, unpredictive giggling, silly behavior and mannerisms, and profound regression.
  paranoid s., a psychotic state marked by illogical and relatively fragmentary delusions of grandeur or persecution or both; usually accompanied by auditory hallucinations.
  simple s., schizophrenia marked by apathy, lack of initiative, and withdrawal.
  undifferentiated s., a form with mixed symptomatology.

schizothemia (skiz″o-the′me-ah) interruption of an argument by reminiscences; regarded as hysterical.

schizotrichia (skiz″o-trik′e-ah) splitting of the hairs at the ends.

Schlatter-Osgood disease (shlat′er oz′good) osteochondrosis of the tuberosity of the tibia.

Schmorl's disease (shmorlz) herniation of the nucleus pulposus.

Schönlein's disease (shān′līnz) nonthrombocytopenic purpura with swelling, pain and tenderness of the joints.

Schüller's disease (shil′erz) 1. Hand-Schüller-Christian disease. 2. osteoporosis circumscripta.

Schwabach test (shvah′bak) a test of hearing made with tuning forks of 256, 512, 1024 and 2048 cycle frequency, the duration of perception of the patient by bone conduction being compared with that of the examiner.

schwannoglioma, schwannoma (shwah″no-gli-o′mah), (shwah-no′mah) a tumor arising from the sheath of a nerve fiber.

sciage (se-ahzh′) [Fr.] a sawing movement in massage.

sciatic (si-at′ik) pertaining to the ischium.
  s. nerve, a nerve extending from the base of the spine down the thigh, with branches throughout the lower leg and foot. It is the widest nerve of the body and one of the longest. Inflammation of the sciatic nerve causes pain along its course, or SCIATICA.

sciatica (si-at′ĭ-kah) neuralgia or neuritis of the sciatic nerve. The term is popularly used to describe a number of disorders directly or indirectly affecting the sciatic nerve. Because of its length, the nerve is exposed to many different kinds of injury, and inflammation of the nerve or injury to it causes pain that travels down from the back or thigh along its course in the leg and into the foot and toes. Certain muscles of the legs may be partly or completely paralyzed by such a disorder.
  True sciatic neuritis is comparatively rare. It can be caused by certain toxic substances, such as lead and alcohol, and occasionally by various other factors. Sciatic pain can be produced by a number of conditions other than inflammation of the nerve. Probably the most common cause is a slipped, or herniated, DISK. A back injury, irritation from arthritis of the spine or pressure on the nerve from certain types of exertion may also be the cause. Occasionally certain diseases such as diabetes mellitus, gout and vitamin deficiencies may be the inciting factor. In rare cases, pain may be referred over

connected nerve pathways to the sciatic nerve from a disorder in another part of the body. Some cases are idiopathic. Because of the long, painful and disabling course of severe sciatica, the underlying cause should be investigated and corrected when possible.

scieropia (si″er-o′pe-ah) a defect of vision in which objects appear in a shadow.

scintigram (sin′tĭ-gram) a graphic record of the particles registered by a scintiscanner, after administration of a radioisotope.

scintillation (sin″tĭ-la′shun) 1. the emission of charged particles. 2. the sensation of sparks before the eyes.

scintiscan (sin′tĭ-skan) a two-dimensional representation (map) of the gamma rays emitted by a radioisotope, revealing its concentration in a specific organ or tissue.

scintiscanner (sin″tĭ-skan′er) an apparatus for recording the concentration of a gamma ray-emitting isotope in tissue.

scirrho- (skir′o) word element [Gr.], *hard.*

scirrhoid (skir′oid) resembling a scirrhus.

scirrhoma (skir-o′mah) scirrhus.

scirrhosarca (skir″o-sar′kah) scleroderma.

scirrhous (skir′us) of the nature of a scirrhus.

scirrhus (skir′us) a hard cancer with predominance of connective tissue.

scissura (sĭ-su′rah), pl. *scissu′rae* [L.] an incisure; a splitting.

scler(o)- (skle′ro) word element [Gr.[, *hard; sclera of the eye.*

sclera (skle′rah) the tough, white covering of approximately the posterior five-sixths of the eyeball, continuous anteriorly with the cornea and posteriorly with the external sheath of the optic nerve. adj., **scle′ral.**
  blue s., abnormal blueness of the sclera, occurring as a hereditary condition transmitted by a dominant gene, and sometimes associated with brittleness of the bones and deafness.

scleradenitis (sklēr″ad-ĕ-ni′tis) inflammation and hardening of a gland.

sclerectasia (sklēr″ek-ta′ze-ah) a bulging state of the sclera.

sclerectomy (sklĕ-rek′to-me) excision of part of the sclera.

scleredema (sklēr″ĕ-de′mah) edematous hardening of the skin.
  s. adulto′rum, Buschke's s., hardening of the skin and subcutaneous tissues, affecting chiefly the head, neck and trunk, rarely the extremities.
  s. neonato′rum, sclerema neonatorum.

sclerema (sklĕ-re′mah) scleredema.
  s. adipo′sum, s. neonato′rum, a condition characterized by diffuse, rapidly spreading, nonedematous, tallow-like hardening of the subcutaneous tissues in the first few weeks of life.

scleriasis (sklĕ-ri′ah-sis) scleroderma.

scleriritomy (skle″rĭ-rit′o-me) incision of the sclera and iris in keratoglobus.

scleritis (sklĕ-ri′tis) inflammation of the sclera. It may be superficial (episcleritis) or deep.
  anterior s., inflammation of the sclera adjoining the limbus of the cornea.
  posterior s., scleritis involving the retina and choroid.

scleroblastema (skle″ro-blas-te′mah) the embryonic tissue from which bone is formed.

sclerochoroiditis (skle″ro-ko″roi-di′tis) inflammation of the sclera and choroid.

sclerocornea (skle″ro-kor′ne-ah) the sclera and cornea regarded as one.

sclerodactylia (skle″ro-dak-til′e-ah) scleroderma of the fingers and toes.

scleroderma (skle″ro-der′mah) an insidious chronic disorder characterized by progressive collagenous fibrosis of many organs and systems, usually beginning with the skin (see also COLLAGEN DISEASES).
  circumscribed s., that affecting only localized areas of the skin, with no apparent visceral involvement.
  s. neonato′rum, sclerema neonatorum.

sclerodermitis (skle″ro-der-mi′tis) inflammation and hardening of the skin.

sclerogenous (sklĕ-roj′ĕ-nus) producing a hard tissue or material.

scleroiritis (skle″ro-i-ri′tis) inflammation of the sclera and iris.

sclerokeratitis (skle″ro-ker″ah-ti′tis) inflammation of the sclera, cornea and iris.
  respiratory s., the presence of bluish-red granulomas on the mucosa of the upper respiratory tract, the involved parts enlarging slowly and becoming hard as ivory.

scleroma (sklĕ-ro′mah) a hardened patch or induration.

scleromalacia (skle″ro-mah-la′she-ah) degeneration (softening) of the sclera, occurring in patients with rheumatoid arthritis.

scleromyxedema (skle″ro-mik″sĕ-de′mah) a variant of lichen myxedematosus characterized by a generalized eruption of the nodules and diffuse thickening of the skin.

scleronyxis (skle″ro-nik′sis) puncture of the sclera.

sclero-oophoritis (skle″ro-o″of-o-ri′tis) sclerosing inflammation of the ovary.

sclerophthalmia (skle″rof-thal′me-ah) encroachment of the sclera upon the cornea, so that only a portion of the latter remains clear.

scleroplasty (skle′ro-plas″te) plastic repair of the sclera.

scleroprotein (skle″ro-pro′te-in) a strong, fibrous protein having structural and protective functions in the organism and insoluble in the usual solvents of proteins.

sclerosarcoma (skle″ro-sar-ko′mah) a firm, fleshy mass or growth.

sclerose (skle′rōs) to become, or cause to become, hardened.

sclerosis (sklĕ-ro′sis) an induration or hardening; especially hardening of a part from inflammation and in diseases of the interstitial substance. The term is used chiefly for such a hardening of the nervous system. adj., **sclerot′ic.**

  amyotrophic lateral s., degeneration of the anterior horn cells and pyramidal tract, with muscular atrophy (see also AMYOTROPHIC LATERAL SCLEROSIS).

  arteriolar s., arteriosclerosis of the minute arterioles.

  disseminated s., multiple sclerosis.

  lateral s., a form seated in the lateral columns of the spinal cord. It may be primary, with spastic paraplegia, rigidity of the limbs and increase of the tendon reflexes but no sensory disturbances, or secondary to myelitis, with paraplegia and sensory disturbance.

  multiple s., sclerosis of the brain and spinal cord occurring in scattered patches, and resulting in a chronic disabling condition characterized by visual disturbances, weakness, tremors and finally paralysis (see also MULTIPLE SCLEROSIS).

  tuberous s., a familial disease with tumors on the surfaces of the lateral ventricles of the brain and sclerotic patches on its surface, and marked by mental deterioration and epileptic attacks.

scleroskeleton (skle″ro-skel′ĕ-ton) the part of the bony skeleton formed by ossification in ligaments, fasciae and tendons.

sclerostenosis (skle″ro-stĕ-no′sis) hardening with contraction.

sclerostomy (sklĕ-ros′to-me) surgical creation of an opening through the sclera for the relief of glaucoma.

sclerotherapy (skle″ro-ther′ah-pe) injection of sclerosing solutions in the treatment of hemorrhoids or other varicose veins.

sclerothrix (skle′ro-thriks) abnormal hardness and dryness of the hair.

sclerotica (sklĕ-rot′ĭ-kah) [L.] sclera.

scleroticopuncture (sklĕ-rot″ĭ-ko-pungk′tūr) puncture of the sclera.

sclerotitis (skle″ro-ti′tis) scleritis.

sclerotium (sklĕ-ro′she-um) a hard mass formed by certain fungi, as ergot.

sclerotome (skle′ro-tōm) 1. one of the masses of diffuse cells formed by the breaking down of the ventromedial wall of each somite, which develop into vertebrae. 2. a knife for incising the sclera.

sclerotomy (sklĕ-rot′o-me) incision of the sclera.

  anterior s., the opening of the anterior chamber of the eye, chiefly done for the relief of glaucoma.

  posterior s., an opening made into the vitreous through the sclera, as for detachment of the retina or the removal of a foreign body.

sclerous (skle′rus) hard; indurated.

S.C.M. State Certified Midwife.

scolecology (sko″le-kol′o-je) helminthology.

scolex (sko′leks), pl. *sco′lices* [Gr.] the attachment organ of a tapeworm, generally considered the anterior, or cephalic, end.

scoli(o)- (sko′le-o) word element [Gr.], *crooked; twisted.*

scoliokyphosis (sko″le-o-ki-fo′sis) combined lateral and posterior curvature of the spine.

scoliorachitic (sko″le-o-rah-kit′ik) affected with scoliosis and rickets.

scoliosiometry (sko″le-o-se-om′ĕ-tre) measurement of spinal curvature.

scoliosis (sko″le-o′sis) lateral curvature of the vertebral column. adj., **scoliot′ic.**

  Scoliosis may begin during infancy, and the curvature usually occurs in the upper part of the infant's spine and grows progressively more marked. More often the condition develops about the age of 12; this form is ten times more common in girls than in boys. The first visible sign is likely to be unevenness of the hips or shoulders. In general, the earlier the condition begins, the more severe the curvature finally becomes. The malformation tends to progress no further once the spine has reached full growth, i.e., about the age of 15 for girls and 17 for boys.

  CAUSES. Habitually poor posture over a long period of time is a common cause of scoliosis; the faulty posture may be accompanied by lack of muscle tone and general physical inactivity. Unevenness in the length of the legs may lead to lateral curvature of the spine. This can usually be corrected by adding a lift to the shoe worn on the foot of the shorter leg. Diseases that affect the spine, such as RICKETS, or that weaken the muscles supporting the vertebral column can bring about scoliosis. In the majority of cases, particularly in adolescents, the original cause is unknown.

  TREATMENT. The type of treatment depends on the cause and degree of the malformation. Corrective exercises may eliminate the condition in some cases; in others, braces, casts or surgery may be necessary.

scolopsia (sko-lop′se-ah) a suture between two bones that allows motion of one upon the other.

scopograph (skop′o-graf) a combined fluoroscope and radiographic unit.

scopolamine (sko-pol′ah-mēn) an alkaloid derived from various plants, used in parasympathetic blockade and as a central nervous system depressant. It is used frequently during labor because of its tendency to cause amnesia.

scopometer (sko-pom′ĕ-ter) an instrument for measuring the turbidity of solutions, i.e., the density of a precipitate.

scopophilia (sko″po-fil′e-ah) 1. the derivation of sexual pleasure from looking at genitalia (active scopophilia). 2. a morbid desire to be seen (passive scopophilia).

scopophobia (sko″po-fo′be-ah) morbid dread of being seen.

scoptophilia (skop″to-fil′e-ah) scopophilia.

-scopy (skop′e) word element [Gr.], *examination of.*

scoracratia (sko″rah-kra′she-ah) fecal incontinence.

scorbutic (skor-bu′tik) pertaining to scurvy.

scorbutigenic (skor-bu″tĭ-jen′ik) causing scurvy.

scorbutus (skor-bu′tus) [L.] scurvy.

scordinemia (skor″dĭ-ne′me-ah) yawning and stretching with a feeling of lassitude.

score (skōr) a rating, usually expressed numerically, based on specific achievement or the degree to which certain qualities are manifest.
  Apgar s., a numerical expression of an infant's condition at birth, based on heart rate, respiratory effort, muscle tone, reflex irritability and color.

scoto- (sko′to) word element [Gr.], *darkness.*

scotochromogen (sko″to-kro′mo-jen) a microorganism whose pigmentation develops in the dark as well as in the light; specifically, a member of a group of the anonymous mycobacteria.

scotodinia (sko″to-din′e-ah) vertigo with headache and dimness of vision.

scotogram, scotograph (sko′to-gram), (sko′to-graf) 1. roentgenogram. 2. the effect produced on a photographic plate in the dark by certain substances.

scotoma (sko-to′mah) an area of depressed vision within the visual field, surrounded by an area of less depressed or of normal vision.
  central s., an area of depressed vision corresponding with the fixation point and interfering with or abolishing central vision.
  centrocecal s., a horizontal defect in the visual field situated between and embracing both the fixation point and the blind spot.
  color s., an isolated area of depressed or defective vision for color in the visual field.
  scintillating s., the sensation of a luminous appearance before the eyes, with a zigzag, wall-like outline; called also teichopsia.

scotomagraph (sko-to′mah-graf) an instrument for recording a scotoma.

scotometry (sko-tom′ĕ-tre) the measurement of isolated areas of depressed vision (scotomas) within the visual field.

scotomization (sko″to-mĭ-za′shun) development of scotomas, or blind spots, especially of mental "blind spots," the patient attempting to deny existence of everything that conflicts with his ego.

scotophilia (sko″to-fil′e-ah) love of darkness.

scotophobia (sko″to-fo′be-ah) morbid fear of darkness.

scotopia (sko-to′pe-ah) the adjustment of the eye for darkness. adj., **scotop′ic.**

scr. scruple.

scratch test (skrach) a test for hypersensitivity in which a minute amount of the substance in question is inserted in small scratches made in the skin. A positive reaction is swelling and reddening at the site within 30 minutes. Used in allergy testing and in testing for tuberculosis (Pirquet's reaction). (See also SKIN TEST.)

screatus (skre-a′tus) paroxysmal attacks of hawking and snorting, due to neurosis.

screen (skrēn) 1. a framework used as a shield or protector. 2. to examine.
  Bjerrum s., tangent screen.
  fluorescent s., a plate in the fluoroscope coated with crystals of a substance that fluoresces, permitting visualization of internal body structures by x-ray.
  tangent s., a large square of black cloth with a central mark for fixation; used in mapping the field of vision.

screening (skrēn′ing) examination of a large number of individuals to disclose certain characteristics, or a certain disease, as tuberculosis or diabetes mellitus.
  multiphasic s., multiple s., simultaneous examination of a population for several different diseases.

scrobiculate (skro-bik′u-lāt) marked with pits.

scrobiculus (skro-bik′u-lus) [L.] pit.
  s. cor′dis, the pit of the stomach.

scrofula (skrof′u-lah) a tuberculous disease of lymph nodes and of bone, with slowly suppurating abscesses. adj., **scrof′ulous.**

scrofuloderma (skrof″u-lo-der′mah) a skin disease of scrofulous nature and marked by irregular superficial ulcers.

scrofulosis (skrof″u-lo′sis) a tendency toward scrofula.

scrotectomy (skro-tek′to-me) excision of part of the scrotum.

scrotitis (skro-ti′tis) inflammation of the scrotum.

scrotocele (skro′to-sēl) scrotal hernia.

scrotoplasty (skro′to-plas″te) plastic reconstruction of the scrotum.

scrotum (skro′tum) the skin-covered pouch that contains the testes and their accessory organs. It is composed of skin, the dartos, fascia and the tunica vaginalis. adj., **scro′tal.** Each TESTIS is connected to a cremaster muscle descending from the abdominal wall. During cold weather these muscles draw the testes closer to the body to maintain their temperature. In hot weather the reverse occurs. The scrotum usually follows this movement.
  The scrotum is subject to the same diseases as the rest of the skin, including cysts and cancer. Edema, whether caused by heart disease or the tropical disease ELEPHANTIASIS, can cause great enlargement of the scrotum by filling its loose tissues with fluid.

scruple (skroo′pl) a unit of weight of the apothecaries' system, equal to 20 grains; the equivalent of 1.296 Gm.

scultetus binder (skul-te′tus) one applied in strips overlapping each other in shingle fashion.

the species *Enterobius vermicularis* (see also WORMS).

scurf (skurf) a branny substance of epidermic origin; dandruff.

scurvy (skur've) a condition due to deficiency of ASCORBIC ACID (vitamin C). Symptoms of infantile scurvy include poor appetite, digestive disturbances, failure to gain weight and increasing irritability. Black and blue spots are scattered over the skin. Severe deficiency may cause changes in bone structure.

The only adults in the United States likely to develop scurvy are older people who live alone and neglect their diet. In adults, scurvy causes swollen and bleeding gums, looseness of the teeth, rupture of small blood vessels and small black and blue spots on the skin. Later symptoms may include anemia, extreme weakness, soreness of the arms and legs, tachycardia and dyspnea.

Treatment of scurvy consists of supplying the missing vitamin in prescribed doses, and supplying the proper diet, including fresh fruits and vegetables. When this is done, the symptoms quickly disappear.

Fruits and vegetables that are rich sources of vitamin C include the following: grapefruit, oranges, lemons, limes, cantaloupes, strawberries, raspberries, turnips, raw cabbage, potatoes (baked) and tomatoes.

scute (skūt) the bony plate separating the upper part of the middle ear from the mastoid cells.

scutiform (sku'tĭ-form) shaped like a shield.

scutum (sku'tum) a protective covering or shield, e.g., a chitin plate in the exoskeleton of an arthropod.

scybalous (sib'ah-lus) of the nature of a scybalum.

scybalum (sib'ah-lum), pl. *scyb'ala* [Gr.] a hard mass of fecal matter in the intestine.

scyphoid (si'foid) shaped like a cup or goblet.

scytoblastema (si"to-blas-te'mah) the rudimentary skin of the embryo.

SD streptodornase.

S.D. skin dose; standard deviation.

Se chemical symbol, *selenium*.

searcher (serch'er) an instrument used in examining the bladder for calculi; called also stone searcher.

seasickness (se'sik-nes) discomfort caused by the motion of a boat under way, a form of MOTION SICKNESS. The unusual motion disturbs the organs of balance located in the inner ear. The symptoms are nausea and vomiting, dizziness, headache, pallor and cold perspiration.

There are a number of ways to help ward off seasickness. It is best to stay in the fresh air instead of in a stuffy room, to eat lightly and to avoid fatty, fried or spicy foods. Antinausea medicines may be effective. If seasickness occurs, the sufferer should rest lying down with his head low, in a comfortable well ventilated place.

seatworm (sēt'werm) pinworm; an individual of

sebaceous (se-ba'shus) 1. pertaining to sebum or suet. 2. secreting a greasy lubricating substance.

s. cyst, a benign retention cyst of a sebaceous gland containing the fatty secretion of the gland; called also wen. Sebaceous cysts may occur anywhere on the body except the palms of the hands and soles of the feet; they are most common on the scalp, back and scrotum. A cyst may be a source of irritation or infection, and should be excised by a physician.

s. gland, one of the thousands of minute glands in the skin that secrete an oily, colorless, odorless fluid (sebum) through the hair follicles.

sebiferous, sebiparous (se-bif'er-us), (se-bip'ah-rus) secreting or producing a fatty substance.

sebocystoma (se"bo-sis-to'mah) a sebaceous cyst.

sebolith (seb'o-lith) a calculus in a sebaceous gland.

seborrhagia, seborrhea (seb"o-ra'je-ah), (seb"-o-re'ah) excessive discharge from the sebaceous glands, forming greasy scales or cheesy plugs on the body; it is generally attended with itching or burning.

s. capillit'ii, seborrhea of the scalp.

s. ni'gricans, seborrhea with a dark-colored crust.

s. sic'ca, the commonest form of seborrhea, characterized by the formation of brownish gray scales.

seborrheic (seb"o-re'ik) affected with or of the nature of seborrhea.

s. dermatitis, an inflammatory condition of the skin of the scalp, with yellowish, greasy scaling of the skin; commonly known as dandruff. It may spread to other areas about the face, neck, central part of the trunk and axillae.

The underlying cause is not known; the sebaceous glands become overactive and the hair and scalp are excessively oily. The scales are greasy, yellowish and crusty. Burning or itching and erythema of the involved areas may occur.

There is also a dry form of the condition, in which the scales are hard, dry and whitish gray in color and the hair is dry and brittle.

Although there is no specific cure for dandruff, various measures are used to control and relieve it. The most imperative point is cleanliness of the hair, scalp, combs and brushes. There are some helpful medical preparations which are prescribed for persistent cases. These usually contain sulfur, tar, salicylic acid, selenium sulfide or steroids.

seborrheid (seb"o-re'id) a seborrheic eruption.

sebum (se'bum) the oily secretion of the sebaceous glands, whose ducts open into the hair follicles. It is composed of fat and epithelial debris from the cells of the malpighian layer, and it lubricates the skin.

secale (se-ka'le) [L.] rye.

s. cornu'tum, ergot.

secobarbital (sek"o-bar'bĭ-tal) a short- to intermediate-acting barbiturate.

sodium s., a hypnotic compound for oral or parenteral use.

Seconal (sek'ŏ-nal) trademark for preparations of secobarbital.

second-set phenomenon the occurrence in a recipient of a more severe immune reaction to a second graft of tissue from the same donor, because of antibodies produced as a result of the first graft.

secreta (se-kre′tah) [L., *pl.*] the secretions.

secretagogue (se-krēt′ah-gog) 1. causing a flow of secretion. 2. an agent that stimulates secretion.

secretin (se-kre′tin) 1. a hormone secreted by the mucosa of the duodenum and jejunum when acid chyme enters the intestine; carried by the blood, it stimulates the secretion of pancreatic juice and bile. 2. a general name for any hormone that stimulates glandular secretion.

secretion (se-kre′shun) 1. the process of elaborating a specific product as a result of the activity of a gland. This activity may range from separating a specific substance of the blood to the elaboration of a new chemical substance. 2. any substance produced by secretion. One example is the fatty substance produced by the sebaceous glands to lubricate the skin. Saliva, produced by the salivary glands, and gastric juice, secreted by specialized glands of the stomach, are both used in digestion. The secretions of the endocrine glands include various hormones and are important in the overall regulation of body processes.

secretoinhibitory (se-kre″to-in-hib′ĭ-tor″e) inhibiting secretion.

secretomotor (se-kre″to-mo′tor) stimulating secretion; said of nerves.

secretor (se-kre′tor) a person having A or B type blood whose saliva and other secretions contain the particular (A or B) substance.

secretory (se-kre′to-re) pertaining to secretion.

sectio (sek′she-o), pl. *sectio′nes* [L.] section.

section (sek′shun) 1. an act of cutting. 2. a cut surface. 3. a segment or subdivision of an organ.
   abdominal s., laparotomy; incision of the abdominal wall.
   cesarean s., delivery of a fetus by incision through the abdominal wall and uterus.
   frontal s., a section through the body passing from left to right at right angles to the median plane.
   frozen s., a specimen cut by microtome from tissue that has been frozen.
   perineal s., external urethrotomy.
   sagittal s., a section through the body coinciding or parallel with the sagittal suture, thus dividing the body into more or less equal right and left halves.
   serial s's, histologic sections of a specimen made in consecutive order and so arranged for the purpose of microscopic examination.
   sigaultian s., symphysiotomy.
   vaginal s., incision through the vaginal wall into the abdominal cavity.

sectioning (sek′shun-ing) the cutting of thin sections of tissue for study under the microscope.

sectorial (sek-to′re-al) cutting.

secundigravida (se-kun″dĭ-grav′ĭ-dah) a woman pregnant the second time; gravida II.

secundines (se-kun′dīnz) afterbirth; the placenta and the membranes expelled after childbirth.

secundipara (se″kun-dip′ah-rah) bipara; a woman who has had two pregnancies that resulted in viable offspring; para II.

Sedamyl (sed′ah-mil) trademark for a preparation of acetylcarbromal, a sedative.

sedation (se-da′shun) the production of a sedative effect; the act or process of calming.

sedative (sed′ah-tiv) 1. allaying activity and excitement. 2. an agent that calms nervousness, irritability and excitement. In general, sedatives depress the central nervous system and tend to cause lassitude and reduced mental activity.

The degree of relaxation produced varies with the kind of sedative, the dose, the means of administration and the mental state of the patient. By causing relaxation, a sedative may help a patient go to sleep, but it does not put him to sleep. Medicines that induce sleep are known as hypnotics. A drug may act as a sedative in small amounts and as a hypnotic in large amounts.

The BARBITURATES, such as phenobarbital, are the best-known sedatives. They are also widely used as hypnotics. Other effective sedatives are the bromides, paraldehyde and chloral hydrate.

Sedatives are useful in the treatment of any condition in which rest and relaxation are important to recovery. Some sedatives are also useful in treatment of convulsive disorders or epilepsy and in counteracting the effect of convulsion-producing drugs. They are used to calm patients before childbirth or surgery. Restlessness in invalids, profound grief in adults and overexcitement in children can be controlled by medically supervised sedation. Because many sedatives are habit-forming, they should be used only under the supervision of a physician.

Among drugs related to sedatives are the TRANQUILIZERS, which also have a calming effect but, unlike sedatives, usually do not suppress body reactions.

sedentary (sed′en-ter″e) of inactive habits; pertaining to a sitting posture.

sediment (sed′ĭ-ment) a precipitate, especially that formed spontaneously.

sedimentation (sed″ĭ-men-ta′shun) the settling out of sediment.
   s. rate, erythrocyte sedimentation rate; the rate at which erythrocytes settle out of unclotted blood in an hour. Abbreviated sed. rate or E.S.R. The test is based on the fact that inflammatory processes cause an alteration in blood proteins, resulting in aggregation of the red cells, which makes them heavier and more likely to fall rapidly when placed in a special vertical test tube. Normal ranges vary according to the type of tube used, each type being of a different size. The most common methods and the normal range for each are: Wintrobe method — 0 to 6.5 mm. per hour for men, 0 to 15 mm. per hour for women; Westergren method — 0 to 15 mm. per hour for men, 0 to 20 mm. per hour for women.

The sedimentation rate is often inconclusive and is not considered specific for any particular disorder. It is most often used as gauge for determining the progress of an inflammatory disease such as rheumatic fever, rheumatoid arthritis and respiratory infections. The information provided by this test must be used in conjunction with results from other tests and clinical evaluations.

seed (sēd) 1. semen. 2. the small body produced by flowering plants containing the embryo of the new individual. 3. a small container of radioactive material used in radiotherapy of certain tumors.

   plantago s., plantain s., psyllium s., cleaned, dried ripe seed of species of Plantago; used as a cathartic.

   radon s., a small sealed container for radon, for insertion into the tissues of the body in radiotherapy.

segment (seg′ment) a demarcated portion of a whole.

   bronchopulmonary s., one of the smaller subdivisions of the lobe of a lung, separated from others by a connective tissue septum and supplied by its own branch of the bronchus leading to the particular lobe.

   uterine s., one of the portions into which the uterus becomes differentiated early in labor; the upper contractile portion, which becomes thicker as labor approaches, and the lower noncontractile portion, which is thin walled and passive in character.

segmentation (seg″men-ta′shun) division into similar parts.

segregation (seg″rĕ-ga′shun) 1. in genetics, the separation of the two genes of a pair in the process of maturation so that only one goes to each germ cell. 2. the progressive restriction of potencies in the zygote to the various regions of the forming embryo.

Seidlitz powders (sīd′litz) a mixture of sodium bicarbonate, potassium sodium tartrate and tartaric acid; used as a cathartic.

seismesthesia (sīz″mes-the′ze-ah) tactile perception of vibrations in a liquid or aerial medium.

seismocardiogram (sīz″mo-kar′de-o-gram″) the record obtained by seismocardiography.

seismocardiography (sīz″mo-kar″de-og′rah-fe) the selective recording of cardiac vibrations and beats.

seismotherapy (sīz″mo-ther′ah-pe) treatment of disease by mechanical vibration.

seizure (se′zhur) 1. a sudden attack, as of a disease. 2. an attack of EPILEPSY.

   focal s., a seizure involving a limited area of the body.

   grand mal s., one involving the entire body.

   petit mal s., one in which there is a period of apparent inattentiveness; usually seen in children under the age of 13.

   psychomotor s., an episode of mental confusion with apparently purposeful but coarse and poorly coordinated muscular movements.

selenium (sĕ-le′ne-um) a chemical element, atomic number 34, atomic weight 78.96, symbol Se. (See table of ELEMENTS.)

   s. sulfide, a bright orange, insoluble powder; used topically in solution in the treatment of seborrheic dermatitis.

self-limited (self-lim′ĭ-ted) limited by its own peculiarities, and not by outside influence; said of a disease that runs a definite limited course.

self-suspension (self″sus-pen′shun) suspension of the body by the head and axillae for the purpose of stretching the vertebral column.

selfwise (self′wīz) developing in a previously determined manner despite transplantation to a new and strange location; said of embryonic cells or tissue.

sella (sel′ah), pl. *sel′lae* [L.] a saddle-shaped depression. adj., **sel′lar.**

   s. tur′cica, a depression on the upper surface of the sphenoid bone, lodging the pituitary gland.

semantics (se-man′tiks) study of the meanings of words and the rules of their use; study of the relation between language and significance.

semeiography (se″mi-og′rah-fe) symptomatology.

semeiotic (se″mi-ot′ik) 1. pertaining to symptoms. 2. pathognomonic.

semel (sem′el) [L.] once.

semelincident (sem″el-in′sĭ-dent) affecting a person only once.

semelparity (sem″el-par′ĭ-te) the state, in an individual organism, of reproducing only once in a lifetime.

semen (se′men) fluid discharged at ejaculation in the male, consisting of spermatozoa in their nutrient plasma, secretions from the prostate, seminal vesicles and various other glands, epithelial cells and minor constituents. adj., **sem′inal.**

semenuria (se″men-u′re-ah) discharge of semen in the urine.

semi- (sem′e) word element [L.], *half.*

semicanal (sem″ĭ-kah-nal′) a trench or furrow open at one side.

semicircular (sem″ĭ-ser′ku-lar) shaped like a half-circle.

   s. canals, the passages in the inner ear, or labyrinth, which control the sense of balance. Each ear has three semicircular canals situated approximately at right angles to each other. The canals are filled with fluid and have enlarged portions at one end, called ampullae, which contain nerve endings.

   The semicircular canals respond to movement of the head. When the head changes position in any direction, the fluid in the canal that lies in the plane of movement also moves but, because of its inertia, the fluid flow lags behind the head movement. Thus the fluid presses against the delicate hairs of the nerves in the ampulla, and these nerves then register the fact that the head is turning in such a direction. This helps the body maintain its equilibrium.

   It is the fluid movement in the semicircular canals that causes the feeling of dizziness or vertigo after spinning. When the spinning stops, the fluid in the horizontal canal continues to move for a moment in the direction of the spin, giving a temporary false reading that the head is turning in the other direction. Motion sickness is caused by the unusual and erratic motions of the head in an airplane, car or ship, and the resulting stimulation of the semicircular canals.

semicoma (sem″ĭ-ko′mah) a mild coma from which the patient may be aroused.

semiflexion (sem″ĭ-flek′shun) the position of a limb midway between flexion and extension.

Semikon (sem′ĭ-kon) trademark for preparations of methapyrilene, an antihistamine.

semilunar (sem″ĭ-lu′nar) shaped like a half-moon.
  s. valves, valves guarding the entrances into the aorta and pulmonary trunk from the cardiac ventricles.

semimicroanalysis (sem″ĭ-mi″kro-ah-nal′ĭ-sis) chemical analysis based on 0.01 to 0.02 Gm. of the substance under study.

semination (sem″ĭ-na′shun) insemination.

seminiferous (sem″ĭ-nif′er-us) producing or carrying semen.

seminoma (sem″ĭ-no′mah) a dysgerminoma of the testis.
  ovarian s., a dysgerminoma of the ovary.

semipermeable (sem″ĭ-per′me-ah-bl) permitting passage only of certain molecules.

semis (se′mis) [L.] half; abbreviated *ss.*

semisulcus (sem″ĭ-sul′kus) a depression that, with an adjoining one, forms a sulcus.

semisupination (sem″ĭ-su″pĭ-na′shun) a position halfway toward supination.

semisynthetic (sem″ĭ-sin-thet′ik) produced partially by natural processes and partially by artificial manipulation.

Semmelweiss (sem′el-vīs) Ignaz Philipp (1818–1865). Hungarian physician and pioneer of antisepsis in obstetrics. He was born at Buda and educated at the universities of Pest and Vienna. As assistant in an obstetrics ward of Allgemeines Krankenhaus in Vienna, where the mortality rate from puerperal fever was extremely high, Semmelweiss recognized that the infection was carried from patient to patient by the physicians, and he instituted preventive measures, such as cleansing of the physicians' hands with chlorinated lime. He met such fierce opposition from many of his colleagues that he left Vienna and returned to Pest, as physician in the maternity department.

Semoxydrine (sem-ok′sĭ-drin) trademark for a preparation of methamphetamine, a central nervous system stimulant.

Senear-Usher disease (se-nēr′ ush′er) pemphigus erythematosus.

senescence (sĕ-nes′ens) the process of growing old. adj., **senes′cent.**

Sengstaken-Blakemore tube (sengz′ta-ken blāk′mōr) a device used for the tamponade of bleeding esophageal varices, consisting of three tubes; one leading to a balloon that is inflated in the stomach, to retain the instrument in place and compress the vessels around the cardia; one leading to a long narrow balloon by which pressure is exerted against the wall of the esophagus; and the third attached to a suction apparatus for aspirating contents of the stomach.

senile (se′nīl) pertaining to old age.

senilism (se′nil-izm) premature old age.

senility (sĕ-nil′ĭ-te) old age; a pronounced and abnormal loss of mental, physical or emotional control in aged people, caused by physical or mental deterioration or a combination of the two. Certain types of psychosis are associated with senility.
  By the age of 70, many people normally experience some degree of physical change, such as a slowing of the reflexes and a greater susceptibility to fatigue. In senility, however, these changes are often extreme in nature. Senility refers to psychologic changes; commonly the patient suffers lapses of memory and confuses the present with the past. Sudden uncontrolled outbursts of joy, rage or despair may occur for no apparent reason. In severe cases, the patient may suffer from delusions of persecution or depression and apathy.
  PSYCHOLOGIC CAUSES. Senility of psychologic origin is the most common type and is believed to be a reaction to loss of interests and stimulation and to the insecurities, frustrations, fears and stresses of old age. There may be no physical damage to the brain. The patient may have reason to feel that he has become worthless or useless in his old age, and as a result he withdraws from everyday life. The period of old age makes necessary great adjustments to new physical conditions and living patterns, adjustments that many people are not able to make without professional help.
  PHYSICAL CAUSES. The most common physical cause of senility is cerebral ARTERIOSCLEROSIS, which can cause slow, progressive brain damage. This may lead to a cerebral hemorrhage or thrombosis. The symptoms depend largely on the area of the brain that is damaged.
  TREATMENT. The treatment for patients with psychologic changes of senility is primarily concerned with helping the patient adjust to his reduced capacities and limited physical activities. Psychotherapy is used to assist the patient in this adjustment. In addition, some effort should be made to reduce the demands and pressures of everyday living so that the patient will be better able to cope with his environment. Senility tends to become progressively worse, with irreversible changes in the patient's physical state and emotional makeup and personality.
  NURSING CARE. The patient with psychologic changes due to senility often is difficult to care for because he is irritable and uncooperative and often lacks good judgment. He must be supervised carefully so that he does not injure himself or wander away from his home or hospital room and become lost.
  Unless his physical condition requires bed rest, a routine should be established for indoor exercise and walks out-of-doors when the weather permits. A schedule also should be established for taking the patient to the bathroom or offering him a bedpan if he is confined to bed. This will help avoid accidental soiling and wetting which can occur frequently because of forgetfulness and poor orientation.

Physical care includes special care of the skin, proper diet in small, frequent feedings and sufficient rest. (See also AGED.) A flexible plan for recreational and diversional activities must take into account the mental capacity and physical abilities of the patient, which may vary from day to day or even from one hour to the next.

senna (sen′ah) the dried leaflets of *Cassia acutiflora;* used in a syrup, fluidextract or compound powder as a cathartic.

senopia (se-no′pe-ah) improvement of the visual power in old people.

sensation (sen-sa′shun) an impression produced by impulses conveyed by an afferent nerve to the sensorium.

  concomitant s., secondary sensation.

  cutaneous s., sensation perceived at or on the skin, as touch, temperature, etc.

  girdle s., zonesthesia.

  gnostic s's, sensations perceived by the more recently developed senses, such as those of light touch and the epicritic sensibility to muscle, joint and tendon vibrations.

  primary s., that resulting immediately and directly from application of a stimulus.

  referred s., reflex s., one felt elsewhere than at the site of application of a stimulus.

  secondary s., one developed, without special stimulation, along with, and resulting from, a primary sensation.

  subjective s., one originating within the organism and not occurring in response to an external stimulus.

sense (sens) a faculty by which the conditions or properties of things are perceived. Hunger, thirst, malaise and pain are varieties of sense; a sense of equilibrium or of well-being (euphoria) and other senses are also distinguished. The five major senses comprise VISION, HEARING, SMELL, TASTE and TOUCH.
The operation of all senses involves the reception of stimuli by sense organs. Each sense organ is sensitive to a particular kind of stimulus. The eyes are sensitive to light; the ears, to sound; the olfactory organs of the nose, to odor; and the taste buds of the tongue, to taste. Various sense organs of the skin and other tissues are sensitive to touch, pain, temperature and other sensations.
On receiving stimuli, the sense organ translates them into nerve impulses that are transmitted along the sensory nerves to the brain. In the cerebral cortex, the impulses are interpreted, or perceived, as sensations. The brain associates them with other information, acts upon them and stores them as memory. (See also NERVOUS SYSTEM and BRAIN.)

  kinesthetic s., the muscular sense.

  light s., the faculty by which degrees of brilliancy are distinguished.

  muscle s., muscular s., the faculty by which muscular movements are perceived.

  posture s., a variety of muscular sense by which the position or attitude of the body or its parts is perceived.

  pressure s., the faculty by which pressure upon the surface of the body is perceived.

  sixth s., the general feeling of consciousness of the entire body.

  space s., the faculty by which relative positions and relations of objects in space are perceived.

  special s., one of the five senses of seeing, feeling, hearing, taste and smell.

  stereognostic s., the sense by which form and solidity are perceived.

  temperature s., the faculty by which differences of temperature are appreciated.

sensibility (sen″sĭ-bil′ĭ-te) 1. capacity for perception or feeling. 2. sensitivity.

  deep s., the sensibility to pressure and movement that exists after the skin area is made completely anesthetic.

  epicritic s., the sensibility to gentle stimulations permitting fine discriminations of touch and temperature, localized in the skin.

  protopathic s., the sensibility to strong stimulations of pain and temperature, which is low in degree and poorly localized, existing in the skin and in the viscera, and acting as a defensive agency against pathologic changes in the tissues.

  somesthetic s., the sensibility to stimuli received by the somatic sensory receptors.

  splanchnesthetic s., the sensibility to stimuli received by splanchnic receptors.

sensibilization (sen″sĭ-bil′ĭ-za′shun) 1. the act of making more sensitive. 2. sensitization.

sensibilizer (sen′sĭ-bil-īz″er) amboceptor.

sensible (sen′sĭ-bl) perceptible to the senses.

sensitinogen (sen″sĭ-tin′o-jen) a general term for an antigen having a sensitizing effect on the body.

sensitive (sen′sĭ-tiv) 1. able to receive or transmit a sensation; capable of responding to a stimulus. 2. unusually susceptible to stimulation; showing an exaggerated response, as to painful stimuli.

sensitivity (sen″sĭ-tiv′ĭ-te) the state or quality of being sensitive; often used to denote a state of abnormal responsiveness to stimulation.

sensitization (sen″sĭ-tĭ-za′shun) 1. the process of becoming sensitive, as the rendering of a cell sensitive by the action of an amboceptor. 2. the process of rendering an individual sensitive to a given protein.

  active s., the sensitization that results from the injection of a dose of antigen into the animal.

  passive s., that which results when some of the blood of a sensitized animal is injected into a normal animal.

  protein s., that bodily state in which the individual is sensitive or hypersusceptible to some foreign protein, so that when there is absorption of that protein a typical reaction is set up.

sensitized (sen′sĭ-tīzd) rendered sensitive.

sensomobile (sen″so-mo′bēl) moving in response to a stimulus.

sensomotor (sen″so-mo′tor) sensorimotor.

sensoparalysis (sen″so-pah-ral′ĭ-sis) paralysis of the sensory nerves of a part.

sensorial (sen-so′re-al) pertaining to the sensorium.

sensorimotor (sen″so-re-mo′tor) both sensory and motor.

sensorium (sen-so're-um) 1. a sensory nerve center. 2. the state of an individual as regards consciousness or mental awareness.

s. **commu'ne,** the part of the cerebral cortex that receives and coordinates all the impulses sent to individual nerve centers.

sensory (sen'so-re) pertaining to sensation.

s. **nerve,** a peripheral nerve that conducts impulses from a sense organ to the spinal cord or brain; called also afferent nerve.

sentient (sen'she-ent) able to feel; sensitive.

sepsis (sep'sis) a morbid condition resulting from the presence of pathogenic bacteria and their products.

puerperal s., sepsis occurring after childbirth, due to putrefactive matter absorbed from the birth canal (see also PUERPERAL FEVER).

septa- (sep'tah) word element [L.], *seven.*

septan (sep'tan) recurring on the seventh day (every six days).

septate (sep'tāt) divided by a septum.

septectomy (sep-tek'to-me) excision of part of the nasal septum.

septic (sep'tik) produced by or due to putrefaction.

septicemia (sep"tĭ-se'me-ah) the presence of bacteria or their toxins in the blood. adj., **septice'-mic.**

cryptogenic s., a septicemia in which the focus of infection is not evident during life.

puerperal s., that in which the focus of infection is a lesion of the mucous membrane received during childbirth.

septicopyemia (sep"tĭ-ko-pi-e'me-ah) septicemia with pyemia.

septipara (sep-tip'ah-rah) a woman who has had seven pregnancies that resulted in living offspring; para VII.

septivalent (sep-tiv'ah-lent) having a valence of seven.

septotomy (sep-tot'o-me) incision of the nasal septum.

septulum (sep'tu-lum), pl. *sep'tula* [L.] a small separating wall or partition.

septum (sep'tum), pl. *sep'ta* [L.] a wall or partition dividing a body space or cavity. adj., **sep'tal.** Some septa are membranous, some are composed of bone and some of cartilage, and each is named according to its location. The wall separating the atria (upper chambers) of the heart, for instance, is called the septum atriorum, or interatrial septum.

Usually, however, the term septum is used to refer to the nasal septum, a plate of bone and cartilage covered with mucous membrane that divides the nasal cavity. An injury or malformation of this septum can produce a deviated septum, in which one part of the cavity is smaller than the other. Occasionally the deviation may handicap breathing, block the normal flow of mucus from the sinuses during a cold and prevent proper drainage of infected sinuses. Deviated septum is fairly common and seldom causes complications. In some cases surgery may be necessary to relieve the obstruction and reduce irritation and infection in the nose and sinuses. The surgical procedure is called a partial or complete submucous resection.

An opening, or defect in the septum dividing the right and left sides of the heart sometimes is present at birth. The most common type is ventricular septal defect, an opening between the ventricles, often described by laymen as "a hole in the heart." (See also CONGENITAL HEART DEFECT.)

s. **lu'cidum,** 1. the partition between the lateral ventricles of the brain; called also septum pellucidum. 2. the stratum corneum of the epidermis.

septuplet (sep-tup'let, sep-too'plet) one of seven offspring produced at one birth.

sequela (se-kwe'lah), pl. *seque'lae* [L.] a morbid condition following or occurring as a consequence of another condition or event.

sequester (se-kwes'ter) to detach or separate abnormally a small portion from the whole.

sequestration (se"kwes-tra'shun) 1. abnormal separation of a part from a whole, as a portion of a bone by a pathologic process, or a portion of the circulating blood in a specific part occurring naturally or produced by application of a tourniquet. 2. isolation of a patient.

pulmonary s., loss of connection of lung tissue with the bronchial tree and the pulmonary veins.

sequestrectomy (se"kwes-trek'to-me) excision of a sequestrum.

sequestrum (se-kwes'trum), pl. *seques'tra* [L.] a piece of dead bone that has become separated during the process of necrosis from sound bone.

serapheresis (se"rah-fĕ-re'sis) the production of serum by permitting the clotting of plasma derived by plasmapheresis.

Serenium (sĕ-re'ne-um) trademark for a preparation of ethoxazene, a urinary analgesic.

Serfin (ser'fin) trademark for a preparation of reserpine, an antihypertensive and tranquilizer.

sericeps (ser'ĭ-seps) a silken bag used in making traction on the fetal head.

series (se'rēz) a group or succession of events, objects or substances arranged in regular order or forming a kind of chain; in electricity, parts of a circuit connected successively end to end to form a single path for the current. adj., **se'rial.**

aliphatic s., the open chain or fatty series of chemical compounds.

aromatic s., the compounds derived from benzene.

erythrocytic s., the succession of developing cells that ultimately culminates in the erythrocyte.

fatty s., methane and its derivatives and the homologous hydrocarbons.

homologous s., a series of compounds each member of which differs from the one preceding it by the radical CH_2.

leukocytic s., the succession of developing cells that ultimately culminates in the leukocyte.

serine (ser'ēn) a naturally occurring amino acid.

serocolitis (se"ro-ko-li'tis) inflammation of the serous coat of the colon.

seroculture (se″ro-kul′tūr) a bacterial culture on blood serum.

serodiagnosis (se″ro-di″ag-no′sis) diagnosis of disease from the serum reactions.

seroenteritis (se″ro-en″tĕ-ri′tis) inflammation of the serous coat of the intestine.

seroenzyme (se″ro-en′zīm) an enzyme in blood serum.

serofibrinous (se″ro-fi′brĭ-nus) marked by both a serous exudate and precipitation of fibrin.

seroflocculation (se″ro-flok″u-la′shun) flocculation produced in blood serum by an antigen.

seroglobulin (se″ro-glob′u-lin) the globulin of blood serum.

serohemorrhagic (se″ro-hem″o-raj′ik) characterized by serum and blood.

serohepatitis (se″ro-hep″ah-ti′tis) inflammation of the peritoneum of the liver.

seroimmunity (se″ro-ĭ-mu′nĭ-te) immunity produced by an antiserum; passive immunity.

serolactescent (se″ro-lak-tes′ent) resembling serum and milk.

serolemma (se″ro-lem′ah) the membrane whence the serosa or chorion is developed.

serolipase (se″ro-li′pās) a lipase from blood serum.

serologist (se-rol′o-jist) a specialist in serology.

serology (se-rol′o-je) the study of antigen-antibody reactions in vitro. adj., **serolog′ic.**

serolysin (se-rol′ĭ-sin) a lysin of the blood serum.

seroma (se-ro′mah) a collection of serosanguineous fluid in the body, producing a tumor-like mass.

seromembranous (se″ro-mem′brah-nus) both serous and membranous.

seromucous (se″ro-mu′kus) both serous and mucous.

seromuscular (se″ro-mus′ku-lar) pertaining to the serous and muscular coats of the intestine.

Seromycin (ser′o-mi″sin) trademark for preparations of cycloserine, an antibiotic.

seronegativity (se″ro-neg″ah-tiv′ĭ-te) the state of showing negative results on serologic examination.

seroperitoneum (se″ro-per″ĭ-to-ne′um) fluid in the peritoneal cavity; ascites.

serophyte (se′ro-fīt) an organism that grows in the body fluids.

seroplastic (se″ro-plas′tik) serofibrinous.

seropneumothorax (se″ro-nu″mo-tho′raks) serous effusion and air or gas in the pleural cavity.

seropositivity (se″ro-poz″ĭ-tiv′ĭ-te) the state of showing positive results on serologic examination.

seroprognosis (se″ro-prog-no′sis) prognosis of disease from the serum reactions.

seroprophylaxis (se″ro-pro″fĭ-lak′sis) the injection of immune serum or convalescent serum for protective purposes.

seropurulent (se″ro-pu′roo-lent) both serous and purulent.

seropus (se″ro-pus′) serum mingled with pus.

seroreaction (se″ro-re-ak′shun) 1. any reaction taking place in serum. 2. serum sickness.

serosa (se-ro′sah) any serous membrane. adj., **sero′sal.**

serosamucin (se-ro″sah-mu′sin) a protein from inflammatory serous exudates.

serosanguineous (se″ro-sang-gwin′e-us) composed of serum and blood.

seroscopy (se-ros′ko-pe) diagnostic examination of serum.

seroserous (se″ro-se′rus) pertaining to two serous surfaces.

serositis (se″ro-si′tis) inflammation of a serous membrane.

serosity (se-ros′ĭ-te) the quality of serous fluids.

serosynovitis (se″ro-sin″o-vi′tis) synovitis with effusion of serum.

serotherapy (se″ro-ther′ah-pe) the treatment of disease by the injection of serum from immune individuals.

serothorax (se″ro-tho′raks) hydrothorax.

serotonin (se″ro-to′nin) a potent vasoconstrictor substance secreted by argentaffin cells of the small intestine, absorbed by blood platelets and circulated in the blood. Its full range of activity in vivo has not yet been completely clarified. Called also hydroxytryptamine.

serotoxin (se″ro-tok′sin) 1. a toxin existing in the blood stream. 2. the hypothetical poisonous substance that is formed in the body and responsible for anaphylactic shock.

serotype (se′ro-tīp) the type of a microorganism determined by its constituent antigens, or a taxonomic subdivision based thereon.

serous (se′rus) 1. pertaining to serum; thin and watery, like serum. 2. producing or containing serum.

serovaccination (se″ro-vak″sĭ-na′shun) injection of serum combined with bacterial vaccination to produce passive and active immunity.

Serpasil (ser′pah-sil) trademark for preparations of reserpine, an antihypertensive and tranquilizer.

serpiginous (ser-pij′ĭ-nus) creeping from part to part.

serpigo (ser-pi′go) any creeping eruption.

serrated (ser′āt-ed) having a sawlike edge or border.

serration (sĕ-ra′shun) a notch like that between two saw teeth.

serrulate (ser'u-lāt) characterized by minute serrations.

serum (se'rum), pl. *se'ra* [L.], *serums* the clear portion of any animal or plant fluid that remains after the solid elements have been separated out. The term usually refers to blood serum, the clear, straw-colored, liquid portion of the plasma that does not contain fibrinogen and remains fluid after clotting of blood.

Blood serum from persons or animals whose bodies have built up antibodies is called antiserum or immune serum. Inoculation with such an antiserum provides temporary, or passive, immunity against the disease, and is used when a person has already been exposed to or has contracted the disease. Diseases in which passive immunization is sometimes used include diphtheria, tetanus, botulism and gas gangrene.

antilymphocyte s., ALS, a substance used as an immunosuppressive agent in organ transplantation; a derivative, antilymphocyte globulin (ALG) is now more commonly used.

convalescent s., blood serum from a patient who is convalescent from an infectious disease: such a serum is used as a prophylactic injection in such diseases as measles, scarlet fever and whooping cough.

s. glutamic oxaloacetic transaminase, SGOT, one of the enzymes that catalyze the transfer of an amino group (NH_2) from an amino acid to an alpha keto acid. The enzyme is found normally in heart, liver, muscle, kidney and pancreas. An elevated SGOT level is seen in disease conditions in which dead or damaged cells leak the transaminase into the serum. The SGOT test is not specific for any one disease condition. Its findings are compared with the results of other diagnostic tests and a physical examination. Normal range is 10 to 40 units.

Several drugs can cause elevated SGOT levels, and for this reason it is best to obtain the blood specimen before any drugs are given. About 5 cc. of venous blood is withdrawn, placed in a test tube and allowed to coagulate. It may be stored in a refrigerator until the testing is done.

s. glutamic pyruvic transaminase, SGPT, an enzyme similar to SGOT and found in several tissues of the body. Testing of SGPT levels is primarily a diagnostic test in liver disease. For example, SGPT levels can reach 4000 units in cases of hepatitis. The normal range is 5 to 40 units. A specimen for testing for SGPT is obtained in the same way as one for SGOT.

pooled s., the mixed serum from a number of individuals.

s. sickness, an allergic reaction to injections of serum (antiserum). It is marked by fever, urticarial eruptions, enlarged glands and joint pains.

Reactions to tetanus antitoxin derived from horse serum are especially common. When the serum-sensitive person is injected for the first time, the reaction usually occurs after a period of 6 to 12 days. Once a person has had a serum reaction, the serum responsible should be avoided, since a second reaction will be more severe.

It is customary to test a patient's sensitivity with a small amount of serum before injecting the full dose. This precaution is especially important for patients who have other allergic susceptiblities.

sesamoid (ses'ah-moid) shaped like a sesame seed, as for example, sesamoid bones, a number of small bones occurring mainly in the hands and feet.

sesqui- (ses'kwe) word element [L.], *one and one-half.*

sesquioxide (ses"kwe-ok'sīd) a compound of three parts of oxygen with two of another element.

sesquisalt (ses'kwĭ-sawlt) a salt containing three parts of an acid with two of a base.

sessile (ses'il) not pedunculated; having a broad base.

setaceous (se-ta'shus) bristle-like.

sex (seks) a distinctive character of most animals and plants, based on the type of gametes produced by the gonads, ova being typical of the female, and sperm of the male, or the category in which the individual is placed on such basis.

s. character, primary, a trait directly concerned in reproductive function of the individual.

s. character, secondary, a trait typical of the sex but not directly concerned in reproductive function of the individual.

s. chromatin, a mass of chromatin situated at the periphery of the nucleus, which is present in the cells of normal females, but not of normal males.

chromosomal s., the category into which an individual is placed, as determined by the presence or absence of the Y chromosome.

s. chromosomes, chromosomes that are associated with the determination of sex, in mammals constituting an unequal pain, called the X and the Y chromosome.

s. glands, the glands that regulate reproduction and manufacture the hormones that control the sex characters—the TESTES in the male, and the OVARIES in the female; called also GONADS.

gonadal s., the sex as determined on the basis of the gonadal tissue present.

s. hormones, glandular secretions involved in the regulation of sexual functions. The principal sex hormone in the male is TESTOSTERONE, produced by the testes. In the female, the ovaries produce ESTROGEN and PROGESTERONE.

These hormones control the secondary sex characters, such as the shape and contour of the body, the distribution of body hair and the pitch of the voice. The male hormones stimulate production of sperm in men and the female hormones control ovulation, pregnancy and the menstrual cycle in women.

morphologic s., that determined on the morphology of the external genitalia.

psychologic s., that determined by the gender role assigned to and played by the growing individual.

sex-linked (seks-linkt') transmitted by a gene located on a sex (X or Y) chromosome.

sexology (sek-sol'o-je) the scientific study of sex and sexual relations from the biologic point of view.

sexopathy (sek-sop'ah-the) abnormality of sexual expression.

sextan (seks'tan) recurring on the sixth day (every five days).

sextipara (seks-tip'ah-rah) a woman who has had six pregnancies that resulted in viable offspring; para VI.

sextuplet (seks-tup'let, seks-too'plet, seks'too-plet) any one of six offspring produced at the same birth.

sexual (seks'u-al) 1. pertaining to sex. 2. a person considered in his sexual relations.

s. **deviation,** an emotional illness that is expressed in a form of sexual behavior of an abnormal sort; called also sexual perversion and paraphilia. The sexual deviate is compelled by his inner drives to seek satisfaction through specific forms of abnormal behavior—sadism, HOMOSEXUALITY, EXHIBITIONISM, nymphomania and many other variations. Sexual deviation is considered an illness with roots in deep emotional conflicts.

In this type of behavior, as in many others, there is no sharp dividing line between the normal and the abnormal. There are many complex factors that can lead to a sexual attitude not acceptable to society as a whole; not all of these are fully understood. In general, however, children who have a full and happy family life and whose parents are an example of a normal and healthy relationship are far less likely to develop emotional conflicts of the sort that can lead to sexual deviation.

Sexual deviation may cause legal as well as personal difficulties. Most types of deviant activity are illegal and punishable by imprisonment. However, an increasing number of judges recognize that deviation is more an illness than a crime and refer offenders to psychiatrists for treatment. Pronounced sexual deviation is treated by PSYCHOTHERAPY, which attempts to uncover and resolve the unconscious sources of the deviation.

Before condemning sexual deviation too hastily one should remember that most sexual deviates are emotionally sick and immature people. Many people today are developing some understanding of the problem, and with it, more sympathetic and flexible attitudes. During successive stages of development in childhood and particularly in adolescence, a certain amount of experimentation is normal and understandable. War experiences and long imprisonments have shown that under certain pressures or circumstances, many people may find themselves capable of an abnormal sexual act.

sexuality (seks"u-al'i-te) 1. the characteristic quality of the male and female reproductive elements. 2. the constitution of an individual in relation to sexual attitudes and behavior.

S.G.O. Surgeon-General's Office.

SGOT serum glutamic oxaloacetic transaminase (see under SERUM).

SGPT serum glutamic pyruvic transaminase (see under SERUM).

shadow-casting (shad"o-kast'ing) application of a coating of gold, chromium or other metal for the purpose of increasing the visibility of ultramicroscopic specimens under the microscope.

shaft (shaft) a long slender part, such as the portion of a long bone between the wider ends or extremities.

shank (shangk) the tibia or shin.

sheath (shēth) a tubular case or envelope.

arachnoid s., the delicate membrane between the pial sheath and the dural sheath of the optic nerve.

carotid s., a portion of the cervical fascia enclosing the carotid artery, internal jugular vein and vagus nerve.

crural s., femoral sheath.

dural s., the external investment of the optic nerve.

femoral s., the fascial sheath of the femoral vessels.

Henle's s., a sheath enveloping an isolated nerve fiber exterior to the neurolemma.

lamellar s., the perineurium.

medullary s., myelin s., the sheath surrounding the axon of some nerve fibers, consisting of myelin alternating with the spirally wrapped neurolemma.

perivascular s., a wide lymphatic tube around the smallest blood vessels.

pial s., an extension of the pia mater partly intersecting the optic nerve.

root s., the epidermic layer of a hair follicle.

s. of Schwann, neurolemma.

synovial s., synovial membrane lining the cavity of a bone through which a tendon moves.

sheep cell agglutination test SCAT, a laboratory test for infectious mononucleosis. When the antibody level of a person with this disease reaches a certain level, a sample of his blood will cause agglutination of sheep erythrocytes. If there is agglutination of these cells in concentrations up to 1:28, the findings are considered positive for infectious mononucleosis. The specimen for the test is 5 cc. of venous blood, placed in a test tube and allowed to coagulate. No special preparation of the patient is necessary.

shelf (shelf) a shelflike structure, normal or abnormal.

Blumer's s., a shelflike structure projecting into the rectum as a result of infiltration of Douglas' cul-de-sac with inflammatory or neoplastic material.

shield (shēld) a protecting tube or structure.

shift (shift) a change or deviation.

chloride s., the exchange of chloride and carbonate between the plasma and the erythrocytes that takes place when the blood gives up oxygen and receives carbon dioxide. It serves to maintain ionic equilibrium between the cell and surrounding fluid.

s. **to the left,** a change in the blood picture, with a preponderance of young neutrophils.

Shigella (shǐ-gel'ah) a genus of Schizomycetes that cause dysentery. They are gram-negative, rod-shaped bacteria.

S. **dysente'riae,** a species that produces a neurotropic exotoxin in addition to the endotoxin common to all members of the Shigella group; it is more common in tropical regions and produces severe dysentery. Called also Shiga bacillus.

S. **son'nei,** one of the commonest causes of bacillary dysentery in temperate climates.

shigella (shǐ-gel'ah), pl. *shigel'lae* an individual organism of the genus Shigella.

shigellosis (shǐ"gel-o'sis) infection with Shigella.

shin (shin) the prominent anterior edge of the tibia and leg.

saber s., marked anterior convexity of the tibia, seen in congenital syphilis.

shingles (shing'gelz) herpes zoster.

shiver (shiv'er) 1. a slight tremor. 2. to tremble slightly, as from cold.

shivering (shiv'er-ing) involuntary shaking of the body, as with cold. It is caused by contraction or twitching of the muscles, and is a physiologic method of heat production in man and other mammals.

shock (shok) disruption of the circulation, which can upset all body functions; sometimes referred to as circulatory shock. It occurs when blood pressure is inadequate to force blood through the vital tissues. Shock is a dangerous condition which may be fatal.

MECHANISMS OF CIRCULATORY SHOCK. The essentials of circulatory shock are easier to understand if the circulatory system is thought of as a four-part mechanical device made up of a pump (the heart), a complex system of flexible tubes (the blood vessels), a circulating fluid (the blood) and a fine regulating system or "computer" (the nervous system) designed to control fluid flow and pressure. The diameter of the blood vessels is controlled by impulses from the nervous system which cause the muscular walls to contract. The nervous system also affects the rapidity and strength of the heartbeat, and thereby the blood pressure as well.

Shock, which is associated with a dangerously low blood pressure, can be produced by factors that attack the strength of the heart as a pump, decrease the volume of the blood in the system or permit the blood vessels to increase in diameter.

TYPES OF CIRCULATORY SHOCK. There are five main types of circulatory shock. Low-volume shock occurs whenever there is insufficient blood to fill the circulatory system. Neurogenic shock is due to disorders of the nervous system. Two types of shock, allergic shock and septic shock, are due to reactions that impair the muscular functioning of the blood vessels. Cardiac shock is caused by impaired function of the heart.

Low-Volume Shock. This is a common form of shock that occurs when blood or plasma is lost in such quantities that the remaining blood cannot fill the circulatory system despite constriction of the blood vessels. The blood loss may be external, as when a vessel is severed by an injury, or the blood may be "lost" into spaces inside the body where it is no longer accessible to the circulatory system, as in severe gastrointestinal bleeding from ulcers, fractures of large bones with hemorrhage into surrounding tissues or major burns that attract large quantities of blood fluids to the burn site outside blood vessels and capillaries. The treatment of low-volume shock requires replacement of the lost blood.

Neurogenic Shock. This form of shock, often called fainting, may be brought on by severe pain, fright, unpleasant sights or other strong stimuli that overwhelm the usual regulatory capacity of the nervous system. The diameter of the blood vessels increases, the heart slows and the blood pressure falls to the point where the supply of oxygen carried by the blood to the brain is insufficient. The patient then faints. Placing the head lower than the body is usually sufficient to relieve this form of shock.

Allergic Shock. Allergic shock, commonly called ANAPHYLACTIC SHOCK, occurs rarely when a person receives an injection of a foreign protein to which he is highly sensitive. The blood vessels and other tissues are affected directly by the allergic reaction. Within a few minutes, the blood pressure falls and the severe dyspnea develops. The sudden deaths that in rare cases follow bee stings or injection of certain medicines are due to anaphylactic reactions.

Septic Shock. Septic shock, resulting from bacterial infection, is being recognized with increasing frequency. Certain organisms contain a toxin that seems to act on the blood vessels when it is released into the bloodstream. The blood eventually pools within parts of the circulatory system that expand easily, causing the blood pressure to drop sharply. Gram-negative shock is a form of septic shock due to infection with gram-negative bacteria.

Cardiac Shock. Cardiac shock may be caused by conditions that interfere with the function of the heart as a pump, such as severe myocardial infarction, severe heart failure and certain disorders of rate and rhythm.

THE PATIENT IN SHOCK. The precise progression to a state of shock depends upon the cause of the disorder and the speed of onset. In hemorrhagic shock, for example, as blood is lost the patient with gradually progressing shock feels very restless at first. He becomes thirsty. His skin takes on a pallor and feels cold. Often he perspires profusely. The pulse speeds up but is weak and indistinct. He gradually feels lethargic and faint, and may show signs of air hunger (labored and difficult breathing). The nail beds and lips take on a bluish hue. As shock deepens and the blood pressure falls, the patient becomes comatose and eventually dies if untreated.

TREATMENT. Shock is an emergency that requires immediate treatment. The diagnosis of shock in an unconscious patient may be difficult for the untrained, but the presence of the signs and symptoms previously described, or a severe injury with suspected bleeding, is sufficient evidence to indicate shock without a blood pressure reading. In all such cases, first aid should be given immediately.

The patient should be placed on his back with his head low to insure that the brain gets as much blood as possible. (If the patient has a severe injury of the head, neck or back, however, he should not be moved without instructions from a physician or other qualified person.) Infliction of pain should be avoided, since severe pain causes neurogenic shock. The patient must be able to breathe; if foreign material is obstructing his airway it should be removed, and if the tongue is in the way, the tongue and jaw should be pulled forward. If the person is still not breathing, as in anaphylactic shock, his lungs should be inflated by mouth-to-mouth resuscitation (see ARTIFICIAL RESPIRATION).

Active bleeding in an injured person should be controlled with pressure or a bandage directly on the site of bleeding. Tourniquets should not be used unless absolutely necessary. They may release a flood of dangerous toxins to the body when they are loosened later. The patient should be kept comfortably warm, but excessive heat should not be used because heat causes dilation of blood vessels and worsens shock. Fluids are not given to anyone who is unconscious. Further treatment includes measures aimed at returning blood volume to normal when indicated, administration of drugs to elevate blood pressure if needed and measures to control the primary cause of shock. In certain cases of shock, especially septic, allergic and low-volume shock, large doses of corticosteroids are sometimes used.

electric s., shock caused by electric current passing through the body (see ELECTRIC SHOCK).

insulin s., a condition of circulatory insufficiency resulting from overdosage with insulin, which causes too sudden reduction of blood sugar. It is marked by tremor, sweating, vertigo, diplopia, convulsions and collapse. Such a condition produced intentionally has been used in treatment of schizophrenia. (See also INSULIN SHOCK.)

shell s., a condition of lost nervous control with numerous psychic symptoms, ranging from extreme fear to actual dementia, produced in soldiers under fire by the noise and concussion of bursting shells.

spinal s., the loss of spinal reflexes after injury of the spinal cord that appears in the muscles enervated by the cord segments situated below the site of the lesion.

s. therapy, a technique used in treating certain severe forms of mental illness. The patient is rendered temporarily unconscious, usually by means of an electric current. This form of psychiatric treatment is now frequently referred to as somatic therapy, rather than shock therapy, because it does not necessarily produce a state of shock in the medical sense. Shock therapy has been a method of treatment since the 1930's, but more recently the development of medicines such as tranquilizers and "mood elevators" has reduced its use.

USES AND EFFECTS.   The different types of shock have somewhat different effects. Electroshock is most useful in cases of severe depression and is sometimes used on patients with involutional reaction, a condition that appears in late middle age. It is also employed in patients who are in the depressive stage of affective psychosis.

Inhalant shock, which makes use of an ether compound, has much the same effect as electroshock. Alleviation of severe symptoms is rapid with these treatments.

Insulin shock, produced by administration of insulin, is a more prolonged form of treatment and is helpful primarily in treating cases of severe schizophrenia. It is rarely used, however.

METHODS OF ADMINISTRATION.   In electroshock therapy, electrodes are placed on either side of the patient's forehead and a brief current is applied. The patient immediately becomes unconscious and retains no memory of a shock. Care is taken to prevent injury during the convulsions that follow treatment.

Inhalant therapy has the same effects, but is often accepted more readily by patients than electroshock therapy. Both treatments may be preceded by the administration of an anesthetic so that the patient is asleep during the entire procedure. Medication to relax the muscles so that the convulsion is very mild may also be employed.

In insulin therapy, a carefully measured quantity of insulin is injected into the patient, with coma and occasionally convulsions following. Sometimes insulin therapy is combined with electric shock for patients unresponsive to either treatment alone.

OBJECTIVE.   The objective of shock therapy is to enable patients who have withdrawn into phantasies or severe depression to reestablish contact with the world. It may then be possible to treat the causes of their mental illness with psychotherapy.

shoulder   (shōl'der) the large joint where the

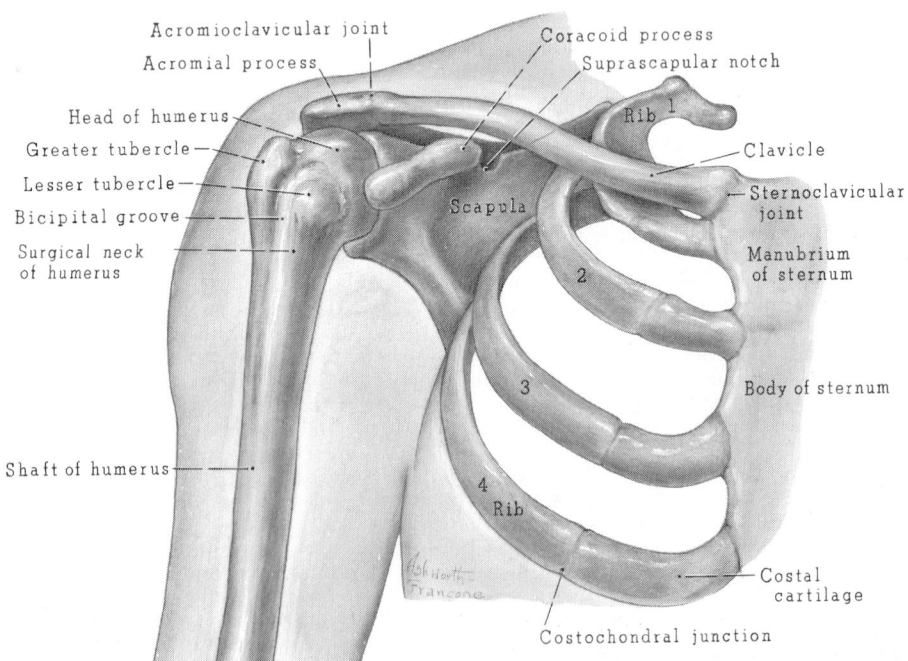

Acromioclavicular joint
Acromial process
Coracoid process
Suprascapular notch
Head of humerus
Greater tubercle
Lesser tubercle
Bicipital groove
Surgical neck of humerus
Scapula
Rib 1
Clavicle
Sternoclavicular joint
Manubrium of sternum
Body of sternum
Shaft of humerus
Rib
Costal cartilage
Costochondral junction

Shoulder. (From Jacob, S. W., and Francone, C. A.: Structure and Function in Man. 2nd ed. Philadelphia, W. B. Saunders Co., 1970.)

humerus joins the scapula. The shoulder is a shallow ball-and-socket joint, similar to the hip joint.

At the shoulder, the smooth, rounded head of the humerus rests against the socket in the scapula. The joint is covered by a tough, flexible protective capsule and is heavily reinforced by ligaments that stretch across the joint. The ends of the bones where they meet at the joint are covered with a layer of cartilage that reduces friction and absorbs shock. A thin membrane, the synovial membrane, lines the socket and lubricates the joint with synovia. Further cushioning and lubrication are provided by fluid-filled sacs called bursae.

DISORDERS OF THE SHOULDER. One of the most common disorders of the shoulder is BURSITIS, or inflammation of the bursa, often caused by excessive use of the joint. The joint becomes painful and difficult to move.

The shoulder is one of the most common sites for a DISLOCATION, in which the ball of the humerus is dislodged from its socket in the scapula. This injures the ligaments and the capsule, and may cause temporary paralysis of the arm as well as pain and swelling. A dislocated shoulder is usually caused by a blow or fall, but sometimes an unusual physical effort may pull the arm from the shoulder socket. A first dislocation often makes the joint more susceptible to future dislocations. Only a doctor should set a dislocated shoulder; inexpert efforts may do far more damage than the original injury.

Frozen shoulder is a disability of the shoulder joint due to chronic inflammation in and around the joint and characterized by pain and limitation of motion.

show (sho) appearance of blood forerunning labor or menstruation.

shunt (shunt) 1. to turn to one side; to divert. 2. an anomalous or artificially created passage connecting two main channels, and diverting (blood) flow from one to the other. 3. a conductor connecting two points in an electric circuit, so as to receive a portion of the current of the main circuit.

left-to-right s., diversion of blood from the systemic to the pulmonary circulation.

portacaval s., diversion of circulation by anastomosis of portal vein and inferior vena cava or by splenectomy and anastomosis of the splenic and left renal veins.

right-to-left s., diversion of blood from the pulmonary to the systemic circulation.

Shwartzman phenomenon (shwarts'man) a local tissue reaction characterized by hemorrhagic necrosis due to an antigen-antibody reaction to certain bacterial substances. Its occurrence in humans is largely theoretical.

Si chemical symbol, *silicon.*

sial(o)- (si″ah-lo) word element [Gr.], *saliva; salivary glands.*

sialadenitis (si″al-ad″ĕ-ni′tis) inflammation of a salivary gland.

sialadenoncus (si″al-ad″ĕ-nong′kus) a tumor of a salivary gland.

sialagogue (si-al′ah-gog) an agent that stimulates the flow of saliva.

sialectasia (si″al-ek-ta′ze-ah) dilatation of a salivary duct.

sialine (si′ah-līn) pertaining to the saliva.

sialismus (si″ah-liz′mus) salivation.

sialoadenectomy (si″ah-lo-ad″ĕ-nek′to-me) excision of a salivary gland.

sialoadenitis (si″ah-lo-ad″ĕ-ni′tis) inflammation of a salivary gland.

sialoadenotomy (si″ah-lo-ad′ĕ-not′o-me) incision of a salivary gland.

sialoaerophagy (si″ah-lo-a″er-of′ah-je) the swallowing of saliva and air.

sialoangiectasis (si″ah-lo-an″je-ek′tah-sis) dilatation of a salivary duct.

sialoangiitis (si″ah-lo-an″je-i′tis) inflammation of a salivary duct.

sialocele (si′ah-lo-sēl) ranula.

sialodochitis (si″ah-lo-do-ki′tis) inflammation of a salivary duct.

sialodochoplasty (si″ah-lo-do′ko-plas″te) plastic repair of a salivary duct.

sialoductitis (si″ah-lo-duk-ti′tis) inflammation of a parotid duct.

sialogenous (si″ah-loj′ĕ-nus) producing saliva.

sialogogue (si-al′o-gog) sialagogue.

sialogram (si-al′o-gram) a roentgenogram obtained by sialography.

sialography (si″ah-log′rah-fe) roentgen demonstration of the salivary ducts by means of the injection of substances opaque to x-rays.

sialolith (si-al′o-lith) a salivary calculus.

sialolithiasis (si″ah-lo-lī-thi′ah-sis) the formation of salivary calculi.

sialolithotomy (si″ah-lo-lī-thot′o-me) excision of a salivary calculus.

sialology (si″ah-lol′o-je) the study of the saliva.

sialoma (si″ah-lo′mah) a tumor of a salivary gland.

sialorrhea (si″ah-lo-re′ah) salivation.

sialoschesis (si″ah-los′kĕ-sis) suppression of secretion of saliva.

sialosis (si″ah-lo′sis) the flow of saliva.

sialostenosis (si″ah-lo-stĕ-no′sis) stenosis of a salivary duct.

sialosyrinx (si″ah-lo-sir′inks) 1. salivary fistula. 2. a syringe for washing out the salivary ducts, or a drainage tube for the salivary ducts.

Siamese twins identical (monozygotic) twins joined together at birth. The connection may be slight or extensive. It involves skin and usually muscles or cartilage of a limited region, such as the head, chest, hip or buttock. The twins may share a single organ, such as an intestine, or occasionally may have parts of the spine in common.

If joined superficially, the twins are easily separated by surgery soon after birth. If more deeply united, they may have to go through life, if they survive, with their handicap. New techniques in surgery, however, are making it possible to separate some Siamese twins whose physical links are highly complex.

sib (sib) a blood relative; one of a group of persons all descended from a common ancestor.

sibilant (sib′ĭ-lant) shrill, whistling or hissing.

sibling (sib′ling) an individual born of the same parents as the person of reference, i.e., a brother or sister.

  half s., an individual one of whose parents was also a parent of the person of reference.

sibship (sib′ship) a group of individuals born of the same parents.

siccative (sik′ah-tiv) 1. drying; removing moisture. 2. an agent that produces drying.

siccus (sik′us) [L.] dry.

sickle cell (sik′l) a crescentic or sickle-shaped erythrocyte, the abnormal shape caused by the presence of varying proportions of hemoglobin S.
  s. c. anemia, a genetically determined defect of hemoglobin synthesis, inherited as an autosomal recessive and confined for the most part to Negroes. In the homozygous state it is characterized by abnormal hemoglobin (hemoglobin S), anemia, reticulocytosis and jaundice. Clinical findings include recurrent attacks of fever, and pain in the arms, legs and abdomen from early childhood; a constant scleral icterus; and, in the crisis period, a tender, rigid abdomen resembling that seen in a surgical illness. Headache, paralysis and convulsions may result from cerebral thrombosis due to increased viscosity of the blood. Treatment is symptomatic. There is a tendency to progressive renal damage in patients who survive the disease beyond the age of 50. (See also ANEMIA for nursing care.)
  s. c. trait, the heterozygous state of sickle cell anemia; it is usually without symptoms.

sicklemia (sik-le′me-ah) sickle cell anemia.

sickling (sik′ling) the development of sickle cells in the blood.

sickness (sik′nes) a condition of deviation from the normal healthy state.

S.I.D. Society for Investigative Dermatology.

side effect (sīd′ ĕ-fekt″) a consequence other than that for which an agent is used, especially an adverse effect on another organ system.

sidero- (sid′er-o) word element [Gr.], *iron.*

siderocyte (sid′er-o-sīt″) a red blood corpuscle containing nonhemoglobin iron.

sideroderma (sid″er-o-der′mah) bronzed coloration of the skin from disordered iron metabolism.

siderodromophobia (sid″er-o-dro″mo-fo′be-ah) morbid dread of railway travel.

siderofibrosis (sid″er-o-fi-bro′sis) fibrosis combined with deposits of iron.

sideropenia (sid″er-o-pe′ne-ah) iron deficiency.

siderophilin (sid″er-of′ĭ-lin) transferrin.

siderophilous (sid″er-of′ĭ-lus) tending to absorb iron.

siderophore (sid′er-o-fōr) a macrophage containing hemosiderin.

siderosis (sid″er-o′sis) 1. a form of PNEUMOCONIOSIS due to the inhalation of iron or other metallic particles. 2. excess of iron in the blood. 3. the deposit of an iron pigment within the eyeball.
  hepatic s., the deposit of an abnormal quantity of iron in the liver.
  urinary s., the presence of hemosiderin granules in the urine.

sig. [L.] *sig′na* (mark).

sight (sīt) the act or faculty of VISION, involving the EYE itself, the visual center in the brain and the optic nerve and nerve fibers in the brain that connect the two.
  far s., long s., hyperopia.
  near s., myopia.
  night s., hemeralopia; day blindness.
  short s., myopia.

sigmatism (sig′mah-tizm) faulty enunciation of *s* sounds.

sigmoid (sig′moid) 1. shaped like the letter C or S. 2. the distal part of the colon, from the level of the iliac crest to the rectum.

sigmoidectomy (sig″moi-dek′to-me) excision of part of the sigmoid colon.

sigmoiditis (sig″moi-di′tis) inflammation of the sigmoid colon.

sigmoidopexy (sig-moi′do-pek″se) fixation of the sigmoid colon in cases of rectal prolapse.

sigmoidoproctostomy,   sigmoidorectostomy (sig-moi″do-prok-tos′to-me),   (sig-moi″do-rek-tos′-to-me) surgical anastomosis of the sigmoid colon to the rectum.

sigmoidoscope (sig-moi′do-skōp) an endoscope for use in sigmoidoscopy.

sigmoidoscopy (sig″moi-dos′ko-pe) direct examination of the interior of the sigmoid colon. (For preparation of the patient, see PROCTOSCOPY.)

sigmoidosigmoidostomy (sig-moi″do-sig″moi-dos′to-me) anastomosis of two previously remote portions of the sigmoid colon.

sigmoidostomy (sig″moi-dos′to-me) surgical creation of an opening from the surface of the body into the sigmoid colon.

sigmoidotomy (sig″moi-dot′o-me) incision of the sigmoid.

sigmoidovesical (sig-moi″do-ves′ĭ-kal) pertaining to or communicating with the sigmoid flexure and the urinary bladder.

sign (sīn) 1. any objective evidence of disease or dysfunction. 2. an observable physical phenomenon so frequently associated with a given condition as to be considered indicative of its presence.
  vital s's, the signs of life, namely pulse, respiration and temperature.

signa (sig'nah) [L.] mark, or write; abbreviated S. or sig. in prescriptions, followed by the signature.

signature (sig'nah-tūr) that part of a drug prescription that gives directions to be followed by the patient in its use.

silica (sil'ĭ-kah) silicon dioxide, a compound occurring naturally as quartz and in other forms, and used in the manufacture of glass.

silicoanthracosis (sil″ĭ-ko-an″thrah-ko'sis) silicosis.

silicon (sil'ĭ-kon) a chemical element, atomic number 14, atomic weight 28.086, symbol Si. (See table of ELEMENTS.)

silicosis (sil″ĭ-ko'sis) a lung disease caused by the prolonged inhalation of silica dust. In the past it was called such colorful names as potter's asthma, stonecutter's cough, miner's mold and grinder's rot, according to the occupation in which it was acquired. Besides silicosis, various other lung diseases result from inhaling industrial substances; together, these "dust diseases" are called PNEU-MOCONIOSES.

Today silicosis is most likely to be contracted in such industrial jobs as sandblasting in tunnels and hardrock mining, but it can occur in anyone who is habitually exposed to the dust of silica, one of the commonest minerals. All types of miners, for example, may be subject to it, from gold miners to coal miners.

Silicosis usually takes about 10 years of fairly constant exposure to develop. It may give few warning symptoms. As time goes on, an affected person experiences progressive shortness of breath, along with steady coughing which in the early stages is dry and unproductive of mucus. Later there may be mucus tinged with blood, loss of appetite, pain in the chest and general weakness. The silica produces a reaction that scars the lungs and makes them receptive to the further complications of bronchitis and emphysema; persons with silicosis are also more susceptible to tuberculosis.

Since silicosis is a serious disease, those who must work near silica should take precautions to breathe as little of it as possible. This can usually be effected by the use of face masks, proper ventilation and other safety devices. The cooperation of industry, labor and government in developing various protective measures has made silicosis a much less common disease today than it used to be.

Regular chest x-rays are recommended for all workers exposed to silica as the quickest and easiest way to detect silicosis. If discovered in its early stages, the disease can usually be arrested by a change of occupation and appropriate therapy. Once fully developed, the disease rarely yields to treatment.

silicotuberculosis (sil″ĭ-ko-tu-ber″ku-lo'sis) tuberculous infection of the lung affected with silicosis.

silkosis (sil-ko'sis) a complication sometimes following use of silk sutures, with formation of sinuses.

silo-filler's disease a chronic inflammatory reaction, principally in interstitial tissues of the lung, due to exposure to dusty, moldy plant materials or to organic fertilizers.

silver (sil'ver) a chemical element, atomic number 47, atomic weight 107.870, symbol Ag. (See table of ELEMENTS.) It is used in medicine for its caustic, astringent and antiseptic effects.

colloidal s., a silver preparation in which the silver exists as free ions to only a small extent.

s. iodide, a yellowish, powdery compound; useful in syphilis and in nervous diseases, and also applied locally in conjunctivitis.

s. nitrate, colorless or white crystals, used as a caustic and local anti-infective, one important use being in prevention of ophthalmia neonatorum.

s. nitrate, toughened, a mixture of silver nitrate and silver chloride, occurring as white crystalline masses molded into pencils or cones; a convenient means of applying silver nitrate locally.

s. protein, silver made colloidal by the presence of, or combination with, protein; an active germicide with a local irritant and astringent effect.

Simmonds' disease (sim'ondz) a rare glandular disorder, marked by extreme weight loss; called also pituitary cachexia. It follows the destruction of the pituitary gland by surgery, infection, injury or tumor; it may also occur after difficult labor in childbirth.

Simmonds' disease was first described by Dr. Morris Simmonds of Hamburg, Germany, in 1914. Symptoms, which vary in intensity, are general debility, pallor, dry and yellowish skin, a slow pulse, hypotension and atrophy of the genitalia and breasts, progressing to premature senility and apathy. Treatment is by regular administration of the various hormones whose release is normally dependent on pituitary function.

Sims (simz) James Marion (1813–1883). American surgeon and pioneer in gynecology. Born in South Carolina and graduated from Jefferson Medical College in Philadelphia, he is known chiefly for the semiprone position and the curved speculum that are named after him, and that contributed to his success in operating for vesicovaginal fistula. He established the State Hospital for Women in New York, and was president of the American Medical Association and honorary president of the International Medical Congress.

simulation (sim″u-la'shun) 1. the act of counterfeiting a disease; malingering. 2. the imitation of one disease by another.

Simulium (sĭ-mu'le-um) a genus of biting gnats, several species of which are the intermediate host of *Onchocerca volvulus*.

Sinaxar (sin'ak-sar) trademark for a preparation of styramate, a skeletal muscle relaxant.

sinciput (sin'sĭ-put) the upper and front part of the head. adj., **sincip'ital.**

sinew (sin'u) a tendon or fibrous cord.

weeping s., an encysted ganglion, chiefly on the back of the hand, containing synovia.

Singoserp (sing'go-serp) trademark for preparations of syrosingopine, an antihypertensive.

singultus (sing-gul'tus) hiccup.

sinister (sin'is-ter) [L.] left; on the left side.

sinistr(o)- (sin′is-tro) word element [L.], *left; left side.*

sinistrad (sin′is-trad) to or toward the left.

sinistral (sin′is-tral) pertaining to the left side.

sinistrality (sin″is-tral′ĭ-te) the preferential use, in voluntary motor acts, of the left member of the major paired organs of the body, as ear, eye, hand and leg.

sinistraural (sin″is-traw′ral) hearing better with the left ear.

sinistrocardia (sin″is-tro-kar′de-ah) displacement of the heart to the left.

sinistrocerebral (sin″is-tro-ser′ĕ-bral) situated in the left hemisphere of the brain.

sinistrocular (sin″is-trok′u-lar) having the left eye dominant.

sinistrocularity (sin″is-trok″u-lar′ĭ-te) dominance of the left eye.

sinistrogyration (sin″is-tro-ji-ra′shun) a turning to the left.

sinistromanual (sin″is-tro-man′u-al) left-handed.

sinistropedal (sin″is-trop′ĕ-dal) using the left foot in preference to the right.

sinistrotorsion (sin″is-tro-tor′shun) a twisting toward the left; used mainly of the eye.

sinoatrial (si″no-a′tre-al) pertaining to the sinus venosus and the atrium of the heart.

s. node, a collection of atypical muscle fibers in the wall of the right atrium where the rhythm of cardiac contraction is usually established; therefore also referred to as the pacemaker of the heart.

sinoauricular (si″no-aw-rik′u-lar) sinoatrial.

sinobronchitis (si″no-brong-ki′tis) chronic paranasal sinusitis with recurrent episodes of bronchitis.

sinopulmonary (si″no-pul′mo-ner″e) pertaining to the sinuses and lungs.

Sintrom (sin′trom) trademark for a preparation of acenocoumarol, an anticoagulant.

sinuitis (sin″u-i′tis) sinusitis.

sinuotomy (si″nu-ot′o-me) sinusotomy.

sinuous (sin′u-us) bending in and out; winding.

sinus (si′nus) 1. a cavity, or hollow space, in a bone or other tissue. 2. an abnormal channel or fistula, permitting escape of pus. In common usage, the word sinus refers to any of the eight cavities in the skull that are connected with the nasal cavity—the paranasal sinuses.

The paranasal sinuses are arranged in four pairs, with members of each pair on the left and right sides of the head. The pairs are the maxillary sinuses, located in the maxillae; the frontal sinuses, in the frontal bone; the sphenoid sinuses, in the sphenoid bone behind the nasal cavity; and the ethmoid sinuses, in the ethmoid bone, behind and below the frontal sinuses.

The functions of the sinuses are not certain. They are believed to help the nose in circulating, warming and moistening the air as it is inhaled, thereby lessening the shock of cold, dry air to the lungs. They also are thought to have a minor role as resonating chambers for the voice.

anal s's, furrows, with pouchlike recesses at the distal end, in the mucous lining of the anal canal.

aortic s's, pouchlike dilatations at the root of the aorta, one opposite each segment of the valve at its opening from the left ventricle.

s. arrhythmia, irregularity of the heartbeat dependent on interference with the impulses originating at the sinoatrial node.

branchial s., a branchial fistula opening on the surface of the body.

carotid s., a dilatation of the proximal portion of the internal carotid or distal portion of the common carotid artery, containing in its wall pressoreceptors that are stimulated by changes in blood pressure.

cavernous s., an irregularly shaped venous channel between the layers of dura mater of the brain, one on either side of the body of the sphenoid bone and communicating across the midline. Several cranial nerves course through this sinus.

cerebral s., one of the ventricles of the brain.

cervical s., a temporary depression in the neck of the embryo containing the branchial arches.

circular s., the venous channel encircling the pituitary gland, formed by the two cavernous sinuses and the anterior and posterior intercavernous sinuses.

coccygeal s., a sinus or fistula just over or close to the tip of the coccyx.

coronary s., the dilated terminal portion of the great cardiac vein, receiving blood from other veins draining the heart muscle and ending in the right atrium.

dermal s., a congenital sinus tract extending from the surface of the body, between the bodies of two adjacent lumbar vertebrae, to the spinal canal.

intercavernous s's, channels connecting the two cavernous sinuses, one passing anterior and the other posterior to the stalk of the pituitary gland.

lymphatic s's, irregular, tortuous spaces within lymphatic tissues through which lymph flows.

marginal s., a venous channel near the edge of the placenta.

occipital s., a venous sinus between the layers of dura mater, passing upward along the midline of the cerebellum.

petrosal s., inferior, a venous channel arising from the cavernous sinus and draining into the internal jugular vein.

petrosal s., superior, one arising from the cavernous sinus and draining into the transverse sinus of the dura mater.

pilonidal s., a suppurating sinus containing hair, occurring chiefly in the coccygeal region.

prostatic s., the posterolateral recess between the seminal colliculus and the wall of the urethra.

s's of pulmonary trunk, spaces between the wall of the pulmonary trunk and cusps of the valve at its opening from the right ventricle.

renal s., a recess in the substance of the kidney, lined by a continuation of the fibrous capsule and occupied by the renal vessels and the expanded upper end of the ureter.

sacrococcygeal s., pilonidal sinus.

sagittal s., inferior, a small venous sinus of the dura mater, opening into the straight sinus.

sagittal s., superior, a venous sinus of the dura mater that ends in the confluence of sinuses.

sigmoid s., a venous sinus of the dura mater on either side, continuous with the straight sinus and draining into the internal jugular vein of the same side.

sphenoparietal s., one of the venous sinuses of the dura mater, emptying into the cavernous sinus.

s's of spleen, dilated venous channels in the substance of the spleen.

straight s., a venous sinus of the dura mater formed by junction of the great cerebral vein and inferior sagittal sinus, and ending in the confluence of sinuses.

tarsal s., a space between the calcaneus and talus.

tentorial s., straight sinus.

transverse s. of dura mater, a large venous sinus on either side of the skull.

transverse s. of pericardium, a passage within the pericardial sac, behind the aorta and pulmonary trunk and in front of the left atrium and superior vena cava.

tympanic s., a deep recess on the medial wall of the middle ear.

urogenital s., a space made by division of the cloaca in the early embryo which ultimately forms most of the vestibule of the vagina in the female, and of the urethra in the male.

uterine s's, venous channels in the wall of the uterus in pregnancy.

uteroplacental s's, blood spaces between the placenta and uterine sinuses.

s. of venae cavae, the posterior portion of the right atrium into which the inferior and the superior vena cava open.

s. veno'sus, the common venous receptacle in the early embryo attached to the posterior wall of the primitive atrium.

venous s's of dura mater, large channels for venous blood forming an anastomosing system between the layers of the dura mater of the brain, receiving blood from the brain and draining into the veins of the scalp or deep veins at the base of the skull.

venous s. of sclera, a circular channel at the junction of the sclera and cornea, into which aqueous humor filters from the anterior chamber of the eye.

sinusitis (si″nŭ-si′tis) inflammation of one or more of the paranasal SINUSES, often occurring during an upper respiratory infection, when infection in the nose spreads to the sinuses (sometimes encouraged by excessively strong blowing of the nose). Sinusitis also may be a complication of tooth infection, allergy or certain infectious diseases, such as pneumonia and measles. There are many other causes of sinusitis, including air pollution, diving and underwater swimming, sudden extremes of temperature and structural defects of the nose that interfere with breathing, such as deviated SEPTUM.

As the mucous membranes of the sinus become inflamed and swollen, the openings that lead from each sinus into the nasal passages become partially or wholly blocked. The mucus that accumulates in the sealed-off sinus causes pressure on the sinus walls, resulting in discomfort, fever, pain and difficult breathing.

SYMPTOMS. The common symptoms of sinusitis are headache, usually located near the sinuses most involved, and nasal discharge. These may be accompanied by a slight rise in temperature, dizziness and a general feeling of weakness and discomfort.

TREATMENT. Steam inhalations and antihistamine nose drops may help relieve the symptoms. An electric heating pad or a hot water bottle may ease pain if applied for 10 minutes every 2 hours over the painful area on the face or forehead. Aspirin will also give some relief.

Since sinusitis, either acute or chronic, can lead to complications of the middle ear or of adjacent bones, it is important to treat the condition early. Antibiotics may be necessary to combat infection.

Plenty of rest and sleep is recommended in acute attacks of sinusitis. Smoke, dust and other irritants to the nasal passages should be avoided, and smoking should be stopped entirely.

When other methods fail to correct troublesome chronic sinusitis of long standing, surgery is sometimes required. The opening to the sinus may be made larger to ensure drainage and ventilation, but such measures cannot always guarantee complete cure.

Though a change of climate can sometimes help cases of chronic sinusitis, it rarely is a necessity. Creating a better indoor climate with such devices as air conditioners and humidifiers often is equally beneficial in reducing the number and severity of sinus attacks.

Psychotherapy may be of help to some patients with disabling, chronic sinusitis because continual emotional strain is one of the factors that can intensify the symptoms.

sinusoid (si′nŭ-soid) 1. resembling a sinus. 2. a form of terminal blood channel consisting of a large, irregular, anastomosing vessel, having a lining of reticuloendothelium but little or no adventitia. Sinusoids are found in the liver, adrenal glands, heart, parathyroid glands, carotid bodies, spleen, hemolymph glands and pancreas.

sinusotomy (si″nŭ-sot′o-me) incision of a sinus.

siphon (si′fon) 1. a bent tube with arms of unequal length, for drawing liquid from one receptacle to another. 2. to draw liquid from one receptacle to another by means of a siphon.

Sippy diet (sip′e) a graduated diet for gastric ulcer. It consists of frequent feedings of milk or cream, followed later by the addition of eggs, custards and other soft foods.

sirenomelus (si″ren-om′ĕ-lus) a fetal monster with fused legs and no feet.

-sis (sis) word element [Gr.], *state; condition.*

sitieirgia (sit″e-īr′je-ah) morbid rejection of food.

sitiology, sitology (sit″e-ol′o-je), (si-tol′o-je) the science of food and nourishment.

sitomania (si″to-ma′ne-ah) excessive hunger, or morbid craving for food.

sitophobia (si″to-fo′be-ah) morbid dread of taking food.

sitosterol (si″tos′ter-ol) one of a group of closely related plant sterols; a preparation of beta-sitosterol and certain saturated sterols is used as an antihypercholesterolemic agent.

sitotherapy (si″to-ther′ah-pe) treatment by food; dietotherapy.

sitotropism (si-tot′ro-pizm) tropism in response to the influence of food.

situs (si′tus), pl. *si′tus* [L.] site or position.
   s. inver′sus, total or partial transposition of the body organs to the side opposite the normal.

sitz bath (sits) immersion in water of only the hips and buttocks, for relief of pain and discomfort following rectal surgery, cystoscopy or vaginal surgery, or for cystitis or infections within the pelvic cavity (see also BATH).

SK streptokinase.

skatole (skat′ōl) a compound formed in the putrefaction of proteins which contributes to the characteristic odor of the feces.

skatoxyl (skah-tok′sil) an oxidation product of skatole found in the urine in certain diseases of the large intestine.

skein (skān) the threadlike figure seen in the earlier stages of mitosis.

skelalgia (ske-lal′je-ah) pain in the leg.

skeletal (skel′ĕ-tal) pertaining to the skeleton.
   s. system, the body's framework of bones; called also the skeleton. The skeleton of an average adult consists of 206 distinct bones.
   FUNCTIONS OF THE SKELETAL SYSTEM. The bones of the skeleton give support and shape to the body and protect delicate internal organs. Muscles attached to the skeleton make motion possible. In addition to supporting the body, the bones store and help maintain the correct level of calcium (see also BONE). The bone marrow manufactures blood cells.
   MAIN PARTS OF THE SKELETON. There are two main parts of the skeleton; the axial skeleton, including the bones of the head and trunk, and the appendicular skeleton, including the bones of the limbs. The axial skeleton has 80 bones; the appendicular skeleton, 126 bones.
   Axial Skeleton. The axial skeleton includes the skull, the spine and the ribs and sternum. The most important of these is the spine, called also the backbone and the vertebral column; it consists of 26 separate bones. Twenty-four vertebrae have holes through them, and the holes are lined up vertically, forming a hollow tube. The spinal cord runs through this bony tube and is protected by it.
   The seven topmost spinal bones, the cervical vertebrae, are the neck bones. They support the skull, which encloses and protects the brain and provides protection for the eyes, the inner ears and the nasal passages. The skull includes the cranium, the facial bones and the auditory ossicles. Of the 28 bones of the skull, only one—the mandible—is movable.
   Below the seven cervical vertebrae of the spine are 12 thoracic vertebrae; attached to them are 12 pairs of ribs, one pair to a vertebra. The ribs curve around to the front of the body, where most of them attach directly to the sternum or are indirectly attached to it by means of cartilage. The two bottom pairs of ribs remain unattached in front and so are called floating ribs. Together, the thoracic vertebrae, the ribs and the sternum form a bony basket, called the thoracic (or rib) cage, that prevents the chest wall from collapsing and protects the heart and the lungs.
   The remaining bones of the spine include five lumbar vertebrae, which support the small of the back, and the sacrum and coccyx.
   The axial skeleton also includes a single bone in the neck, the hyoid bone, to which muscles of the mouth are attached. This is the only bone of the body that does not join with another bone.
   Appendicular Skeleton. The appendicular skeleton includes the shoulder girdle, arm bones, pelvic girdle and leg bones. The shoulder (or pectoral) girdle, from which the arms hang, consists of the two clavicles (collarbones) and two scapulae (shoulder blades). The scapulae are joined to the sternum.
   The arm has three long bones. One end of the upper arm bone, the humerus, fits into a socket in the shoulder girdle; the other end is connected at the elbow to the ulna and the radius, the two long bones of the lower arm. Eight small bones, the carpals, comprise the wrist. Five metacarpals form the palm of the hand, and the finger bones are made up of 14 phalanges in each hand.
   At the lower end of the spine is the pelvic (or hip) girdle. This girdle and the last two bones of the spine, the sacrum and the coccyx, form the pelvis. This part of the skeleton encircles and protects the internal organs of the genitourinary system. In each side of the pelvis is a socket into which a femur fits.
   Leg bones are similar in construction to arm bones, but are heavier and stronger. The thigh bone, or femur, which is the longest bone in the body, extends from the pelvis to the knee, and the tibia and fibula go from knee to ankle. The kneecap is a single bone, the patella. In each leg there are seven ankle bones, or tarsals; five foot bones, or metatarsals; and 14 toe bones, or phalanges.
   JOINTS AND MOVEMENT. Any place in the skeleton where two or more bones come together is known as a JOINT. The way these bones are joined determines whether they can move and how they move. The elbow, for example, is a hinge joint, which allows bending in only one direction. In contrast, both bending and rotary movements are possible in the hip joint, a ball-and-socket joint. Many joints, such as most of those in the skull, are rigid and permit no movement whatsoever.
   The force needed to move the bones is provided by MUSCLES, which are attached to the bones by tendons. A muscle typically spans a joint so that one end is attached by a tendon to one bone, and the other end to a second bone. Usually one bone serves as an anchor for the muscle, and the second bone is free to move. When the muscle contracts, it pulls the second bone. Actually, two sets of muscles that pull in opposite directions take part in any movement. When one set contracts, the opposing set relaxes.

skeletization (skel″ĕ-tī-za′shun) 1. extreme emaciation. 2. removal of the soft parts from the skeleton.

skeletogenous (skel″ĕ-toj′ĕ-nus) producing skeletal structures or tissues.

skeletology (skel″ĕ-tol′o-je) the sum of knowledge regarding the skeleton.

skeleton (skel′ĕ-ton) the hardened tissues forming

the supporting framework of an animal body (see SKELETAL SYSTEM).

skenitis (ske-ni′tis) inflammation of Skene's glands, the mucus-secreting glands within the meatus of the female urethra.

skeocytosis (ske″o-si-to′sis) the presence of immature forms of leukocytes in the blood.

skeptophylaxis (skep″to-fi-lak′sis) production of temporary immunity to a toxic substance by administration of a minute quantity of it.

skia- (ski′ah) word element [Gr.], *shadow* (especially as produced by x-rays).

skiameter (ski-am′ĕ-ter) an instrument for measuring the intensity of x-rays.

skiametry (ski-am′ĕ-tre) observation of the pupil and retina under a beam of light projected into the eye, as a means of determining refractive errors of the eye.

skiascope (ski′ah-skōp) 1. a fluoroscope. 2. an instrument used in skiametry.

skiascopy (ski-as′ko-pe) 1. skiametry. 2. fluoroscopy.

skin (skin) the outer covering of the body. The skin is the largest organ of the body, and it performs a number of vital functions. It serves as a protective barrier against microorganisms. It helps shield the delicate, sensitive tissues underneath from mechanical and other injuries. It acts as an insulator against heat and cold, and helps eliminate body wastes in the form of perspiration. It guards against excessive exposure to the ultraviolet rays of the sun by producing a protective pigmentation, and it helps produce the body's supply of vitamin D. Its sense receptors enable the body to feel pain, cold, heat, touch and pressure.

The skin consists of two main parts: an outer layer, the epidermis, and an inner layer, the corium (dermis, true skin).

EPIDERMIS. The epidermis is thinner than the corium, and is made up of several layers of different kinds of cells. The number of cells varies in different parts of the body; the greatest number is in the palms of the hands and soles of the feet, where the skin is thickest.

The cells in the outer or horny layer of the epidermis are constantly being shed and replaced by new cells from its bottom layers in the lower epidermis. The cells of the protective, horny layer are nonliving and require no supply of blood for nourishment. As long as the horny outer layer remains intact, microorganisms cannot enter.

CORIUM. Underneath the epidermis is the thicker part of the skin, the corium, or dermis, which is made up of connective tissue that contains blood vessels and nerves. The corium projects into the epidermis in ridges called papillae of the corium.

The nerves that extend through the corium end in the papillae. The various skin sensations, such as touch, pain, pressure, heat and cold, are felt through these nerves. The reaction to heat and cold causes the expansion and contraction of the blood capillaries of the corium. This in turn causes more or less blood to flow through the skin, resulting in greater or smaller loss of body heat (see TEMPERATURE).

The sweat glands are situated deep in the corium.

They collect fluid containing water, salt and waste products from the blood and carry it away in canals that end in pores on the skin surface, where it is deposited as sweat. Perspiration helps regulate body temperature as well, because cooling of the skin occurs when sweat evaporates. The sebaceous glands are also in the corium. They secrete the oil that keeps the skin surface lubricated.

Beneath the corium is a layer of subcutaneous tissue. This tissue helps insulate the body against heat and cold, and cushions it against shock.

The hair and nails are outgrowths of the skin. The roots of the hair lie in follicles, or pockets of epidermal cells situated in the corium. Hair grows from the roots, but the hair cells die while still in the follicles, and the closely packed remains that are pushed upward form the hair shaft that is seen on the surface of the skin.

The nails grow in much the same way as the hair. The nail bed, like the hair root, is situated in the corium. The pink color of the nails is due to their translucent quality which allows the blood capillaries of the corium to show through.

DISORDERS OF THE SKIN. The skin reflects the general physical and emotional health. A skin disorder, for instance, may indicate disease within the body. For this reason, it is important that a particular skin condition be diagnosed and treated by a physician rather than by home treatments that may be unnecessary or actually harmful.

It is important to remember that the skin, given the opportunity, tends to heal itself. Overtreatment may be worse than no treatment at all. For common skin ailments, bland treatments, such as cool or warm compresses, lotions and ointments, are usually recommended. Under no circumstances should one scratch, pick or rub an incipient skin irritation or inflammation.

The medical name for an inflammation of the skin is DERMATITIS, and any itching of the skin is called PRURITUS. Dermatitis may occur without pruritus, and vice versa, but often they occur together.

Allergic reactions that may be manifested by skin disorders include URTICARIA (hives), ECZEMA and various forms of contact dermatitis. Fungus infections of the skin include RINGWORM and ATHLETE'S FOOT.

BOILS and CARBUNCLES occur when bacteria gain entrance into the skin and cause the formation of pus. A related condition of the eyelid is a STY.

Streptococci or staphylococci cause IMPETIGO, which is marked by blisters and yellowish crusts and occurs most often in children.

A similar infection that affects the hair follicles at the pore openings of the skin is FOLLICULITIS. When such infection affects the follicles of the beard, it is called SYCOSIS BARBAE, or barber's itch.

ERYSIPELAS, or St. Anthony's fire, is a streptococcal infection of the skin and underlying tissues that can be very serious if not treated. This condition is one of several forms of CELLULITIS that may affect the skin.

COLLAGEN DISEASES, which cause deterioration of the connective tissues, may affect the skin. They include the relatively uncommon LUPUS ERYTHEMATOSUS and scleroderma. PEMPHIGUS is a rare and serious disease that usually begins as a cluster of blisters on the nose or mouth and gradually involves the whole body.

Fever blisters, or coldsores, are caused by the virus of herpes simplex. Another virus disease affecting the skin is HERPES ZOSTER, or shingles, in which an infected nerve causes a skin eruption. WARTS are also caused by a virus.

The skin is subject to a number of pigmentary disorders. Some are congenital; others occur as the result of exposure to sunlight, heat, heavy metals and other products, or as a result of local injury, or in association with various diseases.

Some persons lack pigmentation partially or completely. This condition, which is hereditary, is known as albinism. Vitiligo and leukoderma appear as white spots that occur because of decreased pigmentation. The cause of vitiligo is unknown. Leukoderma may accompany certain infections, or may result from injury or exposure to rubber products.

Excessive pigmentation includes the freckles that light-skinned persons tend to develop from overexposure to sunlight. LIVER SPOTS are brownish patches, somewhat larger and darker than freckles, that sometimes appear on the skin of an older person. Both conditions are harmless.

NEVI, or moles, are dark patches, varying in color from gray to brown to black. On the average, every person has at least 20. Some moles occasionally can become malignant and any change in their appearance should be brought to the attention of a physician.

A HEMANGIOMA is an area in which the blood vessels form an abnormally excessive network in the skin. They usually occur as birthmarks and some disappear with age; others can be treated surgically, with medications or with irradiation. Bronzing of the skin sometimes is associated with ADDISON'S DISEASE and hemochromatosis ("bronze diabetes").

Various kinds of tumors, or growths may be found on the skin. KELOIDS are benign tumors that usually originate in scar tissue. In many cases they

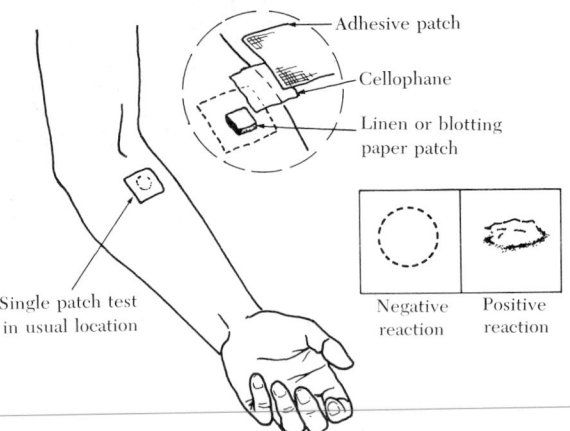

Single patch test in usual location

Adhesive patch

Cellophane

Linen or blotting paper patch

Negative reaction   Positive reaction

Patch test.

can be removed with radium and x-ray therapy. XANTHOMAS are harmless yellow growths caused by deposits of fat in the skin. They may be associated with some underlying disorder of lipid metabolism. They can be eliminated by a physician if they are unsightly. Keratoses are wartlike growths, often brown in color, that appear most frequently in older persons. Because they can develop into cancers, they should receive medical attention. Generally a physician will recommend that they be removed.

CANCER of the skin is the most common of all cancers. Fortunately it is comparatively easy to treat successfully, especially if it is diagnosed early. As protection against skin cancer, sores that persist for more than 2 or 3 weeks and suspicious lumps or growths that suddenly begin to enlarge or change color should be brought to a physician's attention.

s. graft, a bit of skin implanted to replace a lost part of the integument (see also GRAFTING and PLASTIC SURGERY).

s. test, application of a substance to the skin, or intradermal injection of a substance, to permit observation of the body's reaction to it. Such a

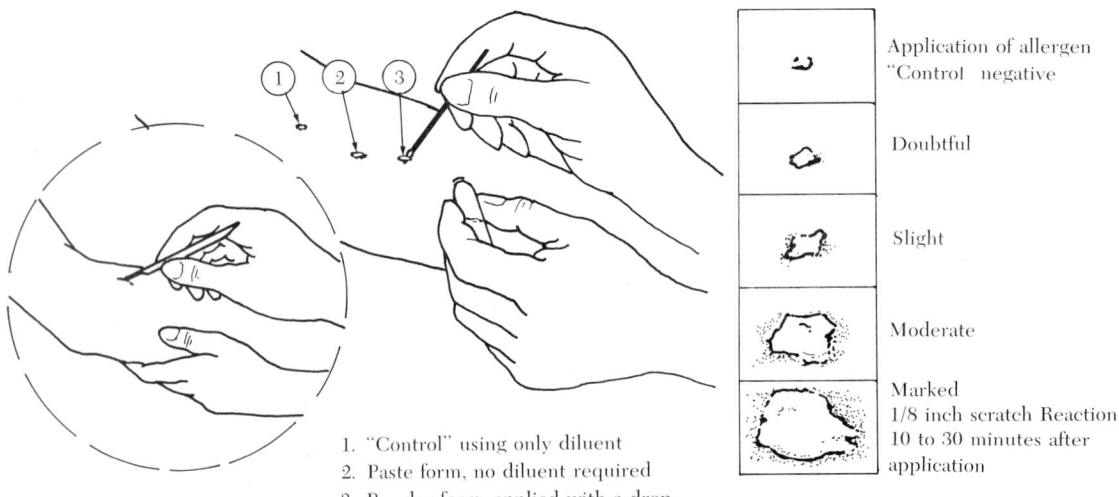

1. "Control" using only diluent
2. Paste form, no diluent required
3. Powder form, applied with a drop of diluent from end of toothpick

Application of allergen "Control" negative

Doubtful

Slight

Moderate

Marked
1/8 inch scratch Reaction 10 to 30 minutes after application

Scratch test.

test detects a person's sensitivity to such allergens as dust and pollen, or to preparations of microorganisms believed to be the cause of a disorder.

There are several types of skin tests, including the patch test, the scratch test and the intradermal test.

PATCH TEST. This is the simplest type of skin test. A small piece of gauze or filter paper is impregnated with a minute quantity of the substance to be tested and is applied to the skin, usually on the forearm. After a certain length of time the patch is removed and the reaction observed. If there is no reaction, the test result is said to be negative; if the skin is reddened or swollen, the result is positive.

The patch test is used most often in testing for skin allergies, especially contact DERMATITIS.

SCRATCH TEST. In this test, one or more small scratches or superficial cuts are made in the skin, and a minute amount of the substance to be tested is inserted in the scratches and allowed to remain there for a short time. If no reaction has occurred after 30 minutes, the substance is removed and the test is considered negative. If there is redness or swelling at the scratch sites, the test is considered positive.

The scratch test is often used in testing for allergies. A complete screening for allergic sensitivity may require numerous skin tests. Only an extremely minute quantity of the substance can be used in each test since severe allergic reactions can occur.

The scratch test is also used in the diagnosis of tuberculosis. In Pirquet's reaction, for example, tuberculin is used, and the local inflammatory reaction that results is more marked in tuberculous persons than in normal ones.

INTRADERMAL TESTS. In these tests, the substance under study is injected between the layers of skin. Intradermal tests are used for diagnosis of infectious diseases and determination of susceptibility to a disease or sensitivity to an allergen.

In the intradermal test for tuberculosis, the Mantoux test, a purified protein derivative (P.P.D.), prepared from tubercle bacilli, is injected. In a positive result, the area becomes reddened or inflamed within 72 hours. This indicates past or present infection. An infection that has been present for at least 2 to 8 weeks will usually be revealed by the test.

The Schick test, used to determine susceptibility to diphtheria, is one of the best-known intradermal skin tests. A very small dose of diphtheria antitoxin is injected into the forearm. In a positive reaction the area becomes red and remains so for about a week. If no reaction occurs, the person is immune to the disease.

The trichophytin test is sometimes used in diagnosing suspected cases of superficial fungus infection of the skin, such as ringworm. In the presence of infection by the fungus Trichophyton, an injection of trichophytin, which is prepared from cultures of the fungus, will produce a reaction similar to the tuberculin reaction. Skin tests, of course, are always made in an area separate from the infected area.

In addition to their frequent use in testing for allergies, intradermal tests are employed in the diagnosis of parasitic infections, such as SCHISTO-SOMIASIS, other fungus diseases besides trichophytosis, and mumps.

Skiodan (ski′o-dan) trademark for preparations of methiodal sodium, used as a radiopaque medium for roentgenography of the urinary tract.

skler(o)- for words beginning thus, see those beginning *scler(o)-*.

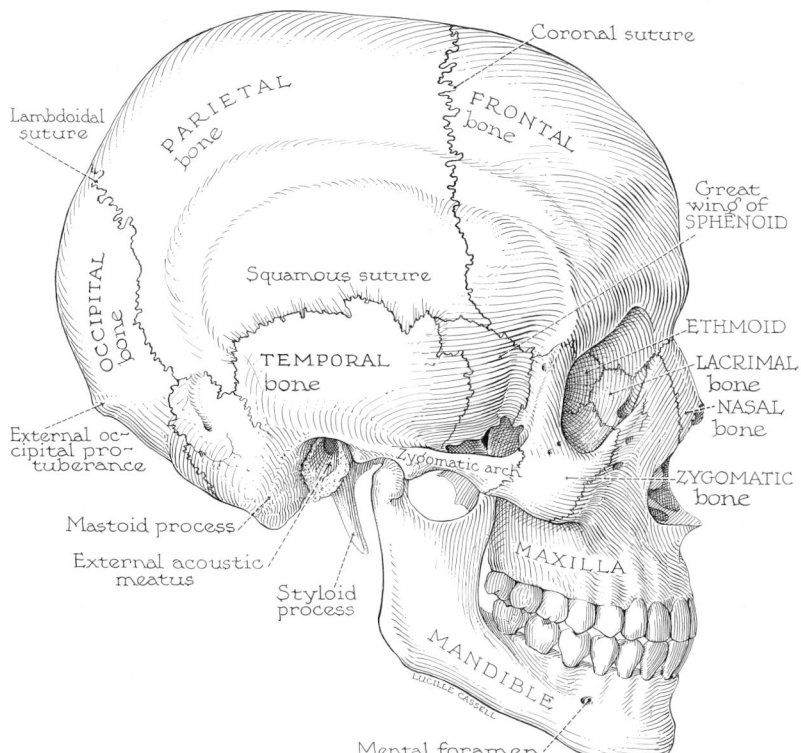

Lateral view of the skull. (From King, B. G., and Showers, M. J.: Human Anatomy and Physiology. 6th ed. Philadelphia, W. B. Saunders Co., 1969.)

skot(o)- for words beginning thus, see those beginning *scot(o)-*.

skull (skul) the bony framework of the head, enclosing and protecting the brain. The skull consists of two parts, the cranium and the facial section.

The cranium is the domed top, back and sides of the skull. It is formed by comparatively large, smooth and gently curved bones connected to each other by dovetailed joints called sutures, which permit no movement and make the mature skull rigid. At birth, however, the skull joints are flexible, so that the infant's head can be compressed as it emerges from the birth canal. The joints remain flexible to allow expansion until the cranial bones are fully formed, around the second year of life. An infant's skull contains soft areas, or FONTANELS, where the bones of the cranium do not meet.

The facial bones are smaller and more complex

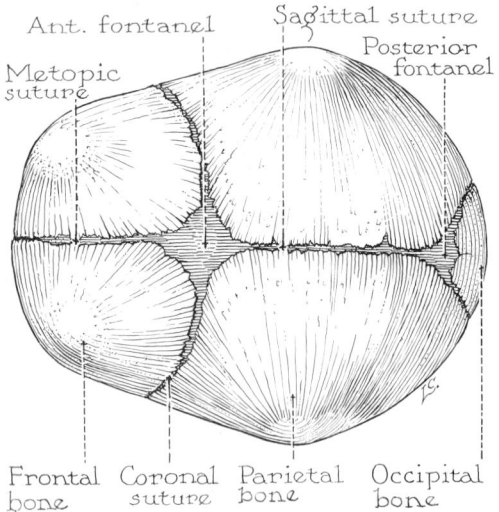

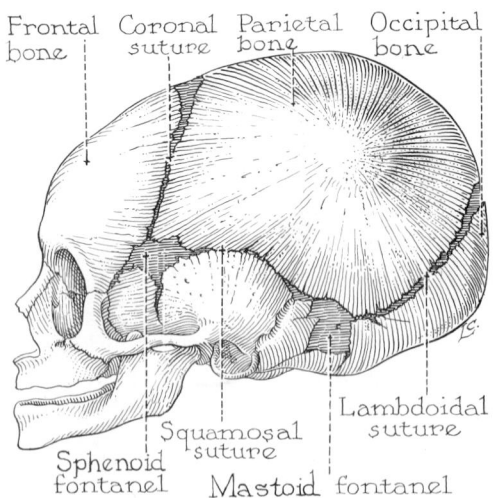

Skull at birth: Above, showing anterior and posterior fontanels; below, lateral view. (From King, B. G., and Showers, M. J.: Human Anatomy and Physiology. 6th ed. Philadelphia, W. B. Saunders Co., 1969.)

than the cranial bones. None of them are movable, except the mandible, which is hinged to the rest of the skull.

The skull protects the brain, the curve of the cranium serving to deflect blows, and it also protects the eyes, ears and nose, which are surrounded by bone and recessed in the skull.

The skull is supported by the highest vertebra, called the atlas. This joint permits a back-and-forth, nodding motion. The atlas turns on the vertebra below it, the axis, which allows the skull to turn from side to side.

DISORDERS OF THE SKULL. The skull is rarely affected by disease. Uncommon ones like OSTEITIS DEFORMANS and ACROMEGALY cause the bones to increase in size. Like other bones, the skull may be fractured by blows, falls or other accidents, but skull fracture can be far more dangerous because of its proximity to the brain. Concussion is almost always present with such fractures. If the fracture is simple, it will usually heal itself. There may be complications, however. If the fracture crosses an artery, surgery may be necessary. Another danger is that a bone or fragment of bone may be pushed in and exert pressure on the brain, possibly causing convulsions. Such a bone intrusion must be corrected by surgery. Open or compound fractures of the skull present the additional danger of infection to the brain. (See also HEAD INJURY.)

During infancy the bones of the skull may unite prematurely, causing the head to be misshapen and sometimes resulting in brain damage because of pressure effects on the growing brain.

sleep (slēp) a natural or artificially induced state of suspension of sensory and motor activity. Sleep is essential to life. During sleep the body processes slow down, so that tissues and organs can recuperate from previous activity. For the brain, sleep is even more vital. Experiments have shown that lack of sleep, which actually has little physical effect on the body if there has been adequate rest, seriously disturbs the mental processes. After 30 to 60 hours of continuous sleeplessness, such reactions as irritation, loss of memory, hallucinations and even symptoms of schizophrenia may begin to appear.

SLEEP REQUIREMENTS. The amount of sleep necessary for good health varies greatly from one person to the next. Sleep requirements are greatest at birth, and a newborn infant will sleep nearly 20 hours a day. Children between the ages of 1 and 4 require about 12 hours daily; those between 4 and 12 should have 10 hours or so of sleep. Adolescents usually need from 8 to 10 hours of sleep, and adults from 6 to 9, although 8 hours seems to be the average. People who are ill or tire easily or engage in strenuous activities may need more than the average amount of sleep.

REM SLEEP. Recent research in sleep physiology has shown that a cyclic phenomenon known as rapid eye movement (REM) sleep occurs in normal persons. The cycle is characterized by periods of neural activity during which the eyes can be observed moving rapidly in all directions under closed eyelids. The period of REM sleep is followed by a period of quiet sleep. The normal adult spends about one-fourth of an 8-hour sleep period in REM sleep, the periods lasting about 20 minutes and occurring every 60 to 90 minutes throughout the time a person is sleeping.

The eye movements have been shown to be associated with dreaming. In laboratory experiments deprivation of REM sleep, and consequently of dreaming, leads to irritability, anxiety, poor motor coordination and difficulty in concentration and remembering. It has been postulated that anxiety, which is thought to reduce REM sleep time, may contribute to the development of a vicious cycle in which the person being deprived of REM sleep time becomes more tense and thus develops anxiety that further deprives him of REM sleep. This could lead to an acute psychotic episode.

Certain drugs have been found to affect the sleep cycle. Amphetamine decreases the REM sleep time, as do the barbiturates, alcohol and the phenothiazine derivatives.

twilight s., a condition of analgesia and amnesia, produced by hypodermic administration of morphine and scopolamine. In this state the patient, while responding to pain, does not retain it in her memory. It is employed in the conduct of labor.

sleeping disease narcolepsy.

sleeping sickness the popular name for EN-CEPHALITIS, an inflammation of the brain and its coverings, the meninges. There are several different forms of the disease, none of which is common in the United States, although a few forms are occasionally epidemic in limited areas of the country. The name sleeping sickness comes from the drowsiness that is often characteristic of the disease.

African s. s., African trypanosomiasis.

sleepwalking walking while asleep; called also somnambulism. Much mystery has been attached to sleepwalking, although it is no more mysterious than dreaming. The principal difference between the two is that the sleepwalker, besides dreaming, is also using a part of his brain that stimulates walking.

The sleepwalker usually seems to be sound asleep; he gets out of bed, walks about and returns to bed without waking; in the morning he has no recollection of having left his bed. The walker often seems to have a purpose, and it is believed that he tends to act according to his subconscious wishes. In some cases the sleepwalker may also speak, or may even see, hear and feel.

Sleepwalking is most likely to happen during periods of emotional stress. Usually it ceases when the source of anxiety is removed. Often it occurs only once or twice and does not happen again. If sleepwalking recurs frequently, it may stem from serious emotional distress.

slide (slīd) a piece of glass or other transparent substance on which material is placed for examination under the microscope.

sling (sling) a bandage or suspensory for supporting a part.

slipped disk the popular name for a rupture of a disk, or pad of cartilage, between vertebrae (see slipped DISK).

slough (sluf) a mass of dead tissue in, or cast out from, living tissue.

sludge (sluj) a suspension of solid or semisolid particles in a fluid.

sludging (sluj′ing) settling out of solid particles from solution.

s. of blood, intravascular agglutination of eryth-rocytes into irregular masses, interfering with circulation of blood.

Sm chemical symbol, *samarium.*

smallpox (smawl′poks) a highly contagious, often fatal viral disease; called also variola. Its most noticeable symptom is the appearance of blisters and pustules on the skin. Smallpox has become rare in most parts of the world because of widespread vaccination against the disease.

Smallpox is one of the most contagious diseases known. The virus that causes the disease is present in the nose and throat of the infected person, in the blisters on his skin and in his excretions throughout the course of the disease.

The incubation period is generally 12 days, although it may vary from 7 to 21 days.

SYMPTOMS. The first symptoms of smallpox are severe headache, chills and high fever. Children may suffer from vomiting and convulsions. Within 3 or 4 days, a rash of small, red pustules appears, first on the face, then on the arms, wrists, hands and legs. A small number of spots appear on the trunk. In a day or two, the spots become blisters and fill with clear fluid. Over the next week, the fluid turns into a yellowish, puslike substance and begins to dry up, leaving a crust or scab on the skin. These scabs fall off after 3 or 4 weeks, leaving disfiguring pits in the skin, particularly on the face.

ISOLATION AND QUARANTINE. A smallpox patient must be rigorously isolated. All those known to have been in contact with the patient are quarantined for 16 days, unless they have just been revaccinated, in which case they may be released from quarantine as soon as the vaccination has "taken." Those in quarantine are kept under careful observation, so that if the disease develops they can be isolated and treated immediately. All contaminated objects are destroyed by burning or sterilized with high-pressure steam or boiling water. The patient's home is thoroughly cleaned and disinfected.

TREATMENT. There is at present no cure for smallpox. One important consideration in treating the disease is the possibility of scarring caused by the blisters or pocks. To avoid this, medications may be given to prevent or soothe itching, and antibiotics are applied to the skin to counteract secondary infection. The patient's fingernails are cut short and his hands kept clean to further reduce the danger of infection.

Other than these measures, treatment consists largely of rest and proper nourishment. Medicines may be given to lower the patient's fever, along with sedatives.

PREVENTION. The smallpox vaccination process takes about 10 days to 2 weeks. A drop of vaccine prepared from cowpox lesions is placed on the skin, usually on the upper arm, and the surface of the skin is lightly scratched with a needle. In a day or two the area becomes reddened and a blister forms, and after several days it hardens and turns brown. The patient may have a slight fever during this period and may feel slightly ill on the eighth or ninth day.

It is recommended that children first be vaccinated against smallpox at the age of 2 or 3 years. Revaccination is given every 5 years, and again if the child is exposed to the disease. Vaccination is to be deferred if the child or those in his immediate family are suffering from eczema. The United States requires that persons entering the country, including Americans returning from abroad, have proof of successful vaccination within the previous 3 years.

smear (smēr) a preparation for microscopic study, the material being spread thinly and unevenly across the slide with a swab or loop, or with the edge of another slide.

smegma (smeg′mah) the secretion, consisting principally of desquamated epithelial cells, found chiefly about the external genitalia.

smell (smel) the sense that enables one to perceive odors. The sense of smell depends on the stimulation of sense organs in the nose by small particles carried in inhaled air. It is important not only for the detection of odors, but also for the enjoyment of food. Flavor is a blend of taste and smell. Taste registers only four qualities: salt, sour, bitter and sweet; other qualities of flavor depend on smell.

The organs of smell are small patches of special (olfactory) cells in the nasal mucosa. One patch is located in each of the two main compartments of the back of the nose. The olfactory cells are connected to the brain by the first cranial (olfactory) nerve. Air currents do not flow directly over the patches in breathing; this is why one must sniff to detect a faint odor or to enjoy a fragrance to the fullest.

When one sniffs, air currents carrying molecules of odorous chemicals enter special compartments, called olfactory chambers, where the chemicals are dissolved in mucus. There they can act on the organs of smell in much the same way that solutions act on the taste buds of the tongue. The endings of the sensory nerves that detect odors, the olfactory receptors, quickly adapt to an odor and cease to be stimulated by it after a few minutes of full exposure.

The sense of smell may be diminished or lost entirely, usually temporarily, as a result of an obstruction of the nose, a nasal infection, injury or deterioration of the nasal tissue, brain tumor or mental illness. In rare instances, injury or disease causes such damage to the olfactory nerve that loss of the sense of smell is permanent. The complete absence of the sense of smell is known as anosmia.

smoking (smōk′ing) the act of drawing into the mouth and puffing out the smoke of tobacco contained in a cigarette, cigar or pipe. For centuries, tobacco smoking has been suspected of being a health hazard. In recent years a close relationship between smoking and lung cancer and heart disease has definitely been established. While smoking is not the only cause of these diseases, its relationship to them and also to other diseases has been so strongly established that no smoker can afford to ignore the evidence. Parents especially owe it to their children to educate them in order that the cigarette habit will never begin.

In 1962 the Surgeon General of the United States organized a committee of experts to review some 8000 statistical studies on the effects of smoking.

The report of this committee, issued in January 1964, stated:

In view of the continuing and mounting evidence from many sources, it is the judgment of the Committee that cigarette smoking contributes substantially to mortality from certain specific diseases and to the overall death rate.

Cigarette smoking is a health hazard of sufficient importance in the United States to warrant appropriate remedial action.

GENERAL EFFECTS ON HEALTH. Tobacco smoke contains a number of harmful substances, including poisons such as NICOTINE, various irritants and carcinogenic compounds. Because cigarette smokers usually inhale this smoke, they are much more subject to its harmful effects than pipe and cigar smokers, who generally do not inhale. In pipe and cigar smoking, however, there is some danger to the heart because of the nicotine that is absorbed by the mouth. There is also the possibility of cancer of the lips, tongue and mouth. Statistically, there is no question that nonsmokers are far less subject to the diseases that affect smokers.

Among the respiratory diseases closely related to cigarette smoking are lung cancer, cancer of the larynx, chronic bronchitis and emphysema. Coronary artery disease and hypertensive heart disease are also closely related to smoking, as are peptic ulcer, Buerger's disease (thromboangiitis obliterans) and cancer of the bladder. Other diseases have been linked with smoking. The risk of incurring any of these diseases increases with the number of cigarettes smoked daily, the length of each cigarette consumed and the length of time the smoking habit has persisted. In general, heavy smokers as a group die younger than do nonsmokers.

S.M.P. Society of Medical Psychoanalysts.

Sn chemical symbol, *tin* (L. *stannum*).

snake (snāk) a limbless reptile, many species of which are poisonous.

s. bite, injury caused by the mouth parts of a snake. Every state in the United States except Alaska and Maine harbors venomous snakes, but only in a few of the southern states do venomous snakes make up an important part of the snake population. There are 19 kinds of venomous snakes in this country. North of a line connecting the northern borders of Virginia, Missouri and Arizona, only two kinds of venomous snakes are found— rattlesnakes and copperheads. Below this line there are, in addition, coral snakes and the cottonmouth, or water moccasin.

A person who is bitten by a venomous snake has about a 98 per cent chance of survival if proper first-aid treatment is given.

RECOGNITION OF VENOMOUS SNAKE BITE. Most snake bites are inflicted by nonvenomous snakes. These bites are usually only small scratches or shallow punctures. Such lacerations should be washed with soap and water, and an antiseptic should be applied.

The bite of a venomous snake usually consists of a pair of well defined deep puncture marks from $1/2$ inch to 1 inch apart. If venom is injected (often it is not), a burning pain is felt almost immediately and within 10 to 15 minutes a puffy and often discolored swelling usually appears at the site.

TREATMENT OF VENOMOUS SNAKE BITE. Modern treatment is based on the formula TISA: tourniquet, incision, suction and antivenin. Speed is essential for the first three steps, in order to remove as much venom as possible, but antivenin should be given only by a physician, preferably in a well equipped hospital. Antivenins are made of horse serum, and the incautious injection of antivenin into a person sensitive to horse serum may cause a serious allergic reaction.

Because activity speeds up the distribution of venom in the body, the victim should remain as quiet and inactive as possible.

Tourniquet. Fortunately, more than 85 per cent of all snake bites are on the limbs. A moderately tight tourniquet, designed to impede the flow of lymph and venous blood but not to stop arterial flow, may be applied between the site of the bite and the trunk before symptoms of poisoning appear. The tourniquet *must* be loosened every 10 minutes for 1 minute.

Incision. Incisions must be made in the bite area as soon as poisoning symptoms appear. A single incision through each fang mark, made lengthwise along the limb, is adequate. The incisions should be about ¼ inch long and just deep enough (also about ¼ inch) to cut through the skin.

Suction. Suction should be started immediately either by mouth or with the suction cups from a snake bite first-aid kit, if available. No danger is involved in mouth suction if there are no cuts or sores in the mouth.

Suction can be discontinued after the first hour but the tourniquet should be kept in use until an adequate amount of antivenin has been injected into the bitten person.

Antivenin. The antivenin used in the United States is a single polyvalent (multipurpose) antivenin designed for the bites of all North American pit vipers (moccasins and rattlesnakes). This antivenin is commonly available in hospitals, drugstores and Poison Control Centers. Some hospitals, major zoos and Poison Control Centers also stock a coral snake antivenin that is manufactured in Brazil.

PREVENTION OF SNAKE BITE. Most snake bites are inflicted on people who handle snakes or are senselessly incautious in localities where venomous snakes are prevalent. Certain common-sense precautions should be taken when visiting an area known to be inhabited by venomous snakes. Keep in mind that most of them are active in the early evening, that they often congregate on rocky south-facing or west-facing slopes to bask in the sunlight (especially in the spring and fall) and that they are not active at temperatures below 50° F.

snap (snap) a short, sharp sound.

   opening s., a short, sharp sound occurring just after the beginning of the second heart sound in mitral stenosis.

snare (snār) a wire loop for removing polyps and other pedunculated growths by cutting them off at the base.

sneeze (snēz) an involuntary, sudden, violent and audible expulsion of air through the mouth and nose. Sneezing is usually caused by the irritation of sensitive nerve endings in the mucous membrane that lines the nose. Allergies, drafts of cold air and even bright light can produce sneezing.

Sneezing and coughing are similar in that both are reflex actions and are preceded by quick inhalations. (However, a cough may also be deliberate, to clear the throat or bronchi.) Sneezing and coughing both involve the glottis. The power for a cough is achieved by closing the glottis and holding the air under pressure for a moment, then suddenly forcing it out by action of the diaphragm and of the muscles of the chest wall and abdomen.

In a sneeze, the glottis is momentarily closed after air is inhaled and the tongue is pressed against the roof of the mouth. When the glottis is suddenly opened, part of the air goes through the nose and, when the tongue is released, part goes through the mouth; in this way mucus and other irritants are expelled from the nose.

Snellen chart (snel'en) a chart printed with block letters in gradually decreasing sizes, used in testing distance vision.

snoring (snōr'ing) breathing during sleep accompanied by harsh sounds. It occurs when inhaled air causes the soft palate to vibrate. Snoring is common among persons who sleep with their mouths open.

Although snoring is a sign of sound sleep, it is sometimes desirable to eliminate or reduce it. If the mouth-breathing is stopped, the snoring will also stop. An obvious reason for mouth-breathing is lying on the back, in which position the mouth tends to hang open. Further, when a person is in deep sleep and lying on his back, his tongue may rest back in his throat, partly blocking the air passage and helping to make the snoring sounds. Gently rolling the snorer on his side can sometimes eliminate the snoring in these cases.

There may be some functional reason for mouth-breathing, such as a common cold or allergy, causing mucus to stop up the nose. Growths, called polyps, may obstruct the nasal passages. A deformity of the nasal SEPTUM, the bony portion that divides the nasal cavity into two compartments, may make nose-breathing difficult.

Correction of sleeping habits and of nose or throat troubles may lessen snoring or reduce it to a minimum. However, if an elderly person has been snoring regularly for many years, there is little that can be done to change his sleeping habits.

snow (sno) a freezing or frozen mixture consisting of discrete particles or crystals.

   carbon dioxide s., the substance formed by rapid evaporation of liquid carbon dioxide; used locally in various skin conditions.

snowblindness (sno'blīnd-nes) temporary loss of sight due to injury to superficial cells of the cornea caused by ultraviolet rays of the sun reinforced by those reflected by snow.

S.N.S. Society of Neurological Surgeons.

snuff (snuf) a medicinal or errhine powder to be inhaled into the nose.

snuffles (snuf'elz) catarrhal discharge from the nasal mucous membrane in congenital syphilis in infants.

soap (sōp) any compound of one or more fatty acids, or their equivalents, with an alkali. Soap is a detergent and is employed in liniments and enemas and in making pills. It is also a mild aperient, antacid and antiseptic.

sociology (so″se-ol′o-je) the scientific study of social relationships and phenomena.

sociometry (so″se-om′ĕ-tre) the branch of sociology concerned with the measurement of human behavior.

sociopathic personality (so″se-o-path′ik) psychopathic personality.

sociopathy (so″se-op′ah-the) a disorder of social behavior.

soda (so′dah) sodium carbonate.
  baking s., sodium bicarbonate.
  caustic s., sodium hydroxide.
  s. lime, calcium hydroxide with sodium or potassium hydroxide, or both; used as adsorbent of carbon dioxide in equipment for metabolism tests, inhalation anesthesia or oxygen therapy.

sodic (so′dik) containing sodium.

sodium (so′de-um) a chemical element, atomic number 11, atomic weight 22.990, symbol Na. (See table of ELEMENTS.) Sodium is the chief cation of extracellular body fluids.
  s. acetate, a systemic and urinary alkalizer.
  s. acetrizoate, a substance used as contrast medium in angiocardiography and in x-ray visualization of the urinary and biliary tracts.
  s. acid phosphate, sodium biphosphate.
  s. alginate, a product derived from brown seaweeds, used in formulating various pharmaceutical preparations as an emulsifier, stabilizer or thickening agent.
  s. aminosalicylate, an antibacterial compound used in tuberculosis.
  s. ascorbate, an antiscorbutic vitamin for parenteral administration.
  s. benzoate, a white, odorless granular or crystalline powder, used chiefly as a test of liver function, and as a preservative for food and various pharmaceuticals.
  s. bicarbonate, a white powder found in most households in the form of baking soda; called also bicarbonate of soda. Taken in water, it is a popular remedy for acid indigestion. It has a rapid and soothing effect on the stomach, but should not be used regularly since when taken in excess it tends to cause ALKALOSIS. It should never be taken by those who have a heart condition or who are on salt-restricted diet, because it is a source of sodium. A teaspoonful of milk of magnesia will usually prove equally effective and is less harmful.
  Sodium bicarbonate can also be mixed with water and applied as a paste for the relief of pain in the treatment of minor BURNS and insect stings. A cupful of bicarbonate of soda in the bath water will sometimes help to relieve itching caused by an allergic reaction. Applied in powder form, bicarbonate of soda is often a more effective deodorant than many commercial preparations.
  s. biphosphate, a colorless or white crystalline compound, used as a urinary acidifier.
  s. bisulfite, an antioxidant compound.
  s. borate, a crystalline compound used in pharmaceutical preparations as an astringent for mucous membranes.
  s. bromide, a central nervous system depressant.
  s. caprylate, a compound used in treatment of fungal infections of the skin.

  s. carbonate, a salt in large, colorless crystals, sometimes used as a mouthwash or vaginal douche, or as a lotion on the skin.
  s. carboxymethyl cellulose, a compound used as a bulk-forming cathartic.
  s. chloride, a white, crystalline compound, a necessary constituent of the body and therefore of the diet; sometimes used parenterally in solution to replenish electrolytes in the body. Called also salt.
  s. citrate, a crystalline compound, largely used as an anticoagulant in blood for transfusion.
  s. colistimethate, an antibacterial compound usually administered intramuscularly.
  s. cyclamate, a compound formerly used as a sweetening agent.
  s. fluoride, a white, odorless powder added to drinking water or applied locally to teeth, in 1 to 2 per cent solution, to reduce the incidence of dental caries.
  s. folate, a compound used in various anemias and in control of diarrhea in sprue.
  s. glucosulfone, a compound used in treatment of leprosy and tuberculosis.
  s. glutamate, the monosodium salt of L-glutamic acid; used in treatment of encephalopathies associated with liver diseases.
  s. hydrate, s. hydroxide, a compound used chiefly in various chemical and pharmaceutical manipulations.
  s. hypochlorite, a compound used in solution as a germicide, deodorant and bleach.
  s. indigotindisulfonate, a compound used in measurement of kidney function and as a test solution.
  s. iodide, a compound used as a source of iodine.
  s. iodipamide, a water-soluble organic iodine compound used in roentgenography of the biliary tract.
  s. iodohippurate, a compound used as a contrast medium in roentgenography of the urinary tract.
  s. iodomethamate, a white, odorless powder used as a contrast medium in roentgenography of the urinary tract.
  s. lactate, a compound used in solution to replenish body fluids and electrolytes.
  s. lauryl sulfate, a surface-active agent used as an ingredient in toothpastes.
  s. liothyronine, the sodium salt of L-3,3′,5-triiodothyronine; used in the treatment of hypothyroidism, metabolic insufficiency and certain gynecologic disorders.
  s. methicillin, a semisynthetic penicillin salt for parenteral administration.
  s. morrhuate, sodium salts of the fatty acids of cod liver oil; used as a sclerosing agent in treatment of varicose veins.
  s. nitrate, a compound used as a reagent and in certain industrial processes.
  s. nitrite, a compound used as an antidote in cyanide poisoning.
  s. oxacillin, a semisynthetic penicillin salt for oral administration.
  s. para-aminohippurate, a compound used in studies for measurement of effective renal plasma flow and determination of the functional capacity of the tubular excretory mechanism.
  s. para-aminosalicylate, sodium aminosalicylate.
  s. perborate, a compound used as an oxidant and local anti-infective.
  s. peroxide, a white powder soluble in water; used as a dental bleach and in ointment form in acne and rosacea.

s. **phosphate,** a colorless or white granular salt, used as a cathartic.

s. **polystyrene sulfonate,** an ion-exchange resin used for removal of potassium ions.

s. **propionate,** a compound used in fungal infections.

s. **psylliate,** the sodium salt of the liquid fatty acids; used as a sclerosing agent.

s. **salicylate,** an analgesic, antipyretic compound (see SALICYLIC ACID).

s. **sulfanilate,** a salt used in acute nasal catarrh.

s. **sulfate,** a salt used as a saline cathartic.

s. **sulfocyanate,** sodium thiocyanate.

s. **sulfoxone,** a compound used in treatment of leprosy.

s. **tetradecyl sulfate,** a white, waxy, odorless solid; used in solution as a sclerosing agent.

s. **thiocyanate,** white or colorless, odorless crystals with a cooling, salty taste; used as a reagent and as a vasodilator.

s. **thiosulfate,** a compound used intravenously as an antidote for cyanide poisoning, to measure extracellular body fluid, and as a fixer in photography.

sodoku (so'do-koo) a relapsing type of infection due to *Spirillum minus,* an organism transmitted by the bite of an infected rat; a form of RATBITE FEVER.

sodomy (sod'o-me) sexual contact between man and animals; sometimes applied to oral-genital or anal contact between humans.

soft palate a fleshy structure at the back of the mouth, which, together with the hard palate, forms the roof of the mouth. From the middle of the free border of the soft palate hangs the fleshy conical body called the uvula. In swallowing, the soft palate is drawn upward against the back of the pharynx and prevents food and fluids from straying into the nasal passage while they pass through the throat.

softening (sof'en-ing) a change of consistency, with loss of firmness or hardness.

  red s., a form of degeneration of brain and spinal cord.

  white s., fatty degeneration of brain substance, the affected area becoming anemic and white.

sol (sol) a liquid colloid solution.

  solid s., a colloid system in which both dispersed phase and disperse medium are solids.

sol. solution.

Solanum (so-la'num) a genus of herbs and shrubs, including the potato, several of the nightshades and many poisonous and medicinal species.

solar plexus (so'lar) a network of ganglia and nerves in the center of the abdomen; it is part of the autonomic nervous system. It is important in the control of the function of the liver, stomach, kidneys and adrenal glands. A blow to it may knock a person out or cause great pain because the organs are momentarily thrown out of gear. Although the plexus recovers quickly, the effects on the body as a whole last longer.

solarization (so"lar-ĭ-za'shun) exposure to sunlight and the effects produced thereby.

solation (so-la'shun) the liquefaction of a gel.

sole (sōl) the bottom of the foot.

solenoid (so'lĕ-noid) a coil of wire each turn of which is equidistant from the next; passage of electric current causes it to act like a magnet.

Solganal (sol'gah-nal) trademark for a preparation of aurothioglucose, an antirheumatic preparation of gold salts.

solid (sol'id) 1. not fluid or gaseous; not hollow. 2. a substance or tissue not fluid or gaseous.

solubility (sol"u-bil'ĭ-te) the quality of being soluble.

soluble (sol'u-bl) susceptible of being dissolved.

solum (so'lum), pl. *so'la* [L.] the bottom or lowest part.

solute (sol'ūt) the substance that is dissolved in a liquid (solvent) to form a solution.

solution (so-loo'shun) 1. a liquid preparation of one or more soluble chemical substances usually dissolved in water. 2. the process of dissolving or disrupting.

PREPARATION OF SOLUTIONS. Formula for preparing solutions from a pure drug:

$$\text{pure drug : finished solution} =$$
$$\text{strength of solution}$$
$$\text{(expressed in percentage or ratio)}$$

For example, to prepare 2000 ml. of a 2 per cent solution from boric acid crystals, the proportion would be

$$\text{X Gm. : 2000 ml.} = \text{2 Gm. : 100 ml.}$$
$$\text{X} = \text{40 Gm. pure drug}$$

Formula for preparing solutions from stock solutions:

$$\text{lesser amount of stock solution : greater amount of}$$
$$\text{stock solution} =$$
$$\text{lesser strength : greater strength}$$

For example, to prepare 1000 ml. of a 2 per cent solution from a 4 per cent stock solution, the proportion would be

$$\text{X ml. : 1000 ml.} = \text{2 per cent : 4 per cent}$$
$$\text{X} = \text{500 ml. stock solution}$$

  aqueous s., one in which water is used as the solvent.

  buffer s., one that resists appreciable change in its hydrogen ion concentration (pH) when acid or alkali is added to it.

  colloid s., colloidal s., a preparation consisting of minute particles of matter suspended in a solvent.

  contrast s., a solution of a substance opaque to the x-ray, used to facilitate x-ray visualization of some organ or structure in the body.

  hyperbaric s., one having a greater specific gravity than a standard of reference.

  hypertonic s., one having an osmotic pressure greater than that of a standard reference.

  hypobaric s., one having a specific gravity less than that of a standard reference.

  hypotonic s., one having an osmotic pressure less than that of standard reference.

  iodine s., a transparent, reddish brown liquid, each 100 ml. of which contains 1.8 to 2.2 Gm. of iodine and 2.1 to 2.6 Gm. of sodium iodide.

isobaric s., a solution having the same specific gravity as a standard of reference.

isosmotic s., isotonic s., one having an osmotic pressure the same as that of a standard of reference.

molar s., a solution each liter of which contains 1 gram-molecule of the active substance.

normal s., a solution each liter of which contains 1 Gm. equivalent weight of the active substance: designated N/1 or 1 N.

ophthalmic s., a sterile solution, free from foreign particles, for instillation into the eye.

physiologic saline s., physiologic salt s., physiologic sodium chloride s., an aqueous solution of sodium chloride and other components, having an osmotic pressure identical to that of blood serum.

saline s., a solution of sodium chloride, or common salt, in purified water.

saturated s., a solution in which the solvent has taken up all of the dissolved substance that it can hold in solution.

sclerosing s., one containing an irritant substance that will cause obliteration of a space, as the lumen of a varicose vein or the cavity of a hernial sac.

standard s., one containing a fixed amount of solute.

supersaturated s., one containing a greater quantity of the solute than the solvent can hold in solution under ordinary conditions.

test s., a standard solution of a specified chemical substance used in performing a certain test procedure.

volumetric s., one that contains a specific quantity of solvent per stated unit of volume.

solvent (sol′vent) 1. capable of dissolving other material. 2. the liquid in which another substance (the solute) is dissolved to form a solution.

Soma (so′mah) trademark for preparations of carisoprodol, an analgesic and skeletal muscle relaxant.

soma (so′mah) the body. adj., **so′mal, somat′ic.**

somasthenia (so″mas-the′ne-ah) bodily weakness with poor appetite and poor sleep.

somat(o)- (so′mah-to) word element [Gr.], *body.*

somatalgia (so″mah-tal′je-ah) bodily pain.

somatesthesia (so″mat-es-the′ze-ah) body consciousness or awareness.

somatic (so-mat′ik) pertaining to or characteristic of the body (soma).

somatization (so″mah-tĭ-za′shun) the conversion of mental experiences or states into bodily symptoms.

somatochrome (so-mat′o-krōm) a nerve cell whose cell body stains readily.

somatodidymus (so″mah-to-did′ĭ-mus) a double fetal monster with fused trunks.

somatogenic (so″mah-to-jen′ik) originating in the body.

somatology (so″mah-tol′o-je) the sum of what is known about the body.

somatome (so′mah-tōm) 1. an appliance for cutting the body of a fetus. 2. a somite.

somatometry (so″mah-tom′ĕ-tre) measurement of the dimensions of the entire body.

somatopagus (so″mah-top′ah-gus) a double fetal monster united at the trunks.

somatopathy (so″mah-top′ah-the) a bodily disorder rather than a mental one.

somatoplasm (so-mat′o-plazm) the body substance.

somatopsychic (so″mah-to-si′kik) pertaining to both mind and body.

somatopsychosis (so″mah-to-si-ko′sis) any mental disease symptomatic of bodily disease.

somatoschisis (so″mah-tos′kĭ-sis) splitting of the bodies of the vertebrae.

somatoscopy (so″mah-tos′ko-pe) examination of the body.

somatosexual (so″mah-to-seks′u-al) pertaining to both body and sex characteristics; physical manifestations of sexual development.

somatotherapy (so″mah-to-ther′ah-pe) treatment aimed at relieving or curing ills of the body.

somatotonia (so″mah-to-to′ne-ah) a group of traits characterized by dominance of muscular activity and vigorous body assertiveness; considered typical of mesomorphy.

somatotopic (so″mah-to-top′ik) related to particular areas of the body; describing the organization of the motor area of the brain, specific regions of the cortex being responsible for the motor control of different areas of the body.

somatotrophin (so″mah-to-tro′fin) growth hormone (see also PITUITARY GLAND). adj., **somatotroph′ic.**

somatotropin (so″mah-to-tro′pin) growth hormone (see also PITUITARY GLAND). adj., **somatotro′pic.**

somatotype (so-mat′o-tīp) a particular type of body build.

somatotyping (so-mat″o-tīp′ing) objective classification of individuals according to type of body build.

Sombulex (som′bu-leks) trademark for a preparation of hexobarbital, an ultra-short-acting barbiturate.

somesthesia (so″mes-the′ze-ah) sensibility to bodily sensations. adj., **somesthet′ic.**

somite (so′mīt) one of the paired segments along the spinal cord of a vertebrate embryo, formed by transverse subdivision of the thickened mesoderm next to the midplane, that develop into the vertebral column and muscles of the body.

somnambule (som-nam′būl) one who sleepwalks.

somnambulism (som-nam′bu-lizm) sleepwalking.

somnifacient (som″nĭ-fa′shent) causing sleep.

somniferous (som-nif′er-us) producing sleep.

somniloquism (som-nil′o-kwizm) habitual talking in one's sleep.

somnipathy (som-nip′ah-the) any disorder of sleep; a condition of hypnotic trance.

somnolence (som′no-lens) sleepiness; also, unnatural drowsiness.

somnolentia (som″no-len′she-ah) 1. incomplete sleep; drowsiness. 2. sleep drunkenness; a condition of incomplete sleep marked by loss of orientation and by excited or violent behavior.

Somnos (som′nos) trademark for preparations of chloral hydrate, a sedative and hypnotic.

sonitus (son′ĭ-tus) tinnitus.

sonometer (so-nom′ĕ-ter) an apparatus for testing acuteness of hearing.

sonorous (so-nōr′us) resonant; sounding.

sophistication (so-fis″tĭ-ka′shun) adulteration of food or medicine.

sophomania (sof″o-ma′ne-ah) an insane belief in one's own great wisdom.

sophoretin (sof″o-re′tin) quercetin, an agent that reduces abnormal capillary fragility.

sophorin (sof′o-rin) rutin.

sopor (so′por) [L.] coma or deep sleep.

soporific (sop″ŏ-rif′ik, so″pŏ-rif′ik) 1. producing deep sleep. 2. a drug or other agent that induces sleep.

soporous (sop′or-us, so′por-us) associated with coma or deep sleep.

sorbefacient (sōr″bĕ-fa′shent) 1. promoting absorption. 2. an agent that promotes absorption.

sordes (sōr′dēz) foul matter collected on the lips and teeth in low fevers, consisting of food, microorganisms and epithelial elements.
 s. gas′tricae, food lying undigested in the stomach.

sore (sōr) a popular term for a lesion of the skin or mucous membrane.
 Baghdad s., cutaneous leishmaniasis.
 bed s., decubitus ulcer.
 cold s., one around the mouth or lips due to herpes simplex virus.
 Delhi s., oriental s., cutaneous leishmaniasis.
 pressure s., decubitus ulcer.

sororiation (so-ro″re-a′shun) development of the breasts at puberty.

sorption (sorp′shun) 1. incorporation of water in a colloid. 2. processes involved in net movement of components of adjoining materials across the boundary separating them; applied to the bidirectional movements of substances across the mucosa of the gastrointestinal tract and the net result of such movements, including absorption, enterosorption, exsorption and insorption.

S.O.S. [L.] *si o′pus sit* (if necessary).

soteria (so-tēr′e-ah) derivation of a sense of security and protection, out of proportion to the stimulus, from an external object, which becomes a neurotic object-source of comfort.

souffle (soo′fl) a soft, blowing auscultatory sound.
 cardiac s., any heart murmur of a blowing quality.
 fetal s., a murmur sometimes heard over the pregnant uterus, supposed to be due to compression of the umbilical cord.
 funic s., funicular s., a hissing souffle synchronous with fetal heart sounds, probably from the umbilical cord.
 mammary s., a murmur sometimes heard in the second, third or fourth intercostal space during pregnancy and the puerperium, attributed to a change of dynamics in blood flow through the internal mammary (thoracic) artery.
 placental s., the sound supposed to be produced by the blood current in the placenta.
 uterine s., a sound made by the blood within the arteries of the gravid uterus.

sound (sownd) 1. percept resulting from stimulation of the ear by mechanical radiant energy of frequency between 20 and 20,000 cycles per second. 2. a slender instrument to be introduced into body passages or cavities, especially for the dilatation of strictures or detection of foreign bodies.
 entotic s., one originating within the ear, as tinnitus.
 friction s., one produced by rubbing of two surfaces.
 heart s's, the sounds produced by the functioning of the heart, the first, a dull, prolonged sound, occurring with ventricular systole, and the second, a sharp, short sound, occurring with closure of the semilunar valves (see also HEART SOUNDS).
 Korotkoff s's, those heard during auscultatory blood pressure determination.
 percussion s., any sound obtained by percussion.
 physiologic s's, those heard when the external acoustic meatus are plugged, caused by the rush of blood through blood vessels in or near the inner ear and by adjacent muscles in continuous low-frequency vibration.
 respiratory s., any sound heard on ausculation over the respiratory tract.
 succussion s's, splashing sounds heard on succussion over a distended stomach or in hydropneumothorax.
 to-and-fro s., a peculiar friction sound heard in pericarditis and pleurisy.
 urethral s., a long, slender instrument for exploring and dilating the urethra.
 white s., that produced by a mixture of all frequencies of mechanical vibration perceptible as sound.

space (spās) 1. a delimited area. 2. an actual or potential cavity of the body. 3. the areas of the universe beyond the earth and its atmosphere.
 arachnoid s., subarachnoid space.
 dead s., 1. space remaining in tissues as a result of failure of proper closure of surgical or other wounds, permitting accumulation of blood or serum. 2. the portions of the respiratory tract (passages and space in the alveoli) occupied by gas not concurrently participating in oxygen-carbon dioxide exchange.

epidural s., the space between the dura mater and the lining of the spinal canal.

intercostal s., the space between two adjacent ribs.

interpleural s., mediastinum.

intervillous s., the cavernous space of the placenta into which the chorionic villi project and through which the maternal blood circulates.

lymph s's, open spaces filled with lymph in connective or other tissue, especially in the brain and meninges.

Meckel's s., a recess in the dura mater that lodges the trigeminal ganglion.

mediastinal s., mediastinum.

medullary s., the central cavity and the intervals between the trabeculae of bone that contain the marrow.

palmar s., a large fascial space in the hand, divided by a fibrous septum into a midpalmar and a thenar space.

parasinoidal s's, spaces in the dura mater along the superior sagittal sinus which receive the venous blood.

perivascular s., a lymph space within the walls of an artery.

plantar s., a fascial space on the sole of the foot, divided by septa into the lateral, middle and median plantar spaces.

pneumatic s., a portion of bone occupied by air-containing cells.

retrobulbar s., the space behind the fascia of the bulb of the eye, containing the eye muscles and the ocular vessels and nerves.

retroperitoneal s., the space between the peritoneum and the posterior abdominal wall.

retropharyngeal s., the space behind the pharynx, containing areolar tissue.

subarachnoid s., the space between the arachnoid and the pia mater, containing cerebrospinal fluid.

subdural s., the space between the dura mater and the arachnoid.

subphrenic s., the space between the diaphragm and subjacent organs.

subumbilical s., somewhat triangular space in the body cavity beneath the umbilicus.

Tenon's s., a lymph space between the sclera and Tenon's capsule.

spanemia (spah-ne′me-ah) poverty or thinness of the blood.

spanogyny (span′o-jin″e) scarcity of women; decrease in female births.

spanomenorrhea (span″o-men″o-re′ah) scanty menstruation.

spanopnea (span″op-ne′ah) a nervous affection with slow, deep breathing and a subjective feeling of dyspnea.

sparganosis (spar″gah-no′sis) infection with spargana, which invade the subcutaneous tissues, causing inflammation and fibrosis. If the lymphatics are involved, elephantiasis results.

sparganum (spar-ga′num), pl. *sparga′na* [Gr.] a migrating larva of a tapeworm.

spargosis (spar-go′sis) 1. distention of a mammary gland with milk. 2. elephantiasis.

Sparine (spar′ēn) trademark for preparations of promazine, a tranquilizer.

spasm (spazm) 1. a sudden involuntary contraction of a muscle or group of muscles. 2. a sudden but transitory constriction of a passage, canal or orifice. Spasms usually occur when the nerve supplying muscles are irritated, and are commonly accompanied by pain. Occasionally a spasm may occur in a blood vessel, and is then called vasospasm.

Spasms vary from mild twitches to severe CONVULSIONS and may be the symptoms of any number of disorders. Usually, spasms will cease when the cause is corrected, although sometimes the only treatment is to suppress the symptoms, as in EPILEPSY.

CLONIC SPASMS. Spasms in which contraction and relaxation of the muscle alternate are called clonic. This is the more common type of spasm and usually is not severe. A typical clonic spasm is the hiccup. Hiccups usually occur when the diaphragm is irritated, as by indigestion; very occasionally they may result from a serious condition, such as a brain tumor. Hiccups generally disappear by themselves or after a drink of water.

Spasms may be repetitive twitching motions, some of which are called tics. Tics often accompany other types of spasm, as in diseases like cerebral palsy and Sydenham's chorea. They may also be seen in neuralgia. In tic douloureux (trigeminal neuralgia) the nerves of the face are involved.

Other types of repetitive twitching movements seem to be purposeless or without a cause and are called habit spasms. They include twitching of the face, blinking of the eyes and grimacing. The movements are rapid and always repeated in the same way, unlike the spasms associated with chorea. The motions are carried out automatically in response to a stimulus that once may have existed but no longer does.

Spasms may also stem from emotional stress. Stuttering that continues after the age of 5 years is generally considered a habit spasm that is caused by emotional conflict or difficulty.

In a convulsive spasm the entire body is jerked by sudden violent movements that may involve almost all the muscles. These spasms may last from a fraction of a second to several seconds, or even minutes. Spasms accompanying epilepsy are usually convulsive. Treatment includes sedatives and any one of several anticonvulsants. In small children convulsions usually indicate a high fever and the onset of infection, or any general illness; at times they may be a symptom of severe disease.

TONIC SPASMS. If the contraction of a spasm is sustained or continuing, it is called tonic, or tetanic, spasm. Tonic spasms are generally severe because they are caused by diseases that affect the central nervous system or brain, as tetanus, rabies and cerebral palsy. Severe tonic spasms can be fatal if not treated in time. Continued spasms can bring on exhaustion or asphyxiation. Treatment varies with the cause. If the disease is caused by a microorganism present in the system, as in tetanus, antiserum must be administered immediately. Antibiotics are also used to help curb infection. In many cases, tranquilizers, sedatives and narcotics must be administered to help ease the spasms.

bronchial s., spasmodic contraction of the muscular coat of the smaller divisions of the bronchi, such as occurs in asthma.

spasmodic (spaz-mod′ik) of the nature of a spasm; occurring in spasms.

spasmolysis (spaz-mol′ĭ-sis) the arrest of spasm.

spasmophemia (spaz″mo-fe′me-ah) stuttering.

spasmophilia (spaz″mo-fil′e-ah) abnormal tendency to convulsions; abnormal sensitivity of motor nerves to stimulation with a resultant tendency to spasm.

spasmotoxin (spaz″mo-tok′sin) a poisonous ptomaine from *Clostridium tetani;* tetanus toxin.

spasmus (spaz′mus) [L.] spasm.
   s. nu′tans, nodding spasm, frequently seen in debilitated children.

spastic (spas′tik) characterized by spasms, or tightening of the muscles, causing stiff and awkward movements and in some cases a scissors-like gait. The term is often used to describe a person suffering from CEREBRAL PALSY.

spasticity (spas-tis′ĭ-te) continuous resistance to stretching by a muscle due to abnormally increased tension.

spatial (spa′shal) pertaining to space.

spatium (spa′she-um), pl. *spa′tia* [L.] space.

spatula (spat′u-lah) a wide, flat, blunt, usually flexible instrument of little thickness, used for spreading material on a smooth surface or mixing.

spatulation (spat″u-la′shun) the combining of materials into a homogeneous mixture by continuously heaping them together and smoothing the mass out on a smooth surface with a spatula.

spay (spa) to deprive of the ovaries.

SPCA serum prothrombin conversion accelerator; clotting factor VII.

specialist (spesh′ah-list) one who is particularly skilled; a physician who has studied extensively and limits his practice to a certain branch of medicine.

specialty (spesh′al-te) a restricted field in which a person is particularly skilled.

species (spe′shēz) a taxonomic category subordinate to a genus (or subgenus) and superior to a subspecies or variety; composed of individuals similar in certain morphologic and physiologic characteristics.
   type s., the original species from which the description of the genus is formulated.

specific (spĕ-sif′ik) 1. pertaining to a species. 2. having a particular effect, or produced by a single kind of microorganism.
   s. gravity, the weight of a substance compared with the weight of an equal amount of some other substance taken as a standard. For liquids the usual standard is water. The specific gravity of water is 1; if a sample of urine shows a specific gravity of 1.025, this means that the urine is 1.025 times heavier than water. Specific gravity is measured by means of a hydrometer.

specificity (spes″ĭ-fis′ĭ-te) the quality of having a certain action, as of affecting only certain organisms or tissues, or reacting only with certain substances, as antibodies with certain antigens (antigen specificity).
   host s., the natural adaptability of a particular parasite to a certain species or group of hosts.

specimen (spes′ĭ-men) a small sample or part taken to show the nature of the whole, as small quantity of urine for urinalysis, or a small fragment of tissue for microscopic study.

spectacles (spek′tĕ-kals) a pair of lenses in a frame to assist vision; called also glasses.

spectrocolorimeter (spek″tro-kul″er-im′ĕ-ter) an instrument for detecting color blindness.

spectrometry (spek-trom′ĕ-tre) determination of the place of lines in a spectrum.

spectrophobia (spek″tro-fo′be-ah) morbid dread of mirrors or of seeing one's reflection in a mirror.

spectrophotometer (spek″tro-fo-tom′ĕ-ter) 1. an apparatus for measuring light sense by means of a spectrum. 2. an apparatus for determining the quantity of coloring matter in a solution by measurement of transmitted light.

spectrophotometry (spek″tro-fo-tom′ĕ-tre) the use of the spectrophotometer.

spectroscope (spek′tro-skōp) an instrument for developing and analyzing the spectrum of a substance.

spectroscopy (spek-tros′ko-pe) examination by means of a spectroscope.

spectrum (spek′trum), pl. *spec′tra* [L.], *spec′trums* 1. the series of images resulting from the refraction of electromagnetic radiation (e.g., light, x-rays) and their arrangement according to frequency or wavelength. 2. range of activity, as of an antibiotic, or of manifestations, as of a disease. adj., **spec′tral.**
   absorption s., one obtained by passing radiation with a continuous spectrum through a selectively absorbing medium.
   antibacterial s., the range of microorganisms against which an antibiotic substance is effective.
   chromatic s., that portion of the electromagnetic spectrum including wavelengths of 7700 to 3900 angstroms, giving rise to the perception of color by the normal eye.
   electromagnetic s., the range of electromagnetic energy from cosmic rays to electric waves, including gamma, x- and ultraviolet rays, visible light and infrared rays and radiowaves, with a range of wavelengths for 10^{11} to 10^{-12} cm.

speculum (spek′u-lum) an instrument for opening or distending a body orifice or cavity to permit visual inspection.
   bivalve s., one having two valves or parts.
   Sims's s., a form of bivalve speculum for examining the vagina and cervix.

speech (spēch) the utterance of vocal sounds conveying ideas. The process is controlled through a speech center located in the frontal lobe of the human brain.
   THE MECHANICS OF SPEECH. The voice originates in the larynx, which is in the upper end of the air passage to the lungs and is located behind

the thyroid cartilage. The larynx, in cooperation with the mouth, throat, trachea and lungs, works on the same principle as an organ or an oboe, in which air is forced over a thin reed to produce sound. The vocal cords, two reedlike bands, are attached at one end to the wall of the larynx behind the Adam's apple; the other ends are attached to movable cartilages. When the voice is not being used, muscles move these cartilages outward and hold the vocal cords against the sides of the larynx so that breathing is not obstructed. When one starts to speak, sing, grunt or shout, the ends of the vocal cords connected to the cartilages are brought across the larynx, so that they partly obstruct it. As air is forced through, the cords vibrate, producing sound waves, the voice.

In speaking, the size and shape of the mouth and pharynx are varied, as the sound goes through, by means of muscles of the mouth, throat and tongue. Vowel sounds are initiated in the throat and are given their distinctive "shapes" by movements of the mouth and tongue. Consonants are formed by controlled interruptions of exhaled air.

VOLUME, PITCH AND TIMBRE. The voice itself has three characteristics—volume, pitch and timbre, or quality. Volume depends on the effort made in forcing air through the vocal cords.

Pitch of the voice depends on the amount of tension placed on the vocal cords, and on the length and thickness of the cords. Children's and women's vocal cords are short, giving them higher-pitched voices. A man's are longer and thicker and his voice is deeper.

Timbre is affected by the size and shape of the individual's various resonating chambers—mouth, pharynx, chest and others—and the way they are used. Bones in the head and chest also contribute to the quality of a voice. By long training in the use of the voice, singers are able to alter and control the mouth, throat and chest cavities to produce a wide range of harmonics or overtones.

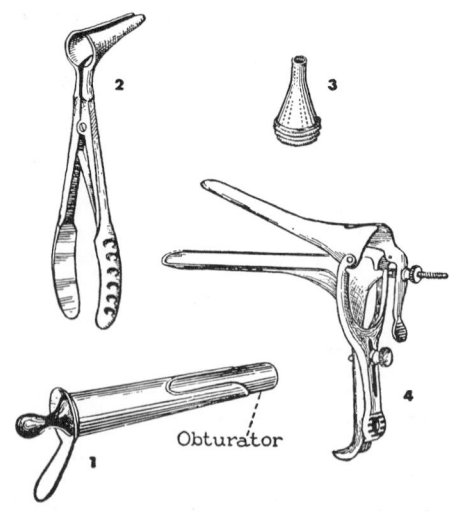

Speculums: 1, rectal (David); 2, nasal (Vienna model); 3, ear (Boucheron); 4, vaginal (Pederson). (From Dorland's Illustrated Medical Dictionary. 24th ed. Philadelphia, W. B. Saunders Co., 1965.)

SPEECH DEFECTS. Over 100 muscles are involved in the utterance of a simple word, and the construction of a simple sentence is a feat so complicated that it is far beyond the capacity of any living thing except man. The process of learning to talk is obviously a difficult task for children, and it is not surprising that 5 to 7 per cent of them reach adulthood with a speech disorder serious enough to be a handicap.

The baby learns to make specific sounds with his voice by babbling and cooing. Gradually he becomes able, more or less unconsciously, to put these sounds together to form intelligible speech in imitation of his parents and other speakers around him. This complicated process is sometimes disturbed if the child is handicapped by congenital physical defects, illness or psychologic difficulties. As a result, speech disorders may occur.

Congenital Causes. Prominent among the congenital defects that may cause speech problems are CLEFT LIP and CLEFT PALATE. These abnormalities are evident at birth and should be corrected by surgery at an early age.

Another congenital defect is tongue-tie, or abnormal shortness of the membrane connecting the base of the tongue to the floor of the mouth. This condition, which if uncorrected may cause lisping and other awkwardness, is easily corrected by surgical cutting of the membrane as soon as the difficulty becomes evident.

Congenital deafness will prevent a child from learning to speak in the usual way and may result in MUTISM. However, if the speech mechanisms are normal, the child can be taught to speak by a speech therapist.

Malformations of the nasal passages, larynx or other parts of the voice-producing tract may cause oddities in the sound of the voice. Such defects also can be corrected in many cases by minor surgery.

Other Causes. By the age of 5 or 6 years, most children have mastered the basic art of talking. Serious difficulties that persist or appear for the first time after this age, and that are not due to congenital defects, are likely to arise from illness, injury or a psychologic disturbance. Damage to speech centers of the brain by multiple sclerosis, syphilis or Parkinson's disease, for example, may cause speech to be singsong, explosive, mechanical or slurred. In such instances improvement of speech follows treatment of the basic disorder.

Poor alignment of the front teeth also may interfere somewhat with proper speech.

Stuttering. Speech defects of psychologic rather than physical origin often appear in the form of stammering, or stuttering. The terms are synonymous. Stuttering may involve involuntary hesitation in starting or finishing a sound, for example, difficulty in starting any word beginning with the letter *t*, or the inability to get beyond a first letter, such as *m* or *s*. There is often the spasmodic repetition of one sound with the apparent inability to pass on to the next one.

These difficulties can have many different specific causes, but generally they arise from feelings of insecurity and anxiety. Once the bad habits are formed, they may endure after the original cause no longer exists.

Various precautions by parents and other grownups in a household can help to encourage clear speech and to prevent the onset of stuttering. A child should be spoken to clearly so that he can learn how words should sound. Baby talk by grownups should be avoided, because it will only tend to prolong baby talk in the child. It is best to avoid criticism of the child's pronunciation and other speech habits—especially criticism in the form of nagging interruptions—that is likely to make him self-conscious, uncertain and awkward.

Stuttering often occurs when a child is addressing an angry or impatient parent or someone else who represents authority. The child's speech may become disorganized by fear of punishment or disapproval, or by an accident or other upsetting event. He is often anxious to get his words out before his listener interrupts or turns away. This anxiety can be especially upsetting in children whose thoughts tend to outrace their ability to form their sentences. Patience and calm will alleviate a child's anxiety and encourage clear speech.

If speech defects persist when a child reaches school age, the help of a speech therapist may be required. Speech disorders resulting from mental illness are best dealt with by a psychiatrist.

ataxic s., intermittent, explosive speech, as in cerebral disorders.

esophageal s., speech produced by expelling swallowed air and modifying the sound by motions of the pharynx, lips and tongue; used after LARYNGECTOMY.

pharyngeal s., speech produced by vibrating air against the roof of the pharynx; used after LARYNGECTOMY.

scanning s., pauses between syllables common in multiple sclerosis or diffuse cerebellar or brain stem disease.

sperm (sperm) the male germ cell, which unites with an ovum in sexual reproduction to produce a new individual (see also SPERMATOZOON).

sperm(o)- (sper'mo) word element [Gr.], *seed;* specifically used to refer to the male germinal element.

spermacrasia (sper″mah-kra′ze-ah) deficiency of sperm in the semen.

spermatemphraxis (sper″mat-em-frak′sis) obstruction to the discharge of semen.

spermatic (sper-mat′ik) pertaining to the spermatozoa or to semen.

s. cord, the structure extending from the abdominal ring to the testis, comprising the pampiniform plexus, nerves, vas deferens, testicular artery and other vessels.

spermatid (sper′mah-tid) a cell produced by meiotic division of a secondary spermatocyte; it develops into the spermatozoon.

spermatitis (sper″mah-ti′tis) inflammation of a vas deferens.

spermato- (sper′mah-to) word element [Gr.], *seed;* specifically used to refer to the male germinal element.

spermatoblast (sper-mat′o-blast) spermatid.

spermatocele (sper-mat′o-sēl) a cystic accumulation of semen in the tunica vaginalis testis.

spermatocelectomy (sper″mah-to-se-lek′to-me) excision of a spermatocele.

spermatocidal (sper″mah-to-si′dal) destructive to spermatozoa.

spermatocyst (sper-mat′o-sist) a seminal vesicle.

spermatocystectomy (sper″mah-to-sis-tek′to-me) excision of a seminal vesicle.

spermatocystitis (sper″mah-to-sis-ti′tis) inflammation of a seminal vesicle.

spermatocystotomy (sper″mah-to-sis-tot′o-me) incision of a seminal vesicle, for the purpose of drainage.

spermatocyte (sper-mat′o-sīt) the mother cell of a spermatid.

primary s., the original large cell into which a spermatogonium develops before the first meiotic division.

secondary s., a cell produced by meiotic division of the primary spermatocyte.

spermatogenesis (sper″mah-to-jen′ĕ-sis) the development of mature spermatozoa from spermatogonia.

spermatogonium (sper″mah-to-go′ne-um), pl. *spermatogo′nia* [Gr.] one of the primitive, unspecialized germ cells that line the seminiferous tubules of the testis.

spermatoid (sper′mah-toid) resembling semen.

spermatolysin (sper″mah-tol′ĭ-sin) a lysin destructive to spermatozoa.

spermatolysis (sper″mah-tol′ĭ-sis) dissolution of spermatozoa.

spermatopathia (sper″mah-to-path′e-ah) abnormality of the semen.

spermatorrhea (sper″mah-to-re′ah) involuntary escape of semen.

spermatoschesis (sper″mah-tos′kĕ-sis) suppression of the semen.

spermatospore (sper-mat′o-spōr) a spermatogonium.

spermatoxin (sper″mah-tok′sin) a toxin that destroys spermatozoa.

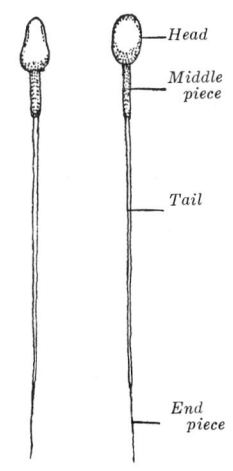

Human spermatozoon, side and flat views. (From Dorland's Illustrated Medical Dictionary. 24th ed. Philadelphia, W. B. Saunders Co., 1965.)

spermatozoicide (sper″mah-to-zo′ĭ-sīd) an agent that destroys spermatozoa.

spermatozoon (sper″mah-to-zo′on), pl. *spermatozo′a* [Gr.] a mature male germ cell, the specific output of the testes. It is the generative element of the semen that serves to impregnate the ovum.

The mature sperm cell is microscopic in size. It looks like a translucent tadpole, and has a flat, elliptical head containing a spherical center section, and a long tail by which it propels itself with a vigorous lashing movement.

Spermatozoa are produced in the testes. When mature, the sperm are carried in the semen. At the climax of coitus, the semen is discharged into the vagina of the female. A single discharge (about a teaspoonful of semen on the average) may contain more than 250 million spermatozoa. Only a few of these will travel as far as the uterine tubes; if an ovum is present there, and if the head of a single sperm penetrates the ovum, fertilization takes place.

spermaturia (sper″mah-tu′re-ah) semen in the urine.

spermectomy (sper-mek′to-me) excision of the spermatic cord.

spermicide (sper′mĭ-sīd) an agent destructive to spermatozoa. adj., **spermici′dal.**

spermiduct (sper′mĭ-dukt) the ejaculatory duct and vas deferens together.

spermiocyte (sper′me-o-sit″) a primary spermatocyte.

spermiogenesis (sper″me-o-jen′ĕ-sis) the second stage in the formation of spermatozoa, in which the spermatids transform into spermatozoa.

spermiogram (sper′me-o-gram″) a diagram or chart of various cells formed in development of the spermatozoon, or of the cells present in a specimen of semen.

spermioteleosis (sper″me-o-te″le-o′sis) progressive development of the spermatogonium through various stages to the mature spermatozoon.

spermoblast (sper′mo-blast) spermatid.

spermolith (sper′mo-lith) a calculus in the vas deferens.

sp. gr. specific gravity.

sphacelate (sfas′ĕ-lāt) to become gangrenous.

sphacelation (sfas″ĕ-la′shun) gangrene.

sphacelism (sfas′ĕ-lizm) a gangrenous state or process.

sphaceloderma (sfas″ĕ-lo-der′mah) gangrene of the skin.

sphacelous (sfas′ĕ-lus) gangrenous; sloughing.

sphacelus (sfas′ĕ-lus) a slough; a mass of gangrenous tissue.

sphenion (sfe′ne-on) the point at the sphenoid angle of the parietal bone.

spheno- (sfe′no) word element [Gr.], *wedge-shaped; sphenoid bone.*

sphenoid (sfe′noid) wedge-shaped; designating especially a very irregular wedge-shaped bone at the base of the skull (sphenoid bone).

sphenoidal (sfe-noi′dal) pertaining to the sphenoid bone.

sphenoiditis (sfe″noi-di′tis) inflammation of the sphenoid sinus.

sphenoidotomy (sfe″noi-dot′o-me) incision of a sphenoid sinus.

sphenomaxillary (sfe″no-mak′sĭ-ler″e) pertaining to the sphenoid bone and the maxilla.

sphenopalatine (sfe″no-pal′ah-tīn) pertaining to the sphenoid and palatine bones.

sphenotresia (sfe″no-tre′ze-ah) craniotomy with perforation of the base of the fetal skull.

sphenotribe (sfe′no-trīb) an instrument used in sphenotresia.

sphere (sfēr) a ball or globe.
  attraction s., centrosome.
  segmentation s., 1. the morula. 2. a blastomere.

sphero- (sfēr′o) word element [Gr.], *round; a sphere.*

spherocyte (sfēr′o-sīt) a small, globular, completely hemoglobinated erythrocyte without the usual central pallor; seen in spherocytosis. adj., **spherocyt′ic.**

spherocytosis (sfēr″o-si-to′sis) a hereditary form of hemolytic anemia with the presence of spherocytes in the blood.

spheroid (sfēr′oid) a spherelike body.

spheroidal (sfe-roi′dal) resembling a sphere.

spherometer (sfe-rom′ĕ-ter) an apparatus for measuring the curvature of a surface.

spheroplast (sfēr′o-plast) a spherical form of a bacterium, produced in a hypertonic medium under conditions that cause partial or complete absence of the cell wall.

sphincter (sfingk′ter) a circular muscle that constricts a passage or closes a natural orifice. When relaxed, a sphincter allows materials to pass through the opening. When contracted, it closes the opening.

There are four sphincter muscles along the alimentary canal that aid in digestion: The cardiac sphincter, between the esophagus and the stomach, opens at the approach of food, which is then swept into the stomach by rhythmic peristaltic waves. The pyloric sphincter controls the opening from the stomach into the duodenum. It is usually closed, opening only for a moment when a peristaltic wave passes over it. The ileocolic sphincter permits passage of digested material from the ileum, the lowest portion of the small intestine, to the colon. Two anal sphincters, internal and external, control the anus, allowing the evacuation of feces.

In addition, there are sphincters in the iris of the eye, the bile duct (sphincter of Oddi), the urinary tract and elsewhere in the body.

sphincteralgia (sfingk″ter-al′je-ah) pain in a sphincter muscle.

sphincterismus (sfingk″ter-iz′mus) spasm of a sphincter.

sphincteritis (sfingk″ter-i′tis) inflammation of a sphincter, particularly the sphincter of Oddi.

sphincterolysis (sfingk″ter-ol′ĭ-sis) separation of the iris from the cornea in anterior synechia.

sphincteroplasty (sfingk′ter-o-plas″te) plastic reconstruction of a sphincter.

sphincterotomy (sfingk″ter-ot′o-me) incision of a sphincter.

sphingolipid (sfing″go-lip′id) a phospholipid containing sphingosine, occurring in high concentrations in the brain and other nerve tissue.

sphingolipidosis (sfing″go-lip′ĭ-do′sis), pl. *sphingolipido′ses* [Gr.] a general designation applied to a disease characterized by abnormal storage of sphingolipids, such as Gaucher's disease, Niemann-Pick disease and amaurotic familial idiocy (Tay-Sachs disease). All are associated with mental retardation and premature death.

sphingomyelin (sfing″go-mi′ĕ-lin) a group of phospholipids that on hydrolysis yield phosphoric acid, choline, sphingosine and a fatty acid.

sphingosine (sfing′go-sin) a basic amino alcohol present in sphingomyelin.

sphygmic (sfig′mik) pertaining to the pulse.

sphygmobolometer (sfig″mo-bo-lom′ĕ-ter) an instrument for recording the energy of the pulse wave, and so, indirectly, the strength of the systole.

sphygmochronograph (sfig″mo-kro′no-graf) a self-registering sphygmograph.

sphygmodynamometer (sfig″mo-di″nah-mom′ĕ-ter) an instrument for measuring the force of the pulse.

sphygmogram (sfig′mo-gram) the record or tracing made by a sphygmograph; called also pulse tracing.

sphygmograph (sfig′mo-graf) an apparatus for registering the movements of the arterial pulse.

sphygmoid (sfig′moid) resembling the pulse.

sphygmology (sfig-mol′o-je) the sum of what is known about the pulse.

sphygmomanometer (sfig″mo-mah-nom′ĕ-ter) an instrument for measuring arterial blood pressure.

sphygmometer (sfig-mom′ĕ-ter) an instrument for measuring the force and frequency of the pulse.

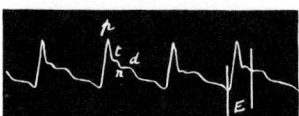

Radial sphygmogram from a healthy person. (From Dorland's Illustrated Medical Dictionary. 24th ed. Philadelphia, W. B. Saunders Co., 1965.)

sphygmoplethysmograph (sfig″mo-plĕ-thiz′mo-graf) an instrument that traces the record of the pulse, together with the curve of fluctuation of volume.

sphygmoscope (sfig′mo-skōp) a device for rendering the pulse beat visible.

sphygmotonometer (sfig″mo-to-nom′ĕ-ter) an instrument for measuring elasticity of arterial walls.

sphyrectomy (sfi-rek′to-me) excision of the malleus, or hammer, of the ear.

sphyrotomy (sfi-rot′o-me) division of the malleus.

spica (spi′kah) a figure-of-8 bandage, with turns crossing each other.

spicule (spik′ūl) a sharp, needle-like body or spike.

spider (spi′der) 1. an arthropod of the class Arachnida. 2. a spider nevus, or nevus arachnoideus.
  black widow s., a poisonous spider, *Latrodectus mactans,* whose bite causes severe poisoning. (For first aid, see INSECT BITES AND STINGS.)

Spielmeyer-Vogt disease (spēl′mi-er fōgt) juvenile amaurotic familial idiocy.

spiloma (spi-lo′mah) a nevus.

spiloplaxia (spi″lo-plak′se-ah) a red spot occurring in leprosy.

spina (spi′nah), pl. *spi′nae* [L.] spine; used in anatomic nomenclature to designate a slender, thornlike process such as occurs on many bones.
  s. bif′ida, a defect of the vertebral column due to imperfect union of the paired vertebral arches at the midline; it may be so extensive (spi′na bif′ida aper′ta) as to allow herniation of the spinal cord and meninges, or it may be covered by intact skin (spi′na bif′ida occul′ta) and evident only on radiologic examination.
  s. vento′sa, tuberculous infection of the bones of the hands or feet, occurring mostly in infants and children, with enlargement of digits, caseation, sequestration and sinus formation.

spinal (spi′nal) pertaining to a spine or to the vertebral column.
  s. cord, that part of the central nervous system lodged in the spinal canal, extending from the foramen magnum to about the level of the third lumbar vertebra.
  s. fusion, surgical creation of ankylosis of contiguous vertebrae; used in treatment of spondylosis and ruptured intervertebral (slipped) disk.
  s. nerve, one of the 31 pairs of nerves arising from the spinal cord and passing out between the vertebrae, including eight cervical, twelve thoracic, five lumbar, five sacral and one coccygeal.
  s. puncture, introduction of a hollow needle into the subarachnoid space of the spinal canal, usually between the fourth and fifth lumbar vertebrae; called also lumbar puncture. In some cases the physician may choose to perform a cisternal puncture, in which the needle is inserted immediately below the occipital bone into the cisterna cerebellomedullaris.

A spinal puncture may be done for diagnostic purposes to determine the pressure within the cerebrospinal cavities, to determine the presence of an obstruction to the flow of CEREBROSPINAL FLUID, to remove a specimen of cerebrospinal fluid for laboratory examination or to inject air or some other contrast medium into the spinal canal for the purpose of obtaining x-ray film of the cerebrospinal system.

NURSING CARE. Before the procedure is begun the patient should be given a simple explanation of the nature and purpose of the test. He should be told that there is no danger of damage to the spinal cord during a lumbar puncture because the spinal cord does not extend below the second lumbar vertebra. For a cisternal puncture, the back of the neck may be shaved.

The patient is positioned so that his knees and head are flexed as much as possible, and he is assisted in maintaining this position during the entire procedure. A local anesthetic such as 1 per cent procaine is injected subcutaneously to anesthetize the skin and underlying tissues. The patient should be warned not to move suddenly and should be told that he will experience slight pressure when the puncture needle is inserted.

Strict adherence to the rules of aseptic technique is necessary to avoid the possibility of introducing microorganisms into the spinal canal. The attendant may be asked to assist in the Queckenstedt test during the spinal puncture. This test involves compression of the veins of the neck, first on one side, then on the other and finally on both sides at once. The cerebrospinal fluid pressure is measured each time the veins are compressed. This test determines whether there is an obstruction in the spinal canal. Care must be taken that the trachea is not constricted while the neck veins are being compressed.

After the procedure the patient is observed for signs of pulse changes, respiratory difficulty or cyanosis. These rarely occur, but headache is common and may be partially relieved by keeping the patient flat in bed for 8 hours after the procedure. An ice cap and aspirin may help alleviate the discomfort.

spinalgia (spi-nal′je-ah) pain in the spinal region.

spinate (spi′nāt) shaped like a thorn.

spindle (spin′del) an elongated structure wider in the middle and tapering at each end, such as the figure formed by protoplasmic fibers extending between either centriole and the equator of a dividing cell.

muscle s., a mechanoreceptor found between the skeletal muscle fibers; the muscle spindles are arranged in parallel with muscle fibers, and respond to passive stretch of the muscle but cease to discharge if the muscle contracts isotonically, thus signaling muscle length. The muscle spindle is the receptor responsible for the stretch or myotatic reflex.

sleep s., a particular wave form in the electroencephalogram during sleep.

spine (spīn) 1. a thornlike process or projection; called also spina. 2. the backbone, or vertebral column. The spine is the axis of the skeleton; the skull and limbs are in a sense appendages. An intricate structure, the spine is composed of the vertebrae. These bones can move to a certain extent and so give flexibility to the spine, allowing it to bend forward, sideways and, to a lesser extent, backward. In the areas of the neck and lower back, the spine also can pivot, which permits the turning of the head and torso.

STRUCTURE OF THE SPINE. Each vertebra consists of two main parts: the body and, behind it, the vertebral arch. The body is a cylinder of bone, separated from the cylinders of neighboring vertebrae by intervertebral disks, layers of cartilage that act as cushions and allow some movement. Projecting backward from each body are two short, thick bony processes (projections) called pedicles. From the ends of these pedicles project two bony plates (laminae), which join together to form the hollow vertebral arch. Through this arch, and protected by it, passes the spinal cord, which is further protected by the meninges and bathed by the cerebrospinal fluid, which serves as a shock absorber.

There are usually 24 movable vertebrae and nine that are fused together. The topmost are the seven cervical vertebrae, which form the back of the neck, supporting the skull and allowing the head to turn from side to side by means of a pivotal motion between the two highest vertebrae. Below these are the 12 thoracic vertebrae, the supports on which the ribs are hinged, and then the five lumbar vertebrae, the largest movable vertebrae (the cervical are the smallest). Below the lumbar vertebrae, the spine terminates with two groups of vertebrae fused into single bones: the sacrum, composed of five vertebrae, and the coccyx, composed of four vertebrae.

Viewed from the side of the body, the spine as a whole has the shape of a double S curve.

SPINAL INJURIES. Fracture, the most serious injury the spine can suffer, has become increasingly common as the number of automobile accidents has increased. When the spine is fractured, the greatest danger comes from the possibility that the spinal cord may be injured by a movement of the fractured vertebrae. Injury to the cord can cause paralysis of all muscles lying below the point of injury. Therefore it is important not to lift or move a person who may have suffered fracture of the spine. If he must be moved before experienced first aid help arrives, he should be drawn carefully backwards or ahead, pulled by both legs or both armpits; any sideways motion must be avoided.

In a slipped DISK, one of the disks of cartilage between the vertebrae is moved partially out of place. The slipped disk may press on the spinal cord or one of the spinal nerves and cause pain, sometimes extremely severe. The disk may slip back into place after a period of bed rest, though sometimes the condition must be corrected surgically.

MALFORMATIONS OF THE SPINE. Of the various types of spinal malformations, some are congenital and others the result of postural defects or injuries. KYPHOSIS (hunchback) may occasionally be congenital, but more often it is caused by one of the diseases that attack the structure of the bones. The most common of these is POTT'S DISEASE, or tuberculosis affecting the vertebrae and soft tissues of the spine. Another is osteitis deformans, a type of bone inflammation in which parts of the bone are replaced by softer tissue.

Less serious malformations include round shoulders, which may sometimes result from poor posture; the condition warrants corrective treatment for it may cause a strain on the heart. A curvature of the spine toward one side (scoliosis) sometimes is caused by a difference in the length of the legs and can be corrected with the use of a built-up shoe. Occasionally the spine is bent backward, perhaps in an effort to correct a heavy abdomen or for the sake of fashion.

Spinal curvature can also result from certain diseases; it can be the cause or symptoms of serious disorders.

OTHER SPINAL DISORDERS. Many of the various forms of arthritis may attack the spine. Among these is rheumatoid spondylitis, or Marie-Strümpell disease, which causes inflammation of cartilage between the vertebrae and eventually can cause the neighboring vertebrae to fuse together, preventing movement. Occasionally the whole spine becomes stiffened, a condition sometimes called poker spine.

Loss of spinal flexibility may also be caused by osteoarthritis, the relatively mild arthritic condition that may develop in the later years. Spinal meningitis is an inflammation of the meninges, the membranes that cover the spinal cord.

spinifugal (spi-nif'u-gal) conducting or moving away from the spinal cord.

spinipetal (spi-nip'ĕ-tal) conducting or moving toward the spinal cord.

spinitis (spi-ni'tis) myelitis.

spinobulbar (spi"no-bul'bar) pertaining to the spinal cord and medulla oblongata.

spinocellular (spi"no-sel'u-lar) pertaining to prickle cells.

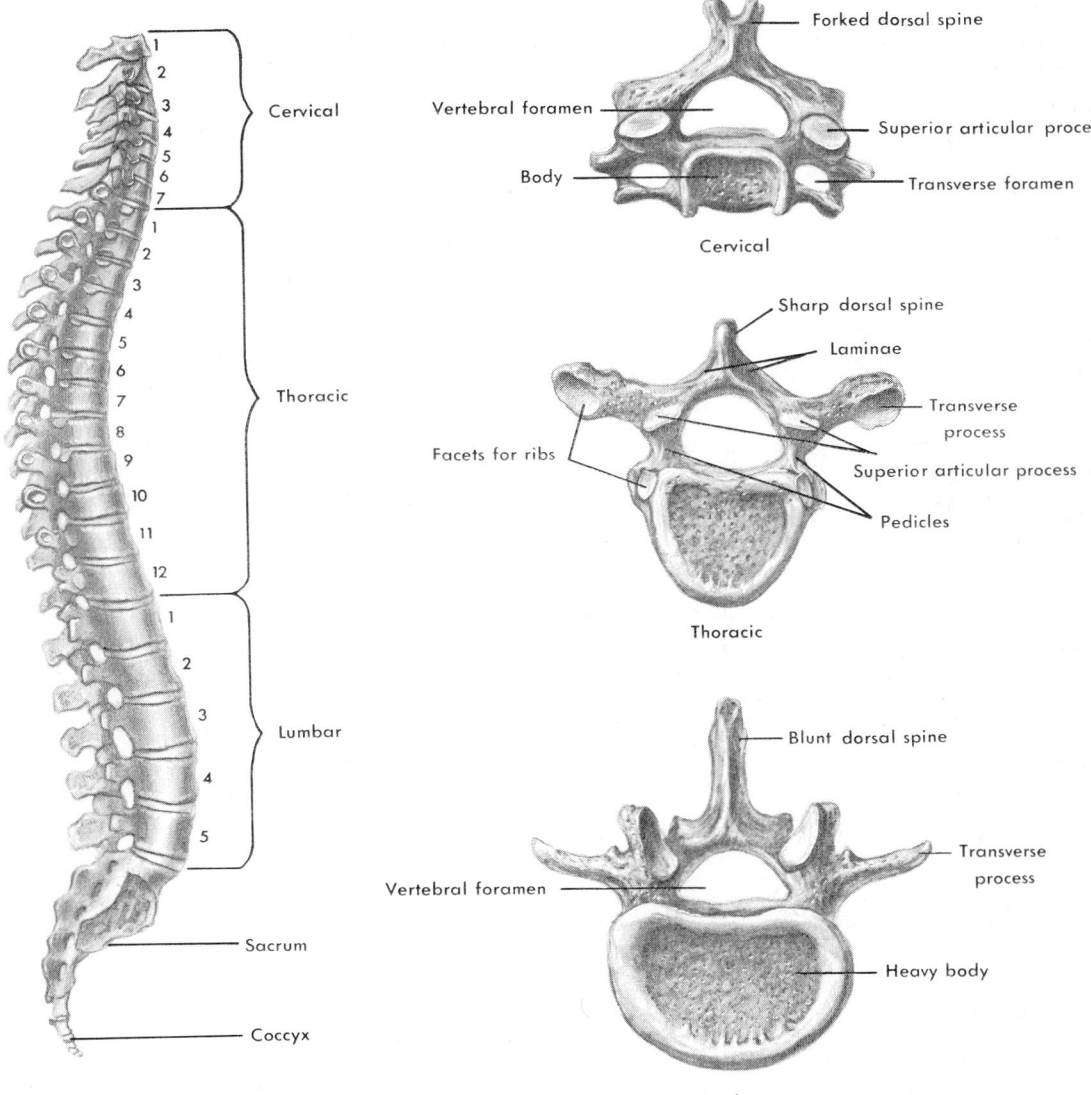

Left: The vertebral column. Right: Typical vertebrae as viewed from above. (From Dienhart, C. M.: Basic Human Anatomy and Physiology. Philadelphia, W. B. Saunders Co., 1967.)

spinocerebellar (spi″no-ser″ĕ-bel′ar) pertaining to the spinal cord and cerebellum.

spinocortical (spi″no-kor′tĭ-kal) pertaining to the spinal cord and cerebral cortex.

spinoneural (spi″no-nu′ral) pertaining to the spinal cord and the peripheral nerves.

spinous (spi′nus) pertaining to or like a spine.

spiradenitis (spi″rad-ĕ-ni′tis) inflammation of the sweat glands.

spiradenoma (spi″rad-ĕ-no′mah) adenoma of the sweat glands.

spiral (spi′ral) 1. winding like the thread of a screw. 2. a structure curving around a central point or axis.
  Curschmann's s's, coiled fibrils of mucin found in the sputum of patients with asthma.

spireme (spi′rēm) the wreath of chromatin fibrils formed in mitosis.

spirillicidal (spi-ril′ĭ-si′dal) destroying spirilla.

spirillicide (spi-ril′ĭ-sīd) an agent that destroys spirilla.

spirilliform (spi-ril′ĭ-form) shaped like a spirillum, or the turn of a screw.

spirillolysis (spi″rĭ-lol′ĭ-sis) the breaking up of spirilla.

spirillosis (spi″rĭ-lo′sis) a disease caused by presence of spirilla, such as ratbite fever.

spirillotropism (spi″rĭ-lot′ro-pizm) the property of having an affinity for spirilla.

spirillum (spi-ril′um), pl. *spiril′la* [L.] spiral-shaped bacterium belonging to the family Spirillaceae. The chief pathogenic organisms belonging to this group are *Spirillum minus*, which causes sodoku, a form of ratbite fever, and *Vibrio comma*, which causes Asiatic cholera. Spirilla are found in stagnant water and decaying animal matter.

spirit (spir′it) 1. a volatile or distilled liquid. 2. a solution of a volatile material in alcohol.
  ammonia s's, aromatic s's of ammonia, a mixture of ammonia, ammonium carbonate and other agents for use as an inhalant to revive a person who has fainted.
  rectified s., alcohol.

Spirochaeta (spi″ro-ke′tah) a genus of Schizomycetes found in fresh-water or sea-water slime.

spirochete (spi′ro-kēt) 1. a highly coiled bacterium; a general term applied to any organism of the order Spirochaetales, which includes the causative organisms of syphilis (*Treponema pallidum*) and yaws (*Treponema pertenue*). 2. an organism of the genus Spirochaeta. adj., **spiroche′tal.**

spirocheticide (spi″ro-ke′tĭ-sīd) an agent that destroys spirochetes.

spirochetolysis (spi″ro-ke-tol′ĭ-sis) the destruction of spirochetes by lysis.

spirochetosis (spi″ro-ke-to′sis) infection with spirochetes.

spirogram (spi′ro-gram) a graph of respiratory movements.

spirograph (spi′ro-graf) an apparatus for measuring and recording respiratory movements.

spiroid (spi′roid) resembling a spiral.

spirometer (spi-rom′ĕ-ter) an instrument for measuring air taken into and expelled from the lungs.

spirometry (spi-rom′ĕ-tre) measurement of the breathing capacity of lungs.

spironolactone (spi-ro″no-lak′tōn) an aldosterone antagonist which, when used with other diuretic drugs, is often successful in relieving edema or ascites in patients who have not responded to other diuretics.

splanchn(o)- (splangk′no) word element [Gr.], *viscus (viscera); splanchnic nerve.*

splanchnapophysis (splangk″nah-pof′ĭ-sis) a skeletal element, such as the lower jaw, connected with the alimentary canal.

splanchnectopia (splangk″nek-to′pe-ah) displacement of a viscus or of the viscera.

splanchnemphraxis (splangk″nem-frak′sis) obstruction of a viscus, particularly of the intestine.

splanchnesthesia (splangk″nes-the′ze-ah) visceral sensation. adj., **splanchnesthet′ic.**

splanchnic (splangk′nik) pertaining to the viscera.
  s. nerves, a group of nerves serving the blood vessels and viscera. (See table of NERVES.)

splanchnicectomy (splangk″nĭ-sek′to-me) excision of part of the greater splanchnic nerve. The operation is combined with sympathectomy for relief of essential hypertension.

splanchnicotomy (splangk″nĭ-kot′o-me) transection of a splanchnic nerve.

splanchnoblast (splangk′no-blast) a rudiment of a viscus.

splanchnocele (splangk′no-sēl) hernial protrusion of a viscus.

splanchnocoele (splangk′no-sēl) the portion of the embryonic body cavity from which the abdominal, pericardial and pleural cavities are formed.

splanchnodiastasis (splangk″no-di-as′tah-sis) displacement of a viscus.

splanchnodynia (splangk″no-din′e-ah) pain in an abdominal organ.

splanchnolith (splangk′no-lith) intestinal calculus.

splanchnology (splangk-nol′o-je) scientific study or description of the organs of the body, as of the digestive, respiratory and genitourinary systems.

splanchnomegaly (splangk″no-meg′ah-le) enlargement of a viscus.

splanchnopathy (splangk-nop'ah-the) disease of the viscera.

splanchnoptosis (splangk″nop-to'sis) prolapse or downward displacement of the viscera.

splanchnosclerosis (splangk″no-sklĕ-ro'sis) hardening of the viscera.

splanchnoskeleton (splangk″no-skel'ĕ-ton) skeletal structures connected with viscera.

splanchnotomy (splangk-not'o-me) anatomy or dissection of the viscera.

splanchnotribe (splangk'no-trīb) an instrument for crushing the intestine to obliterate its lumen.

splayfoot (spla'foot) flatfoot; talipes valgus.

spleen (splēn) a large glandlike organ situated under the ribs in the upper left quadrant of the abdomen. Oblong and flattened in shape, it is dark red in color and weighs about 6 oz. adj., **splen'ic.**

In the unborn child the spleen, with the liver, produces erythrocytes. After birth, this function is taken over by the bone marrow. However, if there is bone marrow failure, the spleen may again produce red blood cells. In the normal adult the spleen is a reservoir for blood, and contains a high concentration of erythrocytes. In times of exertion, emotional stress, pregnancy, severe bleeding, carbon monoxide poisoning or other occasions when the oxygen content of the blood must be increased, the spleen contracts rhythmically to release its store of red cells into the bloodstream.

The spleen also acts to help keep the blood free from unwanted substances, including wastes and infecting organisms. The blood is delivered to the spleen by the splenic artery, and passes through smaller branch arteries into a network of channels lined with leukocytes known as phagocytes (see RETICULOENDOTHELIAL SYSTEM). These clear the blood of old erythrocytes, damaged cells, parasites and other toxic or foreign substances. Hemoglobin from the removed red cells is temporarily stored.

The spleen contains nodules of light-colored lymphatic tissue in which lymphocytes are manufactured. These cells also produce antibodies.

Although its functions are important, the spleen is not an indispensable organ. When ruptured or greatly enlarged because of disease, the spleen can be surgically removed (see SPLENECTOMY). Although this may leave the body less resistant to infection, the spleen's functions are generally taken over by other organs, particularly the liver.

accessory s., a small mass of tissue elsewhere in the body, histologically and functionally identical with that composing the normal spleen.

splen(o)- (sple'no) word element [Gr.], *spleen.*

splenadenoma (splēn″ad-ĕ-no'mah) hyperplasia of the spleen pulp.

splenalgia (sple-nal'je-ah) pain in the spleen.

splenculus (spleng'ku-lus) an accessory spleen.

splenectasis (sple-nek'tah-sis) enlargement of the spleen.

splenectomy (sple-nek'to-me) excision of the SPLEEN. Indications for this procedure include severe trauma to or rupture of the spleen, enlargement (splenomegaly) when the destructive proper-

ties of the organ are greatly accelerated and such blood disorders as idiopathic thrombocytopenic purpura and hereditary spherocytosis. The latter two conditions respond well to splenectomy. In blood dyscrasias in which parts of the reticuloendothelial system other than the spleen are involved, splenectomy may be of little value.

splenectopy (sple-nek'to-pe) displacement of the spleen.

splenemia (sple-ne'me-ah) congestion of the spleen with blood.

splenitis (sple-ni'tis) inflammation of the spleen, a condition that is attended by enlargement of the organ and severe local pain.

splenium (sple'ne-um) a compress or bandage.
   s. cor'poris callo'si, the posterior, rounded end of the corpus callosum.

splenization (splen″ĭ-za'shun) the conversion of a tissue, as of the lung, into tissue resembling that of the spleen, due to engorgement and consolidation.

splenocolic (sple″no-kol'ik) pertaining to the spleen and colon.

splenocyte (splen'o-sīt) the monocyte characteristic of splenic tissue.

splenodynia (sple″no-din'e-ah) pain in the spleen.

splenogenous (sple-noj'ĕ-nus) arising in the spleen.

splenography (sple-nog'rah-fe) 1. roentgenography of the spleen. 2. a description of the spleen.

splenohepatomegaly (sple″no-hep″ah-to-meg'-ah-le) enlargement of the spleen and liver.

splenoid (sple'noid) resembling the spleen.

splenolysin (sple-nol'ĭ-sin) a lysin that destroys spleen tissue.

splenolysis (sple-nol'ĭ-sis) destruction of splenic tissue by a lysin.

splenoma (sple-no'mah) a splenic tumor.

splenomalacia (sple″no-mah-la'she-ah) abnormal softness of the spleen.

splenomegaly (sple″no-meg'ah-le) enlargement of the spleen.
   congestive s., enlargement of the spleen and liver associated with increased pressure in the portal vein. The disorder may be accompanied by anemia and leukopenia.
   hemolytic s., hemolytic jaundice.
   siderotic s., splenomegaly with deposit of iron and calcium.

splenometry (sple-nom'ĕ-tre) determination of the size of spleen.

splenomyelogenous (sple″no-mi″ĕ-loj'ĕ-nus) formed in the spleen and bone marrow.

splenomyelomalacia (sple″no-mi″ĕ-lo-mah-la'-she-ah) softening of the spleen and bone marrow.

splenoncus (sple-nong′kus) splenoma.

splenonephroptosis (sple″no-nef″rop-to′sis) downward displacement of the spleen and kidney.

splenopancreatic (sple″no-pan″kre-at′ik) pertaining to the spleen and pancreas.

splenopathy (sple-nop′ah-the) any disease of the spleen.

splenopexy (sple′no-pek″se) surgical fixation of the spleen.

splenophrenic (splen″o-fren′ik) pertaining to the spleen and diaphragm.

splenoptosis (sple″nop-to′sis) downward displacement of the spleen.

splenorenal (sple″no-re′nal) pertaining to the spleen and kidney, or to splenic and renal veins.

splenorrhagia (sple″no-ra′je-ah) hemorrhage from the spleen.

splenorrhaphy (sple-nor′ah-fe) suture of the spleen.

splenosis (sple-no′sis) the presence of numerous implants of splenic tissue in the peritoneal cavity.

splenotomy (sple-not′o-me) incision of the spleen.

splint (splint) a rigid or flexible appliance for fixation of displaced or movable parts.

Uses. Splints are most commonly used to immobilize broken bones or dislocated joints. When a broken bone has been properly set, a splint permits complete rest at the site of the fracture and thus allows natural healing to take place with the bone in the proper position. Splints are also necessary to immobilize unset fractures when a patient is moved after an accident; they prevent motion of the fractured bone, which might cause greater damage.

In a pelvic or spinal fracture, the effect of splinting is achieved by placing the patient on a stretcher or board. Breaks of the ribs and of face and skull bones usually do not require the use of splints, since these parts are naturally splinted by adjacent bone and tissue.

Making and Applying Splints. A splint can be improvised from a variety of materials, but should usually be light, straight and rigid. It should be long enough to extend beyond the joint above the injury and below the fracture site. A board used as a splint should be at least as wide as the injured part. Tightly rolled newspapers or magazines can be used to splint the arm or lower leg. Ice cream sticks have been used as splints for broken fingers.

Splints should be padded, at least on one side. Thick soft padding permits the injured part to swell and reduces interference with circulation. Bandages or strips of cloth or adhesive tape are used to hold splints in place.

After splinting, frequent examinations are necessary to determine whether the blood supply has been impaired. If the extremity becomes cold, pale or blue, or if the affected part becomes too painful, the splint should be loosened. Splints should never be tight.

Internal Splints. Internal splints, as well as pins, wires and other devices for the fixation of fractures, are among the more spectacular advances in orthopedics. They have worked wonders in the setting of hip fractures, especially in older people. Internal splints are available for almost every type of fracture. Stainless steel and Vitallium are the most commonly used materials. Splints and devices of this type require surgery for insertion, but are less cumbersome than external splints and permit earlier use of the fractured bone.

airplane s., one that holds the splinted limb suspended in the air.

anchor s., one for fracture of the jaw, with metal loops fitting over the teeth and held together by a rod.

coaptation s's, small splints adjusted about a

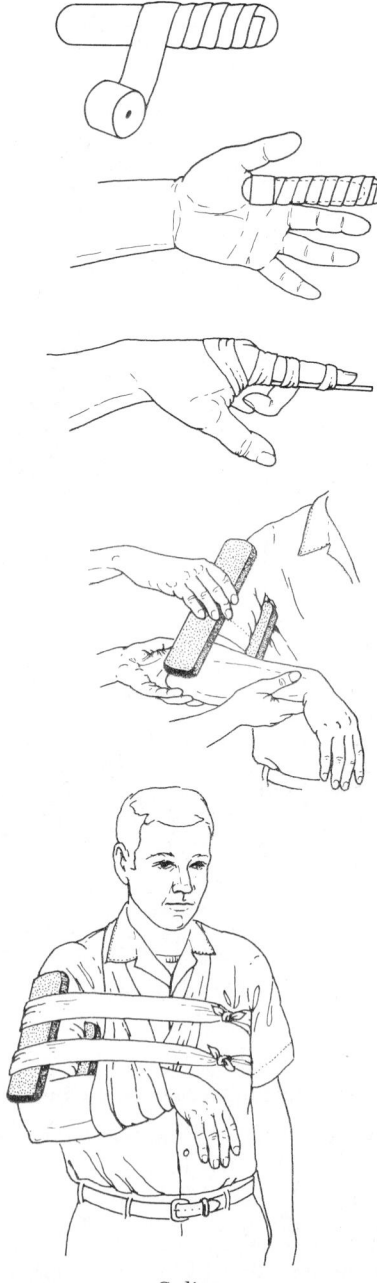

Splints.

fractured limb for the purpose of producing coaptation of fragments.

spodo- (spo′do) word element [Gr.], *waste material.*

spodogenous (spo-doj′ĕ-nus) caused by accumulation of waste material in an organ.

spodophagous (spo-dof′ah-gus) consuming waste material of the body.

spondyl(o)- (spon′dĭ-lo) word element [Gr.], *vertebra; vertebral column.*

spondylalgia (spon″dĭ-lal′je-ah) pain in the vertebrae.

spondylarthritis (spon″dil-ar-thri′tis) inflammation of one or more vertebral joints.

spondylexarthrosis (spon″dil-ek″sar-thro′sis) dislocation of a vertebra.

spondylitis (spon″dĭ-li′tis) inflammation of the vertebrae. Almost always a serious chronic disorder, spondylitis may be associated with tuberculosis of the bones, in which case it is called POTT'S DISEASE. The vertebrae become eroded and collapse, causing KYPHOSIS (hunchback).
　　Spondylitis may also be associated with other infectious diseases, such as brucellosis, or undulant fever. The intervertebral disks and the vertebrae are affected and sometimes destroyed, and permanent stiffening, or ankylosis, of the back results.
　　A particularly serious ailment is rheumatoid spondylitis, called also Marie-Strümpell disease. This is characterized by inflammation of the cartilage in the joints between vertebrae, and inflammation of the gliding joints between the vertebral arches. It affects males almost exclusively. There is stiffening of the spinal joints and ligaments, so that movement becomes increasingly painful and difficult. The stiffening may extend to the ribs and limit the flexibility of the rib cage, so that breathing is impaired.
　　Kümmel's spondylitis is a form of unknown origin or occurring at a great interval after the injury causing it, with collapse of the vertebra and thinning of the intervertebral disks.

spondylizema (spon″dĭ-li-ze′mah) downward displacement of a vertebra because of destruction of the one below it.

spondylocace (spon″dĭ-lok′ah-se) tuberculosis of the vertebrae.

spondylodymus (spon″dĭ-lod′ĭ-mus) a twin monster united by the vertebrae.

spondylodynia (spon″dĭ-lo-din′e-ah) pain in a vertebra.

spondylolisthesis (spon″dĭ-lo-lis-the′sis) forward displacement of a vertebra over a lower segment, usually of the fourth or fifth lumbar, frequently due to spondylolysis.

spondylolysis (spon″dĭ-lol′ĭ-sis) the breaking down of a vertebra, or replacement of a portion of the vertebral arch with cartilage; it frequently results in spondylolisthesis.

spondylopathy (spon″dĭ-lop′ah-the) any disease of the vertebrae.

spondyloptosis (spon″dĭ-lo-to′sis) spondylolisthesis.

spondylopyosis (spon″dĭ-lo-pi-o′sis) suppuration of a vertebra.

spondyloschisis (spon″dĭ-los′kĭ-sis) congenital fissure of a vertebral arch; spina bifida.

spondylosis (spon″dĭ-lo′sis) a condition marked by narrowing of the intervertebral spaces and lipping of the vertebral bodies, impinging on the nerve roots.
　　rhizomelic s., rheumatoid spondylitis affecting the movements of the hips and shoulders.

spondylosyndesis (spon″dĭ-lo-sin′dĕ-sis) surgical creation of ankylosis between contiguous vertebrae; spinal fusion.

sponge (spunj) a porous, absorbent mass, as a pad of gauze or cotton surrounded by gauze, or the elastic fibrous skeleton of certain species of marine animals.
　　gelatin s., absorbable, a sterile, absorbable, water-insoluble, gelatin-base material used in the control of bleeding.

spongi(o)- (spun′je-o) word element [L., Gr.], *sponge; spongelike.*

spongiform (spun′jĭ-form) resembling a sponge.

spongioblast (spon′je-o-blast″) an embryonic cell whose processes form the network from which neuroglia is formed.

spongioblastoma (spun″je-o-blas-to′mah) a tumor containing spongioblasts; gliosarcoma or glioma.

spongioplasm (spun′je-o-plazm″) a network of fibrils pervading the cell substance.

Spontin (spon′tin) trademark for a lyophilized preparation of ristocetins A and B, an antibiotic.

sporadin (spo′rah-din) trophozoite.

spore (spor) the reproductive element of one of the lower organisms, such as a protozoon or certain plants.

sporicide (spor′ĭ-sīd) an agent that kills spores.

sporidium (spo-rid′e-um), pl. *sporid′ia* [L.] a protozoan organism in one of the spore stages of its development.

sporiferous (spo-rif′er-us) bearing spores.

sporocyst (spor′o-sist) 1. any cyst or sac containing spores or reproductive cells; the oocyst of certain protozoa in which sporozoites develop. 2. the larval stages of flukes in snails.

sporogenic (spor′o-jen′ik) producing spores.

sporogony (spo-rog′o-ne) the third phase of the life cycle of a sporozoan parasite, with development of the zygote into one or several haploid spores, each containing a distinctive number of sporozoites.

sporont (spor′ont) a mature protozoon in its sexual cycle.

sporophore (spor′o-fōr) the spore-bearing part of an organism.

sporoplasm   (spōr'o-plazm) the protoplasm of reproductive cells.

sporotrichosis   (spōr″o-trĭ-ko'sis) infection with *Sporotrichum schenckii*, characterized by nodular skin lesions that break down into ulcers and lymphadenopathy.

Sporotrichum   (spo-rot'rĭ-kum) a genus of fungi; *S. schenck'ii* is the causative organism of sporotrichosis.

Sporozoa   (spōr″o-zo'ah) a subphylum of Protozoa, made up exclusively of parasitic forms, which are unable to ingest particulate food or bacteria and depend on the availability of soluble cellular constituents in their environment. adj., **sporozo'an.**

sporozoite   (spōr″o-zo'īt) a spore formed after fertilization; any one of the sickle-shaped nucleated germs formed by division of the protoplasm of a spore of a sporozoan organism. In malaria, the sporozoites are the forms of the plasmodium that are liberated from the oocysts in the mosquito, that accumulate in the salivary glands and that are transferred to man in the act of feeding.

sporozoon   (spōr″o-zo'on), pl. *sporozo'a* [Gr.] an individual organism or species of the subphylum Sporozoa.

spotted fever   a febrile disease characterized by a skin eruption, such as Rocky Mountain spotted fever, boutonneuse fever and other infections due to tick-borne rickettsiae.

sprain   (sprān) wrenching or twisting of a joint, with partial rupture of its ligaments. There may also be damage to the associated blood vessels, muscles, tendons and nerves.

A sprain is more serious than a strain, which is simply the overstretching of a muscle, without swelling. Severe sprains are so painful that the joint cannot be used. There is much swelling, with reddish to blue discoloration owing to hemorrhage from ruptured blood vessels.

First aid for a sprain involves immediate rest and the application of heat or cold by means of compresses. The sprained joint should be kept elevated if possible, and it should not be used.

sprue   (sproo) a chronic disease, affecting the digestive system, that is marked by imperfect absorption of food elements, especially fats but also certain vitamins, from the small intestine. The condition is closely related to CELIAC DISEASE and may be identical with it.

The name sprue derives from a Dutch word describing inflammation of the mouth, which is a frequent symptom. The disease has been recognized for more than 2000 years. It occurs mostly, but not exclusively, in the tropics.

SYMPTOMS AND TREATMENT.   Symptoms are loss of appetite, flatulence, anemia, diarrhea, stomach cramps and extreme loss of weight. Stools are usually pale, greasy, unformed and foul-smelling, but at times become watery. If a deficiency of vitamin B complex is also present, cracks develop at the corners of the mouth and the tongue becomes smooth, glossy and bright red.

Treatment consists of a special diet of foods that are low in fat, high in protein and fairly bland. Diets free of gluten, a viscid grain protein, may be prescribed. Liver preparations, folic acid, calcium lactate tablets, vitamin B$_{12}$ and iron supplements to provide food elements that are not absorbed, as well as skimmed milk and ripe bananas, have produced favorable results. Antibiotics and cortisone have proved temporarily successful, but their prolonged use is not recommended. In critical cases, repeated small blood transfusions have been beneficial.

Cases of sprue that are recognized early respond better to treatment than do cases of long standing. Appetite and weight return rapidly. The time required for complete recovery is prolonged, however, especially in extreme cases.

spur   (sper) a projecting body, as from a bone.

spurious   (spūr'e-us) simulated; not genuine; false.

sputum   (spu'tum) mucous secretion from the lungs, bronchi and trachea which is ejected through the mouth, in contrast to saliva which is the secretion of the salivary glands.

SQ   subcutaneous.

squalene   (skwa'lēn) a compound making up the greater part of liver oil of certain species of sharks.

squama   (skwa'mah), pl. *squa'mae* [L.] a scale, or thin, platelike structure.

squame   (skwām) a scale or scalelike mass.

squamoparietal   (skwa″mo-pah-ri'ĕ-tal) pertaining to the pars squamosa, or squamous portion of the temporal bone, and the parietal bone.

squamous   (skwa'mus) scaly or platelike.
   s. bone, the pars squamosa, or squamous portion of the temporal bone.

squatting   (skwot'ing) a position with the hips and knees flexed, the buttocks resting on the heels; sometimes adopted by the parturient at delivery or by children with certain types of cardiac defects.

squill   (skwill) a plant derivative used as an expectorant and diuretic.

squint   (skwint) strabismus.

S.R.   sedimentation rate.

Sr   chemical symbol, *strontium.*

sRNA   soluble RNA (ribonucleic acid).

ss.   [L.] *se'mis* (one half).

S.T.37   (es″te thir″te-sev'en) trademark for a solution of hexylresorcinol, an anthelmintic.

STA   serum thrombotic accelerator, a factor in serum that has procoagulant properties and the ability to induce blood CLOTTING.

stability   (stah-bil'ĭ-te) the quality of maintaining a constant character despite forces that threaten to disturb it.

stabilization   (sta″bĭ-lĭ-za'shun) the process of making firm and steady.

stable (sta'bl) not readily subject to change.

stactometer (stak-tom'ĕ-ter) a device for measuring drops.

staff (staf) the professional personnel of a hospital.
   attending s., the physicians in regular attendance.
   consulting s., those called in for special consultation.
   house s., the resident physicians of a hospital.

stage (stāj) 1. a definite period or distinct phase, as of development of a disease or of an organism. 2. the platform of a microscope on which the slide containing the object to be studied is placed.

stain (stān) a substance used to impart color to tissues or cells, to facilitate microscopic study and identification.
   acid s., one in which the color is carried by an acid and which has an affinity for basic elements in the specimen.
   basic s., one in which the color is carried by a base and which has an affinity for the acidic elements in the specimen.
   contrast s., a second stain used in preparation of a specimen, which colors other elements than those colored by the first, increasing the contrast between them.
   Gram's s., crystal violet solution and iodine solution, successively applied, followed by washing with ethyl alcohol; a method for classifying bacteria is based on their ability to retain the crystal violet stain (gram positive) or not (gram negative).
   hematoxylin and eosin s., a mixture of hematoxylin in distilled water and aqueous eosin solution, employed almost universally for routine examination of tissues.
   metachromatic s., one that produces in certain elements colors different from that of the stain itself.
   neutral s., one that is neither acid nor basic.
   nuclear s., one that selectively stains cell nuclei, generally a basic stain.
   port-wine s., nevus flammeus.
   protoplasmic s., one that selectively stains cell protoplasm.
   tumor s., an area of increased density in a radiograph, due to collection of contrast material in distorted and abnormal vessels, prominent in the capillary and venous phases of arteriography, and presumed to indicate neoplasm.
   Wright's s., a mixture of eosin and methylene blue, used for demonstrating blood corpuscles and malarial parasites.

staining (stān'ing) artificial coloration of a substance to facilitate examination of tissues, microorganisms or other cells under the microscope.
   intravital s., vital staining.
   supravital s., staining of living tissue removed from the body.
   vital s., staining of a tissue by a dye introduced into a living organism.

stalagmometer (stal"ag-mom'ĕ-ter) an instrument for measuring surface tension by determining the exact number of drops in a given quantity of a liquid.

stammering (stam'er-ing) stuttering.

standard (stan'dard) something established as a measure or model to which other similar things should conform.

standstill (stand'stil) cessation of motion, as of the heart (cardiac standstill) or chest (respiratory standstill).

stannum (stan'um) [L.] tin (symbol Sn).

stanozolol (stan'o-zo-lol") an anabolic steroid compound used to improve appetite and promote gain in weight.

Stanton's disease (stan'tunz) melioidosis.

stapedectomy (sta"pe-dek'to-me) surgical removal of the stapes (stirrup of the middle ear) and replacement with a prosthetic device composed of stainless steel, Teflon or a similar substance. The surgical procedure is performed for the relief of deafness produced by OTOSCLEROSIS, or fixation of the minute bones of the middle ear. Replacement of the fixed stapes with a device capable of vibrating permits the transmission of sound waves from the outer ear to the inner ear, and hearing is thus restored.

   Because the stapes is one of the smallest bones in the body, this procedure is very delicate and must be performed under an operating microscope. Very fine instruments, designed specifically for this procedure, are used.

   The procedure is done under local anesthesia and the patient is allowed out of bed within 48 hours after surgery and usually can go home on the third postoperative day. Vertigo (dizziness) is common following stapedectomy but it is only temporary. The patient must be protected from falls and self-injury until he regains his sense of balance. Care must also be taken to prevent infection and the patient must be cautioned against blowing his nose and getting water in his ear while bathing until the operative site is completely healed. (For additional information on nursing care after stapedectomy, see surgery of the EAR.)

stapedial (stah-pe'de-al) pertaining to the stapes.

stapediolysis (stah-pe"de-ol'ĭ-sis) mobilization of the stapes in the surgical treatment of OTOSCLEROSIS.

stapedioplasty (stah-pe'de-o-plas"te) replacement of the stapes with other material that conducts vibrations from the incus (anvil) in the middle ear to the oval window of the inner ear.

stapediotenotomy (stah-pe"de-o-tĕ-not'o-me) cutting of the tendon of the stapedius muscle.

stapediovestibular (stah-pe"de-o-ves-tib'u-lar) pertaining to the stapes and vestibule.

stapes (sta'pēz) the innermost of the three ossicles of the ear; called also stirrup.

Staphcillin (staf-sil'in) trademark for a preparation of dimethoxyphenyl penicillin sodium, an antibiotic of specific value in treatment of certain penicillin-resistant staphylococci.

staphyl(o)- (staf'ĭ-lo) word element [Gr.], *uvula; like a bunch of grapes.*

staphylectomy (staf"ĭ-lek'to-me) uvulectomy.

staphyledema (staf"il-ĕ-de'mah) edema of the uvula.

staphylin (staf′ĭ-lin) a lysogenic substance produced by active strains of staphylococci that prevents the growth of *Corynebacterium diphtheriae.*

staphyline (staf′ĭ-līn) 1. pertaining to the uvula. 2. shaped like a bunch of grapes.

staphylitis (staf″ĭ-li′tis) inflammation of the uvula.

staphyloangina (staf″ĭ-lo-an′jĭ-nah) mild sore throat with pseudomembrane, due to staphylococcus.

staphylocide (staf′ĭ-lo-sīd″) destructive to staphylococci.

staphylococcemia (staf″ĭ-lo-kok-se′me-ah) staphylococci in the blood.

staphylococcosis (staf″ĭ-lo-kok-o′sis) infection caused by staphylococci.

Staphylococcus (staf″ĭ-lo-kok′us) a genus of Schizomycetes made up of gram-positive, spherical microorganisms, tending to occur in grapelike clusters; there are several species, some of which are pathogenic, including *S. au′reus* and its variant, *S. al′bus.*

staphylococcus (staf″ĭ-lo-kok′us), pl. *staphylococ′ci.* [Gr.] 1. a spherical bacterium that occurs in irregular clumps resembling bunches of grapes. 2. an organism of the genus Staphylococcus. adj., **staphylococ′cal, staphylococ′cic.**

staphylokinase (staf″ĭ-lo-ki′nās) a bacterial kinase produced by certain strains of staphylococci.

staphylolysin (staf″ĭ-lol′ĭ-sin) a substance produced by staphylococci that causes hemolysis.

staphyloma (staf″ĭ-lo′mah) protrusion of the sclera or cornea.
  anterior s., keratoglobus.
  s. cor′neae, bulging and thinning of cornea.
  posterior s., s. posti′cum, backward bulging of sclera at posterior pole of eye.

staphyloncus (staf″ĭ-long′kus) tumor of the uvula.

staphyloptosis (staf″ĭ-lop-to′sis) elongation of the uvula.

staphyloschisis (staf″ĭ-los′kĭ-sis) fissure of the uvula and soft palate.

staphylotomy (staf″ĭ-lot′o-me) excision or incision of the uvula or of a staphyloma.

starch (starch) 1. the form in which carbohydrate is stored in plants. 2. granular material separated from mature corn grain; used as a dusting powder and pharmaceutical aid.
  s. glycerite, a preparation of starch, benzoic acid, purified water and glycerin, used topically as an emollient.
  iodized s., starch that has been treated with iodine.

starvation (star-va′shun) long-continued deprival of food and its morbid effects.

stasibasiphobia (sta″sĭ-ba″sĭ-fo′be-ah) morbid distrust of one's ability to stand or walk.

stasiphobia (sta″sĭ-fo′be-ah) morbid dread of standing erect.

stasis (sta′sis) a stoppage of flow, as of blood or other body fluid, or of intestinal contents.

-stasis (sta′sis) word element [Gr.], *maintenance of (or maintaining) a constant level; preventing increase or multiplication.* adj., **-stat′ic.**

stat. [L.] *sta′tim* (at once).

state (stāt) condition or situation.
  dream s., a state of defective consciousness in which the environment is imperfectly perceived.
  excited s., the condition of a nucleus, atom or molecule produced by the addition of energy to the system as the result of absorption of photons or of inelastic collisions with other particles or systems.
  ground s., the condition of lowest energy of a nucleus, atom or molecule.
  refractory s., a condition of subnormal excitability of muscle and nerve following excitation.
  resting s., the physiologic condition achieved by complete bed rest for at least 1 hour.
  stable s., the condition of a system in which it does not readily undergo change.

static (stat′ik) not in motion; at rest.
  s. electricity, electricity generated by friction, or that does not move in currents.

statim (sta′tim) [L.] at once; abbreviated stat.

station (sta′shun) 1. the manner of standing. 2. a fixed place.

statistics (stah-tis′tiks) 1. numerical facts pertaining to a particular subject or body of objects. 2. the science dealing with the collection, tabulation and analysis of numerical facts.
  vital s., numerical facts pertaining to human natality, morbidity and mortality.

statoconia (stat″o-ko′ne-ah), sing. *statoco′nium* [Gr.] minute calcareous particles in the gelatinous membrane surmounting the macula in the inner ear.

statocyst (stat′o-sist) one of the sacs of the labyrinth to which is attributed an influence in the maintenance of static equilibrium.

statolith (stat′o-lith) a solid or semisolid body occurring in the statocyst.

statometer (stah-tom′ĕ-ter) an apparatus for measuring the degree of exophthalmos.

stature (stat′ūr) the height or tallness of a person standing.

status (sta′tus) [L.] condition or state.
  s. asthmat′icus, asthmatic crisis; asthmatic shock; a continuous and refractory asthmatic attack that may be fatal.
  s. epilep′ticus, rapid succession of epileptic spasms without intervals of consciousness; brain damage may result.
  s. lymphat′icus, a condition marked by enlarged thymus and spleen, hyperplasia of the lymphoid tissues and lowered bodily vitality.
  s. thymicolymphat′icus, a condition resembling

status lymphaticus, with enlargement of lymphadenoid tissue and of the thymus; formerly thought to be the cause of sudden death in children.

s. verruco′sus, a wartlike appearance of the cerebral cortex, produced by disorderly arrangement of the neuroblasts, so that the formation of fissures and sulci is irregular and unpredictable.

steapsin (ste-ap′sin) lipase.

stear(o)- (ste′ah-ro) word element [Gr.], *fat.*

stearate (ste′ah-rāt) any compound of stearic acid.

stearic acid (ste-ar′ik) a saturated fatty acid from animal and vegetable fats.

stearin (ste′ah-rin) a white, solid crystalline substance from fat.

stearodermia (ste″ah-ro-der′me-ah) disease of the skin involving the sebaceous glands.

stearopten (ste″ah-rop′ten) the solid constituent of a volatile oil.

steat(o)- (ste′ah-to) word element [Gr.], *fat; oil.*

steatadenoma (ste″at-ad″ĕ-no′mah) adenoma of the sebaceous glands.

steatitis (ste″ah-ti′tis) inflammation of fatty tissue.

steatocele (ste-at′o-sēl) fatty swelling of the scrotum.

steatocryptosis (ste″ah-to-krip-to′sis) disorder of function of the sebaceous glands.

steatogenous (ste″ah-toj′ĕ-nus) producing fat.

steatolysis (ste″ah-tol′ĭ-sis) the emulsification of fats preparatory to absorption. adj., **steatolyt′ic.**

steatoma (ste″ah-to′mah) 1. lipoma. 2. a fatty mass retained within a sebaceous gland.

steatomatosis (ste″ah-to″mah-to′sis) the presence of numerous sebaceous cysts.

steatonecrosis (ste″ah-to″nĕ-kro′sis) fat necrosis.

steatopathy (ste″ah-top′ah-the) disease of the sebaceous glands.

steatopygia (ste″ah-to-pij′e-ah) excessive fatness of the buttocks.

steatorrhea (ste″ah-to-re′ah) excess fat in the feces due to a malabsorption state caused by disease of the intestinal mucosa (e.g., sprue) or pancreatic enzyme deficiency.

steatosis (ste″ah-to′sis) 1. disease of the sebaceous glands. 2. fatty degeneration.

stechiometry (stek″e-om′ĕ-tre) stoichiometry.

Steclin (stek′lin) trademark for preparations of tetracycline hydrochloride, an antibiotic.

stegnosis (steg-no′sis) 1. stoppage of a secretion. 2. stenosis.

Steinert's disease (sti′nerts) myotonia dystrophica.

Steinmann pin (stīn′man) a pin driven through the distal part of a fractured bone as a means of

applying traction, or used to immobilize the fragments of a broken bone.

Stelazine (stel′ah-zēn) trademark for preparations of trifluoperazine, a tranquilizer.

stella (stel′ah), pl. *stel′lae* [L.] star.

stellate (stel′āt) star-shaped; arranged in rosettes.
s. ganglion, cervicothoracic ganglion.

stellectomy (stel-ek′to-me) excision of a portion of the stellate (cervicothoracic) ganglion.

stem (stem) stalk; a supporting structure.
brain s., the continuation of the spinal cord above the foramen magnum, containing the sensory and motor tracts to and from the cerebrum and cerebellum. It is made up of the medulla oblongata, pons, diencephalon and midbrain and contains a number of vital centers.

Stenediol (sten′di-ol) trademark for preparations of methandriol, an anabolic stimulant.

steno- (sten′o) word element [Gr.], *narrow; contracted; constriction.*

stenocardia (sten″o-kar′de-ah) angina pectoris.

stenocephaly (sten″o-sef′ah-le) narrowness of the head or cranium.

stenochoria (sten″o-ko′re-ah) stenosis.

stenocoriasis (sten″o-ko-ri′ah-sis) contraction of the pupil.

stenopeic (sten″o-pe′ik) having a narrow opening or slit.

stenosed (stĕ-nōst′, stĕ-nōzd′) narrowed; constricted.

stenosis (stĕ-no′sis) narrowing or contraction of a body passage or opening.
aortic s., obstruction to the outflow of blood from the left ventricle into the aorta at the subvalvular, valvular or supravalvular level.
mitral s., a narrowing of the left atrioventricular orifice.
pulmonary s., narrowing of the opening between the pulmonary artery and the right ventricle.
pyloric s., hypertrophic obstruction of the pyloric orifice of the stomach (see also PYLORIC STENOSIS).
tricuspid s., narrowing or stricture of the tricuspid orifice of the heart.

stenostomia (sten″o-sto′me-ah) narrowing of the mouth.

stenothermal, stenothermic (sten″o-ther′mal), (sten″o-ther′mik) pertaining to or characterized by tolerance of only a narrow range of temperature.

stenothorax (sten″o-tho′raks) an abnormally straight, short or narrow thorax.

stenotic (stĕ-not′ik) marked by abnormal narrowing or constriction.

Sterane (ster′ān) trademark for preparations of prednisolone, a glucogenic corticosteroid.

sterco- (ster′ko) word element [L.], *feces.*

stercobilin (ster″ko-bi′lin) a reduction product

of bilirubin excreted in the feces and giving them their brown color.

stercoraceous   (ster″ko-ra′shus) consisting of feces.

stercorolith   (ster′ko-ro-lith″) fecalith; an intestinal concretion composed of fecal matter.

stercoroma   (ster″ko-ro′mah) a tumor-like mass of fecal matter in the rectum.

stercus   (ster′kus) [L.] dung or feces. adj., **ster′coral, ster′corous.**

stereoarthrolysis   (ste″re-o-ar-throl′ĭ-sis) formation of a movable new joint in cases of bony ankylosis.

stereoauscultation   (ste″re-o-aw″skul-ta′shun) auscultation with two stethoscopes, on different parts of the chest.

stereochemistry   (ste″re-o-kem′is-tre) the branch of chemistry treating of the space relations of atoms in molecules. adj., **stereochem′ical.**

stereocinefluorography   (ste″re-o-sin″ĕ-floo″or-og′rah-fe) photographic recording by motion picture camera of images observed by stereoscopic fluoroscopy, affording three-dimensional visualization.

stereognosis   (ste″re-og-no′sis) the sense by which the form of objects is perceived. adj., **stereognos′tic.**

stereoisomer   (ste″re-o-i′so-mer) a compound showing stereoisomerism.

stereoisomerism   (ste″re-o-i-som′ĕ-rizm) isomerism in which the compounds have the same structural formulae, but the atoms are distributed differently in space.

Stereo-orthopter   (ste″re-o-or-thop′ter) a proprietary mirror-reflecting instrument for correcting strabismus.

stereoroentgenography   (ste″re-o-rent″gen-og′-rah-fe) the making of a stereoscopic roentgenogram.

stereoscopic   (ste″re-o-skop′ik) three-dimensional; having depth, as well as height and width.

stereospecific   (ste″re-o-spĕ-sif′ik) pertaining to enzymes that interact only with compounds of very specific structure.

stereotaxic   (ste″re-o-tak′sik) pertaining to or characterized by precise positioning in space.

stereotaxis, stereotropism   (ste″re-o-tak′sis), (ste″re-ot′ro-pizm) movement or growth in response to contact with a solid or rigid surface.

stereotypy   (ste′re-o-ti″pe) persistent repetition of senseless acts or words. It may be a persistent maintaining of a bodily attitude (stereotypy of attitude), repetition of senseless movements (stereotypy of movement) or constant repetition of certain words or phrases (stereotypy of speech).

sterile   (ster′il) 1. free from microorganisms. 2. unable to produce offspring.

sterility   (stĕ-ril′ĭ-te) 1. freedom from microorganisms. 2. inability to produce offspring.

sterilization   (ster″il-ĭ-za′shun) 1. the process of rendering an individual incapable of reproduction, by castration, vasectomy, salpingectomy or other procedure. 2. the process of destroying all microorganisms and their pathogenic products. It is accomplished by heat (wet steam under pressure at 120° C. for 15 minutes, or dry heat at 360 to 380° C. for 3 hours) or by bactericidal chemical compounds.

In sterilizing objects or substances, the high resistance of bacterial spore cells must be taken into account. Most dangerous bacteria are destroyed at a temperature of 50 to 60° C. (122 to 140° F.). Therefore, pasteurization of a fluid, which is the application of heat at about 60° C., destroys disease-causing bacteria. However, temperatures almost twice as high are usually required to destroy the spore cells.

The discovery that heat, in the form of flame, steam or hot water, kills bacteria made possible the advances of modern surgery, which is based on freedom from microorganisms, or asepsis, and prevention of contamination. Sterilization of all equipment used during an operation, and of anything that in any way may touch the operative area, is carried out scrupulously in hospitals. Physicians and nurses wear sterile clothing. Instruments are sterilized by boiling, by chemical antiseptics or by autoclaving.

In a physician's office needles for injections and any instruments used for treatment of wounds or other surgical procedures are also carefully sterilized, and other aseptic techniques are observed.

sterilizer   (ster′ĭ-līz″er) an apparatus used in ridding instruments, dressings, etc., of all microorganisms and their pathogenic products. (See also AUTOCLAVE.)

Sterisol   (ster′ĭ-sol) trademark for a preparation of hexetidine, a local antiseptic.

stern(o)-   (ster′no) word element [L., Gr.], *sternum.*

sternal   (ster′nal) pertaining to the sternum.

   s. puncture, insertion of a hollow needle into the manubrium of the sternum for the purpose of obtaining a sample of bone marrow. The sternum is chosen because of its accessibility and because it is a thin, flat bone. The procedure must be done under surgical asepsis. The physician anesthetizes the skin and periosteum with 1 per cent procaine hydrochloride (Novocaine) before introducing the sternal needle. The needle is designed with a special guard to prevent penetration beyond the desired depth. When the cells are being aspirated into the syringe the patient may experience a sharp pain; otherwise the procedure should not be painful.

The bone marrow samplings are examined for the presence of abnormal cells, for the proportion of cells in their various stages of development and for the characteristics of the blood cells that predominate. This information is used in conjunction with clinical findings and other tests in the diagnosis of blood disorders such as the leukemias and anemia.

sternalgia   (ster-nal′je-ah) pain in the sternum.

sternoclavicular   (ster″no-klah-vik′u-lar) pertaining to the sternum and clavicle.

sternocleidomastoid   (ster″no-kli″do-mas′toid) pertaining to the sternum, clavicle and mastoid process.

sternocostal   (ster″no-kos′tal) pertaining to the sternum and ribs.

sternodymia   (ster″no-dim′e-ah) union of two fetuses by the anterior chest wall.

sternodymus   (ster-nod′ĭ-mus) conjoined twins united at the anterior chest wall.

sternohyoid   (ster″no-hi′oid) pertaining to the sternum and hyoid bone.

sternoid   (ster′noid) resembling the sternum.

sternomastoid   (ster″no-mas′toid) pertaining to the sternum and the mastoid process of the temporal bone.

sternopericardial   (ster″no-per″ĭ-kar′de-al) pertaining to the sternum and pericardium.

sternothyroid   (ster″no-thy′roid) pertaining to the sternum and thyroid cartilage or gland.

sternotomy   (ster-not′o-me) incision of the sternum.

sternum   (ster′num) a plate of bone forming the middle of the anterior wall of the thorax and articulating with the clavicles and the cartilages of the first seven ribs. It consists of three parts, the manubrium, the body and the xiphoid process.

sternutatory   (ster-nu′tah-tor″e) 1. causing sneezing. 2. an agent that causes sneezing.

steroid   (ste′roid) a complex molecule containing carbon atoms in four interlocking rings, three of which contain six carbon atoms each and the fourth of which contains five.

Steroids are important in body chemistry. Among them are the male and female sex hormones, such as testosterone and estrogen, and the hormones of the cortices of the adrenal glands, including cortisone. Vitamins of the D group are steroids involved in calcium metabolism. The cardiac glycosides, a group of compounds derived from certain plants, are partly steroids. Sterols, including cholesterol, are steroids. Cholesterol is the main building block of steroid hormones in the body; it is also converted into bile salts by the liver.

CLASSIFICATION OF STEROIDS

Sterols	Corticosteroids
Bile acids	Vitamins D
Male sex hormones	Saponins
Female sex hormones	Cardiac glycosides

steroidogenesis   (ste-roi″do-jen′ĕ-sis) production of steroids, as by the adrenal glands.

sterol   (ste′rol) a solid alcohol of animal or vegetable origin, having properties like the fats. Cholesterol is the best-known member of the group.

sterolytic   (ster″o-lit′ik) capable of dissolving sterols.

Sterosan   (ster′o-san) trademark for preparations of chlorquinaldol, a bactericide and fungicide.

stertor   (ster′tor) snoring; sonorous respiration, usually due to partial obstruction of the upper airway. adj., **ster′torous.**

steth(o)-   (steth′o) word element [Gr.], *chest.*

stethalgia   (steth-al′je-ah) pain in the chest or chest wall.

stethogoniometer   (steth″o-go″ne-om′ĕ-ter) an apparatus for measuring the curvature of the chest.

stethoscope   (steth′o-skōp) an instrument used to hear and amplify the sounds produced by the heart, lungs and other internal organs. As first introduced by the 19th century French physician, René Laënnec, the stethoscope was a simple wooden tube with a bell-shaped opening at one end. The modern stethoscope is binaural, with two earpieces and flexible rubber tubing leading to them from the two-branched opening of the bell or cone. In this way, sound travels simultaneously through both of the branches to the earpieces.

stethospasm   (steth′o-spazm) spasm of the chest muscles.

STH   somatotropic (growth) hormone.

sthenic   (sthen′ik) characterized by overaction; strong.

sthenophotic   (sthen″o-fo′tik) able to see in a strong light.

stibamine   (stib′ah-min) a compound used in treatment of kala-azar.

stibialism   (stib′e-al-izm″) antimony poisoning.

stibium   (stib′e-um) [L.] antimony (symbol Sb).

stibophen   (stib′o-fen) an antimony-containing agent used against schistosomal and leishmanial infections.

stigma   (stig′mah), pl. *stig′mas, stig′mata* [Gr.] 1. a characteristic abnormality, or an indication of an abnormal or morbid condition. 2. a spot or impression on the skin. adj., **stigmat′ic.**

stigmatization   (stig″mah-tĭ-za′shun) the formation of stigmas.

stigmatosis   (stig″mah-to′sis) a skin disease marked by ulcerated spots.

stilalgin   (stil-al′jin) mephenesin, a muscle relaxant.

stilbestrol   (stil-bes′trol) diethylstilbestrol, a synthetic estrogen.

Stilbetin   (stil-be′tin) trademark for a preparation of diethylstilbestrol, a synthetic estrogen.

stilet   (sti′let) 1. a delicate probe. 2. a wire used to stiffen or clear a catheter.

Still's disease (stilz) juvenile rheumatoid arthritis.

stillbirth (stil′berth) birth of a dead child.

stillborn (stil′born) born dead.

stimulant (stim′u-lant) 1. producing stimulation. 2. an agent that stimulates.

stimulate (stim′u-lāt) to excite functional activity in a part.

stimulation (stim″u-la′shun) the act or process of stimulating; the condition of being stimulated.
   audio-visual-tactile s., the simultaneous rhythmic excitation of the receptors for the senses of hearing, sight and touch.

stimulus (stim′u-lus), pl. *stim′uli* [L.] any agent, act or influence that produces functional or trophic reaction in a receptor or an irritable tissue.

sting (sting) injury caused by a poisonous substance produced by an animal or plant (biotoxin) introduced into an individual or with which he comes in contact, together with mechanical trauma incident to its introduction. (See also INSECT BITES AND STINGS.)

stippling (stip′ling) a spotted condition or appearance, such as an appearance of the retina as if dotted with light and dark points, or the spotted appearance of the erythrocytes in basophilia.

stirrup (stir′up) the stapes, the innermost of the three ossicles of the ear.

stitch (stich) 1. a sudden cutting pain, generally in the flank. 2. a loop made in sewing or suturing.

stochastic (sto-kas′tik) arrived at by skillful conjecturing.

stoichiometry (stoi″ke-om′ĕ-tre) the science of the numerical relations of chemical elements and compounds and the mathematical laws of chemical changes.

Stokes's disease (stōks) exophthalmic goiter.

Stokes-Adams disease (stōks ad′amz) a condition characterized by sudden attacks of unconsciousness, with or without convulsions, that frequently accompanies heart block; called also Adams-Stokes disease or syndrome.

stoma (sto′mah), pl. *sto′mas, sto′mata* [Gr.] 1. a mouthlike opening. 2. an incised opening that is kept open for drainage or other purposes, such as the opening in the abdominal wall established by a colostomy.

stomach (stum′ak) a curved, muscular, saclike structure that is an enlargement of the alimentary canal between the esophagus and the small intestine.
   The wall of the stomach consists of four coats: an outer serous coat; a muscular coat, made up of longitudinal, circular and oblique muscle fibers; a submucous coat; and mucous coat or membrane forming the inner lining. The muscles account for the stomach's ability to expand when food enters it. The muscle fibers slide over one another, reducing the thickness of the stomach wall while increasing its area. When empty, the stomach has practically no cavity at all, since its walls are pressed tightly together. When full, the average stomach holds about 1½ quarts.
   The stomach muscles perform another function. When food enters the stomach, the muscles contract in rhythm. Their combined action sends a

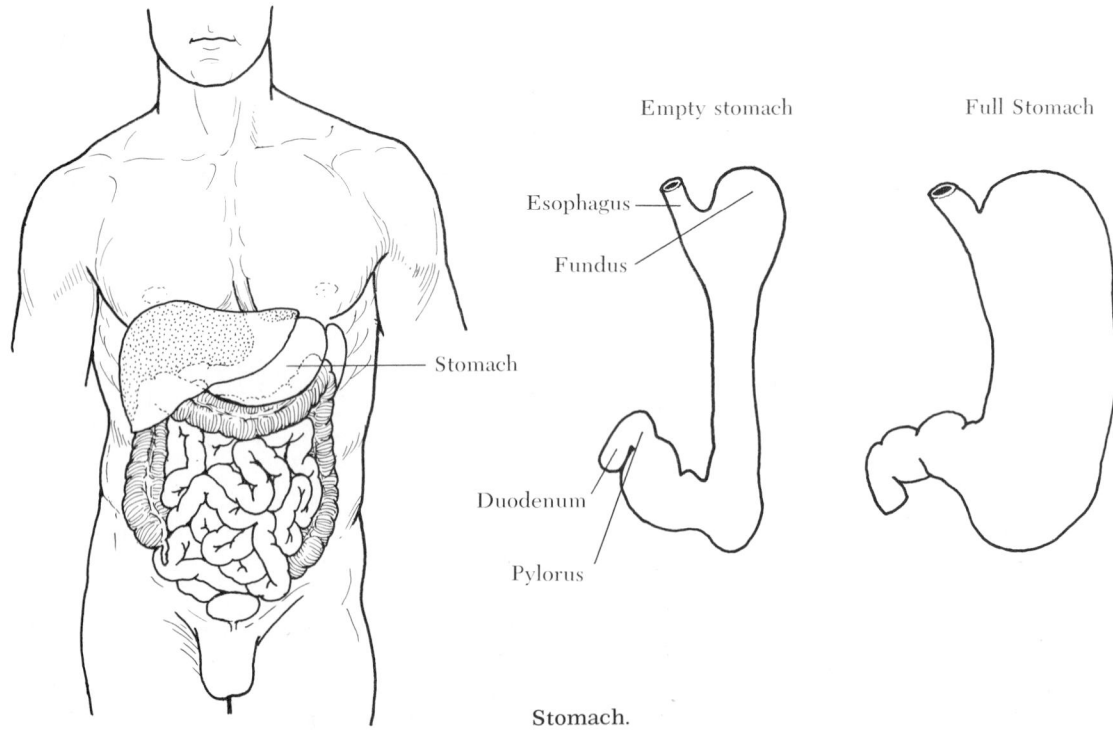

Empty stomach   Full Stomach

Esophagus

Fundus

Stomach

Duodenum

Pylorus

Stomach.

series of wavelike contractions from the upper end of the stomach to the lower end. These contractions, known as peristalsis, mix the partially digested food with the stomach secretions and ingested liquid until it has the consistency of a thick soup; the contractions then push it into the small intestine.

The stomach is emptied of its digested contents in 1 to 4 hours, or longer, depending upon the amount and type of food eaten. Foods rich in carbohydrates leave the stomach more rapidly than proteins, and proteins more rapidly than fats.

The stomach may continue to contract after it is empty. The contraction of the empty stomach stimulates nerves in its wall and may cause hunger pangs.

The mucous membrane lining the stomach contains innumerable gastric glands; their secretion, gastric juice, contains enzymes, mucin and hydrochloric acid. Enzymes help to split the food molecules into smaller parts during digestion. Mucin acts on certain sugars and also protects the mucous lining of the stomach from coarse particles and from the corrosive hydrochloric acid. Hydrochloric acid aids in dissolving the food before the enzymes begin working on it. (See also DIGESTIVE SYSTEM.)

DISORDERS OF THE STOMACH. Disturbances in the functioning of the stomach include indigestion and nausea; organic diseases include peptic ULCER and cancer.

Care given to establishing good eating habits will help to prevent stomach distress. Food should be wholesome, well prepared and properly cooked. Heavy, fried and fatty foods, highly spiced foods, too much roughage and foods to which one has shown a sensitivity should be avoided. When nervous tension and anxiety are the underlying cause of a stomach disorder, an effort should be made to resolve the basic problems causing emotional distress.

Two common forms of gastric discomfort are belching (eructation) and heartburn. Usually belching results from swallowing air while eating, and heartburn, a burning sensation below the sternum, is thought to be caused by distention of the lower part of the esophagus, possibly from gulping food or other faulty eating habits. Both may be associated with peptic ulcer or hiatal hernia.

GASTRITIS, inflammation of the lining of the stomach, is a common disorder. It may be acute, chronic or toxic.

SURGERY OF THE STOMACH. Surgical procedures of the stomach are most often done as treatment for malignant disease or for chronic ulcers that are complicated by hemorrhage or perforation. Surgical removal of the whole stomach is called total gastrectomy; excision of a portion of it is subtotal or partial gastrectomy. When partial gastrectomy is done, the remaining portion of the stomach is anastomosed to a loop of intestine (gastroenterostomy), usually of the jejunum (gastrojejunostomy). This is done to maintain continuity of the digestive tract. When total gastrectomy is performed, continuity is restored by an anastomosis between the end of the esophagus and the jejunum.

Another surgical procedure involving the stomach is GASTROSTOMY. This is a surgical incision into the stomach with the creation of a permanent opening to the surface of the body. Its purpose is the administration of feedings and fluids when strictures or obstruction of the esophagus makes swallowing impossible.

Nursing Care. Unless there is an emergency situation such as hemorrhage, the patient who is to undergo gastric surgery will have several diagnostic tests before the operation, including GASTRIC ANALYSIS, a gastrointestinal series of x-rays (see BARIUM TEST) and GASTROSCOPY.

Before the operation a Levin tube may be inserted and continuous suction used to remove gastric secretions and prevent distention. (For other routine preoperative procedures, see PREOPERATIVE CARE.)

Routine POSTOPERATIVE CARE, including observations of the patient and prevention of complications, is discussed under that heading. Immediately after surgery the patient who has undergone gastric surgery should be checked for tubes and drains that may have been inserted. In most instances the Levin tube will be left in place and suction resumed after surgery. Drainage from this tube will be dark brown at first and may be streaked with bright red blood. The color should gradually become lighter until it is a greenish yellow and the appearance of flecks or streaks of blood should diminish. If there is continued evidence of fresh bleeding the surgeon should be notified at once. The amount and character of drainage through the tube should be observed and recorded on the patient's chart every 8 hours.

Fluids by mouth are restricted until peristalsis resumes and the nasogastric tube is removed. Irrigation of the tube is done as ordered to assure proper drainage. The irrigations should be done gently and only as frequently as ordered because continuous washing can lead to excessive removal of electrolytes from the stomach. Mouth care and care of the nostrils are necessary as long as the tube is in place. Fluids are given intravenously until the patient is able to retain liquids and foods by mouth.

After the tube is removed the surgeon will give written orders regarding liquids and foods permitted. Usually a very small amount of water is given at hourly intervals and the amount increased according to the patient's tolerance. Later, bland liquids and foods are added until the patient has progressed to a full diet. The hospital dietitian usually works closely with the patient in planning his diet so that when he returns home he will have well balanced meals that can be tolerated without difficulty.

Before the patient is discharged from the hospital he may be scheduled for another series of x-rays of the upper intestinal tract. This is done to observe the continuity of the digestive tract and to be sure it is functioning satisfactorily.

A group of symptoms known as the "dumping syndrome" sometimes develops after gastrectomy. They are the result of rapid emptying of gastric contents into the small intestine. These symptoms usually are mild and include palpitation, a feeling of weakness or fainting and sweating; they may last for a few minutes or for as long as an hour. It is believed that meals high in carbohydrates and salt trigger the dumping syndrome because these substances must be diluted in the small intestine before they can be absorbed. To provide for this dilution, the jejunal loop becomes distended and fills with fluids that have shifted from the circulating blood. The symptoms produced by this condition can be relieved somewhat by limiting the intake of salt and carbohydrates and by restricting the amount of liquids taken with each meal.

When the stomach has been removed, the production of intrinsic factor, necessary for the absorption of vitamin B_{12} from the intestinal tract, is brought to a halt. This condition must be corrected by monthly injections of vitamin B_{12} for the rest of the patient's life.

hourglass s., one shaped somewhat like an hourglass.

leather-bottle s., plastic linitis; severe hypertrophy of the stomach wall, usually seen in chronic gastritis or certain forms of carcinoma.

powdered s., dried and powdered defatted wall of the stomach of the hog; used in treatment of pernicious anemia.

s. pump, an apparatus used to remove material from the stomach. It consists of a rubber stomach tube to which a bulb syringe is attached. The tube is inserted into the mouth or nose and passed down the esophagus into the stomach. Suction from the syringe brings the contents of the stomach up through the tube.

A stomach pump can be used either to remove material from the stomach in case of emergency — for example, when a person has swallowed poison — or to obtain a specimen for chemical analysis, as in diagnosis of peptic ulcer or other stomach disorders.

s. tube, a flexible tube used for introducing food, medication or other material directly into the stomach. It can be passed into the stomach by way of either the nose or the mouth. (See also TUBE FEEDING.)

A stomach tube may be employed in emergency feeding, during coma or when patients refuse food. It is also used to dilute the contents of the stomach when a person has swallowed poison, or to lavage the stomach before the contents are pumped out. Stomach tubes are also inserted to decompress the stomach when it becomes abnormally distended after certain abdominal operations.

stomachal (stum'ah-kal) pertaining to the stomach.

stomachalgia (stum″ah-kal'je-ah) pain in the stomach.

stomachic (sto-mak'ik) 1. pertaining to the stomach. 2. a stimulant of gastric activity.

stomat(o)- (sto'mah-to) word element [Gr.], *mouth.*

stomatalgia (sto″mah-tal'je-ah) pain in the mouth.

stomatitis (sto″mah-ti'tis) inflammation of the mucosa of the mouth. It may be caused by one of many diseases of the mouth or it may accompany another disease. Both gingivitis (inflammation of the gums) and glossitis (inflammation of the tongue) are forms of stomatitis.

CAUSES. The causes of stomatitis vary widely, from a mild local irritant to a vitamin deficiency or infection by a possibly dangerous disease-producing organism.

Inflammation may arise from actual injury to the inside of the mouth, as from cheek-biting, jagged teeth, tartar accumulations and badly fitting dentures. Irritating substances, including alcohol, tobacco and excessively hot or spicy food, may also cause stomatitis.

Other causes may be infectious bacteria, such as streptococci and gonococci or those causing TRENCH MOUTH, diphtheria and tuberculosis; the fungus causing THRUSH; or the viruses causing herpes simplex and measles. Extreme vitamin deficiencies can result in mouth inflammation, as can certain blood disorders. Poisoning with heavy metals, such as lead or mercury, can cause stomatitis.

SYMPTOMS. There is generally swelling and redness of the tissues of the mouth, which may become quite sore, particularly during eating. The mouth may have an unpleasant odor. In some types of stomatitis the mouth becomes dry, but in others there is excessive salivation. Ulcerations may appear, and, in extreme cases, gangrene (gangrenous stomatitis).

Other forms of stomatitis may occasionally cause more severe symptoms, including chills, fever and headache. Sometimes bleeding or white patches in the mouth can be seen. In thrush, the symptoms themselves may be slight (white spots in the mouth resembling milk clots) but the disease may give rise to serious infections elsewhere in the body. In some cases, stomatitis causes inflammation of the parotid glands.

Stomatitis resulting from certain diseases presents special identifying symptoms. Syphilitic stomatitis produces patches in the mouth; in scarlet fever the tongue first has a strawberry color, which then deepens to a raspberry hue; in measles, Koplik's spots appear.

TREATMENT AND PREVENTION. The treatment varies according to the cause. When the inflammation is caused by anemia, vitamin deficiency or any infection of the body, both the underlying disease and the infection are treated. Penicillin and various sulfonamide drugs often are effective against the inflammation, and prevent its spreading to the parotid glands. Mouthwashes may be used under a physician's direction after he has determined the cause of the stomatitis. Gentian violet solution may be applied to the lesions of thrush; other forms of stomatitis may be swabbed with sodium bicarbonate, sodium perborate solution or hydrogen peroxide.

With proper care, many cases of stomatitis can be prevented. Cleanliness is essential, especially of the mouth, teeth, dentures and feeding utensils. Infants may acquire mouth infection from dirty bottles or from the mother's nipples. In the case of a prolonged fever or of any severe general illness, dryness of the mouth should be avoided by ingestion of increased amounts of fluids, particularly fruit juices.

aphthous s., an acute infection of the oral mucosa caused by the virus of herpes simplex, with vesicle formation; called also canker sore.

stomatodynia (sto″mah-to-din'e-ah) pain in the mouth.

stomatogastric (sto″mah-to-gas'trik) pertaining to the stomach and mouth.

stomatology (sto″mah-tol'o-je) the sum of what is known about the mouth.

stomatomalacia (sto″mah-to-mah-la'she-ah) softening of the structures of the mouth.

stomatomycosis (sto"mah-to-mi-ko'sis) a fungus disease of the mouth.

stomatonecrosis (sto"mah-to-nĕ-kro'sis) gangrenous stomatitis.

stomatopathy (sto"mah-top'ah-the) any disorder of the mouth.

stomatoplasty (sto'mah-to-plas"te) plastic reconstruction of the mouth.

stomatorrhagia (sto"mah-to-ra'je-ah) hemorrhage from the mouth.

stomocephalus (sto"mo-sef'ah-lus) a fetus with rudimentary jaws and mouth.

stomodeum (sto"mo-de'um) the ectodermal depression at the head end of the embryo, which becomes the front part of the mouth.

-stomy (sto'me) word element [Gr.], *creation of an opening into* or *a communication between.*

stone (stōn) 1. a calculus. 2. a unit of weight, equivalent in the English system to 14 lb. avoirdupois.

stool (stōol) the fecal discharge from the bowels (see also FECES).
  lienteric s., feces containing much undigested food.
  rice water s., the watery stool flecked with fragments of necrotic mucosal epithelium, characteristic of cholera.

stopcock (stop'kok) a valve that regulates the flow of fluid through a tube.

storage disease (stōr'ij) a metabolic disorder in which some substance (e.g., fats, proteins or carbohydrates) accumulates in certain cells in abnormal amounts; called also thesaurismosis.

storax (sto'raks) a balsam obtained from the trunk of trees of the genus Liquidambar; used locally in scabies.

stosstherapy (stos'ther-ah-pe) treatment of a disease by a single massive dose of therapeutic agent or short-term administration of unphysiologically large doses.

strabismometer (strah-biz-mom'ĕ-ter) an apparatus for measuring strabismus.

strabismus (strah-biz'mus) deviation of the eye that the patient cannot overcome, in which the visual axes are not physiologically coordinated; called also crossed eyes and squint. adj., **strabis'-mic.**
  During the first 3 to 6 months of life, the eyes of infants tend to waver and turn either inward or outward independently of one another; this usually corrects itself. If it persists, or if the eyes are continually crossed in the same way, even if the child is less than 6 months old, it may be a sign of strabismus. Children do not outgrow strabismus.
  In an older child, a tendency to tilt the head when reading, or to close or rub one eye, may indicate crossed eyes.
  Strabismus almost always appears at an early age. If not corrected, the condition may impair vision in the nonfocusing eye, as well as marring the child's appearance. In the great majority of cases the eyes can be straightened by proper medical treatment at any age, but vision of the malfunc-

tioning eye may remain impaired. If treated early enough, preferably before 6 years, normal vision can usually be restored in the affected eye.
  CAUSE. Strabismus may result from several factors, including a blow on the head, disease or heredity. Many cases are caused by a malfunction of the muscles that move the eyes. This causes the eyes to focus differently, sending different images to the brain. As the child grows, he learns to ignore the image from one eye with the result that it fails to grow as strong as the eye on which he is depending.
  TREATMENT. Treatment for strabismus varies with the individual case. A patch may be placed over the child's stronger eye for a period, forcing him to use the weaker eye and thus restoring its strength as far as possible, instead of letting it grow worse from lack of use. Eyeglasses or special eye exercises may correct the condition. In some cases, a relatively simple surgical operation on the eye muscles may be necessary. Since these muscles are outside the eye itself, there is no danger to the vision.
  For further information on the functioning of the eyes, see EYE.
  concomitant s., that in which the angle of deviation of the visual axis of the squinting eye is always the same in relation to the other eye, no matter what the direction of the gaze.
  convergent s., that in which the visual axes converge; esotropia.
  divergent s., that in which the visual axes diverge; called also exotropia and walleye.
  horizontal s., that in which the visual axis of the squinting eye deviates in the horizonal plane (esotropia or exotropia).
  nonconcomitant s., that in which the amount of deviation of the squinting eye varies according to the direction in which the eyes are turned.
  vertical s., that in which the visual axis of the squinting eye deviates in the vertical plane (hypertropia or hypotropia).

strabotomy (strah-bot'o-me) cutting of an ocular tendon in treatment of strabismus.

strain (strān) 1. to overexercise. 2 to filter. 3. an overstretching or overexertion of some part of the musculature. 4. excessive effort. 5. a group of organisms within a species or variety, characterized by some particular quality, as rough or smooth strains of bacteria.

strait (strāt) a narrow passage.
  s. jacket, a contrivance for restraining the arms of a violently disturbed person.
  s's of the pelvis, the openings of the true pelvis, distinguished as superior and inferior.

stramonium (strah-mo'ne-um) dried leaves and flowering or fruiting tops of *Datura stramonium;* used in parasympathetic blockade.

strangulated (strang'gu-lat"ed) congested by reason of constriction or hernial restriction, as strangulated HERNIA.

strangulation (strang"gu-la'shun) 1. arrest of respiration by occlusion of the air passages. 2. impairment of the blood supply to a part by mechanical constriction of the vessels.

914

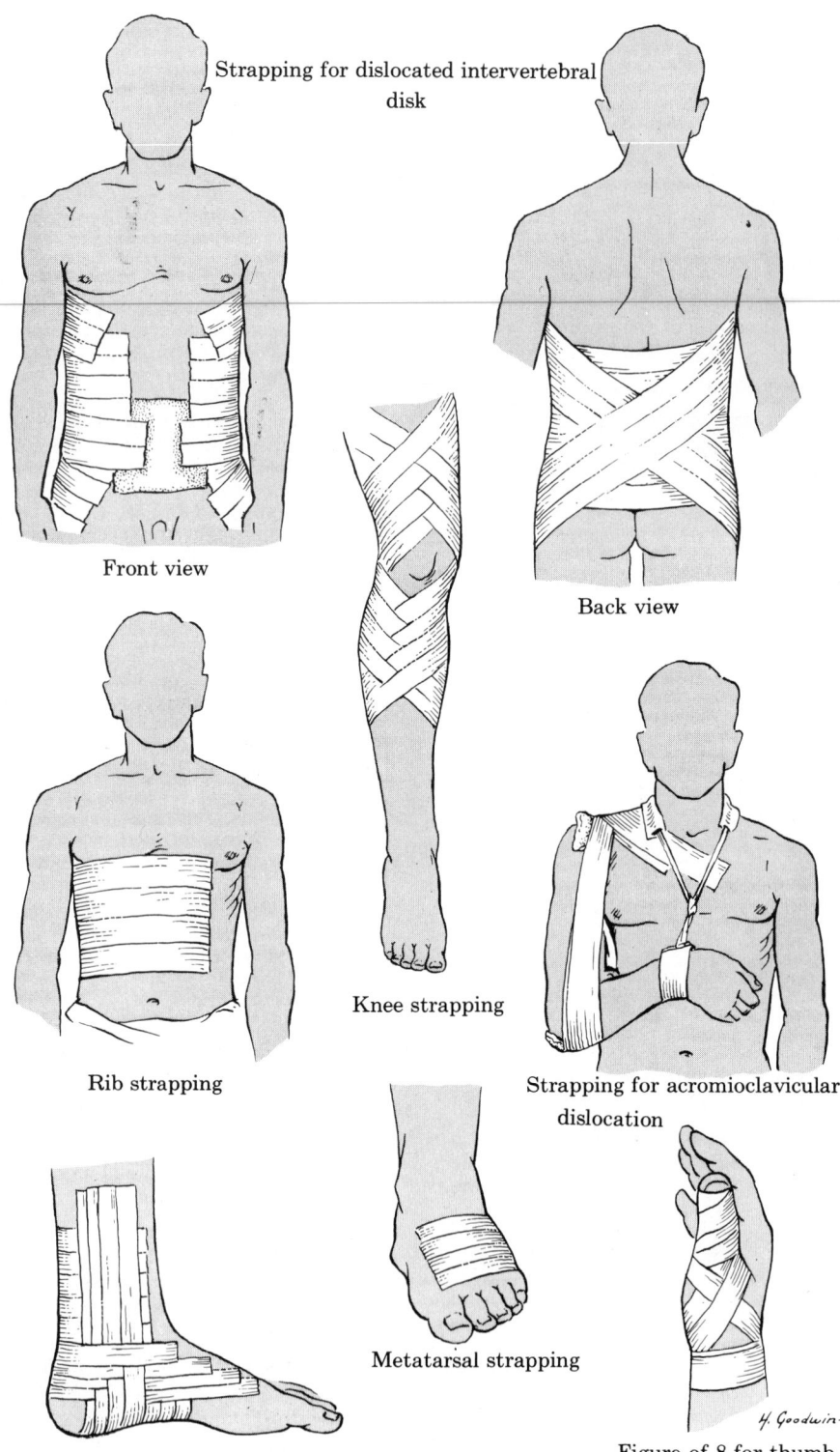

Strapping for dislocated intervertebral
disk

Front view

Back view

Knee strapping

Rib strapping

Strapping for acromioclavicular
dislocation

Basket weave for ankle

Metatarsal strapping

Figure-of-8 for thumb

H. Goodwin-

Types of strapping. (From Dorland's Illustrated Medical Dictionary. 24th ed. Philadelphia, W. B. Saunders Co., 1965.)

strangury (strang'gu-re) slow and painful discharge of urine.

strap (strap) to bind with overlapping strips of adhesive plaster, in order to hold together and prevent movement.

   Montgomery s's, straps made of lengths of adhesive tape, used to secure dressings that must be changed frequently.

stratification (strat"ĭ-fĭ-ca'shun) arrangement in layers.

stratiform (strat'ĭ-form) occurring in layers.

stratigraphy (strah-tig'rah-fe) a method of body-section roentgenography.

stratum (stra'tum), pl. *stra'ta* [L.] a sheetlike mass of tissue of fairly uniform thickness; used in anatomic nomenclature to designate distinct layers making up various tissues or organs, as of the skin, brain, retina.

   s. cor'neum, the outer horny layer of the epidermis, consisting of cells that are dead and desquamating.

   s. germinati'vum, the innermost layer of the epidermis.

   s. granulo'sum, 1. the layer of epidermis next to the stratum lucidum. 2. one of the layers of the retina. 3. a layer of the cortex of the cerebellum. 4. the cellular layer of the wall of an ovarian follicle.

   s. lu'cidum, the clear translucent layer of the skin, just beneath the stratum corneum.

strawberry mark congenital hemangioma.

streak (strēk) a line or stripe.

   angioid s's, pigmented streaks appearing in the retina after hemorrhage.

   primitive s., a thickened axial band appearing caudally on the surface of the embryonic disk.

strephosymbolia (stref"o-sim-bo'le-ah) 1. a reading difficulty inconsistent with a child's general intelligence with confusion between similar but opposite letters (b-d, p-q), and a tendency to read backward. 2. a perceptual disorder in which objects are perceived as mirror images.

strepto- (strep'to) word element [Gr.], *twisted.*

Streptobacillus (strep"to-bah-sil'us) a genus of Schizomycetes.

   s. monilifor'mis, the organism that causes Haverhill fever, a form of RATBITE FEVER.

streptococcal (strep"to-kok'al) pertaining to or due to a streptococcus.

   s. sore throat, "strep throat," a sore throat caused by a streptococcus. The symptoms are more severe than in ordinary sore throat. There may be high fever, swelling of the glands of the neck and a rash. Treatment is usually with penicillin or other antibiotics.

Streptococceae (strep"to-kok'se-e) a tribe of Schizomycetes, occurring as gram-positive spheres in pairs or chains.

streptococcemia (strep"to-kok-se'me-ah) the presence of streptococci in the blood.

streptococcolysin (strep"to-kok-ol'ĭ-sin) streptolysin.

streptococcosis (strep"to-kok-o'sis) infection caused by streptococci.

Streptococcus (strep"to-kok'us) a genus of Schizomycetes. It is separable into the pyogenic group, the viridans group, the enterococcus group and the lactic group. The first group includes the beta-hemolytic human and animal pathogens; the second and third include alpha-hemolytic parasitic forms occurring as normal flora in the upper respiratory tract and the intestinal tract, respectively; and the fourth is made up of saprophytic forms.

   S. pyog'enes, beta-hemolytic, toxigenic pyogenic streptococci of group A, causing septic sore throat, scarlet fever, rheumatic fever, puerperal fever, acute glomerulonephritis and other conditions in man.

streptococcus (strep"to-kok'us), pl. *streptococ'ci* [Gr.] an organism of the genus Streptococcus.

   hemolytic s., any streptococcus that is capable of hemolyzing erythrocytes. The majority of pathogenic streptococci belong to this group.

streptodermatitis (strep"to-der"mah-ti'tis) dermatitis produced by streptococci.

streptodornase (strep"to-dor'nās) a substance produced by hemolytic streptococci that catalyzes the depolymerization of deoxyribonucleic acid (DNA).

streptokinase (strep"to-ki'nās) an enzyme produced by streptococci that catalyzes the conversion of plasminogen to plasmin.

   s.-streptodornase, a mixture of enzymes elaborated by hemolytic streptococci; used as a proteolytic and fibrinolytic agent.

streptoleukocidin (strep"to-lu"ko-si'din) a toxin from streptococci that is destructive to leukocytes.

streptolysin (strep-tol'ĭ-sin) the hemolysin of hemolytic streptococci.

Streptomyces (strep"to-mi'sēz) a genus of Schizomycetes, usually soil forms, but occasionally parasitic on plants and animals, and notable as the source of various antibiotics, e.g., the tetracyclines.

streptomycin (strep"to-mi'sin) an antibiotic substance produced by a species of Streptomyces.

streptonivicin (strep"to-ni'vĭ-sin) novobiocin, an antibiotic.

streptothricin (strep"to-thri'sin) an antibiotic substance active against gram-negative and gram-positive bacteria.

stress (stres) 1. forcibly exerted influence; pressure. 2. any condition or situation that causes strain or tension. Stress may be either physical or psychologic, or both. Just as a bridge is structurally capable of adjusting to certain physical stresses, the human body and mind are normally able to adapt to the stresses of new situations. However, this ability has definite limits beyond which continued stress may cause a breakdown, although this limit varies from person to person.

PHYSICAL STRESS. There are many kinds of physical stress, but they can be divided into two principal types, to which the body reacts in different ways. There is emergency stress, a situation that poses an immediate threat, such as a near accident in an automobile, a wound or an injury. There is also continuing stress, such as that caused by changes in the body during puberty, pregnancy, menopause, acute and chronic diseases and continuing exposure to excessive noise, vibration, fumes or chemicals.

The body's reaction to emergency stress is set off by the adrenal medulla. The medulla of each adrenal gland is directly connected to the nervous system. When an emergency arises, it pours the hormone epinephrine into the bloodstream. This has the effect of speeding up the heart and raising the blood pressure, emptying sugar supplies swiftly into the blood and dilating the blood vessels in the muscles to give them immediate use of this energy. At the same time, the pupils of the eyes dilate. (See also ALARM REACTION.)

The reaction of the body to continuing stress is even more complex. Again the principal organs are the adrenal glands, but after the first phase of alarm, the glands continue to produce a steady supply of hormones that apparently increase the body's resistance. This is in addition to specific defenses such as the production of antibodies to fight infection. If the stress is overwhelming, as in the case of an extensive third-degree burn or an uncontrollable infectious disease, the third phase, exhaustion of the adrenal glands, sets in, sometimes with fatal results.

PSYCHOLOGIC STRESS. The emergency response of the body comes into play when a person merely foresees or imagines danger, as well as in real emergency situations. The thought of danger, or the vicarious experience of danger in a thrilling story, play or film, may be enough to cause the muscles to tense and start the heart pounding. Psychologic situations can have the same effect. One of the best-known examples of this is "stage fright," often characterized by tensed muscles and an increased heart rate. At times the person may not even be aware of the unconscious thought that produces this dramatic reaction.

When stress is prolonged, the response may in fact damage the body. For example, peptic ULCER may result from prolonged nervous tension in response to real or imagined stresses in people who have a predisposition for ulcers. Such reactions to stress are discussed under PSYCHOSOMATIC ILLNESS.

The mind also responds to stress by adaptation. A healthy person can usually "get used" to situations that involve a certain amount of stress.

stretcher (strech'er) a contrivance for carrying the sick or wounded.

stria (stri'ah), pl. *stri'ae* [L.] 1. a streak or line. 2. a narrow, bandlike structure; used in anatomic nomenclature to designate longitudinal collections of nerve fibers in the brain.

  atrophic striae, stri'ae atroph'icae, colorless lines on the abdomen, breasts or thighs, caused by mechanical stretching of the skin, as by a pregnant uterus or a tumor; purple striae occur in adrenocortical hyperactivity (Cushing's syndrome)

or increased corticosteroid levels in the body from whatever cause.

  stri'ae gravida'rum, striae atrophicae occurring in pregnancy.

  stri'ae medulla'res, white lines across the floor of the fourth ventricle.

striate (stri'āt) having streaks or striae.

striation (stri-a'shun) 1. the quality of being streaked. 2. a streak or scratch, or a series of streaks.

Striatran (stri'ah-tran) trademark for a preparation of emylcamate, a tranquilizer.

stricture (strik'tūr) abnormal narrowing of a duct or passage.

stricturotome (strik'tu-ro-tōm″) an instrument for cutting strictures.

stricturotomy (strik″tu-rot'o-me) incision of a stricture.

stridor (stri'dor) a shrill, harsh sound, especially the respiratory sound heard during inspiration in laryngeal obstruction. adj., **strid'ulous.**

  s. den'tium, grinding of the teeth, especially during sleep.

striocerebellar (stri″o-ser″ĕ-bel'ar) pertaining to the corpus striatum and cerebellum.

strobila (stro-bi'lah) the entire adult tapeworm, including the scolex, neck and proglottids.

stroke (strōk) 1. a sudden and severe attack. 2. rupture or blockage of a blood vessel in the brain, depriving parts of the brain of blood supply, resulting in loss of consciousness, paralysis or other symptoms depending on the site and extent of brain damage; called also CEREBRAL VASCULAR ACCIDENT or cerebral apoplexy.

  heat s., a condition caused by exposure to excessive heat; see also SUNSTROKE.

stroma (stro'mah), pl. *stro'mata* [Gr.] the tissue forming the ground substance, framework or matrix of an organ, as opposed to the functioning part or parenchyma. adj., **stro'mal, stromat'ic.**

stromuhr (strōm'oor) an instrument for measuring the velocity of the blood flow.

Strongyloides (stron″jī-loi'dēz) a genus of nematode parasites.

  S. stercora'lis, a species found in the intestine of man and other mammals, primarily in the tropics and subtropics, usually causing diarrhea.

strongyloidiasis, strongyloidosis (stron″jī-loi-di'ah-sis), (stron″jī-loi-do'sis) infection with organisms of the genus Strongyloides.

strontium (stron'she-um) a chemical element, atomic number 38, atomic weight 87.62, symbol Sr. (See table of ELEMENTS.)

strontiuresis (stron″she-u-re'sis) elimination of strontium from the body through the kidneys.

strophulus (strof'u-lus) a papular eruption occurring in infants.

struma (stroo'mah) enlargement of the thyroid gland.

  Hashimoto's s., s. lymphomato'sa, a progressive

disease of the thyroid gland with degeneration of its epithelial elements and replacement by lymphoid and fibrous tissue.

s. malig'na, carcinoma of the thyroid gland.

s. ova'rii, an ovarian tumor containing iodine and histologically resembling thyroid tissue.

Riedel's s., a chronic, proliferating, fibrosing, inflammatory process involving usually one but sometimes both lobes of the thyroid gland, as well as the trachea and other adjacent structures.

strumectomy (stroo-mek'to-me) thyroidectomy.

strumitis (stroo-mi'tis) thyroiditis.

strumous (stroo'mus) scrofulous.

Strümpell's disease (strim'pelz) 1. hereditary spastic spinal paralysis. 2. polioencephalomyelitis.

Strümpell-Leichtenstern disease (strim'pel lĭk'ten-stern) hemorrhagic encephalitis.

Strümpell-Marie disease (strim'pel mah-re') rheumatoid spondylitis.

strychnine (strik'nīn) an alkaloid from seeds of *Strychnos nux-vomica;* used as a central nervous system stimulant.

strychninomania (strik″nin-o-ma'ne-ah) psychosis caused by strychnine.

strychnism (strik'nizm) poisoning by strychnine.

Stryker frame (stri'ker) an apparatus specially designed for care of patients with injuries of the spinal cord or paralysis. It is constructed of pipe and canvas and is designed so that one nurse can turn the patient without difficulty. The frame on which the patient lies while in the supine position is called the posterior frame; the anterior frame is used when the patient is turned on his abdomen. There are perineal openings in both frames for use of a bedpan.

S.T.S. serologic test for syphilis.

Stuart factor (stu'art) clotting factor X.

stump (stump) the distal end of a limb left after amputation.

stupe (stoop) a hot, wet cloth or sponge, charged with a medication for external application.

stupefacient (stu″pĕ-fa'shent) 1. inducing stupor. 2. an agent that induces stupor.

stupefactive (stu″pĕ-fak'tiv) producing narcosis or stupor.

stupor (stu'por) partial or nearly complete unconsciousness; a state of lethargy and immobility with diminished responsiveness to stimulation. adj., **stu'porous.**

Sturge-Weber disease (sterj web'er) telangiectases of the nervous system, with mental defect, focal epilepsy, enlargement of the eye, intracranial calcification and facial nevi, chiefly within the distribution of the ophthalmic nerve.

stuttering (stut'er-ing) a speech problem involving three definitive factors: (1) speech disfluency, most significantly the repetition of parts of words or whole words, prolongation of sounds or words and unduly prolonged pauses; (2) unfavorable reactions of listeners to the speaker's speech defect; and (3) the reactions of the speaker to the listeners' reactions, as well as to his own speech problems and to his conception of himself as a stutterer. (See also SPEECH.)

sty (sti) inflammation of one or more of the sebaceous glands of the eyelid; the lesion resembles a pimple. Called also hordeolum.

Hot compresses applied for 15 minutes every 2 hours may help localize the infection and promote drainage. In some cases a small surgical incision may be necessary. A mild antiseptic may be prescribed to prevent spread of the infection.

styl(o)- (sti'lo) word element [L., Gr.], *stake; pole; styloid process of the temporal bone.*

stylet (sti'let) stilet.

styloid (sti'loid) long and pointed, like a pen or stylus.

s. process, a bony projection, particularly a long spine projecting downward from the inferior surface of the temporal bone.

styloiditis (sti″loi-di'tis) inflammation of tissues around the styloid process.

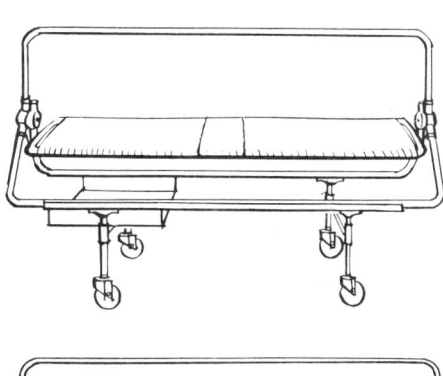

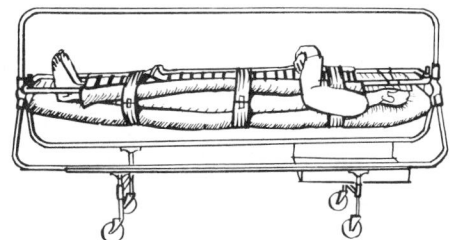

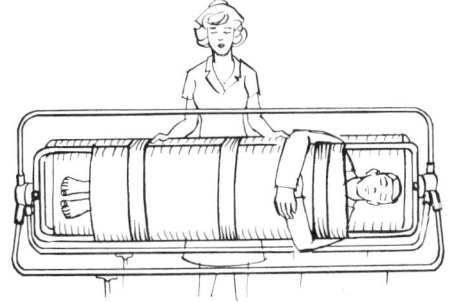

Stryker frame. (From Sutton, A. L.: Bedside Nursing Techniques. 2nd ed. Philadelphia, W. B. Saunders Co., 1969.)

stylomastoid (sti″lo-mas′toid) pertaining to the styloid and mastoid processes of the temporal bone.

stylomaxillary (sti″lo-mak′sĭ-ler″e) pertaining to the styloid process of the temporal bone and the maxilla.

stylus (sti′lus) 1. a stilet. 2. a pencil or stick, as of caustic.

stype (stīp) a tampon or pledget of cotton.

stypsis (stip′sis) 1. astringency; astringent action. 2. use of styptics.

styptic (stip′tik) 1. arresting hemorrhage by means of an astringent quality. 2. a markedly astringent remedy. A chemical styptic works by causing the formation of a blood clot by chemical action. A vascular styptic checks bleeding by causing the blood vessels to contract. A mechanical styptic causes clotting by mechanical means — for example, when one applies a bit of paper or cotton to a slight razor cut.
A styptic pencil is frequently used to stop bleeding from slight cuts. Styptics in various other forms are used by physicians in surgery.

Stypven (stip′ven) trademark for a preparation of Russell's viper venom; used as a hemostatic agent.

styramate (stir′ah-māt) a compound used as a skeletal muscle relaxant.

Suavitil (swav′ĭ-til) trademark for a preparation of benactyzine, used in parasympathetic blockade and as a tranquilizer.

sub (sub) [L.] preposition, *under.*

sub- (sub) word element [L.], *under; less than.*

subabdominal (sub″ab-dom′ĭ-nal) below the abdomen.

subacid (sub-as′id) somewhat acid.

subacromial (sub″ah-kro′me-al) below the acromion.

subacute (sub″ah-kūt′) somewhat acute; between acute and chronic.

subalimentation (sub″al-ĭ-men-ta′shun) insufficient nourishment.

subaponeurotic (sub″ap-o-nu-rot′ik) below an aponeurosis.

subarachnoid (sub″ah-rak′noid) below the arachnoid.

subarachnoiditis (sub″ah-rak″noi-di′tis) inflammation on the lower surface of the arachnoid.

subareolar (sub″ah-re′o-lar) beneath the areola of the nipple.

subastragalar (sub″ah-strag′ah-lar) below the astragalus (talus).

subastringent (sub″ah-strin′jent) moderately astringent.

subaural (sub-aw′ral) below the ear.

subcapsular (sub-kap′su-lar) below a capsule, especially the capsule of the brain.

subcartilaginous (sub-kar″tĭ-laj′ĭ-nus) 1. below a cartilage. 2. partly cartilaginous.

subclavian, subclavicular (sub-kla′ve-an), (sub″klah-vik′u-lar) below the clavicle.

subclinical (sub-klin′ĭ-kal) without clinical manifestations; said of the early stages or a very mild form of a disease.

subconjunctival (sub″kon-jungk-ti′val) beneath the conjunctiva.

subconscious (sub-kon′shus) 1. imperfectly or partially conscious, yet capable of being made conscious by an effort of memory or by association of ideas; called also preconscious. 2. the area of mental activity below the level of conscious perception.

subconsciousness (sub-kon′shus-nes) partial unconsciousness.

subcoracoid (sub-kor′ah-koid) situated under the coracoid process.

subcortex (sub-kor′teks) the brain substance underlying the cortex. adj., **subcor′tical.**

subcostal (sub-kos′tal) below a rib or ribs.

subcostalgia (sub″kos-tal′je-ah) pain over the subcostal nerve, i.e., in the region of the appendix, epigastrium and kidney.

subcranial (sub-kra′ne-al) below the cranium.

subcrepitant (sub-krep′ĭ-tant) somewhat crepitant in nature.

subculture (sub-kul′tūr) a culture of bacteria derived from another culture.

subcutaneous (sub″ku-ta′ne-us) beneath the layers of the skin.
s. injection, an injection made into the subcutaneous tissues (see also subcutaneous INJECTION).

subcuticular (sub″ku-tik′u-lar) below the epidermis.

subdiaphragmatic (sub-di″ah-frag-mat′ik) below the diaphragm.

subdural (sub-du′ral) beneath the dura mater.

subencephalon (sub″en-sef′ah-lon) the pons, medulla oblongata and corpora quadrigemina.

subendocardial (sub″en-do-kar′de-al) below the endocardium.

subendothelial (sub″en-do-the′le-al) beneath an endothelial layer.

subepidermal (sub″ep-ĭ-der′mal) below the epidermis.

subepithelial (sub″ep-ĭ-the′le-al) below the epithelium.

subfamily (sub-fam′ĭ-le) a taxonomic order sometimes established, subordinate to a family and superior to a tribe.

subfascial (sub-fash′al) below a fascia.

subfebrile (sub-feb′ril) somewhat febrile.

subfertility (sub″fer-til′ĭ-te) a state of less than normal fertility.

subfrontal (sub-frun′tal) below the frontal lobe or convolution.

subgenus (sub-je′nus) a taxonomic category sometimes established, subordinate to a genus and superior to a species.

subglenoid (sub-gle′noid) below the glenoid (mandibular) fossa.

subglossal (sub-glos′al) below the tongue.

subgrondation (sub″gron-da′shun) depression of one fragment of bone beneath another.

subhepatic (sub″hĕ-pat′ik) below the liver.

subhyoid (sub-hi′oid) below the hyoid bone.

subiculum (su-bik′u-lum) an underlying or supporting structure.

subiliac (sub-il′e-ak) below the ilium.

subilium (sub-il′e-um) the lowest portion of the ilium.

subinfection (sub″in-fek′shun) 1. a mild infection. 2. infection due to weakening of the resisting cells from constant effort in overcoming pathogenic organisms.

subinvolution (sub″in-vo-lu′shun) incomplete involution; failure of a part to return to its normal size and condition after enlargement from functional activity.

subjacent (sub-ja′sent) located below.

subject (sub′jekt) a person or animal subjected to treatment, observation or experiment.

subjective (sub-jek′tiv) perceived only by the individual involved.

subjugal (sub-ju′gal) below the zygomatic bone.

sublatio retinae (sub-la′she-o ret′ĭ-ne) detachment of the retina of the eye (see DETACHMENT OF RETINA).

sublesional (sub-le′zhun-al) performed or situated beneath a lesion.

sublethal (sub-le′thal) not sufficient to cause death.

sublimate (sub′lĭ-māt) a substance obtained by sublimation (1).

sublimation (sub″lĭ-ma′shun) 1. the conversion of a solid directly into the vapor state. 2. a defense mechanism in which an individual diverts his socially unacceptable instinctive drives into personally approved and socially acceptable channels. Mental conflicts may be resolved by this means although the person achieves only partial satisfaction of his impulses.

subliminal (sub-lim′ĭ-nal) below the threshold of sensation or conscious awareness.

sublingual (sub-ling′gwal) beneath the tongue.
  s. gland, a salivary gland on either side under the tongue.

sublinguitis (sub″ling-gwi′tis) inflammation of the sublingual gland.

sublumbar (sub-lum′bar) below the lumbar region.

subluxation (sub″luk-sa′shun) incomplete or partial DISLOCATION.

submammary (sub-mam′ar-e) below the mammary gland.

submandibular (sub″man-dib′u-lar) below the mandible.

submaxilla (sub″mak-sil′ah) the mandible.

submaxillaritis (sub″mak-sĭ-ler-i′tis) inflammation of the submaxillary gland.

submaxillary (sub-mak′sĭ-ler″e) below the maxilla.
  s. gland, a salivary gland on the inner side of each ramus of the lower jaw.

submental (sub-men′tal) below the chin.

submersion (sub-mer′zhun) the act of placing or the condition of being under the surface of a liquid.

submicron (sub-mi′kron) a small particle invisible with the microscope, but visible with the ultramicroscope.

submicroscopic (sub-mi″kro-skop′ik) too small to be visible with the microscope.

submorphous (sub-mor′fus) neither amorphous nor perfectly crystalline.

submucosa (sub″mu-ko′sah) areolar tissue situated beneath a mucous membrane.

submucous (sub-mu′kus) below mucous membrane.

subnarcotic (sub″nar-kot′ik) moderately narcotic.

subnatant (sub-na′tant) 1. situated below or at the bottom of something. 2. the liquid lying beneath a layer of precipitated insoluble material.

subneural (sub-nu′ral) beneath a nerve or the cerebrospinal axis.

subnormal (sub-nor′mal) below or less than normal.

subnormality (sub″nor-mal′ĭ-te) a state less than normal or that usually encountered, as mental subnormality, generally considered characterized by an intelligence quotient under 69.

suboccipital (sub″ok-sip′ĭ-tal) below the occiput.

suboperculum (sub″o-per′ku-lum) the portion of occipital gyrus overlying the insula.

suborbital (sub-or′bĭ-tal) beneath the orbit.

suborder (sub-or′der) a taxonomic category sometimes established, subordinate to an order and superior to a family.

suboxide (sub-ok′sīd) that oxide in any series which contains the least oxygen.

subpapular (sub-pap′u-lar) indistinctly papular.

subpatellar (sub″pah-tel′ar) below the patella.

subpericardial (sub″per-ĭ-kar′de-al) beneath the pericardium.

subperiosteal (sub″per-e-os′te-al) beneath the periosteum.

subperitoneal (sub″per-ĭ-to-ne′al) beneath the peritoneum.

subpharyngeal (sub″fah-rin′je-al) beneath the pharynx.

subphrenic (sub-fren′ik) beneath the diaphragm.

subphylum (sub-fi′lum), pl. *subphy′la* [L., Gr.] a taxonomic category sometimes established, subordinate to a phylum and superior to a class.

subplacenta (sub″plah-sen′tah) the decidua basalis.

subpleural (sub-ploo′ral) beneath the pleura.

subpontine (sub-pon′tīn) beneath the pons.

subpreputial (sub″pre-pu′shal) beneath the prepuce.

subpubic (sub-pu′bik) beneath the pubic bone.

subpulmonary (sub-pul′mo-ner″e) beneath the lung.

subretinal (sub-ret′ĭ-nal) beneath the retina.

subsalt (sub′sawlt) a basic salt.

subscapular (sub-skap′u-lar) below the scapula.

subscription (sub-skrip′shun) the third chief part of a drug prescription, comprising directions to be followed by the pharmacist in its preparation.

subserous (sub-se′rus) beneath a serous membrane.

subspecies (sub-spe′shēz) a subdivision of a species.

substage (sub′stāj) the part of the microscope underneath the stage.

substance (sub′stans) the material constituting an organ or body.
  agglutinable s., a substance in erythrocytes and bacteria, with which the agglutinin unites to produce specific agglutination.
  agglutinating s., agglutinin.
  depressor s., a substance that tends to decrease activity or blood pressure.
  gray s., nerve tissue composed of nerve cell bodies, unmyelinated nerve fibers and supporting tissue; called also GRAY MATTER.
  ground s., the BASIC homogeneous material of a tissue or organ, in which the specific components occur.
  hemolytic s., the material in a serum that destroys the erythrocytes of a serum added to it.
  medullary s., 1. the white matter of the central nervous system, consisting of axons and their myelin sheaths. 2. the soft, marrow-like substance of such structures as bone marrow, kidney and adrenal gland.
  posterior perforated s., an area on the ventral surface of the brain between the cerebral peduncles that is pierced by numerous branches of the posterior cerebral artery.
  pressor s., a substance that raises blood pressure.
  reaction s., a substance formed in the body of an animal on immunization with cellular products from an animal of another species.
  reticular s., the netlike mass of threads seen in erythrocytes after vital staining.
  transmitter s., a chemical substance that induces activity in an excitable tissue.
  white s., tissue consisting mostly of myelinated nerve fibers and constituting the conducting portion of the brain and spinal cord; called also white matter.

substantia (sub-stan′she-ah), pl. *substan′tiae* [L.] substance; used in anatomic nomenclature in naming various components of various tissues and structures of the body.
  s. gelatino′sa, the substance sheathing the posterior horn of the spinal cord and lining its central canal.
  s. ni′gra, a layer of pigmented gray matter in the brain stem found to undergo pathologic changes in Parkinson's disease.

substernal (sub-ster′nal) below the sternum.

substitution (sub″stī-tu′shun) 1. the act of putting one thing in the place of another, especially the chemical replacement of one substance by another. 2. a defense mechanism in which an individual replaces an unattainable or unacceptable goal, emotion or motive with one that is attainable or acceptable.

substrate (sub′strāt) the compound whose chemical transformation is catalyzed by an enzyme.

substructure (sub′struk-tūr) the underlying or supporting portion of an organ or appliance.

subthalamus (sub-thal′ah-mus) a portion of the hypothalamus situated between the thalamus and the tegmentum of the midbrain.

subtle (sut′l) 1. very fine, as a subtle powder. 2. very acute, as a subtle pain.

subtribe (sub′trīb) a taxonomic category sometimes established, subordinate to a tribe and superior to a genus.

subtrochanteric (sub″tro-kan-ter′ik) below the trochanter.

subtympanic (sub″tim-pan′ik) somewhat tympanic in quality.

subungual (sub-ung′gwal) beneath a nail.

suburethral (sub″u-re′thral) beneath the urethra.

subvaginal (sub-vaj′ĭ-nal) under a sheath, or below the vagina.

subvertebral (sub-ver′tĕ-bral) on the ventral side of the vertebrae.

subvirile (sub-vir′il) having deficient virility.

subvitaminosis (sub-vi″tah-mĭ-no′sis) a vitamin deficiency state.

subvitrinal (sub-vit′rĭ-nal) beneath the vitreous.

subvolution (sub″vo-lu′shun) the operation of turning over a flap to prevent adhesions.

Sucaryl (soo'kah-ril) trademark for a noncaloric sweetening agent.

succagogue (suk'ah-gog) 1. inducing glandular secretion. 2. an agent that induces glandular secretion.

succenturiate (suk″sen-tu're-āt) accessory; serving as a substitute.

succinic acid (suk-sin'ik) a compound formed in the aerobic metabolism of carbohydrate in the body.

succinylcholine (suk″sī-nil-ko'lēn) a compound used as a skeletal muscle relaxant.

succinylsulfathiazole (suk″sī-nil-sul″fah-thi'ah-zōl) an antibacterial agent used in infections of the intestinal tract.

succorrhea (suk″o-re'ah) excessive flow of a natural secretion.

succus (suk'us), pl. *suc'ci* [L.] any fluid derived from living tissue; bodily secretion; juice.

succussion (sŭ-kush'un) a splashing sound elicited when a patient is shaken, indicative of fluid and air in a body cavity.

sucrase (soo'krās) invertin.

sucroclastic (soo″kro-klas'tik) splitting up sugar.

sucrose (soo'krōs) a sugar obtained from sugar cane, sugar beet or other sources; used as a food and sweetening agent.

suction (suk'shun) the withdrawal or uptake of fluid by creation of a partial vacuum.
   post-tussive s., a sucking sound heard over a lung cavity just after a cough.

suctorian (suk-to're-an) a protozoan of the subphylum Ciliophora, characterized by the presence of cilia only during the young developmental stages, the mature organisms having specialized tentacles that serve as locomotor and food-acquiring mechanisms.

sudamen (soo-da'men), pl. *sudam'ina* [L.] a small whitish vesicle caused by retention of sweat in the layers of the epidermis.

Sudan (soo-dan') a substance used as a stain.
   S. red III, a stain that colors fatty tissues red and also is used for tubercle bacilli.

sudanophilia (soo-dan″o-fil'e-ah) a condition in which the leukocytes contain particles staining readily with Sudan red III.

sudarium (soo-da're-um) a sweat bath.

sudation (soo-da'shun) 1. the process of sweating. 2. excessive sweating.

sudatoria (soo″dah-to're-ah) hyperhidrosis.

sudatorium (soo″dah-to're-um), pl. *sudato'ria* [L.] a hot air bath or sweat bath.

Sudeck's disease (soo'deks) acute atrophy of a carpal or tarsal bone, resulting from trauma.

sudogram (soo'do-gram) a graphic representation of the sweating response of different areas of the body after injection of a dye that is excreted by the sweat glands.

sudokeratosis (soo″do-ker″ah-to'sis) keratosis of the sweat ducts.

sudomotor (soo″do-mo'tor) exerting an influence on the sweat glands.

sudor (soo'dor) sweat; perspiration.
   s. an'glicus, miliary fever.
   s. cruen'tus, the excretion of red sweat.

sudoral (soo'dor-al) characterized by profuse sweating.

sudoresis (soo″do-re'sis) profuse sweating.

sudorific (soo″dŏ-rif'ik) an agent causing sweating.

sudoriparous (soo″dŏ-rip'ah-rus) secreting or producing sweat.

suet (soo'et) the hard internal fat of the abdomen of a food animal.
   mutton s., prepared s., the internal fat of the abdomen of sheep; used in formulating ointment bases.

suffocation (suf″ŏ-ka'shun) the stoppage of breathing, or the asphyxia that results from it. If suffocation is complete—that is, no air at all reaches the lungs—the lack of oxygen and excess of carbon dioxide in the blood will cause almost immediate loss of consciousness. Though the heart continues to beat briefly, death will follow in a matter of minutes unless emergency measures are taken to get breathing started again.

Suffocation can be caused by drowning, electric shock, gas or smoke poisoning, strangulation or choking on a foreign body in the trachea. Once the cause of suffocation has been removed, the most important first-aid measure is ARTIFICIAL RESPIRATION, preferably the mouth-to-mouth technique.

FIRST AID IN CASES OF SUFFOCATION. In any emergency when breathing has stopped, have someone get help from the police, a fire department, a nearby hospital or a physician. Meanwhile, give first aid as directed below. Artificial respiration, when called for, should be given preferably by the mouth-to-mouth method.

Drowning
   1. Clear sand and other material from the mouth.
   2. Give artificial respiration.
Gas Poisoning
   1. Drag victim into open air.
   2. Give artificial respiration.
Electric Shock
   1. If victim is in contact with live wire or other electrical source, turn off electric current; if this is impossible, break contact by using a dry board or other nonconductor of electricity.
   2. Give artificial respiration.
Strangulation
   1. Remove whatever is causing strangulation if it is still present.
   2. Give artificial respiration.
Choking on Foreign Body
   1. Slap person on the back; if he is a child, turn him upside down and slap him on back.
   2. Try to remove object with fingers or forceps.

suffusion (sŭ-fu'zhun) 1. the process of overspreading, or diffusion. 2. the condition of being moistened or permeated through.

sugar   (shoog'ar) a simple carbohydrate distributed universally in plants and animal tissues, containing carbon and hydrogen usually in the ratio of 1 to 2.

 cane s., sucrose.

 diabetic s., glucose found in the urine in diabetes mellitus.

 fruit s., levulose.

 invert s., a natural mixture of dextrose and levulose.

 liver s., dextrose from the liver.

 malt s., maltose.

 milk s., lactose.

 starch s., dextrin.

 wood s., xylose.

suggestibility   (sug-jes″ti-bil′i-te) inclination to act on suggestions of others.

suggestible   (sug-jes′ti-bl) inclined to act on the suggestion of another.

suggestion   (sug-jes′chun) impartation of an idea to a subject from without.

 hypnotic s., one imparted to a person in the hypnotic state.

 posthypnotic s., implantation in the mind of a subject during hypnosis of a suggestion to be acted upon after recovery from the hypnotic state.

sugillation   (sug″ji-la′shun) a bruise or ecchymosis.

suicide   (soo′i-sīd) the taking of one's own life. Deaths from suicide total more than 20,000 a year in the United States. These figures do not include the many thousands of people who die each year from complications caused by suicide attempts, or the suicides whose death records are made out as accidental death because the evidence is not clear. The great majority of suicides are preventable.

 Suicide is four times more common among men than women. The suicide rate is four times higher among those over 55 than in the 25 to 34 age group. Adolescent suicides are also shockingly frequent. Every year several hundred persons aged 15 to 19, and a few in younger groups, commit suicide.

 SUICIDAL TENDENCIES. All deeply depressed people are potential suicides. Their depression may be set off by illness or an external event, such as the death of a friend or relative, or there may be no apparent cause. However, depressed people do not always admit their suicidal thoughts, even to a psychiatrist; in fact, they often deny them. The suicidal impulse appears to arise in many cases from a combination of hate, rage, revenge, a sense of guilt and a feeling of unbearable frustration. Suicide often appears to be an act of spite in which the person who takes his own life expresses toward himself the resentment he feels toward other people or the world in general. Simultaneously, he dramatically punishes himself for his own shortcomings. The majority of people who commit suicide suffer from neuroses; some are psychotic. (See NEUROSIS and PSYCHOSIS.)

 Early signs of suicidal tendencies include low moods, with expressions of guilt, tension and agitation; insomnia, early morning awakenings, requests for more sleeping pills; neglected personal appearance in one who is normally tidy; loss of weight and appetite; inability to concentrate; preoccupation with death; crumped copies of tentative suicide notes, left in wastebaskets or on desks; and heavier drinking, to give the person the courage to act.

 TREATMENT AND PREVENTION.   The suicidal person may be treated in the physician's office, in the psychiatric service of a general hospital or in a mental hospital if his condition warrants it. Above all, he should remain under medical supervision until the danger of suicide has passed.

 Any suicide threat must be taken seriously. The widespread belief that no one who talks about suicide is likely to attempt it is false. A suicide threat is perhaps the most important danger signal of all. Of those who commit suicide, at least 80 per cent have discussed it with physicians or relatives.

 Mentally disturbed suicidal persons can often be helped by psychotherapy, which will attempt to discover the actual cause of the person's wish to die. At the same time, the psychiatrist may use other means, such as antidepressant drugs (the opposite of tranquilizers) to help depressed patients out of their suicidal moods.

 The Save-A-Life League, founded about 1902 in New York City, and now also represented in numerous other cities throughout the United States, has helped to rescue more than 50,000 men and women from suicide. Many presuicidal people who are afraid to talk to doctors and clergymen will use this telephone service, maintained around the clock, to listen to the comforting voices of the professional "operators" until a member of the organization can visit the potential suicide and arrange for medical or psychiatric care. Other successful lay antisuicide organizations, relying primarily on telephone service, have been established in the country.

 The Suicide Prevention Center, located in the Los Angeles County General Hospital, is a project set up by psychologists at the University of Southern California in cooperation with the National Institute of Mental Health. The Center refers suicide-inclined people to community agencies, sanitariums, hospitals or state and federal mental institutions for both psychiatric and social care. Further, the Center is gathering data, for the first time in a large community, on the biologic, psychologic and other aspects of suicide.

Sulamyd   (sul′ah-mid) trademark for a preparation of sulfacetamide, a sulfonamide.

sulcate   (sul′kāt) furrowed, or marked with sulci.

sulcation   (sul-ka′shun) the formation of sulci; the state of being marked by sulci.

sulcus   (sul′kus), pl. *sul′ci* [L.] a groove or furrow; used in anatomic nomenclature to designate a linear depression, as one separating the gyri of the brain or one on the surface of another organ.

 sulci cu′tis, fine depressions of the skin between the ridges of the skin.

 gingival s., the groove between the surface of the tooth and the epithelium lining the free gingiva.

sulfa drugs   (sul′fah) a group of chemical compounds used as antibacterial agents; called also sulfonamides.

sulfacetamide   (sul″fah-set′ah-mīd) an antibacterial agent used principally in infections of the urinary tract.

sodium s., an antibacterial compound used topically in ointment or solution.

sulfadiazine (sul″fah-di′ah-zēn) a rapidly absorbed and readily excreted antibacterial agent.
  sodium s., an antibacterial compound used intravenously.

sulfadimethoxine (sul″fah-di″meth-ok′sēn) a rapidly absorbed and slowly excreted antibacterial compound used in urinary tract and other infections.

sulfadimetine (sul″fah-di′mĕ-tēn) sulfisomidine.

sulfadimidine (sul″fah-di′mĭ-dēn) sulfamethazine.

sulfaethidole (sul″fah-eth′ĭ-dōl) a compound used as an antibacterial agent.

sulfafurazole (sul″fah-fu′rah-zōl) sulfisoxazole.

sulfaguanidine (sul″fah-gwan′ĭ-dēn) one of the sulfonamides used especially in intestinal tract infections.

sulfamerazine (sul″fah-mer′ah-zēn) a readily absorbed antibacterial substance.

sulfamethazine (sul″fah-meth′ah-zēn) an antibacterial substance.

sulfamethizole (sul″fah-meth′ĭ-zōl) an antibacterial compound used mainly in urinary tract infections.

sulfamethoxazole (sul″fah-meth-ok′sah-zōl) an antibacterial agent used in both systemic and urinary tract infections.

sulfamethoxypyridazine (sul″fah-meth-ok″se-pi-rid′ah-zēn) an antibacterial agent used in urinary tract and other infections.

sulfamethyldiazine (sul″fah-meth″il-di′ah-zēn) sulfamerazine.

sulfamethylthiadiazole (sul″fah-meth″il-thi″ah-di′ah-zōl) sulfamethizole.

Sulfamezathine (sul″fah-mez′ah-thēn) trademark for a preparation of sulfamethazine.

sulfanemia (sul″fah-ne′me-ah) anemia resulting from use of sulfonamides.

sulfanilamide (sul″fah-nil′ah-mīd) a potent antibacterial compound, the first of the sulfonamides discovered.

sulfapyridine (sul″fah-pir′ĭ-dēn) a sulfonamide effective against pneumococci and staphylococci.

sulfarsphenamine (sulf″ars-fen′ah-min) an arsenic-containing compound formerly used in treatment of syphilis.

Sulfasuxidine (sul″fah-suk′sĭ-dēn) trademark for preparations of succinylsulfathiazole.

sulfatase (sul″fah-tās) an enzyme that catalyzes the hydrolysis of sulfate esters.

sulfate (sul″fāt) a salt of sulfuric acid.
  cupric s., a copper-containing compound used as a fungicide and an emetic.
  ferrous s., an iron-containing compound used in treatment of iron deficiency anemia.

Sulfathalidine (sul″fah-thal′ĭ-dēn) trademark for a preparation of phthalylsulfathiazole, an intestinal antibacterial.

sulfathiazole (sul″fah-thi′ah-zōl) an antibacterial agent.

sulfhemoglobin (sulf″he-mo-glo′bin) sulfmethemoglobin.

sulfhemoglobinemia (sulf″he-mo-glo″bĭ-ne′me-ah) sulfmethemoglobin in the blood.

sulfhydryl (sulf-hi′dril) the univalent radical, −SH.

sulfide (sul′fīd) a compound of sulfur with another element or base.

sulfinpyrazone (sul″fin-pi′rah-zōn) a uricosuric compound used in gout to promote excretion of uric acid.

sulfisomidine (sul″fĭ-som′ĭ-dēn) a compound closely related to sulfamethazine, used in urinary tract infections.

sulfisoxazole (sul″fĭ-sok′sah-zōl) an antibacterial compound used orally, topically and parenterally.

sulfmethemoglobin (sulf″met-he″mo-glo′bin) a compound of hemoglobin and hydrogen sulfide.

sulfobromophthalein (sul″fo-bro″mo-thal′ēn) a sulfur- and bromine-containing compound used in liver function tests (see also BROMSULPHALEIN).

sulfonamide (sul-fon′ah-mīd) a generic name for an antibacterial substance derived from para-aminobenzene-sulfonamide (sulfanilamide).

sulfonamiduria (sul″fōn-am″ĭ-du′re-ah) the presence of a sulfonamide in the urine.

sulfone (sul′fōn) an organic compound produced by oxidation of a sulfide.

sulfonethylmethane (sul″fōn-eth″il-meth′ān) a colorless crystalline substance, a hypnotic somnifacient.

sulfonmethane (sul″fōn-meth′ān) a compound with moderate hypnotic properties.

Sulfonsol (sul-fon′sol) trademark for a suspension of sulfadiazine, sulfamerazine and sulfamethazine for oral use as an antibacterial agent.

sulfoxide (sul-fok′sīd) 1. the divalent radical =SO. 2. an organic compound intermediate between a sulfide and a sulfone.

sulfoxone (sul-fok′sōn) an antibacterial compound derived from dapsone; used in the treatment of leprosy.

sulfur (sul′fer) a chemical element, atomic number 16, atomic weight 32.064, symbol S. (See table of ELEMENTS.)
  s. dioxide, a colorless, noninflammable gas, used as an antioxidant and pharmaceutic aid.
  s. lo′tum, washed sulfur.
  precipitated s., a fine, pale yellow powder; used in an ointment as a scabicide.
  s. sublima′tum, sublimed s., a fine yellow crystalline powder; used as a fungicide, parasiticide and keratolytic agent.

washed s., a fine yellow crystalline powder, without odor or taste; used like sublimed sulfur.

sulfurated (sul′fu-rāt″ed) combined with sulfur.

sulfuret (sul′fu-ret) sulfide.

sulfuric acid (sul-fu′rik) an oily, highly caustic, poisonous compound, H_2SO_4.

sulph- for words beginning thus, see those beginning *sulf-*.

Sul-spansion (sul-span′shun) trademark for a suspension of sulfaethidole, an antibacterial.

sunburn (sun′burn) inflammation – an actual burn – of the skin caused by exposure to ultraviolet rays of the sun. Depending on how severe the burn is, the skin may simply redden or it may become blistered and sore – a second-degree burn. In extreme cases there may be fever.

sunstroke (sun′strōk) a profound disturbance of the body's heat-regulating mechanism, caused by prolonged exposure to excessive heat from the sun, particularly when there is little or no circulation of air. Persons over 40 and those in poor health are most susceptible to it.

The condition is called also heat stroke, a somewhat broader term that covers disorders caused by other forms of intense heat as well as those caused by the sun.

RECOGNITION. Sunstroke is not the same as HEAT EXHAUSTION, a less serious disorder in which the amount of salt and fluid in the body falls below normal. In sunstroke there is a disturbance in the mechanism that controls perspiration. Since sunstroke is much more dangerous than heat exhaustion and is treated differently, it is of the utmost importance to distinguish between the two. The first symptoms of both disorders may be similar: headache, dizziness and weakness. But later symptoms differ sharply. In heat exhaustion, there is perspiration and a normal or below normal temperature, whereas in sunstroke there is extremely high fever and absence of sweating.

Sunstroke also may cause convulsions and sudden loss of consciousness. In extreme cases it may be fatal.

TREATMENT. In treatment of sunstroke, immediate steps must be taken to lower the body temperature, which may rise as high as 108 to 112° F. The patient should be placed in a shady, cool place and most of his clothing should be removed. Cold water is sprinkled on the patient or he is sprayed gently with a garden hose. The arms and legs should be massaged to maintain circulation.

Further treatment consists of measures to lower the body temperature, including ice packs, cold water enemas and iced drinks by mouth. After the temperature has returned to normal, it is best for the patient to rest in bed for several days in a cool, well ventilated room.

super- (soo′per) word element [L.], *above; excessive*.

superalimentation (soo″per-al″ĭ-men-ta′shun) excessive feeding; sometimes used in the treatment of wasting diseases.

superalkalinity (soo″per-al″kah-lin′ĭ-te) excessive alkalinity.

supercilia (soo″per-sil′e-ah) (L., pl.) the hairs on the arching protrusion over either eye, the eyebrow.

supercilium (soo″per-sil′e-um) (L., sing.) eyebrow; the transverse elevation at the junction of the forehead and upper eyelid.

superclass (soo′per-klas) a taxonomic category sometimes established, subordinate to a phylum and superior to a class.

superego (soo″per-e′go) a part of the psyche derived from both the ID and the EGO, which acts, largely unconsciously, as a monitor over the ego. It is that part of the personality concerned with social standards, ethics and conscience. Early in life the superego is formed by the infant's identification with his parents and other significant and esteemed persons in his life. The real or supposed expectations of these persons gradually are accepted as general rules of society and help form the "conscience." The superego tends to be self-critical and in psychotic and neurotic persons strong feelings of guilt and unworthiness can lead to self-punitive measures in an effort to resolve conflicts between the id, ego and superego. (See also NEUROSIS and PSYCHOSIS.)

superexcitation (soo″per-ek″si-ta′shun) excessive excitation.

superfamily (soo″per-fam′ĭ-le) a taxonomic category sometimes established, subordinate to an order and superior to a family.

superfatted (soo″per-fat′ed) containing more fat than can be combined with the quality of alkali present.

superfecundation (soo″per-fe″kun-da′shun) 1. fertilization of two ova, liberated at the same time, by sperm of different fathers. 2. fertilization of an ovum after one has already been fertilized.

superfemale (soo″per-fe′māl) a female organism whose cells contain more than the ordinary number of sex-determining (X) chromosomes. Such an organism is usually infertile.

superfetation (soo″per-fe-ta′shun) fertilization of an ovum when there is already a developing embryo in the uterus.

superficial (soo″per-fish′al) situated on or near the surface.

superficialis (soo″per-fish″e-a′lis) superficial.

superficies (soo″per-fish′e-ēz) an outer surface.

superimpregnation (soo″per-im″preg-na′shun) successive fertilization of two ova.

superinduce (soo″per-in-dūs′) to bring on in addition to an already existing condition.

superinfection (soo″per-in-fek′shun) sudden growth of a type of bacteria different from the original offender in a wound or infection already under treatment.

superinvolution (soo″per-in″vo-lu′shun) excessive involution.

superior (soo-pēr′e-or) situated above, or directed upward; in official anatomic nomenclature, used in reference to the upper surface of an organ or other structure, or to a structure occupying a higher position.

superjacent (soo″per-ja′sent) located above.

superlactation (soo″per-lak-ta′shun) oversecretion of milk.

superlethal (soo″per-le′thal) more than sufficient to cause death.

supermedial (soo″per-me′de-al) situated above the middle.

supermicroscope (soo″per-mi′kro-skōp) electron microscope.

supermotility (soo″per-mo-til′ĭ-te) excessive motility.

supernatant (soo″per-na′tant) 1. situated above or at the top of something. 2. the liquid lying above a layer of precipitated insoluble material.

supernumerary (soo″per-nu′mer-ār″e) in excess of the regular number.

supernutrition (soo″per-nu-trish′un) excessive nutrition.

superphosphate (soo″per-fos′fāt) an acid phosphate.

super-regeneration (soo″per-re-jen″ĕ-ra′shun) the development of superfluous tissue, organs or parts as a result of regeneration.

supersalt (soo′per-sawlt) a salt with excess of acid.

supersaturate (soo″per-sat′u-rāt) to add more of an ingredient than can be held in solution permanently.

superscription (soo″per-skrip′shun) something written above; the first of four chief parts of a drug prescription, the ℞ or prescription sign ("Take thou").

supersecretion (soo″per-se-kre′shun) excess of any secretory function.

supersoft (soo′per-soft) extremely soft; applied to x-rays of extremely long wavelength and low penetrating power.

supertension (soo″per-ten′shun) extreme tension.

supervirulent (soo″per-vir′u-lent) unusually virulent.

supinate (soo′pĭ-nāt) to place in or assume a supine position.

supination (soo′pĭ-na′shun) the act of assuming the supine position; placing or lying on the back. Applied to the hand, the act of turning the palm upward.

supine (soo′pīn) lying with the face upward, or on the dorsal surface.

suppository (sŭ-poz′ĭ-to″re) a cone-shaped mass of solid medicated substance for introduction into the rectum, urethra or vagina.
  glycerin s., one made up of a mixture of glycerin and sodium stearate; used as a rectal evacuant.

suppressant (sŭ-pres′sant) an agent that stops secretion, excretion or normal discharge.

suppression (sŭ-presh′un) 1. sudden stoppage of

a secretion, excretion or normal discharge. 2. the voluntary expulsion of ego-threatening ideas and impulses from the consciousness.

suppurant (sup′u-rant) 1. causing suppuration. 2. an agent causing suppuration.

suppuration (sup″u-ra′shun) formation or discharge of pus. adj., sup′purative.

supra- (soo′prah) word element [L.], above.

supra-acromial (soo″prah-ah-kro′me-al) above the acromion.

supracerebellar (soo″prah-ser″ĕ-bel′ar) on the upper surface of the cerebellum.

supraclavicular (soo″prah-klah-vik′u-lar) above the clavicle.

supracondylar (soo″prah-kon′dĭ-lar) above a condyle.

supracostal (soo″prah-kos′tal) above or upon the ribs.

supracotyloid (soo″prah-kot′ĭ-loid) above the acetabulum.

supracranial (soo″prah-kra′ne-al) on the upper surface of the cranium.

supradiaphragmatic (soo″prah-di″ah-frag-mat′-ik) above the diaphragm.

supraepicondylar (soo″prah-ep″ĭ-kon′dĭ-lar) above the epicondyle.

suprahyoid (soo″prah-hi′oid) above the hyoid bone.

supraliminal (soo″prah-lim′ĭ-nal) above the threshold of sensation.

supralumbar (soo″prah-lum′bar) above the loin.

supramaxillary (soo″prah-mak′sĭ-ler″e) pertaining to the upper jaw.

supranormal (soo″prah-nor′mal) greater than normal; present in or occurring in excess of normal amounts or values.

supraorbital (soo″prah-or′bĭ-tal) above the orbit.

suprapelvic (soo″prah-pel′vik) above the pelvis.

suprapontine (soo″prah-pon′tīn) above or in the upper part of the pons.

suprapubic (soo″prah-pu′bik) above the pubes.

suprarenal (soo″prah-re′nal) above a kidney; adrenal.

Suprarenin (soo″prah-ren′in) trademark for a preparation of epinephrine bitartrate, an adrenergic.

suprascapular (soo″prah-skap′u-lar) above the scapula.

suprascleral (soo″prah-skle′ral) on the outer surface of the sclera.

suprasellar (soo″prah-sel′ar) above the sella turcica.

supravaginal (soo″prah-vaj′ĭ-nal) outside or above a sheath, specifically above the vagina.

sura (soor′ah) [L.] calf of the leg. adj., **su′ral.**

suramin (soor′ah-min) a nonmetallic compound first used in therapy of protozoal infections in Germany.
  sodium s., a compound effective in trypanosomal and filarial infections.

surdimutitas (ser″dĭ-mu′tĭ-tas) deaf-mutism.

surditas (ser′dĭ-tas) deafness.

Surfacaine (ser′fah-kān) trademark for preparations of cyclomethycaine, a surface anesthetic.

surface (ser′fas) the outer part or external aspect of a solid body.
  s.-active agent, any substance capable of altering the physicochemical nature of surfaces and interfaces; an example is a detergent. Called also surfactant.
  anterior s., that surface which is toward the front of the body in man, or toward the head in four-footed animals.
  articular s., that surface of a bone or cartilage which forms a joint with another.
  dorsal s., that surface which is toward the back of the body, or posterior.
  extensor s., the aspect of a joint of a limb (such as the knee or elbow) on the side toward which the movement of extension is directed.
  flexor s., the aspect of a joint of a limb on the side toward which the movement of flexion is directed.
  inferior s., that surface which is lower.
  lateral s., a surface nearer to or directed toward the side of the body.
  medial s., a surface nearer to or directed toward the midline of the body.
  posterior s., that surface which is toward the back of the body in man or directed toward the tail in four-footed animals.
  superior s., that surface which is upper or higher.
  ventral s., the anterior surface in man, and the lower surface nearest the abdominal aspect, in four-footed animals.

surfactant (ser-fak′tant) 1. active on the surface. 2. a surface-active agent. 3. a substance formed in the lungs that helps to keep the small air sacs expanded by virtue of its ability to reduce the surface tension.

surgeon (ser′jun) a practitioner of surgery.

surgery (ser′jer-e) 1. that branch of medicine which treats disease by manual and operative procedures. 2. a place for the performance of surgical operations. adj., **sur′gical.**

Surital (sur′ĭ-tal) trademark for preparations of thiamylal, an ultra-short-acting barbiturate.

surrogate (sur′o-gāt) a substitute; a thing or person that takes the place of something or someone else, as a drug used in place of another, or, in psychiatry, a person who takes the place of another in the subconscious or in dreams.

sursumduction, sursumversion (sur″sum-duk′-shun), (sur″sum-ver′zhun) the turning upward of a part, especially of the eyes.

susceptibility (sŭ-sep″tĭ-bil′ĭ-te) lack of resistance of a body to the deleterious or other effects of an agent, such as a pathogenic microorganism.

susceptible (sŭ-sep′tĭ-bl) capable of being affected; liable to contract a disease.

suscitate (sus′ĭ-tāt) to arouse to great activity.

suscitation (sus″ĭ-ta′shun) arousal to greater activity.

suspension (sus-pen′shun) 1. temporary cessation. 2. a preparation of a finely divided, undissolved substance dispersed in a liquid vehicle.
  colloid s., one in which the suspended particles are very small.

suspensoid (sus-pen′soid) a colloid system resembling a suspension, but in which the particles are so small they do not settle out on standing, but are kept in motion by brownian movement.

suspensory (sus-pen′so-re) 1. serving to hold up a part. 2. a bandage or sling for supporting the testes.

suspirious (sus-pi′re-us) breathing heavily.

sustentacular (sus″ten-tak′u-lar) supporting; sustaining.

sustentaculum (sus″ten-tak′u-lum), pl. *sustentac′uli* [L.] a support.

susurrus (sŭ-sur′us) [L.] murmur.

Sutton's disease (sut′onz) 1. leukoderma acquisitum centrifugum. 2. granuloma fissuratum.

sutura (soo-tu′rah), pl. *sutu′rae* [L.] suture; used in anatomic nomenclature to designate a type of joint in which the apposed bony surfaces are united by fibrous tissue, permitting no movement; found only between bones of the skull.

suturation (soo″tu-ra′shun) the process or act of suturing.

suture (soo′cher) 1. sutura, the line of union of adjoining bones of the skull. 2. a stitch or series of stitches made to secure apposition of the edges of a surgical or accidental wound; used also as a verb to indicate application of such stitches. 3. material used in closing a wound with stitches. adj., **su′tural.**
  absorbable s., a strand of material used for closing wounds, which becomes dissolved in the body fluids and disappears, such as catgut and tendon.
  catgut s., material for wound closure, prepared from submucous connective tissue of the small intestine of healthy sheep.
  coronal s., the line of union between the frontal bone and the parietal bones.
  lambdoid s., the line of union between the upper borders of the occipital and parietal bones, shaped like the Greek letter lambda; called also sutura lambdoidea.
  purse-string s., a type of suture commonly used to bury the stump of the appendix, a continuous running suture being placed about the opening, and then drawn tight.
  sagittal s., the line of union of the two parietal bones, dividing the skull anteroposteriorly into two symmetrical halves; called also sutura sagittalis.
  squamous s., the suture between the pars squamosa of the temporal bone and the parietal bone.

Suvren (suv′ren) trademark for a preparation of captodiamine, a sedative and tranquilizer.

suxamethonium (suk″sah-mĕ-tho′ne-um) succinylcholine, a skeletal muscle relaxant.

swab (swahb) a small pledget of cotton or gauze wrapped around the end of a slender wooden stick or wire for applying medications or obtaining specimens of secretions, etc., from body surfaces or orifices.

swallowing (swahl′o-ing) the taking in of a substance through the mouth and pharynx and into the esophagus. It is a combination of a voluntary act and a series of reflex actions. Once begun, the process operates automatically. Called also deglutition.

THE THREE STAGES OF SWALLOWING. In the first, voluntary, stage of swallowing, the cheeks are sucked in slightly and the tongue is arched against the hard palate, so that the bolus, or ball of chewed food, is moved to the pharynx.

Normally, air is free to pass from the nose or mouth to the lungs and back again. But the moment the bolus approaches the fauces, the passage from the mouth to the pharynx, nerve centers are triggered that control a series of reflex actions. After one quick inhalation, breathing is halted for the brief instant of the next stage.

In this second, involuntary, stage of swallowing, the rear edge of the soft palate, which hangs down from the roof of the mouth, swings up against the back of the pharynx and blocks the passages to the nose. The back of the tongue fits tightly into the space between two muscular pillars at each side of the fauces, sealing the way back to the mouth. Simultaneously, the larynx moves upward against the epiglottis, effectively closing the entrance to the trachea.

Sometimes the larynx does not move up quickly enough and food gets into the air passage, stimulating a coughing reaction. With the one-way route to the stomach firmly established, however, the muscular coat of the pharynx contracts, squeezing the ball of food and forcing its passage into the esophagus.

In the third stage, the rhythmic contraction (peristalsis) of the muscles of the esophagus moves the food on to the stomach. The cardiac sphincter keeps the stomach entrance closed until food is swallowed. As the food approaches, moved by the wavelike contractions of the esophagus, the advancing portion of the wave causes the sphincter to relax and open, while the rear and contracting portion forces the ball of food through the entrance.

DISORDERS OF SWALLOWING. Difficulty in swallowing, dysphagia, is a symptom of most diseases of the esophagus. ACHALASIA is failure of the smooth muscles to relax sufficiently during swallowing. This disorder, found mostly in the elderly, may result in complete or partial esophageal obstruction. Acute and chronic esophagitis can produce difficulty in swallowing, as can esophageal stricture. Although benign tumors of the esophagus may occur, most of them are malignant and are accompanied by progressive difficulty in swallowing.

The feeling that there is a lump in the throat or that food sticks there may also be caused by hysteria, in which case it is known as globus hystericus. It is rare and occurs most often in young girls.

The swallowing process can also be impeded by illnesses such as cerebral palsy, cerebral vascular accident and paralysis.

In diagnosing disorders of swallowing, x-rays and ESOPHAGOSCOPY are used. Treatment may consist of a special diet, dilatation of the esophagus or surgery. With proper care most cases can be cured; early treatment is important.

sweat (swet) the excretion of the sweat (sudoriparous) glands of the skin; PERSPIRATION. Sweating produces an evaporative cooling of the body and also serves an excretory function. Substances eliminated in sweat include water, sodium chloride and small amounts of urea, lactic acid and potassium ions. During maximal sweating, as in extremely hot weather, the amount of water eliminated can account for a loss of as much as 8 lb. of body weight per day.

Excessive sweating is called diaphoresis.

s. gland, one of the glands distributed over the entire body surface that secrete sweat. The sweat gland consists of two main parts: the secretory portion, which is a coiled tube located in the corium, and the duct that acts as a passageway to the surface of the skin. There are about 2 million sweat glands in the body. The largest are in the axillae and groin. The soles of the feet and the palms of the hand contain the greatest number per square inch.

The sweat glands are innervated by cholinergic nerve fibers of the parasympathetic nervous system. They also can be stimulated by the hormones epinephrine and norepinephrine circulating in the blood.

swelling (swel′ing) abnormal enlargement or increase in volume, associated with accumulation in the tissue of a protein-containing exudate.

cloudy s., an early stage of degenerative change characterized by swollen, parboiled-appearing tissues that may revert to normal.

Swift's disease (swifts) acrodynia.

sycephalus (si-sef′ah-lus) syncephalus.

sycoma (si-ko′mah) a condyloma.

sycosiform (si-ko′sī-form) resembling sycosis.

sycosis (si-ko′sis) a pustular inflammation of the hair follicles, usually of the beard.

s. bar′bae, a staphylococcal infection and irritation of the hair follicles in the beard region. It may be associated with other superficial bacterial infections, such as impetigo or furunculosis.

The symptoms include burning, itching and pain, with the formation of small papules and pustules that drain and form crusts. The pustules leave scars when they heal.

Superficial infections are treated with local applications of antibiotics or corticosteroid ointments, or both. Deeper inflammations with bacterial invasion may require incision and drainage of the pustules, removal of the hair from the follicle and systemic antibiotics and corticosteroids. Scrupulous cleanliness and personal hygiene are necessary to prevent reinfection.

lupoid s., a chronic, scarring form of deep sycosis barbae.

Sycotrol (si′ko-trol) trademark for a preparation

of pipethanate hydrochloride, a mild tranquilizer and peripheral anticholinergic.

Sydenham's chorea (sid'en-hamz) a disorder of the central nervous system and one of the clinical manifestations of rheumatic fever; called also Saint Vitus's dance.

The condition is characterized by purposeless, irregular movements of the voluntary muscles that cannot be controlled by the patient. The spasmodic jerking movements may be mild or severe and frequently begin as awkwardness and facial grimaces which can cause the child considerable embarassment since he has no control over them. Emotional instability and extreme nervousness usually accompany the physical symptoms.

Treatment and nursing care are based on relief of symptoms. Complete mental and physical rest are prescribed and mild sedatives such as phenobarbital or one of the tranquilizers may be given to promote relaxation. The prognosis for Sydenham's chorea is good and complete recovery is the rule.

syllepsiology (sĭ-lep'se-ol'o-je) the branch of obstetrics dealing with conception and pregnancy.

syllepsis (sĭ-lep'sis) pregnancy.

symbiont (sim'bi-ont, sim'be-ont) one of the organisms or species associated biologically with an organism of another species.

symbiosis (sim"bi-o'sis) the biologic association of two individuals or populations of different species, classified as mutualism, commensalism, parasitism or predation, depending on the advantage or disadvantage derived from the relationship. adj., **symbiot'ic.**

symblepharon (sim-blef'ah-ron) adhesion of an eyelid to the eyeball.

symblepharopterygium (sim-blef"ah-ro-tĕ-rij'-e-um) symblepharon and pterygium.

symbolism (sim'bo-lizm) 1. an abnormal mental state in which every occurrence is conceived of as a symbol of the patient's own thoughts. 2. in psychoanalysis, a mechanism of unconscious thinking, usually of a sexual nature, whereby the real meaning becomes transformed so as not to be recognized as sexual by the superego.

symbolophobia (sim"bo-lo-fo'be-ah) a morbid fear that one's acts may contain some symbolic meaning.

symmelus (sim'ĕ-lus) a fetal monster with fused legs.

symmetry (sim'ĕ-tre) correspondence in size, form and arrangement of parts on opposite sides of a plane, line or point. adj., **symmet'rical.**

bilateral s., the state of an irregularly shaped body (such as the human body or that of higher animals) that can be divided into equivalent halves by one special cut.

sympathectomize (sim"pah-thek'to-mīz) to deprive of sympathetic innervation.

sympathectomy (sim"pah-thek'to-me) excision or interruption of a sympathetic nerve. The operation produces temporary vasodilation leading to improved nutrition of the part supplied by the vessel. It is used in cases of partial arterial obstruction with resultant trophic changes distally.

chemical s., the interruption of the transmission of impulses through a sympathetic nerve by chemicals.

periarterial s., surgical removal of the sheath of an artery containing the sympathetic nerve fibers.

sympathetic (sim"pah-thet'ik) 1. pertaining to or caused by sympathy. 2. pertaining to the sympathetic nervous system.

s. blockade, block of nerve impulse transmission between a preganglionic sympathetic fiber and the ganglion cell.

s. nervous system, part of the autonomic NERVOUS SYSTEM, the preganglionic fibers of which arise from cell bodies in the thoracic and first three lumbar segments of the spinal cord; postganglionic fibers are distributed to the heart, smooth muscle and glands of the entire body.

sympatheticomimetic (sim"pah-thet"ĭ-ko-mi-met'ik) sympathomimetic.

sympatheticoparalytic (sim"pah-thet"ĭ-ko-par"-ah-lit'ik) caused by paralysis of the sympathetic nervous system.

sympatheticotonia (sim"pah-thet"ĭ-ko-to'ne-ah) sympathicotonia.

sympathicoblast (sim-path'ĭ-ko-blast") an embryonic cell that develops into sympathetic nerve cell.

sympathicoblastoma (sim-path"ĭ-ko-blas-to'-mah) a tumor containing sympathicoblasts.

sympathicolytic (sim-path"ĭ-ko-lit'ik) sympatholytic.

sympathicomimetic (sim-path"ĭ-ko-mi-met'ik) sympathomimetic.

sympathiconeuritis (sim-path"ĭ-ko-nu-ri'tis) inflammation of the sympathetic nerves.

sympathicotonia (sim-path"ĭ-ko-to'ne-ah) a stimulated condition of the sympathetic nervous system, marked by vascular spasm, heightened blood pressure and the dominance of other sympathetic functions.

sympathicotripsy (sim-path"ĭ-ko-trip'se) crushing of a ganglion or plexus of the sympathetic nervous system.

sympathicotropic (sim-path"ĭ-ko-trop'ik) having affinity for or exerting its principal effect on the sympathetic nervous system.

sympathicus (sim-path'ĭ-kus) the sympathetic nervous system.

sympathin (sim'pah-thin) a mediating substance formed at the peripheral ends of sympathetic nerves.

s. E, the excitatory form, which causes vasoconstriction.

s. I, the inhibitory form, which causes vasodilatation.

sympathism (sim'pah-thizm) suggestibility.

sympathogonioma (sim"pah-tho-go"ne-o'ma) a tumor composed of sympathogonia.

sympathogonium (sim"pah-tho-go'ne-um), pl.

sympathogo'nia [Gr.] an embryonic cell that develops into a sympathetic cell.

sympatholytic (sim″pah-tho-lit′ik) blocking transmission of impulses from the adrenergic (sympathetic) postganglionic fibers to effector organs or tissues, inhibiting such sympathetic functions as smooth muscle contraction and glandular secretion.

sympathoma (sim″pah-tho′mah) sympathicoblastoma.

sympathomimetic (sim″pah-tho-mi-met′ik) producing effects resembling those of impulses transmitted by the postganglionic fibers of the sympathetic nervous system.

sympathy (sim′pah-the) the emotional understanding of another person's feelings.

symphalangism (sim-fal′an-jizm) ankylosis of the proximal phalangeal joints.

symphyseal, symphysial (sim-fiz′e-al) pertaining to a symphysis.

symphysiectomy (sim-fiz″e-ek′to-me) resection of the symphysis pubis.

symphysiorrhaphy (sim-fiz″e-or′ah-fe) suture of a divided symphysis.

symphysiotomy (sim-fiz″e-ot′o-me) division of the symphysis pubis to facilitate delivery.

symphysis (sim′fĭ-sis), pl. *sym′physes* [Gr.] a union; a type of joint in which the apposed bony surfaces are firmly united by a plate of fibrocartilage.
  pubic s., s. pu′bis, the line of union of the bodies of the pubic bones in the median plane.

sympodia (sim-po′de-ah) fusion of the lower extremities.

symptom (simp′tom) a change in the physical or mental state of a person that he is able to recognize and frequently bring to a physician's attention. adj., **symptomat′ic.**
  cardinal s's, 1. symptoms of greatest significance to the physician, establishing the identity of the illness. 2. the symptoms shown in the temperature, pulse and respiration.
  dissociation s., anesthesia to pain and to heat and cold, without impairment of tactile sensibility.
  objective s., one perceptible to others than the patient, as pallor, rapid pulse or respiration, restlessness and the like.
  signal s., a peculiar sensation or movement indicative of an impending epileptic attack.
  subjective s., one perceptible only to the patient, as pain, pruritus, vertigo and the like.

symptomatology (simp″to-mah-tol′o-je) the branch of medicine dealing with symptoms.

symptomatolytic (simp″to-mah″to-lit′ik) causing the disappearance of symptoms.

sympus (sim′pus) a fetal monster with feet and legs fused.

syn- (sin) word element [Gr.], *union; association.*

Synalar (sin′ah-lar) trademark for a preparation of fluocinolone acetonide, a steroid used as a topical anti-inflammatory agent.

synalgia (sĭ-nal′je-ah) pain experienced in one place, but caused by stimuli originating in another. adj., **synal′gic.**

synanastomosis (sin″ah-nas″to-mo′sis) the anastomosis of several vessels.

synanthema (sin″an-the′mah) a local or grouped eruption.

synapse (sin′aps) the functional junction between two neurons, where a nerve impulse is transmitted from one neuron to another (see also NEURON).
  axodendritic s., one between the axon of one neuron and the dendrites of another.
  axodendrosomatic s., one between the axon of one neuron and the dendrites and body of another.
  axosomatic s., one between the axon of one neuron and the body of another.

synapsis (sĭ-nap′sis) the pairing off and union of homologous chromosomes from male and female pronuclei at the start of meiosis.

synaptic (sĭ-nap′tik) pertaining to a synapse or to a synapsis.

synaptology (sin″ap-tol′o-je) the study of the synaptic correlations of the nervous system.

synarthrodia (sin″ar-thro′de-ah) synarthrosis. adj., **synarthro′dial.**

synarthrophysis (sin″ar-thro-fi′sis) progressive ankylosis of joints.

synarthrosis (sin″ar-thro′sis), pl. *synarthro′ses* [Gr.] a form of joint in which the bony elements are united by continuous intervening fibrous tissue; called also fibrous joint.

syncanthus (sin-kan′thus) adhesion of the eyeball to the orbital structures.

syncephalus (sin-sef′ah-lus) a twin fetal monster with heads fused into one, there being a single face, with four ears.

synchondrosis (sin″kon-dro′sis), pl. *synchondro′ses* [Gr.] a type of cartilaginous joint, the intervening hyaline cartilage ordinarily being converted into bone before adult life.

synchronous (sing′kro-nus) occurring at the same time.

syncope (sing′ko-pe) 1. a sudden loss of strength. 2. a temporary suspension of consciousness due to cerebral anemia; fainting. adj., **syn′copal.**

syncytium (sin-sish′e-um) a multinuclear mass of protoplasm produced by the merging of cells. adj., **syncyt′ial.**

syndactylia, syndactyly (sin″dak-til′e-ah), (sin-dak′tĭ-le) the most common congenital anomaly of the hand, marked by persistence of the webbing between adjacent digits, so they are more or less completely attached; generally considered an inherited condition, the anomaly may also occur in the foot.

syndesmitis (sin″des-mi′tis) 1. inflammation of a ligament. 2. conjunctivitis.

syndesmography (sin″des-mog′rah-fe) description of the ligaments.

syndesmology (sin″des-mol′o-je) scientific study of the ligaments and joints.

syndesmoma (sin″des-mo′mah) a tumor of connective tissue.

syndesmoplasty (sin-des′mo-plas″te) plastic repair of a ligament.

syndesmorrhaphy (sin″des-mor′ah-fe) suture of a ligament.

syndesmosis (sin″des-mo′sis), pl. *syndesmo′ses* a joint in which the bones are united by fibrous connective tissue forming an interosseous membrane or ligament.

syndesmotomy (sim″des-mot′o-me) incision of a ligament.

syndrome (sin′drōm) a combination of symptoms resulting from a single cause or so commonly occurring together as to constitute a distinct clinical picture. For specific syndromes, see under the specific name, as ADRENOGENITAL SYNDROME.

Syndrox (sin′droks) trademark for preparations of methamphetamine, a central nervous system stimulant.

synechia (sĭ-nek′e-ah), pl. *synech′iae* [Gr.] adhesion, as of the iris to the cornea or the lens.
  annular s., adhesion of the whole rim of the iris to the lens.
  anterior s., adhesion of the iris to the cornea.
  circular a., annular synechia.
  posterior s., adhesion of the iris to the capsule of the lens.
  total s., adhesion of the whole surface of the iris to the lens.
  s. vul′vae, a congenital or acquired condition in which the labia minora are sealed in the midline, with only a small opening below the clitoris through which urination and menstruation may occur.

synechotomy (sin″ĕ-kot′o-me) incision of a synechia.

synencephalus (sin″en-sef′ah-lus) a fetal monster with two bodies and one head.

syneresis (sĭ-ner′ĕ-sis) a drawing together of the particles of the disperse phase of a gel, with separation of some of the disperse medium and shrinkage of the gel, such as occurs in the clotting of blood.

synergism (sin′er-jizm) the joint action of agents so that their combined effect is greater than the algebraic sum of their individual parts. adj., **synergist′ic.**

synergist (sin′er-jist) an agent that acts with or enhances the action of another.

synergy (sin′er-je) correlated action or cooperation by two or more structures or drugs.

synesthesia (sin″es-the′ze-ah) sensation experienced in association with stimuli producing another sensation; or the experience of sensation in one place upon stimulation elsewhere.

synesthesialgia (sin″es-the″ze-al′je-ah) a condition in which a stimulus produces pain on the affected side but no sensation or even a pleasant one on the normal side of the body.

syngamy (sing′gah-me) a method of reproduction in which two individuals (gametes) unite permanently and their nuclei fuse; sexual reproduction.

syngenesis (sin-jen′ĕ-sis) 1. the origin of an individual from a germ derived from both parents and not from either one alone. 2. the state of having descended from a common ancestor.

synkaryon (sin-kar′e-on) a nucleus formed by fusion of two pronuclei, the fertilization nucleus.

Synkavite (sin′ka-vīt) trademark for preparations of menadiol sodium diphosphate, a vitamin K preparation.

synkinesis (sin″ki-ne′sis) an associated movement; an unintentional movement accompanying a volitional movement.

synneurosis (sin″nu-ro′sis) syndesmosis.

synonychia (sin″o-nik′e-ah) fusion of the nails of two or more digits in syndactyly.

synophthalmus (sin″of-thal′mus) cyclops.

Synophylate (sin″o-fi′lāt) trademark for preparations of theophylline sodium glycinate, a smooth muscle relaxant and diuretic.

synorchism (sin′or-kizm) congenital fusion of the testes into one mass.

synosteology (sin″os-te-ol′o-je) the study of joints and articulations.

synosteotomy (sin″os-te-ot′o-me) dissection of the joints.

synostosis (sin″os-to′sis), pl. *synosto′ses* [Gr.] normal or abnormal union of two bones by osseous material.

synotia (sĭ-no′she-ah) a developmental anomaly with fusion of the ears, or their location near the midventral line in the upper part of the neck.

synotus (sĭ-no′tus) a fetal monster exhibiting synotia.

synovectomy (sin″o-vek′to-me) excision of a synovial membrane, as of that lining the capsule of the knee joint, performed in the treatment of rheumatoid arthritis.

synovia (sĭ-no′ve-ah) the transparent, viscid fluid secreted by synovial membrane and found in joint cavities, bursae and tendon sheaths.

synovial (sĭ-no′ve-al) of, pertaining to or secreting synovia.
  s. fluid, synovia.
  s. joint, a specialized form of articulation permitting more or less free movement, the union of the bony elements being surrounded by an articular capsule enclosing a cavity lined by synovial membrane; called also diarthrosis.
  s. membrane, the inner of the two layers of the articular capsule of a synovial joint; composed of loose connective tissue and having a free smooth surface that lines the joint cavity.

synovialis (sĭ-no″ve-a′lis) the synovial membrane.

synovialoma, synovioma (sĭ-no″ve-ah-lo′mah), (sĭ-no″ve-o′mah) a tumor of synovial membrane origin.

synovitis (sin″o-vi′tis) inflammation of a synovial membrane, usually painful, particularly on motion, and characterized by fluctuating swelling, due to effusion in a synovial sac. It may be caused by rheumatic fever, rheumatoid arthritis, tuberculosis, trauma, gout, etc.

　dry s., synovitis with little effusion.

　purulent s., synovitis with effusion of pus in a synovial sac.

　serous s., synovitis with copious nonpurulent effusion.

　s. sic′ca, dry synovitis.

　simple s., synovitis with clear or slightly turbid effusion.

　tendinous s., inflammation of a tendon sheath.

synovium (sĭ-no′ve-um) a synovial membrane.

synthermal (sin-ther′mal) of the same temperature.

synthesis (sin′thĕ-sis) creation of a compound by union of the elements composing it, done artificially or as a result of natural processes. adj., **synthet′ic.**

synthetase (sin′thĕ-tās) an enzyme that catalyzes reactions necessary to the synthesis of a substance in the body.

Synthroid (sin′throid) trademark for a preparation of sodium levothyroxine, used for replacement therapy in hypothyroidism.

Syntocinon (sin-to′sĭ-non) trademark for a solution of synthetic oxytocin, a uterine stimulant.

syntonic (sin-ton′ik) pertaining to a stable, integrated personality.

Syntropan (sin′tro-pan) trademark for a preparation of amprotropine phosphate, an anticholinergic.

syntrophoblast (sin-trof′o-blast) the thick peripheral layer of the trophoblast, in which nuclei lie embedded in a common cytoplasmic mass.

synulotic (sin″u-lot′ik) 1. producing scarring. 2. an agent promoting scarring.

syphilid (sif′ĭ-lid) a skin affection of syphilitic origin. It may be macular, papular, pustular or, in tertiary syphilis, a gumma.

syphilis (sif′ĭ-lis) a contagious venereal disease leading to many structural and cutaneous lesions; called also lues.

Syphilis is caused by a spiral-shaped bacterium (spirochete), *Treponema pallidum.* It is transmitted primarily by coitus. The spirochetes enter the body through a break or abrasion of the skin or a mucous membrane. Since the bacteria can live only for a few minutes outside the body, the disease is seldom spread by contact with drinking or eating utensils previously used by a syphilitic person. It is never contracted from toilet seats.

Syphilis can be readily and completely cured, but if it is untreated or treated improperly, it can cause widespread damage. It is not hereditary but can be transmitted by an affected woman to her unborn child.

PRIMARY SYPHILIS. Within a few hours after the spirochetes penetrate the skin or a mucous membrane, they enter the bloodstream, and usually in about a week they spread throughout the body.

The first sign of primary syphilis is a painless sore, called a chancre, that appears 9 days to 3 months—usually 3 weeks—after infection. Usually firm or hard, the chancre may resemble a blister, pimple or ulcerated open sore. In men, it appears usually on or near the head of the penis. In women, the chancre is commonly found on the labia, but it may be concealed inside the vagina, where it may not be felt or seen. Chancres sometimes develop elsewhere, such as on the lips of the mouth, a breast or a finger. They also may appear in the anal region.

When the material from a chancre is examined under a microscope, the organism may be identified. Blood tests for syphilis, such as the Wassermann test and the Kahn test, may fail to detect the disease during this early stage.

Even though no treatment is given, the chancre will disappear in 10 to 40 days, often leading to the false conclusion that the disease is cured. Occasionally a chancre fails to develop or is too small to be noticed.

Primary syphilis can be cured with penicillin in adequate doses and other antibiotics, such as tetracycline.

SECONDARY SYPHILIS. Two to six months after the primary sore disappears, the secondary stage of syphilis begins; it may last up to 2 years.

A rash is usually one of the first symptoms. It may cover any part of the body and often spreads over the entire skin surface, including the palms of the hands and the soles of the feet. It does not itch and it may resemble that of measles as well as of many other diseases. It can be identified positively as a symptom of syphilis only by a blood test.

During secondary syphilis, thin white sores may appear on the mucosa of the mouth and throat and around the genitalia and rectum. Headache, fever and a general feeling of illness are common. Hair may fall out in patches, bones and joints may be painful and anemia may develop. Sometimes the eyes are affected.

Syphilis is highly contagious in this stage and of great danger to others. If mouth sores are present, the disease may be spread by kissing.

Like primary syphilis, the secondary stage disappears by itself, generally within 3 to 12 weeks, but may return later if the organisms are still present. As in the primary stage, the disease can be cured in the secondary stage by the use of penicillin or other antibiotics.

Together, the primary and secondary stages are known as "early syphilis."

TERTIARY SYPHILIS. The third, or tertiary, stage of the disease is known as "late syphilis." Its symptoms may develop soon after the secondary symptoms have vanished or they may lie hidden for 15 or more years. A person may be unaware that he has the disease. Even a blood test may be negative.

Late syphilis is less contagious to others but is extremely dangerous to the person who has it. It may be fatal, particularly if the central nervous system or heart is affected. The spirochete can invade any cell of the body and can damage any organ or structure of the body, including the internal organs, bones, joints and skin. The characteristic lesion of tertiary syphilis is a soft gummy tumor called a gumma.

If late syphilis attacks the heart, aorta or aortic valve, death may result from rupture of the weakened aorta or from heart failure. When it attacks the central nervous system, general paresis, a severe disease of the brain, may result, which, if not treated promptly, will cause insanity and death. Another serious disorder of the nervous system caused by late syphilis is TABES DORSALIS, or locomotor ataxia, in which there is pain and loss of position sense.

Blindness may result if the infection involves the eyes. Other possible effects are deep ulcers on the legs or elsewhere, chronic inflammation of the bones, which is especially painful at night, and perforation of the soft palate.

Cure of late or tertiary syphilis takes longer and is more difficult than that of primary or secondary syphilis. Sometimes the disease cannot be completely cured. As with early syphilis, however, it may be successfully treated with penicillin and other antibiotics.

CONGENITAL SYPHILIS. Congenital syphilis is transmitted from a diseased mother to her unborn child through the placenta. Often this results in spontaneous abortion or stillbirth.

If the infant is born alive, he may have snuffles, caused by inflammation of the nose, and may be generally weak and sickly. Syphilitic rashes, especially in the genital area, may occur when the baby is 3 to 8 weeks old. Children with congenital syphilis are often born deformed, and may become blind, deaf, paralyzed or insane.

To prevent congenital syphilis, all pregnant women should have a blood test for syphilis during the early months of pregnancy. Treatment before the fifth month will always prevent infection of the unborn child. A syphilitic mother who is not treated early has only one chance in six of having a healthy child. If a child is born with syphilis, immediate treatment may be effective if the disease has not progressed too far.

BLOOD TESTS. Since a person infected with syphilis may not show all or even any of the symptoms of the first, second or third stages of the disease, a routine blood test for syphilis becomes necessary for detection. The best known are the Wassermann test and the Kahn test.

There is no immunization against syphilis at present, but since the disease, if diagnosed and treated early, can be cured with penicillin and other antibiotics, it is advisable to have blood tests for syphilis during routine checkups. The genitalia and rectum should be examined periodically if exposure has occurred. Most states require a blood test for syphilis before marriage.

PREVENTION. The surest method of prevention is the avoidance of exposure to persons who may be infected with syphilis. Those who fail to heed such advice should at least follow recommended precautionary measures—use of a rubber condom during the entire sexual act and the thorough cleansing of genitalia and surrounding parts with soap and water afterward.

In large measure, syphilis can be prevented and controlled through education. Educational campaigns have been effective in reducing the number of cases of syphilis, but the disease is still widespread.

syphilitic (sif″ĭ-lit′ik) affected with, caused by or pertaining to syphilis.

syphiloderm (sif′ĭ-lo-derm″) a syphilitic skin disease.

syphilogenesis (sif″ĭ-lo-jen′ĕ-sis) the development of syphilis.

syphiloid (sif′ĭ-loid) 1. resembling syphilis. 2. a disease like syphilis.

syphilologist (sif″ĭ-lol′o-jist) a specialist in syphilology.

syphilology (sif″ĭ-lol′o-je) the sum of knowledge about syphilis, its pathology and treatment.

syphiloma (sif″ĭ-lo′mah) a tumor of syphilitic origin; a gumma.

syphilopathy (sif″ĭ-lop′ah-the) any syphilitic manifestation.

syphilophobia (sif″ĭ-lo-fo′be-ah) morbid fear of syphilis.

syphilophyma (sif″ĭ-lo-fi′mah) a syphilitic growth or excrescence.

syring(o)- (sĭ-ring′go) word element [Gr.], *tube; fistula.*

syringe (sir′inj) an instrument for introducing fluids into the body or a body cavity.
  hypodermic s., one for introduction of liquids through a hollow needle into subcutaneous tissues.

syringectomy (sir″in-jek′to-me) excision of a fistula.

syringitis (sir″in-ji′tis) inflammation of the eustachian tube.

syringoadenoma (sĭ-ring″go-ad″ĕ-no′mah) tumor of a sweat gland.

syringobulbia (sĭ-ring″go-bul′be-ah) the presence of fluid-filled cavities in the medulla oblongata and pons.

syringocele (sĭ-ring′go-sēl) a cavity-containing herniation of the spinal cord through the bony defect in spina bifida.

syringocoele (sĭ-ring′go-sēl) the central canal of the spinal cord.

syringocystadenoma (sĭ-ring″go-sist″ad-ĕ-no′-mah) adenoma of the sweat glands; called also hidradenoma.

syringocystoma (sĭ-ring″go-sis-to′mah) a cystic tumor of a sweat gland.

syringoma (sir″ing-go′mah) tumor of a sweat gland.

syringomeningocele (sĭ-ring″go-mĕ-ning′go-sēl) meningocele resembling syringomyelocele.

syringomyelia (sĭ-ring″go-mi-e′le-ah) the presence of fluid-filled cavities in the substance of the spinal cord, with destruction of nerve tissue.

syringomyelitis (sĭ-ring″go-mi″ĕ-li′tis) inflammation of the spinal cord with the formation of cavities.

syringomyelocele (si-ring″go-mi′ĕ-lo-sēl″) hernial protrusion of the spinal cord through the bony defect in spina bifida, the mass containing a cavity connected with the central canal of the spinal cord.

syringotomy (sir″ing-got′o-me) incision of a fistula.

syrinx (sir′inks) 1. a tube or pipe; a fistula. 2. the fluid-filled cavity in syringomyelia.

syrosingopine (si″ro-sing′go-pēn) a white or slightly yellowish crystalline powder used as an antihypertensive.

syrup (sir′up) a viscous concentrated solution of a sugar, such as sucrose, in water or other aqueous liquid; combined with other ingredients, such a solution is used as a flavored vehicle for medications.
    simple s., one compounded with purified water and sucrose.

systaltic (sis-tal′tik) alternately contracting and dilating.

system (sis′tem) 1. a set or series of interconnected or interdependent parts or entities (objects, organs or organisms) that act together in a common purpose or produce results impossible by action of one alone. 2. an organized set of principles or ideas. adj., **systemat′ic, system′ic.**
    autonomic nervous s., the portion of the NERVOUS SYSTEM concerned with regulation of activity of cardiac muscle, smooth muscle and glands.
    biologic s., one composed of living material; such systems range from a collection of separate molecules to an assemblage of separate organisms.
    cardiovascular s., the heart and blood vessels, by which blood is pumped and circulated through the body (see also CIRCULATORY SYSTEM).
    central nervous s., the portion of the NERVOUS SYSTEM consisting of the brain and spinal cord.
    centrencephalic s., neurons in the central core of the brain stem from the thalamus down to the medulla oblongata, connecting the two hemispheres of the brain.
    circulatory s., the channels through which nutrient fluids of the body flow (see also CIRCULATORY SYSTEM).
    digestive s., the organs concerned with the ingestion and digestion of food (see also DIGESTIVE SYSTEM).
    endocrine s., the system of glands that elaborate internal secretions, including the pituitary, parathyroid, thyroid and adrenal glands.
    genitourinary s., the organs concerned with production and excretion of urine, together with the organs of reproduction (see also GENITOURINARY SYSTEM).
    haversian s., a haversian canal and its concentrically arranged lamellae, constituting the basic unit of structure in compact bone (osteon).
    hematopoietic s., the tissues concerned in the production of blood.
    heterogeneous s., a system or structure made up of mechanically separable parts, as an emulsion.
    homogeneous s., a system or structure made up of parts that cannot be mechanically separated, as a solution.

    limbic s., a system of brain structures common to the brains of all mammals, comprising the phylogenetically old cortex (archipallium) and its primarily related nuclei. In man its function is thought to be related to emotional response such as anger, fear, etc.
    lymphatic s., the lymphatic vessels and lymphoid tissue, considered collectively (see also CIRCULATORY SYSTEM).
    metric s., a system of weights and measures based on the meter and having all units based on some power of 10 (see also Table of Weights and Measures in the Appendix).
    nervous s., the chief organ system that correlates the adjustments and reactions of an organism to internal and environmental conditions (see also NERVOUS SYSTEM).
    parasympathetic nervous s., part of the autonomic NERVOUS SYSTEM, the preganglionic fibers of which leave the central nervous system with cranial nerves III, VII, IX and X and the first three sacral nerves; postganglionic fibers are distributed to the heart, smooth muscles and glands of the head and neck, and thoracic, abdominal and pelvic viscera.
    peripheral nervous s., the portion of the NERVOUS SYSTEM consisting of the nerves and ganglia outside the brain and spinal cord.
    portal s., an arrangement by which blood collected from one set of capillaries passes through a large vessel or vessels and another set of capillaries before returning to the systemic circulation, as in the pituitary gland and liver.
    respiratory s., the tubular and cavernous organs that allow atmospheric air to reach the membranes across which gases are exchanged with the blood (see also RESPIRATORY SYSTEM).
    reticuloendothelial s., a network of cells and tissues found throughout the body that is concerned in blood cell formation and destruction, storage of fatty materials and the metabolism of iron and pigment, and plays a defensive role in inflammation and immunity (see also RETICULOENDOTHELIAL SYSTEM).
    skeletal s., the body's framework of bones; the skeleton (see also SKELETAL SYSTEM).
    sympathetic nervous s., part of the autonomic NERVOUS SYSTEM, the preganglionic fibers of which arise from cell bodies in the thoracic and first three lumbar segments of the spinal cord; postganglionic fibers are distributed to the heart, smooth muscle and glands of the entire body.
    urinary s., the system formed in the body by the KIDNEYS, the urinary BLADDER, the URETERS and the URETHRA, the organs concerned in the production and excretion of urine.
    urogenital s., genitourinary system.
    vascular s., the vessels of the body, especially the blood vessels.
    vasomotor s., the part of the nervous system that controls the caliber of the blood vessels.

systema (sis-te′mah) [Gr.] system.

systemic (sis-tem′ik) pertaining to or affecting the body as a whole.
    s. circulation, the flow of blood from the left ventricle through the aorta, carrying oxygen and nutrient material to all the tissues of the body, and returning through the superior and inferior venae cavae to the right atrium.

systole (sis'to-le) the contraction, or period of contraction, of the heart, especially of the ventricles, during which blood is forced into the aorta and pulmonary artery. adj., **systol'ic.**

arterial s., the rhythmic contraction of an artery.

atrial s., contraction of the atria by which blood is forced into the ventricles; it precedes the true or ventricular systole.

extra s., an atrial or ventricular contraction occurring prematurely in relation to the basic rhythm of the heart.

ventricular s., contraction of the ventricles, forcing blood into the aorta and pulmonary artery.

systremma (sis-trem'ah) a cramp in the muscles of the calf of the leg.

Sytobex (si'to-beks) trademark for a parenteral preparation of crystalline vitamin B_{12}.

T

T. temperature; tension (of the eyeball); therm (thermal); time.

T − diminished intraocular tension (pressure).

T + increased intraocular tension (pressure).

T.A. toxin-antitoxin.

Ta chemical symbol, *tantalum*.

T.A.B. a vaccine prepared from killed typhoid, paratyphoid A and paratyphoid B bacilli.

tabacism, tabacosis (tab′ah-sizm), (tab″ah-ko′sis) poisoning by tobacco, chiefly by inhaling tobacco dust; a form of PNEUMOCONIOSIS.

Tabanus (tah-ba′nus) a genus of flies of world-wide distribution; commonly known as horseflies, they serve as vectors of various species of Trypanosoma.

tabardillo (tah″bar-dēl′yo) an infectious disease of Mexico, resembling typhoid fever.

tabefaction (tab″ē-fak′shun) wasting of the body; emaciation.

tabes (ta′bēz) 1. a wasting disorder. 2. tabes dorsalis. adj., **tabet′ic.**
cerebral t., general paresis.
cervical t., tabes dorsalis in which the upper extremities are first affected.
t. dorsa′lis, a slowly progressive nervous disorder, from degeneration of the dorsal columns of the spinal cord and sensory nerve trunks, resulting in disturbances of sensation and interference with reflexes and consequently with movements; called also locomotor ataxia. It is caused by syphilis and may appear 5 to 20 years after initial infection. The first symptoms are pain (frequently in the legs although it may occur in the arms or trunk) and loss of position sense. The pupils are uneven and do not react to light (Argyll Robertson pupils). Unless the patient looks down at his legs he does not know where they are and he must depend on his vision for each step. The typical gait of a patient with this condition is jerky and wide-based. There is no cure for tabes dorsalis because there is destruction of nerve cells.

tabescent (tah-bes′ent) growing emaciated; wasting away.

tabetiform (tah-bet′ĭ-form) resembling tabes.

tablature (tab′lah-tūr) separation of the chief cranial bones into inner and outer tables, separated by a diploe.

table (ta′bl) a flat-surface structure.
inner t., the inner compact layer of the bones covering the brain.
outer t., the outer compact layer of the bones covering the brain.

vitreous t., inner table.

tablespoon (ta′bl-spoon) a household unit of capacity, equivalent to about 15 ml. or 4 fluid drams.

tablet (tab′let) a solid dosage form containing a medicinal substance with or without a suitable diluent.
buccal t., a slowly dissolving tablet intended to be held in the mucosal pocket between the cheek and jaw.
coated t., one covered with a thin film of another substance to improve its palatability or delay absorption.
enteric-coated t., one coated with material that delays release of the medication until after it leaves the stomach.
sublingual t., a rapidly dissolving tablet intended to be inserted beneath the tongue.
trisulfapyrimidines t′s, tablets containing sulfadiazine, sulfamerazine and sulfamethazine.

taboparesis (ta″bo-pah-re′sis) tabes with general paresis.

tabophobia (ta″bo-fo′be-ah) a morbid fear of tabes.

tabular (tab′u-lar) resembling a table.

Tacaryl (tak′ah-ril) trademark for preparations of methdilazine, an antihistamine and antipruritic.

Tace (tās) trademark for preparations of chlorotrianisene, a synthetic estrogen.

tache (tahsh) [Fr.] a spot or blemish; applied to various blemishes on the skin, as tache blanche ("white spot"), tache bleuâtre ("blue spot") and tache noir ("black spot"), or to the slight enlargement of the fibril of a motor nerve on a muscle (tache motrice). adj., **tachet′ic.**

tachogram (tak′o-gram) the graphic record produced by tachography.

tachography (tah-kog′rah-fe) the recording of the movement and speed of the blood current.

tachy- (tak′e) word element [Gr.], *rapid; speed.*

tachycardia (tak″e-kar′de-ah) abnormally rapid heart rate, usually taken to be over 100 beats per minute. adj., **tachycar′diac.**
atrial t., a heart rate of 140 to 220 due to impulses arising in an irritable ectopic focus in the atrium.
ectopic t., rapid heart action in response to impulses arising outside the sinoatrial node.
essential t., a paroxysmal form resulting from functional disorder of the cardiac nerves.
orthostatic t., tachycardia occurring on arising from a reclining position.
paroxysmal t., rapid heart action that starts and stops abruptly.
ventricular t., a rapid, regular heart rate due to

stimuli arising in an ectopic focus or ring in the ventricular conduction system.

tachygenesis (tak″e-jen′ĕ-sis) acceleration and compression of ancestral stages in embryonic development.

tachylalia (tak″e-la′le-ah) rapidity of speech.

tachymeter (tah-kim′ĕ-ter) an instrument for measuring rapidity of motion.

tachyphagia (tak″e-fa′je-ah) rapid eating.

tachyphasia (tak″e-fa′ze-ah) rapid speech.

tachyphrasia (tak″e-fra′ze-ah) extreme volubility of speech.

tachyphrenia (tak″e-fre′ne-ah) mental hyperactivity.

tachyphylaxis (tak″e-fi-lak′sis) 1. reduction of reaction to a substance by repeated injection of small quantities of it. 2. reduction of response to a stimulus by repetitive slight stimuli.

tachypnea (tak″ip-ne′ah) rapid respiration; a respiratory neurosis marked by quick, shallow breathing.

tachypragia (tak″e-pra′je-ah) rapidity of action.

tachypsychia (tak″e-si′ke-ah) rapidity of psychic processes.

tachyrhythmia (tak″e-rith′me-ah) tachycardia.

tachysterol (tah-kis′ter-ol) a compound produced by irradiation of ergosterol, an antirachitic substance, vitamin D_2.

tachysystole (tak″e-sis′to-le) abnormally rapid systole.

Tacosal (tak′o-sal) trademark for a preparation of diphenylhydantoin, an anticonvulsant.

tactile (tak′til) pertaining to touch.

tactometer (tak-tom′ĕ-ter) an instrument for measuring the acuteness of the sense of touch.

tactus (tak′tus) [L.] touch. adj., **tac′tual.**
    t. erudi′tus, delicacy of touch acquired by practice.

Taenia (te′ne-ah) a genus of TAPEWORMS.
    T. echinococ′cus, *Echinococcus granulosus.*
    T. sagina′ta, a species 12 to 25 feet long, found in the adult form in the human intestine and in the larval state in muscles and other tissues of the ox. Man acquires it by eating infected meat. Called also beef tapeworm.
    T. so′lium, the pork tapeworm, a common parasite of man where raw or poorly cooked pork is part of the normal diet; adult worms are usually 6 to 10 feet long and composed of 800 to 900 proglottids.

taenia (te′ne-ah) tenia.

taeniacide (te′ne-ah-sīd″) teniacide.

taeniafuge (te′ne-ah-fūj″) teniafuge.

Taeniarhynchus (te″ne-ah-ring′kus) a genus of tapeworms.

Tagathen (tag′ah-then) trademark for a preparation of chlorothen citrate, an antihistamine.

Taka-diastase (tah′kah-di′as-tās) trademark for an amylolytic enzyme produced by the action of a fungus on wheat bran.

talbutal (tal′bu-tal) a short- to intermediate-acting barbiturate.

talc (talk) a native hydrous magnesium silicate, sometimes with a small amount of aluminum silicate; used in pharmaceutical preparations.

talcosis (tal-ko′sis) a condition due to inhalation or implantation in the body of talc.

talcum (tal′kum) talc.

talipes (tal′ĭ-pēz) a congenital deformity of the foot, which is twisted out of shape or position (CLUBFOOT); the foot may have an abnormally high longitudinal arch (talipes ca′vus) or it may be in dorsiflexion (talipes calca′neus) or plantar flexion (talipes equi′nus), abducted, everted (talipes val′gus), abducted, inverted (talipes va′rus) or various combinations of these (talipes calcaneoval′gus, talipes calcaneova′rus, talipes equinoval′gus or talipes equinova′rus).

talipomanus (tal″ĭ-pom′ah-nus) clubhand.

talocalcanean (ta″lo-kal-ka′ne-an) pertaining to the talus and calcaneus.

talocrural (ta″lo-kroo′ral) pertaining to the talus and the leg bones.

talus (ta′lus) a bone of the ankle.

tampon (tam′pon) a pack or plug made of cotton, sponge or other material, variously used in surgery for the control of hemorrhage or the absorption of secretions.

tamponade (tam″po-nād′) 1. the exertion of pressure or compression on a part, occurring as the result of a pathologic process or used as a means of

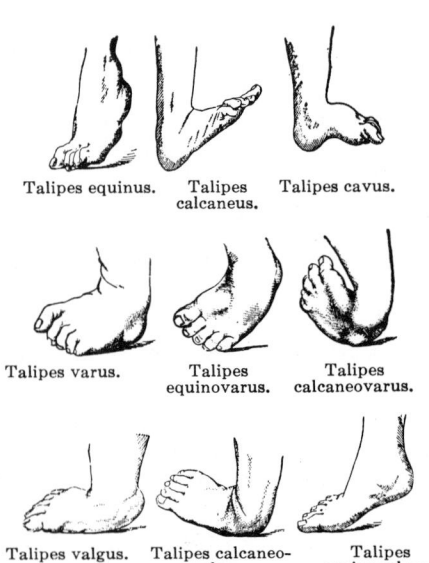

Talipes equinus.   Talipes calcaneus.   Talipes cavus.

Talipes varus.   Talipes equinovarus.   Talipes calcaneovarus.

Talipes valgus.   Talipes calcaneovalgus.   Talipes equinovalgus.

Talipes. (From Dorland's Illustrated Medical Dictionary. 24th ed. Philadelphia, W. B. Saunders Co., 1965.)

arresting hemorrhage. 2. an instrument used in checking internal hemorrhage.

balloon t., a device with a triple-lumen tube and two inflatable balloons, the third lumen providing for aspiration of blood clots, designed for esophagogastric tamponade.

cardiac t., compression of the heart due to collection of fluid or blood in the pericardium.

esophagogastric t., the exertion of pressure against bleeding esophageal varices by means of an inflatable device, with one sausage-shaped balloon in the esophagus and a globular one in the stomach.

Tandearil (tan-de'ah-ril) trademark for a preparation of oxyphenbutazone, an anti-inflammatory agent.

Tangier disease (tan-jēr') a familial disease characterized by a deficiency of high-density lipoproteins in the blood serum, with storage of cholesterol esters in the tonsils and other tissues.

tank (tank) a large artificial receptacle for the storage of fluid substances.

Hubbard t., a tank in which exercises may be performed under water.

tannate (tan'āt) a salt of tannic acid; all tannates are astringent.

tannic acid (tan'ik) a substance obtained from bark and fruit of many plants, used as an astringent.

tannin (tan'in) tannic acid.

tantalum (tan'tah-lum) a chemical element, atomic number 73, atomic weight 180.948, symbol Ta. (See table of ELEMENTS.) It is a noncorrosive and malleable metal used in surgery to repair defects in the skull or other tissues.

tantrum (tan'trum) a violent display of temper.

tap (tap) 1. a quick, light blow. 2. to drain off fluid by paracentesis.

Tapazole (tap'ah-zōl) trademark for a preparation of methimazole, used as a thyroid inhibitor.

tapeinocephaly (tah-pi"no-sef'ah-le) flattening or depression of the skull. adj., **tapeinocephal'ic.**

tapetum (tah-pe'tum), pl. *tape'ta* [L.] a covering structure or layer of cells.

t. lu'cidum, the iridescent epithelium of the choroid of animals that gives their eyes the property of shining in the dark.

tapeworm (tāp'werm) any of a number of parasites of the phylum Platyhelminthes (flatworms) that lodge in the intestines of animals and human beings. They are transmitted to man in larval form, embedded in cysts, in meat or fish that is not properly cooked. In the human they develop to maturity and attach themselves to the wall of the intestine, where they grow and release eggs.

Although a large number of adult tapeworms are considered human parasites, only a few infect man to any great degree. *Taenia saginata,* the beef tapeworm, and *T. solium,* the pork tapeworm, are widespread and quite common. Beef tapeworms grow to a length of 12 to 25 feet, and adult pork tapeworms average 6 to 10 feet in length. Both species release white, egg-containing proglottids, or segments of the body, which make their way to the anus and may be found in clothes or bedding. *Diphyllobothrium latum* is the fish tapeworm, and

is found predominantly in the Great Lakes region of the United States, northern Europe and Japan. It may grow as long as 60 feet. *Hymenolepis nana* and *H. diminuta* are dwarf tapeworms that are common in the tropics and subtropics.

The diagnosis of a tapeworm infection is made when segments of the worm are found in clothing or bedding or when characteristic eggs or segments are found in the stool. Occasionally diarrhea, vague abdominal cramps, flatulence, distention and nausea occur. Mental deterioration and seizures are rare, and occur only when larval forms of the worm invade brain tissue.

Tapeworm infection can be prevented by cooking pork, beef and fish properly. Although most meats and fish are inspected under government supervision, eggs and larvae are not always detectable; the only certain protection is proper cooking.

Once it is inside the body, the tapeworm can be eliminated by specific anthelmintic drugs. The drug of choice is quinacrine hydrochloride (Atabrine). Aspidium oleoresin is just as effective but is toxic in large doses. The patient fasts the evening and night before treatment, and a strong cathartic is given several hours before the drug is administered. No food is permitted until the patient has had at least two copious bowel movements. Cure depends on death or evacuation of the head of the worm. If no head is found, the stools must be examined for 6 months for eggs or segments. If they are found, the treatment must be repeated.

Echinococcus granulosus differs from other tapeworms in that the adult infects the animal host — dogs — and the larval forms are found in man. The larvae develop in the human intestine, penetrate its wall and are carried by the lymphatics to various organs of the body where they form slowly growing cysts (hydatid cysts). The liver is the organ most commonly involved. Treatment is by surgical removal of the cyst. Echinococcosis is uncommon in the United States.

taphophilia (taf"o-fil'e-ah) morbid interest in graves and cemeteries.

taphophobia (taf"o-fo'be-ah) morbid fear of being buried alive.

tapotement (tah-pōt-maw') [Fr.] a tapping manipulation in massage.

tar (tar) a dark, viscid substance obtained from wood of different trees or from bituminous coal.

coal t., a by-product obtained in destructive distillation of bituminous coal; used in ointment or solution in treatment of eczema.

pine t., a product of destructive distillation of the wood of *Pinus Palustris* or other species of pine; used as a local irritant and antibacterial agent.

tarantula (tah-ran'tu-lah) a venomous spider (see also INSECT BITES AND STINGS).

tardive (tar'div) late; applied to a disease in which the characteristic lesion is late in appearing.

tare (tār) 1. the weight of the vessel in which a substance is weighed. 2. to weigh a vessel which is to contain a substance in order to allow for it when the vessel and substance are weighed together.

target (tar'get) an object or area toward which

something is directed, such as that part of the x-ray tube on which the electrons impinge and from which the x-rays are sent out.

tars(o)- (tar′so) word element [Gr.], *edge of eyelid; tarsus of the foot.*

tarsal (tar′sal) 1. pertaining to the tarsus of an eyelid or of the foot. 2. any one of the bones of the tarsus.

tarsalgia (tar-sal′je-ah) pain in a tarsus.

tarsalia (tar-sa′le-ah) the bones of the tarsus.

tarsalis (tar-sa′lis) [L.] tarsal.

tarsectomy (tar-sek′to-me) 1. excision of one or more bones of the tarsus. 2. excision of the cartilage of the eyelid.

tarsitis (tar-si′tis) inflammation of the cartilaginous portion of the eyelid; blepharitis.

tarsoclasis (tar-sok′lah-sis) surgical fracture of the tarsus of the foot.

tarsomalacia (tar″so-mah-la′she-ah) softening of the tarsal cartilage of an eyelid.

tarsometatarsal (tar″so-met″ah-tar′sal) pertaining to the tarsus and metatarsus.

tarsophyma (tar″so-fi′mah) any tumor of the tarsus.

tarsoplasty (tar′so-plas″te) plastic repair of the tarsal cartilage of an eyelid.

tarsoptosis (tar″sop-to′sis) falling of the tarsus; flatfoot.

tarsorrhaphy (tar-sor′ah-fe) suture of the upper and lower tarsal cartilage of an eyelid for the purpose of shortening or closing the palpebral fissure.

tarsotomy (tar-sot′o-me) incision of the tarsal cartilage of an eyelid.

tarsus (tar′sus) 1. the seven bones—talus, calcaneus, navicular, medial, intermediate and lateral cuneiform, and cuboid—composing the articulation between the foot and leg; the ankle. 2. the cartilaginous plate forming the framework of either (upper or lower) eyelid.

tartar (tar′tar) 1. the recrystallized sediment of wine casks; crude potassium bitartrate. 2. a yellowish film formed of calcium phosphate and carbonate, food particles and other organic matter, deposited on the teeth by the saliva; called also dental calculus. Tartar should be removed regularly by a dentist. If neglected, it can cause bacteria to lodge between the gums and the teeth, causing gum infection, dental caries, loosening of the teeth and other disorders.

tartaric acid (tar-tar′ik) a compound used in preparing refrigerant drinks and effervescent powders.

tartrate (tar′trāt) a salt of tartaric acid.

taste (tāst) the peculiar sensation caused by the contact of soluble substances with the tongue; the sense effected by the tongue, the gustatory and other nerves and the gustatory center.

The organs of taste are the taste buds, bundles of slender cells with hairlike branches that are packed together in groups that form the projections called papillae at various places on the tongue. When a substance is introduced into the mouth, its molecules enter the pores of the papillae and stimulate the taste buds directly. In order to do this, the substance has to be dissolved in liquid. If it is not liquid when it enters the mouth, then it melts or is chewed and becomes mixed with saliva.

There are four basic tastes: sweet, salt, sour and bitter. Sometimes alkaline and metallic are also included as basic tastes. All other tastes are combinations of these. The taste buds are specialized, and each responds only to the kind of basic taste that is its specialty. The sweet and salt taste buds are most numerous on the tip and front part of the tongue, sour taste buds are mainly along the edges and bitterness is tasted at the back of the tongue. Bittersweet substances are tasted in two stages, first sweet, then bitter. The solid center of the tongue's surface has very few taste buds.

Other senses, including smell and touch, also play an important role in tasting.

taster (tās′ter) an individual capable of tasting a particular substance, such as phenylthiocarbamide, used in certain genetic studies.

taurine (taw′rēn) a crystallized acid from the bile.

taurocholate (taw″ro-ko′lāt) a salt of taurocholic acid, one of the bile acids.

taurocholemia (taw″ro-ko-le′me-ah) taurocholic acid in the blood.

taurocholic acid (taw″ro-ko′lik) a bile acid; when hydrolyzed it splits into taurine and cholic acid.

tautomer (taw′to-mer) a chemical compound exhibiting, or capable of exhibiting, tautomerism.

tautomeral, tautomeric (taw-tom′er-al), (taw″to-mer′ik) 1. sending axons to the white matter in the same side of the spinal cord; said of nerve cells. 2. exhibiting tautomerism.

tautomerism (taw-tom′er-izm) the dynamic equilibrium between two spontaneously interconvertible isomers.

taxis (tak′sis) 1. an orientation movement of a motile organism in response to a stimulus; it may be either toward (positive) or away from (negative) the source of the stimulus. 2. exertion of force in manual replacement of a displaced organ or part.

  coughing t., manipulation to reduce hernia while the patient coughs.

taxon (tak′son), pl. *tax′a* [Gr.] a particular category into which living organisms are classified on the basis of certain common features, as species, genus, family, order or class.

taxonomy (tak-son′o-me) the orderly classification of organisms into appropriate categories (taxa), with application of suitable and correct names. adj., **taxonom′ic.**

Tay-Sach's disease (ta saks′) amaurotic familial idiocy.

Taylor splint (ta′ler) a horizontal pelvic band and long lateral posterior bars; used to apply traction to the lower extremity.

Tb chemical symbol, *terbium.*

tb tuberculosis; tubercle bacillus.

Tc chemical symbol, *technetium.*

TCID tissue culture infective dose; that amount of a pathogenic agent that will produce pathologic change when inoculated on tissue cultures.

TCID$_{50}$ median tissue culture infective dose; that amount of a pathogenic agent that will produce pathologic change in 50 per cent of cell cultures inoculated.

Te chemical symbol, *tellurium.*

TEA tetraethylammonium, a ganglionic blocking agent, antihypertensive and peripheral vasodilator.

tea (te) an aqueous beverage prepared by infusion of herbs or other substance.
   pectoral t., an aqueous infusion of expectorant and demulcent herbs and aromatics.

TEAB tetraethylammonium bromide.

TEAC tetraethylammonium chloride.

tears (tērz) the watery secretion of the lacrimal glands that moistens the conjunctiva.

tease (tēz) to pull apart gently with fine needles to permit microscopic examination of ultimate structure.

teaspoon (te′spōon) a small spoon containing about 5 ml. or 1 fluid dram.

teat (tēt) the nipple of the mammary gland.

technetium (tek-ne′she-um) a chemical element, atomic number 43, atomic weight 99, symbol Tc. (See table of ELEMENTS.)

technician (tek′nish′an) a person skilled in the performance of technical procedures.

technique (tek-nēk′) the method of procedure and details of a mechanical process or surgical operation.

tectonic (tek-ton′ik) pertaining to plastic surgery.

tectorial (tek-to′re-al) of the nature of a roof or covering.

tectum (tek′tum) a rooflike structure.
   t. of midbrain, the dorsal portion of the midbrain.

teeth (tēth) plural of *tooth.*

teething (tēth′ing) eruption of the teeth through the gums. The average infant cuts his first tooth between the sixth and ninth months. The full set of 20 baby teeth erupt gradually over a period up to about 30 months, the customary pattern being the arrival of two teeth, one on each side of the jaw, at a time.
   Evidence of teething includes drooling, a compulsion to put objects into the mouth and unusual crankiness. Some babies seem to be more bothered by teething than others, and different teeth affect the same baby in different ways.
   It was long fashionable to ascribe any baby ailment to teething, despite the considerable harm such a hasty diagnosis often did by delaying recognition of the real trouble. Although teething sometimes may cause a slight fever, any such symptom should be watched carefully for further developments.

tegmen (teg′men), pl. *teg′mina* [L.] a covering structure or roof.
   t. tym′pani, that part of the petrous bone covering the mastoid antrum.

tegmentum (teg-men′tum), pl. *tegmen′ta* [L.] a covering; used in anatomic nomenclature to designate various structures. adj., **tegmen′tal.**

Tegretol (teg′rĕ-tol) trademark for a preparation of carbamazepine, an anticonvulsant.

tegument (teg′u-ment) the integument or skin.

teichopsia (ti-kop′se-ah) scintillating scotoma; the sensation of a luminous appearance before the eyes, with a zigzag, wall-like outline.

teinodynia (ti″no-din′e-ah) pain in a tendon.

tela (te′lah), pl. *te′lae* [L.] a thin, weblike structure or tissue; used in naming various anatomic structures.
   t. conjuncti′va, connective tissue.
   t. elas′tica, elastic tissue.
   t. subcuta′nea, the subcutaneous connective tissue or superficial fascia.

telalgia (tel-al′je-ah) referred pain; pain occurring in a part distant from the lesion.

telangiectasia (tel-an″je-ek-ta′ze-ah) the presence of small red focal lesions, usually in the skin or mucous membrane, caused by dilation of capillaries, arterioles or venules. adj., **telangiectat′ic.**
   hereditary hemorrhagic t., a hereditary disorder marked by a tendency to bleeding due to local lesions of the capillaries.

telangiectasis (tel-an″je-ek′tah-sis), pl. *telangiec′tases* [Gr.] the small red focal lesion of telangiectasia.
   spider t., a focal network of dilated arterioles, radiating about a central core.

telangiitis (tel-an″je-i′tis) inflammation of capillaries.

telangioma (tel-an″je-o′mah) hemangioma.

telangiosis (tel-an″je-o′sis) any disease of the capillaries.

tele- (tel′e) word element [Gr.], *far away; operating at a distance; an end.*

telecardiography (tel″ĕ-kar″de-og′rah-fe) the recording of changes in the electric potential of the heart, the impulses being transmitted by telephone wires to the receiving apparatus located some distance from the subject.

telecardiophone (tel″ĕ-kar′de-o-fōn″) an apparatus for making heart sounds audible at a distance from the patient.

teleceptor (tel′ĕ-sep″tor) a sensory nerve terminal that is sensitive to stimuli originating at a distance. Such nerve endings exist in the eyes and ears.

telecinesia (tel″ĕ-si-ne′ze-ah) telekinesis.

telecurietherapy (tel″ĕ-ku″re-ther′ah-pe) treatment with radium placed at a distance from the body.

telediastolic (tel″ĕ-di″as-tol′ik) pertaining to the last phase of diastole.

telefluoroscopy (tel″ĕ-floo″or-os′ko-pe) television transmission of images visualized by fluoroscopy for observation and study at a distant location.

telekinesis (tel″ĕ-ki-ne′sis) movement of an object produced without contact.

telemetry (tĕ-lem′ĕ-tre) the making of measurements at a distance from the subject, the measurable evidence of phenomena under investigation being transmitted by radio signals.

telencephalon (tel″en-sef′ah-lon) 1. the larger portion of the forebrain, comprising chiefly the cerebral hemispheres, but including also the area adjacent to the anterior part of the third ventricle and the anterior part of the hypothalamus. 2. the anterior of the two vesicles formed by specialization of the prosencephalon in the developing embryo. adj., **telencephal′ic**.

teleneurite (tel″ĕ-nu′rīt) telodendron.

teleneuron (tel″ĕ-nu′ron) a neuron at which the impulse ceases; a nerve ending.

teleological (te″le-o-loj′ĭ-kal) serving an ultimate purpose in development.

teleology (te″le-ol′o-je) the doctrine that the explanation of phenomena is to be found in terms of their purpose.

teleomitosis (tel″e-o-mi-to′sis) completed mitosis.

teleonomic (tel″e-o-nom′ik) pertaining to or having evolutionary survival value.

teleonomy (tel″e-on′o-me) the doctrine that existence of a structure or function in an organism implies that it has had evolutionary survival value.

teleorganic (tel″e-or-gan′ik) necessary to life.

Telepaque (tel′ĕ-pāk) trademark for a preparation of iopanoic acid, an opaque medium used in cholecystography.

telepathy (tĕ-lep′ah-the) the communication of thought through extrasensory perception.

teleradiography (tel″ĕ-ra″de-og′rah-fe) radiography with the radiation source 6 to 7 feet from the subject.

telergy (tel′er-je) automatism.

teleroentgenography (tel″ĕ-rent″gen-og′rah-fe) roentgenography with the source of x-rays 6 to 7 feet from the subject.

telesthesia (tel″es-the′ze-ah) 1. perception at a distance. 2. extrasensory perception.

telesystolic (tel″ĕ-sis-tol′ik) pertaining to the end of systole.

teletherapy (tel″ĕ-ther′ah-pe) treatment with ionizing radiation whose source is located at a distance from the body.

telethermometer (tel″ĕ-ther-mom′ĕ-ter) a device for registering temperature at a distance from the body being studied.

telluric (tĕ-lu′rik) 1. pertaining to tellurium. 2. pertaining to or originating from the earth.

tellurium (tĕ-lu′re-um) a chemical element, atomic number 52, atomic weight 127.60, symbol Te. (See table of ELEMENTS.)

telo- (tel′o) word element [Gr.], *end*.

telocentric (tel″o-sen′trik) having the centromere at one end of the replicating chromosome.

telodendrion (tel″o-den′dre-on), pl. *teloden′dria* [Gr.] telodendron.

telodendron (tel″o-den′dron) one of the fine terminal branches of an axon.

telognosis (tel″og-no′sis) diagnosis based on facsimiles of roentgenograms transmitted by radio or telephonic communication to a clinical or diagnostic center.

telolecithal (tel″o-les′ĭ-thal) having a yolk concentrated at one of the poles.

telolemma (tel″o-lem′ah) the covering of a motor end-plate, made up of sarcolemma and an extension of Henle's sheath.

telomere (tel′o-mēr) an extremity of a chromosome, which has specific properties, one of which is failure to fuse with other fragments of chromosomes after a chromosome has been broken.

telophase (tel′o-fāz) the last stage of division of the nucleus of a cell in either meiosis or mitosis.

TEM triethylenemelamine, an antineoplastic agent.

Temaril (tem′ah-ril) trademark for preparations of trimeprazine tartrate, a systemic antipruritic.

temperament (tem′per-ah-ment) the peculiar physical character and mental cast of an individual.
  lymphatic t., that characterized by a fair but not ruddy complexion, light hair, and a general softness or laxity of the tissues.
  melancholic t., one characterized by melancholia and moroseness.
  nervous t., that characterized by predominance of the nervous element and by great activity or susceptibility of the brain.
  sanguine t., sanguineous t., that characterized by a fair and ruddy complexion, full, muscular development, large, full veins and an active pulse.

temperature (tem′per-ah-tūr) the degree of sensible heat or cold.
  Body temperature is measured by a clinical thermometer and represents a balance between the heat produced by the body and the heat it loses. Though heat production and heat loss vary with circumstances, the body regulates them, keeping a remarkably constant temperature. An abnormal rise in body temperature is called fever.
  See also Table of Temperature Equivalents in the Appendix.
  NORMAL BODY TEMPERATURE. Body temperature is usually measured by a thermometer placed in the mouth or in the rectum. The normal oral temperature is 98.6 degrees on the Fahrenheit scale; rectally, it is 99.2° F. On the Celsius (centigrade) scale, normal mouth temperature is 37° C. These values are based on a statistical average. Normal temperature varies somewhat from person to person and at different times in each person.

Body temperature is usually slightly higher in the evening than in the morning. It is also somewhat higher during and immediately after eating, exercise or emotional excitement. Temperature in infants and young children tends to vary somewhat more than in adults.

TEMPERATURE REGULATION. To maintain a constant temperature, the body must be able to respond to changes in the temperature of its surroundings. When the outside temperature drops, nerve endings near the skin surface sense the change and communicate it to the hypothalamus. Certain cells of the hypothalamus then signal for an increase in the body's heat production. This heat is conducted to the blood and distributed throughout the body. At the same time, the body acts to conserve its heat. The arterioles constrict so that less blood will flow near the body's surface. The skin becomes pale and cold. Sometimes it takes on a bluish color, the result of a color change in the blood, which occurs when the blood, flowing slowly, gives off more of its oxygen than usual.

Another signal from the brain stimulates muscular activity, which releases heat. Shivering is a form of this activity—a muscular reflex that produces heat.

When the outside temperature goes up, the body's cooling system is ordered into action. Sweat is released from sweat glands beneath the skin, and as it evaporates, the skin is cooled. Heat is also eliminated by the evaporation of moisture in the lungs. This process is accelerated by panting.

An important regulator of body heat is the peripheral capillary system. The vessels of this system form a network just under the skin. When these vessels dilate, they allow more warm blood from the interior of the body to flow through them, where it is cooled by the surrounding air.

ABNORMAL BODY TEMPERATURE. Abnormal temperatures occur when the body's temperature-regulating system is upset by disease or other physical disturbances. FEVER usually accompanies infection and many other disease processes. In most cases when the oral temperature is 100° F. or over, fever is present. Temperatures of 104° F. or over are common in serious illnesses, although occasionally very high fever accompanies an illness that causes little concern. Temperatures as high as 107° F. or higher sometimes accompany diseases in critical stages.

Subnormal temperatures, below 96° F., occur in cases of collapse (see also symptomatic HYPOTHERMIA).

absolute t., that reckoned from absolute zero (−273.15° C. or −459.67° F.).

critical t., that below which a gas may be converted to a liquid by pressure.

normal t., that usually registered by a healthy person (98.6° F. or 37° C.).

template (tem′plāt) a pattern or mold.

temple (tem′pl) the lateral region of the upper part of the head.

tempolabile (tem″po-la′bil) subject to change with the passage of time.

temporal (tem′po-ral) 1. pertaining to the lateral region of the head, above the zygomatic arch. 2. pertaining to time; temporary.

t. bone, one of the two irregular bones forming part of the lateral surfaces and base of the skull, and containing the organs of hearing.

t. lobe, a long, tongue-shaped process constituting the lower lateral portion of the cerebral hemisphere.

temporomandibular (tem″po-ro-man″dib′u-lar) pertaining to the temporal bone and mandible.

temporomaxillary (tem″po-ro-mak′sĭ-ler″e) pertaining to the temporal bone and maxilla.

temporo-occipital (tem″po-ro-ok-sip′ĭ-tal) pertaining to the temporal and occipital bones.

temporospatial (tem″po-ro-spa′shal) pertaining to both time and space.

temporosphenoid (tem″po-ro-sfe′noid) pertaining to the temporal and sphenoid bones.

tempostabile (tem″po-sta′bil) not subject to change with time.

Tempra (tem′prah) trademark for preparations of acetaminophen, an analgesic and antipyretic.

tenacious (tĕ-na′shus) holding fast; adhesive.

tenaculum (tĕ-nak′u-lum) a surgical instrument for grasping and holding parts.

tenalgia (ten-al′je-ah) pain in a tendon.

tenderness (ten′der-nes) a state of unusual sensitivity to touch or pressure.
 rebound t., a state in which pain is felt on the release of pressure over a part.

tendinitis (ten″dĭ-ni′tis) inflammation of a tendon. It is one of the commonest causes of acute pain in the shoulder. Tendinitis is frequently associated with a calcium deposit (calcific tendinitis), which may also involve the bursa around the tendon or near the joint, causing bursitis.

Treatment may consist of the administration of steroids, given orally or by injection into the bursa, or it may take the form of injections of procaine or x-ray therapy. In severe cases, surgical removal of the calcium deposit may be required.

tendinoplasty (ten′dĭ-no-plas″te) tenoplasty.

tendinosuture (ten″dĭ-no-su′tūr) tenorrhaphy.

tendinous (ten′dĭ-nus) pertaining to, or made up of, tendons.

tendo (ten′do), pl. *ten′dines* [L.] tendon; used in anatomic nomenclature.
 t. Achil′lis, t. calca′neus, Achilles tendon.

tendolysis (ten-dol′ĭ-sis) the freeing of a tendon from adhesions.

tendon (ten′don) a cord or band of strong white fibrous tissue that connects a muscle to a bone. When the muscle contracts, or shortens, it pulls on the tendon, which moves the bone. Tendons are so tough they are seldom torn, even when an injury is

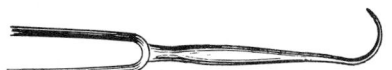

Tenaculum (Da Costa).

Tenaculum. (From Dorland's Illustrated Medical Dictionary. 24th ed. Philadelphia, W. B. Saunders Co., 1965.)

severe enough to break a bone or tear a muscle. One of the most prominent tendons is the Achilles tendon, which can be felt at the back of the ankle just above the heel; it attaches the triceps surae muscle to the calcaneus.

tendovaginal   (ten″do-vaj′ĭ-nal) pertaining to a tendon and its sheath.

tenectomy (tĕ-nek′to-me) excision of a tendon.

tenesmus   (tĕ-nez′mus) ineffectual and painful straining at stool or in urinating.

tenia (te′ne-ah), pl. *te′niae* [L.] 1. a flat band or strip of soft tissue; used in anatomic nomenclature to designate various structures. 2. an individual of the genus Taenia.

  te′niae co′li, the three thickened bands (te′nia li′bera, te′nia mesocol′ica and te′nia omenta′lis) formed by longitudinal fibers in the tunica muscularis of the large intestine, extending from the root of the vermiform appendix to the rectum.

teniacide   (te′ne-ah-sīd″) a medicine for destroying tapeworms.

teniafuge (te′ne-ah-fūj″) a medicine for expelling tapeworms.

teniasis   (te-ni′ah-sis) the presence of tapeworms in the body.

teno- (te′no) word element [Gr.], *tendon*.

tenodesis   (ten-od′ĕ-sis) suture of the end of a tendon to a bone.

tenodynia   (ten″o-din′e-ah) pain in a tendon.

tenomyoplasty (ten″o-mi′o-plas″te) plastic repair of a tendon and muscle, applied especially to an operation for inguinal hernia.

tenomyotomy   (ten″o-mi-ot′o-me) excision of tendon and muscle.

tenonectomy (ten″o-nek′to-me) excision of part of a tendon.

tenonitis   (ten″o-ni′tis) 1. inflammation of a tendon. 2. inflammation of Tenon's capsule, the connective tissue enclosing the eyeball.

tenontitis (ten″on-ti′tis) inflammation of a tendon.

tenonto- (ten-on′to) word element [Gr.], *tendon*.

tenontodynia   (ten″on-to-din′e-ah) pain in the tendons.

tenontography   (ten″on-tog′rah-fe) the written description of tendons.

tenontology   (ten″on-tol′o-je) the sum of what is known about the tendons.

tenontothecitis   (ten-on″to-the-si′tis) tenosynovitis.

tenophyte   (ten′o-fīt) an osseous growth in a tendon.

tenoplasty   (ten′o-plas″te) plastic repair of a tendon.

tenoreceptor   (ten″o-re-sep′tor) a nerve receptor in a tendon.

tenorrhaphy   (ten-or′ah-fe) suture of a tendon.

tenositis (ten″o-si′tis) tenontitis.

tenostosis   (ten″os-to′sis) conversion of a tendon into bone.

tenosuspension (ten″o-sus-pen′shun) attachment of the head of the humerus to the acromion by a strip of tendon; it is done for habitual dislocation of the shoulder.

tenosuture (ten″o-su′tūr) tenorrhaphy.

tenosynovectomy   (ten″o-sin″o-vek′to-me) excision of a tendon sheath.

tenosynovitis   (ten″o-sin″o-vi′tis) inflammation of a tendon and its sheath, the lubricated layer of tissue in which the tendon is housed and through which it moves. Tenosynovitis occurs most frequently in the hands and wrists or feet and ankles, and is often the result of intense and continued use, as with pianists and typists. It is painful, and may temporarily disable the affected part.

  Rheumatoid and other types of arthritis frequently involve tendon sheaths. A less common cause of tenosynovitis is injury to the tendon sheath and subsequent infection. It can also be the result of tuberculous or gonorrheal infection.

  Treatment is by immobilization of the limb or, in severe cases, by surgery for the purpose of draining an infected sheath, or to release a tendon from a constricting sheath.

  villonodular t., a condition marked by exaggerated proliferation of synovial membrane cells, producing a solid tumor-like mass.

tenotomy (ten-ot′o-me) transection of a tendon.
  graduated t., partial transection of a tendon.

tenovaginitis (ten″o-vaj″ĭ-ni′tis) tenosynovitis.

Tensilon (ten′sĭ-lon) trademark for a solution of edrophonium chloride, a parasympathomimetic, muscle stimulant, curare antagonist and diagnostic agent in myasthenia gravis.

tension (ten′shun) the quality of being stretched or strained, or under pressure.
  gaseous t., the elasticity of a gas, or its tendency to expand.
  intraocular t., intraocular pressure.
  premenstrual t., a complex of symptoms, including emotional instability and irritability, sometimes occurring in the 10 days before menstruation; other symptoms include pain in the breasts, headache, nausea, anorexia, constipation and pelvic discomfort (see also PREMENSTRUAL TENSION).
  surface t., tension or resistance that acts to preserve the integrity of a surface.
  tissue t., a state of equilibrium between tissues and cells that prevents overaction of any part.

tensometer (tens-om′ĕ-ter) an apparatus by which the tensile strength of materials can be determined.

tent (tent) 1. a conical, expansible plug for dilating an orifice or for keeping a wound open. 2. a portable shelter to be placed over a patient in bed, to limit dissemination of gases or vapors administered for therapeutic purposes.
  oxygen t., a portable shelter used in administration of OXYGEN.
  sponge t., a conical plug made of compressed sponge.

tentacle (ten′tah-kl) a slender, whiplike organ for receiving stimuli or for motion.

tentigo (ten-ti′go) morbid lasciviousness.

tentorium (ten-to′re-um), pl. *tento′ria* [L.] a covering structure or roof. adj., **tento′rial.**
  t. cerebel′li, that part of the dura mater that forms a partition between the cerebrum and cerebellum and covers the cerebellum.

tephromyelitis (tef″ro-mi″ĕ-li′tis) inflammation of the gray matter of the spinal cord.

tephrosis (tĕ-fro′sis) incineration or cremation.

tepor (te′por) [L.] gentle heat.

ter- (ter) word element [L.], *three.*

tera- (ter′ah) word element [Gr.], *monstrosity;* used in naming units of measurement to designate an amount 10^{12} (a trillion, or million million) times the size of the unit to which it is joined, as teracurie; symbol T.

teracurie (ter″ah-ku′re) a unit of radioactivity, being one trillion (10^{12}) curies.

teras (ter′as), pl. *ter′ata* [L., Gr.] a fetal monster.

teratism (ter′ah-tizm) an anomaly of formation or development; the condition of a fetal monster.

terato- (ter′ah-to) word element [Gr.], *monster; monstrosity.*

teratoblastoma (ter″ah-to-blas-to′mah) teratoma.

teratocarcinoma (ter″ah-to-kar″sĭ-no′mah) teratoma.

teratogen (ter′ah-to-jen) an agent or influence that causes physical defects in the developing embryo. adj., **teratogen′ic.**

teratogenesis (ter″ah-to-jen′ĕ-sis) the production of deformity in the developing embryo, or the production of a fetal monster. adj., **teratogenet′ic.**

teratogenous (ter″ah-toj′ĕ-nus) developed from fetal remains.

teratogeny (ter″ah-toj′ĕ-ne) teratogenesis.

teratoid (ter′ah-toid) like a monster.

teratology (ter″ah-tol′o-je) the branch of embryology that deals with abnormal development and congenital malformations.

teratoma (ter″ah-to′mah) a tumor made up of a number of different types of tissue, none of which is native to the area in which it occurs; a growth containing cellular elements derived from more than one primary germ layer.
  cystic t., a small neoplasm, lined by skin and filled with typical cheesy secretion, derived from the mainly ectodermal proliferation of totipotential cells.

teratophobia (ter″ah-to-fo′be-ah) morbid fear of giving birth to a teratism.

teratosis (ter″ah-to′sis) the condition of a monster.

terbium (ter′be-um) a chemical element, atomic

number 65, atomic weight 158.924, symbol Tb. (See table of ELEMENTS).

terchloride (ter-klo′rīd) trichloride.

terebene (ter′ĕ-bēn) a mixture of hydrocarbons from turpentine oil; antiseptic and expectorant.

terebinth (ter′ĕ-binth) turpentine.

terebration (ter″ĕ-bra′shun) the process of boring or trephining.

teres (te′rēz) [L.] round.

Terfonyl (ter′fo-nil) trademark for preparations of sulfamethazine, sulfadiazine and sulfamerazine (trisulfapyrimidines).

ter in die (ter in de′a) [L.] three times a day.

term (term) 1. a limit or boundary. 2. a definite period, especially the period of gestation, or pregnancy.

terminal (ter′mĭ-nal) 1. pertaining to an end. 2. a termination, end or extremity, especially a nerve ending.

terminatio (ter″mĭ-na′she-o), pl. *terminatio′nes* [L.] an ending; used in anatomic nomenclature to designate free nerve endings (terminationes nervo′rum li′berae).

terminology (ter″mĭ-nol′o-je) nomenclature; a system of scientific or technical terms; the science that deals with the investigation, arrangement and construction of terms.

terminus (ter′mĭ-nus), pl. *ter′mini* [L.] a term; expression. 2. an ending.

ternary (ter′nah-re) 1. third in a series or in order. 2. made up of three elements or radicals.

teroxide (ter-ok′sīd) trioxide.

terpene (ter′pēn) any hydrocarbon of the formula $C_{10}H_{16}$.

terpin (ter′pin) a product obtained by the action of nitric acid on oil of turpentine and alcohol.
  t. hydrate, a bitter, colorless, crystalline compound used as an expectorant.

Terramycin (ter′ah-mi″sin) trademark for preparations of oxytetracycline, an antibiotic.

terror (ter′or) an attack of extreme fear or dread.
  night t., an extreme fear reaction in a child during sleep or at night.

tertian (ter′shan) recurring in 3-day cycles (every second day); applied to the type of fever caused by certain forms of malarial parasites (see also MALARIA).

tertiary (ter′she-a″re) third in order.

tertigravida (ter″she-grav′ĭ-dah) a woman pregnant for the third time; gravida III.

tertipara (ter-tip′ah-rah) tripara; a woman who has had three pregnancies that resulted in viable offspring; para III.

Tessalon (tes′ah-lon) trademark for a preparation of benzonatate, an antitussive.

tessellated (tes'ĕ-lāt″ed) checkered; marked by little squares.

test (test) a procedure designed to demonstrate the existence or nonexistence of a certain quality or condition. See also specific names of tests, as ASCHHEIM-ZONDEK TEST.

acetic acid t., a test for albumin in the urine; acetic acid is added to boiled urine and a white precipitate forms.

agglutination t., one whose results depend on agglutination of bacteria or other cells; used in diagnosing certain infectious diseases and rheumatoid arthritis.

alkali-denaturation t., a spectrophotometric test for measuring the concentration of fetal hemoglobin.

angiotensin-infusion t., one for determining the role of renal artery stenosis in the genesis of a patient's hypertension; it is done by infusing angiotensin and monitoring the patient's blood pressure.

aptitude t., one designed to measure the capacity for developing general or specific skills.

association t., one based on associative reaction, usually by mentioning words to a patient and noting what other words the patient will give as the ones called up in his mind.

autohemolysis t., determination of spontaneous hemolysis in a blood specimen maintained under certain conditions, to detect the presence of certain hemolytic states.

biologic t's, tests involving the use of living organisms to determine the effects of the test material.

chromatin t., determination of chromosomal sex of an individual by examination of body cells for the presence of sex chromatin, which is found in cells of the normal female.

conjunctival t., itching and conjunctival congestion after instillation into the conjunctiva of an antigen to which the person is sensitive.

double-blind t., a study of the effects of a specific agent in which neither the administrator nor the recipient, at the time of administration, knows whether the active or an inert substance is being used.

finger-nose t., a test for coordinated movements of the extremities; the patient is directed to close his eyes, and, with arm extended to one side, slowly endeavor to touch the end of his nose with the point of his index finger.

human erythrocyte agglutination t., one for rheumatoid arthritis, depending on agglutination by the patient's serum of human Rh-positive cells sensitized with incomplete anti-Rh antibody.

intracutaneous t., one that involves introduction of an antigen between the layers of the skin and evaluation of the reaction elicited by it.

latex-fixation t., a serologic test for rheumatoid factor, helpful in the diagnosis of rheumatoid arthritis.

multiple-puncture t., an intracutaneous test in which the material used (e.g., tuberculin) is introduced into the skin by pressure of several needles or pointed tines or prongs.

neutralization t., one for the bacterial neutralization power of a substance by testing its action on the pathogenic properties of the organism concerned.

partial thromboplastin time t., a one-stage clotting test to detect deficiencies of the components of the intrinsic thromboplastin system.

patch t., a test for hypersensitivity, performed by observing the reaction to application to the skin of filter paper or gauze saturated with the substance in question (see also SKIN TEST).

paternity t., one to determine the blood groups of mother, child and alleged father for the purpose of excluding the possibility of paternity.

scratch t., a test for hypersensitivity in which a minute amount of the substance in question is inserted in small scratches made in the skin. A positive reaction is swelling or redness at the site within 30 minutes. Used in ALLERGY testing and in testing for tuberculosis (Pirquet's reaction). (See also SKIN TEST.)

serologic t., one involving examination of blood serum.

sickling t., a method to demonstrate hemoglobin S and the sickling phenomenon in erythrocytes, performed by reducing the oxygen concentration to which the red cells are exposed.

single-blind t., a study of the effects of a specific agent in which the administrator, but not the recipient, knows whether the active or an inert substance is being used.

thematic apperception t., TAT, a psychologic test in which the patient constructs a story from a set of pictures. It is designed to reveal the patient's emotions, drives, sentiments and conflicts.

three-glass t., a test to localize the site of urinary tract infection. The patient voids successively into three containers. In acute anterior urethritis the urine in only the first container will be turbid from pus. In posterior urethritis the urine in all three containers will be turbid.

thromboplastin generation t., a test for delineation of defects in formation of intrinsic thromboplastin and hence deficiencies of the factors involved.

tolerance t., 1. an exercise test to determine the efficiency of the circulation. 2. a test to determine the body's ability to metabolize a substance or to endure administration of a drug.

tourniquet t., one involving the application of a tourniquet to an extremity, as in determination of capillary fragility (denoted by the appearance of petechiae) or of the status of the collateral circulation.

tuberculin t., a test for the presence of active or inactive tuberculosis, consisting in the subcutaneous injection of 5 mg. of tuberculin; a positive test is denoted by redness and induration at the injection site.

two-stage prothrombin t., a method of quantitating prothrombin after tissue thromboplastin and excess clotting factor V have converted it into thrombin.

test meal a portion of food or foods given for the purpose of determining the functioning of the digestive tract.

barium t. m., a meal containing some preparation of barium as the opaque constituent (see also BARIUM TEST).

bismuth t. m., a meal containing some preparation of bismuth as the opaque constituent.

motor t. m., food or drink whose progress through the stomach, pylorus and intestinal tract is observed fluoroscopically.

opaque t. m., a meal containing some substance opaque to x-rays, permitting visualization of the gastrointestinal tract.

test tube a tube of thin glass, closed at one end; used in chemical tests and other laboratory procedures.

test type printed letters of varying size, used in the testing of visual acuity.

testectomy (tes-tek'to-me) removal of a testis; castration.

testes (tes'tēz) [L.] plural of *testis.*

testibrachium (tes"tĭ-bra'ke-um) the superior peduncle of the cerebellum.

testicle (tes'tĭ-kl) testis.

testiculoma (tes-tik"u-lo'mah) a tumor containing testicular tissue.

testis (tes'tis), pl. *tes'tes* [L.] the male gonad, normally situated in the scrotum; called also testicle. The testes produce the spermatozoa, the male reproductive cells, which are ejaculated into the female vagina during coitus, and the male sex hormone, testosterone, which is responsible for the secondary sex characters of the male. adj., **testic'ular.**

If the testes are removed (castration, bilateral ORCHIECTOMY) before puberty, the male is sterile and will never develop all the adult masculine characteristics. If the testes are removed after puberty, the male becomes sterile and his masculine characteristics will diminish unless he receives injections of male hormones. With aging, there is a gradual decrease in the production of testosterone.

In the unborn child, the testes lie close to the kidneys. During approximately the seventh month of fetal life, the testes begin to descend through the abdominal wall at the groin and enter the scrotum. As they descend they are accompanied by blood vessels, nerves and ducts, all contained within the spermatic cord. The passageway through which the testes and spermatic cord descend is called the inguinal canal. Failure of a testis to descend into the scrotum is called CRYPTORCHIDISM.

The testis is divided internally into about 250 compartments or lobules, each of which contains one to three extremely small and convoluted tubules, within which spermatozoa are produced. When mature, the spermatozoa leave the tubules and enter the epididymis situated on top of and behind each testis. The spermatozoa are stored in the epididymis until such time as they are mixed in the semen and ejaculated during coitus. (See also REPRODUCTION and REPRODUCTIVE ORGANS, MALE.)

testitis (tes-ti'tis) inflammation of a testis; called also ORCHITIS.

testoid (tes'toid) 1. resembling a testis. 2. a rudimentary testis.

testosterone (tes-tos'tĕ-rōn) one of the male sex hormones, or ANDROGENS, that are produced by the testes. Its chief function is to stimulate the development of the male reproductive organs, including the prostate, and the secondary sex characters, such as the beard. It encourages growth of bone and muscle, and helps maintain muscle strength.

Testosterone is obtained for therapeutic purposes by extraction from animal testes or by synthesis in a laboratory. It is used generally in all cases of hypogonadism—that is, underfunctioning of the testes. It is also used to relieve some forms of breast cancer. Women normally secrete a certain amount of male hormones; however, if the hormone balance is disturbed and there is overproduction of male hormones in a woman, signs of masculinity may develop.

  ethinyl t., ethisterone, a progestational steroid.

  methyl t., an orally effective form of testosterone.

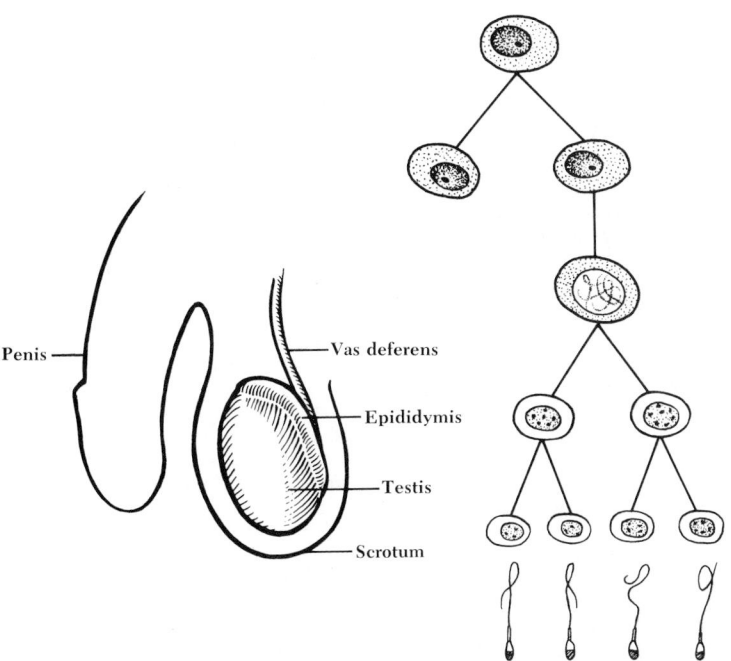

Testis.   Production of spermatozoa.

t. propionate, a creamy white crystalline powder, used as replacement therapy in the male and in treatment of certain conditions in the female, such as palliation of breast cancer.

Testryl (tes′tril) trademark for a suspension of pure crystalline testosterone.

tetaniform (tĕ-tan′ĭ-form) resembling tetanus.

tetanism (tet′ah-nizm) persistent muscular hypertonicity.

tetanization (tet″ah-nĭ-za′shun) the induction of tetanic convulsions or symptoms.

tetanize (tet′ah-nīz) to induce tetanic convulsions or symptoms in the organism or in a muscle.

tetanode (tet′ah-nōd) the unexcited stage of tetany.

tetanoid (tet′ah-noid) resembling tetanus.

tetanolysin (tet″ah-nol′ĭ-sin) a hemotoxin produced by *Clostridium tetani,* the causative organism of tetanus.

tetanophilic (tet″ah-no-fil′ik) having affinity for tetanus toxin.

tetanospasmin (tet″ah-no-spaz′min) the neurotoxic component of the tetanus toxin, of primary importance in the pathogenesis of tetanus.

tetanus (tet′ah-nus) a highly fatal disease caused by the tetanus bacillus (*Clostridium tetani*) and characterized by muscle spasm and convulsions. Because stiffness of the jaw is often the first symptom, it is known also as lockjaw. adj., **tetan′ic.**

Tetanus is a serious illness, but because of widespread immunization, it now strikes only about 500 people in the United States each year.

Tetanus bacilli, which grow in the intestines of animals and man, are prevalent in rural areas. They are found in soil and dust, and are spread by animal and human feces. The organisms enter the body through a break in the skin, particularly in puncture wounds, including those caused by nails, splinters, insect bites or gunshot. Occasionally, the original wound appears trivial and heals quickly; more often, there is obvious infection.

SYMPTOMS. Stiffness of the jaw is usually the first definite indication of tetanus. Difficulty in swallowing, stiffness of the neck, restlessness, irritability, headache, chills, fever and convulsions are also among the early symptoms.

Muscles in the abdomen, back, neck and face may go into spasm. If the infection is severe, convulsions are set off by slight disturbances, such as noises and drafts. During convulsions, there is difficulty in breathing and the possibility of asphyxiation.

TREATMENT. If there is any suspicion of contamination by tetanus bacilli, medical treatment should be obtained. This may include an adequate dose of antitoxin or a booster injection of tetanus toxoid (see below) to counteract any possible tetanus infection. Because of the possible danger of hypersensitivity to horse serum antitoxin, tetanus immune globulin—derived from human instead of horse serum—is preferred when available. In any case, the wound area must be carefully cleaned, and all dead tissue and foreign substances removed.

During a tetanus attack, sedatives are given to reduce the frequency of convulsions. Antibiotics are also used at times to help combat secondary infection. Most recently, hyperbaric oxygenation, providing oxygen under high pressure, has been used in treatment of tetanus.

PREVENTION. The most important weapon against tetanus is immunization. Infants, children and adults should be immunized with tetanus toxoid, which enables the body to manufacture its own antitoxins against future tetanus contamination. A single dose of tetanus toxoid may provide some immunity for life. A series of three toxoid injections, followed by a fourth about a year later, with booster shots at 4-year intervals, provides maximal protection.

By the time he is 6 months old an infant should have had three injections of tetanus toxoid; they are usually given in combination with diphtheria and whooping cough immunization. A fourth combination injection should be given by the time a child is 18 months old.

NURSING CARE. Because the toxin from *Clostridium tetani* attacks the central nervous system, it is extremely important to provide a nonstimulating environment for patients with tetanus. The room must be kept dark and quiet, and drafts of cold air, noises and other external stimuli must be avoided because they may precipitate convulsive muscle spasms. As for any patient subject to convulsions, padded side rails are applied to the bed to prevent injury to the patient during a seizure. The head board is also padded with a cotton blanket or pillow, and a padded tongue depressor is kept at the bedside for insertion during seizures to prevent biting of the tongue. If the jaws are locked in a position that prevents proper insertion of the tongue blade, no attempt should be made to force the jaws open.

Since opening the mouth and swallowing may be very painful or difficult, fluids and nourishment usually are given intravenously during the acute stage of the disease. The patient's intake and output are carefully measured and recorded. Sedatives and antibiotic drugs are administered as ordered to reduce irritability and to combat secondary bacterial infections.

As long as the patient is acutely ill and likely to suffer from convulsive seizures, someone should be in constant attendance. Signs of respiratory difficulty, changes in pulse and blood pressure and frequent and prolonged muscle spasms should be reported immediately to the physician in charge. A tracheostomy set should be readily available in the event severe dyspnea should develop.

t. neonato′rum, tetanus of very young infants, usually due to infection of the umbilicus.

tetany (tet′ah-ne) 1. continuous tonic spasm of a muscle; steady contraction of a muscle without distinct twitching. 2. a syndrome manifested by sharp flexion of the wrist and ankle joints (carpopedal spasm), muscle twitchings, cramps and convulsions, sometimes with attacks of stridor. It is caused by inadequate amounts of ionized calcium in the blood. This shortage of calcium causes irritability of the nerves and muscles, so that they respond to a stimulus with unnatural, violent contractions.

The drop in the calcium level can be caused by any one of several factors. It may occur in women during pregnancy or after childbirth if an excess amount of the mother's body calcium is used.

Tetany in a newborn baby is usually caused by temporarily underactive parathyroid glands. These glands normally keep the calcium and phosphate content of the blood at proper level. In children, tetany is more likely to occur because of an inadequate supply of calcium or vitamin D in the diet. Vitamin D is required for utilization of calcium in the body. Another cause of tetany in children is loss of calcium as a result of constant diarrhea.

An occasional cause of tetany in adults is the accidental removal or destruction of the parathyroid glands during thyroidectomy. This is sometimes unavoidable because the parathyroid glands are small and usually attached to the back of the thyroid gland or embedded in it.

Tetany often accompanies alkalosis, which may occur with prolonged vomiting, resulting in the loss of chlorides, or with excessive use of alkalis such as sodium bicarbonate. Alkalosis is also sometimes produced by hyperventilation.

TREATMENT. Treatment for tetany varies according to the cause and is usually successful. It may include the administration of vitamin D, calcium, parathyroid hormone or other remedies. In chronic cases, as in the loss of the parathyroid glands, treatment may have to be continued indefinitely.

duration t., a continuous tetanic contraction in response to a strong continuous current, occurring especially in degenerated muscles.

gastric t., a severe form due to disease of the stomach, attended by difficult respiration and painful tonic spasms of the extremities.

hyperventilation t., tetany produced by forced inspiration and expiration continued for a considerable time.

latent t., tetany elicited by the application of electrical and mechanical stimulation.

parathyroid t., parathyroprival t., tetany due to removal or hypofunctioning of the parathyroid glands.

thyroprival t., a form due to removal or hypofunctioning of the thyroid gland.

tetartanopia, tetartanopsia (tet″ar-tah-no′pe-ah), (tet″ar-tah-nop′se-ah) 1. quadrantanopia; loss of vision in one-fourth of the visual field. 2. a type of defective color vision.

tetra- (tĕ′trah) word element [Gr.], *four.*

tetrabasic (tĕ″trah-ba′sik) having four replaceable hydrogen atoms.

tetrabrachius (tĕ″trah-bra′ke-us) a fetal monster having four arms.

tetracaine (tĕ′trah-kān) a white or light yellow, waxy solid, used as a local anesthetic; applied topically to the conjunctiva in 0.5 per cent ointment.

t. hydrochloride, a fine white crystalline powder, used as a local anesthetic; administered in solution intraspinally or topically to the conjunctiva or in the nose and throat.

tetrachloride (tĕ″trah-klo′rīd) a compound of a radical with four atoms of chlorine.

tetrachloroethylene (tĕ″trah-klōr″o-eth′ĭ-lēn) a clear, colorless liquid used as an anthelmintic.

tetracrotic (tĕ″trah-krot′ik) having four sphygmographic waves or elevations to one beat of the pulse.

tetracycline (tĕ″trah-si′klēn) an antibiotic substance that is effective against many different microorganisms, including rickettsiae, certain viruses and both gram-negative and gram-positive microorganisms. Preparations include chlortetracycline hydrochloride (Aureomycin), tetracycline hydrochloride (Achromycin) and demethylchlortetracycline (Declomycin).

Tetracyn (tĕ′trah-sin) trademark for preparations of tetracycline.

tetrad (tĕ′trad) 1. an element with a valence of four. 2. a group of four similar bodies or units.

tetradactyly (tĕ″trah-dak′tĭ-le) the presence of four digits on the hand or foot.

tetraethylammonium (tĕ″trah-eth″il-ah-mo′ne-um) a radical that, in various compounds (tetraethylammonium bromide, tetraethylammonium chloride), is used as a ganglionic blocking agent, antihypertensive and peripheral vasodilator.

tetraethylthiuram disulfide (tĕ″trah-eth′il-thi′u-ram di-sul′fīd) a white or slightly yellow powder; used in treatment of alcoholism, because it produces a hypersensitivity reaction to alcohol.

tetragenous (tĕ-traj′ĕ-nus) splitting into groups of four.

tetragonum (tĕ″trah-go′num) [L.] a four-sided figure.

tetrahydrozoline (tĕ″trah-hi-dro′zo-lēn) a sympathomimetic agent used topically as a nasal decongestant.

tetraiodophthalein (tĕ″trah-i″o-do-thal′ēn) iodophthalein.

tetraiodothyronine (tĕ″trah-i″o-do-thi′ro-nēn) thyroxine.

tetralogy (tĕ-tral′o-je) a group or series of four.

t. of Fallot, a congenital defect of the heart that combines four structural anomalies: pulmonary stenosis (narrowing of the pulmonary artery); ventricular septal defect, or abnormal opening between the right and left ventricles; dextroposition of the aorta, in which the aortic opening overrides the septum and receives blood from both the right and left ventricles; and right ventricular hypertrophy, or increase in volume of the myocardium of the right ventricle.

Infants with this condition are sometimes referred to as blue babies because of the presence of cyanosis, an outstanding symptom of tetralogy of Fallot. The cyanosis is due to mixing of poorly oxygenated blood from the systemic circulation with oxygenated blood from the lungs, because of the position of the aorta. Other symptoms include clubbing of the ends of the fingers, hemoptysis, dyspnea on exertion and a slight delay in growth and development.

Diagnosis is confirmed by electrocardiography, angiocardiography and cardiac catheterization. These procedures demonstrate changes in the heart's electric impulses; defects in the ventricles, aorta and pulmonary artery; and, from samplings of blood taken from the various chambers of the heart and great vessels, the oxygen content and pressure of the blood in these various areas.

Treatment of tetralogy of Fallot involves surgical correction whenever possible. Without corrective surgery the prognosis is extremely poor for children who are deeply cyanotic and have dyspnea on slight exertion.

Before surgery medical treatment to avoid complications and to control dyspneic attacks is necessary. Since the hematocrit is high and polycythemia is common, efforts must be made to prevent dehydration and avoid the development of thrombi. Paroxysmal dyspnea, which often follows feeding or a spell of crying, usually can be relieved by placing the infant in knee-chest position, administering oxygen or giving him a mild sedative or morphine.

Surgical procedures for correction of the defects in the heart and great vessels vary according to the severity of symptoms and the age of the patient. In some cases an anastomosis of the arteries may be done as a temporary measure until more extensive surgery is feasible. In most cases open heart surgery is most successful in relieving symptoms and produces the most lasting benefits. The risks of heart surgery have been reduced by the development of machines to provide extracorporeal circulation of the blood while the heart defects are being repaired (see also HEART surgery).

tetrameric (tĕ″trah-mer′ik) having four parts.

tetranopsia (te″trah-nop′se-ah) obliteration of one quadrant of the visual field.

tetraparesis (tĕ″trah-pah-re′sis) muscular weakness affecting all four extremities.

tetrapeptide (tĕ″trah-pep′tīd) a peptide formed from four amino acids.

tetraplegia (tĕ″trah-ple′je-ah) paralysis of all four extremities.

tetraploidy (tĕ′trah-ploi″de) the state of having four sets of chromosomes (4n).

tetrapus (tĕ′trah-pus) a fetal monster with four feet.

tetrasaccharide (tĕ″trah-sak′ah-rīd) a sugar, each molecule of which yields four molecules of monosaccharide on hydrolysis.

tetrascelus (tĕ-tras′ĕ-lus) a fetal monster with four legs.

tetrasomy (tĕ′trah-so″me) the presence of two extra chromosomes of one type in an otherwise diploid cell (2n + 2).

tetraster (tĕ-tras′ter) a figure in mitosis produced by quadruple division of the nucleus.

Tetrastoma (tĕ″trah-sto′mah) a genus of trematodes sometimes found in urine.

tetratomic (tĕ″trah-tom′ik) 1. containing four atoms in the molecule. 2. containing four replaceable hydrogen atoms. 3. containing four hydroxyl groups.

tetravalent (tĕ″trah-va′lent) having a valence of four.

tetroxide (tĕ-trok′sīd) a binary compound containing four oxygen atoms in the molecule.

tetter (tet′er) a popular name for vesicular skin diseases, particularly herpes, eczema, psoriasis and pemphigus.

texis (tek′sis) childbearing.

textiform (teks′tĭ-form) formed like a network.

textoblastic (teks″to-blas′tik) forming adult tissue; regenerative.

textoma (teks-to′mah) a tumor composed of completely differentiated tissue cells.

textural (teks′tūr-al) pertaining to the constitution of tissues.

TGT thromboplastin generation test.

Th chemical symbol, *thorium.*

thalamencephalon (thal″ah-men-sef′ah-lon) that part of the diencephalon including the thalami, metathalamus and epithalamus.

thalamocoele (thal′ah-mo-sēl″) the third ventricle of the brain.

thalamocortical (thal″ah-mo-kor′tĭ-kal) pertaining to the thalamus and cerebral cortex.

thalamolenticular (thal″ah-mo-len-tik′u-lar) pertaining to the thalamus and lenticular nucleus.

thalamotomy (thal″ah-mot′o-me) the production of circumscribed lesions in the thalamus, formerly used in the treatment of certain psychotic states, and now sometimes used in the treatment of Parkinson's disease and certain other disorders of neuromuscular function.

thalamus (thal′ah-mus), pl. *thal′ami* [L.] either of two large ovoid structures composed of gray matter and situated at the base of the cerebrum. adj., **thalam′ic.** The thalamus functions as a relay station in which sensory pathways of the spinal cord and brain stem form synapses on their way to the cerebral cortex. Specific locations in the thalamus are related to specific areas on the body surface and in the cerebral cortex. A sensory impulse from the body surface travels upward to the thalamus, where it is received as a primitive sensation and then is sent on to the cerebral cortex for interpretation as to location, character and duration.

The thalamus has numerous connections to other areas of the brain as well, and these are thought to be important in the integration of cerebral, cerebellar and brain stem activity.

thalassemia (thal″ah-se′me-ah) a term for a group of hereditary hemolytic anemias in which the erythrocytes are extremely thin and fragile. The symptoms are believed to be the result of a defect of hemoglobin synthesis. These anemias occur most often among peoples from the Mediterranean basin, southern Asia and northern and central Africa. Called also erythroblastic anemia, Mediterranean anemia, and Cooley's anemia.

The genetic mechanisms involved in the occurrence of thalassemia are not clearly understood. Thalassemia major is thought to be the homozygous state and thalassemia minor, the heterozygous state.

In thalassemia major, the usual symptoms of anemia are present, and, in addition, the sclera and skin are slightly jaundiced and the spleen may be enlarged. There are bone changes and facial traits like those of Down's syndrome (mongolism). The prognosis in thalassemia major is very poor. Most patients must be given periodic and regular blood transfusions to maintain life. Life expectancy is extremely short; death usually occurs around the age of puberty.

Patients with thalassemia minor have very mild symptoms or none at all and require little or no treatment.

thalassophobia   (thah-las″o-fo′be-ah)   morbid dread of the sea.

thalassoposia   (thah-las″o-po′ze-ah) the drinking of sea water.

thalassotherapy   (thah-las″o-ther′ah-pe)   treatment of disease by sea bathing, sea voyages or sea air.

thalidomide   (thah-lid′o-mīd) a sedative and hypnotic compound whose use during early pregnancy was frequently followed by the birth of infants showing serious developmental deformities, notably malformation of a limb or limbs.

thallium   (thal′e-um) a chemical element, atomic number 81, atomic weight 204.37, symbol Tl. (See table of ELEMENTS.) Its salts are active poisons.

thanato-   (than′ah-to) word element [Gr.], *death.*

thanatobiologic   (than″ah-to-bi″o-loj′ik) pertaining to life and death.

thanatognomonic   (than″ah-tog″no-mon′ik) indicating the approach of death.

thanatoid   (than′ah-toid) resembling death.

thanatomania   (than″ah-to-ma′ne-ah) suicidal or homicidal mania.

thanatophobia   (than″ah-to-fo′be-ah) unfounded apprehension of imminent death.

thassophobia   (thas″o-fo′be-ah) morbid dread of sitting idle.

thebaine   (the-ba′in) a crystalline, poisonous and anodyne alkaloid from opium, having properties similar to those of strychnine.

thebaism   (the′bah-izm) opium poisoning.

theca   (the′kah), pl. *the′cae* [L.] a case or sheath. adj., **the′cal.**
  t. cor′dis, pericardium.
  t. follic′uli, the capsule of a graafian follicle.
  t. vertebra′lis, the membranes or meninges of the spinal cord.

thecoma   (the-ko′mah) a tumor of the ovary containing cells of the theca folliculi.

thecostegnosis   (the″ko-steg-no′sis) contraction of a tendon sheath.

theine   (the′in) the alkaloid of tea, isomeric with caffeine.

thelalgia   (the-lal′je-ah) pain in the nipples.

thelarche   (the-lar′ke) beginning of development of the breast at puberty.

theleplasty   (the′le-plas″te) plastic reconstruction of the nipples.

thelerethism   (thel-er′ĕ-thizm) erection of the nipple.

thelitis   (the-li′tis) inflammation of a nipple.

thelium   (the′le-um) 1. a papilla. 2. a nipple.

thelorrhagia   (the″lo-ra′je-ah) hemorrhage from the nipple.

thelygenic   (thel″ĭ-jen′ik) producing only female offspring.

thelyplasty   (thel′ĭ-plas″te) theleplasty.

thenad   (the′nad) toward the thenar or toward the palm.

thenar   (the′nar) the mound on the palm at the base of the thumb.

thenyldiamine   (then″il-di′ah-mēn) a compound used as an antihistamine.

Thenylene   (then′ĭ-lēn) trademark for a preparation of methapyrilene hydrochloride, an antihistamine.

thenylpyramine   (then″il-pir′ah-mēn) methapyrilene, an antihistamine.

theobromine   (the″o-bro′min) an alkaloid prepared from dried ripe seed of *Theobroma cacao*; used as a diuretic, myocardial stimulant, vasodilator and smooth muscle relaxant; available as theobromine calcium salicylate, theobromine sodium acetate and theobromine sodium salicylate.

Theoglycinate   (the″o-gli′sĭ-nāt) trademark for a preparation of theophylline sodium glycinate, used as a smooth muscle relaxant.

theomania   (the″o-ma′ne-ah) religious insanity; especially mental disorder in which the patient believes himself inspired by or possessed of divinity.

theophobia   (the″o-fo′be-ah) morbid fear of the wrath of God.

theophylline   (the″o-fil′in) an alkaloid derived from tea or produced synthetically; used as a smooth muscle relaxant, myocardial stimulant and diuretic; available as theophylline ethanolamine, theophylline methylglucamine, theophylline sodium acetate and theophylline sodium glycinate.
  t. cholinate, oxtriphylline, a smooth muscle relaxant, myocardial stimulant and diuretic.
  t. ethylenediamine, aminophylline, a smooth muscle relaxant, myocardial stimulant and diuretic.

theory   (the′o-re) a proposition advanced in explanation of an occurrence or condition.
  cell t., all organic matter consists of cells, and cell activity is the essential process of life.
  clonal-selection t. of immunity, immunologic specificity is preformed during embryonic life and mediated through certain cell groups or clones.
  germ t., 1. all organisms are developed from a cell. 2. infectious diseases are of microbic origin.
  unitarian t., a theory of blood cell formation that states that all blood cells (both red and white) derive from a single parental blood cell, the hemocytoblast.

Thephorin   (thef′o-rin) trademark for preparations of phenindamine tartrate, an antihistamine.

therapeutic   (ther″ah-pu′tik) pertaining to or effective in the treatment of disease.

therapeutics (ther″ah-pu′tiks) 1. the science and art of healing. 2. a scientific account of the treatment of disease.

therapeutist, therapist (ther″ah-pu′tist), (ther′-ah-pist) a person skilled in the treatment of disease or other disorder.

physical t., a person skilled in the techniques of physical therapy and qualified to administer treatments prescribed by a physician.

speech t., a person specially trained and qualified to assist patients in overcoming speech and language disorders.

therapy (ther′ah-pe) treatment designated to eliminate disease or other bodily disorder or derangement.

anticoagulant t., the use of drugs to suppress coagulability of the blood and prevent formation of thrombi without incurring the risk of hemorrhage.

collapse t., collapse and immobilization of the lung in treatment of pulmonary disease; artificial pneumothorax.

electroconvulsive t., electroshock t., the induction of convulsions by the passage of an electric current through the brain, as in the treatment of affective psychosis (see also SHOCK THERAPY).

fever t., induction of high body temperature by bacterial or physical means in the treatment of various morbid conditions, such as general paresis.

immunosuppressive t., treatment with agents that depress the formation of antibody, used in patients with autoimmune disease or those receiving organ transplants.

insulin shock t., induction of hypoglycemic coma by the administration of insulin in the treatment of affective psychosis (see also SHOCK THERAPY).

milieu t., in psychiatry, treatment by modification of the life circumstances or immediate environment of the patient.

nonspecific t., treatment of disease by agents that produce a general effect on cellular activity.

occupational t., use during the convalescent period of some type of work or occupation to promote recovery (see also OCCUPATIONAL THERAPY).

physical t., use of physical agents and methods in rehabilitation and restoration of normal bodily function after illness or injury (see also PHYSICAL THERAPY).

replacement t., administration of glandular substance or of hormones to compensate for deficiency of an endocrine secretion in the body.

serum t., serotherapy; treatment of disease by injection of serum from immune individuals.

shock t., the suspension of cerebral function by various means (insulin, electric current or other agent) in the treatment of affective psychosis (see also SHOCK THERAPY).

specific t., treatment by measures that are effective against the organism causing the disease.

speech t., the use of special techniques for correction of speech and language disorders.

substitution t., replacement therapy.

vaccine t., injection of killed cultures of an organism or of its products to produce immunity to or modify the course of a disease.

therm (therm) a unit of heat: (1) the small calorie; (2) British thermal unit.

therm(o)- (ther′mo) word element [Gr.], *heat.*

thermaerotherapy (therm-a″er-o-ther′ah-pe) treatment by application of hot air.

thermal (ther′mal) pertaining to heat.

thermalgesia (ther″mal-je′ze-ah) painful sensation produced by heat.

thermalgia (ther-mal′je-ah) causalgia.

thermanalgesia (therm″an-al-je′ze-ah) absence of sensibility to heat.

thermanesthesia (therm″an-es-the′ze-ah) inability to recognize heat and cold.

thermatology (ther″mah-tol′o-je) the study of heat as a therapeutic agent.

thermelometer (ther″mel-om′ĕ-ter) an electric thermometer.

thermesthesia (therm″es-the′ze-ah) perception of heat or cold.

thermesthesiometer (therm″es-the″ze-om′ĕ-ter) an instrument for measuring sensibility to heat.

thermhyperesthesia (therm″hi-per-es-the′ze-ah) increased sensibility to high temperatures.

thermhypesthesia (therm″hi-pes-the′ze-ah) decreased sensibility to high temperatures.

thermic (ther′mik) pertaining to heat.

thermistor (ther-mis′tor) a special type of resistance thermometer that measures extremely small changes in temperature.

thermobiosis (ther″mo-bi-o′sis) ability to live in a high temperature.

thermocautery (ther″mo-kaw′ter-e) cauterization by a heated wire or point.

thermochemistry (ther″mo-kem′is-tre) the aspect of physical chemistry dealing with temperature changes that accompany chemical reactions.

thermocoagulation (ther″mo-ko-ag″u-la′shun) coagulation of tissue with high-frequency currents.

thermocouple (ther′mo-kup″l) a pair of dissimilar electric conductors so joined that with the application of heat an electromotive force is established; used for measuring small temperature differences.

thermodiffusion (ther″mo-dĭ-fu′zhun) diffusion by heat.

thermoduric (ther″mo-du′rik) able to endure high temperatures.

thermodynamics (ther″mo-di-nam′iks) the branch of science dealing with heat and energy, their interconversion, and problems related thereto.

thermoexcitory (ther″mo-ek-si′tor-e) stimulating production of bodily heat.

thermogenesis (ther″mo-jen′ĕ-sis) the production of heat in organisms. adj., **thermogen′ic.**

thermogenics (ther″mo-jen′iks) the science of heat production.

thermogram (ther′mo-gram) the film produced by thermography.

thermograph (ther'mo-graf) an instrument for registering heat variations.

thermography (ther-mog'rah-fe) a technique of photographically portraying surface temperature of a body, based on self-emanating infrared radiation; sometimes used as a means of diagnosing underlying pathologic processes.

thermohyperalgesia (ther"mo-hi"per-al-je'ze-ah) extreme thermalgesia.

thermohyperesthesia (ther"mo-hi"per-es-the'ze-ah) extreme sensitiveness to heat.

thermoinactivation (ther"mo-in-ak"tĭ-va'shun) destruction of the power to act by exposure to high temperature.

thermoinhibitory (ther"mo-in-hib'ĭ-tor"e) retarding generation of bodily heat.

thermolabile (ther"mo-la'bil) easily affected by heat.

thermology (ther-mol'o-je) the science of heat.

thermoluminescence (ther"mo-lu"mĭ-nes'ens) the production of light by a substance when its temperature is increased.

thermolysis (ther-mol'ĭ-sis) 1. dissociation by means of heat. 2. dissipation of bodily heat by radiation, etc. adj., **thermolyt'ic.**

thermomassage (ther"mo-mah-sahzh') massage with heat.

thermomastography (ther"mo-mas-tog'rah-fe) use of thermography for the detection of lesions of the breast.

thermometer (ther-mom'ĕ-ter) an instrument for determining temperatures, in principle making use of a substance (such as alcohol or mercury) with a physical property that varies with temperature and is susceptible of measurement on some defined scale.

Celsius t., one on which the melting point of ice is 0 and the boiling point of water is 100 degrees. (For equivalents of Celsius and Fahrenheit temperatures, see the Appendix.)

clinical t., one used to determine the temperature of the human body.

Fahrenheit t., one on which the melting point of ice (freezing point of water) is 32 and the boiling point of water is 212 degrees.

oral t., a clinical thermometer whose mercury-containing bulb is placed under the tongue.

Réaumur's t., one on which the freezing point of water is 0 and the boiling point is 80 degrees.

recording t., a temperature-sensitive instrument by which the temperature to which it is exposed is continuously recorded.

rectal t., a clinical thermometer that is inserted in the rectum for determining body temperature.

resistance t., one that uses the electric resistance of metals for determining temperature (thermocouple).

thermometry (ther-mom'ĕ-tre) measurement of temperature.

thermophile (ther'mo-fīl) a microorganism that grows best at temperatures of 55 to 65° C.

thermophobia (ther"mo-fo'be-ah) morbid dread or intolerance of heat.

thermophore (ther'mo-fōr) an apparatus for retaining heat; used in the local application of heat.

thermopile (ther'mo-pīl) a number of thermocouples in series, used to increase sensitivity to change in temperature or for direct conversion of heat into electric energy.

thermoplacentography (ther"mo-plas"en-tog'-rah-fe) use of thermography for determination of the site of placental attachment.

Comparison of the Fahrenheit and Celsius temperature scales. (From Lee, G. L., Van Orden, H. O., and Ragsdale, R. O.: General and Organic Chemistry. Philadelphia, W. B. Saunders Co., 1971.)

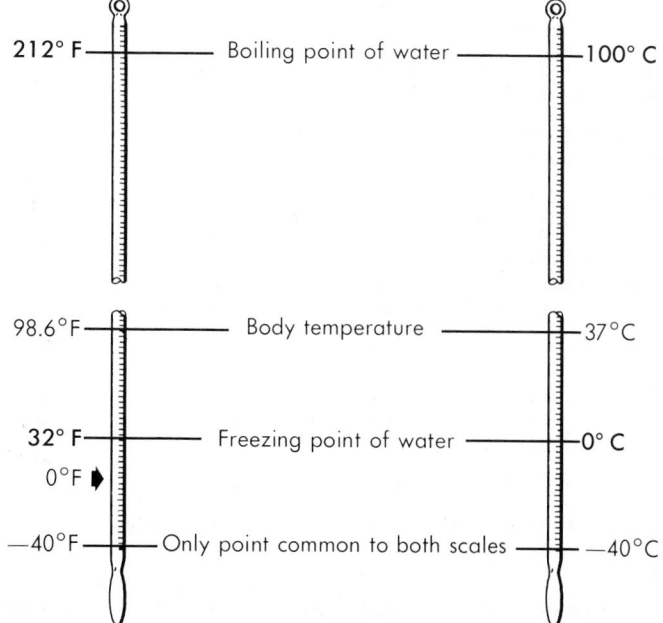

212° F — Boiling point of water — 100° C

98.6°F — Body temperature — 37°C

32° F — Freezing point of water — 0° C

0°F ▶

—40°F — Only point common to both scales — —40°C

thermoplegia (ther″mo-ple′je-ah) heat stroke or sunstroke.

thermopolypnea (ther″mo-pol″ip-ne′ah) quickened breathing due to great heat.

thermoreceptor (ther″mo-re-sep′tor) a nerve ending sensitive to stimulation by heat.

thermoregulation (ther″mo-reg″u-la′shun) heat regulation.

thermoresistance (ther″mo-re-zis′tans) the quality of being neither readily nor greatly affected by heat.

thermostabile (ther″mo-sta′bl) not affected by heat.

thermostasis (ther″mo-sta′sis) maintenance of temperature, as in warm-blooded animals.

thermostat (ther′mo-stat) a device interposed in a heating system by which temperature is automatically maintained between certain levels.

thermosteresis (ther″mo-stē-re′sis) deprivation of heat.

thermosystaltic (ther″mo-sis-tal′tik) contracting under the stimulus of heat.

thermotaxis (ther″mo-tak′sis) 1. normal adjustment of bodily temperature. 2. movement of a freely motile organism in response to an increase in temperature.

thermotherapy (ther″mo-ther′ah-pe) therapeutic use of heat.

thermotics (ther-mot′iks) the science of heat.

thermotolerant (ther″mo-tol′er-ant) capable of enduring heat, as certain bacteria whose activity is not checked by heat.

thermotonometer (ther″mo-to-nom′ĕ-ter) an instrument for measuring the amount of muscular contraction produced by heat.

thermotoxin (ther″mo-tok′sin) a toxic substance formed in the body by heat.

thermotropism (ther″mot′ro-pizm) orientation of growth in response to heat.

Theruhistin (ther″u-his′tin) trademark for preparations of isothipendyl, an antihistamine.

thesaurismosis (the-saw″riz-mo′sis) a metabolic disorder in which some substance accumulates in certain cells in abnormal amounts. The stored substances may be fats, proteins, carbohydrates or other substances.

thesaurosis (the″saw-ro′sis) a condition due to the storing up in the body of unusual amounts of normal or foreign substance.

thi(o)- (thi′o) word element [Gr.], *sulfur.*

thiabendazole (thi″ah-ben′dah-zol) a broad-spectrum anthelmintic found useful in ancylostomiasis and strongyloidiasis.

thiamazole (thi-am′ah-zōl) methimazole, a thyroid inhibitor.

thiamine (thi′ah-min) a vitamin of the B complex; called also vitamin B₁. It is found in high quantities in yeast, pork and whole-grain cereals. Lack of thiamine in the diet can result in beriberi. (See also VITAMIN).

t. hydrochloride, t. mononitrate, preparations used therapeutically as a vitamin supplement.

thiamylal (thi-am′ĭ-lal) an ultra-short-acting barbiturate.

sodium t., a compound used intravenously as a general anesthetic.

thiazide diuretics (thi′ah-zīd) a group of synthetic compounds that effect diuresis by enhancing the excretion of sodium and chloride.

thiemia (thi-e′me-ah) sulfur in the blood.

thigh (thi) the portion of the lower extremity above the knee and below the hip.

thigmesthesia (thig″mes-the′ze-ah) tactile sensibility.

thigmocyte (thig′mo-sīt) a blood platelet.

thigmotaxis (thig″mo-tak′sis) movement of a freely motile organism in response to the stimulation of touch.

thigmotropism (thig-mot′ro-pizm) orientation of growth in response to the stimulation of touch.

thimerosal (thi-mer′o-sal) a mercury-containing compound used as a local antibacterial agent.

thimethaphan (thi-meth′ah-fan) trimethaphan, a compound used in ganglionic blockade and as an antihypertensive.

thiobarbiturate (thi′o-bar-bit′u-rāt) a compound differing from barbiturates by the presence of a sulfur atom.

thiocyanate (thi′o-si′ah-nāt) a salt analogous in composition to a cyanate, but containing sulfur instead of oxygen.

thiodiphenylamine (thi″o-di-fen″il-am′ēn) phenothiazine, a compound whose derivatives are widely used as tranquilizers.

Thiomerin (thi″o-mer′in) trademark for a preparation of mercaptomerin sodium, a mercurial diuretic.

thiomersalate (thi″o-mer′sah-lāt) thimerosal, a local antibacterial.

thionine (thi′o-nin) a purple dye used as a nuclear stain.

thiopental (thi″o-pen′tal) an ultra-short-acting barbiturate.

t. sodium, the sodium salt of thiopental, injected intravenously or rectally as an anesthetic and used also as a sedative and in narcoanalysis.

thiopentone (thi″o-pen′tōn) thiopental.

thiopexy (thi′o-pek″se) the fixation of sulfur.

thiophil (thi′o-fil) an organism that grows successfully in the presence of sulfur or requires sulfur for its growth.

thiopropazate (thi″o-pro′pah-zāt) a phenothiazine compound used as a tranquilizer.

thioridazine (thi″o-rid′ah-zēn) a phenothiazine compound used as a tranquilizer.

thio-tepa (thi″o-te′pah) a compound used as an antineoplastic agent.

thiouracil (thi″o-u′rah-sil) a derivative of thiourea, used in treatment of hyperthyroidism because it suppresses thyroid hormone synthesis.

thiourea (th″o-u-re′ah) urea with its oxygen replaced by sulfur; an antithyroid substance that inhibits thyroid function.

thirst (therst) a sensation, often referred to the mouth and throat, associated with a craving for drink; ordinarily interpreted as a desire for water.

thixotropism, thixotropy (thik-sot′ro-pizm), (thik-sot′ro-pe) the property of certain gels of becoming fluid when shaken and then becoming solid again.

thlipsencephalus (thlip″sen-sef′ah-lus) a fetal monster with a defective skull.

Thomas splint (tom′as) two round iron rods joined at the upper end by an oval iron ring, or half ring, and bent at the lower end to form the letter W; used to give support to the lower extremity and to remove the weight of the body from the knee joint by transferring it to the pelvis.

Thomsen's disease (tom′senz) myotonia congenita.

thonzylamine (thon-zil′ah-min) a compound used as an antihistamine.

thoracalgia (tho″rah-kal′je-ah) pain in the chest.

thoracectomy (tho″rah-sek′to-me) thoracotomy with resection of part of a rib.

thoracentesis (tho″rah-sen-te′sis) surgical puncture and drainage of the thoracic cavity. The procedure may be done as an aid to the diagnosis of inflammatory or neoplastic diseases of the lung or pleura, or it may be used as a therapeutic measure to remove accumulations of fluid from the thoracic cavity.

The patient sits up for this procedure, his arms and head resting on an overbed table. The skin at the site of insertion of the needle is cleansed with an antiseptic, and a local anesthetic is injected. The site most often used is the seventh intercostal space, just below the angle of the scapula.

Equipment needed includes a 50 cc. syringe and an aspirating needle, a stopcock and rubber tubing, a hemostat, sterile gauze dressings, sterile towels and a sterile specimen tube.

After the procedure is completed the wound usually is sealed with collodion and covered with a sterile dressing. The site is checked frequently for signs of leakage, which should be reported to the physician.

The character and amount of fluid obtained is noted and recorded on the patient's chart. The patient is observed for changes in color or respiration, excessive coughing or blood-tinged sputum following the procedure. Frequently a chest x-ray is obtained after thoracentesis to determine whether air has been introduced into the pleural cavity and whether fluid remains.

thoracic (tho-ras′ik) pertaining to the chest.

 t. cage, the bony structure enclosing the thorax, consisting of the ribs, vertebral column and sternum.

 t. duct, a duct beginning in the receptaculum chyli and emptying into the venous system at the junction of the left subclavian and left internal jugular veins. It acts as a channel for the collection of the lymph from the portions of the body below the diaphragm and from the left side of the body above the diaphragm.

 t. surgery, surgical procedures involving entrance into the chest cavity. Until techniques for endotracheal anesthesia were perfected, this type of surgery was extremely dangerous because of the possibility of lung collapse. By administering anesthesia under pressure through an endotracheal tube it is now possible to keep one or both lungs expanded, even when they are subjected to atmospheric pressure.

Surgical procedures involving the lungs, heart and great vessels are included under thoracic surgery. In order to give intelligent care to the patient before and after surgery, one must have adequate knowledge of the anatomy and physiology of the chest and thoracic cavity. It is especially important to know the difference in pressures within and outside the thoracic cavity.

The thorax is like a closed box with an internal pressure of 751 to 754 mm. of mercury. The lungs are elastic sacs, the interiors of which are open to the outside by way of the respiratory tract. This means that their interiors are subjected to atmospheric pressure, about 760 mm. of mercury. The walls of the thoracic cavity, being airtight, protect the lungs from the greater atmospheric pressure, allowing them to inflate and deflate during respiration. Since the pressure within the thoracic cavity and against the exterior of the lungs is less than that of atmospheric pressure, any surgical incision or traumatic puncture of the thoracic wall will result in an inrushing of air into the cavity. These facts are especially important to remember in the care of drainage tubes or catheters inserted during thoracic surgery. It is essential that these catheters be attached to a closed drainage system and that they be clamped off securely whenever emptying of the drainage bottle is necessary.

NURSING CARE. Prior to surgery the nursing care will depend on the specific operation to be done and the particular disorder requiring surgery. (See also surgery of the LUNG, and HEART surgery.) In general, the patient should be given an explanation of the operative procedure anticipated and the type of equipment that will be used in the postoperative period. He will be taught the proper method of coughing to remove secretions accumulated in the lungs. Although coughing may be painful in the immediate postoperative period and may require analgesic medication to relieve the discomfort, if the patient understands the need for coughing up the secretions he will be more cooperative. He may be given special exercises to preserve muscular action of the shoulder on the affected side and to maintain proper alignment of the upper portion of his body and arm. Usually the physical therapist supervises these exercises but the nursing staff must cooperate in seeing that they are done.

Narcotics are rarely given before thoracic surgery because they can depress respiration. Usually the preoperative medication is atropine in combination with a barbiturate.

When the patient returns from the operating room

the drainage catheters are usually protruding from above and below the area of surgery. The upper catheter allows for removal of air and the gradual expansion of the lung. The lower catheter provides for drainage of fluid. These catheters are attached to a closed drainage system.

The purpose of the closed drainage system is not only to keep the thorax free of fluid but also to keep the lung expanded. There are several types of drainage systems. One consists of sterile tubing and two sterile bottles half filled with sterile water. The rubber stopper in the first bottle fits snugly into the bottle neck and has two openings, one for a glass tube to which the tubing and catheter are connected. The end of this glass tube must always be under water as this allows for fluid to flow out of the chest cavity but prevents air from being sucked back into the cavity. The other glass tube is shorter and is connected to the second bottle, called the control bottle. This bottle also has a rubber stopper in its neck and two glass tubes through two holes in the stopper. One long glass tube (the one to which the tubing from the first bottle is attached) must be kept under water. All connections between the drainage catheters and the two bottles must be airtight.

When a patient cannot force out accumulated secretions by coughing, a chest suction machine may be used. These machines incorporate the principle of closed drainage and also provide negative pressure. Whatever the type of equipment used, the nurse should become familiar with its purpose and check frequently to be sure it is in good working order.

Care must be taken that the weight of the patient's body does not press against the drainage tubes and that the tubes are not allowed to kink and obstruct the flow of fluid. Patency of the drainage tubes can be checked by observing the fluctuations of drainage fluid each time the patient breathes. If it rises and falls regularly, the tubes are not obstructed. Should an obstruction occur it must be reported immediately. Damming up of fluids in the chest cavity can cause a change in the position of the heart and great vessels. This is called a mediastinal shift and can be quite serious. Symptoms include a rapid and irregular pulse, dyspnea and signs of shock. Mediastinal shift also can result from a sudden influx of air into the chest cavity. This is spontaneous pneumothorax and can occur when the drainage system is not airtight. It is characterized by dyspnea, sharp pain in the chest and cyanosis. When these complications occur, THORACENTESIS may be necessary to remove secretions or air from the chest cavity and allow for proper position of the heart and great vessels and for adequate expansion of the lung.

Clamps are kept at the bedside to be used if the drainage equipment fails to work properly or if there is a break in the airtight system. Drainage bottles must be kept below the level of the patient's chest so that there will not be a backward flow of fluid or water into the chest cavity. Sterile equipment is used, and when handling the equipment care must be taken not to introduce bacteria into the operative site by contamination of the catheters, rubber tubing or connections.

The amount of drainage fluid in the bottle varies with each patient, and with the type of surgery he has undergone; however, if drainage seems ex-cessive the surgeon should be consulted. Usually the amount is relatively small and the bottle should not require changing more than once in 24 hours If the fluid becomes bright red and seems to indicate fresh bleeding, the surgeon should be notified at once.

If the surgeon permits, the nursing staff may be responsible for measuring and recording the amount of drainage at regular intervals. This requires strict attention to proper clamping and reconnecting of the tubes and catheters before and after the bottles are removed and when they are reattached to the catheters.

As the operative site heals and the lung expands, the catheters can be safely removed. After their removal an airtight bandage is applied to the area. As a precaution against leakage of air into the chest cavity, the physician may apply petrolatum to the edges of the wound before applying the dressing.

t. vertebrae, the 12 vertebrae between the cervical and the lumbar vertebrae, giving attachment to the ribs and forming part of the posterior wall of the thorax.

thoraco- (tho′rah-ko) word element [Gr.], *chest.*

thoracoacromial (tho″rah-ko-ah-kro′me-al) pertaining to the chest and acromion.

thoracobronchotomy (tho″rah-ko-brong-kot′o-me) incision into the bronchus through the thoracic wall.

thoracocautery (tho″rah-ko-kaw′ter-e) division of pulmonary adhesions by cautery.

thoracoceloschisis (tho″rah-ko-se-los′kĭ-sis) fissure of the thorax and abdomen.

thoracocentesis (tho″rah-ko-sen-te′sis) thoracentesis.

thoracocyllosis (tho″rah-ko-sĭ-lo′sis) deformity of the thorax.

thoracocyrtosis (tho″rah-ko-sir-to′sis) abnormal curvature of the thorax.

thoracodelphus (tho″rah-ko-del′fus) a fetal monster with duplication of body parts below the thorax.

thoracodidymus (tho″rah-ko-did′ĭ-mus) thoracopagus.

thoracodynia (tho″rah-ko-din′e-ah) pain in the thorax.

thoracogastroschisis (tho″rah-ko-gas-tros′kĭ-sis) a developmental anomaly resulting from faulty closure of the body wall along the midventral line, involving both thorax and abdomen, i.e., fissure of the thorax and abdomen.

thoracograph (tho-rak′o-graf) an apparatus for recording the chest movements.

thoracolumbar (tho″rah-ko-lum′bar) pertaining to the thoracic and lumbar vertebrae.

thoracolysis (tho″rah-kol′ĭ-sis) pneumonolysis; division of the tissues attaching the lung to the chest wall, to permit collapse of the lung.

thoracomelus (tho″rah-kom′ĕ-lus) a fetal monster with a limb of a twin fetus attached to the thorax.

thoracomyodynia (tho″rah-ko-mi″o-din′e-ah) pain in the muscles of the chest.

thoracopagus (tho"rah-kop'ah-gus) conjoined twins united at the thorax.

thoracopathy (tho"rah-kop'ah-the) any disease of the thoracic organs.

thoracoplasty (tho'rah-ko-plas"te) surgical alteration of the shape of the thoracic cage by removal of ribs, allowing the chest wall and underlying lung to move inward.

thoracopneumoplasty (tho"rah-ko-nu'mo-plas"-te) plastic surgery of the chest and lung.

thoracoschisis (tho"rah-kos'kĭ-sis) fissure of the chest wall.

thoracoscopy (tho"rah-kos'ko-pe) endoscopic examination of the chest.

thoracostenosis (tho"rah-ko-stĕ-no'sis) abnormal contraction of the thorax.

thoracostomy (tho"rah-kos'to-me) incision of the chest wall, with maintenance of the opening for the purpose of drainage.

thoracotomy (tho"rah-kot'o-me) incision of the chest wall.

thorax (tho'raks) the part of the body between the neck and abdomen; the chest. It is separated from the abdomen by the diaphragm. The walls of the thorax are formed by the 12 pairs of ribs, attached to the sides of the spine and curving toward the front. The upper seven ribs are attached to the sternum, the next three connect with cartilage below and the last two (the floating ribs) are unattached in the front. The principal organs in the thoracic cavity are the heart with its major blood vessels, and the lungs with the bronchi, which bring in the body's air supply. The trachea enters the thorax to connect with the lungs, and the esophagus travels through it to connect with the stomach below the diaphragm.

Thorazine (thor'ah-zēn) trademark for preparations of chlorpromazine hydrochloride, an antiemetic and tranquilizer.

thorium (tho're-um) a chemical element, atomic number 90, atomic weight 232.038, symbol Th. (See table of ELEMENTS.) Formerly used as a roentgenographic contrast medium.

thoron (tho'ron) a radioactive isotope of radon.

Thorotrast (tho'ro-trast) a proprietary contrast medium formerly used in roentgenography, but found to be hepatotoxic.

threadworm (thred'werm) any nematode worm, as *Enterobius vermicularis* (See also WORMS).

thremmatology (threm"ah-tol'o-je) the science of the laws of heredity and variation.

threonine (thre'o-nin) a naturally occurring amino acid, one of those essential for human metabolism.

threpsology (threp-sol'o-je) the scientific study of nutrition.

threshold (thresh'old) the level that must be exceeded for an effect to be produced, as the degree of intensity of a stimulus that must be surpassed for a sensation to be produced, or the concentration that must be present in the blood before certain substances are excreted by the kidney (renal threshold).
  auditory t., the slightest perceptible sound.
  t. of consciousness, the lowest limit of sensibility; the point of consciousness at which a stimulus is barely perceived.

thrill (thril) a tremor perceived in auscultation or palpation.
  diastolic t., one felt over the precordium during diastole in advanced aortic insufficiency.
  hydatid t., one felt on percussing over a hydatid cyst.
  presystolic t., one occasionally felt just before the systole over the apex of the heart.
  purring t., a thrill of a quality suggesting the purring of a cat.
  systolic t., one felt over the precordium during systole in aortic stenosis, pulmonary stenosis and aneurysm of the ascending aorta.

thrix (thriks) hair.
  t. annula'ta, a condition in which a hair appears to be marked by alternating bands of white; called also ringed hair.

-thrix (thriks) word element [Gr.], *hair.*

throat (thrōt) 1. the area that includes the LARYNX and PHARYNX, passageways that link the nose and mouth with the respiratory and digestive systems of the body. 2. the fauces. 3. the anterior part of the neck.
  DISORDERS OF THE THROAT. Sore throat is caused by inflammation or irritation of tissue in one or more areas of the pharynx or larynx. The disorder may be a disease in itself (see PHARYNGITIS and LARYNGITIS) or a symptom of a disease affecting other areas of the body. It also may be due to excess smoking or overuse of the voice.
  Streptococcal sore throat, or "strep throat," is more severe than ordinary sore throat and may be accompanied by high fever, swelling of the cervical lymph nodes (swollen glands) and a rash. Penicillin or other antibiotics are usually used in treatment.
  TONSILLITIS is often the cause of inflammation and discomfort in the throat.
  Cancer of the throat, one of the least common forms of cancer, occurs most often in the larynx, and early diagnosis is essential to effective treatment. The first symptoms are persistent hoarseness and the feeling of a lump in the throat (although this feeling is usually caused by emotional stress, and is called globus hystericus).
  CARE OF THE THROAT. Proper care of the throat does not require the use of sprays, gargles or lozenges. On the contrary, nose drops and throat sprays, when inhaled, may irritate the trachea, bronchi or lungs.
  The people most concerned about their throats are usually those who depend on their voices in their occupations or professions. Proper training and use of the vocal muscles, not medications, are the best insurance against loss or change of voice. When muscular exhaustion from strain or overuse of the larynx does bring on laryngitis, rest for the voice muscles is the only real cure.
  In serious cases the physician may recommend medication or the use of steam inhalants, but the essential aspect of treatment is silence, with any

unavoidable talking done in a low voice. This "silent cure," if followed faithfully, is almost certain to result in the return of the normal voice.

thromb(o)- (throm′bo) word element [Gr.], *clot; thrombus.*

thrombase (throm′bās) thrombin.

thrombasthenia (throm″bas-the′ne-ah) a functional disorder of the blood platelets.
   Glanzmann's t., an inherited qualitative disorder of blood platelets, marked by ease of bruising and bleeding from mucous membranes.

thrombectomy (throm-bek′to-me) surgical removal of a clot from a blood vessel.
   medical t., enzymatic dissolution of a blood clot in situ.

thrombin (throm′bin) an enzyme resulting from activation of prothrombin, which catalyzes the conversion of fibrinogen to fibrin; a preparation from prothrombin of bovine origin is used as a clotting agent.

thromboangiitis (throm″bo-an″je-i′tis) intravascular clot formation, with inflammation of the vessel wall.
   t. oblit′erans, thromboangiitis with contraction of the vessel about the clot, leading to diminution of blood flow distal to the site; most frequently the lower extremities are affected. Called also BUERGER'S DISEASE.

thromboarteritis (throm″bo-ar″ter-i′tis) thrombosis with arteritis.

thromboclasis (throm-bok′lah-sis) the dissolution of a thrombus.

thrombocystis (throm″bo-sis′tis) the sac sometimes formed around a clot or thrombus.

thrombocyte (throm′bo-sīt) a blood platelet (see also PLATELET).

thrombocythemia (throm″bo-si-the′me-ah) a fixed increase in the number of circulating blood platelets.
   essential t., hemorrhagic t., a clinical syndrome with repeated spontaneous hemorrhages, either external or into the tissues, and greatly increased number of circulating platelets.

thrombocytin (throm″bo-si′tin) serotonin.

thrombocytocrit (throm″bo-si′to-krit) an instrument for counting thrombocytes.

thrombocytolysin (throm″bo-si-tol′ĭ-sin) clotting factor VIII.

thrombocytolysis (throm″bo-si-tol′ĭ-sis) destruction of thrombocytes.

thrombocytopathy (throm″bo-si-top′ah-the) any qualitative disorder of the blood platelets.

thrombocytopenia (throm″bo-si″to-pe′ne-ah) decrease in number of platelets in circulating blood. adj., **thrombocytope′nic.**

thrombocytopoiesis (throm″bo-si″to-poi-e′sis) the production of thrombocytes.

thrombocytosis (throm″bo-si-to′sis) increase in the number of platelets in the circulating blood.

thromboelastogram (throm″bo-e-las′to-gram) the graphic record of the values determined by thromboelastography.

thromboelastograph (throm″bo-e-las′to-graf) an apparatus used in study of the rigidity of blood or plasma during coagulation.

thromboelastography (throm″bo-e″las-tog′rah-fe) determination of the rigidity of the blood or plasma during coagulation by use of the thromboelastograph.

thromboembolism (throm″bo-em′bo-lizm) obstruction of a blood vessel with a thrombus that has broken loose from its site of formation.

thromboendarterectomy (throm″bo-en″dar-ter-ek′to-me) excision of an obstructing thrombus together with a portion of the inner lining of the obstructed artery.

thromboendarteritis (throm″bo-en″dar-ter-i′tis) inflammation of the innermost coat of an artery, with thrombus formation.

thrombogen (throm′bo-jen) prothrombin.

thrombogenesis (throm″bo-jen′ĕ-sis) clot formation.

thromboid (throm′boid) resembling a thrombus.

thrombokinase (throm″bo-ki′nās) thromboplastin.

thrombokinesis (throm″bo-ki-ne′sis) the clotting of blood.

thrombolymphangitis (throm″bo-lim″fan-ji′tis) inflammation of a lymph vessel due to a thrombus.

thrombolysis (throm-bol′ĭ-sis) dissolution of a thrombus.

thrombon (throm′bon) the circulating thrombocytes and their precursors.

thrombopathy (throm-bop′ah-the) thrombocytopathy.

thrombopenia (throm″bo-pe′ne-ah) thrombocytopenia.

thrombophilia (throm″bo-fil′e-ah) a tendency to the occurrence of thrombosis.

thrombophlebitis (throm″bo-flĕ-bi′tis) the development of venous thrombi in the presence of inflammatory changes in the vessel wall.
   t. mi′grans, a recurrent condition involving different vessels simultaneously or at intervals.

thromboplastic (throm″bo-plas′tik) causing clot formation in the blood.

thromboplastid (throm″bo-plas′tid) thrombocyte.

thromboplastin (throm″bo-plas′tin) a factor essential to production of thrombin and proper hemostasis. Extrinsic and intrinsic thromboplastin are formed as the result of the interaction of different clotting factors; the factors that combine to form extrinsic thromboplastin are not all derived from intravascular sources, whereas those that form intrinsic thromboplastin are. Tissue thromboplastin, called also clotting factor III, is released by or derived from extravascular sources.

thromboplastinogen (throm″bo-plas-tin′o-jen) clotting factor VIII.

thrombopoiesis (throm″bo-poi-e′sis) thrombocytopoiesis.

thrombosed (throm′bōsd) affected with thrombosis.

thrombosin (throm-bo′sin) thrombin.

thrombosinusitis (throm″bo-si″nŭ-si′tis) thrombosis and inflammation of a venous sinus of the dura mater.

thrombosis (throm-bo′sis) formation of blood clots, or thrombi, inside a blood vessel or in one of the chambers of the heart. adj., **thrombot′ic.**

A thrombus may form whenever the flow of blood in the arteries or the veins is impeded. Many factors can interfere with the normal flow of the blood. Sometimes heart failure or physical inactivity retards circulation generally, or a change in the shape or inner surface of a vessel wall impedes the flow of blood, as in atherosclerosis. Any mass that has grown inside the body can exert pressure on a vessel, or the vessel wall can be injured and roughened by an accident, surgery, a burn, cold, inflammation or infection. The blood may thicken in a reaction to the presence of a foreign serum or snake venom.

If the thrombus detaches itself from the wall and is carried along by the bloodstream, the clot is called an embolus. This condition is known as EMBOLISM.

A thrombus may form in the heart chambers. This sometimes occurs after coronary thrombosis (see below) at the place where the wall of the heart is weakened or in the dilated atria in some cases of mitral stenosis.

Because blood normally flows more slowly through the veins than through the arteries, thrombosis is more common in the veins than in the arteries.

VENOUS THROMBOSIS. Venous thrombosis occurs most often in the legs or pelvis. It may be a complication of phlebitis or may result from injury to a vein or from prolonged bed rest. The symptoms of venous thrombosis—a feeling of heaviness, pain, warmth or swelling in the affected part, and possibly chills and fever—do not necessarily indicate its severity. Immediate medical attention is necessary in any case. Under *no* circumstances should the affected limb be massaged.

In a thrombosis of the superficial veins, bed rest with the legs elevated and application of heat to the affected area may be all that is necessary. In a thrombosis of the deep veins, the affected part must

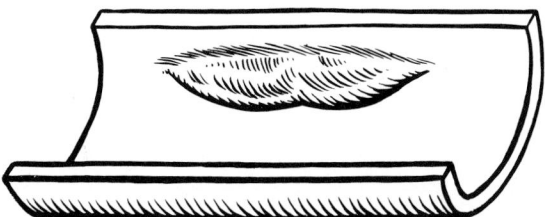

Thrombus on the inner wall of a blood vessel (shown here in section).

be immobilized to prevent the clot from spreading or turning into an embolus, and anticoagulant drugs may be given. With proper treatment, recovery occurs within a short time unless an embolism develops. Occasionally an operation is performed and the veins in which the clots have formed are tied off. Ordinarily, other veins take over their task and the circulation returns to normal.

To prevent venous thrombosis in a bedridden patient, an exercise routine should be followed even if it consists only of contracting and relaxing the muscles. The bedclothes should be loose enough to permit free movement of the legs. Elevating the foot of the bed and wrapping the legs from toe to knee with elastic bandages are also helpful. A board at the foot of the bed against which the patient can press his feet also helps to prevent blood stasis.

ARTERIAL THROMBOSIS. The main types of arterial thrombosis are related to arteriosclerosis, although thrombosis can result from infection or from injury to an artery. Arteriosclerosis may be hereditary or may be brought on by diabetes mellitus.

Coronary thrombosis is a complication of hardening of the coronary arteries. A blood clot in a coronary artery will block off part of the blood supply to the heart muscle and cause a severe heart attack. (See also CORONARY OCCLUSION.) This constitutes a medical emergency.

In cerebral thrombosis, a clot obstructs the supply of blood to the brain and causes a CEREBRAL VASCULAR ACCIDENT (stroke). Besides hardening of the cerebral arteries, cerebral thrombosis can also be caused by hypertension, or may be a complication of syphilis or other infections, dehydration, diabetes mellitus or a violent injury.

In advanced cases of arteriosclerosis, a clot may fill up whatever is left of a passageway, completely blocking off circulation to the area, and may eventually cause gangrene. This condition occurs most frequently in the arteries of the legs and is called peripheral thrombosis. The onset, which is often sudden, is characterized by either a tingling feeling or numbness and coldness in the limb. Pain is not always present. Immediate treatment with anticoagulants to discourage clotting is necessary. If this is not effective, surgery may be required. This condition is most common in the elderly and in diabetics. Modern methods of treatment can often save the limb.

In addition to the surgical removal of a thrombus or an embolus, surgery of the blood vessels also involves the removal of old, narrowed or deteriorated vessels and their replacement with grafts.

thrombostasis (throm-bos′tah-sis) stasis of blood in a part with formation of thrombus.

thrombosthenin (throm″bo-sthe′nin) a substance liberated by blood platelets that is important for clot retraction and firmness of the clot.

thrombus (throm′bus) a solid mass formed in the living heart or vessels from constituents of the blood.

　mural t., one that is attached at only one side to the vessel wall or endocardium and does not entirely obstruct blood flow.

　occluding t., one that occupies the entire lumen of a vessel and obstructs blood flow.

　parietal t., mural thrombus.

thrush (thrush) infection of the oral mucous membrane by a fungus (*Candida albicans*). It is characterized by white patches on a red, moist inflamed surface, occurring anywhere in the mouth, including the tongue, but usually on the inner cheeks. These patches are occasionally accompanied by pain and fever.

Approximately 20 to 30 per cent of the population harbors *Candida albicans*, but the disease develops in only a very small number of this group. Those who are most susceptible are infants and adults who are in a weakened condition from infection, dietary deficiency (malnutrition) or uncontrolled diabetes mellitus, or who have been treated with antibiotics for a long time.

Any baby who has a sore throat and shows discomfort while nursing may have thrush. If the white patches that appear remain untreated, they will become larger and will tend to grow together; they may also spread to other parts of the body. If rubbed or irritated, they will become inflamed or bleed.

Thrush is sometimes regarded as a minor infection, yet it can persist for weeks or even months, especially in young babies. It is important that the cause of the infection be treated. Any dietary deficiency or diabetic condition that may exist must be corrected. Thrush itself is treated with antibiotics and fungicidal drugs. The best preventive measures are good general health, a well balanced diet and good mouth hygiene.

thrypsis (thrip'sis) a comminuted fracture.

thulium (thoo'le-um) a chemical element, atomic number 69, atomic weight 168.934, symbol Tm. (See table of ELEMENTS.)

thumb (thum) the first digit of the hand; it has only two phalanges and is apposable to the four fingers of the hand.

thym(o)- (thi'mo) word element [Gr.], *thymus; mind, soul* or *emotions.*

thymectomy (thi-mek'to-me) excision of the thymus.

thymelcosis (thi″mel-ko'sis) ulceration of the thymus.

thymergasia (thi″mer-ga'ze-ah) affective psychosis.

-thymia (thi'me-ah) word element [Gr.], *condition of mind.* adj., **-thy'mic.**

thymicolymphatic (thi″mǐ-ko-lim-fat'ik) pertaining to the thymus and the lymph nodes.

thymidine (thi'mǐ-dēn) a nucleoside obtained on hydrolysis of deoxyribonucleic acid (DNA).

thymine (thi'min) a pyrimidine base obtained from nucleic acid; used in treatment of pernicious anemia and sprue.

thymitis (thi-mi'tis) inflammation of the thymus.

thymocyte (thi'mo-sīt) a lymphocyte derived from the thymus.

thymogenic (thi″mo-jen'ik) of affective or hysterical origin.

thymol (thi'mol) a colorless or white crystalline compound; used as an anthelmintic, antibacterial and antifungal agent.

t. iodide, a mixture of iodine derivatives of thymol, containing not less than 43 per cent of iodine; mild antiseptic.

thymolysis (thi-mol'ǐ-sis) destruction of thymus tissue.

thymoma (thi-mo'mah) a tumor of the thymus.

thymonucleic acid (thi″mo-nu-kle'ik) a name applied to deoxyribonucleic acid derived from thymus.

thymopathy (thi-mop'ah-the) any disease of the thymus.

thymopsyche (thi″mo-si'ke) the affective processes of the mind.

thymotoxin (thi″mo-tok'sin) an element that exerts a deleterious effect on the thymus.

thymus (thi'mus) a two-lobed ductless gland

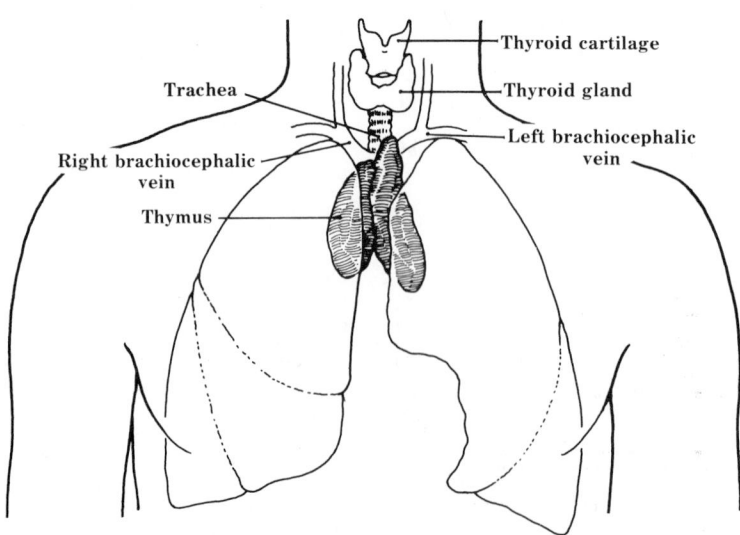

Thyroid cartilage

Thyroid gland

Trachea

Left brachiocephalic vein

Right brachiocephalic vein

Thymus

Thymus.

situated behind the upper part of the sternum and extending into the neck. It is of fairly large size in childhood but usually shrinks in adulthood to little more than a vestigial structure.

Although the thymus is sometimes considered an ENDOCRINE GLAND, it has the structure of a lymph node. It contains a large number of lymphatic follicles and a smaller number of lymphocytes.

The exact functions of the thymus have not been determined. It is believed to play a part in regulation of immune mechanisms of the body. Because it is full size only in childhood, it has been credited with secreting a hormone with youth-prolonging qualities, but there is no evidence that such a hormone exists. The relationship of the thymus to a number of diseases has been noted; in particular, myasthenia gravis has been found to be associated with thymic tumors.

thymusectomy (thi″mus-ek′to-me) excision of the thymus.

thyr(o)- (thi′ro) word element [Gr.], *thyroid.*

thyroadenitis (thi″ro-ad″ĕ-ni′tis) inflammation of the thyroid gland.

thyroaplasia (thi″ro-ah-pla′ze-ah) defective development of the thyroid gland.

thyroarytenoid (thi″ro-ar″ĭ-te′noid) pertaining to the thyroid and arytenoid cartilages.

thyrocardiac (thi″ro-kar′de-ak) pertaining to the thyroid gland and heart.

thyrocarditis (thi″ro-kar-di′tis) any heart disorder occurring with hyperthyroidism.

thyrocele (thi′ro-sēl) goiter.

thyrochondrotomy (thi″ro-kon-drot′o-me) surgical incision of the thyroid cartilage.

thyrocricotomy (thi″ro-kri-kot′o-me) incision of the cricothyroid membrane, the lower part of the fibroelastic membrane of the larynx.

thyrodesmic (thi″ro-dez′mik) thyrotropic.

thyroepiglottic (thi″ro-ep″ĭ-glot′ik) pertaining to the thyroid gland and epiglottis.

thyrogenic (thi″ro-jen′ik) originating in the thyroid gland.

thyroglobulin (thi″ro-glob′u-lin) an iodine-containing glycoprotein characteristically present in the colloid of the thyroid follicles; thyroid hormone is bound to it in the gland.

thyroglossal (thi″ro-glos′al) pertaining to the thyroid gland and tongue.

thyrohyal (thi″ro-hi′al) pertaining to the thyroid cartilage and the hyoid bone.

thyrohyoid (thi″ro-hi′oid) pertaining to the thyroid gland or cartilage and the hyoid bone.

thyroid (thi′roid) 1. resembling a shield. 2. the thyroid gland.
  t. cartilage, the shield-shaped cartilage of the larynx; the prominence it produces on the neck is the Adam's apple.
  t. crisis, a sudden and dangerous increase of the symptoms of thyrotoxicosis.

  t. extract, a pharmaceutical substance derived from thyroid glands from domesticated animals that are used for food by man, the glands having been deprived of connective tissue and fat and then cleaned, dried and powdered. It is used as a specific in hypothyroidism, in doses adjusted to the patient's needs.
  t. gland, the largest of the ENDOCRINE GLANDS, situated in the front and sides of the neck just below the thyroid cartilage. It produces hormones that are vital in maintaining normal growth and metabolism. It also serves as a storehouse for iodine.

Excessive thyroid activity increases metabolism, causing nervousness, heart palpitations, restlessness and insomnia (see also HYPERTHYROIDISM). Deficient thyroid activity produces drowsiness, fatigue and lethargy (see also HYPOTHYROIDISM); marked deficiency can cause weight gain, coarsened features and thick, scaly skin (MYXEDEMA). Enlargement of the thyroid gland is called GOITER, and it often accompanies hyperthyroidism.

  t. hormones, substances manufactured and secreted by the thyroid gland, including thyroxine and triiodothyronine. Together these substances act as a chemical agent or catalyst, stimulating specific organs, tissues and cells. They are mainly responsible for an individual's energy or lack of it, and influence skeletal growth and sexual development, as well as the texture of the skin and luster of the hair.

thyroidectomize (thi″roi-dek′to-mīz) to deprive of the thyroid gland by excision.

thyroidectomy (thi″roi-dek′to-me) surgical excision of the thyroid gland. Total thyroidectomy, removal of the entire gland, may be performed in cases of cancer of the thyroid. Patients with hyperthyroidism that does not respond to the antithyroid drugs may require subtotal thyroidectomy, in which more than half the thyroid gland is removed surgically.
  NURSING CARE. Preoperative care of the patient will depend on the condition for which the surgery is being performed. Hyperthyroid patients will re-

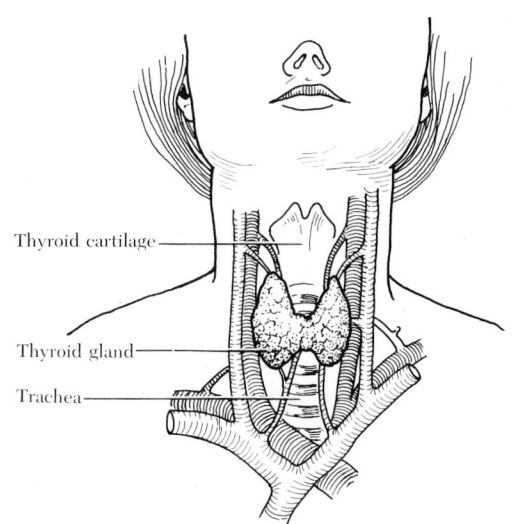

Thyroid cartilage

Thyroid gland

Trachea

Thyroid gland.

quire special physical and emotional preparation for the pending surgery. Since they may be overactive and easily upset they should be approached with an attitude of calm and assurance. Antithyroid drugs should be given as ordered to reduce the symptoms of hyperthyroidism. The patient's pulse, respiration and blood pressure are taken and recorded carefully and used as a guide for comparison during the postoperative period.

Immediately after surgery the patient is placed on his back in a low Fowler's or semi-Fowler's position. Motion of the head, unnecessary talking and strenuous coughing should be discouraged. Temperature, pulse and respirations are taken every 15 minutes until they remain within normal limits for several hours. The dressings are checked frequently for signs of hemorrhage or constriction of the throat. Special note should be made of the back of the neck, where blood may drain unnoticed. Hoarseness and slight difficulty in swallowing can be expected until the local edema subsides, but loss of the voice or severe dyspnea should be reported promptly to the surgeon. A tracheostomy set is kept at the bedside in case of respiratory obstruction.

Other complications to be watched for include tetany and thyroid crisis. Muscular twitching, numbness or tingling of the hands or feet or other signs of irritability may indicate damage to, or accidental removal of, the parathyroid glands, and a resultant decrease in the calcium level of the blood. Thyroid crisis may occur as a result of an increase in the amount of thyroxine released into the blood during manipulation of the gland at the time of its removal. This complication is indicated by a rapid increase in all the vital signs, marked irritability and restlessness and prostration. Death may occur from heart failure. Both tetany and thyroid crisis are rare complications.

thyroidism (thi'roi-dizm) a morbid condition resulting from disorder of functioning of the thyroid gland or excessive use of thyroid extract.

thyroiditis (thi"roi-di'tis) inflammation of the thyroid gland, usually characterized by such symptoms as sore throat, fever and painful enlargement of the gland.

thyroidotomy (thi"roi-dot'o-me) incision of the thyroid gland.

thyroiodine (thi"ro-i'o-dīn) a general term for iodine-containing substances from the thyroid gland.

thyrolysin (thi-rol'ĭ-sin) a substance destructive to thyroid tissue.

thyromegaly (thi"ro-meg'ah-le) enlargement of the thyroid gland.

thyromimetic (thi"ro-mi-met'ik) producing effects similar to those of thyroid hormones or the thyroid gland.

thyroparathyroidectomy (thi"ro-par"ah-thi"roi-dek'to-me) excision of the thyroid and parathyroid glands.

thyropenia (thi"ro-pe'ne-ah) diminished thyroid action.

thyrophyma (thi"ro-fi'mah) tumor of the thyroid gland.

thyroprival (thi"ro-pri'val) due to decreased function or removal of the thyroid gland.

thyroptosis (thi"rop-to'sis) downward displacement of a goitrous thyroid gland.

thyrosis (thi-ro'sis) any disease based on disordered thyroid action.

thyrotomy (thi-rot'o-me) 1. surgical division of the thyroid cartilage. 2. the operation of cutting the thyroid gland.

thyrotoxic (thi"ro-tok'sik) marked by toxic activity of the thyroid gland.

thyrotoxicosis (thi"ro-tok"sĭ-ko'sis) the condition due to excessive thyroid action.

thyrotoxin (thi"ro-tok'sin) a cytotoxin specific for thyroid tissue.

thyrotrophic (thi"ro-trof'ik) thyrotropic.

thyrotrophin (thi"ro-trōf'in) thyrotropin.

thyrotropic (thi"ro-trop'ik) 1. stimulating the thyroid gland. 2. pertaining to thyrotropism.

thyrotropin (thi"ro-trōp'in) a hormone secreted by the anterior lobe of the pituitary gland that stimulates the thyroid gland; called also thyrotropic hormone and thyroid-stimulating hormone (TSH).

thyrotropism (thi-rot'ro-pizm) predominance of the thyroid in the endocrine constitution.

thyroxine (thi-rok'sin) a hormone of the THYROID GLAND that contains iodine and is a derivative of the amino acid tyrosine. The chemical name for thyroxine is tetraiodothyronine; it is formed and stored in the thyroid follicles as thyroglobulin, the storage form. Thyroxine is released from the gland by the action of a proteolytic enzyme.

Thyroxine acts as a catalyst in the body and influences a great variety of effects, including metabolic rate (oxygen consumption); growth and development; metabolism of carbohydrates, fats, proteins, electrolytes and water; vitamin requirements; reproduction; and resistance to infection.

Thyroxine can be extracted from animals or made synthetically; it is prescribed for hypothyroidism and for some types of goiter.

Ti chemical symbol, *titanium.*

tibia (tib'e-ah) the inner and larger bone of the leg below the knee; it articulates with the femur and head of the fibula above and with the talus below. adj., **tib'ial.**
  t. val'ga, a bowing of the leg in which the angulation is away from the midline of the body.
  t. va'ra, a bowing of the leg in which the angulation is toward the midline of the body; bowleg.

tibialis (tib"e-a'lis) [L.] tibial.

tibiofemoral (tib"e-o-fem'o-ral) pertaining to the tibia and femur.

tibiofibular (tib"e-o-fib'u-lar) pertaining to the tibia and fibula.

tibiotarsal (tib"e-o-tar'sal) pertaining to the tibia and tarsus.

tic (tik) a spasmodic twitching movement made involuntarily by muscles that are ordinarily under voluntary control. Twitching of the eyelid, of muscles of the face and of the diaphragm (hiccupping) are examples. In general, tics are of psychologic origin; they tend to develop in young persons of nervous temperament and occasionally persist into adulthood.

t. douloureux (doo-loo-roo'), trigeminal neuralgia, a painful disorder of the trigeminal nerve (the fifth cranial nerve). The disorder is characterized by severe pain in the face and forehead on the affected side. The pain extends to the midline of the face and head and may be triggered by cold drafts, chewing, drinking cold liquids, brushing the hair or washing the face.

TREATMENT. Medical treatment is usually preferred since surgical correction results in complete loss of sensation in the areas served by the nerve. The drugs employed include trichloroethylene administered by inhalation, niacin, potassium chloride, diethazine and most recently carbamazepine (Tegretol).

When surgery is resorted to, the patient must be watched for signs of corneal infection, which frequently occurs. The infection usually develops as a result of loss of the corneal reflex, which normally provides a warning when foreign material or other injurious agents enter the eye. Postoperative instructions must be given the patient so that he can take necessary measures for the protection of his eye after discharge from the hospital.

tick (tik) a blood-sucking arachnid parasite. There are two types, hard and soft. Hard ticks have a smooth, hard cover that shields the entire back of the male but only the anterior portion of the back in the female. Soft ticks lack this shield.

Ticks are visible to the human eye. A hard tick can be seen on the skin, where it burrows into the outer layer with its knifelike tongue; it must be removed from the skin with care. Soft ticks do not bore into the skin. The two varieties carry different diseases but both thrive in the spring and early summer and inhabit wooded areas, brush or grass.

Ticks serve as vectors for viruses causing Colorado tick fever and some forms of encephalitis and for rickettsiae that cause such diseases as ROCKY MOUNTAIN SPOTTED FEVER and boutonneuse fever.

REMOVAL OF HARD TICKS. If hard ticks are extracted from the skin immediately, before they begin to suck blood, the chances of their transmitting disease are lessened; probably the only damage done will be an irritating itch at the site.

Ticks should be extracted whole; if they are carelessly pulled off the body, all or part of the mouth may be left in the skin. To loosen the tick's grasp, heavy oil, gasoline or turpentine is applied to the area and left for half an hour. Once the tick has relinquished its hold, it should be carefully removed with tweezers. The tick should be destroyed, but not with the bare hands. The site should be washed with soap and water and an antiseptic should be applied to prevent infection.

t.i.d. [L.] *ter in di'e* (three times a day).

tidal volume (ti'dal) the amount of gas passing into and out of the lungs in each respiratory cycle.

tide (tīd) a physiologic variation or increase of a certain constituent in body fluids.

acid t., a temporary increase in the acidity of the urine that sometimes follows fasting.

alkaline t., a temporary increase in the alkalinity of the urine during gastric digestion.

fat t., the increase of a fat in the lymph and blood following a meal.

Tigan (ti'gan) trademark for preparations of trimethobenzamide hydrochloride, an antiemetic.

tigrolysis (ti-grol'ĭ-sis) chromatolysis (2).

tilmus (til'mus) carphology; involuntary picking at the bedclothes.

timbre (tim'ber) the musical quality of a tone or sound.

time (tīm) a measure of duration.

bleeding t., the duration of bleeding after puncture of the earlobe (Duke method) or forearm (Ivy method).

circulation t., the time required for blood to flow between two given points, usually from arm to tongue or arm to lung.

clotting t., coagulation t., the time it takes a drop of blood to clot.

inertia t., the time required to overcome the inertia of a muscle after reception of a stimulus from a nerve.

partial thromboplastin t., PTT, a test to detect deficiencies of the components of the intrinsic thromboplastin system.

persistence t., the time following contraction of the ventricle until the occurrence of relaxation.

prothrombin t., a test to detect the deficiency in the blood of clotting factors II (prothrombin), I (fibrinogen), V, VII and X.

reaction t., the time elapsing between the application of a stimulus and the resulting reaction.

timopathy (tim-op'ah-the) a state characterized by abnormal dread or apprehension.

Timovan (tim'o-van) trademark for a preparation of prothipendyl hydrochloride, a tranquilizer.

tin (tin) a chemical element, atomic number 50, atomic weight 118.69, symbol Sn. (See table of ELEMENTS.)

tinct. tincture.

tinctorial (tingk-to're-al) pertaining to dyeing or staining.

tincture (tingk'tūr) an alcoholic or hydroalcoholic solution prepared from an animal or vegetable drug or a chemical substance.

belladonna t., a preparation of belladonna leaf in a menstruum of alcohol and water; used as a parasympatholytic.

benzoin t., compound, a mixture of powdered benzoin and aloe, storax and tolu balsam, with alcohol as the menstruum; applied topically as a protective.

camphorated opium t., paregoric.

digitalis t., finely powdered digitalis in a menstruum of alcohol and water; used as a cardiotonic.

iodine t., a mixture of iodine and sodium iodide in a menstruum of alcohol and water; used topically as an antiseptic.

opium t., an alcoholic solution of opium, each 100 ml. of which yields 0.95 to 1.05 Gm. of anhydrous morphine; used as an intestinal sedative.

Tindal (tin'dal) trademark for a preparation of acetophenazine dimaleate, a tranquilizer.

tinea (tin'e-ah) a name applied to many different kinds of fungal infection of the skin, the specific type (depending on characteristic appearance, etiologic agent and site) usually being designated by a modifying term.

t. **bar'bae**, infection of the bearded parts of the face and neck caused by Trichophyton; called also ringworm of the beard.

t. **cap'itis**, fungal infection of the scalp caused by various species of Microsporum and Trichophyton. Generally it is characterized by one or more small, round, elevated patches, scaling of the scalp and dry and brittle hair. Called also ringworm of the scalp.

t. **cor'poris**, fungal infection of the skin; called also RINGWORM.

t. **cru'ris**, a fungal infection common in males, starting in the perineal folds and extending onto the inner surface of the thighs; called also eczema marginatum, epidermophytosis cruris and jock itch.

t. **imbrica'ta**, a distinctive type of tinea corporis occurring in tropical countries and caused by Trichophyton concentricum; the early lesion is annular, with a circle of scales at the periphery, characteristically attached along one edge. New and larger scaling rings form, sometimes reaching as many as 10 per lesion. Called also Malabar itch and Burmese ringworm.

t. **ke'rion**, a highly inflammatory and suppurative fungal infection of the scalp or beard region.

t. **pe'dis**, a chronic superficial fungal infection of the skin of the foot, especially of that between the toes and on the soles, characterized by maceration, scaling and itching, and caused by species of Trichophyton or by Epidermophyton floccosum or Candida albicans (see also ATHLETE'S FOOT).

t. **un'guium**, onychomycosis; fungal infection of the nails.

t. **versic'olor**, a common, chronic, noninflammatory and usually symptomless disorder caused by Malassezia furfur and characterized by multiple brownish macular patches of all sizes and shapes.

Tinel's sign (tin-elz') a tingling sensation in the distal end of a limb when percussion is made over the site of a divided nerve; it indicates a partial lesion or the beginning regeneration of the nerve.

tingible (tin'jĭ-bl) stainable.

tinnitus (tĭ-ni'tus) a noise in the ears, as ringing, buzzing or roaring, which may at times be heard by others than the patient.

t. **au'rium**, a subjective sensation of noises in the ears.

tintometer (tin-tom'ĕ-ter) an instrument for determining the relative proportion of coloring matter in a liquid, as in blood.

tintometry (tin-tom'ĕ-tre) the use of the tintometer.

tirefond (tēr-faw') [Fr.] an instrument like a corkscrew for raising depressed portions of bone.

tissue (tish'u) a group or layer of similarly specialized cells that together perform certain special functions.

adenoid t., lymphoid tissue.

adipose t., fatty tissue.

areolar t., connective tissue made up largely of interlacing fibers.

bony t., bone.

cancellous t., the spongy tissue of bone.

cartilaginous t., cartilage.

chordal t., the tissue of the notochord.

chromaffin t., tissue that stains yellow or brown with chromium salts, typical of the adrenal medulla and ganglia of the sympathetic nervous system.

cicatricial t., tissue derived directly from granulation tissue.

compact t., the hard, external portion of bone.

connective t., the tissue that binds together and is the support of the various structures of the body; it consists mainly of fibroblasts and collagen and elastic fibrils. (See also CONNECTIVE TISSUE.)

elastic t., connective tissue made up of yellow elastic fibers, frequently massed into sheets.

endothelial t., peculiar connective tissue lining serous and lymph spaces.

epithelial t., a general name for tissues not derived from the mesoderm.

erectile t., spongy tissue that expands and becomes hard when filled with blood.

extracellular t., the total of tissues and body fluids outside the cells.

fatty t., connective tissue made of fat cells in a meshwork of areolar tissue.

fibrous t., the common connective tissue of the body, composed of yellow or white parallel elastic and collagen fibers.

t. fluid, the extracellular fluid that constitutes the environment of the body cells. It is low in protein, is formed by filtration through the capillaries and drains away as lymph.

gelatinous t., mucous tissue.

glandular t., a specialized form of epithelial tissue that elaborates secretions.

granulation t., material formed in repair of wounds of soft tissue, consisting of connective tissue cells and ingrowing young vessels; it ultimately forms cicatrix.

indifferent t., undifferentiated embryonic tissue.

interstitial t., connective tissue between the cellular elements of a structure.

lymphadenoid t., the tissue constituting the lymph nodes, spleen, bone marrow, tonsils and lymph vessels.

lymphoid t., connective tissue with meshes that lodge lymphoid cells.

mesenchymal t., embryonic connective tissue composed of stellate cells and a ground substance of coagulable fluid.

mucous t., embryonic connective tissue, such as occurs in the umbilical cord.

muscular t., muscle.

myeloid t., red bone marrow.

nervous t., the specialized tissue forming the elements of the nervous system.

osseous t., the specialized tissue forming the bones.

reticular t., retiform t., connective tissue composed predominantly of reticulum cells and reticular fibers.

scar t., cicatricial tissue.

sclerous t's, the cartilaginous, fibrous and osseous tissues.

skeletal t., the bony, ligamentous, fibrous and cartilaginous tissue forming the skeleton and its attachments.

subcutaneous t., the layer of loose connective tissue directly under the skin.

titanium (ti-ta'ne-um) a chemical element, atomic number 22, atomic weight 47.90, symbol Ti. (See table of ELEMENTS.)

t. dioxide, a white powder used in ointment or lotion to protect the skin from the rays of the sun.

titer (ti'ter) the quantity of a substance required to react with or to correspond to a given amount of another substance.

titration (ti-tra'shun) analysis by means of comparison with solutions of standard strength, by color, electrical conductivity, etc.

titrimetry (ti-trim'e-tre) analysis by titration.

titubation (tit"u-ba'shun) the act of staggering or reeling; a staggering or stumbling gait, especially one due to a lesion of the spinal system.

Tl chemical symbol, *thallium.*

TLC tender loving care; total lung capacity.

Tm 1. chemical symbol, *thulium.* 2. tubular maximum (in renal excretion).

TNT trinitrotoluene.

tobacco (to-bak'o) the prepared leaves of *Nicotiana tabacum,* an annual plant widely cultivated in the United States, the source of various alkaloids, the principal one being nicotine (see also SMOKING).

Toclase (to'klās) trademark for preparations of carbetapentane citrate, an antitussive.

toco- (to'ko) word element [Gr.], *childbirth; labor.* See also words beginning *toko-.*

tocology (to-kol'o-je) the science of reproduction and the art of obstetrics.

tocomania (to"ko-ma'ne-ah) the mania that sometimes follows childbirth; puerperal mania.

tocometer (to-kom'ĕ-ter) tokodynamometer.

tocopherol (to-kof'er-ol) a compound originally isolated from wheat germ oil; it has the properties of vitamin E. In animals it is needed in the diet to insure reproduction, but its role in humans is unclear.

tocophobia (to"ko-fo'be-ah) abnormal dread of childbirth.

toe (to) a digit of the foot.

hammer t., deformity of a toe in which the proximal phalanx is extended and the second and distal phalanges are flexed, causing a clawlike appearance; it most often affects the second toe.

Morton's t., a painful condition of the third and fourth toes due to thickening of the branch of the sensory nerve supplying them.

pigeon t., a permanent toeing-in position of the feet.

webbed t's, toes abnormally joined by strands of tissue at their base.

Tofranil (to-fra'nil) trademark for preparations of imipramine hydrochloride, an antidepressant.

toilet (toi'let) the cleansing and dressing of a wound.

toko- (to'ko) word element [Gr.], *childbirth; labor.* See also words beginning *toco-.*

tokodynagraph (to"ko-di'nah-graf) a tracing obtained by the tokodynamometer.

tokodynamometer (to"ko-di"nah-mom'ĕ-ter) an instrument for measuring and recording the expulsive force of uterine contractions.

tolazoline (tol-az'o-lēn) a compound used as a sympatholytic agent and a vasodilator.

tolbutamide (tol-bu'tah-mīd) a hypoglycemic agent effective when given orally.

tolerance (tol'er-ans) the ability to endure without effect or injury.

drug t., decrease of susceptibility to the effects of a drug due to its continued administration.

immunologic t., absence of reactivity to a substance normally expected to excite an immunologic response.

work t., the amount of work a chronically ill person can or should do.

tolonium (to-lo'ne-um) a heparin-inhibiting compound used to reduce bleeding tendency in certain hemorrhagic conditions associated with excess of heparinoid substances in the blood.

Tolserol (tol'ser-ol) trademark for preparations of mephenesin, a muscle relaxant.

toluene (tol'u-ēn) the hydrocarbon C_7H_8.

tomatin (to-ma'tin) an antibiotic compound isolated from leaves and roots of common tomato plants.

-tome (-tōm) word element [Gr.], *an instrument for cutting; a segment.*

tomentum (to-men'tum) a network of minute blood vessels of the pia mater and cerebral cortex.

tomo- (to'mo) word element [Gr.], *a section; a cutting.*

tomogram (to'mo-gram) a roentgenogram produced by tomography.

tomography (to-mog'rah-fe) a method of body-section roentgenography with the x-ray tube moved in only one direction, usually an arc.

tomomania (to"mo-ma'ne-ah) 1. a craze for performing needless surgical operations. 2. hysterical desire to undergo surgery.

-tomy (to'me) word element [Gr.], *incision; cutting.*

tone (tōn) 1. normal degree of vigor and tension; in muscle, the resistance to passive elongation or stretch. 2. a particular quality of sound or voice.

tongue (tung) a muscular organ on the floor of the mouth; it aids in chewing, swallowing and speech, and is the location of organs of taste. The taste buds are located in the papillae, which are projections on the upper surface of the tongue.

The condition of the tongue can sometimes be a guide to the general condition of the body. Inflammation of the tongue, or glossitis, can accompany anemia, scarlet fever, nutritional deficiencies and most general infections. Sometimes it is part of an adverse reaction to medication. One form of glossitis causes a smooth tongue, with a red, glazed appearance. A coated or furry tongue may be present in a variety of illnesses, but does not necessarily indicate illness. A dry tongue sometimes indicates insufficiency of fluids in the body, or it may result from fever. When the tongue is extremely dry and has a leathery appearance, the cause may be uremia.

bifid t., a tongue with a lengthwise cleft.

black t., blackening and elongation of the papillae of the tongue.

geographic t., a tongue with denuded patches, surrounded by thickened epithelium.

hairy t., one with the papillae elongated and hairlike.

raspberry t., a diffusely reddened and swollen, uncoated tongue as is seen several days after the onset of scarlet fever.

Sandwith's bald t., an unusually smooth tongue seen in pellagra.

strawberry t., a coated tongue with enlarged red fungiform papillae, seen early in scarlet fever.

trombone t., involuntary movement of the tongue, consisting of vigorous alternating protrusion and retraction.

tongue-tie (tung′ti) abnormal shortness of the frenulum of the tongue, resulting in limitation of its motion; called also ankyloglossia.

tonic (ton′ik) 1. producing and restoring normal tone. 2. characterized by continuous tension. 3. an agent that tends to restore normal tone.

bitter t., a tonic of bitter taste, such as quinine or gentian; used for stimulating the appetite and improving digestion.

cardiac t., an agent that strengthens the heart's action.

general t., an agent that braces up the whole system.

hematic t., an agent that improves the quality of the blood.

intestinal t., an agent that gives tone to intestinal tract.

nervine t., an agent that improves the tone of the nervous system.

stomachic t., an agent that aids digestive functions.

vascular t., an agent that improves the tone of blood vessels.

tonicity (to-nis′ĭ-te) the state of tone or tension.

tono- (to′no) word element [Gr.], *tone; tension.*

tonoclonic (ton″o-klon′ik) both tonic and clonic.

tonofibril (ton′o-fi″bril) one of the fine fibrils in epithelial cells, thought to give a supporting framework to the cell.

tonogram (to′no-gram) the record produced by tonography.

tonograph (to′no-graf) a recording tonometer.

tonography (to-nog′rah-fe) the recording of changes in intraocular pressure due to sustained pressure on the eyeball.

tonometer (to-nom′ĕ-ter) an instrument for measuring tension or pressure, especially for measuring intraocular pressure.

tonometry (to-nom′ĕ-tre) measurement of tension or pressure.

digital t., estimation of the degree of intraocular pressure by pressure exerted on the eyeball by the finger of the examiner.

tonoplast (ton′o-plast) the limiting membrane of an intracellular vacuole, the vacuole membrane.

tonoscope (ton′o-skōp) an instrument for examining the head or cranium by means of sound.

tonsil (ton′sil) a small mass of spongy lymphoid tissue. adj., **ton′sillar.**

There are three different kinds of tonsils. The structures usually referred to as the tonsils are the palatine tonsils, a pair of oval-shaped structures, about the size of almonds, partially embedded in the mucous membrane, one on each side of the back of the throat. Below them, at the base of the tongue, are the lingual tonsils. On the upper rear wall of the mouth cavity are the pharyngeal tonsils, or adenoids, which are of fair size in childhood but which usually shrink after puberty.

These tissues are part of the lymphatic system and help to filter the circulating lymph of bacteria and any other foreign material that may enter the body, especially through the mouth and nose. In the process of fighting infection the palatine tonsils and the adenoids sometimes become enlarged and inflamed (see also TONSILLITIS).

t. of cerebellum, a rounded mass forming part of the cerebellum on its inferior surface.

tonsillectomy (ton″sĭ-lek′to-me) excision of tonsils. The procedure is performed in treatment of chronic infection of the tonsils.

NURSING CARE. Since most patients undergoing tonsillectomy are children, it is important that the preoperative period include adequate emotional preparation of the patient and his family. The child should be told in advance of the admission to the hospital and given some idea of what he can expect. He should not be deceived about the possibility of discomfort, but it is best to stress the positive aspects of surgery, such as the fact that he will not suffer as many colds and attacks of sore throat once the surgery is performed and his throat has healed.

Although tonsillectomy may be considered minor surgery, there is always the possibility of serious hemorrhage after surgery. The child should be placed on his abdomen in bed immediately after surgery, to allow for adequate drainage of blood and mucus from the throat and mouth and avoid their aspiration into the respiratory passages. Signs of excessive bleeding from the operative site include bright red blood from the mouth or nose, frequent swallowing and extreme restlessness. Efforts to keep the child quiet may include holding him, rocking him or otherwise comforting him as he awakens from anesthesia. An ice collar is helpful in preventing edema, reducing blood loss and eliminating nausea.

During the immediate postoperative period the diet is restricted to bland liquids. Citrus fruit juices are not allowed. As the throat heals and edema subsides, more solid foods are gradually added to the diet, but for at least a week after surgery all foods that are chemically, physically or thermally irritating to the throat should be avoided.

tonsillitis (ton″sĭ-li′tis) inflammation and enlargement of a tonsil.

Enlarged tonsils and adenoids need not be a cause

for concern unless they become a source of chronic infection or interfere with swallowing or breathing. They may become enlarged in the process of filtering out frequent, mild infections. Also, the adenoids usually grow larger in children until about the age of 5 years, and then they may cease to be troublesome.

CAUSE. Tonsils are part of the lymphatic system, which aids the body in fighting off infections and "invasions" of foreign matter. Although the exact purpose of the tonsils is unknown, they are believed to act as filters and fighters of bacteria, guarding the entrances to the throat and nasal passages. Sometimes, however, they are overcome by the invading bacteria and become infected. One form of infection sometimes causing tonsillitis is streptococcal infection of the throat.

SYMPTOMS AND TREATMENT. A mild case of tonsillitis may appear to be only a slight sore throat. Symptoms of acute tonsillitis are inflamed, swollen tonsils and a very sore throat, with high fever, rapid pulse and general weakness. Swallowing is difficult and the lymph nodes in the neck may become swollen and painful.

Occasionally in an attack of severe tonsillitis an abscess may form around the tonsil, a condition called quinsy.

Treatment of tonsillitis usually consists of administration of antibiotics, gargles and bed rest. When tonsillitis is recurrent and troublesome, however, it may be necessary to remove the tonsils surgically (see also TONSILLECTOMY).

tonsilloadenoidectomy (ton"sĭ-lo-ad"ĕ-noi-dek'-to-me) excision of lymphoid tissue from the throat and nasopharynx (tonsils and adenoids).

tonsillolith (ton-sil'o-lith) a calculus in a tonsil.

tonsillotomy (ton"sĭ-lot'o-me) incision of a tonsil.

tonus (to'nus) tone, or tonicity; the normal state of slight contraction of all skeletal muscles, maintained as long as innervation to the muscle is intact.

tooth (tōōth), pl. *teeth* one of the small, bonelike structures of the jaws for the biting and mastication of food; the teeth also assist in shaping sounds and forming words in speech.

STRUCTURE. The portion of a tooth that rises above the gum is the crown; the portion below is the root. The crown is covered by enamel, which is related to the epithelial tissue of the skin and is the hardest substance in the human body. The surface of the root is composed of a bonelike tissue called cementum. Underneath the surface enamel and cementum is a substance called dentin, which makes up the main body of the tooth. Within the dentin, in a space in the center of the tooth, is the dental pulp, a soft, sensitive tissue that contains nerves and blood and lymph vessels. The cementum, dentin and pulp are formed from connective tissue.

Covering the root of the tooth and holding it in place in its socket, or alveolus, in the jaw is a fibrous connective tissue called the periodontium. Its many strong fibers are embedded in the cementum and also the wall of the tooth socket. The periodontium not only helps hold the tooth in place but also acts to cushion it against the pressure caused by biting and chewing.

There are 20 deciduous teeth, called also baby teeth or milk teeth, which are eventually replaced by 32 permanent teeth, evenly divided between upper and lower jaw.

Teeth have different shapes because they have different functions. The incisors, in the front of the mouth, are shaped like a cone with a sharp flattened end. They cut the food. There are eight deciduous and permanent incisors, four upper and four lower. The cuspids, at the corners of the mouth, shaped like simple cones, tear and shred food. There are four permanent cuspids; they are called also canines, and the two in the upper jaw are called eyeteeth. The premolars, or bicuspids, flanking the cuspids, consist of two cones, or cusps, fused together. They tear, crush and grind the food. There are eight permanent premolars. The molars are in the back of the mouth. They have between three and five cusps each, and their function is to crush and grind food. There are 12 permanent molars in all, three on each side of both the upper and lower jaw. The hindmost molar in each of these groups, and the last one to emerge, is often called a wisdom tooth.

DEVELOPMENT AND ERUPTION. Both the deciduous teeth and the permanent teeth begin to develop before birth. Because of this, it is vitally important that expectant mothers receive foods that will supply the calcium, phosphorus and vitamins necessary for healthy teeth.

The deciduous teeth begin to form about the sixth week of prenatal life, with calcification beginning about the sixteenth week. A considerable part of the crowns of these teeth is formed by the time the child is born.

Eruption, or cutting of teeth is slower in some children than others, but the deciduous teeth generally begin to appear when the infant is between 6 and 9 months of age, and the process is completed by the time a child is 2 to 2½ years old.

When the child is about 6, the first permanent molar comes in just behind the second molar of the deciduous teeth. About the same time, shedding of the baby teeth begins. The permanent teeth form in the jaw even before the baby teeth have erupted, with the incisors and the cuspids beginning to calcify during the first 6 months of life. Calcification of the others takes place shortly after. As the adult teeth calcify, the roots of the baby teeth gradually disappear, or resorb, and are completely gone by the time the permanent teeth are ready to appear. Occasionally a baby tooth root does not resorb, and as a result the permanent tooth comes in outside its proper position. When resorption does not occur, it is necessary to remove the baby tooth and root.

The first teeth to be shed, about the sixth year, are the central incisors. The permanent incisors erupt shortly afterward. The lateral incisors are lost and replaced during the seventh to ninth years, and the cuspids in the ninth to twelfth years. The first premolars generally appear between the ages of 10 and 12, the second molars between 11 and 13 and the third molars, or wisdom teeth, between 17 and 22. It is not uncommon for the third molars to fail to erupt.

Occasionally there is a partial or total lack of either the deciduous or permanent teeth. In some cases this anodontia is hereditary, or it may be related to endocrine gland disturbances.

TOOTH DECAY AND ITS PREVENTION. Dental CARIES, the most common disease in the United

States, begins on the outside of the teeth in the enamel. Bacteria and food adhere to the tooth surface to form a plaque. The action of the bacteria on starchy and sugary foods produces lactic acid, which is believed to dissolve the enamel. Once there is a breakthrough in the enamel, the decaying process moves on into the dentin and then to the pulp, attacking the nerves and causing toothache.

Brushing the Teeth. Cleanliness is the best weapon against tooth decay. Bacteria and food particles must be removed before the enamel is penetrated. This means thorough brushing regularly each day, preferably after every meal. If it is impossible to brush after every meal, it is helpful to rinse the mouth by swishing water vigorously back and forth between and around the teeth. When the teeth are brushed, food particles that lodge between the teeth should also be removed with dental floss, dental tape or the rubber tips on the ends of some toothbrushes.

Teeth should be brushed down on the upper jaw, and up on the lower, always toward the biting edge. Scrubbing across the teeth does not dislodge food particles and can wear down the enamel or injure the gums. Brushing should be high or low enough to massage the gums. The biting surfaces should be brushed back and forth, with the toothbrush square against them.

There is no essential difference in the cleaning properties of toothpastes and toothpowders, but those containing harsh abrasives or strong antiseptics should be avoided. Bicarbonate of soda mixed with salt and dissolved in a little water is as good as the commercial dentifrices, though it may not taste as pleasant.

Clear drinking water is as effective for rinsing the mouth as the usual commercial mouthwashes. However, a dentist may prescribe a special mouthwash for certain conditions of the gums or tissues of the mouth.

Proper Diet. In order to help maintain healthy teeth, the diet should include all the essential elements of good NUTRITION. Tooth decay can be reduced by limiting the intake of certain forms of sugar, especially the rich or highly concentrated ones such as candy or rich desserts.

Fluoridation. Another important means of preventing caries is through the use of fluoride. Many communities whose water is lacking in an adequate natural supply of fluoride add the chemical to their water supply. FLUORIDATION is effective for children and adolescents, and children raised on fluoridated water retain resistance to tooth decay when they become adults. In communities that do not have fluoridation, dentists may add a fluoride solution directly to the teeth or may suggest other means of obtaining fluoride protection.

Correction of Malocclusion. Another factor leading to tooth decay is poor position of the teeth, resulting in faulty closure of the jaws and uneven meeting of the teeth. This condition is called malocclusion. It should be corrected early because it also can lead to inadequate nutrition because of difficulty in chewing, and if it is severe enough to distort the face, it may have psychologic effects.

accessional teeth, the permanent molars, so called because they have no deciduous predecessors in the dental arch.

impacted t., one so placed in the jaw that it is unable to erupt or to attain its normal position in occlusion.

top(o)- (top'o) word element [Gr.], *particular place or area.*

topagnosia (top″ag-no′ze-ah) 1. loss of touch localization. 2. loss of ability to recognize familiar surroundings.

topectomy (to-pek′to-me) excision of a limited area of brain tissue.

topesthesia (top″es-the′ze-ah) ability to recognize the location of a tactile stimulus.

tophaceous (to-fa′shus) gritty or sandy.

tophus (to′fus), pl. *to′phi* [L.] 1. a deposit of urates in the tissues about the joints or on the ear in GOUT. 2. dental calculus.
   t. syphilit′icus, a syphilitic node.

topical (top′ĭ-kal) pertaining to a particular spot; local.

Topitracin (top″ĭ-tra′sin) trademark for a preparation of bacitracin, an antibiotic.

topoalgia (to″po-al′je-ah) fixed or localized pain.

topoanesthesia (to″po-an″es-the′ze-ah) inability to recognize the location of a tactile stimulus.

topognosis (top″og-no′sis) topesthesia.

topographic (top″o-graf′ik) describing special regions.

topography (to-pog′rah-fe) a special description of a part or region.

toponarcosis (top″o-nar-ko′sis) local anesthesia.

toponeurosis (top″o-nu-ro′sis) neurosis of a limited region.

torcular Herophili (tor′ku-lar he-rof′ĭ-le) a depression in the occipital bone at the confluence of a number of cerebral venous sinuses.

torpid (tor′pid) not acting with normal vigor and facility.

torpor (tor′por) [L.] sluggishness.
   t. ret′inae, sluggish response of the retina to the stimulus of light.

torque (tork) a rotatory force.

torsion (tor′shun) the act of twisting; the state of being twisted.

torsiversion (tor″sĭ-ver′zhun) turning of a tooth on its long axis out of normal position.

torso (tor′so) the body, exclusive of the head and limbs.

torticollis (tor″tĭ-kol′is) wryneck; a contracted state of the cervical muscles, producing torsion of the neck. The deformity may be congenital, hysterical or secondary to pressure on the accessory nerve, to inflammation of glands in the neck or to muscle spasm.

tortipelvis (tor″tĭ-pel′vis) distortions of the spine and hip produced by a disorder marked by irregular muscular contractions of the trunk and extremities.

tortuous (tor'tu-us) twisted; full of turns and twists.

Torula (tor'u-lah) Cryptococcus.
   T. hystolyt'ica. *Cryptococcus neoformans.*

toruloid (tor'u-loid) knotted or beaded, like a yeast cell.

torulosis (tor"u-lo'sis) cryptococcosis.

torulus (tor'u-lus) [L.] a small elevation.
   t. tac'tilis, a tactile elevation in the skin of the palms and soles.

torus (to'rus), pl. *to'ri* [L.] a swelling or bulging projection.

totipotential (to"tĭ-po-ten'shal) characterized by the ability to develop in any direction; said of cells that can give rise to cells of all orders, i.e., the complete individual.

touch (tuch) 1. the sense by which contact of an object with the skin is recognized. 2. palpation with the finger.

Touch is actually not a single sense, but several. There are separate nerves in the skin to register heat, cold, pressure, pain and touch. These thousands of nerves are distributed unevenly over the body, so that some areas are more responsive to cold, others to pain and others to heat or pressure.

Each of these types of nerves has a different structure at the receiving end. A touch nerve has an elongated bulb-shaped end, and a nerve responsive to cold a squat bulb; the nerve that registers warmth has what looks like twisted threads, and the nerve for deep pressure has an egg-shaped end. Pain receptors have no protective sheath.

If the sensory nerves were evenly distributed over the whole body, each square inch of skin would have about 50 heat receptors, 8 for cold, 100 for touch and 800 for pain. The sensitivity of a given

spot depends in part on how thickly receptors of a particular kind are clustered in that spot, and localization of particular sensation depends on the concentration of the particular nerve endings in an area. Touch, pressure and pain are sensations that can be localized quite accurately, but sensations of cold and heat are more diffuse.

The thickness of the skin in a given area and its supply of hairs also contribute to its touch sensitivity. A touch as light as one fifteen-thousandth of an ounce on the thin skin of the forehead can be felt, whereas a touch must be two and a half times as heavy to be felt on a fingertip. Hairs grow almost everywhere on the skin except the palms of the hands and the soles of the feet. They grow at a slant, and touch spots cluster in the skin near each of them. Even a light touch on the tip of a hair bends it back, and like a tiny lever it communicates the touch to the nerve endings.

The tactile sense develops with learning and experience. A simple test is to hold a pea between the first and second fingers. With the eyes closed, it is easy to tell that it is one object. However, if the fingers are crossed first, it will seem that there are two peas, because ordinarily it takes two objects to stimulate the touch receptors on the opposite sides of the fingers.

tourniquet (toor'nĭ-ket) a device for compression of an artery or vein. It is used to stop excessive bleeding, to prevent the spread of snake venom and to facilitate obtaining blood samples or giving intravenous injections.

For hemorrhage, a tourniquet should be used only as a last resort, when the bleeding is so severe that it obviously threatens the life of the injured person and cannot be stopped by direct pressure.

In the case of snake bite, a moderately tight

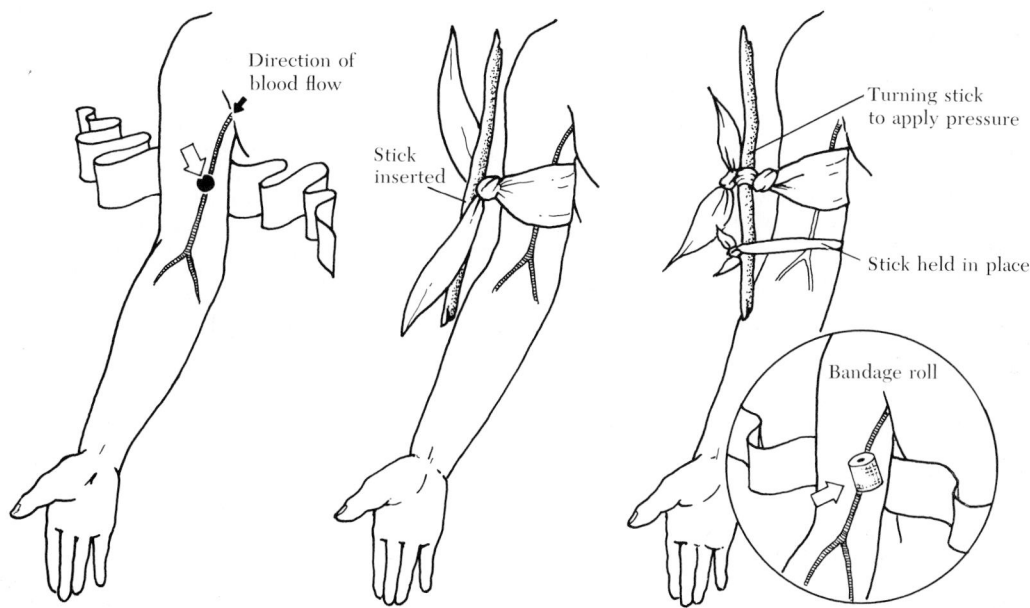

To apply a tourniquet for control of arterial bleeding from the arm: Wrap a gauze pad twice with a strip of cloth just below the armpit and tie with a half knot; tie a stick at the knot with a square knot. Slowly twist stick to tighten. Loosen tourniquet every 10 minutes.

tourniquet that impedes the spread of venom but does not stop arterial blood flow may be applied.

A loosely applied tourniquet inhibits blood flow in the superficial veins, making them more prominent; this is helpful when a vein is being sought for an intravenous injection or for drawing blood.

APPLYING A TOURNIQUET. There are two places on the body where a tourniquet is effective in stopping profuse bleeding from an artery. If blood comes from a wound on the arm, the tourniquet is applied a hand's width below the armpit. If the bleeding is from a leg wound, the tourniquet should be placed a hand's width below the groin.

Any wide, flat piece of cloth long enough to circle the arm or leg twice may be used for a tourniquet. A necktie, scarf or strip of heavy material is suitable. The cloth strip should be placed over a thick pad made of gauze or cloth, then wrapped around the limb and tied with a half knot. A small stick is placed over the half knot, and a square knot is tied over the stick. The tourniquet is tightened by slowly twisting the stick; bleeding will stop suddenly when the tourniquet is twisted tight enough.

Ten minutes after the tourniquet is applied, it should be loosened for exactly 1 minute to permit circulation of the blood in the arm or leg. During this period, a hand should be pressed against the wound. If severe bleeding does not recur during the time the tourniquet is loose, it need not be retightened but should be left in position in case bleeding becomes heavy again.

Tourniquets should never be covered by bandages, clothing or blankets.

A tourniquet applied after snake bite should not be tied with maximum pressure and should be loosened for 1 minute at 10-minute intervals. The tourniquet is always applied above the bite, to prevent flow of the venom toward the heart. If swelling increases, the tourniquet should be moved upward each time it is released (see also SNAKE BITE).

toxalbumin (tok″sal-bu′min) a poisonous albumin of bacterial or other origin.

toxemia (tok-se′me-ah) the presence in the blood of toxic products formed by body cells or bacteria. adj., **toxe′mic.**

t. of pregnancy, a pathologic condition occurring in pregnant women, including hyperemesis gravidarum, preeclampsia and eclampsia. (See also PREGNANCY.)

toxenzyme (tok-sen′zīm) any poisonous enzyme.

toxic (tok′sik) poisonous; pertaining to poisoning.

toxic(o)- (tok′sĭ-ko) word element [Gr.], *poison; poisonous.*

toxicant (tok′sĭ-kant) 1. poisonous. 2. a poison.

toxicide (tok′sĭ-sīd) an agent that overcomes toxins or poisons.

toxicity (tok-sis′ĭ-te) the quality of exerting deleterious effects on an organism or tissue.

Toxicodendron (tok″sĭ-ko-den′dron) a genus name given plants sometimes classified as belonging to the genus Rhus, including poison ivy, etc.

toxicoderma (tok″sĭ-ko-der′mah) a skin disease due to a poison.

toxicogenic (tok″sĭ-ko-jen′ik) giving origin to poisons.

toxicohemia (tok″sĭ-ko-he′me-ah) toxemia.

toxicoid (tok′sĭ-koid) resembling a poison.

toxicologist (tok″sĭ-kol′o-jist) a specialist in toxicology.

toxicology (tok″sĭ-kol′o-je) the science or study of poisons.

toxicomania (tok″sĭ-ko-ma′ne-ah) intense desire for poisons or intoxicants.

toxicomucin (tok″sĭ-ko-mu′sin) a poisonous substance derived from tubercle bacillus (*Mycobacterium tuberculosis*).

toxicopathy (tok″sĭ-kop′ah-the) a morbid condition caused by a poison.

toxicopexy (tok′sĭ-ko-pek″se) the fixation or neutralization of a poison.

toxicophidia (tok″sĭ-ko-fid′e-ah) venomous serpents collectively.

toxicophobia (tok″sĭ-ko-fo′be-ah) morbid dread of poisons.

toxicophylaxin (tok″sĭ-ko-fi-lak′sin) a phylaxin that destroys the poisons produced by microorganisms.

toxicosis (tok″sĭ-ko′sis) a diseased condition due to poisoning.

toxiferous (tok-sif′er-us) conveying or producing a poison.

toxigenic (tok″sĭ-jen′ik) caused by or producing toxins.

toxigenicity (tok″sĭ-jĕ-nis′ĭ-te) the property of producing toxins.

toxi-infection (tok″se-in-fek′shun) toxinfection.

toxin (tok′sin) a poison, especially a poisonous substance produced by certain animals, some plants and pathogenic bacteria.

It is characteristic of bacterial toxins that they do not cause symptoms until after a variable period of incubation while the microbes multiply, or, as is the case in botulism, the preformed toxin reaches and affects the tissue. Usually only a few toxin-producing agents are introduced into the body, and it is not until there are enough of them to overwhelm the leukocytes and other types of antibodies that symptoms occur. In some cases of food poisoning, symptoms are almost immediate because the toxin is taken directly with the food.

Toxins cause antitoxins to form in the body, thus providing a means for establishing IMMUNITY to certain diseases.

bacterial t's, toxins produced by bacteria, including exotoxins, endotoxins and toxic enzymes.

Birkhaug's t., the toxic filtrate of a streptococcus isolated from a patient with endocarditis and rheumatic fever; used in a skin test for rheumatic fever.

botulinus t., one of five type-specific, immunologically differentiable exotoxins (types A to E) produced by *Clostridium botulinum.*

dermonecrotic t., an exotoxin produced by certain bacteria that causes extensive local necrosis on intradermal inoculation.

Dick t., erythrogenic toxin.

diphtheria t., a preparation of toxic products of growth of *Corynebacterium diphtheriae,* used in an intracutaneous test (Schick test) for susceptibility to diphtheria.

dysentery t., one produced by organisms of various species of Shigella.

erythrogenic t., a bacterial toxin from certain strains of *Streptococcus pyogenes* that produces an erythematous reaction when injected intradermally and is responsible for the rash in scarlet fever.

extracellular t., exotoxin.

fatigue t., kenotoxin.

intracellular t., endotoxin.

plant t., phytotoxin.

scarlatinal t., erythrogenic toxin.

soluble t., exotoxin.

tetanus t., the exotoxin of *Clostridium tetani,* consisting of tetanolysin and tetanospasmin.

toxin-antitoxin (tok″sin-an′tĭ-tok″sin) a nearly neutral mixture of diphtheria toxin with its antitoxin; formerly used for vaccination against diphtheria, but now superseded by toxoid.

toxinfection (tok″sin-fek′shun) infection by toxins or other poisonous agents, the causative organism not being recognized.

toxipathic (tok″sĭ-path′ik) pertaining to or caused by the pathogenic action of toxins, of whatever origin.

toxipathy (tok-sip′ah-the) a disease due to poisoning.

toxisterol (tok-sis′ter-ol) a poisonous isomer of ergosterol.

toxitherapy (tok″sĭ-ther′ah-pe) therapeutic use of toxins.

toxo- (tok′so) word element [Gr., L.], *poison.*

Toxocara (tok″so-ka′rah) a genus of nematode parasites found in various animals and sometimes in man.

toxocariasis (tok″so-ka-ri′ah-sis) infection by worms of the genus Toxocara.

toxoid (tok′soid) a toxin treated by heat or chemical agent to destroy its deleterious properties without destroying its ability to stimulate antibody production.

alum-precipitated t., a toxoid of diphtheria or tetanus precipitated with alum.

diphtheria t., a sterile preparation of formaldehyde-treated products of the growth of *Corynebacterium diphtheriae*, used as an active immunizing agent.

tetanus t., a sterile preparation of formaldehyde-treated products of the growth of *Clostridium tetani*, used as an active immunizing agent.

toxopeptone (tok″so-pep′tōn) a poisonous peptone.

toxophilic (tok″so-fil′ik) having affinity for toxins.

toxophore (tok′so-fōr) the group of atoms in a toxin molecule that produces the toxic effect.

toxophorous (tok-sof′o-rus) bearing poison; producing the toxic effect.

toxophylaxin (tok″so-fi-lak′sin) toxicophylaxin.

Toxoplasma (tok″so-plaz′mah) a genus of sporozoan parasites in man, other mammals and some birds; it includes one species, *T. gon′dii,* which is frequently transmitted from an infected mother to an infant in utero or at birth. The infection may be asymptomatic or may produce encephalomyelitis with cerebral calcification and chorioretinitis.

toxoplasmin (tok″so-plaz′min) an antigen that is injected intracutaneously as a test for toxoplasmosis.

toxoplasmosis (tok″so-plaz-mo′sis) infection with toxoplasma.

T.P.R. temperature, pulse, respiration.

tr. tincture.

trabecula (trah-bek′u-lah), pl. *trabec′ulae* [L.] a small beam or supporting structure; used in anatomic nomenclature to designate various fibromuscular bands or cords providing support in various organs, as heart, penis and spleen, adj., **trabec′ular.**

trabeculate (trah-bek′u-lāt) marked with crossbars or trabeculae.

trabeculation (trah-bek″u-la′shun) the formation of trabeculae in a part.

tracer (trās′er) a means by which something may be followed, as (1) a mechanical device by which the outline or movements of an object can be graphically recorded, or (2) a material by which the progress of a compound through the body may be observed.

radioactive t., a radioactive isotope replacing a stable chemical element in a compound introduced into the body, enabling its metabolism, distribution and elimination to be followed.

trachea (tra′ke-ah) the air passage extending from the throat and larynx to the main bronchi; called also the windpipe. adj. **tra′cheal.** This tube, about three-fifths of an inch wide and 4 inches long, is reinforced at the front and sides by a series of C-shaped rings of cartilage that keep the passage uniformly open. The gaps between the rings are bridged by strong fibroelastic membranes.

The trachea is lined with mucous membrane covered with small hairlike processes called cilia. These continously sweep foreign material out of the breathing passages toward the mouth. The process is retarded by cold but speeded by heat.

Although the trachea is closed off during swallowing by the epiglottis, a sort of lid, a foreign body, such as a piece of meat, occasionally becomes lodged in it and causes choking. Surgical incision of the trachea, called tracheotomy, may be necessary for removal of the foreign body.

TRACHEOSTOMY, incision of the trachea with insertion of a tube for passage of air, may be necessary if the trachea is obstructed by swelling due to infection or allergic reaction, by accumulation of tracheobronchial secretions or by a growth such as a polyp or tumor.

tracheaectasy (tra″ke-ah-ek′tah-se) dilatation of the trachea.

trachealgia (tra″ke-al′je-ah) pain in the trachea.

tracheitis   (tra″ke-i′tis) inflammation of the trachea.

trachel(o)- (tra′kĕ-lo) word element [Gr.], *neck; necklike structure*, especially the cervix uteri.

trachelagra (tra″kĕ-lag′rah) gout in the neck.

trachelectomy (tra″kĕ-lek′to-me) excision of the cervix uteri.

trachelematoma (tra″kĕ-lem″ah-to′mah) a hematoma on the sternocleidomastoid muscle.

trachelismus (tra″kĕ-liz′mus) spasm of the neck muscles.

trachelitis (tra″kĕ-li′tis) cervicitis; inflammation of the cervix uteri.

trachelocystitis (tra″kĕ-lo-sis-ti′tis) inflammation of the neck of the bladder.

trachelodynia (tra″kĕ-lo-din′e-ah) pain in the neck.

trachelomyitis (tra″kĕ-lo-mi-i′tis) inflammation of the muscles of the neck.

trachelopexy (tra′kĕ-lo-pek″se) fixation of the cervix uteri.

tracheloplasty (tra′kĕ-lo-plas″te) plastic repair of the cervix uteri.

trachelorrhaphy (tra″kĕ-lor′ah-fe) suture of the cervix uteri.

trachelotomy (tra″kĕ-lot′o-me) incision of the cervix uteri.

tracheo- (tra′ke-o) word element [Gr.], *trachea.*

tracheo-aerocele (tra″ke-o-a′er-o-sēl″) tracheal hernia containing air.

tracheobronchial (tra″ke-o-brong′ke-al) pertaining to the trachea and bronchi.

tracheobronchiomegaly (tra″ke-o-brong″ke-o-meg′ah-le) abnormal dilatation of the trachea and bronchi.

tracheobronchitis (tra″ke-o-brong-ki′tis) inflammation of the trachea and bronchi.

tracheobronchoscopy (tra″ke-o-brong-kos′ko-pe) inspection of the interior of the trachea and bronchus.

tracheocele (tra″ke-o-sēl) 1. hernial protrusion of the tracheal mucous membrane. 2. goiter.

tracheo-esophageal (tra″ke-o-e-sof″ah-je′al) pertaining to the trachea and esophagus.

tracheofissure (tra″ke-o-fish′ūr) incision of the trachea.

tracheolaryngotomy (tra″ke-o-lar″ing-got′o-me) incision of the larynx and trachea.

tracheomalacia (tra″ke-o-mah-la′she-ah) softening of the tracheal cartilages.

tracheopathy (tra″ke-op′ah-the) disease of the trachea.

tracheopharyngeal (tra″ke-o-fah-rin′je-al) pertaining to the trachea and pharynx.

tracheophony (tra″ke-of′o-ne) a sound heard in auscultation over the trachea.

tracheoplasty (tra′ke-o-plas′te) plastic repair of the trachea.

tracheopyosis (tra″ke-o-pi-o′sis) purulent tracheitis

tracheorrhagia (tra″ke-o-ra′je-ah) hemorrhage from the trachea.

tracheorrhaphy (tra″ke-or′ah-fe) suture of the trachea.

tracheoschisis (tra″ke-os′kĭ-sis) fissure of the trachea.

tracheoscopy (tra″ke-os′ko-pe) inspection of the interior of the trachea.

tracheostenosis (tra″ke-o-stĕ-no′sis) constriction of the trachea.

tracheostomize (tra″ke-os′to-mīz) to perform tracheostomy.

tracheostomy (tra″ke-os′to-me) creation of an opening into the trachea through the neck, with insertion of an indwelling tube to facilitate passage of air or evacuation of secretions. The procedure may be an emergency measure or an elective one.

During the operation the patient is placed on his back with a pillow or roll of fabric under his shoulders so that the neck is extended and the trachea is prominent.

TRACHEOSTOMY TRAY.   The number and kinds of instruments available on a tracheostomy tray vary in different institutions, and although a tracheostomy may be done with very few instruments the following list includes those considered to be minimal: a scalpel, a curved blunt bistoury, dissecting scissors, a hemostat, forceps, two retractors, a tracheal dilator, gauze sponges, a pair of sterile gloves and tracheostomy tubes.

The tracheostomy set consists of an outer cannula with an extension on either side of one end, each of which has a strip of cotton tape attached to it. Between the extensions and just above the lumen of the outer cannula there is a small clasp devised to hold the inner cannula in place. The inner cannula fits snugly inside the outer cannula. The obturator is an olive-tipped curved rod that is used to guide the outer cannula as it is inserted into the tracheal incision. After the tracheostomy tube is inserted, the ends of the cotton tape are brought around the neck and tied in place to prevent accidental removal of the outer cannula.

In recent years plastic tracheostomy tubes have gained popularity. They consist of a single tube with one or two balloons affixed to the outer surface at the end of the tube. In the single-balloon type, the balloon is inflated to prevent leakage of air around the tube and aspiration of food or secretions into the trachea. In the tubes with two balloons, each balloon is inflated and deflated at intervals to prevent constant irritation at the site of the incision.

NURSING CARE.   The primary concern of tracheostomy care is maintenance of an adequate airway by keeping the tube free of secretions. During the first 24 hours after the operation the patient should have someone in constant attendance. Because he cannot call for help and will not be able to cough up and expectorate accumulations of secretions in the trachea, the patient may easily panic and feel that he is suffocating.

The patient is observed closely for signs of respiratory difficulty. If there is a change in the respiratory rate or a wheezing or crowing sound on inspiration the tube most likely is obstructed. If suctioning does not relieve the situation a physician should be called immediately. Restlessness, pallor or the development of cyanosis is an indication of inadequate ventilation of the lungs resulting from obstruction of the airway.

Accidental expulsion of the outer cannula due to violent coughing or improperly tied tapes rarely occurs; should it happen, however, a dilator or hemostat must be used to hold open the incision while another tube is inserted.

The mucus will be slightly blood-tinged immediately after the tracheostomy is performed, but it should gradually assume a normal color, If there is evidence of persistent bleeding, this should be reported, as it may indicate internal hemorrhage. The mucus is suctioned as necessary with an electric or wall suction apparatus. The size of the rubber catheter attached to the suction apparatus will depend on the size of the lumen of the tracheostomy tube. It should fit the tube easily without completely obstructing it. A No. 14 or 16 whistle-tip catheter with extra holes cut in the side is usually preferred. Suctioning is done gently and quickly to avoid damage to the mucous membranes and to prevent prolonged obstruction of the airway. It is generally recommended that suctioning be continued not longer than 5 seconds at a time.

A sterile dressing, slit so that it fits around the tube, is applied at the time of the tracheostomy and is changed as often as necessary. If gauze squares are used, care must be taken that the edges are bound so that strings from the dressing will not be aspirated.

The inner cannula is removed and cleaned of secretions as often as needed to prevent encrustation and obstruction. The cannula should be cleaned under cold running water; gauze strips or pipe cleaners are used to clean the inside of the tube. It should be remembered that tubes made of silver are easily bent out of shape and must be handled accordingly.

Secretions are less likely to become dry and the mucus will be less tenacious if some provision is made for moistening the air inhaled through the tracheostomy tube. This can be accomplished by installing a vaporizer at the bedside or, less effectively, by placing a dressing moistened with saline solution over the opening in the tube.

The outer cannula is not removed by the nurse unless the physician specifically writes an order to this effect. If the tracheostomy is permanent and the trachea has been sutured to the opening in the skin, there is less danger in removing the outer cannula because there are no loose flaps of skin to cover the opening while the tube is out of place.

The patient with a permanent tracheostomy must be taught self-care before he leaves the hospital. As he becomes accustomed to breathing through the tube, suctioning it as necessary and replacing the dressings, he will become less apprehensive. He must be cautioned against swimming, and should be warned to use care when taking a shower or bath that water is not aspirated through the tracheostomy.

tracheotome (tra'ke-o-tōm″) an instrument for incising the trachea.

tracheotomy (tra″ke-ot'o-me) incision of the trachea for exploration, for removal of a foreign body or for obtaining a biopsy specimen or removing a local lesion.

trachoma (trah-ko'mah) a chronic communicable disease of the eye, caused by a virus and characterized by inflammation of the conjunctiva. In many parts of the world trachoma is still quite widespread, and is a major cause of blindness. In the United States, however, it is now comparatively rare.

The early symptoms of trachoma are similar to those of conjunctivitis. The eyes become red, and the eyelids swell and stick together in the morning. As trachoma progresses, the eyelids become pocked and scarred, and granules form on the interior surface of the eyelid.

Trachoma can be arrested in the early stages by treatment with tetracycline and sulfonamide preparations. At later stages, these medicines must be supplemented with mild caustics such as silver nitrate to remove the blinding granules from the eyelids.

trachychromatic (tra″ke-kro-mat'ik) having deeply staining chromatin.

trachyphonia (tra″ke-fo'ne-ah) roughness of the voice.

tracing (trās'ing) a graphic record produced by copying another, or scribed by an instrument capable of making a visual record of movements.

tract (trakt) a longitudinal assemblage of tissues or organs, especially a bundle of nerve fibers having a common origin, function and termination, or a number of anatomic structures arranged in series and serving a common function.

 alimentary t., digestive tract.

 biliary t., the liver and gallbladder, and their various ducts.

 digestive t., the passage from the mouth to the anus (see also DIGESTIVE SYSTEM).

 gastrointestinal t., the stomach and intestines; the portion of the digestive tract from the cardia to the anus.

 intestinal t., the small and large intestines in continuity.

 optic t., the central extension of an optic nerve beyond the optic chiasm.

 pyramidal t's, collections of motor nerve fibers arising in the brain and passing down through the spinal cord to motor cells in the anterior horns.

 respiratory t., the organs that allow entrance of air into the lungs and exchange of gases with the blood, from the air passages in the nose to the pulmonary alveoli.

 urinary t., the organs concerned with the elaboration and excretion of urine: the kidneys, ureters, bladder and urethra.

 uveal t., the vascular tunic of the eye, comprising the choroid, ciliary body and iris.

traction (trak'shun) the exertion of a pulling force, as that applied to a fractured bone or dislocated joint to maintain proper position and facilitate healing, or, in obstetrics, that along the axis of the pelvis to assist in delivery of a fetal part.

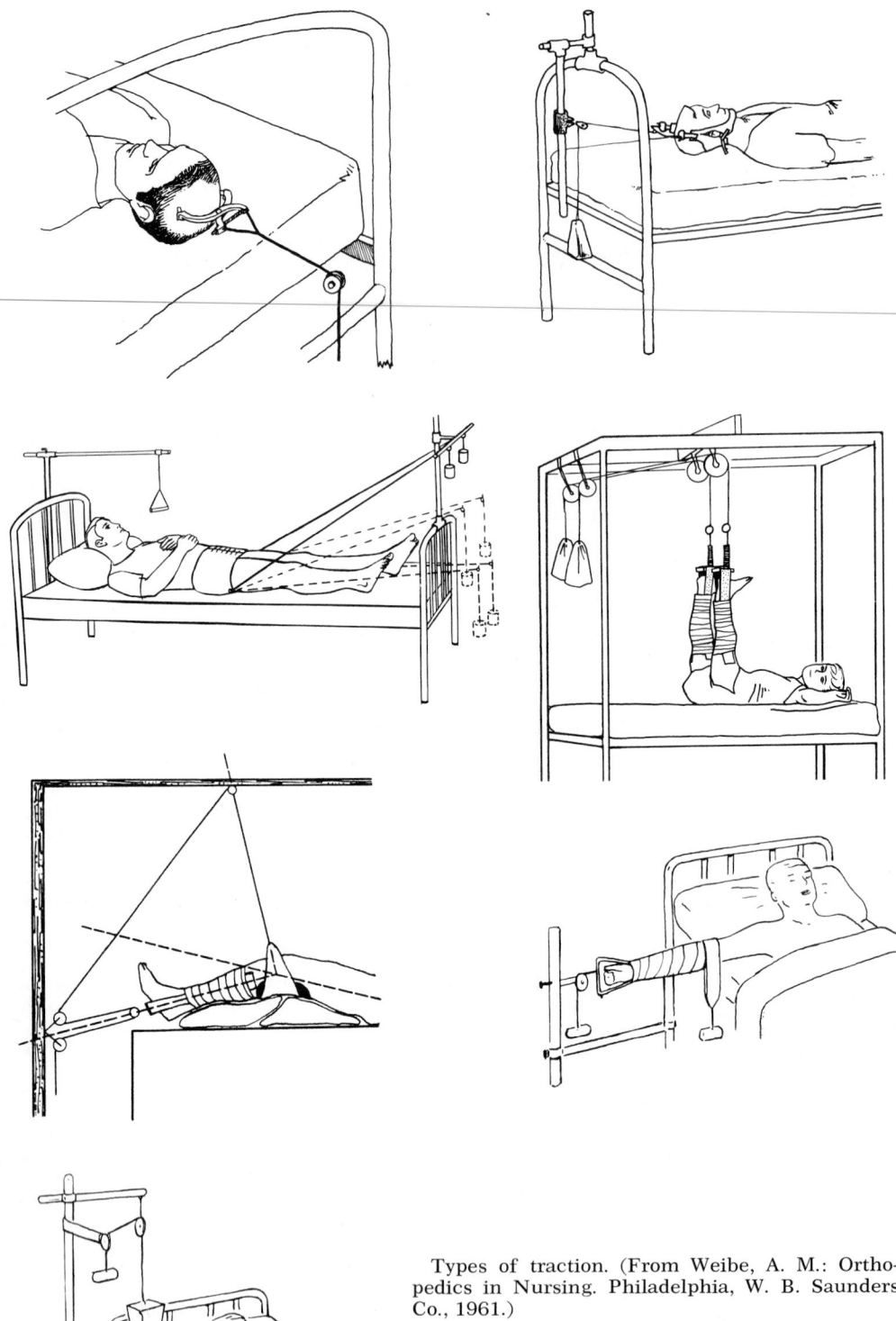

Types of traction. (From Weibe, A. M.: Orthopedics in Nursing. Philadelphia, W. B. Saunders
Co., 1961.)

Traction also may be used to overcome muscle spasms in musculoskeletal disorders, such as "slipped disk," to lessen or prevent contractures and to correct or prevent a deformity.

Traction may be applied by means of a weight connected to a pulley mechanism over the patient's bed; this is known as weight traction. Elastic traction involves the use of an elastic appliance that exerts a pulling force upon the injured limb. In skeletal traction, force is applied directly upon a bone by means of surgically installed pins and wires or tongs. Splints and reinforced garments, such as surgical corsets and collars, also may be employed to provide forms of traction. In skin traction moleskin or some other type of adhesive bandage is used to cover the affected limb, and traction is applied to the bandage.

NURSING CARE. The patient in constant traction must receive special skin care frequently to prevent breakdown of the skin. Since he often cannot move certain parts of his body without help, a regular schedule of changing and alternating positions should be instituted. Bony prominences are checked frequently for signs of pressure and irritation.

When allowed by the physician, the installation of a trapeze bar over the bed can give the patient greater freedom in moving himself about in bed and makes him feel less dependent on the nursing staff. The patient should be instructed to lift himself straight up so as not to alter the position of the affected limb in traction.

The apparatus used for traction must be checked frequently to be sure the weights are hanging free and exerting the required amount of pull. The patient's body weight should counteract the pull of the weights; i.e., his feet should not be resting against the footboard nor should his body position interfere in any way with the tension on the ropes of the traction apparatus.

When traction is applied to the neck with a head halter or other apparatus, it is best to have the patient's head at the foot of the bed. This facilitates observation of the patient, changing of dressings and other treatments and nursing measures that may be necessary.

To disturb the patient as little as possible during the changing of the bottom linen, it is best to start the linen change on the unaffected side. If the limb in traction feels cold to the touch or the patient complains of chilling, a small baby blanket may be used to cover the limb. Care must be taken that other top covers on the bed do not interfere with the traction apparatus.

tractotomy (trak-tot'o-me) transection of a nerve tract in the central nervous system, frequently for the relief of intractable pain.

tractus (trak'tus), pl. *trac'tus* [L.] tract; used in anatomic nomenclature to designate certain collections of nerve fibers in the central nervous system.

tragacanth (trag'ah-kanth) the dried gummy exudation from *Astragalus gummifer* or other species of Astragalus; used as a suspending agent for drugs.

tragomaschalia (trag"o-mas-kal'e-ah) odorous perspiration from the axilla.

tragopodia (trag"o-po'de-ah) knock-knee.

tragus (tra'gus), pl. *tra'gi* [L.] a cartilaginous projection anterior to the external opening of the ear; used also in the plural to designate hairs growing on the pinna of the external ear, especially on the anterior cartilaginous projection.

trait (trāt) 1. a facial line. 2. a distinguishing quality or feature.

Tral (tral) trademark for preparations of hexocyclium methylsulfate, an anticholinergic and antispasmodic.

trance (trans) profound or abnormal sleep from which the patient cannot be aroused easily, and not due to organic disease. It is usually due to hysteria or other psychiatric disturbance and may be induced by hypnotism.

Trancopal (tran'ko-pal) trademark for a preparation of chlormezanone, a muscle relaxant and tranquilizer.

tranquilizer (tran'kwĭ-li"zer) any of a group of compounds that calm or quiet an anxious patient without causing the drowsiness produced by SEDATIVES or the stimulation produced by antidepressants.

Tranquilizers differ in important ways from other drugs used to reduce pain or relieve tension and anxiety. Sedatives, which include barbiturates and chloral hydrate, act as depressants of the nervous system and diminish the response to certain stimuli. They frequently bring about a lessening of anxiety. They may also cause the patient to become drowsy, Alcohol is well known for its effect in relieving emotional tension by a depressant action; it is essentially a sedative.

A tranquilizer has a more direct effect in lessening anxiety. Although it can also cause some drowsiness, the body still reacts to stimuli. A person who has taken a tranquilizer is easily aroused from his drowsiness; this would not usually be possible if he had taken a sedative.

Antidepressants are quite different from tranquilizers. They have the effect of relieving the symptoms of deep depression. Some, such as the amphetamines, act as stimulants and producers of euphoria, or a sense of heightened well-being, and may help relieve lethargy. Others have a more direct antidepressant effect without being stimulants. The antidepressants now available are unfortunately effective in the treatment of only some, not all, forms of depression; other treatments, such as SHOCK THERAPY and PSYCHOTHERAPY, are important.

USES. *In Mental Illness.* Tranquilizers do not cure mental illness. They relieve the intense anxiety of the patient, with the result that the more difficult symptoms of his disease disappear. For this reason, a very important use is in the treatment of highly disturbed psychotics (see PSYCHOSIS). Relieved of their intense anxiety or depression, these patients become more accessible to treatment, with psychotherapy for example. The use of tranquilizers has had a dramatically beneficial effect on the atmosphere of mental hospitals, lessening the need for physical restriction of disturbed patients, and has greatly increased the discharge rate from these hospitals.

In Anxiety and Neurosis. Tranquilizers are sometimes prescribed by physicians to relieve anxiety states from various causes. Chronic alcoholics may benefit from certain tranquilizers which reduce the craving for liquor. The tranquilizers used for these purposes are mild and not so likely to cause serious side effects as the more potent tranquilizers frequently used for more severe disturbances, such as psychosis or delirium.

Although tranquilizers are often useful in the management of NEUROSIS, they serve essentially to ease symptoms. They cannot solve the psychologic conflicts and problems of the neurotic, but by lessening his symptoms they frequently improve his ability to function. Though valuable for this purpose, tranquilizers are sometimes overused by people seeking quick results.

In Physical Illness. Tranquilizers are also effective in the relief of certain physical conditions. They may, for instance, be helpful as antinauseants to stop the vomiting that sometimes accompanies x-ray therapy and certain intestinal disorders. Tranquilizers may be useful in the treatment of hypertension. They may also be used for muscle relaxation.

SIDE EFFECTS. Tranquilizers should never be used except on the advice of a physician. All are potentially habit forming, and most can cause unpleasant side effects in certain cases. Prolonged use can lead to mild discomforts such as headaches, sleeplessness, constipation, dryness of the mouth and nightmares.

Certain tranquilizers are capable of producing more serious side effects. High dosages or sudden withdrawals of the medication may cause tremors or even convulsions. The liver may be affected, producing jaundice. Production of blood cells by the bone marrow may be impaired. Rashes or sensitivity of the skin to sunlight may develop. There may be a possibility of damage to an unborn baby.

It is important to remember that each tranquilizer has its own range of effects and side effects. These are considered when a particular tranquilizer is selected by the physician; his advice should be followed carefully and any side effects should be reported to him.

Some persons take tranquilizers to relieve their tensions and then take stimulants such as amphetamine to give them "pep." These artificial efforts to make the body work both ways are likely to have unfortunate results for both body and mind. For these people, the answer usually is not medication but a return to normal life routines and rhythms — with the aid of a physician or a psychiatrist if necessary.

trans- (trans) word element [L.] *through; across; beyond;* in names of chemical compounds it indicates certain atoms or radicals on opposite sides of the molecule.

transabdominal (trans″ab-dom′ĭ-nal) across the abdominal wall or through the abdominal cavity.

transacetylation (trans-as″ĕ-til-a′shun) a chemical reaction involving the transfer of the acetyl radical.

transamidase (trans-am′ĭ-dās) an enzyme that catalyzes the transfer of an amide group from one molecule to another.

transaminase (trans-am′ĭ-nās) an enzyme that catalyzes the transfer of an amino group from one molecule to another.

    glutamic oxaloacetic t., GOT, an enzyme normally present in serum and various tissues, especially the heart and liver; it is released into serum as a result of tissue injury and is present in increased concentration in myocardial infarction or acute damage to liver cells.

    glutamic pyruvic t., GPT, an enzyme normally present in the body, especially the liver, and observed in higher concentration in the serum of patients with acute damage to liver cells.

transamination (trans″am-ĭ-na′shun) the reversible exchange of amino groups between different amino acids.

transanimation (trans-an″ĭ-ma′shun) resuscitation of an asphyxiated person by mouth-to-mouth breathing (see also ARTIFICIAL RESPIRATION).

transaortic (trans″a-or′tik) performed through the aorta.

transatrial (trans-a′tre-al) performed through the atrium.

transaudient (trans-aw′de-ent) penetrable by sound waves.

transcalent (trans-ka′lent) penetrable by heat rays.

transcervical (trans-ser′vĭ-kal) 1. performed through the cervical opening of the uterus. 2. across or through the neck of a structure.

transduction (trans-duk′shun) the transfer of a genetic fragment from one cell to another.

transduodenal (trans″du-o-de′nal) across or through the duodenum.

transection (tran-sek′shun) a section made across a long axis.

transepidermal (trans″ep-ĭ-der′mal) occurring through or across the epidermis.

transfaunation (trans″faw-na′shun) the transfer of animal parasites from one host organism to another.

transferase (trans′fer-ās) an enzyme that catalyzes the transfer, from one molecule to another, of a chemical group that does not exist in free state during the transfer.

transference (trans-fer′ens) 1. the passage of a symptom or affection from one part to another. 2. in psychiatry, the shifting of an affect from one person to another or from one idea to another; especially the transfer by the patient to the analyst of emotional tones, of either affection or hostility, based on unconscious identification.

transferrin (trans-fer′in) a serum globulin that binds and transports iron.

transfix (trans-fiks′) to pierce through or impale.

transfixion (trans-fik′shun) a piercing through.

transforation (trans″fo-ra′shun) perforation of the fetal skull.

transformer (trans-for′mer) an induction apparatus for changing electrical energy at one voltage and current to electrical energy at another voltage and current, through the medium of magnetic energy, without mechanical motion.

closed-core t., one having a continuous core of magnetic material (usually iron) without any air gap.

step-down t., one for lowering the voltage of the original current.

step-up t., one for raising the voltage of the original current.

transfusion (trans-fu'zhun) introduction into the body circulation of blood or other fluid. Among the solutions employed are whole blood, plasma, serum and various artificial blood substitutes.

Blood transfusions are used to replenish the depleted blood supply of the body in cases of hemorrhage, burns, injuries to blood vessels, shock during surgery and certain blood dyscrasias such as anemia and leukemia.

TRANSFUSION METHODS. There are several different methods of transfusion. Direct transfusion, in which blood from one person is directly transferred to another person, is now rarely used. The usual method is indirect transfusion, in which blood is drawn from a donor, stored in a sterile container and later given to a recipient. Exchange transfusion, in which blood is removed from a person and simultaneously replaced by donor blood, is used mainly in treating ERYTHROBLASTOSIS FETALIS.

In reciprocal transfusion, blood from a person recovering from a contagious disease is transferred into the blood vessels of another person afflicted with the same disease in exchange for an equal amount of blood. This is designed to help the sick person by giving him antibodies developed by the person who is recovering.

Intrauterine Transfusion. Intrauterine transfusion involves direct transfusion of Rh-negative packed blood cells into the fetal peritoneal cavity. It is done to prevent death as a result of maternal-fetal blood incompatibility in which the fetal blood cells are destroyed (ERYTHROBLASTOSIS FETALIS).

The first step in a fetal transfusion is injection of a radiopaque dye into the amniotic fluid. After the fetus ingests the dye, his intestinal tract can be visualized by roentgenography and serves as a guidepost for location of the abdominal cavity. A long pudendal needle is then inserted through the mother's abdomen and guided through the uterine wall, through the fetal abdomen and into the peritoneal cavity. Another x-ray is taken to confirm correct placement of the needle and then the erythrocytes are transfused.

This procedure is obviously not without hazard and is done only if the fetus cannot be expected to survive without it. The treatment may need to be repeated several times before birth.

BLOOD TYPING AND CROSSMATCHING. Transfusions were not practicable until the four main hereditary BLOOD TYPES, A, B, AB and O, were discovered at the beginning of this century. The different blood types are caused by the presence of two substances, A and B, in the erythrocytes, and of their two antibodies, a and b, in the plasma. Various combinations of the substances and antibodies result in the four types. Blood type is readily determined by a simple chemical test of two drops of blood.

A further precaution before transfusion is to mix small samples of the donor's and recipient's blood and to note the reaction; this is known as crossmatching.

Another matter to be considered is the RH FACTOR. Individuals lacking this factor are called Rh negative, and should always receive transfusions of Rh-negative blood.

TRANSFUSION REACTION. If the blood types are not matched correctly for transfusion, the blood of the donor can cause clumping (agglutination) of the recipient's blood cells, making it difficult for the blood to pass through the capillaries and thus endangering his life. Such a situation is called a transfusion reaction. It may also occur in cases of hypersensitivity to serum proteins or to preservatives added to the blood.

Symptoms of a transfusion reaction include rash, itching, chills and fever. In more severe reactions they may be dyspnea, coughing, flushed face, collapse, coma and eventually death. In the event of any symptom of a transfusion reaction the transfusion is stopped immediately.

transiliac (trans-il'e-ak) across the two ilia.

transillumination (trans"-ĭ-lu"mĭ-na'shun) the passage of strong light through a body structure, to permit inspection by an observer on the opposite side.

translateral (trans-lat'er-al) from side to side; in roentgenography, referring to the view obtained with the patient supine and the radiation directed horizontally.

translocation (trans"lo-ka'shun) the attachment of a fragment of one chromosome to a nonhomologous chromosome.

reciprocal t., the mutual exchange of fragments between two broken chromosomes, one part of one uniting with part of the other.

translucent (trans-lu'sent) slightly penetrable by light rays.

transmigration (trans"mi-gra'shun) 1. diapedesis. 2. change of place from one side of the body to the other.

transmission (trans-mish'un) 1. transfer, as of a nerve impulse along a nerve or a disease from one person to another. 2. heredity.

transmutation (trans"mu-ta'shun) 1. evolutionary change of one species into another. 2. the change of one chemical element into another.

transorbital (trans-or'bĭ-tal) performed through the bony socket of the eye.

transovarial (trans"o-va're-al) through the ovary; referring to transmission from the maternal organism through the ovum to individuals of the next generation.

transpalatal (trans-pal'ah-tal) performed through the roof of the mouth, or palate.

transparent (trans-par'ent) permitting the passage of rays of light so that objects may be seen through the substance.

transpeptidase (trans-pep'tĭ-dās) an enzyme that catalyzes the transfer of a peptide group from one molecule to another.

transphosphorylase (trans"fos-for'ĭ-lās) an enzyme that catalyzes the transfer of a phosphate group from one molecule to another.

transpirable (trans-pi′rah-bl) permitting passage of perspiration.

transpiration (trans″pĭ-ra′shun) discharge of air, vapor or sweat through the skin.

transplacental (trans″plah-sen′tal) through the placenta.

transplant 1. (trans′plant) a portion of tissue used in grafting or transplanting. 2. (trans-plant′) to transfer tissue from one part to another.

transplantation (trans″plan-ta′shun) the transfer of living organs from one part of the body to another or from one individual to another. Transplantation and grafting mean the same thing, though the term grafting is more commonly used to refer to the transfer of skin (see GRAFTING).

Occasionally an emergency requires an organ to be transplanted from one place to another within the body. Kidneys, for example, have been relocated to enable them to continue functioning after the ureters have been damaged. Organ transplants within the body, known as autotransplants, require delicate surgery, but otherwise pose no particular problem.

The transplantation of organs from one individual to another (homotransplantation), however, or from a closely related animal such as a chimpanzee to a human being (heterotransplantation), poses far greater problems and is a real challenge to surgeons. Such transplants are still largely experimental, but their numbers increase daily and they show promise of being successful if the problem of rejection can be overcome.

The first successful transplant of a vital organ was made in 1954 when a kidney was removed from one identical twin and implanted in the other to replace his diseased kidney. Since then thousands of kidney transplants have been performed and it is estimated that there will be 5000 renal transplants a year by 1977.

In an effort to save lives, attempts have also been made to transplant livers, spleens, lungs and hearts. So far, such operations have been performed in only a few large medical centers throughout the world, and they have met with limited success in that only a small percentage of the recipients have survived for more than a few months. Nevertheless, the operations have shown that the transplantation of many vital organs is technically feasible and that the transplanted organs are capable of functioning in their new environment.

REJECTION. The major problem to be overcome in transplantation therapy is the immune rejection phenomenon. Organs such as the cornea, skin and bone can be transplanted successfully because, in the case of the cornea, the vascular supply is not involved, or, in skin and bone, the transplant serves as a structural foundation into which the new tissue grows. In the case of intact organs such as the kidney, heart, lung, liver and pancreas, a generous blood supply is essential to their survival in the recipient's body. The blood of the recipient carries in it many of the tools used by the body in defense against foreign substances. As blood is drained from the transplanted organ into the host's general circulation, the body recognizes the transplanted tissue cells as foreign invaders (antigens) and immediately sets up an immune response by producing antibodies. These antibodies are capable of inhibiting metabolism of the cells within the transplanted organ and eventually actively cause their destruction. They also play a role in a delayed inflammatory response that can occur as late as weeks or months after implantation and adds to the destruction of the donor organ.

Control of the immune response in the recipient is attempted by the use of immunosuppressive agents such as antilymphocyte globulin (ALG), and antimetabolites, which tend to suppress the growth of rapidly dividing cells. Corticosteroids also are used because of their anti-inflammatory effect. All of the chemicals used in transplantation therapy interfere in some way with the body's normal defense mechanisms. For this reason a very delicate balance must be maintained in their administration so as to avoid tipping the scales in the direction of rejection of the organ on one side and a fatal infection on the other.

The greatest success in transplantation has been between identical twins. Their tissue pattern and body proteins are sufficiently similar that rejection of the donor organ is not likely. When more is learned about such tissue patterns and protein types, it may be possible to type and match tissues just as blood is typed and matched for transfusion. This seems plausible when we realize that blood transfusions are essentially transplants of blood cells from one person to another.

Other problems of transplantation must be solved. Sometimes, for example, a kidney transplant fails because the new kidney develops the same disease that destroyed the one that was replaced. Another problem that has created much furor among laymen and physicians is that of obtaining healthy organs for transplantation. The problem carries with it many legal and ethical and moral implications that cannot be ignored but that have not yet been solved to everyone's satisfaction.

transport (trans′port) movement of materials in biologic systems, particularly into and out of cells and across epithelial layers.
    active t., movement of materials across cell membranes and epithelial layers resulting directly from expenditure of metabolic energy.

transposition (trans″po-zish′un) displacement to the opposite side; in genetics, the nonreciprocal insertion of material deleted from one chromosome into another, nonhomologous chromosome.
    t. of great vessels, a CONGENITAL HEART DEFECT, in which the position of the chief blood vessels of the heart is reversed.

transsegmental (trans″seg-men′tal) extending across segments.

transseptal (trans-sep′tal) extending or performed through or across a septum.

trans-sexualism (trans-seks′u-al-izm″) conscious desire of a person for an anatomic change of sex.

transsphenoidal (trans″sfe-noi′dal) performed through the sphenoid bone.

transtemporal (trans-tem′po-ral) across the temporal lobe.

transthalamic (trans″thah-lam′ik) across the thalamus.

transthoracic (trans″tho-ras′ik) through the thoracic cavity or across the chest wall.

transthoracotomy (trans″tho-rah-kot′o-me) cutting across the thorax.

transtracheal (trans-tra′ke-al) performed through the wall of the trachea.

transtympanic (trans″tim-pan′ik) across the tympanic membrane or the cavity of the middle ear.

transudate (tran′su-dāt) a substance that has passed through a membrane; in contrast to an exudate, a transudate is characterized by high fluidity and a low content of protein, cells or solid matter derived from cells.

transudation (tran″su-da′shun) passage of serum or other body fluid through a membrane or tissue surface.

transureteroureterostomy (trans″u-re″ter-o-u-re″ter-os′to-me) anastomosis of the distal end of the proximal portion of one ureter to the ureter of the opposite side.

transurethral (trans″u-re′thral) through the urethra.

transvaginal (trans-vaj′ĭ-nal) through the vagina.

transvector (trans-vek′tor) an organism that conveys or transmits a poison derived from another source.

transventricular (trans″ven-trik′u-lar) performed through a ventricle.

transversalis (trans″ver-sa′lis) [L.] transverse.

transverse (trans-vers′) extending from side to side; situated at right angles to the long axis.

transversectomy (trans″ver-sek′to-me) excision of a transverse process of a vertebra.

transversus (trans-ver′sus) [L.] transverse.

transvesical (trans-ves′ĭ-kal) through the bladder.

transvestism (trans-ves′tizm) the wearing of clothes appropriate to the opposite sex.

transvestite (trans-ves′tīt) a person who wears clothing appropriate to the opposite sex, and who desires to be accepted as a member of the opposite sex.

tranylcypromine (tran″il-si′pro-mēn) a compound used as an antidepressant.

trapezium (trah-pe′ze-um) an irregular, four-sided figure.

Trasentine (tras′en-tin) trademark for preparations of adiphenine, an anticholinergic and antispasmodic.

trauma (traw′mah) a wound or injury, especially damage produced by external force.
　psychic t., injury to the subconscious mind by emotional shock, which may produce a lasting effect.

traumat(o)- (traw′mah-to) word element [Gr.], *trauma*.

traumatic (traw-mat′ik) pertaining to external force that damages the organism.

traumatism (traw′mah-tizm) a morbid state resulting from infliction of an injury or wound by external force.

traumatology (traw″mah-tol′o-je) the science, and particularly the surgical specialty, that deals with wounds resulting from external force or violence.

traumatopnea (traw″mah-top-ne′ah) passage of air through a wound in the chest wall.

travail (trah-vāl′) labor; childbirth.

treatment (trēt′ment) management and care of a patient or the combating of the existing disorder.
　active t., treatment directed immediately to counteracting a disease.
　causal t., treatment directed against the cause of a disease.
　conservative t., treatment designed to conserve the vital powers until clear indications develop.
　empiric t., treatment by means that experience has proved to be beneficial.
　expectant t., treatment designed only to relieve untoward symptoms, leaving the cure mainly to nature.
　palliative t., treatment that is designed to relieve pain and distress, but does not attempt a cure.
　preventive t., prophylactic t., that in which the aim is to prevent the occurrence of the disease.
　specific t., treatment particularly adapted to the special disease being treated.

trehalose (tre-ha′lōs) a sugar from mannitol or ergot.

Trematoda (trem″ah-to′dah) a class of animals (phylum Platyhelminthes) characterized by a noncellular layer covering the body, and including the flukes. The trematodes or flukes are parasitic in man and animals, infection resulting from the ingestion of uncooked or insufficiently cooked fish, crustaceans and vegetation which are the intermediate hosts of the trematodes.

trematode (trem′ah-tōd) an individual of the class Trematoda.

tremophobia (trem″o-fo′be-ah, tre″mo-fo′be-ah) morbid fear of trembling.

tremor (trem′or, tre′mor) an involuntary trembling of the body or limbs. It may have either a physical or a psychologic cause.
　Often tremors are associated with Parkinson's disease, in which nerve centers in the brain that control the muscles are affected. Early symptoms include trembling of the hands and nodding of the head. Tremors occur also in cerebral palsy and hyperthyroidism, and in narcotic addicts and alcoholics during withdrawal. They tend to develop as one of the results of aging.
　Tremors are sometimes symptoms of temporary abnormal conditions, as, for example, insulin shock, or of poisoning, especially metallic poisoning. They sometimes appear with a high fever resulting from an infection.
　Tremors of psychologic origin take many forms, some minor and some serious. If there is no physiologic cause, they may be a sign of general tension, as when a person holding a full cup of coffee seems compelled to shake and spill it. Violent, uncon-

trollable trembling is often seen in certain phases of severe mental disorder.

coarse t., that involving large groups of muscle fibers contracting slowly.

fibrillary t., rapidly alternating contraction of small bundles of muscle fibers.

fine t., one in which the vibrations are rapid.

flapping t., asterixis.

forced t., movements persisting after voluntary motion, due to intermittent irritation of the nerve centers.

Hunt's t., tremor associated with every voluntary movement; characteristic of cerebellar lesions.

intention t., one occurring when the patient attempts voluntary movement.

senile t., tremor associated with old age alone.

volitional t., trembling of the entire body during voluntary effort; seen in multiple sclerosis.

tremulous (trem'u-lus) trembling or quivering.

trench fever a louse-borne rickettsial disease marked by sudden fever with pain and soreness in muscles, bones and joints, and by a tendency to relapse.

trench foot a morbid condition resulting from inaction and prolonged exposure to cold and moisture.

trench mouth a disease that affects the gingivae and oral mucous membrane; called also Vincent's angina and necrotizing ulcerative gingivitis. The name trench mouth was given to the disease during World War I, when it was common among soldiers in the trenches.

The cause of the disease and its degree of communicability are not certain. It may be an infection caused by one or more microorganisms, although the suspected bacteria are present in healthy as well as diseased mouths. Trench mouth is more likely to develop in people suffering from poor oral hygiene, nutritional deficiencies or fatigue, and in those who are heavy smokers.

Early symptoms include tenderness and bleeding of the gums. Later there may be sore throat and mouth, swelling of the lymph nodes in the neck, fever and offensive breath. Swallowing may be painful. Prevention depends on good oral hygiene, a balanced diet and sufficient rest.

TREATMENT. Treatment includes the use of antibiotics, which are effective against the disease at all stages but work particularly well when the disorder is discovered and treated early. Mouthwashes of solutions of hydrogen peroxide or sodium perborate also are often prescribed, and a professional cleaning of the teeth usually is essential.

trepan (trĕ-pan') trephine.

trepanation, trephination (trep"ah-na'shun), (tref"ĭ-na'shun) use of the trephine for creating an opening in the skull or in the sclera.

trephine (trĕ-fīn', trĕ-fēn') 1. a small circular saw for removing a circular disk or button of tissue, chiefly from the skull, cornea or sclera. 2. to create an opening with the trephine.

trepidation (trep"ĭ-da'shun) 1. a trembling or oscillatory movement. 2. nervous anxiety and fear. adj., **trep'idant.**

Treponema (trep"o-ne'mah) a genus of Schizo-

mycetes, some of them pathogenic and parasitic for man and other animals, and including *T. pal'-lidum,* the cause of syphilis, and *T. perten'ue,* the cause of yaws in man.

treponema (trep"o-ne'mah) an organism of the genus Treponema. adj., **trepone'mal.**

Treponemataceae (trep"o-ne"mah-ta'se-e) a family of Schizomycetes that commonly occur as parasites in vertebrates, some of them causing disease. They are coarse or slender spiral forms, and are sometimes visible only with a darkfield microscope.

treponematosis (trep"o-ne"mah-to'sis) infection with organisms of the genus Treponema.

treponemicidal (trep"o-ne"mī-si'dal) destroying treponemas.

trepopnea (tre"pop-ne'ah) a condition in which respiration is more comfortable with the patient turned in a definite recumbent position.

treppe (trep'ĕ) [Ger.] the gradual increase in muscular contraction following rapidly repeated stimulation.

tresis (tre'sis) perforation.

tri- (tri) word element [Gr., L.], *three.*

triacetate (tri-as'ĕ-tāt) an acetate that contains three molecules of the acetic acid radical.

triacetin (tri-as'ĕ-tin) glyceryl triacetate; used as a topical antifungal.

triacetyloleandomycin (tri-as"ĕ-til-o"le-an"do-mi'sin) a white, odorless, crystalline powder, used as an antibiotic.

triad (tri'ad) 1. an element with a valence of three. 2. a group of three similar bodies, or a complex composed of three items or units.

triage (tre-ahzh') [Fr.] the sorting out and classification of casualties of war or other disaster, to determine priority of need and proper place of treatment.

triamcinolone (tri"am-sin'o-lōn) a prednisolone compound used topically or by intra-articular injection as an anti-inflammatory steroid.

triangle (tri'ang-gl) a three-cornered object, figure or area, as such an area on the surface of the body capable of fairly precise definition.

carotid t., inferior, that between the median line of the neck in front, the sternocleidomastoid muscle and the anterior belly of the omohyoid muscle.

carotid t., superior, that between the anterior belly of the omohyoid muscle in front, the posterior belly of the digastric muscle above and the sternocleidomastoid muscle behind.

cephalic t., one on the anteroposterior plane of the skull, between lines from the occiput to the forehead and to the chin, and from the chin to the forehead.

digastric t., submaxillary triangle.

t. of elbow, a triangular area on the front of the elbow, bounded by the brachioradial muscle on the outside and the round pronator muscle inside, with the base toward the humerus.

t. of election, superior carotid triangle.

infraclavicular t., that formed by the clavicle

muscle on the inside and the anterior border of the deltoid muscle on the outside.

inguinal t., the triangular area bounded by the inner edge of the sartorius muscle, the inguinal ligament and the outer edge of the long adductor muscle.

lumbocostoabdominal t., that lying between the external oblique muscle of the abdomen, the posterior inferior serratus muscle, the erector muscle of the spine and the internal oblique muscle of the abdomen.

t. of necessity, inferior carotid triangle.

t. of neck, anterior, the two carotid and the submaxillary triangles together.

t. of neck, posterior, the occipital and subclavian triangles together.

occipital t., the area bounded by the sternocleidomastoid muscle in front, the trapezius muscle behind, and the omohyoid muscle below.

subclavian t., a triangular area bounded by the clavicle, the sternocleidomastoid muscle and the omohyoid muscle.

submaxillary t., that bounded by the lower jaw bone above, the posterior belly of the digastric muscle and the stylohyoid muscle below and the median line of the neck in front.

suboccipital t., that lying between the posterior greater rectus muscle of the head and the superior and inferior oblique muscles of the head.

triangular (tri-ang'gu-lar) having three angles or corners.

triangularis (tri-ang″gu-la′ris) [L.] triangular.

Triatoma (tri″ah-to′mah) a genus of arthropods (order Hemiptera), numerous species of which, including *T. protrac′ta* and *T. sanguisu′ga,* are naturally infected by trypanosomes.

triatomic (tri″ah-tom′ik) 1. containing three atoms in the molecule. 2. containing three replaceable hydrogen atoms. 3. containing three hydroxyl groups.

tribe (trīb) a taxonomic category subordinate to a family (or subfamily) and superior to a genus (or subtribe).

triboluminescence (tri″bo-lu″mĭ-nes′ens) the production of light by a substance when it is rubbed to a fine powder.

tribrachius (tri-bra′ke-us) a fetal monster with three arms.

tribromoethanol (tri-bro″mo-eth′ah-nol) a white crystalline powder, administered by rectum, used in the induction phase of general anesthesia.

Triburon (trib′u-ron) trademark for preparations of triclobisonium chloride, a topical and vaginal antiseptic.

tricarboxylic acid cycle (tri″car-bok-sil′ik) a series of biochemical reactions by which carbon chains of sugars, fatty acids and amino acids are metabolized to yield carbon dioxide, water and energy; called also Krebs cycle and citric acid cycle.

tricephalus (tri-sef′ah-lus) a fetal monster with three heads.

triceps (tri′seps) a muscle having three heads; the triceps muscle of the arm extends the forearm.

trich(o)- (trik′o) word element [Gr.], *hair.*

trichangiectasis (trik″an-je-ek′tah-sis) dilatation of the capillaries.

trichiasis (tri-ki′ah-sis) 1. misplacement of the eyelashes so that they impinge on the cornea and conjunctiva covering the eyeball. 2. the appearance of hairlike filaments in the urine.

trichina (tri-ki′nah), pl. *trichi′nae* [Gr.] an individual organism of the genus Trichinella.

Trichinella (trik″ĭ-nel′ah) a genus of nematode parasites.

T. spira′lis, a species found in the striated muscle of various animals, a common cause of infection in man as a result of ingestion of poorly cooked pork.

trichinosis (trik″ĭ-no′sis) infection with the parasitic roundworm *Trichinella spiralis,* which enters the human body in infected pork eaten raw or insufficiently cooked.

The larvae, or early forms, of *T. spiralis* live embedded in tiny capsule-like cysts of muscle tissue of infected pork. When the meat is properly cooked, the larvae are killed by the high temperature. If, however, the pork is undercooked, they survive; when the meat is eaten, digestive juices dissolve the cyst capsules and free the larvae in the intestines, where they grow to maturity.

Carried by the lymphatic system to the lymph nodes and then into the blood, the larvae can travel to any of the body's tissues and organs, including the heart and lungs. In most tissues in which they lodge they cause inflammation, sometimes acute, and eventually they are destroyed by the body's natural defenses. In striated or voluntary muscle tissue, however, they survive. There the larvae coil into spirals; calcium deposits form around them, creating cysts similar to those in which the parent worms entered the body. The larvae do not develop into mature worms but remain encysted in the muscles for several years before dying; or they may even remain there for the lifetime of the host.

It is estimated that about 15 per cent of the adult population of the United States has been infected with trichinosis at some time. In many cases there are no symptoms and the infection is discovered only when Trichinella cysts are found in the muscles. Trichinosis occurs most frequently in areas where pigs are fed on garbage; it is rare in the tropics and in countries such as France where swine are fed root vegetables.

SYMPTOMS AND DEVELOPMENT. Trichinosis develops in stages that correspond to the worms' development in the intestine and, later, the movement of their larvae into other parts of the body. Symptoms and the severity vary according to the stage of the disease, the tissues invaded and the total number of invading parasites.

During the initial stage of the disease, when larvae are developing into mature worms in the intestinal tract, there may be diarrhea, nausea, abdominal pain and fever.

Symptoms that make identification of the disease more certain appear generally after an incubation period of 1 to 2 weeks. By this time, the mature worms have deposited their young in the intestinal wall and these new larvae are beginning to move through the body, causing a variety of reactions in one or several organs and areas. Edema may develop in the eyelids. This may be followed by hemorrhage of the retina, pain in the eyes and extreme sensitivity to light.

As the larvae invade other parts of the body, there may be muscle soreness and pain, fever, thirst, chills, profuse sweating and edema in the infected areas.

For most people there is more discomfort than danger in this most serious phase of trichinosis—the time when the larvae are active in various parts of the body. Often the infection is mild enough for patients to be treated at home. The occasional fatal cases of the disease (fewer than 5 per cent of known cases) usually involve additional infections or disorders in organs weakened by the parasites.

In the usual course of the disease, there is a gradual decrease in symptoms as the larvae in muscle tissue become encysted and dormant and those in other types of tissue are destroyed. After about 3 months, most symptoms disappear, although vague muscular pain and fatigue may still continue for several months. Trichinosis almost never leaves any permanent disability.

TREATMENT AND PREVENTION. With its varying symptoms, trichinosis is sometimes difficult to diagnose, but a skin test has been developed that makes identification of the disease certain in most cases. Chest x-rays and microscopic examination of muscle tissue also can be useful in diagnosis.

There is no specific treatment for trichinosis; recovery is a matter of bed rest and time, which allow the body's natural defenses to overcome the parasites. Medications, including thiabendazol, cortisone and ACTH, may be prescribed to relieve muscular pain and other symptoms.

The only certain safeguard against trichinosis is the thorough cooking of all pork products to ensure destruction of any encysted Trichinella larvae. Pork should be cooked at a temperature of 350° F., with a roasting time of 35 minutes per pound, until the meat is gray in color; if it is pink it is underdone. Pork products such as frankfurters should never be eaten raw.

trichinous (trik'ĭ-nus) affected with Trichinella.

trichloride (tri-klo'rīd) a binary compound containing three chlorine atoms in the molecule.

trichlormethiazide (tri-klōr″mĕ-thi'ah-zīd) a compound used as a diuretic and hypotensive and in the treatment of edema.

trichloroacetic acid (tri-klo″ro-ah-se'tic) colorless deliquescent crystals; germicidal, astringent and caustic.

trichloroethylene (tri″klo-ro-eth'ĭ-lēn) a clear, mobile liquid used as an inhalation analgesic and anesthetic for short operative procedures.

trichlorophenol (tri″klo-ro-fe'nol) a disinfectant and external antiseptic.

trichlorthiazide (tri″klōr-thi'ah-zīd) a compound used as a diuretic and hypotensive and in the treatment of edema.

trichoanesthesia (trik″o-an″es-the'ze-ah) loss of hair sensibility.

trichobacteria (trik″o-bak-te're-ah) bacteria having flagella.

trichobezoar (trik″o-be'zōr) a bezoar composed of hair; hairball.

trichocardia (trik″o-kar'de-ah) a hairy appearance of the heart due to exudative pericarditis.

trichocephaliasis (trik″o-sef″ah-li'ah-sis) trichuriasis.

Trichocephalus (trik″o-sef'ah-lus) Trichuris.

trichoclasia (trik″o-kla'se-ah) brittleness of the hair.

trichocryptosis (trik″o-krip-to'sis) disease of the hair follicles.

trichodynia (trik″o-din'e-ah) painful sensation when the hair is touched.

trichoepithelioma (trik″o-ep″ĭ-the″le-o'mah) a skin tumor originating in the follicles of the lanugo hairs.

trichoesthesia (trik″o-es-the'ze-ah) sensibility of the hair to touch.

trichogenous (trī-koj'ĕ-nus) stimulating the growth of hair.

trichoglossia (trik″o-glos'e-ah) hairy tongue, due to thickening of the papillae.

trichoid (trik'oid) resembling hair.

trichokryptomania (trik″o-krip″to-ma'ne-ah) trichorrhexomania.

trichologia (trik″o-lo'je-ah) the pulling out of the hair by delirious or insane patients.

trichology (trī-kol'o-je) the sum of knowledge about the hair.

trichome (tri'kōm) a filamentous or hairlike structure.

trichomonacide (trik″o-mo'nah-sīd) an agent destructive to trichomonads.

trichomonad (trik″o-mo'nad) a parasite of the genus Trichomonas.

Trichomonas (trik″o-mo'nas) a genus of parasitic protozoa.

    T. hom'inis, a species found in the human mouth and intestines.

    T. te'nax, a species found in the mouth.

    T. vagina'lis, a species occurring in the vaginal secretions; it causes vaginal discharge and pruritis. Trichomonacides such as metronidazole (Flagyl) are used in treatment of trichomonas vaginitis and may be given also to the patient's husband, who may be an asymptomatic carrier of the infection.

trichomoniasis (trik″o-mo-ni'ah-sis) infection by organisms of the genus Trichomonas.

trichomycosis (trik″o-mi-ko'sis) any disease of the hair caused by fungi.

trichonocardiasis (trik″o-no-kar-di'ah-sis) a disease of the pubic and axillary hair caused by *Nocardia tenuis.*

trichonodosis (trik″o-no-do′sis) a condition characterized by apparent or actual knotting of the hair.

trichonosis (trik″o-no′sis) any disease of the hair.

trichopathophobia (trik″o-path″o-fo′be-ah) morbid anxiety with regard to the hair, its growth, disease, etc.

trichopathy (trĭ-kop′ah-the) disease of the hair.

trichophobia (trik″o-fo′be-ah) morbid dread of hair.

trichophytic (trik″o-fit′ik) pertaining to Trichophyton.

trichophytid (trĭ-kof′ĭ-tid) a generalized eruption due to allergy to Trichophyton.

trichophytin (trĭ-kof′ĭ-tin) a filtrate from cultures of Trichophyton; used in testing for Trichophyton infection.

trichophytobezoar (trik″o-fi″to-be′zōr) a bezoar composed of animal hair and vegetable fiber.

Trichophyton (trĭ-kof′ĭ-ton) a genus of fungi that may cause various infections of the skin and its appendages.

trichophytosis (trik″o-fi-to′sis) infection with fungi of the genus Trichophyton.
 t. bar′bae, tinea barbae.
 t. cap′itis, tinea capitis.
 t. cor′poris, tinea corporis.
 t. cru′ris, tinea cruris.
 t. un′guium, fungal infection of the nails due to species of Trichophyton.

trichoptilosis (trik″o-tĭ-lo′sis) splitting of hairs at the end.

trichorrhexis (trik″o-rek′sis) breaking of the hair.
 t. nodo′sa, a condition marked by fracture and splitting of the cortex of a hair into strands, giving the appearance of white nodes at which the hair is easily broken.

trichorrhexomania (trik″o-rek″so-ma′ne-ah) the morbid habit of breaking off one's hair by pinching it with the fingernails.

trichoschisis (trĭ-kos′kĭ-sis) trichoptilosis.

trichoscopy (trĭ-kos′ko-pe) examination of the hair.

trichosiderin (trik″o-sid′er-in) an iron-containing brown pigment found in normal human red hair.

trichosis (trĭ-ko′sis) any disease of the hair.

Trichosporon (trĭ-kos′po-ron) a genus of fungi that may infect the hair.

trichosporosis (trik″o-spo-ro′sis) infection with Trichosporon.

trichostasis spinulosa (trĭ-kos′tah-sis spin″u-lo′-sah) formation of horny plugs containing bundles of hairs in the hair follicles; the skin of the face, arms or trunk may be affected.

trichostrongyliasis, trichostrongylosis (trik″-o-stron″jĭ-li′ah-sis), (trik″o-stron″jĭ-lo′sis) infection by nematodes of the genus Trichostrongylus.

Trichostrongylus (trik″o-stron′jĭ-lus) a genus of nematode parasites infecting animals and man.

trichotillomania (trik″o-til″o-ma′ne-ah) neurotic plucking of the hair.

trichotomous (trĭ-kot′o-mus) divided into three parts.

trichroism (tri′kro-izm) the condition or quality of exhibiting three different colors when viewed from three different aspects.

trichromatopsia (tri″kro-mah-top′se-ah) normal color vision for all three primary colors, red, green and blue.

trichromic (tri-kro′mik) 1. pertaining to or exhibiting three colors. 2. able to distinguish only three of the seven colors of the spectrum.

trichuriasis (trik″u-ri′ah-sis) a morbid condition caused by the presence of Trichuris.

Trichuris (trik-u′ris) a genus of nematodes parasitic in the intestinal tract, including *T. trichiu′ra,* the whipworm, found in man, which may cause vomiting and diarrhea but often produces no symptoms.

tricipital (tri-sip′ĭ-tal) 1. three-headed. 2. pertaining to the triceps.

triclobisonium (tri″klo-bi-so′ne-um) a compound used as a topical and vaginal antiseptic.

Tricofuron (tri″ko-fu′ron) trademark for preparations of furazolidone and nifuroxime, used as an antibacterial and antiprotozoan agent.

Tricoloid (tri′ko-loid) trademark for preparations of tricyclamol, an anticholinergic.

tricornute (tri-kor′nūt) having three cornua or processes.

tricrotism (tri′krŏ-tizm) the quality of having three sphygmographic waves or elevations to one beat of the pulse. adj., **tricrot′ic.**

tricuspid (tri-kus′pid) 1. having three points or cusps. 2. pertaining to the tricuspid valve.
 t. valve, the valve that guards the opening between the right atrium and right ventricle.

tricyclamol (tri-si′klah-mol) a compound used as an anticholinergic.

tridactylism (tri-dak′tĭ-lizm) the presence of only three digits on the hand or foot.

tridentate (tri-den′tāt) having three prongs.

tridermic (tri-der′mik) derived from the ectoderm, entoderm and mesoderm.

tridihexethyl (tri″di-heks-eth′il) a compound used in parasympathetic blockade.

Tridione (tri-di′ōn) trademark for preparations of trimethadione, an anticonvulsant.

triethanolamine (tri″eth-ah-nol′ah-mēn) a compound used as an emulsifier in preparing medicated lotions and ointments.

triethylamine (tri-eth″il-am′in) a ptomaine from putrefying fish.

triethylenemelamine (tri-eth″ĭ-lēn-mel′ah-mēn) a highly poisonous, white, crystalline powder used as an antineoplastic agent.

triethylenethiophosphoramide (tri-eth″ĭ-lēn-thi″o-fos-for′ah-mīd) thio-tepa, an antineoplastic agent.

trifid (tri′fid) split into three parts.

trifluoperazine (tri″floo-o-per′ah-zēn) a phenothiazine compound used as a tranquilizer.

triflupromazine (tri″floo-pro′mah-zēn) a phenothiazine compound used as a tranquilizer.

trifurcation (tri″fur-ka′shun) division or the site of separation into three branches.

trigeminal (tri-jem′ĭ-nal) 1. triple. 2. pertaining to the fifth cranial (trigeminal) nerve.

   t. nerve, the fifth cranial nerve; it arises in the pons, is composed of sensory and motor fibers and has three divisions: ophthalmic, maxillary and mandibular. The ophthalmic division supplies sensory fibers to the skin of the upper eyelid, side of the nose, forehead and anterior half of the scalp. The maxillary division carries sensory impulses from the mucous membranes of the nose, the skin of the cheek and side of the forehead, and the upper lip and upper teeth. The mandibular division carries sensory impulses from the side of the head, chin, mucous membrane of the mouth, lower teeth and anterior two-thirds of the tongue. (One can readily see why this nerve is sometimes called the great sensory nerve of the head.) The motor fibers are part of the mandibular branch and supply several of the muscles of chewing.

   t. neuralgia, pain arising from irritation of the fifth cranial (trigeminal) nerve. The disorder is characterized by brief attacks of severe pain in the face and forehead of the affected side. The cause is unknown. Many patients describe sensitive areas about the nose and mouth which, when touched, excite an attack. Attacks also may be brought on by exposure to cold, eating and drinking and washing the face. Treatment may be palliative or surgical. Called also TIC DOULOUREUX.

trigeminy (tri-jem′ĭ-ne) the condition of occurring in threes, especially the occurrence of three pulse beats in rapid succession.

triglyceride (tri-glis′er-īd) a compound consisting of three molecules of fatty acid esterified to glycerin; a neutral fat that is the usual storage form of lipids in animals.

trigonal (tri′go-nal) 1. triangular. 2. pertaining to a trigone.

trigone (tri′gōn) a triangle.

   t. of bladder, vesical trigone.

   Müller's t., a part of the tuber cinereum that folds over the optic chiasm.

   vesical t., a triangular region of the wall of the urinary bladder, the three angles corresponding with the orifices of the ureters and urethra; it is an area in which the muscle fibers are closely adherent to the mucosa.

trigonectomy (tri″go-nek′to-me) excision of the vesical trigone.

trigonitis (tri″go-ni′tis) inflammation of the trigone of the bladder.

trigonocephaly (tri″go-no-sef′ah-le) triangular shape of the head due to sharp forward angulation at the midline of the frontal bone.

trigonum (tri-go′num), pl. *trigo′na* [L.] trigone, or triangle; used in anatomic nomenclature to designate various regions or structures.

trihexinol (tri-hek′sĭ-nol) a compound used in parasympathetic blockade and in treatment of diarrhea.

trihexyphenidyl (tri-hek″se-fen′ĭ-dil) a compound used as an anticholinergic and in treatment of Parkinson's disease.

trihybrid (tri-hi′brid) a hybrid offspring of parents differing in three mendelian characters.

triiodothyronine (tri″i-o″do-thi′ro-nēn) one of the thyroid hormones; a compound produced by conjugation of monoiodotyrosine and diiodotyrosine. It has several times the biologic activity of thyroxine.

trilabe (tri′lāb) a three-pronged lithotrite.

Trilafon (tri′lah-fon) trademark for preparations of perphenazine, a tranquilizer and antiemetic.

Trilene (tri′lēn) trademark for a preparation of trichloroethylene, an inhalation analgesic and anesthetic.

trilobate (tri-lo′bāt) having three lobes.

trilocular (tri-lok′u-lar) having three loculi or cells.

trilogy (tril′o-je) a group or series of three.

trimanual (tri-man′u-al) accomplished by the use of three hands.

trimensual (tri-men′su-al) occurring every 3 months.

trimeprazine (tri-mep′rah-zēn) a compound used as a systemic antipruritic.

trimester (tri-mes′ter) a period of 3 months.

trimethadione (tri″meth-ah-di′ōn) a white, crystalline compound used as an anticonvulsant.

trimethaphan (tri-meth′ah-fan) a compound used in ganglionic blockade and as an antihypertensive.

trimethidinium (tri-meth″ĭ-din′e-um) a compound used in ganglionic blockade and as an antihypertensive.

trimethobenzamide (tri-meth″o-ben′zah-mīd) a compound used as an antiemetic.

trimethylene (tri-meth′ĭ-lēn) cyclopropane, a general anesthetic.

Trimeton (tri′mĕ-ton) trademark for preparations of pheniramine maleate, an antihistamine.

trimorphous (tri-mor′fus) crystallizing in three different forms.

trinitrate (tri-ni′trāt) a nitrate that contains three radicals of nitric acid.

trinitrin, trinitroglycerol (tri-ni′trin), (tri-ni″tro-glis′er-ol) nitroglycerin.

trinitrophenol (tri-ni″tro-fe′nol) a pale yellow crystalline substance used as an antiseptic, astringent and stimulant of epithelial growth; called also picric acid.

trinitrotoluene (tri-ni″tro-tol′u-ēn) TNT, a highly explosive substance derived from toluene, sometimes a cause of poisoning in those working with it.

triocephalus (tri″o-sef′ah-lus) a fetal monster with no organs of sight, hearing or smell, the head being a nearly shapeless mass.

triolism (tri′o-lizm) sexual interests or practices involving three persons.

triorchidism (tri-or′kĭ-dizm) the presence of three testes.

triose (tri′ōs) a sugar containing three molecules of carbon.

trioxide (tri-ok′sīd) a binary compound containing three oxygen atoms in the molecule.

tripara (trip′ah-rah) tertipara; a woman who has had three pregnancies that resulted in viable offspring; para III.

triparanol (tri-par′ah-nol) a compound used to depress the synthesis of cholesterol.

tripelennamine (tri″pĕ-len′ah-min) a compound used as an antihistamine.

tripeptide (tri-pep′tīd) a peptide formed from three amino acids.

triphalangism (tri-fal′an-jizm) three phalanges in a digit normally having only two.

triphasic (tri-fa′zik) having three phases.

triphosphopyridine nucleotide (tri-fos″fo-pir″ĭ-dēn nu′kle-o-tīd″) a coenzyme that is required in certain enzymatic reactions; called also coenzyme II.

triplegia (tri-ple′je-ah) paralysis of three extremities.

triplet (trip′let) 1. one of three offspring produced at one birth. 2. a combination of three objects or entities acting together, as the three lenses of a microscope.

triplex (tri′pleks) triple or threefold.

triploidy (trip′loi-de) the state of having three sets of chromosomes (3n).

triplokoria (trip″lo-ko′re-ah) the presence of three pupils in an eye.

triplopia (trĭ-plo′pe-ah) defective vision, objects being seen as threefold; usually a hysterical symptom.

tripoding (tri′pod-ing) the use of three points of support, as adopted by paralyzed patients when changing from a sitting or standing position.

tripoli (trip′o-le) a mild abrasive and polishing agent used on the teeth.

triprolidine (tri-pro′lĭ-dēn) a compound used as an antihistamine.

-tripsy (trip′se) word element [Gr.], *crushing;* used to designate a surgical procedure in which a structure is intentionally crushed.

tripus (tri′pus) a fetal monster with three feet.

trisaccharide (tri-sak′ah-rīd) a sugar each molecule of which yields three molecules of monosaccharides on hydrolysis.

triskaidekaphobia (tris″kĭ-dek″ah-fo′be-ah) abnormal dread of the number thirteen.

trismoid (triz′moid) 1. resembling trismus. 2. a condition resembling tetanus neonatorum.

trismus (triz′mus) tonic spasm of the jaw muscles, an early symptom of tetanus.

trisomy (tri′som-e) existence in a cell of three instead of the normal diploid pair of a particular CHROMOSOME. adj., **triso′mic.** Trisomy of chromosome 21, or trisomy 21, results in DOWN'S SYNDROME (mongolism).

trisplanchnic (tri-splangk′nik) pertaining to the three great visceral cavities, the skull, thorax and abdomen.

tristichia (tri-stik′e-ah) the presence of three rows of eyelashes.

tristimania (tris″tĭ-ma′ne-ah) melancholia.

trisulcate (tri-sul′kāt) having three furrows.

trisulfate (tri-sul′fāt) a binary compound containing three sulfate groups in the molecule.

trisulfide (tri-sul′fīd) a binary compound containing three sulfur atoms in the molecule.

tritanopia (tri″tah-no′pe-ah) defective color vision, characterized by perception of only red and green and lacking blue and yellow.

tritiate (trit′e-āt) to treat with tritium.

tritium (trit′e-um, trish′e-um) the mass three isotope of hydrogen, symbol ^3H; used as an indicator or tracer in metabolic studies.

triturable (trit′u-rah-bl) susceptible of being triturated.

triturate (trit′u-rāt) 1. to reduce to powder by rubbing. 2. a substance powdered fine by rubbing.

trituration (trit″u-ra′shun) 1. reduction to powder by friction or grinding. 2. a finely powdered substance.

triturator (trit″u-ra′tor) an apparatus in which substances can be continuously rubbed.

trivalent (tri-va′lent) having a valence of three.

trixenic (tri-zen′ik) associated with only three species of microorganisms, whose names are known.

tRNA transfer RNA (ribonucleic acid).

trocar (tro′kar) a sharp-pointed instrument used with a cannula for piercing a cavity wall.
  Duchenne's t., a trocar for obtaining specimens of deep-seated tissues.

trochanter (tro-kan′ter) a broad, flat process on

the femur, at the upper end of its lateral surface (greater trochanter), or a short conical process on the posterior border of the base of its neck (lesser trochanter). adj., **trochanter'ic.**

troche (tro'ke) a medicinal preparation for solution in the mouth, consisting of an active ingredient incorporated in a mass made of sugar and mucilage or fruit base.

trochlea (trok'le-ah), pl. *troch'leae* [L.] a pulley-shaped part or structure; used in anatomic nomenclature to designate various bony or fibrous structures through or over which tendons pass or with which other structures articulate.

trochlear (trok'le-ar) 1. pertaining to a trochlea. 2. pertaining to the fourth cranial (trochlear) nerve.
    t. nerve, the fourth cranial nerve; it supplies muscle sense and the impulse for movement to the superior oblique muscle of the eyeball.

trochocardia (tro″ko-kar'de-ah) displacement of the heart due to rotation on its axis.

trochocephalia (tro″ko-se-fa'le-ah) abnormal or premature union of the frontal and parietal bones, giving the head a rounded appearance.

trochoid (tro'koid) pivot-like, or pulley-shaped.

trochoides (tro-koi'dēz) a pivot joint.

trolnitrate (trol-ni'trāt) a compound used as a vasodilator, particularly in treatment of angina pectoris.

Trombicula (trom-bik'u-lah) a widely distributed genus of mites, including several frequently encountered species, among them *T. akamu'shi,* which transmits the rickettsia that causes scrub typhus, *T. alfredduge'si,* the chigger, *T. autumna'lis,* whose larvae cause skin lesions, and *T. bata'tas.*

trombiculiasis (trom-bik″u-li'ah-sis) infestation with mites of the genus Trombicula.

Tromexan (tro-mek'san) trademark for a preparation of ethyl biscoumacetate, an anticoagulant.

Tronothane (tron'o-thān) trademark for preparations of pramoxine, a topical anesthetic.

troph(o)- (trof'o) word element [Gr.], *food; nourishment.*

trophectoderm (trof-ek'to-derm) the earliest trophoblast.

trophedema (trof″ĕ-de'mah) a chronic disease with permanent edema of the feet or legs.

trophema (tro-fe'mah) the nourishing blood of the uterine mucosa.

trophesy (trof'ĕ-se) defective nutrition due to disorder of the trophic nerves.

trophic (trof'ik) pertaining to nutrition.

-trophic (trof'ik) word element [Gr.], *nourishing; stimulating.*

trophoblast (trof'o-blast) the extraembryonic

peripheral cells of the blastocyst, which become the placenta and the membranes that nourish and protect the developing organism. The inner cellular layer is the cytotrophoblast and the outer layer is the syntrophoblast.

trophoblastoma (trof″o-blas-to'mah) choriocarcinoma.

trophodermatoneurosis (trof″o-der″mah-to-nu-ro'sis) erythredema polyneuropathy.

trophology (tro-fol'o-je) the science of nutrition of the body.

trophoneurosis (trof″o-nu-ro'sis) 1. any functional nervous disease due to failure of nutrition from defective nerve influence.

trophonosis (trof″o-no'sis) any disease due to nutritional causes.

trophopathy (tro-fop'ah-the) any derangement of nutrition.

trophoplast (trof'o-plast) a granular protoplasmic body.

trophotaxis (trof″o-tak'sis) taxis in relation to food supply.

trophotherapy (trof″o-ther'ah-pe) treatment of disease by dietary measures.

trophotropism (tro-fot'ro-pizm) orientation of cells in relation to food supply.

trophozoite (trof″o-zo'īt) the active, motile feeding stage of a sporozoan parasite.

tropia (tro'pe-ah) heterotropia; deviation of the visual axis of one eye when the other eye is fixing; strabismus, or squint.

-tropic (trop'ik) word element [Gr.], *turning toward.*

tropical (trop'ĭ-kal) pertaining to the tropics, the regions of the earth lying between the tropic of Cancer above the Equator and the tropic of Capricorn below.
    t. anhidrotic asthenia, a condition due to generalized absence of sweating in conditions of high temperature.

tropine (tro'pēn) a crystalline base from atropine.

tropism (tro'pizm) a growth response in a nonmotile organism elicited by an external stimulus, and either toward (positive tropism) or away from (negative tropism) the stimulus; used as a word element combined with a stem indicating nature of the stimulus (e.g., phototropism) or material or entity for which an organism (or substance) shows a special affinity (e.g., neurotropism).

Trousseau's sign (troo-sōz') 1. spontaneous peripheral venous thrombosis, suggestive of visceral carcinoma, especially carcinoma of the pancreas. 2. a sign for tetany in which carpal spasm can be elicited by compressing the upper arm and causing ischemia to the nerves distally.

troxidone (trok'sĭ-dōn) trimethadione, an anticonvulsant.

truncate (trung'kāt) 1. to deprive of limbs or branches. 2. having the end cut squarely off.

truncus (trung'kus), pl. *trun'ci* [L.] trunk; used in anatomic nomenclature.

t. arterio'sus, an artery connected with the fetal heart, developing into the aortic and pulmonary arches.

t. brachiocephal'icus, a vessel arising from the arch of the aorta and giving origin to the right common carotid and right subclavian arteries.

t. celi'acus, celiac trunk.

t. pulmona'lis, pulmonary trunk.

trunk (trungk) the main part, as the part of the body to which the head and limbs are attached, or a larger structure (e.g., vessel or nerve) from which smaller divisions or branches arise, or which is created by their union.

celiac t., a vessel arising from the abdominal aorta and giving origin to the left gastric, common hepatic and splenic arteries.

pulmonary t., a vessel arising from the conus arteriosus of the right ventricle and bifurcating into the right and left pulmonary arteries.

truss (trus) a device for retaining a reduced hernia in its place.

trypaflavine (trip"ah-fla'vin) acriflavine hydrochloride, an antiseptic dye.

trypanocidal (tri-pan"o-si'dal) destructive to trypanosomes.

trypanolysis (tri"pan-ol'ĭ-sis) the destruction of trypanosomes.

Trypanoplasma (tri"pan-o-plaz'mah) a genus of protozoan parasites.

Trypanosoma (tri"pan-o-so'mah) a genus of parasitic protozoa found in the blood of animals and men, including hundreds of species, all of which are parasitic in the blood and lymph of vertebrates and invertebrates. *T. cru'zi* causes South American trypanosomiasis (Chagas' disease). *T. gambien'se* and *T. rhodesien'se* cause African trypanosomiasis (African sleeping sickness).

trypanosome (tri-pan'o-sōm) an individual of the genus Trypanosoma. adj., **trypanoso'mal, trypanoso'mic.**

trypanosomiasis (tri-pan"o-so-mi'ah-sis) infection with trypanosomes, parasitic protozoa found in the blood and lymph of infected animals and humans.

African t., a fatal disease of Africa caused by *Trypanosoma gambiense* or *T. rhodesiense* and involving the central nervous system. The parasites are transmitted to man from cattle or other animals by the bite of the tsetse fly. Usually the first symptom is inflammation at the site of the bite, appearing within 48 hours. Within several weeks the parasites invade the blood and lymph; eventually they attack the central nervous system. Characteristic symptoms include intermittent fever, rapid heartbeat and enlargement of the lymph nodes and spleen. In the advanced stage of the disease there are personality changes, apathy, sleepiness, disturbances of speech and gait and severe emaciation.

Suramin, pentamidine isethionate and tryparsamide are used in the treatment of African trypanosomiasis. Prevention includes injections of pentamidine isethionate or suramin to remove the parasites from the blood or lymph nodes, but the most effective measure is eradication of the tsetse fly.

South American t., a form found in Mexico and Central and South America, caused by *Trypanosoma cruzi;* called also Chagas' disease. It is transmitted from wild animals by means of the feces of a blood-sucking bug. The parasites multiply around the points of entry before entering the blood and eventually attacking the heart, brain and other tissues.

The acute form often attacks children. Early symptoms include swelling of the eyelids and the development of a hard, red, painful nodule on the skin. Enlargement of the lymph nodes, liver and spleen occurs, along with inflammation of the heart muscle, psychic changes and general debility. In adults the chronic form often resembles heart disease.

Preventive measures, such as the wearing of protective clothing and the use of insecticides, are of primary importance since there are no effective drugs for treatment.

trypanosomicide (tri-pan"o-so'mĭ-sīd) an agent destructive to trypanosomes.

trypanosomid (tri-pan"o-so'mid) a skin eruption occurring in trypanosomiasis.

tryparsamide (trip-ar'sah-mīd) a white crystalline powder used in treatment of trypanosomiasis.

trypesis (tri-pe'sis) trephination.

trypsin (trip'sin) a pancreatic enzyme that catalyzes the hydrolysis of practically all types of proteins, produced in the intestine by activation of trypsinogen. adj., **tryp'tic.**

crystallized t., a proteolytic enzyme crystallized from an extract of the pancreas of the ox; used in débridement of necrotic wounds and ulcers, abscesses and fistulas.

trypsinize (trip'sĭ-nīz) to subject to the action of trypsin.

trypsinogen (trip-sin'o-jen) the inactive precursor of trypsin, the form in which it is secreted by the pancreas.

tryptophan (trip'to-fan) a naturally occurring amino acid, one of those essential for human metabolism.

tryptophanase (trip'to-fan"ās) an enzyme that catalyzes the cleavage of tryptophan into indole, pyruvic acid and ammonia.

T.S. test solution.

tsetse (tset'se) an African fly; it is a vector of trypanosomes.

TSH thyroid-stimulating hormone (thyrotropin, thyrotropic hormone).

tsutsugamushi fever (tsoōt"soo-gah-moōsh'e) scrub typhus.

Tuamine (too'ah-min) trademark for preparations of tuaminoheptane.

tuaminoheptane (tu-am"ĭ-no-hep'tān) a compound used as a sympathomimetic agent in congestion of the nasal mucosa.

tuba (tu′bah), pl. *tu′bae* [L.] tube.

Tubadil (too′bah-dil) trademark for a preparation of tubocurarine, a skeletal muscle relaxant.

Tubarine (too′bah-rin) trademark for a preparation of tubocurarine, a skeletal muscle relaxant.

tube (tūb) a hollow cylindrical organ or instrument. adj., **tu′bal.**

   auditory t., the narrow channel connecting the middle ear and nasopharynx; called also eustachian tube.

   Coolidge t., a vacuum tube for the generation of x-rays.

   drainage t., a tube used in surgery to facilitate escape of fluids.

   endotracheal t., a tube inserted into the mouth and passed down into the trachea, for the administration of anesthetics or connection to a mechanical respirator (see also AIRWAY).

   eustachian t., the canal from the nasopharynx to the tympanum, which serves to equalize pressure on either side of the tympanic membrane (eardrum) and may be a route of infection from the pharynx to the middle ear.

   fallopian t., uterine tube.

   Levin t., a nasal gastroduodenal catheter.

   Miller-Abbott t., a double-channel intestinal tube for diagnosing and treating obstructive lesions of the small intestine (see also MILLER-ABBOTT TUBE).

   nasogastric t., a tube of soft rubber or plastic inserted through a nostril and into the stomach, for instilling liquid foods or other substances, or for withdrawing gastric contents.

   nephrostomy t., one inserted through the abdominal wall into the renal pelvis for direct drainage of the urine.

   neural t., the epithelial tube produced by folding of the neural plate in the early embryo.

   otopharyngeal t., eustachian tube.

   safety t., the upper, open portion of the eustachian tube, by which air pressures on each side of the tympanum are equalized.

   Sengstaken-Blakemore t., an instrument used for tamponade of bleeding esophageal varices (see also SENGSTAKEN-BLAKEMORE TUBE).

   stomach t., one that is passed through the esophagus to the stomach, for the introduction of nutrients or gastric lavage (see also STOMACH TUBE).

   test t., a tube of thin glass, closed at one end; used in chemical tests and other laboratory procedures.

   thoracostomy t., one inserted through an opening in the chest wall for application of suction to the pleural cavity to facilitate reexpansion of the lung in spontaneous pneumothorax.

   tracheostomy t., a curved tube that is inserted into the trachea through the opening made in the neck at TRACHEOSTOMY.

   uterine t., a slender tube extending laterally from the uterus toward the ovary on the same side, conveying ova to the cavity of the uterus and permitting passage of spermatozoa in the opposite direction; called also fallopian tube.

tube feeding administration of liquids and semiliquid foods through a nasogastric tube. This type of feeding is most often used for patients who are unconscious or paralyzed and unable to swallow. In some cases it may be necessary to tube-feed a patient who is mentally ill and refuses to take food by mouth. Newborn premature infants are fed a formula by tube until their gag and swallowing reflexes are fully developed.

   NURSING CARE. While the patient is receiving the feeding through the tube he should be sitting in an upright position if at all possible. A 45 degree angle at the hips is best, with the back well supported and the spine in good alignment. The food to be given is warmed and then diluted with water (about half and half) before it is given. If this is done and the feeding is given slowly by gravity flow, there is less possibility of vomiting and diarrhea. The specially prepared formula to be given by tube can be nutritionally adequate with careful planning (see also liquid DIET).

   Tube feedings are usually given every 4 to 6 hours. While a patient is receiving this type of feeding he must have frequent mouth care as there is diminished salivation which leads to dryness and an unpleasant taste in the mouth. Because the tube remains in the stomach for long periods of time, it is necessary to keep the nares clean and well lubricated. It is recommended that the tube be removed and placed in the alternate nostril every other day or so to prevent irritation of the nasal mucosa.

tuber (tu′ber) a swelling or protuberance.

   t. cine′reum, an area of the under surface of the forebrain to which the stalk of the pituitary gland is attached.

tubercle (tu′ber-kl) 1. a nodule, especially a solid elevation of the skin, larger than a papule. 2. a small, rounded nodule produced by the bacillus of tuberculosis (*Mycobacterium tuberculosis*). It is made up of small spherical cells that contain giant cells and are surrounded by spindle-shaped epithelioid cells. 3. a nodule or small eminence, especially one on a bone, for attachment of a tendon. adj., **tuber′cular.**

   caseous t., a tuberculous nodule that has undergone caseation.

   fibrous t., a tubercle of bacillary origin that contains connective tissue elements.

   lymphoid t., a lesion of tuberculosis consisting of lymphoid cells.

   miliary t., a minute tubercle sometimes found in great numbers in various parts and organs in true bacillary tuberculosis.

   supraglenoid t., one on the scapula for attachment of the long head of the biceps muscle.

   zygomatic t., a small eminence of the zygoma, at the junction of its anterior root.

tuberculated (tu-ber′ku-lāt″ed) covered with tubercles.

tuberculid (tu-ber′ku-lid) a skin lesion representing a hypersensitivity reaction in a person with active tuberculosis.

   papulonecrotic t., a condition characterized by crops of deep-seated papules or nodules, with central necrosis or ulceration.

tuberculigenous (tu-ber″ku-lij′ĕ-nus) causing tuberculosis.

tuberculin (tu-ber′ku-lin) a protein or protein

bacterium tuberculosis), used in intradermal tests
for sensitivity to the microorganism.

old t., a sterile solution of concentrated, soluble
products of the growth of the tubercle bacillus, adjusted to standard potency by addition of glycerin
and isotonic sodium chloride solution, final glycerin
content being about 50 per cent.

t. P.P.D., purified protein derivative of t., a sterile,
soluble, partially purified product of the growth of
the tubercle bacillus in a special liquid medium
free from protein.

tuberculitis (tu-ber″ku-li′tis) inflammation of a
tubercle.

tuberculocele (tu-ber′ku-lo-sēl″) tuberculous disease of a testis.

tuberculocide (tu-ber′ku-lo-sīd″) an agent destructive to tubercle bacilli.

tuberculofibroid (tu-ber″ku-lo-fi′broid) characterized by tubercle that has undergone fibroid
degeneration.

tuberculoid (tu-ber′ku-loid) resembling tuberculosis.

tuberculoma (tu-ber″ku-lo′mah) a tumor-like
mass resulting from enlargement of a caseous
tubercle.

tuberculomania (tu-ber″ku-lo-ma′ne-ah) a morbid belief that one is affected with tuberculosis.

tuberculophobia (tu-ber″ku-lo-fo′be-ah) a morbid
fear of tuberculosis.

tuberculosilicosis (tu-ber″ku-lo-sil″ĭ-ko′sis) silicosis with tuberculosis.

tuberculosis (tu-ber′ku-lo′sis) an infectious, inflammatory, communicable disease that commonly
attacks the lungs, although it may occur in almost
any other part of the body. The causative agent is
the tubercle bacillus (*Mycobacterium tuberculosis*).

TRANSMISSION. The tubercle bacilli can enter
the lungs in various ways. The source is usually
the sputum of an infected person. The bacilli may
by spread by droplet infection; they are also carried
in the air, and may be spread by contaminated eating utensils. The bacteria can live for months in
dried sputum, presenting hidden hazards. They can
invade the body through the digestive tract, carried by unpasteurized milk and other dairy products from tuberculous cattle. In the United States,
this means of entry is now rare.

PRIMARY TUBERCULOSIS. When the tuberculosis
bacilli first reach the lungs and begin to multiply
there, the body rushes its defenses to the infected
area and almost always is successful in inactivating
the infection. Some of the bacteria are killed and
the rest are covered with tough scar tissue. Many
normal, healthy people who have never had symptoms of tuberculosis have these scars, which are
visible in chest x-rays. Although the imprisoned
bacilli remain alive, they are powerless. This first
infection usually causes no symptoms.

A simple skin test, called the Mantoux test—in
which tuberculin, a sterile liquid containing
elements of tubercle bacilli, is injected intracutaneously—detects the presence of tubercle bacilli
in the body. If this test is positive, x-ray films are

taken to determine whether the bacilli are safely
contained or are active.

RESISTANCE TO TUBERCULOSIS. Resistance of
the body to tuberculosis depends on two main
factors. One is the condition of the body. Poor
health, fatigue, crowded, poor living conditions,
poor nutrition or another illness can lower the
body's defenses. The second factor is exposure to
tuberculosis bacilli so frequently or in such great
numbers that even a healthy person cannot escape
infection.

A combination of both these conditions is almost
certain to result in tuberculosis. Children are particularly susceptible to the disease.

SYMPTOMS. A child or young person with active
tuberculosis usually suffers from one or more of
the following symptoms: loss of energy, poor appetite, loss of weight and fever. Even though these
symptoms may have other causes than tuberculosis,
they must be regarded as warning signals. The
tuberculin test is helpful in diagnosis.

In adults, listlessness and vague pains in the
chest may go unnoticed, since they are often not
severe enough to attract attention. Unfortunately,
the symptoms that most people associate with
tuberculosis—cough, expectoration of purulent
sputum, fever, night sweats and hemorrhage from
the lungs—do not appear in the early, most easily
curable stage of the disease; often their appearance
is delayed until a year or more after the initial exposure to the bacilli. Annual chest x-rays of all adults
would permit discovery of almost all cases of tuberculosis at an early, easily curable stage.

Chronic pulmonary tuberculosis is often accompanied by pleurisy. Pleurisy with effusion often is
the first symptom of tuberculosis. In certain cases,
complications are possible and each has its characteristic symptoms. At a fairly late stage, the tuberculosis bacillus may cause ulcers or inflammation
around the larynx (tuberculous laryngitis). Less
often, tuberculous ulcers form on the tongue or
tonsils. Sometimes intestinal infections develop;
they are probably caused by swallowed bacteria-
contaminated sputum. A most serious complication is the sudden collapse of a lung, the indication
that a deep tuberculous cavity in the lung has perforated, or opened into the pleural cavity, allowing
air and infected material to flow into it.

When a fairly large and previously walled-off
lesion, or infected area, suddenly discharges its
contents into the bronchial tree, the result is the
infection of a large part of the lung, an acute and
dangerous complication which causes tuberculous
pneumonia.

Tuberculosis bacilli can spread to other parts of
the body by way of the blood, producing the condition called miliary tuberculosis. When a large number of bacilli suddenly enter the circulatory system,
they are carried to all areas of the body and may
lodge in any organ. Minute tubercles form in the
tissues of the organs affected; these lesions are
about the size of a pinhead or millet seed (hence the
name "miliary"). Unless promptly treated, and
occasionally even then, the tiny lesions spread, join
and produce larger areas of infection.

Tuberculous pneumonia can begin in this way, as
can tuberculosis of any other organ. Miliary infections involving the meninges produce a particularly
serious disease; indeed, until the development of

antibiotics and similar medicines, this condition nearly always proved fatal.

Practically all parts and organs of the body can be secondarily invaded by tubercle bacilli, a common type being involvement of the kidneys, which often spreads to the bladder and genitalia. Bone involvement, particularly of the spine (POTT'S DISEASE), was once common, especially among children.

Lupus, or lupus vulgaris, tuberculosis of the skin, is characterized by brown nodules on the corium; another form of tuberculosis of the skin is tuberculosis indurativa, a chronic disease in which indurated nodules form on the skin. When the adrenal glands are affected by tuberculosis, a rare occurrence, the condition can cause ADDISON'S DISEASE.

TREATMENT AND CURE. The majority of tuberculosis patients undergo treatment at home, although in serious cases and in the early treatment of the disease, a stay in a sanatorium may be desirable so that the patient may receive the necessary nursing care, diet, quiet and isolation and learn how to take care of his health and how to prevent himself from infecting others.

Drugs. In recent years, potent new medicines have been developed for the control of tuberculosis. Among the several preparations now in use, the three principal ones are streptomycin, isoniazid and para-aminosalicylic acid (PAS). Prescribed singly or in combination, these drugs have produced rewarding results in many cases. Although usually they are not able to kill all the tubercle bacilli, they often are able to keep them from multiplying and thus aid the body's leukocytes in fighting the disease.

Surgical Procedures. In the past, the sanatorium rest cure frequently was augmented by one of the surgical procedures which aid healing by resting an infected lung for a period of time.

The best-known of these operations, artificial pneumothorax, involves collapsing the lung by injecting air into the pleural cavity. A lung also may be rested by inactivating the phrenic nerve, which carries impulses to the diaphragm from the brain and so helps to control breathing; if the left or right phrenic nerve is inactivated, the diaphragm and lung on the same side will not move.

With the successful treatment of tuberculosis by the new drugs, these operations have become relatively uncommon. In certain cases, however, when the disease is restricted to a lung and medication provides insufficient control, surgical removal of the diseased tissue is necessary.

Depending on the extent of the disease, the surgeon may perform segmental resection (removal of one or more bronchopulmonary segments, of which there are about 20), lobectomy (removal of a lobe, of which there are three in the right lung and two in the left) or pneumonectomy (removal of an entire lung). (See also surgery of the LUNG.)

PREVENTION. Tuberculosis is one of the most easily avoided of all the serious diseases. The best precautions are (1) maintenance of good health, (2) avoidance of unnecessary exposure to tuberculosis organisms and (3) detection of the disease in its earliest stages.

BCG Vaccine. Some success in preventing tuberculosis has been attained by vaccination with BCG (bacille Calmette Guérin)—a vaccine evolved from strains of *Mycobacterium tuberculosis*

taken from cattle. It provides at least partial immunity in most people, although it takes about 2 months to do so. BCG is now usually given to large groups under governmental auspices—for example, to school children living in slum areas in large cities. It has been widely used in many countries, but less widely in the United States. After vaccination with BCG, the patient will have a positive response to the tuberculin test.

Isoniazid. This drug, one of the principal ones used in treating active cases, is given for a year to those who convert from tuberculin negative to tuberculin positive, even though they may be asymptomatic.

bovine t., an infection of cattle caused by *Mycobacterium tuberculosis* var. *bovis,* transmissible to man.

endogenous t., that arising from within the body and transmitted by blood to another organ.

exogenous t., that arising from a source outside the body.

open t., tuberculosis in an active state, capable of transmission.

tuberculostatic (tu-ber″ku-lo-stat′ik) inhibiting the growth of *Mycobacterium tuberculosis.*

tuberculous (tu-ber′ku-lus) pertaining to or affected with tuberculosis.

tuberculum (tu-ber′ku-lum), pl. *tuber′cula* [L.] a nodule or small eminence; used in anatomic nomenclature to designate principally a small eminence on a bone.

tuberosis (tu″ber-o′sis) a condition characterized by the presence of nodules.

tuberositas (tu″bĕ-ros′ĭ-tas), pl. *tuberosita′tes* [L.] tuberosity; used in anatomic nomenclature to designate elevations on bones to which muscles are attached.

tuberosity (tu″bĕ-ros′ĭ-te) an elevation or protuberance; tuberositas.

tuberous (tu′ber-us) covered with tubers; knobby.
  t. sclerosis, a familial disease with tumors on the surfaces of the lateral ventricles of the brain and sclerotic patches on its surface, and marked by mental deterioration and epileptic attacks.

tubo- (tu′bo) word element [L.], *tube.*

tubocurarine (tu″bo-ku-rah′rēn) an alkaloid from the bark and stems of *Chondrodendron tomentosum,* used as a skeletal muscle relaxant.

tuboligamentous (tu″bo-lig″ah-men′tus) pertaining to a uterine tube and a broad ligament.

tubo-ovarian (tu″bo-o-va′re-an) pertaining to a uterine tube and ovary.

tuboperitoneal (tu″bo-per″ĭ-to-ne′al) pertaining to a uterine tube and the peritoneum.

tuborrhea (tu″bo-re′ah) discharge from the eustachian tube.

tubouterine (tu″bo-u′ter-in) pertaining to a uterine tube and the uterus.

tubule (tu′būl) a small tube. adj., **tu′bular.**
  collecting t's, the terminal channels of the nephrons which open on the summits of the renal pyramids in the renal papillae.

convoluted t's, channels that follow a tortuous course; there are convoluted renal tubules and convoluted seminiferous tubules.

dentinal t's, the tubular structures of the teeth.

galactophorous t's, lactiferous t's, small channels for the passage of milk from the secreting cells in the mammary gland.

mesonephric t's, the tubules comprising the mesonephros, or temporary kidney of amniotes.

metanephric t's, the tubules comprising the permanent kidney of amniotes.

renal t's, the minute canals made up of basement membrane and lined with epithelium, composing the substance of the kidney and secreting, collecting and conducting the urine.

segmental t's, the tubules of the mesonephros.

seminiferous t's, the tubules of the testis, in which spermatozoa develop and through which they leave the gland.

uriniferous t's, renal tubules; channels for the passage of urine.

tubulorrhexis (tu″bu-lo-rek′sis) rupture of the tubules of the kidney.

tubulus (tu′bu-lus), pl. *tu′buli* [L.] tubule; a minute canal found in various structures or organs of the body.

tuft (tuft) a small clump, cluster or coil, especially a tassel-like cluster of capillaries.

malpighian t., renal glomerulus.

tularemia (tu″lah-re′me-ah) a disease of rabbits and other rodents, resembling plague, caused by *Pasteurella tularensis* and transmissible to man; called also rabbit fever.

The illness can be contracted by handling diseased animals or their hides, eating infected wild game or being bitten by insects, such as horseflies and deer flies, that have fed on infected animals.

SYMPTOMS AND TREATMENT. Tularemia begins with a sudden onset of chills and fever, accompanied by headache, nausea, vomiting and severe weakness. A day or so later, a small sore usually develops at the site of the infection, and it becomes ulcerated. There may also be enlargement and ulceration of the lymph nodes and a generalized red rash. In untreated cases, the fever may last for weeks or months.

Treatment is with antibiotics, such as tetracycline, streptomycin and chloramphenicol.

PREVENTION. Tularemia is usually thought of as an occupational disease. Those who may be exposed to it, such as game wardens and hunters, should take certain precautions, such as wearing gloves when handling wild animals, particularly rabbits and squirrels, and wearing adequate clothing in the woods to prevent bites by insect vectors of the disease. Wild game must be especially well cooked, in order to kill the tularemia organism.

tumefacient (tu″mĕ-fa′shent) producing tumefaction.

tumefaction (tu″mĕ-fak′shun) a swelling; puffiness.

tumescence (tu-mes′ens) congestion and swelling, especially of sexual organs.

tumid (tu′mid) swollen, edematous.

tumor (tu′mor) 1. swelling, one of the cardinal signs of inflammation. 2. a swelling or enlargement due to pathologic overgrowth of tissue. adj., **tu′-morous.** Tumors are called also neoplasms, which means that they are composed of new and actively growing tissue. Their growth is faster than that of normal tissue, continuing after cessation of the stimuli that evoked the growth, and serving no useful physiologic purpose.

Tumors are classified in a number of ways, one of the simplest being according to their origin and whether they are malignant or benign. Tumors of mesenchymal origin include fibroelastic tumors and those of bone, fat, blood vessels and lymphoid tissue. They may be benign or malignant (sarcoma). Tumors of epithelial origin may be benign or malignant (carcinoma); they are found in glandular tissue or such organs as the breast, stomach, uterus or skin. Mixed tumors contain different types of cells derived from the same primary germ layer, and teratomas contain cells derived from more than one germ layer; both kinds may be benign or malignant.

BENIGN TUMORS. Benign tumors do not endanger life unless they interfere with normal functions of other organs or affect a vital organ. They grow slowly, pushing aside normal tissue but not invading it. They are usually encapsulated, well demarcated growths. They are not metastatic; that is, they do not form secondary tumors in other organs. Benign tumors usually respond favorably to surgical treatment and some forms of RADIO-THERAPY.

MALIGNANT TUMORS. These tumors are composed of embryonic, primitive or poorly differentiated cells. They grow in a disorganized manner and so rapidly that nutrition of the cells becomes a problem. For this reason necrosis and ulceration are characteristic of malignant tumors. They also invade surrounding tissues and are metastatic, initiating the growth of similar tumors in distant organs. (See also CANCER.)

carotid body t., a firm, round mass at the bifurcation of the common carotid artery.

compound t., a teratoma.

cystic t., one containing cavities.

desmoid t., a neoplastic proliferation of fibrous tissue, midway between a benign fibroma and a malignant fibrosarcoma.

erectile t., one composed of erectile tissue.

Ewing's, t., a malignant tumor of bone, arising in medullary tissue and more often in cylindrical bones.

false t., structural enlargement due to extravasation, exudation, echinococcus or retained sebaceous matter.

fibroid t., a common benign tumor of the uterus, properly designated as myoma of the UTERUS.

granulosa t., granulosa cell t., an ovarian tumor originating in the cells of the cumulus oophorus.

heterologous t., one made up of tissue differing from that in which it grows.

homologous t., one made up of tissue resembling that in which it grows.

infiltrating t., one that extends into surrounding tissue.

islet cell t., a tumor of the islands of Langerhans.

Krukenberg's t., a type of carcinoma of the ovary, usually metastatic from cancer of the gastrointestinal tract, especially of the stomach.

organoid t., one composed of complex tissues, resembling an organ.

phantom t., abdominal or other swelling not due to structural change but, usually, to gaseous distention of the intestine.

sand t., psammoma.

sebaceous t., tumor of a sebaceous gland.

theca cell t., a fibroid-like tumor of the ovary containing yellow areas of fatty material.

true t., any tumor produced by proliferation of cells.

turban t's, pink or maroon, grapelike, pedunculated tumors, occurring usually on the scalp, but sometimes on the trunk and extremities.

Wilms' t., a rapidly developing sarcoma of the kidneys, made up of embryonal elements, and occurring chiefly in children before the fifth year; called also embryonal carcinosarcoma.

tumoricidal (tu″mor-ĭ-si′dal) destructive to cancer cells.

tumorigenesis (tu″mor-ĭ-jen′ĕ-sis) the production of tumors.

tumultus (tu-mul′tus) excessive organic action.

Tunga (tung′gah) a genus of fleas native to tropical and subtropical parts of South America.

T. pen′etrans, the chigoe flea, which attacks man, dogs, pigs and other animals, as well as poultry, and causes intense skin irritation.

tungsten (tung′sten) a chemical element, atomic number 74, atomic weight 183.85, symbol W. (See table of ELEMENTS.)

tunic (tu′nik) a covering or coat.

Bichat's t., the intima, or innermost coat, of blood vessels.

tunica (tu′nĭ-kah), pl. *tu′nicae* [L.] a covering or coat; used in anatomic nomenclature to designate a membranous covering of an organ or a distinct layer of the wall of a hollow structure, as a blood vessel.

t. adna′ta oc′uli, the portion of the conjunctiva in contact with the eyeball.

t. adventi′tia, the outermost coat of blood vessels.

t. albugin′ea, 1. the sclera. 2. the fibrous coat of the testis or ovary.

t. ex′tima, tunica adventitia.

t. in′tima, the innermost coat of blood vessels.

t. me′dia, the middle coat of blood vessels.

t. muco′sa, the mucous membrane lining of various tubular structures.

t. pro′pria, the proper coat or layer of a part.

t. sero′sa, the membrane lining the external walls of the body cavities.

t. vagina′lis testis, the serous membrane covering the front and sides of the testis and epididymis.

t. vasculo′sa, a vascular coat, or a layer well supplied with blood vessels.

tunicin (tu′nĭ-sin) a substance resembling cellulose, from the tissues of certain low forms of animal life.

tuning fork (tōōn′ing) a two-pronged forklike instrument of steel, the prongs of which give off a musical note when struck.

tunnel (tun′el) a circumscribed opening through a solid body, or a linear enclosed channel beneath a surface.

carpal t., the osseofibrous passage for the median nerve and the flexor tendons (see also CARPAL TUNNEL SYNDROME).

t. disease, bends.

flexor t., carpal tunnel.

turbid (tur′bid) cloudy.

turbidimeter (tur″bĭ-dim′ĕ-ter) an apparatus for measuring turbidity of a solution.

turbidimetry (tur″bĭ-dim′ĕ-tre) the measurement of the turbidity of a liquid.

turbidity (tur-bid′ĭ-te) cloudiness.

turbinal, turbinate (tur′bĭ-nal), (tur′bĭ-nāt) 1. shaped like a top. 2. nasal concha.

turbinectomy (tur″bĭ-nek′to-me) excision of a nasal concha (turbinate).

turbinotomy (tur″bĭ-not′o-me) incision of a nasal concha.

turgescence (tur-jes′ens) distention or swelling of a part.

turgescent (tur-jes′ent) becoming swollen.

turgid (tur′jid) swollen and congested.

turgor (tur′gor) the condition of being turgid; normal or other fullness.

Turner's syndrome (tur′nerz) a syndrome characterized by retarded growth and sexual development, webbing of the neck, low posterior hair line margin and other deformities; it is associated with absence or structural abnormality of the second sex chromosome. Called also gonadal dysgenesis.

turpentine (tur′pen-tīn) the concrete oleoresin from *Pinus palustris* and other species of pine trees; a local irritant, sometimes used in ointments.

turricephaly (tur″ĭ-sef′ah-le) acrocephaly.

tussis (tus′is) [L.] cough.

tussive (tus′iv) pertaining to or due to a cough.

tutamen (tu-ta′men), pl. *tutam′ina* [L.] a protective covering or structure.

tutam′ina cer′ebri, the hair, scalp, skull and meninges.

tutam′ina oc′uli, the protecting appendages of the eye, as the eyelids, eyelashes, etc.

Tween (twēn) trademark for a sorbitan polyoxyalkalene derivative; used as an emulsifier and detergent.

Tween 80, trademark for polysorbate 80, a surfactant.

twin (twin) one of two offspring produced in the same pregnancy. Twins occur approximately once in every 86 births.

Dizygotic, or fraternal, twins develop from two separate ova fertilized at the same time. They may be of the same sex or of opposite sexes, and are no more similar than any other two children of the same parents. Called also binovular, dichorial, dissimilar and unlike twins.

Monozygotic, or identical, twins develop from a single ovum that divides after fertilization. Because they share the same set of chromosomes, they are always of the same sex, and are remarkably similar in hair color, finger and palm prints, teeth and other respects. Monozygotic twins have exactly the same blood type and can accept tissue or organ transplants from each other. Called also enzygotic, monochorial, mono-ovular, similar or true twins.

Approximately one-third of all twins are identical; the rest are fraternal. It is not clearly understood exactly what causes a single ovum to divide shortly after conception and thereby produce identical twins, although it seems to be a chance occurrence. The reasons for the production and fertilization of two separate ova that result in fraternal twins are not well understood either, but it is thought that a tendency toward fraternal twins runs in families and is transmitted through the genes of the mother. Women are more likely to have fraternal twins in their later childbearing years, between the ages of 30 and 38 years, than earlier. Older age in the father also seems to be a factor with fraternal twins.

conjoined t's, Siamese t's, monozygotic twins whose bodies are joined (see also SIAMESE TWINS).

twinning (twin'ing) 1. the production of symmetrical structures or parts by division. 2. the simultaneous intrauterine production of two or more embryos.

twitch (twich) a brief, contractile response of a skeletal muscle elicited by a single maximal volley of impulses in the neurons supplying it.

twitching (twich'ing) the occurrence of a single contraction or a series of contractions of a muscle.

tychastics (ti-kas'tiks) the study of industrial accidents.

Tylenol (ti'lĕ-nol) trademark for preparations of acetaminophen, an analgesic and antipyretic.

tyloma (ti-lo'ma) a callus or callosity.

tylosis (ti-lo'sis) formation of callosities.

tympanectomy (tim"pah-nek'to-me) excision of the tympanic membrane.

tympanic (tim-pan'ik) 1. pertaining to the tympanum. 2. pertaining to or characterized by tympany.

t. membrane, a thin, semitransparent membrane, nearly oval in shape, that stretches across the ear canal separating the tympanum (middle ear) from the external acoustic meatus (outer ear); called also the eardrum. It is composed of fibrous tissue, covered with skin on the outside and mucous membrane on the inside. It is constructed so that it can vibrate freely with audible sound waves that travel inward from outside. The handle of the malleus (hammer) of the middle ear is attached to the center of the tympanic membrane and receives the vibrations collected by the membrane, transmitting them to other bones of the middle ear (the incus and stapes) and eventually to the fluid of the inner ear.

Perforation of the tympanic membrane can cause some loss of hearing, the degree of loss depending on the size and location of the perforation. Since vibrations can still be transmitted to the inner ear by way of the bones of the skull, even nearly total destruction of the tympanic membrane does not produce total deafness. Surgical incision of the eardrum (myringotomy) may be done to relieve pressure and provide for drainage in an infection of the middle ear (see also OTITIS MEDIA).

tympanism, tympanites (tim'pah-nizm), (tim"-pah-ni'tēz) drumlike distention of the abdomen due to air or gas in the intestine or peritoneal cavity. adj. **tympanit'ic.**

tympanitis (tim"pah-ni'tis) otitis media.

tympanoacryloplasty (tim"pah-no-ah-kril'o-plas"te) surgical obliteration of the mastoid antrum by instillation of an acrylic compound.

tympanomastoiditis (tim"pah-no-mas"toi-di'tis) inflammation of the tympanum and mastoid cells.

tympanoplasty (tim'pah-no-plas"te) plastic reconstruction of the bones of the middle ear, with establishment of ossicular continuity from the tympanic membrane to the oval window. This surgical procedure is performed when chronic infection or tumor has led to destruction of the ossicles, of the pars petrosa of the temporal bone, or both. Because the ossicles are so small, the surgery must be done under magnification with an operating microscope. Tympanoplasty requires great surgical skill and the use of specially designed instruments. It is often done in preference to radical MASTOID-ECTOMY and offers the advantage of greater preservation of hearing. (For nursing care after tympanoplasty, see surgery of the EAR.)

tympanosclerosis (tim"pah-no-sklĕ-ro'sis) a condition characterized by the presence of masses of hard, dense connective tissue around the auditory ossicles in the middle ear.

tympanotomy (tim"pah-not'o-me) myringotomy.

tympanous (tim'pah-nus) distended with gas.

tympanum (tim'pah-num) the part of the cavity of the middle ear, in the temporal bone, just medial to the tympanic membrane.

tympany (tim'pah-ne) a musical note elicited by percussion, of somewhat higher pitch than resonance; the characteristic percussion note of a gas-filled cavity or organ.

type (tīp) 1. the general or prevailing character, as of an individual or a particular case of disease. 2. a block bearing raised letter, or the impression of such a letter registered on a flat surface.

asthenic t., a type of physical constitution, with long limbs, small trunk, flat chest and weak muscles.

athletic t., a type of physical constitution, with broad shoulders, deep chest, flat abdomen, thick neck and good muscular development.

blood t's, categories into which blood can be classified on the basis of agglutinogens in erythrocytes (see also BLOOD TYPE).

pyknic t., a type of physical constitution marked by rounded body, large chest, thick shoulders, broad head and short neck.

sympatheticotonic t., a type of physical constitution characterized by sympathicotonia.

vagotonic t., a physical type characteristic of deficient adrenal activity; there are slow pulse, low blood pressure, localized sweating and high sugar tolerance.

typembryo (ti-pem'bre-o) an embryo in that stage of development at which the characteristics of the type to which it belongs may be seen.

typhl(o)- (tif'lo) word element [Gr.], (1) *cecum;* (2) *blindness.*

typhlectasis (tif-lek'tah-sis) distention of the cecum.

typhlitis (tif-li'tis) inflammation of the cecum.

typhlocolitis (tif"lo-ko-li'tis) colitis in the region of the cecum.

typhlodicliditis (tif"lo-dik"li-di'tis) inflammation of the ileocecal valve.

typhlolexia (tif"lo-lek'se-ah) visual aphasia; loss of ability to comprehend written language.

typhlolithiasis (tif"lo-li-thi'ah-sis) the presence of calculi in the cecum.

typhloptosis (tif"lo-to'sis) downward displacement of the cecum.

typhlosis (tif-lo'sis) blindness.

typhlotomy (tif-lot'o-me) incision of the cecum.

typhoid (ti'foid) 1. resembling typhus. 2. typhoid fever.

    t. fever, a bacterial infection transmitted by contaminated water, milk or other foods, especially shellfish. The causative organism is *Salmonella typhi,* harbored in human excreta.

    Entering the body through the intestinal tract, the typhoid bacillus starts multiplying in the bloodstream, causing fever and diarrhea. The usual incubation period is 7 to 14 days. Later the bacilli localize in the intestinal tract or the gallbladder.

    SYMPTOMS. The first symptoms of typhoid are headache, perhaps sore throat and a fever that may reach 105° F. The temperature rises daily, reaching a peak in 7 to 10 days, maintaining this level for about another week and then subsiding by the end of the fourth week. Periods of chills and sweating may occur, with loss of appetite. A watery, grayish or greenish diarrhea is common, but constipation sometimes occurs instead. After 2 weeks, red spots begin to appear on the chest and abdomen. If the case is severe, the patient may lapse into states of delirious muttering and staring into space. About the third to fourth week an improvement is noticeable, and steady recovery follows. The disease is serious and sometimes fatal.

    TRANSMISSION. A person who has had typhoid fever gains immunity from it but may become a carrier. Although perfectly well, he harbors the bacteria and passes them out in his feces and urine. The typhoid bacillus often lodges in the gallbladder of carriers, and when the gallbladder is removed the person may cease to be a carrier. In cities, food handled by carriers is the principal source of infection. In rural areas carriers may infect food—fruit and fresh vegetables, for example—that they raise. When sewage and sanitation systems are poor, the organisms may enter the water supply. They can also be spread to food and water by flies that have been in contact with body eliminations. Contamination is more likely if human feces are used to fertilize the crops, as they are in some areas.

    PREVENTION AND TREATMENT. Once a widespread disease, typhoid fever has now been virtually eliminated in countries with advanced sanitation. Proper sanitation involves (1) good sewage systems to dispose of human wastes and (2) proper measures for keeping foods uncontaminated. Food should be carefully protected from flies. One should wash his hands carefully before eating and after going to the toilet.

    Effective medicines, such as the antibiotic chloramphenicol, are available for the treatment of the disease.

    A less serious disease whose symptoms resemble those of typhoid fever is paratyphoid, also transmitted by contaminated food or liquids.

    NURSING CARE. Patients with typhoid fever and paratyphoid are placed in isolation until the urine and feces are free of bacilli. (See ISOLATION TECHNIQUE.) If sewage treatment for the community is adequate, the stools and urine need not be disinfected, but if there is danger of incomplete destruction of the bacilli by sewage treatment methods, the urine and feces should be disinfected by chlorinated lime or a 4 per cent Lysol solution before disposal. Other precautionary measures to prevent the spread of the disease include adequate screening of windows and doors so that flies may not come in contact with excreta.

    Many patients with typhoid fever require nursing measures to lower the body temperature when fever is extreme. These include cool sponge baths, application of ice bags and administration of antipyretic drugs as ordered. Fluids should be forced, to prevent dehydration. The diet should consist of soft, bland, easily digested and nourishing foods.

    Observations of the patient include watching for sudden temperature changes, signs of intestinal bleeding and symptoms of intestinal perforation.

    Kaolin or a similar antidiarrheal may be needed to help control diarrhea. If constipation becomes a problem, a low saline enema should be given in preference to a cathartic because of the danger of intestinal perforation.

    Good oral hygiene and care of the lips and mouth are essential, as for any patient with a prolonged febrile condition. In addition, the patient must be kept clean and dry and turned frequently to avoid the development of DECUBITUS ULCERS. During the convalescent period the patient will need adequate rest and a well rounded diet to help him recover from this debilitating illness.

typhoidal (ti-foi'dal) resembling typhoid fever.

typhomalarial fever (ti"fo-mah-lār'e-al) malaria with typhoidal symptoms.

typhomania (ti"fo-ma'ne-ah) the delirium accompanying typhus or typhoid fever.

typhopneumonia (ti"fo-nu-mo'ne-ah) pneumonia with typhoid fever.

typhosepsis (ti"fo-sep'sis) the septic poisoning occurring in typhus.

typhosis (ti-fo'sis) any typhus-like affection; the typhoid state.

typhotoxin (ti"fo-tok'sin) a deadly ptomaine from cultures of typhoid bacillus.

typhus (ti'fus) an acute infectious disease caused by species of the parasitic microorganism Rickettsia. The organisms are usually transmitted from infected rats and other rodents to man by lice, fleas, ticks and mites.

Rickettsiae enter the human body through cuts or breaks in the skin made by the bites of the lice or other pests.

TYPES AND TREATMENT. The principal types of the diseases are louse-borne typhus, murine (flea-borne) typhus, scrub typhus and recrudescent typhus.

Louse-Borne Typhus. Louse-borne typhus (epidemic or classic typhus) occurs after feces of an infected human body are rubbed into a break in the skin. After an incubation period of 6 to 15 days, the symptoms begin to appear—headache, running of the nose, cough, nausea and chest pain. These are followed in a few days by high fever and chills, vomiting, constipation or diarrhea, muscular aching and perhaps delirium or stupor. A red rash, which may bleed, appears on the trunk and spreads to the arms and legs.

After about 2 weeks the symptoms usually subside. Ordinarily louse typhus is not fatal, but it can be, particularly if pneumonia develops or if the afflicted person has heart disease.

Louse typhus is called epidemic typhus because of the devastation it has caused throughout history. It tends to appear where people are crowded together and are weakened by cold, disease and starvation. It has many colloquial names, such as war fever, camp fever or jail fever.

Murine Typhus. Murine typhus is a less common variety. It is called also endemic, rat or flea typhus. As the name "murine" indicates, it is transmitted by the bites of rat or mouse fleas. The symptoms are like those of louse typhus but are less severe, and recovery occurs sooner. Antibiotics are used in treatment.

Scrub Typhus. Scrub typhus, called also Japanese river fever and tsutsugamushi fever, is prevalent in eastern Asia and has been carried to other areas by infected persons. It is transmitted by mites and hence is often called mite fever. The rodent responsible for this illness is the field mouse. The rickettsiae are transferred to humans by the bite of the larval form of the mite, usually in the groin or neck. The fever of scrub typhus and its other symptoms are very similar to those of other forms of typhus. It is treated with chloramphenicol and the tetracyclines.

Recrudescent Typhus. Recrudescent typhus, or Brill-Zinsser disease, is caused by rickettsiae very similar to those that cause louse-borne typhus. These strains, however, remain in the body after a first attack of typhus and can cause a recurrence (a recrudescence) as long as years after the first attack. The recrudescence is milder than the initial infection, however. Treatment is similar to that for epidemic typhus.

Closely related to these forms of typhus are tick-borne rickettsial diseases, such as ROCKY MOUNTAIN SPOTTED FEVER.

PREVENTION. Immunizing vaccines are available if an outbreak of typhus occurs or threatens. They greatly reduce the chance of infection, or modify the effects of the disease. Travelers should be vaccinated before visiting countries where the disease is prevalent. Some countries require proof of such protection before admitting a visitor.

Insect and rodent control are of great importance in the prevention and control of typhus. Adult lice can be destroyed by spraying garments with DDT.

Frequent bathing and changes of underclothes are vital. Outer garments should be sterilized by steam to kill the louse eggs.

Fleas and mites are more difficult to control than lice. The best method is to destroy the rodents on which they live.

NURSING CARE. The patient with typhus is initially isolated until he is free of body lice or mites. He is not capable of transmitting the disease without the aid of these vectors. To accomplish removal of lice or mites the patient should be washed with a 1 per cent solution of Lysol upon admission and his clothing must be disinfected or destroyed. Several shampoos may be necessary to eliminate parasites from the hair. Gentle, thorough cleaning is necessary and every effort must be made to avoid damage to the skin in one's enthusiasm for removing lice or mites.

The patient is given a soft diet and ample fluids, to prevent dehydration. Efforts are made to conserve the patient's strength and to protect him during periods of delirium, which are common.

Typhus is a very debilitating disease and requires a long period of convalescence in which the patient's general health must be improved. Nervous and mental symptoms may persist long after the acute phase of the disease subsides.

typing (tīp′ing) determination of the type of something.

t. of blood, determining the character of the blood on the basis of agglutinogens in the erythrocytes.

tyramine (ti′rah-mēn) a decarboxylation product of tyrosine with a similar (but weaker) action to that of epinephrine and norepinephrine, and capable of releasing stored norepinephrine.

tyrocidin (ti″ro-si′din) a basic cyclic polypeptide present in tyrothricin.

tyrogenous (ti-roj′ĕ-nus) originating in cheese.

tyroid (ti′roid) of cheesy consistency.

tyroma (ti-ro′mah) a caseous mass.

tyromatosis (ti″ro-mah-to′sis) caseation.

tyrosiluria (ti″ro-sĭ-lu′re-ah) the presence in the urine of metabolites of tyrosine.

tyrosine (ti′ro-sēn) a naturally occurring amino acid produced in the body in the metabolism of phenylalanine to melanin, epinephrine and thyroxine.

tyrosinosis (ti″ro-sĭ-no′sis) a condition characterized by a faulty metabolism of tyrosine in which an intermediate product, parahydroxyphenyl pyruvic acid, appears in the urine and gives it an abnormal reducing power.

tyrosinuria (ti″ro-sĭ-nu′re-ah) the presence of tyrosine in the urine.

tyrosis (ti-ro′sis) caseation.

tyrothricin (ti″ro-thri′sin) a substance produced by growth of a soil bacillus, *Bacillus brevis*, consisting principally of gramicidin and tyrocidin; used topically as an antibiotic.

tyrotoxin   (ti″ro-tok′sin) a toxin sometimes developed in cheese and milk by the action of bacilli.

tyrotoxism (ti″ro-tok′sizm) poisoning from a toxin present in milk or cheese.

tysonitis   (ti″son-i′tis) inflammation of Tyson's glands, small sebaceous glands of the corona of the penis and of the labia majora and minora.

Tyvid   (ti′vid) trademark for a preparation of isoniazid, used in treatment of tuberculosis.

Tyzine   (ti′zēn) trademark for preparations of tetrahydrozoline hydrochloride, a nasal decongestant.

tzetze (set′se) tsetse.

U

U chemical symbol, *uranium.*

U. unit.

uberous (u′ber-us) prolific.

uberty (u′ber-te) fertility.

ulalgia (u-lal′je-ah) pain in the gums.

ulatrophia, ulatrophy (u″lah-tro′fe-ah), (u-lat′-ro-fe) shrinkage of the gums.

ulcer (ul′ser) a a local defect, on the body surface or the lining of a mucous surface, produced by sloughing of necrotic inflammatory tissue. As commonly used, the term often refers to a peptic ulcer of the inner wall, or lining, of the stomach (gastric ulcer) or of the duodenum (duodenal ulcer).

Curling′s u., an ulcer of the duodenum seen after severe burns of the body.

decubitus u., an ulceration caused by prolonged pressure on a body area in a patient confined to bed (see also DECUBITUS ULCER).

indolent u., one with an indurated, elevated edge and nongranulating base, usually on the leg.

peptic u., an ulceration of the mucous membrane of the esophagus, stomach or duodenum, caused by the action of the acid gastric juice.

Peptic ulcer is most common among persons who are chronically anxious or irritated, or who otherwise suffer from mental tension. It occurs about three times as often in men as in women. Symptoms include a pain or gnawing sensation in the epigastric region. The pain occurs from 1 to 3 hours after eating, and is usually relieved by eating or taking an antacid drug. Vomiting, sometimes preceded by nausea, usually follows a severe bout of pain.

COMPLICATIONS. If ulcers are untreated, bleeding can occur, leading to anemia and therefore weakness and impaired health. Blood may be vomited, and appears brownish and like coffee grounds because of the digestive effect of gastric secretions on the hemoglobin. There may be blood in the stools, giving them a tarry black color. In acute cases sudden hemorrhage can occur and may be fatal if not treated properly.

The ulcer may become perforated, allowing food to escape from the stomach and intestines into the peritoneal cavity, and causing peritonitis. Pyloric obstruction may result if repeated healing of a peptic ulcer causes stenosis in the pyloric area.

DIAGNOSTIC TESTS. Diagnosis of peptic ulcer is confirmed by x-ray examination of the stomach and duodenum (gastrointestinal series) in which the patient drinks a barium solution that makes the gastrointestinal tract visible to x-ray while it fills. Fluoroscopy may be used to determine the rate at which the stomach and duodenum fill and empty and to locate a defect in either of these organs (see also BARIUM TEST). GASTROSCOPY may be indicated in cases in which the physician wishes to have the advantage of direct visualization of the inner lining of the stomach. Another test often done in the diagnosis of peptic ulcer is GASTRIC ANALYSIS, in which contents of the stomach are withdrawn and analyzed for acidity and cellular content.

TREATMENT. Ulcers frequently can be treated successfully and cured, but there is no easy cure, and complete cooperation of the patient in following a carefully planned regime is necessary. Smoking is usually forbidden, as it tends to irritate the gastric and duodenal mucosa. The patient is usually advised to give up alcohol as well.

Dietary control is important because certain types of food tend to aggravate the ulcer and prevent its healing. Diets vary with the general state

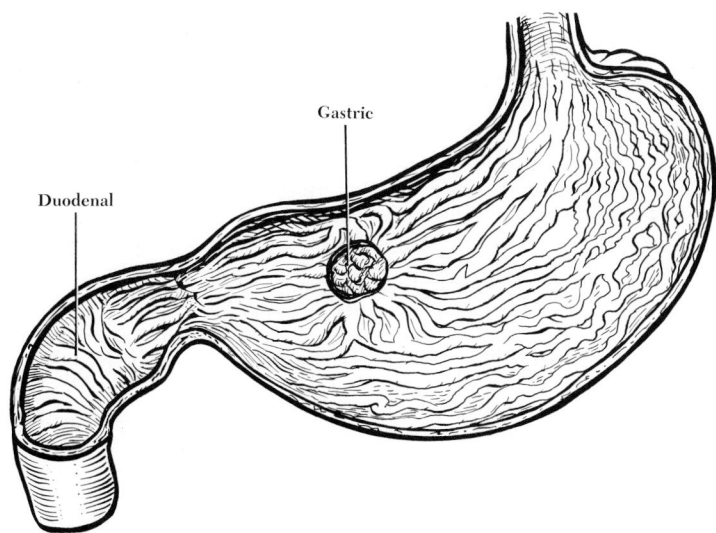

Ulcer.

Gastric

Duodenal

of the patient's health and the stage of progress of the ulcer. Bland liquid and soft foods are recommended. Roughage and highly seasoned foods should be avoided. In the early stages of treatment, meals are small and frequent. Later, the patient progresses to three meals a day.

Medications are administered to relieve the symptoms of peptic ulcer and to help remove some of its causes. Antacids such as aluminum hydroxide gel and magnesium trisilicate are given to counteract the hyperacidity of the stomach and act as a coating for the mucous membranes. Sedatives may be given to reduce tension and nervousness; usually one of the barbiturates is prescribed. Drugs that reduce gastric motility and decrease gastric secretion are beneficial in some cases. These drugs include belladonna, atropine and synthetic preparations such as diphemanil methylsulfate (Prantal) and methantheline bromide (Banthine).

Worry and anxiety can contribute to the development of an ulcer and prevent it from healing. If emotional tensions persist, an ulcer that has been healed by medical treatment can return. Therefore, every effort is made to help the patient relax. Sometimes counseling or psychotherapy is helpful in relieving emotional strain.

Many ulcers can be treated without surgery when patients cooperate fully; however, surgery may be necessary in certain cases—when there is scarring of the ulcer (producing obstruction), recurrent bleeding, extreme pain and perforation. Gastric ulcers are more likely to require surgery than are duodenal ulcers. The operative procedure most frequently done in the treatment of gastric ulcer is subtotal gastrectomy in which the ulcerous portion of the stomach is removed (see also surgery of the STOMACH). This procedure is often done in conjunction with vagotomy, division of the vagus nerve, which eliminates cerebral stimuli of the stomach muscle and glands, thereby reducing gastric motility and secretion.

perforating u., one that involves the entire thickness of an organ, creating an opening on both surfaces.

varicose u., an ulcer due to varicose veins.

venereal u., chancre.

ulcerate (ul'sĕ-rāt) to produce an ulcer or become affected with ulceration.

ulceration (ul"sĕ-ra'shun) 1. formation of an ulcer. 2. an ulcer.

ulcerative (ul'sĕ-ra"tiv, ul'ser-ah-tiv) characterized by ulcer formation.

u. colitis, inflammation of the colon, with formation of ulcers in the intestinal mucosa. It is most likely to occur in young adults, but it can occur at any age. It is potentially serious and may be disabling or even fatal in rare instances.

The cause of ulcerative colitis is unknown. Emotional stress or acute infections frequently precipitate attacks.

SYMPTOMS. The chief symptom is severe diarrhea with as many as 15 or 20 watery stools a day, although none of the usual causes of diarrhea is present. There may be blood and mucus in the stool.

The patient feels weak, loses weight and sometimes has anemia. He may suffer from pains in the joints or from skin disorders. As the disease progresses, it may spread to the covering of the colon, or it may cause intestinal perforation and peritonitis. Malignant degeneration may occur in these patients.

DIAGNOSIS. The lining of the colon can be examined and ulcerations visualized by PROCTOSCOPY. The existence of the disease can be determined also by barium enema (see BARIUM TEST).

TREATMENT. Rest is imperative. This includes not only physical rest in bed but complete freedom from emotional stress. A bland but nutritious diet that omits fruits and vegetables is also required. Antibiotics and cortisone may be prescribed, as well as sedatives and tranquilizers to relieve emotional distress. Counseling or psychotherapy may help the patient to deal with his anxieties and in this way reduce the causes of the disorder.

Treatment is difficult and the prognosis is poor. Advanced cases may respond to surgical procedures such as a colectomy or COLOSTOMY.

NURSING CARE. The emotional aspects of ulcerative colitis are of primary importance in the care of these patients. Although these individuals may assume an outward appearance of calm and resignation to their illness, keeping their anxieties well hidden, they are almost always in need of help in coping with their anxieties and tensions.

The frequency and character of stools must be observed and recorded. Antidiarrheal drugs are administered as ordered and their effectiveness for the individual patient is noted on the chart. Special attention to cleanliness of the anal area will help prevent local irritation and discomfort produced by frequent elimination.

ulcerogangrenous (ul"ser-o-gang'grĕ-nus) characterized by both ulceration and gangrene.

ulcerogenic (ul"ser-o-jen'ik) causing ulceration; leading to the production of ulcers.

ulcerous (ul'ser-us) of the nature of an ulcer.

ulcus (ul'kus) pl. *ul'cera* [L.] ulcer.

ulectomy (u-lek'to-me). 1. excision of scar tissue. 2. excision of the gingiva; gingivectomy.

ulemorrhagia (u"lem-o-ra'je-ah) bleeding from the gums.

ulerythema (u"ler-ĭ-the'mah) an erythematous disease of the skin with formation of cicatrices.

u. ophryog'enes, keratosis pilaris affecting the follicles of the eyebrow hairs.

uletic (u-let'ik) pertaining to the gums.

uliginous (u-lij'ĭ-nus) muddy or slimy.

ulitis (u-li'tis) inflammation of the gums.

ulna (ul'nah), pl. *ul'nae* [L.] the inner and larger bone of the forearm, on the side opposite the thumb. It articulates with the humerus and with the head of the radius and its proximal end; with the radius and bones of the carpus at the distal end. adj., **ul'nar.**

ulnad (ul'nad) toward the ulna.

ulnaris (ul-na'ris) [L.] ulnar.

ulnocarpal (ul"no-kar'pal) pertaining to the ulna and carpus.

ulnoradial (ul"no-ra'de-al) pertaining to the ulna and radius.

ulocace (u-lok′ah-se) ulceration of the gums.

ulocarcinoma (u″lo-kar″sĭ-no′mah) carcinoma of the gums.

uloglossitis (u″lo-glŏ-si′tis) inflammation of the gums and tongue.

uloid (u′loid) resembling a scar, but not due to any lesion of the skin.

uloncus (u-long′kus) swelling of the gums.

ulorrhagia (u″lo-ra′je-ah) free hemorrhage from the gums.

ulorrhea (u″lo-re′ah) bleeding from the gums.

ulosis (u-lo′sis) cicatrization; scar formation.

ulotomy (u-lot′o-me) 1. incision of scar tissue. 2. incision of the gums.

ulotrichous (u-lot′rĭ-kus) having crisp, curly hair.

Ultandren (ul-tan′dren) trademark for a preparation of fluoxymesterone, an androgen.

ultimate (ul′tĭ-mit) the last or farthest.

ultimum (ul′tĭ-mum) [L.] ultimate.

ultra- (ul′trah) word element [L.], *beyond; excess.*

ultrabrachycephalic (ul″trah-brak″e-sĕ-fal′ik) having a cephalic index of more than 90.

ultracentrifugation (ul″trah-sen-trif″u-ga′shun) subjection of material to centrifugal force 200,000 to 400,000 times the force of gravity.

ultracentrifuge (ul″trah-sen′trĭ-fūj) a centrifuge with an exceedingly high rate of rotation that will separate and sediment the molecules of a substance.

ultrafiltration (ul″trah-fil-tra′shun) filtration through a filter capable of removing very minute (ultramiscroscopic) particles.

ultraligation (ul″trah-li-ga′shun) ligation of a vessel beyond the point of origin of a branch.

ultramicropipet (ul″trah-mi-kro-pi-pet′) a pipet designed to handle extremely small quantities of liquid (0.002 to 0.005 ml.).

ultramicroscope (ul″trah-mi′kro-skōp) a special darkfield microscope for examination of particles of colloidal size.

ultramicroscopic (ul″trah-mi″kro-skop′ik) 1. pertraining to the ultramiscroscope. 2. too small to be seen with the ordinary light microscope.

ultramicroscopy (ul″trah-mi-kros′ko-pe) use of an ultramiscroscope.

Ultran (ul′tran) trademark for preparations of phenaglycodol, a tranquilizer.

ultrasonic (ul″trah-son′ik) beyond the audible range; relating to sound waves having a frequency of more than 20,000 cycles per second.

ultrasonics (ul″trah-son′iks) the science dealing with mechanical radiant energy of a frequency greater than 20,000 cycles per second.

ultrasonometry (ul″trah-so-nom′ĕ-tre) measure-

ment of certain physical properties of biologic fluids by means of ultrasound.

ultrasound (ul′trah-sownd) mechanical radiant energy of a frequency greater than 20,000 cycles per second.

ultrastructure (ul′trah-struk″tūr) the structural arrangement of the smallest particles composing a substance.

ultraviolet (ul″trah-vi′o-let) beyond the violet portion of the visible spectrum.
  u. rays, beyond the violet end of the visible spectrum and therefore not visible to man. They are produced by the sun but are absorbed to a large extent by particles of dust and smoke in the earth's atmosphere. They are also produced by the so-called sun lamps.
  Ultraviolet rays can produce sun-burning and affect the pigmentation of the skin, causing tanning. When they strike the skin surface, these rays transform provitamin D, secreted by the glands of the skin, into vitamin D, which is then absorbed into the body.
  Because ultraviolet rays are capable of killing bacteria and other microorganisms, they are sometimes utilized in specially designed cabinets to sterilize objects, and may also be used to sterilize the air in operating rooms and other areas where destruction of bacteria is necessary.

ultravirus (ul″trah-vi′rus) an extremely small pathogenic agent.

ululation (ul″u-la′shun) the loud crying or wailing of hysterical patients.

umb. umbilicus.

umbilectomy (um″bĭ-lek′to-me) excision of the umbilicus; omphalectomy.

umbilical (um-bil′ĭ-kal) pertaining to the umbilicus.
  u. cord, the structure that connects the fetus and placenta. This cord is the lifeline of the fetus in the uterus throughout pregnancy.
  About 2 weeks after conception, the umbilical cord and the PLACENTA are sufficiently developed to begin their functions. Through two arteries and a vein in the cord, nourishment and oxygen pass from the blood vessels in the placenta to the fetus, and waste products pass from the fetus to the placenta.
  Soon after birth, the umbilical cord is clamped or tied and then cut. The length of cord that is attached to the placenta, still in the uterus, is expelled with the placenta. The stump that remains attached to the baby's abdomen is about 2 inches long. After a few days it falls off naturally.
  u. hernia, protrusion of abdominal contents through the abdominal wall at the umbilicus, the defect in the abdominal wall and protruding intestine being covered with skin and subcutaneous tissue.
  During the growth of the fetus, the intestines grow more rapidly than the abdominal cavity. For a period, a portion of the intestines of the unborn child usually lies outside his abdomen in a sac within the umbilical cord. Normally, the intestines return to the abdomen, and the defect is closed by the time of birth. Occasionally the abdominal wall

does not close solidly, and umbilical hernia results. This defect is more likely to be seen in premature infants and in girls rather than boys.

The defect in the abdominal wall usually closes by itself. Coughing, crying and straining temporarily cause the sac to enlarge, but the hernia never bursts and digestion is not affected. The hernia may be strapped with adhesive or elastic tape or a truss may be used, but the effectiveness of these methods is doubtful. If the defect in the abdominal wall has not repaired itself by the time the child is 2 years old, surgery to correct the condition (HERNIOR-RAPHY) can then be performed.

Umbilical hernia should be distinguished from omphalocele, in which the intestines protrude directly into the umbilical cord and are covered only by a thin membrane. Omphalocele is a surgical emergency that must be treated immediately after birth.

umbilicated   (um-bil′ĭ-kāt″ed) marked by depressed spots resembling the umbilicus.

umbilication   (um-bil″ĭ-ka′shun) a depression resembling the umbilicus.

umbilicus   (um-bil′ĭ-kus, um″bĭ-li′kus) the (usually) depressed scar marking the site of entry of the umbilical cord in the fetus.

umbo   (um′bo), pl. *umbo′nes* [L.] a small protuberance at the center of a rounded surface.

unciform   (un′sĭ-form) hooked or shaped like a hook.

Uncinaria   (un″sĭ-na′re-ah) a name formerly given a genus of hookworms.

uncinariasis   (un″sĭ-nah-ri′ah-sis) ancylostomiasis; infection by hookworms.

uncinate   (un′sĭ-nāt) unciform.

uncipressure   (un′sĭ-presh″ur) pressure with a hook to stop hemorrhage.

unconscious   (un-kon′shus) 1. not aware of surrounding environment; not responding to sensory stimulation. 2. the area or activity of the mind in which primitive or unacceptable ideas and impulses are concealed from awareness by the psychic censor.
    collective u., the portion of the unconscious which is theoretically common to mankind.

unconsciousness   (un-kon′shus-nes) an abnormal state of lack of response to sensory stimuli, resulting from injury, illness, shock or some other bodily disorder. A brief loss of consciousness from which the person recovers spontaneously or with slight aid is called fainting. Deep, prolonged unconsciousness is known as coma.

FIRST AID.   Medical help should be summoned. If the unconscious person is not breathing, ARTIFICIAL RESPIRATION should be started immediately, preferably the mouth-to-mouth method. The patient should be given nothing by mouth. He should not be moved if it is possible that he is injured.

The following information on certain kinds and causes of unconsciousness includes measures that can be taken to help the unconscious person.

Alcoholic Excess.   The unconscious person should be turned from side to side at regular intervals while he is lying down. His head should be kept lowered. If unconsciousness is deep and prolonged, a physician should be called.

It should not be assumed that a smell of alcohol on the breath means definitely that unconsciousness is due to intoxication. The person may be a diabetic who has had a few drinks and is in a diabetic coma or insulin shock.

Cerebral Vascular Accident (Stroke).   Stroke is caused by the blocking or rupture of a blood vessel supplying the brain. Consciousness may be lost at once or after a period of dizziness, confusion, stumbling and inability to talk. The patient should be put to bed and the physician called. (See also CEREBRAL VASCULAR ACCIDENT.)

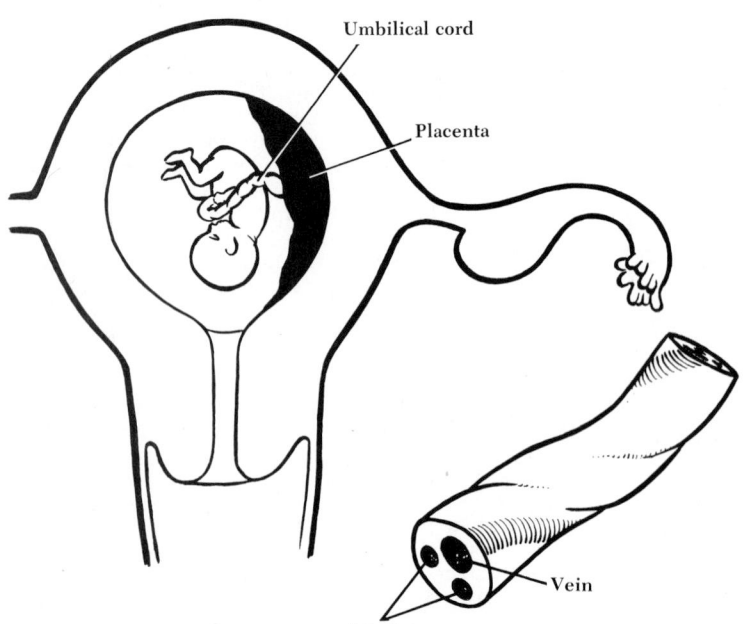

Umbilical cord. Left, in uterus; right, section.

Coronary Occlusion (Heart Attack). When loss of consciousness follows severe pains in the chest, dyspnea and cyanosis, the probable cause is coronary occlusion. A physician should be called immediately. The patient should not be moved without instructions from the physician. He should be covered with a blanket and kept warm, and tight clothing should be loosened. (See also CORONARY OCCLUSION.)

Electric Shock. If the unconscious person is in contact with a live wire or other source of electricity, he should not be touched. If possible, the electric current should be shut off, or an object that does not conduct electricity, such as a dry wooden plank, should be used to separate the person from the electrical source. Then artificial respiration should be given until breathing is regular. Medical help is a must.

Fainting. Fainting may occur as a result of injury, illness or emotional shock. The fainting person should be stretched out, his clothing loosened and his feet raised. Usually, cold water applied to the face, or smelling salts or aromatic spirits of ammonia held under the nose, will restore consciousness within a few minutes. If not, a physician should be called. After regaining consciousness, the person should rest for 10 to 30 minutes.

Head Injury. Head injury is the likely cause of unconsciousness if there is any obvious wound on the head. It also can be suspected in various accidents in which the person may have been "knocked out." In head injuries, the breathing often is unusually rapid and shallow.

Medical aid should be sought at once for anyone with a possible head injury. The injured person should be kept lying down and covered for warmth. He should not be moved to the hospital in a private vehicle unless an ambulance is unavailable. (See also HEAD INJURY.)

Narcotic Overdose. A physician should be called at once if an overdose of barbiturates or other narcotic is suspected. Any information that can be given about the amount or type of drug taken and the patient's behavior before becoming unconscious will be useful to the physician.

It should not be assumed that the unconsciousness is the desired effect of a "sleeping pill," especially if the person cannot be aroused easily. Medical diagnosis should be sought.

Medical treatment may include gastric lavage if the drug was taken a short time before. Stimulants, fluids given intravenously and artificial respiration or oxygen also may be required. Hospital care is often necessary.

Poisoning. In chemical poisoning, an empty container nearby may be a clue to the kind of poison taken and the emergency measures required. Immediate action is vital. If the person has stopped breathing, artificial respiration is given. If he regains consciousness, he should be given large amounts of water or, better still, milk if it is available. For most poisons, it is helpful to induce vomiting by putting a finger down the person's throat or by giving him a glass of warm water with a tablespoonful of salt dissolved in it. Vomiting should not be induced if the poison was lye, kerosene, gasoline or a strong acid or alkali. (See also POISONING.)

In the case of gas poisoning, which is usually cause by carbon monoxide, the person should be taken into fresh air and given artificial respiration. (See also CARBON MONOXIDE POISONING.)

Shock. Massive loss of blood, severe burns or other major injury may cause loss of consciousness as a result of shock. Until medical help arrives, the patient should lie flat, with the feet raised above the head (unless there are head or chest injuries, in which case these parts should be raised). He should be covered with a blanket or coat for warmth. He should not be moved, except that the head may be turned to one side to allow him to vomit without danger of choking. (See also SHOCK.)

Sunstroke. A person found unconscious in direct sunlight on a very hot day may be suffering from sunstroke. If he is, he will have a high fever, dry, hot skin, a red face and a rapid pulse. When these symptoms are present, a physician should be called. The patient is placed in a cool, shady area and his clothing is loosened or removed. Cold water is applied over the whole body in sufficient quantity to reduce the fever. (See also SUNSTROKE.)

unco-osified (un″ko-os′ĭ-fīd) not united into one bone.

unction (ungk′shun) 1. an ointment. 2. application of an ointment.

unctuous (ungk′tu-us) greasy or oily.

uncus (ung′kus) the medial protrusion of the anterior part of the hippocampal gyrus.

undecylenic acid (un″des-ĭ-len′ik) a yellow, liquid, water-insoluble, unsaturated fatty acid. It is used topically, in ointment or powder form, in treatment of certain skin disorders, especially fungus infections. Toxic reactions are rare.

undifferentiation (un″dif-er-en″she-a′shun) lack of normal differentiation.

undine (un′dēn) a small glass flask for irrigating the eye.

undulant fever (un′du-lant) brucellosis.

undulation (un″du-la′shun) a wavelike motion in any medium.

ung. [L.] *unguen′tum* (ointment).

ungual (ung′gwal) pertaining to the nails.

unguent (ung′gwent) an ointment.

unguentum (ung-gwen′tum), pl. *unguen′ta* [L.] ointment.

unguiculate (ung-gwik′u-lāt) having claws; clawlike.

unguinal (ung′gwĭ-nal) pertaining to a nail.

unguis (ung′gwis), pl. *un′gues* [L.] the horny cutaneous plate on the surface of the distal end of finger or toe; a fingernail or toenail. (See also NAIL.)

ungula (ung′gu-lah) an instrument for extracting a dead fetus.

uni- (u′ne) word element [L.], *one.*

uniaxial (u″ne-ak′se-al) having only one axis.

unicellular (u″nĭ-sel′u-lar) made up of a single cell.

unidirectional (u″nĭ-di-rek′shun-al) flowing in only one direction.

uniglandular (u″nĭ-glan′du-lar) affecting only one gland.

unigravida (u″nĭ-grav′ĭ-dah) a woman pregnant for the first time; gravida I.

unilateral (u″nĭ-lat′er-al) affecting only one side.

unilocular (u″nĭ-lok′u-lar) having only one loculus or compartment.

uninucleated (u″nĭ-nu′kle-āt″ed) having a single nucleus.

uniocular (u″ne-ok′u-lar) pertaining to only one eye.

union (ūn′yun) the growing together of tissues separated by injury, as of the ends of a fractured bone, or of the edges of an incision.
  immediate u., healing by first intention.

uniovular (u″ne-ov′u-lar) arising from one ovum.

unipara (u-nip′ah-rah) a woman who has had one pregnancy that resulted in a viable infant; para I. adj., **unip′arous.**

unipolar (u″nĭ-po′lar) having a single pole.

unipotent, unipotential (u-nip′o-tent), (u″nĭ-po-ten′shal) having only one power, as giving rise to cells of one order only.

unit (u′nit) 1. a single thing; one segment of a whole that is made up of identical or similar segments. 2. a specifically defined amount of anything subject to measurement, as of activity, dimension, velocity, volume or the like.
  Angstrom u., the unit of wavelength, being one ten-thousandth of a micron.
  British thermal u., a unit of heat, being the amount necessary to raise the temperature of one pound of water from 39 to 40° F., generally considered the equivalent of 252 calories; abbreviated B.T.U.
  u. of electricity, ampere, coulomb, farad, ohm, volt, watt.
  electrostatic u's, that system of unit which is based on the fundamental definition of a unit charge as one that will repel a similar charge with a force of one dyne when the two charges are 1 cm. apart.
  enzyme u., that amount of an enzyme that will, under defined conditions, transform 1 micromole of substrate per minute, or 1 microequivalent of a substrate in which more than one bond is attached.
  International u., a unit established by the International Conference for the Unification of Formulas; abbreviated I.U.
  Lf u., the amount of diphtheria toxin or toxoid that gives the most rapid flocculation with one standard unit of antitoxin when mixed and incubated in vitro.
  motor u., the unit of motor activity formed by a motor nerve cell and its many innervated muscle fibers.
  U.S.P. u., one used in the United States Pharmacopeia in expressing potency of drugs and other preparations.

unitary (u′nĭ-ter″e) pertaining to a single object or individual.

Unitensen (u″nĭ-ten′sen) trademark for preparations of cryptenamine, a hypotensive.

uniterminal (u″nĭ-ter′mĭ-nal) monoterminal.

univalent (u″nĭ-va′lent) having a valence of one.

Unna's paste boot (oo′nahz) a dressing for varicose ulcers that consists of a gelatin, zinc oxide and glycerin paste and spiral bandages applied in alternate layers on the entire leg to make a rigid boot.

unof. unofficial.

unofficial (un″ŏ-fish′al) not authorized by an established dispensatory or formulary.

unphysiologic (un″fiz-e-o-loj′ik) not in harmony with the laws of physiology.

unsaturated (un-sat′u-rāt″ed) 1. not having all affinities of its elements satisfied (unsaturated compound). 2. not holding all of a solute which can be held in solution by the solvent (unsaturated solution).

unsex (un-seks′) to deprive of the gonads, making reproduction impossible.

urachus (u′rah-kus) a canal in the fetus extending from the bladder to the umbilicus, the lumen usually being obliterated after birth.

uracil (u′rah-sil) a pyrimidine base obtained from nucleic acid.

uracrasia (u″rah-kra′ze-ah) disordered state of the urine.

uracratia (u″rah-kra′she-ah) inability to retain urine.

uragogue (u′rah-gog) an agent that increases urinary secretion.

uraniscolalia (u″rah-nis″ko-la′le-ah) a speech defect characteristic of cleft palate.

uranisconitis (u″rah-nis″ko-ni′tis) inflammation of the palate.

uraniscus (u″rah-nis′kus) the palate.

uranium (u-ra′ne-um) a chemical element, atomic number 92, atomic weight 238.03, symbol U. (See table of ELEMENTS.)

uranophobia (u″rah-no-fo′be-ah) morbid fear of heaven.

uranoplasty (u-ran′o-plas″te) plastic repair of the palate.

uranorrhaphy (u″rah-nor′ah-fe) suture of the palate.

uranoschisis (u″rah-nos′kĭ-sis) cleft palate.

uranostaphyloschisis (u″rah-no-staf″ĭ-los′kĭ-sis) fissure of the soft and hard palates.

urarthritis (u″rar-thri′tis) gouty arthritis.

urate (u′rāt) a salt of uric acid.

uratemia (u″rah-te′me-ah) urates in the blood.

uratic (u-rat′ik) pertaining to urates or to gout.

uratolysis (u″rah-tol′ĭ-sis) the splitting up of urates.

uratoma (u″rah-to′mah) a concretion made up of urates; tophus.

uratosis (u″rah-to′sis) the deposit of urates in the tissues.

uraturia (u″rah-tu′re-ah) urates in the urine.

Urbach-Oppenheim disease (ur″bak op′en-hīm) necrobiosis lipoidica diabeticorum.

urceiform (ur-se′ĭ-form) pitcher-shaped.

ur-defense (ur″de-fens′) a belief essential to the psychologic integrity of the individual. Such beliefs include faith in personal survival, in religious, philosophic or scientific systems and in human succorance.

urea (u-re′ah) a white, crystalline substance, the diamide of carbonic acid. It is one of the chief nitrogenous constituents of urine and is the chief end product of protein metabolism, being the form under which the nitrogen of the body is given off. The amount of urea in the urine increases with the quantity of protein in the diet. This is because urea is an endogenous and exogenous waste product: endogenous because some of it is derived from the breakdown of body protein as the tissues undergo disintegration and repair, and exogenous because some of it is derived from the deamination of amino acids absorbed from the intestinal tract but not utilized by the body.

In severe nephritis or other disorders leading to renal failure, the concentration of urea in the blood may be greatly increased, as revealed by measurement of the blood urea nitrogen (BUN).

u. nitrogen, a compound of urea and nitrogen; a major excretory product of the kidneys. Elevation of urea nitrogen concentration in the blood (blood urea nitrogen, or BUN) indicates a disorder of kidney function. In determination of BUN the nitrogen fraction of the urea nitrogen compound is measured. No special preparation is necessary for the test. Venous blood is used and potassium oxalate is added to the specimen to prevent clotting. Normal range is 8 to 20 mg. per 100 ml. of blood.

ureagenetic (u-re″ah-jĕ-net′ik) forming urea.

ureameter (u″re-am′ĕ-ter) an apparatus for measuring urea in urine.

ureametry (u″re-am′ĕ-tre) measurement of urea in urine.

ureapoiesis (u-re″ah-poi-e′sis) formation of urea.

urease (u′re-ās) a colorless, crystalline globulin found in mucous urine passed during inflammation of the bladder. It is formed by various microorganisms, and is capable of causing the change of urea into carbon dioxide and ammonia and of hippuric acid into benzoic acid and glycine. Called also urea enzyme and urea ferment.

urecchysis (u-rek′ĭ-sis) an effusion of urine into cellular tissue.

Urecholine (u″re-ko′lin) trademark for preparations of bethanechol, a parasympathomimetic agent.

uredema (u″rĕ-de′mah) swelling from extravasated urine.

uredo (u-re′do) urticaria.

ureide (u′re-īd) a compound of urea and an acid or aldehyde formed by the elimination of water.

urelcosis (u″rel-ko′sis) ulceration in the urinary tract.

uremia (u-re′me-ah) accumulation in the blood of substances ordinarily eliminated in the urine. adj., **ure′mic.** The condition develops when the kidneys lose most of their ability to filter out waste products from the blood, because of damage by disease or by severe trauma. It may be the result of a temporary poisoning or of obstruction of the kidneys, or it may occur in the final stage of a severe kidney disease.

ACUTE UREMIA. Acute uraemia is more easily managed than the chronic form, and can usually be treated successfully.

Causes. Acute uremia has a wide range of possible causes, including traumatic or surgical shock, severe transfusion reaction, severe injuries or burns, various kinds of poisoning, administration of sulfonamide drugs and complications of pregnancy. Acute uremia can also occur during an infectious disease, or when the body is severely dehydrated.

Symptoms. The first and most important symptom of acute uremia is always a sudden drop in the volume of urine. In severe cases, the production of urine may stop entirely.

For the first several days there may be few symptoms, and in general no feelings of discomfort. Soon, however, loss of appetite, headache, nausea and vomiting appear. In severe cases, the breath has the ammonia-like odor of urine. There may be drowsiness, and perhaps convulsions.

Treatment. The treatment of acute uremia consists first in treating the original cause of the temporary kidney failure. Beyond this, the treatment attempts to rest the kidneys as much as possible so that they will resume normal function. Therefore, restriction of fluid intake is necessary, and an accurate record intake and output must be kept.

Most cases of acute uremia respond well to treatment, and the kidneys recover satisfactorily within 1 to 6 weeks. If they do not, an artificial KIDNEY may be used. The patient's blood is pumped into this device, which purifies it of the contaminating urine constituents and returns "clean" blood to the body. The nonfunctioning kidneys are thus bypassed and normal blood circulates through the patient's system. At the same time other treatment is continued, to repair the damaged kidneys and restore them to their normal functioning condition.

CHRONIC UREMIA. Chronic uremia can be a grave condition, especially when it occurs as the final stage of a fatal kidney disease.

Causes. Chronic uremia may result from chronic nephritis or an advanced, chronic stage of pyelitis, or it may be caused by hypertensive kidney disease. Many other disorders such as diabetes mellitus, collagen diseases, polycystic kidneys and untreated enlargement of the prostate, kidney stones and other obstructions in the urinary system may cause uremia.

Symptoms. The symptoms of chronic uremia—unlike those of acute uremia—usually make their appearance gradually. Instead of a sudden decrease in the volume of the urine, it is undiminished or may even be increased. But as the kidneys continue to fail, the patient becomes greatly fatigued. Anemia develops and the blood pressure may increase. The vision often becomes dim. Nausea, vomiting and diarrhea occur. The skin is pallid and appears waxy. Frequently there may be periods of hiccupping. The breath and sweat smell of urine; urea frost (a layer of urea crystals) may appear on the face and chest. The patient becomes increasingly drowsy. Finally he lapses into a coma from which he does not awaken.

Treatment. The artificial KIDNEY is used in some cases of chronic uremia. Its disadvantage in chronic uremia is that repeated treatment is necessary. Scientists are working on the construction of a small artificial kidney which can be implanted surgically in the patient.

Some cases of chronic uremia have been treated by kidney TRANSPLANTATION. In the first such case the donor and recipient were identical twins, but increasing success with nontwin transplantation has been achieved.

Nursing Care. Disturbances in the normal fluid balance require strict measuring and recording of the patient's total intake and output. When severe edema is present, the fluid intake may be restricted and oral intake of fluids must then be spaced over a 24-hour period. Nausea and vomiting often present problems of adequate oral intake and should be recorded on the patient's chart so that fluids may be administered intravenously if necessary. The amount of fluid lost by emesis is carefully measured and recorded.

Mouth care is necessary at frequent intervals to prevent drying and cracking of the lips and oral mucosa and to reduce the foul breath which usually carries an odor of urine in uremic patients.

The skin is often dry, and deposits of urea salts cause severe itching. A sponge bath using a mild acid solution of vinegar and water (two tablespoons of vinegar to one pint of warm water) will relieve the irritation and discomfort. The bath should be followed by gentle application of a bland lotion. The presence of edema presents additional problems since edematous tissue breaks down more readily than normal tissue. To avoid rapidly developing decubitus ulcers the patient's position is changed and skin care is given at least every 2 hours. Extreme care must be used to keep the skin intact and to avoid friction against the bed linens when turning the patient.

Observations, in addition to intake and output and vital signs, include frequent checking for signs of developing convulsions. As intracranial pressure due to cerebral edema increases, the patient may exhibit extreme restlessness, irritability and mental confusion. For this reason, and to avoid precipitation of a convulsive seizure, the patient's environment should be as quiet and nonstimulating as possible.

Uremia is often the final phase of severe renal damage. The process is frequently irreversible and death is the inevitable outcome. The patient and his family will need sympathetic understanding, warmth and moral support during this time of emotional crisis.

uremigenic (u-re″mĭ-jen′ik) caused by uremia.

ureolysis (u″re-ol′ĭ-sis) the disintegration or de-

composition of urea into carbon dioxide and ammonia.

ureometer (u″re-om′ĕ-ter) ureameter.

ureometry (u″re-om′ĕ-tre) ureametry.

ureopoiesis (u-re″o-poi-e′sis) unreapoiesis.

ureosecretory (u-re″o-se-kre′tor-e) pertaining to the secretion of urea.

uresis (u-re′sis) secretion and excretion of urine.

-uresis (u-re′sis) word element [Gr.], *urinary excretion of.*

ureter (u-re′ter) a narrow, muscular, foot-long tube that conducts urine from the kidney to the urinary bladder. adj., **ure′teral, ureter′ic.** As urine is produced by each kidney, it passes into the ureter, which, contracting rhythmically, forces the urine along and empties it in spurts into the bladder. After being stored temporarily in the bladder, the urine passes out of the body by way of the urethra.

Rarely, a small calculus, or stone, formed in a kidney, passes into a ureter and obstructs it. The result is the sudden severe pain known as renal or ureteral colic. In such cases the aim of medical treatment is to relieve the pain and obstruction and to eliminate the condition that causes the stone.

ureter(o)- (u-re′ter-o) word element [Gr.], *ureter.*

ureteralgia (u-re″ter-al′je-ah) pain in the ureter.

ureterectasis (u-re″ter-ek′tah-sis) distention of the ureter.

ureterectomy (u-re″ter-ek′to-me) excision of a ureter.

ureteritis (u-re″ter-i′tis) inflammation of a ureter.

ureterocele (u-re′ter-o-sēl″) ballooning of the lower end of the ureter into the bladder.

ureterocelectomy (u-re″ter-o-se-lek′to-me) excision of a ureterocele.

ureterocolostomy (u-re″ter-o-ko-los′to-me) anastomosis of a ureter to the colon.

ureterocutaneostomy (u-re″ter-o-ku-ta″ne-os′to-me) surgical creation of an opening of the ureter on the body surface (skin), permitting drainage of urine directly to the exterior of the body.

ureterocystoneostomy (u-re″ter-o-sis″to-ne-os′to-me) implantation of a ureter at a different site on the bladder wall.

ureterocystoscope (u-re″ter-o-sis′to-skōp) a cystoscope with a catheter for insertion into the ureter.

ureterocystostomy (u-re″ter-o-sis-tos′to-me) ureterocystoneostomy.

ureterodialysis (u-re″ter-o-di-al′ĭ-sis) rupture of a ureter.

ureteroduodenal (u-re″ter-o-du″o-de′nal) pertaining to or communicating with a ureter and the duodenum.

ureteroenterostomy (u-re″ter-o-en″ter-os′to-me) anastomosis of one or both ureters to the wall of the intestine.

ureterography   (u-re″ter-og′rah-fe) roentgenography of the ureter, after injection of a contrast medium.

ureteroheminephrectomy   (u-re″ter-o-hem″ĭ-nefrek′to-me) excision of the diseased portion of a reduplicated kidney and its ureter.

ureteroileostomy   (u-re″ter-o-il″e-os′to-me) anastomosis of the ureters to an isolated loop of the ileum, drained through a stoma on the abdominal wall.

ureterolith   (u-re′ter-o-lith″) a calculus in the ureter.

ureterolithiasis   (u-re″ter-o-lĭ-thi′ah-sis) formation of a calculus in the ureter.

ureterolithotomy   (u-re″ter-o-lĭ-thot′o-me) incision of ureter for removal of calculus; excision of a ureteral calculus.

ureterolysis   (u-re″ter-ol′ĭ-sis) 1. rupture of the ureter. 2. paralysis of the ureter. 3. the operation of freeing the ureter from adhesions.

ureteromeatotomy   (u-re″ter-o-me″ah-tot′o-me) incision of the opening of the ureter in the bladder wall.

ureteroneocystostomy   (u-re″ter-o-ne″o-sis-tos′to-me) ureterocystoneostomy.

ureteroneopyelostomy   (u-re″ter-o-ne″o-pi″ĕ-los′to-me) ureteropyeloneostomy.

ureteronephrectomy   (u-re″ter-o-ne-frek′to-me) excision of a kidney and ureter.

ureteropathy   (u-re″ter-op′ah-the) any disease of the ureter.

ureteropelvioplasty   (u-re″ter-o-pel′ve-o-plas″te) ureteropyeloplasty.

ureteroplasty   (u-re′ter-o-plas″te) plastic repair of a ureter.

ureteropyelitis   (u-re″ter-o-pi″ĕ-li′tis) inflammation of a ureter and kidney pelvis.

ureteropyelography   (u-re″ter-o-pi-ĕ-log′rah-fe) roentgenography of the ureter and pelvis of the kidney.

ureteropyeloneostomy   (u-re″ter-o-pi″ĕ-lo-ne-os′to-me) surgical creation of a new communication between a ureter and the kidney pelvis.

ureteropyelonephritis   (u-re″ter-o-pi″ĕ-lo-nĕ-fri′tis) inflammation of the ureter, renal pelvis and kidney.

ureteropyeloplasty   (u-re″ter-o-pi′ĕ-lo-plas″te) plastic repair of the ureter and renal pelvis.

ureteropyelostomy   (u-re″ter-o-pi″ĕ-los′to-me) ureteropyeloneostomy.

ureteropyosis   (u-re″ter-o-pi-o′sis) suppurative inflammation of the ureter.

ureterorectal   (u-re″ter-o-rek′tal) pertaining to or communicating with a ureter and the rectum.

ureterorrhagia   (u-re″ter-o-ra′je-ah) discharge of blood from the ureter.

ureterorrhaphy   (u-re″ter-or′ah-fe) suture of the ureter.

ureterosigmoidostomy   (u-re″ter-o-sig″moi-dos′to-me) anastomosis of a ureter to the sigmoid colon.

ureterostomy   (u-re″ter-os′to-me) creation of a new outlet for a ureter.
  cutaneous u., external u., the operation of bringing the ureters to the surface of the skin over the abdomen.
  Ureterostomy is necessary when the bladder has been removed surgically. The patient is outfitted with rubber collecting cups that fit over the ureteral stomas ("ureteral buds"). These cups are attached to a bag which is emptied of the urine periodically.

ureterotomy   (u-re″ter-ot′o-me) incision of a ureter.

ureteroureterostomy   (u-re″ter-o-u-re″ter-os′to-me) surgical anastomosis of two previously remote portions of a ureter, or of one ureter and the other.

ureterovaginal   (u-re″ter-o-vaj′ĭ-nal) pertaining to a ureter and the vagina.

ureterovesical   (u-re″ter-o-ves′ĭ-kal) pertaining to a ureter and the bladder.

urethan, urethane   (u′rĕ-thān), a colorless crystalline or granular compound used as an antineoplastic agent.

urethr(o)-   (u-re′thro) word element [Gr.], *urethra*.

urethra   (u-re′thrah) the canal extending from the bladder and opening to the outside of the body. adj., **ure′thral.** The external urinary opening is called the urinary meatus. In men the urethra conveys both urine and the secretions of the reproductive organs. In women its sole function is urination.
  The female urethra is about 1½ inches long. The opening is situated between the clitoris and the opening of the vagina.
  The male urethra is about 8 inches long and is narrower than that of the female. It has three sections—prostatic, membranous, and penile. It extends downward from the bladder through the prostate, which secretes into it a thin fluid. The membranous portion of the urethra receives the secretion of the bulbourethral glands. The urethra then extends down through the main body of the penis to the opening, or meatus, at the tip. Along the entire length of the passage are mucous glands.
  DISORDERS OF THE URETHRA.   Urethritis, inflammation of the urethra, occurs mainly in gonorrhea. Urethral strictures in men, caused by bands of fibrous tissue which obstruct the passage of urine, are also most often caused by neglected gonorrhea but may sometimes be caused by any infection, or by injury. They may be treated surgically or by dilatation. Kidney stones, or calculi, may rarely lodge in the urethra. They usually pass spontaneously but if not, may be removed with forceps or crushed.
  In women, urethral caruncles, small, fleshy, red masses, sometimes form near the opening of the urethra, usually at the time of menopause. Caruncles are not dangerous unless they cause bleeding and painful urination; then surgical removal is required.

urethralgia   (u″re-thral′je-ah) pain in a urethra.

urethratresia   (u-re″thrah-tre′ze-ah) imperforation of the urethra.

urethrectomy (u″re-threk′to-me) excision of the urethra.

urethremphraxis (u″re-threm-frak′sis) obstruction of the urethra.

urethrism (u-re′thrizm) chronic spasm of the urethra.

urethritis (u″re-thri′tis) inflammation of the urethra. The condition is frequently a symptom of gonorrhea but may be caused by other infectious organisms.

In urethritis the urethra swells and narrows, and the flow of urine is impeded. Both urination and the urgency to urinate increase. Urination is accompanied by burning pain. There may be a purulent discharge.

Urethritis usually responds to treatment with antibiotics or sulfonamides.

urethrocele (u-re′thro-sēl) prolapse of the female urethra through the urinary meatus.

urethrocystitis (u-re″thro-sis-ti′tis) inflammation of the urethra and bladder.

urethrocystogram (u-re″thro-sis′to-gram) a roentgenogram of the urethra and bladder.

urethrocystography (u-re″thro-sis-tog′rah-fe) roentgenography of the urethra and bladder after injection of a contrast medium.

urethrodynia (u-re″thro-din′e-ah) urethralgia.

urethrography (u″re-throg′rah-fe) roentgenography of the urethra.

urethrometry (u″re-throm′ĕ-tre) 1. determination of the resistance of various segments of the urethra to retrograde flow of fluid. 2. measurement of the urethra.

urethropenile (u-re″thro-pe′nīl) pertaining to the urethra and penis.

urethroperineal (u-re″thro-per″ĭ-ne′al) pertaining to the urethra and perineum.

urethroperineoscrotal (u-re″thro-per″ĭ-ne″o-skro′tal) pertaining to the urethra, perineum and scrotum.

urethropexy (u-re′thro-pek″se) surgical correction of stress incontinence in the female by fixation of the urethra to the symphysis pubis and fascia of the rectus muscle of the abdomen.

urethrophraxis (u-re″thro-frak′sis) obstruction of the urethra.

urethrophyma (u-re″thro-fi′mah) a tumor in the urethra.

urethroplasty (u-re″thro-plas″te) plastic repair of the urethra.

urethrorectal (u-re″thro-rek′tal) pertaining to the urethra and rectum.

urethrorrhagia (u-re″thro-ra′je-ah) a flow of blood from the urethra.

urethrorrhapy (u″re-thror′ah-fe) suture of a urethral fistula.

urethrorrhea (u-re″thro-re′ah) abnormal discharge from the urethra.

urethroscope (u-re′thro-skōp) an instrument for viewing the interior of the urethra.

urethroscopy (u″re-thros′ko-pe) visual inspection of the urethra.

urethroscrotal (u-re″thro-skro′tal) pertaining to or communicating with the urethra and scrotum.

urethrospasm (u-re′thro-spazm) spasm of the urethral muscular tissue.

urethrostaxis (u-re″thro-stak′sis) oozing of blood from the urethra.

urethrostenosis (u-re″thro-stĕ-no′sis) constriction of the urethra; seen as a complication of gonorrhea.

urethrostomy (u″re-thros′to-me) creation of a new opening in the urethra of the male to facilitate catheter drainage of the bladder.

urethrotome (u-re′thro-tōm) an instrument for cutting a urethral stricture.

urethrotomy (u″re-throt′o-me) incision of the urethra.

urethrotrigonitis (u-re″thro-tri″go-ni′tis) inflammation of the urethra and trigone of the bladder (vesical trigone).

urethrovaginal (u-re″thro-vaj′ĭ-nal) pertaining to the urethra and vagina.

uretic (u-ret′ik) promoting the secretion of urine.

urhidrosis (ur″hĭ-dro′sis) secretion of sweat containing increased amounts of urea and other nitrogenous waste products; seen in uremia.

-uria (u′re-ah) word element [Gr.], *condition of the urine.*

uric (u′rik) pertaining to the urine.
  u. acid, the end product of purine metabolism or oxidation in the body. It is present in blood in a concentration of about 5 mg. per 100 ml. and is excreted in the urine in amounts of a little less than 1 Gm. per day. In GOUT there is an excess of uric acid in the blood, and salts of uric acid—urates— form insoluble stones in the urinary tract, or they may crystallize and form deposits (tophi) in the joints and tissues.
  The presence of high concentrations of uric acid in the urine is significant in the diagnosis of gout, but is of little significance in urinary disorders.

uricacidemia (u″rik-as″ĭ-de′me-ah) uric acid in the blood.

uricaciduria (u″rik-as″ĭ-du′re-ah) excess of uric acid in the urine.

uricemia (u″rĭ-se′me-ah) uricacidemia.

uricocholia (u″rĭ-ko-ko′le-ah) uric acid in the bile.

uricolysis (u″rĭ-kol′ĭ-sis) the splitting up of uric acid. adj., uricolyt′ic.

uricometer (u″rĭ-kom′ĕ-ter) an instrument for measuring uric acid in the urine.

uricopoiesis (u″rĭ-ko-poi-e′sis) the formation of uric acid.

uricosuria (u″rĭ-ko-su′re-ah) excretion of uric acid in the urine. adj., **uricosu′ric.**

uricoxidase (u″rĭ-kok′sĭ-dās) an enzyme that oxidizes uric acid.

uriesthesis (u″re-es-the′sis) the normal impulse to pass the urine.

urin(o)- (u′rĭ-no) word element [Gr., L.], *urine.*

urina (u-ri′nah) [L.] urine.

urinal (u′rĭ-nal) a receptacle for urine.

urinalysis (u″rĭ-nal′ĭ-sis) analysis of the urine as an aid in the diagnosis of disease. Many types of tests are used in analyzing the urine to determine whether it contains abnormal substances indicative of disease. The most significant substances normally absent from urine and detected by urinalysis are protein, glucose, acetone, blood, pus and casts.

urinary (u′rĭ-ner″e) pertaining to the urine; containing or secreting urine.

u. bladder, the musculomembranous sac in the anterior part of the pelvic cavity that serves as a reservoir for urine (see also BLADDER).

u. system, u. tract, the system formed in the body by the KIDNEYS, the urinary BLADDER, the URETERS and the URETHRA, the organs concerned in the production and excretion of urine. Often referred to as the genitourinary or urogenital system because of the proximity and close relationship to the reproductive organs.

urinate (u′rĭ-nāt) to void urine.

urination (u″rĭ-na′shun) passage of urine from the body; called also voiding the urine and micturition. Urine from the kidneys is passed in spurts every few seconds along the ureters to the bladder, where it collects until voided. During the act of urination the urine passes from the bladder to the outside via the urethra.

THE URINARY PROCESS. Urination is a complex process controlled by several sets of muscles, including the internal and external sphincters, which are circular muscles surrounding the urethra; they have the power to contract and prevent flow

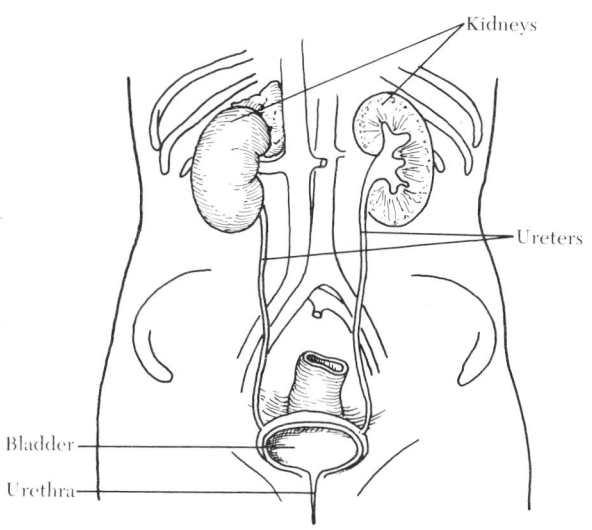

Organs of the urinary system.

through it. The internal sphincter is at the outlet of the bladder and works automatically. The external sphincter, situated along the urethra below the prostate in males and at an equivalent position in females, is controlled voluntarily.

As the bladder fills, the bladder muscle tends to contract automatically. The urge to urinate enters consciousness, but voiding may be controlled consciously to some extent. When the person decides to urinate, the bladder muscle contracts and both sphincters relax.

BED-WETTING AND INCONTINENCE. Control of the sphincters is late in developing. For the first year of life there is no control at all. Conscious control of the external sphincter develops in the second year, but complete control during sleep does not develop until the sphincters can deal automatically with the total amount of urine excreted during the night—about 10 oz. This is why bed-wetting can continue until comparatively late in young children.

Extreme fear in emergency situations may cause automatic relaxation of the sphincters with loss of control of urination, or INCONTINENCE. Incontinence also may occur in epileptic seizures, cerebral vascular accident (stroke) or other neurologic illness. In elderly men it may be due to hypertrophy of the prostate. Infection of the bladder or urethra in both men and women may impair control of urination.

Normally a quart or a quart and a half of urine is passed each day, but the amount is increased by a large intake of liquid or by cold weather. It is decreased in hot weather, when more fluid is eliminated through the skin by perspiration. Urination is usually necessary three or four times a day.

DISORDERS OF URINATION. Excessive secretion of urine (polyuria) may indicate diabetes mellitus, and diminution of urinary secretion (oliguria) may occur in nephritis. Frequent urination is a symptom of cystitis. Painful urination (dysuria) is characteristic of some bladder diseases, inflammation of the prostate and certain infections, including gonorrhea. Nocturia, or excessive urination at night, is a symptom of some urinary system diseases. It often occurs in acute prostatitis.

Urinary suppression is failure of the kidneys to produce urine and results in uremia if not corrected. This condition is brought about by severe disease or injury to the renal cells. Urinary retention is the accumulation of urine within the bladder because of inability to urinate.

urine (u′rin) the fluid containing water and waste products that is secreted by the KIDNEYS, stored in the bladder and discharged by way of the urethra.

CONTENTS OF THE URINE. Several different types of waste products are eliminated in urine—for example, urea, uric acid, ammonia and creatinine—none of which is useful in the blood. The largest component of urine by weight (apart from water) is urea, which is derived from the breakdown of proteins and amino acids in the diet and in the body itself. Its amount varies greatly from person to person, however, depending on the amount of protein in the diet.

Besides waste materials, urine also contains surpluses of products that are necessary for bodily functioning. The kidneys remove not only excess water but also excess sodium chloride and other chemicals. Thus in a typical specimen of urine there will be sodium, potassium, calcium, magnesium, chloride, phosphate and sulfate.

The color of urine is due to the presence of the yellow pigment urochrome. Individual ingredients of urine are not usually visible, but when the urine is alkaline some of the ingredients may form sediments of phosphates and urates. The urine may also become cloudy from the presence of mucus. Persistent cloudiness may indicate the presence of pus or blood.

URINE AS A SIGN OF ILLNESS. Urine can be an important warning of illness. The presence of glucose may signify the development of diabetes mellitus. If the urine is red or brown, this may indicate kidney disease, since the color may be due to blood in the urine (hematuria). A pink hue is not always caused by blood but may be due to certain foods such as beets and rhubarb, and cathartics containing senna, phenolphthalein or cascara. A smoky color may indicate old blood in the urine. With jaundice the urine may become dark or brown-colored.

residual u., urine remaining in the bladder after urination; seen in bladder outlet obstruction (as by prostatic hypertrophy) and disorders affecting nerves controlling bladder function.

urinemia (u″rĭ-ne′me-ah) uremia.

uriniferous (u″rĭ-nif′er-us) transporting or conveying urine.

uriniparous (u″rĭ-nip′ah-rus) secreting urine.

urinogenital (u″rĭ-no-jen′ĭ-tal) urogenital.

urinogenous (u″rĭ-noj′ĕ-nus) of urinary origin.

urinology (u″rĭ-nol′o-je) urology.

urinoma (u″rĭ-no′mah) a cyst containing urine.

urinometer (u″rĭ-nom′ĕ-ter) an instrument for determining the specific gravity of urine.

urinometry (u″rĭ-nom′ĕ-tre) determination of the specific gravity of urine.

urinophilous (u″rĭ-nof′ĭ-lus) having an affinity for urine, as microorganisms that grow best in urine or invade the urinary meatus of bathers in infested waters.

urinous (u′rĭ-nus) containing or resembling urine.

uriposia (u″rĭ-po′ze-ah) the drinking of urine.

urisolvent (u″rĭ-sol′vent) dissolving uric acid.

Uritone (u′rĭ-tōn) trademark for preparations of methenamine, a urinary antiseptic.

uro- (u′ro) word element [Gr.], *urine* (urinary tract, urination).

uroanthelone (u″ro-an′thĕ-lōn) urogastrone.

urobilin (u″ro-bi′lin) a brownish pigment formed by oxidation of urobilinogen; found in the feces and sometimes in the urine after standing in the air.

urobilinicterus (u″ro-bi″lin-ik′ter-us) brownish coloration of the skin from deposit of urobilin.

urobilinogen (u″ro-bi-lin′o-jen) a colorless compound formed in the intestines by the reduction of BILIRUBIN. Normally about 1 per cent of the bilirubin produced in the body by the breakdown of hemoglobin is excreted in the urine as urobilinogen. Increased amounts of urobilinogen in the urine indicate an excessive amount of bilirubin in the blood. Determination of the amount of urobilinogen excreted in a given period makes it possible to evaluate certain types of hemolytic anemia and also is of help in diagnosing liver dysfunction.

Laboratory tests for urobilinogen require collection of urine for a 24-hour period or for a 2-hour period. The 2-hour afternoon collection of urine is most commonly used because it is more convenient and also because it has been found that the excretion of urobilinogen reaches its maximum in the period from midafternoon to late evening. There is no special preparation of the patient for these tests. The exact time period in which the urine has been collected must be noted. The specimen should be taken to the laboratory immediately since bacteria which may be present in the urine can oxidize urobilinogen and change it to urobilin.

urocele (u′ro-sēl) distention of the scrotum with extravasated urine.

urochesia (u″ro-ke′ze-ah) discharge of urine through the rectum.

urochrome (u′ro-krōm) a breakdown product of hemoglobin related to the bile pigments, found in the urine and responsible for its yellow color.

uroclepsia (u″ro-klep′se-ah) the involuntary escape of urine.

urocrisia (u″ro-kriz′e-ah) diagnosis by examining the urine.

urocrisis (u″ro-kri′sis) a crisis marked by copious discharge of urine.

urocriterion (u″ro-kri-te′re-on) an indication of disease observed in examination of urine.

ABNORMAL CONSTITUENTS OF URINE

SUBSTANCE PRESENT	CONDITION INDICATED
Blood	Damage to tissues somewhere along the urinary tract
Pus cells	Infection in the urinary system
Bacteria or other infectious organisms	Local infection of the bladder or urinary tract
Proteins, mainly *albumin*	Kidney disease involving the glomeruli, hypertension, severe heart failure, toxic conditions or abnormal proteins in the blood
Acetone	Diabetes mellitus, ketosis accompanying starvation
Glucose (sugar)	Diabetes mellitus or some other metabolic disorder
Bile	Obstruction of bile ducts from liver or gallbladder; a liver disease that interferes with normal bile removal

urocyanogen (u″ro-si-an′o-jen) a blue pigment of urine, especially of cholera patients.

urocyanosis (u″ro-si″ah-no′sis) blueness of the urine.

urocyst (u′ro-sist) the urinary bladder.

urocystitis (u″ro-sis-ti′tis) inflammation of the urinary bladder.

urodialysis (u″ro-di-al′ĭ-sis) partial suppression of the urine.

urodynia (u″ro-din′e-ah) pain accompanying urination.

uro-edema (u″ro-ĕ-de′mah) edema from infiltration of urine.

uroenterone (u″ro-en′ter-ōn) urogastrone.

uroerythrin (u″ro-er′ĭ-thrin) a reddish pigment of urine.

urofuscohematin (u″ro-fus″ko-hem′ah-tin) a red-brown pigment of urine in certain diseases.

urogastrone (u″ro-gas′trōn) a principle derived from urine of man and other mammals that inhibits gastric secretion.

urogenital (u″ro-jen′ĭ-tal) pertaining to the urinary system and genitalia.

urogenous (u-roj′ĕ-nus) producing urine.

uroglaucin (u″ro-glaw′sin) a blue pigment from urine.

urogram (u′ro-gram) a film obtained by urography.

urography (u-rog′rah-fe) roentgenography of any part of the urinary tract.

   cystoscopic u., retrograde urography.

   descending u., excretion u., excretory u., intravenous u., urography after intravenous injection of an opaque medium which is rapidly excreted in the urine.

   retrograde u., urography after injection of contrast medium into the bladder through the urethra.

urogravimeter (u″ro-grah-vim′ĕ-ter) urinometer.

urohematin (u″ro-hem′ah-tin) the pigments of the urine.

urohematoporphyrin (u″ro-hem″ah-to-por′fĭ-rin) hematoporphyrin found in the urine.

urokinase (u″ro-ki′nās) a principle derived from urine of man and other mammals that acts enzymatically to split plasminogen and activates the fibrinolytic system.

urolith (u′ro-lith) a calculus in the urine or the urinary tract.

urolithiasis (u″ro-lĭ-thi′ah-sis) formation of urinary calculi.

urolithology (u″ro-lĭ-thol′o-je) the sum of knowledge about urinary calculi.

urologist (u-rol′o-jist) a specialist in urology.

urology (u-rol′o-je) the branch of medicine deal-

ing with the urinary system in the female and genitourinary system in the male. adj., **urolog′ic.**

urolutein (u″ro-lu′te-in) a yellow pigment of the urine.

uromancy (u′ro-man″se) prognosis based on examination of urine.

uromelanin (u″ro-mel′ah-nin) a black pigment from urine.

uromelus (u-rom′ĕ-lus) a fetal monster with fused legs and a single foot.

urometer (u-rom′ĕ-ter) urinometer.

uroncus (u-rong′kus) a swelling caused by retention or extravasation of urine.

uronephrosis (u″ro-nĕ-fro′sis) distention of the renal pelvis and tubules with urine.

uropathogen (u″ro-path′o-jen) an agent that causes disease of the urinary tract.

uropathy (u-rop′ah-the) any disease in the urinary tract.

   obstructive u., any disease of the urinary tract caused by obstruction.

uropenia (u″ro-pe′ne-ah) deficiency of urinary secretion.

uropepsin (u″ro-pep′sin) a pepsin-like enzyme occurring in urine.

urophanic (u″ro-fan′ik) appearing in the urine.

uroplania (u″ro-pla′ne-ah) the presence of urine in, or its discharge from, organs not of the genitourinary system.

uropoiesis (u″ro-poi-e′sis) the formation of urine.

uroporphyrin (u″ro-por′fĭ-rin) a porphyrin occurring in urine.

uroporphyrinogen (u″ro-por″fĭ-rin′o-jen) a reduced, colorless compound readily giving rise to uroporphyrin by oxidation.

uropsammus (u″ro-sam′us) urinary gravel.

uropyonephrosis (u″ro-pi″o-nĕ-fro′sis) distention of the renal pelvis and tubules with urine and pus.

uropyoureter (u″ro-pi″o-u-re′ter) collection of urine and pus in the ureter.

urorrhagia (u″ro-ra′je-ah) excessive secretion of urine.

urorrhea (u″ro-re′ah) involuntary flow of urine.

urorrhodin (u″ro-ro′din) a rosy pigment from urine.

urorrhodinogen (u″ro-ro-din′o-jen) a chromogen of the urine that is decomposed into urorrhodin.

urorubin (u″ro-roo′bin) a red pigment from urine.

urorubrohematin (u″ro-roo″bro-hem′ah-tin) a red pigment occasionally found in urine.

urosaccharometry (u″ro-sak″ah-rom′ĕ-tre) estimation of sugar in the urine.

urosacin (u″ro-sa′sin) urorrhodin.

uroscheocele (u-ros′ke-o-sēl″) urocele.

uroschesis (u-ros′kĕ-sis) retention or suppression of the urine.

urosemiology (u″ro-se″me-ol′o-je) diagnostic study of the urine.

urosepsin (u″ro-sep′sin) a septic poison from urine in the tissues.

urosepsis (u″ro-sep′sis) septic poisoning from retained and absorbed urinary substances.

urosis (u-ro′sis) any disease of the urinary organs.

urotoxia (u″ro-tok′se-ah) 1. urosepsis. 2. a poisonous state of the urine. adj., **urotox′ic.**

Urotropin (u-rot′ro-pin) trademark for a preparation of methenamine, a urinary antiseptic.

uroureter (u″ro-u-re′ter) distention of the ureter with urine.

uroxanthin (u″ro-zan′thin) a yellow pigment of the urine.

urticaria (ur″tĭ-ka′re-ah) a vascular reaction of the skin marked by transient appearance of slightly elevated patches that are redder or paler than the surrounding skin and often attended by severe itching; called also hives. It may result from various causes (e.g., allergens, exercise, excitement). adj., **urtica′rial.**

   u. facti′tia, factitious u., a condition in which the lesions are produced by rubbing, pinching or scratching, instead of appearing spontaneously.

    giant u., u. gigan′tea, angioneurotic edema.

    u. medicamento′sa, that due to use of a drug.

    papular u., u. papulo′sa, an allergic reaction to the bite of various insects, with appearance of lesions that evolve into inflammatory, increasingly hard, red or brownish, persistent papules.

    u. pigmento′sa, a highly distinctive dermatosis developing usually in the first year of life, with only one or two or widespread yellowish to reddish brown macules of varying shape, the lesions usually undergoing spontaneous involution.

    solar u., that resulting from exposure to sunlight.

urtication (ur″tĭ-ka′shun) a burning sensation, as of the sting of nettles.

urushiol (u-roo′she-ol) the toxic irritant principle of poison ivy and various related plants.

USAEC United States Atomic Energy Commission.

USAN United States Adopted Name, a nonproprietary designation for any compound used as a drug, established by negotiation between its manufacturer and a council sponsored jointly by the American Medical Association, American Pharmaceutical Association and United States Pharmacopoeial Convention, Inc.

U.S.M.H. United States Marine Hospital.

U.S.P. United States Pharmacopeia, a publication of the United States Pharmacopoeial Convention, first assembled in 1820, revised at regular intervals, to provide authoritative standards for substances and their preparations which are used in the science of medicine.

U.S.P.H.S. United States Public Health Service (see also PUBLIC HEALTH).

ustulation (us″tu-la′shum) the drying of a substance by heat.

ustus (us′tus) [L.] burnt.

uter(o)- (u′ter-o) word element [L.], *uterus.*

uteralgia (u″ter-al′je-ah) pain in the uterus.

uterectomy (u″ter-ek′to-me) hysterectomy.

uterine (u′ter-in, u′ter-īn) pertaining to the uterus.

   u. tube, a slender tube extending laterally from the uterus to the ovary on the same side; called also fallopian tube and oviduct. When the mature ovum leaves the ovary it enters the fringed opening of the uterine tube, through which it travels slowly to the uterus. When conception takes place, the tube is usually the site of fertilization.

   Infertility may be a result of obstruction or infection within the uterine tubes; the principal infections are gonorrhea and tuberculosis. A rare occurrence is the growth of a tumor in a tube. The removal of one tube by surgery, or the failure of a tube to function, ordinarily leaves the other tube intact and able to perform its function in reproduction. Occasionally the fertilized ovum implants in the wall of the uterine tube; this results in an ectopic, or tubal, pregnancy.

uteritis (u″ter-i′tis) inflammation of the uterus.

uteroabdominal (u″ter-o-ab-dom′ĭ-nal) pertaining to the uterus and abdomen.

uterocervical (u″ter-o-ser′vĭ-kal) pertaining to the uterus and cervix uteri.

uterofixation (u″ter-o-fik-sa′shun) hysteropexy; surgical fixation of the uterus.

uterogenic (u″ter-o-jen′ik) formed in the uterus.

uterogestation (u″ter-o-jes-ta′shun) uterine gestation.

uterography (u″ter-og′rah-fe) x-ray examination of the uterus.

uterolith (u′ter-o-lith″) a uterine calculus.

uteromania (u″ter-o-ma′ne-ah) nymphomania.

uterometer (u″ter-om′e-ter) an instrument for measuring the uterus.

utero-ovarian (u″ter-o-o-va′re-an) pertaining to the uterus and ovary.

uteropexy (u′ter-o-pek″se) hysteropexy.

uteroplacental (u″ter-o-plah-sen′tal) pertaining to the placenta and uterus.

uteroplasty (u′ter-o-plas″te) plastic repair of the uterus.

uterorectal (u″ter-o-rek′tal) pertaining to the uterus and rectum, or communicating with the uterine cavity and rectum.

uterosacral (u″ter-o-sa′kral) pertaining to the uterus and sacrum.

uterosalpingography (u″ter-o-sal″ping-gog′rah-fe) roentgenography of the uterus and uterine tubes.

uterosclerosis (u″ter-o-sklĕ-ro′sis) sclerosis of the uterus.

uteroscope (u′ter-o-skōp″) an instrument for viewing the interior of the uterus.

uterotomy (u″ter-ot′o-me) hysterotomy; incision of the uterus.

uterotonic (u″ter-o-ton′ik) increasing the tone of uterine muscle.

uterotropic (u″ter-o-trop′ik) having a special affinity for or exerting its principal influence on the uterus.

uterotubal (u″ter-o-tu′bal) pertaining to the uterus and uterine tubes.

uterovaginal (u″ter-o-vaj′ĭ-nal) pertaining to the uterus and vagina.

uterovesical (u″ter-o-ves′ĭ-kal) pertaining to the uterus and bladder.

uterus (u′ter-us) a hollow muscular organ in the female pelvis; it holds and nourishes the growing fetus. The uterus, or womb, is normally about the size and shape of a pear. The upper part, or fundus, is broad and flattened; the middle portion is the body, or corpus; the lower part, or cervix, is narrow and tubular. The cervix opens downward into the VAGINA. Two UTERINE TUBES enter the uterus at the upper end, one on each side.

The walls of the uterus are composed of muscle;

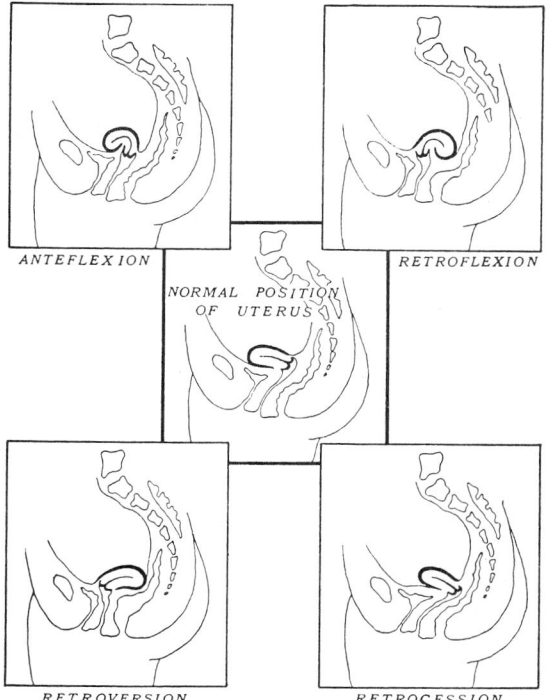

ANTEFLEXION   RETROFLEXION

NORMAL POSITION OF UTERUS

RETROVERSION   RETROCESSION

Types of forward and backward uterine displacements. (From Miller, N. F., and Avery, H.: Gynecology and Gynecologic Nursing. 5th ed. Philadelphia, W. B. Saunders Co., 1965.)

its lining is mucous membrane. The muscular substance of the uterus is called the myometrium; the inner lining is called endometrium. Between puberty and menopause, the lining goes through a monthly cycle of growth and discharge, known as the menstrual cycle. Menstruation occurs when the tissue prepared by the uterus for a possible embryo, or fertilized egg, is unused and passes out through the vagina.

The menstrual cycle is interrupted by pregnancy when a mature ovum is fertilized by a spermatozoon. Fertilization usually takes place in the uterine tube; the fertilized ovum continues moving along the tube and comes to rest in the uterus, where it implants in the endometrium. The endometrium then serves to anchor the placenta, which filters nutrients from the mother's blood into the blood of the growing fetus. (See also REPRODUCTION and REPRODUCTIVE ORGANS, FEMALE.)

DISORDERS OF THE UTERUS. The main organs of the female reproductive system—uterus, uterine tubes and ovaries—are connected to each other by ligaments that normally hold each in its proper place. Occasionally childbirth causes displacement of the uterus. The ligaments may stretch and weaken enough to permit the uterus to bulge into the vagina. This is called a prolapsed uterus. Uterine displacement may give rise to difficulties in urination and at times in conception. Internal supportive pessaries are sometimes prescribed for these conditions. Some can be corrected surgically.

The uterus is a frequent site of cancer, both of the cervix and of the corpus of the uterus. Regular medical examinations help to detect such growths promptly, and early diagnosis makes for successful treatment. Any irregular vaginal bleeding or discharge may be a symptom of such a growth and should have prompt attention.

Benign growths in the uterine walls, called myomas or fibroid tumors, are common, and are not removed unless they produce symptoms or threaten to interfere with a desired pregnancy. Myomas may occur in any part of the uterus, although they are most frequent in the corpus. Occasionally, fibrous tissues are intertwined with the muscle fibers of the tumor, particularly in older women.

Myomas are often numerous, although a single tumor may occur. They are usually small but sometimes grow quite large and may fill the whole uterus. After menopause, their growth usually ceases. Large myomas may cause pressure on neighboring organs, such as the bladder. Symptoms vary according to the location and size of the tumors. As they grow, they may cause painful menstruation, profuse and irregular menstrual bleeding, vaginal discharge or frequent urination, as well as irregular enlargement of the uterus. If the tumor becomes twisted, there may be severe pelvic pain. Myomas may also be the cause of infertility.

In pregnancy, the tumors may interfere with the natural enlargement of the uterus with the growing fetus. They may also cause spontaneous abortion and death of the fetus. Myomas in the lower part of the uterus may block the birth canal, in which case cesarean section may be necessary.

Medical examination is wise if one or more of the symptoms mentioned occur. Small myomas are usually left undisturbed and are checked at frequent intervals. Larger tumors may be removed surgically. In some instances, hysterectomy is performed. It is reassuring that only a small percentage of such tumors ever become malignant, usually in later life.

Other frequent disorders associated with the uterus are menstrual problems, including painful menstruation (DYSMENORRHEA) and excess blood flow (menorrhagia). These disorders are among the most common causes of temporary female disability and are often difficult to correct, but they may also be symptoms of serious conditions. Excessive menstruation may cause anemia.

SURGERY OF THE UTERUS. Surgical procedures involving the uterus include various operations for shortening the ligaments supporting the uterus, for the purpose of correcting uterine displacement, and hysterectomy, or surgical removal of the uterus.

Subtotal (simple) hysterectomy involves removal of all of the uterus except the cervix. This operation is most commonly performed in the case of a large myoma. After the operation pregnancy is no longer possible and menstruation ceases, but glandular functions continue. MENOPAUSE does not occur prematurely, since the ovaries still produce estrogen and progesterone.

If the entire cervix as well as the corpus of the uterus is removed, the operation is called total (complete) hysterectomy. Sometimes one or both of the uterine tubes and the ovaries are removed as well. The operation is sometimes necessary in the case of benign conditions, such as cysts and large myomas, and in malignant conditions.

As long as one ovary remains, menopause is not brought on by the operation. If both ovaries are removed, artificial menopause occurs; hormones or other medications may be given to facilitate this period of hormonal adjustment. Sexual activity is not affected.

Radical hysterectomy is one in which a portion of the vagina, the surrounding lymph nodes and the supporting ligaments of the pelvic organs are removed, in addition to the entire uterus. This operation may be performed in some cases of cancer of the cervix, although radiotherapy is usually preferred.

Usually in a hysterectomy the incision is made in the abdominal wall (abdominal hysterectomy), but in some instances the operation is performed by way of the vagina. A vaginal hysterectomy avoids the discomfort of an abdominal incision. This method may be used in certain benign conditions when other factors are favorable. When the cervix is not removed with the uterus, the procedure usually cannot be performed vaginally.

Nursing Care. Preoperative procedures usually include complete shaving of the lower abdomen and perineum, administration of a cleansing enema and a vaginal douche the evening before surgery and restriction of food and fluids as for any other type of abdominal surgery.

Postoperatively, the patient is observed frequently for signs of hemorrhage. Although some serosanguineous discharge is to be expected, bleeding that exceeds a normal menstrual flow should be reported. The number of perineal pads soiled during an 8-hour period should be noted on the chart. Intra-abdominal bleeding may be recognized by such changes as restlessness, falling blood pressure, pallor, thirst and excessive perspiration.

Complications to be avoided include thrombophlebitis, abdominal distention and urinary retention. To avoid the development of a thrombus in the legs or pelvis the patient is encouraged to exercise her legs and to breathe deeply to improve pelvic circulation. Fowler's position and pillows beneath the knees are not allowed. Any complaint of pain, tenderness or redness in the calf of the leg should be reported immediately. Early ambulation is the best preventive for most complications arising from a hysterectomy.

Abdominal distention is often avoided by insertion of a nasogastric tube prior to surgery. Urinary retention usually is prevented by insertion of a catheter while the patient is anesthetized; this is left in place until the third or fourth postoperative day.

Postoperative infection is relatively rare, but when it does occur the first symptoms develop about the third or fourth postoperative day. Elevation of temperature, malaise and foul vaginal discharge are indicative of this complication.

utricle (u'trĭ-kl) 1. any small sac. 2. the larger of the two divisions of the membranous labyrinth of the inner ear.

  prostatic u., urethral u., a small blind pouch in the substance of the prostate.

utricular (u-trik'u-lar) 1. bladder-like. 2. pertaining to the utricle.

utriculitis (u-trik″u-li′tis) inflammation of the prostatic utricle.

utriculosaccular (u-trik″u-lo-sak′u-lar) pertaining to the utricle and saccule of the membranous labyrinth of the inner ear.

uve(o)- (u′ve-o) word element, *uvea.*

uvea (u′ve-ah) the iris, ciliary body and choroid together. adj., **u′veal.**

uveitis (u″ve-i′tis) inflammation of the uvea. adj., **uveit′ic.**

  heterochromic u., uveitis in which the diseased eye differs in color from the normal one.

  sympathetic u., uveitis following the same affection in the other eye.

uveoparotid fever (u″ve-o-pah-rot′id) an infectious fever marked by inflammation of the parotid gland and uvea.

uveoplasty (u′ve-o-plas″te) plastic repair of the uvea.

uveoscleritis (u″ve-o-sklĕ-ri′tis) inflammation of the uvea and sclera.

uviform (u′vĭ-form) shaped like a grape.

uviofast (u′ve-o-fast″) uvioresistant.

uviometer (u″ve-om′ĕ-ter) an instrument for measuring ultraviolet emanation.

uvioresistant (u″ve-o-re-zis′tant) resistant to ultraviolet rays.

uviosensitive (u″ve-o-sen′sĭ-tiv) sensitive to ultraviolet rays.

uvula (u′vu-lah), pl. *u'vulae* [L.] a pendent, fleshy mass, as the dependent triangular portion of the soft palate (u′vula palati′na or palatine uvula) above the root of the tongue. adj. **u′vular.**

u. of bladder, a rounded elevation at the neck of the bladder, formed by convergence of muscle fibers terminating in the urethra.

u. cerebel′li, a lobule that is the posterior limit of the fourth ventricle of the brain.

uvulectomy (u″vu-lek′to-me) excision of the uvula.

uvulitis (u″vu-li′tis) inflammation of the uvula.

uvuloptosis (u″vu-lop-to′sis) a relaxed, pendulous state of the uvula.

uvulotomy (u″vu-lot′o-me) incision of the uvula.

V

V chemical symbol, *vanadium*.

V. velocity; vision; visual acuity; volt; volume.

V [L.] *ve′na* (vein).

vaccin (vak′sin) vaccine.

vaccina (vak-si′nah) vaccinia.

vaccinal (vak′sĭ-nal) pertaining to vaccinia or to inoculation of vaccinia virus.

vaccinate (vak′sĭ-nāt) to introduce vaccine into.

vaccination (vak″sĭ-na′shun) inoculation with weakened or dead microorganisms to develop immunity to a specific disease. The term vaccination comes from the Latin *vacca,* cow, and was coined when the first inoculations were given with organisms that caused the mild disease cowpox to produce immunity against smallpox. Today the word has the same meaning as inoculation and IMMUNIZATION.

vaccine (vak′sēn) a suspension of attenuated or killed microorganisms (viruses, bacteria or rickettsiae), administered for prevention, amelioration or treatment of infectious diseases.

   autogenous v., a bacterial vaccine prepared from cultures of material derived from a lesion of the patient to be treated.

   BCG v., a preparation for prophylactic inoculation of young infants or other susceptible persons against tuberculosis, consisting of living cultures of bovine tubercle bacilli that have been grown on glycerinated ox bile so that their virulence is greatly reduced (see also BCG VACCINE).

   polyvalent v., one prepared from more than one strain or species of microorganisms.

vaccinia (vak-sin′e-ah) a virus disease of cattle; called also cowpox. When communicated to man, usually by vaccination, it confers immunity to smallpox. Introduction of vaccinia virus for the purpose of immunization against smallpox results in a local reaction—a single lesion at the site of inoculation—or sometimes a general reaction.

In nonimmune patients a papule appears on the third or fourth day after inoculation. The lesion then changes to a vesicle (water-filled blister) and eventually to a pustule which lasts for about 12 days and then dries and forms a crust. During the following 7 days the crust detaches and leaves the characteristic vaccination scar.

Complications of vaccinia are rare. They include autoinoculation, in which other satellite lesions may appear over the body, secondary infection with streptococci or staphylococci and postvaccinal encephalitis. Eczema vaccinatum can occur in persons in whom skin lesions of eczema are present at the time of vaccination. The eruption becomes generalized, particularly in the area where the primary dermatitis was located. To avoid this complication vaccination is contraindicated in patients who have eczema or other skin disorders.

No special treatment or dressing is required for the vaccinia. The lesion should be kept dry and open to the air.

   generalized v., a condition of widespread vaccinal lesions resulting from sensitivity response to smallpox vaccination and delayed production of neutralizing antibodies.

   progressive v., vaccinia in which the patient fails to produce antibodies, with spreading necrosis at the site of the inoculation, metastatic necrotic lesions throughout the body, and eventually death.

vacciniform (vak-sin′ĭ-form) resembling vaccinia.

vacciniola (vak″sĭ-ne-o′lah) secondary eruption of vesicles after vaccination.

vaccinoid (vak′sĭ-noid) spurious or modified vaccinia.

vaccinotherapy (vak″sĭ-no-ther′ah-pe) treatment with bacterial vaccines.

vacuolation (vak″u-o-la′shun) the formation of vacuoles.

vacuole (vak′u-ōl) a space or cavity in the protoplasm of a cell.

   contractile v., a small cavity found in many protozoa that regularly fills with water from the surrounding protoplasm and empties it to the environment.

vacuolization (vak″u-o-lĭ-za′shun) vacuolation.

vacuum (vak′u-um) a space devoid of air or gas; a space from which the air has been exhausted.

vagabond's disease discoloration of the skin from lice.

vagal (va′gal) pertaining to the vagus nerve.

vagina (vah-ji′nah) 1. any sheath or sheathlike structure; used in anatomic nomenclature to designate many enveloping tissues. 2. the canal in the female, from the external genitalia (vulva) to the cervix uteri. The adult vagina is normally about 3 inches long and slopes upward and backward. Internally, the bladder is in front of the vagina and the rectum in back.

The vagina receives the erect penis in coitus. The spermatozoa are discharged into the vagina, swim through the cervical canal and enter the uterus. The vagina is also the passage for menstrual discharge and functions as the birth canal.

The interior lining of the vagina is mucous membrane. Muscles and fibrous tissue form the vaginal walls. In pregnancy, changes occur in these tissues, enabling the vagina to stretch to many times its usual size during labor and childbirth.

In a virgin, the opening of the vagina is usually,

but not necessarily, partially closed by a membrane, the hymen. Usually the hymen breaks at first intercourse; occasionally it ruptures during physical exercise.

In a normal state, the lining of the vagina secretes a fluid that is fermented to an acid by the bacteria that are usually present. This acidity probably helps to protect the vagina from invasion by other organisms. Douching as a regular practice should not be employed except when recommended by a physician.

DISORDERS OF THE VAGINA. Symptoms of vaginal disorders include excessive discharge, soreness and burning, ulceration, pain on intercourse, itching, bleeding, swelling and growths. A physician should be consulted for any of these complaints.

Infection is the most common cause of vaginal disease. A frequent chronic infection is caused by a protozoon called *Trichomonas vaginalis*. A yeast-like organism causes another type of infectious vaginitis (candidiasis). The vagina may also be affected by gonorrhea, syphilis and other venereal diseases. Diabetes mellitus may predispose a woman to vaginal infection.

Trauma during childbirth may damage the vagina. After menopause, the mucous lining tends to dry out and become irritated easily. Cysts and cancers may form in the vagina. Occasionally a fistula, or abnormal passage, may develop between the vagina and the bladder or rectum.

VAGINAL EXAMINATION. Since cancer of the female reproductive organs is a relatively common occurrence and is curable if detected early, physicians recommend that women of reproductive age and beyond have a periodic vaginal or pelvis examination. Such an examination is also necessary during pregnancy and labor and in the postpartum examination 6 to 8 weeks after childbirth. This is a simple procedure that is rarely uncomfortable if the woman understands its purpose.

The patient lies on her back on a special table with her legs raised and spread by stirrups. The physician inserts a speculum to spread the vagina open. He is able to observe the cervix and the lining of the vagina directly, and may take smears for microscopic examination to detect infection or cancer.

After removing the speculum the physician inserts rubber-gloved fingers into the vagina and places the other hand on the abdomen. In this way he is able to palpate the female reproductive organs, including the uterus and ovaries, between his hands. These organs are otherwise difficult or impossible to examine.

Nursing Care. The patient should be prepared physically and emotionally for a vaginal examination. Since relaxation and cooperation of the patient are important to the success of the examination, she should be given a brief explanation of the procedure and encouraged to ask questions before the procedure is begun. The patient is draped with a top sheet so that the legs are covered and only the vulva is exposed. Privacy must be assured immediately before and during the examination. Equipment such as gloves, lubricant and vaginal speculum should be assembled before the physician is summoned to the examining room, and the nurse remains in attendance during the examination. After the physician has completed the examination the patient is assisted from the table.

Ideally, a vaginal examination should be done be-

tween menstrual periods; however, vaginal bleeding is not a contraindication to this procedure. Patients should be told this so that they will not postpone an appointment with the physician when vaginal bleeding persists. They also should be instructed to avoid douching immediately before a vaginal examination as this may remove secretions that can be useful in diagnosis.

vaginal (vaj′ĭ-nal) pertaining to the vagina, the tunica vaginalis testis or any sheath.

vaginalectomy (vaj″ĭ-nal-ek′to-me) excision of the tunica vaginalis testis.

vaginalitis (vaj′ĭ-nal-i′tis) inflammation of the tunica vaginalis testis.

vaginate (vaj′ĭ-nāt) enclosed in a sheath.

vaginismus (vaj″ĭ-niz′mus) painful spasm of the muscles of the vagina.

vaginitis (vaj″ĭ-ni′tis) 1. inflammation of the vagina. 2. inflammation of a sheath.
  v. adhae′siva, senile vaginitis.
  diphtheritic v., diphtheritic inflammation of the vagina.
  emphysematous v., a variety marked by the formation of gas in the meshes of the connective tissue.
  glandular v., a form affecting only the vaginal glands.
  granular v., the most common variety, in which the papillae are enlarged and infiltrated with small cells.
  senile v., vaginitis occurring in old age and marked by the formation of raw patches, which often adhere to apposed surfaces, causing obliteration of the vaginal canal.
  v. tes′tis, perididymitis; inflammation of the tunica vaginalis testis.

vaginoabdominal (vaj″ĭ-no-ab-dom′ĭ-nal) pertaining to the vagina and abdomen.

vaginocele (vaj′ĭ-no-sēl″) colpocele; vaginal hernia.

vaginocutaneous (vaj″ĭ-no-ku-ta′ne-us) pertaining to the vagina and skin, or communicating with the vagina and the cutaneous surface of the body.

vaginodynia (vaj″ĭ-no-din′e-ah) pain in the vagina.

vaginofixation (vaj″ĭ-no-fik-sa′shun) vaginopexy; colpopexy.

vaginogenic (vaj″ĭ-no-jen′ik) originating in the vagina.

vaginogram (vah-ji′no-gram) a roentgenogram of the vagina.

vaginography (vaj″ĭ-nog′rah-fe) roentgenography of the vagina.

vaginolabial (vaj″ĭ-no-la′be-al) pertaining to the vagina and labia.

vaginometer (vaj″ĭ-nom′ĕ-ter) an instrument for measuring the vagina.

vaginomycosis (vaj″ĭ-no-mi-ko′sis) fungus disease of vagina.

vaginopathy (vaj″ĭ-nop′ah-the) any disease of the vagina.

vaginoperineal (vaj″ĭ-no-per″ĭ-ne′al) pertaining to the vagina and perineum.

vaginoperineorrhaphy (vaj″ĭ-no-per″ĭ-ne-or′ah-fe) suture of the vagina and perineum.

vaginoperineotomy (vaj″ĭ-no-per″ĭ-ne-ot′o-me) incision of the vagina and perineum.

vaginoperitoneal (vaj″ĭ-no-per″ĭ-to-ne′al) pertaining to the vagina and peritoneum.

vaginopexy (vah-ji′no-pek″se) colpopexy; suturing of the vagina to the abdominal wall in cases of vaginal relaxation.

vaginoplasty (vah-ji′no-plas″te) colpoplasty; plastic repair of the vagina.

vaginotomy (vaj″ĭ-not′o-me) colpotomy; incision of the vagina.

vaginovesical (vaj″ĭ-no-ves′ĭ-kal) pertaining to the vagina and bladder.

vagitis (va-gi′tis) inflammation of the vagus nerve.

vagitus (vah-ji′tus) the cry of an infant.
   v. uteri′nus, the cry of an infant in the uterus.

vagolysis (va-gol′ĭ-sis) destruction of the esophageal branches of the vagus nerve for cardiospasm.

vagolytic (va″go-lit′ik) having an effect resembling that produced by interruption of impulses transmitted by the vagus nerve; parasympatholytic.

vagomimetic (va″go-mi-met′ik) having an effect resembling that produced by stimulation of the vagus nerve.

vagosympathetic (va″go-sim″pah-thet′ik) pertaining to both the vagus and sympathetic innervation.

vagotomy (va-got′o-me) interruption of the impulses carried by the vagus nerve or nerves; so called because it was first performed by surgical methods. The surgical procedure is done as part of the treatment of gastric or duodenal ULCER and often is performed in combination with gastroenterostomy or partial gastrectomy. The vagus nerve stimulates gastric secretion and affects gastric motility. Vagotomy thus reduces secretion of gastric juices and decreases physical activity of the stomach.
   medical v., interruption of impulses carried by the vagus nerve by administration of suitable drugs.

vagotonia (va″go-to′ne-ah) irritability of the vagus nerve, characterized by vasomotor instability, sweating, disordered peristalsis and muscle spasms. adj., **vagoton′ic.**

vagotonin (va-got′o-nin) a preparation of hormone from the pancreas that increases vagal tone, slows the heart and increases the store of glycogen in the liver.

vagotropic (va″go-trop′ik) having an effect on the vagus nerve.

vagotropism (va-got′ro-pizm) affinity of a drug for the vagus nerve.

vagovagal (va″go-va′gal) arising as a result of afferent and efferent impulses mediated through the vagus nerve.

vagus nerve (va′gus) the tenth cranial nerve; it has the most extensive distribution of the cranial nerves, serving structures of the chest and abdomen as well as the head and neck.
   Afferent fibers of the vagus nerve serve the mucous membrane of larynx, trachea and bronchi, lungs, arch of the aorta, esophagus and stomach. Some of the functions affected by this nerve are coughing, sneezing, reflex inhibitions of the heart rate and the sensation of hunger.
   Motor fibers of the vagus nerve are concerned with swallowing, speech, peristalsis and secretions from the glands of the stomach and the pancreas and contractions of the trachea, bronchi and bronchioles.

valence (va′lens) 1. the power of an atom to combine with other atoms, the combining power of the hydrogen atom being considered unity, and the valence of atoms of other elements being the number of hydrogen atoms they combine with. 2. an expression of the number of reactive sites on the surface of the molecules by which homologous antigens and antibody specifically combine.

valethamate (val-eth′ah-māt) a compound used as an antispasmodic and anticholinergic.

valgus (val′gus) [L.] bent outward; commonly used to designate angulation away from the midline of the body.

valine (va′lēn) a naturally occurring amino acid, one of those essential for optimal growth in infants and for nitrogen equilibrium in human adults.

vallate (val′āt) surrounded with an elevation; cupped.

vallecula (vah-lek′u-lah), pl. *vallec′ulae* [L.] a depression or hollow.
   v. cerebel′li, a longitudinal fissure of the cerebellum.
   v. syl′vii, a depression made by the fissure of Sylvius at the base of the brain.
   v. un′guis, the depression at the root of a nail.

Vallestril (val-les′tril) trademark for a preparation of methallenestril, an estrogenic compound.

Valley fever coccidioidomycosis.

Valmid (val′mid) trademark for a preparation of ethinamate, a hypnotic.

value (val′u) an expression of worth or efficiency, or of other measurable attribute.
   liminal v., threshold v., that intensity of a stimulus which produces a just noticeable impression.

valva (val′vah), pl. *val′vae* [L.] a valve.

valve (valv) a membranous fold in a canal or passage that prevents backward flow of material passing through it.
   aortic v., that guarding the entrance to the aorta from the left ventricle.
   bicuspid v., mitral valve.

cardiac v's, valves that control flow of blood through and from the heart.

coronary v., a valve at entrance of coronary sinus into right atrium.

ileocecal v., ileocolic v., that guarding the opening between the ileum and cecum.

mitral v., that guarding the opening between the left atrium and left ventricle.

pulmonary v., that at the entrance of the pulmonary trunk from the right ventricle.

pyloric v., a prominent fold of mucous membrane at the junction of the stomach and duodenum.

semilunar v's, valves made up of semilunar segments or cusps (valvulae semilunares), guarding the entrances into the aorta and pulmonary trunk from the cardiac ventricles.

thebesian v., a fold of endocardium at the opening of the coronary sinus in the right atrium of the heart.

tricuspid v., that guarding the opening between the right atrium and right ventricle.

valvotomy (val-vot'o-me) incision of a valve; splitting of the commissures of a valve for dilation of the opening.

mitral v., splitting of the commissures of the valve between the left atrium and ventricle, with extension of the opening (see also COMMISS-UROTOMY).

valvula (val'vu-lah), pl. *val'vulae* [L.] a small valve.

val'vulae conniven'tes, transverse mucous folds in the small intestine.

valvular (val'vu-lar) pertaining to, affecting or of the nature of a valve.

valvulectomy (val"vu-lek'to-me) excision of a valve.

valvulitis (val"vu-li'tis) inflammation of a valve, especially of a valve of the heart.

valvuloplasty (val'vu-lo-plas"te) plastic repair of a valve, especially a valve of the heart.

valvulotome (val'vu-lo-tōm") an instrument for cutting a valve.

valvulotomy (val"vu-lot'o-me) valvotomy.

vanadium (vah-na'de-um) a chemical element, atomic number 23, atomic weight 50.942, symbol V. (See table of ELEMENTS.)

vanadiumism (vah-na'de-um-izm") poisoning by vanadium.

Vancocin (van'ko-sin) trademark for a preparation of vancomycin, an antibiotic.

vancomycin (van"ko-mi'sin) an antibiotic used mainly in the treatment of resistant staphylococcal infections. The toxic effects are quite severe and include damage to the eighth cranial (vestibulo-cochlear) nerve and renal disorders.

van den Bergh test (van den berg') a laboratory test done to determine the concentration of BILI-RUBIN in the blood. Blood is obtained by finger prick or venipuncture. Preparation of the patient requires only that he be in a fasting state. Normal range for this test is: direct bilirubin—0.0 to 0.1 mg. per 100 ml. of serum; total bilirubin—0.2 to 1.4 mg. per 100 ml. of serum.

van der Hoeve's syndrome (van der hōvz) a genetically determined condition characterized by blue scleras, deafness and abnormal brittleness of bones.

vanilla (vah-nil'ah) cured, full-grown, unripe fruit of species of Vanilla; used as a flavoring agent.

vanillal (vah-nil'al) ethyl vanillin.

vanillin (vah-nil'in) an aromatic, crystallizable principle used as a flavoring agent.

ethyl v., fine white or slightly yellowish crystals, with a taste and odor similar to those of vanilla; used as a flavoring agent.

vanillism (vah-nil'ism) dermatitis and pruritus from handling vanilla.

vanillylmandelic acid (vah-nil"il-man-del'ik) the major urinary metabolite of both epinephrine and norepinephrine.

Vanogel (van'o-jel) trademark for an aqueous suspension of aluminum hydroxide gel, an antacid.

van't Hoff's law (vant hofs') the velocity of chemical reactions is increased twofold or more for each rise of 10° C. in temperature.

vapor (va'por) a gas, especially of a compound which at ordinary temperatures is a liquid or solid.

vaporization (va"por-ĭ-za'shun) dispersal of a liquid in the form of a gas.

vapotherapy (va"po-ther'ah-pe) treatment by vapor or spray.

Vaquez's disease (vah-kāz') polycythemia vera.

varicella (var"ĭ-sel'ah) chickenpox.

variciform (vah-ris'ĭ-form) having the form of a varix.

varicoblepharon (var"ĭ-ko-blef'ah-ron) a varicose tumor of the eyelid.

varicocele (var'ĭ-ko-sēl") a cystic accumulation of blood in the spermatic cord.

varicocelectomy (var"ĭ-ko-se-lek'to-me) excision of a varicocele.

varicography (var"ĭ-kog'rah-fe) x-ray visualization of varicose veins.

varicomphalos (var"ĭ-kom'fah-los) a varicose tumor of the umbilicus.

varicophlebitis (var"ĭ-ko-flĕ-bi'tis) infection in varicose veins.

varicose (var'ĭ-kōs) of or pertaining to a varix; unnaturally swollen.

v. veins, swollen, distended and knotted veins visible especially in the legs. They result from a stagnated or sluggish flow of the blood, probably in combination with defective valves and weakened walls of the veins.

Varicose veins occur most frequently in those who must stand or sit motionless for long periods of time. Pregnancy is sometimes responsible for the development of the condition. It also appears that a tendency to develop varicose veins may be inherited.

CAUSES. Blood returning to the heart from the legs must flow upward through the veins, against the pull of gravity. This blood is "milked" upward principally by the massaging action of the muscles against the veins. To prevent the blood from flowing backward, the veins contain flaplike valves, located at frequent intervals and operating in pairs. When the blood is flowing toward the heart, the venous valves are open and the blood can move freely. If the blood should attempt to flow backward, the valves close, effectively stopping the reverse movement of the blood.

Prolonged periods of standing or sitting without movement place a heavy strain on the veins. Without the massaging action of the muscles, the blood tends to back up. The weight of blood continually pressing downward against the closed venous valves causes the veins to distend; after a time, they lose their natural elasticity. When a number of valves no longer function efficiently, the blood collects in the veins, which gradually become swollen and more distended.

During pregnancy, more force often is necessary to push the blood through the veins because the pregnant uterus tends to press against the veins coming from the legs and thus prevents the free flow of blood. This increased back pressure can result in varicose veins.

SYMPTOMS. The development of varicose veins is usually gradual. There may be feelings of fatigue in the legs and leg cramps at night; a continual dull ache may develop in the legs, and the ankles may swell.

If the condition is left untreated and allowed to spread, as it often does, the veins become thick and hard to the touch, and dull or stabbing pains may be felt in time. Because of impaired circulation ulcers often develop on the lower legs.

TREATMENT. Treatment of mild cases of varicose veins includes rest periods at intervals during the day; the patient lies flat with his feet raised slightly above his body. Bathing the legs in warm water helps to stimulate the flow of blood, as does exercise. The daily routine should be changed to allow movement and changes in posture; even a brief walk will stimulate circulation grown stagnant during a time of standing or sitting in one position. Stockings lightly reinforced with elastic can be worn to help support the veins in the legs. Heavy elastic stockings, however, should be fitted and worn only under medical supervision, for if they do not fit correctly they may aggravate the condition by further restricting the flow of blood.

Injections. Certain cases of varicose veins that have developed past the stage at which exercise and rest are helpful may be treated by injections of a hardening, or sclerosing, solution into the affected veins. A few hours after this treatment, which usually can be performed in the physician's office, the injected veins become hard, tender to the touch and painful. The pain subsides within a few days, however, and in about 2 months the varicose veins atrophy while the blood is channeled into other veins leading toward the heart.

The number of injections necessary depends upon the extent of the condition, and this form of treatment usually is not recommended for advanced cases because it has been found that in such cases recurrence is likely after a varying period of time following the injections.

Surgery. Varicose veins can cause much discomfort. The poor circulation involved means that any break in the skin of the leg is likely to develop into an ulcer that is painful and heals slowly and with difficulty. Therefore, chronic or well-advanced varicose conditions are best treated surgically. The operation consists of ligating (tying off) the affected vein and removing it.

Prevention. Regular leg exercises or long walks will stimulate the flow of blood through the legs. Those who have a predisposition to varicose veins should make such activities a part of their regular routine. If possible, they should avoid occupations that require them to stand or sit motionless for long periods of time, or should make it a point to walk about and exercise their leg muscles at frequent intervals during working hours. Tight stockings or garters should not be worn, nor should clothing that fits tightly or binds.

Normal veins

Functional valves aid in flow of venous blood back to heart

(see enlargement at left)

Varicose veins

Failure of valves and pooling of blood in superficial veins

Comparison of normal veins and varicose veins in the leg.

varicosity (var″ĭ-kos′ĭ-te) 1. a varix. 2. the quality of being enlarged and tortuous.

varicotomy (var″ĭ-kot′o-me) excision of a varix or of a varicose vein.

varicula (vah-rik′u-lah) a varix of the conjunctiva.

Varidase (var′ĭ-dās) trademark for preparations of streptokinase-streptodornase, used as a proteolytic and fibrinolytic agent, for enzymatic débridement.

variety (vah-ri′ĕ-te) a taxonomic category subordinate to a species.

variola (vah-ri′o-lah) smallpox. adj., **va′riolate.**
  v. mi′nor, a mild form of smallpox having a low fatality rate.

variolation (va″re-o-la′shun) application or ingestion of crusts of dried variola pustules to produce immunity to natural infection by the virus of smallpox.

varioloid (va′re-o-loid″) infection by the virus of smallpox producing no or slight symptoms in a previously vaccinated person, who is capable of transmitting infection that may be fatal to a susceptible person.

variolous (vah-ri′o-lus) pertaining to smallpox.

varix (vār′iks), pl. *var′ices* [L.] an enlarged, tortuous vein. adj., **var′icose.**
  aneurysmal v., a varix due to direct communication with an adjacent artery as a result of a wound.
  arterial v., an enlarged, tortuous artery.
  v. lymphat′icus, an enlarged and tortuous lymphatic vessel.

varolian (vah-ro′le-an) pertaining to the pons varolii.

varus (va′rus) [L.] bent inward; commonly used to indicate angulation toward the midline of the body.

vas (vas), pl. *va′sa* [L.] a vessel. adj., **va′sal.**
  v. aber′rans 1. a blind tube sometimes connected with the epididymis or vas deferens. 2. any anomalous or unusual vessel.
  va′sa afferen′tia, vessels that convey fluid to a structure or part.
  va′sa bre′via, the small branches of the splenic artery going to the stomach.
  v. def′erens, the excretory duct of the testis, which unites with the excretory duct of the seminal vesicle to form the ejaculatory duct; called also ductus deferens.
  va′sa efferen′tia, vessels that convey fluid away from a structure or part.
  v. lymphat′icum, a vessel that conveys lymph.
  va′sa prae′via, appearance of the vessels of the umbilical cord ahead of the presenting part of the fetus at the opening of the uterus.
  va′sa rec′ta, straight tubes formed by the seminiferous tubules.
  va′sa vaso′rum, vessels conveying blood to and from the outer and middle coats of the larger blood vessels.

vas(o)- (vas′o) word element [L.], *blood vessel; vas (ductus) deferens.*

vascular (vas′ku-lar) pertaining to or full of vessels.

vascularity (vas″ku-lar′ĭ-te) the condition of being vascular.

vascularization (vas″ku-lar-ĭ-za′shun) the process of becoming vascular.

vascularize (vas′ku-lar-īz″) to supply with vessels.

vasculature (vas′ku-lah-tūr″) 1. the vascular system of the body, or any part of it. 2. the supply of vessels to a specific region.

vasculitis (vas″ku-li′tis) inflammation of a vessel.

vasectomy (vah-sek′to-me) excision of the vas (ductus) deferens, or a portion of it; bilateral vasectomy results in sterility.

vasifactive (vas′ĭ-fak′tiv) producing new vessels.

vasiform (vas′ĭ-form) resembling a vas or vessel.

vasitis (vas-i′tis) inflammation of the vas (ductus) deferens.

vasoconstriction (vas″o-kon-strik′shun) decrease in the caliber of blood vessels. adj., **vasoconstric′tive.**

vasoconstrictor (vas″o-kon-strik′tor) 1. causing constriction of the blood vessels. 2. an agent (motor nerve or chemical compound) that acts to decrease the caliber of blood vessels.

vasocorona (vas″o-kŏ-ro′nah) the assemblage of arteries passing radially into the spinal cord from its periphery.

vasodentin (vas″o-den′tin) dentin provided with blood vessels.

vasodepression (vas″o-de-presh′un) vasomotor depression or collapse.

vasodepressor (vas″o-de-pres′or) 1. having a depressing effect on the circulation. 2. an agent that causes vasomotor depression.

Vasodilan (vas″o-di′lan) trademark for preparations of isoxsuprine hydrochloride, a vasodilator and uterine relaxant.

vasodilatation (vas″o-dil″ah-ta′shun) dilatation of blood vessels.

vasodilation (vas″o-di-la′shun) increase in the caliber of blood vessels.

vasodilator (vas″o-di-la′tor) 1. causing dilation of blood vessels. 2. a nerve or agent that causes dilation of blood vessels.

vasoepididymostomy (vas″o-ep″ĭ-did″ĭ-mos′to-me) anastomosis of the vas (ductus) deferens and the epididymis.

vasoganglion (vas″o-gang′gle-on) a vascular ganglion or rete.

vasography (vas-og′rah-fe) roentgenography of the blood vessels.

vasohypertonic (vas"o-hi"per-ton'ik) increasing the tone of blood vessels.

vasohypotonic (vas"o-hi"po-ton'ik) decreasing the tone of blood vessels.

vasoinert (vas"o-in-ert') having no effect on the caliber of blood vessels.

vasoinhibitor (vas"o-in-hib'ĭ-tor) 1. inhibiting the vasomotor nerves. 2. an agent that inhibits vaso-motor nerves. adj., **vasoinhib'itory.**

vasoligation (vas"o-li-ga'shun) ligation of the vas (ductus) deferens.

vasomotion (vas"o-mo'shun) the change in caliber of blood vessels.

vasomotor (vas"o-mo'tor) having an effect on the caliber of blood vessels.

vasomotorium (vas"o-mo-to re-um) the vaso-motor system of the body.

vasoneuropathy (vas"o-nu-rop'ah-the) a condi-tion caused by combined vascular and neurologic defect, resulting from simultaneous action or inter-action of the vascular and nervous systems.

vasoneurosis (vas"o-nu-ro'sis) angioneurosis.

vaso-orchidostomy (vas"o-or"kĭ-dos'to-me) anas-tomosis of the epididymis to the severed end of the vas deferens.

vasoparesis (vas"o-pah-re'sis) paralysis of vaso-motor nerves.

vasopressin (vas"o-pres'in) a water-soluble prin-ciple from the posterior lobe of the PITUITARY GLAND which increases blood pressure and in-fluences the reabsorption of water by the kidney tubules. It stimulates contraction of the intestinal musculature and increases peristalsis, and it also exerts some influence on the uterus. Called also antidiuretic hormone.

vasopressor (vas"o-pres'or) an agent that stimu-lates contraction of the muscular tissue of capil-laries and arteries.

vasopuncture (vas"o-pungk'tūr) puncture of the vas (ductus) deferens.

vasoreflex (vas"o-re'fleks) a reflex of blood vessels.

vasorelaxation (vas"o-re"lak-sa'shun) decrease of vascular pressure.

vasoresection (vas"o-re-sek'shun) resection of the vas (ductus) deferens.

vasorrhaphy (vas-or'ah-fe) suture of the vas (ductus) deferens.

vasosection (vas"o-sek'shun) the severing of a vessel or vessels, especially of the vasa deferentia (ductus deferentes).

vasosensory (vas"o-sen'so-re) supplying sensory filaments to the vessels.

vasospasm (vas'o-spazm) spasm of a vessel. adj., **vasospas'tic.**

vasospasmolytic (vas"o-spaz"mo-lit'ik) arresting spasm of the vessels.

vasostimulant (vas"o-stim'u-lant) stimulating vasomotor action.

vasothrombin (vas"o-throm'bin) a fibrin factor formed from the endothelial cells of the vessels, which takes part in the formation of thrombin.

vasotomy (vah-sot'o-me) incision of the vas (ductus) deferens.

vasotonic (vas"o-ton'ik) regulating the tone of a vessel.

vasotrophic (vas"o-trof'ik) affecting nutrition through alterations of the caliber of the blood vessels.

vasotropic (vas"o-trop'ik) exerting an influence on the blood vessels, causing either constriction or dilatation.

vasovasostomy (vas"o-vah-sos'to-me) restoration of the continuity of the divided vas (ductus) def-erens.

vasovesiculectomy (vas"o-vě-sik"u-lek'to-me) excision of the vas (ductus) deferens and seminal vesicle.

vasovesiculitis (vas"o-vě-sik"u-li'tis) inflamma-tion of the vas (ductus) deferens and seminal vesicle.

Vasoxyl (vas-ok'sil) trademark for preparations of methoxamine hydrochloride, a sympathomimetic and vasopressor.

vastus (vas'tus) [L.] great.

V.C. 1. vital capacity. 2. acuity of color vision.

V-cillin (ve-sil'in) trademark for preparations of penicillin V.

V.D. venereal disease.

V.D.G. venereal disease – gonorrhea.

V.D.H. valvular disease of the heart.

VDM vasodepressor material, a substance formed by the liver that stimulates secretion of vasopressin (antidiuretic hormone).

V.D.R.L. Venereal Disease Research Laboratory.

V.D.S. venereal disease – syphilis.

vection (vek'shun) the mechanical transmission of disease germs from an infected person to a well person.

vectis (vek'tis) a curved lever for making traction on the fetal head in labor.

vector (vek'tor) a carrier; an animal (often an arthropod) that transfers an infective agent from one host to another. The mosquito, which carries the malaria parasite, Plasmodium, from man to man, and the tsetse fly, which carries trypanosomes from beast to man, are vectors, as are dogs, bats and other animals that transmit the rabies virus to man. **biologic v.,** an arthropod vector in whose body the infecting organism develops or multiplies be-fore becoming infective to the recipient individual. **mechanical v.,** an arthropod vector that transmits the infective organisms from one host to another but is not essential to the life cycle of the parasite.

vectorcardiogram (vek″tor-kor′de-o-gram″) the record, usually a photograph, of the loop formed on the oscilloscope in vectorcardiography.

vectorcardiography (vek″tor-kar″de-og′rah-fe) the registration, by formation of a loop on an oscilloscope, of the direction and magnitude of the moment-to-moment electromotive forces of the heart during one complete cycle.

vegan (vej′an) a vegetarian who excludes from his diet all protein of animal origin.

veganism (vej′ah-nizm) strict adherence to a vegetable diet, with exclusion of all protein of animal origin.

vegetable (vej′ĕ-tah-bl) pertaining to or derived from plants.

vegetal (vej′ĕ-tal) common to plants.

vegetarian (vej″ĕ-ta′re-an) one who eats only foods of vegetable origin.

vegetarianism (vej″ĕ-ta′re-ah-nizm″) the restriction of man's food to substances of vegetable origin.

vegetation (vej″ĕ-ta′shun) a plantlike neoplasm or growth.

vegetative (vej′ĕ-ta″tiv) concerned with growth and nutrition.

vegetoanimal (vej′ĕ-to-an′ĭ-mal) common to plants and animals.

vehicle (ve′ĭ-kl) a transporting agent, especially the component of a medication (prescription) serving as a solvent or to increase the bulk or decrease the concentration of the mixture.

veil (vāl) 1. a covering structure. 2. a caul or piece of amniotic sac occasionally covering the face of a newborn child. 3. slight huskiness of the voice.

vein (vān) a vessel through which blood passes from various organs or parts back to the heart, in the systemic circulation carrying blood that has given up most of its oxygen. Veins, like arteries, have three coats, an inner, middle and outer, but the coats are not so thick and they collapse when the vessel is cut. Many veins, especially the superficial, have valves formed of reduplication of their lining membrane. (For named veins of the body, see the table.)

    afferent v's, veins that carry blood to an organ.

    allantoic v's paired vessels that accompany the allantois, growing out from the primitive hindgut and entering the body stalk of the early embryo.

    aqueous v's, microscopic, blood vessel-like pathways on the surface of the eye, containing aqueous humor or diluted blood.

    cardinal v's, various (anterior, common and posterior) paired vessels in the early embryo.

    central v., one occupying the axis of an organ.

    emissary v., one passing through a foramen of the skull and draining blood from a cerebral sinus into a vessel outside the skull.

    hypophyseoportal v's, a system of venules connecting capillaries in the hypothalamus with

sinusoidal capillaries in the anterior lobe of the hypophysis (pituitary gland).

    postcardinal v's, paired vessels in the early embryo that return blood from regions caudal to the heart.

    precardinal v's, paired vessels that drain blood from the head region of the embryo.

    pulp v's, vessels draining the venous sinuses of the spleen.

    subcardinal v's, paired vessels in the embryo that replace and supplement the postcardinal veins.

    sublobular v's, tributaries of the hepatic veins that receive the central veins of hepatic lobules.

    supracardinal v's, paired vessels in the embryo developing later than the subcardinal veins and persisting chiefly as the lower segment of the inferior vena cava.

    trabecular v's, vessels coursing in splenic trabeculae, formed by tributary pulp veins.

    umbilical v., a vessel contained in the umbilical cord that conveys blood from the placenta to the fetus.

    varicose v., a permanently distended and tortuous vein, especially one in the leg (see also VARICOSE VEINS).

    vitelline v's, early veins of the developing embryo, communicating with the yolk sac.

Velacycline (val″ah-si′klēn) trademark for preparations of rolitetracycline, an antibiotic.

velamen (ve-la′men), pl. *velam′ina* [L.] a membrane, meninx or tegument. adj., **velamen′tous.**

Velban (vel′ban) trademark for a preparation of vinblastine sulfate, an antineoplastic agent.

vellication (vel″ĭ-ka′shun) a twitching of a muscle.

vellus (vel′us) the coat of fine hairs that appears after the lanugo hairs are cast off and persists until puberty.

velopharyngeal (vel″o-fah-rin′je-al) pertaining to the velum palatinum and pharynx.

velum (ve′lum), pl. *ve′la* [L.] a covering structure or veil. adj., **ve′lar.**

    v. interpos′itum, the membranous roof of the third ventricle of the brain.

    medullary v., one of the two portions (superior medullary velum and inferior medullary velum) of the white matter of the hindbrain that form the roof of the fourth ventricle.

    palatine v., v. palati′num, the dependent portion of the soft palate, including the uvula.

VEM vasoexcitor material.

vena (ve′nah), pl. *ve′nae* [L.] vein.

    v. ca′va, inferior, the vein that returns blood to the heart from the lower part of the body (see table of VEINS).

    v. ca′va, superior, The vein that returns blood to the heart from the upper part of the body (see table of VEINS).

    ve′nae comitan′tes, veins accompanying arteries.

venacavography (ve″nah-ka-vog′rah-fe) roentgenography of a vena cava; usually denoting that of the inferior vena cava.

TABLE OF VEINS

COMMON NAME	NA TERM	REGION	RECEIVES BLOOD FROM	DRAINS INTO
accompanying v. of hypoglossal nerve	v. comitans nervi hypoglossi	accompanies hypoglossal nerve	formed by union of profunda linguae v. and sublingual v.	facial, lingual or internal jugular v.
anastomotic v., inferior	v. anastomotica inferior	interconnects superficial middle cerebral v. and superior sagittal sinus		
anastomotic v., superior	v. anastomotica superior	interconnects superficial middle cerebral v. and transverse sinus		
angular v.	v. angularis	between eye and root of nose	formed by union of supratrochlear v. and supraorbital v.	continues as facial v. behind facial artery
antebrachial v., median	v. mediana antebrachii	forearm between cephalic v. and basilic v.	a palmar venous plexus	cephalic v. and/or basilic v., or median cubital v.
appendicular v.	v. appendicularis	accompanies appendicular artery		joins anterior and posterior cecal vv. to form ileocolic v.
v. of aqueduct of vestibule	v. aqueductus vestibuli	passes through aqueduct of vestibule	internal ear	superior petrosal sinus
arcuate vv. of kidney	vv. arcuatae renis	a series of complete arches across the bases of the renal pyramids, formed by union of interlobular vv. and straight venules of kidney		interlobar vv.
auditory vv., internal. See labyrinthine vv.				
auricular vv., anterior	vv. auriculares anteriores	anterior part of auricle of external ear		superficial temporal v.
auricular v., posterior	v. auricularis posterior	passes down behind auricle	a plexus on side of head	joins retromandibular v. to form external jugular v.
axillary v.	v. axillaris	the upper limb	formed at lower	at lateral border of first rib be-

				comes subclavian v.
azygos v.	v. azygos	intercepting trunk for right intercostal vv. as well as connecting branch between superior and inferior venae cavae; it ascends in front of and on right side of vertebrae	ascending lumbar v.	superior vena cava
azygos v., left. *See* hemiazygos v.				
azygos v., lesser superior. *See* hemiazygos v., accessory				
basal v.	v. basalis	passes from anterior perforated substance backward and around cerebral peduncle	anterior perforated substance	internal cerebral v.
basilic v.	v. basilica	forearm, superficially	ulnar side of dorsal rete of hand	joins brachial vv. to form axillary v.
basilic v., median	v. mediana basilica	sometimes present as medial branch of a bifurcation of median antebrachial v.		basilic v.
basivertebral vv.	vv. basivertebrales	venous sinuses in cancellous tissue of bodies of vertebrae, which communicate with external and internal vertebral plexuses		
brachial vv.	vv. brachiales	accompany brachial artery		join basilic v. to form axillary v.
brachiocephalic vv.	vv. brachiocephalicae (dextra et sinistra)	thorax	head, neck and upper limbs; formed at root of neck by union of ipsilateral internal jugular and subclavian vv.	unite to form superior vena cava

*v. = vein, [L.] vena; vv. = veins, [L.] venae.

TABLE OF VEINS (*Continued*)

COMMON NAME	NA TERM	REGION	RECEIVES BLOOD FROM	DRAINS INTO
bronchial vv.	vv. bronchiales		larger subdivisions of bronchi	azygos v. on left; hemiazygos or superior intercostal v. on right
v. of bulb of penis	v. bulbi penis		bulb of penis	internal pudendal v.
v. of bulb of vestibule	v. bulbi vestibuli		bulb of vestibule of vagina	internal pudendal v.
cardiac vv., anterior	vv. cordis anteriores		anterior wall of right ventricle	right atrium of heart, or lesser cardiac v.
cardiac v., great	v. cordis magna		anterior surface of ventricles	coronary sinus
cardiac v., middle	v. cordis media		diaphragmatic surface of ventricles	coronary sinus
cardiac v., small	v. cordis parva		right atrium and ventricle	corpora cavernosa
"cardiac vv., smallest"	vv. cordis minimae	numerous small veins arising in myocardium, draining independently into cavities of heart and most readily seen in the atria		
carotid v., external. *See* retromandibular v.				
cavernous vv. of penis	vv. cavernosae penis		corpora cavernosa	deep vv. and dorsal v. of penis
central vv. of liver	vv. centrales	in middle of hepatic lobules	liver substance	hepatic v.
central v. of retina	v. centralis retinae	eyeball	retinal vv.	superior ophthalmic v.
central v. of suprarenal gland	v. centralis glandulae suprarenalis	the large single vein into which the various veins within the substance of the gland empty, and which continues at the hilus as the suprarenal v.		

English name	NA term	Location / description	Origin	Drainage / termination
cephalic v.	v. cephalica	winds anteriorly to pass along anterior border of brachioradial muscle; above elbow, ascends along lateral border of biceps muscle	radial side of dorsal rete of hand	axillary v.
cephalic v., accessory	v. cephalica accessoria	forearm	dorsal rete of hand	joins cephalic v. just above elbow
cephalic v., median	v. mediana cephalica	sometimes present as lateral tributary of a bifurcation of median antebrachial v.		cephalic v.
cerebellar vv., inferior	vv. cerebelli inferiores		inferior surface of cerebellum	transverse, sigmoid and inferior petrosal sinuses, or occipital sinus
cerebellar vv., superior	vv. cerebelli superiores		upper surface of cerebellum	straight sinus and great cerebral v., or transverse and superior petrosal sinuses
cerebral v., anterior	v. cerebri anterior	accompanies anterior cerebral artery		basal v.
cerebral v., great	v. cerebri magna	curves around splenium of corpus callosum	formed by union of the 2 internal cerebral veins	straight sinus
cerebral vv., inferior	vv. cerebri inferiores	veins that ramify on inferior surface of brain, those on inferior surface of frontal lobe draining into inferior sagittal sinus and cavernous sinus, those on temporal lobe into superior petrosal sinus and transverse sinus, and those on occipital lobe into straight sinus		
cerebral vv., internal (2)	vv. cerebri internae	pass backward from interventricular foramen through tela choroidea	formed by union of thalamostriate v. and choroid v.; collect blood from basal ganglia	unite at splenium of corpus callosum to form great cerebral v.
cerebral v., middle, deep	v. cerebri media profunda	accompanies middle cerebral artery in floor of fissure of Sylvius		basal v.

TABLE OF VEINS (*Continued*)

COMMON NAME	NA TERM	REGION	RECEIVES BLOOD FROM	DRAINS INTO
cerebral v., middle, superficial	v. cerebri media superficialis	follows lateral cerebral fissure	lateral surface of cerebrum	cavernous sinus
cerebral vv., superior	vv. cerebri superiores	about 12 veins draining superolateral and medial surfaces of cerebrum toward longitudinal fissure		superior sagittal sinus
cervical v., deep	v. cervicalis profunda	accompanies deep cervical artery down neck	a plexus in suboccipital triangle	vertebral v. or brachiocephalic v.
cervical vv., transverse	vv. transversae colli	accompany transverse cervical artery		subclavian v.
choroid v.	v. choroidea	runs whole length of choroid plexus	choroid plexus, hippocampus, fornix, corpus callosum	joins thalamostriate v. to form internal cerebral v.
ciliary vv.	vv. ciliares	anterior vessels follow anterior ciliary arteries; posterior follow posterior ciliary arteries	arise in eyeball by branches from ciliary muscle; anterior ciliary vv. also receive branches from sinus venosus, sclerae, episcleral vv. and conjunctiva of eyeball	superior ophthalmic v.; posterior ciliary vv. empty also into inferior ophthalmic v.
circumflex femoral vv., lateral	vv. circumflexae femoris laterales	accompany lateral circumflex femoral artery		femoral v. or profunda femoris v.
circumflex femoral vv., medial	vv. circumflexae femoris mediales	accompany medial circumflex femoral artery		femoral v. or profunda femoris v.
circumflex iliac v., deep	v. circumflexa ilium profunda	a common trunk formed by veins accompanying deep circumflex iliac artery		external iliac v.

circumflex iliac v., superficial	v. circumflexa illium superficialis	accompanies superficial circumflex iliac artery		great saphenous v.
v. of cochlear canaliculus	v. canaliculi		cochlea	superior bulb of internal jugular v.
colic v., left	v. colica sinistra	accompanies left colic artery		inferior mesenteric v.
colic v., middle	v. colica media	accompanies middle colic artery		superior mesenteric v.
colic v., right	v. colica dextra	accompanies right colic artery		superior mesenteric v.
conjunctival vv.	vv. conjunctivales		conjunctiva	superior ophthalmic v.
coronary vv. *See* entries under cardiac vv.				
cubital v., median	v. mediana cubiti	a large connecting tributary passing obliquely upward across cubital fossa	cephalic v., below elbow	basilic v.
cutaneous v.	v. cutanea	one of the small veins that begin in papillae of skin, from subpapillary plexuses, and open into the subcutaneous veins		
cystic v.	v. cystica	within substance of liver	gallbladder	right branch of portal v.
deep vv. of clitoris	vv. profundae clitoridis		clitoris	vesical venous plexus
deep vv. of penis	vv. profundae penis	accompany deep artery of penis	penis	dorsal v. of penis
digital vv. of foot, dorsal	vv. digitales dorsales pedis	dorsal surfaces of toes		unite at clefts to form dorsal metatarsal vv.
digital vv., palmar	vv. digitales palmares	accompany proper and common palmar digital arteries		superior palmar venous arch
digital vv., plantar	vv. digitales plantares	plantar surfaces of toes		unite at clefts to form plantar metatarsal vv.
diploic v., frontal	v. diploica frontalis		frontal bone	supraorbital v. or superior sagittal sinus

TABLE OF VEINS (*Continued*)

COMMON NAME	NA TERM	REGION	RECEIVES BLOOD FROM	DRAINS INTO
diploic v., occipital	v. diploica occipitalis		occipital bone	occipital v. or transverse sinus
diploic v., temporal, anterior	v. diploica temporalis anterior		lateral portion of frontal bone, anterior part of parietal bone	sphenoparietal sinus or a deep temporal v.
diploic v., temporal, posterior	v. diploica temporalis posterior		parietal bone	transverse sinus
dorsal v. of clitoris	v. dorsalis clitoridis	accompanies dorsal artery of clitoris		vesical plexus
dorsal vv. of clitoris, superficial	vv. dorsales clitoridis superficiales		clitoris, subcutaneously	external pudendal v.
dorsal v. of penis	v. dorsalis penis	a single median vein lying subfascially in penis between the dorsal arteries; it begins in small veins around corona of glans, is joined by deep veins of penis as it passes proximally, and passes between arcuate pubic and transverse perineal ligaments, where it divides into a left and a right vein to join prostatic plexus		
dorsal vv. of penis, superficial	vv. dorsales penis superficiales		penis, subcutaneously	external pudendal v.
dorsal vv. of tongue	vv. dorsales linguae	veins that unite with a small vein accompanying lingual artery and join main lingual trunk		
emissary v., condylar	v. emissaria condylaris	a small vein running through condylar canal of skull, connecting sigmoid sinus with vertebral v. or internal jugular v.		
emissary v., mastoid	v. emissaria mastoidea	a small vein passing through mastoid foramen of skull, connecting sigmoid sinus with occipital v. or posterior auricular v.		

Term	Latin	Location / Description	Drains into
emmissary v., occipital	v. emissaria occipitalis	an occasional small vein running through a minute foramen in occipital protuberance of skull, connecting confluence of sinuses with occipital v.	
emissary v., parietal	v. emissaria parietalis	a small vein passing through parietal foramen of skull, connecting superior sagittal sinus with superficial temporal vv.	
epigastric v., inferior	v. epigastrica inferior	accompanies inferior epigastric artery	external iliac v.
epigastric v., superficial	v. epigastrica superficialis	accompanies superficial epigastric artery	great saphenous v. or femoral v.
epigastric vv., superior	vv. epigastricae superiores	accompany superior epigastric artery	internal thoracic v.
episcleral vv.	vv. episclerales	around cornea	vorticose vv. and ciliary vv.
esophageal vv.	vv. esophageae	esophagus	hemiazygos v. and azygos v., or left brachiocephalic v.
ethmoidal vv.	vv. ethmoidales	accompany anterior and posterior ethmoidal arteries and emerge from ethmoidal foramina	superior ophthalmic v.
facial v.	v. facialis	a vein beginning at medial angle of eye as angular v., descending behind facial artery, and usually ending in internal jugular v.; formerly called anterior facial v., this vessel sometimes joins retromandibular v. to form a common trunk previously known as common facial vein	
facial v., common. *See* facial v.			
facial v., deep	v. faciei profunda	pterygoid plexus	facial v.
facial v., posterior. *See* retromandibular v.			
facial v., transverse	v. transversa faciei	passes backward with transverse facial artery just below zygomatic arch	retromandibular v.

TABLE OF VEINS (*Continued*)

COMMON NAME	NA TERM	REGION	RECEIVES BLOOD FROM	DRAINS INTO
femoral v.	v. femoralis	follows course of femoral artery in proximal two thirds of thigh	continuation of popliteal v.	at inguinal ligament becomes external iliac v.
femoral v., deep. *See* profunda femoris v.				
fibular vv. *See* peroneal vv.	vv. fibulares (official alternative for vv. peroneae)			
gastric v., left	v. gastrica sinistra	accompanies left gastric artery		portal v.
gastric v., right	v. gastrica dextra	accompanies right gastric artery		portal v.
gastric vv., short	vv. gastricae breves		left portion of greater curvature of stomach	splenic v.
gastroepiploic v., left	v. gastroepiploica sinistra	accompanies left gastroepiploic artery		splenic v.
gastroepiploic v., right	v. gastroepiploica dextra	accompanies right gastroepiploic artery		superior mesenteric v.
genicular vv.	vv. genus	accompany genicular arteries		popliteal v.
gluteal vv., inferior	vv. gluteae inferiores	accompany inferior gluteal artery; unite into a single vessel after passing through greater sciatic foramen	subcutaneous tissue of back of thigh, muscles of buttock	internal iliac v.
gluteal vv., superior	vv. gluteae superiores	accompany superior gluteal artery and pass through greater sciatic foramen	muscles of buttock	internal iliac v.
hemiazygos v.	v. hemiazygos	an intercepting trunk for lower	ascending lumbar	azygos v.

			v.	
hemiazygos v., accessory	v. hemiazygos accessoria	left posterior intercostal vv.; ascends on left side of vertebrae to eighth thoracic vertebra, where it may receive accessory tributary, and crosses vertebral column	the descending intercepting trunk for upper left posterior intercostal vv.; it lies on left side and at eighth thoracic vertebra joins hemiazygos v. or crosses to right side to join azygos v. directly; above, it may communicate with left superior intercostal v.	
hemorrhoidal vv. *See* entries under rectal vv.				
hepatic vv.	vv. hepaticae	2 or 3 large veins in an upper group and 6 to 20 small veins in a lower group, forming successively larger vessels	central vv. of liver	inferior vena cava on posterior aspect of liver
hypogastric v. *See* iliac v., internal				
ileal vv.	vv. ilei		walls of ileum	superior mesenteric v.
ileocolic v.	v. ileocolica	accompanies ileocolic artery		superior mesenteric v.
iliac v., common	v. iliaca communis	ascends to right side of fifth lumbar vertebra	arises at sacroiliac joint by union of external and internal iliac vv.	unites with fellow of opposite side to form inferior vena cava
iliac v., external	v. iliaca externa	extends from inguinal ligament to sacroiliac joint	continuation of femoral v.	joins internal iliac v. to form common iliac v.
iliac v., internal	v. iliaca interna	extends from greater sciatic notch to brim of pelvis	formed by union of parietal branches	joins external iliac v. to form common iliac v.
iliolumbar v.	v. iliolumbalis	accompanies iliolumbar artery		internal iliac v. and/or common iliac v.

TABLE OF VEINS (*Continued*)

COMMON NAME	NA TERM	REGION	RECEIVES BLOOD FROM	DRAINS INTO
innominate vv. *See* brachiocephalic vv.				
intercapital vv.	vv. intercapitales	veins at clefts of fingers which pass between heads of metacarpal bones and establish communication between dorsal and palmar venous systems of hand		
intercostal vv., anterior (12 pairs)	vv. intercostales anteriores	accompany anterior thoracic arteries		internal thoracic vv.
intercostal v., highest	v. intercostalis suprema	first posterior intercostal vein of either side, which passes over apex of lung		brachiocephalic, vertebral or superior intercostal v.
intercostal vv., posterior, IV and XI	vv. intercostales posteriores (IV et XI)	accompany posterior intercostal arteries IV and XI		azygos v. on right; hemiazygos or accessory hemiazygos v. on left
intercostal v., superior, left	v. intercostalis superior sinistra	crosses arch of aorta	formed by union of second, third and sometimes fourth posterior intercostal vv.	left brachiocephalic v.
intercostal v., superior, right	v. intercostalis superior dextra		formed by union of second, third and sometimes fourth posterior intercostal vv.	azygos v.
interlobar vv. of kidney	vv. interlobares renis	pass down between renal pyramids	venous arcades of kidney	unite to form renal v.
interlobular vv. of kidney	vv. interlobulares renis		capillary network of renal cortex	venous arcades of kidney
interlobular vv. of liver	vv. interlobulares hepatis	arise between hepatic lobules	liver	portal v.

interosseous vv. of foot, dorsal. *See* metatarsal vv., dorsal				
intervertebral v.	v. intervertebralis	vertebral column	vertebral venous plexuses	
jejunal vv.	vv. jejunales		walls of jejunum	superior mesenteric v.
jugular v., anterior	v. jugularis anterior	arises under chin and passes down neck		external jugular or subclavian v., or jugular venous arch
jugular v., external	v. jugularis externa	begins in parotid gland, passes down neck	formed by union of retromandibular v. and posterior auricular v.	subclavian, internal jugular, or brachiocephalic v.
jugular v., internal	v. jugularis interna	from jugular fossa, descends in neck with internal carotid artery and then with carotid artery	begins as superior bulb, draining much of head and neck	joins subclavian v. to form brachiocephalic v.
labial vv., anterior	vv. labiales anteriores		anterior aspect of labia in female	external pudendal v.
labial vv., inferior	vv. labiales inferiores		region of lower lip	facial v.
labial vv., posterior	vv. labiales posteriores		labia in female	vesical venous plexus
labial v., superior	v. labialis superior		region of upper lip	facial v.
labyrinthine vv.	vv. labyrinthi	pass through internal acoustic meatus	cochlea	inferior petrosal sinus or transverse sinus
lacrimal v.	v. lacrimalis		lacrimal gland	superior ophthalmic v.
laryngeal v., inferior	v. laryngea inferior		larynx	inferior thyroid v.
laryngeal v., superior	v. laryngea superior		larynx	superior thyroid v.

TABLE OF VEINS (*Continued*)

COMMON NAME	NA TERM	REGION	RECEIVES BLOOD FROM	DRAINS INTO
lingual v.	v. lingualis	a deep vein, following distribution of lingual artery		internal jugular v.
lingual v., deep. *See* profunda inguae v.				
lingual vv., dorsal. *See* dorsal vv. of tongue				
lumbar vv., I and II	vv. lumbales (I et II)	accompany first and second lumbar arteries		ascending lumbar v.
lumbar vv., III and IV	vv. lumbales (III et IV)	accompany third and fourth lumbar arteries		usually, inferior vena cava
lumbar v., ascending	v. lumbalis ascendens	an ascending intercepting vein for lumbar vv. of either side; it begins in lateral sacral region and ascends to first lumbar vertebra, where by union with subcostal v. it becomes on right side the azygos v. and on left the hemiazygos v.		
maxillary vv.	vv. maxillares	usually form a single short trunk with pterygoid plexus		joins superficial temporal v. in parotid gland to form retromandibular v.
mediastinal vv.	vv. mediastinales		anterior mediastinum	brachiocephalic v., azygos v. or superior vena cava
meningeal vv.	vv. meningeae	accompany meningeal arteries	dura mater (also communicate with lateral lacunae)	regional sinuses and veins
meningeal vv., middle	vv. meningeae mediae	accompany middle meningeal artery		pterygoid venous plexus
mesenteric v., inferior	v. mesenterica inferior	follows distribution of inferior mesenteric artery		splenic v.

mesenteric v., superior	v. mesenterica superior	follows distribution of superior mesenteric artery		joins splenic v. to form portal v.
metacarpal vv., dorsal	vv. metacarpeae dorsales	veins arising from union of dorsal veins of adjacent fingers and passing proximally to join in forming dorsal venous network of hand		
metacarpal vv., palmar	vv. metacarpeae palmares	accompany palmar metacarpal arteries		deep palmar venous arch
metatarsal vv., dorsal	vv. metatarseae dorsales		arise from dorsal digital vv. of toes at clefts of toes	dorsal venous arch
metatarsal vv., plantar	vv. metatarseae plantares	deep veins of foot	arise from plantar digital veins at clefts of toes	plantar venous arch
musculophrenic vv.	vv. musculophrenicae	accompany musculophrenic artery	parts of diaphragm and wall of thorax and abdomen	internal thoracic vv.
nasal vv., external	vv. nasales externae	small ascending branches from nose		angular v., facial v.
nasofrontal v.	v. nasofrontalis		supraorbital v.	superior ophthalmic v.
oblique v. of left atrium	v. obliqua atrii sinistri	left atrium of heart		coronary sinus
obturator vv.	vv. obturatoriae	enter pelvis though obturator canal	hip joint and regional muscles	internal iliac and/or inferior epigastric v.
occipital v.	v. occipitalis	scalp; follows distribution of occipital artery		opens deep to trapezius muscle into suboccipital venous plexus, or accompanies occipital artery to end in internal jugular v.
ophthalmic v., inferior	v. ophthalmica inferior	a vein formed by confluence of muscular and ciliary tributaries, and running backward either to join superior ophthalmic vein or to open directly into cavernous sinus; it sends a communicating branch through inferior orbital fissure to join pterygoid venous plexus		

TABLE OF VEINS (*Continued*)

COMMON NAME	NA TERM	REGION	RECEIVES BLOOD FROM	DRAINS INTO
ophthalmic v., superior	v. ophthalmica superior	a vein beginning at medial angle of eye, where it communicates with frontal, supraorbital and angular vv.; it follows distribution of ophthalmic artery, and may be joined by inferior ophthalmic v. at superior orbital fissure before opening into cavernous sinus		
ovarian v., left	v. ovarica sinistra		pampiniform plexus of broad ligament on left	left renal v.
ovarian v., right	v. ovarica dextra		pampiniform plexus of broad ligament on right	inferior vena cava
palatine v., external	v. palatina externa		tonsils and soft palate	facial v.
palpebral vv.	vv. palpebrales	small branches from eyelids		superior ophthalmic v.
palpebral vv., inferior	vv. palpebrales inferiores		lower eyelid	facial v.
palpebral vv., superior	vv. palpebrales superiores		upper eyelid	angular v.
pancreatic vv.	vv. pancreaticae		pancreas	splenic v., superior mesenteric v.
pancreaticoduodenal vv.	vv. pancreaticoduodenales	4 veins that drain blood from pancreas and duodenum, closely following pancreaticoduodenal arteries, a superior and an inferior vein originating from an anterior and a posterior venous arcade; anterior superior v. joins right gastroepiploic v., and posterior superior v. joins portal v.; anterior and posterior inferior vv. join, sometimes as one trunk, uppermost jejunal v. or superior mesenteric v.		
paraumbilical vv.	vv. paraumbilicales	veins that communicate with portal v. above and descend to anterior abdominal wall to anastomose		

		with superior and inferior epigastric and superior vesical vv. in region of umbilicus, they form a significant part of collateral circulation of portal v. in event of hepatic obstruction		
parotid vv.	vv. parotideae		parotid gland	superficial temporal v.
perforating vv.	vv. perforantes	accompany perforating arteries of thigh		profunda femoris v.
pericardiac vv.	vv. pericardiaceae		pericardium	brachiocephalic, inferior thyroid and azygos vv., superior vena cava
pericardiacophrenic vv.	vv. pericardiacophrenicae		pericardium and diaphragm	left brachiocephalic v.
peroneal vv.	vv. peroneae	accompany peroneal artery		posterior tibial v.
pharyngeal vv.	vv. pharyngeae		pharyngeal plexus	internal jugular v.
phrenic vv., inferior	vv. phrenicae inferiores	accompany inferior phrenic arteries		on right, enters inferior vena cava; on left, enters left suprarenal or renal v., or inferior vena cava
phrenic vv., superior. *See* pericardiacophrenic vv.				
popliteal v.	v. poplitea	follows popliteal artery	formed by union of anterior and posterior tibial vv.	at adductor hiatus becomes femoral v.
portal v.	v. portae	a short, thick trunk formed by union of superior mesenteric and splenic vv. behind neck of pancreas; it ascends to right end of porta hepatis, where it divides into successively smaller branches, following branches of hepatic artery, until it forms a capillary-like system of sinusoids that permeates entire substance of liver		

TABLE OF VEINS (Continued)

COMMON NAME	NA TERM	REGION	RECEIVES BLOOD FROM	DRAINS INTO
posterior v. of left ventricle	v. posterior ventriculi sinistri cordis		posterior surface of left ventricle	coronary sinus
prepyloric v.	v. prepylorica	accompanies prepyloric artery, passing upward over anterior surface of junction between pylorus and duodenum		right gastric v.
profunda femoris v.	v. profunda femoris	accompanies profunda femoris artery		femoral v.
profunda linguae v.	v. profunda linguae		deep part of tongue	joins sublingual v. to form accompanying v. of hypoglossal nerve
v. of pterygoid canal	v. canalis pterygoidei	passes through pterygoid canal		pterygoid plexus
pudendal vv., external	vv. pudendae externae	follow distribution of external pudendal artery		great saphenous v.
pudendal v., internal	v. pudenda interna	follows course of internal pudendal artery		internal iliac v.
pulmonary v., inferior, left	v. pulmonalis inferior sinistra		lower lobe of left lung (from superior apical branch and common basal v.)	left atrium of heart
pulmonary v., inferior, right	v. pulmonalis inferior dextra		lower lobe of right lung (from apical branch and common, superior and inferior basal vv.)	left atrium of heart
pulmonary v., superior, left	v. pulmonalis		upper lobe of left	left atrium of heart

	superior sinistra		lung (from apicoposterior, anterior and lingular branches)	
pulmonary v., superior, right	v. pulmonalis superior dextra		upper and middle lobes of right lung (from apical, anterior and posterior branches and middle lobar branch)	left atrium of heart
pyloric v. *See* gastric v., right				
radial vv.	vv. radiales	accompany radial artery		brachial vv.
ranine v. *See* profunda linguae v.				
rectal vv., inferior	vv. rectales inferiores		rectal plexus	internal pudendal v.
rectal vv., middle	vv. rectales mediae		rectal plexus	internal iliac and superior rectal vv.
rectal v., superior	v. rectalis superior	establishes connection between portal and systemic systems	upper part of rectal plexus	inferior mesenteric v.
renal vv.	vv. renales	short, thick trunks, one from either kidney, the one on the left being longer than that on the right	kidneys	inferior vena cava
retromandibular v.	v. retromandibularis	a vein formed in upper part of parotid gland behind neck of mandible by union of maxillary and superficial temporal vv.; it passes downward through the gland, communicates with facial v. and, emerging from the gland, joins with posterior auricular v. to form external jugular v.		
sacral vv., lateral	vv. sacrales laterales	follow lateral sacral arteries		help form lateral sacral plexus, empty into internal iliac v. or superior gluteal vv.

COMMON NAME	NA TERM	REGION	RECEIVES BLOOD FROM	DRAINS INTO
sacral v., median	v. sacralis mediana	follows median sacral artery		common iliac v.
saphenous v., accessory	v. saphena accessoria		medial and posterior superficial parts of thigh	great saphenous v.
saphenous v., great	v. saphena magna	extends from dorsum of foot to just below inguinal ligament		femoral v.
saphenous v., long. See saphenous v., great				
saphenous v., short. See saphenous v., small				
saphenous v., small	v. saphena parva	back of ankle and leg		popliteal v.
scrotal vv., anterior	vv. scrotales anteriores		anterior aspect of scrotum	external pudendal v.
scrotal vv., posterior	vv. scrotales posteriores	scrotum		vesical venous plexus
v. of septum pellucidum	v. septi pellucidi	septum pellucidum (septum lucidum)		thalamostriate v.
sigmoid vv.	vv. sigmoideae		sigmoid colon	inferior mesenteric v.
spinal vv.	vv. spinales	anastomosing networks of small veins that drain blood from spinal cord and its pia mater into internal vertebral venous plexuses		
spiral v. of modiolus	v. spiralis modioli	modiolus		labyrinthine vv.
splenic v.	v. lienalis	passes from left to right of neck of pancreas	formed by union of several branches at hilus of spleen	joins superior mesenteric v. to form portal v.
stellate vv. of kidney	venulae stellatae renis		superficial parts of renal cortex	interlobular vv. of kidney

English name	Latin name	Course / description	Origin	Termination
sternocleidomastoid v.	v. sterno-cleidomastoidea	follows course of sternocleido-mastoid artery		internal jugular v.
striate v.	v. striata		anterior perforated substance of brain	basal v.
stylomastoid v.	v. stylomastoidea	follows stylomastoid artery		retromandibular v.
subclavian v.	v. subclavia	follows subclavian artery	continues axillary v. as main venous channel of upper limb	joins internal jugular v. to form brachiocephalic v.
subcostal v.	v. subcostalis	accompanies subcostal artery		joins ascending lumbar v. to form azygos v. on right, hemiazygos v. on left
subcutaneous vv. of abdomen	vv. subcutaneae abdominis	superficial layers of abdominal wall		
sublingual v.	v. sublingualis	follows sublingual artery		lingual v.
submental v.	v. submentalis	follows submental artery		facial v.
supraorbital v.	v. supraorbitalis	passes down forehead lateral to supratrochlear v.		joins supratrochlear vv. to form angular v.
suprarenal v., left	v. suprarenalis sinistra		left suprarenal gland	left renal v.
suprarenal v., right	v. suprarenalis dextra		right suprarenal gland	inferior vena cava
suprascapular v.	v. suprascapularis	accompanies suprascapular artery (sometimes as 2 veins that unite)		usually into external jugular v., occasionally into subclavian v.
supratrochlear vv. (2)	vv. supratrochleares		venous plexuses high up on forehead	join supraorbital v. to form angular v.

TABLE OF VEINS (Continued)

COMMON NAME	NA TERM	REGION	RECEIVES BLOOD FROM	DRAINS INTO
temporal vv., deep	vv. temporales profundae		deep portions of temporal muscle	pterygoid plexus
temporal v., middle	v. temporalis media	descends deep to fascia to zygoma	arises in substance of temporal muscle	superficial temporal v.
temporal vv., superficial	vv. temporales superficiales	veins that drain lateral part of scalp in frontal and parietal regions, the tributaries forming a single superficial temporal v. in front of ear, just above zygoma; this descending vein receives middle temporal and transverse facial vv. and, entering parotid gland, unites with maxillary v. deep to neck of mandible to form retromandibular v.		
testicular v., left	v. testicularis sinistra		left pampiniform plexus	left renal v.
testicular v., right	v. testicularis dextra		right pampiniform plexus	inferior vena cava
thalamostriate v.	v. thalamostriata		corpus striatum and thalamus	joins choroid v. to form internal cerebral v.
thoracic vv., internal	vv. thoracicae internae	2 veins formed by junction of the veins accompanying internal thoracic artery of either side; each continues along the artery to open into brachiocephalic v.		
thoracic v., lateral	v. thoracica lateralis	accompanies lateral thoracic artery		axillary v.
thoracoacromial v.	v. thoraco-acromialis	follows thoracoacromial artery		subclavian v.
thoracoepigastric vv.	vv. thoraco-epigastricae	long, longitudinal, superficial veins in anterolateral subcutaneous tissue of trunk		superiorly into lateral thoracic v.; inferiorly into femoral v.

	Latin	Description	Region/origin	Drains into
thymic vv.	vv. thymicae		thymus	left brachiocephalic v.
thyroid v., inferior	v. thyroidea inferior	either of 2 veins, left and right, that drain thyroid plexus into left and right brachiocephalic vv.; occasionally they may unite into a common trunk to empty, usually, into left brachiocephalic v.		
thyroid vv., middle	vv. thyroideae mediae		thyroid gland	internal jugular v.
thyroid v., superior	v. thyroidea superior	arises from side of upper part of thyroid gland	thyroid gland	internal jugular v., occasionally in common with facial v.
tibial vv., anterior	vv. tibiales anteriores	accompany anterior tibial artery		join posterior tibial vv. to form popliteal v.
tibial vv., posterior	vv. tibiales posteriores	accompany posterior tibial artery		join anterior tibial vv. to form popliteal v.
tracheal vv.	vv. tracheales		trachea	brachiocephalic v.
tympanic vv.	vv. tympanicae	small veins from middle ear that pass through petrotympanic fissure and open into the plexus around temporomandibular joint		retromandibular v.
ulnar vv.	vv. ulnares	accompany ulnar artery		join radial vv. at elbow to form brachial vv.
umbilical v.	v. umbilicalis	in the early embryo, either of the paired veins that carry blood from chorion to sinus venosus and heart; they later fuse and a single vessel persisting in umbilical cord carries all the blood from placenta to ductus venosus of fetus		
uterine vv.	vv. uterinae		uterine plexus	internal iliac vv.
vena cava, inferior	vena cava inferior	the venous trunk for the lower limbs and for pelvic and abdominal viscera; it begins at level of fifth lumbar vertebra by union of common iliac vv. and ascends on right of aorta		right atrium of heart

Table of Veins (Concluded)

COMMON NAME	NA TERM	REGION	RECEIVES BLOOD FROM	DRAINS INTO
vena cava, superior	vena cava superior	the venous trunk draining blood from head, neck, upper limbs and thorax; it begins by union of 2 brachio-cephalic vv. and passes directly downward		right atrium of heart
vertebral v.	v. vertebralis	passes with vertebral artery through transverse foramina of upper 6 cervical vertebrae	suboccipital venous plexus	brachiocephalic v.
vertebral v., accessory	v. vertebralis accessoria	descends with vertebral vein and emerges through transverse foramen of seventh cervical vertebra	a plexus formed around vertebral artery by ver-tebral v.	brachiocephalic v.
vertebral v., anterior	v. vertebralis anterior		venous plexus around transverse pro-cesses of upper cervical vertebrae	vertebral v.
vesical vv.	vv. vesicales		vesical plexus	internal iliac v.
vestibular vv.	vv. vestibulares		vestibule of labyrinth	labyrinthine vv.
vorticose vv. (4)	vv. vorticosae	eyeball	choroid	superior and inferior ophthalmic vv.

venectasia (ve″nek-ta′ze-ah) phlebectasia.

venectomy (ve-nek′to-me) phlebectomy.

venenation (ven″ĕ-na′shun) poisoning; a poisoned condition.

venenific (ven″ĕ-nif′ik) forming poison.

venenosa (ven″ĕ-no′sah) venomous snakes collectively.

venenous (ven′ĕ-nus) poisonous or toxic.

venereal (vĕ-ne′re-al) propagated by coitus.
    v. disease, one of the communicable diseases transmitted through coitus. In addition to SYPHILIS and GONORRHEA, there are three less common venereal diseases: CHANCROID, LYMPHOGRANULOMA VENEREUM and GRANULOMA INGUINALE.

venereologist (vĕ-ne″re-ol′o-jist) a specialist in venereology.

venereology (vĕ-ne″re-ol′o-je) the study and treatment of venereal diseases.

venereophobia (vĕ-ne″re-o-fo′be-ah) morbid fear of contracting venereal disease.

venery (ven′er-e) coitus.

venesection (ven″ĕ-sek′shun) the opening of a vein for letting blood.

veniplex (ven′ĭ-pleks) a venous plexus.

venipuncture (ven″ĭ-pungk′tūr) puncture of a vein for therapeutic purposes or for collection of blood specimens.

venisuture (ven″ĭ-su′tūr) phleborrhaphy.

venoclysis (ve-nok′lĭ-sis) injection of medicinal or nutrient fluid into a vein.

venogram (ve′no-gram) phlebogram.

venography (ve-nog′rah-fe) phlebography.

venom (ve′om) poison, especially a toxic substance normally secreted by a serpent, insect or other animal. adj., **ven′omous.**
    Russell's viper v., the venom of the Russell viper, which acts in vitro as an intrinsic thromboplastin and is useful in defining deficiencies of clotting factor X.

venomization (ven″om-ĭ-za′shun) treatment of a substance with snake venom.

venomotor (ve″no-mo′tor) controlling dilation or contraction of the veins.

veno-occlusive (ve″no-ŏ-kloo′siv) pertaining to or characterized by obstruction of the veins.

venosclerosis (ve″no-sklē-ro′sis) sclerosis of veins.

venosity (ve-nos′ĭ-te) 1. the characteristic quality of venous blood. 2. excess of venous blood in a part.

venostasis (ve″no-sta′sis) checking of return flow of blood by compressing veins in the four extremities.

venostat (ve′no-stat) an instrument for performing venostasis.

venotomy (ve-not′o-me) phlebotomy.

venous (ve′nus) pertaining to the vein.
    v. return, the flow of blood into the heart from the peripheral vessels.

venovenostomy (ve″no-ve-nos′to-me) phlebophlebostomy.

vent (vent) an opening or outlet, such as an opening that discharges pus, or the anus.

venter (ven′ter), pl. *ven′tres* [L.] the belly or any bell-like part; the anterior or inferior surface of the body.

ventilation (ven″tĭ-la′shun) 1. the process of supplying with fesh air, especially the constant supplying of oxygen through the lungs. 2. free discussion, as of one's problems or grievances.

ventr(o)- (ven′tro) word element [L.], *belly; abdomen; ventral aspect.*

ventrad (ven′trad) toward a belly, venter or ventral aspect.

ventral (ven′tral) 1. pertaining to the abdomen or to any venter. 2. directed toward or situated on the belly surface; opposite of dorsal.

ventralis (ven-tra′lis) [L.] ventral.

ventricle (ven′trĭ-kl) a small cavity or chamber, as in the brain or heart.
    v. of Arantius, the lower end of the fourth ventricle of the brain.
    fifth v., a narrow space between the layers of the septum lucidum.
    fourth v., a median cavity in the hindbrain, containing cerebrospinal fluid.
    v. of larynx, the space between the true and false vocal cords.
    lateral v's, cavities in the forebrain, one in each cerebral hemisphere, containing cerebrospinal fluid.
    left v., the lower chamber of the left side of the heart, which pumps oxygenated blood out through the aorta to all the tissues of the body.
    Morgagni's v., ventricle of the larynx.
    v. of myelon, the central canal of spinal cord.
    pineal v., the cavity beneath or within the pineal gland.
    right v., the lower chamber of the right side of the heart, which pumps venous blood through the pulmonary trunk and arteries to the capillaries of the lung.
    third v., a median cavity in the forebrain, containing cerebrospinal fluid.

ventricornu (ven″trĭ-kor′nu) the ventral horn of gray matter in the spinal cord.

ventricular (ven-trik′u-lar) pertaining to a ventricle.
    v. septal defect, a congenital heart defect in which an opening between the ventricles permits flow of blood directly from one ventricle to the other, resulting in bypassing of the pulmonary circulation and producing varying degrees of cyanosis because of oxygen deficiency.

ventriculitis (ven-trik″u-li′tis) inflammation of the cerebral ventricles.

ventriculoatriostomy (ven-trik″u-lo-a″tre-os′to-me) surgical creation of a passage permitting drainage of cerebrospinal fluid from a cerebral ventricle to the right atrium for relief of hydrocephalus.

ventriculocisternostomy (ven-trik″u-lo-sis″ter-nos′to-me) introduction of a catheter for drainage of cerebrospinal fluid from a lateral ventricle of the brain into the cisterna cerebellomedullaris or cervical subarachnoid space.

ventriculogram (ven-trik′u-lo-gram″) a roentgenogram of the cerebral ventricles.

ventriculography (ven-trik″u-log′rah-fe) roentgenography of the cerebral ventricles after introduction of air or other contrast medium.

ventriculomastoidostomy (ven-trik″u-lo-mas″-toi-dos′to-me) surgical provision for drainage of cerebrospinal fluid from the lateral ventricle into the mastoid antrum, in treatment of hydrocephalus.

ventriculometry (ven-trik″u-lom′ĕ-tre) measurement of intracranial pressure.

ventriculomyotomy (ven-trik″u-lo-mi-ot′o-me) incision of the obstructing muscular band in subaortic stenosis.

ventriculonector (ven-trik″u-lo-nek′tor) the bundle of His.

ventriculopuncture (ven-trik″u-lo-pungk′tūr) puncture of a lateral ventricle of the brain.

ventriculoscopy (ven-trik″u-los′ko-pe) endoscopic examination of the cerebral ventricles.

ventriculoseptopexy (ven-trik″u-lo-sep′to-pek″-se) surgical correction of a defect in the interventricular septum.

ventriculoseptoplasty (ven-trik″u-lo-sep′to-plas″te) plastic repair of the interventricular septum of the heart.

ventriculostomy (ven-trik″u-los′to-me) creation of a communication with a cerebral ventricle for drainage of cerebrospinal fluid in hydrocephalus.

ventriculosubarachnoid (ven-trik″u-lo-sub″ah-rak′noid) pertaining to the cerebral ventricles and subarachnoid space.

ventriculotomy (ven-trik″u-lot′o-me) incision of a ventricle of the heart for repair of cardiac defects.

ventriculovenostomy (ven-trik″u-lo-ve-nos′to-me) creation of a communication from a cerebral ventricle to the internal jugular vein, in hydrocephalus.

ventriculus (ven-trik′u-lus), pl. *ventric'uli* [L.] 1. a ventricle. 2. the stomach.

ventricumbent (ven″trĭ-kum′bent) prone; lying on the belly.

ventriduct (ven″trĭ-dukt) to bring or carry ventrad.

ventriflexion (ven″trĭ-flek′shun) flexion toward the ventral aspect.

ventrimeson (ven″trĭ-mes′on) the median line on the ventral surface.

ventrofixation (ven″tro-fik-sa′shun) fixation of a viscus to the abdominal wall.

ventrohysteropexy (ven″tro-his′ter-o-pek″se) ventrofixation of the uterus.

ventroscopy (ven-tros′ko-pe) illumination of the abdominal cavity for purposes of examination.

ventrose (ven′trōs) having a belly.

ventrosuspension (ven″tro-sus-pen′shun) suspension from the abdominal wall, as in fixation of the uterus.

ventrotomy (ven-trot′o-me) celiotomy; opening of the abdominal cavity through an incision in its wall.

venula (ven′u-lah), pl. *ven'ulae* [L.] one of the small vessels receiving blood from capillary plexuses and joining to form veins.

venule (ven′ūl) a small vein.

Veralba (ver-al′bah) trademark for preparations of protoveratrines A and B, used as an antihypertensive.

Veratrum (ver-a′trum) a genus of plants common in North America (*V. vi'ride*) and Europe (*V. al'bum*), which are the source of alkaloids used widely in treatment of hypertensive disorders.

verbigeration (ver-bij″er-a′shun) abnormal repetition of meaningless words and phrases.

verbomania (ver″bo-ma′ne-ah) abnormal talkativeness.

verdigris (ver′dĭ-grēs, ver′dĭ-gris) a mixture of basic copper acetates; an astringent.

verge (verj) a circumference or ring.
  anal v., the opening of the anus on the surface of the body.

vergeture (ver′jĕ-tūr) a stripe or stria, especially on the skin.

vermicide (ver′mĭ-sīd) an agent that destroys worms or intestinal animal parasites.

vermicular (ver-mik′u-lar) wormlike.

vermiculation (ver-mik″u-la′shun) peristaltic motion; peristalsis.

vermiculous (ver-mik′u-lus) 1. wormlike 2. infected with worms.

vermiform (ver′mĭ-form) worm-shaped.
  v. appendix, a small appendage near the juncture of the small intestine and the large intestine (ileocecal valve); often called simply appendix. An apparently useless structure, it can be the source of a serious illness, APPENDICITIS.

vermifugal (ver-mif′u-gal) expelling intestinal worms.

vermifuge (ver′mĭ-fūj) an agent that expels worms or intestinal animal parasites.

vermilion border (ver-mil′yon) the exposed red portion of the upper or lower lip.

vermilionectomy (ver-mil"yon-ek'to-me) excision of the vermilion border of the lip.

vermin (ver'min) an external animal parasite; animal ectoparasites collectively.

vermination (ver"mĭ-na'shun) infection with vermin.

verminosis (ver'mĭ-no'sis) infection with worms.

vermis (ver'mis) [L.] a worm, or wormlike structure.
   v. cerebel'li, the median part of the cerebellum, between the two hemispheres.

vermix (ver'miks) vermiform appendix.

vernix (ver'niks) [L.] varnish.
   v. caseo'sa, the unctuous substance covering the skin of the fetus.

verruca (vĕ-roo'kah) 1. a lesion of the skin of viral origin, commonly small, round and raised, with a rough, dry surface; called also WART. 2. a wartlike growth on any surface, as on the endocardium. adj., **ver'rucose, verru'cous.**
   v. pla'na, one that is only slightly elevated, sometimes occurring in great numbers, most frequently in children (verru'ca pla'na juveni'lis).
   v. planta'ris, a viral epidermal tumor on the sole of the foot.

verruciform (vĕ-roo'sĭ-form) resembling a wart.

verruga (vĕ-roo'gah) wart.
   v. perua'na, a hemangioma-like tumor or nodule occurring in Carrión's disease.

version (ver'zhun) the act of turning; especially the manual turning of the fetus in delivery.
   bipolar v., turning effected by acting upon both poles of the fetus.
   Braxton Hicks v., a combined external and internal method of changing the position of the fetus in utero.
   cephalic v., turning of the fetus so that the head presents.
   combined v., external and internal versions together.
   external v., turning effected by outside manipulation.
   internal v., turning effected by the hand or fingers inserted through the dilated cervix.
   pelvic v., version by manipulation of the breech.
   podalic v., conversion of a more unfavorable presentation into a footling presentation.
   spontaneous v., one that occurs without aid from any extraneous force.

vertebr(o)- (ver'tĕ-bro) word element [L.], *vertebra; spine.*

vertebra (ver'tĕ-brah), pl. *ver'tebrae* [L.] one of the separate segments comprising the spine (vertebral column). adj., **ver'tebral.**
   The vertebrae support the body and provide the protective bony corridor through which the spinal cord passes. The 33 bones that make up the spine differ considerably in size and structure according to location. There are seven cervical (neck) vertebrae, 12 thoracic (high back), five lumbar (low back), five sacral (near the base of the spine) and four coccygeal (at the base). The five sacral vertebrae are fused to form the sacrum, and the four coccygeal vertebrae are fused to form the coccyx.

The weight-bearing portion of a typical vertebra is the vertebral body, the most forward portion. This is a cylindrical structure that is separated from the vertebral bodies above and below by disks of cartilage and fibrous tissue. These intervertebral disks act as cushions to absorb the mechanical shock of walking, running and other activity. Rupture of an intervertebral disk is known popularly as slipped DISK.
   A semicircular arch of bone protrudes from the back of each vertebral body, surrounding the spinal cord. Directly in its midline a bony projection, the spinous process, grows backward from the arch. The spinuous process can be felt on the back as a hard knob. Three pairs of outgrowths project from the arch. One of these protrudes horizontally on each side and in the thorax connects with the ribs. The remaining two form joints with the vertebrae above and below. The joints permit the spine to bend flexibly. The vertebrae are held firmly in place by a series of strong ligaments. (See also SPINE.)
   cranial v., one of the segments that become fused to form the bones of the skull and face.
   v. denta'ta, the second cervical vertebra, or axis.
   dorsal vertebrae, thoracic vertebrae.
   false vertebrae, those vertebrae which normally fuse with adjoining segments: the sacral and coccygeal vertebrae.
   v. mag'num, the sacrum.
   odontoid v., the second cervical vertebra, or axis.
   v. pla'na, a condition of spondylitis in which the body of the vertebra is reduced to a sclerotic disk.
   true vertebrae, those segments of the vertebral column that normally remain unfused throughout life: the cervical, thoracic and lumbar vertebrae.

vertebrarium (ver"tĕ-bra're-um) the vertebral column.

vertebrate (ver'tĕ-brāt) 1. having a vertebral column. 2. an animal with a vertebral column.

vertebrectomy (ver"tĕ-brek'to-me) excision of a vertebra.

vertebrochondral (ver"tĕ-bro-kon'dral) pertaining to a vertebra and a costal cartilage.

vertebrocostal (ver"tĕ-bro-kos'tal) pertaining to a vertebra and a rib.

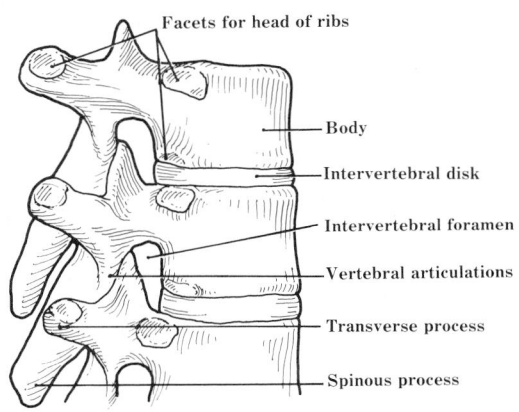

Facets for head of ribs

Body

Intervertebral disk

Intervertebral foramen

Vertebral articulations

Transverse process

Spinous process

Structure of vertebrae.

vertebrosternal (ver″tĕ-bro-ster′nal) pertaining to a vertebra and the sternum.

vertex (ver′teks) the summit or top, especially the crown of the head.

vertical (ver′tĭ-kal) 1. perpendicular to the plane of the horizon. 2. relating to the vertex.

verticalis (ver″tĭ-ka′lis) [L.] vertical.

verticillate (ver-tis′ĭ-lāt) arranged in whorls.

vertigo (ver′tĭ-go) dizziness; a sensation of rotation or movement of one's self (subjective vertigo) or of one's surroundings (objective vertigo) in any plane. adj., **vertig′inous.**

auditory v., aural v., a type of vertigo due to disorder of the inner ear.

central v., that due to disorder of the central nervous system.

labyrinthine v., a form associated with disease of the labyrinth of the ear.

ocular v., a form caused by eye diseases.

organic v., that caused by a lesion of brain or spinal cord.

peripheral v., that due to irritation in some part distant from the brain.

positional v., that occurring when the head is placed in a certain position, due to disorder of the utricle (aural vertigo) or a lesion in the central nervous system, usually the brain stem (central vertigo).

special-sense v., aural or ocular vertigo.

vertigraphy (ver-tig′rah-fe) body-section roentgenography.

verumontanitis (ver″oo-mon″tah-ni′tis) inflammation of the verumontanum.

verumontanum (ver″oo-mon-ta′num) a rounded projection on the floor of the prostatic portion of the urethra, on which are the opening of the prostatic utricle and, on either side of it, the orifices of the ejaculatory ducts; called also seminal colliculus.

ves. [L.] *vesi′ca* (the bladder).

vesalianum (vĕ-sa″le-a′num) a sesamoid bone in the tendon of origin of the gastrocnemius muscle, or in the angle between the cuboid and fifth metatarsal bones.

Vesalius (ve-sa′le-us) Andreas (1514–1564). Flemish anatomist and physician, considered the most eminent anatomist of the 16th century. His *De humani corporis fabrica libri septum* (Seven Books on the Structure of the Human Body) was published in 1543. He was also a pioneer in ethnic craniology and experimental and comparative psychology.

vesic. [L.] *vesic′ula* (a vesicle); [L.] *vesicato′rium* (a blister).

vesic(o)- (ves′ĭ-ko) word element [L.], *blister; bladder.*

vesica (vĕ-si′kah), pl. *vesi′cae* [L.] bladder. adj., **ves′ical.**

vesicant (ves′ĭ-kant) 1. producing blisters. 2. an agent that produces blisters.

vesication (ves″ĭ-ka′shun) the production of blisters or the state of being blistered.

vesicle (ves′ĭ-kl) 1. a small, saclike cavity. 2. a circumscribed, elevated, fluid-containing lesion of the skin, 5 mm. or less in diameter; a blister. adj., **vesic′ular.**

air v., a saccule in lung tissue into which the air is drawn in breathing.

allantoic v., the internal hollow portion of the allantois.

auditory v., an ovoid sac formed by closure of the auditory pit in the early embryo, from which the perceptive parts of the inner ear develop.

brain v's, primary, the three earliest subdivisions of the embryonic neural tube, including the prosencephalon, mesencephalon and rhombencephalon.

brain v's, secondary, the four brain vesicles formed by specialization of the prosencephalon (the telencephalon and diencephalon) and of the rhombencephalon (the metencephalon and myelencephalon) in later embryonic development.

chorionic v., the developing ovum at the time of its invasion of the endometrium of the uterus.

compound v., one that has more than one chamber.

ear v., auditory vesicle.

encephalic v's, brain vesicles.

germinal v., the fluid-filled nucleus of an unripe ovum.

graafian v., graafian follicle.

lens v., the primordium of the lens in the developing eye of the early embryo, formed by invagination of the lens placode.

optic v., a swelling on either side of the anterior of the three primary brain vesicles in the early embryo, from which the perceptive parts of the eye develop.

otic v., auditory vesicle.

seminal v's, paired lobulated structures in close apposition to the bladder in the male, opening into the vas deferens.

umbilical v., the portion of yolk sac outside the body of the embryo.

vesicocele (ves′ĭ-ko-sēl″) hernia of the bladder.

vesicocervical (ves″ĭ-ko-ser′vĭ-kal) pertaining to the bladder and cervix uteri.

vesicoclysis (ves″ĭ-kok′lĭ-sis) introduction of fluid into the bladder.

vesicocolonic (ves″ĭ-ko-ko-lon′ik) pertaining to or communicating with the urinary bladder and the colon.

vesicoenteric, vesicointestinal (ves″ĭ-ko-en-ter′-ik), (ves″ĭ-ko-in-tes′tĭ-nal) pertaining to or communicating with the urinary bladder and intestine.

vesicoperineal (ves″ĭ-ko-per″ĭ-ne′al) pertaining to or communicating with the urinary bladder and the perineum.

vesicoprostatic (ves″ĭ-ko-pros-tat′ik) pertaining to the bladder and prostate.

vesicopubic (ves″ĭ-ko-pu′bik) pertaining to the bladder and pubes.

vesicosigmoidostomy (ves″ĭ-ko-sig″moi-dos′to-me) creation of a permanent communication between the urinary bladder and the sigmoid flexure.

vesicospinal (ves″ĭ-ko-spi′nal) pertaining to the bladder and spine.

vesicotomy (ves″ĭ-kot′o-me) incision of the bladder.

vesicouterine (ves″ĭ-ko-u′ter-in) pertaining to the bladder and uterus.

vesicovaginal (ves″ĭ-ko-vaj′ĭ-nal) pertaining to the bladder and vagina.

vesicula (vĕ-sik′u-lah), pl. *vesic′ulae* [L.] vesicle.

vesiculation (vĕ-sik″u-la′shun) formation of vesicles.

vesiculectomy (vĕ-sik″u-lek′to-me) excision of a vesicle, especially the seminal vesicle.

vesiculiform (vĕ-sik′u-lĭ-form″) shaped like a vesicle.

vesiculitis (vĕ-sik″u-li′tis) inflammation of a seminal vesicle.

vesiculocavernous (vĕ-sik″u-lo-kav′er-nus) both vesicular and cavernous.

vesiculogram (vĕ-sik′u-lo-gram″) a roentgenogram of the seminal vesicles.

vesiculography (vĕ-sik″u-log′rah-fe) roentgenography of the seminal vesicles.

vesiculopapular (vĕ-sik″u-lo-pap′u-lar) marked by vesicles and papules.

vesiculopustular (vĕ-sik″u-lo-pus′tu-lar) marked by vesicles and pustules.

vesiculotomy (vĕ-sik″u-lot′o-me) incision into a vesicle, especially the seminal vesicles.

vesiculotympanic (vĕ-sik″u-lo-tim-pan′ik) both vesicular and tympanic.

Vesprin (ves′prin) trademark for preparations of triflupromazine, tranquilizer.

vessel (ves′el) 1. a channel for carrying a fluid, such as blood (blood vessel) or lymph (lymphatic vessel). 2. a receptacle used in laboratory work, of glass, porcelain or other material.
  absorbent v's, the lacteals and other lymphatic vessels.
  collateral v's, channels other than the principal ones supplying or draining an area which serve in the event of obstruction of the main vessels.
  great v's, the aorta and pulmonary artery.
  nutrient v's, vessels supplying nutritive elements to special tissues, as arteries entering the substance of bone or the walls of large blood vessels.

vestibule (ves′tĭ-būl) a space or cavity at the entrance to another structure. adj., **vestib′ular.**
  v. of aorta, a small space at the root of the aorta.
  v. of ear, a cavity at the entrance to the cochlea in the inner ear.
  v. of mouth, the portion of the oral cavity bounded on the one side by teeth and gingivae and on the other by the lips (labial vestibule) and cheeks (buccal vestibule).
  v. of noise, the anterior part of the nasal cavity.
  v. of pharynx, the fauces.
  v. of vagina, the space between the labia minora into which the urethra and vagina open.

vestibulocochlear nerve (ves-tib″u-lo-kok′le-ar) the eighth cranial nerve, which emerges from the brain between the pons and medulla oblongata, behind the facial nerve. The vestibular division serves the vestibule of the ear and the semicircular canals, carrying impulses for equilibrium. The cochlear division serves the cochlea and carries impulses for the sense of hearing. Called also acoustic nerve and auditory nerve.

vestibuloplasty (ves-tib′u-lo-plas″te) surgical modification of gingiva-mucous membrane relations in the vestibule of the mouth.

vestibulotomy (ves-tib″u-lot′o-me) incision into the vestibule of the ear.

vestibulourethral (ves-tib″u-lo-u-re′thral) pertaining to vestibule of the vagina and the urethra.

vestibulum (ves-tib′u-lum), pl. *vestib′ula* [L.] vestibule.

vestige (ves′tij) the remnant of a structure that functioned in a previous stage of species or individual development. adj., **vestig′ial.**

vestigium (ves-tij′e-um), pl. *vestig′ia* [L.] vestige.

veterinarian (vet″er-ĭ-na′re-an) one who treats diseases and injuries in animals.

veterinary (vet′er-ĭ-ner″e) pertaining to animals.

V.F. visual field; vocal fremitus.

via (vi′ah), pl. *vi′ae* [L.] way; channel.
  pri′mae vi′ae, the alimentary canal.
  secon′dae vi′ae, the lacteals and blood vessels.

viability (vi″ah-bil′ĭ-te) the state or quality of being viable.

viable (vi′ah-bl) able to maintain an independent existence; able to live after birth.

Viadril (vi′ah-dril) trademark for a preparation of hydroxydione sodium, an anesthetic.

vial (vi′al) a small bottle.

vibesate (vi′bĕ-sāt) a modified polyvinyl plastic applied topically as a spray to form an occlusive dressing for surgical wounds and other surface lesions.

vibex (vi′beks), pl. *vib′ices* [L.] a linear ecchymosis or streak of effused blood.

vibratile (vi′brah-tīl) swaying or moving to and fro.

vibration (vi-bra′shun) 1. a rapid movement to and fro; oscillation. 2. a form of massage.
  v. disease, blanching and diminished flexion of the fingers, with loss of perception of cold, heat and pain, and osteoarthritis changes in joints of the arm, due to continued use of vibrating tools.

vibrator (vi′bra-tor) an apparatus used in vibratory treatment.

vibratory (vi′brah-tor″e) having a vibrating or to-and-fro movement.

Vibrio (vib′re-o) a genus of Schizomycetes, consisting of actively motile, gram-negative rods.

V. com'ma, the causative agent of Asiatic cholera in man.

vibrio (vib're-o) an organism of the genus Vibrio, or other spiral motile organism.
   cholera v., the causative agent of cholera.

vibriocidal (vib"re-o-si'dal) destructive to organisms of the genus Vibrio.

vibrissa (vi-bris'ah), pl. *vibris'sae* [L.] one of the hairs growing in the vestibule of the nose in man or about the nose (muzzle) of an animal.

vibrocardiogram (vi"bro-kar'de-o-gram") the record produced by vibrocardiography.

vibrocardiography (vi"bro-kar"de-og'rah-fe) graphic recording of vibrations of the chest wall of relatively high frequency that are produced by the action of the heart.

vibrotherapeutics (vi"bro-ther"ah-pu'tiks) the therapeutic use of vibrating appliances.

Vicia (vish'e-ah) a genus of herbs, including the vetch and broad bean.
   V. fa'ba (V. fa'va), a species whose beans or pollen may cause poisoning.

videognosis (vid"e-og-no'sis) diagnosis in a clinical center based on facsimiles of roentgenograms transmitted by television techniques.

vigilambulism (vij"il-am'bu-lizm) a state resembling somnambulism, but not occurring in sleep; double or multiple personality.

vigor (vig'or) strength or force; a combination of attributes of living organisms expressed in rapid growth, high fertility and fecundity, large size and long life.
   hybrid v., that shown by certain hybrids which exceeds that of either parent.

villi (vil'i) [L.] plural of *villus.*

villiferous (vil-if'er-us) provided with villi.

villikinin (vil"i-ki'nin) a hormone that accelerates any movement of the intestinal villi.

villoma (vi-lo'mah) a papilloma, especially of the rectum.

villose (vil'ōs) shaggy with soft hairs.

villositis (vil"o-si'tis) a bacterial disease with alterations in the villosities of the placenta.

villosity (vĭ-los'ĭ-te) 1. condition of being covered with villi. 2. a villus.

villus (vil'us), pl. *vil'li* [L.] a small vascular process or protrusion, as from the free surface of a membrane.
   chorionic villi, threadlike projections originally occurring uniformly over the external surface of the chorion.
   intestinal villi, multitudinous threadlike projections covering the surface of the mucous membrane lining the small intestine.
   synovial villi, slender projections from the surface of the synovial membrane into the cavity of a joint.

villusectomy (vil"ŭ-sek'to-me) synovectomy; excision of a synovial villus.

Vinactane (vin-ak'tān) trademark for a preparation of viomycin, an antibiotic.

vinbarbital (vin-bar'bĭ-tal) a short- to intermediate-acting barbiturate.
   sodium v., a compound used as a central nervous system depressant.

vinblastine (vin-blas'tēn) an alkaloid derived from *Vinca rosa,* used as an antineoplastic agent.

Vincent's angina (vin'sents) necrotizing ulcerative gingivitis; called also TRENCH MOUTH. It is marked by inflammation of the gums, with bleeding and tenderness, and sometimes with fever and swelling of the lymph nodes of the neck.

vinculum (ving'ku-lum), pl. *vin'cula* [L.] a band or bandlike structure.
   vin'cula ten'dinum, filaments that connect the phalanges with the flexor tendons.

vinegar (vin'ĕ-gar) 1. a weak and impure dilution of acetic acid. 2. a medicinal preparation of dilute acetic acid.

Vinethene (vin'ĕ-thēn) trademark for vinyl ether, an anesthetic.

viocid (vi'o-sid) gentian violet, an anthelmintic and anti-infective.

Viocin (vi'o-sin) trademark for a preparation of viomycin sulfate, used in treatment of tuberculosis.

Vioform (vi'o-form) trademark for preparations of iodochlorhydroxyquin, used in treating amebiasis and trichomoniasis.

violet (vi'o-let) 1. the reddish blue color produced by the shortest rays of the visible spectrum. 2. a dye that produces a reddish blue color.
   crystal v., gentian v., methyl v., a faintly odorous compound used as a dye and in medicine as an anthelmintic and anti-infective; called also methylrosaniline chloride.

viomycin (vi"o-mi'sin) an antibiotic substance produced by a species of Streptomyces and used in treatment of tuberculosis.

viosterol (vi-os'ter-ol) calciferol.

viral (vi'ral) pertaining to or caused by a virus.

viremia (vi-re'me-ah) the presence of viruses in the blood.

virgin (vir'jin) a female who has not had coitus.

viridin (vir'ĭ-din) an alkaloid of *Veratrum viride,* an antihypertensive.

virile (vir'il) characterized by virility.

virilescence (vir"ĭ-les'ens) development of male qualities in women of advanced age.

virilism (vir'ĭ-lizm) 1. masculinity; the development of masculine physical and mental traits in the female. 2. hermaphroditism in which the subject is female, but has male external genitalia.
   prosopopilary v., virilism with the presence of hair on the face.

virility (vĭ-ril'ĭ-te) strength and sexual potency in the male.

virilization (vir"ĭ-lĭ-za'shun) induction or development of male secondary sex characters, especially the appearance of such changes in the female.

virogenetic (vi"ro-jĕ-net'ik) having a viral origin.

virology (vi-rol'o-je) the study of viruses and virus diseases.

virose (vi'rōs) having poisonous qualities.

virosis (vi-ro'sis), pl. *viro'ses* a disease caused by a virus.

virucidal (vi"rŭ-si'dal) capable of neutralizing or destroying a virus.

virucide (vi'rŭ-sīd) an agent that neutralizes or destroys a virus.

virulence (vir'u-lens) competence of a noxious agent to produce its effect. adj., **vir'ulent.**

viruliferous (vir"u-lif'er-us) conveying a virus or infectious agent.

viruria (vi-roo're-ah) the presence of viruses in the urine.

virus (vi'rus) a minute infectious agent, smaller than a bacterium, that requires susceptible host cells for multiplication and activity.

Viruses are so elusive that in most instances they cannot be identified and observed by the conventional methods of microbiology. The electron microscope makes it possible to "see" viruses, and they can be isolated by straining them through the minuscule pores of special filters. Viruses thrive only within the cells of living hosts, so that tissue cultures are used to grow viruses for use in vaccines.

CHARACTERISTICS OF VIRUSES. A virus has no metabolic activity of its own, but it has a very orderly structure, so uniform that some viruses can be crystallized much like common salt. The most important substance in viruses is nucleoprotein, a compound of protein and of nucleic acid, which is a substance common to all living matter. The nucleic acid, either deoxyribonucleic acid (DNA) or ribonucleic acid (RNA), contains the "instructions" and mechanisms that allow the virus to control the metabolic activity of the cells it infects. The nucleoprotein of the virus may be surrounded by one or more protein membranes.

Viruses are parasitic. They attach themselves to a living cell of a plant, animal or human body, inject nucleoprotein into the cell and control the cell's normal metabolic mechanisms. The cell proceeds to make vital structures and assembles the units into complete viruses. The cell bursts, dies and releases countless viruses which can then invade other cells.

In some cases the virus may remain inactive for long periods before taking over control of cellular metabolism. In other cases, the virus may force the cell to make new cells as well as new viruses.

In addition to damaging the host by destroying cells, viruses may produce toxins. Viruses also act as antigens, substances the body recognizes as being foreign and combats by producing antibodies.

Viruses are causative organisms of a variety of infectious diseases, including the common cold, yellow fever, childhood diseases such as chickenpox, measles, mumps and rubella, and certain types of pneumonia and encephalitis. Certain viruses have been shown to cause cancer in laboratory animals, but there is still no evidence that they can cause cancer in man. Viruses have the ability to change their individual characteristics so that they are able to continue to grow and propagate while adapting to new environments. This makes chemical treatment of viral diseases difficult since the viruses surviving an initial dose of a drug can change their characteristics so that they rapidly become resistant to the drug.

arbor (*arthropod-borne*) **v's,** a group of viruses, including the causative agents of yellow fever, viral encephalitis and certain febrile infections such as dengue, which are transmitted to man by various mosquitoes and ticks.

attenuated v., one whose pathogenicity has been reduced by serial animal passage or other means.

bacterial v., one that is capable of producing transmissible lysis of bacteria.

Coxsackie v., one of a heterogeneous group of enteroviruses producing in man a disease resembling poliomyelitis, but without paralysis.

echo (*enteric cytopathogenic human orphan*) **v.,** an orphan virus isolated from intestines of man, sometimes found in association with aseptic meningitis.

encephalomyocarditis v., an arbor virus that causes mild aseptic meningitis and a nonparalytic poliomyelitis-like disease.

enteric v., enterovirus.

v. fixé, rabies virus of maximum virulence obtained by passage through a series of 25 to 40 rabbits.

herpes v., herpesvirus.

latent v., masked v., one that ordinarily occurs in a noninfective state and is demonstrable by indirect methods that activate it.

orphan v., one isolated in tissue culture, but not found specifically associated with any disease.

parainfluenza v., one of a group of viruses isolated from patients with upper respiratory tract disease of varying severity.

plant v., one pathogenic for plants.

respiratory syncytial v., a virus isolated from children with bronchopneumonia and bronchitis, characteristically causing syncytium formation in tissue culture.

street v., virus obtained from a natural case of rabies.

vaccinia v., the virus of cowpox, used in inoculating against smallpox.

vis (vis), pl. *vi'res* [L.] force, energy.

viscera (vis'er-ah) [L.] plural of *viscus.*

viscerad (vis'er-ad) toward the viscera.

visceral (vis'er-al) pertaining to a viscus.

visceralgia (vis"er-al'je-ah) pain in the viscera.

visceralism (vis'er-al-izm") the opinion that the viscera are the main seats of disease.

visceroinhibitory (vis"er-o-in-hib'ĭ-tor"e) arresting the activity of the viscera.

visceromegaly (vis"er-o-meg'ah-le) abnormal enlargement of the viscera.

visceromotor (vis″er-o-mo′tor) conveying motor stimuli to the viscera.

visceroparietal (vis″er-o-pah-ri′ĕ-tal) pertaining to the viscera and the abdominal wall.

visceroperitoneal (vis″er-o-per″ĭ-to-ne′al) pertaining to the viscera and peritoneum.

visceropleural (vis″er-o-ploo′ral) pertaining to the viscera and the pleura.

visceroptosis (vis″er-op-to′sis) splanchnoptosis; prolapse or downward displacement of the viscera.

viscerosensory (vis″er-o-sen′so-re) pertaining to sensation in the viscera.

viscerosomatic (vis″er-o-so-mat′ik) pertaining to the viscera and the body.

viscerotonia (vis″er-o-to′ne-ah) a group of traits characterized by general relaxation, and love of comfort, sociability and conviviality; considered typical of endomorphy.

viscerotropic (vis″er-o-trop′ik) having a special affinity for the abdominal viscera.

viscid (vis′id) having a glutinous consistency.

viscidity (vĭ-sid′ĭ-te) the property of being glutinous.

viscosimeter (vis″ko-sim′ĕ-ter) an apparatus used in measuring viscosity of a substance.

viscosity (vis-kos′ĭ-te) a physical property of a substance that is dependent on the friction of its component molecules as they slide by one another.

viscous (vis′kus) sticky or gummy.

viscus (vis′kus), pl. *vis′cera* [L.] any large interior organ in any of the great body cavities, especially those in the abdomen.

vision (vizh′un) the faculty of seeing; sight. adj., **vis′ual.** The basic components of vision are the eye itself, the visual center in the brain, and the optic nerve, which connects the two.

How the Eye Works. The eye works like a camera. Light rays enter it through the adjustable iris and are focused by the lens onto the retina, a thin light-sensitive layer which corresponds to the film of the camera. The retina converts the light rays into nerve impulses, which are relayed to the visual center. There the brain interprets them as images.

Like a camera lens, the lens of the eye reverses images as it focuses them. The images on the retina are upside down and they are "flipped over" in the visual center. In a psychology experiment, a number of volunteers wore glasses that inverted everything. After 8 days, their visual centers adjusted to this new situation, and when they took off the glasses, the world looked upside down until their brain centers readjusted.

The retina is made up of millions of tiny nerve cells that contain specialized chemicals that are sensitive to light. There are two varieties of these nerve cells, rods and cones. Between them they cover the full range of the eye's adaptation to light. The cones are sensitive in bright light, and the rods in dim light. At twilight, as the light fades, the cones stop operating and the rods go into action. The momentary blindness experienced on going from bright to dim light, or from dim to bright, is the pause needed for the other set of nerve cells to take over.

The rods are spread toward the edges of the retina, so that vision in dim light is general but not very sharp or clear. The cones are clustered thickly in the center of the retina, in the fovea centralis. When the eyes are turned and focused on the object to be seen the image is brought to the central area of the retina. In very dim light, on the other hand, an object is seen more clearly if it is not looked at directly because then its image falls on an area where the rods are thicker.

Color Vision. Color vision is a function of the cones. The most widely accepted theory of color vision is that there are three types of cones, each type containing chemicals that respond to one of the three primary colors—red, green and violet. White light stimulates all three sets of cones; any other color stimulates only one or two sets. The brain can then interpret the impulses from these cones as various colors. Man's color vision is amazingly delicate; a trained expert can distinguish among as many as 300,000 different hues.

Color blindness is the result of a disorder of one or more sets of cones. The great majority of people with some degree of color blindness lack either red or green cones, and cannot distinguish between the two colors. True color blindness, in which none of the sets of color cones works, is very rare. Most color blindness is inherited, and mostly by male children through their mothers from a color-blind grandfather.

Stereoscopic Vision. Stereoscopic vision, or vision in depth, is caused by the way the eyes are placed. Each eye has a slightly different field of vision. The two images are superimposed on one another, but because of the distance between the eyes, the image from each eye goes slightly around its side of the object. From the differences between the images and from other indicators such as the position of the eye muscles when the eyes are focused on the object, the brain can determine the distance of the object.

Stereoscopic vision works best on nearby objects. As the distance increases, the difference between the left-eyed and the right-eyed views becomes less, and the brain must depend on other factors to determine distance. Among these are the relative size of the object, its color and clearness and the receding lines of perspective. These factors may fool the eye; for example, in clear mountain air distant objects may seem to be very close. This is because their sharpness and color are not dulled by the atmosphere as much as they would be in more familiar settings.

Disorders of Vision. Imperfect vision is most commonly caused by abnormal shape of the eyeball. In the normal eye, the lens focuses the image on the retina. This is 20/20 vision. The figures refer to the distance at which a standard object can be recognized. A person who is nearsighted, for example, may only be able to recognize at 20 feet an object that a person with perfect vision can recognize at 100 feet. In this case he is said to have 20/100 vision. For the sake of convenience, eye charts with letters of different sizes are used rather than objects placed at different distances.

Nearsightedness, or myopia, is the result of an eyeball that is longer than usual from front to back, so that the image falls in front of the retina. The lens can bring nearby objects into focus, but not those farther away. Farsightedness, or hyperopia, is caused by an eyeball that is shorter than normal, in which the image focuses behind the retina. ASTIGMATISM is impaired vision caused by irregularities in the curvature of the cornea or lens. All of these conditions can usually be corrected with prescription lenses.

achromatic v., vision characterized by lack of color vision.

binocular v., that resulting from simultaneous stimulation of the receptors of both eyes; termed single binocular vision when the resulting images are properly fused into one.

central v., that produced by stimulation of receptors in the fovea centralis.

daylight v., visual perception in the daylight or under conditions of bright illumination.

dichromatic v., that in which color perception is restricted to a pair of primaries, either blue and yellow or red and green.

double v., diplopia.

finger v., alleged ability to recognize, as a result of stimuli received through the skin of the fingertips, qualities (such as color) ordinarily recognized by sight.

half v., hemianopia.

indirect v., peripheral vision.

monocular v., vision with one eye.

multiple v., polyopia.

night v., visual perception in the darkness of night or under conditions of reduced illumination.

oscillating v., oscillopsia.

peripheral v., that produced by stimulation of receptors in the retina outside the macula lutea.

tunnel v., a condition of great reduction in the visual field, as though the subject were looking through a long tunnel.

visualization (vizh″u-al-ĭ-za′shun) the act of viewing or of achieving a complete visual impression of an object.

visuo-auditory (vizh″u-o-aw′dĭ-to″re) pertaining to sight and hearing.

visuometer (vizh″u-om′ĕ-ter) an instrument for measuring range of vision.

visuopsychic (vizh″u-o-si′kik) pertaining to both visual and psychic processes.

visuosensory (vizh″u-o-sen′so-re) pertaining to perception of visual impressions.

vital (vi′tal) pertaining to life; necessary to life.

v. capacity, the volume of air a person can forcibly expire from the lungs after a maximal inspiration.

v. signs, the signs of life, namely pulse, respiration and temperature.

vitalism (vi′tah-lizm) the theory that bodily functions are produced by a distinct principal called vital force.

vitalist (vi′tah-list) a believer in vitalism.

Vitallium (vi-tal′e-um) a cobalt-chromium alloy used for dentures and surgical appliances.

vitamer (vi′tah-mer) a substance or compound that has vitamin activity.

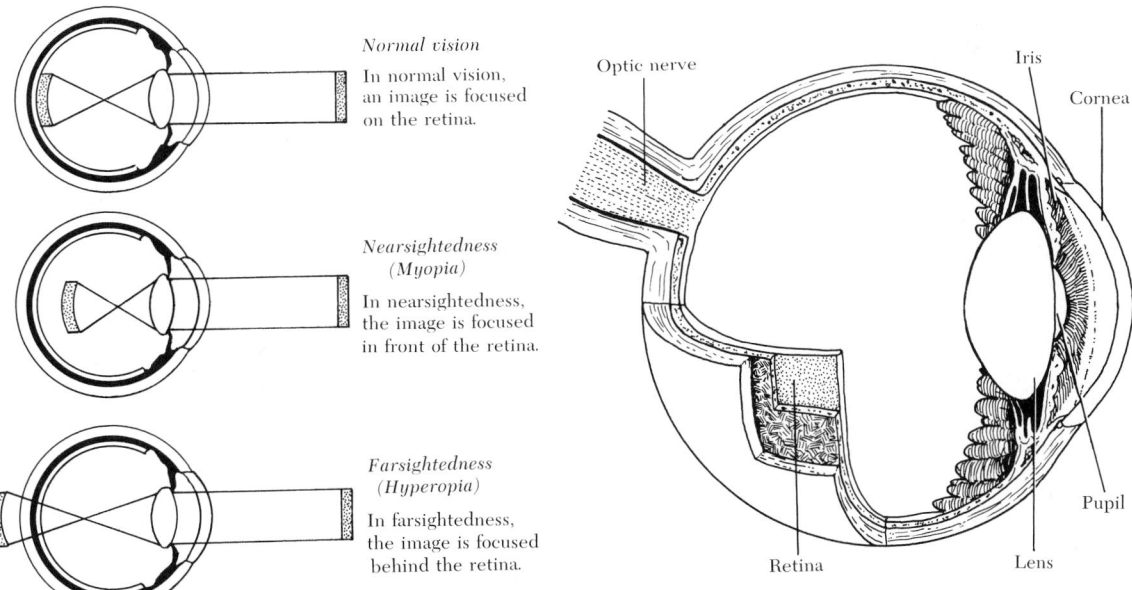

Normal vision
In normal vision, an image is focused on the retina.

Nearsightedness (Myopia)
In nearsightedness, the image is focused in front of the retina.

Farsightedness (Hyperopia)
In farsightedness, the image is focused behind the retina.

Optic nerve

Iris

Cornea

Pupil

Retina

Lens

Right, anatomy of the eye. Vision is the reception of images by the eye as a result of the passage of light into the eye. Light is focused by the lens on the retina where it is converted into nerve impulses which are transmitted to the centers in the brain where images are interpreted.

vitamin (vi'tah-min) an organic substance found in foods and essential in small quantities for growth, health and the preservation of life itself. The body needs vitamins just as it requires other food constituents such as proteins, fats, carbohydrates, minerals and water. Vitamins differ from these in chemical structure, however, and are required only in relatively minute quantities. The absence of one or more vitamins from the diet, or poor absorption of vitamins, can cause deficiency diseases such as rickets, scurvy and beriberi.

Vitamins help transform other food substances into bones, skin, glands, nerves, brain and blood.

The major vitamins are designated by the letters A, C, D, E, K and P, and the term B complex. Some of these, the B vitamins and vitamin C, can be dissolved in water; the rest are soluble in fat. Vitamins do not resemble each other chemically except for their solubility. This quality of solubility is important in absorption of vitamins from the intestinal tract and in certain deficiency diseases.

VITAMIN A. Vitamin A helps to maintain epithelial tissues which cover the body and line certain internal organs. This vitamin also is essential for the proper growth of skeletal and soft tissues, and is necessary for light-sensitive pigments in the eye that make night vision possible. The particular manifestation of vitamin A deficiency depends upon the age of the patient. Among the commonest symptoms of vitamin A deficiency is night blindness. The skin may also be affected, becoming dry and pimply like a toad's skin.

Vitamin A is manufactured by animals and man from carotenes found in green leafy and yellow vegetables, including kale, broccoli, spinach, carrots, squash and sweet potatoes. It is obtained directly by eating animal products such as liver, eggs, whole milk, cream and cheese.

THE B COMPLEX. The original "vitamin B" was found to be a group of vitamins, each differing chemically and each individually important in the body. For convenience, these vitamins are referred to as one group since they are often found together in foods. Deficiency in only one of these vitamins is rare, and the deficiency disease attributed to lack of one vitamin B usually is complicated by deficiencies of the others as well.

Vitamin B₁ (Thiamine). This vitamin is necessary to break down and release energy from carbohydrates. Lack of thiamine can cause loss of appetite, certain types of neuritis and, in severe cases, beriberi, which affects the brain, heart and nerves.

The best sources of thiamine are yeasts, ham and certain pork cuts, liver, peanuts, whole and fortified cereals and milk. The vitamin is easily destroyed by cooking and may also be lost by dissolving in the cooking water. Because the body does not store thiamine well, foods that are good sources of it should be included in each day's diet.

Vitamin B₂ (Riboflavin). This vitamin is believed to play a role in the metabolism of all living cells. Riboflavin deficiency (ariboflavinosis) is believed to be one of the most common vitamin-deficiency diseases in the United States. The symptoms include open sores at the corners of the mouth and on the lips, a purple-red, inflamed tongue, seborrheic dermatitis and corneal and other eye changes.

The main food sources of riboflavin are milk, liver, kidney, heart, green vegetables, dried yeasts and enriched cereals. It is not usually affected by cooking, but is destroyed by light.

Niacin (Nicotinic Acid). This vitamin B appears to act in enzyme systems to utilize carbohydrates, fats and amino acids. Niacin deficiency causes PELLAGRA, once a major deficiency disease in the United States. Symptoms of pellagra involve the skin and digestive and nervous systems.

Food sources of niacin are various high-protein foods such as liver, yeast, bran, peanuts, lean meats, fish and poultry.

Vitamin B₁₂. This vitamin contains a metal, cobalt. It is called also cyanocobalamin and extrinsic factor, and is needed for the efficient production of blood cells and for the health of the nervous system. Only small amounts of B₁₂ are required by the body. The activity of this vitamin is associated with that of another B vitamin, folic acid.

Inability to absorb vitamin B₁₂ occurs in PERNICIOUS ANEMIA, in which a substance normally secreted by the stomach, called intrinsic factor, is missing. Intrinsic factor is needed to absorb vitamin B₁₂ in the small intestine. Injections of vitamin B₁₂ can control pernicious anemia. Poor absorption of vitamin B₁₂ also occurs in sprue.

Vitamin B₁₂ is not found in plant foods. The main sources in the human diet are animal products such as milk, eggs and liver. Probably the ultimate source of B₁₂ is bacterial production in animal intestines. This production occurs in man, and in normal persons probably meets some or perhaps all of the body's requirements.

Other B Vitamins. These include vitamin B₆ (pyridoxine), biotin, folic acid, pantothenic acid, choline, inositol and para-aminobenzoic acid. Vitamin B₆ deficiency can cause convulsions, lethargy, mental changes and retardation, inflammation of the skin and anemia.

These vitamins, like most other members of the B complex, are widely found in fruits, vegetables, meat and whole-grain cereals.

VITAMIN C (ASCORBIC ACID). This vitamin is necessary for the health of the supporting tissues of the body such as bone, cartilage and connective tissue (see also ASCORBIC ACID). Vitamin C deficiency produces SCURVY.

Vitamin C is found in fresh fruits and vegetables, including citrus fruits, tomatoes, brussels sprouts and to some extent whole potatoes. Cooking and storage destroys much of the vitamin C content of foods.

VITAMIN D. The action of sunlight on the skin changes certain substances in the body into vitamin D, a term for any of several active substances required for the utilization of calcium and phosphorus, essential for the growth and maintenance of bone. Vitamin D deficiency in children causes RICKETS, which can sometimes occur in adults as well and is then known as OSTEOMALACIA. Rickets is usually caused either by a diet deficient in vitamin D or by insufficient exposure to sunlight.

Few foods contain vitamin D. The only rich natural sources are fish liver oil and the livers of animals feeding on fish. For this reason vitamin D often is added to milk.

VITAMIN E. The role of this vitamin in human nutrition is uncertain. Experiments with animals indicate that a vitamin E deficiency may be associated with sterility and abortion, and with liver, muscle and kidney disease. Similar diseases have

The Principal Vitamins

Vitamin	Principal Sources	Properties	Physiologic Effects	Deficiency Symptoms	Daily Allowances	Usual Therapeutic Dosage
Vitamin A	Fish liver oils, liver, eggs, milk, butter, vitamin A-fortified margarine, green leafy or yellow vegetables	Oil-soluble; susceptible to oxidation, especially at high temperatures	Essential to normal function of epithelial cells and visual purple	Night blindness Xerophthalmia Hyperkeratosis of skin	Adults: 5,000–8,000 U.S.P. u.† Children: 1,500–5,000 U.S.P. u.‡	Up to 100,000 U.S.P. u./day
Vitamin B₁ (Thiamine)	Yeast, whole grains; meat, especially pork, liver; nuts, egg yolk, legumes, potatoes, most vegetables	Water-soluble; stable to heat, unstable to alkali, but heat-sensitive under neutral and alkaline conditions	Carbohydrate metabolism, nerve function; promotes growth	Beriberi Peripheral neuritis Cardiac disease	All ages: 0.4 mg./1,000 calories	5–30 mg./day
Vitamin B₂ (Riboflavin)	Milk, cheese, liver, organ meats, beef muscle, egg white	Slightly water-soluble; unstable to light and alkali	Promotes growth, general health; essential to cellular oxidation	Cheilosis Angular stomatitis Dermatitis Photophobia	All ages: 0.6 mg./1,000 calories	10–30 mg./day
Niacin (Nicotinic acid)	Yeast, liver, organ meats, peanuts, wheat germ	Water-soluble; stable; intolerance produces flushing, burning, itching (rare with niacinamide)	Essential for health, tissue respiration, tryptophan and carbohydrate metabolism, growth, gastrointestinal function and normal skin	Pellagra (Dermatitis, glossitis, gastrointestinal and nervous system dysfunction)	All ages: 6.6 mg. equivalent/1,000 calories	(Niacinamide) 100–1,000 mg./day
Vitamin B₆ Group (Pyridoxine, Pyridoxal, Pyridoxamine)	Yeast, liver, muscle meats, whole-grain cereals, fish, vegetables, molasses	Water-soluble; heat-, acid- and alkali-stable; sparingly soluble in alcohol; light-sensitive in neutral and alkaline solutions; nontoxic in recommended doses	Essential for cellular function and for metabolism of certain amino and fatty acids	Seborrhea-like skin lesions; nerve inflammation; epileptiform convulsions in infants; anemias	Not established, but thought to be 1.5–2.0 mg./day	25–100 mg./day

1053

The Principal Vitamins (*Continued*)

Vitamin	Principal Sources	Properties	Physiologic Effects	Deficiency Symptoms	Daily Allowances	Usual Therapeutic Dosage
Vitamin B₁₂ (Cyanocobalamin)	Liver; meats, especially beef, pork, organ meats; eggs, milk and milk products	Water- and alcohol-soluble; nontoxic	Maturation of r.b.c.; neural function; may be a growth factor; may be implicated in carbohydrate and fat metabolism	Pernicious anemia; may have a beneficial effect in certain neuritides; tobacco-alcohol amblyopia	Not established, but thought to be about 3–5 (1.0–1.5 absorbed) mcg.	1–2 mcg./day I.M. to maintain remission in pernicious anemia
Vitamin C (Ascorbic acid)	Citrus fruits, tomatoes, potatoes, cabbage, green pepper	Water-soluble; stable in dry state but oxidized by heat and light; nontoxic in recommended doses	Essential to osteoid tissue, collagen formation, vascular function, tissue respiration and wound healing; relationship to adrenocortical hormones suggested	Scurvy (Hemorrhages, loose teeth, gingivitis)	Adults: 70 mg. Children: 30–80 mg.	100–1,000 mg. /day
Vitamin D Ergocalciferol (D₂) Cholecalciferol (D₃)	Fish liver oils, eggs, milk, butter, sunlight and irradiation	Oil-soluble; in large doses may cause hypercalcemia	Metabolism of Ca and K	Infantile rickets Infantile tetany Osteomalacia	Adults and Children: 400 U.S.P. u.	400–1,600 U.S.P. u./day (*see text for higher dosage*)
Folic acid (Pteroylglutamic acid)	Green leafy vegetables, liver and kidney, yeast	Soluble in boiling water or dilute aqueous alkali; nontoxic in recommended doses	Maturation of r.b.c.; may be concerned in synthesis of nucleoproteins	Nutritional macrocytic anemia; may be of value in the treatment of sprue; megaloblastic anemia of infancy	Not established, but 0.05 mg. (0.15 mg. total folic acid activity in foods)/day has been suggested	1–15 mg./day

	Sources	Physical properties	Function	Signs of deficiency	Daily requirement	Therapeutic dose
Pantothenic acid (Calcium pantothenate)	Yeast, liver, kidneys, egg yolk, vegetables	Water-soluble viscous oil; unstable in hot acid or basic solutions	Involved in fat, protein and carbohydrate metabolism by its relation to acetylation processes	Exp'l def'cy in man charact'd by fatigue, malaise, headache, sleep disturbances, nausea, abdominal cramps, vomiting, paresthesias, muscle cramps and impaired coord'n. "Burning feet" syndrome may respond to pantothenate	Not yet established; thought to be about 10 mg./day	Not known; not <50 mg./day should be used for therapeutic trial
Vitamin K (activity)	Intestinal bacterial synthesis and a normal diet		Prothrombin formation; normal blood coagulation	Hemorrhage from prolonged prothrombin time	Undetermined. In situations conducive to neonatal hemorrhage, 2–5 mg. may be given to mothers in labor, or 1–2 mg. to newborn infant	For details on therapeutic dosage, see text
Menadione		Oil-soluble in water; unstable to light				
Menadione sodium bisulfite		Soluble in water; unstable with alkalis				
Phytonadione (Vitamin K₁)		Oily liquid; unstable to heat and light; insoluble in water				
Vitamin E Group (α, β, γ & δ tocopherol)	Vegetable oils, lettuce, eggs, cereal products	Slightly viscous oil; insoluble in water	Intracellular antioxidant	Abnormal fat deposits in muscles; creatinuria; macrocytic anemia when assoc. with protein def'cy	Not firmly established; may range from 10–30 mg. of d-α-tocopherol/day, depending on am't of polyunsaturated fats in diet	Not established. Perhaps between 50–300 mg.

From The Merck Manual. 11th ed. Copyright 1966, Merck & Co., Inc., Rahway, New Jersey.

† 3,000–5,000 U.S.P. u., if all the activity is due to preformed vitamin A.
‡ 900–3,000 U.S.P. u., if all the activity is due to preformed vitamin A.

blue v., copper sulfate.
green v., ferrous sulfate.
white v., zinc sulfate.

not yet been proved to occur in vitamin E deficiency in man.

VITAMIN K. Because this vitamin helps the liver to produce substances important in blood clotting, deficiency of vitamin K delays clotting. Symptoms are excessive bleeding and bruises under the skin. Generally, the bacteria of the intestine produce vitamin K in quantities that are adequate (provided it can be absorbed), except in newborn infants, in whom the deficiency is most frequently found. Vitamin K is also found in green leafy vegetables.

VITAMIN P. The flavone factor in lemon juice is known as vitamin P; deficiency of it causes increased permeability of capillary walls.

VITAMIN SUPPLEMENTS. The exact vitamin requirements for good health often are not known with accuracy; they vary with age, weight, sex and state of health. The need for certain vitamins increases with fever, some diseases, heavy exercise, pregnancy and nursing.

If a person eats an adequate, varied diet of meats, fish, vegetables and dairy products, he will receive enough vitamins to meet his usual requirements. Public health measures such as the addition of vitamin D to milk and the B vitamins to bread and other cereal products have helped to combat deficiency diseases.

The use of vitamin supplements is expensive and in general unnecessary. Specialists in nutrition advise against taking supplementary vitamins unless they are prescribed for a specific reason by a physician. Vitamins should not be used as "tonics." There is a distinct possibility that the indiscriminate use of vitamin preparations may sometimes lead to overdosage, a problem that has arisen in recent years. For example, overdoses of vitamins D, A or K may result in serious disease, the excess vitamins acting like poisons. Also, recent tests suggest that large doses of vitamin D taken by a woman during pregnancy may have undesirable effects on her unborn child. Though these tests are not conclusive, they confirm the need for caution in the use of vitamins.

Vitamins are commonly prescribed in infancy and childhood, during pregnancy and nursing, for elderly patients whose dietary habits are poor and in clearly diagnosed deficiency states. These include not only the more familiar deficiency diseases already described but also alcoholism and chronic wasting diseases.

vitellus (vi-tel′us) the yolk of egg. adj., **vitel′line**.

vitiligo (vit″ĭ-li′go) a condition due to failure of melanin formation in the skin, producing sharply demarcated, milky-white patches with hyperpigmented borders.

vitreocapsulitis (vit″re-o-kap″su-li′tis) inflammation of the membrane that enfolds the vitreous body.

vitreodentin (vit″re-o-den′tin) a dense and glass-like form of dentin.

vitreous (vit′re-us) 1. glasslike or hyaline. 2. the vitreous body; the transparent substance that fills the part of the eyeball between the lens and the retina. Called also vitreous humor.

vitriol (vit′re-ol) any crystalline sulfate.

vitropression (vit′ro-presh′un) exertion of pressure on the skin with a slip of glass, forcing blood from the area.

vitrum (vi′rum) [L.] glass.

vivi- (viv′e) word element [L.], *alive; life.*

vividialysis (viv″ĭ-di-al′ĭ-sis) dialysis through a living membrane (see also PERITONEAL DIALYSIS).

vividiffusion (viv″y-dī-fu′zhun) circulation of the blood through a closed apparatus in which it is passed through a membrane for removal of substances ordinarily removed by the kidneys (see also artificial KIDNEY).

vivification (viv″ĭ-fĭ-ka′shun) conversion of lifeless into living protein matter by assimilation.

viviparous (vi-vip′ah-rus) giving birth to living young that have derived nutrition directly from the maternal organism through a special organ, the placenta, which is an outgrowth of the embryo.

viviperception (viv″ĭ-per-sep′shun) the study of the vital processes of a living organism.

vivisection (viv″ĭ-sek′shun) surgical procedures performed upon a living animal for purpose of physiologic or pathologic investigation.

vivisectionist (viv″ĭ-sek′shun-ist) one who practices or defends vivisection.

Vleminckx's solution (vlem′inks) sulfurated lime; used in treatment of acne.

V.M. voltmeter.

VMA vanillylmandelic acid.

vocal (vo′kal) pertaining to the voice.

v. cords, the thyroarytenoid ligaments of the LARYNX, the superior pair being called the false, and the inferior pair the true, vocal cords. These thin, reedlike bands vibrate to make vocal sounds during speaking, and are capable of producing a vast range of sounds.

One end of each cord is attached to the front wall of the larynx. These ends are close together. The opposite ends are connected to two tiny cartilages near the back wall of the larynx. The cartilages can be rotated so as to swing the cords far apart or bring them together. When the cords are apart, the breath passes through silently, unobstructed. When they are closer together, the cords partly obstruct the air passage, and as the air is forced through them, the cords vibrate like the reeds of a pipe organ, producing sound waves. These waves are what we call the voice. (See also SPEECH.)

Various disorders may affect the larynx and vocal cords. LARYNGITIS may be acute or chronic and is usually caused by continual irritation of the vocal cords by overuse or by inhaled irritants such as tobacco smoke. The voice may be "lost" and then regained after a few days of rest and medication, if the cause has been removed. Prolonged or repeated impairment of the voice requires medical diagnosis.

LARYNGECTOMY, partial or total removal of the larynx, usually is performed as treatment for cancer of the larynx. Once the larynx is removed the patient must learn to speak without his vocal cords, by one of three methods: esophageal speech, pharyngeal speech or use of an electronic voice box.

voice (vois) the sound produced by vibrations of the vocal cords (see also SPEECH).

void (void) to cast out as waste matter, especially the urine.

vol. volume.

vola (vo′lah) a concave or hollow surface.
  v. ma′nus, the palm.
  v. pe′dis, the sole.

volar (vo′lar) pertaining to the sole or palm.

volaris (vo-la′ris) palmar.

volatile (vol′ah-til) evaporating rapidly.

volatilization (vol″ah-til-ĭ-za′shun) conversion into a vapor.

volitional (vo-lish′un-al) pertaining to the will.

Volkmann's contracture (fōlk′mahnz) contraction of the fingers and sometimes of the wrist, with loss of power, after severe injury or improper use of a tourniquet or cast in the region of the elbow.

volley (vol′e) a number of impulses of energy, as nerve impulses, transmitted in rapid succession.

volsella (vol-sel′ah) vulsella.

volt (vōlt) the unit of electromotive force; 1 ampere of current against 1 ohm of resistance.
  electron v., the energy acquired by an electron when accelerated by a potential of one volt, being equivalent to 3.82×10^{-20} calories, or 1.6×10^{-12} ergs.

voltage (vōl′tij) electromotive force measured in volts.

voltmeter (vōlt′me-ter) an instrument for measuring electromotive force in volts.

volume (vol′ūm) the measure of the quantity of a substance.
  blood v., the total quantity of blood in the body.
  circulation v., the amount of blood pumped through the lungs and out to all the organs of the body.
  expiratory reserve v., the maximal amount of gas that can be expired from the end-expiratory level.
  inspiratory reserve v., the maximal amount of gas that can be inspired from the end-inspiratory position.
  minute v., the total flow of blood through the heart per minute, or the total volume of air breathed per minute.
  packed-cell v., the volume of the blood corpuscles in a centrifuged sample of blood, especially the volume of packed red cells in cubic centimeters per 100 cc. of blood.
  residual v., the amount of gas remaining in the lung at the end of a maximal expiration.
  stroke v., the quantity of blood ejected from a ventricle at each beat of the heart.
  tidal v., the amount of gas passing into and out of the lungs in each respiratory cycle.

volumetric (vol″u-met′rik) pertaining to or accompanied by measurement in volumes.

volumometer (vol″u-mom′ĕ-ter) an instrument for measuring volume or changes in volume.

voluntary (vol′un-tār″e) accomplished in accordance with the will.

volute (vo-lūt′) rolled up.

volvulosis (vol″vu-lo′sis) infection with *Onchocerca volvulus*, producing subcutaneous fibrous tumors.

volvulus (vol′vu-lus) [L.] torsion of a loop of intestine, causing obstruction with or without strangulation.

vomer (vo′mer) a bone forming part of the nasal septum. adj., **vo′merine.**

vomica (vom′ĭ-kah) 1. an abnormal cavity in an organ, especially in the lung. 2. profuse and sudden expectoration of pus or putrescent matter.

vomit (vom′it) 1. matter expelled from the stomach by the mouth. 2. to eject stomach contents through the mouth.
  bilious v., vomit stained with bile.
  black v., darkened blood cast up from the stomach in yellow fever.
  coffee-ground v., dark granular material ejected from the stomach, produced by mixture of blood with the gastric contents; it is a sign of bleeding in the upper alimentary canal.

vomiting (vom′it-ing) forcible ejection of contents of stomach through the mouth.
  cyclic v., recurring attacks of vomiting.
  dry v., attempts at vomiting, with the ejection of nothing but gas.
  pernicious v., vomiting in pregnancy so severe as to threaten life.
  v. of pregnancy, vomiting occurring in the morning during the early months of pregnancy (see also MORNING SICKNESS).
  projectile v., vomiting with the material ejected with great force; seen commonly in congenital pyloric obstruction.
  stercoraceous v., vomiting of fecal matter.

vomitory (vom′ĭ-to″re) an emetic.

vomiturition (vom″ĭ-tu-rish′un) repeated ineffectual attempts to vomit; retching.

vomitus (vom′ĭ-tus) 1. vomiting. 2. matter vomited.

von Gierke's disease (von gēr′kez) a disease characterized by abnormal storage of glycogen in children; marked by enlargement of the liver and hypoglycemia and lack of response to epinephrine's glycogen-mobilizing effect. An enzyme deficiency is responsible for the abnormal glycogen metabolism. Called also glycogenosis and glycogen storage disease.

von Jaksch's disease (von yaksh) infantile pseudoleukemia.

von Recklinghausen's disease (von rek′linghow″zenz) 1. neurofibromatosis. 2. osteitis fibrosa cystica.

von Willebrand's disease (von vil′ĕ-brandz) a hereditary familial disease due to a deficiency of antihemophilic globulin and capillary defect, marked by severe epistaxis and bleeding from the gums and genitalia; called also angiohemophilia.

vortex (vor'teks), pl. *vor'tices* [L.] a pattern of curving lines radiating from a common center.

vox (voks) [L.] voice.
  v. choler'ica, the peculiar suppressed voice of true cholera.

voyeurism (voi'yer-izm) a form of sexual aberration in which gratification is derived from looking at another's genital organs.

V.R. vocal resonance.

V.S. volumetric solution.

vuerometer (vu"er-om'ĕ-ter) an instrument for measuring the distance between the eyes.

vulgaris (vul-ga'ris) [L.] ordinary; common.

vulnerary (vul'ner-er"e) an agent that promotes the healing of wounds.

vulnus (vul'nus), pl. *vul'nera* [L.] wound.

vulsella (vul-sel'ah) a forceps with clawlike hooks at the end of each blade.

vulva (vul'vah) the external parts of the female reproductive system that surround the opening of the vagina. adj., **vul'var.**
  Two pairs of skin folds protect the vaginal opening, one on each side. The larger outer folds are the labia majora, and the more delicate inner folds are the labia minora. In a virgin, a thin membrane, the hymen, usually partially covers the opening of the vagina. Normally, the hymen is well perforated, to permit the menstrual flow. Occasionally it is not, and a minor surgical procedure may be necessary.
  The upper or forward ends of the labia minora join around the clitoris, a small projection that is composed of erectile tissue like the male penis and has erotic functions. The opening of the urethra, which empties urine from the bladder, lies between the clitoris and the vagina. (See also REPRODUCTIVE ORGANS, FEMALE.)

vulvectomy (vul-vek'to-me) excision of the vulva.

vulvismus (vul-viz'mus) vaginismus.

vulvitis (vul-vi'tis) inflammation of the vulva.

vulvocrural (vol"vo-kroo'ral) pertaining to the vulva and thigh.

vulvopathy (vul-vop'ah-the) any disease of the vulva.

vulvorectal (vul"vo-rek'tal) pertaining to or communicating with the vulva and rectum.

vulvouterine (vul"vo-u'ter-in) pertaining to the vulva and uterus.

vulvovaginal (vul"vo-vaj'ĭ-nal) pertaining to the vulva and vagina.

vulvovaginitis (vul"vo-vaj"ĭ-ni'tis) inflammation of the vulva and vagina.

vv. [L., pl.] *ve'nae* (veins).

v./v. volume (of solute) per volume (of solvent).

W

W chemical symbol, *tungsten (wolfram)*.

W. watt; weight; work.

Wald (Wawld) Lillian (1867–1940). American nurse; founder of the Henry Street Settlement in Manhattan's Lower East Side, one of the first non-sectarian visiting nurse services in the world.

Waldenström's disease (vahl'den-stremz) 1. (of blood) macroglobulinemia. 2. (of bone) osteochondrosis involving the hip joint.

wall (wawl) a structure bounding or limiting a space or a definitive mass of material.
  cell w., a structure outside of and protecting the cell membrane, present in all plant cells and in many bacteria and other types of cells.
  vessel w., the multiple layers bounding a channel conveying blood or lymph.

walleye (wawl'i) 1. leukoma, a white opacity of the cornea. A common cause is degeneration of the cornea from longstanding, untreated syphilis. Other possible causes include inflammation of the cornea, corneal ulcer and trachoma. 2. exotropia, a congenital defect similar to crossed eyes except that the visual axes diverge outward rather than inward; called also divergent strabismus.

warfarin (wōr'fer-in) a compound used as an anticoagulant.
  potassium w., sodium w., an anticoagulant compound.

wart (wort) a small, hard, abnormal growth on the skin or adjoining mucous membrane, caused by a virus; called also verruca. Warts are generally more common among children and young adults than among older persons. Most warts are less than a quarter of an inch in diameter; they may be flat or raised, dry or moist. Usually they have a rough and pitted surface, either flesh-colored or darker than the surrounding skin.
  Warts develop usually on the exposed parts of the fingers and hands, but also on the elbows, face, scalp and other areas. When on especially vulnerable parts of the body, such as the knee or elbow, they are subject to irritation and may become quite tender. Plantar warts, which occur on the soles of the feet, become very sensitive because of pressure. Anal warts cause itching. Warts can also block a nostril or an external acoustic meatus.
  A wart develops between 1 and 8 months after the virus becomes lodged in the skin. The virus is often spread by scratching, rubbing and slight razor cuts. In more than half the cases, warts disappear without treatment, but some remain for years.
  TREATMENT. Many popular "cures" for warts have been suggested, but are generally useless. Furthermore, self-treatment, by cutting, scraping or using acids or patent medicines, may cause bacterial infection, scarring and other harm—without eliminating the warts.
  A troublesome wart should be removed only by a physician, who may use acids; electrodesiccation, freezing with liquid nitrogen, or x-rays for the purpose. Warts are notoriously stubborn. Often the virus remains in the skin, and the wart grows again.
  It is generally advised that warts on children be removed early. Otherwise they tend to be spread by the child's scratching and other activities. The tendency of warts to spread is less evident in adults.

Wassermann test (wos'er-man) a complement-fixation test used in the diagnosis of syphilis.

Wassermann-fast (wos'er-man-fast") showing a positive reaction to the Wassermann test despite antisyphilitic treatment.

waste (wāst) 1. gradual loss, decay or diminution of bulk. 2. useless and effete material, unfit for further use within the organism. 3. to pine away or dwindle.

water (wot'er) 1. a clear, colorless, odorless, tasteless liquid, H_2O. 2. an aqueous solution of a medicinal substance. 3. (pl.) amniotic fluid.
  distilled w., water that has been purified by distillation.
  lime w., calcium hydroxide solution.

Waterhouse-Friderichsen syndrome (wot'er-hows frid"er-ik'sen) the malignant or fulminating form of meningococcal MENINGITIS, which is marked by sudden onset and short course, fever, coma, collapse, cyanosis, hemorrhages from the skin and mucous membranes and bilateral adrenal hemorrhage.

Watson-Crick helix (wot'son krik) a representation of the structure of deoxyribonucleic acid (DNA), consisting of two coiled chains, each of which contains information completely specifying the other chain.

Watson-Schwartz test (wot'son shwarts) a test for diagnosing acute porphyria, depending on the presence of porphobilinogen in the urine.

watt (wot) the amount of electrical energy developed by 1 volt with 1 ampere of current.

wattage (wot'ij) the output or consumption of an electric device expressed in watts.

wattmeter (wot'me-ter) an instrument for measuring wattage.

wave (wāv) a gradual increase and subsidence, as a progressing disturbance on the surface of a liquid, the rhythmic variation occurring in the transmission of electromagnetic energy, or the sensation of nausea.
  alpha w's, waves in the electroencephalogram having a frequency of 8 to 13 per second.
  beta w's, waves in the electroencephalogram having a frequency of 18 to 30 per second.

brain w's, changes in electric potential of different areas of the brain.

delta w's, waves in the electroencephalogram having a frequency of ½ to 3 per second.

electrical w's, electromagnetic radiation of wavelength between 10^6 and 10^{11} cm. and frequency of 10^4 to 10^{-1} cycles per second.

electromagnetic w's, electromagnetic radiation.

light w's, a form of radiant energy causing the individual particles of the medium to vibrate perpendicularly to the direction of advance of the waves, particularly those of the wavelengths that stimulate the sensation of sight.

P w., a deflection in the normal electrocardiogram produced by the wave of excitation passing over the atria.

pulse w., the elevation of the pulse felt by the finger or shown graphically in the sphygmogram.

Q.w., a deflection of the electrocardiogram corresponding to the early depolarization of the ventricles. It may also be a sign of myocardial damage.

R.w., the upward deflection of the normal electrocardiogram associated with ventricular depolarization.

radio w's, electromagnetic radiation of wavelength between 10^{-1} and 10^6 cm. and frequency of about 10^{11} to 10^4 cycles per second.

S.w., the downward, or negative, deflection of the normal electrocardiogram following the R wave.

sound w's, a form of radiant energy causing the individual particles of the medium to vibrate in the direction of advance of the waves, particularly those of the wavelengths that stimulate the sensation of hearing.

T w., the final deflection of the normal electrocardiogram, recording the potential variations associated with repolarization of the heart.

ultrasonic w's, waves similar to sound waves but of such high frequency that the human ear does not perceive them as sound.

wavelength (wāv'length) the distance between the top of one wave and the identical phase of the succeeding one in the advance of waves of radiant energy.

wax (waks) a plastic solid of plant or animal origin or produced synthetically.
ear w., cerumen.

W.B.C. white blood cell (leukocyte); white blood (cell) count.

wean (wēn) to discontinue the breast feeding of an infant, with substitution of other feeding habits.

weanling (wēn'ling) an animal newly changed from breast feeding to other forms of nourishment.

webbed (webd) connected by a membrane or strand of tissue.

Weber test (va'ber) a hearing test made by placing a vibrating tuning fork at some point on the midline of the head and noting whether it is perceived as heard in the midline (normal) or referred to either ear (middle ear disease).

Weber-Christian disease (web'er kris'chan) nodular nonsuppurative panniculitis.

Wegener's granulomatosis (veg'ĕ-nerz) a progressive disease, with granulomatous lesions of the respiratory tract, focal necrotizing arteriolitis with mainly glomerular renal involvement and, finally, widespread inflammation of all organs of the body.

weight (wāt) heaviness; downward pressure due to gravity. (See also Tables of Weights and Measures in the Appendix.)

apothecaries' w., a system of weight used in compounding prescriptions based on the grain (equivalent 64.8 mg.). Its units are the scruple (20 grains), dram (3 scruples), ounce (8 drams) and pound (12 ounces).

atomic w., the weight of an atom of a chemical element, compared with the weight of an atom of oxygen taken as 16.

avoirdupois w., the system of weight commonly used for ordinary commodities in English-speaking countries. Its units are the dram (27.344 grains), ounce (16 drams) and pound (16 ounces).

equivalent w., the weight in grams of a substance that is equivalent in a chemical reaction to 1.008 Gm. of hydrogen.

molecular w., the weight of a molecule of a chemical compound as compared with the weight of an atom of hydrogen; it is equal to the sum of the weights of its constituent atoms.

weightlessness (wāt'les-nes) absence of downward pressure due to gravity, experienced by bodies in outer space or in certain high-speed flying maneuvers.

Weil's disease (vīlz) leptospiral jaundice.

well (wel) a container for fluid.
atrial w., a device used in open-heart surgery, being attached to the atrium to permit blood to rise within it while the surgeon explores and repairs a defect inside the heart.

wen (wen) a sebaceous cyst.

Westphal-Strümpell disease (vest'fahl strim'-pel) pseudosclerosis.

wet-nurse (wet'nurs) a woman who furnishes breast-feeding for other infants than her own.

wheal (hwēl) a localized area of edema on the body surface, often attended with severe itching and usually evanescent. It is the typical lesion of urticaria, the dermal evidence of allergy.

wheat-germ oil (hwēt'jerm) oil derived from the germ of wheat kernels; it is rich in vitamin E.

wheeze (hwēz) a whistling respiratory sound.

wheezing (hwēz'ing) breathing with a rasp or whistling sound. It results from constriction or obstruction of the throat, pharynx, trachea or bronchi.

Wheezing is commonly a symptom of asthma. In an asthmatic attack, spasm of the bronchi occurs, and air can be forced only with difficulty into and from the lungs through the trachea.

Another cause of wheezing is congestive heart failure, in which there is difficulty in breathing, and frequently the lips have a bluish color and the veins in the neck are distended.

When wheezing is persistent and is not asthmatic, the cause may be an obstruction, such as a foreign body or tumor, somewhere in the breathing passages.

whiplash injury (hwip'lash) injury to the spinal

cord and spine due to rapid acceleration or deceleration of the body, as in sudden stopping or propulsion of a vehicle.

Whipple's disease (hwip'elz) intestinal lipodystrophy.

whipworm (hwip'werm) *Trichuris trichiuria.*

white blood cell leukocyte.

white matter tissue consisting mostly of myelinated nerve fibers and constituting the conducting portion of the brain and spinal cord.

White-Darier disease (hwīt dar'e-a) keratosis follicularis.

Whitfield's ointment (hwit'fēldz) benzoic acid and salicylic acid ointment, used as an adjunct in the treatment of various fungus diseases of the skin. It causes sloughing of the uppermost layers of the skin.

whitlow (hwit'lo) felon.

Whitmore's disease (hwit'mōrz) melioidosis.

W.H.O. World Health Organization.

whoop (hoōp) a sonorous and convulsive inspiration.

whooping cough (hoōp'ing kof) an infectious disease characterized by coryza, bronchitis and violent attacks of coughing; called also pertussis. The causative organism is *Bordetella pertussis.* Whooping cough is a serious and widespread disease, with about 300,000 cases a year reported in the United States. Although it may attack at any age, most cases occur in children under 10, and half of these are in children under 5.

The organisms of whooping cough are spread by the victim's coughing and sneezing and by objects he has touched. The incubation period is usually about 7 days, although it may vary between 2 and 21 days.

SYMPTOMS. Whooping cough frequently starts with a running nose, a slight fever and a persistent cough. This stage usually lasts about 2 weeks. After this, the child feels chilled and begins to vomit. His coughing increases. He begins to cough in spells of eight to ten times in one breath. This forces the air from the lungs, and the face may turn purple or blue from the effort and the shortage of air. Finally he catches his breath in a long, noisy intake, or "whoop." In the very young (under 6 months) the true whoop is often not present, even when paroxysms are severe and frequent.

The coughing stage of the disease usually lasts 4 to 6 weeks, and the coughing may be very severe at night. Then the coughing spells become less frequent and less severe until the disease has run its course. Whooping cough generally lasts about 6 weeks from first symptoms to recovery.

The patient can transmit the disease for about 4 weeks after the first symptoms appear. During this period he should be isolated to prevent the spread of the illness. Isolation continues until the causative organisms are no longer present in the patient's throat, as indicated by a bacterial culture of his sputum.

TREATMENT. A child with whooping cough must be isolated, both to protect others from the disease and to protect the patient. Whooping cough lowers the child's resistance to other diseases, such as pneumonia, and complications can be very dangerous. The patient should be guardêd particularly against people with colds. Antibiotics are often given to prevent secondary bacterial infections, especially in very young children.

Bed rest is advisable as long as fever persists. Cough-provoking factors such as smoke, dust and excitement should be avoided.

In very serious cases, especially in infants, whooping cough may cause severe breathing difficulties. Suction may be necessary at frequent intervals to remove accumulations of mucus from the air passages. Fatalities, particularly in infants, are not uncommon.

A proper diet is essential during whooping cough. Because vomiting may be a problem, small frequent feedings of bland foods are considered best.

IMMUNIZATION. An attack of whooping cough gives immunity, but second attacks are not unknown. A vaccine against whooping cough is available. In the United States, it is usually given in combination with diphtheria and tetanus vaccines. A series of three injections is given, 1 month apart, beginning between the ages of 6 weeks and 2 months. Boosters are usually given at 1 year and again at 4 years. When it is known that a child has been exposed to whooping cough, another booster may be advisable.

whorl (hwerl) a spiral arrangement, as in the ridges on the finger that make up a fingerprint.

Widal test (ve-dahl') a test for the diagnosis of typhoid and paratyphoid fevers, based on agglutination of typhoid bacilli by the patient's serum.

Willebrand's disease (vil'ĕ-brandz) a hereditary familial disease due to a deficiency of antihemophilic globulin and capillary defect, marked by severe epistaxis and bleeding from the gums and genitalia; called also angiohemophilia.

Wilms' tumor (vilmz) a rapidly developing sarcoma of the kidneys, made up of embryonal elements, and occurring chiefly in children before the fifth year; called also embryonal carcinosarcoma.

Wilpo (wil'po) trademark for a preparation of phentermine, an anorexigenic agent.

Wilson's disease (wil'sunz) hepatolenticular degeneration.

window (win'do) a circumscribed opening in a plane surface.
  oval w., an opening in the inner wall of the middle ear, in which the base of the stapes fits; called also fenestra vestibuli.
  round w., an opening in the inner wall of the middle ear, covered by mucous membrane and separating the middle ear from the cochlea; called also fenestra cochleae.

windpipe (wind'pīp) the trachea.

Winstrol (win'strol) trademark for a preparation of stanozolol, an anabolic steroid.

wintergreen oil (win'ter-grēn) methyl salicylate.

witch hazel (wich ha'zel) a liquid extract from the dried leaves or bark of the plant Hamamelis; used as an astringent.

withdrawal (with-draw'al) a group of symptoms brought about by abrupt withdrawal of a narcotic or other drug to which a person has become addicted; called also abstinence syndrome. The usual reactions to alcohol withdrawal are anxiety, weakness, gastrointestinal symptoms, nausea and vomiting, tremor, fever, rapid heartbeat, convulsions and delirium. Similar effects are produced by withdrawal of barbiturates and in this case convulsions occur very frequently, often followed by psychosis with hallucinations.

Morphine withdrawal produces a standard pattern of reactions beginning with restlessness, which later becomes extreme. There may be slight fever, elevated blood pressure and mild hyperglycemia, with lack of appetite and vomiting. The symptoms begin to decline by the third day and usually disappear by about the fourteenth day. The various morphine-like drugs produce similar symptoms, in some instances more acute and in others milder.

TREATMENT consists of providing a substitute drug such as a mild sedative, along with treatment of the symptoms as needed. Parenteral fluids are often required.

W.M.A. World Medical Association.

wolffian body (woolf'e-an) mesonephros.

wolfram (wool'fram) tungsten (symbol W).

womb (woŏm) uterus.

wood alcohol methyl alcohol.

woolsorter's disease pneumonia due to inhalation of spores of *Bacillus anthracis*, the causative organism of ANTHRAX.

World Health Organization WHO; the specialized agency of the United Nations that is concerned with health on an international level. The agency was founded in 1948 and in its constitution are listed the following objectives:

Health is a state of complete physical and social well being, and not merely the absence of disease or infirmity. The enjoyment of the highest attainable standards of health is one of the fundamental rights of every human being without distinction of race, religion, political belief, economic or social condition. The health of all peoples is fundamental to the attainment of peace and security and is dependent upon the fullest cooperation of individuals and States. The achievement of any State in the promotion and protection of health is of value to all.

The major specific aims of the World Health Organization are:

1. To strengthen the health services of member nations, improving the teaching standards in medicine and allied professions, and advising and helping generally in the field of health.
2. To promote better standards for nutrition, housing, recreation, sanitation, economic and working conditions.
3. To improve maternal and child health and welfare.
4. To advance progress in the field of mental health.
5. To encourage and conduct research on problems of public health.

In carrying out these aims and objectives the World Health Organization functions as a directing and coordinating authority on international health. It serves as a center for all types of global and health information, promotes uniform quarantine standards and international sanitary regulations, provides advisory services through public health experts in control of disease and sets up international standards for the manufacture of all important drugs. Through its teams of physicians, nurses and other health personnel it provides modern medical skills and knowledge to communities throughout the world.

worm (werm) a small, slender, elongated, softbodied animal, often found as a parasite in man and other animals. The most common parasitic worms in North America are roundworms and tapeworms. (RINGWORM is not caused by a worm but is a form of fungus infection of the skin.)

Most worm infections are transmitted from person to person via feces that contaminate food and water. Serious worm infections may cause anemia, listlessness, fatigue, irritability, abdominal pain, diarrhea and weight loss. Despite popular belief, worms do not cause convulsions in children.

Parasitic worms usually live in relative balance with their human hosts, taking enough nutrients to survive without destroying the health of the host. However, they reduce the strength and energy of the bodies they inhabit, often produce very uncomfortable symptoms and should never go untreated.

Suspected cases of worms should be brought to the attention of a physician, for self-treatment is likely to be ineffective and can be harmful. Effective medications against worms can be prescribed only by a physician.

ROUNDWORMS (NEMATODA). Roundworms, called also threadworms, somewhat resemble common earthworms in appearance. The varieties most frequently infecting man include *Ascaris lumbricoides*, pinworms, hookworms, filaria and *Trichinella spiralis*, the cause of TRICHINOSIS, which is transmitted through inadequately cooked pork.

Ascaris lumbricoides. The largest of the roundworms that infect man, *Ascaris lumbricoides* is particularly common in the southern mountain regions of the United States. Often it is transmitted in human feces used as fertilizer. The Ascaris eggs develop into larvae in the soil and on growing plants on which the infected feces have been deposited. When vegetables from these areas are eaten without having been properly washed or thoroughly cooked, live larvae are carried into the digestive system along with the food. Migrating from the intestines into the blood, then to the lungs and the esophagus, the larvae finally return to the intestines, where they grow to maturity, reaching a length ranging from 6 to 14 inches.

Ascaris infection may go unsuspected until a worm is passed in the stool. But there may be colic or other abdominal symptoms, and occasionally the worms are vomited during their passage through the esophagus. In children, "wandering worms" may emerge through the skin near the navel, and in adults, near the groin. Infected children usually are thin because the worms consume vital nutrients and inhibit the digestion of proteins. Loss of appetite and angioneurotic edema are common, and the face may be swollen.

Accurate diagnosis of the presence and extent of Ascaris infection usually depends on the detection of eggs in a stool sample examined microscopically. Treatment involves the use of medications such as chenopodium oil and dithiazanine iodide to destroy and expel the parasites, and is completely successful in nearly every case.

Prevention of Ascaris infection depends primarily on the sanitary disposal of human feces and discontinuing their use as fertilizer. Also important are the thorough washing of hands before food is prepared, and the careful cleaning and cooking of possibly infected foods.

Enterobius vermicularis (Pinworm). Enterobius vermicularis, called also pinworm or seatworm, is a spindle-shaped roundworm less than half an inch long that inhabits the upper part of the large intestine, more commonly in children than adults. Pinworms do not produce the fatigue and loss of weight that characterize Ascaris infection, but instead the adult worms migrate to the anal region, usually at night, and deposit eggs, which cause irritation of the skin around the anus, leading to painful scratching and restless sleep.

This irritation is the usual sign of pinworm infection, although there may also be vague intestinal discomfort. Adult worms may appear in the feces, but the infection is transmitted by the eggs, which may be transferred to clothing, bedclothes and toilet seats from the skin around the anus.

In scratching, the infected person is likely to collect the minute eggs on his hands and under his fingernails, and, until he washes thoroughly, he will shed the eggs on anything he touches.

The infection spreads to other persons when the eggs are carried to their mouths either by inhalation or on contaminated food, in beverages or on hands. Widespread pinworm infection is explained by the fact that the eggs, which develop into mature worms only in a human body, can remain dormant but alive and infective for a considerable time in dust or air; they are not killed by most household disinfectants.

Enterobius vermicularis infection is treated by an anthelmintic such as pyrvinium pamoate, piperazine citrate or gentian violet. Equally important, instructions for disinfecting bedclothes and other material that may harbor eggs must be followed carefully to avoid reinfection and spread of pinworms to other members of the family.

Prevention of pinworms is largely a matter of hygiene. Children should be taught to wash their hands well with soap and water before meals and after using the toilet. Care and cleanliness in the preparation of food is essential. If a case of pinworms develops in a family, extra precautions should be taken; toilet seats should be scrubbed daily with soap and water, and the bedding of the infected person should be disinfected by boiling at least twice a week.

Hookworm. Hookworms are small—about half an inch long—and are particularly widespread in the southeastern part of the United States. Their larvae develop in soil contaminated by feces from infected persons and they enter the body through the skin, usually through the sole of the foot. Children who go barefoot are especially susceptible. They travel by way of the blood to the lungs and then to the intestines, where the worms, by now full-grown, attach themselves to the intestinal wall and suck blood from it for nourishment. There may be no symptoms at all, or there may be severe blood loss and anemia, and eventually retardation of growth and mental development and even death. Diagnosis is made by detection of eggs in the feces. The infection is treated by administration of anthelmintic drugs such as hexylresorcinol. It is prevented by improvement in sanitation facilities and wearing shoes out of doors. (See also HOOKWORM.)

Filaria. Another type of threadlike roundworm, often called filaria, causes a tropical disease known as FILARIASIS, which affects lymphoid tissues.

FLATWORMS (PLATYHELMINTHES). Flatworms infecting man include tapeworms, flukes and *Echinococcus granulosus.*

Tapeworm. Several species of tapeworms infect man; all depend on two hosts, one human and one animal, for development through their full life cycle (egg to larva to adult). Usually larvae are found in animal hosts and adult worms in man.

The tapeworms commonly found in the United States enter human bodies in contaminated and insufficiently cooked pork (*Taenia solium*), beef (*T. saginata*) or fish (*Diphyllobothrium latum*). The larvae, embedded in cysts in the meat or fish, develop to maturity in the human intestine and attach themselves to the intestinal wall; from there they release eggs, or, in the case of Taenia species, egg-laden segments of the body called proglottids.

In mild or even moderate infections, tapeworms cause few or no symptoms. In heavy infections there may be diarrhea, abdominal cramps (resembling hunger pains), flatulence, distention and nausea. In most cases, before these symptoms develop, the infected person discovers the tapeworm segments in his clothes or bedding.

Quinacrine hydrochloride (Atabrine) and aspidium oleoresin are used in treatment of tapeworm infection, quinacrine being the drug of choice because it is less toxic. After treatment the stool must be carefully examined for the parasite because if the head is retained in the intestine, the worm will grow again and treatment must be repeated. Prevention depends on thorough cooking of fish and meat. (See also TAPEWORM.)

Flukes (Trematoda). Flukes are not common in the United States but are a serious problem in many Asian, tropical and subtropical countries. The Chinese liver fluke, *Clonorchis sinensis*, enters the body in raw or improperly cooked fish and may cause enlargement of the liver, jaundice, anemia and weakness. Another liver fluke, *Fasciola hepatica*, is occasionally found in man; it causes obstruction of the bile ducts and enlargement of the liver. Blood flukes such as Schistosoma penetrate the skin, make their way to the blood and travel to various parts of the body (see also SCHISTOSOMIASIS).

Treatment varies according to the type of fluke involved and requires careful medical supervision. Proper cooking of fish provides protection against liver fluke infection. Since snails are carriers of flukes, their destruction, usually by poison, is an effective preventive measure in areas where fluke infection is a problem.

Echinococcus granulosus. This tapeworm reverses the usual process of development in human and animal hosts. The adult Echinococcus is found in the intestine of dogs. The larva develops in the human intestine, penetrating the intestinal wall, and settling in various organs—most often the liver—where it forms a cyst (hydatid cyst) that grows slowly. Treatment is by surgical removal of the cyst. This type of worm infection is fortunately not common in the United States.

NURSING CARE. The patient suffering from infection with worms is likely to be malnourished and suffering from anemia. Special attention should be given to the diet so that these conditions can be relieved. The patient also will need adequate rest

Commonly Encountered Intestinal Parasitic Infections

Common Name	Scientific Name (Synonyms or Varieties)	Distribution	Portal of Entry (and Stage)	Diagnostic Stages(s) in Stool (or Other Medium)
ROUNDWORMS: Giant intestinal roundworm	*Ascaris lumbricoides*	Cosmopolitan, more common in warm moist climates	Mouth (embryonated eggs)	Immature eggs in stool. Worms evacuated in stool, occasionally vomited
Hookworm	a) *Ancylostoma duodenale* (Old World type) b) *Necator americanus* (Tropical type)	a) Temperate and warm moist climates b) Warm moist climates	Skin, usually feet, possibly mouth (filariform larvae)	Immature eggs in stool
Threadworm	*Strongyloides stercoralis*	Sou. U.S.A., moist tropics	Skin, usually feet (filariform larvae)	Larvae in stool
Whipworm	*Trichuris trichiura* (*Trichocephalus trichiurus*)	Gulf Coast, U.S.A.; warm moist climates	Mouth (embryonated eggs)	Immature eggs in stool
Pinworm or seatworm	*Enterobius vermicularis* (*Oxyuris vermicularis*)	Cosmopolitan, esp. in children	Mouth (embryonated eggs)	Eggs in perianal swabs; adult worms per anum
TAPEWORMS: Dwarf	*Hymenolepis nana*	Sou. U.S.A., in children	Mouth (eggs)	Eggs in stool
Beef	*Taenia saginata*	Cosmopolitan	Mouth (cysticercus larva in infected beef)	Eggs in stool; proglottids of adult worms per anum
Pork	*Taenia solium*	Rare in U.S.A.; common in Latin America	Mouth (cysticercus larva in infected pork)	Eggs in stool; proglottids of adult worms per anum
Fish	*Diphyllobothrium latum* (*Bothriocephalus latus*)	Northern Minn. and Mich.; Canada	Mouth (larva in infected fresh-water fish flesh)	Immature eggs in stool
Sparganum causing sparganosis	*Spirometra* spp. (*Sparganum mansoni* et al.)	Several areas, incl. Sou. U.S.A.	Usually mouth (larval stages)	Sparganum larva in subcutaneous tissues
PROTOZOA: Dysentery ameba	*Entamoeba histolytica* (*Ent. dysenteriae, Endamoeba histolytica*)	Cosmopolitan; common in warm moist climates	Mouth (cyst)	Vegetative stage or cyst in stool
Giardia	*Giardia lamblia* (*G. intestinalis, Lamblia intestinalis*)	In warm climates, prevalent, especially in children	Mouth (cyst)	Vegetative stage or cyst in stool
FLUKES: Intestinal	a) *Fasciolopsis buski* b) *Heterophyes, Metagonimus* c) *Echinostoma ilocanum* et al.	In U.S.A. only as rare infections imported from Orient or tropics	Mouth (encysted metacercarial larva)	Eggs in stool
Hepatic	*Fasciola hepatica* (sheep) liver fluke)	Cosmopolitan in sheep-raising countries	Mouth (encysted metacercarial larva)	Immature eggs in stool or biliary drainage

Source of Infection	Most Common Symptoms	Therapeutic Agents	Remarks
Fecal contamination of soil (eggs)	Colicky pains, diarrhea "acute abdomen"	Piperazine Hexylresorcinol Dithiazanine iodide	May block intestine, biliary or pancreatic duct; bronchial symptoms (larval stage with eosinophilia*)
Fecal contamination of soil (larvae)	Melena, anemia, cardiac insufficiency, retarded growth	Tetrachloroethylene Hexylresorcinol Bephenium hydroxynaphthoate	Prophylaxis: Use sanitary latrines, wear shoes, treat infected persons
Fecal contamination of soil (larvae)	Radiating pain in pit of stomach, diarrhea	Dithiazanine iodide	Prophylaxis: Use sanitary latrines, wear shoes
Fecal contamination of soil (eggs)	Diarrhea, nausea, retarded growth	Dithiazanine iodide Hexylresorcinol enemas	May produce dysenteric syndrome, acute appendicitis, or prolapse of rectum in children
Eggs from contaminated fomites	Perianal and perineal pruritus, convulsions in children	Piperazine	Often involves entire family
Eggs contaminating environment	Diarrhea, abdominal discomfort, dizziness, inanition in children	Quinacrine hydrochloride Hexylresorcinol	May be symptomless
Poorly cooked or raw infected beef	Systemic toxemia, abdominal distress, "acute appendix"	Quinacrine hydrochloride	Prophylaxis: Thoroughly cook all suspected beef
Poorly cooked infected pork	Similar to T. saginata	Quinacrine hydrochloride	Prophylaxis: Thoroughly cook all pork in infected areas. Ingested eggs may produce human cysticercosis
Infected fresh-water fish	Intestinal toxemia, bowel obstruction, may cause pernicious anemia	Aspidium oleoresin Quinacrine hydrochloride	
Drinking water containing infected Cyclops (primary host)	Inflamed subcutaneous tissue containing sparganum larva	Surgical excision	Adult worm in intestine of various nonhuman mammals
Feces-contaminated water, food, fomites	a) Diarrhea, dysentery, abdominal pain b) Amebic hepatitis	a) Oxytetracycline hydrochloride Diiodohydroxyquin Glycobiarsol b) Emetine hydrochloride Chloroquine phosphate	Amebiasis may be asyndromic in individuals or populations
Human feces	Mucous diarrhea, abdominal pain, loss of weight	Quinacrine hydrochloride	Infection acquired in childhood often spontaneously lost
a) Vegetation b) Fresh-water fish c) Snails	Intestinal toxemia, at times intestinal obstruction	a) Tetrachloroethylene b) Hexylresorcinol c) Aspidium oleoresin	Primary hosts are fresh-water snails
Watercress containing metacercarial cysts	Hepatic colic, cholecystiasis	Emetine hydrochloride	Sheep infected in U.S.A., but only 1 confirmed human infection

COMMONLY ENCOUNTERED INTESTINAL PARASITIC INFECTIONS (*Continued*)

COMMON NAME	SCIENTIFIC NAME (SYNONYMS OR VARIETIES)	DISTRIBUTION	PORTAL OF ENTRY (AND STAGE)	DIAGNOSTIC STAGE(S) IN STOOL (OR OTHER MEDIUM)
Pulmonary	*Paragonimus westermani* (Oriental lung fluke)	Orient, extensive foci	Mouth (encysted metacercarial larva)	Immature eggs in stool or sputum
Blood	a) *Schistosoma japonicum* b) *S. mansoni* c) *S. haematobium*	a) Orient b) Africa, Latin America c) Africa, Near East	Skin (active fork-tailed cercarial)	Embryonated eggs in stool (a, b), or urine (c)

From The Merck Manual. 11th ed. Copyright 1966, Merck & Co., Inc., Rahway, New Jersey.
*Note: Eosinophilia often accompanies intestinal helminthiasis.

and other general measures to improve his state of health.

The anthelmintic drugs prescribed for elimination of worms are often toxic, and the nurse must know the specific drug being administered and the toxic effects that might develop. A special regimen is recommended for the administration of many anthelmintic drugs and includes the following: A purgative or enema is given the night before administration. After a light evening meal (or liquids only), breakfast is withheld. After the drug is given a purgative or enema may be ordered. The stools of the patient must be checked for larvae or worms. It is recommended that toilet paper not be placed in the bedpan with the stool as it may make recognition of the parasite difficult. In the case of tapeworm the head must be passed before the patient can be considered free from infection. If the head is not observed, this should be reported to the physician in charge so that treatment can be repeated as necessary.

The patient should have his own individual bedpan which is thoroughly washed and disinfected after each use. He is not allowed to use the bathroom if it is used by other persons. Some types of worms or eggs must be destroyed before they can be flushed into the sewage system. This will depend on the community's sewage treatment plant and the type of worm involved. If there is any doubt that the worms will be destroyed it is best to disinfect the stool with chlorinated lime before disposal in the sewage system.

Although there are a variety of worms capable of infecting the human body, all are parasites that live at the expense of the human host. The patient and his family may require instruction in the dangers of worm infection and the ways in which this condition can be avoided. It is sometimes a difficult subject to discuss but the nurse must assume a matter-of-fact attitude toward this condition and do all she can to relieve the patient of embarrassment and at the same time help him understand the need for cooperating with the physician, nurses or other health officials.

wound (wŏŏnd) any interruption of the continuity of an external or internal surface caused by physical means.
  contused w., one made by a blunt object.
  incised w., one caused by a cutting instrument.
  lacerated w., one in which the tissues are torn.

  open w., one having a free outward opening.
  penetrating w., one reaching an important cavity of the body.
  puncture w., one made by a pointed instrument, with a very small external opening in the skin.

wreath (rēth) an encircling structure, resembling a circlet of flowers or leaves such as may be worn about the head.
  hippocratic w., the sparse peripheral rim of scalp hair which is the ultimate stage of male-pattern alopecia.

wrist (rist) the region of the joint between the hand and the forearm; called also the carpus.

There are eight carpal bones in the wrist, arranged in two rows. The joint surfaces of these bones glide upon each other in four directions. The carpals join the bones of the forearm, the radius and ulna, and the bones of the hands, the metacarpals. The bones are bound together and protected by tough ligaments and capsules, the enveloping structures. The major arteries, nerves, veins and tendons that serve the hand and fingers run across the wrist. Both tendons and the joint are lined with synovial membrane.

DISORDERS OF THE WRIST. The wrist is a strong but complicated joint and can suffer the same disorders as any other joint. The hands are constantly being used, and any sudden or strong movement or exertion may cause a structure to stretch, tear or become dislocated.

A strained wrist, caused by overstretching or overexertion, is usually treated by rest and the application of heat and light massage. Injury of the joint ligaments is called a SPRAIN and is a common disorder. DISLOCATION, or displacement of the bones of the wrist from their normal relationship, and FRACTURE, which causes swelling and pain on movement, may also occur. Often a fracture is difficult to distinguish from a bad sprain, and x-ray examination may be necessary for diagnosis.

Severe pain, swelling and reddish blue discoloration may be a symptom of any of these cases of wrist injury. An ice pack is often recommended for swelling.

Other disorders of the wrist include ARTHRITIS, infection, ganglion (a form of cystic tumor) and TENOSYNOVITIS.

wristdrop (rist′drop) paralysis of the extensor

SOURCE OF INFECTION	MOST COMMON SYMPTOMS	THERAPEUTIC AGENTS	REMARKS
Crabs or crayfishes containing metacercarial cysts	Peribronchiolar distress, with hemoptysis	Emetine hydrochloride	Related species in wild mammals and hogs in U.S.A.
Infested water containing fork tailed larvae from snail hosts	Dysentery, intestinal and hepatic cirrhosis (a, b), hematuria, urinary fibrosis (c)	Antimony potassium tartrate Stibophen	Related flukes cause "swimmer's itch" in bathers in U.S.A. and elsewhere

muscles of the hand and fingers, mainly due to metallic poisoning.

writing (rīt'ing) the recording of a visible impression, such as the inscription of letters and words on paper.

    automatic w., 1. a dissociative phenomenon in which a person writes while his attention is distracted. 2. that which follows the suggestions made to a patient while he is in a hypnotic trance.

    mirror w., the writing of letters and words in reversed form, as if seen in a mirror.

wryneck (ri'nek) torticollis.

wt. weight.

Wuchereria (voo″ker-e're-ah) a genus of nematode parasites of the superfamily Filarioidea.
    W. bancrof'ti, a species widely distributed in tropical and subtropical countries, producing important pathologic changes in the lymphatic system in human hosts by causing obstruction of the lymphatic ducts (see also FILARIASIS).

wucheriasis (voo″ker-i'ah-sis) infection with worms of the genus Wuchereria.

w./v. weight (of solute) per volume (of solvent).

Wyamine (wi'ah-min) trademark for preparations of mephentermine, used as a sympathomimetic and a pressor substance.

Wycillin (wi-sil'in) trademark for a preparation of procaine penicillin G.

Wydase (wi'dās) trademark for preparations of hyaluronidase for injection, a spreading agent to promote diffusion and enhance absorption.

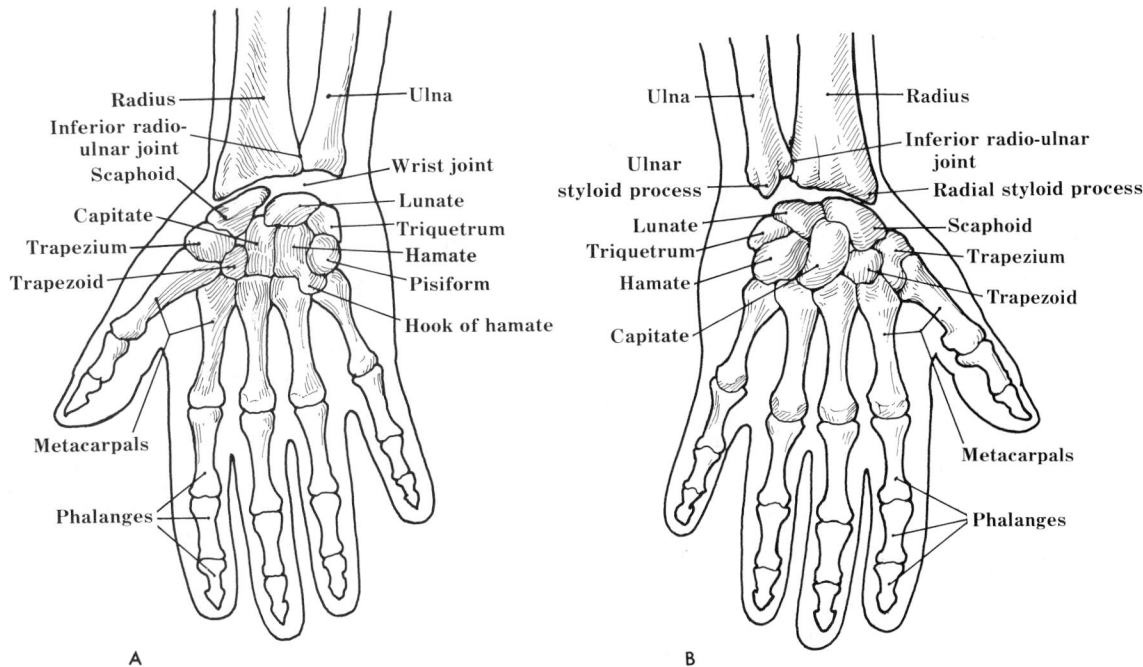

Bones of the wrist (carpal bones). *A,* Anterior view, right arm. *B,* Posterior view, right arm.

X

xanth(o)- (zan′tho) word element [Gr.], *yellow.*

xanthein (zan′the-in) the soluble part of the yellow pigment of flowers.

xanthelasma (zan″thel-az′mah) xanthoma affecting the eyelids and characterized by soft yellow spots.

xanthelasmoidea (zan″thel-az-moi′de-ah) a disease of infants marked by formation of brownish wheals followed by pigmentation.

xanthematin (zan-them′ah-tin) a yellow substance derivable from heme (hematin).

xanthemia (zan-the′me-ah) the presence of yellow coloring matter in the blood.

xanthic (zan′thik) 1. yellow. 2. pertaining to xanthine.

xanthine (zan′thēn) a purine compound found in most bodily tissues; it may be oxidized to uric acid.
  dimethyl x., theobromine.
  trimethyl x., caffeine.

xanthinuria (zan″thin-u′re-ah) excess of xanthine in the urine.

xanthochromatic (zan″tho-kro-mat′ik) yellow-colored.

xanthochromia (zan″tho-kro′me-ah) yellowish discoloration of the skin or spinal fluid. Xanthochromic spinal fluid usually indicates hemorrhage into the central nervous system and is due to the presence of xanthematin.

xanthochrous (zan-thok′ro-us) having a yellowish complexion.

xanthocyanopsia (zan″tho-si″ah-nop′se-ah) inability to perceive red or green tints, vision being limited to yellow and blue.

xanthoderma (zan″tho-der′mah) yellowish discoloration of the skin.

xanthodontous (zan″tho-don′tus) having yellowish teeth.

xanthoma (zan-tho′mah) a tumor-like deposit of fatty substances in the skin. The color of a xanthoma is usually yellow, but may be brown, reddish or cream.

Xanthomas are usually harmless. They range in size from tiny pinheads to large nodules, and the shape may be round, flat or irregular. They are often found around the eyes, the joints, the neck or the palms or over tendons. Often these fatty deposits are not limited to the skin but are found throughout the body in bones, the heart, blood vessels, liver and other organs.

The formation of xanthomas may indicate an underlying disease, usually related to abnormal metabolism of lipids, including cholesterol. Abnormally high levels of blood lipids may be found in diabetes mellitus (xanthoma diabeticorum), in diseases of the liver, kidney and thyroid gland, and in several hereditary metabolic diseases. The excessive lipids carried in the blood may then be deposited as xanthomas.

Another group of diseases producing xanthomas affect the reticuloendothelial system, a widespread system of cells that have several functions, including an influence in the storage of fatty materials. These diseases are thought to have a similar basic mechanism but they have many different manifestations, which may include the formation of xanthomas. The xanthomas are usually found in the reticuloendothelial disorder called Hand-Schüller-Christian disease.

Treatment of xanthomas includes surgery, application of acids directly to the fatty deposits and management of the disease that causes them, as in diabetes mellitus.

xanthomatosis (zan″tho-mah-to′sis) an accumulation of excess lipids in the body due to disturbance of lipid metabolism and marked by the formation of fatty tumors in various parts and sometimes by profound effects on bodily health.
  x. bul′bi, fatty degeneration of the cornea.
  chronic idiopathic x., Hand-Schüller-Christian disease.

xanthomyeloma (zan″tho-mi″ĕ-lo′mah) xanthosarcoma.

xanthophane (zan′tho-fān) a yellow pigment from the retinal cones.

xanthoplasty (zan′tho-plas″te) xanthoderma.

xanthopsia (zan-thop′se-ah) perversion of color vision in which objects are seen as yellow.

xanthopsin (zan-thop′sin) a compound produced by the action of light on rhodopsin.

xanthosarcoma (zan″tho-sar-ko′mah) giant cell sarcoma of tendon sheaths and aponeuroses containing foam cells.

xanthosis (zan-tho′sis) yellowish discoloration.
  x. cu′tis, yellowish pigmentation of the skin, without involvement of the sclera, sometimes resulting from excessive consumption of carotene-rich foods.

xanthurenic acid (zan″thu-ren′ik) a metabolite of L-tryptophan, present in normal urine and in increased amounts in vitamin B_6 deficiency.

Xe chemical symbol, *xenon.*

xenodiagnosis (zen″o-di″ag-no′sis) diagnosis of

disease by finding causative microorganisms in laboratory-bred insects permitted to feed on the patient; used in the diagnosis of South American trypanosomiasis (Chagas' disease).

xenogenesis (zen"o-jen'ĕ-sis) alternation of generation, or heterogenesis.

xenogenous (zĕ-noj'ĕ-nus) caused by a foreign body, or originating outside the organism.

xenomenia (zen"o-me'ne-ah) vicarious menstruation.

xenon (ze'non) a chemical element, atomic number 54, atomic weight 131.30, symbol Xe. (See table of ELEMENTS.)

xenoparasite (zen"o-par'ah-sīt) an organism not usually parasitic on a particular species, but present because of a weakened condition of the individual host.

xenophobia (zen"o-fo'be-ah) morbid dread of strangers.

xenophonia (zen"o-fo'ne-ah) alteration in the quality of the voice.

xenophthalmia (zen"of-thal'me-ah) inflammation caused by a foreign body in the eye.

Xenopsylla (zen"op-sil'ah) a genus of fleas, including more than 30 species, many of which transmit disease-producing microorganisms.
   X. cheo'pis, a species that is a major vector for *Pasteurella pestis,* the causative organism of plague.

xenorexia (zen"o-rek'se-ah) a perversion of appetite leading to the repeated swallowing of foreign bodies not ordinarily ingested.

xer(o)- (ze'ro) word element [Gr.], *dry; dryness.*

xeransis (ze-ran'sis) loss of moisture.

xerasia (ze-ra'ze-ah) a disorder marked by brittleness and dryness of the hair.

xerocheilia (ze"ro-ki'le-ah) dryness of the lips.

xeroderma (ze"ro-der'mah) dryness of the skin.
   x. of Kaposi, x. pigmento'sum, a rare pigmentary and atrophic disease appearing in childhood, progressing to early development of senile changes in the skin and ending in death.

xeroma (ze-ro'mah) abnormal dryness of the conjunctiva; xerophthalmia.

xeromenia (ze"ro-me'ne-ah) the appearance of constitutional symptoms at the menstrual period without any flow of blood.

xerophagia (ze"ro-fa'je-ah) the eating of dry food.

xerophthalmia (ze"rof-thal'me-ah) abnormal dryness of the surface of the conjunctiva; it is due to a definciency of vitamin A.

xeroradiography (ze"ro-ra"de-og'rah-fe) the making of radiographs by a dry, totally photoelectric process, using metal plates coated with a semiconductor.

xerosis (ze-ro'sis) abnormal dryness, as of the conjunctiva (xerophthalmia) or skin (xeroderma).

xerostomia (ze"ro-sto'me-ah) dryness of the mouth from lack of the normal secretion.

xerotocia (ze"ro-to'se-ah) dry labor.

xiph(o)- (zif'o) word element [Gr.], *xiphoid process.*

xiphisternum (zif"ĭ-ster'num) xiphoid process.

xiphocostal (zif"o-kos'tal) pertaining to the xiphoid process and ribs.

xiphoid (zif'oid, zi'foid) sword-shaped.
   x. process, the pointed process of cartilage, supported by a core of bone, connected with the lower end of the body of the sternum.

xiphoiditis (zif"oi-di'tis) inflammation of the xiphoid process.

xiphopagus (zi-fop'ah-gus) symmetrical conjoined twins united in the region of the xiphoid process.

x-rays (ek'rāz) electromagnetic radiation of very short wavelength (0.05 to 5 angstroms) used for diagnosis and treatment of various disorders; called also roentgen rays.
   X-rays are commonly generated by passing a current of high voltage (from 10,000 volts up) through a Coolidge tube. They are able to penetrate most substances to some extent, some much more readily than others, and to affect photographic plate. These qualities make it possible to use them in taking roentgenograms of various parts of the body, thus revealing the presence and position of fractures or foreign bodies or of radiopaque substances that have been purposely introduced. They can also cause certain substances to fluoresce and thus make possible fluoroscopy, by which the size, shape and movements of various organs such as the heart, stomach and intestines can be observed. By reason of the high energy of their quanta, they strongly ionize tissue through which they pass by means of photoelectrons, both primary and secondary, which they liberate. Because of this effect they are used in treating various pathologic conditions. (See also RADIATION and RADIOTHERAPY.)

xylene (zi'lēn) a compound used as a cleaning solvent in microscopy.

xylenol (zi'lĕ-nol) any of a series of colorless crystalline substances resembling phenol.

Xylocaine (zi'lo-kān) trademark for preparations of lidocaine, a regional anesthetic.

xylol (zy'lol) xylene.

xylometazoline (zi"lo-met"ah-zo'lēn) a compound used as a nasal decongestant.

xylose (zi'lōs) a sugar obtained from beechwood and jute.

xylosuria (zi"lo-su're-ah) the presence of xylose in the urine.

xysma (zis'mah) material resembling bits of membrane in stools of diarrhea.

xyster (zis'ter) a filelike instrument used in surgery.

Y

Y chemical symbol, *yttrium*.

yaw (yaw) the raspberry-like excrescence of YAWS.

yawning (yawn'ing) a deep, involuntary inspiration with the mouth open, often accompanied by the act of stretching.

yaws (yawz) a highly infectious disease caused by the spirochete *Treponema pertenue;* called also frambesia.

Although almost nonexistent in the United States, yaws is common among people who live under primitive conditions in equatorial Africa, South America and the East and West Indies.

TRANSMISSION AND SYMPTOMS. Yaws is transmitted by direct contact. The first symptom, appearing usually about a month after exposure, is a single papule, an inflammatory but painless elevation of the skin. Called the "mother yaw," this soon ulcerates. Open, oozing sores appear a few weeks later on the hands, feet, face, scalp and trunk. Eventually, after several years, the disease causes tissue destruction, bone changes and shortening of the fingers or toes, in a cycle that has a resemblance to leprosy and is sometimes mistaken for it.

The causative organism of yaws is closely related to that of syphilis, and both diseases give a positive result in the Wassermann test. Yaws is classified as a nonvenereal disease and is not primarily communicated by coitus.

TREATMENT AND PREVENTION. Effective treatment is afforded by antibiotics, particularly penicillin.

Unsanitary living conditions unquestionably help spread the disease. Ideally, all clothing that has come in contact with yaws lesions should be sterilized and the sores cleaned with antiseptic and covered with clean dressings.

There is as yet no immunizing vaccine for yaws.

Yb chemical symbol, *ytterbium*.

yeast (yēst) a term applied to unicellular, nucleated microorganisms that reproduce by budding and to other organisms that exist usually or predominantly in similar form; some are used in production of various foodstuffs and beverages, and some are pathogenic for man.

    brewer's y., yeast obtained as a by-product from the brewing of beer.

    dried y., dried cells of any suitable strain of *Saccharomyces cerevisiae* or certain other fungi, used as a source of protein and of vitamins of the B complex.

yellow (yel'o) 1. the color produced by stimulation by light waves of wavelength of 571.5 to 578.5 mμ. 2. a dye or stain that produces a yellow color.

    y. fever, an acute infectious viral disease, transmitted by the female of certain types of mosquitoes, and characterized by fever, jaundice and albuminuria.

Yellow fever is less rampant today largely because of vaccination and better control of the mosquito menace, but it is still a danger in most tropical countries. Among native inhabitants who contract the disease there is a mortality rate of about 5 per cent. In visitors from other climates, fatalities once ran as high as 40 per cent, but they are now much lower. With proper immunization precautions, a visitor from a temperate country today takes only a minimal risk.

The mosquito that transmits classic yellow fever is *Aedes aegypti.* In the jungles of Brazil and in parts of Africa, in the absence of *Aedes aegypti*, the disease may be carried by a different type of mosquito, which lives in treetops. These forest mosquitoes can communicate the disease to forest workers and also to certain animals, such as monkeys and marmosets, which then serve as virus reservoirs and as sources of reinfection for man. This form of the disease is called jungle or sylvan yellow fever, and is difficult to control because of the virtual impossibility of eradicating the tropical tree-inhabiting mosquitoes.

SYMPTOMS AND TREATMENT. Yellow fever has an incubation period of 3 to 6 days. It then manifests itself suddenly and intensely with fever, headache, muscular aches and prostration. A few days later, the temperature suddenly falls, only to rise again. The pulse is originally very rapid, but then slows gradually to less than 50 beats per minute. In addition to the characteristic yellowing of the skin, the urine becomes darker. There may be frequent vomiting, and blood may become noticeable in the vomitus (so-called black vomit). There may also be bleeding from the mucous membranes.

The disease runs its course in a little more than a week. Those who survive (and the great majority do) suffer no permanent damage. The jaundice completely disappears. Furthermore, these persons are immune from a second attack. In fatal cases, death is usually due to liver or kidney failure.

There is no specific drug for the cure of yellow fever. The effects of the disease can be mitigated by analgesics, sedatives, bed rest and a high-calorie, high-carbohydrate diet.

NURSING CARE. The patient's fever is controlled with cold or tepid sponges and other nursing measures. The diet consists of liquids and easily digested foods until the vomiting stops, and then is gradually increased. The patient's bed and room should be well screened to prevent transmission of the fever to others via mosquitoes.

    visual y., xanthopsin.

yoghurt (yo'gert) a cheeselike preparation from milk, used as a food.

yoke (yōk) a connecting structure; a depression or ridge connecting two structures.

yolk (yōk) the material of an egg or ovum that serves as food for the developing organism until it obtains nourishment in some other way.

Young's rule (yungz) the dose of a drug for a child is obtained by multiplying the adult dose by the child's age in years and dividing the result by the sum of the child's age plus 12.

Young-Helmholtz theory (yung helm'hōlts) the doctrine that color vision depends on three sets of retinal receptors, corresponding to the colors red, green and violet.

ytterbium (ī-ter'be-um) a chemical element, atomic number 70, atomic weight 173.04, symbol Yb. (See table of ELEMENTS.)

yttrium (ĭ'tre-um) a chemical element, atomic number 39, atomic weight 88.905, symbol Y. (See table of ELEMENTS.)

Z

Z symbol, *atomic number*.

Zactane (zak′tān) trademark for a preparation of ethoheptazine citrate, an analgesic.

Zanchol (zan′kol) trademark for a preparation of florantyrone, a hydrocholeretic.

Zarontin (zah-ron′tin) trademark for a preparation of ethosuximide, an anticonvulsant.

zein (ze′in) a soft yellow protein from maize.

zeismus (ze-is′mus) a skin disease, said to be due to excessive diet of maize.

zeoscope (ze′o-skōp) an apparatus for determining the alcoholic strength of a liquid by means of its boiling point.

Zephiran (zef′i-ran) trademark for preparations of benzalkonium, a topical antiseptic.

zero (ze′ro) the point on a thermometer scale from which the degrees are numbered. The zero of the Celsius (centigrade) and Réaumur thermometers is the freezing point of water; on the Fahrenheit thermometer it is 32 degrees below the freezing point of water.
   absolute z., the lowest possible temperature, the equivalent of $-273.15°$ C. or $-459.67°$ F.
   physiologic z., the temperature at which a thermal stimulus ceases to cause a sensation.

zinc (zingk) a chemical element, atomic number 30, atomic weight 65.37, symbol Zn. (See table of ELEMENTS.)
   z. carbonate, a salt used as a dusting powder.
   z. chloride, a white or nearly white crystalline compound used in dentistry as an astringent or dentin desensitizer.
   z. gelatin, a mixture of zinc oxide, gelatin, glycerin and purified water, used topically as a protectant.
   z. ointment, a preparation of zinc oxide and liquid petrolatum in white ointment; used topically as an astringent and protectant.
   z. oxide, a fine, amorphous, white or yellowish white powder, used as an astringent and protectant.
   z. peroxide, medicinal, a zinc compound used topically as an antiseptic and astringent.
   z. phenolsulfonate, colorless crystals or white granules or powder; used as an antiseptic and astringent.
   z. stearate, a compound of zinc and stearic acid used as a dusting powder.
   z. sulfate, a compound used as an ophthalmic astringent.
   z. undecylenate, a fine white powder used topically in 20 per cent ointment as a fungistatic agent.
   white, z., zinc oxide.

zirconium (zir-ko′ne-um) a chemical element, atomic number 40, atomic weight 91.22, symbol Zr. (See table of ELEMENTS.)

Zn chemical symbol, *zinc*.

zo(o)- (zo′o) word element [Gr.], animal.

zoanthropy (zo-an′thro-pe) the delusion that one has become a wild animal.

zoetic (zo-et′ik) pertaining to life.

Zollinger-Ellison syndrome (zol′in-jer-el′ĭ-sun) a triad comprising intractable, sometimes fulminating and in many ways atypical peptic ulcers; extreme gastric hyperacidity; and nonbeta cell, non-insulin-secreting islet cell tumors, which might be single or multiple, small or large, innocent or malignant.

zona (zo′nah), pl. *zo′nae* [L.] 1. zone. 2. herpes zoster.
   z. facia′lis, herpes zoster of face.
   z. fascicula′ta, the intermediate layer of the adrenal cortex.
   z. glomerulo′sa, the outermost layer of the adrenal cortex.
   z. ophthal′mica, herpetic infection of the cornea.
   z. pellu′cida, the transparent, noncellular, secreted layer surrounding an ovum.
   z. radia′ta, a zona pellucida exhibiting conspicuous radial striations.
   z. reticula′ris, the innermost layer of the adrenal cortex.
   z. stria′ta, a zona pellucida exhibiting conspicuous striations.

zone (zōn) 1. a girdle or belt. 2. a restricted area.
   biokinetic z., the range of temperatures within which the living cell carries on its life activities, lying approximately between 10 and 45° C.
   comfort z., an environmental temperature between 13 and 21° C. (55 and 70° F.) with a humidity of 30 to 55 per cent.
   epileptogenic z., a superficial area, stimulation of which provokes an epileptic seizure.
   erogenous z′s, erotogenic z′s, areas of the body whose stimulation produces erotic desire.
   hypnogenic z., hypnogenous z., an area of the body pressure on which will characteristically induce sleep.
   root z., that part of the white matter of the spinal cord connected with the anterior and posterior nerve roots.
   superficial z., the outermost of the four layers of cortical cells of the cerebrum.

zonesthesia (zo″nes-the′ze-ah) a sensation of constriction, as by a girdle.

zonifugal (zo-nif′u-gal) passing outward from a zone or region.

zonipetal (zo-nip′ĕ-tal) passing toward a zone or region.

zonula (zōn′u-lah), pl. *zon′ulae* [L.] zonule.

zonule (zōn′ūl) a small encircling structure or zone.
   ciliary z., z. of Zinn, a series of fibers connecting

1072

the ciliary body and lens of the eye, holding the lens in place.

zonulitis (zōn″u-li′tis) inflammation of the ciliary zonule.

zonulolysis (zon″u-lol′ĭ-sis) dissolution of the ciliary zonule by use of enzymes, to permit surgical removal of the lens.

zonulotomy (zon″u-lot′o-me) incision of the ciliary zonule.

zoobiology (zo″o-bi-ol′o-je) the biology of animals.

zoochemistry (zo″o-kem′is-tre) chemistry of animal tissues.

zoodermic (zo″o-der′mik) performed with the skin of an animal, especially in reference to skin grafts.

zoodetritus (zo″de-tri′tus) detritus produced by disintegration and decomposition of animal tissues and organisms.

zoodynamics (zo″o-di-nam′iks) animal physiology.

zoogenous (zo-oj′ĕ-nus) acquired from animals.

zoogeny (zo-oj′ĕ-ne) the production or generation of animals.

zoogeography (zo″o-je-og′rah-fe) the scientific study of the distribution of animals.

zoogony (zo-og′o-ne) the production of living young from within the body.

zoograft (zo′o-graft) a graft of tissue from an animal.

zoography (zo-og′rah-fe) a treatise on animals.

zooid (zo′oid) resembling an animal.

zoology (zo-ol′o-je) the science of the form, nature and classification of animals.

zoonosis (zo″o-no′sis) a disease of animals that may secondarily be transmitted to man.

zoonosology (zo″o-no-sol′o-je) the classification of diseases of animals.

zooparasite (zo″o-par′ah-sīt) an animal parasite.

zooparasitic (zo″o-par″ah-sit′ik) living as a parasite on an animal organism.

zoopathology (zo″o-pah-thol′o-je) the science of the diseases of animals.

zoophagous (zo-of′ah-gus) carnivorous.

zoopharmacy (zo″o-far′mah-se) veterinary pharmacy.

zoophilia (zo″o-fil′e-ah) abnormal fondness for animals.

zoophobia (zo″o-fo′be-ah) abnormal fear of animals.

zoophyte (zo′o-fīt) any plantlike animal, such as sponges.

zooplankton (zo″o-plangk′ton) minute animal organisms floating free in practically all natural waters.

zooplasty (zo′o-plas″te) transplantation of tissue from animal to man.

zoopsia (zo-op′se-ah) a hallucination with vision of animals.

zooscopy (zo-os′ko-pe) 1. zoopsia. 2. observation of physiologic phenomena in animals.

zoosis (zo-o′sis) any disease due to animal agents.

zoosmosis (zo″os-mo′sis) passage of living protoplasm from blood vessels into the tissues.

zoospermia (zo″o-sper′me-ah) the presence of live spermatozoa in ejaculated semen.

zoospore (zo′o-spōr) any spore moving by means of cilia.

zoosterol (zo-os′ter-ol) a sterol of animal origin.

zootechnics (zo″o-tek′niks) the breeding and handling of animals in domestication.

zootherapeutics (zo″o-ther″ah-pu′tiks) the treatment of diseases of animals.

zootomy (zo-ot′o-me) the dissection or anatomy of animals.

zootoxin (zo″o-tok′sin) a toxin produced by higher animals, especially snakes, scorpions and spiders, which is usually a mixture of hemotoxin and neurotoxin.

zoster (zos″ter) herpes zoster.

zosteriform (zos-ter′ĭ-form) resembling herpes zoster.

zoxazolamine (zok″sah-zol′ah-mēn) a compound used as a skeletal muscle relaxant and uricosuric agent.

Z-plasty (ze′plas-te) repair of a skin defect by the transposition of two triangular flaps of adjacent skin.

Zr chemical symbol, *zirconium.*

zyg(o)- (zi′go) word element [Gr.], *yoked; joined; a junction.*

zygal (zi′gal) shaped like a yoke, or pertaining to a yoke-shaped structure.

zygion (zij′e-on) the most lateral point on the zygomatic arch.

zygocyte (zi′go-sīt) zygote.

zygodactyly (zi″go-dak′tĭ-le) union of digits by soft tissues (skin), without bony fusion of the phalanges involved.

zygoma (zi-go′mah) the process of the temporal bone that connects with the zygomatic bone.

zygomatic (zi″go-mat′ik) pertaining to the zygoma.
  z. arch, the arch formed by the zygomatic and temporal bones.
  z. bone, the bone forming the hard part of the cheek and the lower, lateral portion of the rim of the orbit.

zygon (zi′gon) the stem connecting the two branches of a zygal fissure.

zygoneure (zi′go-nūr) a nerve cell connecting other nerve cells.

zygosity (zi-gos'ĭ-te) the condition relating to the zygote; specifically, whether derived from one ovum or more than one (monozygotic or dizygotic), or whether having identical or unlike genes in respect to a certain character (homozygous or heterozygous).

zygote (zi'gōt) the cell produced by the union of two gametes; the fertilized ovum. (See also REPRODUCTION.) adj., **zygot'ic.**

zyloprim (zi'lo-prim) trademark for preparations of allopurinol, an inhibitor of uric acid production in the body; used in prevention of acute attacks of gout.

zym(o)- (zi'mo) word element [Gr.], *enzyme; fermentation.*

zymase (zi'mās) enzyme.

zymic (zi'mik) pertaining to enzymes or fermentation.

zymocyte (zi'mo-sīt) an organism that causes fermentation.

zymogen (zi'mo-jen) an inactive material that may be converted into an enzyme by action of an acid or another enzyme or by other means; a proenzyme.

zymogram (zi'mo-gram) a graphic representation of enzymatically active components of a material separated by electrophoresis.

zymoid (zi'moid) any poison from decaying tissue.

zymology (zi-mol'o-je) the sum of knowledge about fermentation.

zymolysis (zi-mol'ĭ-sis) digestion by means of an enzyme.

zymome (zi'mōm) an enzyme.

zymophore (zi'mo-fōr) the group of atoms in a molecule of an enzyme that is responsible for its effect.

zymophyte (zi'mo-fīt) a bacterium causing fermentation.

zymoplastic (zi"mo-plas'tik) forming ferment.

zymoprotein (zi"mo-pro'te-in) a protein having catalytic powers.

zymosan (zi'mo-san) a mixture of lipids, polysaccharides, proteins and ash, derived from the cell walls or the entire cell of yeast.

zymoscope (zi'mo-skōp) an apparatus for determining the fermenting power of yeast.

zymose (zi'mōs) invertin.

zymosis (zi-mo'sis) 1. fermentation. 2. the propagation and development of an infectious disease. 3. any infectious or contagious disease. adj., **zymot'ic.**
    z. gas'trica, the presence of an organic acid in the stomach.

zymosterol (zi-mos'ter-ol) a sterol occurring in fungi and molds.

zymurgy (zi'mur-je) the science of the industrial use of enzymes and fermentation.

Appendix

1. Desirable Weights for Men and Women
Weight in Pounds According to Frame
(in Indoor Clothing)

Men of Ages 25 and Over

Height (with shoes on) 1-inch heels Feet Inches	Small Frame	Medium Frame	Large Frame
5 2	112–120	118–129	126–141
5 3	115–123	121–133	129–144
5 4	118–126	124–136	132–148
5 5	121–129	127–139	135–152
5 6	124–133	130–143	138–156
5 7	128–137	134–147	142–161
5 8	132–141	138–152	147–166
5 9	136–145	142–156	151–170
5 10	140–150	146–160	155–174
5 11	144–154	150–165	159–179
6 0	148–158	154–170	164–184
6 1	152–162	158–175	168–189
6 2	156–167	162–180	173–194
6 3	160–171	167–185	178–199
6 4	164–175	172–190	182–204

Women of Ages 25 and Over

Height (with shoes on) 2-inch heels Feet Inches	Small Frame	Medium Frame	Large Frame
4 10	92– 98	96–107	104–119
4 11	94–101	98–110	106–122
5 0	96–104	101–113	109–125
5 1	99–107	104–116	112–128
5 2	102–110	107–119	115–131
5 3	105–113	110–122	118–134
5 4	108–116	113–126	121–138
5 5	111–119	116–130	125–142
5 6	114–123	120–135	129–146
5 7	118–127	124–139	133–150
5 8	122–131	128–143	137–154
5 9	126–135	132–147	141–158
5 10	130–140	136–151	145–163
5 11	134–144	140–155	149–168
6 0	138–148	144–159	153–173

For girls between 18 and 25, subtract 1 pound for each year under 25.

Courtesy of Metropolitan Life Insurance Company.

2. Ideal Weights for Boys and Girls, According to Height and Age

Boys, Aged 14 to 19 Years

Height Feet Inches	Age 14	15	16	17	18	19
4 6	72					
4 7	74					
4 8	78	80				
4 9	83	83				
4 10	86	87				
4 11	90	90	90			
5 0	94	95	96			
5 1	99	100	103	106		
5 2	103	104	107	111	116	
5 3	108	110	113	118	123	127
5 4	113	115	117	121	126	130
5 5	118	120	122	127	131	134
5 6	122	125	128	132	136	139
5 7	128	130	134	136	139	142
5 8	134	134	137	141	143	147
5 9	137	139	143	146	149	152
5 10	143	144	145	148	151	155
5 11	148	150	151	152	154	159
6 0		153	155	156	158	163
6 1		157	160	162	164	167
6 2		160	164	168	170	171

Girls, Aged 14 to 18 Years

Height Feet Inches	Age 14	15	16	17	18
4 7	78				
4 8	83				
4 9	88	92			
4 10	93	96	101		
4 11	96	100	103	104	
5 0	101	105	108	109	111
5 1	105	108	112	113	116
5 2	109	113	115	117	118
5 3	112	116	117	119	120
5 4	117	119	120	122	123
5 5	121	122	123	125	126
5 6	124	124	125	128	130
5 7	130	131	133	133	135
5 8	133	135	136	138	138
5 9	135	137	138	140	142
5 10	136	138	140	142	144
5 11	138	140	142	144	145

From American Child Health Association.

3. Tables of Weights and Measures

Measures of Mass

Avoirdupois Weight

GRAINS	DRAMS	OUNCES	POUNDS	METRIC EQUIVALENTS, GRAMS
1	0.0366	0.0023	0.00014	0.0647989
27.34	1	0.0625	0.0039	1.772
437.5	16	1	0.0625	28.350
7000	256	16	1	453.5924277

Apothecaries' Weight

GRAINS	SCRUPLES (℈)	DRAMS (ʒ)	OUNCES (℥)	POUNDS(lb.)	METRIC EQUIVALENTS, GRAMS
1	0.05	0.0167	0.0021	0.00017	0.0647989
20	1	0.333	0.042	0.0035	1.296
60	3	1	0.125	0.0104	3.888
480	24	8	1	0.0833	31.103
5760	288	96	12	1	373.24177

Troy Weight

GRAINS	PENNYWEIGHTS	OUNCES	POUNDS	METRIC EQUIVALENTS, GRAMS
1	0.042	0.002	0.00017	0.0647989
24	1	0.05	0.0042	1.555
480	20	1	0.083	31.103
5760	240	12	1	373.24177

TABLES OF WEIGHTS AND MEASURES—*Continued*

MEASURES OF MASS

METRIC WEIGHT

MICROGRAM	MILLIGRAM	CENTIGRAM	DECIGRAM	GRAM	DECAGRAM	HECTOGRAM	KILOGRAM	EQUIVALENTS	
								AVOIRDUPOIS	APOTHECARIES'
1	...	...	...	...	...	...	...		0.000015 grains
10^3	1	...	...	...	...	...	...		0.015432 grains
10^4	10	1	...	...	...	...	...		0.154323 grains
10^5	10^2	10	1	...	...	...	...		1.543235 grains
10^6	10^3	10^2	10	1	...	...	...		15.432356 grains
10^7	10^4	10^3	10^2	10	1	...	...	5.6438 dr.	7.7162 scr.
10^8	10^5	10^4	10^3	10^2	10	1	...	3.527 oz.	3.215 oz.
10^9	10^6	10^5	10^4	10^3	10^2	10	1	2.2046 lb.	2.6792 lb.
10^{12}	10^9	10^8	10^7	10^6	10^5	10^4	10^3	2204.6223 lb.	2679.2285 lb.

MEASURES OF CAPACITY

APOTHECARIES' (WINE) MEASURE

MINIMS	FLUID DRAMS	FLUID OUNCES	GILLS	PINTS	QUARTS	GALLONS	EQUIVALENTS		
							CUBIC INCHES	MILLI-LITERS	CUBIC CENTIMETERS
1	0.0166	0.002	0.0005	0.00013	...	...	0.00376	0.06161	0.06161
60	1	0.125	0.0312	0.0078	0.0039	...	0.22558	3.6966	3.6967
480	8	1	0.25	0.0625	0.0312	0.0078	1.80468	29.5729	29.5737
1920	32	4	1	0.25	0.125	0.0312	7.21875	118.2915	118.2948
7680	128	16	4	1	0.5	0.125	28.875	473.167	473.179
15360	256	32	8	2	1	0.25	57.75	946.333	946.358
61440	1024	128	32	8	4	1	231	3785.332	3785.434

TABLES OF WEIGHTS AND MEASURES—*Continued*

MEASURES OF CAPACITY

METRIC MEASURE

MICROLITER	MILLILITER	CENTILITER	DECILITER	LITER	DEKALITER	HECTOLITER	KILOLITER	MYRIALITER	EQUIVALENTS (APOTHECARIES' FLUID)
1	...	...	...	...	...	...	...	...	0.01623108 min.
10^3	1	...	...	...	...	...	...	...	16.23 min.
10^4	10	1	...	...	...	...	...	...	2.7 fl. dr.
10^5	10^2	10	1	...	...	...	...	...	3.38 fl. oz.
10^6	10^3	10^2	10	1	...	...	...	...	2.11 pts.
10^7	10^4	10^3	10^2	10	1	...	...	...	2.64 gal.
10^8	10^5	10^4	10^3	10^2	10	1	...	...	26.418 gal.
10^9	10^6	10^5	10^4	10^3	10^2	10	1	...	264.18 gal.
10^{10}	10^7	10^6	10^5	10^4	10^3	10^2	10	1	2641.8 gal.

1 liter = 2.113363738 pints (Apothecaries').

Measures of Length

Metric Measure

MICRON	MILLI-METER	CENTI-METER	DECI-METER	METER	DEKA-METER	HECTO-METER	KILO-METER	MYRIA-METER	MEGA-METER	EQUIVALENTS
1	0.001	10^{-4}	...	...	...	...	...	...	...	0.000039 inch
10^3	1	10^{-1}	...	...	...	...	...	...	...	0.03937 inch
10^4	10	1	...	...	...	...	...	...	...	0.3937 inch
10^5	10^2	10	1	...	...	...	...	...	...	3.937 inch
10^6	10^3	10^2	10	1	...	...	...	...	...	39.37 inch
10^7	10^4	10^3	10^2	10	1	...	...	...	...	10.9361 yards
10^8	10^5	10^4	10^3	10^2	10	1	...	...	...	109.3612 yards
10^9	10^6	10^5	10^4	10^3	10^2	10	1	...	...	1093.6121 yards
10^{10}	10^7	10^6	10^5	10^4	10^3	10^2	10	1	...	6.2137 miles
10^{11}	10^8	10^7	10^6	10^5	10^4	10^3	10^2	10	1	62.1370 miles

TABLES OF WEIGHTS AND MEASURES — *Continued*

CONVERSION TABLES

AVOIRDUPOIS — METRIC WEIGHT			APOTHECARIES' — METRIC LIQUID MEASURE	
Ounces	Grams		Minims	Milliliters
1/16	1.772		1	0.06
1/8	3.544		2	0.12
1/4	7.088		3	0.19
1/2	14.175		4	0.25
1	28.350		5	0.31
2	56.699		10	0.62
3	85.049		15	0.92
4	113.398		20	1.23
5	141.748		25	1.54
6	170.097		30	1.85
7	198.447		35	2.16
8	226.796		40	2.46
9	255.146		45	2.77
10	283.495		50	3.08
11	311.845		55	3.39
12	340.194		60 (1 fl.dr.)	3.70
13	368.544			
14	396.893		Fluid drams	
15	425.243		1	3.70
16 (1 lb.)	453.59		2	7.39
			3	11.09
Pounds			4	14.79
			5	18.48
1 (16 oz.)	453.59		6	22.18
2	907.18		7	25.88
3	1360.78 (1.36 kg.)		8 (1 fl.oz.)	29.57
4	1814.37 (1.81 ")			
5	2267.96 (2.27 ")		Fluid ounces	
6	2721.55 (2.72 ")		1	29.57
7	3175.15 (3.18 ")		2	59.15
8	3628.74 (3.63 ")		3	88.72
9	4082.33 (4.08 ")		4	118.29
10	4535.92 (4.54 ")		5	147.87
			6	177.44
			7	207.01
			8	236.58
			9	266.16
			10	295.73
			11	325.30
			12	354.88
METRIC — AVOIRDUPOIS WEIGHT			13	384.45
			14	414.02
GRAMS	OUNCES		15	443.59
0.001 (1 mg.)	0.000035274		16 (1 pt.)	473.17
1	0.035274		32 (1 qt.)	946.33
1000 (1 kg.)	35.274 (2.2046 lb.)		128 (1 gal.)	3785.32

METRIC — APOTHECARIES' LIQUID MEASURE

MILLILITERS	MINIMS		MILLILITERS	FLUID DRAMS	MILLILITERS	FLUID OUNCES
1	16.231		5	1.35	30	1.01
2	32.5		10	2.71	40	1.35
3	48.7		15	4.06	50	1.69
4	64.9		20	5.4	500	16.91
5	81.1		25	6.76	1000 (1 L.)	33.815
			30	7.1		

TABLES OF WEIGHTS AND MEASURES—*Continued*

CONVERSION TABLES

APOTHECARIES'—METRIC WEIGHT		METRIC—APOTHECARIES' WEIGHT	
Grains	Grams	Milligrams	Grains
1/150	0.0004	1	0.015432
1/120	0.0005	2	0.030864
1/100	0.0006	3	0.046296
1/80	0.0008	4	0.061728
1/64	0.001	5	0.077160
1/50	0.0013	6	0.092592
1/48	0.0014	7	0.108024
1/30	0.0022	8	0.123456
1/25	0.0026	9	0.138888
1/16	0.004	10	0.154320
1/12	0.005	15	0.231480
1/10	0.006	20	0.308640
1/9	0.007	25	0.385800
1/8	0.008	30	0.462960
1/7	0.009	35	0.540120
1/6	0.01	40	0.617280
1/5	0.013	45	0.694440
1/4	0.016	50	0.771600
1/3	0.02	100	1.543240
1/2	0.032		
1	0.065	Grams	
1 1/2	0.097 (0.1)	0.1	1.5432
2	0.12	0.2	3.0864
3	0.20	0.3	4.6296
4	0.24	0.4	6.1728
5	0.30	0.5	7.7160
6	0.40	0.6	9.2592
7	0.45	0.7	10.8024
8	0.50	0.8	12.3456
9	0.60	0.9	13.8888
10	0.65	1.0	15.4320
15	1.00	1.5	23.1480
20 (1℈)	1.30	2.0	30.8640
30	2.00	2.5	38.5800
Scruples		3.0	46.2960
1	1.296 (1.3)	3.5	54.0120
2	2.592 (2.6)	4.0	61.728
3 (1ʒ)	3.888 (3.9)	4.5	69.444
Drams		5.0	77.162
1	3.888	10.0	154.324
2	7.776		
3	11.664		Equivalents
4	15.552	10	2.572 drams
5	19.440	15	3.858 "
6	23.328	20	5.144 "
7	27.216	25	6.430 "
8 (1ℨ)	31.103	30	7.716 "
Ounces		40	1.286 oz.
1	31.103	45	1.447 "
2	62.207	50	1.607 "
3	93.310	100	3.215 "
4	124.414	200	6.430 "
5	155.517	300	9.644 "
6	186.621	400	12.859 "
7	217.724	500	1.34 lb.
8	248.828	600	1.61 "
9	279.931	700	1.88 "
10	311.035	800	2.14 "
11	342.138	900	2.41 "
12 (1 lb.)	373.242	1000	2.68 "

TABLES OF WEIGHTS AND MEASURES – *Continued*

METRIC DOSES WITH APPROXIMATE APOTHECARY EQUIVALENTS*

These *approximate* dose equivalents represent the quantities usually prescribed, under identical conditions, by physicians trained, respectively, in the metric or in the apothecary system of weights and measures. In labeling dosage forms in both the metric and the apothecary systems, if one is the approximate equivalent of the other, the approximate figure shall be enclosed in parentheses.

When prepared dosage forms such as tablets, capsules, pills, etc., are prescribed in the metric system, the pharmacist may dispense the corresponding *approximate* equivalent in the apothecary system, and vice versa, as indicated in the following table.

Caution – For the conversion of specific quantities in a prescription which requires compounding, or in converting a pharmaceutical formula from one system of weights or measures to the other, *exact* equivalents must be used.

LIQUID MEASURE		LIQUID MEASURE	
METRIC	APPROX. APOTHECARY EQUIVALENTS	METRIC	APPROX. APOTHECARY EQUIVALENTS
1000 ml.	1 quart	3 ml.	45 minims
750 ml.	1 1/2 pints	2 ml.	30 minims
500 ml.	1 pint	1 ml.	15 minims
250 ml.	8 fluid ounces	0.75 ml.	12 minims
200 ml.	7 fluid ounces	0.6 ml.	10 minims
100 ml.	3 1/2 fluid ounces	0.5 ml.	8 minims
50 ml.	1 3/4 fluid ounces	0.3 ml.	5 minims
30 ml.	1 fluid ounce	0.25 ml.	4 minims
15 ml.	4 fluid drams	0.2 ml.	3 minims
10 ml.	2 1/2 fluid drams	0.1 ml.	1 1/2 minims
8 ml.	2 fluid drams	0.06 ml.	1 minim
5 ml.	1 1/4 fluid drams	0.05 ml.	3/4 minim
4 ml.	1 fluid dram	0.03 ml.	1/2 minim

WEIGHT		WEIGHT	
METRIC	APPROX. APOTHECARY EQUIVALENTS	METRIC	APPROX. APOTHECARY EQUIVALENTS
30 Gm.	1 ounce	30 mg.	1/2 grain
15 Gm.	4 drams	25 mg.	3/8 grain
10 Gm.	2 1/2 drams	20 mg.	1/3 grain
7.5 Gm.	2 drams	15 mg.	1/4 grain
6 Gm.	90 grains	12 mg.	1/5 grain
5 Gm.	75 grains	10 mg.	1/6 grain
4 Gm.	60 grains (1 dram)	8 mg.	1/8 grain
3 Gm.	45 grains	6 mg.	1/10 grain
2 Gm.	30 grains (1/2 dram)	5 mg.	1/12 grain
1.5 Gm.	22 grains	4 mg.	1/15 grain
1 Gm.	15 grains	3 mg.	1/20 grain
0.75 Gm.	12 grains	2 mg.	1/30 grain
0.6 Gm.	10 grains	1.5 mg.	1/40 grain
0.5 Gm.	7 1/2 grains	1.2 mg.	1/50 grain
0.4 Gm.	6 grains	1 mg.	1/60 grain
0.3 Gm.	5 grains	0.8 mg.	1/80 grain
0.25 Gm.	4 grains	0.6 mg.	1/100 grain
0.2 Gm.	3 grains	0.5 mg.	1/120 grain
0.15 Gm.	2 1/2 grains	0.4 mg.	1/150 grain
0.12 Gm.	2 grains	0.3 mg.	1/200 grain
0.1 Gm.	1 1/2 grains	0.25 mg.	1/250 grain
75 mg.	1 1/4 grains	0.2 mg.	1/300 grain
60 mg.	1 grain	0.15 mg.	1/400 grain
50 mg.	3/4 grain	0.12 mg.	1/500 grain
40 mg.	2/3 grain	0.1 mg.	1/600 grain

Note – A milliliter (ml.) is the approximate equivalent of a cubic centimeter (cc.).

*Adopted by the latest Pharmacopeia, National Formulary, and New and Nonofficial Remedies, and approved by the Federal Food and Drug Administration.

4. Milliequivalent Conversion Factors

mEq./L. of:	Divide mg./100 ml. or Vol. % by:	
Calcium	2.0	
Chlorides (from Cl)	3.5	
(from NaCl)	5.85	
CO_2 combining power	2.22	
Magnesium	1.2	
Phosphorus	3.1	(mM.)
Potassium	3.9	
Sodium	2.3	

From Brainerd, H., Margen, S., and Chatton, M. J.: Current Diagnosis and Treatment. Los Altos, Calif., Lange Medical Publications, 1967.

5. Approximate Household Equivalents

	Liquid	Weight
1 teaspoon	5 ml.	5 Gm.
1 tablespoon = 3 teaspoons	15 ml.	15 Gm.
1 cup = 16 tablespoons	237 ml.	240 Gm.
1 pint = 2 cups	473 ml.	480 Gm.
1 quart = 2 pints = 4 cups	946 ml.	960 Gm.

1 pound of butter	=	2 cups
8 average eggs	=	1 cup
4 cups sifted flour	=	1 pound
2 cups granulated sugar	=	1 pound
2⅔ cups confectioner's sugar	=	1 pound
2⅔ cups brown sugar	=	1 pound

6. TABLE OF TEMPERATURE EQUIVALENTS

CELSIUS (CENTIGRADE): FAHRENHEIT SCALE

CELSIUS : FAHRENHEIT $^{\circ}F = (^{\circ}C \times \tfrac{9}{5}) + 32$				FAHRENHEIT : CELSIUS $^{\circ}C = (^{\circ}F - 32) \times \tfrac{5}{9}$					
C°	F°	C°	F°	F°	C°	F°	C°	F°	C°
−50	−58.0	49	120.2	−50	−46.7	99	37.2	157	69.4
−40	−40.0	50	122.0	−40	−40.0	100	37.7	158	70.0
−35	−31.0	51	123.8	−35	−37.2	101	38.3	159	70.5
−30	−22.0	52	125.6	−30	−34.4	102	38.8	160	71.1
−25	−13.0	53	127.4	−25	−31.7	103	39.4	161	71.6
−20	−4.0	54	129.2	−20	−28.9	104	40.0	162	72.2
−15	−5.0	55	131.0	−15	−26.6	105	40.5	163	72.7
−10	14.0	56	132.8	−10	−23.3	106	41.1	164	73.3
−5	23.0	57	134.6	−5	−20.6	107	41.6	165	73.8
0	32.0	58	136.4	0	−17.7	108	42.2	166	74.4
+1	33.8	59	138.2	+1	−17.2	109	42.7	167	75.0
2	35.6	60	140.0	5	−15.0	110	43.3	168	75.5
3	37.4	61	141.8	10	−12.2	111	43.8	169	76.1
4	39.2	62	143.6	15	−9.4	112	44.4	170	76.6
5	41.0	63	145.4	20	−6.6	113	45.0	171	77.2
6	42.8	64	147.2	25	−3.8	114	45.5	172	77.7
7	44.6	65	149.0	30	−1.1	115	46.1	173	78.3
8	46.4	66	150.8	31	−0.5	116	46.6	174	78.8
9	48.2	67	152.6	32	0	117	47.2	175	79.4
10	50.0	68	154.4	33	+0.5	118	47.7	176	80.0
11	51.8	69	156.2	34	1.1	119	48.3	177	80.5
12	53.6	70	158.0	35	1.6	120	48.8	178	81.1
13	55.4	71	159.8	36	2.2	121	49.4	179	81.6
14	57.2	72	161.6	37	2.7	122	50.0	180	82.2
15	59.0	73	163.4	38	3.3	123	50.5	181	82.7
16	60.8	74	165.2	39	3.8	124	51.1	182	83.3
17	62.6	75	167.0	40	4.4	125	51.6	183	83.8
18	64.4	76	168.8	41	5.0	126	52.2	184	84.4
19	66.2	77	170.6	42	5.5	127	52.7	185	85.0
20	68.0	78	172.4	43	6.1	128	53.3	186	85.5
21	69.8	79	174.2	44	6.6	129	53.8	187	86.1
22	71.6	80	176.0	45	7.2	130	54.4	188	86.6
23	73.4	81	177.8	46	7.7	131	55.0	189	87.2
24	75.2	82	179.6	47	8.3	132	55.5	190	87.7
25	77.0	83	181.4	48	8.8	133	56.1	191	88.3
26	78.8	84	183.2	49	9.4	134	56.6	192	88.8
27	80.6	85	185.0	50	10.0	135	57.2	193	89.4
28	82.4	86	186.8	55	12.7	136	57.7	194	90.0
29	84.2	87	188.6	60	15.5	137	58.3	195	90.5
30	86.0	88	190.4	65	18.3	138	58.8	196	91.1
31	87.8	89	192.2	70	21.1	139	59.4	197	91.6
32	89.6	90	194.0	75	23.8	140	60.0	198	92.2
33	91.4	91	195.8	80	26.6	141	60.5	199	92.7
34	93.2	92	197.6	85	29.4	142	61.1	200	93.3
35	95.0	93	199.4	86	30.0	143	61.6	201	93.8
36	96.8	94	201.2	87	30.5	144	62.2	202	94.4
37	98.6	95	203.0	88	31.0	145	62.7	203	95.0
38	100.4	96	204.8	89	31.6	146	63.3	204	95.5
39	102.2	97	206.6	90	32.2	147	63.8	205	96.1
40	104.0	98	208.4	91	32.7	148	64.4	206	96.6
41	105.8	99	210.2	92	33.3	149	65.0	207	97.2
42	107.6	100	212.0	93	33.8	150	65.5	208	97.7
43	109.4	101	213.8	94	34.4	151	66.1	209	98.3
44	111.2	102	215.6	95	35.0	152	66.6	210	98.8
45	113.0	103	217.4	96	35.5	153	67.2	211	99.4
46	114.8	104	219.2	97	36.1	154	67.7	212	100.0
47	116.6	105	221.0	98	36.6	155	68.3	213	100.5
48	118.4	106	222.8	98.6	37.0	156	68.8	214	101.1

7. Pulmonary Function (Normal Values)

Vital Capacity (liters)	Male: = [(27.63 − [0.112 × Age in yr.]) × Ht. in cm.] ÷ 1,000
	Female: = [(21.78 − [0.101 × Age in yr.]) × Ht. in cm.] ÷ 1,000
Tidal Air	0.350–0.500 L.
Residual Volume*	1.0–1.5 L.
Total Lung Capacity	Vital Capacity + Residual Volume
Residual Volume: Total Lung Capacity	20–30%
Maximum Breathing Capacity	Male: 100–150 L./min. (approx. values) Female: 70–120 L./min. Male: L./min. = [86.5 − (0.522 × Age in yr.)] × sq.M. of B.S.A.** Female: L./min. = [71.3 − (0.474 × Age in yr.)] × sq.M. of B.S.A.**
Respiratory Rate (resting)	8–20/min.
Pulmonary Ventilation (resting)	3–4 L./min./sq.M. of B.S.A.
Pulmonary Compliance	0.200 L./cm. of H_2O intrapleural pressure change
O_2 Uptake (resting)	110–140 cc./min.sq.M. of B.S.A.
CO_2 Output (resting)	88–120 cc./min./sq.M. of B.S.A.
Respiratory Exchange Ratio (Resp. Quotient, R.Q.)	$\dfrac{CO_2}{O_2} = 0.77\text{–}0.90$
Bronchospirometric Ratio (% total function)	Rt. lung: 52–58% Lt. lung: 48–42%
Timed Vital Capacity	First sec. = 83 + % of total vital capacity First 2 sec. = 94 + % of total vital capacity First 3 sec. = 97% of total vital capacity

From The Merck Manual. 11th ed. Copyright 1966, Merck & Co., Inc., Rahway, New Jersey.
*Air in lungs at maximal expiration.
**More accurate formulas.

8. Symbols Commonly Used in Pedigree Charts

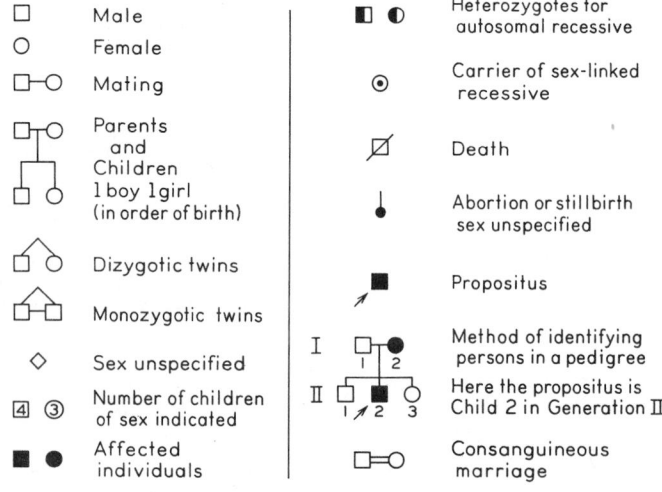

□	Male
○	Female
□—○	Mating
	Parents and Children 1 boy 1 girl (in order of birth)
	Dizygotic twins
	Monozygotic twins
◇	Sex unspecified
4 ③	Number of children of sex indicated
■ ●	Affected individuals
◧ ◑	Heterozygotes for autosomal recessive
⊙	Carrier of sex-linked recessive
⌀	Death
	Abortion or stillbirth sex unspecified
■	Propositus
	Method of identifying persons in a pedigree
	Here the propositus is Child 2 in Generation II
□—○	Consanguineous marriage

From Thompson, J. S., and Thompson, M. W.: Genetics in Medicine. Philadelphia, W. B. Saunders Co., 1966.

9. Voluntary Health and Welfare Agencies

Addicts Anonymous
Box 2000, Lexington, Ky.   40501

Aging, National Council on the
315 Park Ave. South, New York, N.Y.   10010

Alcoholics Anonymous
468 Park Ave. South, New York, N.Y.   10016

Alcoholism, National Council on
2 East 103rd St., New York, N.Y.   10029

Allergy, American Academy of
756 North Milwaukee St., Milwaukee, Wis. 53202

Allergy Foundation of America
801 Second Ave., New York, N.Y.   10017

Arthritis Foundation
1212 Ave. of the Americas, New York, N.Y. 10036

Blind, American Foundation for the
15 West 16th St., New York, N.Y.   10011

Blindness, National Society for the Prevention of
79 Madison Ave., New York, N.Y.   10016

Cancer Research, The Institute for
7701 Burholme Ave., Philadelphia, Pa.   19111

Cancer Society, American
219 East 42nd St., New York, N.Y.   10017

Cerebral Palsy Association, United
66 East 34th Street, New York, N.Y.   10016

Crippled Children and Adults, National Easter Seal
Society for
2023 West Ogden Ave., Chicago, Ill.   60612

Cystic Fibrosis Research Foundation, National
521 Fifth Ave., New York, N.Y.   10017

Deaf, Alexander Graham Bell Association for the
1537 35th St., N.W., Washington, D.C.   20007

Deafness Research Foundation
366 Madison ave., New York, N.Y.   10017

Dental Association, American
211 East Chicago ave., Chicago, Ill.   60611

Diabetes Association, American
18 East 48th St., New York, N.Y.   10017

Dietetic Association, American
620 North Michigan Ave., Chicago, Ill.   60611

Epilepsy Foundation of America
733 15th St., Washington, D.C.   20005

Epilepsy League, National
203 North Wabash Ave., Chicago, Ill.   60601

Family Service Association of America
44 East 23rd St., New York, N.Y.   10010

Geriatrics Society, American
10 Columbus Circle, New York, N.Y.   10019

Hearing and Speech Agencies, National
Association of
919 18th St., N.W., Washington, D.C.   20006

Heart Association, American
44 East 23rd St., New York, N.Y.   10010

Kidney Foundation, National
342 Madison Ave., New York, N.Y.   10017

Leukemia Society
211 East 43rd St., New York, N.Y.   10017

Mental Health, National Association for
10 Columbus Circle, New York, N.Y.   10019

Multiple Sclerosis Society, National
257 Park Ave. South, New York, N.Y.   10010

Muscular Dystrophy Associations of America
1790 Broadway, New York, N.Y.   10019

Narcotics Education
6830 Laurel Ave., Washington, D.C.   20012

Planned Parenthood Federation of America
515 Madison Ave., New York, N.Y.   10022

Rehabilitation Association, National
1522 K St., N.W., Washington, D.C.   20005

Retarded Children, National Association for
420 Lexington Ave., New York, N.Y.   10017

Rheumatism Association, American
1212 Ave. of the Americas, New York, N.Y. 10036

Social Health Association, American
1740 Broadway, New York, N.Y.   10019

Speech and Hearing Association, American
1001 Connecticut Ave., N.W., Washington, D.C.
20006

Tuberculosis and Respiratory Disease Association,
National
1740 Broadway, New York, N.Y.   10019

Volta Bureau
1537 35th St., N.W., Washington, D.C.   20007